W9-APO-423

Basic & Clinical Pharmacology

tenth edition

Edited by

Bertram G. Katzung, MD, PhD
Professor Emeritus
Department of Cellular & Molecular Pharmacology
University of California, San Francisco

Medical

New York   Chicago   San Francisco   Lisbon   London   Madrid   Mexico City
Milan   New Delhi   San Juan   Seoul   Singapore   Sydney   Toronto

McGraw·Hill Companies

Basic & Clinical Pharmacology, Tenth Edition

2 3 4 5 6 7 8 9 0 DOC / DOC 0 9 8 7

ISBN: 978-0-07-145153-6
MHID: 0-07-145153-6

Notice

Medicine is an ever-changing science. As new research and clinical experience broaden our knowledge, changes in treatment and drug therapy are required. The authors and the publisher of this work have checked with sources believed to be reliable in their efforts to provide information that is complete and generally in accord with the standards accepted at the time of publication. However, in view of the possibility of human error or changes in medical sciences, neither the authors nor the publisher nor any other party who has been involved in the preparation or publication of this work warrants that the information contained herein is in every respect accurate or complete, and they disclaim all responsibility for any errors or omissions or for the results obtained from use of the information contained in this work. Readers are encouraged to confirm the information contained herein with other sources. For example and in particular, readers are advised to check the product information sheet included in the package of each drug they plan to administer to be certain that the information contained in this work is accurate and that changes have not been made in the recommended dose or in the contraindications for administration. This recommendation is of particular importance in connection with new or infrequently used drugs.

This book was set in Garamond by Silverchair Science + Communications, Inc.
The editors were Jason O. Malley, Harriet Lebowitz, Donna Frassetto, Alison Kelley, and Karen Davis.
The production supervisor was Sherri Souffrance.
The cover designer was Kelly Parr.
The index was prepared by Barbara S. Littlewood.
RR Donnelley, Crawfordsville, was printer and binder.

This book is printed on acid-free paper.

Contents

Preface

This book is designed to provide a complete, authoritative, current, and readable pharmacology textbook for students in the health sciences. It also offers special features that make it useful to house officers and practicing clinicians.

Information is organized according to the sequence used in many pharmacology courses and in integrated organ system curricula: basic principles; autonomic drugs; cardiovascular-renal drugs; drugs with important actions on smooth muscle; central nervous system drugs; drugs used to treat inflammation, gout, and diseases of the blood; endocrine drugs; chemotherapeutic drugs; toxicology; and special topics. This sequence builds new information on a foundation of information already assimilated. For example, early presentation of autonomic pharmacology allows students to integrate the physiology and neuroscience they know with the pharmacology they are learning and prepares them to understand the autonomic effects of other drugs. This is especially important for the cardiovascular and central nervous system drug groups. However, chapters can be used equally well in courses and curricula that present these topics in a different sequence.

Within each chapter, emphasis is placed on discussion of drug groups and prototypes rather than offering repetitive detail about individual drugs. Selection of the subject matter and the order of its presentation are based on the accumulated experience of teaching this material to thousands of medical, pharmacy, dental, podiatry, nursing, and other health science students.

Major features that make this book especially useful to professional students include sections that specifically address the clinical choice and use of drugs in patients and the monitoring of their effects—in other words, *clinical pharmacology* is an integral part of this text. Lists of the commercial preparations available, including trade and generic names and dosage formulations, are provided at the end of each chapter for easy reference by the house officer or practitioner writing a chart order or prescription.

Significant revisions in this edition include the following:

- Major revisions of the chapters on prostaglandins, nitric oxide, anti-inflammatory drugs, hypothalamic and pituitary hormones, antidiabetic drugs, antiviral drugs, and immunopharmacology
- Many new figures, most in color, that help to clarify important concepts in pharmacology
- Many descriptions of important developments based on genetically modified mice ("knockout" and "knockin" mice), a research tool of great importance in pharmacology
- Continuing expansion of the coverage of general concepts relating to receptors and listings of newly discovered drug transporters and receptors
- Descriptions of important new drugs released through August 2006, including numerous new immunopharmacologic agents

An important related source of information is *Katzung & Trevor's Pharmacology: Examination & Board Review, 7th ed* (Trevor AJ, Katzung BG, & Masters SB: McGraw-Hill, 2005). This book provides a succinct review of pharmacology with one of the largest available collections of sample examination questions and answers. It is especially helpful to students preparing for board-type examinations. A more highly condensed source of information suitable for review purposes is *USMLE Road Map: Pharmacology, 2nd ed* (Katzung BG, Trevor AJ: McGraw-Hill, 2006).

This edition marks the 25th year of publication of *Basic & Clinical Pharmacology*. The widespread acceptance of the first nine editions suggests that this book fills an important need. We believe that the tenth edition will satisfy this need even more successfully. Spanish, Portuguese, Italian, French, Czech, Indonesian, Japanese, and Chinese translations are available. Translations into other languages are under way; the publisher may be contacted for further information.

I wish to acknowledge the prior and continuing efforts of my contributing authors and the major contributions of the staff at Lange Medical Publications, Appleton & Lange, and more recently at McGraw-Hill, and of our editors, Alison Kelley and Donna Frassetto. I also wish to thank my wife, Alice Camp, for her expert proofreading contributions since the first edition.

Special thanks and recognition are due James Ransom, PhD, the long-time Senior Editor at Lange Medical Publications, who provided major inspiration and invaluable guidance through the first eight editions of the book. Without him, this book would not exist.

Suggestions and comments about *Basic & Clinical Pharmacology* are always welcome. They may be sent to me at the Department of Cellular & Molecular Pharmacology, P.O. Box 0450, University of California, San Francisco, CA 94143-0450.

Bertram G. Katzung, MD, PhD
San Francisco
September 2006

Authors

Emmanuel T. Akporiaye, PhD
Professor, Department of Microbiology and Immunology, University of Arizona Health Sciences Center, Tucson

Michael J. Aminoff, MD, DSc, FRCP
Professor, Department of Neurology, University of California, San Francisco

Allan I. Basbaum, PhD
Professor and Chair, Department of Anatomy and W.M. Keck Foundation Center for Integrative Neuroscience, University of California, San Francisco

Neal L. Benowitz, MD
Professor of Medicine, Psychiatry, and Biopharmaceutical Sciences, University of California, San Francisco

Barry A. Berkowitz, PhD
Adjunct Professor, Northeastern University, Boston University; CEO and President, Cetek Corporation, Marlborough, Massachusetts

Daniel D. Bikle, MD, PhD
Professor of Medicine, Department of Medicine, and Co-Director, Special Diagnostic and Treatment Unit, University of California, San Francisco, and Veterans Affairs Medical Center, San Francisco

Henry R. Bourne, MD
Professor, Department of Cellular & Molecular Pharmacology, University of California, San Francisco

Homer A. Boushey, MD
Chief, Asthma Clinical Research Center and Division of Allergy & Immunology; Professor of Medicine, Department of Medicine, University of California, San Francisco

Adrienne D. Briggs, MD
Clinical Director, Bone Marrow Transplant Program, Banner Good Samaritan Hospital, Phoenix

Henry F. Chambers, MD
Professor of Medicine, University of California, San Francisco; Chief of Infectious Diseases, San Francisco General Hospital, San Francisco

Kanu Chatterjee, MB, FRCP, FCCP, FACC, MACP
Ernest Gallo Distinguished Professor of Medicine, University of California, San Francisco

George P. Chrousos, MD
Professor & Chair, First Department of Pediatrics, Athens University Medical School, Athens

Edward Chu, MD
Professor of Medicine and Pharmacology; Director, VACT Cancer Center; Associate Director, Yale Cancer Center; Yale University School of Medicine, New Haven

Robin L. Corelli, PharmD
Associate Clinical Professor, Department of Clinical Pharmacy, School of Pharmacy, University of California, San Francisco

Maria Almira Correia, PhD
Professor of Pharmacology, Pharmaceutical Chemistry and Biopharmaceutical Sciences, Department of Cellular & Molecular Pharmacology, University of California, San Francisco

Cathi E. Dennehy, PharmD
Associate Clinical Professor, Department of Clinical Pharmacy, School of Pharmacy, University of California, San Francisco

Betty J. Dong, PharmD
Professor of Clinical Pharmacy and Clinical Professor of Family and Community Medicine, Department of Clinical Pharmacy and Department of Family and Community Medicine, Schools of Pharmacy and Medicine, University of California, San Francisco

Garret A. FitzGerald, MD
Professor and Chair, Department of Pharmacology, University of Pennsylvania School of Medicine, Philadelphia

Daniel E. Furst, MD
Carl M. Pearson Professor of Rheumatology, Director, Rheumatology Clinical Research Center, Department of Rheumatology, University of California, Los Angeles

Augustus O. Grant, MD, PhD
Professor of Medicine, Cardiovascular Division, Duke University Medical Center, Durham

Francis S. Greenspan, MD, FCAP
Clinical Professor of Medicine and Radiology and Chief, Thyroid Clinic, Division of Endocrinology, Department of Medicine, University of California, San Francisco

Brian B. Hoffman, MD
Visiting Professor of Medicine, Harvard Medical School, Boston; Co-Chief of Medicine, Veterans Administration Boston Health Care System, West Roxbury

Nicholas H. G. Holford, MBChB, MSc, MRCP(UK), FRACP
Professor, Department of Pharmacology and Clinical Pharmacology, University of Auckland Medical School, Auckland

Leo E. Hollister, MD[†]
Professor Emeritus of Psychiatry, University of Texas Medical School, Houston

John R. Horn, PharmD
Professor of Pharmacy, School of Pharmacy, University of Washington, Seattle

Joseph R. Hume, PhD
Professor and Chairman, Department of Pharmacology; Adjunct Professor, Department of Physiology and Cell Biology, University of Nevada School of Medicine, Reno

Harlan E. Ives, MD, PhD
Professor of Medicine, Department of Medicine, University of California, San Francisco

Samie R. Jaffrey, MD, PhD
Associate Professor of Pharmacology, Department of Pharmacology, Cornell University Weill Medical College, New York City

John P. Kane, MD, PhD
Professor of Medicine, Department of Medicine; Professor of Biochemistry and Biophysics; Associate Director, Cardiovascular Research Institute, University of California, San Francisco

John H. Karam, MD[†]
Professor Emeritus, Department of Medicine, University of California, San Francisco

Bertram G. Katzung, MD, PhD
Professor Emeritus, Department of Cellular & Molecular Pharmacology, University of California, San Francisco

Gideon Koren, MD, FABMT, FRCPC
Professor and Chairman, Ivey Chair in Molecular Toxicology, University of Western Ontario; Director, The Motherisk Program, Professor of Pediatrics, Pharmacology, Pharmacy, Medicine, and Medical Genetics, The University of Toronto; Senior Scientist, The Research Institute, The Hospital for Sick Children, Toronto

Michael J. Kosnett, MD, MPH
Associate Clinical Professor of Medicine, Division of Clinical Pharmacology and Toxicology, University of Colorado Health Sciences Center, Denver

Douglas F. Lake, PhD
Associate Professor, The Biodesign Institute, Arizona State University, Tempe

Harry W. Lampiris, MD
Associate Professor of Medicine, School of Medicine, University of California, San Francisco

Paul W. Lofholm, PharmD
Clinical Professor of Pharmacy, School of Pharmacy, University of California, San Francisco

[†]Deceased

Christian Lüscher, MD
Departements des Neurosciences fondamentales et cliniques, University of Geneva

Daniel S. Maddix, PharmD
Associate Clinical Professor of Pharmacy, University of California, San Francisco

Howard I. Maibach, MD
Professor of Dermatology, Department of Dermatology, University of California, San Francisco

Mary J. Malloy, MD
Clinical Professor of Pediatrics and Medicine, Departments of Pediatrics and Medicine, Cardiovascular Research Institute, University of California, San Francisco

Susan B. Masters, PhD
Adjunct Professor of Pharmacology, Department of Cellular & Molecular Pharmacology, University of California, San Francisco

Kenneth R. McQuaid, MD
Professor of Clinical Medicine, Department of Medicine, University of California, San Francisco; Director of Gastrointestinal Endoscopy, San Francisco Veterans Affairs Medical Center, San Francisco

Brian S. Meldrum, MB, PhD
Professor Emeritus, GKT School of Medicine, Guy's Campus, London

Roger A. Nicoll, MD
Professor of Pharmacology and Physiology, Departments of Cellular & Molecular Pharmacology and Physiology, University of California, San Francisco

Martha S. Nolte, MD
Associate Clinical Professor, Department of Medicine, University of California, San Francisco

Kent R. Olson, MD
Clinical Professor, Departments of Medicine, and Pharmacy, University of California, San Francisco; Medical Director, San Francisco Division, California Poison Control System

Achilles J. Pappano, PhD
Professor, Department of Pharmacology, University of Connecticut Health Center, Farmington

William W. Parmley, MD, MACC
Emeritus Professor of Medicine, University of California, San Francisco

Gabriel L. Plaa, PhD
Professeur Émérite de Pharmacologie, Départment de Pharmacologie, Faculté de Médecine, Université de Montréal

Roger J. Porter, MD
Adjunct Professor of Neurology, University of Pennsylvania, Philadelphia; Adjunct Professor of Pharmacology, Uniformed Services University of the Health Sciences, Bethesda

William Z. Potter, MD, PhD
Vice President, Clinical Neuroscience Division, MERCK Research Laboratories, West Point

Ian A. Reid, PhD
Professor Emeritus, Department of Physiology, University of California, San Francisco

Dirk B. Robertson, MD
Professor of Clinical Dermatology, Department of Dermatology, Emory University School of Medicine, Atlanta

Philip J. Rosenthal, MD
Professor, Department of Medicine, San Francisco General Hospital, University of California, San Francisco

Sharon Safrin, MD, FACP
Associate Clinical Professor, Department of Medicine, University of California, San Francisco

Alan C. Sartorelli, PhD
Alfred Gilman Professor of Pharmacology, Department of Pharmacology, Yale University School of Medicine, New Haven

Mark A. Schumacher, PhD, MD
Associate Professor, Department of Anesthesia and Perioperative Care, University of California, San Francisco

Don Sheppard, MD
Assistant Professor, Departments of Medicine, Microbiology and Immunology, McGill University, Montreal

Emer M. Smyth, PhD
Assistant Professor, Department of Pharmacology, University of Pennsylvania School of Medicine, Philadelphia

Anthony J. Trevor, PhD
Professor Emeritus, Department of Cellular & Molecular Pharmacology, University of California, San Francisco

Candy Tsourounis, PharmD
Associate Professor of Clinical Pharmacy, Department of Clinical Pharmacy, School of Pharmacy, University of California, San Francisco

Robert W. Ulrich, PharmD
Associate Professor, School of Medicine, University of California, Los Angeles

Mark von Zastrow, MD, PhD
Associate Professor, Departments of Psychiatry and Cellular & Molecular Pharmacology, University of California, San Francisco

Alice Lee Wang, PhD
Associate Research Chemist, Department of Pharmaceutical Chemistry, University of California, San Francisco

Ching Chung Wang, PhD
Professor of Chemistry and Pharmaceutical Chemistry, Department of Pharmaceutical Chemistry, University of California, San Francisco

Walter L. Way, MD
Professor Emeritus, Departments of Anesthesia and Cellular & Molecular Pharmacology, University of California, San Francisco

Paul F. White, PhD, MD
Professor and Holder of the Margaret Milam McDermott Distinguished Chair of Anesthesiology, Department of Anesthesiology and Pain Management, University of Texas Southwestern Medical Center at Dallas Southwestern Medical School, Dallas

James L. Zehnder, MD
Professor of Pathology and Medicine, Pathology Department, Stanford University School of Medicine, Stanford

SECTION I
Basic Principles

Introduction

Bertram G. Katzung, MD, PhD

Pharmacology can be defined as the study of substances that interact with living systems through chemical processes, especially by binding to regulatory molecules and activating or inhibiting normal body processes. These substances may be chemicals administered to achieve a beneficial therapeutic effect on some process within the patient or for their toxic effects on regulatory processes in parasites infecting the patient. Such deliberate therapeutic applications may be considered the proper role of **medical pharmacology,** which is often defined as the science of substances used to prevent, diagnose, and treat disease. **Toxicology** is that branch of pharmacology which deals with the undesirable effects of chemicals on living systems, from individual cells to complex ecosystems.

THE HISTORY OF PHARMACOLOGY

Prehistoric people undoubtedly recognized the beneficial or toxic effects of many plant and animal materials. Early written records from China and from Egypt list remedies of many types, including a few still recognized as useful drugs today. Most, however, were worthless or actually harmful. In the 1500 years or so preceding the present, there were sporadic attempts to introduce rational methods into medicine, but none was successful owing to the dominance of systems of thought that purported to explain all of biology and disease without the need for experimentation and observation. These schools promulgated bizarre notions such as the idea that disease was caused by excesses of bile or blood in the body, that wounds could be healed by applying a salve to the weapon that caused the wound, and so on.

Around the end of the 17th century, reliance on observation and experimentation began to replace theorizing in medicine, following the example of the physical sciences. As the value of these methods in the study of disease became clear, physicians in Great Britain and on the Continent began to apply them to the effects of traditional drugs used in their own practices. Thus, **materia medica**—the science of drug preparation and the medical use of drugs—began to develop as the precursor to pharmacology. However, any real understanding of the mechanisms of action of drugs was prevented by the absence of methods for purifying active agents from the crude materials that were available and—even more—by the lack of methods for testing hypotheses about the nature of drug actions.

In the late 18th and early 19th centuries, François Magendie, and later his student Claude Bernard, began to develop the methods of **experimental animal physiology** and **pharmacology.** Advances in chemistry and the further development of physiology in the 18th, 19th, and early 20th centuries laid the foundation needed for understanding how drugs work at the organ and tissue levels. Paradoxically, real advances in basic pharmacology during this time were accompanied by an outburst of unscientific promotion by manufacturers and marketers of worthless "patent medicines." Not until the concepts of rational therapeutics, especially that of the **controlled clinical trial,** were reintroduced into medicine—only about 50 years ago—did it become possible to accurately evaluate therapeutic claims.

Around the same time, a major expansion of research efforts in all areas of biology began. As new concepts and new techniques were introduced, information accumulated about drug action and the biologic substrate of that action, the **drug receptor.** During the last half-century, many fundamentally new drug groups and new members of old groups were introduced. The last three decades have seen an even more rapid growth of information and understanding of the molecular basis for drug action. The molecular mechanisms of action of many drugs have now been identified, and numerous receptors have been isolated, structurally characterized, and cloned. In fact, the use of receptor identification methods (described in Chapter 2) has led to the discovery of many orphan receptors—receptors for which no ligand has been discovered and whose function can only be surmised. Studies of the local molecular environment of receptors have shown that receptors and effectors do not function in isolation; they are strongly influenced by companion regulatory proteins. Decoding of the genomes of many species—from bacteria to humans—has led to the recognition of unsuspected relationships between receptor families and the ways that receptor proteins have evolved. **Pharmacogenomics**—the relation of the individual's genetic makeup to his or her response to specific drugs—is close to becoming a practical area of therapy (see Box: Pharmacology & Genetics). Much of that progress is summarized in this book.

The extension of scientific principles into everyday therapeutics is still going on, although the medication-consuming public unfortunately is still exposed to vast amounts of inaccurate, incomplete, or unscientific information regarding the pharmacologic effects of chemicals. This has resulted in the faddish use of innumerable expensive, ineffective, and sometimes harmful remedies and the growth of a huge "alternative health care" industry. Conversely, lack of understanding of basic scientific principles in biology and statistics and the absence of critical thinking about public health issues have led to rejection of medical science by a segment of the public and to a common tendency to assume that all adverse drug effects are the result of malpractice.

Two general principles that the student should always remember are, first, that *all* substances can under certain circumstances be toxic; and second, that all dietary supplements and all therapies promoted as health-enhancing should meet the same standards of efficacy and safety, ie, there should be no artificial separation between scientific medicine and "alternative" or "complementary" medicine.

PHARMACOLOGY & GENETICS

It has been known for centuries that certain diseases are inherited, and we now understand that individuals with such diseases have a heritable abnormality in their DNA. During the last 10 years, the genomes of humans, mice, and many other organisms have been decoded in considerable detail. This has opened the door to a remarkable range of new approaches to research and treatment. It is now possible in the case of some inherited diseases to define exactly which DNA base pairs are anomalous and in which chromosome they appear. In a small number of animal models of such diseases, it has been possible to correct the abnormality by **gene therapy,** ie, insertion of an appropriate "healthy" gene into somatic cells. Human somatic cell gene therapy has been attempted, but the technical difficulties are great.

Studies of a newly discovered receptor or endogenous ligand are often confounded by incomplete knowledge of the exact role of that receptor or ligand. One of the most powerful of the new genetic techniques is the ability to breed animals (usually mice) in which the gene for the receptor or its endogenous ligand has been "knocked out," ie, mutated so that the gene product is absent or nonfunctional. Homozygous **knockout** mice usually have complete suppression of that function, whereas heterozygous animals usually have partial suppression. Observation of the behavior, biochemistry, and physiology of the knockout mice often defines the role of the missing gene product very clearly. When the products of a particular gene are so essential that even heterozygotes do not survive to birth, it is sometimes possible to breed "knockdown" versions with only limited suppression of function. Conversely, "knockin" mice have been bred, which overexpress certain proteins of interest.

Some patients respond to certain drugs with greater than usual sensitivity to standard doses. It is now clear that such increased sensitivity is often due to a very small genetic modification that results in decreased activity of a particular enzyme responsible for eliminating that drug. (Such variations are discussed in Chapter 4.) **Pharmacogenomics** (or pharmacogenetics) is the study of the genetic variations that cause differences in drug response among individuals or populations. Future clinicians may screen every patient for a variety of such differences before prescribing a drug.

PHARMACOLOGY & THE PHARMACEUTICAL INDUSTRY

Much of the recent progress in the application of drugs to disease problems can be ascribed to the pharmaceutical industry and specifically to "big pharma," the multibillion-dollar corporations that specialize in drug discovery and development. These entities deserve great credit for making possible many of the therapeutic advances that we enjoy today. As described in Chapter 5, these companies are uniquely skilled in exploiting discoveries from academic and governmental laboratories and translating these basic findings into commercially successful therapeutic breakthroughs.

Such breakthroughs come at a price, however, and the escalating cost of drugs has become a significant contributor to the inflationary increase in the cost of health care. Development of new drugs is enormously expensive and to survive and prosper, big pharma must pay the costs of drug development and marketing and return a profit to its shareholders. At present, considerable controversy surrounds drug pricing. Critics claim that the costs of development and marketing are grossly inflated by marketing procedures, which may consume as much as 25% or more of a company's budget in advertising and other promotional efforts. Furthermore, profit margins for big pharma have historically exceeded all other industries by a significant factor. Finally, pricing schedules for many drugs vary dramatically from country to country and even within countries, where large organizations can negotiate favorable prices and small ones cannot. Some countries have already addressed these problems, and it seems likely that all countries will have to do so during the next few decades.

GENERAL PRINCIPLES OF PHARMACOLOGY

The Nature of Drugs

In the most general sense, a drug may be defined as any substance that brings about a change in biologic function through its chemical actions. In the great majority of cases, the drug molecule interacts with a specific molecule in the biologic system that plays a regulatory role. This molecule is called a **receptor.** The nature of receptors is discussed more fully in Chapter 2. In a very small number of cases, drugs known as chemical antagonists may interact directly with other drugs, whereas a few drugs (osmotic agents) interact almost exclusively with water molecules. Drugs may be synthesized within the body (eg, **hormones**) or may be chemicals *not* synthesized in the body, ie, **xenobiotics** (from the Greek *xenos,* meaning "stranger"). **Poisons** are drugs that have almost exclusively harmful effects. However, Paracelsus (1493–1541) famously stated that "the dose makes the poison," meaning that almost all substances can be harmful if taken in the wrong dosage. **Toxins** are usually defined as poisons of biologic origin, ie, synthesized by plants or animals, in contrast to inorganic poisons such as lead and arsenic.

To interact chemically with its receptor, a drug molecule must have the appropriate size, electrical charge, shape, and atomic composition. Furthermore, a drug is often administered at a location distant from its intended site of action, eg, a pill given orally to relieve a headache. Therefore, a useful drug must have the necessary properties to be transported from its site of administration to its site of action. Finally, a practical drug should be inactivated or excreted from the body at a reasonable rate so that its actions will be of appropriate duration.

A. THE PHYSICAL NATURE OF DRUGS

Drugs may be solid at room temperature (eg, aspirin, atropine), liquid (eg, nicotine, ethanol), or gaseous (eg, nitrous oxide). These factors often determine the best route of administration. The most common routes of administration are described in Chapter 3. The various classes of organic compounds—carbohydrates, proteins, lipids, and their constituents—are all represented in pharmacology.

A number of useful or dangerous drugs are inorganic elements, eg, lithium, iron, and heavy metals. Many organic drugs are weak acids or bases. This fact has important implications for the way they are handled by the body, because pH differences in the various compartments of the body may alter the degree of ionization of such drugs (see below).

B. DRUG SIZE

The molecular size of drugs varies from very small (lithium ion, MW 7) to very large (eg, alteplase [t-PA], a protein of MW 59,050). However, most drugs have molecular weights between 100 and 1000. The lower limit of this narrow range is probably set by the requirements for specificity of action. To have a good "fit" to only one type of receptor, a drug molecule must be sufficiently unique in shape, charge, and other properties, to prevent its binding to other receptors. To achieve such selective binding, it appears that a molecule should in most cases be at least 100 MW units in size. The upper limit in molecular weight is determined primarily by the requirement that drugs be able to move within the body (eg, from site of administration to site of action). Drugs much larger than MW 1000 do not diffuse readily between compartments of the body (see Permeation, below). Therefore, very large drugs (usually proteins) must often be administered directly into the compartment where they have their effect. In the case of alteplase, a clot-dissolving enzyme, the drug is administered directly into the vascular compartment by intravenous or intra-arterial infusion.

C. Drug Reactivity and Drug-Receptor Bonds

Drugs interact with receptors by means of chemical forces or bonds. These are of three major types: **covalent, electrostatic,** and **hydrophobic.** Covalent bonds are very strong and in many cases not reversible under biologic conditions. Thus, the covalent bond formed between the acetyl group of aspirin and its enzyme target in platelets, cyclooxygenase, is not readily broken. The platelet aggregation–blocking effect of aspirin lasts long after free acetylsalicylic acid has disappeared from the bloodstream (about 15 minutes) and is reversed only by the synthesis of new enzyme in new platelets, a process that takes about 7 days. Other examples of highly reactive, covalent bond-forming drugs are the DNA-alkylating agents used in cancer chemotherapy to disrupt cell division in the tumor.

Electrostatic bonding is much more common than covalent bonding in drug-receptor interactions. Electrostatic bonds vary from relatively strong linkages between permanently charged ionic molecules to weaker hydrogen bonds and very weak induced dipole interactions such as van der Waals forces and similar phenomena. Electrostatic bonds are weaker than covalent bonds.

Hydrophobic bonds are usually quite weak and are probably important in the interactions of highly lipid-soluble drugs with the lipids of cell membranes and perhaps in the interaction of drugs with the internal walls of receptor "pockets."

The specific nature of a particular drug-receptor bond is of less practical importance than the fact that drugs that bind through weak bonds to their receptors are generally more selective than drugs that bind by means of very strong bonds. This is because weak bonds require a very precise fit of the drug to its receptor if an interaction is to occur. Only a few receptor types are likely to provide such a precise fit for a particular drug structure. Thus, if we wished to design a highly selective short-acting drug for a particular receptor, we would avoid highly reactive molecules that form covalent bonds and instead choose molecules that form weaker bonds.

A few substances that are almost completely inert in the chemical sense nevertheless have significant pharmacologic effects. For example, xenon, an "inert" gas, has anesthetic effects at elevated pressures.

D. Drug Shape

The shape of a drug molecule must be such as to permit binding to its receptor site via the bonds just described. Optimally, the drug's shape is complementary to that

Table 1–1. Dissociation constants (K_d) of the enantiomers and racemate of carvedilol.

Form of Carvedilol	Inverse of Affinity for α Receptors (K_d, nmol/L)	Inverse of Affinity for β Receptors (K_d, nmol/L)
R(+) enantiomer	14	45
S(–) enantiomer	16	0.4
R,S(+/–) enantiomers	11	0.9

Note: The K_d is the concentration for 50% saturation of the receptors and is inversely proportionate to the affinity of the drug for the receptors.
Data from Ruffolo RR et al: The pharmacology of carvedilol. Eur J Pharmacol 1990;38:S82.

of the receptor site in the same way that a key is complementary to a lock. Furthermore, the phenomenon of **chirality (stereoisomerism)** is so common in biology that more than half of all useful drugs are chiral molecules; that is, they exist as enantiomeric pairs. Drugs with two asymmetric centers have four diastereomers, eg, ephedrine, a sympathomimetic drug. In most cases, one of these enantiomers is much more potent than its mirror image enantiomer, reflecting a better fit to the receptor molecule. For example, the (S)(+) enantiomer of methacholine, a parasympathomimetic drug, is over 250 times more potent than the (R)(–) enantiomer. If one imagines the receptor site to be like a glove into which the drug molecule must fit to bring about its effect, it is clear why a "left-oriented" drug is more effective in binding to a left-hand receptor than its "right-oriented" enantiomer.

The more active enantiomer at one type of receptor site may not be more active at another type, eg, a receptor type that may be responsible for some other effect. For example, carvedilol, a drug that interacts with adrenoceptors, has a single chiral center and thus two enantiomers (Table 1–1). One of these enantiomers, the (S)(–) isomer, is a potent β-receptor blocker. The (R)(+) isomer is 100-fold weaker at the β receptor. However, the isomers are approximately equipotent as α-receptor blockers. Ketamine is an intravenous anesthetic. The (+) enantiomer is a more potent anesthetic and is less toxic than the (–) enantiomer. Unfortunately, the drug is still used as the racemic mixture.

Finally, because enzymes are usually stereoselective, one drug enantiomer is often more susceptible than the other to drug-metabolizing enzymes. As a result, the duration of action of one enantiomer may be quite different from that of the other.

Unfortunately, most studies of clinical efficacy and drug elimination in humans have been carried out with racemic mixtures of drugs rather than with the separate enantiomers. At present, only about 45% of the chiral drugs used clinically are marketed as the active isomer—the rest are available only as racemic mixtures. As a result, many patients are receiving drug doses of which 50% or more is less active, inactive, or actively toxic. However, there is increasing interest at both the scientific and the regulatory levels in making more chiral drugs available as their active enantiomers.

E. RATIONAL DRUG DESIGN

Rational design of drugs implies the ability to predict the appropriate molecular structure of a drug on the basis of information about its biologic receptor. Until recently, no receptor was known in sufficient detail to permit such drug design. Instead, drugs were developed through random testing of chemicals or modification of drugs already known to have some effect (see Chapter 5). However, during the past three decades, many receptors have been isolated and characterized. A few drugs now in use were developed through molecular design based on a knowledge of the three-dimensional structure of the receptor site. Computer programs are now available that can iteratively optimize drug structures to fit known receptors. As more becomes known about receptor structure, rational drug design will become more common.

F. RECEPTOR NOMENCLATURE

The spectacular success of newer, more efficient ways to identify and characterize receptors (see Chapter 2) has resulted in a variety of differing systems for naming them. This in turn has led to a number of suggestions regarding more rational methods of naming them. The interested reader is referred for details to the efforts of the International Union of Pharmacology (IUPHAR) *Committee on Receptor Nomenclature and Drug Classification* (reported in various issues of *Pharmacological Reviews*) and to Alexander SPH, Mathie A, Peters JA: Guide to receptors and channels. Br J Pharmacol 2006;147(Suppl 3):S1–S180. The chapters in this book mainly use these sources for naming receptors.

Drug-Body Interactions

The interactions between a drug and the body are conveniently divided into two classes. The actions of the drug on the body are termed **pharmacodynamic** processes; the principles of pharmacodynamics are presented in greater detail in Chapter 2. These properties determine the group in which the drug is classified and play the major role in deciding whether that group is appropriate therapy for a particular symptom or disease. The actions of the body on the drug are called **pharmacokinetic** processes and are described in Chapters 3 and 4. Pharmacokinetic processes govern the absorption, distribution, and elimination of drugs and are of great practical importance in the choice and administration of a particular drug for a particular patient, eg, a patient with impaired renal function. The following paragraphs provide a brief introduction to pharmacodynamics and pharmacokinetics.

Pharmacodynamic Principles

Most drugs must bind to a receptor to bring about an effect. However, at the molecular level, drug binding is only the first in what is often a complex sequence of steps.

A. TYPES OF DRUG-RECEPTOR INTERACTIONS

Agonist drugs bind to and *activate* the receptor in some fashion, which directly or indirectly brings about the effect. Some receptors incorporate effector machinery in the same molecule, so that drug binding brings about the effect directly, eg, opening of an ion channel or activation of enzyme activity. Other receptors are linked through one or more intervening coupling molecules to a separate effector molecule. The five major types of drug-receptor-effector coupling systems are discussed in Chapter 2. **Pharmacologic antagonist** drugs, by binding to a receptor, *prevent* binding by other molecules. For example, acetylcholine receptor blockers such as atropine are antagonists because they prevent access of acetylcholine and similar agonist drugs to the acetylcholine receptor and they stabilize the receptor in its inactive state. These agents reduce the effects of acetylcholine and similar molecules in the body.

B. AGONISTS THAT *INHIBIT* THEIR BINDING MOLECULES AND PARTIAL AGONISTS

Some drugs mimic agonist drugs by inhibiting the molecules responsible for terminating the action of an endogenous agonist. For example, acetylcholinesterase *inhibitors*, by slowing the destruction of endogenous acetylcholine, cause cholinomimetic effects that closely resemble the actions of cholinoceptor *agonist* molecules even though cholinesterase inhibitors do not bind or only incidentally bind to cholinoceptors (see Chapter 7, Cholinoceptor-Activating & Cholinesterase-Inhibiting Drugs). Other drugs bind to receptors and activate them but do not evoke as great a response as so-called full agonists. Thus, pindolol, a β adrenoceptor "partial agonist," may act as either an agonist (if no full agonist is present) or as an antagonist (if a full agonist such as epinephrine is present). (See Chapter 2.)

C. DURATION OF DRUG ACTION

Termination of drug action at the receptor level results from one of several processes. In some cases, the effect lasts only as long as the drug occupies the receptor, so that dissociation of drug from the receptor automatically terminates the effect. In many cases, however, the action may persist after the drug has dissociated, because, for example, some coupling molecule is still present in activated form. In the case of drugs that bind covalently to the receptor site, the effect may persist until the drug-receptor complex is destroyed and new receptors or enzymes are synthesized, as described previously for aspirin. Finally, many receptor-effector systems incorporate desensitization mechanisms for preventing excessive activation when agonist molecules continue to be present for long periods. See Chapter 2 for additional details.

D. Receptors and Inert Binding Sites

To function as a receptor, an endogenous molecule must first be **selective** in choosing ligands (drug molecules) to bind; and second, it must **change its function** upon binding in such a way that the function of the biologic system (cell, tissue, etc) is altered. The first characteristic is required to avoid constant activation of the receptor by promiscuous binding of many different ligands. The second characteristic is clearly necessary if the ligand is to cause a pharmacologic effect. The body contains many molecules that are capable of binding drugs, however, and not all of these endogenous molecules are regulatory molecules. Binding of a drug to a nonregulatory molecule such as plasma albumin will result in no detectable change in the function of the biologic system, so this endogenous molecule can be called an inert binding site. Such binding is not completely without significance, however, because it affects the distribution of drug within the body and determines the amount of free drug in the circulation. Both of these factors are of pharmacokinetic importance (see below and Chapter 3).

Pharmacokinetic Principles

In practical therapeutics, a drug should be able to reach its intended site of action after administration by some convenient route. In some cases, a chemical that is readily absorbed and distributed is administered and then converted to the active drug by biologic processes—inside the body. Such a chemical is called a **prodrug.**

In only a few situations is it possible to directly apply a drug to its target tissue, eg, by topical application of an anti-inflammatory agent to inflamed skin or mucous membrane. Most often, a drug is administered into one body compartment, eg, the gut, and must move to its site of action in another compartment, eg, the brain. This requires that the drug be **absorbed** into the blood from its site of administration and **distributed** to its site of action, **permeating** through the various barriers that separate these compartments. For a drug given orally to produce an effect in the central nervous system, these barriers include the tissues that make up the wall of the intestine, the walls of the capillaries that perfuse the gut,

and the "blood-brain barrier," the walls of the capillaries that perfuse the brain. Finally, after bringing about its effect, a drug should be **eliminated** at a reasonable rate by metabolic inactivation, by excretion from the body, or by a combination of these processes.

A. Permeation

Drug permeation proceeds by several mechanisms. Passive diffusion in an aqueous or lipid medium is common, but active processes play a role in the movement of many drugs, especially those whose molecules are too large to diffuse readily.

1. Aqueous diffusion—Aqueous diffusion occurs within the larger aqueous compartments of the body (interstitial space, cytosol, etc) and across epithelial membrane tight junctions and the endothelial lining of blood vessels through aqueous pores that—in some tissues—permit the passage of molecules as large as MW 20,000–30,000.*

Aqueous diffusion of drug molecules is usually driven by the concentration gradient of the permeating drug, a downhill movement described by Fick's law (see below). Drug molecules that are bound to large plasma proteins (eg, albumin) do not permeate most vascular aqueous pores. If the drug is charged, its flux is also influenced by electrical fields (eg, the membrane potential and—in parts of the nephron—the transtubular potential).

2. Lipid diffusion—Lipid diffusion is the most important limiting factor for drug permeation because of the large number of lipid barriers that separate the compartments of the body. Because these lipid barriers separate aqueous compartments, the lipid:aqueous partition coefficient of a drug determines how readily the molecule moves between aqueous and lipid media. In the case of weak acids and weak bases (which gain or lose electrical charge-bearing protons, depending on the pH), the ability to move from aqueous to lipid or vice versa varies with the pH of the medium, because charged molecules attract water molecules. The ratio of lipid-soluble form to water-soluble form for a weak acid or weak base is expressed by the Henderson-Hasselbalch equation (see below).

3. Special carriers—Special carrier molecules exist for certain substances that are important for cell function and too large or too insoluble in lipid to diffuse passively through membranes, eg, peptides, amino acids, glucose. These carriers bring about movement by active transport or facilitated diffusion and, unlike passive diffusion, are saturable and inhibitable. Because many drugs are or resemble such naturally occurring peptides,

---

*The capillaries of the brain, the testes, and some other tissues are characterized by the absence of pores that permit aqueous diffusion. They may also contain high concentrations of drug export pumps (MDR pumps; see text). These tissues are therefore protected or "sanctuary" sites from many circulating drugs.

amino acids, or sugars, they can use these carriers to cross membranes.

Many cells also contain less selective membrane carriers that are specialized for expelling foreign molecules. One large family of such transporters bind adenosine triphosphate (ATP) and is called the ABC (ATP-binding cassette) family. This family includes the **P-glycoprotein** or **multidrug-resistance type 1 (MDR1) transporter** found in the brain, testes, and other tissues, and in some drug-resistant neoplastic cells. Similar transport molecules from the ABC family, the **multidrug resistance-associated protein (MRP1** through **MRP5)** transporters, play important roles in excretion of some drugs or their metabolites into urine and bile and in resistance of some tumors to chemotherapeutic drugs. Several other transporter families have been identified that do not bind ATP but use ion gradients for transport energy. Some of these are particularly important in the uptake of neurotransmitters across nerve ending membranes.

4. Endocytosis and exocytosis—A few substances are so large or impermeant that they can enter cells only by endocytosis, the process by which the substance is engulfed by the cell membrane and carried into the cell by pinching off of the newly formed vesicle inside the membrane. The substance can then be released inside the cytosol by breakdown of the vesicle membrane. This process is responsible for the transport of vitamin B_{12}, complexed with a binding protein (intrinsic factor) across the wall of the gut into the blood. Similarly, iron is transported into hemoglobin-synthesizing red blood cell precursors in association with the protein transferrin. Specific receptors for the transport proteins must be present for this process to work.

The reverse process (exocytosis) is responsible for the secretion of many substances from cells. For example, many neurotransmitter substances are stored in membrane-bound vesicles in nerve endings to protect them from metabolic destruction in the cytoplasm. Appropriate activation of the nerve ending causes fusion of the storage vesicle with the cell membrane and expulsion of its contents into the extracellular space (see Chapter 6).

B. Fick's Law of Diffusion

The passive flux of molecules down a concentration gradient is given by Fick's law:

Flux (molecules per unit time) =

$$(C_1 - C_2) \times \frac{\text{Area} \times \text{Permeability coefficient}}{\text{Thickness}}$$

where C_1 is the higher concentration, C_2 is the lower concentration, area is the area across which diffusion is occurring, permeability coefficient is a measure of the mobility of the drug molecules in the medium of the diffusion path,

and thickness is the thickness (length) of the diffusion path. In the case of lipid diffusion, the lipid:aqueous partition coefficient is a major determinant of mobility of the drug, because it determines how readily the drug enters the lipid membrane from the aqueous medium.

C. Ionization of Weak Acids and Weak Bases; the Henderson-Hasselbalch Equation

The electrostatic charge of an ionized molecule attracts water dipoles and results in a polar, relatively water-soluble and lipid-insoluble complex. Because lipid diffusion depends on relatively high lipid solubility, ionization of drugs may markedly reduce their ability to permeate membranes. A very large fraction of the drugs in use are weak acids or weak bases (Table 1–2). For drugs, a weak acid is best defined as a neutral molecule that can reversibly dissociate into an anion (a negatively charged molecule) and a proton (a hydrogen ion). For example, aspirin dissociates as follows:

$$C_8H_7O_2COOH \rightleftharpoons C_8H_7O_2COO^- + H^+$$

Neutral   Aspirin   Proton
aspirin   anion

A drug that is a weak base can be defined as a neutral molecule that can form a cation (a positively charged molecule) by combining with a proton. For example, pyrimethamine, an antimalarial drug, undergoes the following association-dissociation process:

$$C_{12}H_{11}ClN_3NH_3^+ \rightleftharpoons C_{12}H_{11}ClN_3NH_2 + H^+$$

Pyrimethamine   Neutral   Proton
cation   pyrimethamine

Note that the protonated form of a weak acid is the neutral, more lipid-soluble form, whereas the unprotonated form of a weak base is the neutral form. The law of mass action requires that these reactions move to the left in an acid environment (low pH, excess protons available) and to the right in an alkaline environment. The Henderson-Hasselbalch equation relates the ratio of protonated to unprotonated weak acid or weak base to the molecule's pK_a and the pH of the medium as follows:

$$\log \frac{(\text{Protonated})}{(\text{Unprotonated})} = pK_a - pH$$

This equation applies to both acidic and basic drugs. Inspection confirms that the lower the pH relative to the pK_a, the greater will be the fraction of drug in the protonated form. Because the uncharged form is the more lipid-soluble, more of a weak acid will be in the lipid-soluble form at acid pH, whereas more of a basic drug will be in the lipid-soluble form at alkaline pH.

Table 1–2. Ionization constants of some common drugs.

Drug	pK$_a$[1]	Drug	pK$_a$[1]	Drug	pK$_a$[1]
Weak acids		**Weak bases**		**Weak bases (cont'd)**	
Acetaminophen	9.5	Albuterol (salbutamol)	9.3	Isoproterenol	8.6
Acetazolamide	7.2	Allopurinol	9.4, 12.3[2]	Lidocaine	7.9
Ampicillin	2.5	Alprenolol	9.6	Metaraminol	8.6
Aspirin	3.5	Amiloride	8.7	Methadone	8.4
Chlorothiazide	6.8, 9.4[2]	Amiodarone	6.56	Methamphetamine	10.0
Chlorpropamide	5.0	Amphetamine	9.8	Methyldopa	10.6
Ciprofloxacin	6.1, 8.7[2]	Atropine	9.7	Metoprolol	9.8
Cromolyn	2.0	Bupivacaine	8.1	Morphine	7.9
Ethacrynic acid	2.5	Chlordiazepoxide	4.6	Nicotine	7.9, 3.1[2]
Furosemide	3.9	Chloroquine	10.8, 8.4	Norepinephrine	8.6
Ibuprofen	4.4, 5.2[2]	Chlorpheniramine	9.2	Pentazocine	7.9
Levodopa	2.3	Chlorpromazine	9.3	Phenylephrine	9.8
Methotrexate	4.8	Clonidine	8.3	Physostigmine	7.9, 1.8[2]
Methyldopa	2.2, 9.2[2]	Cocaine	8.5	Pilocarpine	6.9, 1.4[2]
Penicillamine	1.8	Codeine	8.2	Pindolol	8.6
Pentobarbital	8.1	Cyclizine	8.2	Procainamide	9.2
Phenobarbital	7.4	Desipramine	10.2	Procaine	9.0
Phenytoin	8.3	Diazepam	3	Promethazine	9.1
Propylthiouracil	8.3	Diphenhydramine	8.8	Propranolol	9.4
Salicylic acid	3.0	Diphenoxylate	7.1	Pseudoephedrine	9.8
Sulfadiazine	6.5	Ephedrine	9.6	Pyrimethamine	7.0
Sulfapyridine	8.4	Epinephrine	8.7	Quinidine	8.5, 4.4[2]
Theophylline	8.8	Ergotamine	6.3	Scopolamine	8.1
Tolbutamide	5.3	Fluphenazine	8.0, 3.9[2]	Strychnine	8.0, 2.3[2]
Warfarin	5.0	Hydralazine	7.1	Terbutaline	10.1
		Imipramine	9.5	Thioridazine	9.5

[1]The pK$_a$ is that pH at which the concentrations of the ionized and un-ionized forms are equal.
[2]More than one ionizable group.

Application of this principle is made in the manipulation of drug excretion by the kidney. Almost all drugs are filtered at the glomerulus. If a drug is in a lipid-soluble form during its passage down the renal tubule, a significant fraction will be reabsorbed by simple passive diffusion. If the goal is to accelerate excretion of the drug (eg, in a case of drug overdose), it is important to prevent its reabsorption from the tubule. This can often be accomplished by adjusting urine pH to make certain that most of the drug is in the ionized state, as shown in Figure 1–1. As a result of this partitioning effect, the drug will be "trapped" in the urine. Thus, weak acids are usually excreted faster in alkaline urine; weak bases are usually excreted faster in acidic urine. Other body fluids in which pH differences from blood pH may cause trapping or reabsorption are the contents of the stomach and small intestine; breast milk; aqueous humor; and vaginal and prostatic secretions (Table 1–3).

As suggested by Table 1–2, a large number of drugs are weak bases. Most of these bases are amine-containing molecules. The nitrogen of a neutral amine has three atoms associated with it plus a pair of unshared electrons (see the display that follows). The three atoms may consist of one carbon (designated "R") and two hydrogens (a ***primary*** amine), two carbons and one hydrogen (a ***secondary*** amine), or three carbon atoms (a ***tertiary*** amine). Each of these three forms may reversibly bind a proton with the unshared electrons. Some drugs have a fourth carbon-nitrogen bond; these are ***quaternary*** amines. However, the quaternary amine is permanently charged and has no unshared electrons with which to reversibly bind a proton. Therefore, primary, secondary, and tertiary amines may undergo reversible protonation and vary their lipid solubility with pH, but quaternary amines are always in the poorly lipid-soluble charged form.

Primary	Secondary	Tertiary	Quaternary
H	R	R	R
$\overset{\cdot\cdot}{R:N:}$	$\overset{\cdot\cdot}{R:N:}$	$\overset{\cdot\cdot}{R:N:}$	$\overset{\cdot\cdot}{R:N:R}$
H	H	R	R

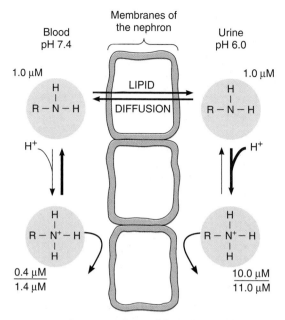

Figure 1–1. Trapping of a weak base (pyrimethamine) in the urine when the urine is more acidic than the blood. In the hypothetical case illustrated, the diffusible uncharged form of the drug has equilibrated across the membrane, but the total concentration (charged plus uncharged) in the urine is almost eight times higher than in the blood.

Drug Groups

To learn each pertinent fact about each of the many hundreds of drugs mentioned in this book would be an impractical goal and, fortunately, is unnecessary. Almost all of the several thousand drugs currently available can be arranged in about 70 groups. Many of the drugs within each group are very similar in pharmacodynamic actions and often in their pharmacokinetic properties as well. For most groups, one or more **prototype drugs** can be identified that typify the most important characteristics of the group. This permits classification of other important drugs in the group as variants of the prototype, so that only the prototype must be learned in detail and, for the remaining drugs, only the differences from the prototype.

Sources of Information

Students who wish to review the field of pharmacology in preparation for an examination are referred to *Pharmacology: Examination and Board Review*, by Trevor, Katzung, and Masters (McGraw-Hill, 2005) or *USMLE Road Map: Pharmacology*, by Katzung and Trevor (McGraw-Hill, 2006).

The references at the end of each chapter in this book were selected to provide reviews, or classic publications, of information specific to those chapters. Specific questions relating to basic or clinical research are best answered by referring to the journals covering general pharmacology and clinical specialties. For the student and the physician, three periodicals can be recommended as especially useful sources of cur-

Table 1–3. Body fluids with potential for drug "trapping" through the pH-partitioning phenomenon.

Body Fluid	Range of pH	Total Fluid: Blood Concentration Ratios for Sulfadiazine (acid, pK$_a$ 6.5)[1]	Total Fluid: Blood Concentration Ratios for Pyrimethamine (base, pK$_a$ 7.0)[1]
Urine	5.0–8.0	0.12–4.65	72.24–0.79
Breast milk	6.4–7.6[2]	0.2–1.77	3.56–0.89
Jejunum, ileum contents	7.5–8.0[3]	1.23–3.54	0.94–0.79
Stomach contents	1.92–2.59[2]	0.11[4]	85,993–18,386
Prostatic secretions	6.45–7.4[2]	0.21	3.25–1.0
Vaginal secretions	3.4–4.2[3]	0.11[4]	2848–452

[1]Body fluid protonated-to-unprotonated drug ratios were calculated using each of the pH extremes cited; a blood pH of 7.4 was used for blood:drug ratio. For example, the steady-state urine:blood ratio for sulfadiazine is 0.12 at a urine pH of 5.0; this ratio is 4.65 at a urine pH of 8.0. Thus, sulfadiazine is much more effectively trapped and excreted in alkaline urine.
[2]Lentner C (editor): *Geigy Scientific Tables*, vol 1, 8th ed. Ciba Geigy, 1981.
[3]Bowman WC, Rand MJ: *Textbook of Pharmacology*, 2nd ed. Blackwell, 1980.
[4]Insignificant change in ratios over the physiologic pH range.

rent information about drugs: *The New England Journal of Medicine,* which publishes much original drug-related clinical research as well as frequent reviews of topics in pharmacology; *The Medical Letter on Drugs and Therapeutics,* which publishes brief critical reviews of new and old therapies, mostly pharmacologic; and *Drugs,* which publishes extensive reviews of drugs and drug groups.

Other sources of information pertinent to the USA should be mentioned as well. The "package insert" is a summary of information that the manufacturer is required to place in the prescription sales package; *Physicians' Desk Reference (PDR)* is a compendium of package inserts published annually with supplements twice a year. The *USP DI* (vol 1, *Drug Information for the Health Care Professional*) is a large annual drug compendium with monthly Internet updates published by the Micromedex Corporation. The package insert consists of a brief description of the pharmacology of the product. While this brochure contains much practical information, it is also used as a means of shifting liability for untoward drug reactions from the manufacturer onto the practitioner. Therefore, the manufacturer typically lists every toxic effect ever reported, no matter how rare. A useful and objective quarterly handbook that presents information on drug toxicity and interactions is *Drug Interactions: Analysis and Management.* Finally, the Food and Drug Administration (FDA) has an Internet website that carries news regarding recent drug approvals, withdrawals, warnings, etc. It can be reached using a personal computer equipped with Internet browser software at http://www.fda.gov.

The following addresses are provided for the convenience of readers wishing to obtain any of the publications mentioned above:

Drug Interactions: Analysis and Management (quarterly)
Wolters Kluwer Publications
111 Westport Plaza, Suite 300
St Louis, MO 63146

Pharmacology: Examination & Board Review, 7th ed.
McGraw-Hill Companies, Inc
2 Penn Plaza 12th Floor
New York, NY 10121-2298

USMLE Road Map: Pharmacology
McGraw-Hill Companies, Inc
2 Penn Plaza 12th Floor
New York, NY 10121-2298

The Medical Letter on Drugs and Therapeutics
56 Harrison Street
New Rochelle, NY 10801

The New England Journal of Medicine
10 Shattuck Street
Boston, MA 02115

Physicians' Desk Reference
Box 2017
Mahopac, NY 10541

United States Pharmacopeia Dispensing Information
Micromedex, Inc.
6200 S. Syracuse Way, Suite 300
Englewood, CO 80111

Drug Receptors & Pharmacodynamics

2

Henry R. Bourne, MD, & Mark von Zastrow, MD, PhD

Therapeutic and toxic effects of drugs result from their interactions with molecules in the patient. Most drugs act by associating with specific macromolecules in ways that alter the macromolecules' biochemical or biophysical activities. This idea, more than a century old, is embodied in the term **receptor**: the component of a cell or organism that interacts with a drug and initiates the chain of events leading to the drug's observed effects.

Receptors have become the central focus of investigation of drug effects and their mechanisms of action (pharmacodynamics). The receptor concept, extended to endocrinology, immunology, and molecular biology, has proved essential for explaining many aspects of biologic regulation. Many drug receptors have been isolated and characterized in detail, thus opening the way to precise understanding of the molecular basis of drug action.

The receptor concept has important practical consequences for the development of drugs and for arriving at therapeutic decisions in clinical practice. These consequences form the basis for understanding the actions and clinical uses of drugs described in almost every chapter of this book. They may be briefly summarized as follows:

(1) Receptors largely determine the quantitative relations between dose or concentration of drug and pharmacologic effects. The receptor's affinity for binding a drug determines the concentration of drug required to form a significant number of drug-receptor complexes, and the total number of receptors may limit the maximal effect a drug may produce.

(2) Receptors are responsible for selectivity of drug action. The molecular size, shape, and electrical charge of a drug determine whether—and with what affinity—it will bind to a particular receptor among the vast array of chemically different binding sites available in a cell, tissue, or patient. Accordingly, changes in the chemical structure of a drug can dramatically increase or decrease a new drug's affinities for different classes of receptors, with resulting alterations in therapeutic and toxic effects.

(3) Receptors mediate the actions of both pharmacologic agonists and antagonists. Some drugs and many natural ligands, such as hormones and neurotransmitters, regulate the function of receptor macromolecules as agonists; ie, they activate the receptor to signal as a direct result of binding to it. Some agonists activate a single kind of receptor to produce all of their biologic functions, whereas others selectively promote one receptor function more than another.

Other drugs act as pharmacologic antagonists; ie, they bind to receptors but do not activate generation of a signal; consequently, they interfere with the ability of an agonist to activate the receptor. The effect of a so-called "pure" antagonist on a cell or in a patient depends entirely on its preventing the binding of agonist molecules and blocking their biologic actions. Other antagonists, in addition to preventing agonist binding, suppress the basal signaling ("constitutive") activity of receptors. Some of the most useful drugs in clinical medicine are pharmacologic antagonists.

MACROMOLECULAR NATURE OF DRUG RECEPTORS

Most receptors are proteins, presumably because the structures of polypeptides provide both the necessary diversity and the necessary specificity of shape and electrical charge. Receptors vary greatly in structure and can be identified in many ways. Traditionally, drug binding was used to identify or purify receptors from tissue extracts; consequently, receptors were discovered more recently than the drugs that bind to them. However, advances in molecular biology and genome sequencing have begun to reverse this order. Now receptors are being discovered by predicted structure or sequence homology to other (known) receptors, and drugs that bind to them are developed later using chemical screening methods. This effort has revealed, for many known drugs, a larger diversity of receptors than previously anticipated. It has also identified a number of "orphan" receptors, so-called because their ligands are presently unknown, which may prove to be useful targets for the development of new drugs.

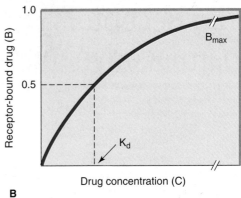

Figure 2–1. Relations between drug concentration and drug effect (panel **A**) or receptor-bound drug (panel **B**). The drug concentrations at which effect or receptor occupancy is half-maximal are denoted EC_{50} and K_d, respectively.

The best-characterized drug receptors are **regulatory proteins,** which mediate the actions of endogenous chemical signals such as neurotransmitters, autacoids, and hormones. This class of receptors mediates the effects of many of the most useful therapeutic agents. The molecular structures and biochemical mechanisms of these regulatory receptors are described in a later section entitled Signaling Mechanisms & Drug Action.

Other classes of proteins that have been clearly identified as drug receptors include **enzymes,** which may be inhibited (or, less commonly, activated) by binding a drug (eg, dihydrofolate reductase, the receptor for the antineoplastic drug methotrexate); **transport proteins** (eg, Na^+/K^+ ATPase, the membrane receptor for cardioactive digitalis glycosides); and **structural proteins** (eg, tubulin, the receptor for colchicine, an anti-inflammatory agent).

This chapter deals with three aspects of drug receptor function, presented in increasing order of complexity: (1) Receptors as determinants of the quantitative relation between the concentration of a drug and the pharmacologic response. (2) Receptors as regulatory proteins and components of chemical signaling mechanisms that provide targets for important drugs. (3) Receptors as key determinants of the therapeutic and toxic effects of drugs in patients.

RELATION BETWEEN DRUG CONCENTRATION & RESPONSE

The relation between dose of a drug and the clinically observed response may be complex. In carefully controlled in vitro systems, however, the relation between concentration of a drug and its effect is often simple and can be described with mathematical precision. This idealized relation underlies the more complex relations between dose and effect that occur when drugs are given to patients.

Concentration-Effect Curves & Receptor Binding of Agonists

Even in intact animals or patients, responses to low doses of a drug usually increase in direct proportion to dose. As doses increase, however, the response increment diminishes; finally, doses may be reached at which no further increase in response can be achieved. In idealized or in vitro systems, the relation between drug concentration and effect is described by a hyperbolic curve (Figure 2–1A) according to the following equation:

$$E = \frac{E_{max} \times C}{C + EC_{50}}$$

where E is the effect observed at concentration C, E_{max} is the maximal response that can be produced by the drug, and EC_{50} is the concentration of drug that produces 50% of maximal effect.

This hyperbolic relation resembles the mass action law, which describes association between two molecules of a given affinity. This resemblance suggests that drug agonists act by binding to ("occupying") a distinct class of biologic molecules with a characteristic affinity for the drug receptor. Radioactive receptor ligands have been used to confirm this occupancy assumption in many drug-receptor systems. In these systems, drug bound to receptors (B) relates to the concentration of free (unbound) drug (C) as depicted in Figure 2–1B and as described by an analogous equation:

Figure 2–2. Logarithmic transformation of the dose axis and experimental demonstration of spare receptors, using different concentrations of an irreversible antagonist. Curve **A** shows agonist response in the absence of antagonist. After treatment with a low concentration of antagonist (curve **B**), the curve is shifted to the right; maximal responsiveness is preserved, however, because the remaining available receptors are still in excess of the number required. In curve **C**, produced after treatment with a larger concentration of antagonist, the available receptors are no longer "spare"; instead, they are just sufficient to mediate an undiminished maximal response. Still higher concentrations of antagonist (curves **D** and **E**) reduce the number of available receptors to the point that maximal response is diminished. The apparent EC$_{50}$ of the agonist in curves **D** and **E** may approximate the K$_d$ that characterizes the binding affinity of the agonist for the receptor.

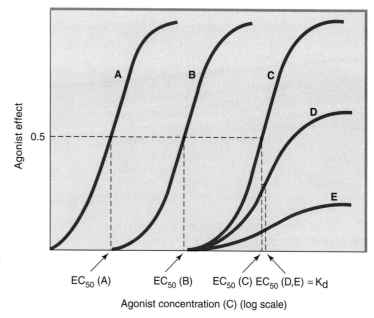

$$B = \frac{B_{max} \times C}{C + K_d}$$

in which B$_{max}$ indicates the total concentration of receptor sites (ie, sites bound to the drug at infinitely high concentrations of free drug). K$_d$ (the equilibrium dissociation constant) represents the concentration of free drug at which half-maximal binding is observed. This constant characterizes the receptor's affinity for binding the drug in a reciprocal fashion: If the K$_d$ is low, binding affinity is high, and vice versa. The EC$_{50}$ and K$_d$ may be identical, but need not be, as discussed below. Dose-response data are often presented as a plot of the drug effect (ordinate) against the *logarithm* of the dose or concentration (abscissa). This mathematical maneuver transforms the hyperbolic curve of Figure 2–1 into a sigmoid curve with a linear midportion (eg, Figure 2–2). This expands the scale of the concentration axis at low concentrations (where the effect is changing rapidly) and compresses it at high concentrations (where the effect is changing slowly), but has no special biologic or pharmacologic significance.

Receptor-Effector Coupling & Spare Receptors

When a receptor is occupied by an agonist, the resulting conformational change is only the first of many steps usually required to produce a pharmacologic response. The transduction process that links drug occupancy of receptors and pharmacologic response is often termed **coupling.** The relative efficiency of occupancy-response coupling is partially determined by the initial conformational change in the receptor; thus, the effects of full agonists can be considered more efficiently coupled to receptor occupancy than can the effects of partial agonists, as described below. Coupling efficiency is also determined by the biochemical events that transduce receptor occupancy into cellular response. Sometimes the biologic effect of the drug is linearly related to the number of receptors bound. This is often true for drug-regulated ion channels, eg, where the ion current produced by the drug is directly proportional to the number of receptors (ion channels) bound. In other cases the biologic response is a more complex function of drug binding to receptors. This is often true for receptors linked to enzymatic signal transduction cascades, eg, where the biologic response often increases disproportionately to the number of receptors occupied by drug.

Many factors can contribute to nonlinear occupancy-response coupling, and often these factors are only partially understood. The concept of "spare" receptors, irrespective of the precise biochemical mechanism involved, can help us to think about these effects. Receptors are said to be "spare" for a given pharmacologic response if it is possible to elicit a maximal biologic response at a concentration of agonist that does not result in occupancy of the full complement of available receptors. Experimentally, spare receptors may be demonstrated by using irreversible antagonists to prevent binding of agonist to a proportion of available receptors and showing that high concentrations of agonist can still produce an undiminished maximal response (Figure 2–2). Thus, the same maximal inotropic response of heart muscle to catecholamines can be elicited even under conditions where 90% of the β-adrenoceptors are occupied by a quasi-irreversible antagonist. Accordingly, myocardial cells are said to contain a large proportion of spare β-adrenoceptors.

How can we account for the phenomenon of spare receptors? In the example of the β-adrenoceptor, receptor activation promotes binding of guanosine triphosphate (GTP) to an intermediate signaling protein, and activation of the signaling intermediate may greatly outlast the agonist-receptor interaction (see the following section on G Proteins & Second Messengers). In such a case, the "spareness" of receptors is *temporal*. Maximal response can be elicited by activation of relatively few receptors because the response initiated by an individual ligand-receptor binding event persists longer than the binding event itself.

In other cases, where the biochemical mechanism is not understood, we imagine that the receptors might be *spare in number*. If the concentration or amount of cellular components other than the receptors limits the coupling of receptor occupancy to response, then a maximal response can occur without occupancy of all receptors. Thus, the sensitivity of a cell or tissue to a particular concentration of agonist depends not only on the *affinity* of the receptor for binding the agonist (characterized by the K_d) but also on the *degree of spareness*—the total number of receptors present compared with the number actually needed to elicit a maximal biologic response.

The concept of spare receptors is very useful clinically because it allows one to think precisely about the effects of drug dosage, without needing to consider biochemical details of the signaling response. The K_d of the agonist-receptor interaction determines what fraction (B/B_{max}) of total receptors will be occupied at a given free concentration (C) of agonist regardless of the receptor concentration:

$$\frac{B}{B_{max}} = \frac{C}{C + K_d}$$

Imagine a responding cell with four receptors and four effectors. Here the number of effectors does not limit the maximal response, and the receptors are *not* spare in number. Consequently, an agonist present at a concentration equal to the K_d will occupy 50% of the receptors, and half of the effectors will be activated, producing a half-maximal response (ie, two receptors stimulate two effectors). Now imagine that the number of receptors increases 10-fold to 40 receptors but that the total number of effectors remains constant. Most of the receptors are now spare in number. As a result, a much lower concentration of agonist suffices to occupy two of the 40 receptors (5% of the receptors), and this same low concentration of agonist is able to elicit a half-maximal response (two of four effectors activated). Thus, it is possible to change the sensitivity of tissues with spare receptors by changing the receptor concentration.

Competitive & Irreversible Antagonists

Receptor antagonists bind to receptors but do not activate them. The primary action of antagonists is to prevent agonists (other drugs or endogenous regulatory molecules) from activating receptors. Some antagonists (so-called "inverse agonists"), also reduce receptor activity below basal levels observed in the absence of bound ligand. Antagonists are divided into two classes depending on whether or not they *reversibly compete* with agonists for binding to receptors.

In the presence of a fixed concentration of agonist, increasing concentrations of a reversible **competitive antagonist** progressively inhibit the agonist response; high antagonist concentrations prevent response completely. Conversely, sufficiently high concentrations of agonist can completely surmount the effect of a given concentration of the antagonist; that is, the E_{max} for the agonist remains the same for any fixed concentration of antagonist (Figure 2–3A). Because the antagonism is competitive, the presence of antagonist increases the agonist concentration required for a given degree of response, and so the agonist concentration-effect curve is shifted to the right.

The concentration (C′) of an agonist required to produce a given effect in the presence of a fixed concentration ([I]) of competitive antagonist is greater than the agonist concentration (C) required to produce the same effect in the absence of the antagonist. The ratio of these two agonist concentrations (the "dose ratio") is related to the dissociation constant (K_i) of the antagonist by the Schild equation:

$$\frac{C'}{C} = 1 + \frac{[I]}{K_i}$$

Pharmacologists often use this relation to determine the K_i of a competitive antagonist. Even without knowledge of the relationship between agonist occupancy of the receptor and response, the K_i can be determined simply and accurately. As shown in Figure 2–3, concentration response curves are obtained in the presence and in

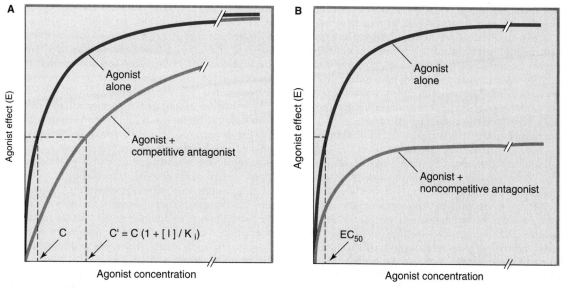

Figure 2–3. Changes in agonist concentration-effect curves produced by a competitive antagonist (Panel **A**) or by an irreversible antagonist (Panel **B**). In the presence of a competitive antagonist, higher concentrations of agonist are required to produce a given effect; thus the agonist concentration (C′) required for a given effect in the presence of concentration [I] of an antagonist is shifted to the right, as shown. High agonist concentrations can overcome inhibition by a competitive antagonist. This is not the case with an irreversible (or noncompetitive) antagonist, which reduces the maximal effect the agonist can achieve, although it may not change its EC_{50}.

the absence of a fixed concentration of competitive antagonist; comparison of the agonist concentrations required to produce identical degrees of pharmacologic effect in the two situations reveals the antagonist's K_i. If C′ is twice C, for example, then [I] = K_i.

For the clinician, this mathematical relation has two important therapeutic implications:

(1) The degree of inhibition produced by a competitive antagonist depends on the concentration of antagonist. Different patients receiving a fixed dose of propranolol, for example, exhibit a wide range of plasma concentrations, owing to differences in clearance of the drug. As a result, the effects of a fixed dose of this competitive antagonist of norepinephrine may vary widely in patients, and the dose must be adjusted accordingly.

(2) Clinical response to a competitive antagonist depends on the concentration of agonist that is competing for binding to receptors. Here also propranolol provides a useful example: When this competitive β-adreno-ceptor antagonist is administered in doses sufficient to block the effect of basal levels of the neurotransmitter norepinephrine, resting heart rate is decreased. However, the increase in release of norepinephrine and epinephrine that occurs with exercise, postural changes, or emotional stress may suffice to overcome competitive antagonism

by propranolol and increase heart rate, and thereby can influence therapeutic response.

Some receptor antagonists bind to the receptor in an **irreversible** or nearly irreversible fashion, either by forming a covalent bond with the receptor or by binding so tightly that, for practical purposes, the receptor is unavailable for binding of agonist. After occupancy of some proportion of receptors by such an antagonist, the number of remaining unoccupied receptors may be too low for the agonist (even at high concentrations) to elicit a response comparable to the previous maximal response (Figure 2–3B). If spare receptors are present, however, a lower dose of an irreversible antagonist may leave enough receptors unoccupied to allow achievement of maximum response to agonist, although a higher agonist concentration will be required (Figures 2–2B and C; see Receptor-Effector Coupling and Spare Receptors, above).

Therapeutically, irreversible antagonists present distinctive advantages and disadvantages. Once the irreversible antagonist has occupied the receptor, it need not be present in unbound form to inhibit agonist responses. Consequently, the duration of action of such an irreversible antagonist is relatively independent of its own rate of elimination and more dependent on the rate of turnover of receptor molecules.

Phenoxybenzamine, an irreversible α-adrenoceptor antagonist, is used to control the hypertension caused by catecholamines released from pheochromocytoma, a tumor of the adrenal medulla. If administration of phenoxybenzamine lowers blood pressure, blockade will be maintained even when the tumor episodically releases very large amounts of catecholamine. In this case, the ability to prevent responses to varying and high concentrations of agonist is a therapeutic advantage. If overdose occurs, however, a real problem may arise. If the α-adrenoceptor blockade cannot be overcome, excess effects of the drug must be antagonized "physiologically," ie, by using a pressor agent that does not act via α receptors.

Antagonists can function noncompetitively in a different way; that is, by binding to a site on the receptor protein separate from the agonist binding site and thereby preventing receptor activation without blocking agonist binding. Although these drugs act noncompetitively, their actions are reversible if they do not bind covalently. Some drugs, often called *allosteric modulators*, bind to a separate site on the receptor protein and alter receptor function without inactivating the receptor. For example, benzodiazepines bind noncompetitively to ion channels activated by the neurotransmitter γ-aminobutyric acid (GABA), enhancing the net activating effect of GABA on channel conductance.

Partial Agonists

Based on the maximal pharmacologic response that occurs when all receptors are occupied, agonists can be divided into two classes: **partial agonists** produce a lower response, at full receptor occupancy, than do **full agonists.** Partial agonists produce concentration-effect curves that resemble those observed with full agonists in the presence of an antagonist that irreversibly blocks some of the receptor sites (compare Figures 2–2 [curve D] and 2–4B). It is important to emphasize that the failure of partial agonists to produce a maximal response is not due to decreased affinity for binding to receptors. Indeed, a partial agonist's inability to cause a maximal pharmacologic response, even when present at high concentrations that saturate binding to all receptors, is indicated by the fact that partial agonists competitively inhibit the responses produced by full agonists (Figure 2–4C). Many drugs used clinically as antagonists are in fact weak partial agonists.

Other Mechanisms of Drug Antagonism

Not all of the mechanisms of antagonism involve interactions of drugs or endogenous ligands at a single type of receptor, and some types of antagonism do not involve a receptor at all. For example, protamine, a protein that is positively charged at physiologic pH, can be used clinically to counteract the effects of heparin, an anticoagulant that is negatively charged; in this case, one drug acts as a **chemical antagonist** of the other simply by ionic binding that makes the other drug unavailable for interactions with proteins involved in blood clotting.

Another type of antagonism is **physiologic antagonism** between endogenous regulatory pathways mediated by different receptors. For example, several catabolic actions of the glucocorticoid hormones lead to increased blood sugar, an effect that is physiologically opposed by insulin. Although glucocorticoids and insulin act on quite distinct receptor-effector systems, the clinician must sometimes administer insulin to oppose the hyperglycemic effects of a glucocorticoid hormone, whether the latter is elevated by endogenous synthesis (eg, a tumor of the adrenal cortex) or as a result of glucocorticoid therapy.

In general, use of a drug as a physiologic antagonist produces effects that are less specific and less easy to control than are the effects of a receptor-specific antagonist. Thus, for example, to treat bradycardia caused by increased release of acetylcholine from vagus nerve endings, the physician could use isoproterenol, a β-adrenoceptor agonist that increases heart rate by mimicking sympathetic stimulation of the heart. However, use of this physiologic antagonist would be less rational—and potentially more dangerous—than would use of a receptor-specific antagonist such as atropine (a competitive antagonist at the receptors at which acetylcholine slows heart rate).

SIGNALING MECHANISMS & DRUG ACTION

Until now we have considered receptor interactions and drug effects in terms of equations and concentration-effect curves. We must also understand the molecular mechanisms by which a drug acts. Such understanding allows us to ask basic questions with important clinical implications:

- Why do some drugs produce effects that persist for minutes, hours, or even days after the drug is no longer present?
- Why do responses to other drugs diminish rapidly with prolonged or repeated administration?
- How do cellular mechanisms for amplifying external chemical signals explain the phenomenon of spare receptors?
- Why do chemically similar drugs often exhibit extraordinary selectivity in their actions?
- Do these mechanisms provide targets for developing new drugs?

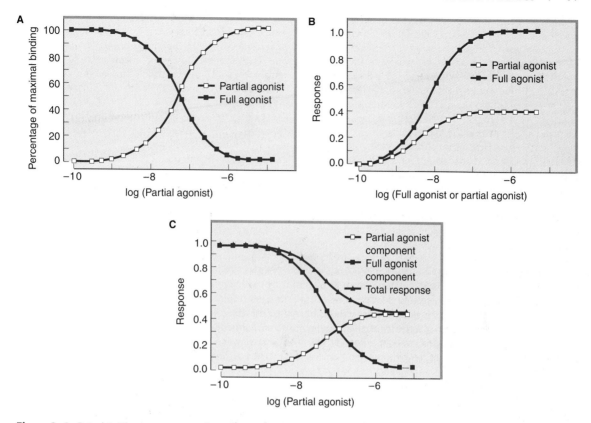

Figure 2–4. Panel **A:** The percentage of receptor occupancy resulting from full agonist (present at a single concentration) binding to receptors in the presence of increasing concentrations of a partial agonist. Because the full agonist (filled squares) and the partial agonist (open squares) compete to bind to the same receptor sites, when occupancy by the partial agonist increases, binding of the full agonist decreases. Panel **B:** When each of the two drugs is used alone and response is measured, occupancy of all the receptors by the partial agonist produces a lower maximal response than does similar occupancy by the full agonist. Panel **C:** Simultaneous treatment with a single concentration of full agonist and increasing concentrations of the partial agonist produces the response patterns shown in the bottom panel. The fractional response caused by a single high concentration of the full agonist (filled squares) decreases as increasing concentrations of the partial agonist compete to bind to the receptor with increasing success; at the same time the portion of the response caused by the partial agonist (open squares) increases, while the total response—ie, the sum of responses to the two drugs (filled triangles)—gradually decreases, eventually reaching the value produced by partial agonist alone (compare panel B).

Most transmembrane signaling is accomplished by a small number of different molecular mechanisms. Each type of mechanism has been adapted, through the evolution of distinctive protein families, to transduce many different signals. These protein families include receptors on the cell surface and within the cell, as well as enzymes and other components that generate, amplify, coordinate, and terminate postreceptor signaling by chemical second messengers in the cytoplasm. This section first discusses the mechanisms for carrying chemical information across the plasma membrane and then outlines key features of cytoplasmic second messengers.

Five basic mechanisms of transmembrane signaling are well understood (Figure 2–5). Each uses a different strategy to circumvent the barrier posed by the lipid bilayer of the plasma membrane. These strategies use (1) a lipid-soluble ligand that crosses the membrane and acts on an intracellular receptor; (2) a transmembrane receptor protein whose intracellular enzymatic activity is allosterically regulated by a ligand that binds to a site on the protein's extracellular domain; (3) a

Figure 2–5. Known transmembrane signaling mechanisms: **1:** A lipid-soluble chemical signal crosses the plasma membrane and acts on an intracellular receptor (which may be an enzyme or a regulator of gene transcription); **2:** the signal binds to the extracellular domain of a transmembrane protein, thereby activating an enzymatic activity of its cytoplasmic domain; **3:** the signal binds to the extracellular domain of a transmembrane receptor bound to a protein tyrosine kinase, which it activates; **4:** the signal binds to and directly regulates the opening of an ion channel; **5:** the signal binds to a cell-surface receptor linked to an effector enzyme by a G protein. (A, C, substrates; B, D, products; R, receptor; G, G protein; E, effector [enzyme or ion channel]; Y, tyrosine; P, phosphate.)

transmembrane receptor that binds and stimulates a protein tyrosine kinase; (4) a ligand-gated transmembrane ion channel that can be induced to open or close by the binding of a ligand; or (5) a transmembrane receptor protein that stimulates a GTP-binding signal transducer protein (G protein), which in turn modulates production of an intracellular second messenger.

While the five established mechanisms do not account for all the chemical signals conveyed across cell membranes, they do transduce many of the most important signals exploited in pharmacotherapy.

Intracellular Receptors for Lipid-Soluble Agents

Several biologic ligands are sufficiently lipid-soluble to cross the plasma membrane and act on intracellular receptors. One class of such ligands includes steroids (corticosteroids, mineralocorticoids, sex steroids, vitamin D), and thyroid hormone, whose receptors stimulate the transcription of genes by binding to specific DNA sequences near the gene whose expression is to be regulated. Many of the target DNA sequences (called **response elements**) have been identified.

These "gene-active" receptors belong to a protein family that evolved from a common precursor. Dissection of the receptors by recombinant DNA techniques has provided insights into their molecular mechanism.

For example, binding of glucocorticoid hormone to its normal receptor protein relieves an inhibitory constraint on the transcription-stimulating activity of the protein. Figure 2–6 schematically depicts the molecular mechanism of glucocorticoid action: In the absence of hormone, the receptor is bound to hsp90, a protein that appears to prevent normal folding of several structural domains of the receptor. Binding of hormone to the ligand-binding domain triggers release of hsp90. This allows the DNA-binding and transcription-activating domains of the receptor to fold into their functionally active conformations, so that the activated receptor can initiate transcription of target genes.

The mechanism used by hormones that act by regulating gene expression has two therapeutically important consequences:

(1) All of these hormones produce their effects after a characteristic lag period of 30 minutes to several hours—the time required for the synthesis of new proteins. This means that the gene-active hormones cannot be expected to alter a pathologic state within minutes (eg, glucocorticoids will not immediately relieve the symptoms of acute bronchial asthma).

(2) The effects of these agents can persist for hours or days after the agonist concentration has been reduced to zero. The persistence of effect is primarily due to the relatively slow turnover of most enzymes and

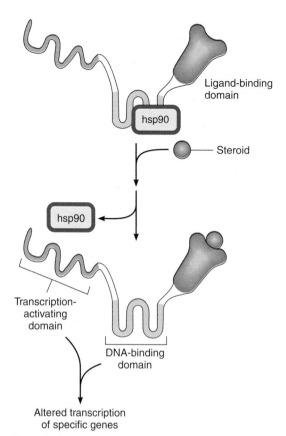

Figure 2–6. Mechanism of glucocorticoid action. The glucocorticoid receptor polypeptide is schematically depicted as a protein with three distinct domains. A heat-shock protein, hsp90, binds to the receptor in the absence of hormone and prevents folding into the active conformation of the receptor. Binding of a hormone ligand (steroid) causes dissociation of the hsp90 stabilizer and permits conversion to the active configuration.

proteins, which can remain active in cells for hours or days after they have been synthesized. Consequently, it means that the beneficial (or toxic) effects of a gene-active hormone will usually decrease slowly when administration of the hormone is stopped.

Ligand-Regulated Transmembrane Enzymes Including Receptor Tyrosine Kinases

This class of receptor molecules mediates the first steps in signaling by insulin, epidermal growth factor (EGF), platelet-derived growth factor (PDGF), atrial natriuretic peptide (ANP), transforming growth factor-β (TGF-β), and many other trophic hormones. These receptors are polypeptides consisting of an extracellular hormone-binding domain and a cytoplasmic enzyme domain, which may be a protein tyrosine kinase, a serine kinase, or a guanylyl cyclase (Figure 2–7). In all these receptors, the two domains are connected by a hydrophobic segment of the polypeptide that crosses the lipid bilayer of the plasma membrane.

The receptor tyrosine kinase signaling pathway begins with binding of ligand, typically a polypeptide hormone or growth factor, to the receptor's extracellular domain. The resulting change in receptor conformation causes receptor molecules to bind to one another, which in turn brings together the tyrosine kinase domains, which become enzymatically active, and phosphorylate one another as well as additional downstream signaling proteins. Activated receptors catalyze phosphorylation of tyrosine residues on different target signaling proteins, thereby allowing a single type of activated receptor to modulate a number of biochemical processes.

Insulin, for example, uses a single class of receptors to trigger increased uptake of glucose and amino acids, and to regulate metabolism of glycogen and triglycerides in the cell. Similarly, each of the growth factors initiates in its specific target cells a complex program of cellular events ranging from altered membrane transport of ions and metabolites to changes in the expression of many genes. Inhibitors of receptor tyrosine kinases are finding increased use in neoplastic disorders where excessive growth factor signaling is often involved. Some of these inhibitors are monoclonal antibodies (eg, trastuzumab, cetuximab), which bind to the extracellular domain of a particular receptor and interfere with binding of growth factor. Other inhibitors are membrane-permeant "small molecule" chemicals (eg, gefitinib, erlotinib), which inhibit the receptor's kinase activity in the cytoplasm.

The intensity and duration of action of EGF, PDGF, and other agents that act via receptor tyrosine kinases are limited by a process called receptor **down-regulation.** Ligand binding often induces accelerated endocytosis of receptors from the cell surface, followed by the degradation of those receptors (and their bound ligands). When this process occurs at a rate faster than de novo synthesis of receptors, the total number of cell-surface receptors is reduced (down-regulated) and the cell's responsiveness to ligand is correspondingly diminished. A well-understood example is the EGF receptor tyrosine kinase, which undergoes rapid endocytosis and is trafficked to lysosomes after EGF binding; genetic mutations that interfere with this process cause excessive growth factor–induced cell proliferation and are associated with an increased susceptibility to certain types of cancer. Endocytosis of other receptor tyrosine kinases, most notably receptors for nerve growth factor,

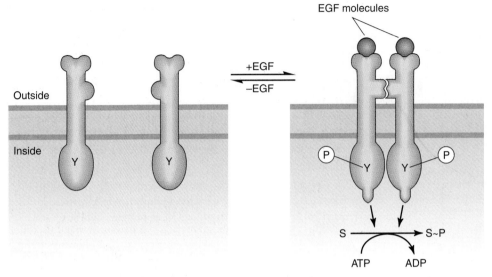

Figure 2–7. Mechanism of activation of the epidermal growth factor (EGF) receptor, a representative receptor tyrosine kinase. The receptor polypeptide has extracellular and cytoplasmic domains, depicted above and below the plasma membrane. Upon binding of EGF (circle), the receptor converts from its inactive monomeric state (left) to an active dimeric state (right), in which two receptor polypeptides bind noncovalently. The cytoplasmic domains become phosphorylated (P) on specific tyrosine residues (Y) and their enzymatic activities are activated, catalyzing phosphorylation of substrate proteins (S).

serves a very different function. Internalized nerve growth factor receptors are not rapidly degraded and are translocated in endocytic vesicles from the distal axon, where receptors are activated by nerve growth factor released from the innervated tissue, to the cell body. In the cell body the growth factor signal is transduced to transcription factors regulating the expression of genes controlling cell survival. This process effectively transports a critical survival signal from its site of release to its site of signaling effect, and does so over a remarkably long distance—more than 1 meter in certain sensory neurons. A number of regulators of growth and differentiation, including TGF-β, act on another class of transmembrane receptor enzymes that phosphorylate serine and threonine residues. ANP, an important regulator of blood volume and vascular tone, acts on a transmembrane receptor whose intracellular domain, a guanylyl cyclase, generates cGMP (see below). Receptors in both groups, like the receptor tyrosine kinases, are active in their dimeric forms.

Cytokine Receptors

Cytokine receptors respond to a heterogeneous group of peptide ligands that includes growth hormone, erythropoietin, several kinds of interferon, and other regulators of growth and differentiation. These receptors use a

mechanism (Figure 2–8) closely resembling that of receptor tyrosine kinases, except that in this case, the protein tyrosine kinase activity is not intrinsic to the receptor molecule. Instead, a separate protein tyrosine kinase, from the Janus-kinase (JAK) family, binds noncovalently to the receptor. As in the case of the EGF-receptor, cytokine receptors dimerize after they bind the activating ligand, allowing the bound JAKs to become activated and to phosphorylate tyrosine residues on the receptor. Tyrosine phosphates on the receptor then set in motion a complex signaling dance by binding another set of proteins, called STATs (signal transducers and activators of transcription). The bound STATs are themselves phosphorylated by the JAKs, two STAT molecules dimerize (attaching to one another's tyrosine phosphates), and finally the STAT/STAT dimer dissociates from the receptor and travels to the nucleus, where it regulates transcription of specific genes.

Ligand-Gated Channels

Many of the most useful drugs in clinical medicine act by mimicking or blocking the actions of endogenous ligands that regulate the flow of ions through plasma membrane channels. The natural ligands include acetylcholine, serotonin, GABA, and glutamate. All of these agents are synaptic transmitters.

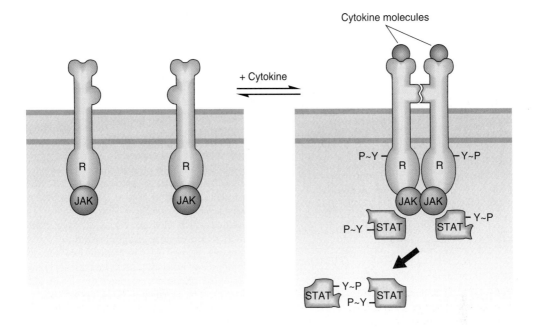

Figure 2–8. Cytokine receptors, like receptor tyrosine kinases, have extracellular and intracellular domains and form dimers. However, after activation by an appropriate ligand, separate mobile protein tyrosine kinase molecules (JAK) are activated, resulting in phosphorylation of signal transducers and activation of transcription (STAT) molecules. STAT dimers then travel to the nucleus, where they regulate transcription.

Each of their receptors transmits its signal across the plasma membrane by increasing transmembrane conductance of the relevant ion and thereby altering the electrical potential across the membrane. For example, acetylcholine causes the opening of the ion channel in the nicotinic acetylcholine receptor (AChR), which allows Na^+ to flow down its concentration gradient into cells, producing a localized excitatory postsynaptic potential—a depolarization.

The AChR (Figure 2–9) is one of the best-characterized of all cell-surface receptors for hormones or neurotransmitters. One form of this receptor is a pentamer made up of four polypeptide subunits (eg, two α chains plus one β, one γ, and one δ chain, all with molecular weights ranging from 43,000 to 50,000). These polypeptides, each of which crosses the lipid bilayer four times, form a cylindric structure 8 nm in diameter. When acetylcholine binds to sites on the α subunits, a conformational change occurs that results in the transient opening of a central aqueous channel through which sodium ions penetrate from the extracellular fluid into the cell.

The time elapsed between the binding of the agonist to a ligand-gated channel and the cellular response can often be measured in milliseconds. The rapidity of this signaling mechanism is crucially important for moment-to-moment transfer of information across synapses. Ligand-gated ion channels can be regulated by multiple mechanisms, including phosphorylation and endocytosis. In the central nervous system, these mechanisms contribute to synaptic plasticity involved in learning and memory.

G Proteins & Second Messengers

Many extracellular ligands act by increasing the intracellular concentrations of second messengers such as cyclic adenosine-3′,5′-monophosphate (cAMP), calcium ion, or the phosphoinositides (described below). In most cases they use a transmembrane signaling system with three separate components. First, the extracellular ligand is specifically detected by a cell-surface receptor. The receptor in turn triggers the activation of a G protein located on the cytoplasmic face of the plasma membrane. The activated G protein then changes the activity of an effector element, usually an enzyme or ion channel. This element then changes the concentration of the intracellular second messenger. For cAMP, the effector enzyme is adenylyl cyclase, a membrane protein that converts intracellular adenosine triphosphate (ATP) to cAMP. The corresponding G protein, G_s, stimulates adenylyl cyclase after being activated by hormones and neurotransmitters that act via specific

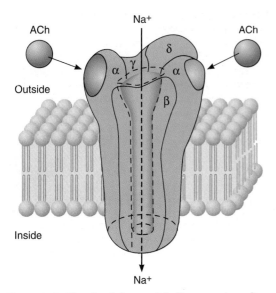

Figure 2–9. The nicotinic acetylcholine receptor, a ligand-gated ion channel. The receptor molecule is depicted as embedded in a rectangular piece of plasma membrane, with extracellular fluid above and cytoplasm below. Composed of five subunits (two α, one β, one γ, and one δ), the receptor opens a central transmembrane ion channel when acetylcholine (ACh) binds to sites on the extracellular domain of its α subunits.

G_s-coupled receptors. There are many examples of such receptors including β-adrenoceptors, glucagon receptors, thyrotropin receptors, and certain subtypes of dopamine and serotonin receptors.

G_s and other G proteins use a molecular mechanism that involves binding and hydrolysis of GTP (Figure 2–10). This mechanism allows the transduced signal to be amplified. For example, a neurotransmitter such as norepinephrine may encounter its membrane receptor for only a few milliseconds. When the encounter generates a GTP-bound G_s molecule, however, the duration of activation of adenylyl cyclase depends on the longevity of GTP binding to G_s rather than on the receptor's affinity for norepinephrine. Indeed, like other G proteins, GTP-bound G_s may remain active for tens of seconds, enormously amplifying the original signal. This mechanism also helps explain how signaling by G proteins produces the phenomenon of spare receptors (described above). The family of G proteins contains several functionally diverse subfamilies (Table 2–1), each of which mediates effects of a particular set of receptors to a distinctive group of effectors. Note that an endogenous ligand (eg, norepinephrine, acetylcholine, serotonin, many others not listed in Table 2–1) may bind and stimulate receptors that couple to different subsets of G proteins. The apparent promiscuity of such a ligand allows it to elicit different G protein-dependent responses in different cells. For instance, the body responds to danger by using catecholamines (norepinephrine and epinephrine) both to increase heart rate and to induce constriction of blood vessels in the skin, by acting on G_s-coupled β-adrenoceptors and G_q-coupled α_1-adrenoceptors, respectively. Ligand promiscuity also offers opportunities in drug development (see Receptor Classes & Drug Development, below).

Receptors coupled to G proteins comprise a family of "seven-transmembrane" (7-TM) or "serpentine" receptors, so called because the receptor polypeptide chain "snakes" across the plasma membrane seven times (Figure 2–11). Receptors for adrenergic amines, serotonin, acetyl-

Table 2–1. G proteins and their receptors and effectors.

G Protein	Receptors for:	Effector/Signaling Pathway
G_s	β-Adrenergic amines, glucagon, histamine, serotonin, and many other hormones	↑ Adenylyl cyclase → ↑ cAMP
G_{i1}, G_{i2}, G_{i3}	α_2-Adrenergic amines, acetylcholine (muscarinic), opioids, serotonin, and many others	Several, including: ↓ Adenylyl cyclase → ↓ cAMP Open cardiac K$^+$ channels → ↓ heart rate
G_{olf}	Odorants (olfactory epithelium)	↑ Adenylyl cyclase → ↑ cAMP
G_o	Neurotransmitters in brain (not yet specifically identified)	Not yet clear
G_q	Acetylcholine (muscarinic), bombesin, serotonin (5-HT$_{1C}$), and many others	↑ Phospholipase C → ↑ IP$_3$, diacylglycerol, cytoplasmic Ca^{2+}
G_{t1}, G_{t2}	Photons (rhodopsin and color opsins in retinal rod and cone cells)	↑ cGMP phosphodiesterase → ↓ cGMP (phototransduction)

Key: cAMP = cyclic adenosine monophosphate; cGMP = cyclic guanosine monophosphate.

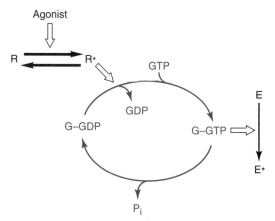

Figure 2–10. The guanine nucleotide-dependent activation-inactivation cycle of G proteins. The agonist activates the receptor (R→R*), which promotes release of GDP from the G protein (G), allowing entry of GTP into the nucleotide binding site. In its GTP-bound state (G-GTP), the G protein regulates activity of an effector enzyme or ion channel (E). The signal is terminated by hydrolysis of GTP, followed by return of the system to the basal unstimulated state. Open arrows denote regulatory effects. (P_i, inorganic phosphate.)

choline (muscarinic but not nicotinic), many peptide hormones, odorants, and even visual receptors (in retinal rod and cone cells) all belong to the serpentine family. All were derived from a common evolutionary precursor. Several serpentine receptors exist as dimers or larger complexes. Serpentine receptors signal by a different mechanism than receptor tyrosine kinases and cytokine receptors, however, and it is thought that dimerization is not essential for activation of many serpentine receptors.

All serpentine receptors transduce signals across the plasma membrane in essentially the same way. Often the agonist ligand—eg, a catecholamine, acetylcholine, or the photon-activated chromophore of retinal photoreceptors—is bound in a pocket enclosed by the transmembrane regions of the receptor (as in Figure 2–11). The resulting change in conformation of these regions is transmitted to cytoplasmic loops of the receptor, which in turn activate the appropriate G protein by promoting replacement of GDP by GTP, as described above. Amino acids in the third cytoplasmic loop of the serpentine receptor polypeptide are generally thought to play a key role in mediating receptor interaction with G proteins (shown by arrows in Figure 2–11).

Receptor Regulation

G protein-mediated responses to drugs and hormonal agonists often attenuate with time (Figure 2–12, top).

After reaching an initial high level, the response (eg, cellular cAMP accumulation, Na^+ influx, contractility, etc) diminishes over seconds or minutes, even in the continued presence of the agonist. This "desensitization" is often rapidly reversible; a second exposure to agonist, if provided a few minutes after termination of the first exposure, results in a response similar to the initial response.

The mechanism mediating rapid desensitization of G protein–coupled receptors often involves receptor phosphorylation, as illustrated by rapid desensitization of the β-adrenoceptor (Figure 2–12, top). The agonist-induced change in conformation of the receptor causes it to bind, activate, and serve as a substrate for a family of specific receptor kinases, called G protein-coupled receptor kinases (GRKs). The activated GRK then phosphorylates serine residues in the receptor's carboxyl terminal tail. The presence of phosphoserines increases the receptor's

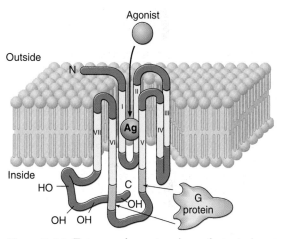

Figure 2–11. Transmembrane topology of a typical serpentine receptor. The receptor's amino (N) terminal is extracellular (above the plane of the membrane), and its carboxyl (C) terminal intracellular. The terminals are connected by a polypeptide chain that traverses the plane of the membrane seven times. The hydrophobic transmembrane segments (light color) are designated by roman numerals (I–VII). The agonist (Ag) approaches the receptor from the extracellular fluid and binds to a site surrounded by the transmembrane regions of the receptor protein. G proteins interact with cytoplasmic regions of the receptor, especially with portions of the third cytoplasmic loop between transmembrane regions V and VI. The receptor's cytoplasmic terminal tail contains numerous serine and threonine residues whose hydroxyl (–OH) groups can be phosphorylated. This phosphorylation may be associated with diminished receptor-G protein interaction.

affinity for binding a third protein, β-arrestin. Binding of β-arrestin to cytoplasmic loops of the receptor diminishes the receptor's ability to interact with G_s, thereby reducing the agonist response (ie, stimulation of adenylyl cyclase). Upon removal of agonist, GRK activation is terminated and the desensitization process can be reversed by cellular phosphatases.

For the β-adrenoceptor, and many other serpentine receptors, β-arrestin binding also accelerates endocytosis of receptors from the plasma membrane. Endocytosis of receptors promotes their dephosphorylation, by a receptor phosphatase that is present at high concentration on endosome membranes, and receptors then return to the plasma membrane. This helps explain the ability of cells to recover receptor-mediated signaling responsiveness very efficiently after agonist-induced desensitization. Several serpentine receptors—including the β-adrenoceptor if it is persistently activated—instead traffic to lysosomes after endocytosis and are degraded. This process effectively attenuates (rather than restores) cellular responsiveness, similar to the process of down-regulation described above for the epidermal growth factor receptor. Thus, depending on the particular receptor and duration of activation, endocytosis can contribute to either rapid recovery or prolonged attenuation of cellular responsiveness (Figure 2–12).

Well-Established Second Messengers

A. Cyclic Adenosine Monophosphate (cAMP)

Acting as an intracellular second messenger, cAMP mediates such hormonal responses as the mobilization of stored energy (the breakdown of carbohydrates in liver or triglycerides in fat cells stimulated by β-adrenomimetic catecholamines), conservation of water by the kidney (mediated by vasopressin), Ca^{2+} homeostasis (regulated by parathyroid hormone), and increased rate and contractile force of heart muscle (β-adrenomimetic catecholamines). It also regulates the production of adrenal and sex steroids (in response to corticotropin or follicle-stimulating hormone), relaxation of smooth muscle, and many other endocrine and neural processes.

cAMP exerts most of its effects by stimulating cAMP-dependent protein kinases (Figure 2–13). These kinases are composed of a cAMP-binding regulatory (R) dimer and two catalytic (C) chains. When cAMP binds to the R dimer, active C chains are released to diffuse through the cytoplasm and nucleus, where they transfer phosphate from ATP to appropriate substrate proteins, often enzymes. The specificity of cAMP's regulatory effects resides in the distinct protein substrates of the kinases that are expressed in different cells. For example, liver is rich in phosphorylase kinase and glycogen synthase, enzymes whose reciprocal regulation by cAMP-dependent phosphorylation governs carbohydrate storage and release.

When the hormonal stimulus stops, the intracellular actions of cAMP are terminated by an elaborate series of enzymes. cAMP-stimulated phosphorylation of enzyme substrates is rapidly reversed by a diverse group of specific and nonspecific phosphatases. cAMP itself is degraded to 5′-AMP by several cyclic nucleotide phosphodiesterases (PDE, Figure 2–13). Competitive inhibition of cAMP degradation is one way caffeine, theophylline, and other methylxanthines produce their effects (see Chapter 20).

B. Calcium and Phosphoinositides

Another well-studied second messenger system involves hormonal stimulation of phosphoinositide hydrolysis (Figure 2–14). Some of the hormones, neurotransmitters, and growth factors that trigger this pathway bind to receptors linked to G proteins, while others bind to receptor tyrosine kinases. In all cases, the crucial step is

Figure 2–12. Rapid desensitization and longer-term down-regulation of β-adrenoceptors. Panel **A:** Response to a β-adrenoceptor agonist (ordinate) versus time (abscissa). Temporal duration of exposure to a constant concentration of agonist is indicated by the light-colored bar. The break in the time axis indicates passage of time in the absence of agonist. Desensitization refers to the reduced cAMP response after several minutes in the continued presence of agonist; restored response is observed after a brief period (typically several more minutes) in the absence of agonist. Panel **B:** Agonist-induced phosphorylation (P) by a G protein–coupled receptor kinase (GRK) of carboxyl terminal hydroxyl groups (–OH) of the β-adrenoceptor. This phosphorylation induces binding of a protein, β-arrestin (β-arr), which prevents the receptor from interacting with G_s. Removal of agonist for a short period of time (on the order of several minutes) allows dissociation of β-arr, removal of phosphate (Pi) from the receptor by phosphatases (P'ase), and restoration of the receptor's normal responsiveness to agonist. Panel **C:** Agonist-induced endocytosis and endocytic membrane trafficking of receptors. Beta-arrestin promotes receptor binding to endocytotic structures in the plasma membrane called coated pits. After short-term agonist exposure, receptors primarily undergo dephosphorylation by phosphatases (P'ase) and recycling, promoting rapid recovery of signaling responsiveness. After longer-term agonist exposure, receptors that have undergone endocytosis traffic to lysosomes, promoting the process of receptor down-regulation.

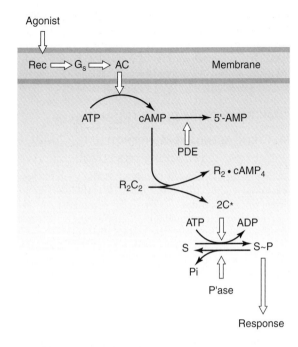

Figure 2–13. The cAMP second messenger pathway. Key proteins include hormone receptors (Rec), a stimulatory G protein (G_s), catalytic adenylyl cyclase (AC), phosphodiesterases (PDE) that hydrolyze cAMP, cAMP-dependent kinases, with regulatory (R) and catalytic (C) subunits, protein substrates (S) of the kinases, and phosphatases (P'ase), which remove phosphates from substrate proteins. Open arrows denote regulatory effects.

stimulation of a membrane enzyme, phospholipase C (PLC), which splits a minor phospholipid component of the plasma membrane, phosphatidylinositol-4,5-bisphosphate (PIP_2), into two second messengers, diacylglycerol (DAG) and inositol-1,4,5-trisphosphate (IP_3 or $InsP_3$). Diacylglycerol is confined to the membrane where it activates a phospholipid- and calcium-sensitive protein kinase called protein kinase C. IP_3 is water-soluble and diffuses through the cytoplasm to trigger release of Ca^{2+} from internal storage vesicles. Elevated cytoplasmic Ca^{2+} concentration promotes the binding of Ca^{2+} to the calcium-binding protein calmodulin, which regulates activities of other enzymes, including calcium-dependent protein kinases.

With its multiple second messengers and protein kinases, the phosphoinositide signaling pathway is much more complex than the cAMP pathway. For example, different cell types may contain one or more specialized calcium- and calmodulin-dependent kinases with limited substrate specificity (eg, myosin light chain kinase) in addition to a general calcium- and calmodu-

lin-dependent kinase that can phosphorylate a wide variety of protein substrates. Furthermore, at least nine structurally distinct types of protein kinase C have been identified.

As in the cAMP system, multiple mechanisms damp or terminate signaling by this pathway. IP_3 is inactivated by dephosphorylation; diacylglycerol is either phosphorylated to yield phosphatidic acid, which is then converted back into phospholipids, or it is deacylated to yield arachidonic acid; Ca^{2+} is actively removed from the cytoplasm by Ca^{2+} pumps.

These and other nonreceptor elements of the calcium-phosphoinositide signaling pathway are now becoming targets for drug development. For example, the therapeutic effects of lithium ion, an established agent for treating manic-depressive disorder, may be mediated by effects on the metabolism of phosphoinositides (see Chapter 29).

C. CYCLIC GUANOSINE MONOPHOSPHATE (cGMP)

Unlike cAMP, the ubiquitous and versatile carrier of diverse messages, cGMP has established signaling roles in only a few cell types. In intestinal mucosa and vascular smooth muscle, the cGMP-based signal transduction mechanism closely parallels the cAMP-mediated

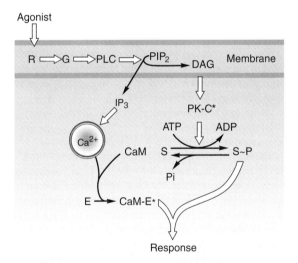

Figure 2–14. The Ca^{2+}-phosphoinositide signaling pathway. Key proteins include hormone receptors (R), a G protein (G), a phosphoinositide-specific phospholipase C (PLC), protein kinase C substrates of the kinase (S), calmodulin (CaM), and calmodulin-binding enzymes (E), including kinases, phosphodiesterases, etc. (PIP_2, phosphatidylinositol-4,5-bisphosphate; DAG, diacylglycerol; IP_3, inositol trisphosphate. Asterisk denotes activated state. Open arrows denote regulatory effects.)

signaling mechanism. Ligands detected by cell surface receptors stimulate membrane-bound guanylyl cyclase to produce cGMP, and cGMP acts by stimulating a cGMP-dependent protein kinase. The actions of cGMP in these cells are terminated by enzymatic degradation of the cyclic nucleotide and by dephosphorylation of kinase substrates.

Increased cGMP concentration causes relaxation of vascular smooth muscle by a kinase-mediated mechanism that results in dephosphorylation of myosin light chains (Figure 12–2). In these smooth muscle cells, cGMP synthesis can be elevated by two different transmembrane signaling mechanisms utilizing two different guanylyl cyclases. Atrial natriuretic peptide, a blood-borne peptide hormone, stimulates a transmembrane receptor by binding to its extracellular domain, thereby activating the guanylyl cyclase activity that resides in the receptor's intracellular domain. The other mechanism mediates responses to nitric oxide (NO; see Chapter 19), which is generated in vascular endothelial cells in response to natural vasodilator agents such as acetylcholine and histamine. After entering the target cell, NO binds to and activates a cytoplasmic guanylyl cyclase. A number of useful vasodilating drugs, such as nitroglycerin and sodium nitroprusside used in treating cardiac ischemia and acute hypertension, act by generating or mimicking NO. Other drugs produce vasodilation by inhibiting specific phosphodiesterases, thereby interfering with the metabolic breakdown of cGMP. One such drug is sildenafil, used in treating erectile dysfunction (see Chapter 12).

Interplay Among Signaling Mechanisms

The calcium-phosphoinositide and cAMP signaling pathways oppose one another in some cells and are complementary in others. For example, vasopressor agents that contract smooth muscle act by IP_3-mediated mobilization of Ca^{2+}, whereas agents that relax smooth muscle often act by elevation of cAMP. In contrast, cAMP and phosphoinositide second messengers act together to stimulate glucose release from the liver.

Phosphorylation: A Common Theme

Almost all second messenger signaling involves reversible phosphorylation, which performs two principal functions in signaling: amplification and flexible regulation. In **amplification,** rather like GTP bound to a G protein, the attachment of a phosphoryl group to a serine, threonine, or tyrosine residue powerfully amplifies the initial regulatory signal by recording a molecular memory that the pathway has been activated; dephosphorylation erases the memory, taking a longer time to do so than is required for dissociation of an allosteric ligand. In **flexible regulation,** differing substrate specificities of the multiple protein kinases regulated by second messengers provide branch points in signaling pathways that may be independently regulated. In this way, cAMP, Ca^{2+}, or other second messengers can use the presence or absence of particular kinases or kinase substrates to produce quite different effects in different cell types. Inhibitors of protein kinases have great potential as therapeutic agents, particularly in neoplastic diseases. Trastuzumab, an antibody that antagonizes growth factor receptor signaling, was discussed earlier and is a useful therapeutic agent for breast cancer. Another example of this general approach is imatinib, a small molecule inhibitor of the cytoplasmic tyrosine kinase Abl, which is activated by growth factor signaling pathways. Imatinib appears to be very effective for treating chronic myelogenous leukemia, which is caused by a chromosomal translocation event that produces an active Bcr/Abl fusion protein in hematopoietic cells.

RECEPTOR CLASSES & DRUG DEVELOPMENT

The existence of a specific drug receptor is usually inferred from studying the **structure-activity relationship** of a group of structurally similar congeners of the drug that mimic or antagonize its effects. Thus, if a series of related agonists exhibits identical relative potencies in producing two distinct effects, it is likely that the two effects are mediated by similar or identical receptor molecules. In addition, if identical receptors mediate both effects, a competitive antagonist will inhibit both responses with the same K_i; a second competitive antagonist will inhibit both responses with its own characteristic K_i. Thus, studies of the relation between structure and activity of a series of agonists and antagonists can identify a species of receptor that mediates a set of pharmacologic responses.

Exactly the same experimental procedure can show that observed effects of a drug are mediated by *different* receptors. In this case, effects mediated by different receptors may exhibit different orders of potency among agonists and different K_i values for each competitive antagonist.

Wherever we look, evolution has created many different receptors that function to mediate responses to any individual chemical signal. In some cases, the same chemical acts on completely different structural receptor classes. For example, acetylcholine uses ligand-gated ion channels (nicotinic AChRs) to initiate a fast excitatory postsynaptic potential (EPSP) in postganglionic neurons. Acetylcholine also activates a separate class of G protein-coupled receptors (muscarinic AChRs), which modulate responsiveness of the same neurons to the fast EPSP. In addition, each structural class usually includes multiple subtypes of receptor, often with significantly different signaling or regulatory properties. For example, many biogenic amines (eg, norepinephrine, acetylcholine, and serotonin) activate more than one receptor, each of which may activate a different G protein, as described above (see also Table 2–1). The existence of multiple receptor classes and subtypes for the same endogenous ligand has created important opportunities for drug development. For example, propranolol, a selective antagonist of β-adrenoceptors, can reduce an accelerated heart rate without preventing the sympathetic nervous system from causing vasoconstriction, an effect mediated by α_1 receptors.

The principle of drug selectivity may even apply to structurally identical receptors expressed in different cells, eg, receptors for steroids such as estrogen (Figure 2–6). Different cell types express different accessory proteins, which interact with steroid receptors and change the functional effects of drug-receptor interaction. For example, tamoxifen acts as an *antagonist* on estrogen receptors expressed in mammary tissue but as an *agonist* on estrogen receptors in bone. Consequently, tamoxifen may be useful not only in the treatment and prophylaxis of breast cancer but also in the prevention of osteoporosis by increasing bone density (see Chapters 40 and 42). Tamoxifen may also create complications in postmenopausal women, however, by exerting an agonist action in the uterus, stimulating endometrial cell proliferation.

New drug development is not confined to agents that act on receptors for extracellular chemical signals. Pharmaceutical chemists are now determining whether elements of signaling pathways distal to the receptors may also serve as targets of selective and useful drugs. For example, clinically useful agents might be developed that act selectively on specific G proteins, kinases, phosphatases, or the enzymes that degrade second messengers.

RELATION BETWEEN DRUG DOSE & CLINICAL RESPONSE

We have dealt with receptors as molecules and shown how receptors can quantitatively account for the relation between dose or concentration of a drug and pharmacologic responses, at least in an idealized system. When faced with a patient who needs treatment, the prescriber must make a choice among a variety of possible drugs and devise a dosage regimen that is likely to produce maximal benefit and minimal toxicity. In order to make rational therapeutic decisions, the prescriber must understand how drug-receptor interactions underlie the relations between dose and response in patients, the nature and causes of variation in pharmacologic responsiveness, and the clinical implications of selectivity of drug action.

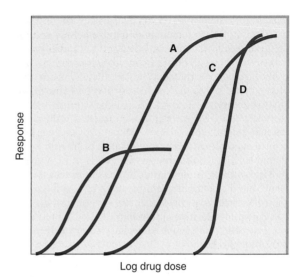

Figure 2–15. Graded dose-response curves for four drugs, illustrating different pharmacologic potencies and different maximal efficacies. (See text.)

Dose & Response in Patients

A. GRADED DOSE-RESPONSE RELATIONS

To choose among drugs and to determine appropriate doses of a drug, the prescriber must know the relative **pharmacologic potency** and **maximal efficacy** of the drugs in relation to the desired therapeutic effect. These two important terms, often confusing to students and clinicians, can be explained by referring to Figure 2–15, which depicts graded dose-response curves that relate dose of four different drugs to the magnitude of a particular therapeutic effect.

1. Potency—Drugs A and B are said to be more potent than drugs C and D because of the relative positions of their dose-response curves along the **dose axis** of Figure 2–15. Potency refers to the concentration (EC_{50}) or dose (ED_{50}) of a drug required to produce 50% of that drug's maximal effect. Thus, the pharmacologic potency of drug A in Figure 2–15 is less than that of drug B, a partial agonist, because the EC_{50} of A is greater than the EC_{50} of B. Potency of a drug depends in part on the affinity (K_d) of receptors for binding the drug and in part on the efficiency with which drug-receptor interaction is coupled to response. Note that some doses of drug A can produce larger effects than any dose of drug B, despite the fact that we describe drug B as pharmacologically more potent. The reason for this is that drug A has a larger maximal efficacy, as described below.

For clinical use, it is important to distinguish between a drug's potency and its efficacy. The clinical effectiveness of a drug depends not on its potency (EC_{50}), but on its maximal efficacy (see below) and its ability to reach the relevant receptors. This ability can depend on its route of administration, absorption, distribution through the body, and clearance from the blood or site of action. In deciding which of two drugs to administer to a patient, the prescriber must usually consider their relative effectiveness rather than their relative potency. Pharmacologic potency can largely determine the administered dose of the chosen drug.

For therapeutic purposes, the potency of a drug should be stated in dosage units, usually in terms of a particular therapeutic end point (eg, 50 mg for mild sedation, 1 mcg/kg/min for an increase in heart rate of 25 beats/min). Relative potency, the ratio of equi-effective doses (0.2, 10, etc), may be used in comparing one drug with another.

2. Maximal efficacy—This parameter reflects the limit of the dose-response relation on the **response axis.** Drugs A, C, and D in Figure 2–15 have equal maximal efficacy, while all have greater maximal efficacy than drug B. The maximal efficacy (sometimes referred to simply as efficacy) of a drug is obviously crucial for making clinical decisions when a large response is needed. It may be determined by the drug's mode of interactions with receptors (as with partial agonists, described above)* or by characteristics of the receptor-effector system involved.

Thus, diuretics that act on one portion of the nephron may produce much greater excretion of fluid and electrolytes than diuretics that act elsewhere. In addition, the practical efficacy of a drug for achieving a therapeutic end point (eg, increased cardiac contractility) may be limited by the drug's propensity to cause a toxic effect (eg, fatal cardiac arrhythmia) even if the drug could otherwise produce a greater therapeutic effect.

B. SHAPE OF DOSE-RESPONSE CURVES

While the responses depicted in curves A, B, and C of Figure 2–15 approximate the shape of a simple Michaelis-Menten relation (transformed to a logarithmic plot), some clinical responses do not. Extremely steep dose-response curves (eg, curve D) may have important clinical consequences if the upper portion of the curve rep-

resents an undesirable extent of response (eg, coma caused by a sedative-hypnotic). Steep dose-response curves in patients can result from cooperative interactions of several different actions of a drug (eg, effects on brain, heart, and peripheral vessels, all contributing to lowering of blood pressure).

C. QUANTAL DOSE-EFFECT CURVES

Graded dose-response curves of the sort described above have certain limitations in their application to clinical decision making. For example, such curves may be impossible to construct if the pharmacologic response is an either-or (quantal) event, such as prevention of convulsions, arrhythmia, or death. Furthermore, the clinical relevance of a quantitative dose-response relationship in a single patient, no matter how precisely defined, may be limited in application to other patients, owing to the great potential variability among patients in severity of disease and responsiveness to drugs.

Some of these difficulties may be avoided by determining the dose of drug required to produce a specified magnitude of effect in a large number of individual patients or experimental animals and plotting the cumulative frequency distribution of responders versus the log dose (Figure 2–16). The specified quantal effect may be chosen on the basis of clinical relevance (eg, relief of headache) or for preservation of safety of experimental subjects (eg, using low doses of a cardiac stimulant and specifying an increase in heart rate of 20 beats/min as the quantal effect), or it may be an inherently quantal event (eg, death of an experimental animal). For most drugs, the doses required to produce a specified quantal effect in individuals are lognormally distributed; that is, a frequency distribution of such responses plotted against the log of the dose produces a gaussian normal curve of variation (colored area, Figure 2–16). When these responses are summated, the resulting cumulative frequency distribution constitutes a quantal dose-effect curve (or dose-percent curve) of the proportion or percentage of individuals who exhibit the effect plotted as a function of log dose (Figure 2–16).

The quantal dose-effect curve is often characterized by stating the **median effective dose (ED_{50}),** the dose at which 50% of individuals exhibit the specified quantal effect. (Note that the abbreviation ED_{50} has a different meaning in this context from its meaning in relation to graded dose-effect curves, described above.) Similarly, the dose required to produce a particular toxic effect in 50% of animals is called the **median toxic dose (TD_{50}).** If the toxic effect is death of the animal, a **median lethal dose (LD_{50})** may be experimentally defined. Such values provide a convenient way of comparing the potencies of drugs in experimental and clinical settings: Thus, if the ED_{50}s of two drugs for producing a specified quantal effect are 5 and 500 mg,

---

*Note that "maximal efficacy," used in a therapeutic context, does not have exactly the same meaning the term denotes in the more specialized context of drug-receptor interactions described earlier in this chapter. In an idealized in vitro system, efficacy denotes the relative maximal efficacy of agonists and partial agonists that act via the same receptor. In therapeutics, efficacy denotes the extent or degree of an effect that can be achieved in the intact patient. Thus, therapeutic efficacy may be affected by the characteristics of a particular drug-receptor interaction, but it also depends on a host of other factors as noted in the text.

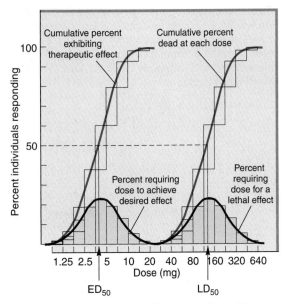

Figure 2–16. Quantal dose-effect plots. Shaded boxes (and the accompanying black curves) indicate the frequency distribution of doses of drug required to produce a specified effect; that is, the percentage of animals that required a particular dose to exhibit the effect. The open boxes (and the corresponding colored curves) indicate the cumulative frequency distribution of responses, which are lognormally distributed.

respectively, then the first drug can be said to be 100 times more potent than the second for that particular effect. Similarly, one can obtain a valuable index of the selectivity of a drug's action by comparing its ED_{50}s for two different quantal effects in a population (eg, cough suppression versus sedation for opioid drugs).

Quantal dose-effect curves may also be used to generate information regarding the margin of safety to be expected from a particular drug used to produce a specified effect. One measure, which relates the dose of a drug required to produce a desired effect to that which produces an undesired effect, is the **therapeutic index.** In animal studies, the therapeutic index is usually defined as the ratio of the TD_{50} to the ED_{50} for some therapeutically relevant effect. The precision possible in animal experiments may make it useful to use such a therapeutic index to estimate the potential benefit of a drug in humans. Of course, the therapeutic index of a drug in humans is almost never known with real precision; instead, drug trials and accumulated clinical experience often reveal a range of usually effective doses and a different (but sometimes overlapping) range of possibly toxic doses. The clinically acceptable risk of toxicity depends critically on the severity of the disease being treated. For

example, the dose range that provides relief from an ordinary headache in the great majority of patients should be very much lower than the dose range that produces serious toxicity, even if the toxicity occurs in a small minority of patients. However, for treatment of a lethal disease such as Hodgkin's lymphoma, the acceptable difference between therapeutic and toxic doses may be smaller.

Finally, note that the quantal dose-effect curve and the graded dose-response curve summarize somewhat different sets of information, although both appear sigmoid in shape on a semilogarithmic plot (compare Figures 2–15 and 2–16). Critical information required for making rational therapeutic decisions can be obtained from each type of curve. Both curves provide information regarding the **potency** and **selectivity** of drugs; the graded dose-response curve indicates the **maximal efficacy** of a drug, and the quantal dose-effect curve indicates the potential **variability** of responsiveness among individuals.

Variation in Drug Responsiveness

Individuals may vary considerably in their responsiveness to a drug; indeed, a single individual may respond differently to the same drug at different times during the course of treatment. Occasionally, individuals exhibit an unusual or **idiosyncratic** drug response, one that is infrequently observed in most patients. The idiosyncratic responses are usually caused by genetic differences in metabolism of the drug or by immunologic mechanisms, including allergic reactions.

Quantitative variations in drug response are in general more common and more clinically important. An individual patient is **hyporeactive** or **hyperreactive** to a drug in that the intensity of effect of a given dose of drug is diminished or increased in comparison to the effect seen in most individuals. (*Note:* The term **hypersensitivity** usually refers to allergic or other immunologic responses to drugs.) With some drugs, the intensity of response to a given dose may change during the course of therapy; in these cases, responsiveness usually decreases as a consequence of continued drug administration, producing a state of relative **tolerance** to the drug's effects. When responsiveness diminishes rapidly after administration of a drug, the response is said to be subject to **tachyphylaxis.**

Even before administering the first dose of a drug, the prescriber should consider factors that may help in predicting the direction and extent of possible variations in responsiveness. These include the propensity of a particular drug to produce tolerance or tachyphylaxis as well as the effects of age, sex, body size, disease state, genetic factors, and simultaneous administration of other drugs.

Four general mechanisms may contribute to variation in drug responsiveness among patients or within an individual patient at different times.

A. Alteration in Concentration of Drug That Reaches the Receptor

Patients may differ in the rate of absorption of a drug, in distributing it through body compartments, or in clearing the drug from the blood (see Chapter 3). By altering the concentration of drug that reaches relevant receptors, such pharmacokinetic differences may alter the clinical response. Some differences can be predicted on the basis of age, weight, sex, disease state, liver and kidney function, and by testing specifically for genetic differences that may result from inheritance of a functionally distinctive complement of drug-metabolizing enzymes (see Chapters 3 and 4). Another important mechanism influencing drug availability is active transport of drug from the cytoplasm, mediated by a family of membrane transporters encoded by the so-called multidrug resistance (*MDR*) genes. For example, up-regulation of *MDR* gene–encoded transporter expression is a major mechanism by which tumor cells develop resistance to anticancer drugs.

B. Variation in Concentration of an Endogenous Receptor Ligand

This mechanism contributes greatly to variability in responses to pharmacologic antagonists. Thus, propranolol, a β-adrenoceptor antagonist, will markedly slow the heart rate of a patient whose endogenous catecholamines are elevated (as in pheochromocytoma) but will not affect the resting heart rate of a well-trained marathon runner. A partial agonist may exhibit even more dramatically different responses: Saralasin, a weak partial agonist at angiotensin II receptors, lowers blood pressure in patients with hypertension caused by increased angiotensin II production and raises blood pressure in patients who produce small amounts of angiotensin.

C. Alterations in Number or Function of Receptors

Experimental studies have documented changes in drug responsiveness caused by increases or decreases in the number of receptor sites or by alterations in the efficiency of coupling of receptors to distal effector mechanisms. In some cases, the change in receptor number is caused by other hormones; for example, thyroid hormones increase both the number of β receptors in rat heart muscle and cardiac sensitivity to catecholamines. Similar changes probably contribute to the tachycardia of thyrotoxicosis in patients and may account for the usefulness of propranolol, a β-adrenoceptor antagonist, in ameliorating symptoms of this disease.

In other cases, the agonist ligand itself induces a decrease in the number (eg, down-regulation) or coupling efficiency (eg, desensitization) of its receptors.

These mechanisms (discussed above, under Signaling Mechanisms & Drug Actions) may contribute to two clinically important phenomena: first, tachyphylaxis or tolerance to the effects of some drugs (eg, biogenic amines and their congeners), and second, the "over-shoot" phenomena that follow withdrawal of certain drugs. These phenomena can occur with either agonists or antagonists. An antagonist may increase the number of receptors in a critical cell or tissue by preventing down-regulation caused by an endogenous agonist. When the antagonist is withdrawn, the elevated number of receptors can produce an exaggerated response to physiologic concentrations of agonist. Potentially disastrous withdrawal symptoms can result for the opposite reason when administration of an agonist drug is discontinued. In this situation, the number of receptors, which has been decreased by drug-induced down-regulation, is too low for endogenous agonist to produce effective stimulation. For example, the withdrawal of clonidine (a drug whose α_2-adrenoceptor agonist activity reduces blood pressure) can produce hypertensive crisis, probably because the drug down-regulates α_2-adrenoceptors (see Chapter 11).

Genetic factors also can play an important role in altering the number or function of specific receptors. For example, a specific genetic variant of the α_{2C}-adrenoceptor—when inherited together with a specific variant of the α_1-adrenoceptor—confers increased risk for developing heart failure, which may be reduced by early intervention using antagonist drugs. The identification of such genetic factors, part of the rapidly developing field of pharmacogenetics, holds promise for clinical diagnosis and in the future may help physicians design the most appropriate pharmacologic therapy for individual patients. Another interesting example of genetic effects on drug response is seen in the treatment of cancers involving excessive growth factor signaling. Somatic mutations affecting the tyrosine kinase domain of the epidermal growth factor receptor confer enhanced sensitivity to kinase inhibitors such as gefitinib in certain lung cancers. This effect enhances the antineoplastic effect of the drug and, because the somatic mutation is specific to the tumor and not present in the host, the therapeutic index of these drugs can be significantly enhanced in patients whose tumors harbor such somatic mutations.

D. Changes in Components of Response Distal to the Receptor

Although a drug initiates its actions by binding to receptors, the response observed in a patient depends on the functional integrity of biochemical processes in the responding cell and physiologic regulation by interacting organ systems. Clinically, changes in these postreceptor processes represent the largest and most important class of mechanisms that cause variation in responsiveness to drug therapy.

Before initiating therapy with a drug, the prescriber should be aware of patient characteristics that may limit the clinical response. These characteristics include the age and general health of the patient and—most importantly—the severity and pathophysiologic mechanism of the disease. The most important potential cause of failure to achieve a satisfactory response is that the diagnosis is wrong or physiologically incomplete. Drug therapy will always be most successful when it is accurately directed at the pathophysiologic mechanism responsible for the disease.

When the diagnosis is correct and the drug is appropriate, an unsatisfactory therapeutic response can often be traced to compensatory mechanisms in the patient that respond to and oppose the beneficial effects of the drug. Compensatory increases in sympathetic nervous tone and fluid retention by the kidney, for example, can contribute to tolerance to antihypertensive effects of a vasodilator drug. In such cases, additional drugs may be required to achieve a useful therapeutic result.

Clinical Selectivity: Beneficial versus Toxic Effects of Drugs

Although we classify drugs according to their principal actions, it is clear that *no drug causes only a single, specific effect.* Why is this so? It is exceedingly unlikely that any kind of drug molecule will bind to only a single type of receptor molecule, if only because the number of potential receptors in every patient is astronomically large. Even if the chemical structure of a drug allowed it to bind to only one kind of receptor, the biochemical processes controlled by such receptors would take place in multiple cell types and would be coupled to many other biochemical functions; as a result, the patient and the prescriber would probably perceive more than one drug effect. Accordingly, drugs are only *selective*—rather than specific—in their actions, because they bind to one or a few types of receptor more tightly than to others and because these receptors control discrete processes that result in distinct effects.

It is only because of their selectivity that drugs are useful in clinical medicine. Selectivity can be measured by comparing binding affinities of a drug to different receptors or by comparing ED_{50}s for different effects of a drug in vivo. In drug development and in clinical medicine, selectivity is usually considered by separating effects into two categories: **beneficial** or **therapeutic effects** versus **toxic effects.** Pharmaceutical advertisements and prescribers occasionally use the term **side effect,** implying that the effect in question is insignificant or occurs via a pathway that is to one side of the principal action of the drug; such implications are frequently erroneous.

A. BENEFICIAL AND TOXIC EFFECTS MEDIATED BY THE SAME RECEPTOR-EFFECTOR MECHANISM

Much of the serious drug toxicity in clinical practice represents a direct pharmacologic extension of the therapeutic actions of the drug. In some of these cases (eg, bleeding caused by anticoagulant therapy; hypoglycemic coma due to insulin), toxicity may be avoided by judicious management of the dose of drug administered, guided by careful monitoring of effect (measurements of blood coagulation or serum glucose) and aided by ancillary measures (avoiding tissue trauma that may lead to hemorrhage; regulation of carbohydrate intake). In still other cases, the toxicity may be avoided by not administering the drug at all, if the therapeutic indication is weak or if other therapy is available.

In certain situations, a drug is clearly necessary and beneficial but produces unacceptable toxicity when given in doses that produce optimal benefit. In such situations, it may be necessary to add another drug to the treatment regimen. In treating hypertension, for example, administration of a second drug often allows the prescriber to reduce the dose and toxicity of the first drug (see Chapter 11).

B. BENEFICIAL AND TOXIC EFFECTS MEDIATED BY IDENTICAL RECEPTORS BUT IN DIFFERENT TISSUES OR BY DIFFERENT EFFECTOR PATHWAYS

Many drugs produce both their desired effects and adverse effects by acting on a single receptor type in different tissues. Examples discussed in this book include: digitalis glycosides, which act by inhibiting Na^+/K^+ ATPase in cell membranes; methotrexate, which inhibits the enzyme dihydrofolate reductase; and glucocorticoid hormones.

Three therapeutic strategies are used to avoid or mitigate this sort of toxicity. First, the drug should always be administered at the lowest dose that produces acceptable benefit. Second, adjunctive drugs that act through different receptor mechanisms and produce different toxicities may allow lowering the dose of the first drug, thus limiting its toxicity (eg, use of other immunosuppressive agents added to glucocorticoids in treating inflammatory disorders). Third, selectivity of the drug's actions may be increased by manipulating the concentrations of drug available to receptors in different parts of the body, for example, by aerosol administration of a glucocorticoid to the bronchi in asthma.

C. BENEFICIAL AND TOXIC EFFECTS MEDIATED BY DIFFERENT TYPES OF RECEPTORS

Therapeutic advantages resulting from new chemical entities with improved receptor selectivity were mentioned earlier in this chapter and are described in detail in later chapters. Such drugs include the α- and β-selective adrenoceptor agonists and antagonists, the H_1 and H_2 antihistamines, nicotinic and muscarinic blocking agents, and receptor-selective steroid hormones. All of these receptors are grouped in functional families, each responsive to a small class of endogenous agonists. The receptors and their associated therapeutic uses were discovered by analyzing effects of the physiologic chemical signals—catecholamines, histamine, acetylcholine, and corticosteroids.

Several other drugs were discovered by exploiting therapeutic or toxic effects of chemically similar agents observed in a clinical context. Examples include quinidine, the sulfonylureas, thiazide diuretics, tricyclic antidepressants, opioid drugs, and phenothiazine antipsychotics. Often the new agents turn out to interact with receptors for endogenous substances (eg, opioids and phenothiazines for endogenous opioid and dopamine receptors, respectively). It is likely that other new drugs will be found to do so in the future, perhaps leading to the discovery of new classes of receptors and endogenous ligands for future drug development.

Thus, the propensity of drugs to bind to different classes of receptor sites is not only a potentially vexing problem in treating patients, it also presents a continuing challenge to pharmacology and an opportunity for developing new and more useful drugs.

REFERENCES

Aaronson DS, Horvath CM: A road map for those who know JAK-STAT. Science 2002;296:1653.

Arteaga CL, Moulder SL, Yakes FM: HER (erbB) tyrosine kinase inhibitors in the treatment of breast cancer. Semin Oncol 2002;29:4.

Berridge MJ, Bootman MD, Roderick HL: Calcium signalling: Dynamics, homeostasis and remodelling. Nat Rev Mol Cell Biol 2003;4:517.

Cabrera-Vera TM et al: Insights into G protein structure, function, and regulation. Endocr Rev 2003;24:765.

Civelli O: GPCR deorphanizations: The novel, the known and the unexpected transmitters. Trends Pharmacol Sci 2005; 26:15.

Dancey JE: Predictive factors for epidermal growth factor receptor inhibitors—The bull's-eye hits the arrow. Cancer Cell 2004; 5:411.

Derynck R, Akhurst RJ, Balmain A: TGF-beta signaling in tumor suppression and cancer progression. Nat Genet 2001;29:117.

Ginty DD, Segal RA: Retrograde neurotrophin signaling: Trk-ing along the axon. Curr Opin Neurobiol 2002;12:268.

Gouaux E, MacKinnon R: Principles of selective ion transport in channels and pumps. Science 2005;310:1461.

Hermiston ML et al: Reciprocal regulation of lymphocyte activation by tyrosine kinases and phosphatases. J Clin Invest 2002; 109:9.

Kenakin T: Efficacy at G-protein-coupled receptors. Nat Rev Drug Discov 2002;1:103.

Mosesson Y, Yarden Y: Oncogenic growth factor receptors: Implications for signal transduction therapy. Semin Cancer Biol 2004;14:262.

Pierce KL, Premont RT, Lefkowitz RJ: Seven-transmembrane receptors. Nat Rev Mol Cell Biol 2002;3:639.

Roden DM, George AL Jr: The genetic basis of variability in drug responses. Nat Rev Drug Discov 2002;1:37.

Rotella DP: Phosphodiesterase 5 inhibitors: Current status and potential applications. Nat Rev Drug Discov 2002;1:674.

Small KM, McGraw DW, Liggett SB: Pharmacology and physiology of human adrenergic receptor polymorphisms. Ann Rev Pharmacol Toxicol 2003;43:381.

Sorkin A, von Zastrow M: Signal transduction and endocytosis-close encounters of many kinds. Nat Rev Mol Cell Biol 2002; 3:600.

Yoshihara HA, Scanlan TS: Selective thyroid hormone receptor modulators. Curr Top Med Chem 2003;3:1601.

Yu FH, Catterall WA: Overview of the voltage-gated sodium channel family. Genome Biol 2003;4:207.

Pharmacokinetics & Pharmacodynamics: Rational Dosing & the Time Course of Drug Action

3

Nicholas H.G. Holford, MB, ChB, FRACP

The goal of therapeutics is to achieve a desired beneficial effect with minimal adverse effects. When a medicine has been selected for a patient, the clinician must determine the dose that most closely achieves this goal. A rational approach to this objective combines the principles of pharmacokinetics with pharmacodynamics to clarify the dose-effect relationship (Figure 3–1). Pharmacodynamics governs the concentration-effect part of the interaction, whereas pharmacokinetics deals with the dose-concentration part. The pharmacokinetic processes of absorption, distribution, and elimination determine how rapidly and for how long the drug will appear at the target organ. The pharmacodynamic concepts of maximum response and sensitivity determine the magnitude of the effect at a particular concentration (see the definitions of E_{max} and EC_{50}, Chapter 2).

Figure 3–1 illustrates a fundamental hypothesis of pharmacology, namely, that a relationship exists between a beneficial or toxic effect of a drug and the concentration of the drug. This hypothesis has been documented for many drugs, as indicated by the Target Concentrations and Toxic Concentrations columns in Table 3–1. The apparent lack of such a relationship for some drugs does not weaken the basic hypothesis but points to the need to consider the time course of concentration at the actual site of pharmacologic effect (see below).

Knowing the relationship between dose, drug concentration, and effects allows the clinician to take into account the various pathologic and physiologic features of a particular patient that make him or her different from the average individual in responding to a drug. The importance of pharmacokinetics and pharmacodynamics in patient care thus rests upon the improvement in therapeutic benefit and reduction in toxicity that can be achieved by application of these principles.

PHARMACOKINETICS

The "standard" dose of a drug is based on trials in healthy volunteers and patients with average ability to absorb, distribute, and eliminate the drug (see Clinical Trials: The IND & NDA in Chapter 5). This dose will not be suitable for every patient. Several physiologic processes (eg, maturation of organ function in infants) and pathologic processes (eg, heart failure, renal failure) dictate dosage adjustment in individual patients. These processes modify specific pharmacokinetic parameters. The two basic parameters are **clearance,** the measure of the ability of the body to eliminate the drug; and **volume of distribution,** the measure of the apparent space in the body available to contain the drug. These parameters are illustrated schematically in Figure 3–2 (p. 39), where the volume of the compartments into which the drugs diffuse represents the volume of distribution and the size of the outflow "drain" in Figures 3–2B and 3–2D represents the clearance.

Volume of Distribution

Volume of distribution (V_d) relates the amount of drug in the body to the concentration of drug (C) in blood or plasma:

$$V_d = \frac{\text{Amount of drug in body}}{C} \qquad (1)$$

The volume of distribution may be defined with respect to blood, plasma, or water (unbound drug), depending on the concentration used in equation (1) (C = C_b, C_p, or C_u).

That the V_d calculated from equation (1) is an *apparent* volume may be appreciated by comparing the volumes of distribution of drugs such as digoxin or chloroquine (Table 3–1) with some of the physical volumes of the body (Table 3–2). Volume of distribution can vastly exceed any physical volume in the body because it is the volume apparently necessary to contain the amount of drug *homogeneously* at the concentration found in the blood, plasma, or water. Drugs with very high volumes of distribution have much higher concentrations in extravascular tissue

Figure 3–1. The relationship between dose and effect can be separated into pharmaco-kinetic (dose-concentration) and pharmacodynamic (concentration-effect) components. Concentration provides the link between pharmacokinetics and pharmacodynamics and is the focus of the target concentration approach to rational dosing. The three primary processes of pharmacokinetics are absorption, distribution, and elimination.

than in the vascular compartment; that is, they are *not* homogeneously distributed. Drugs that are completely retained within the vascular compartment, on the other hand, have a minimum possible volume of distribution equal to the blood component in which they are distributed, eg, 0.04 L/kg body weight or 2.8 L/70 kg (Table 3–2) for a drug that is restricted to the plasma compartment.

Clearance

Drug clearance principles are similar to the clearance concepts of renal physiology. Clearance of a drug is the factor that predicts the rate of elimination in relation to the drug concentration:

$$CL = \frac{\text{Rate of elimination}}{C} \quad (2)$$

Clearance, like volume of distribution, may be defined with respect to blood (CL_b), plasma (CL_p), or unbound in water (CL_u), depending on the concentration measured.

It is important to note the additive character of clearance. Elimination of drug from the body may involve processes occurring in the kidney, the lung, the liver, and other organs. Dividing the rate of elimination at each organ by the concentration of drug presented to

it yields the respective clearance at that organ. Added together, these separate clearances equal total systemic clearance:

$$CL_{renal} = \frac{\text{Rate of elimination}_{kidney}}{C} \quad (3a)$$

$$CL_{liver} = \frac{\text{Rate of elimination}_{liver}}{C} \quad (3b)$$

$$CL_{other} = \frac{\text{Rate of elimination}_{other}}{C} \quad (3c)$$

$$CL_{systemic} = CL_{renal} + CL_{liver} + CL_{other} \quad (3d)$$

"Other" tissues of elimination could include the lungs and additional sites of metabolism, eg, blood or muscle.

The two major sites of drug elimination are the kidneys and the liver. Clearance of unchanged drug in the urine represents renal clearance. Within the liver, drug elimination occurs via biotransformation of parent drug to one or more metabolites, or excretion of unchanged drug into the bile, or both. The pathways of biotransformation are discussed in Chapter 4. For most drugs, clearance is constant over the concentration range encountered in clinical settings, ie, elimination is not saturable,

Table 3–1. Pharmacokinetic and pharmacodynamic parameters for selected drugs.
(See Speight & Holford, 1997, for a more comprehensive listing.)

Drug	Oral Availability (F) (%)	Urinary Excretion (%)	Bound in Plasma (%)	Clearance (L/h/70 kg)[1]	Volume of Distribution (L/70 kg)	Half-Life (h)	Target Concentrations	Toxic Concentrations
Acetaminophen	88	3	0	21	67	2	15 mg/L	>300 mg/L
Acyclovir	23	75	15	19.8	48	2.4	...	...
Amikacin	...	98	4	5.46	19	2.3	...	...
Amoxicillin	93	86	18	10.8	15	1.7	...	...
Amphotericin	...	4	90	1.92	53	18	...	...
Ampicillin	62	82	18	16.2	20	1.3	...	...
Aspirin	68	1	49	39	11	0.25	...	...
Atenolol	56	94	5	10.2	67	6.1	1 mg/L	...
Atropine	50	57	18	24.6	120	4.3	...	...
Captopril	65	38	30	50.4	57	2.2	50 ng/mL	...
Carbamazepine	70	1	74	5.34	98	15	6 mg/L	>9 mg/L
Cephalexin	90	91	14	18	18	0.9	...	...
Cephalothin	...	52	71	28.2	18	0.57	...	...
Chloramphenicol	80	25	53	10.2	66	2.7	...	...
Chlordiazepoxide	100	1	97	2.28	21	10	1 mg/L	...
Chloroquine	89	61	61	45	13000	214	20 ng/mL	250 ng/mL
Chlorpropamide	90	20	96	0.126	6.8	33	...	...
Cimetidine	62	62	19	32.4	70	1.9	0.8 mg/L	...
Ciprofloxacin	60	65	40	25.2	130	4.1	...	...
Clonidine	95	62	20	12.6	150	12	1 ng/mL	...
Cyclosporine	23	1	93	24.6	85	5.6	200 ng/mL	>400 ng/mL
Diazepam	100	1	99	1.62	77	43	300 ng/mL	...
Digitoxin	90	32	97	0.234	38	161	10 ng/mL	>35 ng/mL
Digoxin	70	60	25	7	500	50	1 ng/mL	>2 ng/mL
Diltiazem	44	4	78	50.4	220	3.7	...	...
Disopyramide	83	55	[2]	5.04	41	6	3 mg/mL	>8 mg/mL
Enalapril	95	90	55	9	40	3	>0.5 ng/mL	...
Erythromycin	35	12	84	38.4	55	1.6	...	...
Ethambutol	77	79	5	36	110	3.1	...	>10 mg/L
Fluoxetine	60	3	94	40.2	2500	53	...	...
Furosemide	61	66	99	8.4	7.7	1.5	...	>25 mg/L
Gentamicin	...	90	10	5.4	18	2.5	...	...
Hydralazine	40	10	87	234	105	1	100 ng/mL	...

(continued)

Table 3–1. Pharmacokinetic and pharmacodynamic parameters for selected drugs *(continued)*.

Drug	Oral Availability (F) (%)	Urinary Excretion (%)	Bound in Plasma (%)	Clearance (L/h/70 kg)[1]	Volume of Distribution (L/70 kg)	Half-Life (h)	Target Concentrations	Toxic Concentrations
Imipramine	40	2	90	63	1600	18	200 ng/mL	>1 mg/L
Indomethacin	98	15	90	8.4	18	2.4	1 mg/L	>5 mg/L
Labetalol	18	5	50	105	660	4.9	0.1 mg/L	...
Lidocaine	35	2	70	38.4	77	1.8	3mg/L	>6 mg/L
Lithium	100	95	0	1.5	55	22	0.7 mEq/L	>2 mEq/L
Meperidine	52	12	58	72	310	3.2	0.5 mg/L	...
Methotrexate	70	48	34	9	39	7.2	750 μM-h[3]	>950 μM-h
Metoprolol	38	10	11	63	290	3.2	25 ng/mL	...
Metronidazole	99	10	10	5.4	52	8.5	4 mg/L	...
Midazolam	44	56	95	27.6	77	1.9	...	...
Morphine	24	8	35	60	230	1.9	60 ng/mL	...
Nifedipine	50	0	96	29.4	55	1.8	50 ng/mL	...
Nortriptyline	51	2	92	30	1300	31	100 ng/mL	>500 ng/mL
Phenobarbital	100	24	51	0.258	38	98	15 mg/L	>30 mg/L
Phenytoin	90	2	89	Conc-dependent[4]	45	Conc-dependent[5]	10 mg/L	>20 mg/L
Prazosin	68	1	95	12.6	42	2.9	...	...
Procainamide	83	67	16	36	130	3	5 mg/L	>14 mg/L
Propranolol	26	1	87	50.4	270	3.9	20 ng/mL	...
Pyridostigmine	14	85	...	36	77	1.9	75 ng/mL	...
Quinidine	80	18	87	19.8	190	6.2	3 mg/L	>8 mg/L
Ranitidine	52	69	15	43.8	91	2.1	100 ng/mL	...
Rifampin	?	7	89	14.4	68	3.5	...	...
Salicylic acid	100	15	85	0.84	12	13	200 mg/L	>200 mg/L
Sulfamethoxazole	100	14	62	1.32	15	10	...	...
Terbutaline	14	56	20	14.4	125	14	2 ng/mL	...
Tetracycline	77	58	65	7.2	105	11	...	...
Theophylline	96	18	56	2.8	35	8.1	10 mg/L	>20 mg/L
Tobramycin	...	90	10	4.62	18	2.2	...	...
Tocainide	89	38	10	10.8	210	14	10 mg/L	...
Tolbutamide	93	0	96	1.02	7	5.9	100 mg/L	...
Trimethoprim	100	69	44	9	130	11	...	...
Tubocurarine	...	63	50	8.1	27	2	0.6 mg/L	...
Valproic acid	100	2	93	0.462	9.1	14	75 mg/L	>150 mg/L

(continued)

Table 3–1. Pharmacokinetic and pharmacodynamic parameters for selected drugs *(continued)*.

Drug	Oral Availability (F) (%)	Urinary Excretion (%)	Bound in Plasma (%)	Clearance (L/h/70 kg)[1]	Volume of Distribution (L/70 kg)	Half-Life (h)	Target Concentrations	Toxic Concentrations
Vancomycin	...	79	30	5.88	27	5.6	...	...
Verapamil	22	3	90	63	350	4	...	...
Warfarin	93	3	99	0.192	9.8	37	...	...
Zidovudine	63	18	25	61.8	98	1.1	...	...

[1]Convert to mL/min by multiplying the number given by 16.6.
[2]Varies with concentration.
[3]Target area under the concentration time curve after a single dose.
[4]Can be estimated from measured C_p using $CL = V_{max}/(K_m + C_p)$; $V_{max} = 415$ mg/d, $K_m = 5$ mg/L. See text.
[5]Varies because of concentration-dependent clearance.

and the rate of drug elimination is directly proportional to concentration (rearranging equation [2]):

$$\text{Rate of elimination} = CL \times C \qquad (4)$$

This is usually referred to as **first-order elimination.** When clearance is first-order, it can be estimated by calculating the **area under the curve (AUC)** of the time-concentration profile after a dose. Clearance is calculated from the dose divided by the AUC.

A. Capacity-Limited Elimination

For drugs that exhibit capacity-limited elimination (eg, phenytoin, ethanol), clearance will vary depending on the concentration of drug that is achieved (Table 3–1). Capacity-limited elimination is also known as saturable, dose- or concentration-dependent, nonlinear, and Michaelis-Menten elimination.

Most drug elimination pathways will become saturated if the dose is high enough. When blood flow to an organ does not limit elimination (see below), the relation between elimination rate and concentration (C) is expressed mathematically in equation (5):

$$\text{Rate of elimination} = \frac{V_{max} \times C}{K_m + C} \qquad (5)$$

The maximum elimination capacity is V_{max}, and K_m is the drug concentration at which the rate of elimination is 50% of V_{max}. At concentrations that are high relative to the K_m, the elimination rate is almost independent of concentration—a state of "pseudo-zero order" elimination. If dosing rate exceeds elimination capacity, steady state cannot be achieved: The concentration will keep on rising as long as dosing continues. This pattern of capacity-limited elimination is important for three drugs in common use: ethanol,

phenytoin, and aspirin. Clearance has no real meaning for drugs with capacity-limited elimination, and AUC cannot be used to describe the elimination of such drugs.

B. Flow-Dependent Elimination

In contrast to capacity-limited drug elimination, some drugs are cleared very readily by the organ of elimination, so that at any clinically realistic concentration of the drug, most of the drug in the blood perfusing the organ is eliminated on the first pass of the drug through it. The elimination of these drugs will thus depend primarily on the rate of drug delivery to the organ of elimination. Such drugs (see Table 4–7) can be called "high-extraction" drugs since they are almost completely extracted from the blood by the organ. Blood flow to the organ is the main determinant of drug delivery, but plasma protein binding and blood cell partitioning may also be important for extensively bound drugs that are highly extracted.

Half-Life

Half-life ($t_{1/2}$) is the time required to change the amount of drug in the body by one-half during elimination (or during a constant infusion). In the simplest case—and the most useful in designing drug dosage regimens—the body may be considered as a single compartment (as illustrated in Figure 3–2B) of a size equal to the volume of distribution (V_d). The time course of drug in the body will depend on both the volume of distribution and the clearance:

$$t_{1/2} = \frac{0.7^* \times V_d}{CL} \qquad (6)$$

*The constant 0.7 in equation (6) is an approximation to the natural logarithm of 2. Because drug elimination can be described by an exponential process, the time taken for a twofold decrease can be shown to be proportional to ln(2).

Figure 3–2. Models of drug distribution and elimination. The effect of adding drug to the blood by rapid intravenous injection is represented by expelling a known amount of the agent into a beaker. The time course of the amount of drug in the beaker is shown in the graphs at the right. In the first example **(A)**, there is no movement of drug out of the beaker, so the graph shows only a steep rise to maximum followed by a plateau. In the second example **(B)**, a route of elimination is present, and the graph shows a slow decay after a sharp rise to a maximum. Because the level of material in the beaker falls, the "pressure" driving the elimination process also falls, and the slope of the curve decreases. This is an exponential decay curve. In the third model **(C)**, drug placed in the first compartment ("blood") equilibrates rapidly with the second compartment ("extravascular volume") and the amount of drug in "blood" declines exponentially to a new steady state. The fourth model **(D)** illustrates a more realistic combination of elimination mechanism and extravascular equilibration. The resulting graph shows an early distribution phase followed by the slower elimination phase.

Half-life is useful because it indicates the time required to attain 50% of steady state—or to decay 50% from steady-state conditions—after a change in the rate of drug administration. Figure 3–3 shows the time course of drug accumulation during a constant-rate drug infusion and the time course of drug elimination after stopping an infusion that has reached steady state.

Disease states can affect both of the physiologically related primary pharmacokinetic parameters: volume of

Table 3–2. Physical volumes (in L/kg body weight) of some body compartments into which drugs may be distributed.

Compartment and Volume	Examples of Drugs
Water	
Total body water (0.6 L/kg[1])	Small water-soluble molecules: eg, ethanol.
Extracellular water (0.2 L/kg)	Larger water-soluble molecules: eg, gentamicin.
Blood (0.08 L/kg); plasma (0.04 L/kg)	Strongly plasma protein-bound molecules and very large molecules: eg, heparin.
Fat (0.2–0.35 L/kg)	Highly lipid-soluble molecules: eg, DDT.
Bone (0.07 L/kg)	Certain ions: eg, lead, fluoride.

[1]An average figure. Total body water in a young lean man might be 0.7 L/kg; in an obese woman, 0.5 L/kg.

distribution and clearance. A change in half-life will not necessarily reflect a change in drug elimination. For example, patients with chronic renal failure have decreased renal clearance of digoxin but also a decreased volume of distribution; the increase in digoxin half-life is not as great as might be expected based on the change in renal function. The decrease in volume of distribution is due to the decreased renal and skeletal muscle mass and consequent decreased tissue binding of digoxin to Na^+/K^+ ATPase.

Many drugs will exhibit multicompartment pharmacokinetics (as illustrated in Figures 3–2C and 3–2D). Under these conditions, the "true" terminal half-life, as given in Table 3–1, will be greater than that calculated from equation (6).

Drug Accumulation

Whenever drug doses are repeated, the drug will accumulate in the body until dosing stops. This is because it takes an infinite time (in theory) to eliminate all of a given dose. In practical terms, this means that if the dosing interval is shorter than four half-lives, accumulation will be detectable.

Accumulation is inversely proportional to the fraction of the dose lost in each dosing interval. The fraction lost is 1 minus the fraction remaining just before the next dose. The fraction remaining can be predicted from the dosing interval and the half-life. A convenient index of accumulation is the **accumulation factor.**

$$Accumulation\ factor = \frac{1}{Fraction\ lost\ in\ one\ dosing\ interval}$$

$$= \frac{1}{1 - Fraction\ remaining} \quad (7)$$

For a drug given once every half-life, the accumulation factor is 1/0.5, or 2. The accumulation factor predicts the ratio of the steady-state concentration to that seen at the same time following the first dose. Thus, the peak concentrations after intermittent doses at steady state will be equal to the peak concentration after the first dose multiplied by the accumulation factor.

Bioavailability

Bioavailability is defined as the fraction of unchanged drug reaching the systemic circulation following administration by any route (Table 3–3). The area under the blood concentration-time curve (AUC) is a common measure of the extent of bioavailability for a drug given by a particular route (Figure 3–4). For an intravenous dose of the drug, bioavailability is assumed to be equal to unity. For a drug administered orally, bioavailability

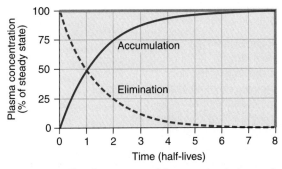

Figure 3–3. The time course of drug accumulation and elimination. **Solid line:** Plasma concentrations reflecting drug accumulation during a constant rate infusion of a drug. Fifty percent of the steady-state concentration is reached after one half-life, 75% after two half-lives, and over 90% after four half-lives. **Dashed line:** Plasma concentrations reflecting drug elimination after a constant rate infusion of a drug had reached steady state. Fifty percent of the drug is lost after one half-life, 75% after two half-lives, etc. The "rule of thumb" that four half-lives must elapse after starting a drug-dosing regimen before full effects will be seen is based on the approach of the accumulation curve to over 90% of the final steady-state concentration.

Table 3–3. Routes of administration, bioavailability, and general characteristics.

Route	Bioavailability (%)	Characteristics
Intravenous (IV)	100 (by definition)	Most rapid onset
Intramuscular (IM)	75 to ≤100	Large volumes often feasible; may be painful
Subcutaneous (SC)	75 to ≤100	Smaller volumes than IM; may be painful
Oral (PO)	5 to <100	Most convenient; first-pass effect may be significant
Rectal (PR)	30 to <100	Less first-pass effect than oral
Inhalation	5 to <100	Often very rapid onset
Transdermal	80 to ≤100	Usually very slow absorption; used for lack of first-pass effect; prolonged duration of action

may be less than 100% for two main reasons—incomplete extent of absorption and first-pass elimination.

A. Extent of Absorption

After oral administration, a drug may be incompletely absorbed, eg, only 70% of a dose of digoxin reaches the systemic circulation. This is mainly due to lack of absorption from the gut. Other drugs are either too hydrophilic (eg, atenolol) or too lipophilic (eg, acyclovir) to be absorbed easily, and their low bioavailability is also due to incomplete absorption. If too hydrophilic, the drug cannot cross the lipid cell membrane; if too lipophilic, the drug is not soluble enough to cross the water layer adjacent to the cell. Drugs may not be absorbed because of a reverse transporter associated with P-glycoprotein. This process actively pumps drug out of gut wall cells back into the gut lumen. Inhibition of P-glycoprotein and gut wall metabolism, eg, by grapefruit juice, may be associated with substantially increased drug absorption.

B. First-Pass Elimination

Following absorption across the gut wall, the portal blood delivers the drug to the liver prior to entry into the systemic circulation. A drug can be metabolized in the gut wall (eg, by the CYP3A4 enzyme system)

or even in the portal blood, but most commonly it is the liver that is responsible for metabolism before the drug reaches the systemic circulation. In addition, the liver can excrete the drug into the bile. Any of these sites can contribute to this reduction in bioavailability, and the overall process is known as first-pass elimination. The effect of first-pass hepatic elimination on bioavailability is expressed as the extraction ratio (ER):

$$ER = \frac{CL_{liver}}{Q} \qquad (8a)$$

where Q is hepatic blood flow, normally about 90 L/h in a person weighing 70 kg.

The systemic bioavailability of the drug (F) can be predicted from the extent of absorption (f) and the extraction ratio (ER):

$$F = f \times (1 - ER) \qquad (8b)$$

A drug such as morphine is almost completely absorbed (f = 1), so that loss in the gut is negligible. However, the hepatic extraction ratio for morphine is 0.67, so (1 – ER) is 0.33. The bioavailability of morphine is therefore expected to be about 33%, which is close to the observed value (Table 3–1).

A: Drug rapidly and completely available

B: Only half of availability of A but rate equal to A

C: Drug completely available but rate only half of A

Figure 3–4. Blood concentration-time curves, illustrating how changes in the rate of absorption and extent of bioavailability can influence both the duration of action and the effectiveness of the same total dose of a drug administered in three different formulations. The dashed line indicates the target concentration (TC) of the drug in the blood.

C. Rate of Absorption

The distinction between rate and extent of absorption is shown in Figure 3–4. The rate of absorption is determined by the site of administration and the drug formulation. Both the rate of absorption and the extent of input can influence the clinical effectiveness of a drug. For the three different dosage forms depicted in Figure 3–4, there would be significant differences in the intensity of clinical effect. Dosage form B would require twice the dose to attain blood concentrations equivalent to those of dosage form A. Differences in rate of availability may become important for drugs given as a single dose, such as a hypnotic used to induce sleep. In this case, drug from dosage form A would reach its target concentration earlier than drug from dosage form C; concentrations from A would also reach a higher level and remain above the target concentration for a longer period. In a multiple dosing regimen, dosage forms A and C would yield the same average blood level concentrations, although dosage form A would show somewhat greater maximum and lower minimum concentrations.

The mechanism of drug absorption is said to be zero-order when the rate is independent of the amount of drug remaining in the gut, eg, when it is determined by the rate of gastric emptying or by a controlled-release drug formulation. In contrast, when the full dose is dissolved in gastrointestinal fluids, the rate of absorption is usually proportional to the gastrointestinal concentration and is said to be first-order.

Extraction Ratio & the First-Pass Effect

Systemic clearance is not affected by bioavailability. However, clearance can markedly affect the extent of availability because it determines the extraction ratio (equation [8a]). Of course, therapeutic blood concentrations may still be reached by the oral route of administration if larger doses are given. However, in this case, the concentrations of the drug *metabolites* will be increased significantly over those that would occur following intravenous administration. Lidocaine and verapamil are both used to treat cardiac arrhythmias and have bioavailability less than 40%, but lidocaine is never given orally because its metabolites are believed to contribute to central nervous system toxicity. Other drugs that are highly extracted by the liver include morphine, propranolol, verapamil, and several tricyclic antidepressants (Table 3–1) as well as isoniazid.

Drugs with high extraction ratios will show marked variations in bioavailability between subjects because of differences in hepatic function and blood flow. These differences can explain the marked variation in drug concentrations that occurs among individuals given similar doses of highly extracted drugs. For drugs that are highly extracted by the liver, shunting of blood past hepatic sites of elimination will result in substantial increases in drug availability, whereas for drugs that are poorly extracted by the liver (for which the difference between entering and exiting drug concentration is small), shunting of blood past the liver will cause little change in availability. Drugs in Table 3–1 that are poorly extracted by the liver include chlorpropamide, diazepam, phenytoin, theophylline, tolbutamide, and warfarin.

Alternative Routes of Administration & the First-Pass Effect

There are several reasons for different routes of administration used in clinical medicine (Table 3–3)—for convenience (eg, oral), to maximize concentration at the site of action and minimize it elsewhere (eg, topical), to prolong the duration of drug absorption (eg, transdermal), or to avoid the first-pass effect.

The hepatic first-pass effect can be avoided to a great extent by use of sublingual tablets and transdermal preparations and to a lesser extent by use of rectal suppositories. Sublingual absorption provides direct access to systemic—not portal—veins. The transdermal route offers the same advantage. Drugs absorbed from suppositories in the lower rectum enter vessels that drain into the inferior vena cava, thus bypassing the liver. However, suppositories tend to move upward in the rectum into a region where veins that lead to the liver predominate. Thus, only about 50% of a rectal dose can be assumed to bypass the liver.

Although drugs administered by inhalation bypass the hepatic first-pass effect, the lung may also serve as a site of first-pass loss by excretion and possibly metabolism for drugs administered by nongastrointestinal ("parenteral") routes.

THE TIME COURSE OF DRUG EFFECT

The principles of pharmacokinetics (discussed in this chapter) and those of pharmacodynamics (discussed in Chapter 2; Holford & Sheiner, 1981) provide a framework for understanding the time course of drug effect.

Immediate Effects

In the simplest case, drug effects are directly related to plasma concentrations, but this does not necessarily mean that effects simply parallel the time course of concentrations. Because the relationship between drug concentration and effect is not linear (recall the E_{max} model described in Chapter 2), the effect will not usually be linearly proportional to the concentration.

Consider the effect of an angiotensin-converting enzyme (ACE) inhibitor, such as enalapril, on plasma ACE. The half-life of enalapril is about 3 hours. After

Figure 3–5. Time course of angiotensin-converting enzyme (ACE) inhibitor concentrations and effects. The black line shows the plasma enalapril concentrations in nanograms per milliliter after a single oral dose. The colored line indicates the percentage inhibition of its target, ACE. Note the different shapes of the concentration-time course (exponentially decreasing) and the effect-time course (linearly decreasing in its central portion).

an oral dose of 10 mg, the plasma concentration at 3 hours is about 50 ng/mL. Enalapril is usually given once a day, so seven half-lives will elapse from the time of peak concentration to the end of the dosing interval. The concentration of enalapril after each half-life and the corresponding extent of ACE inhibition are shown in Figure 3–5. The extent of inhibition of ACE is calculated using the E_{max} model, where E_{max}, the maximum extent of inhibition, is 100% and the EC_{50} is about 1 ng/mL.

Note that plasma concentrations of enalapril change by a factor of 16 over the first 12 hours (four half-lives) after the peak, but ACE inhibition has only decreased by 20%. Because the concentrations over this time are so high in relation to the EC_{50}, the effect on ACE is almost constant. After 24 hours, ACE is still 33% inhibited. This explains why a drug with a short half-life can be given once a day and still maintain its effect throughout the day. The key factor is a high initial concentration in relation to the EC_{50}. Even though the plasma concentration at 24 hours is less than 1% of its peak, this low concentration is still half the EC_{50}. This is very common for drugs that act on enzymes (eg, ACE inhibitors) or compete at receptors (eg, propranolol).

When concentrations are in the range between one fourth and four times the EC_{50}, the time course of effect is essentially a linear function of time—13% of the effect is lost every half-life over this concentration range. At concentrations below one fourth the EC_{50}, the effect becomes almost directly proportional to concentration and the time course of drug effect will follow the exponential decline of concentration. It is only when the concentration is low in relation to the EC_{50} that the concept of a "half-life of drug effect" has any meaning.

Delayed Effects

Changes in drug effects are often delayed in relation to changes in plasma concentration. This delay may reflect the time required for the drug to distribute from plasma to the site of action. This will be the case for almost all drugs. The delay due to distribution is a pharmacokinetic phenomenon that can account for delays of a few minutes. This distributional delay can account for the lag of effects after rapid intravenous injection of central nervous system (CNS)–active agents such as thiopental.

A common reason for more delayed drug effects—especially those that take many hours or even days to occur—is the slow turnover of a physiologic substance that is involved in the expression of the drug effect. For example, warfarin works as an anticoagulant by inhibiting vitamin K epoxidase in the liver. This action of warfarin occurs rapidly, and inhibition of the enzyme is closely related to plasma concentrations of warfarin. The clinical effect of warfarin, eg, on the prothrombin time, reflects a decrease in the concentration of the prothrombin complex of clotting factors. Inhibition of vitamin K epoxidase decreases the synthesis of these clotting factors, but the complex has a long half-life (about 14 hours), and it is this half-life that determines how long it takes for the concentration of clotting factors to reach a new steady state and for a drug effect to become manifest that reflects the warfarin plasma concentration.

Cumulative Effects

Some drug effects are more obviously related to a cumulative action than to a rapidly reversible one. The renal toxicity of aminoglycoside antibiotics (eg, gentamicin) is greater when administered as a constant infusion than with intermittent dosing. It is the accumulation of aminoglycoside in the renal cortex that is thought to cause renal damage. Even though both dosing schemes produce the same average steady-state concentration, the intermittent dosing scheme produces much higher peak concentrations, which saturate an uptake mechanism into the cortex; thus, total aminoglycoside accumulation is less. The difference in toxicity is a predictable consequence of the different patterns of concentration and the saturable uptake mechanism.

The effect of many drugs used to treat cancer also reflects a cumulative action—eg, the extent of binding of a drug to DNA is proportional to drug concentration and is usually irreversible. The effect on tumor growth is therefore a consequence of cumulative exposure to

Figure 3–6. Relationship between frequency of dosing and maximum and minimum plasma concentrations when a steady-state theophylline plasma level of 10 mg/L is desired. The smoothly rising line (solid black) shows the plasma concentration achieved with an intravenous infusion of 28 mg/h. The doses for 8-hourly administration (light color) are 224 mg; for 24-hourly administration (dark color), 672 mg. In each of the three cases, the mean steady-state plasma concentration is 10 mg/L.

the drug. Measures of cumulative exposure, such as AUC, provide a means to individualize treatment.

THE TARGET CONCENTRATION APPROACH TO DESIGNING A RATIONAL DOSAGE REGIMEN

A rational dosage regimen is based on the assumption that there is a **target concentration** that will produce the desired therapeutic effect. By considering the pharmacokinetic factors that determine the dose-concentration relationship, it is possible to individualize the dose regimen to achieve the target concentration. The effective concentration ranges shown in Table 3–1 are a guide to the concentrations measured when patients are being effectively treated. The initial target concentration should usually be chosen from the lower end of this range. In some cases, the target concentration will also depend on the specific therapeutic objective—eg, the control of atrial fibrillation by digoxin often requires a target concentration of 2 ng/mL, while heart failure is usually adequately managed with a target concentration of 1 ng/mL.

Maintenance Dose

In most clinical situations, drugs are administered in such a way as to maintain a steady state of drug in the body, ie, just enough drug is given in each dose to replace the drug eliminated since the preceding dose. Thus, calculation of the appropriate maintenance dose is a primary goal.

Clearance is the most important pharmacokinetic term to be considered in defining a rational steady-state drug dosage regimen. At steady state, the dosing rate ("rate in") must equal the rate of elimination ("rate out"). Substitution of the target concentration (TC) for concentration (C) in equation (4) predicts the maintenance dosing rate:

$$\text{Dosing rate}_{ss} = \text{Rate of elimination}_{ss}$$

$$= \text{CL} \times \text{TC} \qquad (9)$$

Thus, if the desired target concentration is known, the clearance in that patient will determine the dosing rate. If the drug is given by a route that has a bioavailability less than 100%, then the dosing rate predicted by equation (9) must be modified. For oral dosing:

$$\text{Dosing rate}_{oral} = \frac{\text{Dosing rate}}{\text{F}_{oral}} \qquad (10)$$

If intermittent doses are given, the maintenance dose is calculated from:

$$\text{Maintenance dose} =$$

$$\text{Dosing rate} \times \text{Dosing interval} \qquad (11)$$

(See Box, Example: Maintenance Dose Calculation.)

Note that the steady-state concentration achieved by continuous infusion or the *average* concentration following intermittent dosing depends only on clearance. The volume of distribution and the half-life need not be known in order to determine the average plasma concentration expected from a given dosing rate or to predict the dosing rate for a desired target concentration. Figure 3–6 shows that at different dosing intervals, the concentration time curves will have different maximum and minimum values even though the average level will always be 10 mg/L.

Estimates of dosing rate and average steady-state concentrations, which may be calculated using clearance, are independent of any specific pharmacokinetic model. In contrast, the determination of maximum and minimum steady-state concentrations requires further assumptions about the pharmacokinetic model. The accumulation factor (equation [7]) assumes that the drug follows a one-compartment body model (Figure 3–2B), and the peak concentration prediction assumes that the absorption rate is much faster than the elimination rate. For the calculation of estimated maximum and minimum concentrations in a clinical situation, these assumptions are usually reasonable.

Loading Dose

When the time to reach steady state is appreciable, as it is for drugs with long half-lives, it may be desirable to administer a loading dose that promptly raises the concentration of drug in plasma to the target concentration. In theory, only the amount of the loading dose need be computed—not the rate of its administration—and, to a first approximation, this is so. The volume of distribution is the proportionality factor that relates the total amount of drug in the body to the concentration in the plasma (C_p); if a loading dose is to achieve the target concentration, then from equation (1):

$$\text{Loading dose} = \begin{array}{c}\text{Amount in the body}\\ \text{immediately following}\\ \text{the loading dose}\end{array}$$

$$= V_d \times TC \qquad (12)$$

For the theophylline example given in the Box, Example: Maintenance Dose Calculation, the loading dose would be 350 mg (35 L × 10 mg/L) for a 70 kg person. For most drugs, the loading dose can be given as a single dose by the chosen route of administration.

Up to this point, we have ignored the fact that some drugs follow more complex multicompartment pharmacokinetics, eg, the distribution process illustrated by the two-compartment model in Figure 3–2. This is justified in the great majority of cases. However, in some cases the distribution phase may not be ignored, particularly in connection with the calculation of loading doses. If the rate of absorption is rapid relative to distribution (this is always true for intravenous bolus administration), the concentration of drug in plasma that results from an appropriate loading dose—calculated using the apparent volume of distribution—can initially be considerably higher than desired. Severe toxicity may occur, albeit transiently. This may be particularly important, for example, in the administration of antiarrhythmic drugs such as lidocaine, where an almost immediate toxic response may occur. Thus, while the estimation of the *amount* of a loading dose may be quite correct, the *rate of administration* can sometimes be crucial in preventing excessive drug concentrations, and slow administration of an intravenous drug (over minutes rather than seconds) is almost always prudent practice. For intravenous doses of theophylline, initial injections should be given over a 20-minute period to reduce the possibility of high plasma concentrations during the distribution phase.

EXAMPLE: MAINTENANCE DOSE CALCULATION

A target plasma theophylline concentration of 10 mg/L is desired to relieve acute bronchial asthma in a patient. If the patient is a nonsmoker and otherwise normal except for asthma, we may use the mean clearance given in Table 3–1, ie, 2.8 L/h/70 kg. Since the drug will be given as an intravenous infusion, F = 1.

$$\text{Dosing rate} = CL \times TC$$
$$= 2.8\,\text{L/h/70 kg} \times 10\,\text{mg/L}$$
$$= 28\,\text{mg/h/70 kg}$$

Therefore, in this patient, the proper infusion rate would be 28 mg/h/70 kg.

If the asthma attack is relieved, the clinician might want to maintain this plasma level using oral theophylline, which might be given every 12 hours using an extended-release formulation to approximate a continuous intravenous infusion. According to Table 3–1, F_{oral} is 0.96. When the dosing interval is 12 hours, the size of each maintenance dose would be:

$$\begin{array}{c}\text{Maintenance}\\ \text{dose}\end{array} = \frac{\text{Dosing rate}}{F} \times \text{Dosing interval}$$
$$= \frac{28\,\text{mg/h}}{0.96} \times 12\,\text{hours}$$
$$= 350\,\text{mg}$$

A tablet or capsule size close to the ideal dose of 350 mg would then be prescribed at 12-hourly intervals. If an 8-hour dosing interval was used, the ideal dose would be 233 mg; and if the drug was given once a day, the dose would be 700 mg. In practice, F could be omitted from the calculation since it is so close to 1.

When intermittent doses are given, the loading dose calculated from equation (12) will only reach the average steady-state concentration and will not match the peak steady-state concentration (Figure 3–6). To match the peak steady-state concentration, the loading dose can be calculated from equation (13):

$$\text{Loading dose} = \text{Maintenance dose} \times \text{Accumulation factor} \quad (13)$$

THERAPEUTIC DRUG MONITORING: RELATING PHARMACOKINETICS & PHARMACODYNAMICS

The basic principles outlined above can be applied to the interpretation of clinical drug concentration measurements on the basis of three major pharmacokinetic variables: absorption, clearance, and volume of distribution (and the derived variable, half-life); and two pharmacodynamic variables: maximum effect attainable in the target tissue and the sensitivity of the tissue to the drug. Diseases may modify all of these parameters, and the ability to predict the effect of disease states on pharmacokinetic parameters is important in properly adjusting dosage in such cases. (See Box: The Target Concentration Strategy.)

Pharmacokinetic Variables

A. Absorption

The amount of drug that enters the body depends on the patient's compliance with the prescribed regimen and on the rate and extent of transfer from the site of administration to the blood.

Overdosage and underdosage relative to the prescribed dosage—both aspects of failure of compliance—can frequently be detected by concentration measurements when gross deviations from expected values are obtained. If compliance is found to be adequate, absorption abnormalities in the small bowel may be the cause of abnormally low concentrations. Variations in the extent of bioavailability are rarely caused by irregularities in the manufacture of the particular drug formulation. More commonly, variations in bioavailability are due to metabolism during absorption.

B. Clearance

Abnormal clearance may be anticipated when there is major impairment of the function of the kidney, liver, or heart. Creatinine clearance is a useful quantitative indicator of renal function. Conversely, drug clearance may be a useful indicator of the functional consequences of heart, kidney, or liver failure, often with greater precision than clinical findings or other laboratory tests. For example, when renal function is changing rapidly, estimation of the clearance of aminoglycoside antibiotics may be a more accurate indicator of glomerular filtration than serum creatinine.

Hepatic disease has been shown to reduce the clearance and prolong the half-life of many drugs. However, for many other drugs known to be eliminated by hepatic processes, no changes in clearance or half-life have been noted with similar hepatic disease. This reflects the fact that hepatic disease does not always affect the hepatic intrinsic clearance. At present, there is no reliable marker of hepatic drug-metabolizing function that can be used to predict changes in liver clearance in a manner analogous to the use of creatinine clearance as a marker of renal drug clearance.

THE TARGET CONCENTRATION STRATEGY

Recognition of the essential role of concentration in linking pharmacokinetics and pharmacodynamics leads naturally to the target concentration strategy. Pharmacodynamic principles can be used to predict the concentration required to achieve a particular degree of therapeutic effect. This target concentration can then be achieved by using pharmacokinetic principles to arrive at a suitable dosing regimen. The target concentration strategy is a process for optimizing the dose in an individual on the basis of a measured surrogate response such as drug concentration:

1. Choose the target concentration, TC.

2. Predict volume of distribution (V_d) and clearance (CL) based on standard population values (eg, Table 3–1) with adjustments for factors such as weight and renal function.

3. Give a loading dose or maintenance dose calculated from TC, V_d, and CL.

4. Measure the patient's response and drug concentration.

5. Revise V_d and/or CL based on the measured concentration.

6. Repeat steps 3–5, adjusting the predicted dose to achieve TC.

C. Volume of Distribution

The apparent volume of distribution reflects a balance between binding to tissues, which decreases plasma concentration and makes the apparent volume larger, and binding to plasma proteins, which increases plasma concentration and makes the apparent volume smaller. Changes in either tissue or plasma binding can change the apparent volume of distribution determined from plasma concentration measurements. Older people have a relative decrease in skeletal muscle mass and tend to have a smaller apparent volume of distribution of digoxin (which binds to muscle proteins). The volume of distribution may be overestimated in obese patients if based on body weight and the drug does not enter fatty tissues well, as is the case with digoxin. In contrast, theophylline has a volume of distribution similar to that of total body water. Adipose tissue has almost as much water in it as other tissues, so that the apparent total volume of distribution of theophylline is proportional to body weight even in obese patients.

Abnormal accumulation of fluid—edema, ascites, pleural effusion—can markedly increase the volume of distribution of drugs such as gentamicin that are hydrophilic and have small volumes of distribution.

D. Half-Life

The differences between clearance and half-life are important in defining the underlying mechanisms for the effect of a disease state on drug disposition. For example, the half-life of diazepam increases with age. When clearance is related to age, it is found that clearance of this drug does not change with age. The increasing half-life for diazepam actually results from changes in the volume of distribution with age; the metabolic processes responsible for eliminating the drug are fairly constant.

Pharmacodynamic Variables

A. Maximum Effect

All pharmacologic responses must have a maximum effect (E_{max}). No matter how high the drug concentration goes, a point will be reached beyond which no further increment in response is achieved.

If increasing the dose in a particular patient does not lead to a further clinical response, it is possible that the maximum effect has been reached. Recognition of maximum effect is helpful in avoiding ineffectual increases of dose with the attendant risk of toxicity.

B. Sensitivity

The sensitivity of the target organ to drug concentration is reflected by the concentration required to produce 50% of maximum effect, the EC_{50}. Failure of response due to diminished sensitivity to the drug can be detected by measuring—in a patient who is not getting better—drug concentrations that are usually associated with therapeutic response. This may be a result of abnormal physiology—eg, hyperkalemia diminishes responsiveness to digoxin—or drug antagonism—eg, calcium channel blockers impair the inotropic response to digoxin.

Increased sensitivity to a drug is usually signaled by exaggerated responses to small or moderate doses. The pharmacodynamic nature of this sensitivity can be confirmed by measuring drug concentrations that are low in relation to the observed effect.

INTERPRETATION OF DRUG CONCENTRATION MEASUREMENTS

Clearance

Clearance is the single most important factor determining drug concentrations. The interpretation of measurements of drug concentrations depends on a clear understanding of three factors that may influence clearance: the dose, the organ blood flow, and the intrinsic function of the liver or kidneys. Each of these factors should be considered when interpreting clearance estimated from a drug concentration measurement. It must also be recognized that changes in protein binding may lead the unwary to believe there is a change in clearance when in fact drug elimination is not altered (see Box: Plasma Protein Binding: Is It Important?). Factors affecting protein binding include the following:

(1) Albumin concentration: Drugs such as phenytoin, salicylates, and disopyramide are extensively bound to plasma albumin. Albumin levels are low in many disease states, resulting in lower total drug concentrations.

(2) Alpha$_1$-acid glycoprotein concentration: α_1-acid glycoprotein is an important binding protein with binding sites for drugs such as quinidine, lidocaine, and propranolol. It is increased in acute inflammatory disorders and causes major changes in total plasma concentration of these drugs even though drug elimination is unchanged.

(3) Capacity-limited protein binding: The binding of drugs to plasma proteins is capacity-limited. Therapeutic concentrations of salicylates and prednisolone show concentration-dependent protein binding. Because unbound drug concentration is determined by dosing rate and clearance—which is not altered, in the case of these low-extraction-ratio drugs, by protein binding—increases in dosing rate will cause corresponding changes in the pharmacodynamically important unbound concentration. Total drug concentration will increase less rapidly than the dosing rate would suggest as protein binding approaches saturation at higher concentrations.

PLASMA PROTEIN BINDING: IS IT IMPORTANT?

Plasma protein binding is often mentioned as a factor playing a role in pharmacokinetics, pharmacodynamics, and drug interactions. However, there are no clinically relevant examples of changes in drug disposition or effects that can be clearly ascribed to changes in plasma protein binding (Benet & Hoener 2002). The idea that if a drug is displaced from plasma proteins it would increase the unbound drug concentration and increase the drug effect and, perhaps, produce toxicity seems a simple and obvious mechanism. Unfortunately, this simple theory, which is appropriate for a test tube, does not work in the body, which is an open system capable of eliminating unbound drug.

First, a seemingly dramatic change in the unbound fraction from 1% to 10% releases less than 5% of the total amount of drug in the body into the unbound pool because less than one third of the drug in the body is bound to plasma proteins even in the most extreme cases, eg, warfarin. Drug displaced from plasma protein will of course distribute throughout the volume of distribution, so that a 5% increase in the amount of unbound drug in the body produces at most a 5% increase in pharmacologically active unbound drug at the site of action.

Second, when the amount of unbound drug in plasma increases, the rate of elimination will increase (if unbound clearance is unchanged), and after four half-lives the unbound concentration will return to its previous steady-state value. When drug interactions associated with protein binding displacement and clinically important effects have been studied, it has been found that the displacing drug is also an inhibitor of clearance, and it is the change in *clearance* of the *unbound* drug that is the relevant mechanism explaining the interaction.

The clinical importance of plasma protein binding is only to help interpretation of measured drug concentrations. When plasma proteins are lower than normal, then total drug concentrations will be lower but unbound concentrations will not be affected.

Dosing History

An accurate dosing history is essential if one is to obtain maximum value from a drug concentration measurement. In fact, if the dosing history is unknown or incomplete, a drug concentration measurement loses all predictive value.

Timing of Samples for Concentration Measurement

Information about the rate and extent of drug absorption in a particular patient is rarely of great clinical importance. However, absorption usually occurs during the first 2 hours after a drug dose and varies according to food intake, posture, and activity. Therefore, it is important to avoid drawing blood until absorption is complete (about 2 hours after an oral dose). Attempts to measure peak concentrations early after oral dosing are usually unsuccessful and compromise the validity of the measurement, because one cannot be certain that absorption is complete.

Some drugs such as digoxin and lithium take several hours to distribute to tissues. Digoxin samples should be taken at least 6 hours after the last dose and lithium just before the next dose (usually 24 hours after the last dose). Aminoglycosides distribute quite rapidly, but it is still prudent to wait 1 hour after giving the dose before taking a sample.

Clearance is readily estimated from the dosing rate and mean steady-state concentration. Blood samples should be appropriately timed to estimate steady-state concentration. Provided steady state has been approached (at least three half-lives of constant dosing), a sample obtained near the midpoint of the dosing interval will usually be close to the mean steady-state concentration.

Initial Predictions of Volume of Distribution & Clearance

A. VOLUME OF DISTRIBUTION

Volume of distribution is commonly calculated for a particular patient using body weight (70 kg body weight is assumed for the values in Table 3–1). If a patient is obese, drugs that do not readily penetrate fat (eg, gentamicin and digoxin) should have their volumes calculated from ideal body weight as shown below:

$$\text{Ideal body wt (kg)} = 52 + 1.9 \text{ kg/in height}$$
$$\text{over 5 ft (men)}$$
$$= 49 + 1.7 \text{ kg/in height}$$
$$\text{over 5 ft (women)} \qquad (14)$$

Patients with edema, ascites, or pleural effusions offer a larger volume of distribution to the aminoglycoside antibiotics (eg, gentamicin) than is predicted by body weight. In such patients, the weight should be corrected as follows: Subtract an estimate of the weight of the excess fluid accumulation from the measured weight. Use the resultant "normal" body weight to calculate the normal volume of distribution. Finally, this normal volume should be increased by 1 L for each estimated kilogram of excess fluid. This correction is important because of the relatively small volumes of distribution of these water-soluble drugs.

B. CLEARANCE

Drugs cleared by the renal route often require adjustment of clearance in proportion to renal function. This can be conveniently estimated from the creatinine clearance, calculated from a single serum creatinine measurement and the predicted creatinine production rate.

The predicted creatinine production rate in women is 85% of the calculated value, because they have a smaller muscle mass per kilogram and it is muscle mass that determines creatinine production. Muscle mass as a fraction of body weight decreases with age, which is why age appears in the Cockcroft-Gault equation.*

The decrease of renal function with age is independent of the decrease in creatinine production. Because of the difficulty of obtaining complete urine collections, creatinine clearance calculated in this way is at least as reliable as estimates based on urine collections. Ideal body weight should be used for obese patients, and correction should be made for muscle wasting in severely ill patients.

Revising Individual Estimates of Volume of Distribution & Clearance

The commonsense approach to the interpretation of drug concentrations compares predictions of pharmacokinetic parameters and expected concentrations to mea-

---

*The Cockcroft-Gault equation is given in Chapter 61.

sured values. If measured concentrations differ by more than 20% from predicted values, revised estimates of V_d or CL for that patient should be calculated using equation (1) or equation (2). If the change calculated is more than a 100% increase or 50% decrease in either V_d or CL, the assumptions made about the timing of the sample and the dosing history should be critically examined.

For example, if a patient is taking 0.25 mg of digoxin a day, a clinician may expect the digoxin concentration to be about 1 ng/mL. This is based on typical values for bioavailability of 70% and total clearance of about 7 L/h (CL_{renal} 4 L/h, $CL_{nonrenal}$ 3 L/h). If the patient has heart failure, the nonrenal (hepatic) clearance might be halved because of hepatic congestion and hypoxia, so the expected clearance would become 5.5 L/h. The concentration is then expected to be about 1.3 ng/mL. Suppose that the concentration actually measured is 2 ng/mL. Commonsense would suggest halving the daily dose to achieve a target concentration of 1 ng/mL. This approach implies a revised clearance of 3.5 L/h. The smaller clearance compared with the expected value of 5.5 L/h may reflect additional renal functional impairment due to heart failure.

This technique will often be misleading if steady state has not been reached. At least a week of regular dosing (three to four half-lives) must elapse before the implicit method will be reliable.

REFERENCES

Benet LZ, Hoener B: Changes in plasma protein binding have little clinical relevance. Clin Pharmacol Ther 2002;71:115.

Holford NHG: Pharmacokinetic and pharmacodynamic principles. 2003; http://www.health.auckland.ac.nz/courses/Humanbio251/.

Holford NHG, Sheiner LB: Understanding the dose-effect relationship. Clin Pharmacokinet 1981;6:429.

Holford NHG: Target concentration intervention: Beyond Y2K. Br J Clin Pharmacol 1999;48:9.

Speight T, Holford NHG: *Avery's Drug Treatment,* 4th ed. Adis International, 1997.

Drug Biotransformation

4

Maria Almira Correia, PhD

Humans are exposed daily to a wide variety of foreign compounds called **xenobiotics**—substances absorbed across the lungs or skin or, more commonly, ingested either unintentionally as compounds present in food and drink or deliberately as drugs for therapeutic or "recreational" purposes. Exposure to environmental xenobiotics may be inadvertent and accidental or—when they are present as components of air, water, and food—inescapable. Some xenobiotics are innocuous, but many can provoke biologic responses. Such biologic responses often depend on conversion of the absorbed substance into an active metabolite. The discussion that follows is applicable to xenobiotics in general (including drugs) and to some extent to endogenous compounds.

WHY IS DRUG BIOTRANSFORMATION NECESSARY?

Renal excretion plays a pivotal role in terminating the biologic activity of some drugs, particularly those that have small molecular volumes or possess polar characteristics such as functional groups that are fully ionized at physiologic pH. However, many drugs do not possess such physicochemical properties. Pharmacologically active organic molecules tend to be lipophilic and remain unionized or only partially ionized at physiologic pH; these are readily reabsorbed from the glomerular filtrate in the nephron. Certain lipophilic compounds are often strongly bound to plasma proteins and may not be readily filtered at the glomerulus. Consequently, most drugs would have a prolonged duration of action if termination of their action depended solely on renal excretion.

An alternative process that can lead to the termination or alteration of biologic activity is metabolism. In general, lipophilic xenobiotics are transformed to more polar and hence more readily excreted products. The role metabolism plays in the inactivation of lipid-soluble drugs can be quite dramatic. For example, lipophilic barbiturates such as thiopental and pentobarbital would have extremely long half-lives if it were not for their metabolic conversion to more water-soluble compounds.

Metabolic products are often less pharmacodynamically active than the parent drug and may even be inactive. However, some biotransformation products have *enhanced* activity or toxic properties. It is noteworthy that

the synthesis of endogenous substrates such as steroid hormones, cholesterol, active vitamin D congeners, and bile acids involves many pathways catalyzed by enzymes associated with the metabolism of xenobiotics. Finally, drug-metabolizing enzymes have been exploited in the design of pharmacologically inactive prodrugs that are converted to active molecules in the body.

THE ROLE OF BIOTRANSFORMATION IN DRUG DISPOSITION

Most metabolic biotransformations occur at some point between absorption of the drug into the general circulation and its renal elimination. A few transformations occur in the intestinal lumen or intestinal wall. In general, all of these reactions can be assigned to one of two major categories called **phase I** and **phase II reactions** (Figure 4–1).

Phase I reactions usually convert the parent drug to a more polar metabolite by introducing or unmasking a functional group (–OH, –NH$_2$, –SH). Often these metabolites are inactive, although in some instances activity is only modified or even enhanced.

If phase I metabolites are sufficiently polar, they may be readily excreted. However, many phase I products are not eliminated rapidly and undergo a subsequent reaction in which an endogenous substrate such as glucuronic acid, sulfuric acid, acetic acid, or an amino acid combines with the newly incorporated functional group to form a highly polar conjugate. Such conjugation or synthetic reactions are the hallmarks of phase II metabolism. A great variety of drugs undergo these sequential biotransformation reactions, although in some instances the parent drug may already possess a functional group that may form a conjugate directly. For example, the hydrazide moiety of isoniazid is known to form an *N*-acetyl conjugate in a phase II reaction. This conjugate is then a substrate for a phase I type reaction, namely, hydrolysis to isonicotinic acid (Figure 4–2). Thus, phase II reactions may actually precede phase I reactions.

WHERE DO DRUG BIOTRANSFORMATIONS OCCUR?

Although every tissue has some ability to metabolize drugs, the liver is the principal organ of drug metabo-

50

ABSORPTION   **METABOLISM**   **ELIMINATION**

Phase I   Phase II

Drug ———————————————→ Conjugate ———→

Drug metabolite with
modified activity ————→ Conjugate ———→

Drug ⟨

Inactive drug
metabolite ————————→ Conjugate ———→

Drug ————————————————————————→

Lipophilic ——————————————————————→ Hydrophilic

Figure 4–1. Phase I and phase II reactions, and direct elimination, in drug biodisposition. Phase II reactions may also precede phase I reactions.

lism. Other tissues that display considerable activity include the gastrointestinal tract, the lungs, the skin, and the kidneys. Following oral administration, many drugs (eg, isoproterenol, meperidine, pentazocine, morphine) are absorbed intact from the small intestine and transported first via the portal system to the liver, where they undergo extensive metabolism. This process is called the **first-pass effect** (see Chapter 3). Some orally administered drugs (eg, clonazepam, chlorpromazine, cyclosporine) are more extensively metabolized in the intestine

than in the liver, whereas others (eg, midazolam) undergo significant (50%) intestinal metabolism. Thus, intestinal metabolism can contribute to the overall first-pass effect, and individuals with compromised liver function may increasingly rely on such intestinal metabolism for drug elimination. First-pass effects may so greatly limit the bioavailability of orally administered drugs (eg, lidocaine) that alternative routes of administration must be used to achieve therapeutically effective blood levels. Furthermore, the lower gut harbors intestinal microorganisms that are capable of many biotransformation reactions. In addition, drugs may be metabolized by gastric acid (eg, penicillin), by digestive enzymes (eg, polypeptides such as insulin), or by enzymes in the wall of the intestine (eg, sympathomimetic catecholamines).

Although drug biotransformation in vivo can occur by spontaneous, noncatalyzed chemical reactions, the vast majority of transformations are catalyzed by specific cellular enzymes. At the subcellular level, these enzymes may be located in the endoplasmic reticulum (ER), mitochondria, cytosol, lysosomes, or even the nuclear envelope or plasma membrane.

MICROSOMAL MIXED FUNCTION OXIDASE SYSTEM & PHASE I REACTIONS

Many drug-metabolizing enzymes are located in the lipophilic ER membranes of the liver and other tissues. When these lamellar membranes are isolated by homogenization and fractionation of the cell, they re-form into vesicles called **microsomes.** Microsomes retain most of the morphologic and functional characteristics of the intact membranes, including the rough and smooth surface features

Phase II (acetylation)

Phase I (hydrolysis)

Isonicotinic acid

(INH)

(*N*-acetyl INH)

(acetylhydrazine)

Acetylation of
macromolecules
(proteins)

Hepatotoxicity

Figure 4–2. Phase II activation of isoniazid (INH) to a hepatotoxic metabolite.

Figure 4–3. Cytochrome P450 cycle in drug oxidations. (RH, parent drug; ROH, oxidized metabolite; e⁻, electron.)

of the rough (ribosome-studded) and smooth (no ribosomes) ER. Whereas the rough microsomes tend to be dedicated to protein synthesis, the smooth microsomes are relatively rich in enzymes responsible for oxidative drug metabolism. In particular, they contain the important class of enzymes known as the **mixed function oxidases** (MFOs), or **monooxygenases.** The activity of these enzymes requires both a reducing agent (nicotinamide adenine dinucleotide phosphate [NADPH]) and molecular oxygen; in a typical reaction, one molecule of oxygen is consumed (reduced) per substrate molecule, with one oxygen atom appearing in the product and the other in the form of water.

In this oxidation-reduction process, two microsomal enzymes play a key role. The first of these is a flavoprotein, **NADPH-cytochrome P450 reductase.** One mole of this enzyme contains 1 mol each of flavin mononucleotide (FMN) and flavin adenine dinucleotide (FAD). The second microsomal enzyme is a hemoprotein called **cytochrome P450,** which serves as the terminal oxidase. In fact, the microsomal membrane harbors multiple forms of this hemoprotein, and this multiplicity is increased by repeated administration of exogenous chemicals (see below). The name cytochrome P450 (abbreviated as **CYP** or **P450**) is derived from the spectral properties of this hemoprotein. In its reduced (ferrous) form, it binds carbon monoxide to give a complex that absorbs light maximally at 450 nm. The relative abundance of P450s, compared with that of the reductase in the liver, contributes to making P450 heme reduction a rate-limiting step in hepatic drug oxidations.

Microsomal drug oxidations require P450, P450 reductase, NADPH, and molecular oxygen. A simplified scheme of the oxidative cycle is presented in Figure 4–3. Briefly, oxidized (Fe^{3+}) P450 combines with a drug substrate to form a binary complex (step 1). NADPH donates an electron to the flavoprotein P450 reductase, which in turn reduces the oxidized P450-drug complex (step 2). A second electron is introduced from NADPH via the same P450 reductase, which serves to reduce molecular oxygen and to form an "activated oxygen"-P450-substrate complex (step 3). This complex in turn transfers activated oxygen to the drug substrate to form the oxidized product (step 4).

The potent oxidizing properties of this activated oxygen permit oxidation of a large number of substrates. Substrate specificity is very low for this enzyme complex. High lipid solubility is the only common structural feature of the wide variety of structurally unrelated drugs and chemicals that serve as substrates in this system (Table 4–1).

Human Liver P450 Enzymes

Immunoblotting analyses, combined with the use of relatively selective functional markers and selective P450 inhibitors, have identified numerous P450 isoforms (CYP: 1A2, 2A6, 2B6, 2C8, 2C9, 2C18, 2C19, 2D6, 2E1, 3A4, 3A5, 4A11, and 7) in human liver microsomal preparations. Of these, **CYP1A2, CYP2A6, CYP2C9, CYP2D6, CYP2E1, and CYP3A4** appear to be the most important forms, accounting for approximately, 15%, 4%, 20%, 5%, 10%, and 30%, respectively, of the total human liver P450 content. Together, they are responsible for cata-

Table 4–1. Phase I reactions.

REACTION CLASS	STRUCTURAL CHANGE	DRUG SUBSTRATES
Oxidations		
Cytochrome P450- dependent oxidations:		
Aromatic hydroxylations		Acetanilide, propranolol, phenobarbital, phenytoin, phenylbutazone, amphetamine, warfarin, 17α-ethinyl estradiol, naphthalene, benzpyrene
Aliphatic hydroxylations	$RCH_2CH_3 \rightarrow RCH_2CH_2OH$ $RCH_2CH_3 \rightarrow RCHCH_3$ $\quad\quad\quad\quad\quad\quad\quad \underset{OH}{\mid}$	Amobarbital, pentobarbital, secobarbital, chlorpropamide, ibuprofen, meprobamate, glutethimide, phenylbutazone, digitoxin
Epoxidation	$RCH = CHR \rightarrow R - \overset{H}{\underset{}{C}} \overset{O}{\underset{}{\diagup\diagdown}} \overset{H}{\underset{}{C}} - R$	Aldrin
Oxidative dealkylation N-Dealkylation	$RNHCH_3 \rightarrow RNH_2 + CH_2O$	Morphine, ethylmorphine, benzphetamine, aminopyrine, caffeine, theophylline
O-Dealkylation	$ROCH_3 \rightarrow ROH + CH_2O$	Codeine, *p*-nitroanisole
S-Dealkylation	$RSCH_3 \rightarrow RSH + CH_2O$	6-Methylthiopurine, methitural
N-Oxidation Primary amines	$RNH_2 \rightarrow RNHOH$	Aniline, chlorphentermine
Secondary amines	$\underset{R_2}{\overset{R_1}{\diagdown}} NH \rightarrow \underset{R_2}{\overset{R_1}{\diagdown}} N - OH$	2-Acetylaminofluorene, acetaminophen
Tertiary amines	$\underset{R_3}{\overset{R_1}{\diagdown}} R_2 - N \rightarrow \underset{R_3}{\overset{R_1}{\diagdown}} R_2 - N \rightarrow O$	Nicotine, methaqualone
S-Oxidation	$\underset{R_2}{\overset{R_1}{\diagdown}} S \rightarrow \underset{R_2}{\overset{R_1}{\diagdown}} S = O$	Thioridazine, cimetidine, chlorpromazine
Deamination	$RCHCH_3 \rightarrow R - \overset{OH}{\underset{NH_2}{C}} - CH_3 \rightarrow R - \overset{}{\underset{O}{C}}CH_3 + NH_3$ $\underset{NH_2}{\mid}$	Amphetamine, diazepam
Desulfuration	$\underset{R_2}{\overset{R_1}{\diagdown}} C = S \rightarrow \underset{R_2}{\overset{R_1}{\diagdown}} C = O$	Thiopental

(continued)

Table 4–1. Phase I reactions (continued).

REACTION CLASS	STRUCTURAL CHANGE	DRUG SUBSTRATES
Cytochrome P450- dependent oxidations: (continued)	R_1 $P=S \rightarrow$ R_2 / R_1 $P=O$ R_2	Parathion
Dechlorination	$CCl_4 \rightarrow [CCl_3^{\cdot}] \rightarrow CHCl_3$	Carbon tetrachloride
Cytochrome P450-independent oxidations:		
Flavin monooxygenase (Ziegler's enzyme)	$R_3N \longrightarrow R_3N^+ \rightarrow O^- \xrightarrow{H^+} R_3N^+OH$	Chlorpromazine, amitriptyline, benzphetamine
	$RCH_2N—CH_2R \rightarrow RCH_2—N—CH_2R \rightarrow$ $\quad\quad\quad\;$ H $\quad\quad\quad\quad\quad\quad\;$ OH $RCH=N—CH_2R$ $\quad\quad\quad\quad\;$ O$^-$	Desipramine, nortriptyline
	$—N$ $\quad$ $—N$ $\quad$ $—N$ $\;\;\;$ —SH$\rightarrow$ $\;\;\;$ —SOH$\rightarrow$ $\;\;\;$ —SO$_2$H $—N$ $\quad$ $—N$ $\quad$ $—N$	Methimazole, propylthiouracil
Amine oxidases	$RCH_2NH_2 \rightarrow RCHO + NH_3$	Phenylethylamine, epinephrine
Dehydrogenations	$RCH_2OH \rightarrow RCHO$	Ethanol
Reductions		
Azo reductions	$RN=NR_1 \rightarrow RNH—NHR_1 \rightarrow RNH_2 + R_1NH_2$	Prontosil, tartrazine
Nitro reductions	$RNO_2 \rightarrow RNO \rightarrow RNHOH \rightarrow RNH_2$	Nitrobenzene, chloramphenicol, clonazepam, dantrolene
Carbonyl reductions	$RCR' \rightarrow RCHR'$ $\quad\;$ ‖ $\quad\quad$ │ $\quad\;$ O $\quad\quad$ OH	Metyrapone, methadone, naloxone
Hydrolyses		
Esters	$R_1COOR_2 \rightarrow R_1COOH + R_2OH$	Procaine, succinylcholine, aspirin, clofibrate, methylphenidate
Amides	$RCONHR_1 \rightarrow RCOOH + R_1NH_2$	Procainamide, lidocaine, indomethacin

lyzing the bulk of the hepatic drug and xenobiotic metabolism (Table 4–2).

It is noteworthy that CYP3A4 alone is responsible for the metabolism of over 50% of the clinically prescribed drugs metabolized by the liver. The involvement of individual P450s in the metabolism of a given drug may be screened in vitro by means of selective functional markers, selective chemical P450 inhibitors, and anti-P450 antibodies. In vivo, such screening may be accomplished by means of relatively selective noninvasive markers, which include breath tests or urinary analyses of specific metabolites after administration of a P450-selective substrate probe.

Enzyme Induction

Some of the chemically dissimilar P450 substrate drugs, on repeated administration, *induce* P450 by enhancing the rate of its synthesis or reducing its rate of degradation (Table 4–2). Induction results in an acceleration of substrate metabolism and usually in a decrease in the pharma-

Table 4–2. Human liver P450s (CYPs), and some of the drugs metabolized (substrates), inducers, and selective inhibitors.

CYP	Substrates	Inducers	Inhibitors
1A2	Acetaminophen, antipyrine, caffeine, clomipramine, phenacetin, tacrine, tamoxifen, theophylline, warfarin	Smoking, charcoal-broiled foods, cruciferous vegetables, omeprazole	Galangin, furafylline, fluvoxamine
2A6	Coumarin, tobacco nitrosamines, nicotine (to cotinine and 2′-hydroxynicotine)	Rifampin, phenobarbital	Tranylcypromine, menthofuran, methoxsalen
2B6	Artemisinin, bupropion, S-mephobarbital, cyclophosphamide, S-mephenytoin (N-demethylation to nirvanol), propofol, selegiline, sertraline	Phenobarbital, cyclophosphamide	Ticlopidine, clopidogrel
2C8	Taxol, all-*trans*-retinoic acid	Rifampin, barbiturates	Trimethoprim
2C9	Celecoxib, flurbiprofen, hexobarbital, ibuprofen, losartan, phenytoin, tolbutamide, trimethadione, sulfaphenazole, S-warfarin, ticrynafen	Barbiturates, rifampin	Tienilic acid, sulfaphenazole
2C18	Tolbutamide	Phenobarbital	
2C19	Diazepam, S-mephenytoin, naproxen, nirvanol, omeprazole, propranolol	Barbiturates, rifampin	N3-benzylnirvanol, N3-benzylphenobarbital, fluconazole
2D6	Bufuralol, bupranolol, clomipramine, clozapine, codeine, debrisoquin, dextromethorphan, encainide, flecainide, fluoxetine, guanoxan, haloperidol, hydrocodone, 4-methoxy-amphetamine, metoprolol, mexiletine, oxycodone, paroxetine, phenformin, propafenone, propoxyphene, risperidone, selegiline (deprenyl), sparteine, thioridazine, timolol, tricyclic antidepressants	St. John's wort, rifampin	Quinidine, paroxetine
2E1	Acetaminophen, chlorzoxazone, enflurane, halothane, ethanol (a minor pathway)	Ethanol, isoniazid	4-Methylpyrazole, disulfiram
3A4[1]	Acetaminophen, alfentanil, amiodarone, astemizole, cisapride, cocaine, cortisol, cyclosporine, dapsone, diazepam, dihydroergotamine, dihydropyridines, diltiazem, erythromycin, ethinyl estradiol, gestodene, indinavir, lidocaine, lovastatin, macrolides, methadone, miconazole, midazolam, mifepristone (RU 486), nifedipine, paclitaxel, progesterone, quinidine, rapamycin, ritonavir, saquinavir, spironolactone, sulfamethoxazole, sufentanil, tacrolimus, tamoxifen, terfenadine, testosterone, tetrahydrocannabinol, triazolam, troleandomycin, verapamil	Barbiturates, carbamazepine, glucocorticoids, macrolide antibiotics, pioglitazone, phenytoin, rifampin	Azamulin, diltiazem, erythromycin, fluconazole, grapefruit juice (furanocoumarins), itraconazole, ketoconazole, ritonavir, troleandomycin

[1]CYP3A5 has similar substrate and inhibitor profiles, but except for a few drugs is generally less active than CYP3A4.

cologic action of the inducer and also of coadministered drugs. However, in the case of drugs metabolically transformed to reactive metabolites, enzyme induction may exacerbate metabolite-mediated toxicity.

Various substrates induce P450 isoforms having different molecular masses and exhibiting different substrate specificities and immunochemical and spectral characteristics.

Environmental pollutants are also capable of inducing P450 enzymes. As noted above, exposure to benzo[a]pyrene and other polycyclic aromatic hydrocarbons, which are present in tobacco smoke, charcoal-broiled meat, and other organic pyrolysis products, is known to induce

CYP1A enzymes and to alter the rates of drug metabolism. Other environmental chemicals known to induce specific P450s include the polychlorinated biphenyls (PCBs), which were once used widely in industry as insulating materials and plasticizers, and 2,3,7,8-tetrachlorodibenzo-p-dioxin (dioxin, TCDD), a trace byproduct of the chemical synthesis of the defoliant 2,4,5-T (see Chapter 57).

Increased P450 synthesis requires enhanced transcription and translation. A cytoplasmic receptor (termed AhR) for polycyclic aromatic hydrocarbons (eg, benzo[a]pyrene, dioxin) has been identified, and the translocation of the inducer-receptor complex into the nucleus and subsequent activation of regulatory elements of genes have been documented. A pregnane X receptor (PXR), a member of the steroid-retinoid-thyroid hormone receptor family, has recently been shown to mediate CYP3A induction by various chemicals (dexamethasone, rifampin) in the liver and intestinal mucosa. A similar receptor, the constitutive androstane receptor (CAR) has been identified for the phenobarbital class of inducers.

P450 enzymes may also be induced by **substrate stabilization,** ie, decreased degradation, as is the case with troleandomycin- or clotrimazole-mediated induction of CYP3A enzymes and the ethanol-mediated induction of CYP2E1.

Enzyme Inhibition

Certain drug substrates inhibit cytochrome P450 enzyme activity (Table 4–2). Imidazole-containing drugs such as cimetidine and ketoconazole bind tightly to the P450 heme iron and effectively reduce the metabolism of endogenous substrates (eg, testosterone) or other coadministered drugs through competitive inhibition. However, macrolide antibiotics such as troleandomycin, erythromycin, and erythromycin derivatives are metabolized, apparently by CYP3A, to metabolites that complex the cytochrome P450 heme-iron and render it catalytically inactive. Another compound that acts through this mechanism is the inhibitor proadifen (SKF-525-A, used in research), which binds tightly to the heme iron and quasi-irreversibly inactivates the enzyme, thereby inhibiting the metabolism of potential substrates.

Some substrates irreversibly inhibit P450s via covalent interaction of a metabolically generated reactive intermediate that may react with the P450 apoprotein or heme moiety or even cause the heme to fragment and irreversibly modify the apoprotein. The antibiotic chloramphenicol is metabolized by CYP2B1 to a species that modifies its protein and thus also inactivates the enzyme. A growing list of such **suicide inhibitors**—inactivators that attack the heme or the protein moiety—includes certain steroids (ethinyl estradiol, norethindrone, and spironolactone); fluroxene; allobarbital; the analgesic sedatives allylisopropylacetylurea, diethylpentenamide, and ethchlorvynol; carbon disulfide; grapefruit furanocoumarins; deprenyl; phencyclidine; ticlopidine and clopidogrel; ritonavir, and propylthiouracil. On the other hand, the barbiturate secobarbital is found to inactivate CYP2B1 by modification of *both* its heme and protein moieties. Other metabolically activated drugs whose P450 inactivation mechanism is not fully elucidated include mifepristone (RU-486), troglitazone, raloxifene, and tamoxifen.

PHASE II REACTIONS

Parent drugs or their phase I metabolites that contain suitable chemical groups often undergo coupling or conjugation reactions with an endogenous substance to yield **drug conjugates** (Table 4–3). In general, conjugates are polar molecules that are readily excreted and often inactive. Conjugate formation involves high-energy intermediates and specific transfer enzymes. Such enzymes (**transferases**) may be located in microsomes or in the cytosol. They catalyze the coupling of an activated endogenous substance (such as the uridine 5′-diphosphate [UDP] derivative of glucuronic acid) with a drug (or endogenous compound), or of an activated drug (such as the S-CoA derivative of benzoic acid) with an endogenous substrate. Because the endogenous substrates originate in the diet, nutrition plays a critical role in the regulation of drug conjugations.

Drug conjugations were once believed to represent terminal inactivation events and as such have been viewed as "true detoxification" reactions. However, this concept must be modified, because it is now known that certain conjugation reactions (acyl glucuronidation of nonsteroidal anti-inflammatory drugs, O-sulfation of N-hydroxyacetylaminofluorene, and N-acetylation of isoniazid) may lead to the formation of reactive species responsible for the toxicity of the drugs. Furthermore, sulfation is known to activate the orally active prodrug minoxidil into a very efficacious vasodilator and morphine-6-glucuronide is more potent than morphine itself.

METABOLISM OF DRUGS TO TOXIC PRODUCTS

Metabolism of drugs and other foreign chemicals may not always be an innocuous biochemical event leading to detoxification and elimination of the compound. Indeed, as noted above, several compounds have been shown to be metabolically transformed to reactive intermediates that are toxic to various organs. Such toxic reactions may not be apparent at low levels of exposure to parent compounds when alternative detoxification mechanisms are not yet overwhelmed or compromised and the availability of endogenous detoxifying cosubstrates (glutathione [**GSH**], glucuronic acid, sulfate) is not limited. However, when these resources are exhausted, the toxic pathway may prevail, resulting in overt organ toxicity or carcinogenesis. The number of specific examples of such drug-induced toxicity is expanding rapidly. An example is acetaminophen (paracetamol)-induced hepatotoxicity (Figure 4–4). This analgesic antipyretic drug is quite safe in therapeutic doses (1.2 g/d for an adult). It normally undergoes glucuronidation and sulfation to the corresponding conjugates, which together comprise 95% of the total excreted metabolites. The alternative P450-dependent GSH conjugation pathway accounts for the remaining 5%. When acetaminophen intake far exceeds therapeutic doses, the glucuronidation and sulfation pathways are saturated, and the P450-dependent pathway becomes increasingly important. Little or no hepatotoxicity results as long as GSH is available for

Table 4–3. Phase II reactions.

Type of Conjugation	Endogenous Reactant	Transferase (Location)	Types of Substrates	Examples
Glucuronidation	UDP glucuronic acid	UDP glucuronosyl-transferase (microsomes)	Phenols, alcohols, carboxylic acids, hydroxylamines, sulfonamides	Nitrophenol, morphine, acetaminophen, diazepam, *N*-hydroxydapsone, sulfathiazole, meprobamate, digitoxin, digoxin
Acetylation	Acetyl-CoA	*N*-Acetyltransferase (cytosol)	Amines	Sulfonamides, isoniazid, clonazepam, dapsone, mescaline
Glutathione conjugation	Glutathione (GSH)	GSH-*S*-transferase (cytosol, microsomes)	Epoxides, arene oxides, nitro groups, hydroxylamines	Acetminphen, ethacrynic acid, bromobenzene
Glycine conjugation	Glycine	Acyl-CoA glycine-transferase (mitochondria)	Acyl-CoA derivatives of carboxylic acids	Salicylic acid, benzoic acid, nicotinic acid, cinnamic acid, cholic acid, deoxycholic acid
Sulfation	Phosphoadenosyl phosphosulfate	Sulfotransferase (cytosol)	Phenols, alcohols, aromatic amines	Estrone, aniline, phenol, 3-hydroxy-coumarin, acetaminophen, methyldopa
Methylation	*S*-Adenosyl-methionine	Transmethylases (cytosol)	Catecholamines, phenols, amines	Dopamine, epinephrine, pyridine, histamine, thiouracil
Water conjugation	Water	Epoxide hydrolase (microsomes)	Arene oxides, *cis*-di-substituted and mono-substituted oxiranes	Benzopyrene 7,8-epoxide, styrene 1,2-oxide, carbamazepine epoxide
		(cytosol)	Alkene oxides, fatty acid epoxides	Leukotriene A$_4$

conjugation. However, with time, hepatic GSH is depleted faster than it can be regenerated, and a reactive, toxic metabolite accumulates. In the absence of intracellular nucleophiles such as GSH, this reactive metabolite (*N*-acetylbenzoiminoquinone) reacts with nucleophilic groups of cellular proteins, resulting in hepatotoxicity.

The chemical and toxicologic characterization of the electrophilic nature of the reactive acetaminophen metabolite has led to the development of effective antidotes—cysteamine and *N*-acetylcysteine. Administration of *N*-acetylcysteine (the safer of the two) within 8–16 hours following acetaminophen overdosage has been shown to protect victims from fulminant hepatotoxicity and death (see Chapter 59). Administration of GSH is not effective because it does not cross cell membranes readily.

CLINICAL RELEVANCE OF DRUG METABOLISM

The dose and frequency of administration required to achieve effective therapeutic blood and tissue levels vary in different patients because of individual differences in drug distribution and rates of drug metabolism and elimination. These differences are determined by genetic factors and nongenetic variables such as age, sex, liver size, liver function, circadian rhythm, body temperature, and nutritional and environmental factors such as concomitant exposure to inducers or inhibitors of drug metabolism. The discussion that follows summarizes the most important of these variables.

Individual Differences

Individual differences in metabolic rate depend on the nature of the drug itself. Thus, within the same population, steady-state plasma levels may reflect a 30-fold variation in the metabolism of one drug and only a two-fold variation in the metabolism of another.

Genetic Factors

Genetic factors that influence enzyme levels account for some of these differences. Succinylcholine, for example, is metabolized only half as rapidly in persons with genetically determined defects in pseudocholinesterase as in persons with normally functioning pseudocholinesterase. Analo-

Figure 4–4. Metabolism of acetaminophen (top center) to hepatotoxic metabolites. (GSH, glutathione; SG, glutathione moiety).

gous pharmacogenetic differences are seen in the acetylation of isoniazid and the hydroxylation of warfarin. The defect in slow acetylators (of isoniazid and similar amines) appears to be caused by the synthesis of less of the enzyme rather than of an abnormal form of it. Inherited as an autosomal recessive trait, the **slow acetylator phenotype** occurs in about 50% of blacks and whites in the USA, more frequently in Europeans living in high northern latitudes, and much less commonly in Asians and Inuits

(Eskimos). Similarly, genetically determined defects in the oxidative metabolism of debrisoquin, phenacetin, guanoxan, sparteine, phenformin, warfarin, and others have been reported (Table 4–4). The defects are apparently transmitted as autosomal recessive traits and may be expressed at any one of the multiple metabolic transformations that a chemical might undergo.

Of the several recognized genetic varieties of drug metabolism polymorphisms, three have been particularly

Table 4–4. Some examples of genetic polymorphisms in drug metabolism.

Defect	Enzyme Involved	Drug and Therapeutic Use	Clinical Consequences[1]
Oxidation	CYP2D6	Bufuralol (β-adrenoceptor blocker)	Exacerbation of β-blockade, nausea
Oxidation	CYP2D6	Codeine (analgesic)	Reduced analgesia
Oxidation	CYP2D6	Debrisoquin (antihypertensive)	Orthostatic hypotension
Oxidation	Aldehyde dehydro-genase	Ethanol (recreational drug)	Facial flushing, hypotension, tachy-cardia, nausea, vomiting
N-Acetylation	N-acetyl transferase	Hydralazine (antihypertensive)	Lupus erythematosus-like syndrome
N-Acetylation	N-acetyl transferase	Isoniazid (antitubercular)	Peripheral neuropathy
Oxidation	CYP2C19	Mephenytoin (antiepileptic)	Overdose toxicity
S-Methylation	Thiopurine methyl-transferase	Mercaptopurines (cancer chemothera-peutic)	Myelotoxicity
Oxidation	CYP2A6	Nicotine (stimulant)	Lesser toxicity
Oxidation	CYP2D6	Nortriptyline (antidepressant)	Toxicity
O-Demethylation	CYP2C19	Omeprazole (proton pump inhibitor)	Increased therapeutic efficacy
Oxidation	CYP2D6	Sparteine	Oxytocic symptoms
Ester hydrolysis	Plasma cholinesterase	Succinylcholine (neuromuscular blocker)	Prolonged apnea
Oxidation	CYP2C9	S-warfarin (anticoagulant)	Bleeding
Oxidation	CYP2C9	Tolbutamide (hypoglycemic)	Cardiotoxicity

[1]Observed or predictable.

well characterized and afford some insight into possible underlying mechanisms. First is the **debrisoquin-sparteine oxidation** type of polymorphism, which apparently occurs in 3–10% of whites and is inherited as an autosomal recessive trait. In affected individuals, the CYP2D6-dependent oxidations of debrisoquin and other drugs (see Table 4–2; Figure 4–5) are impaired. These defects in oxidative drug metabolism are probably coinherited. The precise molecular basis for the defect appears to be faulty expression of the P450 protein, resulting in little or no isoform-catalyzed drug metabolism. More recently, however, another polymorphic genotype has been reported that results in ultrarapid metabolism of relevant drugs due to the presence of 2D6 allelic variants with up to 13 gene copies in tandem. This genotype is most common in Ethiopians and Saudi Arabians, populations that display it in up to one third of individuals. As a result, these subjects require twofold to threefold higher daily doses of nortriptyline (a 2D6 substrate) to achieve therapeutic plasma levels. Conversely, in these ultrarapidly metabolizing populations, the prodrug codeine (another 2D6 substrate) is metabolized much faster to morphine, often resulting in undesirable adverse effects of morphine, such as abdominal pain.

A second well-studied genetic drug polymorphism involves the stereoselective **aromatic (4)-hydroxylation** of the anticonvulsant mephenytoin, catalyzed by **CYP2C19**. This polymorphism, which is also inherited as an autosomal recessive trait, occurs in 3–5% of Caucasians and 18–23% of Japanese populations. It is genetically independent of the debrisoquin-sparteine polymorphism. In normal "extensive metabolizers," (S)-mephenytoin is extensively hydroxylated by CYP2C19 at the 4 position of the phenyl ring before its glucuronidation and rapid excretion in the urine, whereas (R)-mephenytoin is slowly N-demethylated to nirvanol, an active metabolite. "Poor metabolizers," however, appear to totally lack the stereospecific (S)-mephenytoin hydroxylase activity, so both (S)- and (R)-mephenytoin enantiomers are N-demethylated to nirvanol, which accumulates in much higher concentrations. Thus, poor metabolizers of mephenytoin show signs of profound sedation and ataxia after doses of the drug that are well tolerated by normal metabolizers. The molecular basis for this defect is a single base pair mutation in exon 5 of the CYP2C19 gene that creates an aberrant splice site, a correspondingly altered reading frame of the mRNA, and, finally, a truncated, nonfunctional protein. It is clinically important to

Figure 4–5. Genetic polymorphism in debrisoquin 4-hydroxylation by CYP2D6 in a Caucasian population. The semilog frequency distribution histogram of the metabolic ratio (MR; defined as percent of dose excreted as unchanged debrisoquin divided by the percent of dose excreted as 4-hydroxydebrisoquin metabolite) in the 8-hour urine collected after oral ingestion of 12.8 mg debrisoquin sulfate (equivalent to 10 mg free debrisoquin base). Individuals with MR values > 12.6 were phenotyped as poor metabolizers (PM, *dark gray bars*), and those with MR values < 12.6 but > 0.2 were designated extensive metabolizers (EM, *light color bars*). Those with MR values < 0.2 were designated as ultrarapid metabolizers (URM, *dark color bars*) based on the MR values (0.01–0.1) of individuals with documented multiple copies of CYP2D6 allelic variants resulting from inherited amplification of this gene. (Data from Woolhouse et al: Debrisoquin hydroxylation polymorphism among Ghanians and Caucasians. Clin Pharmacol Ther 1979;26:584.)

recognize that the safety of a drug may be severely reduced in individuals who are poor metabolizers.

The third recently characterized genetic polymorphism is that of **CYP2C9.** Two well-characterized variants of this enzyme exist, each with amino acid mutations that result in altered metabolism. The **CYP2C9*2** allele encodes an Arg144Cys mutation, exhibiting impaired functional interactions with P450 reductase. The other allelic variant, **CYP2C9*3,** encodes an enzyme with an Ile359Leu mutation that has lowered affinity for many substrates. For example, individuals displaying the CYP2C9*3 phenotype have greatly reduced tolerance for the anticoagulant warfarin. The warfarin clearance in CYP2C9*3-homozygous individuals is about 10% of normal values, and these people have a much lower tolerance for the drug than those who are homozygous for the normal wild-type allele. These individuals also have a much

higher risk of adverse effects with warfarin (eg, bleeding) and with other CYP2C9 substrates such as phenytoin, losartan, tolbutamide, and some NSAIDs.

Allelic variants of CYP3A4 have also been reported but their contribution to its well-known interindividual variability in drug metabolism apparently is limited. On the other hand, the expression of **CYP3A5,** another human liver isoform, is markedly polymorphic, ranging from 0% to 100% of the total hepatic CYP3A content. This CYP3A5 protein polymorphism is now known to result from a single nucleotide polymorphism (SNP) within intron 3, which enables normally spliced CYP3A5 transcripts in 5% of Caucasians, 29% of Japanese, 27% of Chinese, 30% of Koreans, and 73% of African Americans. Thus, it can significantly contribute to interindividual differences in the metabolism of preferential CYP3A5 substrates such as midazolam.

Additional genetic polymorphisms in drug metabolism (eg, CYP2B6) that are inherited independently from those already described are being discovered. Studies of theophylline metabolism in monozygotic and dizygotic twins that included pedigree analysis of various families have revealed that a distinct polymorphism may exist for this drug and may be inherited as a recessive genetic trait. Genetic drug metabolism polymorphisms also appear to occur for aminopyrine and carbocysteine oxidations. Regularly updated information on human P450-polymorphisms is available at www.imm.ki.se/CYPalleles/.

Although genetic polymorphisms in drug oxidations often involve specific P450 enzymes, such genetic variations can also occur in other enzymes. Recent descriptions of a polymorphism in the oxidation of trimethylamine, believed to be metabolized largely by the **flavin monooxygenase (Ziegler's enzyme),** suggest that genetic variants of other non-P450-dependent oxidative enzymes may also contribute to such polymorphisms.

Diet & Environmental Factors

Diet and environmental factors contribute to individual variations in drug metabolism. Charcoal-broiled foods and cruciferous vegetables are known to induce CYP1A enzymes, whereas grapefruit juice is known to inhibit the CYP3A metabolism of coadministered drug substrates (Table 4–2). Cigarette smokers metabolize some drugs more rapidly than nonsmokers because of enzyme induction (see previous section). Industrial workers exposed to some pesticides metabolize certain drugs more rapidly than nonexposed individuals. Such differences make it difficult to determine effective and safe doses of drugs that have narrow therapeutic indices.

Age & Sex

Increased susceptibility to the pharmacologic or toxic activity of drugs has been reported in very young and very old patients compared with young adults (see Chapters 60 and 61). Although this may reflect differences in absorption, distribution, and elimination, differences in drug metabolism also play a role. Slower metabolism could be due to reduced activity of metabolic enzymes or reduced availability of essential endogenous cofactors.

Sex-dependent variations in drug metabolism have been well documented in rats but not in other rodents. Young adult male rats metabolize drugs much faster than mature female rats or prepubertal male rats. These differences in drug metabolism have been clearly associated with androgenic hormones. Clinical reports suggest that similar sex-dependent differences in drug metabolism also exist in humans for ethanol, propranolol, some benzodiazepines, estrogens, and salicylates.

Drug-Drug Interactions during Metabolism

Many substrates, by virtue of their relatively high lipophilicity, are retained not only at the active site of the enzyme but remain nonspecifically bound to the lipid ER membrane. In this state, they may induce microsomal enzymes, particularly after repeated use. Acutely, depending on the residual drug levels at the active site, they also may competitively inhibit metabolism of a simultaneously administered drug.

Enzyme-inducing drugs include various sedative-hypnotics, antipsychotics, anticonvulsants, the antitubercular drug rifampin, and insecticides (Table 4–5). Patients who routinely ingest barbiturates, other sedative-hypnotics, or certain antipsychotic drugs may require considerably higher doses of warfarin to maintain a therapeutic effect. On the other hand, discontinuance of the sedative inducer may result in reduced metabolism of the anticoagulant and bleeding—a toxic effect of the ensuing enhanced plasma levels of the anticoagulant. Similar interactions have been observed in individuals receiving various combinations of drug regimens such as rifampin, antipsychotics, or sedatives with contraceptive agents, sedatives with anticonvulsant drugs, and even alcohol with hypoglycemic drugs (tolbutamide).

It must also be noted that an inducer may enhance not only the metabolism of other drugs but also its own metabolism. Thus, continued use of some drugs may result in a pharmacokinetic type of **tolerance**—progressively reduced therapeutic effectiveness due to enhancement of their own metabolism.

Conversely, simultaneous administration of two or more drugs may result in impaired elimination of the more slowly metabolized drug and prolongation or potentiation of its pharmacologic effects (Table 4–6). Both competitive substrate inhibition and irreversible substrate-mediated enzyme inactivation may augment plasma drug levels and lead to toxic effects from drugs with narrow therapeutic indices. Indeed, such acute interactions of terfenadine (a second-generation antihistamine) with a CYP3A4 substrate-inhibitor (ketoconazole, erythromycin, or grapefruit

Table 4–5. Partial list of drugs that enhance drug metabolism in humans.

Inducer	Drug Whose Metabolism Is Enhanced
Benzo[a]pyrene	Theophylline
Carbamazepine	Carbamazepine, clonazepam, itraconazole
Chlorcyclizine	Steroid hormones
Ethchlorvynol	Warfarin
Glutethimide	Antipyrine, glutethimide, warfarin
Griseofulvin	Warfarin
Phenobarbital and other barbiturates[1]	Barbiturates, chloramphenicol, chlorpromazine, cortisol, coumarin anticoagulants, desmethylimipramine, digitoxin, doxorubicin, estradiol, itraconazole, phenylbutazone, phenytoin, quinine, testosterone
Phenylbutazone	Aminopyrine, cortisol, digitoxin
Phenytoin	Cortisol, dexamethasone, digitoxin, itraconazole, theophylline
Rifampin	Coumarin anticoagulants, digitoxin, glucocorticoids, itraconazole, methadone, metoprolol, oral contraceptives, prednisone, propranolol, quinidine, saquinavir
Ritonavir[2]	Midazolam
St. John's wort	Alprazolam, cyclosporine, digoxin, indinavir, oral contraceptives, ritonavir, simvastatin, tacrolimus, warfarin

[1]Secobarbital is an exception. See Table 4–6 and text.
[2]With chronic (repeated) administration; acutely, ritonavir is a potent CYP3A4 *inhibitor/inactivator*.

juice) resulted in fatal cardiac arrhythmias (torsade de pointes) requiring its withdrawal from the market. Similar drug-drug interactions with CYP3A4 substrate-inhibitors (such as the antibiotics erythromycin and clarithromycin, the antidepressant nefazodone, the antifungals itraconazole and ketoconazole, and the HIV protease inhibitors indinavir and ritonavir), and consequent cardiotoxicity led to withdrawal or restricted use of the 5-HT₄ agonist, cisapride. Similarly, allopurinol both prolongs the duration and enhances the chemotherapeutic and toxic actions of mercaptopurine by competitive inhibition of xanthine oxidase. Consequently, to avoid bone marrow toxicity, the dose of mercaptopurine must be reduced in patients receiving allopurinol. Cimetidine, a drug used in the treatment of peptic ulcer, has been shown to potentiate the pharmacologic actions of anticoagulants and sedatives. The metabolism of the sedative chlordiazepoxide has been

Table 4–6. Partial list of drugs that inhibit drug metabolism in humans.

Inhibitor[1]	Drug Whose Metabolism Is Inhibited
Allopurinol, chloramphenicol, isoniazid	Antipyrine, dicumarol, probenecid, tolbutamide
Chlorpromazine	Propranolol
Cimetidine	Chlordiazepoxide, diazepam, warfarin, others
Dicumarol	Phenytoin
Diethylpentenamide	Diethylpentenamide
Disulfiram	Antipyrine, ethanol, phenytoin, warfarin
Ethanol	Chlordiazepoxide (?), diazepam (?), methanol
Grapefruit juice[2]	Alprazolam, atorvastatin, cisapride, cyclosporine, midazolam, triazolam
Itraconazole	Alfentanil, alprazolam, astemizole, atorvastin, buspirone, cisapride, cyclosporine, delavirdine, diazepam, digoxin, felodipine, indinavir, loratidine, lovastatin, midazolam, nisoldipine, phenytoin, quinidine, ritonavir, saquinavir, sildenafil, simvastatin, sirolimus, tacrolimus, triazolam, verapamil, warfarin
Ketoconazole	Astemizole, cyclosporine, terfenadine
Nortriptyline	Antipyrine
Oral contraceptives	Antipyrine
Phenylbutazone	Phenytoin, tolbutamide
Ritonavir	Amiodarone, cisapride, itraconazole, midazolam, triazolam
Saquinavir	Cisapride, ergot derivatives, midazolam, triazolam
Secobarbital	Secobarbital
Spironolactone	Digoxin
Troleandomycin	Theophylline, methylprednisolone

[1]While some inhibitors are selective for a given P450 enzyme, others are more general and can inhibit several P450s concurrently.
[2]Active components in grapefruit juice include furanocoumarins such as 6′, 7′-dihydroxybergamottin (which inactivates both intestinal and liver CYP3A4) as well as other unknown components that inhibit P-glycoprotein-mediated intestinal drug efflux and consequently further enhance the bioavailability of certain drugs such as cyclosporine.

shown to be inhibited by 63% after a single dose of cimetidine; such effects are reversed within 48 hours after withdrawal of cimetidine.

Impaired metabolism may also result if a simultaneously administered drug irreversibly inactivates a common metabolizing enzyme. These inhibitors, in the course of their metabolism by cytochrome P450, inactivate the enzyme and result in impairment of their own metabolism and that of other cosubstrates.

Interactions between Drugs & Endogenous Compounds

As noted previously, some drugs require conjugation with endogenous substrates such as glutathione, glucuronic acid, or sulfate for their inactivation. Consequently, different drugs may compete for the same endogenous substrates, and the faster-reacting drug may effectively deplete endogenous substrate levels and impair the metabolism of the slower-reacting drug. If the latter has a steep dose-response curve or a narrow margin of safety, potentiation of its pharmacologic and toxic effects may result.

Diseases Affecting Drug Metabolism

Acute or chronic diseases that affect liver architecture or function markedly affect hepatic metabolism of some drugs. Such conditions include alcoholic hepatitis, active or inactive alcoholic cirrhosis, hemochromatosis, chronic active hepatitis, biliary cirrhosis, and acute viral or drug-induced hepatitis. Depending on their severity, these conditions may significantly impair hepatic drug-metabolizing enzymes, particularly microsomal oxidases, and thereby markedly affect drug elimination. For example, the half-lives of chlordiazepoxide and diazepam in patients with liver cirrhosis or acute viral hepatitis are greatly increased, with a corresponding prolongation of their effects. Consequently, these drugs may cause coma in patients with liver disease when given in ordinary doses.

Some drugs are metabolized so readily that even marked reduction in liver function does not significantly prolong their action. However, cardiac disease, by limiting blood flow to the liver, may impair disposition of those drugs whose metabolism is flow-limited (Table 4–7). These drugs are so readily metabolized by the liver that hepatic clearance is essentially equal to liver blood flow. Pulmonary disease may also affect drug metabolism as indicated by the impaired hydrolysis of procainamide and procaine in patients with chronic respiratory insufficiency and the increased half-life of antipyrine in patients with lung cancer. The impaired enzyme activity or defective formation of enzymes associated with heavy metal poisoning or porphyria also results in reduced hepatic drug metabolism.

Table 4–7. Rapidly metabolized drugs whose hepatic clearance is blood flow-limited.

Alprenolol	Lidocaine
Amitriptyline	Meperidine
Clomethiazole	Morphine
Desipramine	Pentazocine
Imipramine	Propoxyphene
Isoniazid	Propranolol
Labetalol	Verapamil

Although the effects of endocrine dysfunction on drug metabolism have been well explored in experimental animal models, corresponding data for humans with endocrine disorders are scanty. Thyroid dysfunction has been associated with altered metabolism of some drugs and of some endogenous compounds as well. Hypothyroidism increases the half-life of antipyrine, digoxin, methimazole, and some beta blockers, whereas hyperthyroidism has the opposite effect. A few clinical studies in diabetic patients indicate no apparent impairment of drug metabolism, although impairment has been noted in diabetic rats. Malfunctions of the pituitary, adrenal cortex, and gonads markedly reduce hepatic drug metabolism in rats. On the basis of these findings, it may be supposed that such disorders could significantly affect drug metabolism in humans. However, until sufficient evidence is obtained from clinical studies in patients, such extrapolations must be considered tentative.

REFERENCES

Correia MA: Human and rat liver cytochromes P450: Functional markers, diagnostic inhibitor probes and parameters frequently used in P450 studies. In: Ortiz de Montellano P (editor). *Cytochrome P450: Structure, Mechanism and Biochemistry*, 3rd ed. Kluwer-Academic/Plenum Press, 2005.

Correia MA, Ortiz de Montellano P: Inhibitors of cytochrome P-450 and possibilities for their therapeutic application. In: Ruckpaul K (editor): *Frontiers in Biotransformation*, vol 8. Taylor & Francis, 1993.

Correia MA, Ortiz de Montellano P: Inhibition of cytochrome P450 enzymes. In: Ortiz de Montellano P (editor). *Cytochrome P450: Structure, Mechanism and Biochemistry*, 3rd ed. Kluwer-Academic/Plenum Press, 2005.

Gonzalez F: The molecular biology of cytochrome P450s. Pharmacol Rev 1989;40:243.

Guengerich FP: Human cytochrome P450 enzymes. In: Ortiz de Montellano P (editor). *Cytochrome P450: Structure, Mechanism and Biochemistry*, 3rd ed. Kluwer-Academic/Plenum Press, 2005.

Guengerich FP: Role of cytochrome P450 enzymes in drug-drug interactions. Adv Pharmacol 1997;43:7.

Hustert E et al: The genetic determinants of the CYP3A5 polymorphism. Pharmacogenetics 2001;11:773.

Ingelman-Sundberg M: Pharmacogenetics: An opportunity for a safer and more efficient pharmacotherapy. J Intern Med 2001;250:186.

Kroemer HK, Klotz U: Glucuronidation of drugs: A reevaluation of the pharmacological significance of the conjugates and modulating factors. Clin Pharmacokinet 1992;23:292.

Meyer UA: Pharmacogenetics and adverse drug reactions. Lancet 2000;356:1667.

Nelson DR et al: The P450 superfamily: Update on new sequences, gene mapping, accession numbers, and nomenclature. Pharmacogenetics 1996;6:1.

Nelson DR et al: Updated human P450 sequences available at http://drnelson.utmem.edu/human.P450.seqs.html.

Sueyoshi T, Negishi M: Phenobarbital response elements of cytochrome P450 genes and nuclear receptors. Annu Rev Pharmacol Toxicol 2001;41:123.

Thummel KE, Wilkinson GR: In vitro and in vivo drug interactions involving human CYP3A. Annu Rev Pharmacol Toxicol 1998;38:389.

Willson TM, Kliewer SA: PXR, CAR and drug metabolism. Nat Rev Drug Discov 2002;1:259.

Xu C et al: CYP2A6 genetic variation and potential consequences. Adv Drug Delivery Rev 2002;54:1245.

Development & Regulation of Drugs

5

Barry A. Berkowitz, PhD

New drugs have revolutionized the practice of medicine, converting many once fatal or debilitating diseases into manageable therapeutic exercises. For example, deaths from cardiovascular disease, the main cause of death in the USA, and from stroke have decreased by more than 50% in the USA over the past 30 years. This decline is due—in part—to the discovery and increased use of antihypertensives, cholesterol synthesis inhibitors, drugs that prevent or dissolve blood clots, medical devices, and drug-releasing stents.

Among the first steps in the development of a new drug is the discovery or synthesis of a potential new drug molecule and seeking an understanding of its interaction (mechanism) with the appropriate biologic targets. Repeated application of this approach leads to compounds with increased potency and selectivity (Figure 5–1). By law, the safety and efficacy of drugs must be defined before marketing. In addition to in vitro studies, relevant biologic effects, drug metabolism, and pharmacokinetic profiles and particularly an assessment of the relative safety of the drug must be characterized in animals before human drug trials can be started. With regulatory approval, human testing can then go forward in three phases before the drug can be considered for approval for general use. A fourth phase of data gathering and safety monitoring is becoming increasingly important and follows after approval for general use.

Enormous and increasing costs, with estimates from $150 million to $900 million, are involved in the research and development of a single new drug that reaches the marketplace. Only 3 of 10 marketed drugs return their research and development (R&D) investments, thus providing considerable motivation to develop "blockbusters." Thousands of compounds may be synthesized and hundreds of thousands tested from libraries of compounds for each successful new drug lead, which then generally needs to be further optimized for reasons of potency, selectivity, drug metabolism, and dosing convenience before each drug reaches the market. Because of the economic investment required and the need to efficiently access multiple technologies, most new drugs are developed in pharmaceutical companies.

At the same time, the incentives to succeed in drug development can be equally enormous. The global market for pharmaceuticals in 2006 is estimated at about $640 billion. The 2004 sales of the top-selling drug worldwide (Lipitor) exceeded $10 billion. During the second half of the 20th century, estimates indicate that medications produced by the pharmaceutical industry saved more than 1.5 million lives and $140 billion in the costs of treatment for tuberculosis, poliomyelitis, coronary artery disease, and cerebrovascular disease alone. New drugs played a key role in the post-1995 decline in HIV mortality and the social returns for HIV drug innovation appear to be extremely large. In the USA, approximately 10% of the health care dollar is presently spent on prescription drugs.

DRUG DISCOVERY

Most new drugs or drug products are discovered or developed through one or more of six approaches:

1. Identification or elucidation of a new drug target
2. Rational drug design of a new drug based on an understanding of biologic mechanisms, drug receptor structure, and drug structure
3. Chemical modification of a known molecule
4. Screening for biologic activity of large numbers of natural products, banks of previously discovered chemical entities, and large libraries of peptides, nucleic acids, and other organic molecules
5. Biotechnology and cloning using genes to produce peptides and proteins. Efforts continue to focus on the discovery of new targets and approaches, from studies with genomics, proteomics, nucleic acids and molecular pharmacology for drug therapy. Significantly increasing the number of useful disease targets should be a positive driver for new and improved drugs.
6. Combinations of known drugs to obtain additive or synergistic effects or a repositioning of a known drug for a new therapeutic use.

In vitro studies	Animal testing	Clinical testing		Marketing

Figure 5–1. The development and testing process required to bring a drug to market in the USA. Some of the requirements may be different for drugs used in life-threatening diseases.

Drug Screening

Regardless of the source or the key idea leading to a drug candidate molecule, testing it involves a sequence of iterative experimentation and characterization called **drug screening.** A variety of biologic assays at the molecular, cellular, organ system, and whole animal levels are used to define the activity and selectivity of the drug (Table 5–1). The type and number of initial screening tests depend on the pharmacologic and therapeutic goal. Anti-infective drugs may be tested against a variety of infectious organisms some of which are resistant to standard agents, hypoglycemic drugs for their ability to lower blood sugar, etc. In addition, the molecule will also be studied for a broad array of other actions to establish the mechanism of action and selectivity of the drug. This has the advantage of demonstrating both suspected and unsuspected toxic effects. Occasionally, an unsuspected therapeutic action is serendipitously discovered by the careful observer. The selection of molecules for further study is most efficiently conducted in animal models of human disease. Where good predictive preclinical models exist (eg, antibacterials, hypertension or thrombotic disease), we generally have adequate drugs. Good drugs or breakthough improvements are conspicuously lacking and slow for diseases for which pre-clinical models are poor, or not yet available, eg, Alzheimer's disease.

Studies are performed during drug screening to define the **pharmacologic profile** of the drug at the molecular, cellular, system, organ, and organism levels. For example, a broad range of tests would be performed on a drug designed to act as an antagonist at vascular α-adrenoceptors for the treatment of hypertension.

At the molecular level, the compound would be screened for receptor binding affinity to cell membranes containing α receptors (if possible on human receptors), other receptors, and binding sites on enzymes. If crystal structures of the drug and target are available, structural biology analyses or computer-assisted virtual screening might be done to better understand the drug receptor interaction. Early studies would be done to predict effects that might later cause undesired drug metabolism or toxicologic complications. For example, studies on liver cytochrome P450 enzymes would be performed to determine whether the drug of interest is likely to be a substrate or inhibitor of these enzymes or to interfere with the metabolism of other drugs. Effects on cardiac ion channels such as the hERG potassium channel, possibly predictive of life threatening arrhythmias, would be considered.

Effects on cell function would be studied to determine whether the drug is an agonist, partial agonist, or antagonist at α receptors. Isolated tissues, especially vascular smooth muscle, would be utilized to characterize the pharmacologic activity and selectivity of the new

Table 5–1. Pharmacologic profile tests.

Experimental Method or Target Organ	Species or Tissue	Measurement
Molecular		
Receptor binding (example: β-adrenoceptors)	Cell membrane fractions from organs or cultured cells; cloned receptors	Receptor affinity and selectivity
Enzyme activity (examples: tyrosine hydroxylase, dopamine-3-hydroxy-lase, monoamine oxidase)	Sympathetic nerves; adrenal glands; purified enzymes	Enzyme inhibition and selectivity
Cytochrome P450	Liver	Enzyme inhibition; effects on drug metabolism
Cellular		
Cell function	Cultured cells	Evidence for receptor activity—agonism or antagonism (example: effects on cyclic nucleotides)
Isolated tissue	Blood vessels, heart, lung, ileum (rat or guinea pig)	Effects on vascular contraction and relaxation; selectivity for vascular receptors; effects on other smooth muscles
Systems/disease models		
Blood pressure	Dog, cat (anesthetized)	Systolic-diastolic changes
	Rat, hypertensive (conscious)	Antihypertensive effects
Cardiac effects	Dog (conscious)	Electrocardiography
	Dog (anesthetized)	Inotropic, chronotropic effects, cardiac output, total peripheral resistance
Peripheral autonomic nervous system	Dog (anesthetized)	Effects on response to known drugs and electrical stimulation of central and peripheral autonomic nerves
Respiratory effects	Dog, guinea pig	Effects on respiratory rate and amplitude, bronchial tone
Diuretic activity	Dog	Natriuresis, kaliuresis, water diuresis, renal blood flow, glomerular filtration rate
Gastrointestinal effects	Rat	Gastrointestinal motility and secretions
Circulating hormones, cholesterol, blood sugar	Rat, dog	Serum concentration
Blood coagulation	Rabbit	Coagulation time, clot retraction, prothrombin time
Central nervous system	Mouse, rat	Degree of sedation, muscle relaxation, locomotor activity, stimulation

compound in comparison with reference compounds. Comparison with other drugs would also be undertaken in other in vitro preparations such as gastrointestinal and bronchial smooth muscle. At each step in this process, the compound would have to meet specific performance criteria to be carried further.

Whole animal studies are generally necessary to determine the effect of the drug on organ systems and disease models. Cardiovascular and renal function studies of all new drugs are generally first performed in normal animals. Where appropriate, studies on disease models would be performed. For a candidate antihypertensive drug, animals with hypertension would be treated to see if blood pressure was lowered in a dose-related manner and to characterize other effects of the compound. Evidence would be collected on duration of action and efficacy following oral and parenteral administration. If the agent possessed useful activity, it would be further studied for possible adverse effects on other major organ systems, including the respiratory, gastrointestinal, endocrine, and central nervous systems.

These studies might suggest the need for further chemical modification to achieve more desirable pharmacokinetic or pharmacodynamic properties. For example, oral administration studies might show that the drug was poorly absorbed or rapidly metabolized in the liver; modification to improve bioavailability might be indicated. If the drug was to be administered long-term, an assessment of tolerance development would be made. For drugs related to or having mechanisms of action similar to those known to cause physical dependence, abuse potential would also be studied. For each major action found, a pharmacologic mechanism would be sought.

The desired result of this screening procedure (which may have to be repeated several times with analogs or congeners of the original molecules) is called a **lead compound,** ie, a leading candidate for a successful new drug. A patent application would generally be filed for a novel compound (a composition of matter patent) that is efficacious, or for a new and nonobvious therapeutic use (a use patent) for a previously known chemical entity.

PRECLINICAL SAFETY & TOXICITY TESTING

All drugs are toxic at some dose. Seeking to correctly define the limiting toxicities of drugs and the therapeutic index comparing benefits and risks of a new drug might be argued as the most essential part of the new drug development process. Most drug candidates fail to reach the market, but the art of drug discovery and development is the effective assessment and management of risk and not total risk avoidance.

Candidate drugs that survive the initial screening and profiling procedures must be carefully evaluated for potential risks before and during clinical testing. Depending on the proposed use of the drug, preclinical toxicity testing includes most or all of the procedures shown in Table 5–2. Although no chemical can be certified as completely "safe" (free of risk), the objective is to estimate the risk associated with exposure to the drug candidate and to consider this in the context of therapeutic needs and duration of likely drug use.

The goals of preclinical toxicity studies include identifying potential human toxicities; designing tests to further define the toxic mechanisms; and predicting

Table 5–2. Safety tests.

Type of Test	Approach
Acute toxicity	Acute dose that is lethal in approximately 50% of animals and the maximum tolerated dose. Usually two species, two routes, single dose.
Subacute toxicity	Three doses, two species. 4 weeks to 3 months may be necessary prior to clinical trial. The longer the duration of expected clinical use, the longer the subacute test.
Chronic toxicity	Rodent and non-rodent species. 6 months or longer. Required when drug is intended to be used in humans for prolonged periods. Usually run concurrently with clinical trial.
Effect on reproductive performance	Effects on animal mating behavior, reproduction, parturition, progeny, birth defects, postnatal development.
Carcinogenic potential	Two years, two species. Required when drug is intended to be used in humans for prolonged periods.
Mutagenic potential	Effects on genetic stability and mutations in bacteria (Ames test) or mammalian cells in culture; dominant lethal test and clastogenicity in mice.
Investigative toxicology	Determine sequence and mechanisms of toxic action. Discover the genes, proteins, pathways involved. Develop new methods for assessing toxicity.

the specific and the most relevant toxicities to be monitored in clinical trials. In addition to the studies shown in Tables 5–1 and 5–2, several quantitative estimates are desirable. These include the **"no-effect" dose**—the maximum dose at which a specified toxic effect is not seen; the **minimum lethal dose**—the smallest dose that is observed to kill any experimental animal; and, if necessary, the **median lethal dose (LD_{50})**—the dose that kills approximately 50% of the animals. Presently, the LD_{50} is estimated from the smallest number of animals possible. These doses are used to calculate the initial dose to be tried in humans, usually taken as one hundredth to one tenth of the no-effect dose in animals.

It is important to recognize the limitations of preclinical testing. These include the following:

1. Toxicity testing is time-consuming and expensive. Two to 6 years may be required to collect and analyze data on toxicity and estimates of therapeutic

index (a comparison of the amount that causes the desired therapeutic effect to the amount that causes toxic effects, see Chapter 2) before the drug can be considered ready for testing in humans.

2. Large numbers of animals may be needed to obtain valid preclinical data. Scientists are properly concerned about this situation, and progress has been made toward reducing the numbers required while still obtaining valid data. Cell and tissue culture in vitro methods are increasingly being used, but their predictive value is still severely limited. Nevertheless, some segments of the public attempt to halt all animal testing in the unfounded belief that it has become unnecessary.

3. Extrapolations of therapeutic index and toxicity data from animals to humans are reasonably predictive for many but not for all toxicities. Seeking an improved process, a Predictive Safety Testing Consortium of five of America's largest pharmaceutical companies with an advisory role by the Food and Drug Administration (FDA) has been formed to share internally developed laboratory methods to predict the safety of new treatments before they are tested in humans.

4. For statistical reasons, rare adverse effects are unlikely to be detected.

EVALUATION IN HUMANS

Less than one third of the drugs tested in clinical trials reach the marketplace. Federal law in the USA and ethical considerations require that the study of new drugs in humans be conducted in accordance with stringent guidelines. Scientifically valid results are not guaranteed simply by conforming to government regulations, however, and the design and execution of a good clinical trial require interdisciplinary personnel including basic scientists, clinical pharmacologists, clinician specialists, statisticians, and frequently others. The need for careful design and execution is based on three major confounding factors inherent in the study of any drug in humans.

Confounding Factors in Clinical Trials

A. THE VARIABLE NATURAL HISTORY OF MOST DISEASES

Many diseases tend to wax and wane in severity; some disappear spontaneously, even, on occasion, malignant neoplasms. A good experimental design takes into account the natural history of the disease by evaluating a large enough population of subjects over a sufficient period of time. Further protection against errors of interpretation caused by disease fluctuations is provided by using a crossover design, which consists of alternating periods of administration of test drug, placebo preparation (the control), and the standard treatment (positive control), if any, in each subject. These sequences are systematically varied, so that different subsets of patients receive each of the possible sequences of treatment.

B. THE PRESENCE OF OTHER DISEASES AND RISK FACTORS

Known and unknown diseases and risk factors (including lifestyles of subjects) may influence the results of a clinical study. For example, some diseases alter the pharmacokinetics of drugs (see Chapters 3 and 4). Concentrations of a blood or tissue component being monitored as a measure of the effect of the new agent may be influenced by other diseases or other drugs. Attempts to avoid this hazard usually involve the crossover technique (when feasible) and proper selection and assignment of patients to each of the study groups. This requires obtaining accurate medical and pharmacologic histories (including use of recreational drugs) and the use of statistically valid methods of randomization in assigning subjects to particular study groups.

C. SUBJECT AND OBSERVER BIAS

Most patients tend to respond in a positive way to any therapeutic intervention by interested, caring, and enthusiastic medical personnel. The manifestation of this phenomenon in the subject is the **placebo response** (Latin, "I shall please") and may involve objective physiologic and biochemical changes as well as changes in subjective complaints associated with the disease. The placebo response is usually quantitated by administration of an inert material, with exactly the same physical appearance, odor, consistency, etc, as the active dosage form. The magnitude of the response varies considerably from patient to patient and may also be influenced by the duration of the study. Placebo adverse effects and "toxicity" also occur but usually involve subjective effects: stomach upset, insomnia, sedation, etc.

Subject bias effects can be quantitated—and minimized relative to the response measured during active therapy—by the single-blind design. This involves use of a placebo as described above, administered to the same subjects in a crossover design, if possible, or to a separate control group of subjects. Observer bias can be taken into account by disguising the identity of the medication being used—placebo or active form—from both the subjects and the personnel evaluating the subjects' responses (double-blind design). In this design, a third party holds the code identifying each medication packet, and the code is not broken until all of the clinical data have been collected.

The Food & Drug Administration (FDA)

It is the responsibility of those seeking to market a drug to test it and submit evidence on its relative safety and effectiveness. The FDA is the administrative body that oversees the drug evaluation process in the USA and grants approval for marketing of new drug products.

Outside the USA, the regulatory and drug approval for marketing process is generally similar to that in the USA. For example, the European Agency for the Evaluation of Medical Products (EMEA) is responsible for biologicals and optional for synthetic drugs. In Japan, the marketing and manufacture of drugs is regulated by the Ministry of Health, Labor and Welfare (MHLW) and advised by the Central Pharmaceutical Affairs Council (CPAC), which evaluates scientific data.

The FDA's authority to regulate drugs derives from specific legislation (Table 5–3). If a drug has not been shown through adequately controlled testing to be "safe and effective" for a specific use, it cannot be marketed in interstate commerce for this use.*

Unfortunately, "safe" can mean different things to the patient, the physician, and society. As noted above, complete absence of risk is impossible to demonstrate, but this fact is not well understood by the average member of the public, who frequently assume that any medication sold with the approval of the FDA should indeed be free of serious "side effects." This confusion is a major factor in litigation and dissatisfaction with aspects of drugs and medical care.

The history of drug regulation reflects several medical and public health events that precipitated major shifts in public opinion. The Pure Food and Drug Act of 1906 (Table 5–3) became law mostly in response to revelations of unsanitary and unethical practices in the meat-packing industry. The Federal Food, Drug, and Cosmetic Act of 1938 was largely a reaction to deaths associated with the use of a preparation of sulfanilamide marketed before it and its vehicle were adequately tested. Thalidomide is another example of a drug that altered drug testing methods and stimulated drug regulating legislation. This agent was introduced in Europe in 1957–1958 and, based on animal tests then commonly used, was marketed as a "nontoxic" hypnotic and for morning sickness treatment during pregnancy. In 1961, reports were published suggesting that thalidomide was responsible for a dramatic increase in the incidence of a rare birth defect called phocomelia, a condition involving shortening or complete absence of the limbs. Epidemiologic studies provided strong evidence for the association of this defect with thalidomide use by women during the first trimester of preg-

nancy, and the drug was withdrawn from sale worldwide. An estimated 10,000 children were born with birth defects because of maternal exposure to this one agent. The tragedy led to the requirement for more extensive testing of new drugs for teratogenic effects and played an important role in stimulating passage of the Kefauver-Harris Amendments of 1962, even though the drug was not then approved for use in the USA. In spite of its disastrous fetal toxicity and effects in pregnancy, thalidomide is a relatively safe drug for humans other than the fetus. Even the most serious risk of toxicities may be avoided or managed if understood, and despite its toxicity thalidomide is now allowed by the FDA for limited use as a potent immunoregulatory agent and to treat certain forms of leprosy.

It is impossible to certify that a drug is absolutely safe, ie, free of all risk. It is possible, however, to identify most of the hazards likely to be associated with use of a new drug and to place some statistical limits on frequency of occurrence of such events in the population under study. As a result, an operational and pragmatic definition of "safety" can usually be reached that is based on the nature and incidence of drug-associated hazards compared with the hazard of nontherapy of the target disease.

Clinical Trials: The IND & NDA

Once a drug is judged ready to be studied in humans, a **Notice of Claimed Investigational Exemption for a New Drug (IND)** must be filed with the FDA (Figure 5–1). The IND includes (1) information on the composition and source of the drug, (2) chemical and manufacturing information, (3) all data from animal studies, (4) proposed clinical plans and protocols, (5) the names and credentials of physicians who will conduct the clinical trials, and (6) a compilation of the key data relevant to study the drug in man made available to investigators and their institutional review boards.

It often requires 4–6 years of clinical testing to accumulate and analyze all required data. Testing in humans is begun after sufficient acute and subacute animal toxicity studies have been completed. Chronic safety testing in animals, including carcinogenicity studies, is usually done concurrently with clinical trials. In each of the three formal phases of clinical trials, volunteers or patients must be informed of the investigational status of the drug as well as the possible risks and must be allowed to decline or to consent to participate and receive the drug. These regulations are based on the ethical principles set forth in the Declaration of Helsinki. In addition to the approval of the sponsoring organization and the FDA, an interdisciplinary institutional review board (IRB) at the facility

---

*Although the FDA does not directly control drug commerce within states, a variety of state and federal laws control interstate production and marketing of drugs.

Table 5–3. Major legislation pertaining to drugs in the United States.

Law	Purpose and Effect
Pure Food and Drug Act of 1906	Prohibited mislabeling and adulteration of drugs.
Opium Exclusion Act of 1909	Prohibited importation of opium.
Amendment (1912) to the Pure Food and Drug Act	Prohibited false or fraudulent advertising claims.
Harrison Narcotic Act of 1914	Established regulations for use of opium, opiates, and cocaine (marijuana added in 1937).
Food, Drug, and Cosmetic Act of 1938	Required that new drugs be safe as well as pure (but did not require proof of efficacy). Enforcement by FDA.
Durham-Humphrey Act of 1952	Vested in the FDA the power to determine which products could be sold without prescription.
Kefauver-Harris Amendments (1962) to the Food, Drug, and Cosmetic Act	Required proof of efficacy as well as safety for new drugs and for drugs released since 1938; established guidelines for reporting of information about adverse reactions, clinical testing, and advertising of new drugs.
Comprehensive Drug Abuse Prevention and Control Act (1970)	Outlined strict controls in the manufacture, distribution, and prescribing of habit-forming drugs; established programs to prevent and treat drug addiction.
Orphan Drug Amendments of 1983	Amended Food, Drug, and Cosmetic Act of 1938, providing incentives for development of drugs that treat diseases with less than 200,000 patients in USA.
Drug Price Competition and Patent Restoration Act of 1984	Abbreviated new drug applications for generic drugs. Required bioequivalence data. Patent life extended by amount of time drug delayed by FDA review process. Cannot exceed 5 extra years or extend to more than 14 years post-NDA approval.
Expedited Drug Approval Act (1992)	Allowed accelerated FDA approval for drugs of high medical need. Required detailed postmarketing patient surveillance.
Prescription Drug User Fee Act (1992) Reauthorized 1997 and 2002	Manufacturers pay user fees for certain new drug applications. FDA review time for new chemical entities dropped from 30 months in 1992 to 20 months in 1994.
Dietary Supplement Health and Education Act (1994)	Amended the Federal Food, Drug, and Cosmetic Act of 1938 to establish standards with respect to dietary supplements. Required the establishment of specific ingredient and nutrition information labeling that defines dietary supplements and classifies them as part of the food supply.
Bioterrorism Act of 2002	Enhanced controls on dangerous biologic agents and toxins. Seeks to protect safety of food, water, and drug supply.

where the clinical drug trial will be conducted must review and approve the plans and ethics for testing in humans.

In **phase 1,** the effects of the drug as a function of dosage are established in a small number (25–50) of healthy volunteers. Although a goal is to find the maximum tolerated dose, the study is designed to avoid severe toxicity. If the drug is *expected* to have significant toxicity, as is often the case in cancer and AIDS ther-

apy, volunteer patients with the disease are used in phase 1 rather than normal volunteers. Phase 1 trials are done to determine whether humans and animals show significantly different responses to the drug and to establish the probable limits of the safe clinical dosage range. These trials are nonblind or "open"; that is, both the investigators and the subjects know what is being given. Many predictable toxicities are detected in this phase. Pharmacokinetic measurements of absorption, half-life, and metabolism are often done in phase 1. Phase 1 studies are usually performed in research centers by specially trained clinical pharmacologists.

In **phase 2,** the drug is studied in patients with the target disease to determine its efficacy. A modest number of patients (100–200) are studied in detail. A single-blind design is often used, with an inert placebo medication and an established active drug (positive control) in addition to the investigational agent. Phase 2 trials are usually done in special clinical centers (eg, university hospitals). A broader range of toxicities may be detected in this phase.

In **phase 3,** the drug is evaluated in much larger numbers of patients with the target disease—sometimes thousands—to further establish safety and efficacy. Using information gathered in phases 1 and 2, phase 3 trials are designed to minimize errors caused by placebo effects, variable course of the disease, etc. Therefore, double-blind and crossover techniques are frequently used. Phase 3 trials are usually performed in settings similar to those anticipated for the ultimate use of the drug. Phase 3 studies can be difficult to design and execute and are usually expensive because of the large numbers of patients involved and the masses of data that must be collected and analyzed. The investigators are usually specialists in the disease being treated. Certain toxic effects, especially those caused by immunologic processes, may first become apparent in phase 3.

If phase 3 results meet expectations, application is made for permission to market the new agent. Marketing approval requires submission of a **New Drug Application (NDA)** to the FDA. The application contains, often in hundreds of volumes, full reports of all preclinical and clinical data pertaining to the drug under review. The number of subjects studied in support of the NDA has been increasing and currently averages more than 5000 patients for new drugs of novel structure (new molecular entities). The duration of the FDA review leading to approval (or denial) of the NDA may vary from months to years. Priority approvals are designated for products that represent significant improvements compared with marketed products; in 2004, the median priority approval time was 6 months. Standard approvals, which take longer, are designated for products judged similar to those on the market—in 2004, the median standard approval time was 12.9 months. In cases in which an urgent need is perceived (eg, cancer chemotherapy), the process of preclinical and clinical testing and FDA review may be accelerated. For serious diseases, the FDA may permit extensive but controlled marketing of a new drug before phase 3 studies are completed; for life-threatening diseases, it may permit controlled marketing even before phase 2 studies have been completed.

Once approval to market a drug has been obtained, **phase 4** begins. This constitutes monitoring the safety of the new drug under actual conditions of use in large numbers of patients. The importance of careful and complete reporting of toxicity by physicians after marketing begins can be appreciated by noting that many important drug-induced effects have an incidence of 1 in 10,000 or less and that some side effects may become more apparent after chronic dosing. The sample size required to disclose drug-induced events or toxicities is very large for such rare events. For example, several hundred thousand patients may have to be exposed before the first case is observed of a toxicity that occurs with an average incidence of 1 in 10,000 (see Box: Case Study: Aspirin to COX-2 Inhibitors—From Discovery to Recall). Therefore, low-incidence drug effects are not generally detected before phase 4 no matter how carefully the studies are executed. Phase 4 has no fixed duration.

The time from the filing of a patent application to approval for marketing of a new drug may be 5 years or considerably longer. Since the lifetime of a patent is 20 years in the USA, the owner of the patent (usually a pharmaceutical company) has exclusive rights for marketing the product for only a limited time after approval of the NDA. Because the FDA review process can be lengthy, the time consumed by the review is sometimes added to the patent life. However, the extension (up to 5 years) cannot increase the total life of the patent to more than 14 years after NDA approval. After expiration of the patent, any company may produce the drug, file an ANDA (abbreviated NDA), demonstrate required equivalence, and, with FDA approval, market the drug as a **generic** product without paying license fees to the original patent owner. However, a trademark (the drug's proprietary trade name) may be legally protected indefinitely. Therefore, pharmaceutical companies are motivated to give their new drugs easily remembered trade names. Generic prescribing is described in Chapter 66.

The FDA drug approval process is one of the rate-limiting factors in the time it takes for a drug to be marketed and to reach patients. The Prescription Drug User Fee Act (PDUFA) of 1992, reauthorized in 1997 and 2002, attempts to make more FDA resources available to the drug approval process and increase efficiency through use of fees collected from the drug companies that produce certain human drugs and biologic products. Current PDUFA fees for a new chemical entity are about $1 million.

Orphan Drugs & Treatment of Rare Diseases

Drugs for rare diseases—so-called orphan drugs—can be difficult to research, develop, and market. Proof of drug safety and efficacy in small populations must be established, but doing so is a complex process. For example, for ethical and legal reasons, clinical testing of drugs in children is severely restricted, but a number of rare diseases affect the very young. Furthermore, because basic research in the pathophysiology and mechanisms of rare diseases receives relatively little attention or funding in both academic and industrial settings, recognized rational targets for drug action may be few. In addition, the cost of developing a drug can greatly influence priorities when the target population is relatively small.

The Orphan Drug Act of 1983, which amended the 1938 Federal Food, Drug, and Cosmetic Act, provides incentives for the development of drugs for treatment of a rare disease or condition defined as "any disease or condition which (a) affects less than 200,000 persons in the U.S. or (b) affects more than 200,000 persons in the U.S. but for which there is no reasonable expectation that the cost of developing and making available in the U.S. a drug for such disease or condition will be recovered from sales in the U.S. of such drug." Since 1983, the FDA has approved for marketing 268 orphan drugs to treat more than 82 rare diseases.

CASE STUDY: ASPIRIN TO COX-2 INHIBITORS—FROM DISCOVERY TO RECALL*

The idea. The pain-relieving and fever-reducing effects of willow bark and its extracts have been known for millennia; its main active component, salicin, was identified in 1828. The synthesis of the salicin derivative, aspirin (acetylsalicylic acid) in 1897 and recognition of its anti-inflammatory effect constituted a landmark event. Determining how aspirin worked and might be improved would take another 70 years.

The clinical need. Aspirin has broad therapeutic actions. However, it also has significant adverse effects including stomach pain and gastrointestinal (GI) bleeding. Corticosteroids are too toxic for chronic use. The need and opportunity for improved nonsteroidal anti-inflammatory drugs (NSAIDs) became confluent with improved understanding of mediators of inflammation, especially prostaglandins (PGs) as drug targets. From the 1950s through the 1980s, many NSAIDs were developed that were more potent than aspirin but had similar toxicities, especially GI adverse effects.

The biologic hypothesis. Vane and his colleagues demonstrated that aspirin had a key role in inhibiting PG synthesis. Needleman and others found that the enzyme cyclooxygenase (COX) involved in the synthesis of specific PGs was increased in inflamed tissue and stimulated by certain cytokines. Needleman provided evidence for an inducible COX (COX-2) that is up-regulated in inflammation, which could be differentiated from the other, constitutive, isoform (COX-1) that maintains the integrity of the lining of the stomach. COX-1 also helps maintain normal platelet and kidney functions. Could COX-2 be a new drug target?

The chemical hypothesis. In 1991, scientists cloned and expressed COX-2. Using both screening and rational drug design, an inhibitor much more selective for COX-2 than for COX-1 was discovered and named celecoxib (Celebrex). Soon thereafter, the COX-2-selective drug rofecoxib (Vioxx) was discovered, followed by a third valdecoxib (Bextra).

Development. Celecoxib was approved in December 1998 for treatment of osteoarthritis and rheumatoid arthritis.

The NDA for rofecoxib was filed in 1998. At about the same time, its manufacturer began two large clinical trials with rofecoxib in an attempt to discover whether the drug also protected against colonic polyps and against Alzheimer's disease. In 1999, the FDA approved the rofecoxib NDA for the relief of osteoarthritis symptoms, management of acute pain, and painful menstruation. About 1 year later, the results of the first large comparison trial became available. These showed the benefits of rofecoxib in protecting the stomach, but also showed a fourfold higher risk of heart attacks compared with a nonselective COX inhibitor. In 2002, the FDA approved changes to the rofecoxib label, including noting cardiovascular risks, GI benefits, and a new use to treat rheumatoid arthritis. In 2004, the second large trial showed twice the risk of heart attacks among patients taking rofecoxib for 18 months compared with those who took placebos. The manufacturer then decided to voluntarily withdraw rofecoxib, ceasing marketing and sales.

Postscript. The discovery, development, and marketing of celecoxib and the recall of rofecoxib (and subsequently valdecoxib) are representative of the opportunities, mistakes, and issues facing health care companies and practitioners. However, it is clear that vigorous phase 4 and follow-up drug surveillance efforts are now an increasingly important aspect of the drug R&D process.

---

*Case studies are illustrative and highly condensed. They present key events, but not necessarily all events, contributions, or contributors are noted.

Adverse Drug Reactions (ADRs)

An adverse reaction to a drug is a harmful or unintended response. ADRs are claimed to be the 4th leading cause of death, exceeding pulmonary disease, AIDS, accidents, and automobile deaths. The FDA has further estimated that 300,000 preventable adverse events occur in hospitals, many as a result of confusing medical information. Some adverse reactions, such as overdose, excessive effects, and drug interactions, may occur in anyone. Adverse reactions occurring only in susceptible patients include intolerance, idiosyncrasy (frequently genetic in origin), and allergy (usually immunologically mediated). During the IND and clinical phase 1–3 trials and before FDA approval, all adverse events (serious, life-threatening, disabling, reasonably drug-related, or unexpected) must be reported. Following FDA approval to market, surveillance, evaluation, and reporting must continue for any adverse events in patients that are related to use of the drug, including overdose, accident, failure of expected action, events occurring from drug withdrawal, and unexpected events not listed in labeling. Events that are both serious and unexpected must be reported to the FDA within 15 days. In January 2006, the FDA announced a new prescription drug information format to improve patient safety by implementing improvements in prescription drug labels and inserts so they are less confusing and more concise with respect to prescribing information aiding both patients and health care professionals.

REFERENCES

Angell M: *The Truth about the Drug Companies.* Random House, 2004.

Avorn J: *Powerful Medicines: The Benefits and Risks and Costs of Prescription Drugs*, Alfred A. Knopf, 2004.

Berkowitz BA, Sachs G: Life cycle of a block buster: Discovery and development of omeprazole (Prilosec™). Mol Interv 2002;2:6.

Brown WA: The placebo effect, Sci Am 1998;1:91.

Cutler DM: *Your Money or Your Life.* Oxford University Press, 2004.

DiMasi JA: Risks in new drug development: Approval success rates for investigational drugs. Clin Pharmacol Ther 2001;69:297.

DiMasi JA: Rising research and development costs for new drugs in a cost containment environment. J Health Econ. 2003;22:151.

FDA web site: http://www.fda.gov

Gingrich N: *Saving Lives and Saving Money: Transforming Health and Healthcare.* The Alexis de Tocqueville Institution, 2003.

Grabowski H, Vernon J, DiMasi J: Returns on research and development for 1990's. Pharmacoeconomics 2002;suppl 3:11.

Guarino RA: New drug approval process. In: *Drugs and The Pharmaceutical Sciences,* vol. 100. Marcel Dekker, 2000.

Hoffman GA, Harrington A, Fields, HK: Pain and the placebo response: What have we learned. Perspect Biol Med 2005; 48:248.

Lee C-J et al: *Clinical Trials of Drugs and Biopharmaceuticals.* CRC Publishing, 2005.

Lichtenberg FR: Availability of new drugs and Americans' ability to work. J Occup Envir Med 2005;47:373.

Lichtenberg FR: The effect of new drug approvals on HIV mortality in the US, 1987–1998. Econ Hum Biol 2003;1:259.

Miller RD, Frech HE: *Health Care Matters.* The AEI Press, 2004.

McKinnell H: *A Call to Action: Taking Back the Healthcare for Future Generations.* McGraw Hill, 2005.

Needleman P, Isakson PC: The discovery and function of COX-2. J Rheumatol 1997;49;Suppl:4.

News feature: Painful lessons: Nature Reviews Drug Discovery— News Analysis 2005;4:800 (1 Oct).

Ng R: *Drugs from Discovery to Approval.* Wiley-Liss, 2004.

Pharmaceutical Research and Manufacturers of America web site: www.phrma.org.

Vane JR: The fight against rheumatism from willow bark to COX1-sparing drugs. J Physiol Pharmacol 2000;51(pt 1):573.

Vane JR, Botting RM: The mechanism of action of aspirin: Thromb Res 2003;110:255.

SECTION II
Autonomic Drugs

Introduction to Autonomic Pharmacology

6

Bertram G. Katzung, MD, PhD

The motor (efferent) portion of the nervous system can be divided into two major subdivisions: **autonomic** and **somatic.** The **autonomic nervous system (ANS)** is largely autonomous (independent) in that its activities are not under direct conscious control. It is concerned primarily with visceral functions such as cardiac output, blood flow to various organs, and digestion, which are necessary for life. The somatic division is largely concerned with consciously controlled functions such as movement, respiration, and posture. Both systems have important afferent (sensory) inputs that provide information regarding the internal and external environments and modify motor output through reflex arcs of varying size and complexity.

The nervous system has several properties in common with the endocrine system, which is the other major system for control of body function. These include high-level integration in the brain, the ability to influence processes in distant regions of the body, and extensive use of negative feedback. Both systems use chemicals for the transmission of information. In the nervous system, chemical transmission occurs between nerve cells and their effector cells. Chemical transmission takes place through the release of small amounts of transmitter substances from the nerve terminals into the synaptic cleft. The transmitter crosses the cleft by diffusion and activates or inhibits the postsynaptic cell by binding to a specialized receptor molecule.

By using drugs that mimic or block the actions of chemical transmitters, we can selectively modify many autonomic functions. These functions involve a variety of effector tissues, including cardiac muscle, smooth muscle, vascular endothelium, exocrine glands, and presynaptic nerve terminals. Autonomic drugs are useful in many clinical conditions. However, a very large number of drugs used for other purposes have unwanted effects on autonomic function.

ANATOMY OF THE AUTONOMIC NERVOUS SYSTEM

The autonomic nervous system lends itself to division on anatomic grounds into two major portions: the **sympathetic (thoracolumbar)** division and the **parasympathetic (craniosacral)** division (Figure 6–1). Both divisions originate in nuclei within the central nervous system and give rise to preganglionic efferent fibers that exit from the brain stem or spinal cord and terminate in motor ganglia. The sympathetic preganglionic fibers leave the central nervous system through the thoracic and lumbar spinal nerves. The parasympathetic preganglionic fibers leave the central nervous system through the cranial nerves (especially the third, seventh, ninth, and tenth) and the third and fourth sacral spinal roots.

Most of the sympathetic preganglionic fibers terminate in ganglia located in the paravertebral chains that lie on either side of the spinal column. The remaining sympathetic preganglionic fibers terminate in prevertebral ganglia, which lie in front of the vertebrae, usually on the surface of the aorta. From the ganglia, postganglionic sympathetic fibers run to the tissues innervated. Some preganglionic parasympathetic fibers terminate in para-

Figure 6–1. Schematic diagram comparing some anatomic and neurotransmitter features of autonomic and somatic motor nerves. Only the primary transmitter substances are shown. Parasympathetic ganglia are not shown because most are in or near the wall of the organ innervated. Cholinergic nerves are shown in color. Note that some sympathetic postganglionic fibers release acetylcholine or dopamine rather than norepinephrine. The adrenal medulla, a modified sympathetic ganglion, receives sympathetic preganglionic fibers and releases epinephrine and norepinephrine into the blood. (ACh, acetylcholine; D, dopamine; Epi, epinephrine; NE, norepinephrine; N, nicotinic receptors; M, muscarinic receptors.)

sympathetic ganglia located outside the organs innervated: the ciliary, pterygopalatine, submandibular, otic, and several pelvic ganglia. The majority of parasympathetic preganglionic fibers terminate on ganglion cells distributed diffusely or in networks in the walls of the innervated organs. Note that the terms "sympathetic" and "parasympathetic" are anatomic designations and do not depend on the type of transmitter chemical released from the nerve endings nor on the kind of effect—excitatory or inhibitory—evoked by nerve activity.

In addition to these clearly defined peripheral motor portions of the ANS, large numbers of afferent fibers run from the periphery to integrating centers, including the enteric plexuses in the gut, the autonomic ganglia, and the central nervous system. Many of the sensory neurons that end in the central nervous system terminate in the integrating centers of the hypothalamus and medulla and evoke reflex motor activity that is carried to the effector cells by the efferent fibers described above. There is increasing evidence that some of these

sensory fibers also have peripheral motor functions (see Nonadrenergic, Noncholinergic Neurons, below).

The **enteric nervous system (ENS)** is a large and highly organized collection of neurons located in the walls of the gastrointestinal system (Figure 6–2). It is sometimes considered a third division of the ANS. The ENS includes the myenteric plexus (the plexus of Auerbach) and the submucous plexus (the plexus of Meissner). These neuronal networks receive preganglionic fibers from the parasympathetic system and postganglionic sympathetic axons. They also receive sensory input from within the wall of the gut. Fibers from the cell bodies in these plexuses travel to the smooth muscle of the gut to control motility and to secretory cells in the mucosa. Sensory fibers transmit information from the mucosa and from stretch receptors to motor neurons in the plexuses and to postganglionic neurons in the sympathetic ganglia. The parasympathetic and sympathetic fibers that synapse on enteric plexus neurons appear to play a modulatory role, as indicated by the observation

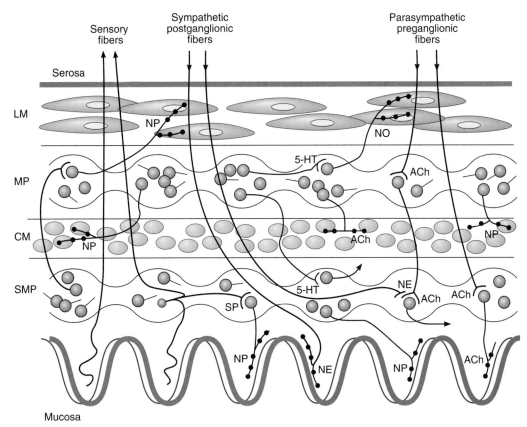

Figure 6–2. A highly simplified diagram of the intestinal wall and some of the circuitry of the enteric nervous system (ENS). The ENS receives input from both the sympathetic and the parasympathetic systems and sends afferent impulses to sympathetic ganglia and to the central nervous system. Many transmitter or neuromodulator substances have been identified in the ENS; see Table 6–1. (LM, longitudinal muscle layer; MP, myenteric plexus; CM, circular muscle layer; SMP, submucosal plexus; ACh, acetylcholine; NE, norepinephrine; NO, nitric oxide; NP, neuropeptides; SP, substance P; 5-HT, serotonin.)

that deprivation of input from both ANS divisions does not completely halt activity in the plexuses nor in the smooth muscle and glands innervated by them.

NEUROTRANSMITTER CHEMISTRY OF THE AUTONOMIC NERVOUS SYSTEM

An important traditional classification of autonomic nerves is based on the primary transmitter molecules—acetylcholine or norepinephrine—released from their terminal boutons and varicosities. A large number of peripheral ANS fibers synthesize and release acetylcholine; they are **cholinergic** fibers, ie, they act by releasing acetylcholine. As shown in Figure 6–1, these include all preganglionic efferent autonomic fibers and the somatic (nonautonomic) motor fibers to skeletal muscle as well. Thus, almost all efferent fibers leaving the central nervous sys-

tem are cholinergic. In addition, most parasympathetic postganglionic and a few sympathetic postganglionic fibers are cholinergic. A significant number of parasympathetic postganglionic neurons utilize nitric oxide or peptides for transmission. Most postganglionic sympathetic fibers release norepinephrine (also known as noradrenaline); they are **noradrenergic** (often called simply "adrenergic") fibers; that is, they act by releasing norepinephrine. These transmitter characteristics are presented schematically in Figure 6–1. As noted above, a few sympathetic fibers release acetylcholine. Dopamine is a very important transmitter in the central nervous system, and there is evidence that it may be released by some peripheral sympathetic fibers. Adrenal medullary cells, which are embryologically analogous to postganglionic sympathetic neurons, release a mixture of epinephrine and norepinephrine. Finally, most autonomic nerves also release several transmitter substances, or *cotransmitters,* in addition to the primary transmitters described above.

Five key features of neurotransmitter function provide potential targets for pharmacologic therapy: synthesis, storage, release, and termination of action of the transmitter, and functions of the receptor. These processes are discussed in detail below.

Cholinergic Transmission

The terminals of cholinergic neurons contain large numbers of small membrane-bound vesicles concentrated near the synaptic portion of the cell membrane (Figure 6–3) as well as a smaller number of large dense-cored vesicles located farther from the synaptic membrane. The large vesicles contain a high concentration of peptide cotransmitters (Table 6–1), whereas the smaller clear vesicles contain most of the acetylcholine. Vesicles are initially synthesized in the neuron soma and transported to the terminal. They may also be recycled several times within the terminal. Vesicles are provided with **vesicle-associated membrane proteins (VAMPs),** which serve to align them with release sites on the inner neuronal cell membrane and participate in triggering the release of transmitter. The corresponding release site on the inner surface of the nerve terminal membrane contains **synaptosomal nerve-associated proteins (SNAPs).**

Acetylcholine is synthesized in the cytoplasm from acetyl-CoA and choline through the catalytic action of the enzyme choline acetyltransferase (ChAT). Acetyl-CoA is synthesized in mitochondria, which are present in large numbers in the nerve ending. Choline is transported from the extracellular fluid into the neuron terminal by a sodium-dependent membrane **choline transporter** (Figure 6–3, **CHT**). This symporter can be blocked by a group of research drugs called **hemicholiniums.** Once synthesized, acetylcholine is transported from the cytoplasm into the vesicles by a **vesicle-associated transporter** that is driven by proton efflux (Figure 6–3, carrier **VAT**). This antiporter can be blocked by the research drug **vesamicol.** Acetylcholine synthesis is a rapid process capable of supporting a very high rate of transmitter release. Storage of acetylcholine is accomplished by the packaging of "quanta" of acetylcholine molecules (usually 1000–50,000 molecules in each vesicle).

Vesicles are concentrated on the inner surface of the nerve terminal facing the synapse through the interaction of so-called SNARE proteins on the vesicle (VAMPs called v-SNAREs, especially synaptobrevin) and on the inside of the neuronal cell membrane (SNAPs called t-SNAREs, especially syntaxin and SNAP-25). Release of transmitter from the vesicles is dependent on extracellular calcium and occurs when an action potential reaches the terminal and triggers sufficient influx of calcium ions. Calcium interacts with the VAMP synaptotagmin on the vesicle membrane and

triggers fusion of the vesicle membrane with the terminal membrane and opening of a pore into the synapse. The opening of the pore results in exocytotic expulsion—in the case of somatic motor nerves—of several hundred quanta of acetylcholine into the synaptic cleft. The amount of transmitter released by one depolarization of an autonomic postganglionic nerve terminal is probably smaller. In addition to acetylcholine, several cotransmitters are released at the same time (Table 6–1). The acetylcholine vesicle release process is blocked by botulinum toxin through the enzymatic removal of two amino acids from one or more of the fusion proteins.

After release from the presynaptic terminal, acetylcholine molecules may bind to and activate an acetylcholine receptor (**cholinoceptor**). Eventually (and usually very rapidly), all of the acetylcholine released diffuses within range of an **acetylcholinesterase** (AChE) molecule. AChE very efficiently splits acetylcholine into choline and acetate, neither of which has significant transmitter effect, and thereby terminates the action of the transmitter (Figure 6–3). Most cholinergic synapses are richly supplied with acetylcholinesterase; the half-life of acetylcholine in the synapse is therefore very short (seconds). Acetylcholinesterase is also found in other tissues, eg, red blood cells. (Another cholinesterase with a lower specificity for acetylcholine, butyrylcholinesterase [pseudocholinesterase], is found in blood plasma, liver, glia, and many other tissues.)

Adrenergic Transmission

Adrenergic neurons (Figure 6–4) also transport a precursor molecule into the nerve ending, then synthesize the catecholamine transmitter, and finally store it in membrane-bound vesicles, but, as indicated in Figure 6–5, the synthesis of the catecholamine transmitters is more complex than that of acetylcholine. In most sympathetic postganglionic neurons, norepinephrine is the final product. In the adrenal medulla and certain areas of the brain, norepinephrine is further converted to epinephrine. In dopaminergic neurons, synthesis terminates with dopamine. Several processes in these nerve terminals are potential sites of drug action. One of these, the conversion of tyrosine to dopa, is the rate-limiting step in catecholamine transmitter synthesis. It can be inhibited by the tyrosine analog **metyrosine** (Figure 6–4). A high-affinity carrier for catecholamines located in the wall of the storage vesicle (**vesicular monoamine transporter, VMAT**) can be inhibited by the **reserpine** alkaloids (Figure 6–4, carrier VMAT). Reserpine causes depletion of transmitter stores. Another transporter (**norepinephrine transporter, NET**) carries norepinephrine and similar molecules back into the cell cytoplasm from the synaptic cleft (Figure 6–4, NET). NET is also commonly called uptake 1 or reuptake 1. NET can be inhibited by **cocaine** and **tricyclic antidepressant** drugs, resulting in

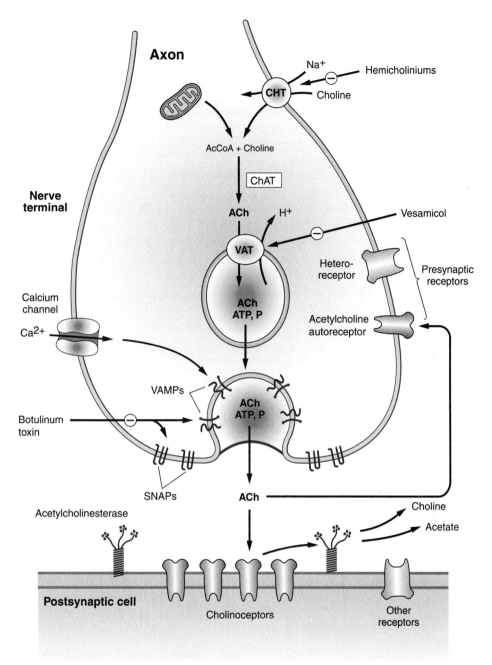

Figure 6–3. Schematic illustration of a generalized cholinergic junction (not to scale). Choline is transported into the presynaptic nerve terminal by a sodium-dependent choline transporter (CHT). This transporter can be inhibited by hemicholinium drugs. In the cytoplasm, acetylcholine is synthesized from choline and acetyl Co-A (AcCoA) by the enzyme choline acetyltransferase (ChAT). ACh is then transported into the storage vesicle by a second carrier, the vesicle-associated transporter (VAT), which can be inhibited by vesamicol. Peptides (P), adenosine triphosphate (ATP), and proteoglycan are also stored in the vesicle. Release of transmitter occurs when voltage-sensitive calcium channels in the terminal membrane are opened, allowing an influx of calcium. The resulting increase in intracellular calcium causes fusion of vesicles with the surface membrane and exocytotic expulsion of ACh and cotransmitters into the junctional cleft (see text). This step can be blocked by botulinum toxin. Acetylcholine's action is terminated by metabolism by the enzyme acetylcholinesterase. Receptors on the presynaptic nerve ending regulate transmitter release. (SNAPs, synaptosome-associated proteins; VAMPs, vesicle-associated membrane proteins.)

Table 6-1. Some of the transmitter substances found in autonomic nervous system (ANS), enteric nervous system (ENS), and nonadrenergic, noncholinergic neurons.[1]

Substance	Probable Roles
Acetylcholine (ACh)	The primary transmitter at ANS ganglia, at the somatic neuromuscular junction, and at parasympathetic postganglionic nerve endings. A primary excitatory transmitter to smooth muscle and secretory cells in the ENS. Probably also the major neuron-to-neuron ("ganglionic") transmitter in the ENS.
Adenosine triphosphate (ATP)	Acts as a transmitter or cotransmitter at many ANS-effector synapses.
Calcitonin gene-related peptide (CGRP)	Found with substance P in cardiovascular sensory nerve fibers. Present in some secretomotor ENS neurons and interneurons. A cardiac stimulant.
Cholecystokinin (CCK)	May act as a cotransmitter in some excitatory neuromuscular ENS neurons.
Dopamine	A modulatory transmitter in some ganglia and the ENS. Probably a postganglionic sympathetic transmitter in renal blood vessels.
Enkephalin and related opioid peptides	Present in some secretomotor and interneurons in the ENS. Appear to inhibit ACh release and thereby inhibit peristalsis. May *stimulate* secretion.
Galanin	Present in secretomotor neurons; may play a role in appetite-satiety mechanisms.
GABA (γ-aminobutyric acid)	May have presynaptic effects on excitatory ENS nerve terminals. Has some relaxant effect on the gut. Probably not a major transmitter in the ENS.
Gastrin-releasing peptide (GRP)	Extremely potent excitatory transmitter to gastrin cells. Also known as mammalian bombesin.
Neuropeptide Y (NPY)	Found in many noradrenergic neurons. Present in some secretomotor neurons in the ENS and may inhibit secretion of water and electrolytes by the gut. Causes long-lasting vasoconstriction. It is also a cotransmitter in some parasympathetic postganglionic neurons.
Nitric oxide (NO)	A cotransmitter at inhibitory ENS neuromuscular junctions; may be especially important at sphincters.
Norepinephrine (NE)	The primary transmitter at most sympathetic postganglionic nerve endings.
Serotonin (5-HT)	An important transmitter or cotransmitter at excitatory neuron-to-neuron junctions in the ENS.
Substance P (and related "tachykinins")	Substance P is an important sensory neuron transmitter in the ENS and elsewhere. Tachykinins appear to be excitatory cotransmitters with ACh at ENS neuromuscular junctions. Found with CGRP in cardiovascular sensory neurons. Substance P is a vasodilator (probably via release of nitric oxide).
Vasoactive intestinal peptide (VIP)	Excitatory secretomotor transmitter in the ENS; may also be an inhibitory ENS neuromuscular cotransmitter. A probable cotransmitter in many cholinergic neurons. A vasodilator (found in many perivascular neurons) and cardiac stimulant.

[1]See Chapter 21 for transmitters found in the central nervous system.

an increase of transmitter activity in the synaptic cleft. Similar transporters (**DAT, SERT**) are responsible for the reuptake of dopamine and 5-HT (serotonin), respectively, into the neurons that release these transmitters.

Release of the vesicular transmitter store from noradrenergic nerve endings is similar to the calcium-dependent process described above for cholinergic terminals. In addition to the primary transmitter (norepinephrine), adenosine triphosphate (ATP), dopamine-β-hydroxylase, and peptide cotransmitters are also released into the synaptic cleft. Indirectly acting and mixed sympathomimetics, eg, **tyramine, amphetamines,** and **ephedrine,** are capable of releasing stored transmitter from noradrenergic nerve endings by a calcium-independent process. These drugs are poor agonists (some are inactive) at adrenoceptors, but they are excellent substrates for monoamine transporters. As a result, they are avidly taken up into noradrenergic nerve endings by NET. In the nerve ending, they are then transported by VMAT into the vesicles, displacing norepinephrine, which is subsequently expelled into the synaptic space by reverse transport via NET. Amphetamines also inhibit monoamine oxidase and have other effects that result in increased norepinephrine activity in the synapse. Their action does not require vesicle exocytosis.

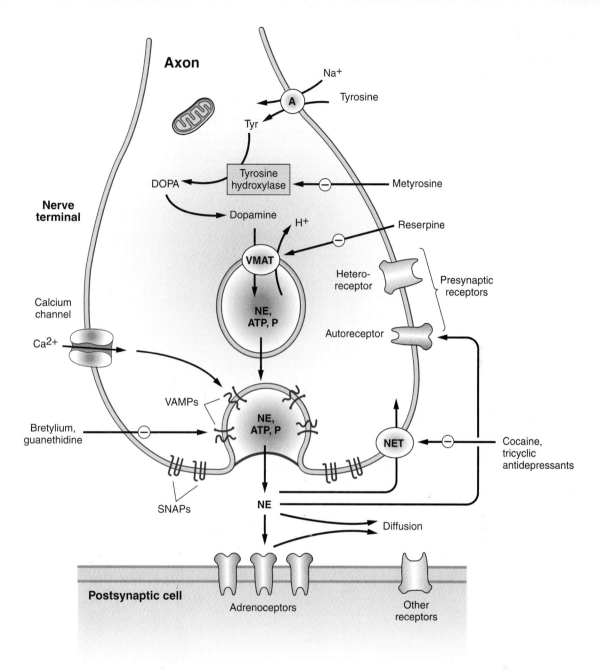

Figure 6–4. Schematic diagram of a generalized noradrenergic junction (not to scale). Tyrosine is transported into the noradrenergic ending or varicosity by a sodium-dependent carrier (A). Tyrosine is converted to dopamine (see Figure 6–5 for details), which is transported into the vesicle by the vesicular monoamine transporter (VMAT), which can be blocked by reserpine. The same carrier transports norepinephrine (NE) and several other amines into these granules. Dopamine is converted to NE in the vesicle by dopamine-β-hydroxylase. Physiologic release of transmitter occurs when an action potential opens voltage-sensitive calcium channels and increases intracellular calcium. Fusion of vesicles with the surface membrane results in expulsion of norepinephrine, cotransmitters, and dopamine-β-hydroxylase. Release can be blocked by drugs such as guanethidine and bretylium. After release, norepinephrine diffuses out of the cleft or is transported into the cytoplasm of the terminal by the norepinephrine transporter (NET), which can be blocked by cocaine and tricyclic antidepressants, or into postjunctional or perijunctional cells. Regulatory receptors are present on the presynaptic terminal. (SNAPs, synaptosome-associated proteins; VAMPs, vesicle-associated membrane proteins.)

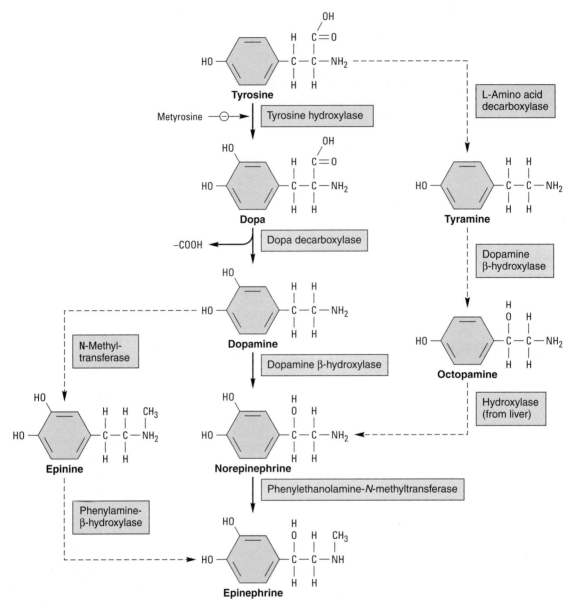

Figure 6–5. Biosynthesis of catecholamines. The rate-limiting step, conversion of tyrosine to dopa, can be inhibited by metyrosine (α-methyltyrosine). The alternative pathways shown by the dashed arrows have not been found to be of physiologic significance in humans. However, tyramine and octopamine may accumulate in patients treated with monoamine oxidase inhibitors. (Reproduced, with permission, from Greenspan FS, Gardner DG (editors): *Basic and Clinical Endocrinology*, 7th ed. McGraw-Hill, 2003.)

Norepinephrine and epinephrine can be metabolized by several enzymes, as shown in Figure 6–6. Because of the high activity of monoamine oxidase in the mitochondria of the nerve terminal, there is significant turnover of norepinephrine even in the resting terminal. Since the metabolic products are excreted in the urine, an estimate of catechol-amine turnover can be obtained from laboratory analysis of total metabolites (sometimes referred to as "VMA and metanephrines") in a 24-hour urine sample. However, metabolism is not the primary mechanism for termination of action of norepinephrine physiologically released from noradrenergic nerves. Termination of noradrenergic trans-

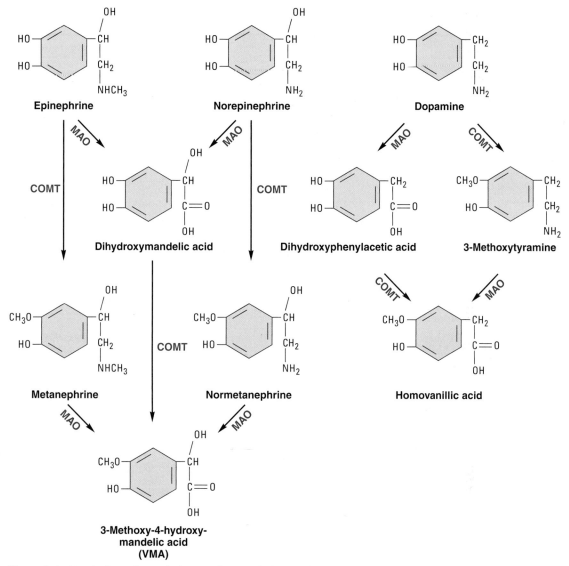

Figure 6–6. Metabolism of catecholamines by catechol-*O*-methyltransferase (COMT) and monoamine oxidase (MAO). (Modified and reproduced, with permission, from Greenspan FS, Gardner DG (editors): *Basic and Clinical Endocrinology,* 7th ed. McGraw-Hill, 2003.)

mission results from two processes, simple diffusion away from the receptor site (with eventual metabolism in the plasma or liver), and reuptake into the nerve terminal by NET (Figure 6–4) or into perisynaptic glia or other cells.

Cotransmitters in Cholinergic & Adrenergic Nerves

As previously noted, the vesicles of both cholinergic and adrenergic nerves contain other substances in addition to the primary transmitter. Some of the substances identified to date are listed in Table 6–1. Many of these substances are also *primary* transmitters in the nonadrenergic, noncholinergic nerves described in the text that follows. Their roles in the function of nerves that release acetylcholine or norepinephrine are not yet fully understood. In some cases, they provide a faster or slower action to supplement or modulate the effects of the primary transmitter. They also participate in feedback inhibition of the same and nearby nerve terminals.

Table 6–2. Major autonomic receptor types.

Receptor Name	Typical Locations	Result of Ligand Binding
Cholinoceptors		
Muscarinic M_1	CNS neurons, sympathetic postganglionic neurons, some presynaptic sites	Formation of IP_3 and DAG, increased intracellular calcium
Muscarinic M_2	Myocardium, smooth muscle, some presynaptic sites; CNS neurons	Opening of potassium channels, inhibition of adenylyl cyclase
Muscarinic M_3	Exocrine glands, vessels (smooth muscle and endothelium); CNS neurons	Like M_1 receptor-ligand binding
Muscarinic M_4	CNS neurons; possibly vagal nerve endings	Like M_2 receptor-ligand binding
Muscarinic M_5	Vascular endothelium, especially cerebral vessels; CNS neurons	Like M_1 receptor-ligand binding
Nicotinic N_N	Postganglionic neurons, some presynaptic cholinergic terminals	Opening of Na^+, K^+ channels, depolarization
Nicotinic N_M	Skeletal muscle neuromuscular endplates	Opening of Na^+, K^+ channels, depolarization
Adrenoceptors		
$Alpha_1$	Postsynaptic effector cells, especially smooth muscle	Formation of IP_3 and DAG, increased intracellular calcium
$Alpha_2$	Presynaptic adrenergic nerve terminals, platelets, lipocytes, smooth muscle	Inhibition of adenylyl cyclase, decreased cAMP
$Beta_1$	Postsynaptic effector cells, especially heart, lipocytes, brain; presynaptic adrenergic and cholinergic nerve terminals, juxtaglomerular apparatus of renal tubules, ciliary body epithelium	Stimulation of adenylyl cyclase, increased cAMP
$Beta_2$	Postsynaptic effector cells, especially smooth muscle and cardiac muscle	Stimulation of adenylyl cyclase and increased cAMP. Activates cardiac G_i under some conditions.
$Beta_3$	Postsynaptic effector cells, especially lipocytes; heart	Stimulation of adenylyl cyclase and increased cAMP[1]
Dopamine receptors		
D_1 (DA_1), D_5	Brain; effector tissues, especially smooth muscle of the renal vascular bed	Stimulation of adenylyl cyclase and increased cAMP
D_2 (DA_2)	Brain; effector tissues, especially smooth muscle; presynaptic nerve terminals	Inhibition of adenylyl cyclase; increased potassium conductance
D_3	Brain	Inhibition of adenylyl cyclase
D_4	Brain, cardiovascular system	Inhibition of adenylyl cyclase

[1]Cardiac $beta_3$-receptor function is poorly understood, but activation does *not* appear to result in stimulation of rate or force.

AUTONOMIC RECEPTORS

Historically, structure-activity analyses, with careful comparisons of the potency of series of autonomic agonist and antagonist analogs, led to the definition of different autonomic receptor subtypes, including muscarinic and nicotinic cholinoceptors, and α, β, and dopamine adrenoceptors (Table 6–2). Subsequently, binding of isotope-labeled ligands permitted the purifi-

cation and characterization of several of the receptor molecules. Molecular biology now provides techniques for the discovery and expression of genes that code for related receptors within these groups (see Chapter 2).

The primary acetylcholine receptor subtypes were named after the alkaloids originally used in their identification: muscarine and nicotine. These nouns are readily converted into adjectives—thus, **muscarinic** and **nicotinic receptors.** In the case of receptors associated with noradrenergic nerves, the coining of simple adjectives from the names of the agonists (noradrenaline, phenylephrine, isoproterenol, etc) was not practicable. Therefore, the term **adrenoceptor** is widely used to describe receptors that respond to catecholamines such as norepinephrine. By analogy, the term **cholinoceptor** denotes receptors (both muscarinic and nicotinic) that respond to acetylcholine. In North America, receptors were colloquially named after the nerves that usually innervate them; thus, **adrenergic** (or noradrenergic) **receptors** and **cholinergic receptors**. The general class of adrenoceptors can be further subdivided into α-**adrenoceptor,** β-**adrenoceptor,** and **dopamine-receptor** types on the basis of both agonist and antagonist selectivity and on genomic grounds. Development of more selective blocking drugs has led to the naming of subclasses within these major types; for example, within the α-adrenoceptor class, α_1 and α_2 receptors differ in both agonist and antagonist selectivity. Specific examples of such selective drugs are given in the chapters that follow.

NONADRENERGIC, NONCHOLINERGIC (NANC) NEURONS

It has been known for many years that autonomic effector tissues (eg, gut, airways, bladder) contain nerve fibers that do not show the histochemical characteristics of either cholinergic or adrenergic fibers. Both motor and sensory nonadrenergic, noncholinergic fibers are present. Although peptides are the most common transmitter substances found in these nerve endings, other substances, eg, nitric oxide synthase and purines, are also present in many nerve terminals (Table 6–1). Capsaicin, a neurotoxin derived from chili peppers, can cause the release of transmitter (especially substance P) from such neurons and, if given in high doses, destruction of the neuron.

The enteric system in the gut wall (Figure 6–2) is the most extensively studied system containing nonadrenergic, noncholinergic neurons in addition to cholinergic and adrenergic fibers. In the small intestine, for example, these neurons contain one or more of the following: nitric oxide synthase, calcitonin gene-related peptide, cholecystokinin, dynorphin, enkephalins, gastrin-releasing peptide, 5-hydroxytryptamine (serotonin), neuropeptide Y, somatostatin, substance P, and vasoactive intestinal peptide. Some neurons contain as many as five different transmitters. The ENS functions in a semiautonomous manner, utilizing input from the motor outflow of the ANS for modulation of gastrointestinal activity and sending sensory information back to the central nervous system. The ENS provides the necessary synchronization of impulses that, for example, ensures forward, not backward, propulsion of

gut contents and relaxation of sphincters when the gut wall contracts.

The sensory fibers in the nonadrenergic, noncholinergic systems are probably better termed "sensory-efferent" or "sensory-local effector" fibers because, when activated by a sensory input, they are capable of releasing transmitter peptides from the sensory ending itself, from local axon branches, and from collaterals that terminate in the autonomic ganglia. These peptides are potent agonists at many autonomic effector tissues.

FUNCTIONAL ORGANIZATION OF AUTONOMIC ACTIVITY

A basic understanding of the interactions of autonomic nerves with each other and with their effector organs is essential for an appreciation of the actions of autonomic drugs, especially because of the significant reflex (compensatory) effects that may be evoked by these agents.

Central Integration

At the highest level—midbrain and medulla—the two divisions of the ANS and the endocrine system are integrated with each other, with sensory input, and with information from higher central nervous system centers. These interactions are such that early investigators called the parasympathetic system a **trophotropic** one (ie, leading to growth) used to "rest and digest" and the sympathetic system an **ergotropic** one (ie, leading to energy expenditure), which is activated for "fight or flight." Although such terms offer little insight into the mechanisms involved, they do provide simple descriptions applicable to many of the actions of the systems (Table 6–3). For example, slowing of the heart and stimulation of digestive activity are typical energy-conserving actions of the parasympathetic system. In contrast, cardiac stimulation, increased blood sugar, and cutaneous vasoconstriction are responses produced by sympathetic discharge that are suited to fighting or surviving attack.

At a more subtle level of interactions in the brain stem, medulla, and spinal cord, there are important cooperative interactions between the parasympathetic and sympathetic systems. For some organs, sensory fibers associated with the parasympathetic system exert reflex control over motor outflow in the sympathetic system. Thus, the sensory carotid sinus baroreceptor fibers in the glossopharyngeal nerve have a major influence on sympathetic outflow from the vasomotor center. This example is described in greater detail below. Similarly, parasympathetic sensory fibers in the wall of the urinary bladder significantly influence sympathetic inhibitory outflow to that organ. Within the enteric

Table 6–3. Direct effects of autonomic *nerve* activity on some organ systems. Autonomic *drug* effects are similar but not identical (see text).

| Organ | Effect of | | | |
| | Sympathetic Activity | | Parasympathetic Activity | |
	Action[1]	Receptor[2]	Action	Receptor[2]
Eye				
Iris radial muscle	Contracts	α_1	...	...
Iris circular muscle	...	...	Contracts	M_3
Ciliary muscle	[Relaxes]	β	Contracts	M_3
Heart				
Sinoatrial node	Accelerates	β_1, β_2	Decelerates	M_2
Ectopic pacemakers	Accelerates	β_1, β_2	...	...
Contractility	Increases	β_1, β_2	Decreases (atria)	M_2
Blood vessels				
Skin, splanchnic vessels	Contracts	α	...	...
Skeletal muscle vessels	Relaxes	β_2	...	...
	[Contracts]	α	...	...
	Relaxes	M^3	...	...
Endothelium			Releases EDRF[4]	$M_3, M_5{}^5$
Bronchiolar smooth muscle	Relaxes	β_2	Contracts	M_3
Gastrointestinal tract				
Smooth muscle				
Walls	Relaxes	$\alpha_2{}^6, \beta_2$	Contracts	M_3
Sphincters	Contracts	α_1	Relaxes	M_3
Secretion	...	...	Increases	M_3
Genitourinary smooth muscle				
Bladder wall	Relaxes	β_2	Contracts	M_3
Sphincter	Contracts	α_1	Relaxes	M_3
Uterus, pregnant	Relaxes	β_2	...	...
	Contracts	α	Contracts	M_3
Penis, seminal vesicles	Ejaculation	α	Erection	M
Skin				
Pilomotor smooth muscle	Contracts	α	...	...
Sweat glands			...	...
Thermoregulatory	Increases	M	...	...
Apocrine (stress)	Increases	α	...	...
Metabolic functions				
Liver	Gluconeogenesis	β_2, α	...	...
Liver	Glycogenolysis	β_2, α	...	...
Fat cells	Lipolysis	β_3	...	...
Kidney	Renin release	β_1	...	...

[1]Less important actions are shown in brackets.
[2]Specific receptor type: α = alpha, β = beta, M = muscarinic.
[3]Vascular smooth muscle in skeletal muscle has sympathetic cholinergic dilator fibers.
[4]The endothelium of most blood vessels releases EDRF (endothelium-derived relaxing factor), which causes marked vasodilation, in response to muscarinic stimuli. However, unlike the receptors innervated by sympathetic cholinergic fibers in skeletal muscle blood vessels, these muscarinic receptors are not innervated and respond only to circulating muscarinic agonists.
[5]Cerebral blood vessels dilate in response to M_5 receptor activation.
[6]Probably through presynaptic inhibition of parasympathetic activity.

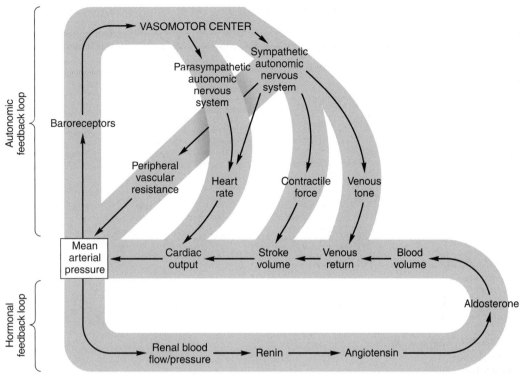

Figure 6–7. Autonomic and hormonal control of cardiovascular function. Note that two feedback loops are present: the autonomic nervous system loop and the hormonal loop. The sympathetic nervous system directly influences four major variables: peripheral vascular resistance, heart rate, force, and venous tone. It also directly modulates renin production (not shown). The parasympathetic nervous system directly influences heart rate. In addition to its role in stimulating aldosterone secretion, angiotensin II directly increases peripheral vascular resistance and facilitates sympathetic effects (not shown). The net feedback effect of each loop is to compensate for changes in arterial blood pressure. Thus, decreased blood pressure due to blood loss would evoke increased sympathetic outflow and renin release. Conversely, elevated pressure due to the administration of a vasoconstrictor drug would cause reduced sympathetic outflow, reduced renin release, and increased parasympathetic (vagal) outflow.

nervous system, sensory fibers from the wall of the gut synapse on both preganglionic and postganglionic motor cells that control intestinal smooth muscle and secretory cells (Figure 6–2).

Integration of Cardiovascular Function

Autonomic reflexes are particularly important in understanding cardiovascular responses to autonomic drugs. As indicated in Figure 6–7, the primary controlled variable in cardiovascular function is **mean arterial pressure.** Changes in any variable contributing to mean arterial pressure (eg, a drug-induced increase in peripheral vascular resistance) evoke powerful **homeostatic** secondary responses that tend to compensate for the directly evoked change. The homeostatic response may be sufficient to reduce the change in mean arterial pressure and to reverse

the drug's effects on heart rate. A slow infusion of norepinephrine provides a useful example. This agent produces direct effects on both vascular and cardiac muscle. It is a powerful vasoconstrictor and, by increasing peripheral vascular resistance, increases mean arterial pressure. In the absence of reflex control—in a patient who has had a heart transplant, for example—the drug's effect on the heart is also stimulatory; that is, it increases heart rate and contractile force. However, in a subject with intact reflexes, the negative feedback baroreceptor response to increased mean arterial pressure causes decreased sympathetic outflow to the heart and a powerful increase in parasympathetic (vagus nerve) discharge at the cardiac pacemaker. As a result, the *net* effect of ordinary pressor doses of norepinephrine in a normal subject is to produce a marked increase in peripheral vascular resistance, an increase in mean arterial pressure, and a consistent *slowing*

Table 6–4. Autoreceptor, heteroreceptor, and modulatory effects in peripheral synapses.[1]

Transmitter/Modulator	Receptor Type	Neuron Terminals Where Found
Inhibitory effects		
Acetylcholine	M_2, M_1	Adrenergic, enteric nervous system
Norepinephrine	Alpha$_2$	Adrenergic
Dopamine	D_2; less evidence for D_1	Adrenergic
Serotonin (5-HT)	5-HT$_1$, 5-HT$_2$, 5-HT$_3$	Cholinergic preganglionic
ATP and adenosine	P_2 (ATP), P_1 (adenosine)	Adrenergic autonomic and ENS cholinergic neurons
Histamine	H_3, possibly H_2	H_3 type identified on CNS adrenergic and serotonergic neurons
Enkephalin	Delta (also mu, kappa)	Adrenergic, ENS cholinergic
Neuropeptide Y	Y_1, Y_2 (NPY)	Adrenergic, some cholinergic
Prostaglandin E_1, E_2	EP$_3$	Adrenergic
Excitatory effects		
Epinephrine	Beta$_2$	Adrenergic, somatic motor cholinergic
Acetylcholine	N_M	Somatic motor cholinergic
Angiotensin II	AT$_1$	Adrenergic

[1]A provisional list. The number of transmitters and locations will undoubtedly increase with additional research.

of heart rate. Bradycardia, the reflex compensatory response elicited by this agent, is the *exact opposite* of the drug's direct action; yet it is completely predictable if the integration of cardiovascular function by the ANS is understood.

Presynaptic Regulation

The principle of negative feedback control is also found at the presynaptic level of autonomic function. Important presynaptic feedback inhibitory control mechanisms have been shown to exist at most nerve endings. A well-documented mechanism involves the α_2 receptor located on noradrenergic nerve terminals. This receptor is activated by norepinephrine and similar molecules; activation diminishes further release of norepinephrine from these nerve endings (Table 6–4). Conversely, a presynaptic β receptor appears to facilitate the release of norepinephrine from some adrenergic neurons. Presynaptic receptors that respond to the primary transmitter substance released by the nerve ending are called **autoreceptors.** Autoreceptors are usually inhibitory, but many cholinergic fibers, especially somatic motor fibers, have excitatory nicotinic autoreceptors.

Control of transmitter release is not limited to modulation by the transmitter itself. Nerve terminals also carry regulatory receptors that respond to many other substances. Such **heteroreceptors** may be activated by substances released from other nerve terminals that synapse with the nerve ending. For example, some vagal fibers in the myocardium synapse on sympathetic noradrenergic nerve terminals and inhibit norepinephrine release. Alternatively, the ligands for these receptors may diffuse to the receptors from the blood or from nearby tissues. Some of the transmitters and receptors identified to date are listed in Table 6–4. Presynaptic regulation by a variety of endogenous chemicals probably occurs in all nerve fibers.

Postsynaptic Regulation

Postsynaptic regulation can be considered from two perspectives: modulation by the history of activity at the primary receptor (which may up- or down-regulate receptor number or desensitize receptors; see Chapter 2) and modulation by other temporally associated events.

The first mechanism has been well documented in several receptor-effector systems. Up- and down-regulation are known to occur in response to decreased or increased activation, respectively, of the receptors. An extreme form of up-regulation occurs after denervation of some tissues, resulting in **denervation supersensitivity** of the tissue to activators of that receptor type. In skeletal muscle, for example, nicotinic receptors are

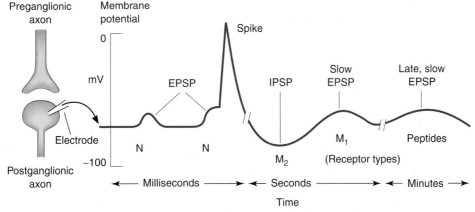

Figure 6–8. Excitatory and inhibitory postsynaptic potentials (EPSP and IPSP) in an autonomic ganglion cell. The postganglionic neuron shown at the left with a recording electrode might undergo the membrane potential changes shown schematically in the recording. The response begins with two EPSP responses to nicotinic (N) receptor activation, the first not reaching threshold. The action potential is followed by an IPSP, probably evoked by M_2 receptor activation (with possible participation from dopamine receptor activation). The IPSP is, in turn, followed by a slower, M_1-dependent EPSP, and this is sometimes followed by a still slower peptide-induced excitatory postsynaptic potential.

normally restricted to the end plate regions underlying somatic motor nerve terminals. Surgical denervation results in marked proliferation of nicotinic cholinoceptors over all parts of the fiber, including areas not previously associated with any motor nerve junctions. A pharmacologic supersensitivity related to denervation supersensitivity occurs in autonomic effector tissues after administration of drugs that deplete transmitter stores and prevent activation of the postsynaptic receptors for a sufficient period of time. For example, prolonged administration of large doses of reserpine, a norepinephrine depleter, can cause increased sensitivity of the smooth muscle and cardiac muscle effector cells served by the depleted sympathetic fibers.

The second mechanism involves modulation of the primary transmitter-receptor event by events evoked by the same or other transmitters acting on different postsynaptic receptors. Ganglionic transmission is a good example of this phenomenon (Figure 6–8). The postganglionic cells are activated (depolarized) as a result of binding of an appropriate ligand to a neuronal nicotinic (N_N) acetylcholine receptor. The resulting fast excitatory postsynaptic potential (EPSP) evokes a propagated action potential if threshold is reached. This event is often followed by a small and slowly developing but longer-lasting hyperpolarizing afterpotential—a slow inhibitory postsynaptic potential (IPSP). The hyperpolarization involves opening of potassium channels by M_2 cholinoceptors. The IPSP is followed by a small, slow excitatory postsynaptic potential caused by closure of potassium channels linked to M_1 cholinoceptors. Finally, a

late, very slow EPSP may be evoked by peptides released from other fibers. These slow potentials serve to modulate the responsiveness of the postsynaptic cell to subsequent primary excitatory presynaptic nerve activity. (See Chapter 21 for additional examples.)

PHARMACOLOGIC MODIFICATION OF AUTONOMIC FUNCTION

Because transmission involves different mechanisms in different segments of the ANS, some drugs produce highly specific effects, whereas others are much less selective in their actions. A summary of the steps in transmission of impulses, from the central nervous system to the autonomic effector cells, is presented in Table 6–5. Drugs that block action potential propagation (local anesthetics) are very nonselective in their action, since they act on a process that is common to all neurons. On the other hand, drugs that act on the biochemical processes involved in transmitter synthesis and storage are more selective, since the biochemistry of adrenergic transmission is very different from that of cholinergic transmission. Activation or blockade of effector cell receptors offers maximum flexibility and selectivity of effect: adrenoceptors are easily distinguished from cholinoceptors. Furthermore, individual subgroups can often be selectively activated or blocked within each major type. Some examples are given in the Box, Pharmacology of the Eye.

The next four chapters provide many more examples of this useful diversity of autonomic control processes.

Table 6–5. Steps in autonomic transmission: effects of drugs.

Process Affected	Drug Example	Site	Action
Action potential propagation	Local anesthetics, tetrodotoxin,[1] saxitoxin[2]	Nerve axons	Block sodium channels; block conduction
Transmitter synthesis	Hemicholinium	Cholinergic nerve terminals: membrane	Blocks uptake of choline and slows synthesis
	α-Methyltyrosine (metyrosine)	Adrenergic nerve terminals and adrenal medulla: cytoplasm	Blocks synthesis
Transmitter storage	Vesamicol	Cholinergic terminals vesicles	Prevents storage, depletes
	Reserpine	Adrenergic terminals vesicles	Prevents storage, depletes
Transmitter release	Many[3]	Nerve terminal membrane receptors	Modulate release
	ω-Conotoxin GVIA[4]	Nerve terminal calcium channels	Reduces transmitter release
	Botulinum toxin	Cholinergic vesicles	Prevents release
	α-Latrotoxin[5]	Cholinergic and adrenergic vesicles	Causes explosive transmitter release
	Tyramine, amphetamine	Adrenergic nerve terminals	Promote transmitter release
Transmitter uptake after release	Cocaine, tricyclic antidepressants	Adrenergic nerve terminals	Inhibit uptake; increase transmitter effect on postsynaptic receptors
Receptor activation or blockade	Norepinephrine	Receptors at adrenergic junctions	Binds α receptors; causes contraction
	Phentolamine	Receptors at adrenergic junctions	Binds α receptors; prevents activation
	Isoproterenol	Receptors at adrenergic junctions	Binds β receptors; activates adenylyl cyclase
	Propranolol	Receptors at adrenergic junctions	Binds β receptors; prevents activation
	Nicotine	Receptors at nicotinic cholinergic junctions (autonomic ganglion, neuromuscular end plates)	Binds nicotinic receptors; opens ion channel in postsynaptic membrane
	Tubocurarine	Neuromuscular end plates	Prevents activation
	Bethanechol	Receptors, parasympathetic effector cells (smooth muscle, glands)	Binds and activates muscarinic receptors
	Atropine	Receptors, parasympathetic effector cells	Binds muscarinic receptors; prevents activation
Enzymatic inactivation of transmitter	Neostigmine	Cholinergic synapses (acetylcholinesterase)	Inhibits enzyme; prolongs and intensifies transmitter action
	Tranylcypromine	Adrenergic nerve terminals (monoamine oxidase)	Inhibits enzyme; increases stored transmitter pool

[1]Toxin of puffer fish, California newt.
[2]Toxin of *Gonyaulax* (red tide organism).
[3]Norepinephrine, dopamine, acetylcholine, angiotenisn II, various prostaglandins, etc.
[4]Toxin of marine snails of the genus *Conus*.
[5]Black widow spider venom.

PHARMACOLOGY OF THE EYE

The eye is a good example of an organ with multiple autonomic nervous system (ANS) functions, controlled by several different autonomic receptors. As shown in Figure 6–9, the anterior chamber is the site of several tissues controlled by the ANS. These tissues include three different muscles (pupillary dilator and constrictor muscles in the iris and the ciliary muscle) and the secretory epithelium of the ciliary body.

Parasympathetic nerve activity and muscarinic cholinomimetics mediate contraction of the circular pupillary constrictor muscle and of the ciliary muscle. Contraction of the pupillary constrictor muscle causes **miosis,** a reduction in pupil size. Miosis is usually present in patients exposed to large systemic or small topical doses of cholinomimetics, especially organophosphate cholinesterase inhibitors. Ciliary muscle contraction causes **accommodation of focus** for near vision. Marked contraction of the ciliary muscle, which often occurs with cholinesterase inhibitor intoxication, is called *cyclospasm.* Ciliary muscle contraction also puts tension on the trabecular meshwork, opening its pores and facilitating outflow of the aqueous humor into the canal of Schlemm. Increased outflow reduces intraocular pressure, a very useful result in patients with glaucoma. All of these effects are prevented or reversed by muscarinic blocking drugs such as atropine.

Alpha adrenoceptors mediate contraction of the radially oriented pupillary dilator muscle fibers in the iris and result in **mydriasis.** This occurs during sympathetic discharge and when alpha agonist drugs such as phenylephrine are placed in the conjunctival sac. Beta-adrenoceptors on the ciliary epithelium facilitate the secretion of aqueous humor. Blocking these receptors (with β-blocking drugs) reduces the secretory activity and reduces intraocular pressure, providing another therapy for glaucoma.

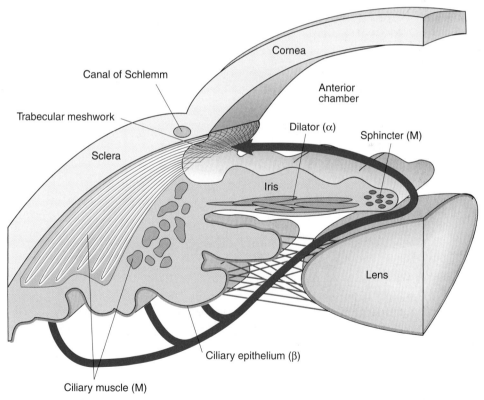

Figure 6–9. Structures of the anterior chamber of the eye. Tissues with significant autonomic functions and the associated ANS receptors are shown in this schematic diagram. Aqueous humor is secreted by the epithelium of the ciliary body, flows into the space in front of the iris, through the trabecular meshwork, and exits via the canal of Schlemm (arrow). Blockade of the β adrenoceptors associated with the ciliary epithelium causes decreased secretion of aqueous. Blood vessels (not shown) in the sclera are also under autonomic control and influence aqueous drainage.

REFERENCES

Andersson K-E, Wein AJ: Pharmacology of the lower urinary tract: Basis for current and future treatments of urinary incontinence. Pharmacol Rev 2004;56:581.

Bivalacqua TJ et al: Pharmacotherapy for erectile dysfunction. Trends Pharmacol Sci 2000;21:484.

Boehm S, Kubista H: Fine tuning of sympathetic transmitter release via ionotropic and metabotropic presynaptic receptors. Pharmacol Rev 2002;54:43.

Burnstock G: Cotransmission. Curr Opin Pharmacol 2004;4:47.

Chang HY, Mashimo H, Goyal RK: Musings on the wanderer: What's new in our understanding of the vago-vagal reflex? IV. Current concepts of vagal efferent projections to the gut. Am J Physiol Gastrointest Liver Physiol 2003;284:G357.

Furchgott RF: Role of endothelium in responses of vascular smooth muscle to drugs. Annu Rev Pharmacol Toxicol 1984;24:175.

Galligan JJ: Ligand-gated ion channels in the enteric nervous system. Neurogastroenterol Motil 2002;14:611.

Goldstein DS et al: Dysautonomias: Clinical disorders of the autonomic nervous system. Ann Intern Med 2002;137:753.

Miller RJ: Presynaptic receptors. Annu Rev Pharmacol Toxicol 1998;38:201.

Toda N, Herman AG: Gastrointestinal function regulation by nitrergic efferent nerves. Pharmacol Rev 2005;57:315.

Toda N, Okamura T: The pharmacology of nitric oxide in the peripheral nervous system of blood vessels. Pharmacol Rev 2003;55:271.

Westfall DP, Todorov LD, Mihaylova-Todorova ST: ATP as a cotransmitter in sympathetic nerves and its inactivation by releasable enzymes. J Pharmacol Exp Ther 2002;303:439.

Wilson RF et al: Regional differences in sympathetic reinnervation after human orthotopic cardiac transplantation. Circulation 1993;88:165.

Cholinoceptor-Activating & Cholinesterase-Inhibiting Drugs

7

Achilles J. Pappano, PhD

Acetylcholine receptor stimulants and cholinesterase inhibitors together comprise a large group of drugs that mimic acetylcholine (cholinomimetic agents) (Figure 7–1). Cholinoceptor stimulants are classified pharmacologically by their spectrum of action depending on the type of receptor—muscarinic or nicotinic—that is activated. They are also classified by their mechanism of action because some cholinomimetic drugs bind directly to (and activate) cholinoceptors while others act indirectly by inhibiting the hydrolysis of endogenous acetylcholine.

SPECTRUM OF ACTION OF CHOLINOMIMETIC DRUGS

Early studies of the parasympathetic nervous system showed that the alkaloid **muscarine** mimicked the effects of parasympathetic nerve discharge, ie, the effects were **parasympathomimetic.** Application of muscarine to ganglia and to autonomic effector tissues (smooth muscle, heart, exocrine glands) showed that the parasympathomimetic action of the alkaloid occurred through an action on receptors at effector cells, not those in ganglia. The effects of acetylcholine itself and of other cholinomimetic drugs at autonomic neuroeffector junctions are called parasympathomimetic effects, and are mediated by muscarinic receptors. In contrast, low concentrations of the alkaloid **nicotine** stimulated autonomic ganglia and skeletal muscle neuromuscular junctions but not autonomic effector cells. The ganglion and skeletal muscle receptors were therefore labeled nicotinic. When acetylcholine was later identified as the physiologic transmitter at both muscarinic and nicotinic receptors, both receptors were recognized as cholinoceptor subtypes.

Cholinoceptors are members of either G protein–linked (muscarinic) or ion channel (nicotinic) families on the basis of their transmembrane signaling mechanisms. Muscarinic receptors contain seven transmembrane domains whose third cytoplasmic loop is coupled to G proteins that function as transducers (see Figure 2–11). These receptors regulate the production of intra-cellular second messengers and modulate certain ion channels via their G proteins. Agonist selectivity is determined by the subtypes of muscarinic receptors and G proteins that are present in a given cell (Table 7–1). Muscarinic receptors are located on plasma membranes of cells in the central nervous system, in organs innervated by parasympathetic nerves as well as on some tissues that are not innervated by these nerves, eg, endothelial cells (Table 7–1), and on those tissues innervated by postganglionic sympathetic cholinergic nerves.

Nicotinic receptors are part of a transmembrane polypeptide whose subunits form cation-selective ion channels (see Figure 2–9). These receptors are located on plasma membranes of postganglionic cells in all autonomic ganglia, of muscles innervated by somatic motor fibers, and of some central nervous system neurons (see Figure 6–1).

Unselective cholinoceptor stimulants in sufficient dosage can produce very diffuse and marked alterations in organ system function because acetylcholine has multiple sites of action where it initiates both excitatory and inhibitory effects. Fortunately, drugs are available that have a degree of selectivity, so that desired effects can often be achieved while avoiding or minimizing adverse effects. Selectivity of action is based on several factors. Some drugs stimulate either muscarinic receptors or nicotinic receptors selectively. Some agents stimulate nicotinic receptors at neuromuscular junctions preferentially and have less effect on nicotinic receptors in ganglia. Organ selectivity can also be achieved by using appropriate routes of administration ("pharmacokinetic selectivity"). For example, muscarinic stimulants can be administered topically to the surface of the eye to modify ocular function while minimizing systemic effects.

MODE OF ACTION OF CHOLINOMIMETIC DRUGS

Direct-acting cholinomimetic agents bind to and activate muscarinic or nicotinic receptors (Figure 7–1). Indirect-acting agents produce their primary effects by

Figure 7–1. The major groups of cholinoceptor-activating drugs, receptors, and target tissues.

inhibiting acetylcholinesterase, which hydrolyzes acetylcholine to choline and acetic acid (see Figure 6–3). By inhibiting acetylcholinesterase, the indirect-acting drugs increase the endogenous acetylcholine concentration in synaptic clefts and neuroeffector junctions. The excess acetylcholine, in turn, stimulates cholinoceptors to evoke increased responses. These drugs act primarily where acetylcholine is physiologically released and are thus *amplifiers* of endogenous acetylcholine.

Some cholinesterase inhibitors also inhibit butyrylcholinesterase (pseudocholinesterase). However, inhibition of butyrylcholinesterase plays little role in the action of indirect-acting cholinomimetic drugs because this enzyme is not important in the physiologic termination of synaptic acetylcholine action. Some quaternary cholinesterase inhibitors also have a modest direct action as well, eg, neostigmine, which activates neuromuscular nicotinic cholinoceptors directly in addition to blocking cholinesterase.

Table 7–1. Subtypes and characteristics of cholinoceptors.

Receptor Type	Other Names	Location	Structural Features	Postreceptor Mechanism
M_1		Nerves	Seven transmembrane segments, $G_{q/11}$ protein-linked	IP_3, DAG cascade
M_2	Cardiac M_2	Heart, nerves, smooth muscle	Seven transmembrane segments, $G_{i/o}$ protein-linked	Inhibition of cAMP production, activation of K^+ channels
M_3	.	Glands, smooth muscle, endothelium	Seven transmembrane segments, $G_{q/11}$ protein-linked	IP_3, DAG cascade
M_4		CNS	Seven transmembrane segments, $G_{i/o}$ protein-linked	Inhibition of cAMP production
M_5		CNS	Seven transmembrane segments, $G_{q/11}$ protein-linked	IP_3, DAG cascade
N_M	Muscle type, end plate receptor	Skeletal muscle neuromuscular junction	Pentamer $(\alpha_2\beta\delta\gamma)$[1]	Na^+, K^+ depolarizing ion channel
N_N	Neuronal type, ganglion receptor	Postganglionic cell body, dendrites	α and β subunits only as $\alpha_2\beta_2$ or $\alpha_3\beta_3$	Na^+, K^+ depolarizing ion channel

[1]Structure in *Torpedo* electric organ and fetal mammalian muscle. In adult muscle, the γ subunit is replaced by an ϵ subunit. Several different α and β subunits have been identified in different mammalian tissues (Lukas et al, 1999).

■ I. BASIC PHARMACOLOGY OF THE DIRECT-ACTING CHOLINOCEPTOR STIMULANTS

The direct-acting cholinomimetic drugs can be divided on the basis of chemical structure into esters of choline (including acetylcholine) and alkaloids (such as muscarine and nicotine). A few of these drugs are highly selective for the muscarinic or for the nicotinic receptor. Many have effects on both receptors; acetylcholine is typical.

Chemistry & Pharmacokinetics

A. STRUCTURE

Four important choline esters that have been studied extensively are shown in Figure 7–2. Their permanently charged quaternary ammonium group renders them relatively insoluble in lipids. Many naturally occurring and synthetic cholinomimetic drugs that are not choline esters have been identified; a few of these are shown in Figure 7–3. The muscarinic receptor is strongly stereoselective: *(S)*-bethanechol is almost 1000 times more potent than *(R)*-bethanechol.

B. ABSORPTION, DISTRIBUTION, AND METABOLISM

Choline esters are poorly absorbed and poorly distributed into the central nervous system because they are hydrophilic. Although all are hydrolyzed in the gastrointestinal tract (and less active by the oral route), they differ markedly in their susceptibility to hydrolysis by cholinesterase. Acetylcholine is very rapidly hydrolyzed (see Chapter 6); large amounts must be infused intravenously to achieve concentrations sufficient to produce detectable effects. A large intravenous bolus injection has a brief effect, typically 5–20 seconds, whereas intramuscular and subcutaneous injections produce only local effects. Methacholine is more resistant to hydrolysis, and the carbamic acid esters carbachol and bethanechol are still more resistant to hydrolysis by cholinesterase and have correspondingly longer durations of action. The β-methyl group (methacholine, bethanechol) reduces the potency of these drugs at nicotinic receptors (Table 7–2).

The tertiary natural cholinomimetic alkaloids (pilocarpine, nicotine, lobeline; Figure 7–3) are well absorbed from most sites of administration. Nicotine, a liquid, is sufficiently lipid-soluble to be absorbed across the skin. Muscarine, a quaternary amine, is less completely absorbed from the gastrointestinal tract than the

Figure 7–2. Molecular structures of four choline esters and carbamic acid. Acetylcholine and methacholine are acetic acid esters of choline and β-methylcholine, respectively. Carbachol and bethanechol are carbamic acid esters of the same alcohols.

tertiary amines but is nevertheless toxic when ingested, eg, in certain mushrooms, and even enters the brain. Lobeline is a plant derivative similar to nicotine. These amines are excreted chiefly by the kidneys. Acidification of the urine accelerates clearance of the tertiary amines.

Pharmacodynamics

A. MECHANISM OF ACTION

Activation of the parasympathetic nervous system modifies organ function by two major mechanisms. First, acetylcholine released from parasympathetic nerves acti-

ACTION CHIEFLY
MUSCARINIC

ACTION CHIEFLY
NICOTINIC

Muscarine

Nicotine

Pilocarpine

Lobeline

Figure 7–3. Structures of some cholinomimetic alkaloids.

vates muscarinic receptors on effector cells to alter organ function directly. Second, acetylcholine released from parasympathetic nerves interacts with muscarinic receptors on nerve terminals to inhibit the release of their neurotransmitter. By this mechanism, acetylcholine release and circulating muscarinic agonists indirectly alter organ function by modulating the effects of the parasympathetic and sympathetic nervous systems and perhaps nonadrenergic, noncholinergic (NANC) systems.

As indicated in Chapter 6, muscarinic receptor subtypes have been characterized by binding studies and cloned. Several cellular events occur when muscarinic receptors are activated, one or more of which might serve as second messengers for muscarinic activation. All muscarinic receptors appear to be of the G-protein

coupled type (see Chapter 2 and Table 7–1). Muscarinic agonist binding activates the inositol trisphosphate (IP_3), diacylglycerol (DAG) cascade. Some evidence implicates DAG in the opening of smooth muscle calcium channels; IP_3 releases calcium from endoplasmic and sarcoplasmic reticulum. Muscarinic agonists also increase cellular cGMP concentrations. Activation of muscarinic receptors also increases potassium flux across cardiac cell membranes and decreases it in ganglion and smooth muscle cells. This effect is mediated by the binding of an activated G protein directly to the channel. Finally, muscarinic receptor activation in some tissues (eg, heart, intestine) inhibits adenylyl cyclase activity. Moreover, muscarinic agonists attenuate the activation of adenylyl cyclase and modulate the increase in cAMP levels induced by hormones such as catecholamines. These muscarinic effects on cAMP generation reduce the physiologic response of the organ to stimulatory hormones.

The mechanism of nicotinic receptor activation has been studied in great detail, taking advantage of three factors: (1) the receptor is present in extremely high concentration in the membranes of the electric organs of electric fish; (2) α-bungarotoxin, a component of certain snake venoms, binds tightly to the receptors and is readily labeled as a marker for isolation procedures; and (3) receptor activation results in easily measured electrical and ionic changes in the cells involved. The nicotinic receptor in muscle tissues is a pentamer of four types of glycoprotein subunits (one monomer occurs twice) with a total molecular weight of about 250,000 (see Figure 2–9). The neuronal nicotinic

Table 7–2. Properties of choline esters.

Choline Ester	Susceptibility to Cholinesterase	Muscarinic Action	Nicotinic Action
Acetylcholine chloride	++++	+++	+++
Methacholine chloride	+	++++	None
Carbachol chloride	Negligible	++	+++
Bethanechol chloride	Negligible	++	None

receptor consists of α and β subunits only (Table 7–1). Each subunit has four transmembrane segments. Each α subunit has a receptor site that, when occupied by a nicotinic agonist, causes a conformational change in the protein (channel opening) that allows sodium and potassium ions to diffuse rapidly down their concentration gradients. Binding of an agonist molecule by one of the two α subunit receptor sites only modestly increases the probability of channel opening; simultaneous binding of agonist by both of the receptor sites greatly enhances opening probability. Nicotinic receptor activation causes depolarization of the nerve cell or neuromuscular end plate membrane.

Prolonged agonist occupancy of the nicotinic receptor abolishes the effector response; that is, the postganglionic neuron stops firing (ganglionic effect), and the skeletal muscle cell relaxes (neuromuscular end plate effect). Furthermore, the continued presence of the nicotinic agonist prevents electrical recovery of the postjunctional membrane. Thus, a state of "depolarizing blockade" is induced that is refractory to reversal by other agonists. As noted below, this effect can be exploited for producing muscle paralysis.

B. ORGAN SYSTEM EFFECTS

Most of the direct organ system effects of muscarinic cholinoceptor stimulants are readily predicted from a knowledge of the effects of parasympathetic nerve stimulation (see Table 6–3) and the distribution of muscarinic receptors. Effects of a typical agent such as acetylcholine are listed in Table 7–3. The effects of nicotinic agonists are similarly predictable from a knowledge of the physiology of the autonomic ganglia and skeletal muscle motor end plate.

1. Eye—Muscarinic agonists instilled into the conjunctival sac cause contraction of the smooth muscle of the iris sphincter (resulting in miosis) and of the ciliary muscle (resulting in accommodation). As a result, the iris is pulled away from the angle of the anterior chamber, and the trabecular meshwork at the base of the ciliary muscle is opened. Both effects facilitate aqueous humor outflow into the canal of Schlemm, which drains the anterior chamber.

2. Cardiovascular system—The primary cardiovascular effects of muscarinic agonists are reduction in peripheral vascular resistance and changes in heart rate. The direct effects listed in Table 7–3 are modified by important homeostatic reflexes, as described in Chapter 6 and depicted in Figure 6–7. Intravenous infusions of minimally effective doses of acetylcholine in humans (eg, 20–50 mcg/min) cause vasodilation, resulting in a reduction in blood pressure, often accompanied by a reflex increase in heart rate. Larger doses of acetylcholine produce bradycardia and decrease atrioventricular node conduction velocity in addition to hypotension.

Table 7–3. Effects of direct-acting cholinoceptor stimulants. Only the direct effects are indicated; homeostatic responses to these direct actions may be important (see text).

Organ	Response
Eye	
Sphincter muscle of iris	Contraction (miosis)
Ciliary muscle	Contraction for near vision
Heart	
Sinoatrial node	Decrease in rate (negative chronotropy)
Atria	Decrease in contractile strength (negative inotropy). Decrease in refractory period
Atrioventricular node	Decrease in conduction velocity (negative dromotropy). Increase in refractory period
Ventricles	Small decrease in contractile strength
Blood vessels	
Arteries	Dilation (via EDRF). Constriction (high-dose direct effect)
Veins	Dilation (via EDRF). Constriction (high-dose direct effect)
Lung	
Bronchial muscle	Contraction (bronchoconstriction)
Bronchial glands	Stimulation
Gastrointestinal tract	
Motility	Increase
Sphincters	Relaxation
Secretion	Stimulation
Urinary bladder	
Detrusor	Contraction
Trigone and sphincter	Relaxation
Glands	
Sweat, salivary, lacrimal, nasopharyngeal	Secretion

The direct cardiac actions of muscarinic stimulants include the following: (1) an increase in a potassium current ($I_{K(ACh)}$) in atrial muscle cells and in the cells of the sinoatrial and atrioventricular nodes as well; (2) a decrease in the slow inward calcium current (I_{Ca}) in heart cells; and (3) a reduction in the hyperpolarization-activated current (I_f) that underlies diastolic depolarization. All of these actions are mediated by M_2 receptors and

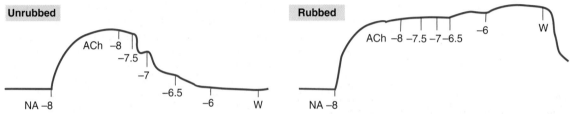

Figure 7–4. Activation of endothelial cell muscarinic receptors by acetylcholine releases endothelium-derived relaxing factor (nitric oxide) (EDRF [NO]), which causes relaxation of vascular smooth muscle precontracted with norepinephrine. Removal of the endothelium by rubbing eliminates the relaxant effect and reveals contraction caused by direct action of acetylcholine on vascular smooth muscle. (NA, noradrenaline [norepinephrine]; ACh, acetylcholine. Numbers indicate the log concentration applied at the time indicated.) (Modified and reproduced, with permission, from Furchgott RF, Zawadzki JV: The obligatory role of endothelial cells in the relaxation of arterial smooth muscle by acetylcholine. Nature 1980;288:373.)

contribute to slowing the pacemaker rate. Effects (1) and (2) cause hyperpolarization and decrease the contractility of atrial cells. Predictably, carbachol does not inhibit sinoatrial rate in animals with mutated M_2 receptors.

The direct slowing of sinoatrial rate and atrioventricular conduction that is produced by muscarinic agonists is often opposed by reflex sympathetic discharge, elicited by the decrease in blood pressure. The resultant sympathetic-parasympathetic interaction is complex because of the muscarinic modulation of sympathetic influences that occurs by inhibition of norepinephrine release and by postjunctional cellular effects. Muscarinic receptors that are present on postganglionic parasympathetic nerve terminals allow neurally released acetylcholine to inhibit its own secretion. The neuronal muscarinic receptors need not be the same subtype as found on effector cells. Therefore, the net effect on heart rate depends on local concentrations of the agonist in the heart and in the vessels and on the level of reflex responsiveness.

Parasympathetic innervation of the ventricles is much less extensive than that of the atria; activation of ventricular muscarinic receptors causes much less physiologic effect than that seen in atria. However, during sympathetic nerve stimulation, the effects of muscarinic agonists on ventricular function are clearly evident because of muscarinic modulation of sympathetic effects ("accentuated antagonism").

In the intact organism, muscarinic agonists produce marked vasodilation. However, earlier studies of isolated blood vessels often showed a contractile response to these agents. It is now known that acetylcholine-induced vasodilation requires the presence of intact endothelium (Figure 7–4). Muscarinic agonists release endothelium-derived relaxing factor (EDRF) from the endothelial cells that relaxes smooth muscle. Isolated vessels prepared with the endothelium preserved consistently reproduce the vasodilation seen in the intact organism. EDRF appears to be largely nitric oxide (NO). This substance activates

guanylyl cyclase and increases cGMP in smooth muscle, resulting in relaxation (see Figure 12–2).

The cardiovascular effects of all of the choline esters are similar to those of acetylcholine, the main difference being in their potency and duration of action. Because of the resistance of methacholine, carbachol, and bethanechol to acetylcholinesterase, lower doses given intravenously are sufficient to produce effects similar to those of acetylcholine, and the duration of action of these synthetic choline esters is longer. The cardiovascular effects of most of the cholinomimetic natural alkaloids and the synthetic analogs are also generally similar to those of acetylcholine.

Pilocarpine is an interesting exception to the above statement. If given intravenously (an experimental exercise), it may produce hypertension after a brief initial hypotensive response. The longer-lasting hypertensive effect can be traced to sympathetic ganglionic discharge caused by activation of postganglionic cell membrane M_1 receptors, which close K^+ channels and elicit slow excitatory (depolarizing) postsynaptic potentials. This effect, like the hypotensive effect, can be blocked by atropine, an antimuscarinic drug.

3. Respiratory system—Muscarinic stimulants contract the smooth muscle of the bronchial tree. In addition, the glands of the tracheobronchial mucosa are stimulated to secrete. This combination of effects can occasionally cause symptoms, especially in individuals with asthma.

4. Gastrointestinal tract—Administration of muscarinic agonists, like parasympathetic nervous system stimulation, increases the secretory and motor activity of the gut. The salivary and gastric glands are strongly stimulated; the pancreas and small intestinal glands less so. Peristaltic activity is increased throughout the gut, and most sphincters are relaxed. Stimulation of contraction in this organ system involves depolarization of the smooth muscle cell membrane and increased calcium influx. Muscarinic agonists do not cause contraction of the ileum in mutant mice lacking M_2 and M_3 receptors. The M_3 receptor is required for direct activation of smooth muscle contraction while the M_2 receptor reduces cAMP formation and relaxation caused by sympathomimetic drugs.

5. Genitourinary tract—Muscarinic agonists stimulate the detrusor muscle and relax the trigone and sphincter muscles of the bladder, thus promoting voiding. The function of M_2 and M_3 receptors in the urinary bladder appears to be the same as in intestinal smooth muscle. The human uterus is not notably sensitive to muscarinic agonists.

6. Miscellaneous secretory glands—Muscarinic agonists stimulate secretion by thermoregulatory sweat, lacrimal, and nasopharyngeal glands.

7. Central nervous system—The central nervous system contains both muscarinic and nicotinic receptors, the brain being relatively richer in muscarinic sites and the spinal cord containing a preponderance of nicotinic sites. The physiologic roles of these receptors are discussed in Chapter 21.

The role of muscarinic receptors in the central nervous system has been confirmed by experiments in knockout mice. The central nervous system effects of the synthetic muscarinic agonist oxotremorine (tremor, hypothermia, and antinociception) were also lacking in mice with homozygously mutated M_2 receptors. Animals lacking M_3 receptors, especially those in the hypothalamus, had reduced appetite and diminished body fat mass. Knockout of M_1 receptors was associated with different changes in the peripheral and central nervous systems. Oxotremorine did not suppress M current in sympathetic ganglia, and pilocarpine did not induce epileptic seizures in M_1 mutant mice.

In spite of the smaller ratio of nicotinic to muscarinic receptors in the brain, nicotine and lobeline (Figure 7–3) have important effects on the brainstem and cortex. The mild alerting action of nicotine absorbed from inhaled tobacco smoke is the best-known of these effects. In high concentrations, nicotine induces tremor, emesis, and stimulation of the respiratory center. At still higher levels, nicotine causes convulsions, which may terminate in fatal coma. The lethal effects on the central nervous system and the fact that nicotine is readily absorbed form the basis for the use of nicotine as an insecticide.

8. Peripheral nervous system—Autonomic ganglia are important sites of nicotinic synaptic action. The nicotinic agents shown in Figure 7–3 cause marked activation of these nicotinic receptors and initiate action potentials in postganglionic neurons (see Figure 6–8). Nicotine itself has a somewhat greater affinity for neuronal than for skeletal muscle nicotinic receptors. The action is the same on both parasympathetic and sympathetic ganglia. The initial response therefore often resembles simultaneous discharge

of both the parasympathetic and the sympathetic nervous systems. In the case of the cardiovascular system, the effects of nicotine are chiefly sympathomimetic. Dramatic hypertension is produced by parenteral injection of nicotine; sympathetic tachycardia may alternate with a bradycardia mediated by vagal discharge. In the gastrointestinal and urinary tracts, the effects are largely parasympathomimetic: nausea, vomiting, diarrhea, and voiding of urine are commonly observed. Prolonged exposure may result in depolarizing blockade of the ganglia.

Neuronal nicotinic receptors are present on sensory nerve endings—especially afferent nerves in coronary arteries and the carotid and aortic bodies as well as on the glomus cells of the latter. Activation of these receptors by nicotinic stimulants and of muscarinic receptors on glomus cells by muscarinic stimulants elicits complex medullary responses, including respiratory alterations and vagal discharge.

9. Neuromuscular junction—The nicotinic receptors on the neuromuscular end plate apparatus are similar but not identical to the receptors in the autonomic ganglia (Table 7–1). Both types respond to acetylcholine and nicotine. (However, as discussed in Chapter 8, the receptors differ in their structural requirements for nicotinic blocking drugs.) When a nicotinic agonist is applied directly (by iontophoresis or by intra-arterial injection), an immediate depolarization of the end plate results, caused by an increase in permeability to sodium and potassium ions. The contractile response varies from disorganized fasciculations of independent motor units to a strong contraction of the entire muscle depending on the synchronization of depolarization of end plates throughout the muscle. Depolarizing nicotinic agents that are not rapidly hydrolyzed (like nicotine itself) cause rapid development of depolarization blockade; transmission blockade persists even when the membrane has repolarized (discussed further in Chapters 8 and 27). This block is manifested as flaccid paralysis in the case of skeletal muscle.

■ II. BASIC PHARMACOLOGY OF THE INDIRECT-ACTING CHOLINOMIMETICS

The actions of acetylcholine released from autonomic and somatic motor nerves are terminated by enzymatic hydrolysis of the molecule. Hydrolysis is accomplished by the action of acetylcholinesterase, which is present in high concentrations in cholinergic synapses. The indirect-acting cholinomimetics have their primary effect at the active site of this enzyme, although some also have direct actions at nicotinic receptors. The chief differences between mem-

Figure 7–5. Cholinesterase inhibitors. Neostigmine exemplifies the typical ester composed of carbamic acid ([1]) and a phenol bearing a quaternary ammonium group ([2]). Physostigmine, a naturally occurring carbamate, is a tertiary amine. Edrophonium is not an ester but binds to the active site of the enzyme.

bers of the group are chemical and pharmacokinetic—their pharmacodynamic properties are almost identical.

Chemistry & Pharmacokinetics

A. STRUCTURE

There are three chemical groups of cholinesterase inhibitors: (1) simple alcohols bearing a quaternary ammonium group, eg, edrophonium; (2) carbamic acid esters of alcohols bearing quaternary or tertiary ammonium groups (carbamates, eg, neostigmine); and (3) organic derivatives of phosphoric acid (organophosphates, eg, echothiophate). Examples of the first two groups are shown in Figure 7–5. Edrophonium, neostigmine, and pyridostigmine are synthetic quaternary ammonium agents used in medicine. Physostigmine (eserine) is a naturally occurring tertiary amine of greater lipid solubility that is also used in therapeutics. Carbaryl (carbaril) is typical of a large group of carbamate insecticides designed for very high lipid solubility, so that absorption into the insect and distribution to its central nervous system are very rapid.

A few of the estimated 50,000 organophosphates are shown in Figure 7–6. Many of the organophosphates (echothiophate is an exception) are highly lipid-soluble liquids. Echothiophate, a thiocholine derivative, is of clinical value because it retains the very long duration of action of other organophosphates but is more stable in aqueous solution. Soman is an extremely potent "nerve gas." Parathion and malathion are thiophos-phate prodrugs that are inactive as such; they are converted to the phosphate derivatives in animals and plants and are used as insecticides.

B. ABSORPTION, DISTRIBUTION, AND METABOLISM

Absorption of the quaternary carbamates from the conjunctiva, skin, and lungs is predictably poor, since their permanent charge renders them relatively insoluble in lipids. Thus, much larger doses are required for oral administration than for parenteral injection. Distribution into the central nervous system is negligible. Physostigmine, in contrast, is well absorbed from all sites and can be used topically in the eye (see Table 7–4). It is distributed into the central nervous system and is more toxic than the more polar quaternary carbamates. The carbamates are relatively stable in aqueous solution but can be metabolized by nonspecific esterases in the body as well as by cholinesterase. However, the duration of their effect is determined chiefly by the stability of the inhibitor-enzyme complex (see Mechanism of Action, below), not by metabolism or excretion.

The organophosphate cholinesterase inhibitors (except for echothiophate) are well absorbed from the skin, lung, gut, and conjunctiva—thereby making them dangerous to humans and highly effective as insecticides. They are relatively less stable than the carbamates when dissolved in water and thus have a limited half-life in the environment (compared with the other major class of insecticides, the halogenated hydrocarbons, eg, DDT). Echothiophate is highly polar and more stable than most

Figure 7–6. Structures of some organophosphate cholinesterase inhibitors. The dashed lines indicate the bond that is hydrolyzed in binding to the enzyme. The shaded ester bonds in malathion represent the points of detoxification of the molecule in mammals and birds.

other organophosphates. When prepared in aqueous solution for ophthalmic use, it retains activity for weeks.

The thiophosphate insecticides (parathion, malathion, and related compounds) are quite lipid-soluble and are rapidly absorbed by all routes. They must be activated in the body by conversion to the oxygen analogs (Figure 7–6), a process that occurs rapidly in both insects and vertebrates. Malathion and a few other organophosphate insecticides are also rapidly metabolized by other pathways to inactive products in birds and mammals but not in insects; these agents are therefore considered safe enough for sale to the general public. Unfortunately, fish cannot detoxify malathion, and significant numbers of fish have died from the heavy use of this agent on and near waterways. Parathion is not detoxified effectively in vertebrates; thus, it is considerably more dangerous than malathion to humans and livestock and is not available for general public use.

All of the organophosphates except echothiophate are distributed to all parts of the body, including the central nervous system. Poisoning with these agents therefore includes an important component of central nervous system toxicity.

Pharmacodynamics

A. MECHANISM OF ACTION

Acetylcholinesterase is the primary target of these drugs, but butyrylcholinesterase is also inhibited. Acetylcholinesterase is an extremely active enzyme. In the initial catalytic step, acetylcholine binds to the enzyme's active site and is hydrolyzed, yielding free choline and the acetylated enzyme. In the second step, the covalent acetyl-enzyme bond is split, with the addition of water (hydration). The entire process takes place in approximately 150 microseconds.

All of the cholinesterase inhibitors increase the concentration of endogenous acetylcholine at cholinoceptors by inhibiting acetylcholinesterase. However, the molecular details of their interaction with the enzyme vary according to the three chemical subgroups mentioned above.

The first group, of which edrophonium is the major example, consists of quaternary alcohols. These agents reversibly bind electrostatically and by hydrogen bonds to the active site, thus preventing access of acetylcholine. The enzyme-inhibitor complex does not involve a covalent bond and is correspondingly short-lived (on the order of 2–10 minutes). The second group consists of carbamate esters, eg, neostigmine and physostigmine. These agents undergo a two-step hydrolysis sequence analogous to that described for acetylcholine. However, the covalent bond of the *carbamoylated* enzyme is considerably more resistant to the second (hydration) process, and this step is correspondingly prolonged (on the order of 30 minutes to 6 hours). The third group consists of the organophosphates. These agents also undergo initial binding and hydrolysis by the enzyme, resulting in a *phosphorylated* active site. The covalent phosphorus-enzyme bond is extremely stable and hydrolyzes in water at a very slow rate (hundreds of hours). After the initial binding-hydrolysis step, the phosphorylated enzyme complex may undergo a process called **aging.** This process apparently involves the breaking of one of the oxygen-phosphorus bonds of the inhibitor and further strengthens the phosphorus-enzyme bond. The rate of aging varies with the particular organophosphate compound. If given before aging has occurred, strong nucleophiles like pralidoxime are able to break the phosphorus-enzyme bond and can be used as "cholinesterase regenerator" drugs for organophosphate insecticide poisoning (see Chapter 8). Once aging has occurred, the enzyme-inhibitor complex is even more stable and is more difficult to break, even with oxime regenerator compounds.

The organophosphate inhibitors are sometimes referred to as "irreversible" cholinesterase inhibitors, and edrophonium and the carbamates are considered "reversible" inhibitors because of the marked differences in duration of action. However, the molecular mechanisms of action of the three groups do not support this simplistic description.

B. ORGAN SYSTEM EFFECTS

The most prominent pharmacologic effects of cholinesterase inhibitors are on the cardiovascular and gastrointestinal systems, the eye, and the skeletal muscle neuromuscular junction. Because the primary action is to amplify the actions of endogenous acetylcholine, the effects are similar (but not always identical) to the effects of the direct-acting cholinomimetic agonists.

1. Central nervous system—In low concentrations, the lipid-soluble cholinesterase inhibitors cause diffuse activation on the electroencephalogram and a subjective alerting response. In higher concentrations, they cause generalized convulsions, which may be followed by coma and respiratory arrest.

2. Eye, respiratory tract, gastrointestinal tract, urinary tract—The effects of the cholinesterase inhibitors on these organ systems, all of which are well innervated by the parasympathetic nervous system, are qualitatively quite similar to the effects of the direct-acting cholinomimetics (Table 7–3).

3. Cardiovascular system—The cholinesterase inhibitors can increase activity in both sympathetic and parasympathetic ganglia supplying the heart and at the acetylcholine receptors on neuroeffector cells (cardiac and vascular smooth muscles) that receive cholinergic innervation.

In the heart, the effects on the parasympathetic limb predominate. Thus, cholinesterase inhibitors such as edrophonium, physostigmine, or neostigmine mimic the effects of vagal nerve activation on the heart. Negative chronotropic, dromotropic, and inotropic effects are produced, and cardiac output falls. The fall in cardiac output is attributable to bradycardia, decreased atrial contractility, and some reduction in ventricular contractility. The latter effect occurs as a result of prejunctional inhibition

of norepinephrine release as well as inhibition of postjunctional cellular sympathetic effects.

Cholinesterase inhibitors have less marked effects on vascular smooth muscle and on blood pressure than direct-acting muscarinic agonists. This is because indirect-acting drugs can modify the tone of only those vessels that are innervated by cholinergic nerves and because the net effects on vascular tone may reflect activation of both the parasympathetic and sympathetic nervous systems. The cholinomimetic effect at the smooth muscle effector tissue is minimal since few vascular beds receive cholinergic innervation. Activation of sympathetic ganglia may increase vascular resistance.

The *net* cardiovascular effects of moderate doses of cholinesterase inhibitors therefore consist of modest bradycardia, a fall in cardiac output, and no change or a modest fall in blood pressure. Large (toxic) doses of these drugs cause more marked bradycardia (occasionally tachycardia) and hypotension.

4. Neuromuscular junction—The cholinesterase inhibitors have important therapeutic and toxic effects at the skeletal muscle neuromuscular junction. Low (therapeutic) concentrations moderately prolong and intensify the actions of physiologically released acetylcholine. This increases strength of contraction, especially in muscles weakened by curare-like neuromuscular blocking agents or by myasthenia gravis. At higher concentrations, the accumulation of acetylcholine may result in fibrillation of muscle fibers. Antidromic firing of the motor neuron may also occur, resulting in fasciculations that involve an entire motor unit. With marked inhibition of acetylcholinesterase, depolarizing neuromuscular blockade occurs and that may be followed by a phase of nondepolarizing blockade as seen with succinylcholine (see Table 27–2 and Figure 27–7).

Some quaternary carbamate cholinesterase inhibitors, eg, neostigmine, have an additional *direct* nicotinic agonist effect at the neuromuscular junction. This may contribute to the effectiveness of these agents as therapy for myasthenia.

■ III. CLINICAL PHARMACOLOGY OF THE CHOLINOMIMETICS

The major therapeutic uses of the cholinomimetics are for diseases of the eye (glaucoma, accommodative esotropia), the gastrointestinal and urinary tracts (postoperative atony, neurogenic bladder), the neuromuscular junction (myasthenia gravis, curare-induced neuromuscular paralysis), and very rarely, the heart (certain atrial arrhythmias). Cholinesterase inhibitors are occasionally used in the treatment of atropine overdosage. Several newer cholinesterase inhibitors are being used to treat patients with Alzheimer's disease.

Clinical Uses

A. THE EYE

Glaucoma is a disease characterized by increased intraocular pressure. Muscarinic stimulants and cholinesterase inhibitors reduce intraocular pressure by causing contraction of the ciliary body so as to facilitate outflow of aqueous humor and perhaps also by diminishing the rate of its secretion (see Figure 6–9). In the past, glaucoma was treated with either direct agonists (pilocarpine, methacholine, carbachol) or cholinesterase inhibitors (physostigmine, demecarium, echothiophate, isoflurophate). For chronic glaucoma, these drugs have been largely replaced by topical β-blockers and prostaglandin derivatives.

Acute angle-closure glaucoma is a medical emergency that is frequently treated initially with drugs but usually requires surgery for permanent correction. Initial therapy often consists of a combination of a direct muscarinic agonist and a cholinesterase inhibitor (eg, pilocarpine plus physostigmine) as well as other drugs. Once the intraocular pressure is controlled and the danger of vision loss is diminished, the patient can be prepared for corrective surgery (iridectomy). Open-angle glaucoma and some cases of secondary glaucoma are chronic diseases that are not amenable to traditional surgical correction although newer laser techniques appear to be useful. Other treatments for glaucoma are described in the Box, Treatment of Glaucoma in Chapter 10.

Accommodative esotropia (strabismus caused by hypermetropic accommodative error) in young children is sometimes diagnosed and treated with cholinomimetic agonists. Dosage is similar to or higher than that used for glaucoma.

B. GASTROINTESTINAL AND URINARY TRACTS

In clinical disorders that involve depression of smooth muscle activity without obstruction, cholinomimetic drugs with direct or indirect muscarinic effects may be helpful. These disorders include postoperative ileus (atony or paralysis of the stomach or bowel following surgical manipulation) and congenital megacolon. Urinary retention may occur postoperatively or postpartum or may be secondary to spinal cord injury or disease (neurogenic bladder). Cholinomimetics are also sometimes used to increase the tone of the lower esophageal sphincter in patients with reflux esophagitis. Of the choline esters, bethanechol is the most widely used for these disorders. For gastrointestinal problems, it is usually administered orally in a dose of 10–25 mg three or four times daily. In patients with urinary retention,

bethanechol can be given subcutaneously in a dose of 5 mg and repeated in 30 minutes if necessary. Of the cholinesterase inhibitors, neostigmine is the most widely used for these applications. For paralytic ileus or atony of the urinary bladder, neostigmine can be given subcutaneously in a dose of 0.5–1 mg. If patients are able to take the drug by mouth, neostigmine can be given orally in a dose of 15 mg. In all of these situations, the clinician must be certain that there is no mechanical obstruction to outflow prior to using the cholinomimetic. Otherwise, the drug may exacerbate the problem and may even cause perforation as a result of increased pressure.

Pilocarpine has long been used to increase salivary secretion. Cevimeline, a quinuclidine derivative of acetylcholine, is a new direct-acting muscarinic agonist used for the treatment of dry mouth associated with Sjögren's syndrome.

C. NEUROMUSCULAR JUNCTION

Myasthenia gravis is a disease affecting skeletal muscle neuromuscular junctions. An autoimmune process causes production of antibodies that bind to the α subunits of the nicotinic receptor. This effect causes accelerated degradation of the receptor and blockade of acetylcholine binding to receptors on muscle end plates. Frequent findings are ptosis, diplopia, difficulty in speaking and swallowing, and extremity weakness. Severe disease may affect all the muscles, including those necessary for respiration. The disease resembles the neuromuscular paralysis produced by d-tubocurarine and similar nondepolarizing neuromuscular blocking drugs (see Chapter 27). Patients with myasthenia are exquisitely sensitive to the action of curariform drugs and other drugs that interfere with neuromuscular transmission, eg, aminoglycoside antibiotics.

Cholinesterase inhibitors—but not direct-acting acetylcholine receptor agonists—are extremely valuable as therapy for myasthenia. Almost all patients are also treated with immunosuppressant drugs and some with thymectomy.

Edrophonium is sometimes used as a diagnostic test for myasthenia. A 2 mg dose is injected intravenously after baseline measurements of muscle strength have been obtained. If no reaction occurs after 45 seconds, an additional 8 mg may be injected. If the patient has myasthenia gravis, an improvement in muscle strength that lasts about 5 minutes will usually be observed.

Edrophonium is also used to assess the adequacy of treatment with the longer-acting cholinesterase inhibitors in patients with myasthenia gravis. If excessive amounts of cholinesterase inhibitor have been used, patients may become paradoxically weak because of nicotinic depolarizing blockade of the motor end plate.

These patients may also exhibit symptoms of excessive stimulation of muscarinic receptors (abdominal cramps, diarrhea, increased salivation, excessive bronchial secretions, miosis, bradycardia). Small doses of edrophonium (1–2 mg intravenously) will produce no relief or even worsen weakness if the patient is receiving excessive cholinesterase inhibitor therapy. On the other hand, if the patient improves with edrophonium, an increase in cholinesterase inhibitor dosage may be indicated. Clinical situations in which severe myasthenia (myasthenic crisis) must be distinguished from excessive drug therapy (cholinergic crisis) usually occur in very ill myasthenic patients and must be managed in hospital with adequate emergency support systems (eg, mechanical ventilators) available.

Long-term therapy for myasthenia gravis is usually accomplished with pyridostigmine; neostigmine or ambenonium are alternatives. The doses are titrated to optimum levels based on changes in muscle strength. These agents are relatively short-acting and therefore require frequent dosing (every 6 hours for pyridostigmine and ambenonium and every 4 hours for neostigmine; Table 7–4). Sustained-release preparations are available but should be used only at night and if needed. Longer-acting cholinesterase inhibitors such as the organophosphate agents are not used, because the dose requirement in this disease changes too rapidly to permit smooth control with long-acting drugs.

If muscarinic effects of such therapy are prominent, they can be controlled by the administration of antimuscarinic drugs such as atropine. Frequently, tolerance to the muscarinic effects of the cholinesterase inhibitors develops, so atropine treatment is not required.

Neuromuscular blockade is frequently produced as an adjunct to surgical anesthesia, using nondepolarizing neuromuscular relaxants such as pancuronium and newer agents (see Chapter 27). Following surgery, it is usually desirable to reverse this pharmacologic paralysis promptly. This can be easily accomplished with cholinesterase inhibitors; neostigmine and edrophonium are the drugs of choice. They are given intravenously or intramuscularly for prompt effect.

D. HEART

The short-acting cholinesterase inhibitor edrophonium was used to treat supraventricular tachyarrhythmias, particularly paroxysmal supraventricular tachycardia. In this application, edrophonium has been replaced by newer drugs (adenosine and the calcium channel blockers verapamil and diltiazem).

E. ANTIMUSCARINIC DRUG INTOXICATION

Atropine intoxication is potentially lethal in children (see Chapter 8) and may cause prolonged severe behavioral disturbances and arrhythmias in adults. The tricyclic antidepressants, when taken in overdosage (often with suicidal intent), also cause severe muscarinic blockade (see Chapter 30). The muscarinic receptor blockade produced by all these agents is competitive in nature and can be overcome by increasing the amount of endogenous acetylcholine present at the neuroeffector junctions. Theoretically, a cholinesterase inhibitor could be used to reverse these effects. Physostigmine has been used for this application, because it enters the central nervous system and reverses the central as well as the peripheral signs of muscarinic blockade. However, as noted previously, physostigmine itself can produce dangerous central nervous system effects, and such therapy is therefore used only in patients with dangerous elevation of body temperature or very rapid supraventricular tachycardia.

F. CENTRAL NERVOUS SYSTEM

Tacrine is a drug with anticholinesterase and other cholinomimetic actions that has been used for the treatment of mild to moderate Alzheimer's disease. Tacrine's efficacy is modest and hepatic toxicity is significant. Donepezil, galantamine, and rivastigmine are newer, more selective acetylcholinesterase inhibitors that appear to have the same modest clinical benefit as tacrine in treatment of cognitive dysfunction in Alzheimer's patients. Donepezil may be given once daily because of its long half-life, and it lacks the hepatotoxic effect of tacrine. However, no comparative trials of these newer drugs and tacrine have been reported. These drugs are discussed in Chapter 61.

Table 7–4. Therapeutic uses and durations of action of cholinesterase inhibitors.

	Uses	Approximate Duration of Action
Alcohols		
Edrophonium	Myasthenia gravis, ileus, arrhythmias	5–15 minutes
Carbamates and related agents		
Neostigmine	Myasthenia gravis, ileus	0.5–2 hours
Pyridostigmine	Myasthenia gravis	3–6 hours
Physostigmine	Glaucoma	0.5–2 hours
Ambenonium	Myasthenia gravis	4–8 hours
Demecarium	Glaucoma	4–6 hours
Organophosphates		
Echothiophate	Glaucoma	100 hours

Varenicline is a new direct-acting nicotinic agonist that is approved for use in smoking cessation treatment. It appears to have some selectivity for the $\alpha_4\beta_2$ isoform of the N_N receptor. It is orally active and has a half-life of 14–20 hours. Toxicity includes nausea, headache, and sleep disturbances.

Toxicity

The toxic potential of the cholinoceptor stimulants varies markedly depending on their absorption, access to the central nervous system, and metabolism.

A. DIRECT-ACTING MUSCARINIC STIMULANTS

Drugs such as pilocarpine and the choline esters cause predictable signs of muscarinic excess when given in overdosage. These effects include nausea, vomiting, diarrhea, urinary urgency, salivation, sweating, cutaneous vasodilation, and bronchial constriction. The effects are all blocked competitively by atropine and its congeners.

Certain mushrooms, especially those of the genus *Inocybe,* contain muscarinic alkaloids. Ingestion of these mushrooms causes typical signs of muscarinic excess within 15–30 minutes. Treatment is with atropine, 1–2 mg parenterally. (*Amanita muscaria,* the first source of muscarine, contains very low concentrations of the alkaloid.)

B. DIRECT-ACTING NICOTINIC STIMULANTS

Nicotine itself is the only common cause of this type of poisoning. The acute toxicity of the alkaloid is well-defined but much less important than the chronic effects associated with smoking. In addition to tobacco products, nicotine is also used in insecticides.

1. Acute toxicity—The fatal dose of nicotine is approximately 40 mg, or 1 drop of the pure liquid. This is the amount of nicotine in two regular cigarettes. Fortunately, most of the nicotine in cigarettes is destroyed by burning or escapes via the "sidestream" smoke. Ingestion of nicotine insecticides or of tobacco by infants and children is usually followed by vomiting, limiting the amount of the alkaloid absorbed.

The toxic effects of a large dose of nicotine are simple extensions of the effects described previously. The most dangerous are (1) central stimulant actions, which cause convulsions and may progress to coma and respiratory arrest; (2) skeletal muscle end plate depolarization, which may lead to depolarization blockade and respiratory paralysis; and (3) hypertension and cardiac arrhythmias.

Treatment of acute nicotine poisoning is largely symptom-directed. Muscarinic excess resulting from parasympathetic ganglion stimulation can be controlled with atropine. Central stimulation is usually treated with parenteral anticonvulsants such as diazepam. Neuromuscular blockade is not responsive to pharmacologic treatment and may require mechanical respiration.

Fortunately, nicotine is metabolized and excreted relatively rapidly. Patients who survive the first 4 hours usually recover completely if hypoxia and brain damage have not occurred.

2. Chronic nicotine toxicity—The health costs of tobacco smoking to the smoker and its socioeconomic costs to the general public are still incompletely understood. However, the 1979 *Surgeon General's Report on Health Promotion and Disease Prevention* stated that "cigarette smoking is clearly the largest single preventable cause of illness and premature death in the United States." This statement has been supported by numerous subsequent studies. Unfortunately, the fact that the most important of the tobacco-associated diseases are delayed in onset reduces the health incentive to stop smoking.

Clearly, the addictive power of cigarettes is directly related to their nicotine content. It is not known to what extent nicotine per se contributes to the other well-documented adverse effects of chronic tobacco use. It appears highly probable that nicotine contributes to the increased risk of vascular disease and sudden coronary death associated with smoking. Also, nicotine probably contributes to the high incidence of ulcer recurrences in smokers with peptic ulcer.

C. CHOLINESTERASE INHIBITORS

The acute toxic effects of the cholinesterase inhibitors, like those of the direct-acting agents, are direct extensions of their pharmacologic actions. The major source of such intoxications is pesticide use in agriculture and in the home. Approximately 100 organophosphate and 20 carbamate cholinesterase inhibitors are available in pesticides and veterinary vermifuges used in the USA.

Acute intoxication must be recognized and treated promptly in patients with heavy exposure. The dominant initial signs are those of muscarinic excess: miosis, salivation, sweating, bronchial constriction, vomiting, and diarrhea. Central nervous system involvement usually follows rapidly, accompanied by peripheral nicotinic effects, especially depolarizing neuromuscular blockade. Therapy always includes (1) maintenance of vital signs—respiration in particular may be impaired; (2) decontamination to prevent further absorption—this may require removal of all clothing and washing of the skin in cases of exposure to dusts and sprays; and (3) atropine parenterally in large doses, given as often as required to control signs of muscarinic excess. Therapy often also includes treatment with pralidoxime as described in Chapter 8.

Chronic exposure to certain organophosphate compounds, including some organophosphate cholinesterase inhibitors, causes neuropathy associated with demyelination of axons. **Triorthocresylphosphate,** an additive in lubricating oils, is the prototype agent of this class. The effects are not caused by cholinesterase inhibition.

PREPARATIONS AVAILABLE

DIRECT-ACTING CHOLINOMIMETICS

Acetylcholine (Miochol-E)
Ophthalmic: 1% intraocular solution

Bethanechol (generic, Urecholine)
Oral: 5, 10, 25, 50 mg tablets
Parenteral: 5 mg/mL for SC injection

Carbachol
Ophthalmic (topical, Isopto Carbachol, Carboptic): 0.75, 1.5, 2.25, 3% solution
Ophthalmic (intraocular, Miostat, Carbastat): 0.01% solution

Cevimeline (Evoxac)
Oral: 30 mg capsules

Pilocarpine (generic, Isopto Carpine)
Ophthalmic (topical): 0.5, 1, 2, 3, 4, 6, 8, 10% solutions, 4% gel
Ophthalmic sustained-release inserts (Ocusert Pilo-20, Ocusert Pilo-40): release 20 and 40 mcg pilocarpine per hour for 1 week, respectively
Oral (Salagen): 5 mg tablets

Varenicline (Chantix)
Oral: 0.5, 1 mg tablets

CHOLINESTERASE INHIBITORS

Ambenonium (Mytelase)
Oral: 10 mg tablets

Demecarium (Humorsol)
Ophthalmic: 0.125, 0.25% drops

Donepezil (Aricept)
Oral: 5, 10 mg tablets

Echothiophate (Phospholine)
Ophthalmic: 1.5 mg (0.03%) powder to reconstitute for solution; 0.06, 0.125, 0.25% drops

Edrophonium (generic, Tensilon)
Parenteral: 10 mg/mL for IM or IV injection

Galantamine (Reminyl)
Oral: 4, 8, 12 mg tablets; 4 mg/mL solution

Neostigmine (generic, Prostigmin)
Oral: 15 mg tablets
Parenteral: 0.2, 0.5, 1, 2.5 mg/mL solution

Physostigmine, eserine (generic)
Ophthalmic: 0.25% ointment; 0.25, 0.5% solution
Parenteral: 1 mg/mL for IM or slow IV injection

Pyridostigmine (Mestinon, Regonol)
Oral: 30, 60 mg tablets; 180 mg sustained-release tablets; 12 mg/mL syrup
Parenteral: 5 mg/mL for IM or slow IV injection

Rivastigmine (Exelon)
Oral: 1.5, 3, 4.5, 6 mg tablets; 2 mg/mL solution

Tacrine (Cognex)
Oral: 10, 20, 30, 40 mg tablets

REFERENCES

Boehm S, Kubista H: Fine tuning of sympathetic transmitter release via ionotropic and metabotropic presynaptic receptors. Pharmacol Rev 2002;54:43.

Brodde OE et al: Presence, distribution and physiological function of adrenergic and muscarinic receptor subtypes in the human heart. Basic Res Cardiol 2001;96:528.

Celie PH et al: Nicotine and carbamylcholine binding to nicotinic acetylcholine receptors as studied in AChBP crystal structures. Neuron 2004;41:907.

Eglen RM, Choppin A, Watson N: Therapeutic opportunities from muscarinic receptor research. Trends Pharmacol Sci 2001;22:409.

Ehlert FJ: Contractile role of M2 and M3 muscarinic receptors in gastrointestinal, airway and urinary bladder smooth muscle. Life Sci 2003;74:355.

Fox RI, Konttinen Y, Fisher A: Use of muscarinic agonists in the treatment of Sjögren's syndrome. Clin Immunol 2001;101:249.

Furchgott RF, Zawadzki JV: The obligatory role of endothelial cells in the relaxation of arterial smooth muscle by acetylcholine. Nature 1980;288:373.

Gerthoffer WT: Signal-transduction pathways that regulate visceral smooth muscle function. III. Coupling of muscarinic receptors to signaling kinases and effector proteins in gastrointestinal smooth muscles. Am J Physiol 2005;288:G849.

Harvey RD, Belevych AE: Muscarinic regulation of cardiac ion channels. Br J Pharmacol 2003;139:1074.

Hobbiger F: Pharmacology of anticholinesterase drugs. In: Zaimis E (editor): *Handbook of Experimental Pharmacology. Vol. 42: Neuromuscular Junction.* Springer, 1976.

Hogg RC, Raggenbass M, Bertrand D: Nicotinic acetylcholine receptors: From structure to brain function. Rev Physiol Biochem Pharmacol 2003;147:1.

Irvine RF, Schell MJ: Back in the water: The return of the inositol phosphates. Nat Rev Mol Cell Biol 2001;2:327.

Lukas RJ et al: International Union of Pharmacology. XX. Current status of the nomenclature for nicotinic acetylcholine receptors and their subunits. Pharmacol Rev 1999;51:397.

Matsui M et al: Increased relaxant action of forskolin and isoproterenol against muscarinic agonist-induced contractions in smooth muscle from M_2 receptor knockout mice. J Pharmacol Exp Ther 2003;305:106.

Molitor H: A comparative study of the effects of five choline compounds used in therapeutics: Acetylcholine chloride, acetyl-beta-methylcholine chloride, carbaminoyl choline, ethyl ether beta-methylcholine chloride, carbaminoyl beta-methylcholine chloride. J Pharmacol Exp Ther 1936; 58:337.

Okamoto H et al: Muscarinic agonist potencies at three different effector systems linked to the M(2) or M(3) receptor in longitudinal smooth muscle of guinea-pig small intestine. Br J Pharmacol 2002;135:1765.

Smulders CJ et al: Selective effects of carbamate pesticides on rat neuronal nicotinic acetylcholine receptors and rat brain acetylcholinesterase. Toxicol Appl Pharmacol 2003;193:139.

The Surgeon General: Smoking and Health. US Department of Health and Human Services, 1979.

Unwin N: Structure and action of the nicotinic acetylcholine receptor explored by electron microscopy. FEBS Lett 2003;555:91.

Vincent A, Drachman DB: Myasthenia gravis. Adv Neurol 2002; 88:159.

Wess J: Muscarinic acetylcholine receptor knockout mice: novel phenotypes and clinical implications. Annu Rev Pharmacol Toxicol 2004;44:423.

Cholinoceptor-Blocking Drugs

8

Achilles J. Pappano, PhD

Cholinoceptor antagonists, like agonists, are divided into muscarinic and nicotinic subgroups on the basis of their specific receptor affinities. Ganglion-blockers and neuromuscular junction blockers comprise the antinicotinic drugs. The ganglion-blocking drugs have little clinical use and are discussed at the end of this chapter. The neuromuscular blockers are discussed in Chapter 27. This chapter emphasizes drugs that block muscarinic cholinoceptors.

Five subtypes of muscarinic receptors have been identified, primarily on the basis of data from ligand-binding and cDNA-cloning experiments (see Chapters 6 and 7). A standard terminology (M_1 through M_5) for these subtypes is now in common use, and evidence, based mostly on selective agonists and antagonists, indicates that functional differences exist between several of these subtypes.

As suggested in Chapter 6, the M_1 receptor subtype is located on central nervous system neurons, sympathetic postganglionic cell bodies, and many presynaptic sites. M_2 receptors are located in the myocardium, smooth muscle organs, and some neuronal sites. M_3 receptors are most common on effector cell membranes, especially glandular and smooth muscle cells.

■ I. BASIC PHARMACOLOGY OF THE MUSCARINIC RECEPTOR-BLOCKING DRUGS

Muscarinic antagonists are sometimes called parasympatholytic because they block the effects of parasympathetic autonomic discharge. However, they do not "lyse" parasympathetic nerves, and they have some effects that are not predictable from block of the parasympathetic nervous system. For these reasons, the term "antimuscarinic" is preferable.

Naturally occurring compounds with antimuscarinic effects have been known and used for millennia as medicines, poisons, and cosmetics. Atropine is the prototype of these drugs. Many similar plant alkaloids are

known, and hundreds of synthetic antimuscarinic compounds have been prepared.

Chemistry & Pharmacokinetics

A. SOURCE AND CHEMISTRY

Atropine and its naturally occurring congeners are tertiary amine alkaloid esters of tropic acid (Figure 8–1). Atropine (hyoscyamine) is found in the plant *Atropa belladonna*, or deadly nightshade, and in *Datura stramonium*, also known as jimsonweed (Jamestown weed), sacred Datura, or thorn apple. Scopolamine (hyoscine) occurs in *Hyoscyamus niger*, or henbane, as the *l*(−) stereoisomer. Naturally occurring atropine is *l*(−)-hyoscyamine, but the compound readily racemizes, so the commercial material is racemic *d,l*-hyoscyamine. The *l*(−) isomers of both alkaloids are at least 100 times more potent than the *d*(+) isomers.

A variety of semisynthetic and fully synthetic molecules have antimuscarinic effects.

The tertiary members of these classes (Figure 8–2) are often used for their effects on the eye or the central nervous system. Many antihistaminic (see Chapter 16), antipsychotic (see Chapter 29), and antidepressant (see Chapter 30) drugs have similar structures and, predictably, significant antimuscarinic effects.

Quaternary amine antimuscarinic agents (Figure 8–2) have been developed to produce more peripheral effects with reduced central nervous system effects.

B. ABSORPTION

The natural alkaloids and most tertiary antimuscarinic drugs are well absorbed from the gut and conjunctival membranes. When applied in a suitable vehicle, some (eg, scopolamine) are even absorbed across the skin (transdermal route). In contrast, only 10–30% of a dose of a quaternary antimuscarinic drug is absorbed after oral administration, reflecting the decreased lipid solubility of the charged molecule.

C. DISTRIBUTION

Atropine and the other tertiary agents are widely distributed in the body. Significant levels are achieved in the central nervous system within 30 minutes to 1

Figure 8–1. The structure of atropine (oxygen at *[1]* is missing) or scopolamine (oxygen present). In homatropine, the hydroxymethyl at *[2]* is replaced by a hydroxyl group, and the oxygen at *[1]* is absent.

hour, and this can limit the dose tolerated when the drug is taken for its peripheral effects. Scopolamine is rapidly and fully distributed into the central nervous system where it has greater effects than most other antimuscarinic drugs. In contrast, the quaternary derivatives are poorly taken up by the brain and therefore are relatively free—at low doses—of central nervous system effects.

D. Metabolism and Excretion

After administration, atropine disappears rapidly from the blood with a half-life of 2 hours. About 60% of the dose is excreted unchanged in the urine. Most of the rest appears in the urine as hydrolysis and conjugation products. The drug's effect on parasympathetic function declines rapidly in all organs except the eye. Effects on the iris and ciliary muscle persist for ≥ 72 hours.

Pharmacodynamics

A. Mechanism of Action

Atropine causes reversible (surmountable) blockade (see Chapter 2) of cholinomimetic actions at muscarinic receptors—ie, blockade by a small dose of atropine can be overcome by a larger concentration of acetylcholine or equivalent muscarinic agonist. Mutation experiments suggest that aspartate in the receptor forms the characteristic bond with the nitrogen atom of acetylcholine; this amino acid is also required for binding of antimuscarinic drugs. When atropine binds to the muscarinic receptor, it prevents actions such as the release of inositol trisphosphate (IP_3) and the inhibition of adenylyl cyclase that are caused by muscarinic agonists (see Chapter 7).

The effectiveness of antimuscarinic drugs varies with the tissue and with the source of agonist. Tissues most sensitive to atropine are the salivary, bronchial, and sweat glands. Secretion of acid by the gastric parietal cells is the least sensitive. In most tissues, antimuscarinic agents block exogenously administered cholinoceptor agonists more effectively than endogenously released acetylcholine.

Atropine is highly selective for muscarinic receptors. Its potency at nicotinic receptors is much lower, and actions at nonmuscarinic receptors are generally undetectable clinically.

Atropine does not distinguish between the M_1, M_2, and M_3 subgroups of muscarinic receptors. In contrast, other antimuscarinic drugs are moderately selective for one or another of these subgroups (Table 8–1). Most synthetic antimuscarinic drugs are considerably less selective than atropine in interactions with nonmuscarinic receptors. For example, some quaternary amine antimuscarinic agents have significant ganglion-blocking actions, and others are potent histamine receptor blockers. The antimuscarinic effects of other agents, eg, antipsychotic and antidepressant drugs, have been mentioned. Their relative selectivity for muscarinic receptor subtypes has not been defined.

B. Organ System Effects

1. Central nervous system—In the doses usually used, atropine has minimal stimulant effects on the central nervous system, especially the parasympathetic medullary centers, and a slower, longer-lasting sedative effect on the brain. Scopolamine has more marked central effects, producing drowsiness when given in recommended dosages and amnesia in sensitive individuals. In toxic doses, scopolamine and to a lesser degree atropine can cause excitement, agitation, hallucinations, and coma.

The tremor of Parkinson's disease is reduced by centrally acting antimuscarinic drugs, and atropine—in the form of belladonna extract—was one of the first drugs used in the therapy of this disease. As discussed in Chapter 28, parkinsonian tremor and rigidity seem to result from a *relative* excess of cholinergic activity because of a deficiency of dopaminergic activity in the basal ganglia-striatum system. The combination of an antimuscarinic agent with a dopamine precursor drug (levodopa) can sometimes provide more effective therapy than either drug alone.

Vestibular disturbances, especially motion sickness, appear to involve muscarinic cholinergic transmission. Scopolamine is often effective in preventing or reversing these disturbances.

2. Eye—The pupillary constrictor muscle (see Figure 6–9) depends on muscarinic cholinoceptor activation. This activation is blocked by topical atropine and other tertiary antimuscarinic drugs and results in unopposed sympathetic dilator activity and mydriasis (Figure 8–3). Dilated pupils were considered cosmetically desirable during the Renaissance and account for the name bella-

Quaternary amines for gastrointestinal applications (peptic disease, hypermotility):

Propantheline

Glycopyrrolate

Tertiary amines for peripheral applications:

Pirenzepine
(peptic disease)

Dicyclomine
(peptic disease, hypermotility)

Tropicamide
(mydriatic, cycloplegic)

Quaternary amine for use in asthma:

Tertiary amine for Parkinson's disease:

Ipratropium

Benztropine

Figure 8–2. Structures of some semisynthetic and synthetic antimuscarinic drugs.

Table 8–1. Muscarinic receptor subgroups and their antagonists.

Property	Subgroup		
	M_1	M_2	M_3
Primary locations	Nerves	Heart, nerves, smooth muscle	Glands, smooth muscle, endothelium
Dominant effector system	↑IP$_3$, ↑DAG	↓cAMP, ↑K$^+$ channel current	↑IP$_3$, ↑DAG
Antagonists	Pirenzepine, telenzepine, dicyclomine,[2] trihexyphenidyl[3]	Gallamine,[1] methoctramine, AF-DX 116[4]	4-DAMP, darifenacin, solifenacin, oxybutynin, tolterodine
Approximate dissociation constant[5]			
Atropine	1	1	1
Pirenzepine	25	300	500
AF-DX 116	2000	65	4000
Darifenacin	70	55	8

[1]In clinical use as a neuromuscular blocking agent.
[2]In clinical use as an intestinal antispasmodic agent.
[3]In clinical use in the treatment of Parkinson's disease.
[4]Compound used in research only.
[5]Relative to atropine. Smaller numbers indicate higher affinity.
AF-DX 116, 11-({2-[(diethylamino)methyl]-1-piperidinyl}acetyl)-5,11-dihydro-6H-pyrido-[2,3-b](1,4)benzodiazepine-6-one; DAG, diacylglycerol; IP$_3$, inositol trisphosphate; 4-DAMP, 4-diphenylacetoxy-N-methylpiperidine.

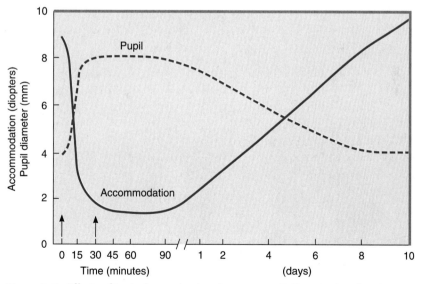

Figure 8–3. Effects of topical scopolamine drops on pupil diameter (mm) and accommodation (diopters) in the normal human eye. One drop of 0.5% solution of drug was applied at zero time, and a second drop was administered at 30 minutes (*arrows*). The responses of 42 eyes were averaged. Note the extremely slow recovery. (Redrawn from Marron J: Cycloplegia and mydriasis by use of atropine, scopolamine, and homatropine-paredrine. Arch Ophthalmol 1940;23:340.)

donna (Italian, "beautiful lady") applied to the plant and its active extract because of the use of the extract as eye drops during that time.

The second important ocular effect of antimuscarinic drugs is to weaken contraction of the ciliary muscle, or **cycloplegia.** Cycloplegia results in loss of the ability to accommodate; the fully atropinized eye cannot focus for near vision (Figure 8–3).

Both mydriasis and cycloplegia are useful in ophthalmology. They are also potentially hazardous, since acute glaucoma may be induced in patients with a narrow anterior chamber angle.

A third ocular effect of antimuscarinic drugs is to reduce lacrimal secretion. Patients occasionally complain of dry or "sandy" eyes when receiving large doses of antimuscarinic drugs.

3. Cardiovascular system—The sinoatrial node is very sensitive to muscarinic receptor blockade. Moderate to high therapeutic doses of atropine cause tachycardia in the innervated and spontaneously beating heart by blockade of vagal slowing. However, lower doses often result in initial bradycardia before the effects of peripheral vagal block become manifest (Figure 8–4). This slowing may be due to block of prejunctional M_1 receptors (autoreceptors, see Chapter 6) on vagal postganglionic fibers that normally limit acetylcholine release in the sinus node and other tissues. The same mechanisms operate in the atrioventricular node; in the presence of high vagal tone, atropine can significantly

reduce the PR interval of the electrocardiogram by blocking muscarinic receptors in the atrioventricular node. Muscarinic effects on atrial muscle are similarly blocked, but these effects are of no clinical significance except in atrial flutter and fibrillation. The ventricles are less affected by antimuscarinic drugs at therapeutic levels because of a lesser degree of muscarinic control. In toxic concentrations, the drugs can cause intraventricular conduction block that has been attributed to a local anesthetic action.

Most blood vessels receive no direct innervation from the parasympathetic system. However, parasympathetic nerve stimulation dilates coronary arteries, and sympathetic cholinergic nerves cause vasodilation in the skeletal muscle vascular bed (see Chapter 6). Atropine can block this vasodilation. Furthermore, almost all vessels contain endothelial muscarinic receptors that mediate vasodilation (see Chapter 7). These receptors are readily blocked by antimuscarinic drugs. At toxic doses, and in some individuals at normal doses, antimuscarinic agents cause cutaneous vasodilation, especially in the upper portion of the body. The mechanism is unknown.

The net cardiovascular effects of atropine in patients with normal hemodynamics are not dramatic: tachycardia may occur, but there is little effect on blood pressure. However, the cardiovascular effects of administered direct-acting muscarinic agonists are easily prevented.

4. Respiratory system—Both smooth muscle and secretory glands of the airway receive vagal innerva-

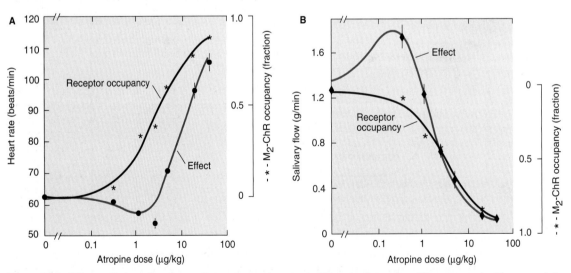

Figure 8–4. Effects of increasing doses of atropine on heart rate (**A**) and salivary flow (**B**) compared with muscarinic receptor occupancy in humans. The parasympathomimetic effect of low-dose atropine is attributed to blockade of prejunctional muscarinic receptors that suppress acetylcholine release. (Modified and reproduced, with permission, from Wellstein A, Pitschner HF: Complex dose-response curves of atropine in man explained by different functions of M_1 and M_2 cholinoceptors. Naunyn Schmiedebergs Arch Pharmacol 1988;338:19.)

tion and contain muscarinic receptors. Even in normal individuals, administration of atropine can cause some bronchodilation and reduce secretion. The effect is more significant in patients with airway disease, although the antimuscarinic drugs are not as useful as the β-adrenoceptor stimulants in the treatment of asthma (see Chapter 20). The effectiveness of unselective antimuscarinic drugs in treating chronic obstructive pulmonary disease (COPD) is limited because block of autoinhibitory M_2 receptors on postganglionic parasympathetic nerves can oppose the bronchodilation caused by block of M_3 receptors on airway smooth muscle. Nevertheless, antimuscarinic agents are valuable in some patients with asthma or COPD.

Antimuscarinic drugs are frequently used prior to administration of inhalant anesthetics to reduce the accumulation of secretions in the trachea and the possibility of laryngospasm.

5. Gastrointestinal tract—Blockade of muscarinic receptors has dramatic effects on motility and some of the secretory functions of the gut. However, even complete muscarinic block cannot totally abolish activity in this organ system since local hormones and noncholinergic neurons in the enteric nervous system (see Chapters 6 and 63) also modulate gastrointestinal function. As in other tissues, exogenously administered muscarinic stimulants are more effectively blocked than the effects of parasympathetic (vagal) nerve activity. The removal of autoinhibition, a negative feedback mechanism by which neural acetylcholine suppresses its own release, might explain the greater efficacy of antimuscarinic drugs against exogenous muscarinic stimulants.

Antimuscarinic drugs have marked effects on salivary secretion; dry mouth occurs frequently in patients taking antimuscarinic drugs for Parkinson's disease or urinary conditions (Figure 8–5). Gastric secretion is blocked less effectively: the volume and amount of acid, pepsin, and mucin are all reduced, but large doses of atropine may be required. Basal secretion is blocked more effectively than that stimulated by food, nicotine, or alcohol. Pirenzepine and a more potent analog, telenzepine, reduce gastric acid secretion with fewer adverse effects than atropine and other less selective agents. This results from a selective blockade of presynaptic excitatory muscarinic receptors on vagal nerve endings as suggested by their high ratio of M_1 to M_3 affinity (Table 8–1). Pirenzepine and telenzepine are investigational in the USA. Pancreatic and intestinal secretion are little affected by atropine; these processes are primarily under hormonal rather than vagal control.

Gastrointestinal smooth muscle motility is affected from the stomach to the colon. In general, the walls of

Figure 8–5. Effects of subcutaneous injection of atropine on salivation, speed of micturition (voiding), heart rate, and accommodation in normal adults. Note that salivation is the most sensitive of these variables, accommodation the least. (Data from Herxheimer A: Br J Pharmacol 1958;13:184.)

the viscera are relaxed, and both tone and propulsive movements are diminished. Therefore, gastric emptying time is prolonged, and intestinal transit time is lengthened. Diarrhea due to overdosage with parasympathomimetic agents is readily stopped, and even that caused by nonautonomic agents can usually be temporarily controlled. However, intestinal "paralysis" induced by antimuscarinic drugs is temporary; local mechanisms within the enteric nervous system will usually reestablish at least some peristalsis after 1–3 days of antimuscarinic drug therapy.

6. Genitourinary tract—The antimuscarinic action of atropine and its analogs relaxes smooth muscle of the ureters and bladder wall and slows voiding (Figure 8–5). This action is useful in the treatment of spasm induced by mild inflammation, surgery, and certain neurologic conditions, but it can precipitate urinary retention in men who have prostatic hyperplasia (see following section, Clinical Pharmacology of the Muscarinic Receptor-Blocking Drugs). The antimuscarinic drugs have no significant effect on the uterus.

7. Sweat glands—Atropine suppresses thermoregulatory sweating. Sympathetic cholinergic fibers innervate eccrine sweat glands, and their muscarinic receptors are readily accessible to antimuscarinic drugs. In adults, body temperature is elevated by this effect only if large doses are administered, but in infants and children even ordinary doses may cause "atropine fever."

■ II. CLINICAL PHARMACOLOGY OF THE MUSCARINIC RECEPTOR-BLOCKING DRUGS

Therapeutic Applications

A. CENTRAL NERVOUS SYSTEM DISORDERS

1. Parkinson's disease—As described in Chapter 28, the treatment of Parkinson's disease is often an exercise in polypharmacy, since no single agent is fully effective over the course of the disease. Most antimuscarinic drugs promoted for this application (see Table 28–1) were developed before levodopa became available. Their use is accompanied by all of the adverse effects described below, but the drugs remain useful as adjunctive therapy in some patients.

2. Motion sickness—Certain vestibular disorders respond to antimuscarinic drugs (and to antihistaminic agents with antimuscarinic effects). Scopolamine is one of the oldest remedies for seasickness and is as effective as any more recently introduced agent. It can be given by injection, by mouth, or as a transdermal patch. The patch formulation produces significant blood levels over 48–72 hours. Unfortunately, useful doses by any route usually cause significant sedation and dry mouth.

B. OPHTHALMOLOGIC DISORDERS

Accurate measurement of refractive error in uncooperative patients, eg, young children, requires ciliary paralysis. Also, ophthalmoscopic examination of the retina is greatly facilitated by mydriasis. Therefore, antimuscarinic agents, administered topically as eye drops or ointment, are very helpful in doing a complete examination. For adults and older children, the shorter-acting drugs are preferred (Table 8–2). For younger children, the greater efficacy of atropine is sometimes necessary,

Table 8–2. Antimuscarinic drugs used in ophthalmology.

Drug	Duration of Effect (days)	Usual Concentration (%)
Atropine	7–10	0.5–1
Scopolamine	3–7	0.25
Homatropine	1–3	2–5
Cyclopentolate	1	0.5–2
Tropicamide	0.25	0.5–1

but the possibility of antimuscarinic poisoning is correspondingly increased. Drug loss from the conjunctival sac via the nasolacrimal duct into the nasopharynx can be diminished by the use of the ointment form instead of drops. Formerly, ophthalmic antimuscarinic drugs were selected from the tertiary amine subgroup to ensure good penetration after conjunctival application. Recent experiments in animals, however, suggest that glycopyrrolate, a quaternary agent, is as rapid in onset and as long-lasting as atropine.

Antimuscarinic drugs should never be used for mydriasis unless cycloplegia or prolonged action is required. Alpha-adrenoceptor stimulant drugs, eg, phenylephrine, produce a short-lasting mydriasis that is usually sufficient for funduscopic examination (see Chapter 9).

A second ophthalmologic use is to prevent synechia (adhesion) formation in uveitis and iritis. The longer-lasting preparations, especially homatropine, are valuable for this indication.

C. RESPIRATORY DISORDERS

The use of atropine became part of routine preoperative medication when anesthetics such as ether were used, because these irritant anesthetics markedly increased airway secretions and were associated with frequent episodes of laryngospasm. Preanesthetic injection of atropine or scopolamine could prevent these hazardous effects. Scopolamine also produces significant amnesia for the events associated with surgery and obstetric delivery, a side effect that was considered desirable. On the other hand, urinary retention and intestinal hypomotility following surgery were often exacerbated by antimuscarinic drugs. Newer inhalational anesthetics are far less irritating to the airways.

As described in Chapter 20, the hyperactive neural bronchoconstrictor reflex present in most individuals with asthma is mediated by the vagus, acting on muscarinic receptors on bronchial smooth muscle cells. **Ipratropium** (Figure 8–2), a synthetic analog of atropine, is used as an inhalational drug in asthma. The aerosol route of administration has the advantages of maximal concentration at the bronchial target tissue with reduced systemic effects. This application is discussed in greater detail in Chapter 20. Ipratropium has also proved useful in COPD, a condition that occurs with higher frequency in older patients, particularly chronic smokers. Patients with COPD benefit from bronchodilators, especially antimuscarinic agents such as ipratropium and the recently approved **tiotropium.** In contrast to ipratropium, tiotropium has a longer bronchodilator action and can be given once daily. Tiotropium reduces the incidence of COPD exacerbations and is a useful adjunct to pulmonary rehabilitation in increasing exercise tolerance.

D. CARDIOVASCULAR DISORDERS

Marked reflex vagal discharge sometimes accompanies the pain of myocardial infarction (eg, vasovagal attack) and may depress sinoatrial or atrioventricular node function sufficiently to impair cardiac output. Parenteral atropine or a similar antimuscarinic drug is appropriate therapy in this situation. Rare individuals without other detectable cardiac disease have hyperactive carotid sinus reflexes and may experience faintness or even syncope as a result of vagal discharge in response to pressure on the neck, eg, from a tight collar. Such individuals may benefit from the judicious use of atropine or a related antimuscarinic agent.

Pathophysiology can influence muscarinic activity in other ways as well. Circulating autoantibodies against the second extracellular loop of cardiac muscarinic receptors have been detected in some patients with idiopathic dilated cardiomyopathy. These antibodies exert parasympathomimetic actions on the heart that are prevented by atropine. Although their role in the pathology of heart failure is unknown, they should provide clues to the molecular basis of receptor activation.

E. GASTROINTESTINAL DISORDERS

Antimuscarinic agents are now rarely used for peptic ulcer disease in the USA (see Chapter 63). Antimuscarinic agents can provide some relief in the treatment of common traveler's diarrhea and other mild or self-limited conditions of hypermotility. They are often combined with an opioid antidiarrheal drug, an extremely effective therapy. In this combination, however, the very low dosage of the antimuscarinic drug functions primarily to discourage abuse of the opioid agent. The classic combination of atropine with diphenoxylate, a nonanalgesic congener of meperidine, is available under many names (eg, Lomotil) in both tablet and liquid form (see Chapter 63).

F. URINARY DISORDERS

Atropine and other antimuscarinic drugs have been used to provide symptomatic relief in the treatment of urinary urgency caused by minor inflammatory bladder disorders (Table 8–3). However, specific antimicrobial therapy is essential in bacterial cystitis. In the human urinary bladder, M_2 and M_3 receptors are expressed predominantly with the M_3 subtype mediating direct activation of contraction. As in intestinal smooth muscle, the M_2 subtype appears to act indirectly by inhibiting relaxation by norepinephrine and epinephrine.

Oxybutynin, which is somewhat selective for M_3 receptors, is used to relieve bladder spasm after urologic surgery, eg, prostatectomy. It is also valuable in reducing involuntary voiding in patients with neurologic disease, eg, children with meningomyelocele. Oral oxybutynin or instillation of the drug by catheter into the

Table 8–3. Antimuscarinic drugs used in gastrointestinal and genitourinary conditions.

Drug	Usual Dosage
Quaternary amines	
Anisotropine	50 mg tid
Clidinium	2.5 mg tid–qid
Glycopyrrolate	1 mg bid–tid
Isopropamide	5 mg bid
Mepenzolate	25–50 mg qid
Methantheline	50–100 mg qid
Methscopolamine	2.5 mg qid
Oxyphenonium	5–10 mg qid
Propantheline	15 mg qid
Tridihexethyl	25–50 mg tid–qid
Trospium	20 mg bid
Tertiary amines	
Atropine	0.4 mg tid–qid
Darifenacin	7.5 mg qd
Dicyclomine	10–20 mg qid
Oxybutynin	5 mg tid
Oxyphencyclimine	10 mg bid
Propiverine	15 mg bid–tid
Scopolamine	0.4 mg tid
Solifenacin	5 mg qd
Tolterodine	2 mg bid

bladder in such patients appears to improve bladder capacity and continence and to reduce infection and renal damage. **Trospium,** an unselective antagonist, has recently been approved and is comparable in efficacy and side effects with oxybutynin. **Darifenacin** and **solifenacin** are recently approved antagonists that have greater selectivity for M_3 receptors than oxybutynin or trospium. Their advantages include once daily dosing because of their long half-lives and a reduced incidence of xerostomia and constipation. **Tolterodine,** another M_3-selective antimuscarinic, is available for use in adults with urinary incontinence. It has many of the qualities of darifenacin and solifenacin. The reason for the reduced incidence of dry mouth with these drugs as compared with oxybutynin is not known.

Imipramine, a tricyclic antidepressant drug with strong antimuscarinic actions, has long been used to reduce incontinence in institutionalized elderly patients. It is moderately effective but causes significant central nervous system toxicity. Propiverine, a newer antimuscarinic agent, has been approved for this purpose.

Antimuscarinic agents have also been used in urolithiasis to relieve the painful ureteral smooth muscle spasm caused by passage of the stone. However, their usefulness in this condition is debatable.

G. CHOLINERGIC POISONING

Severe cholinergic excess is a medical emergency, especially in rural communities where cholinesterase inhibitor insecticides are commonly used and in cultures where wild mushrooms are commonly eaten. The potential use of cholinesterase inhibitors as chemical warfare "nerve gases" also requires an awareness of the methods for treating acute poisoning (see Chapter 59).

1. Antimuscarinic therapy—As noted in Chapter 7, both the nicotinic and the muscarinic effects of the cholinesterase inhibitors can be life-threatening. Unfortunately, there is no effective method for directly blocking the nicotinic effects of cholinesterase inhibition, because nicotinic agonists *and* antagonists cause blockade of transmission (see Chapter 27). To reverse the muscarinic effects, a tertiary (not quaternary) amine drug must be used (preferably atropine) to treat the central nervous system effects as well as the peripheral effects of the organophosphate inhibitors. Large doses of atropine may be needed to oppose the muscarinic effects of extremely potent agents like parathion and chemical warfare nerve gases: 1–2 mg of atropine sulfate may be given intravenously every 5–15 minutes until signs of effect (dry mouth, reversal of miosis) appear. The drug may have to be repeated many times, since the acute effects of the anticholinesterase agent may last for 24–48 hours or longer. In this life-threatening situation, as much as 1 g of atropine per day may be required for as long as 1 month for full control of muscarinic excess.

2. Cholinesterase regenerator compounds—A second class of compounds, capable of regenerating active enzyme from the organophosphorus-cholinesterase complex, is also available to treat organophosphorus poisoning. These oxime agents include pralidoxime (PAM), diacetylmonoxime (DAM), and others.

The oxime group (=NOH) has a very high affinity for the phosphorus atom, and these drugs can hydrolyze the phosphorylated enzyme if the complex has not "aged" (see Chapter 7). Pralidoxime is the most extensively studied—in humans—of the agents shown and the only one available for clinical use in the USA. It is most effective in regenerating the cholinesterase associated with skeletal muscle neuromuscular junctions. Pralidoxime is ineffective in reversing the central effects of organophosphate poisoning because its positive charge prevents entry into the central nervous system. Diacetylmonoxime, on the other hand, crosses the blood-brain barrier and, in experimental animals, can regenerate some of the central nervous system cholinesterase.

Pralidoxime is administered by intravenous infusion, 1–2 g given over 15–30 minutes. In spite of the likelihood of aging of the phosphate-enzyme complex, recent reports suggest that administration of multiple doses of pralidoxime over several days may be useful in severe poisoning. In excessive doses, pralidoxime can induce neuromuscular weakness and other adverse effects. Pralidoxime is *not* recommended for the reversal of inhibition of acetylcholinesterase by carbamate inhibitors. Further details of treatment of anticholinesterase toxicity are given in Chapter 59.

A third approach to protection against excessive AChE inhibition is *pretreatment* with reversible enzyme inhibitors to prevent binding of the irreversible organophosphate inhibitor. This prophylaxis can be achieved with pyridostigmine or physostigmine but is reserved for situations in which possibly lethal poisoning is anticipated, eg, chemical warfare. Simultaneous use of atropine is required to control muscarinic excess.

Mushroom poisoning has traditionally been divided into rapid-onset and delayed-onset types. The rapid-onset type is usually apparent within 15–30 minutes following ingestion of the mushrooms. It is often characterized entirely by signs of muscarinic excess: nausea, vomiting, diarrhea, urinary urgency, vasodilation, reflex tachycardia (occasionally bradycardia), sweating, salivation, and sometimes bronchoconstriction. Although *Amanita muscaria* contains muscarine (the alkaloid was named after the mushroom), numerous other alkaloids, including antimuscarinic agents, are found in this fungus. In fact, ingestion of *A muscaria* may produce signs of atropine poisoning, not muscarine excess. Other mushrooms, especially those of the *Inocybe* genus, cause rapid-onset poisoning of the muscarinic excess type. Parenteral atropine, 1–2 mg, is effective treatment in such intoxications.

Delayed-onset mushroom poisoning, usually caused by *Amanita phalloides, A virosa, Galerina autumnalis,* or *G marginata,* manifests its first symptoms 6–12 hours after ingestion. Although the initial symptoms usually include nausea and vomiting, the major toxicity involves

Pralidoxime   **Diacetylmonoxime**

hepatic and renal cellular injury by amatoxins that inhibit RNA polymerase. Atropine is of no value in this form of mushroom poisoning (see Chapter 59).

H. OTHER APPLICATIONS

Hyperhidrosis (excessive sweating) is sometimes reduced by antimuscarinic agents. However, relief is incomplete at best, probably because apocrine rather than eccrine glands are usually involved.

Adverse Effects

Treatment with atropine or its congeners directed at one organ system almost always induces undesirable effects in other organ systems. Thus, mydriasis and cycloplegia are adverse effects when an antimuscarinic agent is used to reduce gastrointestinal secretion or motility, even though they are therapeutic effects when the drug is used in ophthalmology.

At higher concentrations, atropine causes block of all parasympathetic functions. However, atropine is a remarkably safe drug *in adults*. Atropine poisoning has occurred as a result of attempted suicide, but most cases are due to attempts to induce hallucinations. Poisoned individuals manifest dry mouth, mydriasis, tachycardia, hot and flushed skin, agitation, and delirium for as long as a week. Body temperature is frequently elevated. These effects are memorialized in the adage, "dry as a bone, blind as a bat, red as a beet, mad as a hatter."

Unfortunately, children, especially infants, are very sensitive to the hyperthermic effects of atropine. Although accidental administration of over 400 mg has been followed by recovery, deaths have followed doses as small as 2 mg. Therefore, atropine should be considered a highly dangerous drug when overdose occurs in infants or children.

Overdoses of atropine or its congeners are generally treated symptomatically (see Chapter 59). In the past, physostigmine or another cholinesterase inhibitor was recommended, but most poison control experts now consider physostigmine more dangerous and no more effective in most patients than symptomatic management. When physostigmine is deemed necessary, *small* doses are given *slowly* intravenously (1–4 mg in adults, 0.5–1 mg in children). Symptomatic treatment may require temperature control with cooling blankets and seizure control with diazepam.

Poisoning caused by high doses of quaternary antimuscarinic drugs is associated with all of the peripheral signs of parasympathetic blockade but few or none of the central nervous system effects of atropine. These more polar drugs may cause significant ganglionic blockade, however, with marked orthostatic hypotension (see below). Treatment of the antimuscarinic effects, if required, can be carried out with a quaternary cholinesterase inhibitor such as neostigmine. Control of hypotension may require the administration of a sympathomimetic drug such as phenylephrine.

Contraindications

Contraindications to the use of antimuscarinic drugs are relative, not absolute. Obvious muscarinic excess, especially that caused by cholinesterase inhibitors, can always be treated with atropine.

Antimuscarinic drugs are contraindicated in patients with glaucoma, especially angle-closure glaucoma. Even systemic use of moderate doses may precipitate angle closure (and acute glaucoma) in patients with shallow anterior chambers.

In elderly men, antimuscarinic drugs should always be used with caution and should be avoided in those with a history of prostatic hyperplasia.

Because the antimuscarinic drugs slow gastric emptying, they may *increase* symptoms in patients with gastric ulcer. Nonselective antimuscarinic agents should never be used to treat acid-peptic disease (see Chapter 63).

■ III. BASIC & CLINICAL PHARMACOLOGY OF THE GANGLION-BLOCKING DRUGS

These agents competitively block the action of acetylcholine and similar agonists at nicotinic receptors of both parasympathetic and sympathetic autonomic ganglia. Some members of the group also block the ion channel that is gated by the nicotinic cholinoceptor. The ganglion-blocking drugs are important and used in pharmacologic and physiologic research because they can block all autonomic outflow. However, their lack of selectivity confers such a broad range of undesirable effects that they have limited clinical use.

Chemistry & Pharmacokinetics

All ganglion-blocking drugs of interest are synthetic amines. **Tetraethylammonium (TEA),** the first to be recognized as having this action, has a very short duration of action. **Hexamethonium ("C6")** was developed and was introduced clinically as the first drug effective for management of hypertension. As shown in Figure 8–6, there is an obvious relationship between the structures of the agonist acetylcholine and the nicotinic antagonists tetraethylammonium and hexamethonium. Decamethonium, the "C10" analog of hexamethonium, is a depolarizing neuromuscular blocking agent.

CH$_3$
CH$_3$—N$^+$—CH$_2$—CH$_2$—CH$_2$—CH$_2$—CH$_2$—CH$_2$—$^+$N—CH$_3$
CH$_3$
CH$_3$
CH$_3$

Hexamethonium

CH$_3$
CH$_3$
CH$_3$
NH—CH$_3$

Mecamylamine

CH$_2$—CH$_3$
CH$_3$—CH$_2$—N$^+$—CH$_2$—CH$_3$
CH$_2$—CH$_3$

Tetraethylammonium

CH$_3$ O
CH$_3$—N$^+$—CH$_2$—CH$_2$—O—C—CH$_3$
CH$_3$

Acetylcholine

Figure 8–6. Some ganglion-blocking drugs. Acetylcholine is shown for reference.

Mecamylamine, a secondary amine, was developed to improve the degree and extent of absorption from the gastrointestinal tract because the quaternary amine ganglion-blocking compounds were poorly and erratically absorbed after oral administration. **Trimethaphan,** a short-acting ganglion blocker, is inactive orally and is given by intravenous infusion.

Pharmacodynamics

A. MECHANISM OF ACTION

Ganglionic nicotinic receptors, like those of the skeletal muscle neuromuscular junction, are subject to both depolarizing and nondepolarizing blockade (see Chapters 7 and 27). Nicotine itself, carbamoylcholine, and even acetylcholine (if amplified with a cholinesterase inhibitor) can produce depolarizing ganglion block.

Drugs now used as ganglion blockers are classified as nondepolarizing competitive antagonists. However, hexamethonium actually produces most of its blockade by occupying sites in or on the nicotinic ion channel, not by occupying the cholinoceptor itself. In contrast, trimethaphan appears to block the nicotinic receptor, not the channel. Blockade can be surmounted by increasing the concentration of an agonist, eg, acetylcholine.

B. ORGAN SYSTEM EFFECTS

1. Central nervous system—Mecamylamine, unlike the quaternary amine agents and trimethaphan, crosses the blood-brain barrier and readily enters the central nervous system. Sedation, tremor, choreiform movements, and mental aberrations have been reported as effects of mecamylamine.

2. Eye—The ganglion-blocking drugs cause a predictable cycloplegia with loss of accommodation because the ciliary muscle receives innervation primarily from the parasympathetic nervous system. The effect on the pupil is not so easily predicted, since the iris receives both sympathetic innervation (mediating pupillary dilation) and parasympathetic innervation (mediating pupillary constriction). Ganglionic blockade often causes moderate dilation of the pupil because parasympathetic tone usually dominates this tissue.

3. Cardiovascular system—Blood vessels receive chiefly vasoconstrictor fibers from the sympathetic nervous system; therefore, ganglionic blockade causes a marked decrease in arteriolar and venomotor tone. The blood pressure may fall precipitously, because both peripheral vascular resistance and venous return are decreased (see Figure 6–7). Hypotension is especially marked in the upright position (orthostatic or postural hypotension), because postural reflexes that normally prevent venous pooling are blocked.

Cardiac effects include diminished contractility and, because the sinoatrial node is usually dominated by the parasympathetic nervous system, a moderate tachycardia.

4. Gastrointestinal tract—Secretion is reduced, although not enough to effectively treat peptic disease. Motility is profoundly inhibited, and constipation can be marked.

5. Other systems—Genitourinary smooth muscle is partially dependent on autonomic innervation for normal function. Therefore, ganglionic blockade causes hesitancy in urination and may precipitate urinary retention in men with prostatic hyperplasia. Sexual function is impaired in that both erection and ejaculation may be prevented by moderate doses.

Thermoregulatory sweating is reduced by the ganglion-blocking drugs. However, hyperthermia is not a problem except in very warm environments, because cutaneous vasodilation is usually sufficient to maintain a normal body temperature.

6. Response to autonomic drugs—Patients receiving ganglion-blocking drugs are fully responsive to autonomic drugs acting on muscarinic, α-, and β-adrenergic receptors because these effector cell receptors are not blocked. In fact, responses may be exaggerated or even reversed (eg, norepinephrine may cause tachycardia rather than bradycardia), because homeostatic reflexes, which normally moderate autonomic responses, are absent.

Clinical Applications & Toxicity

Use of the ganglion blockers is infrequent because more selective autonomic blocking agents are available. Mecamylamine is being studied for possible use in reducing nicotine craving in patients attempting to quit smoking and for some other central indications. Trimethaphan is occasionally used in the treatment of hypertensive emergencies and dissecting aortic aneurysm; to produce controlled hypotension, which can be of value in neurosurgery to reduce bleeding in the operative field; and in patients undergoing electroconvulsive therapy. The toxicity of the ganglion-blocking drugs is limited to the autonomic effects already described. For most patients, these effects are intolerable except for acute use.

PREPARATIONS AVAILABLE

ANTIMUSCARINIC ANTICHOLINERGIC DRUGS*

Atropine (generic)
Oral: 0.4, 0.6 mg tablets
Parenteral: 0.05, 0.1, 0.3, 0.4, 0.5, 0.8, 1 mg/mL for injection
Ophthalmic (generic, Isopto Atropine): 0.5, 1, 2% drops; 0.5, 1% ointments

Belladonna alkaloids, extract or tincture (generic)
Oral: 0.27–0.33 mg/mL liquid

Clidinium (generic, Quarzan, others)
Oral: 2.5, 5 mg capsules

Cyclopentolate (generic, Cyclogyl, others)
Ophthalmic: 0.5, 1, 2% drops

Darifenacin (Enablex)
Oral: 7.5, 15 mg tablets (extended release)

Dicyclomine (generic, Bentyl, others)
Oral: 10, 20 mg capsules; 20 mg tablets; 10 mg/5 mL syrup
Parenteral: 10 mg/mL for injection

Flavoxate (Urispas)
Oral: 100 mg tablets

Glycopyrrolate (generic, Robinul)
Oral: 1, 2 mg tablets
Parenteral: 0.2 mg/mL for injection

Homatropine (generic, Isopto Homatropine, others)
Ophthalmic: 2, 5% drops

l-Hyoscyamine (Anaspaz, Cystospaz-M, Levsinex)
Oral: 0.125, 0.15 mg tablets; 0.375 mg timed-release capsules; 0.125 mg/5 mL oral elixir and solution
Parenteral: 0.5 mg/mL for injection

Ipratropium (generic, Atrovent)
Aerosol: 200 dose metered-dose inhaler
Solution for nebulizer: 0.02%
Nasal spray: 0.03, 0.06%

Mepenzolate (Cantil)
Oral: 25 mg tablets

Methantheline (Banthine)
Oral: 50 mg tablets

Methscopolamine (Pamine)
Oral: 2.5 mg tablets

Oxybutynin (generic, Ditropan)
Oral: 5 mg tablets; 5, 10, 15 mg extended-release tablets; 5 mg/5 mL syrup

Propantheline (generic, Pro-Banthine, others)
Oral: 7.5, 15 mg tablets

Scopolamine (generic)
Oral: 0.25 mg tablets
Parenteral: 0.3, 0.4, 0.86, 1 mg/mL for injection
Ophthalmic (Isopto Hyoscine): 0.25% solution
Transdermal (Transderm Scop): 1.5 mg (delivers 0.5 mg) patch

Solifenacin (Vesicare)
Oral: 5, 10 mg tablets

Tiotropium (Spiriva)
Aerosol: 18 mcg tablet for inhaler

Tolterodine (Detrol)
Oral: 1, 2 mg tablets; 2, 4 mg extended-release capsules

Tridihexethyl (Pathilon)
Oral: 25 mg tablets

Tropicamide (generic, Mydriacyl Ophthalmic, others)
Ophthalmic: 0.5, 1% drops

Trospium (Spasmex)
Oral: 5, 15, 30 mg tablets
Suppository: 0.75, 1.0 mg
Parenteral: 0.6 mg/mL

GANGLION BLOCKERS

Mecamylamine (Inversine)
Oral: 2.5 mg tablets

Trimethaphan (Arfonad)
Parenteral: 50 mg/mL

CHOLINESTERASE REGENERATOR

Pralidoxime (generic, Protopam)
Parenteral: 1 g vial with 20 mL diluent for IV administration; 600 mg in 2 mL autoinjector

*Antimuscarinic drugs used in parkinsonism are listed in Chapter 28.

REFERENCES

Andersson KE: Antimuscarinics for treatment of overactive bladder. Lancet Neurol 2004;3:46.

Brodde OE et al: Presence, distribution and physiological function of adrenergic and muscarinic receptor subtypes in the human heart. Basic Res Cardiol 2001;96:528.

Campbell SC: Clinical aspects of inhaled anticholinergic therapy. Respir Care 2001;46:275.

Casaburi R et al: Improvement in exercise tolerance with the combination of tiotropium and pulmonary rehabilitation in patients with COPD. Chest 2005;127:809.

Chapple CR et al: A comparison of the efficacy and tolerability of solifenacin succinate and extended release tolterodine at treating overactive bladder syndrome: Results of the STAR trial. Eur Urol 2005;48:464.

Chapple CR, Abrams P: Comparison of darifenacin and oxybutynin in patients with overactive bladder: assessment of ambulatory urodynamics and impact on salivary flow. Eur Urol 2005;48:102.

Coulson FR, Fryer AD: Muscarinic acetylcholine receptors and airway diseases. Pharmacol Ther 2003;98:59.

Disse B: Antimuscarinic treatment for lung diseases from research to clinical practice. Life Sci 2001;68:2557.

Fukusaki M et al: Effects of controlled hypotension with sevoflurane anesthesia on hepatic function of surgical patients. Eur J Anaesthesiol 1999;16:111.

Gurney AM, Rang HP: The channel-blocking action of methonium compounds on rat submandibular ganglion cells. Br J Pharmacol 1984;82:623.

Kranke P et al: The efficacy and safety of transdermal scopolamine for the prevention of postoperative nausea and vomiting: A quantitative systematic review. Anesth Analg 2002;95:133.

Matsui S et al: Beneficial effect of muscarinic-2 antagonist on dilated cardiomyopathy induced by autoimmune mechanism against muscarinic-2 receptor. J Cardiovasc Pharmacol 2001; 38(suppl 1):S43.

Moreland RB et al: Emerging pharmacologic approaches for the treatment of lower urinary tract disorders. J Pharm Exp Ther 2004;308:797.

Olson K: Mushrooms. In: Olson K (editor). *Poisoning & Drug Overdose,* 4th ed. McGraw-Hill, 2003.

Petrides G et al: Trimethaphan (Arfonad) control of hypertension and tachycardia during electroconvulsive therapy: A double-blind study. J Clin Anesth 1996;8:104.

Wess J: Muscarinic acetylcholine receptor knockout mice: Novel phenotypes and clinical implications. Annu Rev Pharmacol Toxicol 2004;44:423.

Young JM et al: Mecamylamine: New therapeutic uses and toxicity/risk profile. Clin Ther 2001;23:532.

Treatment of Anticholinesterase Poisoning

Loke WK, Simm MK, Go ML: O-substituted derivatives of pralidoxime: Muscarinic properties and protection against soman effects in rats. Eur J Pharmacol 2002;442:279.

Newmark J: Nerve agents: Pathophysiology and treatment of poisoning. Semin Neurol 2004;24:185.

Weinbroum AA: Pathophysiological and clinical aspects of combat anticholinesterase poisoning. Br Med Bull 2005; 72:119.

Worek F et al: Kinetic analysis of interactions between human acetylcholinesterase, structurally different organophosphorus compounds and oximes. Biochem Pharmacol 2004; 68:2237.

Adrenoceptor-Activating & Other Sympathomimetic Drugs

9

Brian B. Hoffman, MD

The sympathetic nervous system is an important regulator of the activities of organs such as the heart and peripheral vasculature, especially in responses to stress (see Chapter 6). The ultimate effects of sympathetic stimulation are mediated by release from nerve terminals of norepinephrine that serves to activate the adrenoceptors on postsynaptic sites. Also, in response to a variety of stimuli such as stress, the adrenal medulla releases epinephrine, which is transported in the blood to target tissues; in other words, epinephrine acts as a hormone. Drugs that mimic the actions of epinephrine or norepinephrine—**sympathomimetic drugs**—would be expected to have a wide range of effects. An understanding of the pharmacology of these agents is thus a logical extension of what we know about the physiologic role of the catecholamines.

The Mode & Spectrum of Action of Sympathomimetic Drugs

Like the cholinomimetic drugs, the sympathomimetics can be grouped by mode of action and by the spectrum of receptors that they activate. Some of these drugs (eg, norepinephrine and epinephrine) act by a *direct* mode; that is, they directly interact with and activate adrenoceptors. Others act *indirectly*; their actions are dependent on the release of endogenous catecholamines. These indirect agents may have either of two different mechanisms: (1) displacement of stored catecholamines from the adrenergic nerve ending (eg, amphetamine and tyramine) or (2) inhibition of reuptake of catecholamines already released (eg, cocaine and tricyclic antidepressants). Some drugs have both direct and indirect actions. Both types of sympathomimetics, direct and indirect, ultimately cause activation of adrenoceptors, leading to some or all of the characteristic effects of endogenous catecholamines. The selectivity of different sympathomimetics for various types of adrenoceptors is discussed below.

■ I. BASIC PHARMACOLOGY OF SYMPATHOMIMETIC DRUGS

IDENTIFICATION OF ADRENOCEPTORS

The effort to understand the molecular mechanisms by which catecholamines act has a long and rich history. A great conceptual debt is owed to the work done by John Langley and Paul Ehrlich 100 years ago in developing the hypothesis that drugs have their effects by interacting with specific "receptive" substances. Raymond Ahlquist in 1948 rationalized a large body of observations by his conjecture that catecholamines acted via two principal receptors. He termed these receptors α and β. Alpha receptors are those that have the comparative potencies epinephrine $\geq$ norepinephrine $\gg$ isoproterenol. Beta receptors have the comparative potencies isoproterenol > epinephrine $\geq$ norepinephrine. Ahlquist's hypothesis was dramatically confirmed by the development of drugs that selectively antagonize β receptors but not α receptors (see Chapter 10). More recent evidence suggests that α receptors comprise two major families. At present, therefore, it appears appropriate to classify adrenoceptors into three major groups, namely, β, α_1, and α_2 receptors. Each of these major groups of receptors also has three subtypes. Considerable effort has been expended in elucidating structure-function relationships that determine ligand binding properties and the molecular signaling characteristics of the various adrenergic receptors.

A. BETA ADRENOCEPTORS

Soon after the demonstration of separate α and β receptors, it was found that there were at least two *subtypes* of β receptors, designated β_1 and β_2. These subtypes are operationally defined by their affinities for epinephrine and norepinephrine: β_1 receptors have approximately equal affinity for epinephrine and norepinephrine,

Table 9–1. Adrenoceptor types and subtypes.

Receptor	Agonist	Antagonist	Effects	Gene on Chromosome
α_1 type	Phenylephrine	Prazosin	↑ IP_3, DAG common to all	
α_{1A}				C5
α_{1B}				C8
α_{1D}				C20
α_2 type	Clonidine	Yohimbine	↓ cAMP common to all	
α_{2A}	Oxymetazoline			C10
α_{2B}		Prazosin		C2
α_{2C}		Prazosin		C4
β type	Isoproterenol	Propranolol	↑ cAMP common to all	
β_1	Dobutamine	Betaxolol		C10
β_2	Albuterol	Butoxamine		C5
β_3				C8
Dopamine type	Dopamine			
D_1	Fenoldopam		↑ cAMP	C5
D_2	Bromocriptine		↓ cAMP	C11
D_3			↓ cAMP	C3
D_4		Clozapine	↓ cAMP	C11
D_5			↑ cAMP	C4

whereas β_2 receptors have a higher affinity for epinephrine than for norepinephrine. Subsequently, β_3 receptors were identified as a novel and distinct third β-adrenoceptor subtype. These receptor types are listed in Table 9–1.

B. Alpha Adrenoceptors

Following the demonstration of the β subtypes, two major groups of α receptors were found: α_1 and α_2. These receptors were originally identified with antagonist drugs that distinguished between α_1 and α_2 receptors. For example, α adrenoceptors were identified in a variety of tissues by measuring the binding of radiolabeled antagonist compounds that are considered to have a high affinity for these receptors, eg, dihydroergocryptine (α_1 and α_2), prazosin (α_1), and yohimbine (α_2). These radioligands were used to measure the number of receptors in tissues and to determine the affinity (by displacement of the radiolabeled ligand) of other drugs that interact with the receptors.

The concept of subtypes *within* the α_1 group emerged out of pharmacologic experiments that demonstrated complex shapes of agonist dose-response curves of smooth muscle contraction as well as differ-

ences in antagonist affinities in inhibiting contractile responses in various tissues. These experiments demonstrated the existence of two subtypes of α_1 receptor that could be distinguished on the basis of their reversible affinities for a variety of drugs and experimental compounds. A third α_1-receptor subtype was subsequently identified by molecular cloning techniques. These α_1 receptors are termed α_{1A}, α_{1B}, and α_{1D} receptors. There is evidence that the α_{1A} receptor has splice variants. A major current area of investigation is determining the importance of each of these various subtypes in mediating α_1-receptor responses in a variety of organs.

The hypothesis that there are subtypes of α_2 receptors emerged from pharmacologic experiments and molecular cloning. It is now known that there are three subtypes of α_2 receptors, termed α_{2A}, α_{2B}, and α_{2C}, which are products of distinct genes.

C. Dopamine Receptors

The endogenous catecholamine dopamine produces a variety of biologic effects that are mediated by interactions with specific dopamine receptors (Table 9–1). These receptors are distinct from α and β receptors and are particularly important in the brain (see Chapters 21 and 29) and in the splanchnic and renal vasculature. There is now considerable evidence for the existence of at least five subtypes of dopamine receptors. Pharmacologically distinct dopamine receptor subtypes, termed D_1 and D_2, have been known for some time. Molecular cloning has identified several distinct genes encoding each of these subtypes. Further complexity occurs because of the presence of introns within the coding region of the D_2-like receptor genes, which allows for alternative splicing of the exons in this major subtype. There is extensive polymorphic variation in the D_4 human receptor gene. The terminology of the various subtypes is D_1, D_2, D_3, D_4, and D_5. They comprise two D_1-like receptors (D_1 and D_5) and three D_2-like (D_2, D_3, and D_4). These subtypes may have importance for understanding the efficacy and adverse effects of novel antipsychotic drugs (see Chapter 29).

Receptor Selectivity

Examples of clinically useful sympathomimetic agonists that are relatively selective for α_1-, α_2-, and β-adrenoceptor subgroups are compared with some nonselective agents in Table 9–2. Selectivity means that a drug may preferentially bind to one subgroup of receptors at concentrations too low to interact extensively with another subgroup. For example, norepinephrine preferentially activates β_1 receptors compared with β_2 receptors. However, selectivity is not usually absolute (nearly absolute selectivity has been termed "specificity"), and at higher concentrations related classes of receptor may also interact with the drug. As a result, the "numeric" subclassification of adrenoceptors is clinically important mainly for drugs that have relatively marked selectivity. Given interpatient variations in drug kinetics and dynamics, the extent of a drug's selectivity should be kept in mind if this property is viewed as clinically important in the treatment of an individual patient.

The exact number of adrenoceptor subtypes that are actually expressed in human tissues is uncertain, but expression of subtypes has been demonstrated in tissues in which the physiologic or pharmacologic importance of the subtype is not yet known. These results suggest the possibility of designing novel drugs to exploit the expression of a particular receptor subtype in a single target tissue. For example, determining which blood vessels express which subtypes of α_1 and α_2 receptors could lead to design of drugs having selectivity for certain vascular beds such as the splanchnic or coronary vessels. Similarly, there has been extensive investigation into the α_1-receptor subtypes mediating pharmacologic responses in the human prostate (see Box: Receptor Selectivity and Physiologic Functions of Adrenoceptor Subtypes).

MOLECULAR MECHANISMS OF SYMPATHOMIMETIC ACTION

The effects of catecholamines are mediated by cell surface receptors. As described in Chapter 2, these GPCRs (G protein-coupled receptors) are coupled by G proteins to the various effector proteins whose activities are regulated by those receptors. Each G protein is a heterotrimer consisting of α, β, and γ subunits. G proteins are classified on the basis of their distinctive α subunits. G proteins of particular importance for adrenoceptor function include G_s, the stimulatory G protein of adenylyl cyclase; G_i, the inhibitory G protein of adenylyl cyclase; and G_q, the protein coupling α receptors to phospholipase C. The activation of G protein-coupled receptors by catecholamines promotes the dissociation of GDP from the α subunit of the appropriate G protein. GTP then binds to this G protein, and the α subunit dissociates from the β-γ unit. The activated GTP-bound α subunit then regulates the activity of its effector. Effectors of adrenoceptor-activated α subunits include adenylyl cyclase, cGMP phosphodiesterase, phospholipase C, and ion channels. The α subunit is inactivated by hydrolysis of the bound GTP to GDP and phosphate, and the subsequent reassociation of the α subunit with the β-γ subunit. The β-γ subunits have additional independent effects, acting on a variety of effectors such as ion channels and enzymes.

RECEPTOR SELECTIVITY AND PHYSIOLOGIC FUNCTIONS OF ADRENOCEPTOR SUBTYPES: LESSONS FROM KNOCKOUT MICE

Since pharmacologic tools used to evaluate the function of adrenoceptor subtypes have some limitations, a number of knockout mice have been developed with one or more adrenoceptor genes subjected to loss of function mutations, as described in Chapter 1 (see Box: Pharmacology & Genetics). These models have their own complexities and extrapolations from mice to humans may be uncertain. Nonetheless, these studies have yielded some novel insights. For example, α-adrenoceptor subtypes play an important role in cardiac responses, the α_{2A}-adrenoceptor subtype is critical in transducing the effects of α_2 agonists on blood pressure control, and β_1 receptors play a predominant role in directly increasing heart rate in mouse heart.

Table 9–2. Relative selectivity of adrenoceptor agonists.

	Relative Receptor Affinities
Alpha agonists	
Phenylephrine, methoxamine	$\alpha_1 > \alpha_2 >>>>> \beta$
Clonidine, methylnorepinephrine	$\alpha_2 > \alpha_1 >>>>> \beta$
Mixed alpha and beta agonists	
Norepinephrine	$\alpha_1 = \alpha_2; \beta_1 >> \beta_2$
Epinephrine	$\alpha_1 = \alpha_2; \beta_1 = \beta_2$
Beta agonists	
Dobutamine[1]	$\beta_1 > \beta_2 >>>> \alpha$
Isoproterenol	$\beta_1 = \beta_2 >>>> \alpha$
Terbutaline, metaproterenol, albuterol, ritodrine	$\beta_2 >> \beta_1 >>>> \alpha$
Dopamine agonists	
Dopamine	$D_1 = D_2 >> \beta >> \alpha$
Fenoldopam	$D_1 >> D_2$

[1]See text.

Receptor Types

A. Alpha Receptors

Alpha$_1$ receptors are coupled to polyphosphoinositide hydrolysis, leading to the formation of **inositol 1,4,5-trisphosphate (IP_3)** and **diacylglycerol (DAG)** (Table 9–1, Figure 9–1). G proteins in the G_q family couple α_1 receptors to phospholipase C. IP_3 promotes the release of sequestered Ca^{2+} from intracellular stores, which increases the cytoplasmic concentration of free Ca^{2+} and the activation of various calcium-dependent protein kinases. Activation of these receptors may also increase influx of calcium across the cell's plasma membrane. IP_3 is sequentially dephosphorylated, which ultimately leads to the formation of free inositol. DAG activates protein kinase C, which modulates activity of many signaling pathways. In addition, α_1 receptors activate signal transduction pathways that were originally described for peptide growth factor receptors that activate tyrosine kinases. For example, α_1 receptors have been found to activate mitogen-activated kinases (MAP kinases) and polyphosphoinositol-3-kinase (PI-3-kinase). These pathways may have importance for the α_1-receptor-mediated stimulation of cell growth and proliferation through the regulation of gene expression. The physiologic significance of this "cross talk" between major signaling pathways remains to be determined.

Alpha$_2$ receptors inhibit adenylyl cyclase activity and cause intracellular cyclic adenosine monophosphate (cAMP) levels to decrease. In addition to this well-documented effect, α_2 receptors utilize other signaling pathways, including regulation of ion channel activities and the activities of important enzymes involved in signal transduction. α_2-receptor–mediated inhibition of adenylyl cyclase activity is transduced by the inhibitory regulatory protein, G_i (Figure 9–2). How the activation of G_i leads to the inhibition of adenylyl cyclase is unclear, but it is likely that both α and the β-γ subunits of G_i contribute to this response. In addition, some of the effects of α_2 adrenoceptors are independent of their ability to inhibit adenylyl cyclase; for example, α_2-receptor agonists cause platelet aggregation and a decrease in platelet cAMP levels, but it is not clear whether aggregation is the result of the decrease in cAMP or other mechanisms involving G_i-regulated effectors.

B. Beta Receptors

The mechanism of action of β agonists has been studied in considerable detail. Activation of all three receptor subtypes (β_1, β_2, and β_3) results in activation of adenylyl cyclase and increased conversion of adenosine triphosphate (ATP) to cAMP (Table 9–1, Figure 9–2). Activation of the cyclase enzyme is mediated by the stimulatory coupling protein G_s. cAMP is the major second messenger of β-receptor activation. For example, in the liver of many species, β-receptor activation increases cAMP synthesis, which leads to a cascade of events culminating in the activation of glycogen phosphorylase. In the heart, β-receptor activation increases the influx of calcium across the cell membrane and its sequestration inside the cell. Beta-receptor activation also promotes the relaxation of smooth muscle. Although the mechanism of the smooth muscle effect is uncertain, it may involve the phosphorylation of myosin light-chain kinase to an inactive form (see Figure 12–1). Beta adrenoceptors may activate voltage-sensitive calcium channels in the heart via G_s-mediated enhancement independently of changes in cAMP concentration. Under certain circumstances, β_2 receptors may couple to G_q proteins. These receptors have been demonstrated to activate additional kinases, such as MAP kinases, by forming multi-subunit complexes within cells, which contain multiple signaling molecules. In addition, recent evidence suggests that formation of dimers of β receptors themselves (both homodimers and heterodimers of β_1 and β_2 receptors) is prominently involved in their signaling mechanisms. Moreover, agonist activation of β receptors promotes the association of several different proteins with these receptors, leading to activation of novel, additional signal pathways that regulate complex intracellular functions. Similarly, additional proteins interact directly with α_1 and α_2 receptors, leading to further physiologic responses at a cellular level.

Figure 9–1. Activation of α_1 responses. Stimulation of α_1 receptors by catecholamines leads to the activation of a G_q-coupling protein. The activated α subunit (α_q*) of this G protein activates the effector, phospholipase C, which leads to the release of IP_3 (inositol 1,4,5-trisphosphate) and DAG (diacylglycerol) from phosphatidylinositol 4,5-bisphosphate *(PtdIns 4,5-P_2)*. IP_3 stimulates the release of sequestered stores of calcium, leading to an increased concentration of cytoplasmic Ca^{2+}. Ca^{2+} may then activate Ca^{2+}-dependent protein kinases, which in turn phosphorylate their substrates. DAG activates protein kinase C (PKC). See text for additional effects of α_1-receptor activation.

C. DOPAMINE RECEPTORS

The D_1 receptor is typically associated with the stimulation of adenylyl cyclase (Table 9–1); for example, D_1-receptor-induced smooth muscle relaxation is presumably due to cAMP accumulation in the smooth muscle of those vascular beds in which dopamine is a vasodilator. D_2 receptors have been found to inhibit adenylyl cyclase activity, open potassium channels, and decrease calcium influx.

Receptor Regulation

Responses mediated by adrenoceptors are not fixed and static. The number and function of adrenoceptors on the cell surface and their responses may be regulated by catecholamines themselves, other hormones and drugs, age, and a number of disease states (see Chapter 2). These changes may modify the magnitude of a tissue's physiologic response to catecholamines and can be important clinically during the course of treatment. One of the best-studied examples of receptor regulation is the **desensitization** of adrenoceptors that may occur after exposure to catecholamines and other sympathomimetic drugs. After a cell or tissue has been exposed for a period of time to an agonist, that tissue often becomes less responsive to further stimulation by that agent. Other terms such as tolerance, refractoriness, and tachyphylaxis have also been used to denote desensitization. This process has potential clinical significance because it may limit the therapeutic response to sympathomimetic agents.

Many mechanisms have been found to contribute to desensitization. Operating at transcriptional, translational, and protein levels, some mechanisms function relatively slowly—over the course of hours or days. Other mechanisms of desensitization occur quickly, within minutes. Rapid modulation of receptor function

Figure 9–2. Activation and inhibition of adenylyl cyclase by agonists that bind to catecholamine receptors. Binding to β adrenoceptors stimulates adenylyl cyclase by activating the stimulatory G protein, G_s, which leads to the dissociation of its α subunit charged with GTP. This activated α_s subunit directly activates adenylyl cyclase, resulting in an increased rate of synthesis of cAMP. Alpha$_2$-adrenoceptor ligands inhibit adenylyl cyclase by causing dissociation of the inhibitory G protein, G_i, into its subunits; ie, an activated α_i subunit charged with GTP and a βγ unit. The mechanism by which these subunits inhibit adenylyl cyclase is uncertain. cAMP binds to the regulatory subunit *(R)* of cAMP-dependent protein kinase, leading to the liberation of active catalytic subunits *(C)* that phosphorylate specific protein substrates and modify their activity. These catalytic units also phosphorylate the cAMP response element binding protein (CREB), which modifies gene expression. See text for other actions of β and α_2 adrenoceptors.

in desensitized cells may involve critical covalent modification of the receptor, especially by phosphorylation on specific amino acid residues, association of these receptors with other proteins, or changes in their subcellular location.

There are two major categories of desensitization of responses mediated by G protein-coupled receptors. **Homologous** desensitization refers to loss of responsiveness exclusively of the receptors that have been exposed to repeated or sustained activation by a drug. **Heterologous** desensitization refers to loss of responsiveness of some cell surface receptors that have not been directly activated by the drug in question.

A major mechanism of desensitization that occurs rapidly involves phosphorylation of receptors by members of the **G protein-coupled receptor kinase (GRK)** family, of which there are at least seven members. Specific adrenoceptors are substrates for these kinases only when they are bound to an agonist. This mechanism is an example of homologous desensitization because it specifically involves only agonist-occupied receptors.

Phosphorylation of these receptors enhances their affinity for β **arrestins;** upon binding of a β-arrestin molecule, the capacity of the receptor to activate G proteins is blunted, presumably due to steric hindrance (see

Figure 2–12). Arrestins constitute another large family of widely expressed proteins. Receptor phosphorylation followed by β-arrestin binding has been linked to subsequent endocytosis of the receptor. This response may be facilitated by the capacity of β arrestins to bind to the structural protein clathrin. In addition to blunting responses requiring the presence of the receptor on the cell surface, these regulatory processes may also contribute to novel mechanisms of receptor signaling via intracellular pathways.

Receptor desensitization may also be mediated by second-messenger feedback. For example, β adrenoceptors stimulate cAMP accumulation, which leads to activation of protein kinase A; protein kinase A can phosphorylate residues on β receptors, resulting in inhibition of receptor function. For the β_2 receptor, phosphorylation occurs on serine residues both in the third cytoplasmic loop and in the carboxyl terminal tail of the receptor. Similarly, activation of protein kinase C by G_q-coupled receptors may lead to phosphorylation of this class of G protein-coupled receptors. This second-messenger feedback mechanism has been termed heterologous desensitization because activated protein kinase A or protein kinase C may phosphorylate any structurally similar receptor with the appropriate consensus sites for phosphorylation by these enzymes.

ADRENOCEPTOR POLYMORPHISMS

Since elucidation of the sequences of the genes encoding the α_1, α_2, and β subtypes of adrenoceptors, it has become clear that there are relatively common genetic polymorphisms for many of these receptor subtypes in humans. Some of these may lead to changes in critical amino acid sequences that have pharmacologic importance. There is evidence that some of these polymorphisms may change the susceptibility to diseases such as heart failure, alter the propensity of a receptor to desensitize, and alter therapeutic responses to drugs in diseases such as asthma.

CHEMISTRY & PHARMACOKINETICS OF SYMPATHOMIMETIC DRUGS

Phenylethylamine may be considered the parent compound from which sympathomimetic drugs are derived (Figure 9–3). This compound consists of a benzene ring with an ethylamine side chain. Substitutions may be made (1) on the terminal amino group, (2) on the benzene ring, and (3) on the α or β carbons. Substitution by –OH groups at the 3 and 4 positions yields sympathomimetic drugs collectively known as catecholamines. The effects of modification of phenylethylamine are to change the affinity of the drugs for α and β receptors as well as to influence the intrinsic ability to activate the receptors.

In addition, chemical structure determines the pharmacokinetic properties of these molecules. Sympathomimetic drugs may activate both α and β receptors; however, the relative α-receptor versus β-receptor activity spans the range from almost pure α activity (methoxamine) to almost pure β activity (isoproterenol).

A. SUBSTITUTION ON THE AMINO GROUP

Increasing the size of alkyl substituents on the amino group tends to increase β-receptor activity. For example, methyl substitution on norepinephrine, yielding epinephrine, enhances activity at β_2 receptors. Beta activity is further enhanced with isopropyl substitution at the amino nitrogen (isoproterenol). Beta$_2$-selective agonists generally require a large amino substituent group. The larger the substituent on the amino group, the lower the activity at α receptors; for example, isoproterenol is very weak at α receptors.

B. SUBSTITUTION ON THE BENZENE RING

Maximal α and β activity is found with catecholamines (drugs having –OH groups at the 3 and 4 positions). The absence of one or the other of these groups, particularly the hydroxyl at C_3, without other substitutions on the ring may dramatically reduce the potency of the drugs. For example, phenylephrine (Figure 9–4) is much less potent than epinephrine; indeed, α-receptor affinity is decreased about 100-fold and β activity is almost negligible except at very high concentrations. However, catecholamines are subject to inactivation by catechol-*O*-methyltransferase (COMT), an enzyme found in gut and liver (see Chapter 6). Therefore, absence of one or both –OH groups on the phenyl ring increases the bioavailability after oral administration and prolongs the duration of action. Furthermore, absence of ring –OH groups tends to increase the distribution of the molecule to the central nervous system. For example, ephedrine and amphetamine (Figure 9–4) are orally active, have a prolonged duration of action, and produce central nervous system effects not typically observed with the catecholamines.

C. SUBSTITUTION ON THE ALPHA CARBON

Substitutions at the α carbon block oxidation by monoamine oxidase (MAO) and prolong the action of such drugs, particularly the noncatecholamines. Ephedrine and amphetamine are examples of α-substituted compounds (Figure 9–4). Alpha-methyl compounds are also called phenylisopropylamines. In addition to their resistance to oxidation by MAO, some phenylisopropylamines have an enhanced ability to displace catecholamines from storage sites in noradrenergic nerves (see Chapter 6). Therefore, a portion of their activity is

Catechol

Phenylethylamine

Norepinephrine

Epinephrine

Isoproterenol

Dopamine

Figure 9–3. Phenylethylamine and some important catecholamines. Catechol is shown for reference.

dependent on the presence of normal norepinephrine stores in the body; they are indirectly acting sympathomimetics.

D. SUBSTITUTION ON THE BETA CARBON

Direct-acting agonists typically have a β-hydroxyl group, though dopamine does not. In addition to facilitating activation of adrenoceptors, this hydroxyl group

may be important for storage of sympathomimetic amines in neural vesicles.

ORGAN SYSTEM EFFECTS OF SYMPATHOMIMETIC DRUGS

General outlines of the cellular actions of sympathomimetics are presented in Tables 6–3 and 9–3. The net

Phenylephrine

Methoxamine

Ephedrine

Amphetamine

Figure 9–4. Some examples of noncatecholamine sympathomimetic drugs. The isopropyl group is shown in gray.

Table 9–3. Distribution of adrenoceptor subtypes.

Type	Tissue	Actions
α_1	Most vascular smooth muscle (innervated)	Contraction
	Pupillary dilator muscle	Contraction (dilates pupil)
	Pilomotor smooth muscle	Erects hair
	Prostate	Contraction
	Heart	Increases force of contraction
α_2	Postsynaptic CNS adrenoceptors	Probably multiple
	Platelets	Aggregation
	Adrenergic and cholinergic nerve terminals	Inhibition of transmitter release
	Some vascular smooth muscle	Contraction
	Fat cells	Inhibition of lipolysis
β_1	Heart	Increases force and rate of contraction
β_2	Respiratory, uterine, and vascular smooth muscle	Promotes smooth muscle relaxation
	Skeletal muscle	Promotes potassium uptake
	Human liver	Activates glycogenolysis
β_3	Fat cells	Activates lipolysis
D_1	Smooth muscle	Dilates renal blood vessels
D_2	Nerve endings	Modulates transmitter release

effect of a given drug in the intact organism depends on its relative receptor affinity (α or β), intrinsic activity, and the compensatory reflexes evoked by its direct actions.

Cardiovascular System

A. Blood Vessels

Vascular smooth muscle tone is regulated by adrenoceptors; consequently, catecholamines are important in controlling peripheral vascular resistance and venous capacitance. Alpha receptors increase arterial resistance, whereas β_2 receptors promote smooth muscle relaxation. There are major differences in receptor types in the various vascular beds (Table 9–4). The skin vessels have predominantly α receptors and constrict in response to epinephrine and norepinephrine, as do the splanchnic vessels. Vessels in skeletal muscle may constrict or dilate depending on whether α or β receptors are activated. Consequently, the overall effects of a sympathomimetic drug on blood vessels depend on the relative activities of that drug at α and β receptors and the anatomic sites of the vessels affected. In addition, D_1 receptors promote vasodilation of renal, splanchnic, coronary, cerebral, and perhaps other resistance vessels. Activation of the D_1 receptors in the renal vasculature may play a major role in the natriuresis induced by pharmacologic administration of dopamine.

B. Heart

Direct effects on the heart are determined largely by β_1 receptors, although β_2 and to a lesser extent α receptors are also involved, especially in heart failure. Beta-receptor activation results in **increased calcium influx** in cardiac cells. This has both electrical (Figure 9–5) and mechani-

Table 9–4. Cardiovascular responses to sympathomimetic amines.[1]

	Phenyl-ephrine	Epi-nephrine	Isopro-terenol
Vascular resistance (tone)			
Cutaneous, mucous membranes (α)	↑↑	↑↑	0
Skeletal muscle (β_2, α)	↑	↓ or ↑	↓↓
Renal (α, D_1)	↑	↑	↓
Splanchnic (α, β)	↑↑	↓ or ↑[2]	↓
Total peripheral resistance	↑↑↑	↓ or ↑[2]	↓↓
Venous tone (α, β)	↑	↑	↓
Cardiac			
Contractility (β_1)	0 or ↑	↑↑↑	↑↑↑
Heart rate (predominantly β_1)	↓↓ (vagal reflex)	↑ or ↓	↑↑↑
Stroke volume	0, ↓, ↑	↑	↑
Cardiac output	↓	↑	↑↑
Blood pressure			
Mean	↑↑	↑	↓
Diastolic	↑↑	↓ or ↑[2]	↓↓
Systolic	↑↑	↑↑	0 or ↓
Pulse pressure	0	↑↑	↑↑

[1] ↑ = increase; ↓ = decrease; 0 = no change.
[2] Small doses decrease, large doses increase.

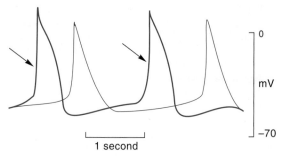

Figure 9–5. Effect of epinephrine on the transmembrane potential of a pacemaker cell in the frog heart. The arrowed trace was recorded after the addition of epinephrine. Note the increased slope of diastolic depolarization and decreased interval between action potentials. This pacemaker acceleration is typical of β_1-stimulant drugs. (Modified and reproduced, with permission, from Brown H, Giles W, Noble S: Membrane currents underlying rhythmic activity in frog sinus venosus. In: Bonke FIM [editor]: *The Sinus Node: Structure, Function, and Clinical Relevance.* Martinus Nijhoff, 1978.)

cal consequences. Pacemaker activity, both normal (sinoatrial node) and abnormal (eg, Purkinje fibers), is increased **(positive chronotropic effect).** Conduction velocity in the atrioventricular node is increased, and the refractory period is decreased. Intrinsic contractility is increased **(positive inotropic effect),** and relaxation is accelerated. As a result, the twitch response of isolated cardiac muscle is increased in tension but abbreviated in duration. In the intact heart, intraventricular pressure rises and falls more rapidly, and ejection time is decreased. These direct effects are easily demonstrated in the absence of reflexes evoked by changes in blood pressure, eg, in isolated myocardial preparations and in patients with ganglionic blockade. In the presence of normal reflex activity, the direct effects on heart rate may be dominated by a reflex response to blood pressure changes. Physiologic stimulation of the heart by catecholamines tends to increase coronary blood flow.

C. BLOOD PRESSURE

The effects of sympathomimetic drugs on blood pressure can be explained on the basis of their effects on the heart, the peripheral vascular resistance, and the venous return (see Figure 6–7 and Table 9–4). A relatively pure α agonist such as phenylephrine increases peripheral arterial resistance and decreases venous capacitance. The enhanced arterial resistance usually leads to a dose-dependent rise in blood pressure (Figure 9–6). In the presence of normal cardiovascular reflexes, the rise in blood pressure elicits a baroreceptor-mediated increase in vagal tone with slowing of the heart rate, which may

be quite marked. However, cardiac output may not diminish in proportion to this reduction in rate, since increased venous return may increase stroke volume. Furthermore, direct α-adrenoceptor stimulation of the heart may have a modest positive inotropic action. While these are the expected effects of pure α agonists in normal subjects, their use in hypotensive patients usually does not lead to brisk reflex responses because in this situation blood pressure is returning to normal, not exceeding normal.

The blood pressure response to a pure β-adrenoceptor agonist is quite different. Stimulation of β receptors in the heart increases cardiac output. A relatively pure β agonist such as isoproterenol also decreases peripheral resistance by activating β_2 receptors, leading to vasodilation in certain vascular beds (Table 9–4). The net effect is to maintain or slightly increase systolic pressure while permitting a fall in diastolic pressure owing to enhanced diastolic runoff (Figure 9–6). The actions of drugs with both α and β effects (eg, epinephrine and norepinephrine) are discussed below.

Eye

The radial pupillary dilator muscle of the iris contains α receptors; activation by drugs such as phenylephrine causes mydriasis (see Figure 6–9). Alpha stimulants also have important effects on intraocular pressure. Present evidence suggests that α agonists increase the outflow of aqueous humor from the eye and reduce intraocular pressure. In contrast, β agonists have little effect, but β *antagonists* decrease the production of aqueous humor. These effects are important in the treatment of glaucoma (see Chapter 10), a leading cause of blindness. Beta stimulants relax the ciliary muscle to a minor degree, causing an insignificant decrease in accommodation. In addition, adrenergic drugs may directly protect neuronal cells in the retina.

Respiratory Tract

Bronchial smooth muscle contains β_2 receptors that cause relaxation. Activation of these receptors results in bronchodilation (see Chapter 20 and Table 9–3). The blood vessels of the upper respiratory tract mucosa contain α receptors; the decongestant action of adrenoceptor stimulants is clinically useful (see Clinical Pharmacology).

Gastrointestinal Tract

Relaxation of gastrointestinal smooth muscle can be brought about by both α- and β-stimulant agents. Beta receptors appear to be located directly on the smooth muscle cells and mediate relaxation via hyperpolarization and decreased spike activity in these cells. Alpha

Figure 9–6. Effects of an α-selective (phenylephrine), β-selective (isoproterenol), and nonselective (epinephrine) sympathomimetic, given as an intravenous bolus injection to a dog. (BP, blood pressure; HR, heart rate.) Reflexes are blunted but not eliminated in this anesthetized animal.

stimulants, especially α_2-selective agonists, decrease muscle activity *indirectly* by presynaptically reducing the release of acetylcholine and possibly other stimulants within the enteric nervous system (see Chapter 6). The α-receptor-mediated response is probably of greater pharmacologic significance than the β-stimulant response. Alpha$_2$ receptors may also decrease salt and water flux into the lumen of the intestine.

Genitourinary Tract

The human uterus contains α and β_2 receptors. The fact that the β receptors mediate relaxation may be clinically useful in pregnancy (see Clinical Pharmacology). The bladder base, urethral sphincter, and prostate contain α receptors that mediate contraction and therefore promote urinary continence. The specific subtype of α_1 receptor involved in mediating constriction of the bladder base and prostate is uncertain, but α_{1A} receptors probably play an important role. The β_2 receptors of the bladder wall mediate relaxation. Ejaculation depends on normal α-receptor (and possibly purinergic receptor)

activation in the ductus deferens, seminal vesicles, and prostate. The detumescence of erectile tissue that normally follows ejaculation is also brought about by norepinephrine (and possibly neuropeptide Y) released from sympathetic nerves. Alpha activation appears to have a similar detumescent effect on erectile tissue in female animals.

Exocrine Glands

The salivary glands contain adrenoceptors that regulate the secretion of amylase and water. However, certain sympathomimetic drugs, eg, clonidine, produce symptoms of dry mouth. The mechanism of this effect is uncertain; it is likely that central nervous system effects are responsible, though peripheral effects may contribute.

The apocrine sweat glands, located on the palms of the hands and a few other areas, respond to adrenoceptor stimulants with increased sweat production. These are the apocrine nonthermoregulatory glands usually associated with psychologic stress. (The diffusely distributed thermoregulatory eccrine sweat glands are regulated by *sympathetic cholinergic* postganglionic nerves that activate muscarinic cholinoceptors; see Chapter 6.)

Metabolic Effects

Sympathomimetic drugs have important effects on intermediary metabolism. Activation of β adrenoceptors in fat cells leads to increased lipolysis with enhanced release of free fatty acids and glycerol into the blood. Beta$_3$ adrenoceptors play a role in mediating this response. There is considerable interest in developing β$_3$-receptor-selective agonists, which could be useful in some metabolic disorders. Human lipocytes also contain α$_2$ receptors that inhibit lipolysis by decreasing intracellular cAMP. Sympathomimetic drugs enhance glycogenolysis in the liver, which leads to increased glucose release into the circulation. In the human liver, the effects of catecholamines are probably mediated mainly by β receptors, though α$_1$ receptors may also play a role. Catecholamines in high concentration may also cause metabolic acidosis. Activation of β$_2$ adrenoceptors by endogenous epinephrine or by sympathomimetic drugs promotes the uptake of potassium into cells, leading to a fall in extracellular potassium. This may lead to a fall in the plasma potassium concentration during stress or protect against a rise in plasma potassium during exercise. Blockade of these receptors may accentuate the rise in plasma potassium that occurs during exercise. Beta receptors and α$_2$ receptors that are expressed in pancreatic islets tend to increase and decrease, respectively, insulin secretion, although the major regulator of insulin release is the plasma concentration of glucose.

Effects on Endocrine Function & Leukocytosis

Catecholamines are important endogenous regulators of hormone secretion from a number of glands. As mentioned above, insulin secretion is stimulated by β receptors and inhibited by α$_2$ receptors. Similarly, renin secretion is stimulated by β$_1$ and inhibited by α$_2$ receptors; indeed, β-receptor antagonist drugs may lower plasma renin and blood pressure in patients with hypertension at least in part by this mechanism. Adrenoceptors also modulate the secretion of parathyroid hormone, calcitonin, thyroxine, and gastrin; however, the physiologic significance of these control mechanisms is probably limited. In high concentrations, epinephrine and related agents cause leukocytosis, in part by promoting demargination of white blood cells sequestered away from the general circulation.

Effects on the Central Nervous System

The action of sympathomimetics on the central nervous system varies dramatically, depending on their ability to cross the blood-brain barrier. The catecholamines are almost completely excluded by this barrier, and subjective central nervous system effects are noted only at the highest rates of infusion. These effects have been described as ranging from "nervousness" to "a feeling of impending disaster," sensations that are undesirable. Furthermore, peripheral effects of β-adrenoceptor agonists such as tachycardia and tremor are similar to the somatic manifestations of anxiety. In contrast, noncatecholamines with indirect actions, such as amphetamines, which readily enter the central nervous system from the circulation, produce qualitatively very different central nervous system effects. These actions vary from mild alerting, with improved attention to boring tasks; through elevation of mood, insomnia, euphoria, and anorexia; to full-blown psychotic behavior. These effects are not readily assigned to either α- or β-mediated actions and may represent enhancement of dopamine-mediated processes or other effects of these drugs in the central nervous system.

SPECIFIC SYMPATHOMIMETIC DRUGS

Catecholamines

Epinephrine (adrenaline) is a very potent vasoconstrictor and cardiac stimulant. The rise in systolic blood pressure that occurs after epinephrine release or administration is caused by its positive inotropic and chronotropic actions on the heart (predominantly β$_1$ receptors) and the vasoconstriction induced in many vascular beds (α receptors). Epinephrine also activates β$_2$ receptors in some vessels (eg, skeletal muscle blood vessels), leading to their dilation. Consequently, total peripheral resistance may actually fall, explaining the fall in diastolic pressure that is sometimes seen with epinephrine injection (Figure 9–6; Table 9–4). Activation of these β$_2$ receptors in skeletal muscle contributes to increased blood flow during exercise. Under physiologic conditions, epinephrine functions largely as a hormone; after release from the adrenal medulla into the blood, it acts on distant cells.

Norepinephrine (levarterenol, noradrenaline) and epinephrine have similar effects on β$_1$ receptors in the heart and similar potency at α receptors. Norepinephrine has relatively little effect on β$_2$ receptors. Consequently, norepinephrine increases peripheral resistance and both diastolic and systolic blood pressure. Compensatory vagal reflexes tend to overcome the direct positive chronotropic effects of norepinephrine; however, the positive inotropic effects on the heart are maintained (Table 9–4).

Isoproterenol (isoprenaline) is a very potent β-receptor agonist and has little effect on α receptors. The drug has positive chronotropic and inotropic actions; because isoproterenol activates β receptors almost exclusively, it is a potent vasodilator. These actions lead to a marked increase in cardiac output associated with a fall in diastolic and mean arterial pressure and a lesser decrease or a slight increase in systolic pressure (Table 9–4; Figure 9–6).

Dopamine, the immediate metabolic precursor of norepinephrine, activates D_1 receptors in several vascular beds, which leads to vasodilation. The effect this has on renal blood flow can be of clinical value. The activation of presynaptic D_2 receptors, which suppress norepinephrine release, contributes to these effects to an unknown extent. In addition, dopamine activates β_1 receptors in the heart. At low doses, peripheral resistance may decrease. At higher rates of infusion, dopamine activates vascular α receptors, leading to vasoconstriction, including in the renal vascular bed. Consequently, high rates of infusion of dopamine may mimic the actions of epinephrine.

Fenoldopam is a D_1-receptor agonist that selectively leads to peripheral vasodilation in some vascular beds. The primary indication for fenoldopam is in the intravenous treatment of severe hypertension (Chapter 11). Continuous infusions of the drug have prompt effects on blood pressure.

Dopamine agonists with central actions are of considerable value for the treatment of Parkinson's disease and prolactinemia. These agents are discussed in Chapters 28 and 37.

Dobutamine is a relatively β_1-selective synthetic catecholamine. As discussed below, dobutamine also activates α_1 receptors.

Other Sympathomimetics

These agents are of interest because of pharmacokinetic features (oral activity, distribution to the central nervous system) or because of relative selectivity for specific receptor subclasses.

Phenylephrine was previously described as an example of a relatively pure α agonist (Table 9–2). It acts directly on the receptors. Because it is not a catechol derivative (Figure 9–4), it is not inactivated by COMT and has a much longer duration of action than the catecholamines. It is an effective mydriatic and decongestant and can be used to raise the blood pressure (Figure 9–6).

Methoxamine acts pharmacologically like phenylephrine, since it is predominantly a direct-acting α_1-receptor agonist. It may cause a prolonged increase in blood pressure due to vasoconstriction; it also causes a vagally mediated bradycardia. Methoxamine is available for parenteral use, but clinical applications are rare and limited to hypotensive states.

Midodrine is a prodrug that is enzymatically hydrolyzed to desglymidodrine, an α_1-receptor-selective agonist. The peak concentration of desglymidodrine is achieved about 1 hour after midodrine is administered. The primary indication for midodrine is the treatment of postural hypotension, typically due to impaired autonomic nervous system function. Although the drug has efficacy in diminishing the fall of blood pressure when the patient is standing, it may cause hypertension when the subject is supine.

Ephedrine occurs in various plants and has been used in China for over 2000 years; it was introduced into Western medicine in 1924 as the first orally active sympathomimetic drug. It is found in ma-huang, a popular herbal medication (see Chapter 65). Ma-huang contains multiple ephedrine-like alkaloids in addition to ephedrine. Because ephedrine is a noncatechol phenylisopropylamine (Figure 9–4), it has high bioavailability and a relatively long duration of action—hours rather than minutes. As is the case with many other phenylisopropylamines, a significant fraction of the drug is excreted unchanged in the urine. Since it is a weak base, its excretion can be accelerated by acidification of the urine.

Ephedrine has not been extensively studied in humans in spite of its long history of use. Its ability to activate β receptors probably accounted for its earlier use in asthma. Because it gains access to the central nervous system, it is a mild stimulant. Ingestion of ephedrine alkaloids contained in ma-huang has raised important safety concerns. Pseudoephedrine, one of four ephedrine enantiomers, has been available over the counter as a component of many decongestant mixtures. However, the use of pseudoephedrine as a precursor in the illicit manufacture of methamphetamine has led to restrictions on its sale.

Xylometazoline and **oxymetazoline** are direct-acting α agonists. These drugs have been used as topical decongestants because of their ability to promote constriction of the nasal mucosa. When taken in large doses, oxymetazoline may cause hypotension, presumably because of a central clonidine-like effect (Chapter 11). Oxymetazoline has significant affinity for α_{2A} receptors.

Amphetamine is a phenylisopropylamine (Figure 9–4) that is important chiefly because of its use and misuse as a central nervous system stimulant (see Chapter 32). Its pharmacokinetics are similar to those of ephedrine; however, amphetamine even more readily enters the central nervous system, where it has marked stimulant effects on mood and alertness and a depressant effect on appetite. Its peripheral actions are mediated primarily through the release of catecholamines. **Methamphetamine** (*N*-methylamphetamine) is very similar to amphetamine with an even higher ratio of central to peripheral actions. **Phenmetrazine** is a variant phenylisopropylamine with amphetamine-like effects. It has been promoted as an

Figure 9–7. Examples of β_1- and β_2-selective agonists.

anorexiant and is also a popular drug of abuse. **Methyl-phenidate** and **pemoline** are amphetamine variants whose major pharmacologic effects and abuse potential are similar to those of amphetamine. These two drugs appear to have efficacy in some children with attention deficit hyperactivity disorder (see Clinical Pharmacology). Pemoline has been withdrawn from use in the USA because of an association with life-threatening hepatic failure. **Modafinil** is a new drug with both similarities to and differences from amphetamine. It has significant effects on central α_{1B} receptors but in addition appears to affect GABAergic, glutaminergic, and serotonergic synapses (see Clinical Pharmacology).

Receptor-Selective Sympathomimetic Drugs

Alpha$_2$-selective agonists have an important ability to decrease blood pressure through actions in the central nervous system even though direct application to a blood vessel may cause vasoconstriction. Such drugs (eg, clonidine, methyldopa, guanfacine, guanabenz) are useful in the treatment of hypertension (and some other conditions) and are discussed in Chapter 11. **Dexmedetomidine** is a centrally acting α_2-selective agonist that is indicated for sedation of initially intubated and mechanically ventilated patients during treatment in an intensive care setting.

Beta-selective agonists are very important because of the separation of β_1 and β_2 effects that has been achieved (Table 9–2). Although this separation is incomplete, it is sufficient to reduce adverse effects in several clinical applications.

Beta$_1$-selective agents include dobutamine and a partial agonist, prenalterol (Figure 9–7). Because they are less effective in activating vasodilator β_2 receptors, they may increase cardiac output with less reflex tachycardia than occurs with nonselective β agonists such as isoproterenol. Dobutamine consists of two isomers, administered as a racemic mixture. The (+) isomer is a potent β_1 agonist and an α_1 receptor antagonist. The (–) isomer is a potent α_1 agonist, capable of causing significant vasoconstriction when given alone. This action tends to reduce vasodilation and may also contribute to the positive inotropic action caused by the isomer with predominantly β-receptor activity. A major limitation with these drugs—as with other direct-acting sympathomimetic agents—is that tolerance to their effects may develop with prolonged use and the likelihood that chronic cardiac stimulation in patients with heart failure may worsen long-term outcome.

Beta$_2$-selective agents have achieved an important place in the treatment of asthma and are discussed in Chapter 20. An additional application is to achieve uterine relaxation in premature labor (ritodrine; see below). Some examples of β_2-selective drugs currently in use are shown in Figures 9–7 and 20–4; many more are available or under investigation.

Special Sympathomimetics

Cocaine is a local anesthetic with a peripheral sympathomimetic action that results from inhibition of transmitter reuptake at noradrenergic synapses (see Chapter 6). It readily enters the central nervous system and produces an amphetamine-like effect that is shorter lasting and more intense. The major action of cocaine in the central nervous system is to inhibit dopamine reuptake into neurons in the "pleasure centers" of the brain. These properties and the fact that it can be smoked, "snorted" into the nose, or injected for rapid onset of effect have made it a heavily abused drug (see Chapter 32). Interestingly, dopamine-transporter knockout mice still self-administer cocaine, suggesting that cocaine may have additional pharmacologic targets.

Tyramine (see Figure 6–5) is a normal by-product of tyrosine metabolism in the body and is also found in high concentrations in some fermented foods such as cheese (Table 9–5). It is readily metabolized by MAO in the liver and is normally inactive when taken orally because of a very high first-pass effect, ie, low bioavailability. If administered parenterally, it has an indirect sympathomimetic action caused by the release of stored catecholamines. Consequently, its spectrum of action is similar to that of norepinephrine. In patients treated with MAO inhibitors—particularly inhibitors of the MAO-A isoform—this effect of tyramine may be greatly intensified, leading to marked increases in blood pressure. This occurs because of increased bioavailability of tyramine and increased neuronal stores of catecholamines. Patients taking MAO inhibitors must be very careful to avoid tyramine-containing foods. There are differences in the effects of various MAO inhibitors on tyramine bioavailability, and isoform-specific or reversible enzyme antagonists may be safer (see Chapters 28 and 30).

■ II. CLINICAL PHARMACOLOGY OF SYMPATHOMIMETIC DRUGS

The rationale for the use of sympathomimetic drugs in therapy rests on a knowledge of the physiologic effects of catecholamines on tissues. Selection of a particular sympathomimetic drug from the host of compounds available depends upon such factors as whether activation of α, β_1, or β_2 receptors is desired; the duration of action desired; and the preferred route of administration. Sympathomimetic drugs are very potent and can have pro-

Table 9–5. Foods reputed to have a high content of tyramine or other sympathomimetic agents.

Food	Tyramine Content of an Average Serving
Beer	(No data)
Broad beans, fava beans	Negligible (but contains dopamine)
Cheese, natural or aged	Nil to 130 mg (cheddar, Gruyère, and Stilton especially high)
Chicken liver	Nil to 9 mg
Chocolate	Negligible (but contains phenylethylamine)
Sausage, fermented (eg, salami, pepperoni, summer sausage)	Nil to 74 mg
Smoked or pickled fish (eg, pickled herring)	Nil to 198 mg
Snails	(No data)
Wine (red)	Nil to 3 mg
Yeast (eg, dietary brewer's yeast supplements)	2–68 mg

Note: In a patient taking an irreversible MAO inhibitor drug, 20–50 mg of tyramine in a meal may increase the blood pressure significantly (see also Chapter 30: Antidepressant Agents). Note that only cheese, sausage, pickled fish, and yeast supplements contain sufficient tyramine to be consistently dangerous. This does not rule out the possibility that some preparations of other foods might contain significantly greater than average amounts of tyramine.

found effects on a variety of organ systems, particularly the heart and peripheral circulation. Therefore, great caution is indicated when these agents are used parenterally. In most cases, rather than using fixed doses of the drugs, careful monitoring of pharmacologic response is required to determine the appropriate dosage, especially if the drug is being infused. Generally, it is desirable to use the minimum dose required to achieve the desired response. The adverse effects of these drugs are generally understandable in terms of their known physiologic effects.

Cardiovascular Applications

A. CONDITIONS IN WHICH BLOOD FLOW OR PRESSURE IS TO BE ENHANCED

Hypotension may occur in a variety of settings such as decreased blood volume, cardiac arrhythmias, neurologic disease or accidents, adverse reactions to medications such as antihypertensive drugs, and infection. If cerebral, renal, cardiac perfusion is maintained, hypotension itself does not usually require vigorous direct treatment. Rather, placing the patient in the recumbent position and ensuring adequate fluid volume, while the primary problem is determined and treated, is usually the correct course of action. The use of sympathomimetic drugs merely to elevate a blood pressure that is not an immediate threat to the patient may increase morbidity (see Toxicity of Sympathomimetic Drugs, below). Sympathomimetic drugs may be used in a hypotensive emergency to preserve cerebral and coronary blood flow. Such situations might arise in severe hemorrhage, spinal cord injury, or overdoses of antihypertensive or central nervous system depressant medications. The treatment is usually of short duration while the appropriate intravenous fluid or blood is being administered. Direct-acting α agonists such as **norepinephrine, phenylephrine,** or **methoxamine** have been utilized in this setting if vasoconstriction is desired. For the treatment of chronic orthostatic hypotension, oral **ephedrine** has been the traditional therapy. **Midodrine,** an orally active α agonist, may be the preferred sympathomimetic in this application if further studies confirm its long-term safety and efficacy.

Shock is a complex acute cardiovascular syndrome that results in a critical reduction in perfusion of vital tissues and a wide range of systemic effects. Shock is usually associated with hypotension, an altered mental state, oliguria, and metabolic acidosis. If untreated, shock usually progresses to a refractory deteriorating state and death. The three major mechanisms responsible for shock are hypovolemia, cardiac insufficiency, and altered vascular resistance. **Volume replacement** and treatment of the underlying disease are the mainstays of the treatment of shock. Although sympathomimetic drugs have been used in the treatment of virtually all forms of shock, their efficacy is unclear.

In most forms of shock, vasoconstriction mediated by the sympathetic nervous system is already intense. Indeed, efforts aimed at reducing rather than increasing peripheral resistance may be more fruitful if cerebral, coronary, and renal perfusion are improved. A decision to use vasoconstrictors or vasodilators is best made on the basis of information about the underlying cause, which may require invasive monitoring.

Cardiogenic shock, usually due to massive myocardial infarction, has a poor prognosis. Mechanically assisted perfusion and emergency cardiac surgery have been utilized in some settings. Optimal fluid replacement requires monitoring of pulmonary capillary wedge pressure and other parameters of cardiac function. Positive inotropic agents such as **dopamine** or **dobutamine** may have a role in this situation. In low to moderate doses, these drugs may increase cardiac output and, compared with norepinephrine, cause relatively little peripheral

vasoconstriction. Isoproterenol increases heart rate and work more than either dopamine or dobutamine. See Chapter 13 and Table 13–4 for a discussion of shock associated with myocardial infarction.

Unfortunately, the patient with shock may not respond to any of these therapeutic maneuvers; the temptation is then great to use vasoconstrictors to maintain adequate blood pressure. Coronary perfusion may be improved, but this gain may be offset by increased myocardial oxygen demands as well as more severe vasoconstriction in blood vessels to the abdominal viscera. Therefore, the goal of therapy in shock should be to optimize tissue perfusion, not blood pressure.

B. CONDITIONS IN WHICH BLOOD FLOW IS TO BE REDUCED

Reduction of local or regional blood flow is desirable for achieving hemostasis in surgery, for reducing diffusion of local anesthetics away from the site of administration, and for reducing mucous membrane congestion. In each instance, α-receptor activation is desired, and the choice of agent depends upon the maximal efficacy required, the desired duration of action, and the route of administration.

Effective pharmacologic hemostasis, often necessary for facial, oral, and nasopharyngeal surgery, requires drugs of high efficacy that can be administered in high concentration by local application. **Epinephrine** is usually applied topically in nasal packs (for epistaxis) or in a gingival string (for gingivectomy). **Cocaine** is still sometimes used for nasopharyngeal surgery, because it combines a hemostatic effect with local anesthesia. Occasionally, cocaine is mixed with epinephrine for maximum hemostasis and local anesthesia.

Combining α agonists with some local anesthetics greatly prolongs the duration of infiltration nerve block; the total dose of local anesthetic (and the probability of toxicity) can therefore be reduced. **Epinephrine,** 1:200,000, is the favored agent for this application, but norepinephrine, phenylephrine, and other α agonists have also been used. Systemic effects on the heart and peripheral vasculature may occur even with local drug administration.

Mucous membrane decongestants are α agonists that reduce the discomfort of hay fever and, to a lesser extent, the common cold by decreasing the volume of the nasal mucosa. These effects are probably mediated by α_1 receptors. Unfortunately, rebound hyperemia may follow the use of these agents, and repeated topical use of high drug concentrations may result in ischemic changes in the mucous membranes, probably as a result of vasoconstriction of nutrient arteries. Constriction of these vessels may involve activation of α_2 receptors. For example, **phenylephrine** is often used in nasal decongestant sprays. A longer duration of action—at the cost of much lower local concentrations and greater potential for cardiac and central nervous system effects—can be achieved by the oral administration of agents such as **ephedrine** or one of its isomers, **pseudoephedrine.** Long-acting topical decongestants include **xylometazoline** and **oxymetazoline.** Most of these mucous membrane decongestants are available as over-the-counter products.

C. CARDIAC APPLICATIONS

Catecholamines such as isoproterenol and epinephrine have been used in the temporary emergency management of complete heart block and cardiac arrest. Epinephrine may be useful in cardiac arrest in part by redistributing blood flow during cardiopulmonary resuscitation to coronaries and to the brain. However, electronic pacemakers are both safer and more effective in heart block and should be inserted as soon as possible if there is any indication of continued high-degree block.

Heart failure may respond to the positive inotropic effects of drugs such as dobutamine. These applications are discussed in Chapter 13. The development of tolerance or desensitization is a major limitation to the use of catecholamines in heart failure.

Pulmonary Applications

One of the most important uses of sympathomimetic drugs is in the therapy of bronchial asthma. This use is discussed in Chapter 20. Nonselective drugs (epinephrine), β-selective agents (isoproterenol), and β_2-selective agents (metaproterenol, terbutaline, albuterol) are all available for this indication. Sympathomimetics other than the β_2-selective drugs are now rarely used because they are likely to have more adverse effects than the selective drugs.

Anaphylaxis

Anaphylactic shock and related immediate (type I) IgE-mediated reactions affect both the respiratory and the cardiovascular systems. The syndrome of bronchospasm, mucous membrane congestion, angioedema, and severe hypotension usually responds rapidly to the parenteral administration of **epinephrine,** 0.3–0.5 mg (0.3–0.5 mL of 1:1000 epinephrine solution). Intramuscular injection may be the preferred route of administration, since skin blood flow (and hence systemic drug absorption from subcutaneous injection) is unpredictable in hypotensive patients. In some patients with impaired cardiovascular function, intravenous injection of epinephrine may be required. Extensive experimental and clinical experience with the drug in anaphylaxis supports epinephrine as the agent of choice, presumably because epinephrine activates α, β_1, and β_2 receptors, all of which may be important in reversing the pathophysiologic processes underlying anaphylaxis. Glucocorticoids and antihistamines (both H_1- and H_2-receptor antagonists) may be useful as secondary therapy in anaphylaxis; however, epinephrine is the initial treatment.

Ophthalmic Applications

Phenylephrine is an effective mydriatic agent frequently used to facilitate examination of the retina. It is also a useful decongestant for minor allergic hyperemia and itching of the conjunctival membranes. Sympathomimetics administered as ophthalmic drops are also useful in localizing the lesion in Horner's syndrome. (See Box: An Application of Basic Pharmacology to a Clinical Problem.)

AN APPLICATION OF BASIC PHARMACOLOGY TO A CLINICAL PROBLEM

Horner's syndrome is a condition—usually unilateral—that results from interruption of the sympathetic nerves to the face. The effects include vasodilation, ptosis, miosis, and loss of sweating on the side affected. The syndrome can be caused by either a preganglionic or a postganglionic lesion, such as a tumor. Knowledge of the location of the lesion (preganglionic or postganglionic) helps determine the optimal therapy.

An understanding of the effects of denervation on neurotransmitter metabolism permits the clinician to use drugs to localize the lesion. In most situations, a localized lesion in a nerve causes degeneration of the distal portion of that fiber and loss of transmitter contents from the degenerated nerve ending—without affecting neurons innervated by the fiber. Therefore, a preganglionic lesion leaves the postganglionic adrenergic neuron intact, whereas a postganglionic lesion results in degeneration of the adrenergic nerve endings and loss of stored catecholamines from them. Because indirectly acting sympathomimetics require normal stores of catecholamines, such drugs can be used to test for the presence of normal adrenergic nerve endings. The iris, because it is easily visible and responsive to topical sympathomimetics, is a convenient assay tissue in the patient.

If the lesion of Horner's syndrome is postganglionic, indirectly acting sympathomimetics (eg, cocaine, hydroxyamphetamine) will not dilate the abnormally constricted pupil because catecholamines have been lost from the nerve endings in the iris. In contrast, the pupil dilates in response to phenylephrine, which acts directly on the α receptors on the smooth muscle of the iris. A patient with a preganglionic lesion, on the other hand, shows a normal response to both drugs, since the postganglionic fibers and their catecholamine stores remain intact in this situation.

Glaucoma responds to a variety of sympathomimetic and sympathoplegic drugs. (See Box in Chapter 10: The Treatment of Glaucoma.) Epinephrine and its prodrug dipivefrin are now rarely used, but β-blocking agents are among the most important therapies. **Apraclonidine** and **brimonidine** are α_2-selective agonists that also lower intraocular pressure and are approved for use in glaucoma. The mechanism of action of these drugs in treating glaucoma is still uncertain; direct neuroprotective effects may be involved in addition to the benefits of lowering intraocular pressure.

Genitourinary Applications

As noted above, β_2-selective agents relax the pregnant uterus. **Ritodrine, terbutaline,** and similar drugs have been used to suppress premature labor. The goal is to defer labor long enough to ensure adequate maturation of the fetus. These drugs may delay labor for several days. This may afford time to administer corticosteroid drugs, which decrease the incidence of neonatal respiratory distress syndrome. However, meta-analysis of older trials and a randomized study suggest that β-agonist therapy may have no significant benefit on perinatal infant mortality and may increase maternal morbidity.

Oral sympathomimetic therapy is occasionally useful in the treatment of stress incontinence. Ephedrine or pseudoephedrine may be tried.

Central Nervous System Applications

The **amphetamines** have a mood-elevating (euphoriant) effect; this effect is the basis for the widespread abuse of this drug and some of its analogs (see Chapter 32). The amphetamines also have an alerting, sleep-deferring action that is manifested by improved attention to repetitive tasks and by acceleration and desynchronization of the electroencephalogram. A therapeutic application of this effect is in the treatment of narcolepsy. **Modafinil,** a new amphetamine substitute, is approved for use in narcolepsy and is claimed to have fewer disadvantages (excessive mood changes, insomnia, abuse potential) than amphetamine in this condition. The appetite-suppressing effect of these agents is easily demonstrated in experimental animals. In obese humans, an encouraging initial response may be observed, but there is no evidence that long-term improvement in weight control can be achieved with amphetamines alone, especially when administered for a relatively short course. A final application of the CNS-active sympathomimetics is in the attention-deficit hyperactivity disorder (ADHD) of children, a poorly defined and overdiagnosed behavioral syndrome consisting of short attention span, hyperkinetic physical behavior, and learning problems. Some patients with this syndrome respond well to low doses of methylphenidate and related agents or to clonidine. Extended-release formulations of methylphenidate may simplify dosing regimens and increase adherence to therapy, especially in school-age children. Evidence from several clinical trials suggests that modafinil may also be useful in ADHD.

Additional Therapeutic Uses

Although the primary use of the α_2 agonist **clonidine** is in the treatment of hypertension (Chapter 11), the drug has been found to have efficacy in the treatment of diarrhea in diabetics with autonomic neuropathy, perhaps because of its ability to enhance salt and water absorption from the intestines. In addition, clonidine has efficacy in diminishing craving for narcotics and alcohol during withdrawal and may facilitate cessation of cigarette smoking. Clonidine has also been used to diminish menopausal hot flushes and is being used experimentally to reduce hemodynamic instability during general anesthesia. **Dexmedetomidine** is indicated for sedation under intensive care circumstances.

TOXICITY OF SYMPATHOMIMETIC DRUGS

The adverse effects of adrenoceptor agonists are primarily extensions of their pharmacologic effects in the cardiovascular and central nervous systems.

Adverse cardiovascular effects seen with intravenously infused pressor agents include marked elevations in blood pressure that cause increased cardiac work, which may precipitate cardiac ischemia and failure. Systemically administered β-receptor-stimulant drugs may cause sinus tachycardia and may even provoke serious ventricular arrhythmias. Sympathomimetic drugs may lead to myocardial damage, particularly after prolonged infusion. Special caution is indicated in elderly patients and those with hypertension or coronary artery disease. To avoid excessive pharmacologic responses, it is essential to monitor the blood pressure when administering sympathomimetic drugs parenterally.

If an adverse sympathomimetic effect requires urgent reversal, a specific adrenoceptor antagonist can be used (see Chapter 10).

Central nervous system toxicity is rarely observed with catecholamines or drugs such as phenylephrine. In moderate doses, amphetamines commonly cause restlessness, tremor, insomnia, and anxiety; in high doses, a paranoid state may be induced. Cocaine may precipitate convulsions, cerebral hemorrhage, arrhythmias, or myocardial infarction. Therapy is discussed in Chapter 59.

PREPARATIONS AVAILABLE[1]

Amphetamine, racemic mixture (generic)
Oral: 5, 10 mg tablets
Oral (Adderall): 1:1:1:1 mixtures of amphetamine sulfate, amphetamine aspartate, dextroamphetamine sulfate, and dextroamphetamine saccharate, formulated to contain a total of 5, 7.5, 10, 12.5, 15, 20, or 30 mg in tablets; or 10, 20, or 30 mg in capsules

Apraclonidine (Iopidine)
Topical: 0.5, 1% solutions

Brimonidine (Alphagan)
Topical: 0.15, 0.2% solution

Dexmedetomidine (Precedex)
Parenteral: 100 mcg/mL

Dexmethylphenidate (Focalin)
Oral: 2.5, 5, 10 mg tablets

Dextroamphetamine (generic, Dexedrine)
Oral: 5, 10 mg tablets
Oral sustained-release: 5, 10, 15 mg capsules
Oral mixtures with amphetamine: see Amphetamine (Adderall)

Dipivefrin (generic, Propine)
Topical: 0.1% ophthalmic solution

Dobutamine (generic, Dobutrex)
Parenteral: 12.5 mg/mL in 20 mL vials for injection

Dopamine (generic, Intropin)
Parenteral: 40, 80, 160 mg/mL for injection; 80, 160, 320 mg/100 mL in 5% D/W for injection

Ephedrine (generic)
Oral: 25 mg capsules
Parenteral: 50 mg/mL for injection

Epinephrine (generic, Adrenalin Chloride, others)
Parenteral: 1:1000 (1 mg/mL), 1:2000 (0.5 mg/mL), 1:10,000 (0.1 mg/mL), 1:100,000 (0.01 mg/mL) for injection
Parenteral autoinjector (Epipen): 1:1000 (1 mg/mL), 1:2000 (0.5 mg/mL)
Ophthalmic: 0.1, 0.5, 1, 2% drops
Nasal: 0.1% drops and spray
Aerosol for bronchospasm (Primatene Mist, Bronkaid Mist): 0.22 mg/spray
Solution for aerosol: 1:100

Fenoldopam (Corlopam)
Parenteral: 10 mg/mL for IV infusion

Hydroxyamphetamine (Paredrine)
Ophthalmic: 1% drops

Isoproterenol (generic, Isuprel)
Parenteral: 1:5000 (0.2 mg/mL), 1:50,000 (0.02 mg/mL) for injection

Mephentermine (Wyamine Sulfate)
Parenteral: 15, 30 mg/mL for injection

Metaraminol (Aramine)
Parenteral: 10 mg/mL for injection

Methamphetamine (Desoxyn)
Oral: 5 mg tablets

Methoxamine (Vasoxyl)
Parenteral: 20 mg/mL for injection

Methylphenidate (generic, Ritalin, Ritalin-SR)
Oral: 5, 10, 20 mg tablets
Oral sustained-release: 10, 18, 20, 27, 36, 54 mg tablets; 20, 30, 40 mg capsules

Midodrine (ProAmatine)
Oral: 2.5, 5, 10 mg tablets

Modafinil (Provigil)
Oral: 100, 200 mg tablets

Naphazoline (generic, Privine)
Nasal: 0.05% drops and spray
Ophthalmic: 0.012, 0.02, 0.03, 0.1% drops

Norepinephrine (generic, Levophed)
Parenteral: 1 mg/mL for injection

Oxymetazoline (generic, Afrin, Neo-Synephrine 12 Hour, Visine LR)
Nasal: 0.05% spray
Ophthalmic: 0.025% drops

Phenylephrine (generic, Neo-Synephrine)
Oral: 10 mg chewable tablets
Parenteral: 10 mg/mL for injection
Nasal: 0.125, 0.16, 0.25, 0.5, 1% drops and spray
Ophthalmic: 0.12, 2.5, 10% solution

Pseudoephedrine (generic, Sudafed)
Oral: 30, 60 mg tablets; 30, 60 mg capsules; 15, 30 mg/5 mL syrups; 7.5 mg/0.8 mL drops
Oral extended-release: 120, 240 mg tablets, capsules

Tetrahydrozoline (generic, Tyzine)
Nasal: 0.05, 0.1% drops
Ophthalmic: 0.05% drops

Xylometazoline (generic, Otrivin)
Nasal: 0.05, 0.1% drops

---

[1]α_2-Agonists used in hypertension are listed in Chapter 11. β_2-Agonists used in asthma are listed in Chapter 20.

REFERENCES

Brown SG: Cardiovascular aspects of anaphylaxis: implications for treatment and diagnosis. Curr Opin Allergy Clin Immunol 2005;5:359.

Collins S, Cao W, Robidoux J: Learning new tricks from old dogs: Beta-adrenergic receptors teach new lessons on firing up adipose tissue metabolism. Mol Endocrinol 2004;18:2123.

Evans WE, McLeod HL: Pharmacogenomics—drug disposition, drug targets, and side effects. N Engl J Med 2003;348:538.

Gainetdinov RR et al: Desensitization of G protein-coupled receptors and neuronal functions. Annu Rev Neurosci 2004;27:107.

Hawrylyshyn KA et al: Update on human alpha1-adrenoceptor subtype signaling and genomic organization. Trends Pharmacol Sci 2004;25:449.

Holmes A, Lachowicz JE, Sibley DR: Phenotypic analysis of dopamine receptor knockout mice; recent insights into the functional specificity of dopamine receptor subtypes. Neuropharmacology 2004;47:1117.

Koch WJ: Genetic and phenotypic targeting of beta-adrenergic signaling in heart failure. Mol Cell Biochem 2004;263:5.

Koshimizu T et al: Recent progress in alpha$_1$-adrenoceptor pharmacology. Biol Pharm Bull 2002;25:401.

Lefkowitz RJ, Shenoy SK: Transduction of receptor signals by beta-arrestins. Science 2005;308:512.

Mitler MM, Hayduk R: Benefits and risks of pharmacotherapy for narcolepsy. Drug Saf 2002;25:791.

Oldenburg O et al: Treatment of orthostatic hypotension. Curr Opin Pharmacol 2002;2:740.

Philipp M, Hein L: Adrenergic receptor knockout mice: Distinct functions of 9 receptor subtypes. Pharmacol Ther 2004; 101:65.

Rockman HA, Koch WJ, Lefkowitz RJ: Seven-transmembrane-spanning receptors and heart function. Nature 2002; 415:206.

Sandilands AJ, O'Shaughnessy KM: The functional significance of genetic variation within the beta-adrenoceptor. Br J Clin Pharmacol 2005;60:235.

Small KM, McGraw DW, Liggett SB: Pharmacology and physiology of human adrenergic receptor polymorphisms. Ann Rev Pharmacol Toxicol 2003;43:381.

Soltau JB, Zimmerman TJ: Changing paradigms in the medical treatment of glaucoma. Surv Ophthalmol 2002;47(Suppl 1):S2.

Wechsler ME, Israel E: How pharmacogenomics will play a role in the management of asthma. Am J Respir Crit Care Med 2005;172:12.

Wechsler ME et al: Beta-adrenergic receptor polymorphisms and response to salmeterol. Am J Respir Crit Care Med 2006; 173:519.

Adrenoceptor Antagonist Drugs

10

Brian B. Hoffman, MD

Since catecholamines play a role in a variety of physiologic and pathophysiologic responses, drugs that block adrenoceptors have important effects, some of which are of great clinical value. These effects vary dramatically according to the drug's selectivity for α and β receptors. The classification of adrenoceptors into α_1, α_2, and β subtypes and the effects of activating these receptors are discussed in Chapters 6 and 9. Blockade of peripheral dopamine receptors is of no recognized clinical importance at present. In contrast, blockade of central nervous system dopamine receptors is very important; drugs that act on these receptors are discussed in Chapters 21 and 29. This chapter deals with pharmacologic antagonist drugs whose major effect is to occupy either α_1, α_2, or β receptors outside the central nervous system and prevent their activation by catecholamines and related agonists.

For pharmacologic research, α_1- and α_2-adrenoceptor antagonist drugs have been very useful in the experimental exploration of autonomic nervous system function. In clinical therapeutics, nonselective α antagonists are used in the treatment of pheochromocytoma (tumors that secrete catecholamines), and α_1-selective antagonists are used in primary hypertension and benign prostatic hyperplasia. Beta-receptor antagonist drugs have been found useful in a much wider variety of clinical conditions and are firmly established in the treatment of hypertension, ischemic heart disease, arrhythmias, endocrinologic and neurologic disorders, glaucoma, and other conditions.

■ I. BASIC PHARMACOLOGY OF THE ALPHA-RECEPTOR ANTAGONIST DRUGS

Mechanism of Action

Alpha-receptor antagonists may be reversible or irreversible in their interaction with these receptors. Reversible antagonists dissociate from receptors and the block can be surmounted with sufficiently high concentrations of agonists; irreversible drugs do not dissociate and cannot be surmounted. Phentolamine (Figure 10–1) and prazosin are examples of reversible antagonists. Prazosin (and analogs) and labetalol—drugs used primarily for their antihypertensive effects—as well as several ergot derivatives (see Chapter 16) are also reversible α-adrenoceptor antagonists or partial agonists. Phenoxybenzamine, an agent related to the nitrogen mustards, forms a reactive ethyleneimonium intermediate (Figure 10–1) that covalently binds to α receptors, resulting in irreversible blockade. Figure 10–2 illustrates the effects of a reversible drug in comparison with those of an irreversible agent.

As discussed in Chapters 1 and 2, the duration of action of a reversible antagonist is largely dependent on the half-life of the drug in the body and the rate at which it dissociates from its receptor: The shorter the half-life of the drug in the body, the less time it takes for the effects of the drug to dissipate. In contrast, the effects of an irreversible antagonist may persist long after the drug has been cleared from the plasma. In the case of phenoxybenzamine, the restoration of tissue responsiveness after extensive α-receptor blockade is dependent on synthesis of new receptors, which may take several days. The rate of return of α_1-adrenoceptor responsiveness may be particularly important in patients having a sudden cardiovascular event or who become candidates for urgent surgery.

Pharmacologic Effects

A. CARDIOVASCULAR EFFECTS

Because arteriolar and venous tone are determined to a large extent by α receptors on vascular smooth muscle, α-receptor antagonist drugs cause a lowering of peripheral vascular resistance and blood pressure (Figure 10–3). These drugs can prevent the pressor effects of usual doses of α agonists; indeed, in the case of agonists with both α and β_2 effects (eg, epinephrine), selective α-receptor antagonism may convert a pressor to a depressor response (Figure 10–3). This change in response is called **epinephrine reversal**; it illustrates

Figure 10–1. Structure of several α-receptor-blocking drugs.

how the activation of both α and β receptors in the vasculature may lead to opposite responses. Alpha-receptor antagonists often cause postural hypotension and reflex tachycardia; nonselective ($\alpha_1 = \alpha_2$, Table 10–1) blockers usually cause significant tachycardia if blood pressure is lowered below normal. Postural hypotension is due to antagonism of sympathetic nervous system stimulation of α_1 receptors in venous smooth muscle; contraction of veins is an important component of the normal capacity to maintain blood pressure in the upright position since it decreases venous pooling in the periphery. Constriction of arterioles in the legs may also contribute to the postural response. Tachycardia may be more marked with agents that block α_2-presynaptic receptors in the heart, since the augmented release of norepinephrine will further stimulate β receptors in the heart.

B. OTHER EFFECTS

Minor effects that signal the blockade of α receptors in other tissues include miosis and nasal stuffiness. Alpha$_1$-receptor blockade of the base of the bladder and the prostate is associated with decreased resistance to the flow of urine. Individual agents may have other important effects in addition to α-receptor antagonism (see below).

SPECIFIC AGENTS

Phentolamine, an imidazoline derivative, is a potent competitive antagonist at both α_1 and α_2 receptors (Table 10–1). Phentolamine causes a reduction in peripheral resistance through blockade of α_1 receptors and possibly α_2 receptors on vascular smooth muscle. The cardiac stimulation induced by phentolamine is due to sympathetic stimulation of the heart resulting from baroreflex mechanisms. Furthermore, since phentolamine potently blocks α_2 receptors, antagonism of presynaptic α_2 receptors may lead to enhanced release of norepinephrine from sympathetic nerves. In addition to being an α_1- and α_2-receptor antagonist, phentolamine also has minor inhibitory effects at serotonin receptors and agonist effects at muscarinic and H$_1$ and H$_2$ histamine receptors.

Phentolamine has limited absorption after oral administration. Its pharmacokinetic properties are not well known; it may reach peak concentrations within an hour after oral administration and has a half-life of 5–7 hours. The principal adverse effects are related to

Figure 10–2. Dose-response curves to norepinephrine in the presence of two different α-adrenoceptor-blocking drugs. The tension produced in isolated strips of cat spleen, a tissue rich in α receptors, was measured in response to graded doses of norepinephrine. **Left:** Tolazoline, a reversible blocker, shifted the curve to the right without decreasing the maximum response when present at concentrations of 10 and 20 μmol/L. **Right:** Dibenamine, an analog of phenoxybenzamine and irreversible in its action, reduced the maximum response attainable at both concentrations tested. (Modified and reproduced, with permission, from Bickerton RK: The response of isolated strips of cat spleen to sympathomimetic drugs and their antagonists. J Pharmacol Exp Ther 1963;142:99.)

cardiac stimulation, which may cause severe tachycardia, arrhythmias, and myocardial ischemia, especially after intravenous administration. With oral administration, adverse effects include tachycardia, nasal congestion, and headache.

Phentolamine has been used in the treatment of pheochromocytoma—especially intraoperatively—as well as for male erectile dysfunction by injection intracavernosally and when taken orally (see below).

Phenoxybenzamine binds covalently to α receptors, causing irreversible blockade of long duration (14–48 hours or longer). It is somewhat selective for α_1 receptors but less so than prazosin (Table 10–1). The drug also inhibits reuptake of released norepinephrine by presynaptic adrenergic nerve terminals. Phenoxybenzamine blocks histamine (H_1), acetylcholine, and serotonin receptors as well as α receptors (see Chapter 16).

The pharmacologic actions of phenoxybenzamine are primarily related to antagonism of α-receptor–mediated events. Most significant is that phenoxybenzamine attenuates catecholamine-induced vasoconstriction. While phenoxybenzamine causes relatively little fall in blood pressure in normal supine individuals, it reduces blood pressure when sympathetic tone is high, eg, as a result of

upright posture or because of reduced blood volume. Cardiac output may be increased because of reflex effects and because of some blockade of presynaptic α_2 receptors in cardiac sympathetic nerves.

Phenoxybenzamine is absorbed after oral administration, although bioavailability is low and its kinetic properties are not well known. The drug is usually given orally, starting with low doses of 10–20 mg/d and progressively increasing the dose until the desired effect is achieved. A dosage of less than 100 mg/d is usually sufficient to achieve adequate α-receptor blockade. The major use of phenoxybenzamine is in the treatment of pheochromocytoma (see below).

Many of the adverse effects of phenoxybenzamine derive from its α-receptor–blocking action; the most important are postural hypotension and tachycardia. Nasal stuffiness and inhibition of ejaculation also occur. Since phenoxybenzamine enters the central nervous system, it may cause less specific effects, including fatigue, sedation, and nausea. Because phenoxybenzamine is an alkylating agent, it may have other adverse effects that have not yet been characterized. Phenoxybenzamine causes tumors in animals, but the clinical implications of this observation are unknown.

BP 135/85   128/50

HR 160   200

Phentolamine

BP 135/90   190/124   160/82   175/110

HR 180   210

Epinephrine before phentolamine

BP 125/85   100/35

HR 190   210

Epinephrine after phentolamine

Figure 10–3. **Top:** Effects of phentolamine, an α-receptor-blocking drug, on blood pressure in an anesthetized dog. Epinephrine reversal is demonstrated by tracings showing the response to epinephrine before **(middle)** and after **(bottom)** phentolamine. All drugs given intravenously. (BP, blood pressure; HR, heart rate.)

Table 10–1. Relative selectivity of antagonists for adrenoceptors.

	Receptor Affinity
α Antagonists	
Prazosin, terazosin, doxazosin	$\alpha_1 >>>> \alpha_2$
Phenoxybenzamine	$\alpha_1 > \alpha_2$
Phentolamine	$\alpha_1 = \alpha_2$
Rauwolscine, yohimbine, tolazoline	$\alpha_2 >> \alpha_1$
Mixed antagonists	
Labetalol, carvedilol	$\beta_1 = \beta_2 \geq \alpha_1 > \alpha_2$
β Antagonists	
Metoprololol, acebutolol, alprenolol, atenolol, betaxolol, celiprolol, esmolol	$\beta_1 >>> \beta_2$
Propranolol, carteolol, penbutolol, pindolol, timolol	$\beta_1 = \beta_2$
Butoxamine	$\beta_2 >>> \beta_1$

Tolazoline is an obsolete agent similar to phentolamine. **Ergot derivatives,** eg, ergotamine, dihydroergotamine, cause reversible α-receptor blockade, probably via a partial agonist action (Chapter 16).

Prazosin is a piperazinyl quinazoline effective in the management of hypertension (see Chapter 11). It is highly selective for α_1 receptors and typically 1000-fold less potent at α_2 receptors. This may partially explain the relative absence of tachycardia seen with prazosin compared with that reported with phentolamine and phenoxybenzamine. Prazosin leads to relaxation of both arterial and venous vascular smooth muscle, as well as smooth muscle in the prostate, due to blockade of α_1 receptors. Prazosin is extensively metabolized in humans; because of metabolic degradation by the liver, only about 50% of the drug is available after oral administration. The half-life is normally about 3 hours.

Terazosin is another reversible α_1-selective antagonist that is effective in hypertension (Chapter 11); it is also approved for use in men with urinary symptoms due to benign prostatic hyperplasia (BPH). Terazosin has high bioavailability but is extensively metabolized in the liver, with only a small fraction of unchanged drug excreted in the urine. The half-life of terazosin is 9–12 hours.

Doxazosin is efficacious in the treatment of hypertension and BPH. It differs from prazosin and terazosin in having a longer half-life of about 22 hours. It has moderate bioavailability and is extensively metabolized, with very little parent drug excreted in urine or feces. Doxazosin has active metabolites, although their contribution to the drug's effects is probably small.

Tamsulosin is a competitive α_1 antagonist with a structure quite different from that of most other α_1-receptor blockers. It has high bioavailability and a long half-life of 9–15 hours. It is metabolized extensively in the liver. Tamsulosin has higher affinity for α_{1A} and α_{1D} receptors than for the α_{1B} subtype. Evidence suggests that tamsulosin has relatively greater potency in inhibiting contraction in *prostate* smooth muscle versus *vascular* smooth muscle compared with other α_1-selective antagonists. The drug's efficacy in BPH suggests that the α_{1A} subtype may be the most important α subtype mediating prostate smooth muscle contraction. Furthermore, compared with other antagonists, tamsulosin has less effect on standing blood pressure in patients. Nevertheless, caution is appropriate in using any α antagonist in patients with diminished sympathetic nervous system function.

OTHER ALPHA-ADRENOCEPTOR ANTAGONISTS

Alfuzosin is an α_1-selective quinazoline derivative that is approved for use in BPH. It has a bioavailability of about 60%, is extensively metabolized, and has an elimination half-life of about 5 hours. **Indoramin** is another α_1-selective antagonist that also has efficacy as an antihypertensive. **Urapidil** is an α_1 antagonist (its primary effect) that also has weak α_2-agonist and 5-HT$_{1A}$-agonist actions and weak antagonist action at β_1 receptors. It is used in Europe as an antihypertensive agent and for benign prostatic hyperplasia. **Labetalol** has both α_1-selective and β-antagonistic effects; it is discussed below. **Neuroleptic drugs** such as chlorpromazine and haloperidol are potent dopamine receptor antagonists but are also antagonists at α receptors. Their antagonism of α receptors probably contributes to some of their adverse effects, particularly hypotension. Similarly, the antidepressant **trazodone** has the capacity to block α_1 receptors.

Yohimbine, an indole alkaloid, is an α_2-selective antagonist. It has no established clinical role. Theoretically, it could be useful in autonomic insufficiency by promoting neurotransmitter release through blockade of presynaptic α_2 receptors. It has been suggested that

yohimbine improves male sexual function; however, evidence for this effect in humans is limited. Yohimbine can abruptly reverse the antihypertensive effects of an α_2-adrenoceptor agonist such as clonidine—a potentially serious adverse drug interaction.

■ II. CLINICAL PHARMACOLOGY OF THE ALPHA-RECEPTOR– BLOCKING DRUGS

Pheochromocytoma

The major clinical use of both phenoxybenzamine and phentolamine is in the management of pheochromocytoma. This tumor is usually found in the adrenal medulla; it typically releases a mixture of epinephrine and norepinephrine. Patients have many symptoms and signs of catecholamine excess, including intermittent or sustained hypertension, headaches, palpitations, and increased sweating.

The diagnosis of pheochromocytoma is usually made on the basis of chemical assay of circulating catecholamines and urinary excretion of catecholamine metabolites, especially 3-hydroxy-4-methoxymandelic acid, metanephrine, and normetanephrine (see Chapter 6). Measurement of plasma metanephrines is also an effective diagnostic tool. A variety of diagnostic techniques are available to localize a pheochromocytoma diagnosed biochemically, including CT and MRI scans as well as scanning with various radioisotopes.

Unavoidable release of stored catecholamines sometimes occurs during operative manipulation of pheochromocytoma; the resulting hypertension may be controlled with phentolamine or nitroprusside. Nitroprusside has many advantages, particularly since its effects can be more readily titrated and it has a shorter duration of action.

Alpha-receptor antagonists are most useful in the preoperative management of patients with pheochromocytoma (Figure 10–4). Administration of phenoxybenzamine in the preoperative period will help control hypertension and will tend to reverse chronic changes resulting from excessive catecholamine secretion such as plasma volume contraction, if present. Furthermore, the patient's operative course may be simplified. Oral doses of 10–20 mg/d can be increased at intervals of several days until hypertension is controlled. Some physicians give phenoxybenzamine to patients with pheochromocytoma for 1–3 weeks before surgery. Other surgeons prefer to operate on patients in the absence of treatment with phenoxybenzamine, counting on modern anesthetic techniques to control blood pressure and

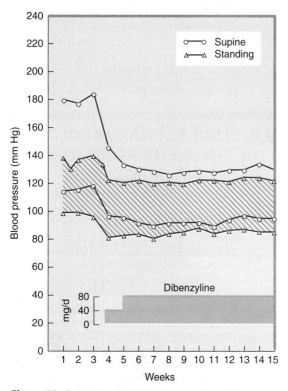

Figure 10–4. Effects of phenoxybenzamine (Dibenzyline) on blood pressure in a patient with pheochromocytoma. Dosage of the drug was begun in the third week as shown by the shaded bar. Supine systolic and diastolic pressures are indicated by the circles, the standing pressures by triangles and the hatched area. Note that the α-blocking drug dramatically reduced blood pressure. The reduction in orthostatic hypotension, which was marked before treatment, is probably due to normalization of blood volume, a variable that is sometimes markedly reduced in patients with long-standing pheochromocytoma-induced hypertension. (Redrawn and reproduced, with permission, from Engelman E, Sjoerdsma A: Chronic medical therapy for pheochromocytoma. Ann Intern Med 1961;61:229.)

heart rate during surgery. Phenoxybenzamine can be very useful in the chronic treatment of inoperable or metastatic pheochromocytoma. Although there is less experience with alternative drugs, hypertension in patients with pheochromocytoma may also respond to reversible α₁-selective antagonists or to conventional calcium channel antagonists. Beta-receptor antagonists may be required after α-receptor blockade has been instituted to reverse the cardiac effects of excessive catecholamines. Beta antagonists should not be used prior to establishing effective α-receptor blockade, since unopposed β-receptor blockade could theoretically cause blood pressure elevation from increased vasoconstriction.

Pheochromocytoma is rarely treated with **metyrosine** (α-methyltyrosine), the α-methyl analog of tyrosine. This agent is a competitive inhibitor of tyrosine hydroxylase and interferes with synthesis of dopamine, norepinephrine, and epinephrine (see Figure 6–5). Metyrosine is especially useful in symptomatic patients with inoperable or metastatic pheochromocytoma.

Hypertensive Emergencies

The α-adrenoceptor antagonist drugs have limited application in the management of hypertensive emergencies, although labetalol has been used in this setting (see Chapter 11). In theory, α-adrenoceptor antagonists are most useful when increased blood pressure reflects excess circulating concentrations of α agonists, eg, in pheochromocytoma, overdosage of sympathomimetic drugs, or clonidine withdrawal. However, other drugs are generally preferable, since considerable experience is necessary to use phentolamine safely in these settings and few physicians have such experience.

Chronic Hypertension

Members of the prazosin family of α₁-selective antagonists are efficacious drugs in the treatment of mild to moderate systemic hypertension (see Chapter 11). They are generally well tolerated by most patients. However, their efficacy in preventing heart failure when used as monotherapy for hypertension has been questioned in the ALLHAT study. Their major adverse effect is postural hypotension, which may be severe after the first doses but is otherwise uncommon. Nonselective α antagonists are not used in primary systemic hypertension. Prazosin and related drugs may also be associated with feelings of dizziness. This symptom may not be due to a fall in blood pressure, but postural changes in blood pressure should be checked routinely in any patient being treated for hypertension.

It is interesting that the use of α-adrenoceptor antagonists such as prazosin has been found to be associated with either no changes in plasma lipids or increased concentrations of high-density lipoproteins (HDL), which could be a favorable alteration. The mechanism for this effect is not known.

Peripheral Vascular Disease

Although α-receptor-blocking drugs have been tried in the treatment of peripheral vascular occlusive disease, there is no evidence that the effects are significant when morphologic changes limit flow in the vessels. Occasionally, individuals with Raynaud's phenomenon and other conditions involving excessive reversible vasospasm in the peripheral circulation do benefit from phentolamine, prazosin, or phenoxybenzamine, although calcium channel blockers may be preferable for many patients.

Local Vasoconstrictor Excess

Phentolamine has been used to reverse the intense local vasoconstriction caused by inadvertent infiltration of α agonists (eg, norepinephrine) into subcutaneous tissue during intended intravenous administration. The α antagonist is administered by local infiltration into the ischemic tissue.

Urinary Obstruction

Benign prostatic hyperplasia is a prevalent disorder in elderly men. A variety of surgical treatments are effective in relieving the urinary symptoms of BPH; however, drug therapy is efficacious in many patients. The mechanism of action in improving urine flow involves partial reversal of smooth muscle contraction in the enlarged prostate and in the bladder base. It has been suggested that some α_1-receptor antagonists may have additional effects on cells in the prostate that help improve symptoms.

A number of well-controlled studies have demonstrated reproducible efficacy of several α_1-receptor antagonists in patients with BPH. Prazosin, doxazosin, and terazosin are efficacious. These drugs are particularly useful in patients who also have hypertension. Considerable interest has focused on which α_1-receptor subtype is most important for smooth muscle contraction in the prostate: *subtype-selective* α_{1A}-receptor antagonists might lead to improved efficacy and safety in treating this disease. As indicated above, tamsulosin is also efficacious in BPH and has little if any effect on blood pressure at a low dose. This drug may be preferred in patients who have experienced postural hypotension with other α_1-receptor antagonists.

Erectile Dysfunction

A combination of phentolamine with the nonspecific smooth muscle relaxant papaverine, when injected directly into the penis, may cause erections in men with sexual dysfunction. Fibrotic reactions may occur, especially with long-term administration. Systemic absorption may lead to orthostatic hypotension; priapism may require direct treatment with an α-adrenoceptor agonist such as phenylephrine. Alternative therapies include prostaglandins (see Chapter 18), sildenafil and other cGMP phosphodiesterase inhibitors (see Chapter 12), and apomorphine.

Applications of Alpha$_2$ Antagonists

Alpha$_2$ antagonists have relatively little clinical usefulness. There has been experimental interest in the development of highly selective antagonists for use in Raynaud's phenomenon to inhibit smooth muscle contraction, for treatment of type 2 diabetes (α_2 receptors inhibit insulin secretion), and for treatment of psychiatric depression. It is not known to what extent the recognition of multiple subtypes of α_2 receptors will lead to development of clinically useful subtype-selective new drugs.

■ III. BASIC PHARMACOLOGY OF THE BETA-RECEPTOR ANTAGONIST DRUGS

Beta-receptor antagonists share the common feature of antagonizing the effects of catecholamines at β adrenoceptors. Beta-blocking drugs occupy β receptors and competitively reduce receptor occupancy by catecholamines and other β agonists. (A few members of this group, used only for experimental purposes, bind irreversibly to β receptors.) Most β-blocking drugs in clinical use are pure antagonists; that is, the occupancy of a β receptor by such a drug causes no activation of the receptor. However, some are partial agonists; that is, they cause partial activation of the receptor, albeit less than that caused by the full agonists epinephrine and isoproterenol. As described in Chapter 2, partial agonists inhibit the activation of β receptors in the presence of high catecholamine concentrations but moderately activate the receptors in the absence of endogenous agonists. Finally, evidence suggests that some β blockers (eg, betaxolol, metoprolol) are *inverse agonists*—drugs that reduce constitutive activity of β receptors—in some tissues. The clinical significance of this property is not known.

Another major difference among the many β-receptor-blocking drugs concerns their relative affinities for β_1 and β_2 receptors (Table 10–1). Some of these antagonists have a higher affinity for β_1 than for β_2 receptors, and this selectivity may have important clinical implications. Since none of the clinically available β-receptor antagonists are absolutely specific for β_1 receptors, the selectivity is dose-related; it tends to diminish at higher drug concentrations. Other major differences among β antagonists relate to their pharmacokinetic characteristics and local anesthetic membrane-stabilizing effects.

Chemically, the β-receptor-antagonist drugs (Figure 10–5) resemble isoproterenol (see Figure 9–3), a potent β-receptor agonist.

$O-CH_2-CH-CH_2-NH-CH(CH_3)_2$
OH

Propranolol

$O-CH_2-CH-CH_2-NH-CH(CH_3)_2$
OH
$CH_2-CH_2-O-CH_3$

Metoprolol

$O-CH_2-CH-CH_2-NH-C(CH_3)_3$
OH
HO
HO

Nadolol

O
N
$N \quad N$
S
$O-CH_2-CH-CH_2-NH-C(CH_3)_3$
OH

Timolol

$O-CH_2-CH-CH_2-NH-CH(CH_3)_2$
OH
N
H

Pindolol

$O-CH_2-CH-CH_2-NH-CH(CH_3)_2$
OH
O
CH_2-C-NH_2

Atenolol

O
CH_3-C
$O-CH_2-CH-CH_2-NH-CH(CH_3)_2$
OH
O
$NH-C-CH_2-CH_2-CH_3$

Acebutolol

$HO-CH-CH_2-NH-CH-CH_2-CH_2$
CH_3
O
$C-NH_2$
OH

Labetalol

Figure 10–5. Structures of some β-receptor antagonists.

Pharmacokinetic Properties of the Beta-Receptor Antagonists

A. Absorption

Most of the drugs in this class are well absorbed after oral administration; peak concentrations occur 1–3 hours after ingestion. Sustained-release preparations of propranolol and metoprolol are available.

B. Bioavailability

Propranolol undergoes extensive hepatic (first-pass) metabolism; its bioavailability is relatively low (Table 10–2). The proportion of drug reaching the systemic circulation increases as the dose is increased, suggesting that hepatic extraction mechanisms may become saturated. A major consequence of the low bioavailability of propranolol is that oral administration of the drug leads to much lower drug concentrations than are achieved after intravenous injection of the same dose. Because the first-pass effect varies among individuals, there is great individual variability in the plasma concentrations achieved after oral propranolol. For the same reason, bioavailability is limited to varying degrees for most β antagonists with the exception of betaxolol, penbutolol, pindolol, and sotalol.

Table 10–2. Properties of several beta-receptor-blocking drugs.

	Selectivity	Partial Agonist Activity	Local Anesthetic Action	Lipid Solubility	Elimination Half-Life	Approximate Bioavailability
Acebutolol	β_1	Yes	Yes	Low	3–4 hours	50
Atenolol	β_1	No	No	Low	6–9 hours	40
Betaxolol	β_1	No	Slight	Low	14–22 hours	90
Bisoprolol	β_1	No	No	Low	9–12 hours	80
Carteolol	None	Yes	No	Low	6 hours	85
Carvedilol[1]	None	No	No	High	7–10 hours	25–35
Celiprolol	β_1	Yes	No	Low	4–5 hours	70
Esmolol	β_1	No	No	Low	10 minutes	0
Labetalol[1]	None	Yes	Yes	Moderate	5 hours	30
Metoprolol	β_1	No	Yes	Moderate	3–4 hours	50
Nadolol	None	No	No	Low	14–24 hours	33
Penbutolol	None	Yes	No	High	5 hours	>90
Pindolol	None	Yes	Yes	Moderate	3–4 hours	90
Propranolol	None	No	Yes	High	3.5–6 hours	30[2]
Sotalol	None	No	No	Low	12 hours	90
Timolol	None	No	No	Moderate	4–5 hours	50

[1]Carvedilol and labetalol also cause α_1 adrenoceptor blockade.
[2]Bioavailability is dose-dependent.

C. DISTRIBUTION AND CLEARANCE

The β antagonists are rapidly distributed and have large volumes of distribution. Propranolol and penbutolol are quite lipophilic and readily cross the blood-brain barrier (Table 10–2). Most β antagonists have half-lives in the range of 3–10 hours. A major exception is esmolol, which is rapidly hydrolyzed and has a half-life of approximately 10 minutes. Propranolol and metoprolol are extensively metabolized in the liver, with little unchanged drug appearing in the urine. The cytochrome P450 2D6 (CYP2D6) genotype is a major determinant of interindividual differences in metoprolol plasma clearance (see Chapter 4). Poor metabolizers exhibit threefold to tenfold higher plasma concentrations after administration of metoprolol than extensive metabolizers. Atenolol, celiprolol, and pindolol are less completely metabolized. Nadolol is excreted unchanged in the urine and has the longest half-life of any available β antagonist (up to 24 hours). The half-life of nadolol is prolonged in

renal failure. The elimination of drugs such as propranolol may be prolonged in the presence of liver disease, diminished hepatic blood flow, or hepatic enzyme inhibition. It is notable that the pharmacodynamic effects of these drugs are often prolonged well beyond the time predicted from half-life data.

Pharmacodynamics of the Beta-Receptor-Antagonist Drugs

Most of the effects of these drugs are due to occupancy and blockade of β receptors. However, some actions may be due to other effects, including partial agonist activity at β receptors and local anesthetic action, which differ among the β blockers (Table 10–2).

A. EFFECTS ON THE CARDIOVASCULAR SYSTEM

Beta-blocking drugs given chronically lower blood pressure in patients with hypertension (see Chapter 11). The mechanisms involved are not fully understood but

Figure 10–6. The effect in an anesthetized dog of the injection of epinephrine before and after propranolol. In the presence of a β-receptor–blocking agent, epinephrine no longer augments the force of contraction (measured by a strain gauge attached to the ventricular wall) nor increases cardiac rate. Blood pressure is still elevated by epinephrine because vasoconstriction is not blocked. (Reproduced, with permission, from Shanks RG: The pharmacology of β sympathetic blockade. Am J Cardiol 1966;18:312.)

probably include effects on the heart and blood vessels, suppression of the renin-angiotensin system, and perhaps effects in the central nervous system or elsewhere. In contrast, conventional doses of these drugs do *not* usually cause hypotension in healthy individuals with normal blood pressure.

Beta-receptor antagonists have prominent effects on the heart (Figure 10–6) and are very valuable in the treatment of angina (see Chapter 12) and chronic heart failure (see Chapter 13) and following myocardial infarction (see Chapter 14). The negative inotropic and chronotropic effects are predictable from the role of adrenoceptors in regulating these functions. Slowed atrioventricular conduction with an increased PR interval is a related result of adrenoceptor blockade in the atrioventricular node. In the vascular system, β-receptor blockade opposes β_2-mediated vasodilation. This may acutely lead to a rise in peripheral resistance from unopposed α-receptor-mediated effects as the sympathetic nervous system discharges in response to lowered blood pressure due to the fall in cardiac output. Nonselective and β_1-blocking drugs antagonize the release of renin caused by the sympathetic nervous system.

Overall, although the acute effects of these drugs may include a rise in peripheral resistance, chronic drug administration leads to a fall in peripheral resistance in patients with hypertension. How this adjustment occurs is not yet clear.

B. EFFECTS ON THE RESPIRATORY TRACT

Blockade of the β_2 receptors in bronchial smooth muscle may lead to an increase in airway resistance, particu-

larly in patients with asthma. Beta$_1$-receptor antagonists such as metoprolol and atenolol may have some advantage over nonselective β antagonists when blockade of β_1 receptors in the heart is desired and β_2-receptor blockade is undesirable. However, no currently available β_1-selective antagonist is sufficiently specific to *completely* avoid interactions with β_2 adrenoceptors. Consequently, these drugs should generally be avoided in patients with asthma. On the other hand, many patients with chronic obstructive pulmonary disease (COPD) may tolerate these drugs quite well and the benefits, for example in patients with concomitant ischemic heart disease, may outweigh the risks.

C. EFFECTS ON THE EYE

Several β-blocking agents reduce intraocular pressure, especially in glaucomatous eyes. The mechanism usually reported is decreased aqueous humor production. (See Clinical Pharmacology and Box: The Treatment of Glaucoma.)

D. METABOLIC AND ENDOCRINE EFFECTS

Beta-receptor antagonists such as propranolol inhibit sympathetic nervous system stimulation of lipolysis. The effects on carbohydrate metabolism are less clear, though glycogenolysis in the human liver is at least partially inhibited after β_2-receptor blockade. However, glucagon is the primary hormone used to combat hypoglycemia. It is unclear to what extent β antagonists impair recovery from hypoglycemia, but they should be used with caution in insulin-dependent diabetic patients. This may be particularly important in diabetic patients with inadequate glucagon reserve and in pancreatectomized patients since catecholamines may be the major factors in stimulating glucose release from the liver in response to hypoglycemia. Beta$_1$-receptor–selective drugs may be less prone to inhibit recovery from hypoglycemia. Beta-receptor antagonists are much safer in those type 2 diabetic patients who do not have hypoglycemic episodes.

The chronic use of β-adrenoceptor antagonists has been associated with increased plasma concentrations of very-low-density lipoproteins (VLDL) and decreased concentrations of HDL cholesterol. Both of these changes are potentially unfavorable in terms of risk of cardiovascular disease. Although low-density lipoprotein (LDL) concentrations generally do not change, there is a variable decline in the HDL cholesterol/LDL cholesterol ratio that may increase the risk of coronary artery disease. These changes tend to occur with both selective and nonselective β-blockers, though they are perhaps less likely to occur with β-blockers possessing intrinsic sympathomimetic activity (partial agonists). The mechanisms by which β-receptor antagonists cause these changes are not understood, though changes in sensitivity to insulin action may contribute.

E. EFFECTS NOT RELATED TO BETA-BLOCKADE

Partial β-agonist activity was significant in the first β-blocking drug synthesized, dichloroisoproterenol. It has been suggested that retention of some intrinsic sympathomimetic activity is desirable to prevent untoward effects such as precipitation of asthma or excessive bradycardia. Pindolol and other partial agonists are noted in Table 10–2. It is not yet clear to what extent partial agonism is clinically valuable. Furthermore, these drugs may not be as effective as the pure antagonists in secondary prevention of myocardial infarction. However, they may be useful in patients who develop symptomatic bradycardia or bronchoconstriction in response to pure antagonist β-adrenoceptor drugs, but only if they are strongly indicated for a particular clinical indication.

Local anesthetic action, also known as "membrane-stabilizing" action, is a prominent effect of several β blockers (Table 10–2). This action is the result of typical local anesthetic blockade of sodium channels and can be demonstrated experimentally in isolated neurons, heart muscle, and skeletal muscle membrane. However, it is unlikely that this effect is important after systemic administration of these drugs, since the concentration in plasma usually achieved by these routes is too low for the anesthetic effects to be evident. These membrane-stabilizing β-blockers are not used topically on the eye, where local anesthesia of the cornea would be highly undesirable. Sotalol is a nonselective β-receptor antagonist that lacks local anesthetic action but has marked class III antiarrhythmic effects, reflecting potassium channel blockade (see Chapter 14).

THE TREATMENT OF GLAUCOMA

Glaucoma is a major cause of blindness and of great pharmacologic interest because the chronic form often responds to drug therapy. The primary manifestation is increased intraocular pressure not initially associated with symptoms. Without treatment, increased intraocular pressure results in damage to the retina and optic nerve, with restriction of visual fields and, eventually, blindness. Intraocular pressure is easily measured as part of the routine ophthalmologic examination. Two major types of glaucoma are recognized: open-angle and closed-angle (or narrow-angle). The closed-angle form is associated with a shallow anterior chamber, in which a dilated iris can occlude the outflow drainage pathway at the angle between the cornea and the ciliary body (see Figure 6–9). This form is associated with acute and painful increases of pressure, which must be controlled on an emergency basis with drugs or prevented by surgical removal of part of the iris (iridectomy). The open-angle form of glaucoma is a chronic condition, and treatment is largely pharmacologic. Because intraocular pressure is a function of the balance between fluid input and drainage out of the globe, the strategies for the treatment of open-angle glaucoma fall into two classes: reduction of aqueous humor secretion and enhancement of aqueous outflow. Five general groups of drugs—cholinomimetics, α agonists, β blockers, prostaglandin F$_{2\alpha}$ analogs, and diuretics—have been found to be useful in reducing intraocular pressure and can be related to these strategies as shown in Table 10–3. Of the five drug groups listed in Table 10–3, the prostaglandin analogs and the β blockers are the most popular. This popularity results from convenience (once- or twice-daily dosing) and relative lack of adverse effects (except, in the case of β blockers, in patients with asthma or cardiac pacemaker or conduction pathway disease). Other drugs that have been reported to reduce intraocular pressure include prostaglandin E$_2$ and marijuana. The use of drugs in acute closed-angle glaucoma is limited to cholinomimetics, acetazolamide, and osmotic agents preceding surgery. The onset of action of the other agents is too slow in this situation.

Table 10–3. Drugs used in open-angle glaucoma.

	Mechanism	Methods of Administration
Cholinomimetics		
Pilocarpine, carbachol, physostigmine, echothiophate, demecarium	Ciliary muscle contraction, opening of trabecular meshwork; increased outflow	Topical drops or gel; plastic film slow-release insert
Alpha agonists		
Unselective	Increased outflow	Topical drops
Epinephrine, dipivefrin		
Alpha$_2$-selective	Decreased aqueous secretion	
Apraclonidine		Topical, postlaser only
Brimonidine		Topical
Beta-blockers		
Timolol, betaxolol, carteolol, levobunolol, metipranolol	Decreased aqueous secretion from the ciliary epithelium	Topical drops
Diuretics		
Dorzolamide, brinzolamide	Decreased aqueous secretion due to lack of HCO_3^-	Topical
Acetazolamide, dichlorphenamide, methazolamide		Oral
Prostaglandins		
Latanoprost, bimatoprost, travoprost, unoprostone	Increased outflow	Topical

SPECIFIC AGENTS (SEE TABLE 10–2.)

Propranolol is the prototypical β-blocking drug. As noted above, it has low and dose-dependent bioavailability. A long-acting form of propranolol is available; prolonged absorption of the drug may occur over a 24-hour period. The drug has negligible effects at α and muscarinic receptors; however, it may block some serotonin receptors in the brain, though the clinical significance is unclear. It has no detectable partial agonist action at β receptors.

Metoprolol, atenolol, and several other drugs (see Table 10–2) are members of the β$_1$-selective group. These agents may be safer in patients who experience bronchoconstriction in response to propranolol. Since their β$_1$ selectivity is rather modest, they should be used with great caution, if at all, in patients with a history of asthma. However, in selected patients with chronic obstructive lung disease the benefits may exceed the risks, eg, in patients with myocardial infarction. Beta$_1$-selective antagonists may be preferable in patients with diabetes or peripheral vascular disease when therapy with a β blocker is required, since β$_2$ receptors are probably important in liver (recovery from hypoglycemia) and blood vessels (vasodilation).

Nadolol is noteworthy for its very long duration of action; its spectrum of action is similar to that of timolol.

Timolol is a nonselective agent with no local anesthetic activity. It has excellent ocular hypotensive effects when administered topically in the eye. **Levobunolol** (nonselective) and **betaxolol** (β$_1$-selective) are also used for topical ophthalmic application in glaucoma; the latter drug may be less likely to induce bronchoconstriction than nonselective antagonists. **Carteolol** is a nonselective β-receptor antagonist.

Pindolol, acebutolol, carteolol, bopindolol, * **oxprenolol,** * **celiprolol,** * and **penbutolol** are of interest because they have partial β-agonist activity.

They are effective in the major cardiovascular applications of the β-blocking group (hypertension and angina). Although these partial agonists may be less likely to cause bradycardia and abnormalities in plasma lipids than are antagonists, the overall clinical significance of intrinsic sympathomimetic activity remains uncertain. Pindolol, perhaps as a result of actions on serotonin signaling, may potentiate the action of traditional antidepressant medications. Celiprolol is a β$_1$-selective antagonist with a modest capacity to activate β$_2$ receptors.

There is limited evidence suggesting that celiprolol may have less adverse bronchoconstrictor effect in

---

*Not available in the USA.

asthma and may even promote bronchodilation. Acebutolol is also a β_1-selective antagonist.

Labetalol is a reversible adrenoceptor antagonist available as a racemic mixture of two pairs of chiral isomers (the molecule has two centers of asymmetry). The *(S,S)-* and *(R,S)-*isomers are nearly inactive, *(S,R)-* is a potent α blocker, and the *(R,R)*-isomer is a potent β blocker. Labetalol's affinity for α receptors is less than that of phentolamine, but labetalol is α_1-selective. Its β-blocking potency is somewhat lower than that of propranolol. Hypotension induced by labetalol is accompanied by less tachycardia than occurs with phentolamine and similar α blockers.

Carvedilol, medroxalol,* and **bucindolol*** are nonselective β-receptor antagonists with some capacity to block α_1-adrenergic receptors.

Carvedilol antagonizes the actions of catecholamines more potently at β receptors than at α receptors. The drug has a half-life of 6–8 hours. It is extensively metabolized in the liver, and stereoselective metabolism of its two isomers is observed. Since metabolism of *(R)*-carvedilol is influenced by polymorphisms in cytochrome P450 2D6 activity and by drugs that inhibit this enzyme's activity (such as quinidine and fluoxetine), drug interactions may occur. Carvedilol also appears to attenuate oxygen free radical–initiated lipid peroxidation and to inhibit vascular smooth muscle mitogenesis independently of adrenoceptor blockade. These effects may contribute to the clinical benefits of the drug in chronic heart failure (see Chapter 13).

Esmolol is an ultra-short–acting β_1-selective adrenoceptor antagonist. The structure of esmolol contains an ester linkage; esterases in red blood cells rapidly metabolize esmolol to a metabolite that has a low affinity for β receptors. Consequently, esmolol has a short half-life (about 10 minutes). Therefore, during continuous infusions of esmolol, steady-state concentrations are achieved quickly, and the therapeutic actions of the drug are terminated rapidly when its infusion is discontinued. Esmolol is potentially safer to use than longer-acting antagonists in critically ill patients who require a β-adrenoceptor antagonist. Esmolol is useful in controlling supraventricular arrhythmias, arrhythmias associated with thyrotoxicosis, perioperative hypertension, and myocardial ischemia in acutely ill patients.

Butoxamine is a research drug selective for β_2 receptors. Selective β_2-blocking drugs have not been actively sought because there is no obvious clinical application for them; none is available for clinical use.

---

*Not available in the USA.

■ IV. CLINICAL PHARMACOLOGY OF THE BETA-RECEPTOR–BLOCKING DRUGS

Hypertension

The β-adrenoceptor-blocking drugs have proved to be effective and well tolerated in hypertension. Although many hypertensive patients respond to a β blocker used alone, the drug is often used with either a diuretic or a vasodilator. In spite of the short half-life of many β antagonists, these drugs may be administered once or twice daily and still have an adequate therapeutic effect. Labetalol, a competitive α and β antagonist, is effective in hypertension, though its ultimate role is yet to be determined. Use of these agents is discussed in detail in Chapter 11. There is some evidence that drugs in this class may be less effective in blacks and the elderly. However, these differences are relatively small and may not apply to an individual patient. Indeed, since effects on blood pressure are easily measured, the therapeutic outcome for this indication can be readily detected in any patient.

Ischemic Heart Disease

Beta-adrenoceptor blockers reduce the frequency of anginal episodes and improve exercise tolerance in many patients with angina (see Chapter 12). These actions relate to the blockade of cardiac β receptors, resulting in decreased cardiac work and reduction in oxygen demand. Slowing and regularization of the heart rate may contribute to clinical benefits (Figure 10–7). Multiple large-scale prospective studies indicate that the long-term use of **timolol, propranolol,** or **metoprolol** in patients who have had a myocardial infarction prolongs survival (Figure 10–8). At the present time, data are less compelling for the use of other than the three mentioned β-adrenoceptor antagonists for this indication. It is significant that surveys in many populations have indicated that β-receptor antagonists are underused, leading to unnecessary morbidity and mortality. In addition, β-adrenoceptor antagonists are strongly indicated in the acute phase of a myocardial infarction. In this setting, relative contraindications include bradycardia, hypotension, moderate or severe left ventricular failure, shock, heart block, and active airways disease. It has been suggested that certain polymorphisms in β_2-adrenoceptor genes may influence survival among patients receiving antagonists after acute coronary syndromes.

Cardiac Arrhythmias

Beta antagonists are often effective in the treatment of both supraventricular and ventricular arrhythmias (see

Figure 10–7. Heart rate in a patient with ischemic heart disease measured by telemetry while watching television. Measurements were begun 1 hour after receiving placebo (upper line, black) or 40 mg of oxprenolol (color), a nonselective β-antagonist with partial agonist activity. Not only was the heart rate decreased by the drug under the conditions of this experiment; it also varied much less in response to stimuli. (Modified and reproduced, with permission, from Taylor SH: Oxprenolol in clinical practice. Am J Cardiol 1983;52:34D.)

Chapter 14). It has been suggested that the improved survival following myocardial infarction in patients using β antagonists (Figure 10–8) is due to suppression of arrhythmias, but this has not been proved. By increasing the atrioventricular nodal refractory period, β antagonists slow ventricular response rates in atrial flutter and fibrillation. These drugs can also reduce ventricular ectopic beats, particularly if the ectopic activity has been precipitated by catecholamines. Sotalol has additional antiarrhythmic effects involving ion channel blockade in addition to its β-blocking action; these are discussed in Chapter 14.

Heart Failure

Clinical trials have demonstrated that at least three β antagonists—metoprolol, bisoprolol, and carvedilol—are effective in treating chronic heart failure in selected patients. Although administration of these drugs may worsen acute congestive heart failure, cautious long-term use with gradual dose increments in patients who tolerate them may prolong life. Although mechanisms are uncertain, there appear to be beneficial effects on myocardial remodeling and in decreasing the risk of sudden death (see Chapter 13).

Other Cardiovascular Disorders

Beta-receptor antagonists have been found to increase stroke volume in some patients with obstructive cardiomyopathy. This beneficial effect is thought to result from the slowing of ventricular ejection and decreased outflow resistance. Beta antagonists are useful in dissecting aortic aneurysm to decrease the rate of development of systolic pressure. Beta antagonists are also useful in selected at-risk patients in the prevention of adverse cardiovascular outcomes resulting from noncardiac surgery.

Glaucoma
(See Box: The Treatment of Glaucoma)

Systemic administration of β-blocking drugs for other indications was found serendipitously to reduce intraocular pressure in patients with glaucoma. Subsequently, it was found that topical administration also reduces intraocular pressure. The mechanism appears to involve reduced production of aqueous humor by the ciliary body, which is physiologically activated by cAMP. Timolol and related β antagonists are suitable for local use in the eye because they lack local anesthetic properties. Beta antagonists appear

Figure 10–8. Effects of β-blocker therapy on life-table cumulated rates of mortality from all causes over 6 years among 1884 patients surviving myocardial infarctions. Patients were randomly assigned to treatment with placebo (dashed line) or timolol (color). (Reproduced, with permission, from Pederson TR: Six-year follow-up of the Norwegian multicenter study on timolol after acute myocardial infarction. N Engl J Med 1985;313:1055.)

to have an efficacy comparable to that of epinephrine or pilocarpine in open-angle glaucoma and are far better tolerated by most patients. While the maximal daily dose applied locally (1 mg) is small compared with the systemic doses commonly used in the treatment of hypertension or angina (10–60 mg), sufficient timolol may be absorbed from the eye to cause serious adverse effects on the heart and airways in susceptible individuals. Topical timolol may interact with orally administered verapamil and increase the risk of heart block.

Betaxolol, carteolol, levobunolol, and metipranolol are β-receptor antagonists approved for the treatment of glaucoma. Betaxolol has the potential advantage of being β_1-selective; to what extent this potential advantage might diminish systemic adverse effects remains to be determined. The drug apparently has caused worsening of pulmonary symptoms in some patients.

Hyperthyroidism

Excessive catecholamine action is an important aspect of the pathophysiology of hyperthyroidism, especially in relation to the heart (see Chapter 38). The β antagonists have salutary effects in this condition. These beneficial effects presumably relate to blockade of adrenoceptors and perhaps in part to the inhibition of peripheral conversion of thyroxine to triiodothyronine. The latter action may vary from one β antagonist to

another. Propranolol has been used extensively in patients with thyroid storm (severe hyperthyroidism); it is used cautiously in patients with this condition to control supraventricular tachycardias that often precipitate heart failure.

Neurologic Diseases

Several studies show a beneficial effect of propranolol in reducing the frequency and intensity of migraine headache. Other β-receptor antagonists with preventive efficacy include metoprolol and probably also atenolol, timolol, and nadolol. The mechanism is not known. Since sympathetic activity may enhance skeletal muscle tremor, it is not surprising that β antagonists have been found to reduce certain tremors (see Chapter 28). The somatic manifestations of anxiety may respond dramatically to low doses of propranolol, particularly when taken prophylactically. For example, benefit has been found in musicians with performance anxiety ("stage fright"). Propranolol may contribute to the symptomatic treatment of alcohol withdrawal in some patients.

Miscellaneous

Beta-receptor antagonists have been found to diminish portal vein pressure in patients with cirrhosis. There is evidence that both propranolol and nadolol decrease the incidence of the first episode of bleeding from esophageal varices and decrease the mortality rate associated with bleeding in patients with cirrhosis. Nadolol in combination with isosorbide mononitrate appears to be more efficacious than sclerotherapy in preventing re-bleeding in patients who have previously bled from esophageal varices. Variceal band ligation in combination with a β antagonist may be more efficacious.

CHOICE OF A BETA-ADRENOCEPTOR ANTAGONIST DRUG

Propranolol is the standard against which newer β antagonists developed for systemic use have been compared. In many years of very wide use, propranolol has been found to be a safe and effective drug for many indications. Since it is possible that some actions of a β-receptor antagonist may relate to some other effect of the drug, these drugs should not be considered interchangeable for all applications. For example, only β antagonists known to be effective in stable heart failure or in prophylactic therapy after myocardial infarction should be used for those indications. It is possible that the beneficial effects of one drug in these settings might not be shared by another drug in the same class. The possible advantages and disadvantages of β-receptor antagonists that are partial agonists have not been clearly defined in clinical settings, although current evidence suggests that they are probably less efficacious in secondary prevention after a myocardial infarction compared to pure antagonists.

CLINICAL TOXICITY OF THE BETA-RECEPTOR ANTAGONIST DRUGS

A variety of minor toxic effects have been reported for propranolol. Rash, fever, and other manifestations of drug allergy are rare. Central nervous system effects include sedation, sleep disturbances, and depression. Rarely, psychotic reactions may occur. Discontinuing the use of β blockers in any patient who develops a depression should be seriously considered if clinically feasible. It has been claimed that β-receptor antagonist drugs with low lipid solubility are associated with a lower incidence of central nervous system adverse effects than compounds with higher lipid solubility (see Table 10–2). Further studies designed to compare the central nervous system adverse effects of various drugs are required before specific recommendations can be made, though it seems reasonable to try the hydrophilic drugs nadolol or atenolol in a patient who experiences unpleasant central nervous system effects with other β blockers.

The major adverse effects of β-receptor antagonist drugs relate to the predictable consequences of β blockade. Beta$_2$-receptor blockade associated with the use of nonselective agents commonly causes worsening of pre-existing asthma and other forms of airway obstruction without having these consequences in normal individuals. Indeed, relatively trivial asthma may become severe after β blockade. However, because of their life-saving possibilities in cardiovascular disease, strong consideration should be given to individualized therapeutic trials in some classes of patients, eg, those with chronic obstructive pulmonary disease who have appropriate indications for β blockers. While β$_1$-selective drugs may have less effect on airways than nonselective β antagonists, they must be used very cautiously, if at all, in patients with reactive airways. Beta$_1$-selective antagonists are generally well tolerated in patients with mild to moderate peripheral vascular disease, but caution is required in patients with severe peripheral vascular disease or vasospastic disorders.

Beta-receptor blockade depresses myocardial contractility and excitability. In patients with abnormal myocardial function, cardiac output may be dependent on sympathetic drive. If this stimulus is removed by β blockade, cardiac decompensation may ensue. Thus, caution must be exercised in starting a β-receptor antagonist in patients with compensated heart failure even though long-term use of these drugs in these patients may prolong life. A life-threatening adverse cardiac effect of a β antagonist may be overcome directly with isoproterenol or with glucagon (glucagon stimulates the heart via glucagon receptors, which are not blocked by β antagonists), but neither of these methods is without hazard. A very small dose of a β antagonist (eg, 10 mg of propranolol) may provoke severe cardiac failure in a susceptible individual. Beta blockers may interact with the calcium antagonist verapamil; severe hypotension, bradycardia, heart failure, and cardiac conduction abnormalities have all been described. These adverse effects may even arise in susceptible patients taking a topical (ophthalmic) β blocker and oral verapamil.

Some hazards are associated with abruptly discontinuing β-antagonist therapy after chronic use. Evidence suggests that patients with ischemic heart disease may be at increased risk if β blockade is suddenly interrupted. The mechanism of this effect is uncertain but might involve up-regulation of the number of β receptors. Until better evidence is available regarding the magnitude of the risk, prudence dictates the gradual tapering rather than abrupt cessation of dosage when these drugs are discontinued, especially drugs with short half-lives, such as propranolol and metoprolol.

The incidence of hypoglycemic episodes in diabetics that are exacerbated by β-blocking agents is unknown. Nevertheless, it is inadvisable to use β antagonists in insulin-dependent diabetic patients who are subject to frequent hypoglycemic reactions if alternative therapies are available. Beta$_1$-selective antagonists offer some advantage in these patients, since the rate of recovery from hypoglycemia may be faster compared with diabetics receiving nonselective β-adrenoceptor antagonists. There is considerable potential benefit from these drugs in diabetics after a myocardial infarction, so the balance of risk versus benefit must be evaluated in individual patients.

PREPARATIONS AVAILABLE

Alpha Blockers

Alfuzosin (Uroxatral)
Oral: 10 mg tablets (extended-release)
Doxazosin (generic, Cardura)
Oral: 1, 2, 4, 8 mg tablets
Phenoxybenzamine (Dibenzyline)
Oral: 10 mg capsules
Phentolamine (generic, Regitine)
Parenteral: 5 mg/vial for injection
Prazosin (generic, Minipress)
Oral: 1, 2, 5 mg capsules
Tamsulosin (Flomax)
Oral: 0.4 mg capsule
Terazosin (generic, Hytrin)
Oral: 1, 2, 5, 10 mg tablets, capsules
Tolazoline (Priscoline)
Parenteral: 25 mg/mL for injection

Beta Blockers

Acebutolol (generic, Sectral)
Oral: 200, 400 mg capsules
Atenolol (generic, Tenormin)
Oral: 25, 50, 100 mg tablets
Parenteral: 0.5 mg/mL for IV injection
Betaxolol
Oral (Kerlone): 10, 20 mg tablets
Ophthalmic (generic, Betoptic): 0.25%, 0.5% drops
Bisoprolol (Zebeta)
Oral: 5, 10 mg tablets
Carteolol
Oral (Cartrol): 2.5, 5 mg tablets
Ophthalmic (generic, Ocupress): 1% drops
Carvedilol (Coreg)
Oral: 3.125, 6.25, 12.5, 25 mg tablets
Esmolol (Brevibloc)
Parenteral: 10 mg/mL for IV injection; 250 mg/mL for IV infusion

Labetalol (generic, Normodyne, Trandate)
Oral: 100, 200, 300 mg tablets
Parenteral: 5 mg/mL for injection
Levobunolol (Betagan Liquifilm, others)
Ophthalmic: 0.25, 0.5% drops
Metipranolol (Optipranolol)
Ophthalmic: 0.3% drops
Metoprolol (generic, Lopressor, Toprol)
Oral: 50, 100 mg tablets
Oral sustained-release: 25, 50, 100, 200 mg tablets
Parenteral: 1 mg/mL for injection
Nadolol (generic, Corgard)
Oral: 20, 40, 80, 120, 160 mg tablets
Penbutolol (Levatol)
Oral: 20 mg tablets
Pindolol (generic, Visken)
Oral: 5, 10 mg tablets
Propranolol (generic, Inderal)
Oral: 10, 20, 40, 60, 80, 90 mg tablets; 4, 8, 80 mg/mL solutions
Oral sustained-release: 60, 80, 120, 160 mg capsules
Parenteral: 1 mg/mL for injection
Sotalol (generic, Betapace)
Oral: 80, 120, 160, 240 mg tablets
Timolol
Oral (generic, Blocadren): 5, 10, 20 mg tablets
Ophthalmic (generic, Timoptic): 0.25, 0.5% drops, gel

Synthesis Inhibitor

Metyrosine (Demser)
Oral: 250 mg capsules

REFERENCES

Becker AJ et al: Oral phentolamine as treatment for erectile dysfunction. J Urol 1998;159:1214.

Blaufarb I, Pfeifer TM, Frishman WH: Beta-blockers: Drug interactions of clinical significance. Drug Saf 1995;13:359.

Boyer TD: Primary prophylaxis for variceal bleeding: Are we there yet? Gastroenterology 2005;128:1120.

Brantigan CO, Brantigan TA, Joseph N: Effect of beta blockade and beta stimulation on stage fright. Am J Med 1982;72:88.

Bristow M: Antiadrenergic therapy of chronic heart failure: surprises and new opportunities. Circulation 2003;107:1100.

Cheng J, Kamiya K, Kodama I: Carvedilol: Molecular and cellular basis for its multifaceted therapeutic potential. Cardiovasc Drug Rev 2001;19:152.

Cleland JG: Beta-blockers for heart failure: Why, which, when, and where. Med Clin North Am 2003;87:339.

Cooper KL, McKiernan JM, Kaplan SA: Alpha-adrenoceptor antagonists in the treatment of benign prostatic hyperplasia. Drugs 1999;57:9.

Ellison KE, Gandhi G: Optimising the use of beta-adrenoceptor antagonists in coronary artery disease. Drugs 2005;65:787.

Fitzgerald JD: Do partial agonist beta-blockers have improved clinical utility? Cardiovasc Drugs Ther 1993;7:303.

Freemantle N et al: Beta blockade after myocardial infarction: Systematic review and meta regression analysis. BMJ 1999;318:1730.

Gold EH et al: Synthesis and comparison of some cardiovascular properties of the stereoisomers of labetalol. J Med Chem 1982;25:1363.

Harada K, Ohmori M, Fujimura A: Comparison of the antagonistic activity of tamsulosin and doxazosin at vascular α_1-adrenoceptors in humans. Naunyn Schmiedebergs Arch Pharmacol 1996;354:557.

Kaplan SA et al: Combination therapy using oral α-blockers and intracavernosal injection in men with erectile dysfunction. Urology 1998;52:739.

Kyprianou N: Doxazosin and terazosin suppress prostate growth by inducing apoptosis: Clinical significance. J Urol 2003;169:1520.

Lanfear et al: β_2-Adrenergic receptor genotype and survival among patients receiving β-blocker therapy after an acute coronary syndrome. JAMA 2005;294:1526.

Lepor H et al: The efficacy of terazosin, finasteride, or both in benign prostate hyperplasia. N Engl J Med 1996; 335:533.

Maggio PM, Taheri PA: Perioperative issues: Myocardial ischemia and protection—beta-blockade. Surg Clin North Am 2005;85:1091.

Marquis RE, Whitson JT: Management of glaucoma: Focus on pharmacological therapy. Drugs Aging 2005;22:1.

McKeage K, Plosker GL: Alfuzosin: A review of the therapeutic use of the prolonged-release formulation given once daily in the management of benign prostatic hyperplasia. Drugs 2002;62:633.

McVary KT: Alfuzosin for symptomatic benign prostatic hyperplasia: Long-term experience. J Urol 2006;175:35.

Nickerson M: The pharmacology of adrenergic blockade. Pharmacol Rev 1949;1:27.

Padma-Nathan H et al: Long-term safety and efficacy of oral phentolamine mesylate (Vasomax) in men with mild to moderate erectile dysfunction. Int J Impot Res 2002;14:266.

Roehrborn CG, Schwinn DA: Alpha$_1$-adrenergic receptors and their inhibitors in lower urinary tract symptoms and benign prostatic hyperplasia. J Urol 2004;171:1029.

Wespes E: Intracavernous injection as an option for aging men with erectile dysfunction. Aging Male 2002;5:177.

Wilt TJ, MacDonald R, Rutks I: Tamsulosin for benign prostatic hyperplasia. Cochrane Database Syst Rev 2003;(1):CD002081.

Wuttke H et al: Increased frequency of cytochrome P450 2D6 poor metabolizers among patients with metoprolol-associated adverse effects. Clin Pharmacol Ther 2002;72:429.

SECTION III
Cardiovascular-Renal Drugs

Antihypertensive Agents

11

Neal L. Benowitz, MD

Hypertension is the most common cardiovascular disease. In a survey carried out in 2000, hypertension was found in 28% of American adults. According to a Framingham study of blood pressure trends in middle-aged and older individuals, approximately 90% of Caucasian Americans will develop hypertension in their lifetime. The prevalence varies with age, race, education, and many other variables. Sustained arterial hypertension damages blood vessels in kidney, heart, and brain and leads to an increased incidence of renal failure, coronary disease, cardiac failure, and stroke. Effective pharmacologic lowering of blood pressure has been shown to prevent damage to blood vessels and to substantially reduce morbidity and mortality rates. Unfortunately, several surveys indicate that only one third of Americans with hypertension have adequate blood pressure control. Many effective drugs are available. Knowledge of their antihypertensive mechanisms and sites of action allows accurate prediction of efficacy and toxicity. As a result, rational use of these agents, alone or in combination, can lower blood pressure with minimal risk of serious toxicity in most patients.

HYPERTENSION & REGULATION OF BLOOD PRESSURE

Diagnosis

The diagnosis of hypertension is based on repeated, reproducible measurements of elevated blood pressure. The diagnosis serves primarily as a prediction of consequences for the patient; it seldom includes a statement about the cause of hypertension.

Epidemiologic studies indicate that the risks of damage to kidney, heart, and brain are directly related to the extent of blood pressure elevation. Even mild hypertension (blood pressure 140/90 mm Hg) increases the risk of eventual end organ damage. Starting at 115/75 mm Hg cardiovascular disease risk doubles with each increment of 20/10 mm Hg throughout the blood pressure range. The risks—and therefore the urgency of instituting therapy—increase in proportion to the magnitude of blood pressure elevation. The risk of end organ damage at any level of blood pressure or age is greater in African-Americans and relatively less in premenopausal women than in men. Other positive risk factors include smoking, hyperlipidemia, diabetes, manifestations of end organ damage at the time of diagnosis, and a family history of cardiovascular disease.

It should be noted that the diagnosis of hypertension depends on measurement of blood pressure and not on symptoms reported by the patient. In fact, hypertension is usually asymptomatic until overt end organ damage is imminent or has already occurred.

Etiology of Hypertension

A specific cause of hypertension can be established in only 10–15% of patients. It is important to consider specific causes in each case, however, because some of them are amenable to definitive surgical treatment: renal artery constriction, coarctation of the aorta, pheochromocytoma, Cushing's disease, and primary aldosteronism.

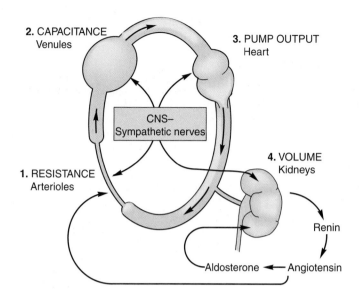

Figure 11–1. Anatomic sites of blood pressure control.

Patients in whom no specific cause of hypertension can be found are said to have essential hypertension.*

In most cases, elevated blood pressure is associated with an overall increase in resistance to flow of blood through arterioles, while cardiac output is usually normal. Meticulous investigation of autonomic nervous system function, baroreceptor reflexes, the renin-angiotensin-aldosterone system, and the kidney has failed to identify a primary abnormality as the cause of increased peripheral vascular resistance in essential hypertension.

Elevated blood pressure is usually caused by a combination of several (multifactorial) abnormalities. Epidemiologic evidence points to genetic inheritance, psychological stress, and environmental and dietary factors (increased salt and decreased potassium or calcium intake) as perhaps contributing to the development of hypertension. Increase in blood pressure with aging does not occur in populations with low daily sodium intake. Patients with labile hypertension appear more likely than normal controls to have blood pressure elevations after salt loading.

The heritability of essential hypertension is estimated to be about 30%. Mutations in several genes have been linked to various rare causes of hypertension. Functional variations of the genes for angiotensinogen, angiotensin-converting enzyme (ACE), the β_2 adrenoceptor, and α adducin (a cytoskeletal protein) appear to contribute to some cases of essential hypertension.

Normal Regulation of Blood Pressure

According to the hydraulic equation, arterial blood pressure (BP) is directly proportionate to the product of the blood flow (cardiac output, CO) and the resistance to passage of blood through precapillary arterioles (peripheral vascular resistance, PVR):

$$BP = CO \times PVR$$

Physiologically, in both normal and hypertensive individuals, blood pressure is maintained by moment-to-moment regulation of cardiac output and peripheral vascular resistance, exerted at three anatomic sites (Figure 11–1): arterioles, postcapillary venules (capacitance vessels), and heart. A fourth anatomic control site, the kidney, contributes to maintenance of blood pressure by regulating the volume of intravascular fluid. Baroreflexes, mediated by autonomic nerves, act in combination with humoral mechanisms, including the renin-angiotensin-aldosterone system, to coordinate function at these four control sites and to maintain normal blood pressure. Finally, local release of vasoactive substances from vascular endothelium may also be involved in the regulation of vascular resistance. For example, endothelin-1 (see Chapter 17) constricts and nitric oxide (see Chapter 19) dilates blood vessels.

Blood pressure in a hypertensive patient is controlled by the same mechanisms that are operative in normotensive subjects. Regulation of blood pressure in hypertensive patients differs from healthy patients in that the baroreceptors and the renal blood volume-pressure control systems appear to be "set" at a higher level of blood pressure. All antihypertensive drugs act by interfering with these normal mechanisms, which are reviewed below.

---

*The adjective originally was intended to convey the now abandoned idea that blood pressure elevation was essential for adequate perfusion of diseased tissues.

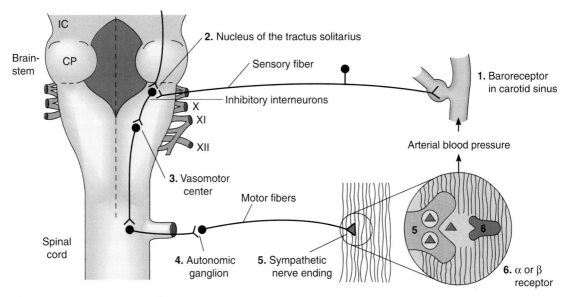

IC

Brain-stem

CP

2. Nucleus of the tractus solitarius

Sensory fiber

Inhibitory interneurons

X
XI
XII

1. Baroreceptor in carotid sinus

Arterial blood pressure

3. Vasomotor center

Motor fibers

Spinal cord

4. Autonomic ganglion

5. Sympathetic nerve ending

5   6

6. α or β receptor

Figure 11–2. Baroreceptor reflex arc.

A. POSTURAL BAROREFLEX (FIGURE 11–2)

Baroreflexes are responsible for rapid, moment-to-moment adjustments in blood pressure, such as in transition from a reclining to an upright posture. Central sympathetic neurons arising from the vasomotor area of the medulla are tonically active. Carotid baroreceptors are stimulated by the stretch of the vessel walls brought about by the internal pressure (arterial blood pressure). Baroreceptor activation inhibits central sympathetic discharge. Conversely, reduction in stretch results in a reduction in baroreceptor activity. Thus, in the case of a transition to upright posture, baroreceptors sense the reduction in arterial pressure that results from pooling of blood in the veins below the level of the heart as reduced wall stretch, and sympathetic discharge is disinhibited. The reflex increase in sympathetic outflow acts through nerve endings to increase peripheral vascular resistance (constriction of arterioles) and cardiac output (direct stimulation of the heart and constriction of capacitance vessels, which increases venous return to the heart), thereby restoring normal blood pressure. The same baroreflex acts in response to any event that lowers arterial pressure, including a primary reduction in peripheral vascular resistance (eg, caused by a vasodilating agent) or a reduction in intravascular volume (eg, due to hemorrhage or to loss of salt and water via the kidney).

B. RENAL RESPONSE TO DECREASED BLOOD PRESSURE

By controlling blood volume, the kidney is primarily responsible for long-term blood pressure control. A reduction in renal perfusion pressure causes intrarenal redistribution of blood flow and increased reabsorption of salt and water. In addition, decreased pressure in renal arterioles as well as sympathetic neural activity (via β adrenoceptors) stimulates production of renin, which increases production of angiotensin II (see Figure 11–1 and Chapter 17). Angiotensin II causes (1) direct constriction of resistance vessels and (2) stimulation of aldosterone synthesis in the adrenal cortex, which increases renal sodium absorption and intravascular blood volume. Vasopressin released from the posterior pituitary gland also plays a role in maintenance of blood pressure through its ability to regulate water reabsorption by the kidney (see Chapters 15 and 17).

■ I. BASIC PHARMACOLOGY OF ANTIHYPERTENSIVE AGENTS

All antihypertensive agents act at one or more of the four anatomic control sites depicted in Figure 11–1 and produce their effects by interfering with normal mechanisms of blood pressure regulation. A useful classification of these agents categorizes them according to the principal regulatory site or mechanism on which they act (Figure 11–3). Because of their common mechanisms of action, drugs within each category tend to produce a similar spectrum of toxicities. The categories include the following:

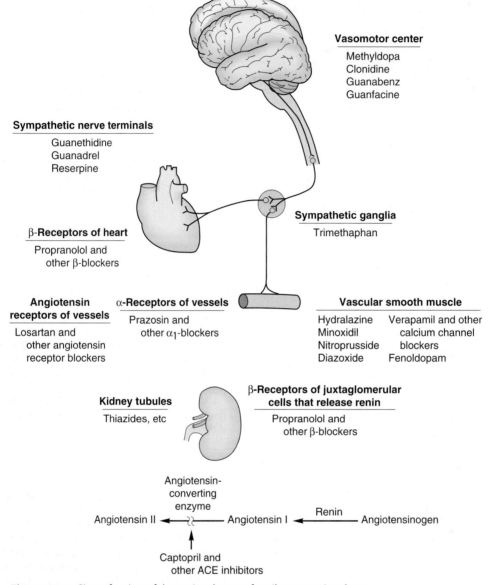

Figure 11–3. Sites of action of the major classes of antihypertensive drugs.

(1) Diuretics, which lower blood pressure by depleting the body of sodium and reducing blood volume and perhaps by other mechanisms.

(2) Sympathoplegic agents, which lower blood pressure by reducing peripheral vascular resistance, inhibiting cardiac function, and increasing venous pooling in capacitance vessels. (The latter two effects reduce cardiac output.) These agents are further subdivided according to their putative sites of action in the sympathetic reflex arc (see below).

(3) Direct vasodilators, which reduce pressure by relaxing vascular smooth muscle, thus dilating resistance vessels and—to varying degrees—increasing capacitance as well.

(4) Agents that block production or action of angiotensin and thereby reduce peripheral vascular resistance and (potentially) blood volume.

The fact that these drug groups act by different mechanisms permits the combination of drugs from two or more groups with increased efficacy and, in some cases, decreased toxicity. (See Box: Monotherapy Versus Polypharmacy in Hypertension, p. 172.)

DRUGS THAT ALTER SODIUM & WATER BALANCE

Dietary sodium restriction has been known for many years to decrease blood pressure in hypertensive patients. With the advent of diuretics, sodium restriction was thought to be less important. However, there is now general agreement that dietary control of blood pressure is a relatively nontoxic therapeutic measure and may even be preventive. Several studies have shown that even modest dietary sodium restriction lowers blood pressure (although to varying extents) in many hypertensive individuals.

Mechanisms of Action & Hemodynamic Effects of Diuretics

Diuretics lower blood pressure primarily by depleting body sodium stores. Initially, diuretics reduce blood pressure by reducing blood volume and cardiac output; peripheral vascular resistance may increase. After 6–8 weeks, cardiac output returns toward normal while peripheral vascular resistance declines. Sodium is believed to contribute to vascular resistance by increasing vessel stiffness and neural reactivity, possibly related to increased sodium-calcium exchange with a resultant increase in intracellular calcium. These effects are reversed by diuretics or sodium restriction.

Some diuretics have direct vasodilating effects in addition to their diuretic action. Indapamide is a nonthiazide sulfonamide diuretic with both diuretic and vasodilator activity. As a consequence of vasodilation, cardiac output remains unchanged or increases slightly. Amiloride inhibits smooth muscle responses to contractile stimuli, probably through effects on transmembrane and intracellular calcium movement that are independent of its action on sodium excretion.

Diuretics are effective in lowering blood pressure by 10–15 mm Hg in most patients, and diuretics alone often provide adequate treatment for mild or moderate essential hypertension. In more severe hypertension, diuretics are used in combination with sympathoplegic and vasodilator drugs to control the tendency toward sodium retention caused by these agents. Vascular responsiveness—ie, the ability to either constrict or dilate—is diminished by sympathoplegic and vasodilator drugs, so that the vasculature behaves like an inflexible tube. As a consequence, blood pressure becomes exquisitely sensitive to blood volume. Thus, in severe hypertension, when multiple drugs are used, blood pressure may be well controlled when blood volume is 95% of normal but much too high when blood volume is 105% of normal.

Use of Diuretics

The sites of action within the kidney and the pharmacokinetics of various diuretic drugs are discussed in Chapter 15. Thiazide diuretics are appropriate for most patients with mild or moderate hypertension and normal renal and cardiac function. More powerful diuretics (eg, those acting on the loop of Henle) are necessary in severe hypertension, when multiple drugs with sodium-retaining properties are used; in renal insufficiency, when glomerular filtration rate is less than 30 or 40 mL/min; and in cardiac failure or cirrhosis, where sodium retention is marked.

Potassium-sparing diuretics are useful both to avoid excessive potassium depletion, particularly in patients taking digitalis, and to enhance the natriuretic effects of other diuretics. Aldosterone receptor antagonists in particular also have a favorable effect on cardiac function in people with heart failure.

Some pharmacokinetic characteristics and the initial and usual maintenance dosages of hydrochlorothiazide are listed in Table 11–1. Although thiazide diuretics are more natriuretic at higher doses (up to 100–200 mg of hydrochlorothiazide), when used as a single agent, lower doses (25–50 mg) exert as much antihypertensive effect as do higher doses. In contrast to thiazides, the blood pressure response to loop diuretics continues to increase at doses many times greater than the usual therapeutic dose.

Toxicity of Diuretics

In the treatment of hypertension, the most common adverse effect of diuretics (except for potassium-sparing diuretics) is potassium depletion. Although mild degrees of hypokalemia are tolerated well by many patients, hypokalemia may be hazardous in persons taking digitalis, those who have chronic arrhythmias, or those with acute myocardial infarction or left ventricular dysfunction. Potassium loss is coupled to reabsorption of sodium, and restriction of dietary sodium intake will therefore minimize potassium loss. Diuretics may also cause magnesium depletion, impair glucose tolerance, and increase serum lipid concentrations. Diuretics increase uric acid concentrations and may precipitate gout. The use of low doses minimizes these adverse metabolic effects without impairing the antihypertensive action. Several case-control studies have reported a small but significant excess risk of renal cell carcinoma associated with diuretic use. Potassium-sparing diuretics may produce hyperkalemia, particularly in patients with renal insufficiency and those taking ACE inhibi-

Table 11–1. Pharmacokinetic characteristics and dosage of selected oral antihypertensive drugs.

Drug	Half-life (h)	Bioavailability (percent)	Suggested Initial Dose	Usual Maintenance Dose Range	Reduction of Dosage Required in Moderate Renal Insufficiency[1]
Amlodipine	35	65	2.5 mg/d	5.5–10 mg/d	No
Atenolol	6	60	50 mg/d	50–100 mg/d	Yes
Benazepril	0.6[2]	35	5–10 mg/d	20–40 mg/d	Yes
Captopril	2.2	65	50–75 mg/d	75–150 mg/d	Yes
Clonidine	8–12	95	0.2 mg/d	0.2–1.2 mg/d	Yes
Diltiazem	3.5	40	120–140 mg/d	240–360 mg/d	No
Guanethidine	5 d	3–50	10 mg/d	25–50 mg/d	Possible
Hydralazine	1.5–3	25	40 mg/d	40–200 mg/d	No
Hydrochlorothiazide	12	70	25 mg/d	25–50 mg/d	No
Lisinopril	12	25	10 mg/d	10–80 mg/d	Yes
Losartan	1–2[3]	36	50 mg/d	25–100 mg/d	No
Methyldopa	2	25	1 g/d	1–2 g/d	No
Metoprolol	3–7	40	50–100 mg/d	200–400 mg/d	No
Minoxidil	4	90	5–10 mg/d	40 mg/d	No
Nifedipine	2	50	30 mg/d	30–60 mg/d	No
Prazosin	3–4	70	3 mg/d	10–30 mg/d	No
Propranolol	3–5	25	80 mg/d	80–480 mg/d	No
Reserpine	24–48	50	0.25 mg/d	0.25 mg/d	No
Verapamil	4–6	22	180 mg/d	240–480 mg/d	No

[1]Creatinine clearance ≥ 30 mL/min. Many of these drugs do require dosage adjustment if creatinine clearance falls below 30 mL/min.
[2]The active metabolite of benazepril has a half-life of 10 h.
[3]The active metabolite of losartan has a half-life of 3–4 hours.

tors or angiotension receptor blockers; spironolactone (a steroid) is associated with gynecomastia.

DRUGS THAT ALTER SYMPATHETIC NERVOUS SYSTEM FUNCTION

In patients with moderate to severe hypertension, most effective drug regimens include an agent that inhibits function of the sympathetic nervous system. Drugs in this group are classified according to the site at which they impair the sympathetic reflex arc (Figure 11–2). This neuroanatomic classification explains prominent differences in cardiovascular effects of drugs and allows the clinician to predict interactions of these drugs with one another and with other drugs.

Most importantly, the subclasses of drugs exhibit different patterns of potential toxicity. Drugs that lower blood pressure by actions on the central nervous system tend to cause sedation and mental depression and may produce disturbances of sleep, including nightmares. Drugs that act by inhibiting transmission through autonomic ganglia produce toxicity from inhibition of parasympathetic regulation, in addition to profound sympathetic blockade. Drugs that act chiefly by reducing release of norepinephrine from sympathetic nerve endings cause effects that are similar to those of surgical sympathectomy, including inhibition of ejaculation, and hypotension that is increased by upright posture and after exercise. Drugs that block postsynaptic adrenoceptors produce a more selective spectrum of effects depending on the class of receptor to which they bind.

Finally, one should note that *all* of the agents that lower blood pressure by altering sympathetic function can elicit compensatory effects through mechanisms that are not dependent on adrenergic nerves. Thus, the antihypertensive effect of any of these agents used alone may be limited by retention of sodium by the kidney and expansion of blood volume. For these reasons, sympathoplegic antihypertensive drugs are most effective when used concomitantly with a diuretic.

CENTRALLY ACTING SYMPATHOPLEGIC DRUGS

Mechanisms & Sites of Action

These agents reduce sympathetic outflow from vasopressor centers in the brainstem but allow these centers to retain or even increase their sensitivity to baroreceptor control. Accordingly, the antihypertensive and toxic actions of these drugs are generally less dependent on posture than are the effects of drugs that act directly on peripheral sympathetic neurons.

Methyldopa (L-α-methyl-3,4-dihydroxyphenylalanine) is an analog of L-dopa and is converted to α-methyldopamine and α-methylnorepinephrine; this pathway directly parallels the synthesis of norepinephrine from dopa illustrated in Figure 6–5. Alpha-methylnorepinephrine is stored in adrenergic nerve vesicles, where it stoichiometrically replaces norepinephrine, and is released by nerve stimulation to interact with postsynaptic adrenoceptors. However, this replacement of norepinephrine by a false transmitter in peripheral neurons is *not* responsible for methyldopa's antihypertensive effect, because the α-methylnorepinephrine released is an effective agonist at the α adrenoceptors that mediate peripheral sympathetic constriction of arterioles and venules. Direct electrical stimulation of sympathetic nerves in methyldopa-treated animals produces sympathetic responses similar to those observed in untreated animals.

In fact, methyldopa's antihypertensive action appears to be due to stimulation of *central* α adrenoceptors by α-methylnorepinephrine or α-methyldopamine, based on the following evidence: (1) Much lower doses of methyldopa are required to lower blood pressure in animals when the drug is administered centrally by injection into the cerebral ventricles rather than intravenously. (2) Alpha-receptor antagonists, especially α_2-selective antagonists, administered centrally, block the antihypertensive effect of methyldopa, whether the latter is given centrally or intravenously. (3) Potent inhibitors of dopa decarboxylase, administered centrally, block methyldopa's antihypertensive effect, thus showing that metabolism of the parent drug in the central nervous system is necessary for its action.

The antihypertensive action of **clonidine**, a 2-imidazoline derivative, was discovered in the course of testing the drug for use as a topically applied nasal decongestant.

After intravenous injection, clonidine produces a brief rise in blood pressure followed by more prolonged hypotension. The pressor response is due to direct stimulation of α adrenoceptors in arterioles. The drug is classified as a partial agonist at α receptors because it also inhibits pressor effects of other α agonists.

Considerable evidence indicates that the hypotensive effect of clonidine is exerted at α adrenoceptors in the medulla of the brain. In animals, the hypotensive effect of clonidine is prevented by central administration of α antagonists. Clonidine reduces sympathetic and increases parasympathetic tone, resulting in blood pressure lowering and bradycardia. The reduction in pressure is accompanied by a decrease in circulating catecholamine levels. These observations suggest that clonidine sensitizes brainstem pressor centers to inhibition by baroreflexes.

Thus, studies of clonidine and methyldopa suggest that normal regulation of blood pressure involves central adrenergic neurons that modulate baroreceptor reflexes. Clonidine and α-methylnorepinephrine bind more tightly to α_2 than to α_1 adrenoceptors. As noted in Chapter 6, α_2 receptors are located on presynaptic adrenergic neurons as well as some postsynaptic sites. It is possible that clonidine and α-methylnorepinephrine act in the brain to reduce norepinephrine release onto relevant receptor sites. Alternatively, these drugs may act on postsynaptic α_2 adrenoceptors to inhibit activity of appropriate neurons. Finally, clonidine also binds to a nonadrenoceptor site, the **imidazoline receptor**, which may also mediate antihypertensive effects.

Methyldopa and clonidine produce slightly different hemodynamic effects: clonidine lowers heart rate and cardiac output more than does methyldopa. This difference suggests that these two drugs do not have identical sites of action. They may act primarily on different populations of neurons in the vasomotor centers of the brainstem.

Guanabenz and **guanfacine** are centrally active antihypertensive drugs that share the central α-adrenoceptor-stimulating effects of clonidine. They do not appear to offer any advantages over clonidine.

METHYLDOPA

Methyldopa is useful in the treatment of mild to moderately severe hypertension. It lowers blood pressure chiefly by reducing peripheral vascular resistance, with a variable reduction in heart rate and cardiac output.

Most cardiovascular reflexes remain intact after administration of methyldopa, and blood pressure reduction is not markedly dependent on maintenance of upright posture. Postural (orthostatic) hypotension sometimes occurs, particularly in volume-depleted patients.

One potential advantage of methyldopa is that it causes reduction in renal vascular resistance.

α-Methyldopa
(α-methyl group in color)

Pharmacokinetics & Dosage

Pharmacokinetic characteristics of methyldopa are listed in Table 11–1. Methyldopa enters the brain via an aromatic amino acid transporter. The usual oral dose of methyldopa produces its maximal antihypertensive effect in 4–6 hours, and the effect can persist for up to 24 hours. Because the effect depends on accumulation and storage of a metabolite (α-methylnorepinephrine) in the vesicles of nerve endings, the action persists after the parent drug has disappeared from the circulation.

Toxicity

The most frequent undesirable effect of methyldopa is overt sedation, particularly at the onset of treatment. With long-term therapy, patients may complain of persistent mental lassitude and impaired mental concentration. Nightmares, mental depression, vertigo, and extrapyramidal signs may occur but are relatively infrequent. Lactation, associated with increased prolactin secretion, can occur both in men and in women treated with methyldopa. This toxicity is probably mediated by inhibition of dopaminergic mechanisms in the hypothalamus.

Other important adverse effects of methyldopa are development of a positive Coombs test (occurring in 10–20% of patients undergoing therapy for longer than 12 months), which sometimes makes cross-matching blood for transfusion difficult and rarely is associated with hemolytic anemia, as well as hepatitis and drug fever. Discontinuation of the drug usually results in prompt reversal of these abnormalities.

CLONIDINE

Hemodynamic studies indicate that blood pressure lowering by clonidine results from reduction of cardiac output due to decreased heart rate and relaxation of capacitance vessels, with a reduction in peripheral vascular resistance, particularly when patients are upright (when sympathetic tone is normally increased).

Reduction in arterial blood pressure by clonidine is accompanied by decreased renal vascular resistance and maintenance of renal blood flow. As with methyldopa, clonidine reduces blood pressure in the supine position and only rarely causes postural hypotension. Pressor effects of clonidine are not observed after ingestion of therapeutic doses of clonidine, but severe hypertension can complicate a massive overdose.

Clonidine

Pharmacokinetics & Dosage

Typical pharmacokinetic characteristics are listed in Table 11–1.

Clonidine is lipid-soluble and rapidly enters the brain from the circulation. Because of its relatively short half-life and the fact that its antihypertensive effect is directly related to blood concentration, oral clonidine must be given twice a day (or as a patch, below) to maintain smooth blood pressure control. However, as is not the case with methyldopa, the dose-response curve of clonidine is such that increasing doses are more effective (but also more toxic).

A transdermal preparation of clonidine that reduces blood pressure for 7 days after a single application is also available. This preparation appears to produce less sedation than clonidine tablets but is often associated with local skin reactions.

Toxicity

Dry mouth and sedation are frequent and may be severe. Both effects are centrally mediated and dose-dependent and coincide temporally with the drug's antihypertensive effect.

The drug should not be given to patients who are at risk for mental depression and should be withdrawn if depression occurs during therapy. Concomitant treatment with tricyclic antidepressants may block the antihypertensive effect of clonidine. The interaction is believed to be due to α-adrenoceptor-blocking actions of the tricyclics.

Withdrawal of clonidine after protracted use, particularly with high dosages (greater than 1 mg/d), can result in life-threatening hypertensive crisis mediated by increased sympathetic nervous activity. Patients exhibit nervousness, tachycardia, headache, and sweating after omitting one or two doses of the drug. Although the incidence of severe hypertensive crisis is unknown, it is high enough to require that all patients who take clonidine be carefully warned of the possibility. If the drug must be stopped, this should be done gradually while other antihypertensive agents are being substituted. Treatment of the hypertensive crisis consists of reinstitution of clonidine therapy or administration of α- and β-adrenoceptor–blocking agents.

GANGLION-BLOCKING AGENTS

Historically, drugs that block stimulation of postganglionic autonomic neurons by acetylcholine were among the first agents used in the treatment of hypertension. Most such drugs are no longer available clinically because of intolerable toxicities related to their primary action (see below).

Ganglion blockers competitively block nicotinic cholinoceptors on postganglionic neurons in both sympathetic and parasympathetic ganglia. In addition, these drugs may directly block the nicotinic acetylcholine channel, in the same fashion as neuromuscular nicotinic blockers (see Figure 27–6).

The adverse effects of ganglion blockers are direct extensions of their pharmacologic effects. These effects include both sympathoplegia (excessive orthostatic hypotension and sexual dysfunction) and parasympathoplegia (constipation, urinary retention, precipitation of glaucoma, blurred vision, dry mouth, etc). These severe toxicities are the major reason for the abandonment of ganglion blockers for the therapy of hypertension.

ADRENERGIC NEURON–BLOCKING AGENTS

These drugs lower blood pressure by preventing normal physiologic release of norepinephrine from postganglionic sympathetic neurons.

GUANETHIDINE

In high enough doses, guanethidine can produce profound sympathoplegia. The resulting high maximal efficacy of this agent made it the mainstay of outpatient therapy of severe hypertension for many years. For the same reason, guanethidine can produce all of the toxicities expected from "pharmacologic sympathectomy," including marked postural hypotension, diarrhea, and impaired ejaculation. Because of these adverse effects, guanethidine is now rarely used.

Guanethidine is too polar to enter the central nervous system. As a result, this drug has none of the central effects seen with many of the other antihypertensive agents described in this chapter.

Guanadrel is a guanethidine-like drug that is available in the USA. **Bethanidine** and **debrisoquin,** antihypertensive agents not available for clinical use in the

USA, are similar to guanethidine in mechanism of antihypertensive action.

Mechanism & Sites of Action

Guanethidine inhibits the release of norepinephrine from sympathetic nerve endings (see Figure 6–4). This effect is probably responsible for most of the sympathoplegia that occurs in patients. Guanethidine is transported across the sympathetic nerve membrane by the same mechanism that transports norepinephrine itself (NET, uptake 1), and uptake is essential for the drug's action. Once guanethidine has entered the nerve, it is concentrated in transmitter vesicles, where it replaces norepinephrine. Because it replaces norepinephrine, the drug causes a gradual depletion of norepinephrine stores in the nerve ending.

Inhibition of norepinephrine release is probably caused by guanethidine's local anesthetic properties on sympathetic nerve terminals. Although the drug does not impair axonal conduction in sympathetic fibers, local blockade of membrane electrical activity may occur in nerve endings because the nerve endings specifically take up and concentrate the drug.

Because neuronal uptake is necessary for the hypotensive activity of guanethidine, drugs that block the catecholamine uptake process or displace amines from the nerve terminal (see Chapter 6) block its effects. These include cocaine, amphetamine, tricyclic antidepressants, phenothiazines, and phenoxybenzamine.

Guanethidine increases sensitivity to the hypertensive effects of exogenously administered sympathomimetic amines. This results from inhibition of neuronal uptake of such amines and, after long-term therapy with guanethidine, supersensitivity of effector smooth muscle cells, in a fashion analogous to the process that follows surgical sympathectomy (see Chapter 6).

The hypotensive action of guanethidine early in the course of therapy is associated with reduced cardiac output, due to bradycardia and relaxation of capacitance vessels. With long-term therapy, peripheral vascular resistance decreases. Compensatory sodium and water retention may be marked during guanethidine therapy.

Pharmacokinetics & Dosage

Because of its long half-life (5 days) the onset of sympathoplegia is gradual (maximal effect in 1–2 weeks), and sympathoplegia persists for a comparable period after cessation of therapy. The dose should not ordinarily be increased at intervals shorter than 2 weeks.

Toxicity

Therapeutic use of guanethidine is often associated with symptomatic postural hypotension and hypotension following exercise, particularly when the drug is given in high doses, and may produce dangerously decreased blood flow to heart and brain or even overt shock. Guanethidine-induced sympathoplegia in men may be associated with delayed or retrograde ejaculation (into the bladder). Guanethidine commonly causes diarrhea, which results from increased gastrointestinal motility due to parasympathetic predominance in controlling the activity of intestinal smooth muscle.

Interactions with other drugs may complicate guanethidine therapy. Sympathomimetic agents, at doses available in over-the-counter cold preparations, can produce hypertension in patients taking guanethidine. Similarly, guanethidine can produce hypertensive crisis by releasing catecholamines in patients with pheochromocytoma. When tricyclic antidepressants are administered to patients taking guanethidine, the drug's antihypertensive effect is attenuated, and severe hypertension may follow.

RESERPINE

Reserpine, an alkaloid extracted from the roots of an Indian plant, *Rauwolfia serpentina,* was one of the first effective drugs used on a large scale in the treatment of hypertension. At present, it is considered an effective and relatively safe drug for treating mild to moderate hypertension.

Mechanism & Sites of Action

Reserpine blocks the ability of aminergic transmitter vesicles to take up and store biogenic amines, probably by interfering with the vesicular membrane-associated transporter (VMAT, see Figure 6–4). This effect occurs throughout the body, resulting in depletion of norepinephrine, dopamine, and serotonin in both central and peripheral neurons. Chromaffin granules of the adrenal medulla are also depleted of catecholamines, although to a lesser extent than are the vesicles of neurons. Reserpine's effects on adrenergic vesicles appear irreversible; trace amounts of the drug remain bound to vesicular membranes for many days. Although sufficiently high doses of reserpine in animals can reduce catecholamine stores to zero, lower doses cause inhibition of neurotransmission that is roughly proportionate to the degree of amine depletion.

Depletion of peripheral amines probably accounts for much of the beneficial antihypertensive effect of reserpine, but a central component cannot be ruled out. The effects of low but clinically effective doses resemble those of centrally acting agents (eg, methyldopa) in that sympathetic reflexes remain largely intact, blood pressure is reduced in supine as well as in standing patients, and postural hypotension is mild. Reserpine readily enters the brain, and depletion of cerebral amine stores causes sedation, mental depression, and parkinsonism symptoms.

At lower doses used for treatment of mild hypertension, reserpine lowers blood pressure by a combination of decreased cardiac output and decreased peripheral vascular resistance.

Pharmacokinetics & Dosage

See Table 11–1.

Toxicity

At the low doses usually administered, reserpine produces little postural hypotension. Most of the unwanted effects of reserpine result from actions on the brain or gastrointestinal tract.

High doses of reserpine characteristically produce sedation, lassitude, nightmares, and severe mental depression; occasionally, these occur even in patients receiving low doses (0.25 mg/d). Much less frequently, ordinary low doses of reserpine produce extrapyramidal effects resembling Parkinson's disease, probably as a result of dopamine depletion in the corpus striatum. Although these central effects are uncommon, it should be stressed that they may occur at any time, even after months of uneventful treatment. Patients with a history of mental depression should not receive reserpine, and the drug should be stopped if depression appears.

Reserpine rather often produces mild diarrhea and gastrointestinal cramps and increases gastric acid secretion. The drug should probably not be given to patients with a history of peptic ulcer.

ADRENOCEPTOR ANTAGONISTS

The pharmacology of α- and β-adrenoceptor blockers is presented in Chapter 10. This chapter will concentrate on two prototypical drugs, propranolol and prazosin, primarily in relation to their use in treatment of hypertension. Other adrenoceptor antagonists will be considered only briefly.

PROPRANOLOL

Propranolol was the first β blocker shown to be effective in hypertension and ischemic heart disease. It is now clear that all β-adrenoceptor-blocking agents are very useful for lowering blood pressure in mild to moderate hypertension. In severe hypertension, β blockers are especially useful in preventing the reflex tachycardia that often results from treatment with direct vasodilators. Beta blockers have been shown to reduce mortality in patients with heart failure, and they are particularly advantageous for treating hypertension in that population (see Chapter 13).

Mechanism & Sites of Action

Propranolol's efficacy in treating hypertension as well as most of its toxic effects result from nonselective β blockade. Propranolol decreases blood pressure primarily as a result of a decrease in cardiac output. Other β blockers may decrease cardiac output or decrease peripheral vascular resistance to various degrees, depending on cardioselectivity and partial agonist activities.

Beta blockade in brain, kidney, and peripheral adrenergic neurons has been proposed as contributing to the antihypertensive effect observed with β-receptor blockers. In spite of conflicting evidence, the brain appears unlikely to be the primary site of the hypotensive action of these drugs, because some β blockers that do not readily cross the blood-brain barrier (eg, nadolol, described below) are nonetheless effective antihypertensive agents.

Propranolol inhibits the stimulation of renin production by catecholamines (mediated by β_1 receptors). It is likely that propranolol's effect is due in part to depression of the renin-angiotensin-aldosterone system. Although most effective in patients with high plasma renin activity, propranolol also reduces blood pressure in hypertensive patients with normal or even low renin activity. Beta blockers might also act on peripheral presynaptic β adrenoceptors to reduce sympathetic vasoconstrictor nerve activity.

In mild to moderate hypertension, propranolol produces a significant reduction in blood pressure without prominent postural hypotension.

Pharmacokinetics & Dosage

See Table 11–1. Resting bradycardia and a reduction in the heart rate during exercise are indicators of propranolol's β-blocking effect. Measures of these responses may be used as guides in regulating dosage. Propranolol can be administered once or twice daily and slow-release preparations are available.

Toxicity

The principal toxicities of propranolol result from blockade of cardiac, vascular, or bronchial β receptors and are described in more detail in Chapter 10. The most important of these predictable extensions of the β-blocking action occur in patients with bradycardia or cardiac conduction disease, asthma, peripheral vascular insufficiency, and diabetes.

When propranolol is discontinued after prolonged regular use, some patients experience a withdrawal syndrome, manifested by nervousness, tachycardia, increased intensity of angina, or increase of blood pressure. Myocardial infarction has been reported in a few patients. Although the incidence of these complications is probably low, propranolol should not be discontinued abruptly. The withdrawal syndrome may involve up-regulation or supersensitivity of β adrenoceptors.

OTHER BETA-ADRENOCEPTOR–BLOCKING AGENTS

Of the large number of β blockers tested, most have been shown to be effective in lowering blood pressure. The pharmacologic properties of several of these agents differ from those of propranolol in ways that may confer therapeutic benefits in certain clinical situations.

1. Metoprolol

Metoprolol is approximately equipotent to propranolol in inhibiting stimulation of β_1 adrenoceptors such as those in the heart but 50- to 100-fold less potent than propranolol in blocking β_2 receptors. Although metoprolol is in other respects very similar to propranolol, its relative cardioselectivity may be advantageous in treating hypertensive patients who also suffer from asthma, diabetes, or peripheral vascular disease. Studies of small numbers of asthmatic patients have shown that metoprolol causes less bronchial constriction than propranolol at doses that produce equal inhibition of β_1 adrenoceptor responses. The cardioselectivity is not complete, however, and asthmatic symptoms have been exacerbated by metoprolol. See Table 11–1.

2. Nadolol, Carteolol, Atenolol, Betaxolol, & Bisoprolol

Nadolol and carteolol, nonselective β-receptor antagonists, and atenolol, a β_1-selective blocker, are not appreciably metabolized and are excreted to a considerable extent in the urine. Betaxolol and bisoprolol are β_1-selective blockers that are primarily metabolized in the liver but have long half-lives. Because of these relatively long half-lives, these drugs can be administered once daily. Nadolol is usually begun at a dosage of 40 mg/d, atenolol at 50 mg/d, carteolol at 2.5 mg/d, betaxolol at 10 mg/d, and bisoprolol at 5 mg/d. Increases in dosage to obtain a satisfactory therapeutic effect should take place no more often than every 4 or 5 days. Patients with reduced renal function should receive correspondingly reduced doses of nadolol, carteolol, and atenolol. It is claimed that atenolol produces fewer central nervous system-related effects than other more lipid-soluble β antagonists.

3. Pindolol, Acebutolol, & Penbutolol

Pindolol, acebutolol, and penbutolol are partial agonists, ie, β blockers with some intrinsic sympathomimetic activity. They lower blood pressure by decreasing vascular resistance and appear to depress cardiac output or heart rate less than other β blockers, perhaps because of significantly greater agonist than antagonist effects at β_2 receptors. This may be particularly beneficial for patients with bradyarrhythmias or peripheral vascular disease. Daily doses of pindolol start at 10 mg; of acebutolol, at 400 mg; and of penbutolol, at 20 mg.

4. Labetalol & Carvedilol

Labetalol is formulated as a racemic mixture of four isomers (it has two centers of asymmetry). Two of these isomers—the (S,S)- and (R,S)-isomers—are relatively inactive, a third (S,R)- is a potent α blocker, and the last (R,R)- is a potent β blocker. The β-blocking isomer is thought to have selective β_2 agonist and nonselective β antagonist action. Labetalol has a 3:1 ratio of β:α antagonism after oral dosing. Blood pressure is lowered by reduction of systemic vascular resistance without significant alteration in heart rate or cardiac output. Because of its combined α- and β-blocking activity, labetalol is useful in treating the hypertension of pheochromocytoma and hypertensive emergencies. Oral daily doses of labetalol range from 200 to 2400 mg/d. Labetalol is given as repeated intravenous bolus injections of 20–80 mg to treat hypertensive emergencies.

Carvedilol, like labetalol, is administered as a racemic mixture. The S(–) isomer is a nonselective β-adrenoceptor blocker, but both S(–) and R(+) isomers have approximately equal α-blocking potency. The isomers are stereoselectively metabolized in the liver, which means that their elimination half-lives may differ. The average half-life is 7–10 hours. The usual starting dosage of carvedilol for ordinary hypertension is 6.25 mg twice daily.

5. Esmolol

Esmolol is a β_1-selective blocker that is rapidly metabolized via hydrolysis by red blood cell esterases. It has a short half-life (9–10 minutes) and is administered by constant intravenous infusion. Esmolol is generally administered as a loading dose (0.5–1 mg/kg), followed by a constant infusion. The infusion is typically started at 50–150 mcg/kg/min, and the dose increased every 5 minutes, up to 300 mcg/kg/min, as needed to achieve the desired therapeutic effect. Esmolol is used for management of intraoperative and postoperative hypertension, and sometimes for hypertensive emergencies, particularly when hypertension is associated with tachycardia.

PRAZOSIN & OTHER ALPHA₁ BLOCKERS

Mechanism & Sites of Action

Prazosin, terazosin, and doxazosin produce most of their antihypertensive effect by selectively blocking α_1 receptors in arterioles and venules. These agents produce less reflex tachycardia when lowering blood pressure than do nonselective α antagonists such as phentolamine. Alpha₁ receptor selectivity allows norepinephrine to exert unopposed negative feedback (mediated by presynaptic α_2 receptors) on its own release (see Chapter 6); in contrast, phentolamine blocks both presynaptic and postsynaptic α receptors, with the result that reflex activation of sympathetic neurons produces greater release of transmitter onto β receptors and correspondingly greater cardioacceleration.

Alpha blockers reduce arterial pressure by dilating both resistance and capacitance vessels. As expected, blood pressure is reduced more in the upright than in the supine position. Retention of salt and water occurs when these drugs are administered without a diuretic. The drugs are more effective when used in combination with other agents, such as a β blocker and a diuretic, than when used alone.

Pharmacokinetics & Dosage

Pharmacokinetic characteristics of prazosin are listed in Table 11–1. Terazosin is also extensively metabolized but undergoes very little first-pass metabolism and has a half-life of 12 hours. Doxazosin has an intermediate bioavailability and a half-life of 22 hours.

Terazosin can often be given once daily, with doses of 5–20 mg/d. Doxazosin is usually given once daily starting at 1 mg/d and progressing to 4 mg/d or more as needed. Although long-term treatment with these α blockers causes relatively little postural hypotension, a precipitous drop in standing blood pressure develops in some patients shortly after the first dose is absorbed. For this reason, the first dose should be small and should be administered at bedtime. While the mechanism of this first-dose phenomenon is not clear, it occurs more commonly in patients who are salt- and volume-depleted.

Aside from the first-dose phenomenon, the reported toxicities of the α_1 blockers are relatively infrequent and mild. These include dizziness, palpitations, headache, and lassitude. Some patients develop a positive test for antinuclear factor in serum while on prazosin therapy, but this has not been associated with rheumatic symptoms. The α_1 blockers do not adversely and may even beneficially affect plasma lipid profiles but this action has not been shown to confer any benefit on clinical outcomes.

OTHER ALPHA-ADRENOCEPTOR– BLOCKING AGENTS

The nonselective agents, **phentolamine** and **phenoxybenzamine,** are useful in diagnosis and treatment of pheochromocytoma and in other clinical situations associated with exaggerated release of catecholamines (eg, phentolamine may be combined with propranolol to treat the clonidine withdrawal syndrome, described above). Their pharmacology is described in Chapter 10.

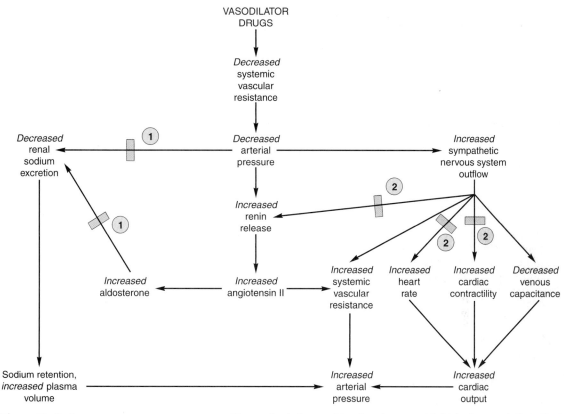

Figure 11–4. Compensatory responses to vasodilators; basis for combination therapy with β blockers and diuretics. ① Effect blocked by diuretics. ② Effect blocked by β blockers.

VASODILATORS

Mechanism & Sites of Action

Within this class of drugs are the oral vasodilators, hydralazine and minoxidil, which are used for long-term outpatient therapy of hypertension; the parenteral vasodilators, nitroprusside, diazoxide, and fenoldopam, which are used to treat hypertensive emergencies; and the calcium channel blockers, which are used in both circumstances.

Chapter 12 contains a general discussion of vasodilators. All of the vasodilators useful in hypertension relax smooth muscle of arterioles, thereby decreasing systemic vascular resistance. Sodium nitroprusside also relaxes veins. Decreased arterial resistance and decreased mean arterial blood pressure elicit compensatory responses, mediated by baroreceptors and the sympathetic nervous system (Figure 11–4), as well as renin, angiotensin, and aldosterone. Because sympathetic reflexes are intact, vasodilator therapy does not cause orthostatic hypotension or sexual dysfunction.

Vasodilators work best in combination with other antihypertensive drugs that oppose the compensatory cardiovascular responses. (See Box: Monotherapy Versus Polypharmacy in Hypertension, p. 172.)

HYDRALAZINE

Hydralazine, a hydrazine derivative, dilates arterioles but not veins. It has been available for many years, although it was initially thought not to be particularly effective because tachyphylaxis to its antihypertensive effects developed rapidly. The benefits of combination therapy are now recognized, and hydralazine may be used more effectively, particularly in severe hypertension.

Hydralazine

MONOTHERAPY VERSUS POLYPHARMACY IN HYPERTENSION

Monotherapy of hypertension (treatment with a single drug) is desirable because compliance is likely to be better, cost is lower, and because in some cases adverse effects are fewer. However, most patients with hypertension require two or more drugs, each acting by a different mechanism (polypharmacy). The rationale for polypharmacy is that each of the drugs acts on one of a set of interacting, mutually compensatory regulatory mechanisms for maintaining blood pressure (see Figures 6–7 and 11–1).

For example, because an adequate dose of hydralazine causes a significant decrease in peripheral vascular resistance, there will initially be a drop in mean arterial blood pressure, evoking a strong response in the form of compensatory tachycardia and salt and water retention (Figure 11–4). The result is an increase in cardiac output that is capable of almost completely reversing the effect of hydralazine. The addition of a β blocker prevents the tachycardia; addition of a diuretic (eg, hydrochlorothiazide) prevents the salt and water retention. In effect, all three drugs increase the sensitivity of the cardiovascular system to each other's actions. Thus, partial impairment of one regulatory mechanism (sympathetic discharge to the heart) increases the antihypertensive effect of impairing regulation by another mechanism (peripheral vascular resistance). Finally, in some circumstances, a normal compensatory response accounts for the toxicity of an antihypertensive agent, and the toxic effect can be prevented by administering a second type of drug. In the case of hydralazine, compensatory tachycardia and increased cardiac output may precipitate angina in patients with coronary atherosclerosis. Addition of the β blocker and diuretic can prevent this toxicity in many patients.

In practice, when hypertension does not respond adequately to a regimen of one drug, a second drug from a different class with a different mechanism of action and different pattern of toxicity is added. If the response is still inadequate and compliance is known to be good, a third drug may be added. The drugs least likely to be successful as monotherapy are the vasodilators hydralazine and minoxidil. It is not completely clear why other vasodilators such as calcium channel blockers cause less marked compensatory responses for the same amount of blood pressure lowering.

Pharmacokinetics & Dosage

Hydralazine is well absorbed and rapidly metabolized by the liver during the first pass, so that bioavailability is low (averaging 25%) and variable among individuals. It is metabolized in part by acetylation at a rate that appears to be bimodally distributed in the population (see Chapter 4). As a consequence, rapid acetylators have greater first-pass metabolism, lower bioavailability, and less antihypertensive benefit from a given dose than do slow acetylators. The half-life of hydralazine ranges from 1.5 to 3 hours, but vascular effects persist longer than do blood concentrations, possibly due to avid binding to vascular tissue.

Usual dosage ranges from 40 mg/d to 200 mg/d. The higher dosage was selected as the dose at which there is a small possibility of developing the lupus erythematosus-like syndrome described in the next section. However, higher dosages result in greater vasodilation and may be used if necessary. Dosing two or three times daily provides smooth control of blood pressure.

Toxicity

The most common adverse effects of hydralazine are headache, nausea, anorexia, palpitations, sweating, and flushing. In patients with ischemic heart disease, reflex tachycardia and sympathetic stimulation may provoke angina or ischemic arrhythmias. With dosages of 400 mg/d or more, there is a 10–20% incidence—chiefly in persons who slowly acetylate the drug—of a syndrome characterized by arthralgia, myalgia, skin rashes, and fever that resembles lupus erythematosus. The syndrome is not associated with renal damage and is reversed by discontinuance of hydralazine. Peripheral neuropathy and drug fever are other serious but uncommon adverse effects.

MINOXIDIL

Minoxidil is a very efficacious orally active vasodilator. The effect results from the opening of potassium channels in smooth muscle membranes by minoxidil sulfate, the active metabolite. Increased potassium permeability stabilizes the membrane at its resting potential and makes contraction less likely. Like hydralazine, minoxidil dilates arterioles but not veins. Because of its greater potential antihypertensive effect, minoxidil should replace hydralazine when maximal doses of the latter are not effective or in patients with renal failure and severe hypertension, who do not respond well to hydralazine.

Minoxidil

Pharmacokinetics & Dosage

Pharmacokinetic parameters of minoxidil are listed in Table 11–1. Even more than with hydralazine, the use of minoxidil is associated with reflex sympathetic stimulation and sodium and fluid retention. Minoxidil must be used in combination with a β blocker and a loop diuretic.

Toxicity

Tachycardia, palpitations, angina, and edema are observed when doses of β blockers and diuretics are inadequate. Headache, sweating, and hirsutism, which is particularly bothersome in women, are relatively common. Minoxidil illustrates how one person's toxicity may become another person's therapy. Topical minoxidil (as Rogaine) is used as a stimulant to hair growth for correction of baldness.

SODIUM NITROPRUSSIDE

Sodium nitroprusside is a powerful parenterally administered vasodilator that is used in treating hypertensive emergencies as well as severe heart failure. Nitroprusside dilates both arterial and venous vessels, resulting in reduced peripheral vascular resistance and venous return. The action occurs as a result of activation of guanylyl cyclase, either via release of nitric oxide or by direct stimulation of the enzyme. The result is increased intracellular cGMP, which relaxes vascular smooth muscle (see Figure 12-2).

In the absence of heart failure, blood pressure decreases, owing to decreased vascular resistance, while cardiac output does not change or decreases slightly. In patients with heart failure and low cardiac output, output often increases owing to afterload reduction.

Nitroprusside

Pharmacokinetics & Dosage

Nitroprusside is a complex of iron, cyanide groups, and a nitroso moiety. It is rapidly metabolized by uptake into red blood cells with liberation of cyanide. Cyanide in turn is metabolized by the mitochondrial enzyme rhodanase, in the presence of a sulfur donor, to the less toxic thiocyanate. Thiocyanate is distributed in extracellular fluid and slowly eliminated by the kidney.

Nitroprusside rapidly lowers blood pressure, and its effects disappear within 1–10 minutes after discontinuation. The drug is given by intravenous infusion. Sodium nitroprusside in aqueous solution is sensitive to light and must therefore be made up fresh before each administration and covered with opaque foil. Infusion solutions should be changed after several hours. Dosage typically begins at 0.5 mcg/kg/min and may be increased up to 10 mcg/kg/min as necessary to control blood pressure. Higher rates of infusion, if continued for more than an hour, may result in toxicity. Because of its efficacy and rapid onset of effect, the drug should be administered by infusion pump and arterial blood pressure continuously monitored via intra-arterial recording.

Toxicity

Other than excessive blood pressure lowering, the most serious toxicity is related to accumulation of cyanide; metabolic acidosis, arrhythmias, excessive hypotension, and death have resulted. In a few cases, toxicity after relatively low doses of nitroprusside suggested a defect in cyanide metabolism. Administration of sodium thiosulfate as a sulfur donor facilitates metabolism of cyanide. Hydroxocobalamin combines with cyanide to form the nontoxic cyanocobalamin. Both have been advocated for prophylaxis or treatment of cyanide poisoning during nitroprusside infusion. Thiocyanate may accumulate over the course of prolonged administration, usually several days or more, particularly in patients with renal insufficiency who do not excrete thiocyanate at a normal rate. Thiocyanate toxicity is manifested as weakness, disorientation, psychosis, muscle spasms, and convulsions, and the diagnosis is confirmed by finding serum concentrations greater than 10 mg/dL. Rarely, delayed hypothyroidism occurs, owing to thiocyanate inhibition of iodide uptake by the thyroid. Methemoglobinemia during infusion of nitroprusside has also been reported.

DIAZOXIDE

Diazoxide is an effective and relatively long-acting parenterally administered arteriolar dilator that is occasionally used to treat hypertensive emergencies. Injection of diazoxide results in a rapid fall in systemic vascular resistance and mean arterial blood pressure associated with substantial tachycardia and increase in cardiac output. Studies of its mechanism suggest that it prevents vascular smooth muscle contraction by opening potassium channels and stabilizing the membrane potential at the resting level.

Diazoxide

Pharmacokinetics & Dosage

Diazoxide is similar chemically to the thiazide diuretics but has no diuretic activity. It is bound extensively to serum albumin and to vascular tissue. Diazoxide is partially metabolized; its metabolic pathways are not well characterized. The remainder is excreted unchanged. Its half-life is approximately 24 hours, but the relationship between blood concentration and hypotensive action is not well established. The blood pressure-lowering effect after a rapid injection is established within 5 minutes and lasts for 4–12 hours.

When diazoxide was first marketed, a dose of 300 mg by rapid injection was recommended. It appears, however, that excessive hypotension can be avoided by beginning with smaller doses (50–150 mg). If necessary, doses of 150 mg may be repeated every 5 minutes until blood pressure is lowered satisfactorily. Nearly all patients respond to a maximum of three or four doses. Alternatively, diazoxide may be administered by intravenous infusion at rates of 15–30 mg/min. Because of reduced protein binding, hypotension occurs after smaller doses in persons with chronic

renal failure, and smaller doses should be administered to these patients. The hypotensive effects of diazoxide are also greater if patients are pretreated with β blockers to prevent the reflex tachycardia and associated increase in cardiac output.

Toxicity

The most significant toxicity from diazoxide has been excessive hypotension, resulting from the recommendation to use a fixed dose of 300 mg in all patients. Such hypotension has resulted in stroke and myocardial infarction. The reflex sympathetic response can provoke angina, electrocardiographic evidence of ischemia, and cardiac failure in patients with ischemic heart disease, and diazoxide should be avoided in this situation.

Diazoxide inhibits insulin release from the pancreas (probably by opening potassium channels in the β cell membrane) and is used to treat hypoglycemia secondary to insulinoma. Occasionally, hyperglycemia complicates diazoxide use, particularly in persons with renal insufficiency.

In contrast to the structurally related thiazide diuretics, diazoxide causes renal salt and water *retention*. However, because the drug is used for short periods only, this is rarely a problem.

FENOLDOPAM

Fenoldopam is a peripheral arteriolar dilator used for hypertensive emergencies and postoperative hypertension. It acts primarily as an agonist of dopamine D_1 receptors, resulting in dilation of peripheral arteries and natriuresis. The commercial product is a racemic mixture with the *(R)*-isomer mediating the pharmacologic activity.

Fenoldopam is rapidly metabolized, primarily by conjugation. Its half-life is 10 minutes. The drug is administered by continuous intravenous infusion. Fenoldopam is initiated at a low dosage (0.1 mcg/kg/min), and the dose is then titrated upward every 15 or 20 minutes up to a maximum dose of 1.6 mcg/kg/min or until the desired blood pressure reduction is achieved.

As with other direct vasodilators, the major toxicities are reflex tachycardia, headache, and flushing. Fenoldopam also increases intraocular pressure and should be avoided in patients with glaucoma.

CALCIUM CHANNEL BLOCKERS

In addition to their antianginal (see Chapter 12) and antiarrhythmic effects (see Chapter 14), calcium channel blockers also reduce peripheral resistance and blood pressure. The mechanism of action in hypertension (and, in part, in angina) is inhibition of calcium influx into arterial smooth muscle cells.

Verapamil, diltiazem, and the **dihydropyridine** family **(amlodipine, felodipine, isradipine, nicardipine, nifedipine,** and **nisoldipine)** are all equally effective in lowering blood pressure, and many formulations are currently approved for this use in the USA. Hemodynamic differences among calcium channel blockers may influence the choice of a particular agent. Nifedipine and the other dihydropyridine agents are more selective as vasodilators and have less cardiac depressant effect than verapamil and diltiazem. Reflex sympathetic activation with slight tachycardia maintains or increases cardiac output in most patients given dihydropyridines. Verapamil has the greatest depressant effect on the heart and may decrease heart rate and cardiac output. Diltiazem has intermediate actions. The pharmacology and toxicity of these drugs is discussed in more detail in Chapter 12. Doses of calcium channel blockers used in treating hypertension are similar to those used in treating angina. Some epidemiologic studies reported an increased risk of myocardial infarction or mortality in patients receiving short-acting nifedipine for hypertension. It is therefore recommended that short-acting dihydropyridines not be used for hypertension. Sustained-release calcium blockers or calcium blockers with long half-lives provide smoother blood pressure control and are more appropriate for treatment of chronic hypertension. Intravenous nicardipine is available for the treatment of hypertension when oral therapy is not feasible, although parenteral verapamil and diltiazem could be used for the same indication. Nicardipine is typically infused at rates of 2–15 mg/h. Oral short-acting nifedipine has been used in emergency management of severe hypertension.

INHIBITORS OF ANGIOTENSIN

Renin, angiotensin, and aldosterone play important roles in at least some individuals with essential hypertension. Approximately 20% of patients with essential hypertension have inappropriately low and 20% have inappropriately high plasma renin activity. Blood pressure of patients with high-renin hypertension responds well to β-adrenoceptor blockers, which lower plasma renin activity, and to angiotensin inhibitors—supporting a role for excess renin and angiotensin in this population.

Mechanism & Sites of Action

Renin release from the kidney cortex is stimulated by reduced renal arterial pressure, sympathetic neural stimulation, and reduced sodium delivery or increased sodium concentration at the distal renal tubule (see Chapter 17). Renin acts upon angiotensinogen to split off the inactive precursor decapeptide angiotensin I. Angiotensin I is then converted, primarily by endothelial ACE, to the arterial vasoconstrictor octapeptide angiotensin II (Figure 11–5), which is in turn converted in the adrenal gland to angiotensin III. Angiotensin II has vasoconstrictor and sodium-retaining activity. Angiotensin II and III both stimulate aldosterone release. Angiotensin may contribute to maintaining high vascular resistance in hypertensive states associated with high plasma renin activity, such as renal arterial stenosis, some types of intrinsic renal disease, and malignant hypertension, as well as in essential hypertension after treatment with sodium restriction, diuretics, or vasodilators. However, even in low-renin hypertensive states, these drugs can lower blood pressure (see below).

A parallel system for angiotensin generation exists in several other tissues (eg, heart) and may be responsible for trophic changes such as cardiac hypertrophy. The converting enzyme involved in tissue angiotensin II synthesis is also inhibited by the ACE inhibitors.

Two classes of drugs act specifically on the renin-angiotensin system: the ACE inhibitors and the competitive inhibitors of angiotensin at its receptors, including losartan and other nonpeptide antagonists, and the peptide saralasin. (Saralasin is no longer in clinical use.) An orally active renin antagonist (aliskiren, see Chapter 17) is currently under study.

ANGIOTENSIN-CONVERTING ENZYME (ACE) INHIBITORS

Captopril (see Figure 17–2) and other drugs in this class inhibit the converting enzyme peptidyl dipeptidase that hydrolyzes angiotensin I to angiotensin II and (under the name plasma kininase) inactivates bradykinin, a potent vasodilator, which works at least in part by stimulating release of nitric oxide and prostacyclin. The hypotensive activity of captopril results both from an inhibitory action on the renin-angiotensin system and a stimulating action on the kallikrein-kinin system (Figure 11–5). The latter mechanism has been demonstrated by showing that a bradykinin receptor antagonist, **icatibant** (see Chapter 17), blunts the blood pressure-lowering effect of captopril.

Enalapril (see Figure 17–3) is an oral prodrug that is converted by hydrolysis to a converting enzyme inhibitor, enalaprilat, with effects similar to those of captopril. Enalaprilat itself is available only for intravenous use, primarily for hypertensive emergencies. **Lisinopril** is a lysine derivative of enalaprilat. **Benazepril, fosinopril, moexipril, perindopril, quinapril, ramipril,** and **trandolapril** are other long-acting members of the class. All are prodrugs, like enalapril, and are converted to the active agents by hydrolysis, primarily in the liver.

Angiotensin II inhibitors lower blood pressure principally by decreasing peripheral vascular resistance. Cardiac

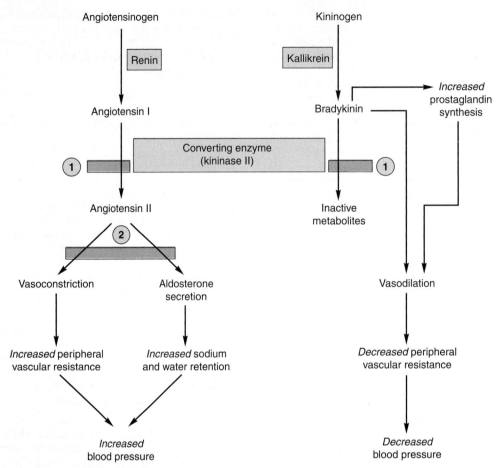

Figure 11–5. Sites of action of ACE inhibitors and angiotensin II receptor blockers. ① Site of angiotensin-converting enzyme blockade. ② Site of receptor blockade.

output and heart rate are not significantly changed. Unlike direct vasodilators, these agents do not result in reflex sympathetic activation and can be used safely in persons with ischemic heart disease. The absence of reflex tachycardia may be due to downward resetting of the baroreceptors or to enhanced parasympathetic activity.

Although converting enzyme inhibitors are most effective in conditions associated with high plasma renin activity, there is no good correlation among subjects between plasma renin activity and antihypertensive response. Accordingly, renin profiling is unnecessary.

ACE inhibitors have a particularly useful role in treating patients with chronic kidney disease because they diminish proteinuria and stabilize renal function (even in the absence of lowering of blood pressure). These benefits probably result from improved intrarenal hemodynamics, with decreased glomerular efferent arteriolar resistance and a resulting reduction of intraglomerular capillary pressure. ACE inhibitors have also

proved to be extremely useful in the treatment of heart failure, and after myocardial infarction, and there is recent evidence that ACE inhibitors reduce the incidence of diabetes in patients with high cardiovascular risk (see Chapter 13).

Pharmacokinetics & Dosage

Captopril's pharmacokinetic parameters and dosing recommendations are set forth in Table 11–1. Peak concentrations of enalaprilat, the active metabolite, occur 3–4 hours after dosing with enalapril. The half-life of enalaprilat is about 11 hours. Typical doses of enalapril are 10–20 mg once or twice daily. Lisinopril has a half-life of 12 hours. Doses of 10–80 mg once daily are effective in most patients. All of the ACE inhibitors except fosinopril and moexipril are eliminated primarily by the kidneys; doses of these drugs should be reduced in patients with renal insufficiency.

Toxicity

Severe hypotension can occur after initial doses of any ACE inhibitor in patients who are hypovolemic due to diuretics, salt restriction, or gastrointestinal fluid loss. Other adverse effects common to all ACE inhibitors include acute renal failure (particularly in patients with bilateral renal artery stenosis or stenosis of the renal artery of a solitary kidney), hyperkalemia, dry cough sometimes accompanied by wheezing, and angioedema. Hyperkalemia is more likely to occur in patients with renal insufficiency or diabetes. Bradykinin and substance P seem to be responsible for the cough and angioedema seen with ACE inhibition.

The use of ACE inhibitors is contraindicated during the second and third trimesters of pregnancy because of the risk of fetal hypotension, anuria, and renal failure, sometimes associated with fetal malformations or death. Recent evidence also implicates first trimester exposure to ACE inhibitors in increased teratogenic risk. Captopril, particularly when given in high doses to patients with renal insufficiency, may cause neutropenia or proteinuria. Minor toxic effects seen more typically include altered sense of taste, allergic skin rashes, and drug fever, which may occur in as many as 10% of patients.

Important drug interactions include those with potassium supplements or potassium-sparing diuretics, which can result in hyperkalemia. Nonsteroidal anti-inflammatory drugs may impair the hypotensive effects of ACE inhibitors by blocking bradykinin-mediated vasodilation, which is at least in part, prostaglandin mediated.

ANGIOTENSIN RECEPTOR–BLOCKING AGENTS

Losartan and **valsartan** were the first marketed blockers of the angiotensin II type 1 (AT_1) receptor. More recently, **candesartan, eprosartan, irbesartan,** and **telmisartan** have been released. They have no effect on bradykinin metabolism and are therefore more selective blockers of angiotensin effects than ACE inhibitors. They also have the potential for more complete inhibition of angiotensin action compared with ACE inhibitors because there are enzymes other than ACE that are capable of generating angiotensin II. Angiotensin receptor blockers provide benefits similar to those of ACE inhibitors in patients with heart failure and chronic kidney disease. Losartan's pharmacokinetic parameters are listed in Table 11–1. The adverse effects are similar to those described for ACE inhibitors, including the hazard of use during pregnancy. Cough and angioedema can occur but are less common with angiotensin receptor blockers than with ACE inhibitors.

■ II. CLINICAL PHARMACOLOGY OF ANTIHYPERTENSIVE AGENTS

Hypertension presents a unique problem in therapeutics. It is usually a lifelong disease that causes few symptoms until the advanced stage. For effective treatment, medicines that may be expensive and often produce adverse effects must be consumed daily. Thus, the physician must establish with certainty that hypertension is persistent and requires treatment and must exclude secondary causes of hypertension that might be treated by definitive surgical procedures. Persistence of hypertension, particularly in persons with mild elevation of blood pressure, should be established by finding an elevated blood pressure on at least three different office visits. Ambulatory blood pressure monitoring may be the best predictor of risk and therefore of need for therapy in mild hypertension. Isolated systolic hypertension and hypertension in the elderly also benefit from therapy.

Once the presence of hypertension is established, the question of whether or not to treat and which drugs to use must be considered. The level of blood pressure, the age and sex of the patient, the severity of organ damage (if any) due to high blood pressure, and the presence of cardiovascular risk factors must all be considered. At this stage, the patient must be educated about the nature of hypertension and the importance of treatment so that he or she can make an informed decision regarding therapy.

Once the decision is made to treat, a therapeutic regimen must be developed. Selection of drugs is dictated by the level of blood pressure, the presence and severity of end organ damage, and the presence of other diseases. Severe high blood pressure with life-threatening complications requires more rapid treatment with more efficacious drugs. Most patients with essential hypertension, however, have had elevated blood pressure for months or years, and therapy is best initiated in a gradual fashion.

Education about the natural history of hypertension and the importance of treatment compliance as well as potential side effects of drugs is essential. Follow-up visits should be frequent enough to convince the patient that the physician thinks the illness is serious. With each follow-up visit, the importance of treatment should be reinforced and questions concerning dosing or side effects of medication encouraged. Other factors that may improve compliance are simplifying dosing regimens and having the patient monitor blood pressure at home.

OUTPATIENT THERAPY OF HYPERTENSION

The initial step in treating hypertension may be non-pharmacologic. As discussed previously, sodium restriction may be effective treatment for many patients with mild hypertension. The average American diet contains about 200 mEq of sodium per day. A reasonable dietary goal in treating hypertension is 70–100 mEq of sodium per day, which can be achieved by not salting food during or after cooking and by avoiding processed foods that contain large amounts of sodium. Eating a diet rich in fruits, vegetables, and low-fat dairy products with a reduced content of saturated and total fat, and moderation of alcohol intake (no more than two drinks per day) also lower blood pressure.

Weight reduction even without sodium restriction has been shown to normalize blood pressure in up to 75% of overweight patients with mild to moderate hypertension. Regular exercise has been shown in some but not all studies to lower blood pressure in hypertensive patients.

For pharmacologic management of mild hypertension, blood pressure can be normalized in many patients with a single drug. However, most patients with hypertension require two or more antihypertensive medications. Thiazide diuretics, β blockers, ACE inhibitors, angiotensin receptor blockers, and calcium channel blockers have all been shown to reduce complications of hypertension and may be used for initial drug therapy. There has been concern that diuretics, by adversely affecting the serum lipid profile or impairing glucose tolerance, may add to the risk of coronary disease, thereby offsetting the benefit of blood pressure reduction. However a recent large clinical trial comparing different classes of antihypertensive mediations for initial therapy found that chlorthalidone (a thiazide diuretic) was as effective as other agents in reducing coronary heart disease death and nonfatal myocardial infarction, and was superior to amlodipine in preventing heart failure and superior to lisinopril in preventing stroke.

The presence of concomitant disease should influence selection of antihypertensive drugs because two diseases may benefit from a single drug. For example, ACE inhibitors are particularly useful in patients with evidence of chronic kidney disease. Beta blockers or calcium channel blockers are useful in patients who also have angina; diuretics, ACE inhibitors, angiotension receptor blockers, or β blockers in patients who also have heart failure; and α_1 blockers in men who have benign prostatic hyperplasia. Race may also affect drug selection: African-Americans respond better to diuretics and calcium channel blockers than to β blockers and ACE inhibitors. Chinese are more sensitive to the effects of β blockers and may require lower doses.

If a single drug does not adequately control blood pressure, drugs with different sites of action can be combined to effectively lower blood pressure while minimizing toxicity ("stepped care"). If a diuretic is not used initially, it is often selected as the second drug. If three drugs are required, combining a diuretic, a sympathoplegic agent or an ACE inhibitor, and a direct vasodilator (eg, hydralazine or a calcium channel blocker) is often effective. In the USA, fixed-dose drug combinations containing a β blocker, an ACE inhibitor, or an angiotensin receptor blocker plus a thiazide, and a calcium channel blocker plus an ACE inhibitor are available. Fixed-dose combinations have the drawback of not allowing for titration of individual drug doses but have the advantage of allowing fewer pills to be taken, potentially enhancing compliance.

Assessment of blood pressure during office visits should include measurement of recumbent, sitting, and standing pressures. An attempt should be made to normalize blood pressure in the posture or activity level that is customary for the patient. The recent large Hypertension Optimal Treatment study suggests that the optimal blood pressure end point is 138/83 mm Hg. Lowering blood pressure below this level produces no further benefit. In diabetic patients, however, there is a continued reduction of event rates with progressively lower blood pressures. Systolic hypertension (> 140 mm Hg in the presence of normal diastolic blood pressure) is a strong cardiovascular risk factor in people older than 50 years of age and should be treated. In addition to noncompliance with medication, causes of failure to respond to drug therapy include excessive sodium intake and inadequate diuretic therapy with excessive blood volume (this can be measured directly), and drugs such as tricyclic antidepressants, nonsteroidal anti-inflammatory drugs, over-the-counter sympathomimetics, abuse of stimulants (amphetamine or cocaine), or excessive doses of caffeine and oral contraceptives that can interfere with actions of some antihypertensive drugs or directly raise blood pressure.

MANAGEMENT OF HYPERTENSIVE EMERGENCIES

Despite the large number of patients with chronic hypertension, hypertensive emergencies are relatively rare. Marked or sudden elevation of blood pressure may be a serious threat to life, however, and prompt control of blood pressure is indicated. Most commonly, hypertensive emergencies occur in patients whose hypertension is severe and poorly controlled and in those who suddenly discontinue antihypertensive medications.

Clinical Presentation & Pathophysiology

Hypertensive emergencies include hypertension associated with vascular damage (termed malignant hypertension) and hypertension associated with hemodynamic complications such as heart failure, stroke, or dissecting aneurysm. The underlying pathologic process in malignant hypertension is a progressive arteriopathy with inflammation and necrosis of arterioles. Vascular lesions occur in the kidney, which releases renin, which in turn stimulates production of angiotensin and aldosterone, which further increase blood pressure.

Hypertensive encephalopathy is a classic feature of malignant hypertension. Its clinical presentation consists of severe headache, mental confusion, and apprehension. Blurred vision, nausea and vomiting, and focal neurologic deficits are common. If untreated, the syndrome may progress over a period of 12–48 hours to convulsions, stupor, coma, and even death.

Treatment of Hypertensive Emergencies

The general management of hypertensive emergencies requires monitoring the patient in an intensive care unit with continuous recording of arterial blood pressure. Fluid intake and output must be monitored carefully and body weight measured daily as an indicator of total body fluid volume during the course of therapy.

Parenteral antihypertensive medications are used to lower blood pressure rapidly (within a few hours); as soon as reasonable blood pressure control is achieved, oral antihypertensive therapy should be substituted, because this allows smoother long-term management of hypertension. The goal of treatment in the first few hours or days is not complete normalization of blood pressure because chronic hypertension is associated with autoregulatory changes in cerebral blood flow. Thus, rapid normalization of blood pressure may lead to cerebral hypoperfusion and brain injury. Rather, blood pressure should be lowered by about 25%, maintaining diastolic blood pressure at no less than 100–110 mm Hg. Subsequently, blood pressure can be reduced to normal levels using oral medications over several weeks. The drug most commonly used to treat hypertensive emergencies is the vasodilator sodium nitroprusside. Other parenteral drugs that may be effective include fenoldopam, nitroglycerin, labetalol, calcium channel blockers, diazoxide, and hydralazine. Esmolol is often used to manage intraoperative and postoperative hypertension. Diuretics such as furosemide are administered to prevent the volume expansion that typically occurs during administration of powerful vasodilators.

Chapter continues on next page.

PREPARATIONS AVAILABLE

Beta-Adrenoceptor Blockers

Acebutolol (generic, Sectral)
Oral: 200, 400 mg capsules
Atenolol (generic, Tenormin)
Oral: 25, 50, 100 mg tablets
Parenteral: 0.5 mg/mL for injection
Betaxolol (Kerlone)
Oral: 10, 20 mg tablets
Bisoprolol (Zebeta)
Oral: 5, 10 mg tablets
Carteolol (Cartrol)
Oral: 2.5, 5 mg tablets
Carvedilol (Coreg)
Oral: 3.125, 6.25, 12.5, 25 mg tablets
Esmolol (BreviBloc)
Parenteral: 10, 250 mg/mL for injection
Labetalol (generic, Normodyne, Trandate)
Oral: 100, 200, 300 mg tablets
Parenteral: 5 mg/mL for injection
Metoprolol (generic, Lopressor)
Oral: 50, 100 mg tablets
Oral extended-release (Toprol-XL): 25, 50, 100, 200 mg tablets
Parenteral: 1 mg/mL for injection
Nadolol (generic, Corgard)
Oral: 20, 40, 80, 120, 160 mg tablets
Penbutolol (Levatol)
Oral: 20 mg tablets
Pindolol (generic, Visken)
Oral: 5, 10 mg tablets
Propranolol (generic, Inderal)
Oral: 10, 20, 40, 60, 80, 90 mg tablets; 4, 8 mg/mL oral solution; Intensol, 80 mg/mL solution
Oral sustained-release (generic, Inderal LA): 60, 80, 120, 160 mg capsules
Parenteral: 1 mg/mL for injection
Timolol (generic, Blocadren)
Oral: 5, 10, 20 mg tablets

Centrally Acting Sympathoplegic Drugs

Clonidine (generic, Catapres)
Oral: 0.1, 0.2, 0.3 mg tablets
Transdermal (Catapres-TTS): patches that release 0.1, 0.2, 0.3 mg/24 h
Guanabenz (generic, Wytensin)
Oral: 4, 8 mg tablets
Guanfacine (Tenex)
Oral: 1, 2 mg tablets
Methyldopa (generic)
Oral: 250, 500 mg tablets
Parenteral (Methyldopate HCl): 50 mg/mL for injection

Postganglionic Sympathetic Nerve Terminal Blockers

Guanadrel (Hylorel)
Oral: 10, 25 mg tablets
Guanethidine (Ismelin)
Oral: 10, 25 mg tablets
Reserpine (generic)
Oral: 0.1, 0.25 mg tablets

Alpha$_1$-Selective Adrenoceptor Blockers

Doxazosin (generic, Cardura)
Oral: 1, 2, 4, 8 mg tablets
Prazosin (generic, Minipress)
Oral: 1, 2, 5 mg capsules
Terazosin (generic, Hytrin)
Oral: 1, 2, 5, 10 mg capsules and tablets

Ganglion-Blocking Agents

Mecamylamine (Inversine)
Oral: 2.5 mg tablets

Vasodilators Used in Hypertension

Diazoxide (Hyperstat IV)
Parenteral: 15 mg/mL ampule
Oral (Proglycem): 50 mg capsule; 50 mg/mL oral suspension (for insulinoma)
Fenoldopam (Corlopam)
Parenteral: 10 mg/mL for IV infusion
Hydralazine (generic, Apresoline)
Oral: 10, 25, 50, 100 mg tablets
Parenteral: 20 mg/mL for injection
Minoxidil (generic, Loniten)
Oral: 2.5, 10 mg tablets
Topical (generic, Rogaine): 2% lotion
Nitroprusside (generic, Nitropress)
Parenteral: 50 mg/vial

Calcium Channel Blockers

Amlodipine (Amvaz, Norvasc)
Oral 2.5, 5, 10 mg tablets
Diltiazem (generic, Cardizem)
Oral: 30, 60, 90, 120 mg tablets (unlabeled in hypertension)
Oral sustained-release (Cardizem CD, Cardizem SR, Dilacor XL): 60, 90, 120, 180, 240, 300, 360, 420 mg capsules
Parenteral: 5 mg/mL for injection
Felodipine (Plendil)
Oral extended-release: 2.5, 5, 10 mg tablets
Isradipine (DynaCirc)
Oral: 2.5, 5 mg capsules; 5, 10 mg controlled-release tablets

(continued)

Nicardipine (generic, Cardene)
Oral: 20, 30 mg capsules
Oral sustained-release (Cardene SR): 30, 45, 60 mg capsules
Parenteral (Cardene I.V.): 2.5 mg/mL for injection
Nisoldipine (Sular)
Oral extended-release: 10, 20, 30, 40 mg tablets
Nifedipine (generic, Adalat, Procardia)
Oral: 10, 20 mg capsules (unlabeled in hypertension)
Oral extended-release (Adalat CC, Procardia-XL): 30, 60, 90 mg tablets
Verapamil (generic, Calan, Isoptin)
Oral: 40, 80, 120 mg tablets
Oral sustained-release (generic, Calan SR, Verelan): 120, 180, 240 mg tablets; 100, 120, 180, 200, 240, 300, 360 mg capsules
Parenteral: 2.5 mg/mL for injection

ANGIOTENSIN-CONVERTING ENZYME INHIBITORS

Benazepril (generic, Lotensin)
Oral: 5, 10, 20, 40 mg tablets
Captopril (generic, Capoten)
Oral: 12.5, 25, 50, 100 mg tablets
Enalapril (generic, Vasotec)
Oral: 2.5, 5, 10, 20 mg tablets
Parenteral (Enalaprilat): 1.25 mg/mL for injection
Fosinopril (generic, Monopril)
Oral: 10, 20, 40 mg tablets

Lisinopril (generic, Prinivil, Zestril)
Oral: 2.5, 5, 10, 20, 40 mg tablets
Moexipril (generic, Univasc)
Oral: 7.5, 15 mg tablets
Perindopril (Aceon)
Oral: 2, 4, 8 mg tablets
Quinapril (Accupril)
Oral: 5, 10, 20, 40 mg tablets
Ramipril (Altace)
Oral: 1.25, 2.5, 5, 10 mg capsules
Trandolapril (Mavik)
Oral: 1, 2, 4 mg tablets

ANGIOTENSIN RECEPTOR BLOCKERS

Candesartan (Atacand)
Oral: 4, 8, 16, 32 mg tablets
Eprosartan (Teveten)
Oral: 400, 600 mg tablets
Irbesartan (Avapro)
Oral; 75, 150, 300 mg tablets
Losartan (Cozaar)
Oral: 25, 50, 100 mg tablets
Olmesartan (Benicar)
Oral: 5, 20, 40 mg tablets
Telmisartan (Micardis)
Oral: 20, 40, 80 mg tablets
Valsartan (Diovan)
Oral: 40, 80, 160, 320 mg tablet

REFERENCES

ACE Inhibitors in Diabetic Nephropathy Trialist Group: Should all patients with type 1 diabetes mellitus and microalbuminuria receive angiotensin-converting enzyme inhibitors? A meta-analysis of individual patient data. Ann Intern Med 2001;134:370.

ALLHAT Officers and Coordinators for the ALLHAT Collaborative Research Group: Major outcomes of high-risk hypertensive patients randomized to angiotensin-converting enzyme inhibitor or calcium channel blockers vs diuretic: The antihypertensive and lipid-lowering treatment to prevent heart attack trial. JAMA 2002;288:2981.

Appel LJ et al: Effects of comprehensive lifestyle modification on blood pressure control: Main results of the PREMIER clinical trial. JAMA 2003;289:2083.

August P: Initial treatment of hypertension. N Engl J Med 2003; 348:610.

Boehm M, Nabel EG: Angiotensin-converting enzyme 2—a new cardiac regulator. N Engl J Med 2002;347:1795.

Burnier M: Cardiovascular Drugs: Angiotensin II type 1 receptor blockers. Circulation 2001;103:904.

Chobanian AV et al: The Seventh report of the Joint National Committee on Prevention, Detection, Evaluation, and Treatment of High Blood Pressure. JAMA 2003;289:2560.

Garg J, Messerli AW, Bakris GL: Evaluation and treatment of patients with systemic hypertension. Circulation 2002;105:2458.

Garovic VD, Textor SC: Renovascular hypertension and ischemic nephropathy. Circulation 2005;112:1362.

Kaplan NM: Management of hypertension in patients with type 2 diabetes mellitus: Guidelines based on current evidence. Ann Intern Med 2001;135:1079.

Ko DT et al: β-Blocker therapy and symptoms of depression, fatigue, and sexual dysfunction. JAMA 2002;288:351.

Murphy MB, Murray C, Shorten GD: Fenoldopam—a selective peripheral dopamine-receptor agonist for the treatment of severe hypertension. N Engl J Med 2001;345:1548.

Palmer BF: Renal dysfunction complicating the treatment of hypertension. N Engl J Med 2002;347:1256.

Psaty BM et al: Health outcomes associated with various antihypertensive therapies used as first-line agents: A network meta-analysis. JAMA 2003;289:2534.

Remuzzi G, Ruggenenti P, Perico N: Chronic renal diseases: Renoprotective benefits of renin-angiotensin-system inhibition. Ann Intern Med 2002;136:604.

Stevens VJ et al: Long-term weight loss and changes in blood pressure: Results of the trials of hypertension prevention, phase II. Ann Intern Med 2001;134:1.

Verdecchia P et al: Angiotensin-converting enzyme inhibitors and calcium channel blockers for coronary heart disease and stroke prevention. Hypertension 2005;46:386.

Vermes E et al: Enalapril reduces the incidence of diabetes in patients with chronic heart failure: Insight from the Studies Of Left Ventricular Dysfunction (SOLVD). Circulation 2003; 107:1291.

Vollmer WM et al: Effects of diet and sodium intake on blood pressure: Subgroup analysis of the DASH-Sodium trial. Ann Intern Med 2001;135:1019.

Wang TJ, Ramachandran SV: Epidemiology of uncontrolled hypertension in the United States. Circulation 2005; 112:1651.

Wing LMH et al: A comparison of outcomes with angiotensin-converting-enzyme inhibitors and diuretics for hypertension in the elderly. N Engl J Med 2003;348:583.

Wright JT Jr et al: Effect of blood pressure lowering and antihypertensive drug class on progression of hypertensive kidney disease. Results from AASK Trial. JAMA 2002; 288:2421.

Vasodilators & the Treatment of Angina Pectoris

Bertram G. Katzung, MD, PhD, & Kanu Chatterjee, MB, FRCP

Angina pectoris is the most common condition involving tissue ischemia in which vasodilator drugs are used. The name denotes chest pain caused by accumulation of metabolites resulting from myocardial ischemia. The organic nitrates, eg, **nitroglycerin,** are the mainstay of therapy for the immediate relief of angina. Another group of vasodilators, the **calcium channel blockers,** is also important, especially for prophylaxis, and the β **blockers,** which are *not* vasodilators, are also useful in prophylaxis. New groups of drugs under investigation include fatty acid oxidation inhibitors and selective cardiac rate inhibitors.

Ischemic heart disease is the most common serious health problem in many Western societies. By far the most frequent cause of angina is atheromatous obstruction of the large coronary vessels **(atherosclerotic angina, classic angina).** However, transient spasm of localized portions of these vessels, which is usually associated with underlying atheromas, can also cause significant myocardial ischemia and pain **(vasospastic** or **variant angina).**

The primary cause of angina pectoris is an imbalance between the oxygen requirement of the heart and the oxygen supplied to it via the coronary vessels. In classic angina, the imbalance occurs when the myocardial oxygen requirement increases, as during exercise, and coronary blood flow does not increase proportionately. The resulting ischemia usually leads to pain. Classic angina is therefore "angina of effort." (In some individuals, the ischemia is not always accompanied by pain, resulting in "silent" or "ambulatory" ischemia.) In variant angina, oxygen delivery decreases as a result of reversible coronary vasospasm. Variant angina is also called **Prinzmetal's** angina.

In theory, the imbalance between oxygen delivery and myocardial oxygen demand can be corrected by **decreasing oxygen demand** or by **increasing delivery** (by increasing coronary flow). In effort angina, oxygen demand can be reduced by decreasing cardiac work or, according to recent studies, by shifting myocardial metabolism to substrates that require less oxygen per unit of ATP produced. In variant angina, on the other hand, spasm of

coronary vessels can be reversed by nitrates or calcium channel blockers. Lipid-lowering drugs, especially the "statins," have become extremely important in the long-term treatment of atherosclerotic disease (see Chapter 35).

Unstable angina, an acute coronary syndrome, is said to be present when there are episodes of angina at rest and when there is a change in the character, frequency, and duration of chest pain as well as precipitating factors in patients with previously stable angina. Unstable angina is caused by episodes of increased epicardial coronary artery tone or small platelet clots occurring in the vicinity of an atherosclerotic plaque. In most cases, formation of labile nonocclusive thrombi at the site of a fissured or ulcerated plaque is the mechanism for reduction in flow. The course and the prognosis of unstable angina are variable, but this subset of acute coronary syndrome is associated with a high risk of myocardial infarction and death.

PATHOPHYSIOLOGY OF ANGINA

Determinants of Myocardial Oxygen Demand

The major determinants of myocardial oxygen requirement are set forth in Table 12–1. As a consequence of its continuous activity, the heart's oxygen needs are relatively high, and it extracts approximately 75% of the available oxygen even in the absence of stress. The myocardial oxygen requirement increases when there is an increase in heart rate, contractility, arterial pressure, or ventricular volume. These hemodynamic alterations frequently occur during physical exercise and sympathetic discharge, which often precipitate angina in patients with obstructive coronary artery disease.

The heart favors fatty acids as a substrate for energy production. However, oxidation of fatty acids requires more oxygen per unit of ATP generated than oxidation of carbohydrates. Therefore, drugs that shift myocardial metabolism toward greater use of glucose (fatty acid oxidation inhibitors) have the potential of reducing the oxygen demand without altering hemodynamics.

Table 12–1. Determinants of myocardial oxygen consumption.

Wall stress
Intraventricular pressure
Ventricular radius (volume)
Wall thickness
Heart rate
Contractility

Determinants of Coronary Blood Flow & Myocardial Oxygen Supply

Increased myocardial demands for oxygen in the normal heart are met by augmenting coronary blood flow. Coronary blood flow is directly related to the perfusion pressure (aortic diastolic pressure) and the duration of diastole. Because coronary flow drops to negligible values during systole, the duration of diastole becomes a limiting factor for myocardial perfusion during tachycardia. Coronary blood flow is inversely proportional to coronary vascular bed resistance. Resistance is determined mainly by intrinsic factors—including metabolic products and autonomic activity—and by various pharmacologic agents. Damage to the endothelium of coronary vessels has been shown to alter their ability to dilate and to increase coronary vascular resistance.

Determinants of Vascular Tone

Arteriolar and venous tone (smooth muscle tension) both play a role in determining myocardial wall stress (Table 12–1). Arteriolar tone directly controls peripheral vascular resistance and thus arterial blood pressure. In systole, intraventricular pressure must exceed aortic pressure to eject blood; arterial blood pressure thus determines the *systolic* wall stress in an important way. Venous tone determines the capacity of the venous circulation and controls the amount of blood sequestered in the venous system versus the amount returned to the heart. Venous tone thereby determines the *diastolic* wall stress.

The regulation of smooth muscle contraction and relaxation is shown schematically in Figure 12–1. As shown in Figures 12–1 and 12–2, drugs may relax vascular smooth muscle in several ways:

(1) Increasing cGMP: As indicated in Figure 12–2, cGMP facilitates the dephosphorylation of myosin light chains, preventing the interaction of myosin with actin. Nitric oxide is an effective activator of soluble guanylyl cyclase and acts mainly through this mechanism. Important molecular donors of nitric oxide include nitroprusside (see Chapter 11) and the organic nitrates used in angina.

(2) Decreasing intracellular Ca^{2+}: Calcium channel blockers predictably cause vasodilation because they reduce intracellular Ca^{2+}, a major modulator of the activation of myosin light chain kinase. (Beta blockers and calcium channel blockers reduce Ca^{2+} influx in cardiac muscle, thereby reducing rate, contractility, and oxygen requirement unless reversed by compensatory responses.)

(3) Stabilizing or preventing depolarization of the vascular smooth muscle cell membrane: The membrane potential of excitable cells is stabilized near the resting potential by increasing potassium permeability. Potassium channel openers, such as minoxidil sulfate, (see Chapter 11) increase the permeability of K^+ channels, probably ATP-dependent K^+ channels. Certain newer agents under investigation for use in angina (eg, nicorandil) may act, in part, by this mechanism.

(4) Increasing cAMP in vascular smooth muscle cells: As shown in Figure 12–1, an increase in cAMP increases the rate of inactivation of myosin light chain kinase, the enzyme responsible for triggering the interaction of actin with myosin in these cells. This appears to be the mechanism of vasodilation caused by β_2 agonists, drugs that are *not* used in angina.

Figure 12–1. Control of smooth muscle contraction and site of action of calcium channel-blocking drugs. Contraction is triggered by influx of calcium (which can be blocked by calcium channel blockers) through transmembrane calcium channels. The calcium combines with calmodulin to form a complex that converts the enzyme myosin light chain kinase to its active form (*MLCK**). The latter phosphorylates the myosin light chains, thereby initiating the interaction of myosin with actin. Beta$_2$ agonists (and other substances that increase cAMP) may cause relaxation in smooth muscle by accelerating the inactivation of MLCK (heavy arrows) and by facilitating the expulsion of calcium from the cell (not shown).

Figure 12–2. Mechanism of action of nitrates, nitrites, and other substances that increase the concentration of nitric oxide (NO) in smooth muscle cells. (MLCK*, activated myosin light chain kinase [see Figure 12–1]; guanylyl cyclase*, activated guanylyl cyclase; ?, unknown intermediate steps. Steps leading to relaxation are shown with heavy arrows.)

■ I. BASIC PHARMACOLOGY OF DRUGS USED TO TREAT ANGINA

Drug Action in Angina

Three of the four drug groups currently approved for use in angina (organic nitrates, calcium channel blockers, and β blockers) *decrease myocardial oxygen requirement* by decreasing the determinants of oxygen demand (heart rate, ventricular volume, blood pressure, and contractility). In some patients, a redistribution of coronary flow may increase oxygen delivery to ischemic tissue. In variant angina, the nitrates and the calcium channel blockers may also *increase myocardial oxygen delivery* by reversing coronary arterial spasm. The fourth group, represented by ranolazine, is discussed later.

NITRATES & NITRITES

Chemistry

These agents are simple nitric and nitrous acid esters of polyalcohols. **Nitroglycerin** may be considered the prototype of the group. Although nitroglycerin is used in the manufacture of dynamite, the formulations used in medicine are not explosive. The conventional sublingual tablet form of nitroglycerin may lose potency when stored as a result of volatilization and adsorption to plastic surfaces. Therefore, it should be kept in tightly closed glass containers. It is not sensitive to light.

All therapeutically active agents in the nitrate group have identical mechanisms of action and similar toxicities. Therefore, pharmacokinetic factors govern the choice of agent and mode of therapy when using the nitrates.

$$H_2C - O - NO_2$$
$$|$$
$$HC - O - NO_2$$
$$|$$
$$H_2C - O - NO_2$$

Nitroglycerin (glyceryl trinitrate)

Pharmacokinetics

The liver contains a high-capacity organic nitrate reductase that removes nitrate groups in a stepwise fashion from the parent molecule and ultimately inactivates the drug. Therefore, oral bioavailability of the traditional organic nitrates (eg, nitroglycerin and **isosorbide dinitrate**) is very low (typically < 10–20%). For this reason, the sublingual route, which avoids the first-pass effect, is preferred for achieving a therapeutic blood level rapidly. Nitroglycerin and isosorbide dinitrate are both absorbed efficiently by this route and reach therapeutic blood levels within a few minutes. However, the total dose administered by this route must be limited to avoid excessive effect; therefore, the total duration of effect is brief (15–30 minutes). When much longer duration of action is needed, oral preparations can be given that contain an amount of drug sufficient to result in sustained systemic blood levels of the parent drug plus active metabolites. Other routes of administration available for nitroglycerin include transdermal and buccal absorption from slow-release preparations; these are described below.

Amyl nitrite and related nitrites are highly volatile liquids. Amyl nitrite is available in fragile glass ampules packaged in a protective cloth covering. The ampule can be crushed with the fingers, resulting in rapid release of inhalable vapors through the cloth covering. The inhalation route provides very rapid absorption and, like the sublingual route, avoids the hepatic first-pass effect. Because of its unpleasant odor and short duration of action, amyl nitrite is now obsolete for angina.

Once absorbed, the unchanged nitrate compounds have half-lives of only 2–8 minutes. The partially denitrated metabolites have much longer half-lives (up to 3 hours). Of the nitroglycerin metabolites (two dinitroglycerins and two mononitro forms), the dinitro derivatives have significant vasodilator efficacy; they probably provide most of the therapeutic effect of orally administered nitroglycerin. The 5-mononitrate metabolite of isosorbide dinitrate is an active metabolite of the latter drug and is available for clinical use as **isosorbide mononitrate.** It has a bioavailability of 100%.

Excretion, primarily in the form of glucuronide derivatives of the denitrated metabolites, is largely by way of the kidney.

Pharmacodynamics

A. MECHANISM OF ACTION IN SMOOTH MUSCLE

Nitroglycerin is denitrated by glutathione S-transferase. Free nitrite ion is released, which is then converted to **nitric oxide** (see Chapter 19). A different unknown enzymatic reaction releases nitric oxide directly from the parent drug molecule. As shown in Figure 12–2, nitric oxide (or an S-nitrosothiol derivative) causes activation of guanylyl cyclase and an increase in cGMP, which are the first steps toward smooth muscle relaxation. The production of prostaglandin E or prostacyclin (PGI_2) and membrane hyperpolarization may also be involved. There is no evidence that autonomic receptors are involved in the primary nitrate response (although autonomic *reflex* responses are evoked when hypotensive doses are given).

As described below, tolerance is an important consideration in the use of nitrates. While tolerance may be caused in part by a decrease in tissue sulfhydryl groups, it can be only partially prevented or reversed with a sulfhydryl-regenerating agent. Increased generation of oxygen free radicals during nitrate therapy may be another important mechanism of tolerance.

Nicorandil and several other investigational antianginal agents appear to combine the activity of nitric oxide release with potassium channel-opening action, thus providing an additional mechanism for causing vasodilation.

B. ORGAN SYSTEM EFFECTS

Nitroglycerin relaxes all types of smooth muscle irrespective of the cause of the preexisting muscle tone (Figure 12–3). It has practically no direct effect on cardiac or skeletal muscle.

1. Vascular smooth muscle—All segments of the vascular system from large arteries through large veins relax in response to nitroglycerin. Veins respond at the lowest concentrations, arteries at slightly higher ones. Arterioles and precapillary sphincters are dilated less than the large arteries and the veins, partly because of reflex responses and partly because different vessels vary in their ability to release nitric oxide. The primary direct result of an effective dose of nitroglycerin is marked relaxation of veins with increased venous capacitance and decreased ventricular preload. Pulmonary vascular pressures and heart size are significantly reduced. In the absence of heart failure, cardiac output is reduced. Because venous capacitance is increased, orthostatic hypotension may be marked and syncope can result. Dilation of some large arteries (including the aorta) may be significant because of their large increase in compliance. Temporal artery pulsations and a throbbing headache associated with meningeal artery pulsations are frequent effects of nitroglycerin and amyl nitrite. In heart failure, preload is often abnormally high; the nitrates and other vasodilators, by reducing preload, may have a beneficial effect on cardiac output in this condition (see Chapter 13).

The indirect effects of nitroglycerin consist of those compensatory responses evoked by baroreceptors and hormonal mechanisms responding to decreased arterial pressure (see Figure 6–7); this consistently results in tachycardia and increased cardiac contractility. Retention of salt and water may also be significant, especially with intermediate- and long-acting nitrates. These compensatory responses contribute to the development of tolerance.

In normal subjects without coronary disease, nitroglycerin can induce a significant, if transient, increase in total coronary blood flow. In contrast, there is no evidence that total coronary flow is increased in patients with angina due to atherosclerotic obstructive coronary artery disease. However, some studies suggest that *redistribution* of coronary flow from normal to ischemic regions may play a role in nitroglycerin's therapeutic effect. Nitroglycerin also exerts a weak negative inotropic effect via nitric oxide.

2. Other smooth muscle organs—Relaxation of smooth muscle of the bronchi, gastrointestinal tract (including biliary system), and genitourinary tract has been demonstrated experimentally. Because of their brief duration, these actions of the nitrates are rarely of any clinical value. During recent years, the use of amyl nitrite and isobutyl nitrite by inhalation as purported recreational (sex-enhancing) drugs has become popular with

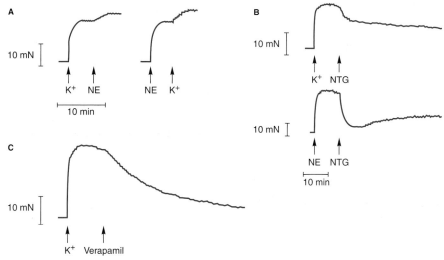

Figure 12–3. Effects of vasodilators on contractions of human vein segments studied in vitro. Panel **A** shows contractions induced by two vasoconstrictor agents, norepinephrine (NE) and potassium (K+). Panel **B** shows the relaxation induced by nitroglycerin (NTG), 4 μmol/L. The relaxation is prompt. Panel **C** shows the relaxation induced by verapamil, 2.2 μmol/L. The relaxation is slower but more sustained. (Modified and reproduced, with permission, from Mikkelsen E, Andersson KE, Bengtsson B: Effects of verapamil and nitroglycerin on contractile responses to potassium and noradrenaline in isolated human peripheral veins. Acta Pharmacol Toxicol 1978;42:14.)

some segments of the population. Nitrites release nitric oxide in erectile tissue as well as vascular smooth muscle and activate guanylyl cyclase. The resulting increase in cGMP causes dephosphorylation of myosin light chains and relaxation (Figure 12–2), which enhances erection. Drugs used in the treatment of erectile dysfunction are discussed in the Box, Drugs Used in the Treatment of Erectile Dysfunction.

3. Action on platelets—Nitric oxide released from nitroglycerin stimulates guanylyl cyclase in platelets as in smooth muscle. The increase in cGMP that results is responsible for a decrease in platelet aggregation. Unfortunately, recent prospective trials have established no survival benefit when nitroglycerin is used in acute myocardial infarction.

4. Other effects—*Nitrite* ion reacts with hemoglobin (which contains ferrous iron) to produce methemoglobin (which contains ferric iron). Because methemoglobin has a very low affinity for oxygen, large doses of nitrites can result in pseudocyanosis, tissue hypoxia, and death. Fortunately, the plasma level of *nitrite* resulting from even large doses of organic and inorganic *nitrates* is too low to cause significant methemoglobinemia in adults. However, sodium nitrite is used as a curing agent for meats. In nursing infants, the intestinal flora is capable of converting significant amounts of

inorganic nitrate, eg, from well water, to nitrite ion. Thus, inadvertent exposure to large amounts of nitrite ion can occur and may produce serious toxicity.

One therapeutic application of this otherwise toxic effect of nitrite has been discovered. Cyanide poisoning results from complexing of cytochrome iron by the CN⁻ ion. Methemoglobin iron has a very high affinity for CN⁻; thus, administration of sodium nitrite ($NaNO_2$) soon after cyanide exposure will regenerate active cytochrome. The cyanmethemoglobin produced can be further detoxified by the intravenous administration of sodium thiosulfate ($Na_2S_2O_3$); this results in formation of thiocyanate ion (SCN⁻), a less toxic ion that is readily excreted. Methemoglobinemia, if excessive, can be treated by giving methylene blue intravenously.

Toxicity & Tolerance

A. ACUTE ADVERSE EFFECTS

The major acute toxicities of organic nitrates are direct extensions of therapeutic vasodilation: orthostatic hypotension, tachycardia, and throbbing headache. Glaucoma, once thought to be a contraindication, does not worsen, and nitrates can be used safely in the presence of increased intraocular pressure. Nitrates are contraindicated, however, if intracranial pressure is elevated.

DRUGS USED IN THE TREATMENT OF ERECTILE DYSFUNCTION

Erectile dysfunction in men has long been the subject of research (by both amateur and professional scientists). Among the substances used in the past and generally discredited are "Spanish Fly" (a bladder and urethral irritant), yohimbine (an α_2 antagonist; see Chapter 10), nutmeg, and mixtures containing lead, arsenic, or strychnine. Substances currently favored by practitioners of herbal medicine include ginseng and kava.

Scientific studies of the process have shown that erection requires *relaxation* of the nonvascular smooth muscle of the corpora cavernosa. This relaxation permits inflow of blood at nearly arterial pressure into the sinuses of the cavernosa, and it is the pressure of the blood that causes erection. Physiologic erection occurs in response to the release of nitric oxide from nonadrenergic-noncholinergic nerves (see Chapter 6) associated with parasympathetic discharge. Thus, parasympathetic innervation must be intact and nitric oxide synthesis must be active. (It appears that a similar process occurs in female erectile tissues.) Certain other smooth muscle relaxants—eg, PGE_1 analogs or α antagonists—if present in high enough concentration, can independently cause sufficient cavernosal relaxation to result in erection. As noted in the text, nitric oxide activates guanylyl cyclase, which increases the concentration of cGMP, and the latter messenger stimulates the dephos-phorylation of myosin light chains (see Figure 12–2) and relaxation of the smooth muscle. Thus, any drug that increases cGMP might be of value in erectile dysfunction if normal innervation is present. **Sildenafil** (Viagra) acts to increase cGMP by inhibiting its breakdown by phosphodiesterase isoform 5. The drug has been very successful in the marketplace because it can be taken orally. However, sildenafil is of little or no value in men with loss of potency due to cord injury or other damage to innervation and in men lacking libido. Furthermore, sildenafil potentiates the action of nitrates used for angina, and severe hypotension and a few myocardial infarctions have been reported in men taking both drugs. It is recommended that at least 6 hours pass between use of a nitrate and the ingestion of sildenafil. Sildenafil also has effects on color vision, causing difficulty in blue-green discrimination. Two similar PDE-5 inhibitors, **tadalafil** and **vardenafil,** are available.

The drug most commonly used in patients who do not respond to sildenafil is **alprostadil,** a PGE_1 analog (see Chapter 18) that can be injected directly into the cavernosa or placed in the urethra as a minisuppository, from which it diffuses into the cavernosal tissue. Phentolamine can be used by injection into the cavernosa. These drugs will cause erection in most men who do not respond to sildenafil.

B. TOLERANCE

With continuous exposure to nitrates, isolated smooth muscle may develop complete tolerance (tachyphylaxis), and the intact human becomes progressively more tolerant when long-acting preparations (oral, transdermal) or continuous intravenous infusions are used for more than a few hours without interruption.

Continuous exposure to high levels of nitrates can occur in the chemical industry, especially where explosives are manufactured. When contamination of the workplace with volatile organic nitrate compounds is severe, workers find that upon starting their work week (Monday), they suffer headache and transient dizziness. After a day or so, these symptoms disappear owing to the development of tolerance. Over the weekend, when exposure to the chemicals is reduced, tolerance disappears, so symptoms recur each Monday. Other hazards of industrial exposure, including dependence, have been reported. There is no evidence that physical dependence develops as a result of the therapeutic use of short-acting nitrates for angina, even in large doses.

The mechanisms by which tolerance develops are not completely understood. As noted above, dimin-ished release of nitric oxide resulting from depletion of tissue thiol compounds may be partly responsible for tolerance to nitroglycerin. Systemic compensation also plays a role in tolerance in the intact human. Initially, significant sympathetic discharge occurs and after one or more days of therapy with long-acting nitrates, retention of salt and water may reverse the favorable hemodynamic changes normally caused by nitroglycerin.

C. CARCINOGENICITY OF NITRATE AND NITRATE DERIVATIVES

Nitrosamines are small molecules with the structure R_2–N–NO formed from the combination of nitrates and nitrites with amines. Some nitrosamines are powerful carcinogens in animals, apparently through conversion to reactive derivatives. While there is no direct proof that these agents cause cancer in humans, there is a strong epidemiologic correlation between the incidence of esophageal and gastric carcinoma and the nitrate content of food in different cultures. Nitrosamines are also found in tobacco and in cigarette smoke. There is no evidence that the small doses of nitrates used in the treatment of angina result in significant body levels of nitrosamines.

Mechanisms of Clinical Effect

The beneficial and deleterious effects of nitrate-induced vasodilation are summarized in Table 12–2.

A. NITRATE EFFECTS IN ANGINA OF EFFORT

Decreased venous return to the heart and the resulting reduction of intracardiac volume are the principal hemodynamic effects. Arterial pressure also decreases. Decreased intraventricular pressure and left ventricular volume are associated with decreased wall tension (Laplace relation) and decreased myocardial oxygen requirement. In rare instances, a paradoxical increase in myocardial oxygen demand may occur as a result of excessive reflex tachycardia and increased contractility.

Intracoronary, intravenous, or sublingual nitrate administration consistently increases the caliber of the large epicardial coronary arteries. Coronary arteriolar resistance tends to decrease, although to a lesser extent. However, nitrates administered by the usual systemic routes also consistently *decrease* overall coronary blood flow and myocardial oxygen consumption. The reduction in oxygen consumption is the major mechanism for the relief of effort angina.

B. NITRATE EFFECTS IN VARIANT ANGINA

Nitrates benefit patients with variant angina by relaxing the smooth muscle of the epicardial coronary arteries and relieving coronary artery spasm.

C. NITRATE EFFECTS IN UNSTABLE ANGINA

Nitrates are also useful in the treatment of this acute coronary syndrome, but the precise mechanism for their beneficial effects is not clear. Because both increased coronary vascular tone and increased myocardial oxygen demand can precipitate rest angina in these patients, nitrates may exert their beneficial effects both by dilating the epicardial coronary arteries and by simultaneously reducing myocardial oxygen demand. As noted above, nitroglycerin also decreases platelet aggregation, and this effect may be of importance in unstable angina.

Clinical Use of Nitrates

Some of the forms of nitroglycerin and its congeners are listed in Table 12–3. Because of its rapid onset of action (1–3 minutes), sublingual nitroglycerin is the most frequently used agent for the immediate treatment of angina. Because its duration of action is short (not exceeding 20–30 minutes), it is not suitable for maintenance therapy. The onset of action of intravenous nitroglycerin is also rapid (minutes), but its hemodynamic

Table 12–2. Beneficial and deleterious effects of nitrates in the treatment of angina.

Effect	Result
Potential beneficial effects	
Decreased ventricular volume	Decreased myocardial oxygen requirement
Decreased arterial pressure	
Decreased ejection time	
Vasodilation of epicardial coronary arteries	Relief of coronary artery spasm
Increased collateral flow	Improved perfusion to ischemic myocardium
Decreased left ventricular diastolic pressure	Improved subendocardial perfusion
Potential deleterious effects	
Reflex tachycardia	Increased myocardial oxygen requirement
Reflex increase in contractility	
Decreased diastolic perfusion time due to tachycardia	Decreased coronary perfusion

effects are quickly reversed by stopping its infusion. Clinical application of intravenous nitroglycerin, therefore, is restricted to the treatment of severe, recurrent rest angina. Slowly absorbed preparations of nitroglycerin include a buccal form, oral preparations, and several transdermal forms. These formulations have been shown to provide blood concentrations for long periods but, as noted above, this leads to the development of tolerance.

The hemodynamic effects of sublingual or chewable isosorbide dinitrate and other organic nitrates are similar to those of nitroglycerin. The recommended dosage schedules for commonly used long-acting nitrate preparations, along with their durations of action, are listed in Table 12–3. Although transdermal administration may provide blood levels of nitroglycerin for 24 hours or longer, the full hemodynamic effects usually do not persist for more than 6–8 hours. The clinical efficacy of slow-release forms of nitroglycerin in maintenance therapy of angina is thus limited by the development of significant tolerance. Therefore, a nitrate-free period of at least 8 hours between doses should be observed to reduce or prevent tolerance.

OTHER NITRO-VASODILATORS

Nicorandil is a nicotinamide nitrate ester that has vasodilating properties in normal coronary arteries but more complex effects in patients with angina. Clinical

Table 12–3. Nitrate and nitrite drugs used in the treatment of angina.

Drug	Dose	Duration of Action
"Short-acting"		
Nitroglycerin, sublingual	0.15–1.2 mg	10–30 minutes
Isosorbide dinitrate, sublingual	2.5–5 mg	10–60 minutes
Amyl nitrite, inhalant	0.18–0.3 mL	3–5 minutes
"Long-acting"		
Nitroglycerin, oral sustained-action	6.5–13 mg per 6–8 hours	6–8 hours
Nitroglycerin, 2% ointment, transdermal	1–1.5 inches per 4 hours	3–6 hours
Nitroglycerin, slow-release, buccal	1–2 mg per 4 hours	3–6 hours
Nitroglycerin, slow-release patch, transdermal	10–25 mg per 24 hours (one patch per day)	8–10 hours
Isosorbide dinitrate, sublingual	2.5–10 mg per 2 hours	1.5–2 hours
Isosorbide dinitrate, oral	10–60 mg per 4–6 hours	4–6 hours
Isosorbide dinitrate, chewable oral	5–10 mg per 2–4 hours	2–3 hours
Isosorbide mononitrate, oral	20 mg per 12 hours	6–10 hours

studies suggest that it reduces both preload and afterload. It also provides some myocardial protection via preconditioning by activation of cardiac K_{ATP} channels. One large trial showed a significant reduction in relative risk of fatal and nonfatal coronary events in patients receiving the drug. Nicorandil is currently approved for use in the treatment of angina in Europe and Japan and has been submitted for approval in the USA.

CALCIUM CHANNEL-BLOCKING DRUGS

It has been known since the late 1800s that calcium influx was necessary for the contraction of smooth and cardiac muscle. The discovery of a calcium channel in cardiac muscle was followed by the finding of several different types of calcium channels in different tissues (Table 12–4). The discovery of these channels made possible the development of clinically useful blocking drugs. Although the successful therapeutic blockers developed to date have been exclusively L-type channel blockers, selective blockers of other types of calcium channels are under intensive investigation.

Chemistry & Pharmacokinetics

Verapamil, the first clinically useful member of this group, was the result of attempts to synthesize more active analogs of papaverine, a vasodilator alkaloid

Table 12–4. Properties of several recognized voltage-activated calcium channels.

Type	Channel Name	Where Found	Properties of the Calcium Current	Blocked By
L	CaV1.1–CaV1.3	Muscle, neurons (CaV1.4 is found in retina)	Long, large, high threshold	Verapamil, DHPs, Cd^{2+}
T	CaV3.1–CaV3.3	Heart, neurons	Short, small, low threshold	sFTX, flunarizine, Ni^{2+}
N	CaV2.2	Neurons	Short, high threshold	ω-CTX-GVIA, Cd^{2+}
P/Q	CaV2.1	Cerebellar Purkinje neurons	Long, high threshold	ω-CTX-MVIIC, ω-Aga-IVA
R	CaV2.3	Neurons	Pacemaking	SNX-482

DHPs, dihydropyridines (eg, nifedipine); sFTX, synthetic funnel web spider toxin; ω-CTX, conotoxins extracted from several marine snails of the genus *Conus;* ω-Aga-IVA, a toxin of the funnel web spider, *Agelenopsis aperta*; SNX-482, a toxin of the African tarantula, *Hysterocrates gigas.*

Table 12–5. Clinical pharmacology of some calcium channel-blocking drugs.

Drug	Oral Bioavailability (%)	Half-Life (hours)	Indication	Dosage
Dihydropyridines				
Amlodipine	65–90	30–50	Angina, hypertension	5–10 mg orally once daily
Felodipine	15–20	11–16	Hypertension, Raynaud's phenomenon	5–10 mg orally once daily
Isradipine	15–25	8	Hypertension	2.5–10 mg orally twice daily
Nicardipine	35	2–4	Angina, hypertension	20–40 mg orally every 8 hours
Nifedipine	45–70	4	Angina, hypertension, Raynaud's phenomenon	3–10 mcg/kg IV; 20–40 mg orally every 8 hours
Nimodipine	13	1–2	Subarachnoid hemorrhage	40 mg orally every 4 hours
Nisoldipine	< 10	6–12	Hypertension	20–40 mg orally once daily
Nitrendipine	10–30	5–12	Investigational	20 mg orally once or twice daily
Miscellaneous				
Diltiazem	40–65	3–4	Angina, hypertension, Raynaud's phenomenon	75–150 mcg/kg IV; 30–80 mg orally every 6 hours
Verapamil	20–35	6	Angina, hypertension, arrhythmias, migraine	75–150 mcg/kg IV; 80–160 mg orally every 8 hours

found in the opium poppy. Since then, dozens of agents of varying structure have been found to have the same fundamental pharmacologic action (Table 12–5). Three chemically dissimilar calcium channel blockers are shown in Figure 12–4. Nifedipine is the prototype of the dihydropyridine family of calcium channel blockers; dozens of molecules in this family have been investigated, and seven are currently approved in the USA for angina and other indications. Nifedipine is the most extensively studied of this group, but the properties of the other dihydropyridines can be assumed to be similar to it unless otherwise noted.

The calcium channel blockers are orally active agents and are characterized by high first-pass effect, high plasma protein binding, and extensive metabolism. Verapamil and diltiazem are also used by the intravenous route.

Pharmacodynamics

A. MECHANISM OF ACTION

The L-type calcium channel is the dominant type in cardiac and smooth muscle and is known to contain several drug receptors. It has been demonstrated that nifedipine and other dihydropyridines bind to one site, while verapamil and diltiazem appear to bind to closely related but not identical receptors in another region. Binding of a drug to the verapamil or diltiazem receptors also affects dihydropyridine binding. These receptor regions are stereoselective, since marked differences in both stereoisomer-binding affinity and pharmacologic potency are observed for enantiomers of verapamil, diltiazem, and optically active nifedipine congeners.

Blockade by these drugs resembles that of sodium channel blockade by local anesthetics (see Chapters 14 and 26). The drugs act from the inner side of the membrane and bind more effectively to channels in depolarized membranes. Binding of the drug reduces the frequency of opening in response to depolarization. The result is a marked decrease in transmembrane calcium current, resulting in smooth muscle with a long-lasting relaxation (Figure 12–3), and in cardiac muscle with a reduction in contractility throughout the heart and decreases in sinus node pacemaker rate and in atrioventricular node conduction velocity.*

Smooth muscle responses to calcium influx through *receptor*-operated calcium channels are also reduced by these drugs but not as markedly. The block can be partially reversed by elevating the concentration of cal-

---

*At very low doses and under certain circumstances, some dihydropyridines *increase* calcium influx. Some special dihydropyridines, eg, Bay K 8644, actually increase calcium influx over most of their dose range.

Figure 12–4. Chemical structures of several calcium channel-blocking drugs.

cium, although the levels of calcium required are not easily attainable. Block can also be partially reversed by the use of drugs that increase the transmembrane flux of calcium, such as sympathomimetics.

Other types of calcium channels are less sensitive to blockade by these calcium channel blockers (Table 12–4). Therefore, tissues in which these other channel types play a major role—neurons and most secretory glands—are much less affected by these drugs than are cardiac and smooth muscle.

B. Organ System Effects

1. Smooth muscle—Most types of smooth muscle are dependent on transmembrane calcium influx for normal resting tone and contractile responses. These cells are relaxed by the calcium channel blockers (Figure 12–3). Vascular smooth muscle appears to be the most sensitive, but similar relaxation can be shown for bronchiolar, gastrointestinal, and uterine smooth muscle. In the vascular system, arterioles appear to be more sensitive than veins; orthostatic hypotension is not a common adverse effect. Blood pressure is reduced with all calcium channel blockers. Women may be more sensitive than men to the hypotensive action of diltiazem. The reduction in peripheral vascular resistance is one mechanism by which these agents may benefit the patient with angina of effort. Reduction of coronary arterial tone has been demonstrated in patients with variant angina.

Important differences in vascular selectivity exist among the calcium channel blockers. In general, the dihydropyridines have a greater ratio of vascular smooth muscle effects relative to cardiac effects than do diltiazem and verapamil. Furthermore, the dihydropyridines may differ in their potency in different vascular beds. For example, nimodipine is claimed to be particularly selective for cerebral blood vessels.

2. Cardiac muscle—Cardiac muscle is highly dependent upon calcium influx for normal function. Impulse generation in the sinoatrial node and conduction in the atrioventricular node—so-called slow response, or calcium-dependent, action potentials—may be reduced or blocked by all of the calcium channel blockers. Excitation-contraction coupling in all cardiac cells requires calcium influx, so these drugs reduce cardiac contractility in a dose-dependent fashion. In some cases, cardiac output may also decrease. This reduction in cardiac mechanical function is another mechanism by which the calcium channel blockers can reduce the oxygen requirement in patients with angina.

Important differences between the available calcium channel blockers arise from the details of their interactions with cardiac ion channels and, as noted above, differences in their relative smooth muscle versus cardiac effects. Sodium channel block is modest with verapamil and still less marked with diltiazem. It is negligible with nifedipine and other dihydropyridines. Verapamil and diltiazem interact kinetically with the calcium channel receptor in a different manner than the dihydropyridines; they block tachycardias in calcium-dependent cells, eg, the atrioventricular node, more selectively than do the dihydropyridines. (See Chapter 14 for additional details.) On the other hand, the dihydropyridines appear to block smooth muscle calcium channels at concentrations below those required for significant cardiac effects; they are therefore less depressant on the heart than verapamil or diltiazem.

3. Skeletal muscle—Skeletal muscle is not depressed by the calcium channel blockers because it uses intracellular pools of calcium to support excitation-contraction coupling and does not require as much transmembrane calcium influx.

4. Cerebral vasospasm and infarct following subarachnoid hemorrhage—Nimodipine, a member of the dihydropyridine group of calcium channel blockers, has a high affinity for cerebral blood vessels and appears to reduce morbidity following a subarachnoid hemorrhage. Nimodipine is therefore labeled for use in patients who have had a hemorrhagic stroke. Although evidence suggests that calcium channel blockers may also reduce cerebral damage following thromboembolic stroke in experimental animals, there is no evidence that this occurs in humans.

5. Other effects—Calcium channel blockers minimally interfere with stimulus-secretion coupling in glands and nerve endings because of differences between calcium channels in different tissues, as noted above. Verapamil has been shown to inhibit insulin release in humans, but the dosages required are greater than those used in management of angina.

A significant body of evidence suggests that the calcium channel blockers may interfere with platelet aggregation in vitro and prevent or attenuate the development of atheromatous lesions in animals. Clinical studies have not established their role in human blood clotting and atherosclerosis.

Verapamil has been shown to block the P-glycoprotein responsible for the transport of many foreign drugs out of cancer (and other) cells; other calcium channel blockers appear to have a similar effect. This action is not stereospecific. Verapamil has been shown to partially reverse the resistance of cancer cells to many chemotherapeutic drugs in vitro. Some clinical results suggest similar effects in patients (see Chapter 55).

Toxicity

The most important toxic effects reported for the calcium channel blockers are direct extensions of their therapeutic action. Excessive inhibition of calcium influx can cause serious cardiac depression, including cardiac arrest, bradycardia, atrioventricular block, and heart failure. These effects have been rare in clinical use.

Retrospective case control studies reported that immediate-acting nifedipine increased the risk of myocardial infarction in patients with hypertension. Slow-release and long-acting vasoselective calcium channel blockers are usually well tolerated. However, dihydropyridines, compared with angiotensin-converting enzyme inhibitors, have been reported to increase the risk of adverse cardiac events in patients with hypertension with or without diabetes. These results suggest that relatively short-acting calcium channel blockers have the potential to enhance the risk of adverse cardiac events and should be avoided. Patients receiving β-adrenoceptor-blocking drugs are more sensitive to the cardiodepressant effects of calcium channel blockers. Minor toxicity (troublesome but not usually requiring discontinuance of therapy) includes flushing, dizziness, nausea, constipation, and peripheral edema.

Mechanisms of Clinical Effects

Calcium channel blockers decrease myocardial contractile force, which reduces myocardial oxygen requirements. Inhibition of calcium entry into arterial smooth muscle is associated with decreased arteriolar tone and systemic vascular resistance, resulting in decreased arterial and intraventricular pressure. Some of these drugs (eg, verapamil, diltiazem) also possess a nonspecific antiadrenergic effect, which may contribute to peripheral vasodilation. As a result of all of these effects, left ventricular wall stress declines, which reduces myocardial oxygen requirements. Decreased heart rate with the use of verapamil or diltiazem causes a further decrease in myocardial oxygen demand. Calcium channel-blocking agents also relieve and prevent the primary cause of variant angina—focal coronary artery spasm. Use of these agents has thus emerged as the most effective prophylactic treatment for this form of angina pectoris.

Sinoatrial and atrioventricular nodal tissues, which are mainly composed of calcium-dependent, slow response cells, are affected markedly by verapamil, moderately by diltiazem, and much less by dihydropyridines. Thus, verapamil and diltiazem decrease atrioventricular nodal conduction and are effective in the management of supraventricular reentry tachycardia and in decreasing ventricular responses in atrial fibrillation or flutter. Nifedipine does not affect atrioventricular conduction. Nonspecific sympathetic antagonism is most marked with diltiazem and much less with verapamil. Nifedipine does not appear to have this effect. Thus, significant reflex tachycardia in response to hypotension occurs most frequently with nifedipine and less so with diltiazem and verapamil. These differences in pharmacologic effects should be considered in selecting calcium channel-blocking agents for the management of angina.

Clinical Uses of Calcium Channel–Blocking Drugs

In addition to angina, calcium channel blockers have well-documented efficacy in hypertension (see Chapter

11) and supraventricular tachyarrhythmias (see Chapter 14). They also show promise in a variety of other conditions, including hypertrophic cardiomyopathy, migraine, and Raynaud's phenomenon.

The pharmacokinetic properties of these drugs are set forth in Table 12–5. The choice of a particular calcium channel-blocking agent should be made with knowledge of its specific potential adverse effects as well as its pharmacologic properties. Nifedipine does not decrease atrioventricular conduction and therefore can be used more safely than verapamil or diltiazem in the presence of atrioventricular conduction abnormalities. A combination of verapamil or diltiazem with β blockers may produce atrioventricular block and depression of ventricular function. In the presence of overt heart failure, all calcium channel blockers can cause further worsening of heart failure as a result of their negative inotropic effect. Amlodipine, however, does not increase the mortality of patients with heart failure due to left ventricular systolic dysfunction and can be used safely in these patients. In the presence of relatively low blood pressure, dihydropyridines can cause further deleterious lowering of pressure. Verapamil and diltiazem appear to produce less hypotension and may be better tolerated in these circumstances. In patients with a history of atrial tachycardia, flutter, and fibrillation, verapamil and diltiazem provide a distinct advantage because of their antiarrhythmic effects. In the patient receiving digitalis, verapamil should be used with caution, because it may increase digoxin blood levels through a pharmacokinetic interaction. Although increases in digoxin blood level have also been demonstrated with diltiazem and nifedipine, such interactions are less consistent than with verapamil.

In patients with unstable angina, immediate-release short-acting calcium channel blockers can increase the risk of adverse cardiac events and therefore are contraindicated (see Toxicity, above). However, in patients with non-Q-wave myocardial infarction, diltiazem can decrease the frequency of postinfarction angina and may be used.

BETA-ADRENORECEPTOR–BLOCKING DRUGS

Although they are not vasodilators, β-blocking drugs (see Chapter 10) are extremely useful in the management of angina pectoris associated with effort. The beneficial effects of β-blocking agents are related primarily to their hemodynamic effects—decreased heart rate, blood pressure, and contractility—which decrease myocardial oxygen requirements at rest and during exercise. Lower heart rate is also associated with an increase in diastolic perfusion time that may increase coronary perfusion. However, reduction of heart rate and blood pressure and consequently decreased myocardial oxygen consumption appear to be the most important mechanisms for relief of angina and improved exercise tolerance. Beta blockers may also be valuable in treating silent or ambulatory ischemia. Because this condition causes no pain, it is usually detected by the appearance of typical electrocardiographic signs of ischemia. The total amount of "ischemic time" per day is reduced by long-term therapy with a β blocker. Beta-blocking agents decrease mortality of patients with recent myocardial infarction and improve survival and prevent stroke in patients with hypertension. Randomized trials in patients with stable angina have shown better outcome and symptomatic improvement with β blockers compared with calcium channel blockers.

Undesirable effects of β-blocking agents in angina include an increase in end-diastolic volume and an increase in ejection time. Increased myocardial oxygen requirements associated with increased diastolic volume partially offset the beneficial effects of β-blocking agents. These potentially deleterious effects of β-blocking agents can be balanced by the concomitant use of nitrates as described below.

The contraindications to the use of β blockers are asthma and other bronchospastic conditions, severe bradycardia, atrioventricular blockade, bradycardia-tachycardia syndrome, and severe unstable left ventricular failure. Potential complications include fatigue, impaired exercise tolerance, insomnia, unpleasant dreams, worsening of claudication, and erectile dysfunction.

NEWER ANTIANGINAL DRUGS

Because of the high incidence of angina, new drugs are actively sought for its treatment. Some of the drugs or drug groups currently under investigation are listed in Table 12–6.

The metabolic modulators (eg, **ranolazine,** trimetazidine) are known as **pFOX inhibitors** because they partially inhibit the fatty acid oxidation pathway

Table 12–6. Drugs or drug groups under investigation for use in angina.

Metabolic modulators, eg, ranolazine
Direct bradycardic agents, eg, ivabradine
Potassium channel activators, eg, nicorandil
Rho-kinase inhibitors, eg, fasudil
Sulfonylureas, eg, glibenclamide
Thiazolidinediones
Vasopeptidase inhibitors
Nitric oxide donors, eg, L-arginine
Capsaicin
Amiloride

in myocardium. Because metabolism shifts to oxidation of fatty acids in ischemic myocardium, the oxygen requirement per unit of ATP produced increases. Partial inhibition of the enzyme required for fatty acid oxidation (long chain 3-ketoacyl thiolase, LC-3KAT) appears to improve the metabolic status of ischemic tissue. However, blockade of a late sodium current that facilitates calcium entry may play a larger role in the action of ranolazine.

So-called bradycardic drugs, relatively selective I_f sodium channel blockers (eg, **ivabradine**), reduce cardiac rate by inhibiting the hyperpolarization-activated sodium channel in the sinoatrial node. No other significant hemodynamic effects have been reported. Ivabradine appears to reduce anginal attacks with an efficacy similar to that of calcium channel blockers and blockers.

Figure 12–5. Effects of diltiazem on the double product (heart rate times systolic blood pressure) in a group of 20 patients with angina of effort. In a double-blind study using a standard protocol, patients were tested on a treadmill during treatment with placebo and three doses of the drug. Heart rate (HR) and systolic blood pressure (BP) were recorded at 180 seconds of exercise (midpoints of lines) and at the time of onset of anginal symptoms (rightmost points). Note that the drug treatment decreased the double product at all times during exercise and prolonged the time to appearance of symptoms. (Data from Lindenberg BS et al: Efficacy and safety of incremental doses of diltiazem for the treatment of angina. J Am Coll Cardiol 1983;2:1129. Used with permission of the American College of Cardiology.)

■ II. CLINICAL PHARMACOLOGY OF DRUGS USED TO TREAT ANGINA

Because the most common cause of angina is atheroclerotic disease of the coronaries (CAD), therapy must address the underlying causes of CAD as well as the immediate symptoms of angina. In addition to reducing the need for antianginal therapy, such primary management has been shown to reduce major cardiac events such as myocardial infarction.

First-line therapy of CAD depends on modification of risk factors such as smoking, hypertension (Chapter 11), hyperlipidemia (Chapter 35), obesity, and clinical depression. In addition, antiplatelet drugs (Chapter 34) are very important.

Specific pharmacologic therapy to prevent myocardial infarction and death consists of antiplatelet agents (aspirin, clopidogrel) and lipid-lowering agents, especially statins. Aggressive therapy with statins has been shown to reduce the incidence and severity of ischemia in patients during exercise testing and the incidence of cardiac events (including infarction and death) in clinical trials. Angiotensin-converting enzyme inhibitors also reduce the risk of adverse cardiac events in patients at high risk for CAD although they have not been consistently shown to exert antianginal effects. In patients with unstable angina and non-ST-segment elevation myocardial infarction, aggressive therapy consisting of coronary stenting, antilipid drugs, heparin, and antiplatelet agents is recommended.

The treatment of established angina and other manifestations of myocardial ischemia includes the corrective measures described above as well as treatment to prevent or relieve symptoms. Treatment of symptoms is based on reduction of myocardial oxygen demand and increase of coronary blood flow to the potentially ischemic myocardium to restore the balance between myocardial oxygen supply and demand.

Angina of Effort

Many studies have demonstrated that nitrates, calcium channel blockers, and β blockers increase time to onset of angina and ST depression during treadmill tests in patients with angina of effort (Figure 12–5). Although exercise tolerance increases, there is usually no change in the angina threshold, ie, the rate-pressure product at which symptoms occur.

For maintenance therapy of chronic stable angina, long-acting nitrates, calcium channel-blocking agents, or β blockers may be chosen; the best choice of drug will depend on the individual patient's response. In hypertensive patients, monotherapy with either slow-release or long-acting calcium channel blockers or β blockers may be adequate. In normotensive patients, long-acting nitrates may be suitable. The combination

Table 12–7. Effects of nitrates alone and with β blockers or calcium channel blockers in angina pectoris. (Undesirable effects are shown in italics.)

	Nitrates Alone	Beta Blockers or Calcium Channel Blockers	Combined Nitrates with Beta Blockers or Calcium Channel Blockers
Heart rate	*Reflex[1] increase*	Decrease	Decrease
Arterial pressure	Decrease	Decrease	Decrease
End-diastolic volume	Decrease	*Increase*	None or decrease
Contractility	*Reflex[1] increase*	Decrease	None
Ejection time	Decrease[1]	*Increase*	None

[1]Baroreceptor reflex.

of a β blocker with a calcium channel blocker (eg, propranolol with nifedipine) or two different calcium channel blockers (eg, nifedipine and verapamil) has been shown to be more effective than individual drugs used alone. If response to a single drug is inadequate, a drug from a different class should be added to maximize the beneficial reduction of cardiac work while minimizing undesirable effects (Table 12–7). Some patients may require therapy with all three drug groups.

Surgical revascularization (ie, coronary artery bypass grafting [CABG]) and catheter-based revascularization (ie, percutaneous coronary intervention [PCI]) are the primary methods for promptly restoring coronary blood flow and increasing oxygen supply to the myocardium.

Vasospastic Angina

Nitrates and the calcium channel blockers are effective drugs for relieving and preventing ischemic episodes in patients with variant angina. In approximately 70% of patients treated with nitrates plus calcium channel blockers, angina attacks are completely abolished; in another 20%, marked reduction of frequency of anginal episodes is observed. Prevention of coronary artery spasm (in the presence or absence of fixed atheroscle-

rotic coronary artery lesions) is the principal mechanism for this beneficial response. All presently available calcium channel blockers appear to be equally effective, and the choice of a particular drug should depend on the patient, as indicated above. Surgical revascularization and angioplasty are not indicated in patients with variant angina.

Unstable Angina & Acute Coronary Syndromes

In patients with unstable angina with recurrent ischemic episodes at rest, recurrent platelet-rich nonocclusive thrombus formation is the principal mechanism. Aggressive antiplatelet therapy with a combination of aspirin and clopidigrel is indicated. Intravenous heparin or subcutaneous low-molecular-weight heparin is also indicated in most patients. If PCI with stenting is required, glycoprotein IIb/IIIa inhibitors such as abciximab should be added. In addition, therapy with nitroglycerin and β blockers should be considered; calcium channel blockers should be added in refractory cases for relief of myocardial ischemia. Primary lipid-lowering and ACE-inhibitor therapy should also be initiated.

PREPARATIONS AVAILABLE

NITRATES & NITRITES

Amyl nitrite (generic)
Inhalant: 0.3 mL capsules

Isosorbide dinitrate (generic, Isordil)
Oral: 5, 10, 20, 30, 40 mg tablets; 5, 10 mg chewable tablets
Oral sustained-release (Isochron, Dilatrate SR): 40 mg tablets and capsules
Sublingual: 2.5, 5 mg sublingual tablets

Isosorbide mononitrate (Ismo, others)
Oral: 10, 20 mg tablets; extended-release 30, 60, 120 mg tablets

Nitroglycerin
Sublingual or buccal: 0.3, 0.4, 0.6 mg tablets; 0.4 mg/metered dose aerosol spray
Oral sustained-release (generic, Nitro-Time): 2.5, 6.5, 9 mg capsules
Parenteral (generic): 5 mg/mL for IV administration; 100, 200, 400 mcg/mL in dextrose for IV infusion
Transdermal patches (generic, Nitrek, Nitro-Dur, Transderm-Nitro): to release at rates of 0.1, 0.2, 0.3, 0.4, 0.6, or 0.8 mg/h
Topical ointment (generic, Nitro-Bid): 20 mg/mL ointment (1 inch, or 25 mm, of ointment contains about 15 mg nitroglycerin)

CALCIUM CHANNEL BLOCKERS

Amlodipine (Norvasc, Amvaz)
Oral: 2.5, 5, 10 mg tablets

Diltiazem (Cardizem, generic)
Oral: 30, 60, 90, 120 mg tablets
Oral sustained-release (Cardizem SR, Dilacor XL, others): 60, 90, 120, 180, 240, 300, 360, 420 mg capsules, tablets
Parenteral: 5 mg/mL for injection

Felodipine (Plendil)
Oral extended-release: 2.5, 5, 10 mg tablets

Isradipine (DynaCirc)
Oral: 2.5, 5 mg capsules
Oral controlled-release: 5, 10 mg tablets

Nicardipine (Cardene, others)
Oral: 20, 30 mg capsules
Oral sustained-release (Cardene SR): 30, 45, 60 mg capsules)
Parenteral (Cardene I.V.): 2.5 mg/mL

Nifedipine (Adalat, Procardia, others)
Oral: 10, 20 mg capsules
Oral extended-release (Procardia XL, Adalat CC): 30, 60, 90 mg tablets

Nimodipine (Nimotop)
Oral: 30 mg capsules. (Labeled for use in subarachnoid hemorrhage, not angina.)

Nisoldipine (Sular)
Oral extended-release: 10, 20, 30, 40 mg tablets

Verapamil (generic, Calan, Isoptin)
Oral: 40, 80, 120 mg tablets
Oral sustained-release: 100, 120, 180, 240 mg tablets or capsules
Parenteral: 2.5 mg/mL for injection

BETA BLOCKERS

See Chapter 10.

METABOLISM MODIFIERS

Ranolazine (Ranexa)
Oral: 500 mg extended-release tablets

REFERENCES

Belardinelli L, Shyrock JC, Fraser H: Inhibition of the late sodium current as a potential cardioprotective principle. Heart 2006; 92(Suppl 4):iv6.

Borer JS et al: Antianginal and antiischemic effects of ivabradine, an I(f) inhibitor, in stable angina: A randomized, double-blind, multicentered, placebo-controlled trial. Circulation 2003;107:817.

Braunwald E et al: ACC/AHA Guideline update for the management of patients with unstable angina and non-ST-segment elevation myocardial infarction—2002. Circulation 2002; 106:1893.

Carmichael P, Lieben J: Sudden death in explosives workers. Arch Environ Health 1963;7:50.

Chaitman BR: Efficacy and safety of a metabolic modulator drug in chronic stable angina: Review of evidence from clinical trials. J Cardiovasc Pharmacol Ther 2004;9(Suppl 1):S47.

Chaitman BR: Ranolazine for the treatment of chronic angina and potential use in other cardiovascular conditions. Circulation 2006;113:2462.

Chatterjee K: Ischemic heart disease. In: Stein JH (editor). *Internal Medicine*, 5th ed. Little, Brown, 1998.

DeWitt CR, Waksman JC: Pharmacology, pathophysiology and management of calcium channel blocker and beta-blocker toxicity. Toxicol Rev 2004;23:223.

Gibbons RJ et al: ACC/AHA 2002 guideline update for the management of patients with chronic stable angina—summary article: A report of the American College of Cardiology/American Heart Association Task Force on practice guidelines (Committee on the Management of Patients With Chronic Stable Angina). J Am Coll Cardiol 2003;41:159.

Lacinova L: Voltage-dependent calcium channels. Gen Physiol Biophys 2005;24(Suppl 1):1.

LaPorte R, Hui A, Laher I: Pharmacological modulation of sarcoplasmic reticulum function in smooth muscle. Pharmacol Rev 2004;56:439.

Drugs Used in Heart Failure

13

Bertram G. Katzung, MD, PhD, & William W. Parmley, MD

Heart failure occurs when cardiac output is inadequate to provide the oxygen needed by the body. It is a highly lethal condition, with a 5-year mortality rate conventionally said to be about 50%. The most common cause of heart failure in the USA is coronary artery disease. Two major types of failure may be distinguished. In **systolic failure,** the mechanical pumping action (contractility) and the ejection fraction of the heart are reduced. In **diastolic failure** stiffening and loss of adequate relaxation plays a major role in reducing cardiac output and ejection fraction may be normal. Because other cardiovascular conditions are now being treated more effectively (especially myocardial infarction), more patients are surviving long enough for heart failure to develop, making this one of the cardiovascular conditions that is actually increasing in prevalence.

Although it is believed that the primary defect in early heart failure resides in the excitation-contraction coupling machinery of the heart, the clinical condition also involves many other processes and organs, including the baroreceptor reflex, the sympathetic nervous system, the kidneys, angiotensin II and other peptides, aldosterone, and apoptosis of cardiac cells. Recognition of these factors has resulted in evolution of a variety of treatment strategies (Table 13–1).

Clinical research has shown that therapy directed at noncardiac targets is more valuable in the long-term treatment of heart failure than traditional positive inotropic agents (cardiac glycosides [digitalis]). Careful clinical trials have shown that angiotensin-converting enzyme (ACE) inhibitors, angiotensin receptor blockers, β blockers, aldosterone receptor antagonists, and combined hydralazine-nitrate therapy are the only agents in current use that actually prolong life in patients with chronic heart failure. Positive inotropic drugs, on the other hand, can be very helpful in acute failure. They also reduce symptoms in chronic failure.

Control of Normal Cardiac Contractility

The vigor of contraction of heart muscle is determined by several processes that lead to the movement of actin and myosin filaments in the cardiac sarcomere (Figure 13–1). Ultimately, contraction results from the interaction of *activator* calcium (during systole) with the actin-

troponin-tropomyosin system, thereby releasing the actin-myosin interaction. This calcium is released from the sarcoplasmic reticulum (SR). The amount released depends on the amount stored in the SR and on the amount of *trigger* calcium that enters the cell during the plateau of the action potential.

A. Sensitivity of the Contractile Proteins to Calcium

The determinants of calcium sensitivity, ie, the curve relating the shortening of cardiac myofibrils to the cytoplasmic calcium concentration, are incompletely understood, but several types of drugs can be shown to affect it in vitro. **Levosimendan** is the most recent example of a drug that increases calcium sensitivity (it may also inhibit phosphodiesterase) and reduces symptoms in models of heart failure.

B. The Amount of Calcium Released from the Sarcoplasmic Reticulum

A small rise in free cytoplasmic calcium, brought about by calcium influx during the action potential, triggers the opening of ryanodine-sensitive calcium channels (RyR2) in the membrane of the cardiac SR and the rapid release of a large amount of the ion into the cytoplasm in the vicinity of the actin-troponin-tropomyosin complex. The amount released is proportional to the amount stored in the SR and the amount of trigger calcium that enters the cell through the cell membrane. (Ryanodine is a potent negative inotropic plant alkaloid that interferes with the release of calcium through cardiac SR channels.)

C. The Amount of Calcium Stored in the Sarcoplasmic Reticulum

The SR membrane contains a very efficient calcium uptake transporter, known as the sarcoplasmic endoplasmic reticulum Ca^{2+}-ATPase (SERCA). This pump maintains free cytoplasmic calcium at very low levels during diastole by pumping calcium into the SR. The amount of calcium sequestered in the SR is thus determined, in part, by the amount accessible to this transporter. This in turn is dependent on the balance of calcium influx (primarily through the voltage-gated membrane calcium

Table 13–1. Drug groups commonly used in heart failure.

Diuretics
Aldosterone receptor antagonists
Angiotensin-converting enzyme inhibitors
Angiotensin receptor blockers
Beta blockers
Cardiac glycosides
Vasodilators
Beta agonists, dopamine
Bipyridines
Natriuretic peptide

---

channels) and calcium efflux, the amount removed from the cell (primarily via the sodium-calcium exchanger, a transporter in the cell membrane).

D. THE AMOUNT OF TRIGGER CALCIUM

The amount of trigger calcium that enters the cell depends on the availability of membrane calcium channels (primarily the L type) and the duration of their opening. As described in Chapters 6 and 9, sympathomimetics cause an increase in calcium influx through an action on these channels. Conversely, the calcium channel blockers (see Chapter 12) reduce this influx and depress contractility.

E. ACTIVITY OF THE SODIUM-CALCIUM EXCHANGER

This antiporter uses the sodium gradient to move calcium against its concentration gradient from the cyto-

Figure 13–1. Schematic diagram of a cardiac muscle sarcomere, with sites of action of several drugs that alter contractility (numbered structures). Site *1* is Na⁺/K⁺ ATPase, the sodium pump. Site *2* (NaxC) is the sodium/calcium exchanger. Site *3* is the voltage-gated calcium channel. Site *4* (SERCA) is a calcium transporter that pumps calcium into the sarcoplasmic reticulum (SR). Site *5* (RyR) is a calcium channel in the membrane of the SR that is triggered to release stored calcium by trigger calcium. Site *6* is the actin-troponin-tropomyosin complex at which activator calcium brings about the contractile interaction of actin and myosin.

plasm to the extracellular space. Extracellular concentrations of these ions are much less labile than intracellular concentrations under physiologic conditions. The sodium-calcium exchanger's ability to carry out this transport is thus strongly dependent on the intracellular concentrations of both ions, especially sodium.

F. Intracellular Sodium Concentration and Activity of Na⁺/K⁺ ATPase

Na^+/K^+ ATPase, by removing intracellular sodium, is the major determinant of sodium concentration in the cell. The sodium influx through voltage-gated channels, which occurs as a normal part of almost all cardiac action potentials, is another determinant although the amount of sodium that enters with each action potential is much less than 1% of the total intracellular sodium. As described below, Na^+/K^+ ATPase appears to be the primary target of cardiac glycosides.

Pathophysiology of Heart Failure

Heart failure is a syndrome with multiple causes that may involve the right ventricle, the left ventricle, or both. Cardiac output in heart failure is usually below the normal range. Systolic dysfunction, with reduced cardiac output and significantly reduced ejection fraction (< 45%), is typical of acute failure, especially that resulting from myocardial infarction. Diastolic dysfunction often occurs as a result of hypertrophy and stiffening of the myocardium, and although cardiac output is reduced, ejection fraction may be normal. Heart failure due to diastolic dysfunction does not usually respond optimally to positive inotropic drugs.

Rarely, "high-output" failure may occur. In this condition, the demands of the body are so great that even increased cardiac output is insufficient. High-output failure can result from hyperthyroidism, beriberi, anemia, and arteriovenous shunts. This form of failure responds poorly to the drugs discussed in this chapter and should be treated by correcting the underlying cause.

The primary signs and symptoms of all types of heart failure include tachycardia, decreased exercise tolerance, shortness of breath, peripheral and pulmonary edema, and cardiomegaly. Decreased exercise tolerance with rapid muscular fatigue is the major direct consequence of diminished cardiac output. The other manifestations result from the attempts by the body to compensate for the intrinsic cardiac defect.

Neurohumoral (extrinsic) compensation involves two major mechanisms previously presented in Figure 6–7: the sympathetic nervous system and the renin-angiotensin-aldosterone hormonal response. Some of the pathologic as well as beneficial features of these compensatory responses are illustrated in Figure 13–2. The baroreceptor reflex appears to be reset, with a lower

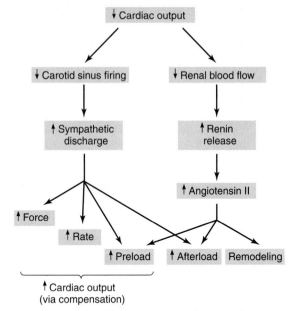

Figure 13–2. Some compensatory responses that occur during congestive heart failure. In addition to the effects shown, angiotensin II increases sympathetic effects by facilitating norepinephrine release.

sensitivity to arterial pressure, in patients with heart failure. As a result, baroreceptor sensory input to the vasomotor center is reduced even at normal pressures; sympathetic outflow is increased, and parasympathetic outflow is decreased. Increased sympathetic outflow causes tachycardia, increased cardiac contractility, and increased vascular tone.

While the increased preload, force, and heart rate initially increase cardiac output, increased arterial tone results in increased afterload and decreased ejection fraction, cardiac output, and renal perfusion. After a relatively short time, complex down-regulatory changes in the β_1-adrenoceptor-G protein-effector system take place that result in diminished stimulatory effects. Beta₂ receptors are *not* down-regulated and may develop increased coupling to the IP_3-DAG cascade. It has also been suggested that cardiac β_3 receptors (which do not appear to be down-regulated in failure) may mediate negative inotropic effects. Excessive beta activation can lead to leakage of calcium from the SR via RyR2 channels and contributes to stiffening of the ventricles and arrhythmias. Increased angiotensin II production leads to increased aldosterone secretion (with sodium and water retention), to increased afterload, and to remodeling of both heart and vessels (discussed below). Other hormones may also be released, including natriuretic peptide and endothelin (see Chapter 17).

The most important intrinsic compensatory mechanism is **myocardial hypertrophy.** This increase in muscle mass helps maintain cardiac performance. However, after an initial beneficial effect, hypertrophy can lead to ischemic changes, impairment of diastolic filling, and alterations in ventricular geometry. **Remodeling** is the term applied to dilation (other than that due to passive stretch) and other slow structural changes that occur in the stressed myocardium. It may include proliferation of connective tissue cells as well as abnormal myocardial cells with some biochemical characteristics of fetal myocytes. Ultimately, myocytes in the failing heart die at an accelerated rate through apoptosis, leaving the remaining myocytes subject to even greater stress.

The severity of heart failure is usually described according to a scale devised by the New York Heart Association. Class I failure is associated with no limitations on ordinary activities and symptoms that occur only with greater than ordinary exercise. Class II is characterized by slight limitation of ordinary activities, which result in fatigue and palpitations with ordinary physical activity. Class III failure results in no symptoms at rest, but fatigue, etc, with less than ordinary physical activity. Class IV is associated with symptoms even when the patient is at rest.

Pathophysiology of Cardiac Performance

Cardiac performance is a function of four primary factors:

(1) Preload: When some measure of left ventricular performance such as stroke volume or stroke work is plotted as a function of left ventricular filling pressure or end-diastolic fiber length, the resulting curve is termed the left ventricular function curve (Figure 13–3). The ascending limb (< 15 mm Hg filling pressure) represents the classic Frank-Starling relation. Beyond approximately 15 mm Hg, there is a plateau of performance. Preloads greater than 20–25 mm Hg result in pulmonary congestion. As noted above, preload is usually increased in heart failure because of increased blood volume and venous tone. Because the curve of the failing heart is lower, the plateau is reached at much lower values of stroke work or output. Increased fiber length or filling pressure increases oxygen demand in the myocardium. Reduction of high filling pressure is the goal of salt restriction and diuretic therapy in heart failure. Venodilator drugs (eg, nitroglycerin) also reduce preload by redistributing blood away from the chest into peripheral veins.

(2) Afterload: Afterload is the resistance against which the heart must pump blood and is represented by aortic impedance and systemic vascular resistance. As cardiac output falls in chronic failure, there is a reflex increase in systemic vascular resistance, mediated in part

Figure 13–3. Relation of left ventricular (LV) performance to filling pressure in patients with acute myocardial infarction, an important cause of heart failure. The upper line indicates the range for normal, healthy individuals. If acute heart failure occurs, function is shifted down and to the right. Similar depression is observed in patients with chronic heart failure. (Modified and reproduced with permission, from Swan HJC, Parmley WW: Congestive heart failure. In: Sodeman WA Jr, Sodeman TM [editors]. *Pathologic Physiology.* Saunders, 1979.)

by increased sympathetic outflow and circulating catecholamines and in part by activation of the renin-angiotensin system. Endothelin, a potent vasoconstrictor peptide, may also be involved. This sets the stage for the use of drugs that reduce arteriolar tone in heart failure.

(3) Contractility: Heart muscle obtained by biopsy from patients with chronic low-output failure demonstrates a reduction in intrinsic contractility. As contractility decreases in the patient, there is a reduction in the velocity of muscle shortening, the rate of intraventricular pressure development (dP/dt), and the stroke output achieved (Figure 13–3). However, the heart is still capable of some increase in all of these measures of contractility in response to inotropic drugs.

(4) Heart rate: The heart rate is a major determinant of cardiac output. As the intrinsic function of the heart decreases in failure and stroke volume diminishes, an increase in heart rate—through sympathetic activation of β adrenoceptors—is the first compensatory mechanism that comes into play to maintain cardiac output.

■ I. BASIC PHARMACOLOGY OF DRUGS USED IN HEART FAILURE

Although digitalis is not the first drug and never the only drug used in heart failure, we begin our discussion with this group because other drugs are discussed in more detail in other chapters. For a more detailed discussion of the cardiac glycosides the reader is referred to earlier editions of this book.

DIGITALIS

Digitalis is the genus name for the family of plants that provide most of the medically useful cardiac glycosides, eg, digoxin. Such plants have been known for thousands of years but were used erratically and with variable success until 1785, when William Withering, an English physician and botanist, published a monograph describing the clinical effects of an extract of the purple foxglove plant (*Digitalis purpurea*, a major source of these agents).

Chemistry

All of the cardiac glycosides, or cardenolides—of which **digoxin** is the prototype—combine a steroid nucleus linked to a lactone ring at the 17 position and a series of sugars at carbon 3 of the nucleus. Because they lack an easily ionizable group, their solubility is not pH-dependent. Digoxin is obtained from *Digitalis lanata*, the white foxglove, but many common plants contain cardiac glycosides.

Pharmacokinetics

A. ABSORPTION AND DISTRIBUTION

Digoxin, the only cardiac glycoside used in the USA, is 65–80% absorbed after oral administration. Absorption of other glycosides varies from zero to nearly 100%.

Once present in the blood, all cardiac glycosides are widely distributed to tissues, including the central nervous system.

B. METABOLISM AND EXCRETION

Digoxin is not extensively metabolized in humans; almost two thirds is excreted unchanged by the kidneys. Its renal clearance is proportionate to creatinine clearance. Equations and nomograms are available for adjusting digoxin dosage in patients with renal impairment.

Pharmacodynamics

Digoxin has multiple direct and indirect cardiovascular effects, with both therapeutic and toxic consequences. In addition, it has undesirable effects on the central nervous system and gut.

At the molecular level, all therapeutically useful cardiac glycosides **inhibit Na$^+$/K$^+$ ATPase,** the membrane-bound transporter often called the *sodium pump*. Inhibition of this transporter over most of the dose range has been extensively documented in all tissues studied. It is probable that this inhibitory action is largely responsible for the therapeutic effect (positive inotropy) as well as a major portion of the toxicity of digitalis. Other molecular-level effects of digitalis have been studied in the heart and are discussed below. The fact that a receptor for cardiac glycosides exists on the sodium pump has prompted some investigators to propose that an endogenous "digitalis-like" steroid, possibly ouabain, must exist.

A. CARDIAC EFFECTS

1. Mechanical effects—Cardiac glycosides increase contraction of the cardiac sarcomere (Figure 13–1) by increasing the free calcium concentration in the vicinity of the contractile proteins during systole. The increase in calcium concentration is the result of a two-step process: first, an increase of intracellular sodium concentration because of Na$^+$/K$^+$ ATPase inhibition (*1* in Figure 13–1); and second, a relative reduction of calcium expulsion from the cell by the sodium-calcium exchanger (NaxC in Figure 13–1) caused by the increase in intracellular sodium. The increased cytoplasmic calcium is sequestered by the SERCA in the SR for later release. Other mechanisms have been proposed but are not well supported.

The net result of the action of therapeutic concentrations of a cardiac glycoside is a distinctive increase in cardiac contractility (Figure 13–4, bottom trace). In isolated myocardial preparations, the rate of development of tension and of relaxation are both increased, with little or no change in time to peak tension. This effect occurs in both normal and failing myocardium, but in the intact animal or patient the responses are

Figure 13–4. Effects of a cardiac glycoside, ouabain, on isolated cardiac tissue. The top tracing shows action potentials evoked during the control period, early in the "therapeutic" phase, and later, when toxicity is present. The middle tracing shows the light (L) emitted by the calcium-detecting protein aequorin (relative to the maximum possible, L_{max}) and is roughly proportionate to the free intracellular calcium concentration. The bottom tracing records the tension elicited by the action potentials. The early phase of ouabain action **(A)** shows a slight shortening of action potential and a marked increase in free intracellular calcium concentration and contractile tension. The toxic phase **(B)** is associated with depolarization of the resting potential, a marked shortening of the action potential, and the appearance of an oscillatory depolarization, calcium increment, and contraction (*arrows*). (Unpublished data kindly provided by P Hess and H Gil Wier.)

modified by cardiovascular reflexes and the pathophysiology of heart failure.

2. Electrical effects—The effects of digitalis on the electrical properties of the heart are a mixture of direct and autonomic actions. Direct actions on the membranes of cardiac cells follow a well-defined progression: an early, brief prolongation of the action potential, followed by shortening (especially the plateau phase). The decrease in action potential duration is probably the result of increased potassium conductance that is caused by increased intracellular calcium (see Chapter 14). All of these effects can be observed at therapeutic concentrations in the absence of overt toxicity (Table 13–2).

At higher concentrations, resting membrane potential is reduced (made less negative) as a result of inhibition of the sodium pump and reduced intracellular potassium. As toxicity progresses, oscillatory depolarizing afterpotentials appear following normally evoked action potentials (Figure 13–4, panel B). The afterpotentials (also known as *delayed afterdepolarizations, DADs*) are associated with overloading of the intracellular calcium stores and oscillations in the free intracellular calcium ion concentration. When afterpotentials reach threshold, they elicit action potentials (premature depolarizations or ectopic "beats") that are coupled to the preceding normal action potentials. If afterpotentials in the Purkinje conducting system regularly reach threshold in this way, bigeminy will be recorded on the electrocardiogram (Figure 13–5). With further intoxication, each afterpotential-evoked action potential will itself elicit a suprathreshold afterpotential, and a self-sustaining tachycardia will be established. If allowed to progress, such a tachycardia may deteriorate into fibrillation; in the case of ventricular fibrillation, the arrhythmia will be rapidly fatal unless corrected.

Autonomic actions of cardiac glycosides on the heart involve both the parasympathetic and the sympathetic systems. In the lower portion of the dose range, cardioselective parasympathomimetic effects predominate. In fact, these atropine-blockable effects account for a significant portion of the early electrical effects of digitalis (Table 13–2). This action involves sensitization of the baroreceptors, central vagal stimulation, and facilitation of muscarinic transmission at the cardiac muscle cell. Because cholinergic innervation is much richer in the atria, these actions affect atrial and atrioventricular nodal function more than Purkinje or ventricular function. Some of the cholinomimetic effects are useful in the treatment of certain arrhythmias. At toxic levels, sympathetic outflow is increased by digitalis. This effect is not essential for typical digitalis toxicity but sensitizes the myocardium and exaggerates all the toxic effects of the drug.

Table 13–2. Effects of digoxin on electrical properties of cardiac tissues.

Tissue or Variable	Effects at Therapeutic Dosage	Effects at Toxic Dosage
Sinus node	↓ Rate	↓ Rate
Atrial muscle	↓ Refractory period	↓ Refractory period, arrhythmias
Atrioventricular node	↓ Conduction velocity, ↑ refractory period	↑ Refractory period, arrhythmias
Purkinje system, ventricular muscle	Slight ↓ refractory period	Extrasystoles, tachycardia, fibrillation
Electrocardiogram	↑ PR interval, ↓ QT interval	Tachycardia, fibrillation, arrest at extremely high dosage

The most common cardiac manifestations of digitalis toxicity include atrioventricular junctional rhythm, premature ventricular depolarizations, bigeminal rhythm, and second-degree atrioventricular blockade. However, it is claimed that digitalis can cause virtually any arrhythmia.

B. EFFECTS ON OTHER ORGANS

Cardiac glycosides affect all excitable tissues, including smooth muscle and the central nervous system. The gastrointestinal tract is the most common site of digitalis toxicity outside the heart. The effects include anorexia, nausea, vomiting, and diarrhea. This toxicity may be partially caused by direct effects on the gastrointestinal tract but is also the result of central nervous system actions.

Central nervous system effects include vagal and chemoreceptor trigger zone stimulation. Less often, disorientation and hallucinations—especially in the elderly—and visual disturbances are noted. The latter effect may include aberrations of color perception. Gynecomastia is a rare effect reported in men taking digitalis.

Figure 13–5. Electrocardiographic record showing digitalis-induced bigeminy. The complexes marked NSR are normal sinus rhythm beats; an inverted T wave and depressed ST segment are present. The complexes marked PVB are premature ventricular beats and are the electrocardiographic manifestations of depolarizations evoked by delayed oscillatory afterpotentials as shown in Figure 13–4. (Modified and reproduced, with permission, from Goldman MJ: *Principles of Clinical Electrocardiography,* 12th ed. Lange, 1986.)

C. INTERACTIONS WITH POTASSIUM, CALCIUM, AND MAGNESIUM

Potassium and digitalis interact in two ways. First, they inhibit each other's binding to Na^+/K^+ ATPase; therefore, hyperkalemia reduces the enzyme-inhibiting actions of cardiac glycosides, whereas hypokalemia facilitates these actions. Second, abnormal cardiac automaticity is inhibited by hyperkalemia (see Chapter 14). Moderately increased extracellular K^+ therefore reduces the effects of digitalis, especially the toxic effects.

Calcium ion facilitates the toxic actions of cardiac glycosides by accelerating the overloading of intracellular calcium stores that appears to be responsible for digitalis-induced abnormal automaticity. Hypercalcemia therefore increases the risk of a digitalis-induced arrhythmia. The effects of magnesium ion appear to be opposite to those of calcium. These interactions mandate careful evaluation of serum electrolytes in patients with digitalis-induced arrhythmias.

OTHER POSITIVE INOTROPIC DRUGS USED IN HEART FAILURE

Drugs that inhibit **phosphodiesterases,** the family of enzymes that inactivate cAMP and cGMP, have long been used in therapy of heart failure. Although they have positive inotropic effects, most of their benefits appear to derive from vasodilation, as discussed below. The bipyridines **inamrinone** and **milrinone** are the most successful of these agents found to date, but their usefulness is quite limited. Levosimendan, an investigational drug that sensitizes the troponin system to calcium, also appears to inhibit phosphodiesterase and cause some vasodilation in addition to its inotropic effects. Some early clinical trials suggest that this drug may be useful in patients with heart failure. A group of β-adrenoceptor stimulants has also been used as digitalis substitutes, but they may increase mortality (see below).

BIPYRIDINES

Inamrinone (previously called amrinone) and milrinone are bipyridine compounds that inhibit phosphodiesterase isozyme 3 (PDE-3). They are active orally as well as parenterally but are only available in parenteral forms. They have elimination half-lives of 3–6 hours, with 10–40% being excreted in the urine.

Pharmacodynamics

The bipyridines increase myocardial contractility by increasing inward calcium flux in the heart during the action potential; they may also alter the intracellular movements of calcium by influencing the sarcoplasmic reticulum. They also have an important vasodilating effect. Inhibition of phosphodiesterase results in an increase in cAMP and the increase in contractility and vasodilation.

The toxicity of inamrinone includes nausea and vomiting; arrhythmias, thrombocytopenia, and liver enzyme changes have also been reported in a significant number of patients. This drug has been withdrawn in some countries. Milrinone appears less likely to cause bone marrow and liver toxicity than inamrinone, but it does cause arrhythmias. Inamrinone and milrinone are now used only intravenously and only for acute heart failure or for severe exacerbation of chronic heart failure.

BETA-ADRENOCEPTOR STIMULANTS

The general pharmacology of these agents is discussed in Chapter 9. The selective β_1 agonist that has been most widely used in patients with heart failure is **dobutamine.** This parenteral drug produces an increase in cardiac output together with a decrease in ventricular filling pressure. Some tachycardia and an increase in myocardial oxygen consumption have been reported. Therefore, the potential for producing angina or arrhythmias in patients with coronary artery disease must be considered, as well as the tachyphylaxis that accompanies the use of any β stimulant. Intermittent dobutamine infusion may benefit some patients with chronic heart failure.

Dopamine has also been used in acute heart failure and may be particularly helpful if there is a need to raise blood pressure.

DRUGS WITHOUT POSITIVE INOTROPIC EFFECTS USED IN HEART FAILURE

Paradoxically, these agents—not positive inotropic drugs—are the first-line therapies for chronic heart failure. The drugs most commonly used are diuretics, ACE inhibitors, angiotensin receptor antagonists, and β blockers (see Table 13–1). In acute failure, diuretics and vasodilators play important roles.

DIURETICS

The diuretics are discussed in detail in Chapter 15. Their major mechanism of action in heart failure is to reduce venous pressure and ventricular preload. This results in reduction of edema and its symptoms, and reduction of cardiac size, which leads to improved pump efficiency. Spironolactone and eplerenone, the aldosterone antagonist diuretics (see Chapter 15), have the additional benefit of decreasing morbidity and mortality in patients with severe heart failure who are also receiving ACE inhibitors and other standard therapy. One possible mechanism for this benefit lies in accumulating evidence that aldosterone may also cause myocardial and vascular fibrosis and baroreceptor dysfunction in addition to its renal effects.

ANGIOTENSIN-CONVERTING ENZYME INHIBITORS, ANGIOTENSIN RECEPTOR BLOCKERS, & RELATED AGENTS

The ACE inhibitors such as **captopril** are introduced in Chapter 11 and discussed again in Chapter 17. These versatile drugs reduce peripheral resistance and thereby reduce afterload; they also reduce salt and water retention (by reducing aldosterone secretion) and in that way reduce preload. The reduction in tissue angiotensin levels also reduces sympathetic activity, probably through diminution of angiotensin's presynaptic effects on norepinephrine release. Finally, these drugs reduce the long-term remodeling of the heart and vessels, an effect that may be responsible for the observed reduction in mortality and morbidity (see Section II, Clinical Pharmacology).

Angiotensin AT_1 receptor-blockers such as **losartan** (see Chapters 11 and 17) appear to have similar but more limited beneficial effects. Angiotensin receptor blockers should be considered in patients intolerant of ACE inhibitors. In some trials, candesartan was beneficial when *added* to an ACE inhibitor.

VASODILATORS

The vasodilators are effective in acute heart failure because they provide a reduction in preload (through venodilation), or reduction in afterload (through arteriolar dilation), or both. Some evidence suggests that long-term use of hydralazine and isosorbide dinitrate can also reduce damaging remodeling of the heart.

A synthetic form of the endogenous peptide **brain natriuretic peptide (BNP)** is approved for use in acute cardiac failure as **nesiritide.** This recombinant product increases cGMP in smooth muscle cells and reduces venous and arteriolar tone in experimental preparations. It also causes diuresis. The peptide has a short half-life of about 18 minutes and is administered as a bolus intravenous dose followed by continuous infusion. Excessive hypotension is the most common adverse effect. Reports of significant renal damage and deaths have resulted in application of extra warnings regarding this agent and it should be used with great caution.

Measurement of *endogenous* BNP has been proposed as a diagnostic test because plasma concentrations rise in most patients with heart failure.

Bosentan, an orally active competitive inhibitor of endothelin (see Chapter 17), has been shown to have some benefits in experimental animal models of heart failure, but results in human trials have been disappointing. This drug is approved for use in pulmonary hypertension (see Chapter 11). It has significant teratogenic and hepatotoxic effects.

BETA-ADRENOCEPTOR BLOCKERS

Most patients with chronic heart failure respond favorably to certain β blockers in spite of the fact that these drugs can precipitate acute decompensation of cardiac function (see Chapter 10). Studies with bisoprolol, carvedilol, and metoprolol showed a reduction in mortality in patients with stable severe heart failure but this effect was not observed with another β blocker, bucindolol. A full understanding of the beneficial action of β blockade is lacking, but suggested mechanisms include attenuation of the adverse effects of high concentrations of catecholamines (including apoptosis), up-regulation of β receptors, decreased heart rate, and reduced remodeling through inhibition of the mitogenic activity of catecholamines.

■ II. CLINICAL PHARMACOLOGY OF DRUGS USED IN HEART FAILURE

In the past, prescription of a diuretic plus digitalis was almost automatic in every case of chronic heart failure, and other drugs were rarely considered. At present, diuretics are still considered as first-line therapy, but digitalis is reserved for patients who do not respond adequately to diuretics, ACE inhibitors, and β blockers (see Table 13–1).

MANAGEMENT OF CHRONIC HEART FAILURE

The major steps in the management of patients with chronic heart failure are outlined in Table 13–3. Reduction of cardiac workload is helpful in most cases. This can be accomplished by reducing activity and weight, and—especially important—control of hypertension.

Table 13–3. Steps in the treatment of chronic heart failure.

1. Reduce workload of the heart
   a. Limit activity, put on bed rest
   b. Reduce weight
   c. Control hypertension
2. Restrict sodium intake
3. Restrict water (rarely required)
4. Give diuretics
5. Give ACE inhibitor or angiotensin receptor blocker
6. Give digitalis if systolic dysfunction with 3rd heart sound or atrial fibrillation is present
7. Give β blockers to patients with stable class II–IV heart failure
8. Give vasodilators
9. Cardiac resynchronization if wide QRS interval is present in normal sinus rhythm

SODIUM REMOVAL

Sodium removal is the next important step—by dietary salt restriction or a diuretic—especially if edema is present. In mild failure, it is reasonable to start with a thiazide diuretic, switching to agents such as furosemide as required. Sodium loss causes secondary loss of potassium, which is particularly hazardous if the patient is to be given digitalis. Hypokalemia can be treated with potassium supplementation or through the addition of an ACE inhibitor or a potassium-sparing diuretic such as spironolactone. As noted above, spironolactone or eplerenone should probably be considered in all patients with moderate or severe heart failure since they appear to reduce both morbidity and mortality. Serum potassium should be monitored in patients receiving any of these agents.

ACE INHIBITORS & ANGIOTENSIN RECEPTOR BLOCKERS

In patients with left ventricular dysfunction but no edema, an ACE inhibitor should be used first. Several large studies have compared ACE inhibitors with digoxin or with other traditional therapies for chronic heart failure. The results show clearly that ACE inhibitors are superior to both placebo and to vasodilators and must be considered, along with diuretics, as first-line therapy for chronic failure. However, ACE inhibitors cannot replace digoxin in patients already receiving that drug because patients withdrawn from the cardiac glycoside deteriorate while on ACE inhibitor therapy.

By reducing preload and afterload in asymptomatic patients, ACE inhibitors appear to slow the progress of ventricular dilation and thus delay the onset of clinical heart failure. Thus, ACE inhibitors are beneficial in all subsets of patients, from those who are asymptomatic to those in severe chronic failure. This benefit appears to be a class effect, ie, all ACE inhibitors appear to be effective.

The angiotensin II AT$_1$ receptor blockers (ARBs, eg, losartan, candesartan, etc) produce beneficial hemodynamic effects similar to those of the ACE inhibitors. However, large clinical trials suggest that the angiotensin receptor blockers should only be used in patients who are intolerant of ACE inhibitors (usually because of cough).

VASODILATORS

Vasodilator drugs can be divided into selective arteriolar dilators, venous dilators, and drugs with nonselective vasodilatory effects. For this purpose, the ACE inhibitors may be considered nonselective arteriolar and venous dilators. The choice of agent should be based on the patient's signs and symptoms and hemodynamic measurements. Thus, in patients with high filling pressures in whom the principal symptom is dyspnea, venous dilators such as long-acting nitrates will be most helpful in reducing filling pressures and the symptoms of pulmonary congestion. In patients in whom fatigue due to low left ventricular output is a primary symptom, an arteriolar dilator such as hydralazine may be helpful in increasing forward cardiac output. In most patients with severe chronic failure that responds poorly to other therapy, the problem usually involves both elevated filling pressures and reduced cardiac output. In these circumstances, dilation of both arterioles and veins is required. In a trial in African-American patients already receiving ACE inhibitors, addition of hydralazine and isosorbide dinitrate reduced mortality.

BETA BLOCKERS & CALCIUM CHANNEL BLOCKERS

Trials of β-blocker therapy in patients with heart failure are based on the hypothesis that excessive tachycardia and adverse effects of high catecholamine levels on the heart contribute to the downward course of heart failure patients. The results clearly indicate that such therapy is beneficial if initiated very cautiously at low doses, even though acutely blocking the supportive effects of catecholamines can worsen heart failure. Several months of therapy may be required before improvement is noted; this usually consists of a slight rise in ejection fraction, slower heart rate, and reduction in symptoms. As noted above, bisoprolol, carvedilol, and metoprolol have been shown to reduce mortality.

In contrast, the calcium-blocking drugs appear to have no role in the treatment of patients with heart failure. Their depressant effects on the heart may worsen heart failure.

DIGITALIS

Digoxin is indicated in patients with heart failure and atrial fibrillation. It is also most helpful in patients with a dilated heart and third heart sound. It is usually given only if diuretics and ACE inhibitors have failed to control symptoms. Only about 50% of patients with normal sinus rhythm (usually those with documented systolic dysfunction) will have documentable relief of heart failure from digitalis. Better results are obtained in patients with atrial fibrillation. If the decision is made to use a cardiac glycoside, digoxin is the one chosen in the great majority of cases (and the only one available in the USA). When symptoms are mild, slow loading (digitalization) with 0.125–0.25 mg per day is safer and just as effective as the rapid method (0.5–0.75 mg every 8 hours for 3 doses, followed by 0.125–0.25 mg per day).

Determining the optimal level of digitalis effect may be difficult. In patients with atrial fibrillation, reduction of ventricular rate is the best measure of glycoside effect. In patients in normal sinus rhythm, symptomatic improvement and reductions in heart size, heart rate during exercise, venous pressure, or edema may signify optimum drug levels in the myocardium. Unfortunately, toxic effects may occur before the therapeutic end point is detected. If digitalis is being loaded slowly, simple omission of one dose and halving the maintenance dose will often bring the patient to the narrow range between suboptimal and toxic concentrations. Measurement of plasma digoxin levels is useful in patients who appear unusually resistant or sensitive; a level of 1 ng/mL or less is appropriate.

Because it has a moderate but persistent positive inotropic effect, digitalis can, in theory, reverse all the signs and symptoms of heart failure. Although the drug has no net effect on mortality, it reduces hospitalization and deaths from progressive heart failure at the expense of an increase in sudden death. It is important to note that the mortality rate is reduced in patients with serum digoxin concentrations of less than 0.9 ng/mL but increased in those with digoxin levels greater than 1.5 ng/mL.

Other Clinical Uses of Digitalis

Digitalis is useful in the management of atrial arrhythmias because of its cardioselective parasympathomimetic effects. In atrial flutter and fibrillation, the depressant effect of the drug on atrioventricular conduction will help control an excessively high ventricular rate. Digitalis has also been used in the control of paroxysmal atrial and atrioventricular nodal tachycardia. At present, calcium channel blockers and adenosine are preferred for this application.

Digitalis should be avoided in the therapy of arrhythmias associated with Wolff-Parkinson-White syndrome because it increases the probability of conduction of arrhythmic atrial impulses through the alternative rapidly conducting atrioventricular pathway. It is explicitly contraindicated in patients with Wolff-Parkinson-White syndrome and atrial fibrillation (see Chapter 14).

Table 13–4. Therapeutic classification of subsets in acute myocardial infarction.

Subset	Systolic Arterial Pressure (mm Hg)	Left Ventricular Filling Pressure (mm Hg)	Cardiac Index (L/min/m²)	Therapy
1. Hypovolemia	< 100	< 10	< 2.5	Volume replacement
2. Pulmonary congestion	100–150	> 20	> 2.5	Diuretics
3. Peripheral vasodilation	< 100	10–20	> 2.5	None or vasoactive drugs
4. Power failure	< 100	> 20	< 2.5	Vasodilators, inotropic drugs
5. Severe shock	< 90	> 20	< 2.0	Vasoactive drugs, inotropic drugs, circulatory assist devices
6. Right ventricular infarct	< 100	RVFP > 10 LVFP < 15	< 2.5	Volume replacement for LVFP, inotropic drugs. Avoid diuretics.
7. Mitral regurgitation, ventricular septal defect	< 100	> 20	< 2.5	Vasodilators, inotropic drugs, circulatory assist, surgery

The numeric values are intended to serve as general guidelines and not as absolute cutoff points. Arterial pressures apply to patients who were previously normotensive and should be adjusted upward for patients who were previously hypertensive. (RVFP and LVFP = right and left ventricular filling pressures.)

Toxicity

In spite of its limited benefits and recognized hazards, digitalis is still heavily used and toxicity is common. Therapy of toxicity manifested as visual changes or gastrointestinal disturbances generally requires no more than reducing the dose of the drug. If cardiac arrhythmia is present and can definitely be ascribed to digitalis, more vigorous therapy may be necessary. Serum digitalis and potassium levels and the electrocardiogram should always be monitored during therapy of significant digitalis toxicity. Electrolyte status should be corrected if abnormal (see above).

In severe digitalis intoxication, serum potassium will already be elevated at the time of diagnosis (because of potassium loss from the intracellular compartment of skeletal muscle and other tissues). Furthermore, automaticity is usually depressed, and antiarrhythmic agents administered in this setting may lead to cardiac arrest. Such patients are best treated with prompt insertion of a temporary cardiac pacemaker catheter and administration of digitalis antibodies **(digoxin immune fab).** These antibodies recognize digitoxin and cardiac glycosides from many other plants in addition to digoxin. They are extremely useful in reversing severe intoxication with most glycosides.

Digitalis-induced arrhythmias are frequently made worse by cardioversion; this therapy should be reserved for ventricular fibrillation if the arrhythmia is glycoside-induced.

Cardiac Resynchronization Therapy

Patients with normal sinus rhythm and a wide QRS interval have some dyssynchronization of ventricular contraction. Poor synchronization of left ventricular contraction results in diminished cardiac output. Resynchronization, with left ventricular or biventricular pacing, has been shown to reduce mortality in patients with chronic heart failure who were already receiving optimal medical therapy.

■ MANAGEMENT OF ACUTE HEART FAILURE

Acute heart failure occurs frequently in patients with chronic failure. Such episodes are usually associated with increased exertion, emotion, salt in the diet, noncompliance with medical therapy, or increased metabolic demand occasioned by fever, anemia, etc. A particularly common and important cause of acute failure—with or without chronic failure—is acute myocardial infarction.

Patients with acute myocardial infarction are best treated with emergency revascularization using either coronary angioplasty and a stent or a thrombolytic agent. Even with revascularization, acute failure may develop in such patients. Many of the signs and symptoms of acute and chronic failure are identical, but their therapies diverge because of the need for more rapid response and the relatively greater frequency and severity of pulmonary vascular congestion in the acute form.

Measurements of arterial pressure, cardiac output, stroke work index, and pulmonary capillary wedge pressure are particularly useful in patients with acute myocardial infarction and acute heart failure. Such patients can be usefully characterized on the basis of three hemodynamic measurements: arterial pressure, left ventricular filling pressure, and cardiac index. One such classification and therapies that have proved most effective are set forth in Table 13–4. When filling pressure is greater than 15 mm Hg and stroke work index is less than 20 gm/m^2, the mortality rate is high. Intermediate levels of these two variables imply a much better prognosis.

Among patients with acute decompensation, a small subset is found to have hyponatremia, presumably due to increased vasopressin activity. A new V_{1a} and V_2 receptor antagonist, **conivaptan,** has recently been approved for the parenteral treatment of euvolemic hyponatremia. Several clinical trials have indicated that this drug and related V_2 antagonists may have a beneficial effect in some patients with acute heart failure and hyponatremia.

 PREPARATIONS AVAILABLE

(DIURETICS: SEE CHAPTER 15.)

DIGITALIS

Digoxin (generic, Lanoxicaps, Lanoxin)
Oral: 0.125, 0.25 mg tablets; 0.05, 0.1, 0.2 mg capsules*; 0.05 mg/mL elixir
Parenteral: 0.1, 0.25 mg/mL for injection

DIGITALIS ANTIBODY

Digoxin immune fab (ovine) (digibind, digifab)
Parenteral: 38 or 40 mg per vial with 75 mg sorbitol lyophilized powder to reconstitute for IV injection. Each vial will bind approximately 0.5 mg digoxin or digitoxin.

SYMPATHOMIMETICS MOST COMMONLY USED IN CONGESTIVE HEART FAILURE

Dobutamine (generic, Dobutrex)
Parenteral: 12.5 mg/mL for IV infusion
Dopamine (generic, Intropin)
Parenteral: 40, 80, 160 mg/mL for IV injection; 80, 160, 320 mg/dL in 5% dextrose for IV infusion

ANGIOTENSIN-CONVERTING ENZYME INHIBITORS

Benazepril (generic, Lotensin)
Oral: 5, 10, 20, 40 mg tablets
Captopril (generic, Capoten)
Oral: 12.5, 25, 50, 100 mg tablets
Enalapril (Vasotec, Vasotec I.V.)
Oral: 2.5, 5, 10, 20 mg tablets
Parenteral: 1.25 mg enalaprilat/mL
Fosinopril (generic, Monopril)
Oral: 10, 20, 40 mg tablets
Lisinopril (generic, Prinivil, Zestril)
Oral: 2.5, 5, 10, 20, 30, 40 mg tablets
Moexipril (generic, Univasc)
Oral: 7.5, 15 mg tablets
Perindopril (Aceon)
Oral: 2, 4, 8 mg tablets

Quinapril (Accupril)
Oral: 5, 10, 20, 40 mg tablets
Ramipril (Altace)
Oral: 1.25, 2.5, 5, 10 mg capsules
Trandolapril (Mavik)
Oral: 1, 2, 4 mg tablets

ANGIOTENSIN RECEPTOR BLOCKERS

Candesartan (Atacand)
Oral: 4, 8, 16, 32 mg tablets
Eprosartan (Teveten)
Oral: 400, 800 mg tablets
Irbesartan (Avapro)
Oral: 75, 150, 300 mg tablets
Losartan (Cozaar)
Oral: 25, 50, 100 mg tablets
Olmesartan (Benicar)
Oral: 5, 20, 40 mg tablets
Telmisartan (Micardis)
Oral: 20, 40, 80 mg tablets
Valsartan (Diovan)
Oral: 40, 80, 160, 320 mg tablets

BETA BLOCKERS THAT HAVE REDUCED MORTALITY IN HEART FAILURE

Bisoprolol (Zebeta, unlabeled use)
Oral: 5, 10 mg tablets
Carvedilol (Coreg)
Oral: 3.125, 6.25, 12.5, 25 mg tablets
Metoprolol (Lopressor, Toprol XL)
Oral: 50, 100 mg tablets; 25, 50, 100, 200 mg extended-release tablets
Parenteral: 1 mg/mL for IV injection

OTHER DRUGS

Inamrinone
Parenteral: 5 mg/mL for IV injection
Milrinone (generic, Primacor)
Parenteral: 1 mg/mL for IV injection; 200 mcg/mL premixed for IV infusion
Nesiritide (Natrecor)
Parenteral: 1.58 mg powder for IV injection
Bosentan (Tracleer)
Oral: 62.5, 125 mg tablets

---

*Digoxin capsules (Lanoxicaps) have greater bioavailability than digoxin tablets.

REFERENCES

Cleland JCF et al: The effect of cardiac resynchronization on morbidity and mortality in heart failure. N Engl J Med 2005; 352:1539.

Cohn J et al: A randomized trial of the angiotensin receptor blocker valsartan in heart failure. N Engl J Med 2002; 345:1667.

CONSENSUS Trial Study Group: Effects of enalapril on mortality in severe congestive heart failure. N Engl J Med 1987; 316:1429.

Dec GW: Digoxin remains useful in the management of chronic heart failure. Med Clin North Am 2003;87:317.

Foody JM, Farrell MH, Krumholtz H: Beta blocker therapy in heart failure. JAMA 2002;287:883.

Hunt SA et al: ACC/AHA 2005 guideline update for the diagnosis and management of chronic heart failure in the adult: Summary article: A report of the American College of Cardiology/ American Heart Association Task Force on Practice Guidelines. J Am Coll Cardiol 2005;46:1116.

Klein L et al: Pharmacologic therapy for patients with chronic heart failure and reduced systolic function: Review of trials and practical considerations. Am J Cardiol 2003;91(Suppl 9A):18F.

Mann DL et al: New therapeutics for chronic heart failure. Annu Rev Med 2002;53:59.

McMurray JJ et al: Effects of candesartan in patients with chronic heart failure and reduced left ventricular systolic function taking ACE inhibitors: The CHARM-Added Trial. Lancet 2003;362:767.

Pitt B et al: Eplerenone, a selective aldosterone blocker, in patients with left ventricular dysfunction after myocardial infarction. N Engl J Med 2003;348:1309.

Post SR, Hammond HK, Insel PA: β-Adrenergic receptors and receptor signaling in heart failure. Annu Rev Pharmacol Toxicol 1999;39:343.

Rathbone SS et al: Association of serum digoxin concentration and outcomes in patients with heart failure. JAMA 2003;289:871.

Ryan TJ et al: 1999 Update ACC/AHA Guidelines for the management of acute myocardial infarction. Circulation 1999; 100:1016.

Schrier RW, Abraham WT: Hormones and hemodynamics in heart failure. N Engl J Med 1999;341:577.

Taur Y, Frishman WH: The cardiac ryanodine receptor (RyR2) and its role in heart disease. Cardiol Rev 2005;13:142.

Taylor AL et al: Combination of isosorbide dinitrate and hydralazine in blacks with heart failure. N Engl J Med 2004; 351:2049.

Agents Used in Cardiac Arrhythmias 14

Joseph R. Hume, PhD, & Augustus O. Grant, MD, PhD

Cardiac arrhythmias are a frequent problem in clinical practice, occurring in up to 25% of patients treated with digitalis, 50% of anesthetized patients, and over 80% of patients with acute myocardial infarction. Arrhythmias may require treatment because rhythms that are too rapid, too slow, or asynchronous can reduce cardiac output. Some arrhythmias can precipitate more serious or even lethal rhythm disturbances—eg, early premature ventricular depolarizations can precipitate ventricular fibrillation. In such patients, antiarrhythmic drugs may be lifesaving. On the other hand, the hazards of antiarrhythmic drugs—and in particular the fact that they can *precipitate* lethal arrhythmias in some patients—has led to a reevaluation of their relative risks and benefits. In general, treatment of asymptomatic or minimally symptomatic arrhythmias should be avoided for this reason.

Arrhythmias can be treated with the drugs discussed in this chapter and with nonpharmacologic therapies such as pacemakers, cardioversion, catheter ablation, and surgery. This chapter describes the pharmacology of drugs that suppress arrhythmias by a direct action on the cardiac cell membrane. Other modes of therapy are discussed briefly (see Box, The Nonpharmacologic Therapy of Cardiac Arrhythmias).

■ ELECTROPHYSIOLOGY OF NORMAL CARDIAC RHYTHM

The electrical impulse that triggers a normal cardiac contraction originates at regular intervals in the sinoatrial node (Figure 14–1), usually at a frequency of 60–100 beats per minute. This impulse spreads rapidly through the atria and enters the atrioventricular node, which is normally the only conduction pathway between the atria and ventricles. Conduction through the atrioventricular node is slow, requiring about 0.15 s. (This delay provides time for atrial contraction to propel blood into the ventricles.) The impulse then propagates over the His-Purkinje system and invades all parts of the ventricles, beginning with the endocardial surface near the apex and ending with the epicardial surface at the base of the heart. Ventricular activation is complete in less than 0.1 s;

therefore, contraction of all of the ventricular muscle is normally synchronous and hemodynamically effective.

Arrhythmias consist of cardiac depolarizations that deviate from the above description in one or more aspects— ie, there is an abnormality in the site of origin of the impulse, its rate or regularity, or its conduction.

Ionic Basis of Membrane Electrical Activity

The transmembrane potential of cardiac cells is determined by the concentrations of several ions—chiefly sodium (Na^+), potassium (K^+), calcium (Ca^{2+}), and chloride (Cl^-)—on either side of the membrane and the permeability of the membrane to each ion. These water-soluble ions are unable to freely diffuse across the lipid cell membrane in response to their electrical and concentration gradients; they require aqueous channels (specific pore-forming proteins) for such diffusion. Thus, ions move across cell membranes in response to their gradients only at specific times during the cardiac cycle when these ion channels are open. The movements of the ions produce currents that form the basis of the cardiac action potential. Individual channels are relatively ion-specific, and the flux of ions through them is thought to be controlled by "gates" (probably flexible peptide chains or energy barriers). Each type of channel has its own type of gate (sodium, calcium, and some potassium channels are each thought to have two types of gates), and each type of gate is opened and closed by specific transmembrane voltage, ionic, or metabolic conditions.

At rest, most cells are not significantly permeable to sodium, but at the start of each action potential, they become quite permeable (see below). In electrophysiologic terms, the conductance of the fast sodium channel suddenly increases in response to a depolarizing stimulus. Similarly, calcium enters and potassium leaves the cell with each action potential. Therefore, in addition to ion channels, the cell must have mechanisms to maintain stable transmembrane ionic conditions by establishing and maintaining ion gradients. The most important of these active mechanisms is the sodium pump, Na^+/K^+ ATPase, described in Chapter 13. This pump and other active ion carriers contribute indirectly to the transmembrane potential by maintaining the gradients necessary for diffusion through channels. In addition, some pumps and exchangers produce net current flow (eg, by exchanging three Na^+ for two K^+ ions) and hence are termed "electrogenic."

THE NONPHARMACOLOGIC THERAPY OF CARDIAC ARRHYTHMIAS

It was recognized over 100 years ago that reentry in simple in vitro models (eg, rings of conducting tissues) was permanently interrupted by transecting the reentry circuit. This concept is now applied in cardiac arrhythmias with defined anatomic pathways—eg, atrioventricular reentry using accessory pathways, atrioventricular node reentry, atrial flutter, and some forms of ventricular tachycardia—by treatment with **radiofrequency catheter ablation.** Recent studies have shown that paroxysmal and persistent atrial fibrillation may arise from one of the pulmonary veins. Both forms of atrial fibrillation can be cured by electrically isolating the pulmonary veins by radiofrequency catheter ablation or during concomitant cardiac surgery.

Another form of nonpharmacologic therapy is the **implantable cardioverter-defibrillator (ICD),** a device that can automatically detect and treat potentially fatal arrhythmias such as ventricular fibrillation. ICDs are now widely used in patients who have been resuscitated from such arrhythmias, and several trials have shown that ICD treatment reduces mortality in patients with coronary artery disease who have an ejection fraction $\leq 30\%$ and in patients with class 2 or 3 heart failure and no prior history of arrhythmias. The increasing use of nonpharmacologic antiarrhythmic therapies reflects both advances in the relevant technologies and an increasing appreciation of the dangers of long-term therapy with currently available drugs.

When the cardiac cell membrane becomes permeable to a specific ion (ie when the channels selective for that ion are open), movement of that ion across the cell membrane is determined by Ohm's law: current = voltage ÷ resistance, or current = voltage × conductance. Conductance is determined by the properties of the individual ion channel protein. The voltage term is the difference between the actual membrane potential and the reversal potential for that ion (the membrane potential at which no current would flow even if channels were open). For example, in the case of sodium in a cardiac cell at rest, there is a substantial concentration gradient (140 mmol/L Na^+ outside; 10–15 mmol/L Na^+ inside) and an electrical gradient (0 mV outside; −90 mV inside) that would drive Na^+ into cells. Sodium does not enter the cell at rest because sodium channels are closed; when sodium channels open, the very large influx of Na^+ ions accounts for phase 0 depolarization. The situation for K^+ ions in the resting cardiac cell is quite different. Here, the concentration gradient (140 mmol/L inside; 4 mmol/L outside) would drive the ion out of the cell, but the electrical gradient would drive it in; that is, the inward gradient is in equilibrium with the outward gradient. In fact, certain potassium channels ("inward rectifier" channels) are open in the resting cell, but little current flows through them because of this balance. The equilibrium, or **reversal potential,** for ions is determined by the **Nernst equation:**

$$E_{ion} = 61 \times \log\left(\frac{C_e}{C_i}\right)$$

where C_e and C_i are the extracellular and intracellular concentrations, respectively, multiplied by their activity coefficients. Note that raising extracellular potassium makes E_K less negative. When this occurs, the membrane depolarizes until the new E_K is reached. Thus, extracellular potassium concentration and inward rectifier channel function are the major factors determining the membrane potential of the resting cardiac cell. The conditions required for application of the Nernst equation are approximated at the peak of the overshoot (using sodium concentrations) and during rest (using potassium concentrations) in most nonpacemaker cardiac cells. If the permeability is significant for both potassium and sodium, the Nernst equation is not a good predictor of membrane potential, but the **Goldman-Hodgkin-Katz equation** may be used:

$$E_{mem} = 61 \times \log\left(\frac{P_K \times K_e + P_{Na} \times Na_e}{P_K \times K_i + P_{Na} \times Na_i}\right)$$

In pacemaker cells (whether normal or ectopic), spontaneous depolarization (the pacemaker potential) occurs during diastole (phase 4, Figure 14–1). This depolarization results from a gradual increase of depolarizing current through special hyperpolarization-activated ion channels in pacemaker cells. The effect of changing extracellular potassium is more complex in a pacemaker cell than it is in a nonpacemaker cell because the effect on permeability to potassium is much more important in a pacemaker (see Box, Effects of Potassium). In a pacemaker—especially an ectopic one—the end result of an increase in extracellular potassium will usually be to slow or stop the

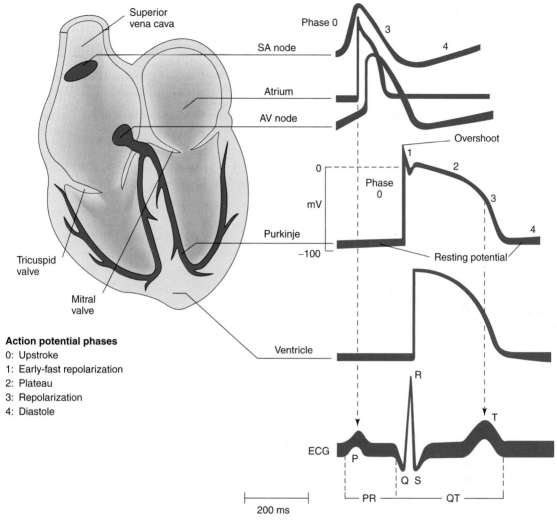

Figure 14–1. Schematic representation of the heart and normal cardiac electrical activity (intracellular recordings from areas indicated and ECG). Sinoatrial node, atrioventricular node, and Purkinje cells display pacemaker activity (phase 4 depolarization). The ECG is the body surface manifestation of the depolarization and repolarization waves of the heart. The P wave is generated by atrial depolarization, the QRS by ventricular muscle depolarization, and the T wave by ventricular repolarization. Thus, the PR interval is a measure of conduction time from atrium to ventricle, and the QRS duration indicates the time required for all of the ventricular cells to be activated (ie, the intraventricular conduction time). The QT interval reflects the duration of the ventricular action potential.

pacemaker. Conversely, hypokalemia will often facilitate ectopic pacemakers.

The Active Cell Membrane

In normal atrial, Purkinje, and ventricular cells, the action potential upstroke (phase 0) is dependent on sodium current. From a functional point of view, it is convenient to describe the behavior of the sodium current in terms of three channel states (Figure 14–2). The cardiac sodium channel protein has been cloned, and it is now recognized that these channel states actually represent different protein conformations. In addition, regions of the protein that confer specific behaviors, such as voltage sensing, pore formation, and inactivation, are now being identified. The gates described below and in Figure 14–2 represent such regions.

EFFECTS OF POTASSIUM

The effects of changes in serum potassium on cardiac action potential duration, pacemaker rate, and arrhythmias can appear somewhat paradoxical if changes are predicted based solely on a consideration of changes in the potassium *electrochemical gradient*. In the heart, however, changes in serum potassium concentration have the additional effect of altering potassium *conductance* (increased extracellular potassium increases potassium conductance) independent of simple changes in electrochemical driving force, and this effect often predominates. As a result, the actual observed effects of **hyperkalemia** include reduced action potential duration, slowed conduction, decreased pacemaker rate, and decreased

pacemaker arrhythmogenesis. Conversely, the actual observed effects of **hypokalemia** include prolonged action potential duration, increased pacemaker rate, and increased pacemaker arrhythmogenesis. Furthermore, pacemaker rate and arrhythmias involving ectopic pacemaker cells appear to be more sensitive to changes in serum potassium concentration, compared with cells of the sinoatrial node. These effects of serum potassium on the heart probably contribute to the observed increased sensitivity to potassium channel-blocking antiarrhythmic agents (quinidine or sotalol) during hypokalemia, eg, accentuated action potential prolongation and tendency to cause torsade de pointes.

Depolarization to the threshold voltage results in opening of the activation (*m*) gates of sodium channels (Figure 14–2, middle). If the inactivation (*h*) gates of these channels have not already closed, the channels are now open or activated, and sodium permeability is markedly increased, greatly exceeding the permeability for any other ion. Extracellular sodium therefore diffuses down its electrochemical gradient into the cell, and the membrane potential very rapidly approaches the sodium equilibrium potential, E_{Na} (about +70 mV when Na_e = 140 mmol/L and Na_i = 10 mmol/L). This

intense sodium current is very brief because opening of the *m* gates upon depolarization is promptly followed by closure of the *h* gates and inactivation of the sodium channels (Figure 14–2, right).

Most calcium channels become activated and inactivated in what appears to be the same way as sodium channels, but in the case of the most common type of cardiac calcium channel (the "L" type), the transitions occur more slowly and at more positive potentials. The action potential plateau (phases 1 and 2) reflects the turning off of most of the sodium current, the waxing

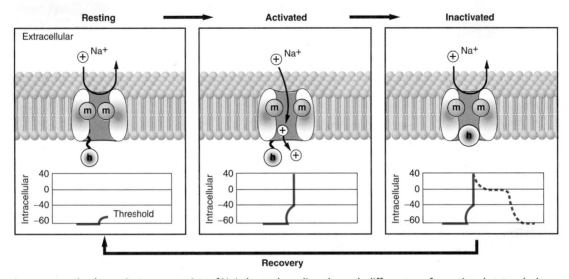

Figure 14–2. A schematic representation of Na^+ channels cycling through different conformational states during the cardiac action potential. Transitions between resting, activated, and inactivated states are dependent on membrane potential and time. The activation gate is shown as *m* and the inactivation gate as *h*. Potentials typical for each state are shown under each channel schematic as a function of time. The dashed line indicates that part of the action potential during which most Na^+ channels are completely or partially inactivated and unavailable for reactivation.

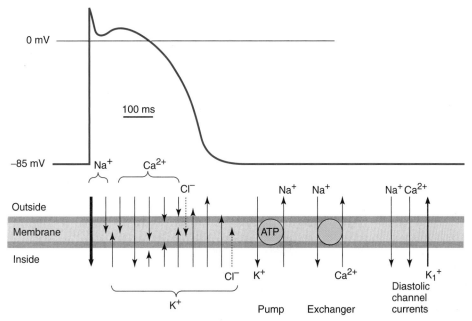

Figure 14–3. Schematic diagram of the ion permeability changes and transport processes that occur during an action potential and the diastolic period following it. The size and weight of the arrows indicate approximate magnitudes of the ion channel currents; arrows pointing down indicate inward (depolarizing) membrane currents, arrows pointing up indicate outward (repolarizing) membrane currents. Multiple subtypes of potassium and calcium currents, with different sensitivities to blocking drugs, have been identified. Chloride currents (dotted arrows) produce both inward and outward membrane currents during the cardiac action potential.

and waning of calcium current, and the slow development of a repolarizing potassium current.

Final repolarization (phase 3) of the action potential results from completion of sodium and calcium channel inactivation and the growth of potassium permeability, so that the membrane potential once again approaches the potassium equilibrium potential. The major potassium currents involved in phase 3 repolarization include a rapidly activating potassium current (I_{Kr}) and a slowly activating potassium current (I_{Ks}). These two potassium currents are sometimes discussed together as "I_K." These processes are diagrammed in Figure 14–3. It is noteworthy that a different potassium current, distinct from I_{Kr} and I_{Ks}, may control repolarization in sinoatrial nodal cells. This explains why some drugs that block either I_{Kr} or I_{Ks} may prolong repolarization in Purkinje and ventricular cells, but have little effect on sinoatrial nodal repolarization (see Box, Molecular & Genetic Basis of Cardiac Arrhythmias).

The Effect of Resting Potential on Action Potentials

A key factor in the pathophysiology of arrhythmias and the actions of antiarrhythmic drugs is the relationship between the resting potential of a cell and the action potentials that can be evoked in it (Figure 14–4, left panel). Because the inactivation gates of sodium channels in the resting membrane close over the potential range –75 to –55 mV, fewer sodium channels are "available" for diffusion of sodium ions when an action potential is evoked from a resting potential of –60 mV than when it is evoked from a resting potential of –80 mV. Important consequences of the reduction in peak sodium permeability include reduced maximum upstroke velocity (called V_{max}, for maximum rate of change of membrane voltage), reduced action potential amplitude, reduced excitability, and reduced conduction velocity.

During the plateau of the action potential, most sodium channels are inactivated. Upon repolarization, recovery from inactivation takes place (in the terminology of Figure 14–2, the *h* gates reopen), making the channels again available for excitation. The time between phase 0 and sufficient recovery of sodium channels in phase 3 to permit a new propagated response to an external stimulus is the **refractory period.** Changes in refractoriness (determined by either altered recovery from inactivation or altered action potential duration) can be important in the genesis or suppression of certain arrhythmias. Another important effect of less negative resting potential is pro-

Figure 14–4. Dependence of sodium channel function on the membrane potential preceding the stimulus. **Left:** The fraction of sodium channels available for opening in response to a stimulus is determined by the membrane potential immediately preceding the stimulus. The decrease in the fraction available when the resting potential is depolarized in the absence of a drug (control curve) results from the voltage-dependent closure of *h* gates in the channels. The curve labeled *Drug* illustrates the effect of a typical local anesthetic antiarrhythmic drug. Most sodium channels are inactivated during the plateau of the action potential. **Right:** The time constant for recovery from inactivation after repolarization also depends on the resting potential. In the absence of drug, recovery occurs in less than 10 ms at normal resting potentials (–85 to –95 mV). Depolarized cells recover more slowly (note logarithmic scale). In the presence of a sodium channel-blocking drug, the time constant of recovery is increased, but the increase is far greater at depolarized potentials than at more negative ones.

longation of this recovery time, as shown in Figure 14–4 (right panel). The prolongation of recovery time is reflected in an increase in the effective refractory period.

A brief, sudden, depolarizing stimulus, whether caused by a propagating action potential or by an external electrode arrangement, causes the opening of large numbers of activation gates before a significant number of inactivation gates can close. In contrast, slow reduction (depolarization) of the resting potential, whether brought about by hyperkalemia, sodium pump blockade, or ischemic cell damage, results in depressed sodium currents during the upstrokes of action potentials. Depolarization of the resting potential to levels positive to –55 mV abolishes sodium currents, since all sodium channels are inactivated. However, such severely depolarized cells have been found to support special action potentials under circumstances that increase calcium permeability or decrease potassium permeability. These "slow responses"—slow upstroke velocity and slow conduction—depend on a calcium inward current and constitute the normal electrical activity in the sinoatrial and atrioventricular nodes, since these tissues have a normal resting potential in the range of –50 to –70 mV. Slow responses may also be important for certain arrhythmias. Modern techniques of molecular biology and electrophysiology can identify multiple subtypes of calcium and potassium channels. One way in which such subtypes may differ is in sensitivity to drug effects, so drugs targeting specific channel subtypes may be developed in the future.

■ MECHANISMS OF ARRHYTHMIAS

Many factors can precipitate or exacerbate arrhythmias: ischemia, hypoxia, acidosis or alkalosis, electrolyte abnormalities, excessive catecholamine exposure, autonomic influences, drug toxicity (eg, digitalis or antiarrhythmic drugs), overstretching of cardiac fibers, and the presence of scarred or otherwise diseased tissue. However, all arrhythmias result from (1) disturbances in impulse formation, (2) disturbances in impulse conduction, or (3) both.

Disturbances of Impulse Formation

The interval between depolarizations of a pacemaker cell is the sum of the duration of the action potential and the duration of the diastolic interval. Shortening of either duration results in an increase in pacemaker rate. The more important of the two, diastolic interval, is determined primarily by the slope of phase 4 depolarization (pacemaker potential). Vagal discharge and β-receptor-blocking drugs slow normal pacemaker rate by reducing the phase 4 slope (acetylcholine also makes the maximum diastolic potential more negative). Acceleration of pacemaker discharge is often brought about by increased phase 4 depolarization slope, which can be caused by hypokalemia, β-adrenoceptor stimulation, positive chro-

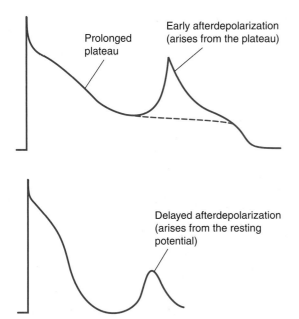

Figure 14–5. Two forms of abnormal activity, early **(top)** and delayed after depolarizations **(bottom).** In both cases, abnormal depolarizations arise during or after a normally evoked action potential. They are therefore often referred to as "triggered" automaticity; that is, they require a normal action potential for their initiation.

notropic drugs, fiber stretch, acidosis, and partial depolarization by currents of injury.

Latent pacemakers (cells that show slow phase 4 depolarization even under normal conditions, eg, some Purkinje fibers) are particularly prone to acceleration by the above mechanisms. However, all cardiac cells, including normally quiescent atrial and ventricular cells, may show repetitive pacemaker activity when depolarized under appropriate conditions, especially if hypokalemia is also present.

Afterdepolarizations (Figure 14–5) are depolarizations that interrupt phase 3 **(early afterdepolarizations, EADs)** or phase 4 **(delayed afterdepolarizations, DADs).** EADs are usually exacerbated at slow heart rates and are thought to contribute to the development of long QT-related arrhythmias (see Box, Molecular & Genetic Basis of Cardiac Arrhythmias). DADs on the other hand, discussed in Chapter 13, often occur when intracellular calcium is increased. They are exacerbated by fast heart rates and are thought to be responsible for some arrhythmias related to digitalis excess, to catecholamines, and to myocardial ischemia.

Disturbances of Impulse Conduction

Severely depressed conduction may result in simple **block,** eg, atrioventricular nodal block or bundle branch block. Because parasympathetic control of atrioventricular conduction is significant, partial atrioventricular block is sometimes relieved by atropine. Another common abnormality of conduction is **reentry** (also known as "circus movement"), in which one impulse reenters and excites areas of the heart more than once (Figure 14–6).

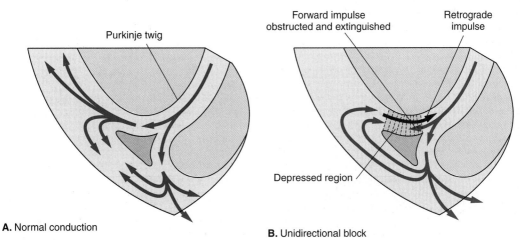

A. Normal conduction

B. Unidirectional block

Figure 14–6. Schematic diagram of a reentry circuit that might occur in small bifurcating branches of the Purkinje system where they enter the ventricular wall. **A:** Normally, electrical excitation branches around the circuit, is transmitted to the ventricular branches, and becomes extinguished at the other end of the circuit due to collision of impulses. **B:** An area of unidirectional block develops in one of the branches, preventing anterograde impulse transmission at the site of block, but the retrograde impulse may be propagated through the site of block if the impulse finds excitable tissue; that is, the refractory period is shorter than the conduction time. This impulse will then reexcite tissue it had previously passed through, and a reentry arrhythmia will be established.

The path of the reentering impulse may be confined to very small areas, eg, within or near the atrioventricular node, or it may involve large portions of the atrial or ventricular walls. Some forms of reentry are strictly anatomically determined; for example, in the Wolff-Parkinson-White syndrome, the reentry circuit consists of atrial tissue, the AV node, ventricular tissue, and an accessory atrioventricular connection (a "bypass tract"). In other cases (eg, atrial or ventricular fibrilla-tion), multiple reentry circuits, determined by the properties of the cardiac tissue, may meander through the heart in apparently random paths. Furthermore, the circulating impulse often gives off "daughter impulses" that can spread to the rest of the heart. Depending on how many round trips through the pathway the impulse makes before dying out, the arrhythmia may be manifest as one or a few extra beats or as a sustained tachycardia.

MOLECULAR & GENETIC BASIS OF CARDIAC ARRHYTHMIAS

It is now possible to define the molecular basis of several congenital and acquired cardiac arrhythmias. The best example is the polymorphic ventricular tachycardia known as torsade de pointes (shown in Figure 14–7), which is associated with prolongation of the QT interval (especially at the onset of the tachycardia), syncope, and sudden death. This must represent prolongation of the action potential of at least some ventricular cells (Figure 14–1). The effect can, in theory, be attributed either to increased inward current (gain of function) or decreased outward current (loss of function) during the plateau of the action potential. In fact, recent molecular genetic studies have identified up to 300 different mutations in at least eight ion channel genes that produce the congenital long QT (LQT) syndrome (Table 14–1), and each mutation may have different clinical implications. Loss of function mutations in potassium channel genes produce decreases in outward repolarizing current and are responsible for LQT subtypes 1, 2, 5, 6, and 7. HERG and KCNE2 (MiRP1) genes encode subunits of the the rapid delayed rectifier potassium current (I_{Kr}), whereas KCNQ1 and KCNE1 (minK) encode subunits of the slow delayed rectifier potassium current (I_{Ks}). KCNJ2 encodes an inwardly rectifying potassium current (I_{Kir}). In contrast, gain of function mutations in the sodium channel gene (SCN5A) or calcium channel gene (CACNA1c) cause increases in inward plateau current and are responsible for LQT subtypes 3 and 8, respectively.

Molecular genetic studies have identified the reason why congenital and acquired cases of torsades de pointes can be so strikingly similar. The potassium channel I_{Kr} (encoded by HERG) is blocked or modified by many drugs (eg, quinidine, sotalol) or electrolyte abnormalities (hypokalemia, hypomagnesemia, hypocalcemia) that also produce torsades de pointes. Thus, the identification of the precise molecular mechanisms underlying various forms of the LQT syndromes now raises the possibility that specific therapies may be developed for individuals with defined molecular abnormalities. Indeed, preliminary reports suggest that the sodium channel blocker mexiletine can correct the clinical manifestations of congenital LQT subtype 3 syndrome. It is likely that torsade de pointes originates from triggered upstrokes arising from early afterdepolarizations (Figure 14–5). Thus, therapy is directed at correcting hypokalemia, eliminating triggered upstrokes (eg, by using β blockers or magnesium), or shortening the action potential (eg, by increasing heart rate with isoproterenol or pacing)—or all of these.

The molecular basis of several other congenital cardiac arrhythmias associated with sudden death has also recently been identified. Three forms of short QT syndrome have been identified that are linked to gain of function mutations in three different potassium channel genes (KCNH2, KCNQ1, and KCNJ2). Catecholaminergic polymorphic ventricular tachycardia, a disease that is characterized by stress- or emotion-induced syncope, can be caused by genetic mutations in two different proteins in the sarcoplasmic reticulum that control intracellular calcium homeostasis. Mutations in two different ion channel genes (HCN4 and SCN5A) have been linked to congenital forms of sick sinus syndrome. The Brugada syndrome, which is characterized by ventricular fibrillation associated with persistent ST-segment elevation, and progressive cardiac conduction disorder (PCCD), characterized by impaired conduction in the His-Purkinje system and right or left bundle block leading to complete atrioventricular block, have both been linked to several loss-of-function mutations in the sodium channel gene, SCN5A. At least one form of familial atrial fibrillation is caused by a gain-of-function mutation in the potassium channel gene, KCNQ1.

Table 14–1. Molecular and genetic basis of some cardiac arrhythmias.

Type	Chromosome Involved	Defective Gene	Ion Channel or Proteins Affected	Result[1]
LQT-1[2]	11	KCNQ1	I_{Ks}	LF
LQT-2	7	KCNH2 (HERG)	I_{Kr}	LF
LQT-3	3	SCN5A	I_{Na}	GF
LQT-4	4	Ankyrin-B	[3]	LF
LQT-5	21	KCNE1 (minK)	I_{Ks}	LF
LQT-6	21	KCNE2 (MiRP1)	I_{Kr}	LF
LQT-7[4]	17	KCNJ2	I_{Kir}	LF
LQT-8[5]	12	CACNA1c	I_{Ca}	GF
SQT-1[6]	7	KCNH2	I_{Kr}	GF
SQT-2	11	KCNQ1	I_{Ks}	GF
SQT-3	17	KCNJ2	I_{Kir}	GF
CPVT-1[7]	1	hRyR2	Ryanodine receptor	GF
CPVT-2	1	CASQ2	Calsequestrin	LF
Sick sinus syndrome	15 or 3	HCN4 or SCN5A	[8]	LF
Brugada syndrome	3	SCN5A	I_{Na}	LF
PCCD[9]	3	SCN5A	I_{Na}	LF
Familial atrial fibrillation	11	KCNQ1	I_{Ks}	GF

[1]LF, loss of function; GF, gain of function.
[2]LQT, long QT syndrome.
[3]Ankyrins are intracellular proteins that associate with a variety of transport proteins including Na^+ channels, Na^+/K^+ ATPase, Na^+/Ca^{2+} exchange, Ca^{2+} release channels.
[4]Also known as Andersen syndrome.
[5]Also known as Timothy syndrome; multiple organ dysfunction, including autism.
[6]SQT, short QT syndrome.
[7]CPVT, catecholaminergic polymorphic ventricular tachycardia; mutations in intracellular ryanodine Ca^{2+} release channel or the Ca^{2+} buffer protein, calsequestrin, may result in enhanced sarcoplasmic reticulum Ca^{2+} leakage or enhanced Ca^{2+} release during adrenergic stimulation, causing triggered arrhythmogenesis.
[8]HCN4 encodes a pacemaker current in sinoatrial nodal cells; mutations in sodium channel gene (SCN5A) cause conduction defects.
[9]PCCD, progressive cardiac conduction disorder.

In order for reentry to occur, three conditions must coexist, as indicated in Figure 14–6: (1) There must be an obstacle (anatomic or physiologic) to homogeneous conduction, thus establishing a circuit around which the reentrant wavefront can propagate; (2) there must be unidirectional block at some point in the circuit, ie conduction must die out in one direction but continue in the opposite direction (as shown in Figure 14–6, the impulse can gradually decrease as it invades progressively more depolarized tissue until it finally blocks—a process known as decremental conduction); and (3) conduction time around the circuit must be long enough so that the retrograde impulse does not enter refractory tissue as it travels around the obstacle, ie the conduction time must exceed the effective refractory period. Importantly, reentry depends on conduction that has been depressed by some critical amount, usually as a result of injury or ischemia. If conduction velocity is too slow, bidirectional block rather than unidirectional block occurs; if the reentering impulse is too weak, conduction may fail, or the impulse may arrive so late that it collides with the next regular impulse. On the other hand, if conduction is too rapid, ie almost normal, bidirectional conduction rather than unidirectional block will occur. Even in the presence of unidirec-

Figure 14–7. Electrocardiogram from a patient with the long QT syndrome during two episodes of torsade de pointes. The polymorphic ventricular tachycardia is seen at the start of this tracing and spontaneously halts at the middle of the panel. A single normal sinus beat (NSB) with an extremely prolonged QT interval follows, succeeded immediately by another episode of ventricular tachycardia of the torsade type. The usual symptoms would be dizziness or transient loss of consciousness.

tional block, if the impulse travels around the obstacle too rapidly, it will reach tissue that is still refractory.

Slowing of conduction may be due to depression of sodium current, depression of calcium current (the latter especially in the atrioventricular node), or both. Drugs that abolish reentry usually work by further slowing depressed conduction (by blocking the sodium or calcium current) and causing bidirectional block. In theory, accelerating conduction (by increasing sodium or calcium current) would also be effective, but only under unusual circumstances does this mechanism explain the action of any available drug.

Lengthening (or shortening) of the refractory period may also make reentry less likely. The longer the refractory period in tissue near the site of block, the greater the chance that the tissue will still be refractory when reentry is attempted. (Alternatively, the shorter the refractory period in the depressed region, the less likely it is that unidirectional block will occur.) Thus, increased dispersion of refractoriness is one contributor to reentry, and drugs may suppress arrhythmias by reducing such dispersion.

■ I. BASIC PHARMACOLOGY OF THE ANTIARRHYTHMIC AGENTS

Mechanisms of Action

Arrhythmias are caused by abnormal pacemaker activity or abnormal impulse propagation. Thus, the aim of ther-

apy of the arrhythmias is to reduce ectopic pacemaker activity and modify conduction or refractoriness in reentry circuits to disable circus movement. The major mechanisms currently available for accomplishing these goals are (1) sodium channel blockade, (2) blockade of sympathetic autonomic effects in the heart, (3) prolongation of the effective refractory period, and (4) calcium channel blockade.

Antiarrhythmic drugs decrease the automaticity of ectopic pacemakers more than that of the sinoatrial node. They also reduce conduction and excitability and increase the refractory period to a greater extent in depolarized tissue than in normally polarized tissue. This is accomplished chiefly by selectively blocking the sodium or calcium channels of depolarized cells (Figure 14–8). Therapeutically useful channel-blocking drugs bind readily to activated channels (ie, during phase 0) or inactivated channels (ie, during phase 2) but bind poorly or not at all to rested channels. Therefore, these drugs block electrical activity when there is a fast tachycardia (many channel activations and inactivations per unit time) or when there is significant loss of resting potential (many inactivated channels during rest). This type of drug action is often described as **use-dependent** or **state-dependent;** that is, channels that are being used frequently, or in an inactivated state, are more susceptible to block. Channels in normal cells that become blocked by a drug during normal activation-inactivation cycles will rapidly lose the drug from the receptors during the resting portion of the cycle (Figure 14–8). Channels in

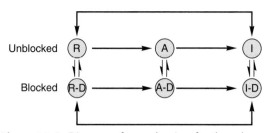

Unblocked   R ——→ A ——→ I
Blocked   R-D ——→ A-D ——→ I-D

Figure 14–8. Diagram of a mechanism for the selective depressant action of antiarrhythmic drugs on sodium channels. The upper portion of the figure shows the population of channels moving through a cycle of activity during an action potential in the absence of drugs: R (rested) → A (activated) → I (inactivated). Recovery takes place via the I → R pathway. Antiarrhythmic drugs (D) that act by blocking sodium channels can bind to their receptors in the channels, as shown by the vertical arrows, to form drug-channel complexes, indicated as R-D, A-D, and I-D. Binding of the drugs to the receptor varies with the state of the channel. The data available for a variety of sodium channel blockers indicate that the binding of the drugs to the active and inactivated channel receptor is much greater than the binding to the rested channel. Furthermore, recovery from the I-D state to the R-D state is much slower than from I to R. As a result, rapid activity (more activations and inactivations) and depolarization of the resting potential (more channels in the I state) will favor blockade of the channels and selectively suppress arrhythmic cells.

myocardium that is chronically depolarized (ie, has a resting potential more positive than −75 mV) will recover from block very slowly if at all (see also right panel, Figure 14–4).

In cells with abnormal automaticity, most of these drugs reduce the phase 4 slope by blocking either sodium or calcium channels, thereby reducing the ratio of sodium (or calcium) permeability to potassium permeability. As a result, the membrane potential during phase 4 stabilizes closer to the potassium equilibrium potential. In addition, some agents may increase the threshold (make it more positive). Beta-adrenoceptor–blocking drugs indirectly reduce the phase 4 slope by blocking the positive chronotropic action of norepinephrine in the heart.

In reentry arrhythmias, which depend on critically depressed conduction, most antiarrhythmic agents slow conduction further by one or both of two mechanisms: (1) steady-state reduction in the number of available unblocked channels, which reduces the excitatory currents to a level below that required for propagation (Figure 14–4, left); and (2) prolongation of recovery time of the channels still able to reach the rested and available state, which increases the effective refractory period (Figure 14–4, right). As a result, early extrasystoles are unable to propagate at all; later impulses propagate more slowly and are subject to bidirectional conduction block.

By these mechanisms, antiarrhythmic drugs can suppress ectopic automaticity and abnormal conduction occurring in depolarized cells—rendering them electrically silent—while minimally affecting the electrical activity in normally polarized parts of the heart. However, as dosage is increased, these agents also depress conduction in normal tissue, eventually resulting in *drug-induced* arrhythmias. Furthermore, a drug concentration that is therapeutic (antiarrhythmic) under the initial circumstances of treatment may become "proarrhythmic" (arrhythmogenic) during fast heart rates (more development of block), acidosis (slower recovery from block for most drugs), hyperkalemia, or ischemia.

■ II. SPECIFIC ANTIARRHYTHMIC AGENTS

The most widely used scheme for the classification of antiarrhythmic drug actions recognizes four classes:

1. Class 1 action is sodium channel blockade. Subclasses of this action reflect effects on the action potential duration (APD) and the kinetics of sodium channel blockade. Drugs with class 1A action prolong the APD and dissociate from the channel with intermediate kinetics; drugs with class 1B action shorten the APD in some tissues of the heart and dissociate from the channel with rapid kinetics; and drugs with class 1C action have minimal effects on the APD and dissociate from the channel with slow kinetics.

2. Class 2 action is sympatholytic. Drugs with this action reduce β-adrenergic activity in the heart.

3. Class 3 action is manifest by prolongation of the APD. Most drugs with this action block the rapid component of the delayed rectifier potassium current, I_{Kr}.

4. Class 4 action is blockade of the cardiac calcium current. This action slows conduction in regions where the action potential upstroke is calcium dependent, eg, the sinoatrial and atrioventricular nodes.

A given drug may have multiple classes of action as indicated by its membrane and electrocardiographic

Table 14–2. Membrane actions of antiarrhythmic drugs.

Drug	Block of Sodium Channels		Refractory Period		Calcium Channel Blockade	Effect on Pacemaker Activity	Sympatholytic Action
	Normal Cells	Depolarized Cells	Normal Cells	Depolarized Cells			
Adenosine	0	0	0	0	+	0	+
Amiodarone	+	+++	↑↑	↑↑	+	↓↓	+
Bretylium	0	0	↑↑↑	↑↑↑	0	↑↓[1]	++
Diltiazem	0	0	0	0	+++	↓↓	0
Disopyramide	+	+++	↑	↑↑	+	↓	0
Dofetilide	0	0	↑	?	0	0	0
Esmolol	0	+	0	NA[2]	0	↓↓	+++
Flecainide	+	+++	0	↑	0	↓↓	0
Ibutilide	0	0	↑	?	0	0	0
Lidocaine	0	+++	↓	↑↑	0	↓↓	0
Mexiletine	0	+++	0	↑↑	0	↓↓	0
Moricizine	+	++	↓	↓	0	↓↓	0
Procainamide	+	+++	↑	↑↑↑	0	↓	+
Propafenone	+	++	↑	↑↑	+	↓↓	+
Propranolol	0	+	↓	↑↑	0	↓↓	+++
Quinidine	+	++	↑	↑↑	0	↓↓	+
Sotalol	0	0	↑↑	↑↑↑	0	↓↓	++
Verapamil	0	+	0	↑	+++	↓↓	+

[1]Bretylium may transiently increase pacemaker rate by causing catecholamine release.
[2]Data not available.

(ECG) effects (Tables 14–2 and 14–3). For example, amiodarone shares all four classes of action. Drugs are usually discussed according to the predominant class of action. Certain antiarrhythmic agents, eg, adenosine and magnesium, do not fit readily into this scheme and are described separately.

SODIUM CHANNEL-BLOCKING DRUGS (CLASS 1)

PROCAINAMIDE (SUBGROUP 1A)

Cardiac Effects

By blocking sodium channels, procainamide slows the upstroke of the action potential, slows conduction, and prolongs the QRS duration of the ECG. The drug also prolongs the action potential duration by nonspecific blockade of potassium channels. The drug may be somewhat less effective than quinidine (see below) in suppressing abnormal ectopic pacemaker activity but more effective in blocking sodium channels in depolarized cells.

Procainamide

Procainamide has directly depressant actions on sinoatrial and atrioventricular nodes that are only slightly counterbalanced by drug-induced vagal block.

Extracardiac Effects

Procainamide has ganglion-blocking properties. This action reduces peripheral vascular resistance and can

Table 14–3. Clinical pharmacologic properties of antiarrhythmic drugs.

Drug	Effect on SA Nodal Rate	Effect on AV Nodal Refractory Period	PR Interval	QRS Duration	QT Interval	Usefulness in Arrhythmias Supra–ventricular	Ventricular	Half-Life
Adenosine	↓,↑	↑↑↑	↑↑↑	0	0	++++	?	< 10 s
Amiodarone	↓↓[1]	↑	Variable	↑	↑↑↑↑	+++	+++	(weeks)
Bretylium	↑↓[2]	↑↓[2]	0	0	0	0	+	
Diltiazem	↑↓	↑↑	↑	0	0	+++	–	4–8 h
Disopyramide	↑↓[1,3]	↑↓[3]	↑↓[3]	↑↑	↑↑	+	+++	7–8 h
Dofetilide	↓(?)	0	0	0	↑↑	++	None	7 h
Esmolol	↓↓	↑↑	↑↑	0	0	+	+	10 min
Flecainide	None,↓	↑	↑	↑↑↑	0	+[4]	++++	20 h
Ibutilide	↓(?)	0	0	0	↑↑	++	?	6 h
Lidocaine	None[1]	None	0	0	0	None[5]	+++	1–2 h
Mexiletine	None[1]	None	0	0	0	None	+++	12 h
Moricizine	None	None	↑	↑↑	0	None	+++	2–6 h[6]
Procainamide	↓[1]	↑↓[3]	↑↓[3]	↑↑	↑↑	+	+++	3–4 h
Propafenone	0,↓	↑	↑	↑↑↑	0	+	+++	5–7 h
Propranolol	↓↓	↑↑	↑↑	0	0	+	+	5 h
Quinidine	↑↓[1,3]	↑↓[3]	↑↓[3]	↑↑	↑↑	+	+++	6 h
Sotalol	↓↓	↑↑	↑↑	0	↑↑↑	+++	+++	7 h
Verapamil	↓↓	↑↑	↑↑	0	0	+++	–	7 h

[1]May suppress diseased sinus nodes.
[2]Initial stimulation by release of endogenous norepinephrine followed by depression.
[3]Anticholinergic effect and direct depressant action.
[4]Especially in Wolff-Parkinson-White syndrome.
[5]May be effective in atrial arrhythmias caused by digitalis.
[6]Half-life of active metabolites much longer.

cause hypotension, particularly with intravenous use. However, in therapeutic concentrations, its peripheral vascular effects are less prominent than those of quinidine. Hypotension is usually associated with excessively rapid procainamide infusion or the presence of severe underlying left ventricular dysfunction.

Toxicity

A. CARDIAC

Procainamide's cardiotoxic effects include excessive action potential prolongation, QT interval prolongation, and induction of torsade de pointes arrhythmia and syncope. Excessive slowing of conduction can also occur. New arrhythmias can be precipitated.

B. EXTRACARDIAC

The most troublesome adverse effect of long-term procainamide therapy is a syndrome resembling lupus erythematosus and usually consisting of arthralgia and arthritis. In some patients, pleuritis, pericarditis, or parenchymal pulmonary disease also occurs. Renal lupus is rarely induced by procainamide. During long-term therapy, serologic abnormalities (eg, increased antinuclear antibody titer) occur in nearly all patients, and in the absence of symptoms these are not an indication to stop drug therapy. Approximately one third of patients receiving long-term procainamide therapy develop these reversible lupus-related symptoms.

Other adverse effects include nausea and diarrhea (about 10% of cases), rash, fever, hepatitis (< 5%), and agranulocytosis (approximately 0.2%).

Pharmacokinetics & Dosage

Procainamide can be administered safely by the intravenous and intramuscular routes and is well absorbed orally. A metabolite (*N*-acetylprocainamide, NAPA) has class 3 activity. Excessive accumulation of NAPA has been implicated in torsade de pointes during procainamide therapy, especially in patients with renal failure. Some individuals rapidly acetylate procainamide and develop high levels of NAPA. The lupus syndrome appears to be less common in these patients.

Procainamide is eliminated by hepatic metabolism to NAPA and by renal elimination. Its half-life is only 3–4 hours, which necessitates frequent dosing or use of a slow-release formulation (the usual practice). NAPA is eliminated by the kidneys. Thus, procainamide dosage must be reduced in patients with renal failure. The reduced volume of distribution and renal clearance associated with heart failure also require reduction in dosage. The half-life of NAPA is considerably longer than that of procainamide, and it therefore accumulates more slowly. Thus, it is important to measure plasma levels of both procainamide and NAPA, especially in patients with circulatory or renal impairment.

If a rapid procainamide effect is needed, an intravenous loading dose of up to 12 mg/kg can be given at a rate of 0.3 mg/kg/min or less rapidly. This dose is followed by a maintenance dosage of 2–5 mg/min, with careful monitoring of plasma levels. The risk of gastrointestinal or cardiac toxicity rises at plasma concentrations greater than 8 mcg/mL or NAPA concentrations greater than 20 mcg/mL.

In order to control ventricular arrhythmias, a total procainamide dosage of 2–5 g/d is usually required. In an occasional patient who accumulates high levels of NAPA, less frequent dosing may be possible. This is also possible in renal disease, where procainamide elimination is slowed.

Therapeutic Use

Procainamide is effective against most atrial and ventricular arrhythmias. However, many clinicians attempt to avoid long-term therapy because of the requirement for frequent dosing and the common occurrence of lupus-related effects. Procainamide is the drug of second choice (after lidocaine) in most coronary care units for the treatment of sustained ventricular arrhythmias associated with acute myocardial infarction.

QUINIDINE (SUBGROUP 1A)

Cardiac Effects

Quinidine has actions similar to those of procainamide: it slows the upstroke of the action potential and con-

duction, and prolongs the QRS duration of the ECG, by blockade of sodium channels. The drug also prolongs the action potential duration by nonspecific blockade of potassium channels. It has more pronounced cardiac antimuscarinic effects than procainamide. Its toxic cardiac effects include excessive QT interval prolongation and induction of torsade de pointes arrhythmia. Toxic concentrations of quinidine also produce excessive sodium channel blockade with slowed conduction throughout the heart.

Quinidine

Extracardiac Effects

Gastrointestinal side effects of diarrhea, nausea, and vomiting are observed in one third to one half of patients. A syndrome of headache, dizziness, and tinnitus (**cinchonism**) is observed at toxic drug concentrations. Idiosyncratic or immunologic reactions, including thrombocytopenia, hepatitis, angioneurotic edema, and fever, are observed rarely.

Pharmacokinetics

Quinidine is absorbed readily following oral administration, bound to albumin and α_1-acid glycoprotein, and eliminated primarily by hepatic metabolism. The elimination half-life is 6–8 hours. Quinidine is usually administered in a slow release formulation, eg, that of the gluconate salt.

Therapeutic Use

Quinidine is used only occasionally to maintain normal sinus rhythm in patients with atrial flutter/fibrillation. Because of its cardiac and extracardiac side effects, its use is now largely restricted to patients with normal (but arrhythmic) hearts. In randomized, controlled clinical trials, quinidine-treated patients are twice as likely to remain in normal sinus rhythm compared with controls, but the risk of death is increased two- to threefold. Quinidine is used rarely in patients with ventricular tachycardia. Quinidine is the optical isomer of quinine and is sometimes used intravenously for the treatment of acute, severe malaria (see Chapter 53).

DISOPYRAMIDE (SUBGROUP 1A)

Cardiac Effects

The effects of disopyramide are very similar to those of procainamide and quinidine. Its cardiac antimuscarinic effects are even more marked than those of quinidine. Therefore, a drug that slows atrioventricular conduction should be administered with disopyramide when treating atrial flutter or fibrillation.

Disopyramide

Toxicity

A. CARDIAC

Toxic concentrations of disopyramide can precipitate all of the electrophysiologic disturbances described under quinidine. As a result of its negative inotropic effect, disopyramide may precipitate heart failure de novo or in patients with preexisting depression of left ventricular function. Because of this effect, disopyramide is not used as a first-line antiarrhythmic agent in the USA. It should not be used in patients with heart failure.

B. EXTRACARDIAC

Disopyramide's atropine-like activity accounts for most of its symptomatic adverse effects: urinary retention (most often, but not exclusively, in male patients with prostatic hyperplasia), dry mouth, blurred vision, constipation, and worsening of preexisting glaucoma. These effects may require discontinuation of the drug.

Pharmacokinetics & Dosage

In the USA, disopyramide is only available for oral use. The usual oral dosage of disopyramide is 150 mg three times a day, but as much as 1 g/d has been used. In patients with renal impairment, dosage must be reduced. Because of the danger of precipitating heart failure, the use of loading doses is not recommended.

Therapeutic Use

Although disopyramide has been shown to be effective in a variety of supraventricular arrhythmias, in the USA it is approved only for the treatment of ventricular arrhythmias.

LIDOCAINE (SUBGROUP 1B)

Lidocaine has a low incidence of toxicity and a high degree of effectiveness in arrhythmias associated with acute myocardial infarction. It is used only by the intravenous route.

Lidocaine

Cardiac Effects

Lidocaine blocks activated and inactivated sodium channels with rapid kinetics (Figure 14–9); the inactivated state block ensures greater effects on cells with long action potentials such as Purkinje and ventricular cells, compared with atrial cells. The rapid kinetics at normal resting potentials result in recovery from block between action potentials and no effect on conduction. The increased inactivation and slower unbinding kinetics result in the selective depression of conduction in depolarized cells.

Toxicity

A. CARDIAC

Lidocaine is one of the least cardiotoxic of the currently used sodium channel blockers. Proarrhythmic effects, including sinoatrial node arrest, worsening of impaired conduction, and ventricular arrhythmias, are uncommon with lidocaine use. In large doses, especially in patients with preexisting heart failure, lidocaine may cause hypotension—partly by depressing myocardial contractility.

B. EXTRACARDIAC

Lidocaine's most common adverse effects—like those of other local anesthetics—are neurologic: paresthesias, tremor, nausea of central origin, lightheadedness, hearing disturbances, slurred speech, and convulsions. These occur most commonly in elderly or otherwise vulnerable patients or when a bolus of the drug is given too rapidly. The effects are dose-related and usually short-lived; seizures respond to intravenous diazepam. In general, if plasma levels above 9 mcg/mL are avoided, lidocaine is well tolerated.

Figure 14–9. Computer simulation of the effect of resting membrane potential on the blocking and unblocking of sodium channels by lidocaine. **Upper tracing:** Action potentials in a ventricular muscle cell. **Lower tracing:** Percentage of channels blocked by the drug. As the membrane depolarizes through -80, -75, and -70 mV, an 800 ms time segment is shown. Extra passage of time is indicated by breaks in the traces. **Left side:** At the normal resting potential of -85 mV, the drug combines with open (activated) and inactivated channels during each action potential, but block is rapidly reversed during diastole because the affinity of the drug for its receptor is so low when the channel recovers to the resting state at -85 mV. **Middle:** Metabolic injury has occurred, eg, ischemia due to coronary occlusion, that causes gradual depolarization over time. With subsequent action potentials arising from more depolarized potentials, the fraction of channels blocked increases because more channels remain in the inactivated state at less negative potentials (Figure 14–4, left), and the time constant for unblocking during diastole rapidly increases at less negative resting potentials (Figure 14–4, right). **Right:** Because of marked drug binding, conduction block and loss of excitability in this tissue result; that is, the "sick" (depolarized) tissue is selectively suppressed.

Pharmacokinetics & Dosage

Because of its extensive first-pass hepatic metabolism, only 3% of orally administered lidocaine appears in the plasma. Thus, lidocaine must be given parenterally. Lidocaine has a half-life of 1–2 hours. In adults, a loading dose of 150–200 mg administered over about 15 minutes (as a single infusion or as a series of slow boluses) should be followed by a maintenance infusion

of 2–4 mg/min to achieve a therapeutic plasma level of 2–6 mcg/mL. Determination of lidocaine plasma levels is of great value in adjusting the infusion rate. Occasional patients with myocardial infarction or other acute illness require (and tolerate) higher concentrations. This may be due to increased plasma α_1-acid glycoprotein, an acute phase reactant protein that binds lidocaine, making less free drug available to exert its pharmacologic effects.

In patients with heart failure, lidocaine's volume of distribution and total body clearance may both be decreased. Thus, both loading and maintenance doses should be decreased. Since these effects counterbalance each other, the half-life may not be increased as much as predicted from clearance changes alone. In patients with liver disease, plasma clearance is markedly reduced and the volume of distribution is often increased; the elimination half-life in such cases may be increased threefold or more. In liver disease, the maintenance dose should be decreased, but usual loading doses can be given. Elimination half-life determines the time to steady state. Thus, while steady-state concentrations may be achieved in 8–10 hours in normal patients and patients with heart failure, 24–36 hours may be required in those with liver disease. Drugs that decrease liver blood flow (eg, propranolol, cimetidine) reduce lidocaine clearance and so increase the risk of toxicity unless infusion rates are decreased. With infusions lasting more than 24 hours, clearance falls and plasma concentrations rise. Renal disease has no major effect on lidocaine disposition.

Therapeutic Use

Lidocaine is the agent of choice for termination of ventricular tachycardia and prevention of ventricular fibrillation after cardioversion in the setting of acute ischemia. However, routine *prophylactic* use of lidocaine in this setting may actually increase total mortality, possibly by increasing the incidence of asystole, and is not the standard of care. Most physicians administer IV lidocaine only to patients with arrhythmias.

MEXILETINE (SUBGROUP 1B)

Mexiletine is an orally active congener of lidocaine. Its electrophysiologic and antiarrhythmic actions are similar to those of lidocaine. (The anticonvulsant phenytoin [see Chapter 24] also exerts similar electrophysiologic effects and has been used as an antiarrhythmic.) Mexiletine is used in the treatment of ventricular arrhythmias. The elimination half-life is 8–20 hours and permits administration two or three times a day. The usual daily dosage of mexiletine is 600–1200 mg/d. Dose-related adverse effects are seen frequently at therapeutic dosage. These are predominantly neurologic, including tremor, blurred vision, and lethargy. Nausea is also a common effect.

Mexiletine

Mexiletine has also shown significant efficacy in relieving chronic pain, especially pain due to diabetic neuropathy and nerve injury. The usual dosage is 450–750 mg/d orally. This application is unlabeled.

FLECAINIDE (SUBGROUP 1C)

Flecainide is a potent blocker of sodium and potassium channels with slow unblocking kinetics. (Note that although it does block certain potassium channels, it does not prolong the action potential or the QT interval.) It is currently used for patients with otherwise normal hearts who have supraventricular arrhythmias. It has no antimuscarinic effects.

Flecainide

Flecainide is very effective in suppressing premature ventricular contractions. However, it may cause severe exacerbation of arrhythmia even when normal doses are administered to patients with preexisting ventricular tachyarrhythmias and those with a previous myocardial infarction and ventricular ectopy. This was dramatically demonstrated in the Cardiac Arrhythmia Suppression Trial (CAST), which was terminated prematurely because of a two and one-half-fold increase in mortality in the patients receiving flecainide and similar Group 1c drugs. Flecainide is well absorbed and has a half-life of approximately 20 hours. Elimination is both by hepatic metabolism and by the kidney. The usual dosage of flecainide is 100–200 mg twice a day.

PROPAFENONE (SUBGROUP 1C)

Propafenone has some structural similarities to propranolol and possesses weak β-blocking activity. Its spectrum of action is very similar to that of quinidine. Its sodium channel blocking kinetics are similar to that of flecainide. Propafenone is metabolized in the liver, with an average half-life of 5–7 hours. The usual daily dosage of propafenone is 450–900 mg in three doses. The drug is used primarily for supraventricular arrhythmias. The most common adverse effects are a metallic taste and constipation; arrhythmia exacerbation can occur.

MORICIZINE (SUBGROUP 1C)

Moricizine is an antiarrhythmic phenothiazine derivative that is used for treatment of ventricular arrhythmias. It is a relatively potent sodium channel blocker that does not prolong action potential duration.

Moricizine has multiple metabolites, some of which are probably active and have long half-lives. Its most common adverse effects are dizziness and nausea. Like other potent sodium channel blockers, it can exacerbate arrhythmias. The usual dosage of moricizine is 200–300 mg by mouth three times a day.

BETA-ADRENOCEPTOR–BLOCKING DRUGS (CLASS 2)

Cardiac Effects

Propranolol and similar drugs have antiarrhythmic properties by virtue of their β-receptor–blocking action and direct membrane effects. As described in Chapter 10, some of these drugs have selectivity for cardiac β_1 receptors, some have intrinsic sympathomimetic activity, some have marked direct membrane effects, and some prolong the cardiac action potential. The relative contributions of the β-blocking and direct membrane effects to the antiarrhythmic effects of these drugs are not fully known. Although β blockers are fairly well tolerated, their efficacy for suppression of ventricular ectopic depolarizations is lower than that of sodium channel blockers. However, there is good evidence that these agents can prevent recurrent infarction and sudden death in patients recovering from acute myocardial infarction (see Chapter 10).

Esmolol is a short-acting β blocker used primarily as an antiarrhythmic drug for intraoperative and other acute arrhythmias. See Chapter 10 for more information. **Sotalol** is a nonselective β-blocking drug that prolongs the action potential (class 3 action).

DRUGS THAT PROLONG EFFECTIVE REFRACTORY PERIOD BY PROLONGING ACTION POTENTIAL (CLASS 3)

These drugs prolong action potentials, usually by blocking potassium channels in cardiac muscle or by enhancing inward current, eg, through sodium channels. Action potential prolongation by most of these drugs often exhibits the undesirable property of "reverse use-dependence": action potential prolongation is least marked at fast rates (where it is desirable) and most marked at slow rates, where it can contribute to the risk of torsade de pointes.

AMIODARONE

In the USA, amiodarone is approved for oral and intravenous use to treat serious ventricular arrhythmias. However, the drug is also highly effective for the treatment of supraventricular arrhythmias such as atrial fibrillation. Amiodarone has a broad spectrum of cardiac actions, unusual pharmacokinetics, and important extracardiac adverse effects. Dronedarone, an analog that lacks iodine atoms, is under investigation.

Amiodarone

Cardiac Effects

Amiodarone markedly prolongs the action potential duration (and the QT interval on the ECG) by blockade of I_{Kr}. During chronic administration, I_{Ks} is also blocked. The action potential duration is prolonged uniformly over a wide range of heart rates; that is, the drug does not have reverse use-dependent action. In spite of its present classification as a class 3 agent, amiodarone also significantly blocks inactivated sodium channels. Its action potential prolonging action reinforces this effect. Amiodarone also has weak adrenergic and calcium channel blocking actions. Consequences of these actions include slowing of the heart rate and atrioventricular node conduction. The broad spectrum of actions may account for its relatively high efficacy and low incidence of torsade de pointes despite significant QT interval prolongation.

Extracardiac Effects

Amiodarone causes peripheral vasodilation. This action is prominent following intravenous administration and may be related to the action of the vehicle.

Toxicity

A. CARDIAC

Amiodarone may produce symptomatic bradycardia and heart block in patients with preexisting sinus or atrioventricular node disease.

B. EXTRACARDIAC

Amiodarone accumulates in many tissues, including the heart (10–50 times greater than plasma), lung, liver, and skin, and is concentrated in tears. Dose-related pulmonary toxicity is the most important adverse effect. Even on a low dose of $\leq$ 200 mg/d, fatal pulmonary fibrosis may be observed in 1% of patients. Abnormal liver function tests and hepatitis may develop during amiodarone treatment. The skin deposits result in a photodermatitis and a gray-blue skin discoloration in sun-exposed areas, eg, the malar regions. After a few weeks of treatment, asymptomatic corneal microdeposits are present in virtually all patients treated with amiodarone. Halos develop in the peripheral visual fields of some patients. Drug discontinuation is usually not required. Rarely, an optic neuritis may progress to blindness.

Amiodarone blocks the peripheral conversion of thyroxine (T_4) to triiodothyronine (T_3). It is also a potential source of large amounts of inorganic iodine. Amiodarone may result in hypothyroidism or hyperthyroidism. Thyroid function should be evaluated prior to initiation of treatment and monitored periodically. Because effects have been described in virtually every organ system, amiodarone treatment should be reevaluated whenever new symptoms develop in a patient, including arrhythmia aggravation.

Pharmacokinetics

Amiodarone is variably absorbed with a bioavailability of 35–65%. It undergoes hepatic metabolism, and the major metabolite, desethylamiodarone, is bioactive. The elimination half-life is complex, with a rapid component of 3–10 days (50% of the drug) and a slower component of several weeks. Following discontinuation of the drug, effects are maintained for 1–3 months. Measurable tissue levels may be observed up to 1 year after discontinuation. A total loading dose of 10 g is usually achieved with 0.8–1.2 g daily doses. The maintenance dose is 200–400 mg daily. Pharmacologic effects may be achieved rapidly by intravenous loading. QT-prolonging effect is modest with this route of administration, whereas bradycardia and atrioventricular block may be significant.

Amiodarone has many important drug interactions and all medications should be reviewed during drug initiation or dose adjustments. Amiodarone is a substrate for the liver cytochrome metabolizing enzyme CYP3A4 and its levels are increased by drugs that inhibit this enzyme, eg, the histamine H_2 blocker cimetidine. Drugs that induce CYP3A4, eg, rifampin, decrease amiodarone concentration when coadministered. Amiodarone inhibits the other liver cytochrome metabolizing enzymes and may result in high levels of drugs that are substrates for these enzymes, eg, digoxin and warfarin.

Therapeutic Use

Low doses (100–200 mg/d) of amiodarone are effective in maintaining normal sinus rhythm in patients with atrial fibrillation. The drug is effective in the prevention of recurrent ventricular tachycardia. Its use is not associated with an increase in mortality in patients with coronary artery disease or heart failure. In many centers, the implanted cardioverter-defibrillator (ICD) has succeeded drug therapy as the primary treatment modality for ventricular tachycardia, but amiodarone may be used for ventricular tachycardia as adjuvant therapy to decrease the frequency of uncomfortable ICD discharges. The drug increases the pacing and defibrillation threshold and these devices require retesting after a maintenance dose has been achieved.

BRETYLIUM

Bretylium was first introduced as an antihypertensive agent. It interferes with the neuronal release of catecholamines but also has direct antiarrhythmic properties.

Cardiac & Extracardiac Effects

Bretylium lengthens the ventricular (but not the atrial) action potential duration and effective refractory period. This effect is most pronounced in ischemic cells, which have shortened action potential durations. Thus, bretylium may reverse the shortening of action potential duration caused by ischemia.

Since bretylium causes an initial release of catecholamines, it has some positive inotropic actions when first administered. This action may also *precipitate* ventricular arrhythmias and must be watched for at the onset of therapy with the drug.

The drug's sympathoplegic actions may result in postural hypotension. This effect can be almost totally prevented by concomitant administration of a tricyclic antidepressant agent such as protriptyline. Nausea and vomiting may occur after the intravenous administration of a bolus of bretylium.

Pharmacokinetics & Dosage

Bretylium is available only for intravenous use in the USA. In adults, an intravenous bolus of bretylium tosylate, 5 mg/kg, is administered over a 10-minute period. This dosage may be repeated after 30 minutes. Maintenance therapy is achieved by a similar bolus every 4–6 hours or by a constant infusion of 0.5–2 mg/min.

Therapeutic Use

Bretylium is rarely used and then only in an emergency setting, often during attempted resuscitation from ventricular fibrillation when lidocaine and cardioversion have failed. In most centers amiodarone is preferred for this indication.

SOTALOL

Sotalol has both β-adrenergic receptor-blocking (class 2) and action potential prolonging (class 3) actions. The drug is formulated as a racemic mixture of *d*- and *l*-sotalol. All the β-adrenergic blocking activity resides in the *l*-isomer; the *d*- and *l*-isomers share action potential prolonging actions. Beta-adrenergic blocking action is not cardioselective and is maximal at doses below those required for action potential prolongation.

Sotalol

Sotalol is well absorbed orally with bioavailability of approximately 100%. It is not metabolized in the liver and it is not bound to plasma proteins. Excretion is predominantly by the kidneys in the unchanged form with a half-life of approximately 12 hours. Because of its relatively simple pharmacokinetics, it exhibits few direct drug interactions. Its most significant cardiac adverse effect is an extension of its pharmacologic action: a dose-related incidence of torsade de pointes that approaches 6% at the highest recommended daily dose. Patients with overt heart failure may experience further depression of left ventricular function during treatment with sotalol.

Sotalol is approved for the treatment of life-threatening ventricular arrhythmias and the maintenance of sinus rhythm in patients with atrial fibrillation. It is also approved for treatment of supraventricular and ventricular arrhythmias in the pediatric age group. Sotalol decreases the threshold for cardiac defibrillation.

DOFETILIDE

Dofetilide has class 3 action potential prolonging action. This action is effected by a dose-dependent blockade of the rapid component of the delayed rectifier potassium current, I_{Kr}. Dofetilide block of I_{Kr} increases in hypokalemia. Dofetilide produces no relevant blockade of the other potassium channels or the sodium channel. Because of the slow rate of recovery from blockade, the extent of blockade shows little dependence on stimulation frequency. However, dofetilide does show less action potential prolongation at rapid rates because of the increased importance of other potassium channels such as I_{Ks} at higher frequencies.

Dofetilide is 100% bioavailable. Verapamil increases peak plasma dofetilide concentration by increasing intestinal blood flow. Eighty percent of an oral dose is eliminated by the kidneys unchanged; the remainder is eliminated in the urine as inactive metabolites. Inhibitors of the renal cation secretion mechanism, eg, cimetidine, prolong the half-life of dofetilide. Since the QT-prolonging effects and risks of ventricular proarrhythmia are directly related to plasma concentration, dofetilide dosage must be based on the estimated creatinine clearance. Treatment with dofetilide should be initiated in hospital after baseline measurement of the rate-corrected QT interval (QT_C) and serum electrolytes. A baseline QT_C of > 450 ms (500 ms in the presence of an intraventricular conduction delay), bradycardia of < 50 beats/min, and hypokalemia are relative contraindications to its use.

Dofetilide is approved for the maintenance of normal sinus rhythm in patients with atrial fibrillation. It is also effective in restoring normal sinus rhythm in patients with atrial fibrillation.

IBUTILIDE

Ibutilide slows cardiac repolarization by blockade of the rapid component of the delayed rectifier potassium current. Activation of slow inward sodium current has also been suggested as an additional mechanism of action. After intravenous administration, ibutilide is rapidly cleared from the plasma by hepatic metabolism. The metabolites are excreted by the kidney. The elimination half-life averages 6 hours.

Intravenous ibutilide is used for the acute conversion of atrial flutter and atrial fibrillation to normal sinus rhythm. The drug is more effective in atrial flutter than fibrillation, with a mean time to termination of 20 minutes. The most important adverse effect is excessive QT interval prolongation and torsade de pointes. Patients require continuous ECG monitoring for 4 hours following ibutilide infusion or until QT_C returns to baseline.

CALCIUM CHANNEL–BLOCKING DRUGS (CLASS 4)

These drugs, of which verapamil is the prototype, were first introduced as antianginal agents and are discussed in greater detail in Chapter 12. Verapamil and diltiazem also have antiarrhythmic effects.

VERAPAMIL

Cardiac Effects

Verapamil blocks both activated and inactivated L-type calcium channels. Thus, its effect is more marked in tissues that fire frequently, those that are less completely polarized at rest, and those in which activation depends exclusively on the calcium current, such as the sinoatrial and atrioventricular nodes. Atrioventricular nodal conduction time and effective refractory period are invariably prolonged by therapeutic concentrations. Verapamil usually slows the sinoatrial node by its direct action, but its hypotensive action may occasionally result in a small reflex increase of sinoatrial nodal rate.

Verapamil can suppress both early and delayed afterdepolarizations and may antagonize slow responses arising in severely depolarized tissue.

Extracardiac Effects

Verapamil causes peripheral vasodilation, which may be beneficial in hypertension and peripheral vasospastic disorders. Its effects upon smooth muscle produce a number of extracardiac effects (see Chapter 12).

Toxicity

A. CARDIAC

Verapamil's cardiotoxic effects are dose-related and usually avoidable. A common error has been to administer intravenous verapamil to a patient with ventricular tachycardia misdiagnosed as supraventricular tachycardia. In this setting, hypotension and ventricular fibrillation can occur. Verapamil's negative inotropic effects may limit its clinical usefulness in diseased hearts (see Chapter 12). Verapamil can induce atrioventricular block when used in large doses or in patients with atrioventricular nodal disease. This block can be treated with atropine and β-receptor stimulants. In patients with sinus node disease, verapamil can precipitate sinus arrest.

B. EXTRACARDIAC

Adverse effects include constipation, lassitude, nervousness, and peripheral edema.

Pharmacokinetics & Dosage

The half-life of verapamil is approximately 7 hours. It is extensively metabolized by the liver; after oral administration, its bioavailability is only about 20%. Therefore, verapamil must be administered with caution in patients with hepatic dysfunction.

In adult patients without heart failure or sinoatrial or atrioventricular nodal disease, parenteral verapamil can be used to terminate supraventricular tachycardia, although adenosine is the agent of first choice. Verapamil dosage is an initial bolus of 5 mg administered over 2–5 minutes, followed a few minutes later by a second 5 mg bolus if needed. Thereafter, doses of 5–10 mg can be administered every 4–6 hours, or a constant infusion of 0.4 mcg/kg/min may be used.

Effective oral dosages are higher than intravenous dosage because of first-pass metabolism and range from 120 to 640 mg daily, divided into three or four doses.

Therapeutic Use

Supraventricular tachycardia is the major arrhythmia indication for verapamil. Adenosine or verapamil are preferred over older treatments (propranolol, digoxin, edrophonium, vasoconstrictor agents, and cardioversion) for termination. Verapamil can also reduce the ventricular rate in atrial fibrillation and flutter. It only rarely converts atrial flutter and fibrillation to sinus rhythm. Verapamil is occasionally useful in ventricular arrhythmias. However, the use of intravenous verapamil in a patient with sustained ventricular tachycardia can cause hemodynamic collapse.

DILTIAZEM

Diltiazem appears to be similar in efficacy to verapamil in the management of supraventricular arrhythmias, including rate control in atrial fibrillation. An intravenous form of diltiazem is available for the latter indication and causes hypotension or bradyarrhythmias relatively infrequently.

MISCELLANEOUS ANTIARRHYTHMIC AGENTS

Certain agents used for the treatment of arrhythmias do not fit the conventional class 1–4 organization. These include digitalis (discussed in Chapter 13), adenosine, magnesium, and potassium.

ADENOSINE

Mechanism & Clinical Use

Adenosine is a nucleoside that occurs naturally throughout the body. Its half-life in the blood is less than 10 seconds. Its mechanism of action involves activation of an inward rectifier K^+ current and inhibition of calcium current. The results of these actions are marked hyperpolarization and suppression of calcium-dependent action potentials. When given as a bolus dose, adenosine directly inhibits atrioventricular nodal conduction and increases the atrioventricular nodal refractory period but has lesser effects on the sinoatrial node. Adenosine is currently the drug of choice for prompt conversion of paroxysmal supraventricular tachycardia to sinus rhythm because of its high efficacy (90–95%) and very short duration of action. It is usually given in a bolus dose of 6 mg followed, if necessary, by a dose

of 12 mg. An uncommon variant of ventricular tachycardia is adenosine sensitive. The drug is less effective in the presence of adenosine receptor blockers such as theophylline or caffeine, and its effects are potentiated by adenosine uptake inhibitors such as dipyridamole.

Toxicity

Adenosine causes flushing in about 20% of patients and shortness of breath or chest burning (perhaps related to bronchospasm) in over 10%. Induction of high-grade atrioventricular block may occur but is very short-lived. Atrial fibrillation may occur. Less common toxicities include headache, hypotension, nausea, and paresthesias.

MAGNESIUM

Originally used for patients with digitalis-induced arrhythmias who were hypomagnesemic, magnesium infusion has been found to have antiarrhythmic effects in some patients with normal serum magnesium levels. The mechanisms of these effects are not known, but magnesium is recognized to influence Na^+/K^+ ATPase, sodium channels, certain potassium channels, and calcium channels. Magnesium therapy appears to be indicated in patients with digitalis-induced arrhythmias if hypomagnesemia is present; it is also indicated in some patients with torsade de pointes even if serum magnesium is normal. The usual dosage is 1 g (as sulfate) given intravenously over 20 minutes and repeated once if necessary. A full understanding of the action and indications of magnesium as an antiarrhythmic drug awaits further investigation.

POTASSIUM

The significance of the potassium ion concentrations inside and outside the cardiac cell membrane has been discussed earlier in this chapter. The effects of increasing serum K^+ can be summarized as (1) a resting potential depolarizing action and (2) a membrane potential stabilizing action, the latter caused by increased potassium permeability. Hypokalemia results in an increased risk of early and delayed afterdepolarizations, and ectopic pacemaker activity, especially in the presence of digitalis; hyperkalemia depresses ectopic pacemakers (severe hyperkalemia is required to suppress the sinoatrial node) and slows conduction. Because both insufficient and excess potassium are potentially arrhythmogenic, potassium therapy is directed toward normalizing potassium gradients and pools in the body.

ANTIARRHYTHMIC DRUG-USE PRINCIPLES APPLIED TO ATRIAL FIBRILLATION

Atrial fibrillation is the most common sustained arrhythmia observed clinically. Its prevalence increases from ~ 0.5% in individuals younger than 65 years of age to 10% in individuals older than 80. Diagnosis is usually straightforward by means of an ECG. The ECG may also enable the identification of a prior myocardial infarction, left ventricular hypertrophy, and ventricular pre-excitation. Hyperthyroidism is an important treatable cause of atrial fibrillation, and a thyroid panel should be obtained at the time of diagnosis to exclude this possibility. With the clinical history and physical examination as a guide, the presence and extent of the underlying heart disease should be evaluated, preferably using noninvasive techniques such as echocardiography.

Treatment of atrial fibrillation is initiated to relieve patient symptoms and prevent the complications of thromboembolism and tachycardia-induced heart failure, the result of prolonged uncontrolled heart rates. The initial treatment objective is control of the ventricular response. This is usually achieved by use of a calcium channel blocking drug alone or in combination with a β-adrenergic blocker. Digoxin may be of value in the presence of heart failure. A second objective is a restoration and maintenance of normal sinus rhythm. Several studies show that rate control (maintenance of ventricular rate in the range of 60–80 beats/min) has a better benefit-to-risk outcome than rhythm control (conversion to normal sinus rhythm) in the long-term health of patients with atrial fibrillation. If rhythm control is deemed desirable, sinus rhythm is usually restored by DC cardioversion in the USA; in some countries, a class 1 antiarrhythmic drug is used initially. For patients with paroxysmal atrial fibrillation, normal sinus rhythm may be restored with a single large oral dose of propafenone or flecainide, provided that safety is initially documented in a monitored setting. Intravenous ibutilide can restore sinus rhythm promptly. For restoration of sinus rhythm in an emergency, eg, atrial fibrillation associated with hypotension or angina, DC cardioversion is the preferred modality. A class 1 or class 3 antiarrhythmic drug is used to maintain normal sinus rhythm.

■ III. PRINCIPLES IN THE CLINICAL USE OF ANTIARRHYTHMIC AGENTS

The margin between efficacy and toxicity is particularly narrow for antiarrhythmic drugs. Risks and benefits must be carefully considered (see Box, Antiarrhythmic Drug-Use Principles Applied to Atrial Fibrillation).

Pretreatment Evaluation

Several important determinations must be made prior to initiation of any antiarrhythmic therapy:

(1) Eliminate the cause if possible. Precipitating factors must be recognized and eliminated if possible. These include not only abnormalities of internal homeostasis, such as hypoxia or electrolyte abnormalities (especially hypokalemia or hypomagnesemia), but also drug therapy and underlying disease states such as hyperthyroidism or underlying cardiac disease. It is important to separate this abnormal substrate from triggering factors, such as myocardial ischemia or acute cardiac dilation, which may be treatable and reversible.

(2) Make a firm diagnosis. A firm arrhythmia diagnosis should be established. For example, the misuse of verapamil in patients with ventricular tachycardia mistakenly diagnosed as supraventricular tachycardia can lead to catastrophic hypotension and cardiac arrest. As increasingly sophisticated methods to characterize underlying arrhythmia mechanisms become available and are validated, it may be possible to direct certain drugs toward specific arrhythmia mechanisms.

(3) Determine the baseline condition. A reliable baseline should be established against which to judge the efficacy of any subsequent antiarrhythmic intervention. Several methods are now available for such baseline quantitation. These include prolonged ambulatory monitoring, electrophysiologic studies that reproduce a target arrhythmia, reproduction of a target arrhythmia by treadmill exercise, or the use of transtelephonic monitoring for recording of sporadic but symptomatic arrhythmias.

(4) Question the need for therapy. The mere identification of an abnormality of cardiac rhythm does not necessarily require that the arrhythmia be treated. An excellent justification for conservative treatment was provided by the Cardiac Arrhythmia Suppression Trial (CAST) referred to earlier.

Benefits & Risks

The benefits of antiarrhythmic therapy are actually relatively difficult to establish. Two types of benefits can be envisioned: reduction of arrhythmia-related symptoms, such as palpitations, syncope, or cardiac arrest; or reduction in long-term mortality in asymptomatic patients. Among drugs discussed here, only β blockers have been definitely associated with reduction of mortality in relatively asymptomatic patients, and the mechanism underlying this effect is not established (see Chapter 10).

Antiarrhythmic therapy carries with it a number of risks. In some cases, the risk of an adverse reaction is clearly related to high dosages or plasma concentrations. Examples include lidocaine-induced tremor or quinidine-induced cinchonism. In other cases, adverse reactions are unrelated to high plasma concentrations (eg, procainamide-induced agranulocytosis). For many serious adverse reactions to antiarrhythmic drugs, the *combination* of drug therapy and the underlying heart disease appears important.

Several specific syndromes of arrhythmia provocation by antiarrhythmic drugs have also been identified, each with its underlying pathophysiologic mechanism and risk factors. Drugs such as quinidine, sotalol, ibutilide, and dofetilide, which act—at least in part—by slowing repolarization and prolonging cardiac action potentials, can result in marked QT prolongation and torsade de pointes. Treatment of torsade de pointes requires recognition of the arrhythmia, withdrawal of any offending agent, correction of hypokalemia, and treatment with maneuvers to increase heart rate (pacing or isoproterenol); intravenous magnesium also appears effective, even in patients with normal magnesium levels.

Drugs that markedly slow conduction, such as flecainide, or high concentrations of quinidine, can result in an increased frequency of reentry arrhythmias, notably ventricular tachycardia in patients with prior myocardial infarction in whom a potential reentry circuit may be present. Treatment here consists of recognition, withdrawal of the offending agent, and intravenous sodium.

Conduct of Antiarrhythmic Therapy

The urgency of the clinical situation determines the route and rate of drug initiation. When immediate drug action is required, the intravenous route is preferred. Therapeutic drug levels can be achieved by administration of multiple intravenous boluses. Drug therapy can be considered effective when the target arrhythmia is suppressed (according to the measure used to quantify at baseline) and toxicities are absent. Conversely, drug therapy should not be considered ineffective unless toxicities occur at a time when arrhythmias are not suppressed.

Monitoring plasma drug concentrations can be a useful adjunct to managing antiarrhythmic therapy. Plasma drug concentrations are also important in establishing compliance during long-term therapy as well as in detecting drug interactions that may result in very high concentrations at low drug dosages or very low concentrations at high dosages.

Chapter continues on next page.

PREPARATIONS AVAILABLE

SODIUM CHANNEL BLOCKERS

Disopyramide (generic, Norpace)
Oral: 100, 150 mg capsules
Oral controlled-release (generic, Norpace CR): 100, 150 capsules

Flecainide (Tambocor)
Oral: 50, 100, 150 mg tablets

Lidocaine (generic, Xylocaine)
Parenteral: 100 mg/mL for IM injection; 10, 20 mg/mL for IV injection; 40, 100, 200 mg/mL for IV admixtures; 2, 4, 8 mg/mL premixed IV (5% D/W) solution

Mexiletine (Mexitil)
Oral: 150, 200, 250 mg capsules

Moricizine (Ethmozine)
Oral: 200, 250, 300 mg tablets

Procainamide (generic, Pronestyl, others)
Oral: 250, 375, 500 mg tablets and capsules
Oral sustained-release (generic, Procan-SR): 250, 500, 750, 1000 mg tablets
Parenteral: 100, 500 mg/mL for injection

Propafenone (Rythmol)
Oral: 150, 225, 300 mg tablets

Quinidine sulfate [83% quinidine base] (generic)
Oral: 200, 300 mg tablets
Oral sustained-release (Quinidex Extentabs): 300 mg tablets

Quinidine gluconate [62% quinidine base] (generic)
Oral sustained-release: 324 mg tablets
Parenteral: 80 mg/mL for injection

Quinidine polygalacturonate [60% quinidine base] (Cardioquin)
Oral: 275 mg tablets

β-BLOCKERS LABELED FOR USE AS ANTIARRHYTHMICS

Acebutolol (generic, Sectral)
Oral: 200, 400 mg capsules

Esmolol (Brevibloc)
Parenteral: 10 mg/mL, 250 mg/mL for IV injection

Propranolol (generic, Inderal)
Oral: 10, 20, 40, 60, 80, 90 mg tablets
Oral sustained-release: 60, 80, 120, 160 mg capsules
Oral solution: 4, 8 mg/mL
Parenteral: 1 mg/mL for injection

ACTION POTENTIAL–PROLONGING AGENTS

Amiodarone (Cordarone)
Oral: 200, 400 mg tablets
Parenteral: 150 mg/3 mL for IV infusion

Bretylium (generic)
Parenteral: 2, 4, 50 mg/mL for injection

Dofetilide (Tikosyn)
Oral: 125, 250, 500 mcg capsules

Ibutilide (Corvert)
Parenteral: 0.1 g/mL solution for IV infusion

Sotalol (generic, Betapace)
Oral: 80, 120, 160, 240 mg capsules

CALCIUM CHANNEL BLOCKERS

Diltiazem (generic, Cardizem, Dilacor)
Oral: 30, 60, 90, 120 mg tablets; 60, 90, 120, 180, 240, 300, 340, 420 mg extended- or sustained-release capsules (*not labeled for use in arrhythmias*)
Parenteral: 5 mg/mL for IV injection

Verapamil (generic, Calan, Isoptin)
Oral: 40, 80, 120 mg tablets
Oral sustained-release (Calan SR, Isoptin SR): 100, 120, 180, 240 mg capsules
Parenteral: 5 mg/2 mL for injection

MISCELLANEOUS

Adenosine (Adenocard)
Parenteral: 3 mg/mL for injection

Magnesium sulfate
Parenteral: 125, 500 mg/mL for IV infusion

REFERENCES

Antzelevitch C, Shimizu W: Cellular mechanisms underlying the long QT syndrome. Curr Opin Cardiol 2002;17:43.

Chen YH et al: KCNQ1 gain-of-function mutation in familial atrial fibrillation. Science 2003;299:251.

Cho H-S, Takano M, Noma A: The electrophysiological properties of spontaneously beating pacemaker cells isolated from mouse sinoatrial node. J Physiol 2003;550:169.

Duan D et al: Functional role of anion channels in cardiac diseases. Acta Pharmacol Sin 2005;26:265.

Dumaine R, Antzelevitch C: Molecular mechanisms underlying the long QT syndrome. Curr Opin Cardiol 2002;17:36.

Echt DS et al for the CAST Investigators: Mortality and morbidity in patients receiving encainide, flecainide, or placebo. The Cardiac Arrhythmia Suppression Trial. N Engl J Med 1991; 324:781.

Fuster V et al: ACC/AHA/ESC Guidelines for the management of patients with atrial fibrillation. Circulation 2001;104:2118.

Gollob MH, Seger JJ: Current status of the implantable cardio-verter-defibrillator. Chest 2001;119:1210.

Grant AO: Molecular biology of sodium channels and their role in cardiac arrhythmias. Am J Med 2001;110:296.

Grant AO: Recent advances in the treatment of arrhythmias. Circ J 2003;67:651.

Hohnloser SH, Woosley RL: Sotalol. N Engl J Med 1994;331:31.

IRCCS Fondazione Salvatore Maugeri: Gene connection for the heart 2005. Available at: http://pc4.fsm.it:81/cardmoc.

Keating MT, Sanguinetti MC: Molecular and cellular mechanisms of cardiac arrhythmias. Cell 2001;104:569.

Khan IA: Clinical and therapeutic aspects of congenital and acquired long QT syndrome. Am J Med 2002;112:58.

Mohler PJ, Gramolini AO, Bennett V: Ankyrins. J Cell Biol 2002; 115:1565.

Morady F: Catheter ablation of supraventricular arrhythmias: state of the art. J Cardiovasc Electrophysiol 2004;15:124.

Nattel S: New ideas about atrial fibrillation 50 years on. Nature 2002;415:219.

Priori SG, Napolitano C: Genetics of cardiac arrhythmias and sudden cardiac death. NY Acad Sci 2004;1015:96.

Splawski I, Tomothy KW, Decher N et al: Severe arrhythmia disorder caused by cardiac L-type calcium channel mutations. Proc Natl Acad Sci USA 2005;102:8089.

Splawski I et al: Variant of SCN5A sodium channel implicated in risk of cardiac arrhythmia. Science 2002;297:1333.

Srivatsa U, Wadhani N, Singh AB: Mechanisms of antiarrhythmic drug actions and their clinical relevance for controlling disorders of cardiac rhythm. Curr Cardiol Rep 2002;4:401.

Subbiah RN, Campbell TJ, Vandenberg JI: Inherited cardiac arrhythmia syndromes: What have they taught us about arrhythmias and anti-arrhythmic therapy? Clin Exp Pharmacol Physiol 2004;31:906.

Tristani-Firouzi M et al: Molecular biology of K(+) channels and their role in cardiac arrhythmias. Am J Med 2001;110:50.

van Gelder I et al: A comparison of rate control and rhythm control in patients with recurrent persistent atrial fibrillation, N Engl J Med 2002;347:1834.

Wyse DG et al: A comparison of rate control and rhythm control in patients with atrial fibrillation. N Engl J Med 2002; 347:1825.

Wehrens XHT, Lehnart SE, Marks AR: Ryanodine receptor-targeted anti-arrhythmic therapy. NY Acad Sci 2005;1047:366.

Diuretic Agents

15

Harlan E. Ives, MD, PhD

Abnormalities in fluid volume and electrolyte composition are common and important clinical disorders. Drugs that block specific transport functions of the renal tubules are valuable clinical tools in the treatment of these disorders. Although various agents that increase urine volume (diuretics) have been described since antiquity, it was not until 1957 that a practical and powerful diuretic agent (chlorothiazide) became available for widespread use.

Technically, a "diuretic" is an agent that increases urine volume, while a "natriuretic" causes an increase in renal sodium excretion. Because natriuretics almost always also increase water excretion, they are usually called diuretics.

The nephron is divided structurally and functionally into several segments (Figure 15–1, Table 15–1), which are discussed in the first part of this chapter. Many diuretics exert their effects on specific membrane transport proteins in renal tubular epithelial cells. Other diuretics exert osmotic effects that prevent water reabsorption (mannitol), inhibit enzymes (acetazolamide), or interfere with hormone receptors in renal epithelial cells (aldosterone receptor blockers). These effects are discussed in the second part of the chapter. The physiology of each segment is closely linked to the pharmacology of the drugs acting there.

■ I. RENAL TUBULE TRANSPORT MECHANISMS

PROXIMAL TUBULE

Sodium bicarbonate ($NaHCO_3$), sodium chloride (NaCl), glucose, amino acids, and other organic solutes are reabsorbed via specific transport systems in the early proximal tubule (proximal convoluted tubule, PCT). Potassium ions (K^+) are reabsorbed via the paracellular pathway. Water is reabsorbed passively, maintaining the osmolality of proximal tubular fluid at a nearly constant level. As tubule fluid is processed along the length of the proximal tubule, the luminal concentrations of these solutes decrease relative to the concentration of inulin, a marker that is filtered but neither secreted nor absorbed by renal tubules. Approximately 66% of total sodium ions (Na^+, but 85% of the filtered $NaHCO_3$), 65% of the K^+, 60% of the water, and virtually all of the filtered glucose and amino acids are reabsorbed in the proximal tubule.

Of the various solutes reabsorbed in the proximal tubule, the most relevant to diuretic action are $NaHCO_3$ and NaCl. Of the currently available diuretics, only one group (carbonic anhydrase inhibitors, which block $NaHCO_3$ reabsorption) acts predominantly in the PCT. In view of the large quantity of NaCl absorbed in this segment, a drug that specifically blocked proximal tubular absorption of NaCl would be a particularly powerful diuretic. No such drug is currently available.

Sodium bicarbonate reabsorption by the PCT is initiated by the action of a Na^+/H^+ exchanger (NHE3) located in the luminal membrane of the proximal tubule epithelial cell (Figure 15–2). This transport system allows Na^+ to enter the cell from the tubular lumen in exchange for a proton (H^+) from inside the cell. As in all portions of the nephron, Na^+/K^+ ATPase in the basolateral membrane pumps the reabsorbed Na^+ into the interstitium so as to maintain a low intracellular Na^+ concentration. The H^+ secreted into the lumen combines with bicarbonate (HCO_3^-) to form H_2CO_3 (carbonic acid), which is rapidly dehydrated to CO_2 and H_2O by carbonic anhydrase. Carbon dioxide produced by dehydration of H_2CO_3 enters the proximal tubule cell by simple diffusion where it is then rehydrated back to H_2CO_3, facilitated by intracellular carbonic anhydrase. After dissociation of H_2CO_3, the H^+ is available for transport by the Na^+/H^+ exchanger, and the HCO_3^- is transported out of the cell by a basolateral membrane transporter (Figure 15–2). Bicarbonate reabsorption by the proximal tubule is thus dependent on carbonic anhydrase. This enzyme can be inhibited by acetazolamide and related agents.

In the late proximal tubule, as HCO_3^- and organic solutes have been largely removed from the tubular fluid, the residual luminal fluid contains predominantly NaCl. Under these conditions, Na^+ reabsorption continues, but the H^+ secreted by the Na^+/H^+ exchanger can no longer bind to HCO_3^-. Free H^+ causes luminal

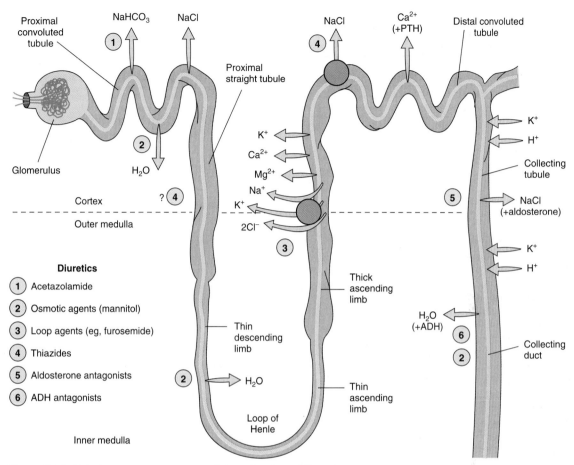

Figure 15–1. Tubule transport systems and sites of action of diuretics.

pH to fall, activating a still poorly defined Cl⁻/base exchanger (Figure 15–2). The net effect of parallel Na^+/H^+ exchange and Cl^-/base exchange is NaCl reabsorption. As yet, there are no diuretic agents that are known to act on this conjoint process.

Because water is reabsorbed in direct proportion to salt reabsorption in the proximal tubule, luminal fluid osmolality remains nearly constant along its length and an impermeant solute like inulin rises in concentration as water is reabsorbed. If large amounts of an impermeant solute such as mannitol (an osmotic diuretic, see below) are present in the tubular fluid, water reabsorption causes the concentration of the solute and osmolality of tubular fluid to rise, eventually preventing further water reabsorption.

Organic acid secretory systems are located in the middle third of the straight part of the proximal tubule (S_2 segment). These systems secrete a variety of organic acids (uric acid, nonsteroidal anti-inflammatory drugs [NSAIDs], diuretics, antibiotics, etc) into the luminal fluid from the blood. These systems thus help deliver diuretics to the luminal side of the tubule, where most of them act. Organic base secretory systems (creatinine, choline, etc) are also present, in the early (S_1) and middle (S_2) segments of the proximal tubule.

LOOP OF HENLE

At the boundary between the inner and outer stripes of the outer medulla, the proximal tubule empties into the thin descending limb of Henle's loop. Water is extracted from the descending limb of this loop by osmotic forces found in the hypertonic medullary interstitium. As in the proximal tubule, impermeant luminal solutes such as mannitol oppose this water extraction. The thin *ascending* limb is relatively water-impermeable.

The thick ascending limb (TAL) of the loop of Henle actively reabsorbs NaCl from the lumen (about

Table 15–1. Major segments of the nephron and their functions.

Segment	Functions	Water Permeability	Primary Transporters and Drug Targets at Apical Membrane	Diuretic with Major Action
Glomerulus	Formation of glomerular filtrate	Extremely high	None	None
Proximal convoluted tubule (PCT)	Reabsorption of 65% of filtered Na^+, K^+, CA^{2+}, and Mg^+; 85% of $NaHCO_3$, and nearly 100% of glucose and amino acids. Isosmotic reabsorption of water.	Very high	Na/H[1] (NHE3), carbonic anhydrase	Carbonic anhydrase inhibitors
Proximal tubule, straight segments	Secretion and reabsorption of organic acids and bases, including uric acid and most diuretics	Very high	Acid (eg, uric acid) and base transporters	None
Thin descending limb of Henle's loop	Passive reabsorption of water	High	Aquaporins	None
Thick ascending limb of Henle's loop (TAL)	Active reabsorption of 15–25% of filtered Na^+, K^+, Cl^-; secondary reabsorption of Ca^{2+} and Mg^+	Very low	Na/K/2Cl (NKCC2)	Loop diuretics
Distal convoluted tubule (DCT)	Active reabsorption of 4–8% of filtered Na^+ and Cl^-; Ca^{2+} reabsorption under parathyroid hormone control	Very low	Na/Cl (NCC)	Thiazides
Cortical collecting tubule (CCT)	Na^+ reabsorption (2–5%) coupled to K^+ and H^+ secretion	Variable[2]	Na channels (ENaC), K channels,[1] H transporter,[1] aquaporins	K^+-sparing diuretics
Medullary collecting duct	Water reabsorption under vasopressin control	Variable[2]	Aquaporins	Vasopressin antagonist

[1]Not a target of currently available drugs.
[2]Controlled by vasopressin activity.

25% of the filtered sodium), but unlike the proximal tubule and the thin limb of Henle's loop, it is nearly impermeable to water. Salt reabsorption in the TAL therefore dilutes the tubular fluid, and it is called a "diluting segment." Medullary portions of the thick ascending limb contribute to medullary hypertonicity and thereby also play an important role in concentration of urine by the collecting duct.

The NaCl transport system in the luminal membrane of the TAL is a $Na^+/K^+/2Cl^-$ cotransporter (called NKCC2 or NK2CL) (Figure 15–3). This transporter is selectively blocked by diuretic agents known as "loop" diuretics (see below). Although the $Na^+/K^+/2Cl^-$ transporter is itself electrically neutral (two cations and two anions are cotransported), the action of the transporter contributes to excess K^+ accumulation within the cell. Back diffusion of this K^+ into the tubular lumen causes a lumen-positive electrical potential that provides the driving force for reabsorption of cations—including magnesium and calcium—via the paracellular pathway. Thus, inhibition of salt transport in the thick ascending limb by loop diuretics, which reduces the lumen-positive potential, causes an increase in urinary excretion of divalent cations in addition to NaCl.

DISTAL CONVOLUTED TUBULE

Only about 10% of the filtered NaCl is reabsorbed in the distal convoluted tubule (DCT). Like the thick ascending limb of Henle's loop, this segment is relatively impermeable to water and NaCl reabsorption further dilutes the tubular fluid. The mechanism of NaCl transport in the DCT is an electrically neutral thiazide-sensitive Na^+ and Cl^- cotransporter (NCC, Figure 15–4).

Because K^+ does not recycle across the apical membrane of the DCT as it does in the TAL, there is no lumen-positive potential in this segment, and Ca^{2+} and Mg^{2+} are not driven out of the tubular lumen by electrical forces. Instead, Ca^{2+} is actively reabsorbed by the DCT epithelial cell via an apical Ca^{2+} channel and

Figure 15–2. Apical membrane Na^+/H^+ exchange (via NHE3) and bicarbonate reabsorption in the proximal convoluted tubule cell. Na^+/K^+ ATPase is present in the basolateral membrane to maintain intracellular sodium and potassium levels within the normal range. Because of rapid equilibration, concentrations of the solutes are approximately equal in the interstitial fluid and the blood. Carbonic anhydrase (CA) is found in other locations in addition to the brush border of the luminal membrane.

Figure 15–3. Ion transport pathways across the luminal and basolateral membranes of the thick ascending limb cell. The lumen positive electrical potential created by K^+ back diffusion drives divalent (and monovalent) cation reabsorption via the paracellular pathway. NKCC2 is the primary transporter in the luminal membrane.

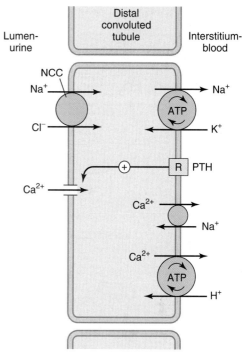

Figure 15–4. Ion transport pathways across the luminal and basolateral membranes of the distal convoluted tubule cell. As in all tubular cells, Na^+/K^+ ATPase is present in the basolateral membrane. NCC is the primary sodium and chloride transporter in the luminal membrane. (R, parathyroid hormone [PTH] receptor.)

basolateral Na^+/Ca^{2+} exchanger (Figure 15–4). This process is regulated by parathyroid hormone.

COLLECTING TUBULE

The collecting tubule (CCT) is responsible for only 2–5% of NaCl reabsorption by the kidney. Despite this small contribution, the CCT plays an important role in renal physiology and in diuretic action. As the final site of NaCl reabsorption, the collecting tubule is responsible for tight regulation of body fluid volume and for determining the final Na^+ concentration of the urine. Furthermore, the collecting tubule is a site at which mineralocorticoids exert a significant influence. Lastly, the collecting tubule is the most important site of K^+ secretion by the kidney and the site at which virtually all diuretic-induced changes in K^+ balance occur.

The mechanism of NaCl reabsorption in the CCT is distinct from the mechanisms found in other tubule segments. The **principal cells** are the major sites of Na^+, K^+, and water transport (Figure 15–5), and the

Figure 15–5. Ion transport pathways across the luminal and basolateral membranes of collecting tubule and collecting duct cells. Inward diffusion of Na^+ via the epithelial sodium channel (ENaC) leaves a lumen-negative potential, which drives reabsorption of Cl^- and efflux of K^+. (R, aldosterone receptor; ADH, antidiuretic hormone.)

intercalated cells are the primary sites of H^+ secretion. Unlike cells in other nephron segments, the principal cells do not contain cotransport systems for Na^+ and other ions in their apical membranes. Principal cell membranes exhibit separate ion channels for Na^+ and K^+. Since these channels exclude anions, transport of Na^+ or K^+ leads to a net movement of charge across the membrane. Because Na^+ entry into the principal cell predominates over K^+ secretion, a 10–50 mV lumen-negative electrical potential develops. Na^+ that enters the principal cell from the tubular fluid is then transported back to the blood via the basolateral Na^+/K^+ ATPase (Figure 15–5). The 10–50 mV lumen-negative electrical potential drives the transport of Cl^- back to the blood via the paracellular pathway and draws K^+ out of cells through the apical membrane K^+ channel. Thus, there is an important relationship between Na^+ delivery to the CCT and the resulting secretion of K^+. Diuretics that act upstream of the CCT will increase Na^+ delivery to this site and will enhance K^+ secretion. If the Na^+ is delivered with an anion that cannot be reabsorbed as readily as Cl^- (eg, HCO_3^-), the lumen-negative potential is increased, and K^+ secretion will be

enhanced. This mechanism, combined with enhanced aldosterone secretion due to volume depletion, is the basis for most diuretic-induced K^+ wasting.

Reabsorption of Na^+ via the epithelial Na channel (ENaC) and its coupled secretion of K^+ is regulated by aldosterone. This steroid hormone, through its actions on gene transcription, increases the activity of both apical membrane channels and the basolateral Na^+/K^+ ATPase. This leads to an increase in the transepithelial electrical potential and a dramatic increase in both Na^+ reabsorption and K^+ secretion.

The collecting tubule is also the site at which the final urine concentration is determined. Antidiuretic hormone (ADH, also called arginine vasopressin, AVP) controls the permeability of this segment to water by regulating the insertion of preformed water channels (aquaporin-2, AQP2) into the apical membrane via a G protein-coupled cAMP-mediated process (Figure 15–6). In the absence of

Figure 15–6. Water transport across the luminal and basolateral membranes of collecting duct cells. Above, low water permeability exists in the absence of antidiuretic hormone (ADH). Below, in the presence of ADH, aquaporins are inserted into the apical membrane, greatly increasing water permeability. (V_2, vasopressin V_2 receptor; AQP2, apical aquaporin water channels; AQP3, 4, basolateral aquaporin water channels.)

ADH, the collecting tubule (and duct) is impermeable to water and dilute urine is produced. ADH markedly increases water permeability and this leads to the formation of a more concentrated final urine. ADH also stimulates the insertion of urea transporter UT1 molecules into the apical membranes of medullary collecting tubule cells. Urea concentration in the medulla plays an important role maintaining the high osmolarity of the medulla and in the concentration of urine. ADH secretion is regulated by serum osmolality and by volume status.

II. BASIC PHARMACOLOGY OF DIURETIC AGENTS

CARBONIC ANHYDRASE INHIBITORS

Carbonic anhydrase is present in many nephron sites, but the predominant location of this enzyme is the luminal membrane of the PCT (Figure 15–2), where it catalyzes the dehydration of H_2CO_3 as described above. By blocking carbonic anhydrase, inhibitors block $NaHCO_3$ reabsorption and cause diuresis.

Carbonic anhydrase inhibitors were the forerunners of modern diuretics. They were discovered when it was found that bacteriostatic sulfonamides caused an alkaline diuresis and hyperchloremic metabolic acidosis. With the development of newer agents, carbonic anhydrase inhibitors are now rarely used as diuretics, but they still have several specific applications that are discussed below. The prototypical carbonic anhydrase inhibitor is **acetazolamide.**

Pharmacokinetics

The carbonic anhydrase inhibitors are well absorbed after oral administration. An increase in urine pH from the HCO_3^- diuresis is apparent within 30 minutes, maximal at 2 hours, and persists for 12 hours after a single dose. Excretion of the drug is by secretion in the proximal tubule S_2 segment. Therefore, dosing must be reduced in renal insufficiency.

Pharmacodynamics

Inhibition of carbonic anhydrase activity profoundly depresses HCO_3^- reabsorption in the PCT. At its maximal safely administered dosage, 85% of the HCO_3^- reabsorptive capacity of the superficial PCT is inhibited. Some HCO_3^- can still be absorbed at other nephron sites by carbonic anhydrase–independent mechanisms, so the overall effect of maximal acetazolamide dosage is only about 45% inhibition of whole kidney

Table 15–2. Changes in urinary electrolyte patterns and body pH in response to diuretic drugs.

Group	Urinary Electrolytes			Body pH
	NaCl	NaHCO₃	K⁺	
Carbonic anhydrase inhibitors	+	+++	+	–
Loop agents	++++	0	+	+
Thiazides	++	+	+	+
Loop agents plus thiazides	+++++	+	++	+
K⁺-sparing agents	+	(+)	–	–

+, increase; –, decrease; 0, no change.

HCO_3^- reabsorption. Nevertheless, carbonic anhydrase inhibition causes significant HCO_3^- losses and hyperchloremic metabolic acidosis (Table 15–2). Because of reduced HCO_3^- in the glomerular filtrate and the fact that HCO_3^- depletion leads to enhanced NaCl reabsorption by the remainder of the nephron, the diuretic efficacy of acetazolamide decreases significantly with use over several days.

At present, the major clinical applications of acetazolamide involve carbonic anhydrase–dependent HCO_3^- and fluid transport at sites other than the kidney. The ciliary body of the eye secretes HCO_3^- from the blood into the aqueous humor. Likewise, formation of cerebrospinal fluid by the choroid plexus involves HCO_3^- secretion. Although these processes remove HCO_3^- from the blood (the direction opposite to that in the proximal tubule), they are similarly inhibited by carbonic anhydrase inhibitors.

Clinical Indications & Dosage (Table 15–3)

A. GLAUCOMA

The reduction of aqueous humor formation by carbonic anhydrase inhibitors decreases the intraocular

Table 15–3. Carbonic anhydrase inhibitors used orally in the treatment of glaucoma.

Drug	Usual Oral Dosage
Acetazolamide	250 mg 1–4 times daily
Dichlorphenamide	50 mg 1–3 times daily
Methazolamide	50–100 mg 2–3 times daily

pressure. This effect is valuable in the management of glaucoma, making it the most common indication for use of carbonic anhydrase inhibitors. Topically active carbonic anhydrase inhibitors (dorzolamide, brinzolamide) are also available. These topical compounds reduce intraocular pressure, but plasma levels are undetectable. Thus, diuretic and systemic metabolic effects are eliminated for the topical agents.

B. URINARY ALKALINIZATION

Uric acid, cystine, and other weak acids are most easily reabsorbed from acidic urine. Therefore, renal excretion of cystine (in cystinuria) and other weak acids can be enhanced by increasing urinary pH with carbonic anhydrase inhibitors. In the absence of continuous HCO_3^- administration, these effects of acetazolamide last only 2–3 days. Prolonged therapy requires HCO_3^- administration.

C. METABOLIC ALKALOSIS

Metabolic alkalosis is generally treated by correction of abnormalities in total body K^+, intravascular volume, or mineralocorticoid levels. However, when the alkalosis is due to excessive use of diuretics in patients with severe heart failure, replacement of intravascular volume may be contraindicated. In these cases, acetazolamide can be useful in correcting the alkalosis as well as producing a small additional diuresis for correction of volume overload. Acetazolamide can also be used to rapidly correct the metabolic alkalosis that may develop in the setting of respiratory acidosis.

D. ACUTE MOUNTAIN SICKNESS

Weakness, dizziness, insomnia, headache, and nausea can occur in mountain travelers who rapidly ascend above 3000 m. The symptoms are usually mild and last for a few days. In more serious cases, rapidly progressing pulmonary or cerebral edema can be life-threatening. By decreasing cerebrospinal fluid formation and by decreasing the pH of the cerebrospinal fluid and brain, acetazolamide can increase ventilation and diminish symptoms of mountain sickness.

E. OTHER USES

Carbonic anhydrase inhibitors have been used as adjuvants in the treatment of epilepsy, in some forms of hypokalemic periodic paralysis, and to increase urinary phosphate excretion during severe hyperphosphatemia.

Toxicity

A. HYPERCHLOREMIC METABOLIC ACIDOSIS

Acidosis predictably results from chronic reduction of body HCO_3^- stores by carbonic anhydrase inhibitors (Table 15–2) and limits the diuretic efficacy of these drugs to 2 or 3 days. Unlike the diuretic effect, acidosis persists as long as the drug is continued.

B. RENAL STONES

Phosphaturia and hypercalciuria occur during the bicarbonaturic response to inhibitors of carbonic anhydrase. Renal excretion of solubilizing factors (eg, citrate) may also decline with chronic use. Calcium salts are relatively insoluble at alkaline pH, which means that the potential for renal stone formation from these salts is enhanced.

C. RENAL POTASSIUM WASTING

Potassium wasting can occur because Na^+ presented to the collecting tubule is partially reabsorbed, increasing the lumen-negative electrical potential in that segment and enhancing K^+ secretion. This effect can be counteracted by simultaneous administration of potassium chloride.

D. OTHER TOXICITIES

Drowsiness and paresthesias are common following large doses of acetazolamide. Carbonic anhydrase inhibitors may accumulate in patients with renal failure, leading to nervous system toxicity. Hypersensitivity reactions (fever, rashes, bone marrow suppression, and interstitial nephritis) may also occur.

Contraindications

Carbonic anhydrase inhibitor-induced alkalinization of the urine will decrease urinary excretion of NH_4^+ and may contribute to the development of **hyperammonemia** and **hepatic encephalopathy** in patients with cirrhosis.

LOOP DIURETICS

Loop diuretics selectively inhibit NaCl reabsorption in the TAL. Due to the large NaCl absorptive capacity of this segment and the fact that the diuretic action of these drugs is not limited by development of acidosis, as is the case with the carbonic anhydrase inhibitors, loop diuretics are among the most efficacious diuretic agents available.

Chemistry

The two prototypical drugs of this group are **furosemide** and **ethacrynic acid.** The structures of these diuretics are shown in Figure 15–7. In addition to furosemide, bumetanide and torsemide are sulfonamide loop diuretics.

Ethacrynic acid—not a sulfonamide derivative—is a phenoxyacetic acid derivative containing an adjacent ketone and methylene group (Figure 15–7). The methylene group (shaded) forms an adduct with the

Figure 15–7. Two loop diuretics. The shaded methylene group on ethacrynic acid is reactive and may combine with free sulfhydryl groups.

free sulfhydryl group of cysteine. The cysteine adduct appears to be an active form of the drug.

Organic **mercurial diuretics** also inhibit salt transport in the TAL but are no longer used because of their toxicity.

Pharmacokinetics

The loop diuretics are rapidly absorbed. They are eliminated by the kidney by glomerular filtration and tubular secretion. Absorption of oral torsemide is more rapid (1 hour) than that of furosemide (2–3 hours) and is nearly as complete as with intravenous administration. The duration of effect for furosemide is usually 2–3 hours and that of torsemide is 4–6 hours. Half-life depends on renal function. Since loop agents act on the luminal side of the tubule, their diuretic activity correlates with their secretion by the proximal tubule. Reduction in the secretion of loop diuretics may result from simultaneous administration of agents such as NSAIDs or probenecid, which compete for weak acid secretion in the proximal tubule. Metabolites of ethacrynic acid and furosemide have been identified, but it is not known if they have any diuretic activity. Torsemide has at least one active metabolite with a half-life considerably longer than that of the parent compound.

Pharmacodynamics

These drugs inhibit NKCC2, the luminal $Na^+/K^+/2Cl^-$ transporter in the thick ascending limb of Henle's loop. By inhibiting this transporter, the loop diuretics reduce the reabsorption of NaCl and also diminish the lumen-

positive potential that comes from K^+ recycling (Figure 15–3). This positive potential normally drives divalent cation reabsorption in the loop (Figure 15–3), and by reducing this potential, loop diuretics cause an increase in Mg^{2+} and Ca^{2+} excretion. Prolonged use can cause significant hypomagnesemia in some patients. Since vitamin D-induced intestinal absorption of Ca^{2+} can be increased and Ca^{2+} is actively reabsorbed in the DCT, loop diuretics do not generally cause hypocalcemia. However, in disorders that cause *hypercalcemia*, Ca^{2+} excretion can be usefully enhanced by treatment with loop diuretics combined with saline infusions.

Loop diuretics induce synthesis of renal prostaglandins, which participate in the renal actions of these diuretics. NSAIDs (eg, indomethacin) can interfere with the actions of the loop diuretics by reducing prostaglandin synthesis in the kidney. This interference is minimal in otherwise normal subjects but may be significant in patients with nephrotic syndrome or hepatic cirrhosis.

In addition to their diuretic activity, loop agents have direct effects on blood flow through several vascular beds. Furosemide increases renal blood flow. Both furosemide and ethacrynic acid have also been shown to reduce pulmonary congestion and left ventricular filling pressures in heart failure before a measurable increase in urinary output occurs, and in anephric patients.

Clinical Indications & Dosage (Table 15–4)

The most important indications for the use of the loop diuretics include acute pulmonary edema, other edematous conditions, and acute hypercalcemia. The use of loop diuretics in these conditions is discussed in Section III, Clinical Pharmacology. Other indications for loop diuretics include hyperkalemia, acute renal failure, and anion overdose.

A. HYPERKALEMIA

In mild hyperkalemia—or after acute management of severe hyperkalemia by other measures—loop diuretics can significantly enhance urinary excretion of K^+. This response is enhanced by simultaneous NaCl and water administration.

Table 15–4. Typical dosages of loop diuretics.

Drug	Total Daily Oral Dose[1]
Bumetanide	0.5–2 mg
Ethacrynic acid	50–200 mg
Furosemide	20–80 mg
Torsemide	5–20 mg

[1]As single dose or in two divided doses.

B. Acute Renal Failure

Loop agents can increase the rate of urine flow and enhance K^+ excretion in acute renal failure. However, they do not shorten the duration of renal failure. If a large pigment load has precipitated acute renal failure (or threatens to), loop agents may help flush out intratubular casts and ameliorate intratubular obstruction. On the other hand, loop agents can theoretically worsen cast formation in myeloma and light chain nephropathy.

C. Anion Overdose

Loop diuretics are useful in treating toxic ingestions of bromide, fluoride, and iodide, which are reabsorbed in the thick ascending limb. Saline solution must be administered to replace urinary losses of Na^+ and to provide Cl^-, so as to avoid extracellular fluid volume depletion.

Toxicity

A. Hypokalemic Metabolic Alkalosis

By inhibiting salt reabsorption in the TAL, loop diuretics increase delivery to the collecting duct. Increased delivery leads to increased secretion of K^+ and H^+ by the duct, causing hypokalemic metabolic alkalosis (Table 15–2). This toxicity is a function of the magnitude of the diuresis and can be reversed by K^+ replacement and correction of hypovolemia.

B. Ototoxicity

Loop diuretics occasionally cause dose-related hearing loss that is usually reversible. It is most common in patients who have diminished renal function or who are also receiving other ototoxic agents such as aminoglycoside antibiotics.

C. Hyperuricemia

Loop diuretics can cause hyperuricemia and precipitate attacks of gout. This is caused by hypovolemia-associated enhancement of uric acid reabsorption in the proximal tubule. It may be prevented by using lower doses to avoid development of hypovolemia.

D. Hypomagnesemia

Magnesium depletion is a predictable consequence of the chronic use of loop agents and occurs most often in patients with dietary magnesium deficiency. It can be reversed by administration of oral magnesium preparations.

E. Allergic & Other Reactions

Except for ethacrynic acid, the loop diuretics are sulfonamides. Therefore skin rash, eosinophilia and, less often, interstitial nephritis are occasional side effects of these drugs. This toxicity usually resolves rapidly after drug withdrawal. Allergic reactions are much less common with ethacrynic acid.

Because Henle's loop is normally responsible for so much salt and water reabsorption, loop diuretics can cause severe dehydration. Hyponatremia is less common than with the thiazides (see below), but patients who increase water intake in response to hypovolemia-induced thirst can become severely hyponatremic with loop agents. Loop agents are sometimes used for their calciuric effect, but hypercalcemia can occur in volume-depleted patients who have another—previously occult—cause for hypercalcemia, such as metastatic breast or squamous cell lung carcinoma.

Contraindications

Furosemide, bumetanide, and torsemide may exhibit allergic cross-reactivity in patients who are sensitive to other sulfonamides but this appears to be very rare. Overzealous use of any diuretic is dangerous in hepatic cirrhosis, borderline renal failure, or heart failure (see below).

THIAZIDES

The thiazide diuretics emerged from efforts to synthesize more potent carbonic anhydrase inhibitors. It subsequently became clear that the thiazides inhibit NaCl transport predominantly in the DCT. However, some members of this group retain significant carbonic anhydrase inhibitory activity. The prototypical thiazide is **hydrochlorothiazide.**

Chemistry & Pharmacokinetics

Like carbonic anhydrase inhibitors and many loop diuretics, all of the thiazides have an unsubstituted sulfonamide group (Figure 15–8).

All of the thiazides can be administered orally, but there are differences in their metabolism. Chlorothiazide, the parent of the group, is not very lipid-soluble and must be given in relatively large doses. It is the only thiazide available for parenteral administration. Chlorthalidone is slowly absorbed and has a longer duration of action. Although indapamide is excreted primarily by the biliary system, enough of the active form is cleared by the kidney to exert its diuretic effect in the DCT.

All of the thiazides are secreted by the organic acid secretory system in the proximal tubule and compete with the secretion of uric acid by that system. As a result, thiazide use may blunt uric acid secretion and elevate serum uric acid level.

Pharmacodynamics

Thiazides inhibit NaCl reabsorption from the luminal side of epithelial cells in the DCT by blocking the

Hydrochlorothiazide

Indapamide

Metolazone

Figure 15–8. Hydrochlorothiazide and related agents.

Na$^+$/Cl$^-$ transporter (NCC). In contrast to the situation in the TAL, where loop diuretics inhibit Ca^{2+} reabsorption, thiazides actually enhance Ca^{2+} reabsorption. This enhancement has been postulated to result from effects in both the proximal and distal convoluted tubules. In the proximal tubule, thiazide-induced volume depletion leads to enhanced Na$^+$ and passive Ca^{2+} reabsorption. In the DCT, lowering of intracellular Na$^+$ by thiazide-induced blockade of Na$^+$ entry enhances Na$^+$/Ca^{2+} exchange in the basolateral membrane (Figure 15–4), and increases overall reabsorption of Ca^{2+}. While thiazides rarely cause hypercalcemia as the result of this enhanced reabsorption, they can unmask hypercalcemia due to other causes (eg, hyperparathyroidism, carcinoma, sarcoidosis). Thiazides are useful in the treatment of kidney stones caused by hypercalciuria.

The action of thiazides depends in part on renal prostaglandin production. As described above for the loop diuretics, the actions of thiazides can also be inhibited by NSAIDs under certain conditions.

Clinical Indications & Dosage (Table 15–5)

The major indications for thiazide diuretics are (1) hypertension, (2) heart failure, (3) nephrolithiasis due to idiopathic hypercalciuria, and (4) nephrogenic diabetes insipidus. Use of the thiazides in each of these conditions is described in Section III, Clinical Pharmacology.

Toxicity

A. HYPOKALEMIC METABOLIC ALKALOSIS AND HYPERURICEMIA

These toxicities are similar to those observed with loop diuretics (see above and Table 15–2).

B. IMPAIRED CARBOHYDRATE TOLERANCE

Hyperglycemia may occur in patients who are overtly diabetic or who have even mildly abnormal glucose tolerance tests. The effect is due to both impaired pancreatic release of insulin and diminished tissue utilization of glucose. Hyperglycemia may be partially reversible with correction of hypokalemia.

C. HYPERLIPIDEMIA

Thiazides cause a 5–15% increase in total serum cholesterol and low-density lipoproteins (LDL). These levels may return toward baseline after prolonged use.

D. HYPONATREMIA

Hyponatremia is an important adverse effect of thiazide diuretics. It is due to a combination of hypovolemia-

Table 15–5. Thiazides and related diuretics.

Drug	Total Daily Oral Dose	Frequency of Administration
Bendroflumethiazide	2.5–10 mg	Single dose
Chlorothiazide	0.5–2 g	Two divided doses
Chlorthalidone[1]	25–50 mg	Single dose
Hydrochlorothiazide	25–100 mg	Single dose
Hydroflumethiazide	12.5–50 mg	Two divided doses
Indapamide[1]	2.5–10 mg	Single dose
Methyclothiazide	2.5–10 mg	Single dose
Metolazone[1]	2.5–10 mg	Single dose
Polythiazide	1–4 mg	Single dose
Quinethazone[1]	25–100 mg	Single dose
Trichlormethiazide	1–4 mg	Single dose

[1]Not a thiazide but a sulfonamide qualitatively similar to the thiazides.

induced elevation of ADH, reduction in the diluting capacity of the kidney, and increased thirst. It can be prevented by reducing the dose of the drug or limiting water intake.

E. ALLERGIC REACTIONS

The thiazides are sulfonamides and share cross-reactivity with other members of this chemical group. Photosensitivity or generalized dermatitis occurs rarely. Serious allergic reactions are extremely rare but do include hemolytic anemia, thrombocytopenia, and acute necrotizing pancreatitis.

F. OTHER TOXICITIES

Weakness, fatigability, and paresthesias similar to those of carbonic anhydrase inhibitors may occur. Impotence has been reported but is probably related to volume depletion.

Contraindications

Excessive use of any diuretic is dangerous in hepatic cirrhosis, borderline renal failure, or heart failure (see below).

POTASSIUM-SPARING DIURETICS

These diuretics prevent K$^+$ secretion by antagonizing the effects of aldosterone at the late distal and cortical collecting tubules. Inhibition may occur by direct pharmacologic antagonism of mineralocorticoid receptors (**spironolactone, eplerenone**) or by inhibition of Na$^+$ influx through ion channels in the luminal membrane (**amiloride, triamterene**).

Chemistry & Pharmacokinetics

The structures of spironolactone and amiloride are shown in Figure 15–9.

Spironolactone is a synthetic steroid that acts as a competitive antagonist to aldosterone. Onset and duration of its action are determined by the kinetics of the aldosterone response in the target tissue. Substantial inactivation of spironolactone occurs in the liver. Overall, spironolactone has a rather slow onset of action, requiring several days before full therapeutic effect is achieved. Eplerenone is a spironolactone analog with greater selectivity for the aldosterone receptor.

Amiloride and triamterene are direct inhibitors of Na$^+$ influx in the CCT. Triamterene is metabolized in the liver, but renal excretion is a major route of elimination for the active form and the metabolites. Because triamterene is extensively metabolized, it has a shorter half-life and must be given more frequently than amiloride (which is not metabolized).

Figure 15–9. Potassium-sparing diuretics.

Pharmacodynamics

Potassium-sparing diuretics reduce Na$^+$ absorption in the collecting tubules and ducts. Na$^+$ absorption (and K$^+$ secretion) at this site is regulated by aldosterone, as described above. Aldosterone antagonists interfere with this process. Similar effects are observed with respect to H$^+$ handling by the intercalated cells of the collecting tubule, in part explaining the metabolic acidosis seen with aldosterone antagonists (Table 15–2).

Spironolactone and eplerenone bind to aldosterone receptors and may also reduce the intracellular formation of active metabolites of aldosterone. Amiloride and triamterene do not block the aldosterone receptor but instead directly interfere with Na$^+$ entry through the epithelial sodium ion channels (ENaC) in the apical membrane of the collecting tubule. Since K$^+$ secretion is coupled with Na$^+$ entry in this segment, these agents are also effective potassium-sparing diuretics.

The actions of the aldosterone antagonists depend on renal prostaglandin production. As described above for loop diuretics and thiazides, the actions of K$^+$-sparing diuretics can be inhibited by NSAIDs under certain conditions.

Clinical Indications & Dosage (Table 15–6)

Potassium-sparing diuretics are most useful in states of mineralocorticoid excess or hyperaldosteronism (also called aldosteronism), due either to primary hypersecretion (Conn's syndrome, ectopic adrenocorticotropic hormone production) or to secondary hyper-

Table 15–6. Potassium-sparing diuretics and combination preparations.

Trade Name	Potassium-Sparing Agent	Hydrochloro-thiazide
Aldactazide	Spironolactone 25 mg	50 mg
Aldactone	Spironolactone 25, 50, or 100 mg	...
Dyazide	Triamterene 37.5 mg	25 mg
Dyrenium	Triamterene 50 or 100 mg	...
Inspra[1]	Eplerenone 25, 50, or 100 mg	...
Maxzide	Triamterene 75 mg	50 mg
Maxzide-25 mg	Triamterene 37.5 mg	25 mg
Midamor	Amiloride 5 mg	...
Moduretic	Amiloride 5 mg	50 mg

[1]Eplerenone is currently approved for use only in hypertension.

aldosteronism (evoked by heart failure, hepatic cirrhosis, nephrotic syndrome, or other conditions associated with diminished effective intravascular volume). Use of diuretics such as thiazides or loop agents can cause or exacerbate volume contraction and may cause secondary hyperaldosteronism. In the setting of enhanced mineralocorticoid secretion and excessive delivery of Na^+ to distal nephron sites, renal K^+ wasting occurs. Potassium-sparing diuretics of either type may be used in this setting to blunt the K^+ secretory response.

Toxicity

A. HYPERKALEMIA

Unlike other diuretics, K^+-sparing diuretics can cause mild, moderate, or even life-threatening hyperkalemia (Table 15–2). The risk of this complication is greatly increased by renal disease (in which maximal K^+ excretion may be reduced) or by the use of other drugs that reduce renin (β blockers, NSAIDs) or angiotensin II activity (angiotensin-converting enzyme inhibitors, angiotensin receptor inhibitors). Since most other diuretic agents lead to K^+ losses, hyperkalemia is more common when K^+-sparing diuretics are used as the sole diuretic agent, especially in patients with renal insufficiency. With fixed-dosage combinations of K^+-sparing and thiazide diuretics, the thiazide-induced hypokalemia and metabolic alkalosis are ameliorated. However, owing to variations in the bio-

availability of the components of fixed-dosage forms, the thiazide-associated adverse effects often predominate. Therefore, it is generally preferable to adjust the doses of the two drugs separately.

B. HYPERCHLOREMIC METABOLIC ACIDOSIS

By inhibiting H^+ secretion in parallel with K^+ secretion, the K^+-sparing diuretics can cause acidosis similar to that seen with type IV renal tubular acidosis.

C. GYNECOMASTIA

Synthetic steroids may cause endocrine abnormalities by actions on other steroid receptors. Gynecomastia, impotence, and benign prostatic hyperplasia have all been reported with spironolactone. Such effects have not been reported with eplerenone.

D. ACUTE RENAL FAILURE

The combination of triamterene with indomethacin has been reported to cause acute renal failure. This has not been reported with other K^+-sparing diuretics.

E. KIDNEY STONES

Triamterene is only slightly soluble and may precipitate in the urine, causing kidney stones.

Contraindications

These agents can cause severe, even fatal hyperkalemia in susceptible patients. Oral K^+ administration should be discontinued if K^+-sparing diuretics are administered. Patients with chronic renal insufficiency are especially vulnerable and should rarely be treated with these diuretics. Concomitant use of other agents that blunt the renin-angiotensin system (β blockers or ACE inhibitors) increases the likelihood of hyperkalemia. Patients with liver disease may have impaired metabolism of triamterene and spironolactone, so dosing must be carefully adjusted. Strong CYP3A4 inhibitors (eg, ketoconazole, itraconazole) can markedly increase blood levels of eplerenone.

AGENTS THAT ALTER WATER EXCRETION

1. Osmotic Diuretics

The proximal tubule and descending limb of Henle's loop are freely permeable to water (Table 15–1). Any osmotically active agent that is filtered by the glomerulus but not reabsorbed causes water to be retained in these segments and promotes a water diuresis. Such agents can be used to reduce intracranial pressure and to promote prompt removal of renal toxins. The prototypic osmotic diuretic is **mannitol.**

Pharmacokinetics

Osmotic diuretics are poorly absorbed, which means that they must be given parenterally. If administered orally, mannitol causes osmotic diarrhea. Mannitol is not metabolized and is excreted by glomerular filtration within 30–60 minutes, without any important tubular reabsorption or secretion.

Pharmacodynamics

Osmotic diuretics have their major effect in the proximal tubule and the descending limb of Henle's loop. Through osmotic effects, they also oppose the action of ADH in the collecting tubule. The presence of a nonreabsorbable solute such as mannitol prevents the normal absorption of water by interposing a countervailing osmotic force. As a result, urine volume increases. The increase in urine flow rate decreases the contact time between fluid and the tubular epithelium, thus reducing Na^+ as well as water reabsorption. The resulting natriuresis is of lesser magnitude than the water diuresis, leading eventually to excessive water loss and hypernatremia.

Clinical Indications & Dosage

A. TO INCREASE URINE VOLUME

Osmotic diuretics are used to increase water excretion in preference to sodium excretion. This effect can be useful when avid Na^+ retention limits the response to conventional agents. It can be used to maintain urine volume and to prevent anuria that might otherwise result from presentation of large pigment loads to the kidney (eg, from hemolysis or rhabdomyolysis). Some oliguric patients do not respond to osmotic diuretics. Therefore, a test dose of mannitol (12.5 g intravenously) should be given prior to starting a continuous infusion. Mannitol should not be continued unless there is an increase in urine flow rate to more than 50 mL/h during the 3 hours following the test dose. Mannitol (12.5–25 g) can be repeated every 1–2 hours to maintain urine flow rate greater than 100 mL/h. Prolonged use of mannitol is not advised.

B. REDUCTION OF INTRACRANIAL AND INTRAOCULAR PRESSURE

Osmotic diuretics alter Starling forces so that water leaves cells and reduces intracellular volume. This effect is used to reduce intracranial pressure in neurologic conditions and to reduce intraocular pressure before ophthalmologic procedures. A dose of 1–2 g/kg mannitol is administered intravenously. Intracranial pressure, which must be monitored, should fall in 60–90 minutes.

Toxicity

A. EXTRACELLULAR VOLUME EXPANSION

Mannitol is rapidly distributed in the extracellular compartment and extracts water from cells. Prior to the diuresis, this leads to expansion of the extracellular volume and hyponatremia. This effect can complicate heart failure and may produce florid pulmonary edema. Headache, nausea, and vomiting are commonly observed in patients treated with osmotic diuretics.

B. DEHYDRATION, HYPERKALEMIA, AND HYPERNATREMIA

Excessive use of mannitol without adequate water replacement can ultimately lead to severe dehydration, free water losses, and hypernatremia. As water is extracted from cells, intracellular K^+ concentration rises, leading to cellular losses and hyperkalemia. These complications can be avoided by careful attention to serum ion composition and fluid balance.

2. Antidiuretic Hormone (ADH) Agonists

Vasopressin and **desmopressin** are used in the treatment of central diabetes insipidus. They are discussed in Chapter 37. Their renal action appears to be mediated primarily via V_2 receptors although V_{1a} receptors may also be involved.

3. Antidiuretic Hormone (ADH) Antagonists

A variety of medical conditions, including congestive heart failure and syndrome of inappropriate ADH (SIADH), cause water retention as the result of ADH excess. Dangerous hyponatremia can result. Several nonpeptide ADH receptor antagonists (vaptans) have been studied, with encouraging clinical results, but only **conivaptan** has been approved for use. Two nonselective agents, lithium and demeclocycline (a tetracycline antimicrobial drug), also have anti-ADH effects.

Pharmacokinetics

Conivaptan, lithium, and demeclocycline are orally active. Conivaptan and demeclocycline have half-lives of 5–10 hours. Lithium (discussed in detail in Chapter 29) is never used as an ADH antagonist.

Pharmacodynamics

Antidiuretic hormone antagonists inhibit the effects of ADH in the collecting tubule. Conivaptan is a pharmacologic antagonist at V_{1a} and V_2 receptors. Both lithium and demeclocycline appear to reduce the formation of cyclic adenosine monophospate (cAMP) in response to ADH and also to interfere with the actions of cAMP in the collecting tubule cells, but the mechanisms of these effects is not known.

Clinical Indications & Dosage

A. SYNDROME OF INAPPROPRIATE ADH SECRETION (SIADH)

Antidiuretic hormone antagonists are used to manage SIADH when water restriction has failed to correct the abnormality. This generally occurs in the outpatient setting, where water restriction cannot be enforced, or in the hospital when large quantities of intravenous fluid are needed for other purposes. Lithium carbonate has been used to treat this syndrome, but the response is unpredictable. Demeclocycline, in dosages of 600–1200 mg/d, yields a more predictable result and is less toxic. Appropriate plasma levels (2 mcg/mL) should be maintained by monitoring. Unlike demeclocycline, conivaptan is administered by IV injection, so it is not suitable for chronic use in outpatients.

B. OTHER CAUSES OF ELEVATED ANTIDIURETIC HORMONE (ADH)

Antidiuretic hormone is also elevated in response to diminished effective circulating blood volume, as often occurs in congestive heart failure. When treatment by volume replacement is not desirable, hyponatremia may result. As for SIADH, water restriction is the treatment of choice, but if it is not successful, demeclocycline or conivaptan may be used.

Toxicity

A. NEPHROGENIC DIABETES INSIPIDUS

If serum Na^+ is not monitored closely, ADH antagonists can cause severe hypernatremia and nephrogenic diabetes insipidus. If lithium is being used for a psychiatric disorder, nephrogenic diabetes insipidus can be treated with a thiazide diuretic or amiloride (see below).

B. RENAL FAILURE

Both lithium and demeclocycline have been reported to cause acute renal failure. Long-term lithium therapy may also cause chronic interstitial nephritis.

C. OTHER

Adverse effects associated with lithium therapy are discussed in Chapter 29. Demeclocycline should be avoided in patients with liver disease (see Chapter 44) and in children younger than 12 years.

DIURETIC COMBINATIONS

LOOP AGENTS & THIAZIDES

Some patients are refractory to the usual dose of loop diuretics or become refractory after an initial response. Since these agents have a short half-life (2–6 hrs), refractoriness may be due to an excessive interval between doses. Renal Na^+ retention may be greatly increased during the time period when the drug is no longer active. After the dosing interval for loop agents is minimized or the dose is maximized, the use of two drugs acting at different nephron sites may exhibit dramatic synergy. Loop agents and thiazides in combination will often produce diuresis when neither agent acting alone is even minimally effective. There are several reasons for this phenomenon. First, salt and water reabsorption in either the TAL or the DCT can increase when the other is blocked. Inhibition of both can therefore produce more than an additive diuretic response. Second, thiazide diuretics often produce a mild natriuresis in the proximal tubule that is usually masked by increased reabsorption in the TAL. The combination of loop diuretics and thiazides can therefore block Na^+ reabsorption, to some extent, from all three segments.

Metolazone is the usual thiazide-like drug used in patients refractory to loop agents alone, but it is likely that other thiazides would be as effective as metolazone. Moreover, metolazone is available only in an oral preparation, while chlorothiazide can be given parenterally.

The combination of loop diuretics and thiazides can mobilize large amounts of fluid, even in patients who have not responded to single agents. Therefore, close hemodynamic monitoring is essential. Routine outpatient use is not recommended. Furthermore, K^+-wasting is extremely common and may require parenteral K^+ administration with careful monitoring of fluid and electrolyte status.

POTASSIUM-SPARING DIURETICS & LOOP AGENTS OR THIAZIDES

Hypokalemia eventually develops in many patients who are placed on loop diuretics or thiazides. This can usually be managed with dietary NaCl restriction or with dietary KCl supplements. When hypokalemia cannot be managed in this way, the addition of a K^+-sparing diuretic can significantly lower K^+ excretion. While this approach is generally safe, it should be avoided in patients with renal insufficiency and in those receiving angiotensin antagonists such as ACE inhibitors, in whom life-threatening hyperkalemia can develop in response to K^+-sparing diuretics.

■ III. CLINICAL PHARMACOLOGY OF DIURETIC AGENTS

A summary of the effects of diuretics on urinary electrolyte excretion is shown in Table 15–2.

EDEMATOUS STATES

A common reason for diuretic use is for reduction of peripheral or pulmonary edema that has accumulated as a result of cardiac, renal, or vascular diseases that reduce blood delivery to the kidney. This reduction is sensed as insufficient "effective" arterial blood volume and leads to salt and water retention and edema formation. Judicious use of diuretics can mobilize this interstitial edema without significant reductions in plasma volume. However, excessive diuretic therapy may lead to further compromise of the effective arterial blood volume with reduction in perfusion of vital organs. Therefore, the use of diuretics to mobilize edema requires careful monitoring of the patient's hemodynamic status and an understanding of the pathophysiology of the underlying illness.

HEART FAILURE

When cardiac output is reduced by heart failure, the resultant changes in blood pressure and blood flow to the kidney are sensed as hypovolemia and lead to renal retention of salt and water. This physiologic response initially increases intravascular volume and venous return to the heart and may partially restore the cardiac output toward normal (see Chapter 13).

If the underlying disease causes cardiac output to deteriorate despite expansion of plasma volume, the kidney continues to retain salt and water, which then leaks from the vasculature and becomes interstitial or pulmonary edema. At this point, diuretic use becomes necessary to reduce the accumulation of edema, particularly in the lungs. Reduction of pulmonary vascular congestion with diuretics may actually improve oxygenation and thereby improve myocardial function. Reduction of preload can reduce the size of the heart, allowing it to work at a more efficient fiber length. Edema associated with heart failure is generally managed with loop diuretics. In some instances, salt and water retention may become so severe that a combination of thiazides and loop diuretics is necessary.

In treating the heart failure patient with diuretics, it must always be remembered that cardiac output in these patients is being maintained in part by high filling pressures and that excessive use of diuretics may diminish venous return and further impair cardiac output. This is especially critical in right ventricular heart failure. Systemic, rather than pulmonary vascular, congestion is the hallmark of this disorder. Diuretic-induced volume contraction will predictably reduce venous return and can severely compromise cardiac output if left ventricular filling pressure is reduced below 15 mm Hg (see Chapter 13).

Diuretic-induced metabolic alkalosis is another adverse effect that may further compromise cardiac function. While this complication can be treated with replacement of K^+ and restoration of intravascular volume with saline, severe heart failure may preclude the use of saline even in patients who have received excessive diuretic therapy. In these cases, adjunctive use of acetazolamide will help correct the alkalosis.

Another serious toxicity of diuretic use, particularly in the cardiac patient, is hypokalemia. Hypokalemia can exacerbate underlying cardiac arrhythmias and contribute to digitalis toxicity. This can usually be avoided by having the patient reduce Na^+ intake, thus decreasing Na^+ delivery to the K^+-secreting collecting tubule. Patients who are noncompliant with a low Na^+ diet must take oral KCl supplements or a K^+-sparing diuretic.

KIDNEY DISEASE

A variety of renal diseases interfere with the kidney's critical role in volume homeostasis. Although some renal disorders cause salt wasting, most kidney diseases cause retention of salt and water. When loss of renal function is severe, diuretic agents are of little benefit, because there is insufficient glomerular filtration to sustain a natriuretic response. However, a large number of patients with milder degrees of renal insufficiency can be treated with diuretics when they retain sodium.

Many glomerular diseases, such as those associated with diabetes mellitus or systemic lupus erythematosus, exhibit renal retention of salt and water. The cause of this sodium retention is not precisely known, but it probably involves disordered regulation of the renal microcirculation and tubular function through release of vasoconstrictors, prostaglandins, cytokines, and other mediators. When edema or hypertension develops in these patients, diuretic therapy can be very effective. If heart failure is also present, see the warnings mentioned above.

Certain forms of renal disease, particularly diabetic nephropathy, are frequently associated with development of hyperkalemia at a relatively early stage of renal failure. In these cases, a thiazide or loop diuretic will enhance K^+ excretion by increasing delivery of salt to the K^+-secreting collecting tubule.

Patients with renal diseases leading to the nephrotic syndrome often present complex problems in volume management. These patients may exhibit fluid retention in the form of ascites or edema but have reduced plasma volume due to reduced plasma oncotic pressures. This is very often the case in patients with "minimal change" nephropathy. In these patients, diuretic use may cause further reductions in plasma volume that can impair glomerular filtration rate and may lead to orthostatic hypotension. Most other causes of nephrotic syndrome are associated with primary retention of salt and water by the kidney, leading to expanded plasma volume and hypertension despite the low plasma oncotic pressure. In these cases, diuretic therapy may be beneficial in controlling the volume-dependent component of hypertension.

In choosing a diuretic for the patient with kidney disease, there are a number of important limitations. Acetazolamide must usually be avoided because it can exacerbate acidosis. Potassium-sparing diuretics may cause hyperkalemia. Thiazide diuretics are generally ineffective when glomerular filtration rate falls below 30 mL/min. Thus, loop diuretics are often the best choice in treating edema associated with kidney failure. Lastly, although excessive use of diuretics can impair renal function in all patients, the consequences are more serious in those with underlying renal disease.

HEPATIC CIRRHOSIS

Liver disease is often associated with edema and ascites in conjunction with elevated portal hydrostatic pressures and reduced plasma oncotic pressures. Mechanisms for retention of Na^+ by the kidney in this setting include diminished renal perfusion (from systemic vascular alterations), diminished plasma volume (due to ascites formation), and diminished oncotic pressure (hypoalbuminemia). In addition, there may be primary Na^+ retention due to elevated plasma aldosterone levels.

When ascites and edema become severe, diuretic therapy can be very useful. However, cirrhotic patients are often resistant to loop diuretics because of decreased secretion of the drug into the tubular fluid and because of high aldosterone levels. In contrast, cirrhotic edema is unusually responsive to spironolactone and eplerenone. The combination of loop diuretics and an aldosterone receptor antagonist may be useful in some patients.

It is important to note that, even more than in heart failure, overly aggressive use of diuretics in this setting can be disastrous. Vigorous diuretic therapy can cause marked depletion of intravascular volume, hypokalemia, and metabolic alkalosis. Hepatorenal syndrome and hepatic encephalopathy are the unfortunate consequences of excessive diuretic use in the cirrhotic patient.

IDIOPATHIC EDEMA

Despite intensive study, the pathophysiology of this disorder (fluctuating salt retention and edema) still remains obscure. Some studies, but not all, suggest that intermittent diuretic use may actually contribute to the syndrome. Idiopathic edema should probably be managed with moderate salt restriction alone if possible.

NONEDEMATOUS STATES

HYPERTENSION

The diuretic and mild vasodilator actions of the thiazides are useful in treating virtually all patients with essential hypertension, and may be sufficient in many. Loop diuretics are usually reserved for patients with renal insufficiency or heart failure. Moderate restriction of dietary Na^+ intake (60–100 mEq/d) has been shown to potentiate the effects of diuretics in essential hypertension and to lessen renal K^+ wasting.

A recent very large study (over 30,000 participants) has shown that inexpensive diuretics like thiazides result in similar or superior outcomes to those found with ACE inhibitor or calcium channel blocker therapy. This important result reinforces the importance of thiazide therapy in hypertension.

Although diuretics are often successful as monotherapy, they also play an important role in patients who require multiple drugs to control blood pressure. Diuretics enhance the efficacy of many agents, particularly the ACE inhibitors. Patients being treated with powerful vasodilators such as hydralazine or minoxidil usually require simultaneous diuretics because the vasodilators cause significant salt and water retention.

NEPHROLITHIASIS

Approximately two thirds of kidney stones contain Ca^{2+} phosphate or Ca^{2+} oxalate. Many patients with such stones exhibit a defect in proximal tubular Ca^{2+} reabsorption that causes hypercalciuria. This can be treated with thiazide diuretics, which enhance Ca^{2+} reabsorption in the distal convoluted tubule and thus reduce the urinary Ca^{2+} concentration. Salt intake must be reduced in this setting, as excess dietary NaCl will overwhelm the hypocalciuric effect of thiazides. Calcium stones may also be caused by increased intestinal absorption of Ca^{2+}, or they may be idiopathic. In these situations, thiazides are also effective, but should be used as adjunctive therapy with decreased Ca^{2+} intake and other measures.

HYPERCALCEMIA

Hypercalcemia can be a medical emergency. Because loop diuretics reduce Ca^{2+} reabsorption significantly, they can be quite effective in promoting Ca^{2+} diuresis. However, loop diuretics alone can cause marked volume contraction. If this occurs, loop diuretics are ineffective (and potentially counterproductive) because Ca^{2+} reabsorption in the proximal tubule would be enhanced. Thus, saline must be administered simultaneously with loop diuretics if an effective Ca^{2+} diuresis is to be maintained. The usual approach is to infuse normal saline and furosemide (80–120 mg) intravenously. Once the diuresis begins, the rate of saline infusion can be matched with the urine flow rate to avoid volume depletion. Potassium chloride may be added to the saline infusion as needed.

DIABETES INSIPIDUS

Diabetes insipidus is due either to deficient production of ADH (neurogenic or central diabetes insipidus) or inadequate responsiveness to ADH (nephrogenic diabetes insipidus). Administration of supplementary ADH or one of its analogs is only effective in central diabetes insipidus. Thiazide diuretics can reduce polyuria and polydipsia in both types of diabetes insipidus. This seemingly paradoxic beneficial effect is mediated through plasma volume reduction, with an associated fall in glomerular filtration rate, enhanced proximal reabsorption of NaCl and water, and decreased delivery of fluid to the downstream diluting segments. Thus, the maximum volume of dilute urine that can be produced is lowered and thiazides can significantly reduce urine flow in the polyuric patient. Dietary sodium restriction can potentiate the beneficial effects of thiazides on urine volume in this setting. Lithium (Li^+), used in the treatment of manic-depressive disorder, is a common cause of nephrogenic diabetes insipidus and thiazide diuretics have been found to be helpful in treating it. Serum Li^+ levels must be carefully monitored in these patients, because diuretics may *reduce* renal clearance of Li^+ and raise plasma Li^+ levels into the toxic range (see Chapter 29). Lithium-induced polyuria can also be partially reversed by amiloride, which blocks Li^+ entry into collecting duct cells, much as it blocks Na^+ entry.

PREPARATIONS AVAILABLE

Acetazolamide (generic, Diamox)
Oral: 125, 250 mg tablets
Oral sustained-release: 500 mg capsules
Parenteral: 500 mg powder for injection
Amiloride (generic, Midamor, combination drugs)
Oral: 5 mg tablets
Bendroflumethiazide (Naturetin, combination drugs)
Oral: 5, 10 mg tablets
Brinzolamide (Azopt) (For ocular conditions)
Ophthalmic: 1% suspension
Bumetanide (generic, Bumex)
Oral: 0.5, 1, 2 mg tablets
Parenteral: 0.5 mg/2 mL ampule for IV or IM injection
Chlorothiazide (generic, Diuril)
Oral: 250, 500 mg tablets; 250 mg/5 mL oral suspension
Parenteral: 500 mg for injection
Chlorthalidone (generic, Hygroton, Thalitone, combination drugs)
Oral: 25, 50, 100 mg tablets
Conivaptan (Vaprisol)
Parenteral: 5 mg/mL for IV injection
Demeclocycline (Declomycin)
Oral: 150 mg tablets and capsules; 300 mg tablets
Dichlorphenamide (Daranide)
Oral: 50 mg tablets
Dorzolamide (Trusopt) (For ocular conditions)
Ophthalmic: 2% solution
Eplerenone (Inspra)
Oral: 25, 50 mg tablets
Ethacrynic acid (Edecrin)
Oral: 25, 50 mg tablets
Parenteral: 50 mg IV injection
Furosemide (generic, Lasix, others)

Oral: 20, 40, 80 mg tablets; 8, 10 mg/mL oral solutions
Parenteral: 10 mg/mL for IM or IV injection
Hydrochlorothiazide (generic, Esidrix, Hydro-DIURIL, combination drugs)
Oral: 12.5 mg capsules; 25, 50, 100 mg tablets; 10, 100 mg/mL solution
Hydroflumethiazide (generic, Saluron)
Oral: 50 mg tablets
Indapamide (generic, Lozol)
Oral: 1.25, 2.5 mg tablets
Mannitol (generic, Osmitrol)
Parenteral: 5, 10, 15, 20, for injection
Methazolamide (generic, Neptazane) (For ocular conditions)
Oral: 25, 50 mg tablets
Methyclothiazide (generic, Aquatensen, Enduron)
Oral: 2.5, 5 mg tablets
Metolazone (Mykrox, Zaroxolyn) (Note: Bioavailability of Mykrox is greater than that of Zaroxolyn.)
Oral: 0.5 (Mykrox); 2.5, 5, 10 mg (Zaroxolyn) tablets
Polythiazide (Renese, combination drugs)
Oral: 1, 2, 4 mg tablets
Quinethazone (Hydromox)
Oral: 50 mg tablets
Spironolactone (generic, Aldactone)
Oral: 25, 50, 100 mg tablets
Torsemide (Demadex)
Oral: 5, 10, 20, 100 mg tablets
Parenteral: 10 mg/mL for injection
Triamterene (Dyrenium)
Oral: 50, 100 mg capsules
Trichlormethiazide (generic, Diurese, Naqua, others)
Oral: 2, 4 mg tablets

REFERENCES

Abdallah JG et al: Loop diuretic infusion increases thiazide-sensitive Na(+)/Cl(-)-cotransporter abundance: Role of aldosterone. J Am Soc Nephrol 2001;12:1335.

ALLHAT Officers and Coordinators for the ALLHAT Collaborative Research Group: Major outcomes in high-risk hypertensive patients randomized to angiotensin-converting enzyme inhibitor or calcium channel blocker vs diuretic: The Antihypertensive and Lipid-Lowering Treatment to Prevent Heart Attack Trial (ALLHAT). JAMA 2002;288:2981.

Alvarez-Guerra M, Garay RC: Renal Na-K-Cl transporter NKCC2 in Dahl salt-sensitive rats. J Hypertens 2002;20:721.

Brenner BM (editor): *Brenner & Rector's The Kidney,* 7th ed. Saunders, 2003.

Costello-Boerrigter LC, Boerrigter G, Burnett JC Jr: Revisiting salt and water retention: New diuretics, aquaretics, and natriuretics. Med Clin North Am 2003;87:475.

Fall PJ: Hyponatremia and hypernatremia. A systematic approach to causes and their correction. Postgrad Med 2000;107:75.

Gottlieb SS et al: BG9719 (CVT-124), an A1 adenosine receptor antagonist, protects against the decline in renal function observed with diuretic therapy. Circulation 2002;105:1348.

Greenberg A: Diuretic complications. Am J Med Sci 2000;319:10.

Hackett PH, Roach RC: High-altitude illness. N Engl J Med 2001; 345:107.

Kalra PR et al: The regulation and measurement of plasma volume in heart failure. J Am Coll Cardiol 2002;39:1901.

Kaplan NM: The place of diuretics in preventing cardiovascular events. J Hum Hypertens 2004;18:S29.

Knepper MA, Brooks HL: Regulation of the sodium transporters NHE3, NKCC2, and NCC in the kidney. Curr Opin Nephrol Hypertens 2001;10:655.

Na KY et al: Upregulation of Na^+ transporter abundance in response to chronic thiazide or loop diuretic treatment in rats. Am J Physiol 2003;284:F133.

Nijenhuis T et al: Enhanced passive Ca^{2+} reabsorption and reduced Mg^{2+} channel abundance explains thiazide-induced hypocalciuria and hypomagnesemia. J Clin Invest 2005; 115:1651.

Rejnmark L et al: Effects of long-term treatment with loop diuretics on bone mineral density, calciotropic hormones and bone turnover. J Intern Med 2005;257:176.

Schrot RJ, Muizelaar JP: Mannitol in acute traumatic brain injury. Lancet 2002;359:1633.

Shlipak MG, Massie BM: The clinical challenge of cardiorenal syndrome. Circulation 2004;110:1514.

Sica DA, Gehr TWB: Diuretic use in stage 5 chronic kidney disease and end-stage renal disease. Curr Opin Nephrol Hypertens 2003;12:483.

Tovar-Palacio C et al: Ion and diuretic specificity of chimeric proteins between apical $Na^+-K^+-2CL^-$ and Na^+-Cl^- cotransporters. Am J Physiol 2004;287:F570.

Wilcox C: New insights into diuretic use in patients with chronic renal disease. J Am Soc Nephrol 2002;13:798.

SECTION IV
Drugs with Important Actions on Smooth Muscle

Histamine, Serotonin, & the Ergot Alkaloids

Bertram G. Katzung, MD, PhD

16

Histamine and serotonin (5-hydroxytryptamine) are biologically active amines that function as neurotransmitters and are found in non-neural tissues, have complex physiologic and pathologic effects through multiple receptor subtypes, and are often released locally. Together with endogenous peptides (see Chapter 17), prostaglandins and leukotrienes (see Chapter 18), and cytokines (see Chapter 56), they are sometimes called *autacoids* (Greek, "self-remedy") or local hormones in recognition of these properties.

Because of their broad and largely undesirable effects, neither histamine nor serotonin has any clinical application in the treatment of disease. However, compounds that *selectively* activate certain receptor subtypes or selectively antagonize the actions of these amines are of considerable clinical usefulness. This chapter therefore emphasizes the basic pharmacology of the agonist amines and the clinical pharmacology of the more selective agonist and antagonist drugs. The ergot alkaloids, compounds with partial agonist activity at serotonin and several other receptors, are discussed at the end of the chapter.

■ I. HISTAMINE

Histamine was synthesized in 1907 and later isolated from mammalian tissues. Early hypotheses concerning

the possible physiologic roles of tissue histamine were based on similarities between the effects of intravenously administered histamine and the symptoms of anaphylactic shock and tissue injury. Marked species variation is observed, but in humans histamine is an important mediator of immediate allergic and inflammatory reactions, although it plays only a modest role in anaphylaxis. Histamine plays an important role in gastric acid secretion (see Chapter 63) and functions as a neurotransmitter and neuromodulator (see Chapters 6, 21). Newer evidence indicates that histamine also plays a role in chemotaxis of white blood cells.

BASIC PHARMACOLOGY OF HISTAMINE

Chemistry & Pharmacokinetics

Histamine occurs in plants as well as in animal tissues and is a component of some venoms and stinging secretions.

Histamine is formed by decarboxylation of the amino acid *l*-histidine, a reaction catalyzed in mammalian tissues by the enzyme histidine decarboxylase. Once formed, histamine is either stored or rapidly inactivated. Very little histamine is excreted unchanged. The major metabolic pathways involve conversion to *N*-methylhistamine, methylimidazoleacetic acid, and imidazoleacetic acid (IAA). Certain neoplasms (systemic mastocytosis, urticaria pigmentosa, gastric carcinoid, and occasionally myelogenous leukemia) are associated with increased numbers of mast cells or basophils and with increased excretion of histamine and its metabolites.

$$\text{HN} \diagdown \text{N} — CH_2 — CH_2 — NH_2$$

Histamine

Most tissue histamine is sequestered and bound in granules (vesicles) in mast cells or basophils; the histamine content of many tissues is directly related to their mast cell content. The bound form of histamine is biologically inactive, but many stimuli, as noted below, can trigger the release of mast cell histamine, allowing the free amine to exert its actions on surrounding tissues. Mast cells are especially rich at sites of potential tissue injury—nose, mouth, and feet; internal body surfaces; and blood vessels, particularly at pressure points and bifurcations.

Non-mast cell histamine is found in several tissues, including the brain, where it functions as a neurotransmitter. Endogenous neurotransmitter histamine may play a role in many brain functions such as neuroendocrine control, cardiovascular regulation, thermal and body weight regulation, and arousal (see Chapter 21).

A second important nonneuronal site of histamine storage and release is the enterochromaffin-like (ECL) cells of the fundus of the stomach. ECL cells release histamine, one of the primary gastric acid secretagogues, to activate the acid-producing parietal cells of the mucosa (see Chapter 63).

Storage & Release of Histamine

The stores of histamine in mast cells can be released through several mechanisms.

A. IMMUNOLOGIC RELEASE

Immunologic processes account for the most important pathophysiologic mechanism of mast cell and basophil histamine release. These cells, if sensitized by IgE antibodies attached to their surface membranes, degranulate "explosively" when exposed to the appropriate antigen (see Figure 56–5, effector phase). This type of release also requires energy and calcium. Degranulation leads to the simultaneous release of histamine, adenosine triphosphate (ATP), and other mediators that are stored together in the granules. Histamine released by this mechanism is a mediator in immediate (type I) allergic reactions. Substances released during IgG- or IgM-mediated immune reactions that activate the complement cascade also release histamine from mast cells and basophils.

By a negative feedback control mechanism mediated by H_2 receptors, histamine appears to modulate its own

release and that of other mediators from sensitized mast cells in some tissues. In humans, mast cells in skin and basophils show this negative feedback mechanism; lung mast cells do not. Thus, histamine may act to limit the intensity of the allergic reaction in the skin and blood.

Endogenous histamine has a modulating role in a variety of inflammatory and immune responses. Upon injury to a tissue, released histamine causes local vasodilation and leakage of plasma containing mediators of acute inflammation (complement, C-reactive protein), and antibodies. Histamine has an active chemotactic attraction for inflammatory cells (neutrophils, eosinophils, basophils, monocytes, and lymphocytes). Histamine inhibits the release of lysosome contents and several T- and B-lymphocyte functions. Most of these actions are mediated by H_2 or H_4 receptors. Release of peptides from nerves in response to inflammation is also probably modulated by histamine, in this case acting through presynaptic H_3 receptors.

B. CHEMICAL AND MECHANICAL RELEASE

Certain amines, including drugs such as morphine and tubocurarine, can displace histamine from the heparin-protein complex within cells. This type of release does not require energy and is not associated with mast cell injury or degranulation. Loss of granules from the mast cell also releases histamine, since sodium ions in the extracellular fluid rapidly displace the amine from the complex. Chemical and mechanical mast cell injury causes degranulation and histamine release. **Compound 48/80,** an experimental drug, selectively releases histamine from tissue mast cells by an exocytotic degranulation process requiring energy and calcium.

Pharmacodynamics

A. MECHANISM OF ACTION

Histamine exerts its biologic actions by combining with specific cellular receptors located on the surface membrane. The four different histamine receptors thus far characterized are designated H_1–H_4 and are described in Table 16–1. Unlike the other amine transmitter receptors discussed previously, no subfamilies have been found within these major types, although different splice variants of several receptor types have been found.

All four receptor types have been cloned and belong to the large superfamily of receptors having seven membrane-spanning regions and coupled with G proteins (GPCR). The structures of the H_1 and H_2 receptors differ significantly and appear to be more closely related to muscarinic and 5-HT$_1$ receptors, respectively, than to each other. The H_4 receptor has about 40% homology with the H_3 receptor but does not seem to be closely related to any other histamine receptor. All four histamine receptors have been shown to have constitutive activity in some sys-

Table 16–1. Histamine receptor subtypes.

Receptor Subtype	Distribution	Postreceptor Mechanism	Partially Selective Agonists	Partially Selective Antagonists
H_1	Smooth muscle, endothelium, brain	G_q, ↑ IP_3, DAG	Histaprodifen	Mepyramine, triprolidine
H_2	Gastric mucosa, cardiac muscle, mast cells, brain	G_s, ↑ cAMP	Amthamine	Ranitidine, tiotidine
H_3	Presynaptic: brain, myenteric plexus, other neurons	G_i, ↓ cAMP	R-α-Methylhistamine, imetit, immepip	Thioperamide, iodophenpropit, clobenpropit[1]
H_4	Eosinophils, neutrophils, CD4 T cells	G_i, ↓ cAMP	Clobenpropit, imetit, clozapine	Thioperamide

[1]Inverse agonist.

tems; thus, some "antihistamines" previously considered to be traditional pharmacologic antagonists must now be considered to be possible inverse agonists (Chapter 2). Indeed, many first- and second-generation H_1 blockers (see below) are probably inverse agonists. Furthermore, a single molecule may be an agonist at one histamine receptor and an antagonist at another. For example, clobenprobit, an agonist at H_4 receptors, is an antagonist or inverse agonist at H_3 receptors (Table 16–1).

In the brain, H_1 and H_2 receptors are located on postsynaptic membranes, whereas H_3 receptors are predominantly presynaptic. Activation of H_1 receptors, which are present in endothelium, smooth muscle cells, and nerve endings, usually elicits an increase in phosphoinositol hydrolysis and an increase in intracellular calcium. Activation of H_2 receptors, present in gastric mucosa, cardiac muscle cells, and some immune cells, increases intracellular cyclic adenosine monophosphate (cAMP) via G_s. Like the β_2 adrenoceptor, under certain circumstances the H_2 receptor may couple to G_q, activating the IP_3-DAG (inositol 1,4,5-trisphosphate-diacylglycerol) cascade. Activation of H_3 receptors decreases transmitter release from histaminergic and other neurons, probably mediated by a decrease in calcium influx through N-type calcium channels in nerve endings. H_4 receptors are mainly found on leukocytes in the bone marrow and circulating blood. H_4 receptors appear to have very important chemotactic effects on eosinophils and mast cells. In this role, they may play an important part in inflammation and allergy. They may also modulate production of these cell types and they may mediate, in part, the previously recognized effects of histamine on cytokine production.

B. TISSUE AND ORGAN SYSTEM EFFECTS OF HISTAMINE

Histamine exerts powerful effects on smooth and cardiac muscle, on certain endothelial and nerve cells, and on the secretory cells of the stomach. However, sensitivity to histamine varies greatly among species. Guinea pigs are exquisitely sensitive, humans, dogs, and cats somewhat less so, and mice and rats very much less so.

1. Nervous system—Histamine is a powerful stimulant of sensory nerve endings, especially those mediating pain and itching. This H_1-mediated effect is an important component of the urticarial response and reactions to insect and nettle stings. Some evidence suggests that local high concentrations can also depolarize efferent (axonal) nerve endings (see paragraph 8, below). In the mouse, and probably in humans, respiratory neurons signaling inspiration and expiration are modulated by H_1 receptors. Presynaptic H_3 receptors play important roles in modulating transmitter release in the nervous system. H_3 agonists reduce the release of acetylcholine, amine, and peptide transmitters in various areas of the brain and in peripheral nerves.

2. Cardiovascular system—In humans, injection or infusion of histamine causes a decrease in systolic and diastolic blood pressure and an increase in heart rate. The blood pressure changes are caused by the direct vasodilator action of histamine on arterioles and precapillary sphincters; the increase in heart rate involves both stimulatory actions of histamine on the heart and a reflex tachycardia. Flushing, a sense of warmth, and headache may also occur during histamine administration, consistent with the vasodilation. Vasodilation elicited by small doses of histamine is caused by H_1-receptor activation and is mediated primarily by release of nitric oxide from the endothelium (see Chapter 19). The decrease in blood pressure is usually accompanied by a reflex tachycardia. Higher doses of histamine activate the H_2-mediated cAMP process of vasodilation and direct cardiac stimulation. In humans, the cardiovascular effects of small doses of histamine can usually be antagonized by H_1-receptor antagonists alone.

Histamine-induced edema results from the action of the amine on H_1 receptors in the vessels of the microcirculation, especially the postcapillary vessels. The effect is associated with the separation of the endothelial cells, which permits the transudation of fluid and molecules as large as small proteins into the perivascular tissue. This effect is responsible for the urticaria (hives) that signals the release of histamine in the skin. Studies of endothelial cells suggest that actin and myosin within these cells contract, resulting in separation of the endothelial cells and increased permeability.

Direct cardiac effects of histamine include both increased contractility and increased pacemaker rate. These effects are mediated chiefly by H_2 receptors. In human atrial muscle, histamine can also decrease contractility; this effect is mediated by H_1 receptors. The physiologic significance of these cardiac actions is not clear. Some of the cardiovascular signs and symptoms of anaphylaxis are due to released histamine, though several other mediators are involved and appear to be more important than histamine in humans.

3. Bronchiolar smooth muscle—In both humans and guinea pigs, histamine causes bronchoconstriction mediated by H_1 receptors. In the guinea pig, this effect is the cause of death from histamine toxicity, but in humans with normal airways, bronchoconstriction following small doses of histamine is not marked. However, patients with asthma are very sensitive to histamine. The bronchoconstriction induced in these patients probably represents a hyperactive neural response, since such patients also respond excessively to many other stimuli, and the response to histamine can be blocked by autonomic blocking drugs such as ganglionic blocking agents as well as by H_1-receptor antagonists (see Chapter 20). Although methacholine provocation is more commonly used, tests using increasing doses of inhaled histamine have been used in the diagnosis of bronchial hyperreactivity in patients with suspected asthma or cystic fibrosis. Such individuals may be 100- to 1000-fold more sensitive to histamine (and methacholine) than are normal subjects. Curiously, a few species (eg, rabbit) respond to histamine with broncho*dilation*, reflecting the dominance of the H_2 receptor in their airways.

4. Gastrointestinal tract smooth muscle—Histamine causes contraction of intestinal smooth muscle, and histamine-induced contraction of guinea pig ileum is a standard bioassay for this amine. The human gut is not as sensitive as that of the guinea pig, but large doses of histamine may cause diarrhea, partly as a result of this effect. This action of histamine is mediated by H_1 receptors.

5. Other smooth muscle organs—In humans, histamine generally has insignificant effects on the smooth muscle of the eye and genitourinary tract. However, pregnant women suffering anaphylactic reactions may abort as a result of histamine-induced contractions, and in some species the sensitivity of the uterus is sufficient to form the basis for a bioassay.

6. Secretory tissue—Histamine has long been recognized as a powerful stimulant of gastric acid secretion and, to a lesser extent, of gastric pepsin and intrinsic factor production. The effect is caused by activation of H_2 receptors on gastric parietal cells and is associated with increased adenylyl cyclase activity, cAMP concentration, and intracellular Ca^{2+} concentration. Other stimulants of gastric acid secretion such as acetylcholine and gastrin do not increase cAMP even though their maximal effects on acid output can be reduced—but not abolished—by H_2-receptor antagonists. These actions are discussed in detail in Chapter 63. Histamine also stimulates secretion in the small and large intestine. In contrast, H_3-selective histamine agonists *inhibit* acid secretion stimulated by food or pentagastrin in several species.

Histamine has much smaller effects on the activity of other glandular tissue at ordinary concentrations. Very high concentrations can cause adrenal medullary discharge.

7. Metabolic effects—Recent studies of H_3-receptor knockout mice demonstrate that absence of this receptor results in animals with increased food intake, decreased energy expenditure, and obesity. They also show insulin resistance and increased blood levels of leptin and insulin. It is not yet known whether the H_3 receptor has a similar role in humans.

8. The "triple response"—Intradermal injection of histamine causes a characteristic red spot, edema, and flare response that was first described over 60 years ago. The effect involves three separate cell types: smooth muscle in the microcirculation, capillary or venular endothelium, and sensory nerve endings. At the site of injection, a reddening appears owing to dilation of small vessels, followed soon by an edematous wheal at the injection site and a red irregular flare surrounding the wheal. The flare is said to be caused by an axon reflex. A sensation of itching may accompany these effects.

Similar local effects may be produced by injecting histamine liberators (compound 48/80, morphine, etc) intradermally or by applying the appropriate antigens to the skin of a sensitized person. Although most of these local effects can be blocked by prior administration of an H_1-receptor-blocking agent, H_2 and H_3 receptors may also be involved.

9. Other effects possibly mediated by histamine receptors—In addition to the local stimulation of peripheral pain nerve endings via H_3 and H_1 receptors, histamine may play a role in nociception in the central nervous system. **Burimamide,** an early candidate for H_2 blocking action, and newer analogs with no effect on H_1, H_2, or H_3 receptors, have been shown to have significant analgesic action in rodents when administered into the central nervous system. The analgesia is said to be comparable to that produced by opioids, but tolerance, respiratory depression, and constipation have not been reported. Although the mechanism of this action is not known, these compounds may represent an important new class of analgesics.

Other Histamine Agonists

Small substitutions on the imidazole ring of histamine significantly modify the selectivity of the compounds for the histamine receptor subtypes. Some of these are listed in Table 16–1.

CLINICAL PHARMACOLOGY OF HISTAMINE

Clinical Uses

In pulmonary function laboratories, histamine aerosol has been used as a provocative test of **bronchial hyperreactivity.** Histamine has no other current clinical applications.

Toxicity & Contraindications

Adverse effects of histamine release, like those following administration of histamine, are dose-related. Flushing, hypotension, tachycardia, headache, wheals, bronchoconstriction, and gastrointestinal upset are noted. These effects are also observed after the ingestion of spoiled fish (scombroid fish poisoning), and there is evidence that histamine produced by bacterial action in the flesh of the fish is the major causative agent.

Histamine should not be given to patients with asthma (except as part of a carefully monitored test of pulmonary function) or to patients with active ulcer disease or gastrointestinal bleeding.

HISTAMINE ANTAGONISTS

The effects of histamine released in the body can be reduced in several ways. **Physiologic antagonists,** especially epinephrine, have smooth muscle actions opposite to those of histamine, but they act at different receptors. This is important clinically because injection of epinephrine can be lifesaving in systemic **anaphylaxis** and in other conditions in which massive release of histamine—and other mediators—occurs.

Release inhibitors reduce the degranulation of mast cells that results from immunologic triggering by antigen-IgE interaction. Cromolyn and nedocromil appear to have this effect (see Chapter 20) and are used in the treatment of asthma, though the molecular mechanism underlying their action is presently unknown. Beta$_2$-adrenoceptor agonists also appear capable of reducing histamine release.

Histamine **receptor antagonists** represent a third approach to the reduction of histamine-mediated responses. For over 60 years, compounds have been available that competitively antagonize many of the actions of histamine

on smooth muscle. However, not until the H$_2$-receptor antagonist burimamide was described in 1972 was it possible to antagonize the gastric acid-stimulating activity of histamine. The development of selective H$_2$-receptor antagonists has led to more effective therapy for peptic disease (see Chapter 63). Selective H$_3$ and H$_4$ antagonists are not yet available for clinical use. However, potent and selective experimental H$_3$-receptor antagonists, thioperamide and clobenpropit, have been developed.

■ II. H$_1$-RECEPTOR ANTAGONISTS

Compounds that competitively block histamine at H$_1$ receptors have been used in the treatment of allergic conditions for many years, and many H$_1$ antagonists are currently marketed in the USA. Many are available without prescription, both alone and in combination formulations such as "cold pills" and sleep aids (see Chapter 64).

BASIC PHARMACOLOGY OF H$_1$-RECEPTOR ANTAGONISTS

Chemistry & Pharmacokinetics

The H$_1$ antagonists are conveniently divided into first-generation and second-generation agents. These groups are distinguished by the relatively strong sedative effects of most of the first-generation drugs. The first-generation agents are also more likely to block autonomic receptors. The relatively less sedating characteristic of the second-generation H$_1$ blockers is due in part to their less complete distribution into the central nervous system. All of the H$_1$ antagonists are stable amines with the general structure illustrated in Figure 16–1. Several chemical subgroups, and the structures of compounds representing different subgroups are shown in the figure. Doses of some of these drugs are given in Table 16–2.

These agents are rapidly absorbed following oral administration, with peak blood concentrations occurring in 1–2 hours. They are widely distributed throughout the body, and the first-generation drugs enter the central nervous system readily. Some of them are extensively metabolized, primarily by microsomal systems in the liver. Several of the second-generation agents are metabolized by the CYP3A4 system and thus are subject to important interactions when other drugs (such as ketoconazole) inhibit this subtype of P450 enzymes. Most of the drugs have an effective duration of action of 4–6 hours following a single dose, but meclizine and several second-generation agents are longer-acting, with a duration of action of 12–24 hours. The newer agents are considerably less lipid-soluble than the first-generation drugs and are substrates of the P-glycoprotein transporter in the blood-brain barrier; as a

X—Y—C—C—N

X is: C or N
Y is: C, O, or omitted

GENERAL STRUCTURE

ETHERS OR ETHANOLAMINE DERIVATIVE

$CH-O-CH_2-CH_2-N$ with CH_3, CH_3

Diphenhydramine or dimenhydrinate

ETHYLENEDIAMINE DERIVATIVE

CH_2

$N-CH_2-CH_2-N$ with CH_3, CH_3

Tripelennamine

PIPERAZINE DERIVATIVE

$CH-N$ $N-CH_3$

Cyclizine

ALKYLAMINE DERIVATIVE

Cl—

$CH-CH_2-CH_2-N$ with CH_3, CH_3

Chlorpheniramine

PHENOTHIAZINE DERIVATIVE

S

$N-CH_2-CH-N$ with CH_3, CH_3; CH_3

Promethazine

PIPERIDINE DERIVATIVES

OH
C

N
$CH_2-CH_2-CH_2-CH-R$ with OH

R: $C-CH_3$ with CH_3, CH_3

Terfenadine

R: $C-COOH$ with CH_3, CH_3

Fexofenadine

Figure 16–1. General structure of H_1 antagonist drugs and examples of the major subgroups.

result they enter the central nervous system with difficulty or not at all. Many H_1 antagonists have active metabolites. The active metabolites of hydroxyzine, terfenadine, and loratadine are available as drugs (cetirizine, fexofenadine, and desloratadine, respectively).

Pharmacodynamics

A. HISTAMINE-RECEPTOR BLOCKADE

H_1-receptor antagonists block the actions of histamine by reversible competitive antagonism at the H_1 receptor. They have negligible potency at the H_2 receptor and little at the H_3 receptor. For example, histamine-

Table 16–2. Some H_1 antihistaminic drugs in clinical use.

Drugs	Usual Adult Dose	Anticholinergic Activity	Comments
FIRST-GENERATION ANTIHISTAMINES			
Ethanolamines			
Carbinoxamine (Clistin)	4–8 mg	+++	Slight to moderate sedation
Dimenhydrinate (salt of diphenhydramine) (Dramamine)	50 mg	+++	Marked sedation; anti-motion sickness activity
Diphenhydramine (Benadryl, etc)	25–50 mg	+++	Marked sedation; anti-motion sickness activity
Ethylaminediamine			
Tripelennamine (PBZ, etc)	25–50 mg	+	Moderate sedation
Piperazine derivatives			
Hydroxyzine (Atarax, etc)	15–100 mg	nd	Marked sedation
Cyclizine (Marezine)	25–50 mg	–	Slight sedation; anti-motion sickness activity
Meclizine (Bonine, etc)	25–50 mg	–	Slight sedation; anti-motion sickness activity
Alkylamines			
Brompheniramine (Dimetane, etc)	4–8 mg	+	Slight sedation
Chlorpheniramine (Chlor-Trimeton, etc)	4–8 mg	+	Slight sedation; common component of OTC "cold" medication
Phenothiazine derivative			
Promethazine (Phenergan, etc)	10–25 mg	+++	Marked sedation; antiemetic; α block
Miscellaneous			
Cyproheptadine (Periactin, etc)	4 mg	+	Moderate sedation; also has antiserotonin activity
SECOND-GENERATION ANTIHISTAMINES			
Piperidine			
Fexofenadine (Allegra)	60 mg	–	
Miscellaneous			
Loratadine (Claritin)	10 mg	–	Longer action
Cetirizine (Zyrtec)	5–10 mg	–	

nd, no data found.

induced contraction of bronchiolar or gastrointestinal smooth muscle can be completely blocked by these agents, but the effects on gastric acid secretion and the heart are unmodified.

B. ACTIONS NOT CAUSED BY HISTAMINE RECEPTOR BLOCKADE

The first-generation H_1-receptor antagonists have many actions not ascribable to blockade of the actions of histamine. The large number of these actions probably results from the similarity of the general structure (Figure 16–1) to the structure of drugs that have effects at muscarinic cholinoceptor, α adrenoceptor, serotonin, and local anesthetic receptor sites. Some of these actions are of therapeutic value and some are undesirable.

1. Sedation—A common effect of first-generation H_1 antagonists is sedation, but the intensity of this effect varies among chemical subgroups (Table 16–2) and among patients as well. The effect is sufficiently prominent with some agents to make them useful as "sleep aids" (see Chapter 64) and unsuitable for daytime use. The effect resembles that of some antimuscarinic drugs and is considered very unlike the disinhibited sedation produced by sedative-hypnotic drugs. Compulsive use has not been reported. At ordinary dosages, children occasionally (and adults rarely) manifest excitation rather than sedation. At very high toxic dose levels, marked stimulation, agitation, and even convulsions may precede coma. Second-generation H_1 antagonists have little or no sedative or stimulant actions. These drugs (or their active metabolites) also have far fewer autonomic effects than the first-generation antihistamines.

2. Antinausea and antiemetic actions—Several first-generation H_1 antagonists have significant activity in preventing motion sickness (Table 16–2). They are less effective against an episode of motion sickness already present. Certain H_1 antagonists, notably doxylamine (in Bendectin), were used widely in the past in the treatment of nausea and vomiting of pregnancy (see below).

3. Antiparkinsonism effects—Some of the H_1 antagonists, especially diphenhydramine, have significant acute suppressant effects on the extrapyramidal symptoms associated with certain antipsychotic drugs. This drug is given parenterally for acute dystonic reactions to antipsychotics.

4. Anticholinoceptor actions—Many of the first-generation agents, especially those of the ethanolamine and ethylenediamine subgroups, have significant atropine-like effects on peripheral muscarinic receptors. This action may be responsible for some of the (uncertain) benefits reported for nonallergic rhinorrhea but may also cause urinary retention and blurred vision.

5. Adrenoceptor-blocking actions—Alpha-receptor–blocking effects can be demonstrated for many H_1 antagonists, especially those in the phenothiazine subgroup, eg, promethazine. This action may cause orthostatic hypotension in susceptible individuals. Beta-receptor blockade is not observed.

6. Serotonin-blocking action—Strong blocking effects at serotonin receptors have been demonstrated for some first-generation H_1 antagonists, notably cyproheptadine. This drug is promoted as an antiserotonin agent and is discussed with that drug group. Nevertheless, its structure resembles that of the phenothiazine antihistamines, and it is a potent H_1-blocking agent.

7. Local anesthesia—Several first-generation H_1 antagonists are potent local anesthetics. They block sodium channels in excitable membranes in the same fashion as procaine and lidocaine. Diphenhydramine and promethazine are actually more potent than procaine as local anesthetics. They are occasionally used to produce local anesthesia in patients allergic to conventional local anesthetic drugs. A small number of these agents also block potassium channels; this action is discussed below (see Toxicity).

8. Other actions—Certain H_1 antagonists, eg, cetirizine, inhibit mast cell release of histamine and some other mediators of inflammation. This action is not due to H_1-receptor blockade. The mechanism is not understood but could play a role in the beneficial effects of these drugs in the treatment of allergies such as rhinitis. A few H_1 antagonists (eg, terfenadine, acrivastine) have been shown to inhibit the P-glycoprotein transporter found in cancer cells, the epithelium of the gut, and the capillaries of the brain. The significance of this effect is not known.

CLINICAL PHARMACOLOGY OF H_1-RECEPTOR ANTAGONISTS

Clinical Uses

A. ALLERGIC REACTIONS

The H_1 antihistaminic agents are often the first drugs used to prevent or treat the symptoms of allergic reactions. In allergic rhinitis and urticaria, in which histamine is the primary mediator, the H_1 antagonists are the drugs of choice and are often quite effective. However, in bronchial asthma, which involves several mediators, the H_1 antagonists are largely ineffective.

Angioedema may be precipitated by histamine release but appears to be maintained by peptide kinins that are not affected by antihistaminic agents. For atopic dermatitis, antihistaminic drugs such as diphenhydramine are used mostly for their sedative side effect, which reduces awareness of itching.

The H_1 antihistamines used for treating allergic conditions such as hay fever are usually selected with the goal of minimizing sedative effects; in the USA, the drugs in widest use are the alkylamines and the second-generation nonsedating agents. However, the sedative effect and the therapeutic efficacy of different agents vary widely among individuals. In addition, the clinical effectiveness of one group may diminish with continued use, and switching to another group may restore drug effectiveness for as yet unexplained reasons.

The second-generation H_1 antagonists are used mainly for the treatment of allergic rhinitis and chronic urticaria. Several double-blind comparisons with older agents (such as chlorpheniramine) indicated about equal therapeutic efficacy. However, sedation and interference with safe operation of machinery, which occur in about 50% of subjects taking first-generation antihistamines, occurred in only about 7% of subjects taking second-generation agents. The newer drugs are much more expensive.

B. MOTION SICKNESS AND VESTIBULAR DISTURBANCES

Scopolamine (Chapter 8) and certain first-generation H_1 antagonists are the most effective agents available for the prevention of motion sickness. The antihistaminic drugs with the greatest effectiveness in this application are diphenhydramine and promethazine. Dimenhydrinate, which is promoted almost exclusively for the treatment of motion sickness, is a salt of diphenhydramine. The piperazines (cyclizine and meclizine) also have significant activity in preventing motion sickness and are less sedating than diphenhydramine in most patients. Dosage is the same as that recommended for allergic disorders (Table 16–2). Both scopolamine and the H_1 antagonists are more effective in preventing motion sickness when combined with ephedrine or amphetamine.

It has been claimed that the antihistaminic agents effective in prophylaxis of motion sickness are also useful in Ménière's syndrome, but efficacy in the latter application is not established.

C. NAUSEA AND VOMITING OF PREGNANCY

Several H_1-antagonist drugs have been studied for possible use in treating "morning sickness." The piperazine derivatives were withdrawn from such use when it was demonstrated that they have teratogenic effects in rodents. Doxylamine, an ethanolamine H_1 antagonist, was promoted for this application as a component of Bendectin, a prescription medication that also contained pyridoxine. Possible teratogenic effects of doxylamine were widely publicized in the lay press after 1978 as a result of a few case reports of fetal malformation associated with maternal ingestion of Bendectin. However, several large prospective studies involving over 60,000 pregnancies, of which more than 3000 involved maternal Bendectin ingestion, disclosed no increase in the incidence of birth defects. However, because of the continuing controversy, adverse publicity, and lawsuits, the manufacturer of Bendectin withdrew the product from the market.

Toxicity

The wide spectrum of nonantihistaminic effects of the H_1 antihistamines is described in the previous text. Several of these effects (sedation, antimuscarinic action) have been used for therapeutic purposes, especially in over-the-counter (OTC) remedies (see Chapter 64). Nevertheless, these two effects constitute the most common undesirable actions when these drugs are used to block histamine receptors.

Less common toxic effects of systemic use include excitation and convulsions in children, postural hypotension, and allergic responses. Drug allergy is relatively common after topical use of H_1 antagonists. The effects of severe systemic overdosage of the older agents resemble those of atropine overdosage and are treated in the same way (see Chapters 8 and 59). Overdosage of astemizole or terfenadine may induce cardiac arrhythmias, but these drugs are no longer marketed in the USA; the same effect may be caused at normal dosage by interaction with enzyme inhibitors (see Drug Interactions, below).

Drug Interactions

Lethal ventricular arrhythmias occurred in several patients taking either of the early second-generation agents, terfenadine or astemizole, in combination with ketoconazole, itraconazole, or macrolide antibiotics such as erythromycin. These antimicrobial drugs inhibit the metabolism of many drugs by CYP3A4 and cause significant increases in blood concentrations of the antihistamines. The mechanism of this toxicity involves blockade of the HERG (I_{Kr}) potassium channels in the heart that are responsible for repolarization of the action potential (see Chapter 14). The result is prolongation of the action potential, and excessive prolongation leads to arrhythmias. Both terfenadine and astemizole were withdrawn from the United States market in recognition of these problems. Where still available, terfenadine and astemizole should be considered to be contraindicated in patients taking ketoconazole, itraconazole, or macrolides and in patients with liver disease. Grapefruit juice also inhibits CYP3A4 and has been shown to increase terfenadine's blood levels significantly.

For those H_1 antagonists that cause significant sedation, concurrent use of other drugs that cause central nervous system depression produces additive effects and is contraindicated while driving or operating machinery. Similarly, the autonomic blocking effects of older antihistamines are additive with those of muscarinic and α-blocking drugs.

■ III. H_2-RECEPTOR ANTAGONISTS

The development of H_2-receptor antagonists was based on the observation that H_1 antagonists had no effect on histamine-induced acid secretion in the stomach. Molecular manipulation of the histamine molecule resulted in drugs that blocked acid secretion and had no H_1-agonist or antagonist effects. The high incidence of peptic ulcer disease and related gastrointestinal complaints created great interest in the therapeutic potential of these H_2-receptor antagonists. Because of the ability of this class of drugs to reduce gastric acid secretion and their low toxicity, they are now among the most frequently used drugs in the USA and have become OTC items. These drugs are discussed in Chapter 63.

■ IV. H_3- & H_4-RECEPTOR ANTAGONISTS

Although no selective H_3 or H_4 ligands are presently available for clinical use, there is great interest in their therapeutic potential. H_3-selective ligands may be of value in sleep disorders, obesity, and cognitive and psychiatric disorders. H_4 blockers have potential in chronic inflammatory conditions such as asthma, in which eosinophils and mast cells play a prominent role.

■ V. SEROTONIN (5-HYDROXYTRYPTAMINE)

Before the identification of 5-hydroxytryptamine (5-HT), it was known that when blood is allowed to clot, a vasoconstrictor (tonic) substance is released from the clot into the serum; this substance was called serotonin. Independent studies established the existence of a smooth muscle stimulant in intestinal mucosa; this was called enteramine. The synthesis of 5-hydroxytryptamine in 1951 permitted the identification of serotonin and enteramine as the same metabolite of 5-hydroxytryptophan.

Serotonin is an important neurotransmitter, a local hormone in the gut, a component of the platelet clotting process, and is thought to play a role in migraine headache. Serotonin is also one of the mediators of the signs and symptoms of *carcinoid syndrome*, an unusual manifestation of carcinoid tumor, a neoplasm of enterochromaffin cells. In patients whose tumor is not operable, a serotonin antagonist may constitute a useful treatment.

BASIC PHARMACOLOGY OF SEROTONIN

Chemistry & Pharmacokinetics

Like histamine, serotonin is widely distributed in nature, being found in plant and animal tissues, venoms, and stings. It is an indoleethylamine formed in biologic systems from the amino acid L-tryptophan by hydroxylation of the indole ring followed by decarboxylation of the amino acid (Figure 16–2). Hydroxylation at C5 is the rate-limiting step and can be blocked by *p*-chlorophenylalanine (PCPA; fenclonine) and by *p*-chloroamphetamine. These agents have been used experimentally to reduce serotonin synthesis in carcinoid syndrome but are too toxic for clinical use.

After synthesis, the free amine is stored or is rapidly inactivated, usually by oxidation catalyzed by the enzyme monoamine oxidase. In the pineal gland, serotonin serves as a precursor of melatonin, a melanocyte-stimulating hormone. In mammals (including humans), over 90% of the serotonin in the body is found in enterochromaffin cells in the gastrointestinal tract. In the blood, serotonin is found in platelets, which are able to concentrate the

Figure 16–2. Structures of serotonin and two 5-HT-receptor blockers.

amine by means of an active serotonin transporter mechanism (SERT) similar to that in the membrane of serotonergic nerve endings. Once transported into the platelet or nerve ending, 5-HT is concentrated in vesicles by a vesicle-associated transporter (VAT) that is blocked by reserpine. Serotonin is also found in the raphe nuclei of the brainstem, which contain cell bodies of serotonergic neurons that synthesize, store, and release serotonin as a transmitter. Brain serotonergic neurons are involved in numerous diffuse functions such as mood, sleep, appetite, and temperature regulation, as well as the perception of pain, the regulation of blood pressure, and vomiting (see Chapter 21). Serotonin also appears to be involved in clinical conditions such as depression, anxiety, and migraine. Serotonergic neurons are also found in the enteric nervous system of the gastrointestinal tract and around blood vessels. In rodents (but not in humans), serotonin is found in mast cells.

The function of serotonin in enterochromaffin cells is not fully understood. These cells synthesize serotonin, store the amine in a complex with ATP and with other substances in granules, and release serotonin in response to mechanical and neuronal stimuli. Some of the released serotonin diffuses into blood vessels and is taken up and stored in platelets.

Table 16–3. Serotonin receptor subtypes. See also Chapter 21.

Receptor Subtype	Distribution	Postreceptor Mechanism	Partially Selective Agonists	Partially Selective Antagonists
5-HT$_{1A}$	Raphe nuclei, hippocampus	G$_i$, ↓ cAMP	8-OH-DPAT	WAY100635
5-HT$_{1B}$	Substantia nigra, globus pallidus, basal ganglia	G$_i$, ↓ cAMP	Sumatriptan, CP93129	
5-HT$_{1Da,b}$	Brain	G$_i$, ↓ cAMP	Sumatriptan	
5-HT$_{1E}$	Cortex, putamen	G$_i$, ↓ cAMP		
5-HT$_{1F}$	Cortex, hippocampus	G$_i$, ↓ cAMP	LY334370	
5-HT$_{1P}$	Enteric nervous system	G$_o$, slow EPSP	5-Hydroxyindalpine	Renzapride
5-HT$_{2A}$	Platelets, smooth muscle, cerebral cortex	G$_q$, ↑ IP$_3$	α-Methyl-5-HT	Ketanserin
5-HT$_{2B}$	Stomach fundus	G$_q$, ↑ IP$_3$	α-Methyl-5-HT	SB204741
5-HT$_{2C}$	Choroid, hippocampus, substantia nigra	G$_q$, ↑ IP$_3$	α-Methyl-5-HT	Mesulergine
5-HT$_3$	Area postrema, sensory and enteric nerves	Receptor is a Na$^+$-K$^+$ ion channel	2-Methyl-5-HT, m-chlorophenylbiguanide	Granisetron, ondansetron, tropisetron
5-HT$_4$	CNS and myenteric neurons, smooth muscle	G$_s$, ↑ cAMP	5-Methoxytryptamine, renzapride, metoclopramide	
5-HT$_{5A,B}$	Brain	↓ cAMP		
5-HT$_{6,7}$	Brain	G$_s$, ↑ cAMP		Clozapine (5-HT$_7$)

Key: 8-OH-DPAT = 8-Hydroxy-2-(di-*n*-propylamine)tetralin
CP93129 = 5-Hydroxy-3(4-1,2,5,6-tetrahydropyridyl)-4-azaindole
LY334370 = 5-(4-fluorobenzoyl)amino-3-(1-methylpiperidin-4-yl)-1*H*-indole fumarate
SB204741 = *N*-(1-methyl-5-indolyl)-*N'*-(3-methyl-5-isothiazolyl)urea
WAY100635 = *N-tert*-Butyl 3-4-(2-methoxyphenyl)piperazin-1-yl-2-phenylpropanamide

Stored serotonin can be depleted by **reserpine** in much the same manner as this drug depletes catecholamines from vesicles in adrenergic nerves (see Chapter 6).

Serotonin is metabolized by monoamine oxidase, and the intermediate product, 5-hydroxyindoleacetaldehyde, is further oxidized by aldehyde dehydrogenase to 5-hydroxyindoleacetic acid (5-HIAA). In humans consuming a normal diet, the excretion of 5-HIAA is a measure of serotonin synthesis. Therefore, the 24-hour excretion of 5-HIAA can be used as a diagnostic test for tumors that synthesize excessive quantities of serotonin, especially carcinoid tumor. A few foods (eg, bananas) contain large amounts of serotonin or its precursors and must be prohibited during such diagnostic tests.

Pharmacodynamics

A. MECHANISMS OF ACTION

Serotonin exerts many actions and, like histamine, has many species differences, making generalizations difficult.

The actions of serotonin are mediated through a remarkably large number of cell membrane receptors. The serotonin receptors that have been characterized thus far are listed in Table 16–3. Seven families of 5-HT-receptor subtypes (those given numeric subscripts 1 through 7) have been identified, six involving G protein-coupled receptors of the usual 7-transmembrane serpentine type and one a ligand-gated ion channel. Among these receptor subtypes, a few still lack a well-documented physiologic function. Discovery of these functions awaits the development of more subtype-selective drugs or the knockout mutation of genes encoding these receptors from the mouse genome.

B. TISSUE AND ORGAN SYSTEM EFFECTS

1. Nervous system—Serotonin is present in a variety of sites in the brain. Its role as a neurotransmitter and its relation to the actions of drugs acting in the central nervous system are discussed in Chapters 21 and 30. Serotonin is also a precursor of melatonin in the pineal gland (see Box: Melatonin Pharmacology, and Chapter 65).

MELATONIN PHARMACOLOGY

Melatonin is *N*-acetyl-5-methoxytryptamine, a simple methoxylated and *N*-acetylated product of serotonin found in the pineal gland. It is produced and released primarily at night and has long been suspected of playing a role in diurnal cycles of animals and the sleep-wake behavior of humans.

Melatonin receptors have been characterized in the central nervous system and several peripheral tissues. In the brain, MT_1 and MT_2 receptors are found in membranes of neurons in the suprachiasmatic nucleus of the hypothalamus, an area associated—from lesioning experiments—with circadian rhythm. MT_1 and MT_2 are seven-transmembrane G_i protein-coupled receptors. The result of receptor binding is inhibition of adenylyl cyclase. A third receptor, MT_3, is an enzyme; binding to this site has a poorly defined physiologic role, possibly related to intraocular pressure. Activation of the MT_1 receptor results in sleepiness, whereas the MT_2 receptor may be related to the light-dark synchronization of the biologic circadian clock.

Melatonin itself is promoted commercially as a sleep aid by the food supplement industry (see Chapter 65). **Ramelteon** is a selective MT_1 and MT_2 agonist that has recently been approved for the medical treatment of insomnia. This drug has no addiction liability (it is not a controlled substance), and it appears to be distinctly more efficacious than melatonin (but less efficacious than benzodiazepines) as a hypnotic. It is metabolized by P450 enzymes and should not be used in individuals taking CYP1A2 inhibitors. It has a half-life of 1–3 hours and an active metabolite with a half-life of up to 5 hours. The toxicity of ramelteon is as yet poorly defined, but prolactin levels were elevated in one clinical trial.

$5\text{-}HT_3$ receptors in the gastrointestinal tract and in the vomiting center of the medulla participate in the vomiting reflex (see Chapter 63). They are particularly important in vomiting caused by chemical triggers such as cancer chemotherapy drugs. $5\text{-}HT_{1P}$ and $5\text{-}HT_4$ receptors also play a role in enteric nervous system function.

Like histamine, serotonin is a potent stimulant of pain and itch sensory nerve endings and is responsible for some of the symptoms caused by insect and plant stings. In addition, serotonin is a powerful activator of chemosensitive endings located in the coronary vascular bed. Activation of $5\text{-}HT_3$ receptors on these afferent vagal nerve endings is associated with the **chemoreceptor reflex** (also known as the Bezold-Jarisch reflex). The reflex response consists of marked bradycardia and hypotension. The bradycardia is mediated by vagal outflow to the heart and can be blocked by atropine. The hypotension is a consequence of the decrease in cardiac output that results from bradycardia. A variety of other agents can activate the chemoreceptor reflex. These include nicotinic cholinoceptor agonists and some cardiac glycosides, eg, ouabain.

2. Respiratory system—Serotonin has a small direct stimulant effect on bronchiolar smooth muscle in normal humans. It also appears to facilitate acetylcholine release from bronchial vagal nerve endings. In patients with carcinoid syndrome, episodes of bronchoconstriction occur in response to elevated levels of the amine or peptides released from the tumor. Serotonin may also cause hyperventilation as a result of the chemoreceptor reflex or stimulation of bronchial sensory nerve endings.

3. Cardiovascular system—Serotonin directly causes the contraction of vascular smooth muscle, mainly through $5\text{-}HT_2$ receptors. In humans, serotonin is a powerful vasoconstrictor except in skeletal muscle and heart, where it dilates blood vessels. At least part of this 5-HT-induced vasodilation requires the presence of vascular endothelial cells. When the endothelium is damaged, coronary vessels constrict. As noted previously, serotonin can also elicit reflex bradycardia by activation of $5\text{-}HT_3$ receptors on chemoreceptor nerve endings. A triphasic blood pressure response is often seen following injection of serotonin in experimental animals. Initially, there is a decrease in heart rate, cardiac output, and blood pressure caused by the chemoreceptor response. Following this decrease, blood pressure increases as a result of vasoconstriction. The third phase is again a decrease in blood pressure attributed to vasodilation in vessels supplying skeletal muscle. Pulmonary and renal vessels seem especially sensitive to the vasoconstrictor action of serotonin.

Serotonin also constricts veins, and venoconstriction with a resulting increased capillary filling appears to be responsible for the flush that is observed following serotonin administration or release from a carcinoid tumor. Serotonin has small direct positive chronotropic and inotropic effects on the heart, which are probably of no clinical significance. However, prolonged elevation of the blood level of serotonin (which occurs in carcinoid syndrome) is associated with pathologic alterations in the endocardium (subendocardial fibroplasia), which may result in valvular or electrical malfunction.

Table 16–4. Characteristics of serotonin syndrome and other hyperthermic syndromes.

Syndrome	Precipitating Drugs	Clinical Presentation	Therapy[1]
Serotonin syndrome	SSRIs, second generation antidepressants, MAOIs, linezolid, tramadol, meperidine, fentanyl, ondansetron, sumatriptan, MDMA, LSD, St. John's wort, ginseng	Hypertension, hyperreflexia, tremor, clonus, hyperthermia, hyperactive bowel sounds, diarrhea, mydriasis, agitation, coma; onset within hours	**Sedation (benzodiazepines), paralysis, intubation and ventilation;** consider 5-HT$_2$ block with cyproheptadine or chlorpromazine
Neuroleptic malignant syndrome	D$_2$-blocking antipsychotics	Acute severe parkinsonism; hypertension, hyperthermia, normal or reduced bowel sounds, onset over 1–3 days	**Diphenhydramine** (parenteral), cooling if temperature is very high, sedation with benzodiazepines
Malignant hyperthermia	Volatile anesthetics, succinylcholine	Hyperthermia, muscle rigidity, hypertension, tachycardia; onset within minutes	**Dantrolene,** cooling

[1]Precipitating drugs should be discontinued immediately. First-line therapy is in **bold** font.
MAOIs, monoamine oxidase inhibitors; MDMA, methylenedioxy-methamphetamine (ecstasy); SSRIs, selective serotonin reuptake inhibitors.

Serotonin causes blood platelets to aggregate by activating surface 5-HT$_2$ receptors. This response, in contrast to aggregation induced during clot formation, is not accompanied by the release of serotonin stored in the platelets. The physiologic role of this effect is unclear.

4. Gastrointestinal tract—Serotonin is a powerful stimulant of gastrointestinal smooth muscle, increasing tone and facilitating peristalsis. This action is caused by the direct action of serotonin on 5-HT$_2$ smooth muscle receptors plus a stimulating action on ganglion cells located in the enteric nervous system (see Chapter 6). Activation of 5-HT$_4$ receptors in the enteric nervous system causes increased acetylcholine release and thereby mediates a motility-enhancing or "prokinetic" effect of selective serotonin agonists such as cisapride. These agents are useful in several gastrointestinal disorders

(see Chapter 63). Overproduction of serotonin (and other substances) in carcinoid tumor is associated with severe diarrhea. Serotonin has little effect on secretions, and what effects it has are generally inhibitory.

5. Skeletal muscle—5-HT$_2$ receptors are present on skeletal muscle membranes, but their physiologic role is not understood. **Serotonin syndrome** is a condition precipitated when MAO inhibitors are given with serotonin agonists, especially antidepressants of the selective serotonin reuptake inhibitor class (SSRIs; see Chapter 30). Although associated with skeletal muscle contractions and the hyperthermia resulting from excessive muscle contraction, serotonin syndrome is probably the result of a central nervous system effect of these drugs (see Table 16–4 and Box: Serotonin Syndrome and Similar Syndromes).

SEROTONIN SYNDROME AND SIMILAR SYNDROMES

Excess synaptic serotonin causes a serious, potentially fatal syndrome that is diagnosed on the basis of a history of administration of a serotonergic drug within recent weeks and physical findings (Table 16–4). It has some characteristics in common with neuroleptic malignant syndrome (NMS) and malignant hyperthermia (MH), but its pathophysiology and management are quite different.

As suggested by the drugs that precipitate it, serotonin syndrome occurs when overdose with a single drug, or concurrent use of several drugs, results in excess serotonergic activity in the central nervous system. It is predictable and not idiosyncratic, but milder

forms may easily be misdiagnosed. In experimental animal models, many of the signs of the syndrome can be reversed by administration of 5-HT$_2$ antagonists; however, other 5-HT receptors may be involved as well. Dantrolene is of no value, unlike the treatment of MH. NMS is idiosyncratic rather than predictable and appears to be associated with hypersensitivity to the parkinsonism-inducing effects of D$_2$-blocking antipsychotics in certain individuals. MH is associated with a genetic defect in the RyR1 calcium channel of skeletal muscle sarcoplasmic reticulum that permits uncontrolled calcium release from the SR when precipitating drugs are given (Chapter 27).

CLINICAL PHARMACOLOGY OF SEROTONIN

Serotonin Agonists

Serotonin has no clinical applications as a drug. However, several receptor subtype-selective agonists have proved to be of value. **Buspirone,** a 5-HT_{1A} agonist, has received wide attention for its usefulness as an effective nonbenzodiazepine anxiolytic (see Chapter 22). **Dexfenfluramine,** another selective 5-HT agonist, was widely used as an appetite suppressant but was withdrawn because of toxicity. Appetite suppression appears to be associated with agonist action at 5-HT_{2C} receptors in the central nervous system. **Sumatriptan** and its congeners are agonists effective in the treatment of acute migraine and cluster headache attacks (see below).

5-$HT_{1D/1B}$ Agonists & Migraine Headache

The 5-$HT_{1D/1B}$ agonists **(triptans)** are used almost exclusively in migraine headache. Migraine in its "classic" form is characterized by an aura of variable duration that may involve nausea, vomiting, and visual scotomas or even hemianopsia and speech abnormalities; followed by a severe throbbing unilateral headache that lasts for a few hours to 1–2 days. "Common" migraine lacks the aura phase, but the headache is similar. Although the symptom pattern varies among patients, the severity of migraine headache justifies vigorous therapy in the great majority of cases.

Migraine involves the trigeminal nerve distribution to intracranial (and possibly extracranial) arteries. These nerves release peptide neurotransmitters, especially **calcitonin gene-related peptide** (CGRP; see Chapter 17), an extremely powerful vasodilator. Substance P and neurokinin A may also be involved. Extravasation of plasma and plasma proteins into the perivascular space appears to be a common feature of animal migraine models and biopsy specimens from migraine patients and probably represents the effect of the neuropeptides on the vessels. The mechanical stretching caused by this perivascular edema may be the immediate cause of activation of pain nerve endings in the dura. The onset of headache is sometimes associated with a marked increase in amplitude of temporal artery pulsations, and relief of pain by administration of effective therapy is sometimes accompanied by diminution of the arterial pulsations.

The mechanisms of action of drugs used in migraine are poorly understood, in part because they include such a wide variety of drug groups and actions. In addition to the triptans, these include ergot alkaloids, nonsteroidal anti-inflammatory analgesic agents, β-adrenoceptor blockers, calcium channel blockers, tricyclic antidepressants and SSRIs, and several antiseizure agents. Furthermore, some of these drug groups are effective only for prophylaxis and not for the acute attack.

Two primary hypotheses have been proposed to explain the actions of these drugs. First, the triptans, the ergot alkaloids, and antidepressants may activate 5-$HT_{1D/1B}$ receptors on presynaptic trigeminal nerve endings to inhibit the release of vasodilating peptides, and antiseizure agents may suppress excessive firing of these nerve endings. Second, the vasoconstrictor actions of direct 5-HT agonists (the triptans and ergot) may prevent vasodilation and stretching of the pain endings. It is possible that both mechanisms contribute in the case of some drugs. Sumatriptan and its congeners are currently first-line therapy for acute severe migraine attacks in most patients. However, they should not be used in patients at risk for coronary artery disease. Anti-inflammatory analgesics such as aspirin and ibuprofen are often helpful in controlling the pain of migraine. Rarely, parenteral opioids may be needed in refractory cases. For patients with very severe nausea and vomiting, parenteral metoclopramide may be helpful.

Propranolol, amitriptyline, and some calcium channel blockers have been found to be effective for the prophylaxis of migraine in some patients. They are of no value in the treatment of acute migraine. The anticonvulsants valproic acid and topiramate (see Chapter 24) have recently been found to have good prophylactic efficacy in many migraine patients. **Flunarizine,** a calcium channel blocker used in Europe, has been reported in clinical trials to effectively reduce the severity of the acute attack and to prevent recurrences. **Verapamil** appears to have modest efficacy as prophylaxis against migraine.

Sumatriptan and the other triptans are selective agonists for 5-HT_{1D} and 5-HT_{1B} receptors; the similarity of the triptan structure to that of 5-HT can be seen in the structure below. These receptor types are found in cerebral and meningeal vessels and mediate vasoconstriction. They are also found on neurons and probably function as presynaptic inhibitory receptors.

Sumatriptan

The efficacy of triptan 5-HT_1 agonists in migraine is equal to or greater than that of other acute drug treatments, eg, parenteral, oral, or rectal ergot alkaloids. The pharmacokinetics of the triptans are set forth in Table 16–5. Most adverse effects are mild and include altered sensations (tingling, warmth, etc), dizziness, muscle

Table 16–5. Pharmacokinetics of triptans.

Drug	Routes	Time to Onset (h)	Single Dose (mg)	Maximum Dose Per Day (mg)	Half-Life (h)
Almotriptan	Oral	2.6	6.25–12.5	25	3.3
Eletriptan	Oral	2	20–40	80	4
Frovatriptan	Oral	3	2.5	7.5	27
Naratriptan	Oral	2	1–2.5	5	5.5
Rizatriptan	Oral	1–2.5	5–10	30	2
Sumatriptan	Oral, nasal, subcutaneous	1.5 (0.2 for subcutaneous)	25–100 (PO)	200	2
Zolmitriptan	Oral, nasal	1.5–3	1.25–2.5	10	2.8

weakness, neck pain, and for parenteral sumatriptan, injection site reactions. Chest discomfort occurs in 1–5% of patients, and chest pain has been reported, probably because of the ability of these drugs to cause coronary vasospasm. They are therefore contraindicated in patients with coronary artery disease and in patients with angina. Another disadvantage is the fact that their duration of effect (especially that of almotriptan, sumatriptan, rizatriptan, and zolmitriptan, Table 16–5) is often shorter than the duration of the headache. As a result, several doses may be required during a prolonged migraine attack, but their adverse effects limit the maximum safe daily dosage. In addition, these drugs are extremely expensive. Naratriptan and eletriptan are contraindicated in patients with severe hepatic or renal impairment or peripheral vascular syndromes; frovatriptan in patients with peripheral vascular disease; and zolmitriptan in patients with Wolff-Parkinson-White syndrome.

Other Serotonin Agonists in Clinical Use

Cisapride, a 5-HT_4 agonist, was used in the treatment of gastroesophageal reflux and motility disorders. Because of toxicity, it is now available only for compassionate use in the USA. **Tegaserod,** a newer 5-HT_4 partial agonist, is used for irritable bowel syndrome with constipation. These drugs are discussed in Chapter 63.

Compounds such as fluoxetine and other SSRIs, which modulate serotonergic transmission by blocking reuptake of the transmitter, are among the most widely prescribed drugs for the management of depression and similar disorders. These drugs are discussed in Chapter 30.

SEROTONIN ANTAGONISTS

The actions of serotonin, like those of histamine, can be antagonized in several ways. Such antagonism is clearly desirable in those rare patients who have carcinoid tumor and may also be valuable in certain other conditions.

As noted above, serotonin synthesis can be inhibited by *p*-chlorophenylalanine and *p*-chloroamphetamine. However, these agents are too toxic for general use. Storage of serotonin can be inhibited by the use of reserpine, but the sympatholytic effects of this drug (see Chapter 11) and the high levels of circulating serotonin that result from release prevent its use in carcinoid. Therefore, receptor blockade is the major approach to therapeutic limitation of serotonin effects.

SEROTONIN-RECEPTOR ANTAGONISTS

A wide variety of drugs with actions at other receptors (α adrenoceptors, H_1-histamine receptors, etc) are also serotonin receptor-blocking agents. **Phenoxybenzamine** (see Chapter 10) has a long-lasting blocking action at 5-HT_2 receptors. In addition, the ergot alkaloids discussed in the last portion of the chapter are partial agonists at serotonin receptors.

Cyproheptadine resembles the phenothiazine antihistaminic agents in chemical structure and has potent H_1-receptor-blocking as well as 5-HT_2-blocking actions. The actions of cyproheptadine are predictable from its H_1 histamine and serotonin receptor affinities. It prevents the smooth muscle effects of both amines but has no effect on the gastric secretion stimulated by histamine. It also has significant antimuscarinic effects and causes sedation.

The major clinical applications of cyproheptadine are in the treatment of the smooth muscle manifestations of carcinoid tumor and in cold-induced urticaria. The usual dosage in adults is 12–16 mg/d in three or four divided doses. It is of some value in serotonin syndrome, but because it is available only in tablet form, it must be crushed and administered by stomach tube in unconscious patients.

Ketanserin (Figure 16–2) blocks 5-HT_{1c} and 5-HT_2 receptors and has little or no reported antagonist activity at other 5-HT or H_1 receptors. However, this drug potently blocks vascular α_1 adrenoceptors. The drug blocks 5-HT$_2$ receptors on platelets and antagonizes platelet aggregation promoted by serotonin. The mechanism involved in ketanserin's hypotensive action is not clear but probably involves α_1 adrenoceptors more than 5-HT$_2$ receptor blockade. Ketanserin is available in Europe for the treatment of hypertension and vasospastic conditions but has not been approved in the USA.

Ritanserin, another 5-HT$_2$ antagonist, has little or no α-blocking action. It has been reported to alter bleeding time and to reduce thromboxane formation, presumably by altering platelet function.

Ondansetron (Figure 16–2) is the prototypical 5-HT$_3$ antagonist. This drug and its analogs are very important in the prevention of nausea and vomiting associated with surgery and cancer chemotherapy. They are discussed in Chapter 63.

Considering the diverse effects attributed to serotonin and the heterogeneous nature of 5-HT receptors, other selective 5-HT antagonists may prove to be clinically useful.

■ VI. THE ERGOT ALKALOIDS

Ergot alkaloids are produced by *Claviceps purpurea,* a fungus that infects grain—especially rye—under damp growing or storage conditions. This fungus synthesizes histamine, acetylcholine, tyramine, and other biologically active products in addition to a score or more of unique ergot alkaloids. These alkaloids affect α adrenoceptors, dopamine receptors, 5-HT receptors, and perhaps other receptor types. Similar alkaloids are produced by fungi parasitic to a number of other grass-like plants.

The accidental ingestion of ergot alkaloids in contaminated grain can be traced back more than 2000 years from descriptions of epidemics of ergot poisoning **(ergotism).** The most dramatic effects of poisoning are dementia with florid hallucinations; prolonged vasospasm, which may result in gangrene; and stimulation of uterine smooth muscle, which in pregnancy may result in abortion. In medieval times, ergot poisoning was called **St. Anthony's fire** after the saint whose help was sought in relieving the burning pain of vasospastic ischemia. Identifiable epidemics have occurred sporadically up to modern times (see Box: Ergot Poisoning: Not Just an Ancient Disease) and mandate continuous surveillance of all grains used for food. Poisoning of grazing animals is common in many areas because the fungi may grow on pasture grasses.

In addition to the effects noted above, the ergot alkaloids produce a variety of other central nervous system and peripheral effects. Detailed structure-activity analysis and appropriate semisynthetic modifications have yielded a large number of agents with documented or potential clinical value.

BASIC PHARMACOLOGY OF ERGOT ALKALOIDS

Chemistry & Pharmacokinetics

Two major families of compounds that incorporate the tetracyclic **ergoline** nucleus may be identified; the amine alkaloids and the peptide alkaloids (Table 16–6). Drugs of therapeutic and toxicologic importance are found in both groups.

The ergot alkaloids are variably absorbed from the gastrointestinal tract. The oral dose of ergotamine is about ten times larger than the intramuscular dose, but the speed of absorption and peak blood levels after oral administration can be improved by administration with caffeine (see below). The amine alkaloids are also absorbed from the rectum and the buccal cavity and after administration by aerosol inhaler. Absorption after intramuscular injection is slow but usually reliable. Bromocriptine and the amine derivative cabergoline are well absorbed from the gastrointestinal tract.

ERGOT POISONING: NOT JUST AN ANCIENT DISEASE

As noted in the text, epidemics of ergotism, or poisoning by ergot-contaminated grain, are known to have occurred sporadically in ancient times and through the Middle Ages. It is easy to imagine the social chaos that might result if fiery pain, gangrene, hallucinations, convulsions, and abortions occurred simultaneously throughout a community in which all or most of the people believed in witchcraft, demonic possession, and the visitation of supernatural punishments upon humans for their misdeeds. Such beliefs are uncommon in most cultures today. However, ergotism has not disappeared. A most convincing demonstration of ergotism occurred in the small French village of Pont-Saint-Esprit in 1951. It was described in the *British Medical Journal* in 1951 (Gabbai et al, 1951) and in a later book-length narrative account (Fuller, 1968). Several hundred individuals suffered symptoms of hallucinations, convulsions, and ischemia—and several died—after eating bread made from contaminated flour. Similar events have occurred even more recently when poverty, famine, or incompetence resulted in the consumption of contaminated grain. Ergot toxicity caused by excessive self-medication with pharmaceutical ergot preparations is still occasionally reported.

Table 16–6. Major ergoline derivatives (ergot alkaloids).

Amine alkaloids	Peptide alkaloids

	R_1	R_8		R_2	R_2'	R_5'
6-Methylergoline	—H	—H				
Lysergic acid	—H	—COOH	Ergotamine[1]	—H	—CH$_3$	—CH$_2$— (benzyl group)
Lysergic acid diethylamide (LSD)	—H	—C(=O)—N(CH$_2$—CH$_3$)$_2$	α-Ergocryptine	—H	—CH(CH$_3$)$_2$	—CH$_2$—CH(CH$_3$)$_2$
Ergonovine (ergometrine)	—H	—C(=O)—NHCHCH$_3$ with CH$_2$OH	Bromocriptine	—Br	—CH(CH$_3$)$_2$	—CH$_2$—CH(CH$_3$)$_2$
Methysergide[2]	—CH$_3$	—C(=O)—NH—CH—CH$_2$—CH$_3$ with CH$_2$OH				

[1]Dihydroergotamine lacks the double bond between carbons 9 and 10.
[2]Methysergide withdrawn in the USA.

The ergot alkaloids are extensively metabolized in the body. The primary metabolites are hydroxylated in the A ring, and peptide alkaloids are also modified in the peptide moiety.

Pharmacodynamics

A. MECHANISM OF ACTION

As suggested, the ergot alkaloids act on several types of receptors. Their effects include agonist, partial agonist, and antagonist actions at α-adrenoceptors and serotonin receptors (especially 5-HT$_{1A}$ and 5-HT$_{1D}$; less for 5-HT$_{1C}$, 5-HT$_2$, and 5-HT$_3$); and agonist or partial agonist actions at central nervous system dopamine receptors (Table 16–7). Furthermore, some members of the ergot family have a high affinity for presynaptic recep-

tors, whereas others are more selective for postjunctional receptors. There is a powerful stimulant effect on the uterus that seems to be most closely associated with agonist or partial agonist effects at 5-HT$_2$ receptors. Structural variations increase the selectivity of certain members of the family for specific receptor types.

B. ORGAN SYSTEM EFFECTS

1. Central nervous system—As indicated by traditional descriptions of ergotism, certain of the naturally occurring alkaloids are powerful hallucinogens. Lysergic acid diethylamide (LSD; "acid") is a synthetic ergot compound that clearly demonstrates this action. The drug has been used in the laboratory as a potent peripheral 5-HT$_2$ antagonist, but good evidence suggests that its behavioral effects are mediated by *agonist* effects at

Table 16–7. Effects of ergot alkaloids at several receptors.[1]

Ergot Alkaloid	α Adrenoceptor	Dopamine Receptor	Serotonin Receptor (5-HT$_2$)	Uterine Smooth Muscle Stimulation
Bromocriptine	–	+++	–	0
Ergonovine	+	+	– (PA)	+++
Ergotamine	– – (PA)	0	+ (PA)	+++
Lysergic acid diethylamide (LSD)	0	+++	– – ++ in CNS	+
Methysergide	+/0	+/0	– – – (PA)	+/0

[1]Agonist effects are indicated by +, antagonist by –, no effect by 0. Relative affinity for the receptor is indicated by the number of + or – signs. PA means partial agonist (both agonist and antagonist effects can be detected).

prejunctional or postjunctional 5-HT$_2$ receptors in the central nervous system. In spite of extensive research, no clinical value has been discovered for LSD's dramatic central nervous system effects. Abuse of this drug has waxed and waned but is still widespread. It is discussed in Chapter 32.

Dopamine receptors in the central nervous system play important roles in extrapyramidal motor control and the regulation of pituitary prolactin release. The actions of the peptide ergoline **bromocriptine** on the extrapyramidal system are discussed in Chapter 28. Of all the currently available ergot derivatives, bromocriptine, **cabergoline,** and **pergolide** have the highest selectivity for the pituitary dopamine receptors. These drugs directly suppress prolactin secretion from pituitary cells by activating regulatory dopamine receptors (Chapter 37). They compete for binding to these sites with dopamine itself and with other dopamine agonists such as apomorphine.

2. Vascular smooth muscle—The action of ergot alkaloids on vascular smooth muscle is drug-, species-, and vessel-dependent, so few generalizations are possible. Ergotamine and related compounds potently constrict most human blood vessels in a predictable, and prolonged manner (Figure 16–3). This response is partially blocked by conventional α-blocking agents. However, ergotamine's effect is also associated with "epinephrine reversal" (see Chapter 10) and with *blockade* of the response to other α agonists. This dual effect represents partial agonist action (Table 16–7). Because ergotamine dissociates very slowly from the α receptor, it produces very long-lasting agonist and antagonist effects at this receptor. There is little or no effect at β adrenoceptors.

While much of the vasoconstriction elicited by ergot alkaloids can be ascribed to partial agonist effects at α adrenoceptors, some may be the result of effects at 5-

HT receptors. Ergotamine, ergonovine, and methysergide all have partial agonist effects at 5-HT$_2$ vascular receptors. The remarkably specific antimigraine action of the ergot derivatives was originally thought to be related to their actions on vascular serotonin receptors. Current hypotheses, however, emphasize their action on prejunctional neuronal 5-HT receptors.

After overdosage with ergotamine and similar agents, vasospasm is severe and prolonged (see Toxicity, below). This vasospasm is not easily reversed by α antagonists, serotonin antagonists, or combinations of both.

Ergotamine is typical of the ergot alkaloids that have a strong vasoconstrictor spectrum of action. The hydrogenation of ergot alkaloids at the 9 and 10 positions (Table 16–6) yields dihydro derivatives that have reduced serotonin partial agonist effects and increased selective α receptor-blocking actions.

3. Uterine smooth muscle—The stimulant action of ergot alkaloids on the uterus, as on vascular smooth muscle, appears to combine α agonist, serotonin, and other effects. Furthermore, the sensitivity of the uterus to the stimulant effects of ergot increases dramatically during pregnancy, perhaps because of increasing dominance of α$_1$ receptors as pregnancy progresses. As a result, the uterus at term is more sensitive to ergot than earlier in pregnancy and far more sensitive than the nonpregnant organ.

In very small doses, ergot preparations can evoke rhythmic contraction and relaxation of the uterus. At higher concentrations, these drugs induce powerful and prolonged contracture. Ergonovine is more selective than other ergot alkaloids in affecting the uterus and is the agent of choice in obstetric applications of these drugs.

4. Other smooth muscle organs—In most patients, the ergot alkaloids have little or no significant effect on bronchiolar or urinary smooth muscle. The gastrointestinal tract, on the other hand, is quite sensitive in most

Figure 16–3. Effects of ergot derivatives on contraction of isolated segments of human basilar artery strips removed at surgery. All of the ergot derivatives are partial agonists, and all are more potent than the full agonists, norepinephrine and serotonin. (NE, norepinephrine; 5-HT, serotonin; ERG, ergotamine; MT, methylergometrine; DHE, dihydroergotamine; MS, methysergide.) (Modified and reproduced, with permission, from Müller-Schweinitzer E. In: *5-Hydroxytryptamine Mechanisms in Primary Headaches.* Oleson J, Saxena PR [editors]. Raven Press, 1992.)

patients. Nausea, vomiting, and diarrhea may be induced even by low doses in some patients. The effect is consistent with action on the central nervous system emetic center and on gastrointestinal serotonin receptors.

CLINICAL PHARMACOLOGY OF ERGOT ALKALOIDS

Clinical Uses

A. MIGRAINE

Ergot derivatives are highly specific for migraine pain; they are not analgesic for any other condition. Although the triptan drugs discussed above are preferred by most clinicians and patients, traditional therapy with **ergotamine** can also be quite effective when given during the prodrome of an attack; it becomes progressively less effective if delayed. Ergotamine tartrate is available for oral, sublingual, rectal suppository, and inhaler use. It is often combined with caffeine (100 mg caffeine for each 1 mg ergotamine tartrate) to facilitate absorption of the ergot alkaloid.

The vasoconstriction induced by ergotamine is long-lasting and cumulative when the drug is taken repeatedly, as in a severe migraine attack. Therefore, patients must be carefully informed that no more than 6 mg of the oral preparation may be taken for each attack and

no more than 10 mg per week. For very severe attacks, ergotamine tartrate, 0.25–0.5 mg, may be given intravenously or intramuscularly. **Dihydroergotamine,** 0.5–1 mg intravenously, is favored by some clinicians for treatment of intractable migraine. Intranasal dihydroergotamine may also be effective.

B. HYPERPROLACTINEMIA

Increased serum levels of the anterior pituitary hormone prolactin are associated with secreting tumors of the gland and also with the use of centrally acting dopamine antagonists, especially the D_2-blocking antipsychotic drugs. Because of negative feedback effects, hyperprolactinemia is associated with amenorrhea and infertility in women as well as galactorrhea in both sexes.

Bromocriptine is extremely effective in reducing the high levels of prolactin that result from pituitary tumors and has even been associated with regression of the tumor in some cases. The usual dosage of bromocriptine is 2.5 mg two or three times daily. **Cabergoline** is similar but more potent. Bromocriptine has also been used in the same dosage to suppress physiologic lactation. However, serious postpartum cardiovascular toxicity has been reported in association with the latter use of bromocriptine or pergolide, and this application is discouraged (Chapter 37).

C. POSTPARTUM HEMORRHAGE

The uterus at term is extremely sensitive to the stimulant action of ergot, and even moderate doses produce a prolonged and powerful spasm of the muscle quite unlike natural labor. Therefore, ergot derivatives should be used only for control of late uterine bleeding and should never be given before delivery. Oxytocin is the preferred agent for control of postpartum hemorrhage, but if this peptide agent is ineffective, ergonovine maleate, 0.2 mg usually given intramuscularly, can be tried. It is usually effective within 1–5 minutes and is less toxic than other ergot derivatives for this application. It is given at the time of delivery of the placenta or immediately afterward if bleeding is significant.

D. DIAGNOSIS OF VARIANT ANGINA

Ergonovine given intravenously produces prompt vasoconstriction during coronary angiography to diagnose variant angina if reactive segments of the coronaries are present.

E. SENILE CEREBRAL INSUFFICIENCY

Dihydroergotoxine, a mixture of dihydro-α-ergocryptine and three similar dihydrogenated peptide ergot alkaloids (ergoloid mesylates), has been promoted for many years for the relief of senility and more recently for the treatment of Alzheimer's dementia. There is no useful evidence that this drug has significant benefit.

Toxicity & Contraindications

The most common toxic effects of the ergot derivatives are gastrointestinal disturbances, including diarrhea, nausea, and vomiting. Activation of the medullary vomiting center and of the gastrointestinal serotonin receptors is involved. Since migraine attacks are often associated with these symptoms before therapy is begun, these adverse effects are rarely contraindications to the use of ergot.

A more dangerous toxic effect of overdosage with agents like ergotamine and ergonovine is prolonged vasospasm. As described above, this sign of vascular smooth muscle stimulation may result in gangrene and require amputation. Bowel infarction has also been reported and may require resection. Peripheral vascular vasospasm caused by ergot is refractory to most vasodilators, but infusions of large doses of nitroprusside or nitroglycerin have been successful in some cases.

Chronic therapy with methysergide was associated with connective tissue proliferation in the retroperitoneal space, the pleural cavity, and the endocardial tissue of the heart. These changes occurred insidiously over months and presented as hydronephrosis (from obstruction of the ureters) or a cardiac murmur (from distortion of the valves of the heart). In some cases, valve damage required surgical replacement. As a result, this drug was withdrawn. Similar fibrotic change has resulted from the chronic use of 5-HT agonists promoted in the past for weight loss (fenfluramine, desfenfluramine).

Other toxic effects of the ergot alkaloids include drowsiness and, in the case of methysergide, occasional instances of central stimulation and hallucinations. In fact, methysergide was sometimes used as a substitute for LSD by members of the "drug culture."

Contraindications to the use of ergot derivatives consist of the obstructive vascular diseases and collagen diseases.

There is no evidence that ordinary use of ergotamine for migraine is hazardous in pregnancy. However, most clinicians counsel restraint in the use of the ergot derivatives by pregnant patients.

PREPARATIONS AVAILABLE

ANTIHISTAMINES (H$_1$ BLOCKERS)*

Azelastine
Nasal (Astelin): 137 mcg/puff nasal spray
Ophthalmic (Optivar): 0.5 mg/mL solution
Brompheniramine (generic, Brovex)
Oral: 6, 12 mg extended release tablets; 12 mg chewable tablets; 8, 12 mg/5 mL suspension
Buclizine (Bucladin-S Softabs)
Oral: 50 mg tablets

*Several other antihistamines are available only in combination products with, for example, phenylephrine.

Carbinoxamine (Histex, Pediatex)
Oral: 4 mg tablets; 8 mg timed-release tablets; 10 mg extended release capsules; 1.5, 4 mg/5 mL liquid; 3.6 mg/5 mL oral suspension
Cetirizine (Zyrtec)
Oral: 5, 10 mg tablets; 5, 10 mg chewable tablets; 5 mg/5 mL syrup
Chlorpheniramine (generic, Chlor-Trimeton)
Oral: 2 mg chewable tablets; 4 mg tablets; 2 mg/5 mL syrup
Oral sustained-release: 8, 12, 16 mg tablets; 8, 12 mg capsules

(continued)

Clemastine (generic, Tavist)
Oral: 1.34, 2.68 mg tablets; 0.67 mg/5 mL syrup

Cyclizine (Marezine)
Oral: 50 mg tablets

Cyproheptadine (generic)
Oral: 4 mg tablets; 2 mg/5 mL syrup

Desloratadine (Clarinex)
Oral: 5 mg regular or rapidly disintegrating tablets; 2.5 mg/5 mL syrup

Dexchlorpheniramine (generic)
Oral: 4, 6 mg extended release tablets; 2 mg/5 mL syrup

Dimenhydrinate[†](Dramamine, others)
Oral: 50 mg tablets; 50 mg chewable tablets; 12.5/5 mL, 12.5 mg/4 mL, 15.62 mg/5 mL liquid
Parenteral: 50 mg/mL for IM or IV injection

Diphenhydramine (generic, Benadryl)
Oral: 12.5 mg chewable tablets; 25, 50 mg tablets, capsules; 12.5 mg/5 mL elixir and syrup
Parenteral: 50 mg/mL for injection

Emedastine (Emadine)
Ophthalmic: 0.05% solution

Epinastine (Elestat)
Ophthalmic: 0.05% solution

Fexofenadine (Allegra)
Oral: 30, 60, 180 mg tablets; 60 mg capsules

Hydroxyzine (generic, Vistaril)
Oral: 10, 25, 50 mg tablets; 25, 50, 100 mg capsules; 10 mg/5 mL syrup; 25 mg/5 mL suspension
Parenteral: 25, 50 mg/mL for injection

Ketotifen (Zaditor)
Ophthalmic: 0.025% solution

Levocabastine (Livostin)
Ophthalmic: 0.05% solution

Loratadine (generic, Claritin, Tavist)
Oral: 10 mg tablets; 10 mg rapidly disintegrating tablets; 1 mg/mL syrup

Meclizine (generic, Antivert)
Oral: 12.5, 25, 50 mg tablets; 25 mg capsules; 25 mg chewable tablets

Olopatadine (Patanol)
Ophthalmic: 0.1% solution

Phenindamine (Nolahist)
Oral: 25 mg tablets

Promethazine (generic, Phenergan)
Oral: 25, 50 mg tablets; 6.25 mg/5 mL syrups
Parenteral: 25, 50 mg/mL for injection
Rectal: 12.5, 25, 50 mg suppositories

Triprolidine (Zymine)
Oral: 1.25 mg/5 mL liquid

H$_2$ BLOCKERS

See Chapter 63.

5-HT AGONISTS

Almotriptan (Axert)
Oral: 6.25, 12.5 mg tablets

Eletriptan (Relpax)
Oral: 24.2, 48.5 mg tablets (equivalent to 20, 40 mg base)

Frovatriptan (Frova)
Oral: 2.5 mg tablets

Naratriptan (Amerge)
Oral: 1, 2.5 mg tablets

Rizatriptan
Oral: 5, 10 mg tablets (Maxalt); 5, 10 mg orally disintegrating tablets (Maxalt-MLT)

Sumatriptan (Imitrex)
Oral: 25, 50, 100 mg tablets
Nasal: 5, 20 mg unit dose spray devices
Parenteral: 6 mg/0.5 mL in SELFdose autoinjection units for subcutaneous injection

Zolmitriptan (Zomig)
Oral: 2.5, 5 mg tablets
Nasal: 5 mg

5-HT ANTAGONISTS

See Chapter 63.

MELATONIN RECEPTOR AGONISTS

Ramelteon (Rozarem)
Oral: 8 mg tablets

ERGOT ALKALOIDS

Dihydroergotamine
Nasal (Migranal): 4 mg/mL nasal spray
Parenteral (D.H.E. 45): 1 mg/mL for injection

Ergonovine (Ergotrate)
Parenteral: 0.2 mg/mL for injection
Oral: 0.2 mg tablets

Ergotamine mixtures (generic, Cafergot)
Oral: 1 mg ergotamine/100 mg caffeine tablets
Rectal: 2 mg ergotamine/100 mg caffeine suppositories

Ergotamine tartrate (Ergomar)
Sublingual: 2 mg sublingual tablets

Methylergonovine (Methergine)
Oral: 0.2 mg tablets
Parenteral: 0.2 mg/mL for injection

---

†Dimenhydrinate is the chlorotheophylline salt of diphenhydramine.

REFERENCES

Histamine

Bakker RA: Histamine H_3-receptor isoforms. Inflamm Res 2004; 53:509.

Barnes PJ: Histamine and serotonin. Pulm Pharmacol Ther 2001; 14:329.

Izzo AA et al: The role of histamine H_1, H_2, and H_3 receptors on enteric ascending synaptic transmission in the guinea pig ileum. J Pharmacol Exp Ther 1998;287:952.

Leurs R et al: Therapeutic potential of histamine H_3-receptor agonists and antagonists. Trends Pharmacol Sci 1998; 19:177.

Lieberman P: Anaphylaxis. Med Clin North Am 2006;90:77.

Schneider E et al: Trends in histamine research: New functions during immune responses and hematopoiesis. Trends Immunol 2002;23:255.

Shin N et al: Molecular modeling and site-specific mutagenesis of the histamine-binding site of the histamine H_4 receptor. Mol Pharmacol 2002;62:38.

Simons FE: Advances in H_1-antihistamines. N Engl J Med 2004; 351:2203.

Takahashi K et al: Targeted disruption of H3 receptors results in changes in brain histamine tone leading to an obese phenotype. J Clin Invest 2002;110:1791.

Serotonin

Boyer EW, Shannon M: The serotonin syndrome. N Engl J Med 2005;352:1112.

Durham PL, Russo AF: New insights into the molecular actions of serotonergic antimigraine drugs. Pharmacol Ther 2002; 94:77.

Egermayer P: Epidemics of vascular toxicity and pulmonary hypertension: What can be learned? J Intern Med 2000;247:11.

Michel K et al: Subpopulations of gastric myenteric neurons are differentially activated via distinct serotonin receptors: Projection, neurochemical coding, and functional implications. J Neurosci 1997;17:8009.

Raymond JR et al: Multiplicity of mechanisms of serotonin receptor signal transduction. Pharmacol Therap 2001;92:179.

Ergot Alkaloids: Historical

Fuller JG: *The Day of St. Anthony's Fire.* Macmillan, 1968; Signet, 1969.

Gabbai Dr, Lisbonne Dr, Pourquier Dr: Ergot poisoning at Pont St. Esprit. Br Med J 1951;Sept. 15:650.

Ergot Alkaloids: Pharmacology

DeGroot ANJA et al: Ergot alkaloids. Current status and review of clinical pharmacology and therapeutic use compared with other oxytocics in obstetrics and gynaecology. Drugs 1998;56:523.

Dierckx RA et al: Intraarterial sodium nitroprusside infusion in the treatment of severe ergotism. Clin Neuropharmacol 1986;9:542.

Dildy GA: Postpartum hemorrhage: New management options. Clin Obstet Gynecol 2002;45:330.

Lake AE, Saper JR: Chronic headache. New advances in treatment strategies. Neurology 2002;59:S8

Mantegani S, Brambilla E, Varasi M: Ergoline derivatives: receptor affinity and selectivity. Farmaco 1999;54:288.

Porter JK, Thompson FN Jr: Effects of fescue toxicosis on reproduction in livestock. J Animal Sci 1992;70:1594.

Snow V et al: Pharmacologic management of acute attacks of migraine and prevention of migraine headache. Ann Intern Med 2002;137:840.

Vasoactive Peptides

17

Ian A. Reid, PhD

Peptides are used by most tissues for cell-to-cell communication. As noted in Chapters 6 and 21, they play important roles in the autonomic and central nervous systems. Several peptides exert important direct effects on vascular and other smooth muscles. These peptides include vasoconstrictors (**angiotensin II, vasopressin, endothelins, neuropeptide Y,** and **urotensin**) and vasodilators (**bradykinin** and related **kinins, natriuretic peptides, vasoactive intestinal peptide, substance P, neurotensin, calcitonin gene-related peptide,** and **adrenomedullin**). This chapter focuses on the smooth muscle actions of the peptides.

■ ANGIOTENSIN

BIOSYNTHESIS OF ANGIOTENSIN

The pathway for the formation and metabolism of angiotensin II is summarized in Figure 17–1. The principal steps include enzymatic cleavage of angiotensin I from angiotensinogen by renin, conversion of angiotensin I to angiotensin II by converting enzyme, and degradation of angiotensin II by several peptidases.

Renin & Factors Controlling Renin Secretion

Renin is an aspartyl protease that specifically catalyzes the hydrolytic release of the decapeptide angiotensin I from angiotensinogen. It is synthesized as a preprohormone that is processed to prorenin, which is inactive, and then to active renin, a glycoprotein consisting of 340 amino acids.

Renin in the circulation originates in the kidneys. Enzymes with renin-like activity are present in several extrarenal tissues, including blood vessels, uterus, salivary glands, and adrenal cortex, but no physiologic role for these enzymes has been established. Within the kidney, renin is synthesized and stored in the juxtaglomerular apparatus of the nephron. Specialized granular cells called juxtaglomerular cells are the site of synthesis, storage, and release of renin. The macula densa is a specialized segment of the nephron that is closely associated with the vascular components of the juxtaglomerular apparatus. The vascular and tubular components of the juxtaglomerular apparatus, including the juxtaglomerular cells, are innervated by noradrenergic neurons.

The rate at which renin is secreted by the kidney is the primary determinant of activity of the renin-angiotensin system. Active renin is released immediately upon stimulation of the juxtaglomerular apparatus. Prorenin is released constitutively and, for unknown reasons, circulates at levels that can be considerably higher than those of active renin. Active renin secretion is controlled by a variety of factors, including a renal vascular receptor, the macula densa, the sympathetic nervous system, and angiotensin II.

A. RENAL VASCULAR RECEPTOR

The renal vascular receptor functions as a stretch receptor, with decreased stretch leading to increased renin release and vice versa. The receptor is apparently located in the afferent arteriole, possibly in the juxtaglomerular cells. Stretch-induced changes in renin release are mediated by changes in Ca^{2+} concentration in the juxtaglomerular cells.

B. MACULA DENSA

The macula densa contains a different type of receptor, sensitive to changes in the rate of delivery of sodium or chloride to the distal tubule. Decreases in distal delivery result in stimulation of renin secretion and vice versa. Potential candidates for signal transmission between the macula densa and the juxtaglomerular cells include adenosine, prostaglandins, and nitric oxide.

C. SYMPATHETIC NERVOUS SYSTEM

Maneuvers that increase renal nerve activity cause stimulation of renin secretion, whereas renal denervation results in suppression of renin secretion. Norepinephrine stimulates renin secretion by a direct action on the juxtaglomerular cells. In humans, this effect is mediated by β_1 adrenoceptors.

Circulating epinephrine and norepinephrine may act via the same mechanisms as the norepinephrine released locally from the renal sympathetic nerves, but there is evidence that a major component of the renin

277

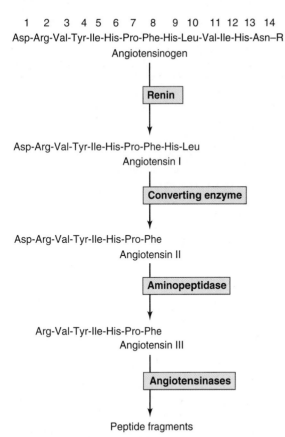

```
 1  2  3  4  5  6  7  8   9 10  11 12 13  14
Asp-Arg-Val-Tyr-Ile-His-Pro-Phe-His-Leu-Val-Ile-His-Asn–R
```
Angiotensinogen

Renin

Asp-Arg-Val-Tyr-Ile-His-Pro-Phe-His-Leu
Angiotensin I

Converting enzyme

Asp-Arg-Val-Tyr-Ile-His-Pro-Phe
Angiotensin II

Aminopeptidase

Arg-Val-Tyr-Ile-His-Pro-Phe
Angiotensin III

Angiotensinases

Peptide fragments

Figure 17–1. Chemistry of the renin-angiotensin system. The amino acid sequence of the amino terminal of human angiotensinogen is shown. R denotes the remainder of the protein molecule. See text for additional steps in the formation and metabolism of angiotensin peptides.

secretory response to circulating catecholamines is mediated by extrarenal β receptors.

D. ANGIOTENSIN

Angiotensin II inhibits renin secretion. The inhibition, which results from a direct action of the peptide on the juxtaglomerular cells, forms the basis of a short-loop negative feedback mechanism controlling renin secretion. Interruption of this feedback with inhibitors of the renin-angiotensin system (see below) results in stimulation of renin secretion.

E. PHARMACOLOGIC ALTERATION OF RENIN RELEASE

The release of renin is altered by a wide variety of pharmacologic agents. Renin release is stimulated by vasodilators (hydralazine, minoxidil, nitroprusside), β-adrenoceptor agonists (isoproterenol), α-adrenoceptor antagonists, phosphodiesterase inhibitors (theophylline, milrinone, rolipram), and most diuretics and anesthetics. This stimulation can be accounted for by the control mechanisms just described. Drugs that inhibit renin release are discussed below in the section on inhibition of the renin-angiotensin system.

Angiotensinogen

Angiotensinogen is the circulating protein substrate from which renin cleaves angiotensin I. It is synthesized in the liver. Human angiotensinogen is a glycoprotein with a molecular weight of approximately 57,000. The 14 amino acids at the amino terminal of the molecule are shown in Figure 17–1. In humans, the concentration of angiotensinogen in the circulation is less than the K_m of the renin-angiotensinogen reaction and is therefore an important determinant of the rate of formation of angiotensin.

The production of angiotensinogen is increased by corticosteroids, estrogens, thyroid hormones, and angiotensin II. It is also elevated during pregnancy and in women taking estrogen-containing oral contraceptives. The increased plasma angiotensinogen concentration is thought to contribute to the hypertension that may occur in these situations.

Angiotensin I

Although angiotensin I contains the peptide sequences necessary for all of the actions of the renin-angiotensin system, it has little or no biologic activity. Instead, it must be converted to angiotensin II by converting enzyme (Figure 17–1). Angiotensin I may also be acted on by plasma or tissue aminopeptidases to form [des-Asp^1]angiotensin I; this in turn is converted to [des-Asp^1]angiotensin II (commonly known as angiotensin III) by converting enzyme.

Converting Enzyme (ACE, Peptidyl Dipeptidase, Kininase II)

Converting enzyme is a dipeptidyl carboxypeptidase that catalyzes the cleavage of dipeptides from the carboxyl terminal of certain peptides. Its most important substrates are angiotensin I, which it converts to angiotensin II, and bradykinin, which it inactivates (see below). It also cleaves enkephalins and substance P, but the physiologic significance of these effects has not been established. The action of converting enzyme is prevented by a penultimate prolyl residue, and angiotensin II is therefore not hydrolyzed by converting enzyme. Converting enzyme is distributed widely in the body. In most tissues, converting enzyme is located on the luminal surface of vascular endothelial cells and is thus in close contact with the circulation.

A homolog of converting enzyme known as ACE2 was recently discovered. ACE2 is highly expressed in vascular endothelial cells of the kidneys, heart, and testes. Unlike converting enzyme, ACE2 has only one active site and functions as a carboxypeptidase rather than a dipeptidyl carboxypeptidase. It removes a single amino acid from the C-terminal of angiotensin I and II forming angiotensin (1-9), which has no known function, and angiotensin (1-7), which has vasodilator activity and may serve to counteract the vasoconstrictor activity of angiotensin II. ACE2 also differs from converting enzyme in that it does not hydrolyze bradykinin and is not inhibited by converting enzyme inhibitors (see below). Thus, the enzyme might better be regarded as an angiotensinase rather than a converting enzyme. (An interesting recent finding is that ACE2 is a functional receptor for coronaviruses including the virus that causes severe acute respiratory syndrome.)

Angiotensinase

Angiotensin II, which has a plasma half-life of 15–60 seconds, is removed rapidly from the circulation by a variety of peptidases collectively referred to as angiotensinase. It is metabolized during passage through most vascular beds (a notable exception being the lung). Most metabolites of angiotensin II are biologically inactive, but the initial product of aminopeptidase action—[des-Asp^1]angiotensin II—retains considerable biologic activity.

ACTIONS OF ANGIOTENSIN II

Angiotensin II exerts important actions at vascular smooth muscle, adrenal cortex, kidney, heart, and brain. Through these actions, the renin-angiotensin system plays a key role in the regulation of fluid and electrolyte balance and arterial blood pressure. Excessive activity of the renin-angiotensin system can result in hypertension and disorders of fluid and electrolyte homeostasis.

Blood Pressure

Angiotensin II is a very potent pressor agent—on a molar basis, approximately 40 times more potent than norepinephrine. The pressor response to intravenous angiotensin II is rapid in onset (10–15 seconds) and sustained during long-term infusions. A large component of the pressor response is due to direct contraction of vascular—especially arteriolar—smooth muscle. In addition, however, angiotensin II can also increase blood pressure through actions on the brain and autonomic nervous system. The pressor response to angiotensin is usually accompanied by little or no reflex bradycardia because the peptide acts on the brain to reset the baroreceptor reflex control of heart rate to a higher pressure.

Angiotensin II also interacts with the autonomic nervous system. It stimulates autonomic ganglia, increases the release of epinephrine and norepinephrine from the adrenal medulla, and—what is most important—facilitates sympathetic transmission by an action at adrenergic nerve terminals. The latter effect involves both increased release and reduced reuptake of norepinephrine. Angiotensin II also has a less important direct positive inotropic action on the heart.

Adrenal Cortex

Angiotensin II acts directly on the zona glomerulosa of the adrenal cortex to stimulate aldosterone biosynthesis. At higher concentrations, angiotensin II also stimulates glucocorticoid biosynthesis.

Kidney

Angiotensin II acts on the kidney to cause renal vasoconstriction, increase proximal tubular sodium reabsorption, and inhibit the secretion of renin.

Central Nervous System

In addition to its central effects on blood pressure, angiotensin II acts on the central nervous system to stimulate drinking (dipsogenic effect) and increase the secretion of vasopressin and adrenocorticotropic hormone (ACTH). The physiologic significance of the effects of angiotensin II on drinking and pituitary hormone secretion is not known.

Cell Growth

Angiotensin II is mitogenic for vascular and cardiac muscle cells and may contribute to the development of cardiovascular hypertrophy. It also exerts a variety of important effects on the vascular endothelium. Considerable evidence now indicates that ACE inhibitors and angiotensin II receptor antagonists (see below) slow or prevent morphologic changes (remodeling) following myocardial infarction that would otherwise lead to heart failure.

ANGIOTENSIN RECEPTORS & MECHANISM OF ACTION

Angiotensin II receptors are widely distributed in the body. Like the receptors for other peptide hormones, angiotensin II receptors are located on the plasma membrane of target cells, and this permits rapid onset of the various actions of angiotensin II.

Two distinct subtypes of angiotensin II receptors, termed **AT$_1$** and **AT$_2$**, have been identified on the basis of their differential affinity for antagonists, and their sensitivity to sulfhydryl-reducing agents. AT_1 receptors have a high affinity for losartan and a low affinity for PD 123177 (an experimental nonpeptide antagonist), whereas AT_2 receptors have a high affinity for PD 123177 and a low affinity for losartan. Angiotensin II and saralasin (see below) bind equally to both subtypes. The relative proportion of the two subtypes varies from tissue to tissue: AT_1 receptors predominate in vascular smooth muscle.

Most of the known actions of angiotensin II are mediated by the AT_1 receptor, a G_q protein-coupled receptor. Binding of angiotensin II to AT_1 receptors in vascular smooth muscle results in activation of phospholipase C and generation of inositol trisphosphate and diacylglycerol (see Chapter 2). These events, which occur within seconds, result in smooth muscle contraction.

The stimulation of vascular and cardiac growth by angiotensin II is mediated by other pathways, probably receptor and nonreceptor tyrosine kinases such as the Janus tyrosine kinase Jak2 and increased transcription of specific genes (see Chapter 2).

The AT_2 receptor has a structure and affinity for angiotensin II similar to those of the AT_1 receptor. In contrast, however, stimulation of AT_2 receptors causes vasodilation that may serve to counteract the vasoconstriction resulting from AT_1 receptor stimulation. AT_2 receptor-mediated vasodilation appears to be nitric oxide (NO)-dependent and may involve the bradykinin B_2 receptor-NO-cGMP pathway.

AT_2 receptors are present at high density in all tissues during fetal development, but they are much less abundant in the adult where they are expressed at high concentration only in the adrenal medulla, reproductive tissues, vascular endothelium, and parts of the brain. AT_2 receptors are up-regulated in pathologic conditions including heart failure and myocardial infarction. The functions of the AT_2 receptor appear to include fetal tissue development, inhibition of growth and proliferation, cell differentiation, apoptosis, and vasodilation.

INHIBITION OF THE RENIN-ANGIOTENSIN SYSTEM

A wide variety of agents are now available that block the formation or actions of angiotensin II. These drugs block renin secretion, the enzymatic action of renin, the conversion of angiotensin I to angiotensin II, or angiotensin II receptors.

Drugs That Block Renin Secretion

Several drugs that interfere with the sympathetic nervous system inhibit the secretion of renin. Examples are clonidine and propranolol. Clonidine inhibits renin secretion by causing a centrally mediated reduction in

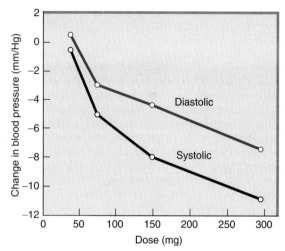

Figure 17–2. Effect of the renin inhibitor aliskiren on blood pressure in patients with essential hypertension. (Data from Stanton A et al: Blood pressure lowering in essential hypertension with an oral renin inhibitor, aliskiren. Hypertension 2003;42:1137.)

renal sympathetic nerve activity, and it may also exert a direct intrarenal action. Propranolol and other β-adrenoceptor–blocking drugs act by blocking the intrarenal and extrarenal β receptors involved in the neural control of renin secretion.

Renin Inhibitors

Drugs that inhibit renin have been available for many years but have been limited by low potency, bioavailability, and duration of action. However, a new class of nonpeptide, low-molecular weight, orally active inhibitors has recently been developed.

Aliskiren is the most advanced of these. In healthy subjects, aliskiren produces a dose-dependent reduction in plasma renin activity and angiotensin I and II and aldosterone concentrations. In patients with essential hypertension, aliskiren suppresses plasma renin activity and causes dose-related reductions in blood pressure similar to those produced by angiotensin II receptor antagonists (Figure 17–2). The safety and tolerability of aliskiren appear to be comparable to angiotensin antagonists and placebo. Renin inhibition thus has considerable promise for the treatment of hypertension and other cardiovascular and renal diseases.

Angiotensin-Converting Enzyme Inhibitors

An important class of orally active **ACE** inhibitors, directed against the active site of ACE, is now extensively used. **Captopril** and **enalapril** (Figure 17–3) are

Captopril

Enalapril

Figure 17–3. Two orally active converting enzyme inhibitors. Enalapril is a prodrug ethyl ester that is hydrolyzed in the body.

examples of the many potent ACE inhibitors that are available. These drugs differ in their structure and pharmacokinetics, but in clinical use, they are interchangeable. ACE inhibitors decrease systemic vascular resistance without increasing heart rate, and they promote natriuresis. As described in Chapters 11 and 13, they are effective in the treatment of hypertension, decrease morbidity and mortality in heart failure and left ventricular dysfunction after myocardial infarction, and delay the progression of diabetic nephropathy.

ACE inhibitors not only block the conversion of angiotensin I to angiotensin II but also inhibit the degradation of other substances, including bradykinin, substance P, and enkephalins. The action of ACE inhibitors to inhibit bradykinin metabolism contributes significantly to their hypotensive action (see Figure 11–5) and is apparently responsible for some adverse side effects, including cough and angioedema.

Recent evidence suggests that some of the beneficial effects of ACE inhibitors can be attributed to activation of a distinct ACE-signaling cascade in addition to the changes in angiotensin II and bradykinin levels.

Angiotensin Receptor Antagonists

Potent peptide antagonists of the action of angiotensin II have been developed. The best-known of these is the partial agonist, **saralasin.** Saralasin lowers blood pressure in hypertensive patients but may elicit pressor responses, particularly when circulating angiotensin II levels are low. Because it must be administered intravenously, saralasin is used only for investigation of renin-dependent hypertension and other hyperreninemic states.

The *non*peptide angiotensin II antagonists are of much greater interest. **Losartan** (Figure 17–4), **valsartan, eprosartan, irbesartan, candesartan, olmesartan,** and **telmesartan** are orally active, potent, and specific competitive antagonists of angiotensin AT_1 receptors. The efficacy of these drugs in hypertension is similar to that of ACE inhibitors, but they are associated with a lower incidence of cough. Like ACE inhibitors, *non*peptide angiotensin II antagonists slow the progression of diabetic nephropathy. The antagonists are also effective in the treatment of heart failure and provide a useful alternative when ACE inhibitors are not well tolerated. Like ACE inhibitors, they are well tolerated but should not be used by patients with nondiabetic renal disease or in pregnancy.

The current angiotensin II receptor antagonists are selective for the AT_1 receptor. Since prolonged treatment with the drugs disinhibits renin secretion and increases circulating angiotensin II levels, there may be increased stimulation of AT_2 receptors. This may be significant in view of the evidence that activation of the AT_2 receptor causes vasodilation and other beneficial effects. AT_2 receptor antagonists such as PD 123177 are available for research but have no clinical applications at this time.

The clinical benefits of AT_1 receptor antagonists are similar to those of ACE inhibitors, and it is not clear if one group of drugs has significant advantages over the other. Combination therapy with both an ACE inhibitor and an angiotensin receptor antagonist has a number of potential advantages and is currently being investigated.

Losartan

Figure 17–4. Structure of an angiotensin AT_1 receptor antagonist.

■ KININS

BIOSYNTHESIS OF KININS

Kinins are potent vasodilator peptides formed enzymatically by the action of enzymes known as kallikreins or kininogenases acting on protein substrates called kininogens. The kallikrein-kinin system has several features in common with the renin-angiotensin system.

Kallikreins

Kallikreins are present in plasma and in several tissues, including the kidneys, pancreas, intestine, sweat glands, and salivary glands. Plasma prekallikrein can be activated to kallikrein by trypsin, Hageman factor, and possibly kallikrein itself. In general, the biochemical properties of tissue kallikreins are different from those of plasma kallikreins. Kallikreins can convert prorenin to active renin, but the physiologic significance of this action has not been established.

Kininogens

Kininogens—the precursors of kinins and substrates of kallikreins—are present in plasma, lymph, and interstitial fluid. Two kininogens are known to be present in plasma: a low-molecular-weight form (LMW kininogen) and a high-molecular-weight form (HMW kininogen). About 15–20% of the total plasma kininogen is in the HMW form. It is thought that LMW kininogen crosses capillary walls and serves as the substrate for tissue kallikreins, whereas HMW kininogen is confined to the bloodstream and serves as the substrate for plasma kallikrein.

FORMATION OF KININS IN PLASMA & TISSUES

The pathway for the formation and metabolism of kinins is shown in Figure 17–5. Three kinins have been identified in mammals: **bradykinin, lysylbradykinin** (also known as **kallidin**), and **methionyllysylbradykinin.** Each contains bradykinin in its structure.

Each kinin is formed from a kininogen by the action of a different enzyme. Bradykinin is released by plasma kallikrein, lysylbradykinin by tissue kallikrein, and methionyllysylbradykinin by pepsin and pepsin-like enzymes. The three kinins have been found in plasma and urine. Bradykinin is the predominant kinin in plasma, whereas lysylbradykinin is the major urinary form.

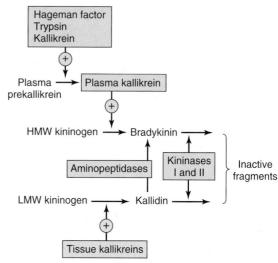

Figure 17–5. The kallikrein-kinin system. Kininase II is identical to converting enzyme peptidyl dipeptidase.

ACTIONS OF KININS

Effects on the Cardiovascular System

Kinins produce marked vasodilation in several vascular beds, including the heart, kidney, intestine, skeletal muscle, and liver. In this respect, kinins are approximately 10 times more potent on a molar basis than histamine. The vasodilation may result from a direct inhibitory effect of kinins on arteriolar smooth muscle or may be mediated by the release of nitric oxide or vasodilator prostaglandins such as PGE_2 and PGI_2. In contrast, the predominant effect of kinins on veins is contraction; again, this may result from direct stimulation of venous smooth muscle or from the release of venoconstrictor prostaglandins such as $PGF_{2\alpha}$. Kinins also produce contraction of most visceral smooth muscle.

When injected intravenously, kinins produce a rapid but brief fall in blood pressure that is due to their arteriolar vasodilator action. Intravenous infusions of the peptide fail to produce a sustained decrease in blood pressure; prolonged hypotension can only be produced by progressively increasing the rate of infusion. The rapid reversibility of the hypotensive response to kinins is due primarily to reflex increases in heart rate, myocardial contractility, and cardiac output. In some species, bradykinin produces a biphasic change in blood pressure—an initial hypotensive response followed by an increase above the preinjection level. The increase in blood pressure may be due to a reflex activation of the sympathetic nervous system, but under some conditions, bradykinin can directly release catecholamines from the adrenal medulla and stimulate sympathetic ganglia. Bradykinin also increases blood pressure when injected into the central nervous system, but the physiologic significance of this effect is not clear, since it is unlikely that kinins cross the blood-brain barrier. Kinins have no consistent effect on sympathetic or parasympathetic nerve endings.

The arteriolar dilation produced by kinins causes an increase in pressure and flow in the capillary bed, thus favoring efflux of fluid from blood to tissues. This effect may be facilitated by increased capillary permeability resulting from contraction of endothelial cells and widening of intercellular junctions, and by increased venous pressure secondary to constriction of veins. As a result of these changes, water and solutes pass from the blood to the extracellular fluid, lymph flow increases, and edema may result.

Effects on Endocrine & Exocrine Glands

As noted earlier, prekallikreins and kallikreins are present in several glands, including the pancreas, kidney, intestine, salivary glands, and sweat glands, and they can be released into the secretory fluids of these glands. The function of the enzymes in these tissues is not known. The enzymes (or active kinins) may diffuse from the organs to the blood and act as local modulators of blood flow. Since kinins have such marked effects on smooth muscle, they may also modulate the tone of salivary and pancreatic ducts and help regulate gastrointestinal motility. Kinins also influence the transepithelial transport of water, electrolytes, glucose, and amino acids, and may regulate the transport of these substances in the gastrointestinal tract and kidney. Finally, kallikreins may play a role in the physiologic activation of various prohormones, including proinsulin and prorenin.

Role in Inflammation

Kinins play an important role in the inflammatory process. Kallikreins and kinins can produce redness, local heat, swelling, and pain, and the production of kinins is increased in inflammatory lesions produced by a variety of methods.

Effects on Sensory Nerves

Kinins are potent pain-producing substances when applied to a blister base or injected intradermally. They elicit pain by stimulating nociceptive afferents in the skin and viscera.

KININ RECEPTORS & MECHANISMS OF ACTION

The biologic actions of kinins are mediated by specific receptors located on the membranes of the target tis-

sues. Two types of kinin receptors, termed B_1 and B_2, have been defined based on the rank orders of agonist potencies. (Note that B here stands for bradykinin, not for β-adrenoceptor.) Bradykinin displays the highest affinity in most B_2 receptor systems, followed by Lys-bradykinin and then by Met-Lys-bradykinin. One exception is the B_2 receptor that mediates contraction of venous smooth muscle; this appears to be most sensitive to Lys-bradykinin. Recent evidence suggests the existence of two B_2-receptor subtypes, which have been termed B_{2A} and B_{2B}.

B_1 receptors appear to have a very limited distribution in mammalian tissues and have few known functional roles. Studies with knockout mice that lack functional B_1 receptors suggest that these receptors participate in the inflammatory response and may also be important in long-lasting kinin effects such as collagen synthesis and cell multiplication. By contrast, B_2 receptors have a widespread distribution that is consistent with the multitude of biologic effects that are mediated by this receptor type. B_2 receptors are G protein–coupled and agonist binding sets in motion multiple signal transduction events, including calcium mobilization, chloride transport, formation of nitric oxide, and activation of phospholipase C, phospholipase A_2, and adenylyl cyclase.

METABOLISM OF KININS

Kinins are metabolized rapidly (half-life < 15 seconds) by nonspecific exopeptidases or endopeptidases, commonly referred to as kininases. Two plasma kininases have been well characterized. Kininase I, apparently synthesized in the liver, is a carboxypeptidase that releases the carboxyl terminal arginine residue. Kininase II is present in plasma and vascular endothelial cells throughout the body. It is identical to angiotensin-converting enzyme (ACE, peptidyl dipeptidase), discussed above. Kininase II inactivates kinins by cleaving the carboxyl terminal dipeptide phenylalanyl-arginine. Like angiotensin I, bradykinin is almost completely hydrolyzed during a single passage through the pulmonary vascular bed.

DRUGS AFFECTING THE KALLIKREIN-KININ SYSTEM

Drugs that modify the activity of the kallikrein-kinin system are available, though none are in wide clinical use. Considerable effort has been directed toward developing kinin receptor antagonists, since such drugs have considerable therapeutic potential as anti-inflammatory and antinociceptive agents. Competitive antagonists of both B_1 and B_2 receptors are available for research use. Examples of B_1 receptor antagonists are the peptides [Leu^8-des-Arg^9]bradykinin and Lys[Leu^8-

des Arg^9]bradykinin. Nonpeptide B$_1$ receptor antagonists are not yet available. The first B$_2$ receptor antagonists to be discovered were also peptide derivatives of bradykinin. These first-generation antagonists were used extensively in animal studies of kinin receptor pharmacology. However, their half-life is short, and they are almost inactive on the human B$_2$ receptor.

Icatibant is a second-generation B$_2$ receptor antagonist. It is orally active, potent, and selective, has a long duration of action (> 60 minutes), and displays high B$_2$-receptor affinity in humans and all other species in which it has been tested. Icatibant has been used extensively in animal studies to block exogenous and endogenous bradykinin and in human studies to evaluate the role of kinins in pain, hyperalgesia, and inflammation.

Recently, a third generation of B$_2$-receptor antagonists was developed; examples are FR 173657, FR 172357, and NPC 18884. These antagonists block both human and animal B$_2$ receptors and are orally active. They have been reported to inhibit bradykinin-induced bronchoconstriction in guinea pigs, carrageenin-induced inflammatory responses in rats, and capsaicin-induced nociception in mice. These antagonists have promise for the treatment of inflammatory pain in humans.

SSR240612 is a new, potent, and orally active selective antagonist of B$_1$ receptors in humans and several animal species. It exhibits analgesic and anti-inflammatory activities in mice and rats and is currently in preclinical development for the treatment of inflammatory and neurogenic pain.

The synthesis of kinins can be inhibited with the kallikrein inhibitor aprotinin. Actions of kinins mediated by prostaglandin generation can be blocked nonspecifically with inhibitors of prostaglandin synthesis such as aspirin. Conversely, the actions of kinins can be enhanced with ACE inhibitors, which block the degradation of the peptides. Indeed, as noted above, inhibition of bradykinin metabolism by ACE inhibitors contributes significantly to their antihypertensive action.

There is evidence that by acting on B$_2$ receptors, bradykinin may play a beneficial, protective role in cardiovascular disease. Selective B$_2$ agonists are available and have been shown to be effective in some animal models of human cardiovascular disease. These drugs may have potential for the treatment of hypertension and myocardial hypertrophy.

■ VASOPRESSIN

Vasopressin (**antidiuretic hormone, ADH**) plays an important role in the long-term control of blood pressure through its action on the kidney to increase water reabsorption. This and other aspects of the physiology of vasopressin are discussed in Chapters 15 and 37 and will not be reviewed here.

Vasopressin also plays an important role in the short-term regulation of arterial pressure by its vasoconstrictor action. It increases total peripheral resistance when infused in doses less than those required to produce maximum urine concentration. Such doses do not normally increase arterial pressure because the vasopressor activity of the peptide is buffered by a reflex decrease in cardiac output. When the influence of this reflex is removed, eg, in shock, pressor sensitivity to vasopressin is greatly increased. Pressor sensitivity to vasopressin is also enhanced in patients with idiopathic orthostatic hypotension. Higher doses of vasopressin increase blood pressure even when baroreceptor reflexes are intact.

VASOPRESSIN RECEPTORS & ANTAGONISTS

Three subtypes of vasopressin receptors have been identified. **V$_{1a}$ receptors** mediate the vasoconstrictor action of vasopressin; **V$_{1b}$ receptors** potentiate the release of ACTH by pituitary corticotropes; and **V$_2$ receptors** mediate the antidiuretic action. V$_{1a}$ effects are mediated by activation of phospholipase C, formation of inositol trisphosphate, and increased intracellular calcium concentration. V$_2$ effects are mediated by activation of adenylyl cyclase.

Vasopressin-like peptides selective for either vasoconstrictor or antidiuretic activity have been synthesized. The most specific V$_1$ vasoconstrictor agonist synthesized to date is [Phe^2, Ile^3, Orn^8]vasotocin. Selective V$_2$ antidiuretic analogs include 1-deamino[D-Arg^8]arginine vasopressin (dDAVP) and 1-deamino[Val^4,D-Arg^8]arginine vasopressin (dVDAVP).

Specific antagonists of the vasoconstrictor action of vasopressin are also available. The peptide antagonist [1-(β-mercapto-β,β-cyclopentamethylenepropionic acid)-2-(O-methyl)tyrosine] arginine vasopressin also has antioxytocic activity but does not antagonize the antidiuretic action of vasopressin. Recently, nonpeptide, orally active V$_{1a}$ receptor antagonists have been discovered, examples being OPC-21268 and SR49059.

The vasopressor antagonists of vasopressin have been particularly useful in revealing the important role that vasopressin plays in blood pressure regulation in situations such as dehydration and hemorrhage. They have potential for the treatment of hypertension and heart failure. To date, most studies have focused on heart failure in which promising results have been obtained with V$_2$ antagonists. However, V$_{1a}$ antagonists also have potential, and **conivaptan** (YM087), a drug with both V$_{1a}$ and V$_2$ antagonist effects, has been approved for treatment of hyponatremia (see Chapter 15).

■ NATRIURETIC PEPTIDES

Synthesis & Structure

The atria and other tissues of mammals contain a family of peptides with natriuretic, diuretic, vasorelaxant, and other properties. The family consists of atrial natriuretic peptide (ANP), brain natriuretic peptide (BNP) and C-type natriuretic peptide (CNP). The structures of the three peptides are similar (Figure 17–6), but there are differences in their biologic effects. ANP is derived from the carboxyl terminal end of a common precursor termed preproANP. ANP is synthesized primarily in cardiac atrial cells, but small amounts are synthesized in ventricular cells. It is also synthesized by neurons in the central and peripheral nervous systems and in the lungs. ANP circulates as a 28-amino-acid peptide with a single disulfide bridge that forms a 17-residue ring.

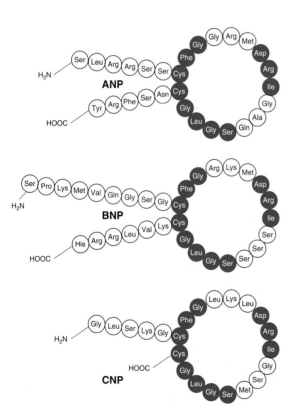

Figure 17–6. Structures of atrial natriuretic peptide (ANP), brain natriuretic peptide (BNP), and C-type natriuretic peptide (CNP). Sequences common to the peptides are indicated in blue.

Several factors increase the release of ANP from the heart, but the most important one appears to be atrial stretch via mechanosensitive ion channels. ANP release is also increased by volume expansion, head-out water immersion, changing from the standing to the supine position, and exercise. ANP release can also be increased by sympathetic stimulation via α_{1A}-adrenoceptors, endothelins (see below) via the ET_A-receptor subtype, glucocorticoids, and vasopressin. Finally, plasma ANP concentration increases in various pathologic states, including heart failure, primary aldosteronism, chronic renal failure, and inappropriate ADH secretion syndrome.

Administration of ANP produces prompt and marked increases in sodium excretion and urine flow. Glomerular filtration rate increases, with little or no change in renal blood flow, so that the filtration fraction increases. The ANP-induced natriuresis is apparently due to both the increase in glomerular filtration rate and a decrease in proximal tubular sodium reabsorption. ANP also inhibits the secretion of renin, aldosterone, and vasopressin; these changes may also increase sodium and water excretion. Finally, ANP decreases arterial blood pressure. This hypotensive action is due to vasodilation, which results from stimulated particulate guanylyl cyclase activity, increased cGMP levels, and decreased cytosolic free calcium concentration. ANP also reduces sympathetic tone to the peripheral vasculature and antagonizes the vasoconstrictor action of angiotensin II and other vasoconstrictors. These actions may contribute to the hypotensive action of the peptide.

There is considerable evidence that ANP participates in the physiologic regulation of sodium excretion and blood pressure. For example, suppression of ANP production or blockade of its action impairs the natriuretic response to volume expansion, and increases blood pressure.

BNP was originally isolated from porcine brain but, like ANP, is synthesized primarily in the heart. It exists in two forms, having either 26 or 32 amino acids (Figure 17–6). Like ANP, the release of BNP appears to be volume-related; indeed, the two peptides may be co-secreted. BNP exhibits natriuretic, diuretic, and hypotensive activities similar to those of ANP but circulates at a lower concentration.

CNP consists of 22 amino acids (Figure 17–6). It is located predominantly in the central nervous system but is also present in several other tissues including the vascular endothelium, kidneys, and intestine. It has not been found in significant concentrations in the circulation. CNP has less natriuretic and diuretic activity than ANP and BNP but is a potent vasodilator. Its physiologic role is unclear.

Pharmacodynamics & Pharmacokinetics

The biologic actions of the natriuretic peptides are mediated through association with specific high-affinity receptors located on the surface of the target cells. Three receptor subtypes termed **ANP$_A$**, **ANP$_B$**, and **ANP$_C$** have been identified. The ANP$_A$ receptor consists of a 120 kDa protein; its primary ligands are ANP and BNP. The ANP$_B$ receptor is similar in structure to the ANP$_A$ receptor, but its primary ligand appears to be CNP. The ANP$_A$ and ANP$_B$ receptors, but not the ANP$_C$ receptor, are coupled to guanylyl cyclase.

The natriuretic peptides have a short half-life in the circulation. They are metabolized in the kidneys, liver, and lungs by the neutral endopeptidase NEP 24.11. Inhibition of this endopeptidase results in increases in circulating levels of the natriuretic peptides, natriuresis, and diuresis. The peptides are also removed from the circulation by binding to ANP$_C$ receptors in the vascular endothelium. This receptor binds the three natriuretic peptides with equal affinity. The receptor and bound peptide are internalized, the peptide is degraded enzymatically, and the receptor is returned to the cell surface.

Administration of BNP as **nesiritide** (see Chapter 13) in patients with severe heart failure increases sodium excretion and improves hemodynamics. However, the peptide has to be given by constant intravenous infusion and has caused fatal renal damage. A more promising approach may be the use of drugs that inhibit the neutral endopeptidase responsible for the breakdown of ANP. This is discussed below under Vasopeptidase Inhibitors. Patients with heart failure have high plasma levels of ANP and BNP; the latter has emerged as a diagnostic and prognostic marker in this condition.

■ VASOPEPTIDASE INHIBITORS

Vasopeptidase inhibitors are a new class of cardiovascular drugs that inhibit two metalloprotease enzymes, NEP 24.11 and ACE. They thus simultaneously increase the levels of natriuretic peptides and decrease the formation of angiotensin II. As a result, they enhance vasodilation, reduce vasoconstriction, and increase sodium excretion, in turn reducing peripheral vascular resistance and blood pressure.

Recently developed vasopeptidase inhibitors include **omapatrilat, sampatrilat,** and **fasidotrilat.** Omapatrilat, which has received the most attention, lowers blood pressure in animal models of hypertension as well as in hypertensive patients, and improves cardiac function in patients with heart failure. Unfortunately, omapatrilat causes a significant incidence of angioedema in addition to cough and dizziness and has not been approved for clinical use.

■ ENDOTHELINS

The endothelium is the source of a variety of substances with vasodilator (PGI$_2$ and nitric oxide) and vasoconstrictor activities. The latter include the endothelin family, potent vasoconstrictor peptides that were first isolated from aortic endothelial cells.

Biosynthesis, Structure, & Clearance

Three isoforms of endothelin have been identified: the originally described endothelin (**ET-1**) and two similar peptides, **ET-2** and **ET-3.** Each isoform is a product of a different gene and is synthesized as a prepro form that is processed to a propeptide and then to the mature peptide. Processing to the mature peptides occurs through the action of endothelin-converting enzyme. Each endothelin is a 21-amino-acid peptide containing two disulfide bridges (Figure 17–7).

Endothelins are widely distributed in the body. ET-1 is the predominant endothelin secreted by the vascular endothelium. It is also produced by neurons and astrocytes in the central nervous system and in endometrial, renal mesangial, Sertoli, breast epithelial, and other cells. ET-2 is produced predominantly in the kidneys and intestine, whereas ET-3 is found in highest concentration in the brain but is also present in the gastrointestinal tract, lungs, and kidneys. Endothelins are

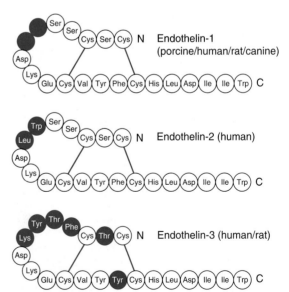

Figure 17–7. Structures of the endothelin peptides endothelin-1, endothelin-2, and endothelin-3. Sequences different in the three peptides are shown in blue.

present in the blood but in low concentration; they apparently act locally in a paracrine or autocrine fashion rather than as circulating hormones.

The expression of the ET-1 gene is increased by growth factors and cytokines, including transforming growth factor-β (TGF-β) and interleukin 1 (IL-1), vasoactive substances including angiotensin II and vasopressin, and mechanical stress. Expression is inhibited by nitric oxide, prostacyclin, and atrial natriuretic peptide.

Clearance of endothelins from the circulation is rapid and involves both enzymatic degradation by NEP 24.11 and clearance by the ET_B receptor.

Actions

Endothelins exert widespread actions in the body. In particular, they cause dose-dependent vasoconstriction in most vascular beds. Intravenous administration of ET-1 causes a rapid and transient decrease in arterial blood pressure followed by a prolonged increase. The depressor response results from release of prostacyclin and nitric oxide from the vascular endothelium, whereas the pressor response is due to direct contraction of vascular smooth muscle. Endothelins also exert direct positive inotropic and chronotropic actions on the heart and are potent coronary vasoconstrictors. They act on the kidneys to cause vasoconstriction and decrease glomerular filtration rate and sodium and water excretion. In the respiratory system, they cause potent contraction of tracheal and bronchial smooth muscle. Endothelins interact with several endocrine systems, increasing the secretion of renin, aldosterone, vasopressin, and atrial natriuretic peptide. They exert a variety of actions on the central and peripheral nervous systems, the gastrointestinal system, the liver, the urinary tract, the male and female reproductive systems, the eye, the skeletal system, and the skin. Finally, ET-1 is a potent mitogen for vascular smooth muscle cells, cardiac myocytes, and glomerular mesangial cells.

Endothelin receptors are widespread in the body. Two endothelin receptor subtypes, termed ET_A and ET_B, have been cloned and sequenced. ET_A receptors have a high affinity for ET-1 and a low affinity for ET-3 and are located on smooth muscle cells, where they mediate vasoconstriction. ET_B receptors have approximately equal affinities for ET-1 and ET-3 and are located on vascular endothelial cells, where they mediate release of PGI_2 and nitric oxide. Both receptor subtypes belong to the G protein-coupled seven-transmembrane domain family of receptors.

The signal transduction mechanisms triggered by binding of ET-1 to its receptors include stimulation of phospholipase C, formation of inositol trisphosphate, and release of calcium from the endoplasmic reticulum, which results in vasoconstriction. Stimulation of PGI_2 and nitric oxide synthesis results in decreased intracellular calcium concentration and vasodilation.

INHIBITORS OF ENDOTHELIN SYNTHESIS & ACTION

The endothelin system can be blocked with receptor antagonists and drugs that block endothelin-converting enzyme. Endothelin ET_A or ET_B receptors can be blocked selectively, or both can be blocked with nonselective ET_A-ET_B antagonists.

Bosentan is a nonselective antagonist. This drug is active intravenously and orally, and blocks both the initial transient depressor (ET_B) and the prolonged pressor (ET_A) responses to intravenous endothelin. Many orally active endothelin receptor antagonists with increased selectivity have been developed and are available for research use.

Bosentan

The formation of endothelins can be blocked by inhibiting endothelin-converting enzyme with phosphoramidon. Phosphoramidon is not specific for endothelin-converting enzyme, but several potent and more selective inhibitors are now available. The therapeutic potential of these drugs may be similar to that of the endothelin receptor antagonists (see below).

PHYSIOLOGIC & PATHOLOGIC ROLES OF ENDOTHELIN: EFFECTS OF ENDOTHELIN ANTAGONISTS

Systemic administration of endothelin receptor antagonists or endothelin-converting enzyme inhibitors causes vasodilation and decreases arterial pressure in humans and experimental animals. Intra-arterial administration of the drugs also causes slow-onset forearm vasodilation in humans. These observations provide evidence that the endothelin system participates in the regulation of vascular tone, even under resting conditions.

There is increasing evidence that endothelins participate in a variety of cardiovascular diseases, including hypertension, cardiac hypertrophy, heart failure, atherosclerosis, coronary artery disease, and myocardial infarction. Endothelins have also been implicated in pulmonary diseases, including asthma and pulmonary hypertension, as well as in several renal diseases.

Endothelin antagonists have considerable potential in the treatment of these diseases. In clinical trials, bosentan and other nonselective antagonists as well as ET_A-selective antagonists (sitaxentan, ambrisentan) have produced beneficial effects on hemodynamics and other symptoms in heart failure, pulmonary hypertension, and essential hypertension. Bosentan is currently approved for use in pulmonary hypertension (see Chapter 11), and a related antagonist, tezosentan, is under investigation for the treatment of acute heart failure.

Endothelin antagonists occasionally cause systemic hypotension, increased heart rate, facial flushing or edema, and headaches. Potential gastrointestinal effects include nausea, vomiting, and constipation. Because of their teratogenic effects, ET antagonists are contraindicated in pregnancy. Bosentan has been associated with fatal hepatotoxicity, and patients taking this drug must have monthly liver function tests. Negative pregnancy test results are required for women of child-bearing age to take this drug.

■ VASOACTIVE INTESTINAL PEPTIDE

Vasoactive intestinal peptide (VIP) is a 28-amino-acid peptide related structurally to secretin and glucagon. VIP is widely distributed in the central and peripheral nervous systems, where it functions as a neurotransmitter or neuromodulator. It is also present in the gastrointestinal tract, heart, lungs, kidneys, and thyroid gland. Many blood vessels are innervated by VIP neurons. VIP is found in blood but does not appear to function as a hormone.

VIP exerts significant effects on the cardiovascular system. It produces marked vasodilation in most vascular beds and in this regard is more potent on a molar basis than acetylcholine. In the heart, VIP causes coronary vasodilation and exerts positive inotropic and chronotropic effects. It may thus participate in the regulation of coronary blood flow, cardiac contraction, and heart rate.

The effects of VIP are mediated by G protein-coupled receptors; two subtypes, **VPAC1** and **VPAC2,** have been cloned from human tissues. Both subtypes are widely distributed in the central ner-

vous system and in the heart, blood vessels, and other tissues. Binding of VIP to its receptors results in activation of adenylyl cyclase and formation of cAMP, which is responsible for the vasodilation and many other effects of the peptide. Other actions may be mediated by nitric oxide and cGMP.

Specific VIP receptor agonists and antagonists are currently available for research use.

■ SUBSTANCE P

Substance P belongs to the **tachykinin** family of peptides, which share the common carboxyl terminal sequence Phe-X-Gly-Leu-Met. Other members of this family are **neurokinin A** and **neurokinin B.** Substance P is an undecapeptide, while neurokinins A and B are decapeptides.

Substance P is present in the central nervous system, where it is a neurotransmitter (see Chapter 21), and in the gastrointestinal tract, where it may play a role as a transmitter in the enteric nervous system and as a local hormone (see Chapter 6).

Substance P exerts a variety of incompletely understood central actions that implicate the peptide in behavior, anxiety, depression, nausea, and emesis. It is a potent arteriolar vasodilator, producing marked hypotension in humans and several animal species. The vasodilation is mediated by release of nitric oxide from the endothelium. Conversely, substance P causes contraction of venous, intestinal, and bronchial smooth muscle. It also stimulates secretion by the salivary glands and causes diuresis and natriuresis by the kidneys.

The actions of substance P and neurokinins A and B are mediated by three G protein-coupled tachykinin receptors designated NK_1, NK_2, and NK_3. Substance P is the preferred ligand for the NK_1 receptor, the predominant tachykinin receptor in the human brain. However, neurokinins A and B also possess considerable affinity for this receptor. In humans, most of the central and peripheral effects of substance P are mediated by NK_1 receptors.

Several nonpeptide NK_1 receptor antagonists have been developed. These compounds are highly selective and orally active, and enter the brain. Recent clinical trials have shown that these antagonists may be useful in treating depression and other disorders and in preventing chemotherapy-induced emesis. The first of these to be approved for the prevention of chemotherapy-induced nausea and vomiting is **aprepitant** (Chapter 63).

■ NEUROTENSIN

Neurotensin is a tridecapeptide that was first isolated from the central nervous system but subsequently was found to be present in the gastrointestinal tract and in the circulation. It is synthesized as part of a larger precursor that also contains **neuromedin N,** a six-amino-acid neurotensin-like peptide.

In the brain, processing of the precursor leads primarily to the formation of neurotensin and neuromedin N; these are released together from nerve endings. In the gut, processing leads mainly to the formation of neurotensin and a larger peptide that contains the neuromedin N sequence at the carboxyl terminal. Both peptides are secreted into the circulation after ingestion of food.

Like many other neuropeptides, neurotensin serves a dual function as a neurotransmitter or neuromodulator in the central nervous system and as a local hormone in the periphery. When administered centrally, neurotensin exerts potent effects including hypothermia, antinociception, and modulation of dopamine neurotransmission. When administered into the peripheral circulation, it causes vasodilation, hypotension, increased vascular permeability, increased secretion of several anterior pituitary hormones, hyperglycemia, inhibition of gastric acid and pepsin secretion, and inhibition of gastric motility.

In the central nervous system, there are close associations between neurotensin and dopamine systems, and neurotensin may be involved in clinical disorders involving dopamine pathways such as schizophrenia, Parkinson's disease, and drug abuse. Consistent with this, it has been shown that central administration of neurotensin produces effects in rodents similar to those produced by antipsychotic drugs.

Three subtypes of neurotensin receptors, designated NT_1, NT_2, and NT_3, have been cloned. NT_1 and NT_2 receptors belong to the G protein-coupled superfamily with seven transmembrane domains; the NT_3 receptor is a single transmembrane domain protein that belongs to a family of sorting proteins.

Neurotensin agonists that cross the blood-brain barrier have been developed and may have potential as therapeutic agents for diseases such as schizophrenia and Parkinson's disease.

Neurotensin receptors can be blocked with the nonpeptide antagonists SR142948A and SR48692. SR142948A is a potent antagonist of the hypothermia and analgesia produced by centrally administered neurotensin. It also blocks the cardiovascular effects of systemic neurotensin.

■ CALCITONIN GENE– RELATED PEPTIDE

Calcitonin gene–related peptide (**CGRP**) is a member of the calcitonin family of peptides, which also includes calcitonin, adrenomedullin and amylin. CGRP consists of 37 amino acids and displays approximately 30% structural homology with salmon calcitonin.

Like calcitonin, CGRP is present in large quantities in the C cells of the thyroid gland. It is also distributed widely in the central and peripheral nervous systems, in the cardiovascular system, the gastrointestinal tract, and the urogenital system. CGRP is found with substance P (see above) in some of these regions and with acetylcholine in others.

When CGRP is injected into the central nervous system, it produces a variety of effects, including hypertension and suppression of feeding. When injected into the systemic circulation, the peptide causes hypotension and tachycardia. The hypotensive action of CGRP results from the potent vasodilator action of the peptide; indeed, CGRP is the most potent vasodilator yet discovered. It dilates multiple vascular beds, but the coronary circulation is particularly sensitive.

The actions of CGRP are mediated by two receptors named $CGRP_1$ and $CGRP_2$. Peptide and nonpeptide antagonists of these receptors have been developed. Of the nonpeptide antagonists now available, the best characterized is BIBN4096BS, which has a high affinity and specificity for the human CGRP receptor.

Evidence is accumulating that release of CGRP from trigeminal nerves plays a central role in the pathophysiology of migraine. The peptide is released during migraine attacks, and successful treatment of migraine with a selective serotonin agonist normalizes cranial CGRP levels. BIBN4096BS has recently been shown to be an effective, well-tolerated treatment for migraine.

■ ADRENOMEDULLIN

Adrenomedullin was first discovered in human adrenal medullary pheochromocytoma tissue. It is a 52-amino acid peptide with a six-amino acid ring and a C-terminal amidation sequence. Like CGRP, adrenomedullin is a member of the calcitonin family of peptides.

Adrenomedullin is widely distributed in the body. The highest concentrations are found in the adrenal glands, hypothalamus, and anterior pituitary, but high levels are also present in the kidneys, lungs, cardiovascular system, and gastrointestinal tract. Adrenomedullin in plasma apparently originates in the heart and vasculature.

In animals, adrenomedullin dilates resistance vessels in the kidney, brain, lung, hind limbs, and mesentery, resulting in a marked, long-lasting hypotension. The hypotension in turn causes reflex increases in heart rate and cardiac output. These responses also occur during intravenous infusion of the peptide in healthy human subjects. Adrenomedullin also acts on the kidneys to increase sodium excretion, and it exerts several endocrine effects including inhibition of aldosterone and insulin secretion. Finally, it acts on the central nervous system to increase sympathetic outflow.

The diverse actions of adrenomedullin are mediated both by CGRP receptors and by specific adrenomedullin receptors termed AM_1 and AM_2. The major second messenger for both receptors is cAMP.

Circulating adrenomedullin levels increase during intense exercise. They also increase in a number of pathologic states, including essential hypertension, cardiac and renal failure, and septic shock. The roles of adrenomedullin in these states remain to be defined, but it is currently thought that the peptide functions as a physiologic antagonist of the actions of vasoconstrictors including endothelin 1 and angiotensin II. By virtue of these actions, adrenomedullin may protect against cardiovascular overload and injury.

■ NEUROPEPTIDE Y

Neuropeptide Y is a member of the family that also includes peptide YY and pancreatic polypeptide. Each peptide consists of 36 amino acids.

Neuropeptide Y is one of the most abundant neuropeptides in both the central and peripheral nervous systems. In the sympathetic nervous system, neuropeptide Y is frequently localized in noradrenergic neurons and apparently functions both as a vasoconstrictor and as a cotransmitter with norepinephrine. Peptide YY and pancreatic polypeptide are both gut endocrine peptides.

Neuropeptide Y produces a variety of central nervous system effects, including increased feeding (it is one of the most potent orexigenic molecules in the brain), hypotension, hypothermia, and respiratory depression. Other effects include vasoconstriction of cerebral blood vessels, positive chronotropic and inotropic actions on the heart, and hypertension. The peptide is a potent renal vasoconstrictor and suppresses renin secretion, but can cause diuresis and natriuresis. Prejunctional neuronal actions include inhibition of transmitter release from sympathetic and parasympathetic nerves. Vascular actions include direct vasoconstriction, potentiation of the action of vasoconstrictors, and inhibition of the action of vasodilators.

These diverse effects are mediated by multiple receptors designated Y_1 through Y_6. All receptors except Y_3 have been cloned and shown to be G protein-coupled receptors linked to mobilization of Ca^{2+} and inhibition of adenylyl cyclase. Y_1 and Y_2 receptors are of major importance in the cardiovascular and other peripheral effects of the peptide. Y_4 receptors have a high affinity for pancreatic polypeptide and may be a receptor for the pancreatic peptide rather than for neuropeptide Y. Y_5 receptors are found mainly in the central nervous system and may be involved in the control of food intake. Y_6 receptors do not appear to contribute significantly to the physiologic effects of neuropeptide Y in humans.

Selective nonpeptide neuropeptide Y receptor antagonists are now available for research. The first nonpeptide Y_1 receptor antagonist, BIBP3226, is also the most thoroughly studied. It has a short half-life in vivo. In animal models, it blocks the vasoconstrictor and pressor responses to neuropeptide Y. Structurally related Y_1 antagonists include BIB03304, and H409/22, which has been tested in humans. SR120107A and SR120819A are orally active Y_1 antagonists and have a long duration of action. BIIE0246 is the first nonpeptide antagonist selective for the Y_2 receptor.

These antagonists have been useful in analyzing the role of neuropeptide Y in cardiovascular regulation. It now appears that the peptide is not important in the regulation of hemodynamics under normal resting conditions, but may be of increased importance in cardiovascular disorders including hypertension and heart failure. Other studies have implicated neuropeptide Y in feeding disorders, seizures, anxiety, and diabetes, and Y_1 and Y_5 receptor antagonists have potential as antiobesity agents.

■ UROTENSIN

Urotensin II was originally identified in fish, but isoforms are now known to be present in mammalian species including the human, mouse, rat and pig. Human urotensin II is an 11-amino acid peptide. Major sites of urotensin II expression in humans include the brain, spinal cord, and kidneys. Urotensin II is also present in plasma, and the kidneys may be a major source of this circulating peptide.

In vitro, urotensin II is a potent constrictor of vascular smooth muscle; its activity depends on the type of blood vessel and the species from which it was obtained. Vasoconstriction occurs primarily in arterial vessels, where urotensin II can be more potent than endothelin 1, making it the most potent known vasoconstrictor. However, under some conditions, urotensin II may cause vasodilation. In vivo, urotensin II has complex hemodynamic effects, the most prominent being regional vasoconstriction and cardiac depression. In some ways, these effects resemble those produced by endothelin 1. Nevertheless, the extent to which the peptide is involved in the regulation of vascular tone and blood pressure in humans is not clear; recent studies have produced conflicting results.

The actions of urotensin II are mediated by a G protein-coupled receptor referred to as the UT receptor. UT receptors are widely distributed in the brain, spinal cord, heart, vascular smooth muscle, skeletal muscle, and pancreas. Some effects of the peptide including vasoconstriction are mediated by the phospholipase C, IP_3-DAG signal transduction pathway.

Modifications of the disulfide bridge of urotensin II have yielded UT-receptor antagonists. A nonpeptide antagonist, palosuran, has also been developed.

Evidence is accumulating that urotensin II is involved in cardiovascular and other diseases. In particular, it has been reported that plasma urotensin II levels are increased in hypertension, heart failure, diabetes mellitus, and renal failure. UT-receptor antagonists will be valuable in studies of the pathophysiologic role of this peptide.

PREPARATIONS AVAILABLE[1]

Aprepitant (Emend)
   Oral: 80, 125 mg capsules
Bosentan (Tracleer)
   Oral: 62.5, 125 mg tablets

[1]Preparations of angiotensin-converting enzyme inhibitors and angiotensin receptor antagonists are found in Chapter 11; preparations of vasopressin are found in Chapter 37.

REFERENCES

Angiotensin

Batenburg WW et al: Angiotensin II type 2 receptor-mediated vasodilation. Focus on bradykinin, NO and endothelium-derived hyperpolarizing factor(s). Vascul Pharmacol 2005;42:109.

Danser AH, Deinum J: Renin, prorenin and the putative (pro)renin receptor. Hypertension 2005;46:1069.

Dinh DT et al: Angiotensin receptors: Distribution, signalling and function. Clin Sci 2001;100:481.

Fleming I, Kohlstedt K, Busse R: New fACEs to the renin-angiotensin system. Physiology (Bethesda) 2005;20:91.

Gradman AH et al: Aliskiren, a novel orally effective renin inhibitor, provides dose-dependent antihypertensive efficacy and placebo-like tolerability in hypertensive patients. Circulation 2005;111:1012.

Kelly DJ, Wilkinson-Berka JL, Gilbert RE: Renin inhibition: New potential for an old therapeutic target. Hypertension 2005; 46:471.

McMurray JJ et al: Which inhibitor of the renin-angiotensin system should be used in chronic heart failure and acute myocardial infarction? Circulation 2004;110:3281.

Sica DA: Combination angiotensin-converting enzyme inhibitor and angiotensin receptor blocker therapy: Its role in clinical practice. J Clin Hypertens (Greenwich) 2003;5:414.

Watanabe T, Barker TA, Berk BC: Angiotensin II and the endothelium: Diverse signals and effects. Hypertension 2005;45:163.

Yan AT, Yan RT, Liu PP: Narrative review: Pharmacotherapy for chronic heart failure: Evidence from recent clinical trials. Ann Intern Med 2005;142:132.

Kinins

Couture R et al: Kinin receptors in pain and inflammation. Eur J Pharmacol 2001;429:161.

Ferreira J et al: The use of kinin B1 and B2 receptor knockout mice and selective antagonists to characterize the nociceptive responses caused by kinins at the spinal level. Neuropharmacology 2002;43:1188.

Leeb-Lundberg LM et al: International union of pharmacology. XLV. Classification of the kinin receptor family: From molecular mechanisms to pathophysiological consequences. Pharmacol Rev 2005;57:27.

Vasopressin

Goldsmith SR, Gheorghiade M: Vasopressin antagonism in heart failure. J Am Coll Cardiol 2005;46:1785.

Thibonnier M et al: The basic and clinical pharmacology of nonpeptide vasopressin receptor antagonists. Annu Rev Pharmacol Toxicol 2001;41:175.

Natriuretic Peptides

Boomsma F, van den Meiracker AH: Plasma A- and B-type natriuretic peptides: Physiology, methodology and clinical use. Cardiovasc Res 2001;51:442.

Munagala VK, Burnett JC, Jr, Redfield MM: The natriuretic peptides in cardiovascular medicine. Curr Probl Cardiol 2004; 29:707.

Vasopeptidase Inhibitors

Campbell DJ: Vasopeptidase inhibition: A double-edged sword? Hypertension 2003;41:383.

Packer M et al: Comparison of omapatrilat and enalapril in patients with chronic heart failure: The Omapatrilat Versus Enalapril Randomized Trial of Utility in Reducing Events (OVERTURE). Circulation 2002;106:920.

Worthley MI, Corti R, Worthley SG: Vasopeptidase inhibitors: Will they have a role in clinical practice? Br J Clin Pharmacol 2004;57:27.

Endothelins

Channick RN et al: Endothelin receptor antagonists in pulmonary arterial hypertension. J Am Coll Cardiol 2004; 43:62S.

Ertl G, Bauersachs J: Endothelin receptor antagonists in heart failure: Current status and future directions. Drugs 2004; 64:1029.

Galie N, Manes A, Branzi A: The endothelin system in pulmonary arterial hypertension. Cardiovasc Res 2004;61:227.

Vasoactive Intestinal Peptide

Henning RJ, Sawmiller DR: Vasoactive intestinal peptide: Cardiovascular effects. Cardiovasc Res 2001;49:27.

Substance P

Aprepitant (emend) for prevention of nausea and vomiting due to cancer chemotherapy. Med Lett Drug Ther 2003;45:620.

Hokfelt T, Pernow B, Wahren J: Substance P: A pioneer amongst neuropeptides. J Intern Med 2001;249:27.

Neurotensin

Kinkead B, Nemeroff CB: Neurotensin, schizophrenia, and antipsychotic drug action. Int Rev Neurobiol 2004;59:327.

Calcitonin Gene–Related Peptide

Olesen J et al: Calcitonin gene-related peptide receptor antagonist BIBN 4096 BS for the acute treatment of migraine. N Engl J Med 2004;350:1104.

Poyner DR et al: International Union of Pharmacology. XXXII. The mammalian calcitonin gene-related peptides, adrenomedullin, amylin, and calcitonin receptors. Pharmacol Rev 2002;54:233.

Adrenomedullin

Hamid SA, Baxter GF: Adrenomedullin: Regulator of systemic and cardiac homeostasis in acute myocardial infarction. Pharmacol Ther 2005;105:95.

Smith DM et al: Adrenomedullin: Receptor and signal transduction. Biochem Soc Trans 2002;30:432.

Neuropeptide Y

DiBona GF: Neuropeptide Y. Am J Physiol 2002;282:R635.

Malmstrom RE: Pharmacology of neuropeptide Y receptor antagonists: Focus on cardiovascular functions. Eur J Pharmacol 2002;447:11.

Urotensin

Douglas SA, Dhanak D, Johns DG: From 'gills to pills': Urotensin-II as a regulator of mammalian cardiorenal function. Trends Pharmacol Sci 2004;25:76.

Ong KL, Lam KS, Cheung BM: Urotensin II: Its function in health and its role in disease. Cardiovasc Drugs Ther 2005;19:65.

The Eicosanoids: Prostaglandins, Thromboxanes, Leukotrienes, & Related Compounds

18

Emer M Smyth, PhD, & Garret A FitzGerald, MD*

The eicosanoids are oxygenation products of polyunsaturated long-chain fatty acids. They are ubiquitous in the animal kingdom and are also found—together with their precursors—in a variety of plants. They constitute a very large family of compounds that are highly potent and display an extraordinarily wide spectrum of biologic activity. Because of their biologic activity, the eicosanoids, their specific receptor antagonists and enzyme inhibitors, and their plant and fish oil precursors have great therapeutic potential. Their short half-lives, which are seconds to minutes, make special delivery systems or synthesis of stable analogs mandatory for their clinical use.

ARACHIDONIC ACID & OTHER POLYUNSATURATED PRECURSORS

Arachidonic acid, the most abundant and important of the eicosanoid precursors, is a 20-carbon (C20) fatty acid that contains four double bonds beginning at the omega-6 position to yield a 5,8,11,14-eicosatetraenoic acid (designated C20:4–6). For eicosanoid synthesis to occur, arachidonate must first be released or mobilized from membrane phospholipids by one or more lipases of the phospholipase A_2 (PLA_2) type (Figure 18–1). At least three phospholipases mediate arachidonate release from membrane lipids: cytosolic (c) PLA_2, secretory (s) PLA_2, and calcium-independent (i) PLA_2. In addition, arachidonate is also released by a combination of phospholipase C and diglyceride lipase.

Following mobilization, arachidonic acid is oxygenated by four separate routes: the cyclooxygenase (COX), lipoxygenase, P450 epoxygenase, and isoprostane pathways (Figure 18–1). A number of factors determine the type of eicosanoid synthesized: (1) the species, (2) the type of cell, and (3) the cell's particular phenotype. The pattern of eicosanoids synthesized also frequently reflects (4) the manner in which the cell is stimulated. Finally, an important factor governing the pattern of eicosanoid release is (5) the nature of the precursor polyunsaturated fatty acid that has been esterified in specific membrane phospholipids. For example, homo-γ-linoleic acid (C20:3–6), which is trienoic, yields products that differ from those derived from arachidonate (C20:4–6), which has four double bonds. Similarly, the products derived from eicosapentaenoic acid (C20:5–3), which has five double bonds, are also quantitatively different. This is the basis for using as nutritional supplements in humans the structurally different fatty acids obtained from cold water fish or from plants. An example of the significance of the polyunsaturated fatty acid precursors is evident when one considers thromboxane A (TXA) derived from the COX pathway. TXA_2 is synthesized from arachidonate, a tetraenoic acid, and is a powerful vaso-

*The authors acknowledge the contributions of the previous authors of this chapter, Drs. Marie L. Foegh and Peter W. Ramwell.

Figure 18–1. Pathways of arachidonic acid (AA) release and metabolism.

constrictor and aggregator of platelets. However 5,8,11,14,17-eicosapentaenoic acid yields TXA$_3$, which is relatively inactive. In theory, dietary eicosapentaenoate substitution for arachidonate should minimize thrombotic events due to the displacement of tetraenoic arachidonate in the membrane by a pentaenoic acid.

SYNTHESIS OF EICOSANOIDS

Products of Prostaglandin Endoperoxide Synthases (Cyclooxygenases)

Two unique COX isozymes convert arachidonic acid into prostaglandin endoperoxide. PGH synthase-1 (**COX-1**) is expressed constitutively in most cells. In contrast, PGH synthase-2 (**COX-2**) is inducible; its expression varies markedly depending on the stimulus. COX-2 is an immediate early-response gene product that is markedly up-regulated by shear stress, growth factors, tumor promoters, and cytokines. COX-1 generates prostanoids for "housekeeping" such as gastric epithelial cytoprotection, whereas COX-2 is the major source of prostanoids in inflammation and cancer. This distinction is overly simplistic, however; there are both physiologic and pathophysiologic processes in which each enzyme is uniquely involved and others in which they function coordinately. For example, endothelial COX-2 is the primary source of vascular pros-

tacyclin, whereas renal COX-2-derived prostanoids are important for normal renal development and maintenance of function. An additional COX-1 variant termed "COX-3" has been described in dogs, but it does not appear functionally relevant in other species.

The synthases are important because it is at this step that the nonsteroidal anti-inflammatory drugs (NSAIDs) exert their therapeutic effects (see Chapter 36). Indomethacin and sulindac are slightly selective for COX-1. Meclofenamate and ibuprofen are approximately equipotent on COX-1 and COX-2, whereas celecoxib, diclofenac, rofecoxib, lumiracoxib, and etoricoxib inhibit COX-2 with increasing selectivity. Aspirin acetylates and inhibits both enzymes covalently. Low doses (< 100 mg/day) inhibit preferentially, but not exclusively, COX-1, whereas higher doses inhibit both COX-1 and COX-2.

Both COX-1 and COX-2 promote the uptake of two molecules of oxygen by cyclization of arachidonic acid to yield a C_9–C_{11} endoperoxide C_{15} hydroperoxide (Figure 18–2). This product is PGG$_2$, which is then rapidly modified by the peroxidase moiety of the COX enzyme to add a 15-hydroxyl group that is essential for biologic activity. This product is PGH$_2$. Both endoperoxides are highly unstable. Analogous families—PGH$_1$ and PGH$_3$ and all their subsequent products—are derived from homo-γ-linolenic acid and eicosapentaenoic acid, respectively.

Figure 18–2. Prostanoid biosynthesis. Compound names are enclosed in boxes

The prostaglandins, thromboxane, and prostacy-clin, collectively termed the prostanoids, are generated from PGH_2 through the action of isomerases and synthases. These terminal enzymes are expressed in a relatively cell-specific fashion, such that most cells make one or two dominant prostanoids. The prostaglandins differ from each other in two ways: (1) in the substituents of the pentane ring (indicated by the last letter, eg, E and F in PGE and PGF) and (2) in the number of double bonds in the side chains (indicated by the subscript, eg, PGE_1, PGE_2). Several products of the arachidonate series are of current clinical importance. **Alprostadil** (PGE_1) may be used for its smooth muscle relaxing effects to maintain the ductus arterosus patent in some neonates awaiting cardiac surgery and in the treatment of impotence. **Misoprostol,** a PGE_1 derivative, is a cytoprotective prosta-glandin used in preventing peptic ulcer and in combi-nation with mifepristone (RU486) for terminating early pregnancies. **PGE_2** and **$PGF_{2\alpha}$** are used in obstetrics to induce labor. **Latanoprost** and several similar compounds are topically active $PGF_{2\alpha}$ deriva-tives used in ophthalmology to treat open angle glau-coma. **Prostacyclin** (PGI_2, epoprostenol) is synthe-sized mainly by the vascular endothelium and is a powerful vasodilator and inhibitor of platelet aggrega-tion. It is used clinically to treat pulmonary hyperten-sion and portopulmonary hypertension. In contrast, **thromboxane** **(TXA_2)** has undesirable properties (aggregation of platelets, vasoconstriction). Therefore TXA_2-receptor antagonists and synthesis inhibitors have been developed for cardiovascular indications, although these (except for aspirin) have yet to estab-lish a place in clinical usage.

All the naturally occurring COX products undergo rapid metabolism either initially by hydration to inactive products, which are then metabolized (PGI$_2$, TXA$_2$), or by oxidation of the key 15-hydroxyl group to the corresponding ketone by prostaglandin 15-OH dehydrogenase. Further metabolism is by Δ^{13} reduction, β-oxidation, and ω-oxidation. The inactive metabolites can be determined in blood and urine by immunoassay or mass spectrometry as a measure of the in vivo synthesis of their parent compounds.

Products of Lipoxygenase

The metabolism of arachidonic acid by the **5-, 12-, and 15-lipoxygenases (LOX)** results in the production of hydroperoxyeicosatetraenoic acids (HPETEs), which rapidly convert to hydroxy derivatives (HETEs) and leukotrienes (Figure 18–3). The most actively investigated leukotrienes are those produced by the 5-lipoxygenase present in inflammatory cells (polymorphonuclear leukocytes [PMNs], basophils, mast cells, eosinophils, macrophages). This pathway is of great interest since it is associated with asthma, anaphylactic shock, and cardiovascular disease. Stimulation of these cells elevates intracellular Ca^{2+} and releases arachidonate; incorporation of moleular oxygen by 5-LOX, in association with **5-LOX-activating protein (FLAP)**, then yields the unstable epoxide leukotriene A$_4$ (LTA$_4$). This intermediate either converts to the dihydroxy leukotriene B$_4$ (LTB$_4$) or conjugates with glutathione to yield leukotri-

Figure 18–3. Leukotriene (LT) biosynthesis. LTC$_4$, LTD$_4$ and LTE$_4$ are known collectively as the Cysteinyl (Cys) LTs. GT, glutamyl transpeptidase; GL, glutamyl leukotrienase.

ene C_4 (LTC_4), which undergoes sequential degradation of the glutathione moiety by peptidases to yield LTD_4 and LTE_4. These three products are called cysteinyl leukotrienes or peptidoleukotrienes.

LTC_4 and **LTD_4** are potent bronchoconstrictors and are recognized as the primary components of the **slow-reacting substance of anaphylaxis (SRS-A)** that is secreted in asthma and anaphylaxis. There are four current approaches to anti-leukotriene drug development: 5-lipoxygenase enzyme inhibitors, leukotriene-receptor antagonists, inhibitors of FLAP, and phospholipase A_2 inhibitors. Selective leukotriene-receptor antagonists (zafirlukast, montelukast, and pranlukast) are currently used or in trials for treatment of asthma.

LTA_4, the primary product of 5-LOX, can be converted via 12-LOX in platelets to the **lipoxins** LXA_4 and LXB_4. These mediators can also arise through 5-LOX metabolism of 15-HETE, the product of 15-LOX-2 metabolism of arachidonic acid. 15-LOX-1 prefers linoleic acid as a substrate forming 15S-hydroxyoctadecadienoic acid. The stereochemical isomer, 15R-HETE, may be derived from the action of aspirin-acetylated COX-2 and further transformed in leukocytes by 5-LOX to 15-epi-LXA_4 or 15-epi-LXB_4, the so-called aspirin-triggered lipoxins. 12-HETE can also undergo a catalyzed molecular rearrangement to epoxy-hydroxyeicosatrienoic acids called **hepoxilins.** The biologic roles of these mediators remain ill-defined.

The LOX located in epidermal cells are distinct from "conventional" enzymes—arachidonic acid and linoleic acid are apparently not the natural substrates for epidermal LOX. Epidermal accumulation of 12R-HETE is a feature of psoriasis and ichthyosis and inhibitors of 12R-LOX are under investigation for the treatment of these proliferative skin disorders.

Epoxygenase Products

Specific isozymes of microsomal cytochrome P450 monooxygenases convert arachidonic acid to four epoxyeicosatrienoic acids (EETs) (Figure 18–1). These are the 5,6-, 6,9-, 11,12-, and 14,15-oxido products. Each EET has two stereoisomers (R and S). Their biosynthesis can be altered by pharmacologic, nutritional, and genetic factors that affect P450 expression. These epoxides are unstable and rapidly form the corresponding dihydroxyeicosatrienoic (DHET) acid, eg, 5,6-DHET. Unlike the prostaglandins, both the EETs and the DHETs can be incorporated into phospholipids, which then act as storage sites. Intracellular fatty acid-binding proteins may differentially bind EETs and DHETs, thus modulating their metabolism, activities, and targeting. The epoxygenase products are synthesized in endothelial cells, and cause vasodilation in a number of vascular beds by activating the smooth muscle large conductance Ca^{2+}-activated K^+ channels. This results in smooth muscle cell hyperpolarization and vasodilation, leading to reduced blood pressure. Substantial evidence indicates that EETs may function as endothelium-derived hyperpolarizing factors, particularly in the coronary circulation.

Isoprostanes

The generation of isoprostanes from arachidonic acid is another potentially important pathway. The isoprostanes are prostaglandin stereoisomers. Because prostaglandins have many asymmetric centers, they have a large number of potential stereoisomers. COX is not needed for the formation of the isoprostanes, and its inhibition with aspirin or other NSAIDs should not affect the isoprostane pathway. The primary epimerization mechanism is peroxidation of arachidonate by free radicals. Peroxidation occurs while arachidonic acid is still esterified to the membrane phospholipids. Thus, unlike prostaglandins, these stereoisomers are "stored" as part of the membrane. They are then cleaved, presumably by phospholipases, circulate, and are excreted in urine. Isoprostanes are present in relatively large amounts (ten-fold greater in blood and urine than the COX-derived prostaglandins). They have potent vasoconstrictor effects when infused into renal and other vascular beds and may activate prostanoid receptors. It has been speculated that they may contribute to the pathophysiology of inflammatory responses in a manner insensitive to COX inhibitors.

■ I. BASIC PHARMACOLOGY OF EICOSANOIDS

MECHANISMS & EFFECTS OF EICOSANOIDS

Receptor Mechanisms

As a result of their short half-lives, the eicosanoids act in an autocrine and paracrine fashion, ie, close to the site of their synthesis. These ligands bind to receptors on the cell surface, and pharmacologic specificity is determined by receptor density and type on different cells. A single gene product has been identified for the PGI_2 receptor (IP receptor), $PGF_{2\alpha}$ (FP), and TXA_2 (TP), while four distinct PGE_2 receptors (EPs 1-4) and two PGD_2 receptors (DP_1 and DP_2) have been cloned. Additional isoforms of the TP (α and β), FP (A and B), and EP_3 (A-D) receptors can arise through differential mRNA splicing. Two receptors exist for both LTB_4

Table 18–1. Eicosanoid receptors.

Receptor	Endogenous Ligand	Secondary Ligands	G protein, Second Messenger	Major Phenotype(s) in Knockout Mice
DP_1	PGD_2		G_s, ↑cAMP	↓Allergic asthma
DP_2,CRTH2	PGD_2	$15d\text{-}PGJ_2$	G_i, ↑Ca^{2+}_i	↑Allergic airway inflammation
EP_1	PGE_2	PGI_2	G_q, ↑Ca^{2+}_i	↓Colon carcinogenesis
EP_2	PGE_2		G_s, ↑cAMP	Impaired ovulation and fertilization Salt-sensitive hypertension
$EP_{3A–D}$	PGE_2		G_i, ↓cAMP G_s, ↑cAMP G_q, ↑PLC	Resistance to pyrogens ↓Acute cutaneous inflammation
EP_4	PGE_2		G_s ↑cAMP	Patent ductus arteriosus ↓Bone mass/density in aged mice ↑Bowel inflammatory/immune response ↓Colon carcinogenesis
$FP_{A,B}$	$PGF_{2\alpha}$	isoPs	G_q, ↑PLC	Parturition failure
IP	PGI_2	PGE_2	G_s, ↑cAMP	↑Thrombotic response ↑Response to vascular injury ↑Atherosclerosis ↑Cardiac fibrosis Salt-sensitive hypertension ↓Joint inflammation
$TP_{\alpha,\beta}$	TXA_2	isoPs	G_q, G_i, $G_{12/13}$, G_{16}, ↑PLC	↑Bleeding time ↓Response to vascular injury ↓Atherosclerosis ↑Survival after cardiac allograft
BLT_1	LTB_4		G_{16}, G_i	Some suppression of inflammatory response
BLT_2	LTB_4	12S-HETE 12R-HETE	G_q-like, G_i-like, G_z-like	?
$CysLT_1$	LTD_4	LTC_4/LTE_4	G_q, ↑PLC	↓Innate and adaptive immune vascular permeability response ↑Pulmonary inflammatory and fibrotic response
$CysLT_2$	LTC_4/LTD_4	LTE_4	G_q, ↑PLC	↓Pulmonary inflammatory and fibrotic response

Splice variants for the eicosanoid receptors are indicated where appropriate.
Ca^{2+}_i, intracellular calcium; cAMP, adenosine 3',5'-monophosphate; PLC, phospholipase C; isoPs, isoprostanes; $15d\text{-}PGJ_2$, 15-deoxy-$\Delta^{12,14}$-PGJ_2.

(BLT$_1$ and BLT$_2$) and the cysteinyl-leukotrienes (cysLT$_1$ and cysLT$_2$). A single lipoxin receptor termed ALX was found to be the same as the formyl peptide (fMPL)-1 receptor. All of these receptors are G protein-coupled; properties of the best-studied receptors are listed in Table 18–1.

EP$_2$, EP$_4$, IP and DP$_1$ receptors activate adenylyl cyclase via G$_s$. This leads to increased intracellular cAMP levels, which in turn activates specific protein kinases (see Chapter 2). These kinases phosphorylate internal calcium pump proteins, an action that decreases free intracellular calcium concentration. In contrast, EP$_1$, FP, and TP receptors activate phosphatidylinositol metabolism, leading to the formation of InsP$_3$ (IP$_3$), with subsequent mobilization of Ca^{2+} stores and an increase of free intracellular calcium. Activation of the TP-receptor isoforms may activate or inhibit adenylyl cyclase via G$_s$ (TP$_\alpha$) or G$_i$ (TP$_\beta$), respectively, and signal via G$_q$ and related proteins to membrane associated protein (MAP) kinase signaling pathways. EP_3 receptors can couple to both elevation of intracellular calcium and a decrease in cAMP. The DP_2 receptor, which is unrelated to the other prostanoid receptors, is a member of the fMLP receptor superfamily. This receptor couples through to a G_i-type G protein and leads to inhibition of cAMP synthesis and increases in intracellular calcium in a variety of cell types.

LTB_4 also generates $InsP_3$ release via the BLT_1 receptor, causing activation, degranulation, and superoxide anion generation in PMNs. The BLT_2 receptor, the low-affinity receptor for LTB_4, is bound with reasonable affinity by 12S- and 12R-HETE, although the biologic relevance of this observation is not clear. $CysLT_1$ receptors couple to G_q, leading to increased intracellular Ca^{2+}.

The contractile effects of eicosanoids on smooth muscle are mediated by the release of calcium, while their relaxing effects are mediated by the generation of cAMP. The effects of eicosanoids on many target systems, including the immune system, can be similarly explained (see below). Many of the eicosanoids' contractile effects on smooth muscle can be inhibited by lowering extracellular calcium or by using calcium channel blocking drugs.

Although prostanoids can activate peroxisome proliferator-activated receptors (PPARs) if added in sufficient concentration in vitro, it is questionable whether these compounds attain concentrations sufficient to function as endogenous nuclear-receptor ligands in vivo.

Effects of Prostaglandins & Thromboxanes

The prostaglandins and thromboxanes have major effects on four types of smooth muscle: vascular, gastrointestinal, airway, and reproductive. Other important targets include platelets and monocytes, kidneys, the central nervous system, autonomic presynaptic nerve terminals, sensory nerve endings, endocrine organs, adipose tissue, and the eye (the effects on the eye may involve smooth muscle).

A. SMOOTH MUSCLE

1. Vascular—TXA_2 is a potent vasoconstrictor. It is also a smooth muscle cell mitogen and is the only eicosanoid that has convincingly been shown to have this effect. The mitogenic effect is potentiated by exposure of smooth muscle cells to testosterone, which up-regulates smooth muscle cell TP receptors. $PGF_{2\alpha}$ is also a vasoconstrictor but is not a mitogen for smooth muscle cells. Another vasoconstrictor is the isoprostane 8-iso-$PGF_{2\alpha}$, also known as $iPF_{2\alpha}$III, which may act via the TP receptor. In patients with cirrhosis, it is produced in large amounts in the liver and is thought to play a pathophysiologic role as an

important vasoconstrictor substance in the hepatorenal syndrome.

Vasodilator prostaglandins, especially PGI_2 and PGE_2, promote vasodilation by increasing cAMP and decreasing smooth muscle intracellular calcium, primarily via IP and EP_4 receptors. Vascular prostacyclin is synthesized by both smooth muscle and endothelial cells, with the latter being the major contributor. In the microcirculation, PGE_2 is a vasodilator produced by endothelial cells.

2. Gastrointestinal tract—Most of the prostaglandins and thromboxanes activate gastrointestinal smooth muscle. Longitudinal muscle is contracted by PGE_2 (via EP_3) and $PGF_{2\alpha}$ (via FP receptors), whereas circular muscle is contracted strongly by $PGF_{2\alpha}$ and weakly by PGI_2, and relaxed by PGE_2 (via EP_4 receptors). Administration of either PGE_2 or $PGF_{2\alpha}$ results in colicky cramps (see Clinical Pharmacology of Eicosanoids, below). The leukotrienes also have powerful contractile effects.

3. Airways—Respiratory smooth muscle is relaxed by PGE_2 and PGI_2 and contracted by PGD_2, TXA_2, and $PGF_{2\alpha}$. Studies of DP_1 knockout mice suggest an important role of this receptor in asthma. The cysteinyl leukotrienes are bronchoconstrictors. They act principally on smooth muscle in peripheral airways and are a thousand times more potent than histamine both in vitro and in vivo. They also stimulate bronchial mucus secretion and cause mucosal edema. Bronchospasm occurs in about 10% of people taking NSAIDs, probably because of a shift in arachidonate metabolism from COX-1 metabolism to leukotriene formation.

4. Reproductive—The actions of prostaglandins on reproductive smooth muscle are discussed below under D. Reproductive Organs.

B. PLATELETS

Platelet aggregation is markedly affected by eicosanoids. Low concentrations of PGE_2 enhance, whereas higher concentrations inhibit, platelet aggregation. Both PGD_2 and PGI_2 inhibit aggregation. TXA_2 is the major product of platelet COX-1, is a platelet aggregator, and amplifies the effects of other more potent platelet agonists such as thrombin. The platelet actions of TXA_2 are restrained in vivo by PGI_2, which inhibits platelet aggregation by all recognized agonists. Platelets release TXA_2 during activation and aggregation. Urinary metabolites of TXA_2 increase in patients experiencing a myocardial infarction; this increment is suppressed substantially by low-dosage aspirin, but a variable contribution, presumably from macrophage COX-2, may be insensitive to such a regimen. Comparative trials of the cardioprotective actions of low- and high-dose aspirin have not been performed. However, indirect comparisons across placebo controlled trials do not suggest an increasing benefit with dose; in fact, they suggest an inverse dose-response relationship, perhaps reflecting increasing inhibition of PGI_2 synthesis at higher doses of aspirin. Platelet COX-1-derived thromboxane synthesis is irreversibly inhibited by chronic dosing with aspirin in low doses. Macrophage COX-2 appears to contribute roughly 10% of the increment in TX biosynthesis observed in smokers, while the rest is derived from platelets.

C. KIDNEY

Both the medulla and the cortex of the kidney synthesize prostaglandins, the medulla substantially more than the cortex. The kidney also synthesizes several hydroxyeicosatetraenoic acids, leukotrienes, cytochrome P450 products, and epoxides. These compounds play important autoregulatory roles in renal function by modifying renal hemodynamics and glomerular and tubular function. This regulatory role is especially important in marginally functioning kidneys, as shown by the decline in kidney function caused by COX inhibitors in elderly patients and those with renal disease.

The major eicosanoid products of the renal cortex are PGE_2 and PGI_2. Both compounds increase renin release; normally, however, renin release is more directly under β_1-adrenoceptor control.

PGE_2 and PGI_2 increase glomerular filtration through their vasodilating effects. These prostaglandins also increase water and sodium excretion. The increase in water clearance probably results from an attenuation of the action of antidiuretic hormone (ADH) on adenylyl cyclase. It is uncertain whether the natriuretic effect is caused by the direct inhibition of sodium reabsorption in the distal tubule or by increased medullary blood flow. Loop diuretics, eg, furosemide, produce some of their effect by stimulating COX activity. In the normal kidney, this increases the synthesis of the vasodilator prostaglandins. Therefore, patient response to a loop diuretic is diminished if a COX inhibitor is administered concurrently (see Chapter 15).

TXA_2 causes intrarenal vasoconstriction (and perhaps an ADH-like effect), resulting in a decline in renal function. The normal kidney synthesizes only small amounts of TXA_2. However, in renal conditions involving inflammatory cell infiltration (such as glomerulonephritis and renal transplant rejection), the inflammatory cells (monocyte-macrophages) release substantial amounts of TXA_2. Theoretically, TXA_2 synthase inhibitors or receptor antagonists should improve renal function in these patients, but no such drug is clinically available.

Hypertension is associated with increased TXA_2 and decreased PGE_2 and PGI_2 synthesis in some animal models, eg, the Goldblatt kidney model. It is not known whether these changes are primary contributing factors or secondary responses. Similarly, increased TXA_2 formation has been reported in cyclosporine-induced nephrotoxicity, but no causal relationship has been established.

D. REPRODUCTIVE ORGANS

1. Female reproductive organs—Uterine muscle is contracted by $PGF_{2\alpha}$, TXA_2, and low concentrations of PGE_2; PGI_2 and high concentrations of PGE_2 cause relaxation. $PGF_{2\alpha}$, together with oxytocin, is essential for the onset of parturition. The effects of prostaglandins on uterine function are discussed below. (See Clinical Pharmacology of Eicosanoids.)

2. Male reproductive organs—The role of prostaglandins in semen is still conjectural. The major source of these prostaglandins is the seminal vesicle; the prostate—despite the name "prostaglandin"—and the testes synthesize only small amounts. The factors that regulate the concentration of prostaglandins in human seminal plasma are not known in detail, but testosterone does promote prostaglandin production. Thromboxane and leukotrienes have not been found in seminal plasma. Men with a low seminal fluid concentration of prostaglandins are relatively infertile.

Smooth muscle–relaxing prostaglandins such as PGE_1 enhance penile erection by relaxing the smooth muscle of the corpora cavernosa. (See Clinical Pharmacology of the Eicosanoids.)

E. CENTRAL AND PERIPHERAL NERVOUS SYSTEMS

1. Fever—PGE_2 increases body temperature, probably via EP_3 receptors, especially when administered directly into the cerebral ventricles. Exogenous $PGF_{2\alpha}$ and PGI_2 induce fever, whereas PGD_2 and TXA_2 do not, but none of these contributes to the natural pyretic response. Instead, pyrogens release interleukin-1, which in turn promotes the synthesis and release of PGE_2. This synthesis is blocked by aspirin and other antipyretic compounds.

2. Sleep—When infused into the cerebral ventricles, PGD_2 induces natural sleep (as determined by electro-encephalographic analysis) via activation of DP_1 receptors and secondary release of adenosine.

3. Neurotransmission—PGE compounds inhibit the release of norepinephrine from postganglionic sympathetic nerve endings. Moreover, NSAIDs increase norepinephrine release in vivo, suggesting that the prostaglandins play a physiologic role in this process. Thus, vasoconstriction observed during treatment with COX inhibitors may be due, in part, to increased release of norepinephrine as well as to inhibition of the endothelial synthesis of the vasodilators PGE_2 and PGI_2. PGE_2 and PGI_2 sensitize the peripheral nerve endings to painful stimuli by lowering the threshold of nociceptors. Centrally, PGE_2 can increase excitability in neuronal pain transmission pathways in the spinal cord. Hyperalgesia is also produced by LTB_4. The release of these eicosanoids during the inflammatory process thus serves to amplify nociception.

F. Neuroendocrine Organs

Both in vitro and in vivo tests have shown that some of the eicosanoids affect the secretion of anterior pituitary hormones. PGE_2 promotes the release of growth hormone, prolactin, TSH, ACTH, FSH, and LH. However, endocrine changes reflecting significant release of these hormones have not been reported in patients receiving PGE compounds. In parturition $PGF_{2\alpha}$ induces an oxytocin-dependent decline in progesterone levels. LOX metabolites also have endocrine effects. LTC_4 and LTD_4 stimulate LHRH and LH secretion (see below). 12-HETE stimulates the release of aldosterone from the adrenal cortex and mediates a portion of the aldosterone release stimulated by angiotensin II but not that by ACTH.

G. Bone Metabolism

Prostaglandins are abundant in skeletal tissue and are produced by osteoblasts and adjacent hematopoietic cells. The major effect of prostaglandins (especially PGE_2, acting on EP_4 receptors) in vivo is to increase bone turnover, ie, stimulation of bone resorption and formation. Deletion of the EP_4 receptors in mice results in an imbalance between bone resorption and formation, leading to a negative balance of bone mass and density in older animals. Prostaglandins may mediate the effects of mechanical forces on bones and changes in bone during inflammation. EP_4-receptor deletion and inhibition of prostaglandin biosynthesis have both been associated with impaired fracture healing in animal models. COX inhibitors can also slow skeletal muscle healing by interfering with prostaglandin effects on myocyte proliferation, differentiation, and fibrosis in response to injury. Prostaglandins may contribute to the bone loss that occurs at menopause; it has been speculated that NSAIDs may be of therapeutic value in osteoporosis and bone loss prevention in older women. However, controlled evaluation of such therapeutic interventions remains to be carried out.

H. Eye

PGE and PGF derivatives lower intraocular pressure. The mechanism of this action is unclear but probably involves increased outflow of aqueous humor from the anterior chamber via the uveoscleral pathway (see Clinical Applications).

Effects of Lipoxygenase & Cytochrome P450-Derived Metabolites

The actions of lipoxygenases generate compounds that can regulate specific cellular responses important in inflammation and immunity. Cytochrome P450-derived metabolites affect nephron transport functions either directly or via metabolism to active compounds (see below). The biologic functions of the various forms of hydroxy- and hydroperoxyeicosaenoic acids are largely unknown, but their pharmacologic potency is impressive.

A. Blood Cells and Inflammation

LTB_4 is a potent chemoattractant for PMNs, eosinophils, and monocytes; LTC_4 and LTD_4 are potent chemoattractants for eosinophils. At higher concentrations, these leukotrienes also promote eosinophil adherence, degranulation, and oxygen radical formation.

The leukotrienes have been strongly implicated in the pathogenesis of inflammation, especially in chronic diseases such as asthma and inflammatory bowel disease. Prostaglandins, on the other hand, generally inhibit lymphocyte function and proliferation, suppressing the immunological response. PGE_2 inhibits the differentiation of B lymphocytes into antibody-secreting plasma cells and depress the humoral antibody response. It also inhibits mitogen-stimulated proliferation of T lymphocytes and the release of lymphokines by sensitized T lymphocytes. PGE_2 and TXA_2 may also play a role in T-lymphocyte development by regulating apoptosis of immature thymocytes. PGD_2, a major product of mast cells, is a potent chemoattractant for eosinophils and induces chemotaxis and migration of $TH2$ lymphocytes. Its degradation product, 15d-PGJ_2, at concentrations actually formed in vivo, may also activate eosinophils via the DP_2 ($CRTH2$) receptor.

Lipoxins have diverse effects on leukocytes, including activation of monocytes and macrophages and inhibition of neutrophil, eosinophil, and lymphocyte activation. Both lipoxin A and lipoxin B inhibit natural killer cell cytotoxicity.

B. Heart and Smooth Muscle

1. Cardiovascular—12(S)-HETE is a potent chemoattractant for smooth muscle cells, causing migration at low concentrations; it may play a role in myointimal proliferation that occurs after vascular injury such as that caused by angioplasty. Its stereoisomer, 12(R)-HETE, is not a chemoattractant, but is a potent inhibitor of the Na^+/K^+ ATPase in the cornea. LTC_4 and LTD_4 reduce myocardial contractility and coronary blood flow, leading to cardiac depression. Lipoxin A and lipoxin B exert coronary vasoconstrictor effects in vitro.

2. Gastrointestinal—Human colonic epithelial cells synthesize LTB_4, a chemoattractant for neutrophils. The colonic mucosa of patients with inflammatory bowel disease contains substantially increased amounts of LTB_4.

3. Airways—The cysteinyl leukotrienes, particularly LTC_4 and LTD_4, are potent bronchoconstrictors and cause increased microvascular permeability, plasma exudation, and mucus secretion in the airways. Controversies exist over whether the pattern and specificity of the leukotriene receptors differ in animal models and humans. LTC_4-specific receptors have not been found in human lung tissue, whereas both high- and low-affinity LTD_4 receptors are present.

C. Renal System

The roles of leukotrienes and cytochrome P450 products in the human kidney are currently speculative, but the 5,6-epoxide has been shown to be a powerful vasodilator in animal experiments.

D. Cancer

There has been significant interest in the role of prostaglandins and COX-2 in the development of malignancies. Angiogenesis, which is required for multistage carcinogenesis, is promoted by COX-2-derived TXA_2, as well as PGE_2 and PGI_2. COX inhibitors reduce colon tumor formation in experimental animals. In large epidemiologic studies, the incidental use of NSAIDs is associated with a 40–50% reduction in relative risk for developing colon cancer. Furthermore, in patients with familial polyposis coli, COX inhibitors significantly decrease polyp formation. A polymorphism in COX-2 has been associated with increased risk of colon cancer. Several studies have suggested that COX-2 expression is associated with markers of tumor progression in breast cancer. In mouse mammary tissue, COX-2 is pro-oncogenic whereas aspirin use is associated with a reduced risk of breast cancer in women, especially for hormone receptor-positive tumors.

E. Miscellaneous

The effects of these products on the reproductive organs remain to be elucidated. Similarly, actions on the nervous system have been suggested but not confirmed. 12-HETE stimulates the release of aldosterone from the adrenal cortex and mediates a portion of the aldosterone release stimulated by angiotensin II but not that by ACTH. Very low concentrations of LTC_4 increase and higher concentrations of arachidonate-derived epoxides augment LH and LHRH release from isolated rat anterior pituitary cells.

INHIBITION OF EICOSANOID SYNTHESIS

Corticosteroids block all the known pathways of eicosanoid synthesis, perhaps by stimulating the synthesis of several inhibitory proteins collectively called **annexins** or **lipocortins.** They inhibit phospholipase A_2 activity, probably by interfering with phospholipid binding and thus preventing the release of arachidonic acid.

The NSAIDs (eg, indomethacin, ibuprofen) block both prostaglandin and thromboxane formation by reversibly inhibiting COX activity. The traditional NSAIDs are not selective for COX-1 or COX-2. Selective COX-2 inhibitors, which were developed more recently, vary in their degree of selectivity. Aspirin is an irreversible COX inhibitor. In platelets, which are anuclear, COX cannot be restored via protein biosynthesis resulting in extended inhibition of TXA_2 biosynthesis.

EP-receptor agonists and antagonists are under evaluation in the treatment of bone fracture and osteoporosis, whereas TP-receptor antagonists are being investigated for usefulness in treatment of cardiovascular syndromes.

Selective inhibitors of the lipoxygenase pathway are also mainly investigational. With a few exceptions, NSAIDs do not inhibit lipoxygenase activity at concentrations that markedly inhibit COX activity. In fact, by preventing arachidonic acid conversion via the COX pathway, NSAIDs may cause more substrate to be metabolized through the lipoxygenase pathways, leading to an increased formation of the inflammatory leukotrienes. Even among the COX-dependent pathways, inhibiting the synthesis of one derivative may increase the synthesis of an enzymatically related product. Therefore, drugs that inhibit both COX and lipoxygenase are being developed.

■ II. CLINICAL PHARMACOLOGY OF EICOSANOIDS

Several approaches have been used in the clinical application of eicosanoids. First, stable oral or parenteral long-acting analogs of the naturally occurring prostaglandins have been developed. Several such compounds have been approved for clinical use overseas and are being introduced in the USA (Figure 18–4). Second, enzyme inhibitors and receptor antagonists have been developed to interfere with the synthesis or effects of the eicosanoids. The discovery of COX-2 as a major source of inflammatory prostanoids

Figure 18–4. Chemical structures of some prostaglandins and prostaglandin analogs currently in clinical use.

led to the development of selective COX-2 inhibitors in an effort to preserve the gastrointestinal and renal functions directed through COX-1, thereby reducing toxicity. Third, dietary manipulation—to change the polyunsaturated fatty acid precursors in the cell membrane phospholipids and so change eicosanoid synthesis—is used extensively in over-the-counter products and in diets emphasizing increased consumption of cold water fish.

Female Reproductive System

Studies with knockout mice have confirmed a role for prostaglandins in reproduction and parturition. COX-1-derived $PGF_{2\alpha}$ appears important for luteolysis, consistent with delayed parturition in COX-1-deficient mice. A complex interplay between $PGF_{2\alpha}$ and oxytocin is critical to the onset of labor. EP_2 receptor-deficient mice demonstrate a preimplantation defect, which under-

lies some of the breeding difficulties seen in COX-2 knockouts.

A. ABORTION

PGE_2 and $PGF_{2\alpha}$ have potent oxytocic actions. The ability of the E and F prostaglandins and their analogs to terminate pregnancy at any stage by promoting uterine contractions has been adapted to common clinical use. Many studies worldwide have established that prostaglandin administration efficiently terminates pregnancy. The drugs are used for first- and second-trimester abortion and for priming or ripening the cervix before abortion. These prostaglandins appear to soften the cervix by increasing proteoglycan content and changing the biophysical properties of collagen.

Dinoprostone, a synthetic preparation of PGE_2, is administered vaginally for oxytocic use. In the USA, it is approved for inducing abortion in the second trimester of pregnancy, for missed abortion, for benign hydatidiform mole, and for ripening of the cervix for induction of labor in patients at or near term.

Dinoprostone stimulates the contraction of the uterus throughout pregnancy. As the pregnancy progresses, the uterus increases its contractile response, and the contractile effect of oxytocin is potentiated as well. Dinoprostone also directly affects the collagenase of the cervix, resulting in softening. The vaginal dose enters the maternal circulation, and a small amount is absorbed directly by the uterus via the cervix and the lymphatic system. Dinoprostone is metabolized in local tissues and on the first pass through the lungs (about 95%). The metabolites are mainly excreted in the urine. The plasma half-life is 2.5–5 minutes.

For the induction of labor, dinoprostone is used either as a gel (0.5 mg PGE_2) or as a controlled-release formulation (10 mg PGE_2) that releases PGE_2 in vivo at a rate of about 0.3 mg/h over 12 hours. An advantage of the controlled-release formulation is a lower incidence of gastrointestinal side effects (< 1%).

For abortifacient purposes, the recommended dosage is a 20-mg dinoprostone vaginal suppository repeated at 3- to 5-hour intervals depending on the response of the uterus. The mean time to abortion is 17 hours, but in more than 25% of cases the abortion is incomplete and requires additional intervention.

For softening of the cervix at term, the preparations used are either a single vaginal insert containing 10 mg PGE_2 or a vaginal gel containing 0.5 mg PGE_2 administered every 6 hours. The softening of the cervix for induction of labor substantially shortens the time to onset of labor and the delivery time.

The use of PGE analogs for "menstrual regulation" or very early abortions—within 1–2 weeks after the last menstrual period—has been explored extensively. There are two problems: prolonged vaginal bleeding and severe menstrual cramps.

Antiprogestins (eg, **mifepristone, RU486**) have been combined with an oral oxytocic prostaglandin (eg, **misoprostol**) to produce early abortion. This regimen is available in the USA and Europe (see Chapter 39). The ease of use and the effectiveness of the combination have aroused considerable opposition in some quarters. The major toxicities are cramping pain and diarrhea. The oral and vaginal routes of administration of misoprostol are equally effective, but the vaginal route has been associated with an increased incidence of sepsis, so the oral route is now recommended by all authorities.

$PGF_{2\alpha}$ is available for clinical gynecologic use. This drug, **carboprost tromethamine** (15-methyl-$PGF_{2\alpha}$; the 15-methyl group prolongs the duration of action) is used to induce second-trimester abortions and to control postpartum hemorrhage that is not responding to conventional methods of management. The success rate is approximately 80%. It is administered as a single 250-mcg intramuscular injection, repeated if necessary. Vomiting and diarrhea occur commonly, probably because of gastrointestinal smooth muscle stimulation. Transient elevations in temperature are seen in approximately one eighth of patients.

B. FACILITATION OF LABOR

Numerous studies have shown that PGE_2, $PGF_{2\alpha}$, and their analogs effectively initiate and stimulate labor, but $PGF_{2\alpha}$ is one tenth as potent as PGE_2. There appears to be no difference in the efficacy of PGE_2 and $PGF_{2\alpha}$ when they are administered intravenously; however, they may be of more use locally to promote labor through ripening of the cervix. These agents and oxytocin have similar success rates and comparable induction-to-delivery intervals. The adverse effects of the prostaglandins are moderate, with a slightly higher incidence of nausea, vomiting, and diarrhea than that produced by oxytocin. $PGF_{2\alpha}$ has more gastrointestinal toxicity than PGE_2. Neither drug has significant maternal cardiovascular toxicity in the recommended doses. In fact, PGE_2 must be infused at a rate about 20 times faster than that used for induction of labor to decrease blood pressure and increase heart rate. $PGF_{2\alpha}$ is a bronchoconstrictor and should be used with caution in women with asthma; however, neither asthma attacks nor bronchoconstriction have been observed during the induction of labor. Although both PGE_2 and $PGF_{2\alpha}$ pass the fetoplacental barrier, fetal toxicity is uncommon.

The effects of oral PGE_2 administration (0.5–1.5 mg/h) have been compared with those of intravenous oxytocin and oral demoxytocin, an oxytocin derivative, in the induction of labor. Oral PGE_2 is superior to the oral oxytocin derivative and in most studies is as efficient as intravenous oxytocin. Oral $PGF_{2\alpha}$ causes too much gastrointestinal toxicity to be useful by this route.

Theoretically, PGE_2 and $PGF_{2\alpha}$ should be superior to oxytocin for inducing labor in women with preeclampsia-eclampsia or cardiac and renal diseases because, unlike oxytocin, they have no antidiuretic effect. In addition, PGE_2 has natriuretic effects. However, the clinical benefits of these effects have not been documented. In cases of intrauterine fetal death, the prostaglandins alone or with oxytocin seem to cause delivery effectively.

C. DYSMENORRHEA

Primary dysmenorrhea is attributable to increased endometrial synthesis of PGE_2 and $PGF_{2\alpha}$ during menstruation, with contractions of the uterus that lead to ischemic pain. NSAIDs successfully inhibit the formation of these prostaglandins (see Chapter 36) and so relieve dysmenorrhea in 75–85% of cases. Some of these drugs are available over the counter. Aspirin is also effective in dysmenorrhea, but because it has low potency and is quickly hydrolyzed, large doses and frequent administration are necessary. In addition, the acetylation of platelet COX, causing irreversible inhibition of platelet TXA_2 synthesis, may increase the amount of menstrual bleeding.

Male Reproductive System

Intracavernosal injection or urethral suppository therapy with **alprostadil** (PGE_1) is a second line treatment for erectile dysfunction. Doses of 2.5–25 mcg are used. Penile pain is a frequent side effect, which may be related to the algesic effects of PGE derivatives; however, only a few patients discontinue the use because of pain. Prolonged erection and priapism are less frequent side effects that occur in less than 4% of patients and are minimized by careful titration to the minimal effective dose. When given by injection, alprostadil may be used as monotherapy or in combination with either papaverine or phentolamine.

Renal System

Increased biosynthesis of prostaglandins has been associated with one form of Bartter's syndrome. This is a rare disease characterized by low-to-normal blood pressure, decreased sensitivity to angiotensin, hyperreninemia, hyperaldosteronism, and excessive loss of K^+. There also is an increased excretion of prostaglandins, especially PGE, in the urine. After long-term administration of COX inhibitors, sensitivity to angiotensin, plasma renin values, and the concentration of aldosterone in plasma return to normal. Although plasma K^+ rises, it remains low, and urinary wasting of K^+ persists. Whether an increase in prostaglandin biosynthesis is the cause of Bartter's syndrome or a reflection of a more basic physiologic defect is not yet known.

Cardiovascular System

The vasodilator effects of PGE compounds have been studied extensively in hypertensive patients. These compounds also promote sodium diuresis. Practical application will require derivatives with oral activity, longer half-lives, and fewer adverse effects.

A. PULMONARY HYPERTENSION

Prostacyclin lowers peripheral, pulmonary, and coronary resistance. It has been used to treat both primary pulmonary hypertension and secondary pulmonary hypertension, which sometimes occurs after mitral valve surgery. In addition, prostacyclin has been used successfully to treat portopulmonary hypertension, which arises secondary to liver disease. A commercial preparation of prostacyclin (epoprostenol) is approved for treatment of primary pulmonary hypertension, in which it appears to improve symptoms, prolong survival, and delay or prevent the need for lung or lung-heart transplantation. However, because of its

extremely short plasma half-life, the drug must be administered as a continuous intravenous infusion through a central line. Several prostacyclin analogs with longer half-lives have been developed, and **treprostinil** is approved for use in pulmonary hypertension. This drug is administered by continuous subcutaneous infusion.

B. PERIPHERAL VASCULAR DISEASE

A number of studies have investigated the use of PGE and PGI_2 compounds in Raynaud's phenomenon and peripheral atherosclerosis. In the latter case, prolonged infusions have been used to permit remodeling of the vessel wall and to enhance regression of ischemic ulcers.

C. PATENT DUCTUS ARTERIOSUS

Patency of the fetal ductus arteriosus depends on COX-2–derived PGE_2 acting on the EP_4 receptor. At birth, reduced PGE_2 levels, a consequence of increased PGE_2 metabolism, allow ductus arteriosus closure. In certain types of congenital heart disease (eg, transposition of the great arteries, pulmonary atresia, pulmonary artery stenosis), it is important to maintain the patency of the neonate's ductus arteriosus before corrective surgery. This is done with alprostadil, PGE_1. Like PGE_2, PGE_1 is a vasodilator and an inhibitor of platelet aggregation, and it contracts uterine and intestinal smooth muscle. Adverse effects include apnea, bradycardia, hypotension, and hyperpyrexia. Because of rapid pulmonary clearance, the drug must be continuously infused at an initial rate of 0.05–0.1 mcg/kg/min, which may be increased to 0.4 mcg/kg/min. Prolonged treatment has been associated with ductal fragility and rupture.

In delayed closure of the ductus arteriosus, COX inhibitors are often used to inhibit synthesis of PGE_2 and so close the ductus. Premature infants in whom respiratory distress develops due to failure of ductus closure can be treated with a high degree of success with indomethacin. This treatment often precludes the need for surgical closure of the ductus.

Blood

As noted above, eicosanoids are involved in thrombosis because TXA_2 promotes platelet aggregation and PGI_2 inhibits it. Low-dose aspirin selectively inhibits platelet COX-1. TXA_2, in addition to activating platelets amplifies the response to other platelet agonists; hence inhibition of its synthesis inhibits secondary aggregation of platelets induced by ADP, by low concentrations of thrombin and collagen, and by epinephrine.

Overview analyses have shown that low-dose aspirin reduces the secondary incidence of heart attack and stroke by about 25%. It elevates the low risk of serious GI bleeds about twofold over placebo. Low-dose aspirin also reduces the incidence of first myocardial infarction.

However, in this case, the benefit versus risk of GI bleeding is less clear. The effects of aspirin on platelet function are discussed in greater detail in Chapter 34.

Respiratory System

PGE_2 is a powerful bronchodilator when given in aerosol form. Unfortunately, it also promotes coughing, and an analog that possesses only the bronchodilator properties has been difficult to obtain.

$PGF_{2\alpha}$ and TXA_2 are both strong bronchoconstrictors and were once thought to be primary mediators in asthma. Polymorphisms in the genes for PGD_2 synthase and the TP have been linked with asthma in humans, and deletion of DP_1 sharply reduces allergen-induced infiltration of lymphocytes and eosinophils and airway hyperreactivity. However, the cysteinyl leukotrienes—LTC_4, LTD_4, and LTE_4—probably dominate during asthmatic constriction of the airway. As described in Chapter 20, leukotriene-receptor inhibitors (eg, **zafirlukast, montelukast**) are effective in asthma. A lipoxygenase inhibitor (**zileuton**) has also been used in asthma but is not as popular as the receptor inhibitors. It remains unclear whether leukotrienes are partially responsible for the acute respiratory distress syndrome.

Corticosteroids and cromolyn are also useful in asthma. Corticosteroids inhibit eicosanoid synthesis and thus limit the amounts of eicosanoid mediator available for release. Cromolyn appears to inhibit the release of eicosanoids and other mediators such as histamine and platelet-activating factor from mast cells.

Gastrointestinal System

The word "cytoprotection" was coined to signify the remarkable protective effect of the E prostaglandins against peptic ulcers in animals at doses that do not reduce acid secretion. Since then, numerous experimental and clinical investigations have shown that the PGE compounds and their analogs protect against peptic ulcers produced by either steroids or NSAIDs. **Misoprostol** is an orally active synthetic analog of PGE_1. The FDA-approved indication is for prevention of NSAID-induced peptic ulcers. The drug is administered at a dosage of 200 mcg four times daily. This and other PGE analogs (eg, enprostil) are cytoprotective at low doses and inhibit gastric acid secretion at higher doses. The adverse effects are abdominal discomfort and occasional diarrhea; both effects are dose-related. More recently, dose-dependent bone pain and hyperostosis have been described in patients with liver disease who were given long-term PGE treatment.

Selective COX-2 inhibitors were developed in an effort to spare gastric COX-1 so that the natural cytoprotection by locally synthesized PGE_2 and PGI_2 is undisturbed (see Chapter 36). However, this benefit is seen only with highly selective inhibitors and may be offset by increased cardiovascular toxicity.

Immune System

Cells of the immune system contribute substantially to eicosanoid biosynthesis during an immune reaction. T and B lymphocytes are not primary synthetic sources; however, they may supply arachidonic acid to monocyte-macrophages for eicosanoid synthesis. In addition, there is evidence for eicosanoid-mediated cell-cell interaction by platelets, erythrocytes, PMNs, and endothelial cells.

The eicosanoids modulate the effects of the immune system, as illustrated by the cell-mediated immune response. PGE_2 and PGI_2 limit T-cell proliferation in vitro as corticosteroids do. T-cell clonal expansion is attenuated through inhibition of interleukin-1 and interleukin-2 and class II antigen expression by macrophages or other antigen-presenting cells. The leukotrienes, TXA_2, and platelet-activating factor stimulate T-cell clonal expansion. These compounds stimulate the formation of interleukin-1 and interleukin-2 as well as the expression of interleukin-2 receptors. The leukotrienes also promote interferon-γ release and can replace interleukin-2 as a stimulator of interferon-γ. These in vitro effects of the eicosanoids agree with in vivo findings in animals with acute organ transplant rejection, as described below.

A. CELL-MEDIATED ORGAN TRANSPLANT REJECTION

Acute organ transplant rejection is a cell-mediated immune response (Chapter 56). Administration of PGI_2 to renal transplant patients has reversed the rejection process in some cases. Experimental in vitro and in vivo data show that PGE_2 and PGI_2 can attenuate T-cell proliferation and rejection, which can also be seen with drugs that inhibit TXA_2 and leukotriene formation. In organ transplant patients, urinary excretion of metabolites of TXA_2 increases during acute rejection. Corticosteroids, the first-line drugs used for treatment of acute rejection because of their lymphotoxic effects, inhibit both phospholipase and COX-2 activity.

B. INFLAMMATION

Aspirin has been used to treat arthritis for approximately 100 years, but its mechanism of action—inhibition of COX activity—was not discovered until 1971. Aspirin and other anti-inflammatory agents that inhibit COX are discussed in Chapter 36. COX-2 appears to be the form of the enzyme most associated with cells involved in the inflammatory process. With the exception of PGD_2, the prostanoids are not chemoattractants, but the leukotrienes and some of the HETEs (eg, 12-HETE) are strong chemoattractants. PGE_2 inhibits both antigen-driven and mitogen-induced B-lymphocyte proliferation and differentiation to plasma cells, resulting in inhibition of IgM synthesis. The concomitant elevation of serum IgE and monocyte PGE_2 synthesis, seen in patients with severe trauma and patients with Hodgkin's disease, is explained by the ability of PGE_2 to enhance immunoglobulin class switching to IgE.

C. RHEUMATOID ARTHRITIS

In rheumatoid arthritis, immune complexes are deposited in the affected joints, causing an inflammatory response that is amplified by eicosanoids. Lymphocytes and macrophages accumulate in the synovium, whereas PMNs localize mainly in the synovial fluid. The major eicosanoids produced by PMNs are leukotrienes, which facilitate T-cell proliferation and act as chemoattractants. Human macrophages synthesize the COX products PGE_2 and TXA_2 and large amounts of leukotrienes.

D. INFECTION

The relationship of eicosanoids to infection is not well defined. The association between the use of the anti-inflammatory steroids and increased risk of infection is well established. However, NSAIDs do not seem to alter patient responses to infection.

Glaucoma

Latanoprost, a stable long-acting $PGF_{2\alpha}$ derivative, was the first prostanoid used for glaucoma. The success of latanoprost has stimulated development of similar prostanoids with ocular hypotensive effects, and **bimatoprost, travaprost,** and **unoprostone** are now available. These drugs act at the FP receptor and are administered as drops into the conjunctival sac once or twice daily. Adverse effects include irreversible brown pigmentation of the iris and eyelashes, drying of the eyes, and conjunctivitis.

DIETARY MANIPULATION OF ARACHIDONIC ACID METABOLISM

Because arachidonic acid is derived from dietary linoleic and α-linolenic acids, which are essential fatty acids, the effects of dietary manipulation on arachidonic acid metabolism have been extensively studied. Two approaches have been used. The first adds corn, safflower, and sunflower oils, which contain linoleic acid (C18:2), to the diet. The second approach adds oils containing eicosapentaenoic (C20:5) and docosahexaenoic acids (C22:6), so-called omega-3 fatty acids, from cold water fish. Both types of diet change the phospholipid composition of cell membranes by replacing arachidonic acid with the dietary fatty acids. It has been claimed that the synthesis of both TXA_2 and PGI_2 is reduced and that changes in platelet aggregation, vasomotor spasm, and cholesterol metabolism follow.

As indicated previously, there are many possible oxidation products of the different polyenoic acids. It is probably naive to ascribe the effects of dietary intervention reported thus far to such metabolites. However, subjects on diets containing highly saturated fatty acids clearly show increased platelet aggregation when compared with other study groups. Such diets (eg, in Finland and the USA) are associated with higher rates of myocardial infarction than are more polyunsaturated diets (eg, in Italy).

PREPARATIONS AVAILABLE

NONSTEROIDAL ANTI-INFLAMMATORY DRUGS ARE LISTED IN CHAPTER 36.

Alprostadil
Penile injection (Caverject, Edex): 5, 10, 20, 40 mcg sterile powder for reconstitution
Penile pellet (Muse): 125, 250, 500, 1000 mcg
Parenteral (Prostin VR Pediatric): 500 mcg/mL ampules

Bimatoprost (Lumigan)
Ophthalmic drops: 0.03% solution

Carboprost tromethamine (Hemabate)
Parenteral: 250 mcg carboprost and 83 mcg tromethamine per mL ampules

Dinoprostone [prostaglandin E_2] (Prostin E2, Prepidil, Cervidil)
Vaginal: 20 mg suppositories, 0.5 mg gel, 10 mg controlled-release system

Epoprostenol [prostacyclin] (Flolan)
Intravenous: 0.5, 1.5 mg powder to reconstitute

Latanoprost (Xalatan)
Topical: 0.005% ophthalmic solution

Misoprostol (generic, Cytotec)
Oral: 100 and 200 mcg tablets

Monteleukast (Singulair)
Oral: 4, 5 mg chewable tablets, 10 mg tablets, 4 mg granules

Travaprost (Travatan)
Ophthalmic solution: 0.004%

Treprostinil (Remodulin)
Parenteral: 1, 2.5, 5, 10 mg/mL for continuous subcutaneous infusion

Unoprostone (Rescula)
Ophthalmic solution 0.15%

Zafirleukast (Accolate)
Oral: 10, 20 mg tablets

Zileuton (Zyflo)
Oral: 600 mg tablets

REFERENCES

Berger J, Moller DE: The mechanisms of action of PPARs. Annu Rev Med 2002;53:409.

Breyer RM et al: Prostanoid receptors: Subtypes and signaling. Annu Rev Pharmacol Toxicol 2001;41:661.

Brink C et al: International Union of Pharmacology XXXVII. Nomenclature for leukotriene and lipoxin receptors. Pharmacol Rev 2003;55:195.

Cheng HF, Harris RC: Cyclooxygenases, the kidney, and hypertension. Hypertension 2004;43:525.

Christin-Maitre S, Bouchard P, Spitz IM: Medical termination of pregnancy. N Engl J Med 2000;342:946.

Grosser T, Fries S, Fitzgerald GA: Biological basis for the cardiovascular consequences of COX-2 inhibition: Therapeutic challenges and opportunities. J Clin Invest 2006;116:4.

Leonhardt A et al: Expression of prostanoid receptors in human ductus arteriosus. Br J Pharmacol 2003;138:655.

Martel-Pelletier J et al: Therapeutic role of dual inhibitors of 5-LOX and COX, selective and non-selective non-steroidal anti-inflammatory drugs. Ann Rheum Dis 2003;62:501.

Maxey KM: Eicosanoids acting via nuclear receptors: The 15-deoxy PGJ compounds and congeners. Prostaglandins Other Lipid Mediat 2000;62:1.

McAdam BF et al: Systemic biosynthesis of prostacyclin by cyclo-oxygenase (COX)-2: The human pharmacology of a selective inhibitor of COX-2. Proc Natl Acad Sci U S A 1999;96:272.

Narumiya S, FitzGerald GA: Genetic and pharmacological analysis of prostanoid receptor function. J Clin Invest 2001;108:25.

Olschewski H et al: Inhaled Iloprost for severe pulmonary hypertension. N Engl J Med 2002;347:322.

Rocca B, FitzGerald GA: Cyclooxygenases and prostaglandins: shaping up the immune response. Int Immunopharmacol 2002;2:603.

Smith WL, Dewitt DL, Garavito MR: Cyclooxygenases: Structural, cellular, and molecular biology. Annu Rev Biochem 2000;69:145.

Smyth EM, FitzGerald GA: Prostaglandin mediators. In: Bradshaw RD, Dennis EA (editors): *Handbook of Cell Signaling*. Academic Press, 2003:265.

Tilley SL, Coffman TM, Koller BH: Mixed messages: Modulation of inflammation and immune responses by prostaglandins and thromboxanes. J Clin Invest 2001;108:15.

Wang D, Dubois RN: Prostaglandins and cancer. Gut 2006;55:115.

Wang D, Mann JR, DuBois RN: The role of prostaglandins and other eicosanoids in the gastrointestinal tract. Gastroenterology 2005;128:1445.

Nitric Oxide[*]

Samie R. Jaffrey, MD, PhD

19

Nitric oxide (NO) is a gaseous signaling molecule that readily diffuses across cell membranes and regulates a wide range of physiologic and pathophysiologic processes including cardiovascular, inflammation, immune, and neuronal functions. Nitric oxide should not be confused with nitrous oxide (N_2O), an anesthetic gas.

■ DISCOVERY OF ENDOGENOUSLY GENERATED NITRIC OXIDE

The first observations of the biologic role of endogenously generated NO were made in rodent macrophages and neutrophils: In vitro exposure of these cells to endotoxin lipopolysaccharide resulted in the accumulation of significant amounts of nitrite and nitrate in the cell culture medium. Furthermore, injection of endotoxin in animals elevated urinary nitrite and nitrate, the two oxidation products of NO.

The second observation was made by investigators in 1980 who found that the ability of acetylcholine to elicit relaxation of isolated strips of rabbit aorta was entirely dependent on the presence of the endothelium. If the endothelium was removed, the vessel still exhibited normal relaxation responses to nitroglycerin, but not to acetylcholine or carbachol. They discovered that following stimulation with acetylcholine or carbachol, the endothelium released a short-lived molecule that resulted in relaxation and dilation of surrounding vascular smooth muscle. The synthesis of this factor was not affected by cyclooxygenase inhibitors, indicating that it was distinct from endothelium-derived prostacyclin. They named this vasodilator **endothelium-derived relaxing factor (EDRF),** since it promoted relaxation of precontracted smooth muscle preparations. In 1987, by comparing the pharmacologic and biochemical properties of the suspect molecule, three independent groups reported that EDRF and NO are the same molecule. It was later reported that other vasodilator molecules may be a part of EDRF, but it is clear that NO provides the major part of its activity. Subsequent studies revealed that NO was generated by many cells and was, like the eicosanoids (see Chapter 18), found in almost all tissues. The finding that NO is endogenously generated and elicits specific biologic effects explains why pharmacologic reagents that release NO (nitrates, nitrites, nitroprusside; see Chapters 11 and 12) are potent vasodilators.

■ NITRIC OXIDE SYNTHESIS, SIGNALING MECHANISMS, & INACTIVATION

Synthesis

NO, written as NO$^{\bullet}$ to indicate an unpaired electron in its chemical structure, or simply NO, is a highly reactive signaling molecule that is made in a wide variety of cells, most prominently neurons, skeletal muscle, endothelial cells, and certain immune system cells. In these cells, NO is synthesized by one or more of three closely related NO synthase (NOS, EC 1.14.13.49) isoenzymes, each of which is encoded by a separate gene and named for the initial cell type in which it was isolated (Table 19–1). These enzymes, neuronal NOS (nNOS or NOS-1), macrophage or inducible NOS (iNOS or NOS-2), and endothelial NOS (eNOS or NOS-3), despite their names, are each expressed in a wide variety of cell types, often with an overlapping distribution. These isoforms generate NO from the amino acid L-arginine in an O_2- and NADPH-dependent reaction (Figure 19–1). This enzymatic reaction involves enzyme-bound cofactors, including heme, tetrahydrobiopterin, and flavin adenine dinucleotide. In the case of nNOS and eNOS, NO synthesis is evoked by agents and processes that increase cytosolic calcium concentrations. Binding of calcium-calmodulin complexes to eNOS and nNOS leads to enzyme activation. On the other hand, iNOS is not regulated by calcium, but is inducible. In macrophages and several other cell types, inflammatory mediators induce

[*]The author acknowledges the contribution of the previous authors of this chapter, George Thomas, PhD, & Peter Ramwell, PhD.

Table 19-1. Properties of the three isoforms of nitric oxide synthase (NOS).

Property	Isoform Names		
	NOS-1	NOS-2	NOS-3
Other names	nNOS (neuronal NOS)	iNOS (inducible NOS)	eNOS (endothelial NOS)
Tissue	Neuronal, epithelial cells	Macrophages, smooth muscle cells	Endothelial cells
Expression	Constitutive	Transcriptional induction	Constitutive
Calcium regulation	Yes	No	Yes
Chromosome	12	17	7
Approximate mass	150–160 kDa	125–135 kDa	133 kDa

the transcriptional activation of the *iNOS* gene, resulting in accumulation of iNOS and generation of increased quantities of NO.

Signaling Mechanisms

NO mediates its effects by covalent modification of proteins. There are three major effector targets of NO (Figure 19–1):

1. **Metalloproteins**—NO interacts with metals, especially iron in heme. Soluble guanylyl cyclase (sGC), an enzyme that generates cyclic GMP from guanosine triphosphate (GTP), contains heme, which binds readily to NO. NO binding to heme results in activation of sGC and elevation in intracellular cGMP levels. cGMP activates protein kinase G (PKG), which phosphorylates specific proteins. NO exerts vasodilatory effects (Chapter 12), which are largely mediated by

Figure 19–1. Nitric oxide generation from L-arginine and nitric oxide donors and the formation of cGMP. L-NMMA inhibits nitric oxide synthase. Some of the nitric oxide donors such as furoxans and organic nitrates and nitrites require a thiol cofactor such as cysteine or glutathione to form nitric oxide.

Table 19–2. Oxides of nitrogen.

Name	Symbol	Known Function
Nitric oxide	$NO^{\bullet}$	Vasodilator, platelet inhibitor, immune regulator, neurotransmitter
Nitroxyl anion	NO^{-}	Smooth muscle relaxant
Nitrogen dioxide	$NO_2^{\bullet}$	Free radical, nitrosating agent, lung irritant
Nitrous oxide	N_2O	Anesthetic
Dinitrogen trioxide	N_2O_3	Nitrosating agent
Dinitrogen tetraoxide	N_2O_4	Nitrosating agent
Nitrite	NO_2^{-}	Produces $NO^{\bullet}$ at acidic pH
Nitrate	NO_3^{-}	Stable oxidation product of $NO^{\bullet}$

NO-dependent elevations in cGMP and PKG activity. Several other metalloproteins are targets of NO. The affinity of NO for iron is also responsible for its inhibitory effect on enzymes that contain iron-sulfur clusters such as the tricarboxylic acid cycle enzyme aconitase. NO inhibits mitochondrial respiration by inhibition of cytochrome oxidase. Inhibition of the heme-containing cytochrome P450 enzymes by NO is a major pathogenic mechanism in inflammatory liver disease.

2. Thiols—NO reacts with thiols (compounds containing the –SH group) to form nitrosothiols. In proteins, the thiol moiety is found in the amino acid cysteine. Upon exposure to NO, certain proteins are found to accumulate nitrosothiols, which can activate or inhibit the activity of these proteins. This posttranslational modification, termed *S*-nitrosylation, is reversed by chemical reduction by intracellular reducing agents. The formation of nitrosothiols is not mediated by direct reaction of NO with thiols, but rather requires either metals or oxygen to catalyze the formation of this adduct. Indeed, NO undergoes both oxidative and reductive reactions, resulting in the formation of a variety of oxides of nitrogen that can nitrosylate thiols, nitrate tyrosines (below), or which are stable oxidation products (Table 19–2). H-ras, a regulator of cell proliferation, is activated by *S*-nitrosylation, while the metabolic enzyme glyceraldehyde-3-phosphate dehydrogenase is inhibited when it is *S*-nitrosylated. Glutathione, a major intracellular sulfhydryl-containing compound, also interacts with NO under physiologic conditions to generate *S*-nitrosoglutathione, a more stable form of NO. Nitrosoglutathione may serve as an endogenous long-lived adduct or carrier of NO. Vascular glutathione is decreased in diabetes mellitus and atherosclerosis, and this may account for the increased incidence of cardiovascular complications in these conditions.

3. Tyrosine nitration—NO reacts very efficiently with superoxide to form peroxynitrite ($ONOO^{-}$), a powerful oxidant that leads to DNA damage, irreversible nitration of tyrosine, and oxidation of cysteine to disulfides or to various oxides (SO_X). In several diseases, cellular degeneration, due to apoptotic mechanisms or due to ischemia, leads to excess superoxide production, and a consequent increase in peroxynitrite levels. Numerous proteins have been found to contain nitrotyrosines, and this modification can be associated with either activation or inhibition of protein function. However, it is not yet clear whether tyrosine nitration has essential roles in either physiologic signaling or in the pathology of any disease. Protein tyrosine nitration is also used as a marker for the presence of oxidative and nitrosative stress. Peroxynitrite-mediated protein modification is regulated by the cellular content of glutathione, which can protect against tissue damage by scavenging peroxynitrite. Factors that regulate the biosynthesis and decomposition of glutathione may have important consequences on the toxicity of NO.

Inactivation

The lability of NO is related to its rapid reactions with metals and reactive oxygen species. Thus, NO reacts with heme and hemoproteins, including oxyhemoglobin, which catalyzes NO oxidation to nitrate. NO reactions with hemoglobin may also result in partial *S*-nitrosylation of hemoglobin, resulting in transport of NO throughout the vasculature. NO is also inactivated by superoxide, and scavengers of superoxide anion such as superoxide dismutase may protect NO, enhancing its potency and prolonging its duration of action.

PHARMACOLOGIC MANIPULATION OF NITRIC OXIDE

Inhibitors of Nitric Oxide Synthesis

The primary strategy to inhibit the generation of NO in cells is to use NOS inhibitors. The majority of these inhibitors are arginine analogs that bind to the NOS arginine-binding site. Since each of the NOS isoforms has high sequence similarity, most of these inhibitors do not exhibit selectivity for any of the NOS isoforms. In many disorders, such as inflammation and sepsis (see below), inhibition of the iNOS isoform is desired, whereas in neurodegenerative conditions, nNOS-specific inhibitors are needed. However, administration of nonselective NOS inhibitors leads to concurrent inhibition of eNOS, which impairs its homeostatic signaling and also results in vasoconstriction and potential ischemic damage. Thus, newer NOS isoform-selective inhibitors are being designed that exploit subtle differences in substrate-binding sites between the isoforms, as well as newer inhibitors that prevent NOS dimerization, the conformation required for enzymatic activity. The efficacy of NOS isoform-selective inhibitors in medical conditions is under investigation.

Nitric Oxide Donors

NO donors, which release NO or related NO species, are used to elicit smooth muscle relaxation. Different classes of NO donors have differing biologic properties, related to the nature of the NO species that is released and the mechanism that relates to their release.

1. **Organic nitrates**—Nitroglycerin, which dilates veins and coronary arteries, is metabolized to NO by mitochondrial aldehyde reductase, an enzyme enriched in venous smooth muscle, accounting for the potent venodilating activity of this molecule. Other organic nitrates, such as isosorbide dinitrate are metabolized to an NO-releasing species through a currently unidentified enzyme. Organic nitrates have less significant effects on aggregation of platelets, which appear to lack the enzymatic pathways necessary for rapid metabolic activation. Organic nitrates are limited by the loss of therapeutic effect during continuous administration. This nitrate tolerance may derive from NO-mediated inhibition of mitochondrial aldehyde reductase.

2. **Organic nitrites**—Organic nitrites, such as the volatile antianginal isoamylnitrite, also require metabolic activation to elicit vasorelaxation, although the responsible enzyme has not been identified. Nitrites are arterial vasodilators and do not exhibit the rapid tolerance seen with nitrates.

3. **Sodium nitroprusside**—Sodium nitroprusside, which is used for rapid pressure reduction in arterial hypertension, generates NO in response to light as well as chemical or enzymatic mechanisms in cell membranes. See Chapter 11 for additional details.

4. **Hybrid NO donors**—A new strategy involves the incorporation of NO-donating moieties onto currently available cardiovascular drugs. This approach is being tested with drugs such as aspirin and the angiotensin-converting enzyme inhibitor captopril. SNOCap, which incorporates a nitrosothiol moiety on captopril, is currently being examined for its efficacy in cardiovascular disorders.

5. **NO gas inhalation**—NO itself can be used therapeutically. Inhalation of NO results in reduced pulmonary artery pressure and improved perfusion of ventilated areas of the lung. Inhaled NO has been used for acute respiratory distress syndrome, acute hypoxemia, and cardiopulmonary resuscitation with evidence for short-term improvements in pulmonary function.

6. **Alternate strategies**—Another mechanism to enhance the activity of NO is to enhance the downstream NO signaling pathway. Sildenafil, an inhibitor of type 5 phosphodiesterase, results in prolongation of the duration of NO-induced cGMP elevations in a variety of tissues (see Chapter 12).

NITRIC OXIDE IN DISEASE

VASCULAR EFFECTS

NO has a significant effect on vascular smooth muscle tone and blood pressure. Numerous endothelium-dependent vasodilators, such as acetylcholine and bradykinin, act by increasing intracellular calcium levels, which induces NO synthesis. Mice with a knockout mutation in the *eNOS* gene display increased vascular tone and elevated mean arterial pressure, indicating that eNOS is a fundamental regulator of blood pressure. The effects of vasopressor drugs are increased by inhibition of NOS.

Apart from being a vasodilator, NO protects against thrombosis and atherogenesis through several mechanisms. A major mechanism involves the inhibition of proliferation and migration of vascular smooth muscle. In animal models, myointimal proliferation following angioplasty can be blocked by NO donors, by NOS gene transfer, and by NO inhalation.

The antithrombotic effects of NO are also mediated by NO-dependent inhibition of platelet aggregation. Both endothelial cells and platelets themselves contain eNOS, which acts to regulate thrombus formation. Thus, endothelial dysfunction and the associated decrease in NO generation may result in abnormal platelet function. As in vascular smooth muscle, cGMP mediates the effect of NO in platelets. NO may have an additional inhibitory effect on blood coagulation by enhancing fibrinolysis via an effect on plasminogen.

NO also reduces endothelial adhesion of monocytes and leukocytes, key features of the early development of atheromatous plaques. This effect is due to the inhibitory effect of NO on the expression of adhesion molecules on the endothelial surface. In addition, NO may act as an antioxidant, blocking the oxidation of low-density lipoproteins and thus preventing or reducing the formation of foam cells in the vascular wall. Plaque formation is also affected by NO-dependent reduction in endothelial cell permeability to lipoproteins. The importance of eNOS in cardiovascular disease is supported by experiments showing increased atherosclerosis in animals deficient in eNOS by pharmacologic inhibition. Atherosclerosis risk factors, such as smoking, hyperlipidemia, diabetes, and hypertension, are associated with decreased endothelial NO production, and thus enhance atherogenesis.

SEPTIC SHOCK

As mentioned previously, increased urinary excretion of nitrate, the oxidative product of NO, is a feature of gram-negative bacterial infection. Lipopolysaccharide components from the bacterial wall induce synthesis of iNOS, resulting in exaggerated hypotension, shock, and, in some cases, death. This hypotension is reversed by NOS inhibitors such as L-NMMA (Table 19–3) in humans as well as in animal models. A similar reversal of hypotension is produced by compounds that prevent the action of NO (such as methylene blue), as well as by scavengers of NO (such as hemoglobin). Furthermore, knockout mice lacking a functional *iNOS* gene are more resistant to endotoxin than wild-type mice. However, thus far there has been no correlation between the hemodynamic effects of relatively nonselective NOS inhibitors and survival rate in gram-negative sepsis. The absence of benefit may reflect the inability of the NOS inhibitors to differentiate between NOS isoforms or may reflect concurrent inhibition of beneficial aspects of iNOS signaling.

INFLAMMATION

The host response to infection or injury involves the recruitment of leukocytes and the release of inflammatory mediators, including NO. Numerous cytokines, such as tumor necrosis factor and interleukin-1, as well as bacterial-derived mediators, induce the transcription of iNOS in leukocytes, fibroblasts, and other cell types, accounting for enhanced levels of NO. NO is an important microbicide and may have important roles in tissue adapting to inflammatory states. However, overproduction of NO may exacerbate tissue injury in both acute and chronic inflammatory conditions. NO generated during inflammation is involved in the vasodilation associated with acute inflammation and can interact with superoxide to generate peroxynitrite and subsequently modify proteins, lipids, and nucleotides. In experimental models of acute inflammation, inhibitors of iNOS have a dose-dependent protective effect, suggesting that NO promotes edema and vascular permeability. NO has a detrimental effect in chronic models of arthritis; dietary L-arginine supplementation exacerbates arthritis, whereas protection is seen with iNOS inhibitors. Psoriasis lesions, airway epithelium in asthma, and inflammatory bowel lesions in humans all demonstrate elevated levels of NO and iNOS. Synovial fluid from patients with arthritis contains increased oxidation products of NO,

Table 19–3. Some inhibitors of nitric oxide synthesis or action.

Inhibitor	Mechanism	Comment
N^G–Monomethyl–L–arginine (L–NMMA)	NOS inhibition	May act as substrate in some tissues
N^G–Nitro–L–arginine methyl ester (L–NAME)	NOS inhibition	Less selective NOS inhibitor
7–Nitroindazole	NOS inhibition	Markedly selective for NOS–1 in vivo
S–Methylthiocitrulline	NOS inhibition	Partially selective for NOS–1
Heme	Nitric oxide scavenger	

NOS, nitric oxide synthase.

particularly peroxynitrite. Recent studies have shown that NO stimulates the synthesis of inflammatory prostaglandins by activating cyclooxygenase isoenzyme II (COX-2). Thus, inhibition of the NO pathway may have a beneficial effect on inflammatory diseases, including joint diseases.

However, NO also appears to play an important protective role in the body via immune cell function. When challenged with foreign antigens, TH1 cells (see Chapter 56) respond by synthesizing NO. Inhibition of NOS and knockout of the *iNOS* gene can markedly impair the protective response to injected parasites in animal models.

THE CENTRAL NERVOUS SYSTEM

NO has been proposed to have a major role in the central nervous system—as a neurotransmitter, as a modulator of ligand-gated receptors, or both. NO synthesis is induced at postsynaptic sites in neurons upon activation of the NMDA subtype of glutamate receptor, which results in calcium influx and activation of nNOS. In several neuronal subtypes, eNOS is also present and activated by neurotransmitter pathways that lead to calcium influx. NO synthesized postsynaptically may function as a retrograde messenger and diffuse to the presynaptic terminal to enhance the efficiency of neurotransmitter release through a cGMP or *S*-nitrosylation-dependent mechanism. It has been suggested that a major role for NO is in the regulation of synaptic plasticity, the molecular process that underlies learning and behavior.

THE PERIPHERAL NERVOUS SYSTEM

Nonadrenergic, noncholinergic (NANC) neurons are widely distributed in peripheral tissues, especially the gastrointestinal and reproductive tracts (see Chapter 6). Considerable evidence implicates NO as a mediator of certain NANC actions, and some NANC neurons appear to release NO. Penile erection is thought to be caused by the release of NO from NANC neurons; it is well documented that NO promotes relaxation of the smooth muscle in the corpora cavernosa—the initiating factor in penile erection—and inhibitors of NOS have been shown to prevent erection caused by pelvic nerve stimulation in the rat. Thus, impotence is a possible clinical indication for the use of a NO donor, and trials have been carried out with nitroglycerin ointment and the nitroglycerin patch. An established approach is to inhibit the breakdown of cGMP by the phosphodiesterase (PDE isoform 5) present in the smooth muscle of the corpora cavernosa with drugs such as sildenafil (see Chapter 12).

RESPIRATORY DISORDERS

NO has been shown to improve cardiopulmonary function in adult patients with pulmonary artery hypertension and is approved for this indication (see Preparations Available). It is administered by inhalation. It has also been administered by inhalation to newborns with pulmonary hypertension and acute respiratory distress syndrome. The current treatment for severely defective gas exchange in the newborn is with extracorporeal membrane oxygenation (ECMO), which does not directly affect pulmonary vascular pressures. NO inhalation decreases pulmonary arterial pressure and improves blood oxygenation. Thus, when pulmonary resistance is elevated, it is possible to exploit the vasodilator properties of NO by administering it via inhalation of a few parts per million. Adults with respiratory distress syndrome also appear—in open trials—to benefit from NO inhalation. NO may have an additional role in relaxing airway smooth muscle and thus acting as a bronchodilator. For these reasons, NO inhalation therapy is being widely tested in both infants and adults with acute respiratory distress syndrome. The adverse effects of this use of NO are being assessed.

 PREPARATIONS AVAILABLE

Nitric Oxide (INOmax)
Inhalation: 100, 800 ppm gas

REFERENCES

Blum A et al: Oral L-arginine in patients with coronary artery disease on medical management. Circulation 2000;101:2160.

Chen Z et al: An essential role for mitochondrial aldehyde dehydrogenase in nitroglycerin bioactivation. Proc Natl Acad Sci U S A 2005;102:12159.

Davis KL et al: Novel effects of nitric oxide. Annu Rev Pharmacol Toxicol 2001;41:203.

Derry F et al: Efficacy and safety of sildenafil citrate (Viagra) in men with erectile dysfunction and spinal cord injury: A review. Urology 2002;20(2 Suppl 2):49.

Furchgott RF: Endothelium-derived relaxing factor: Discovery, early studies, and identification as NO. Biosci Rep 1999;19:235.

Hofseth LJ et al: Nitric oxide-induced cellular stress and p53 activation in chronic inflammation. Proc Natl Acad Sci U S A 2003;100:143.

Napoli C, Ignarro LJ: Nitric oxide-releasing drugs. Annu Rev Pharmacol Toxicol 2003;43:97.

Toda N, Okamura T: The pharmacology of nitric oxide in the peripheral nervous system of blood vessels. Pharmacol Rev 2003;55:271.

Drugs Used in Asthma

Homer A. Boushey, MD

Asthma is characterized clinically by recurrent bouts of coughing, shortness of breath, chest tightness, and wheezing; physiologically by widespread, reversible narrowing of the bronchial airways and a marked increase in bronchial responsiveness to inhaled stimuli; and pathologically by lymphocytic, eosinophilic inflammation of the bronchial mucosa. It is also characterized pathologically by remodeling of the bronchial mucosa, with deposition of collagen beneath the epithelium's lamina reticularis and hyperplasia of the cells of all structural elements—vessels, smooth muscle, and secretory glands and goblet cells.

In mild asthma, symptoms occur only occasionally, as on exposure to allergens or certain pollutants, on exercise, or after a viral upper respiratory infection. More severe forms of asthma are associated with frequent attacks of wheezing dyspnea, especially at night, and may be associated with chronic airway narrowing, causing chronic respiratory impairment. These consequences of asthma are regarded as largely preventable, because effective treatments for relief of acute bronchoconstriction ("short term relievers") and for reduction in symptoms and prevention of attacks ("long-term controllers") are available (but underutilized).

The causes of airway narrowing in acute asthmatic attacks include contraction of airway smooth muscle, inspissation of thick, viscid mucus plugs in the airway lumen, and thickening of the bronchial mucosa from edema, cellular infiltration, and hyperplasia of secretory, vascular, and smooth muscle cells. Of these causes of airway obstruction, contraction of smooth muscle is most easily reversed by current therapy; reversal of the edema and cellular infiltration requires sustained treatment with anti-inflammatory agents.

Short-term relief is thus most effectively achieved by agents that relax airway smooth muscle, of which β-adrenoceptor stimulants (see Chapter 9) are the most effective and most widely used. Theophylline, a methylxanthine drug, and antimuscarinic agents (see Chapter 8) are also used for reversal of airway constriction.

Long-term control is most effectively achieved with an anti-inflammatory agent such as an inhaled corticosteroid. It can also be achieved, though less effectively, with a leukotriene pathway antagonist or an inhibitor of mast cell degranulation, such as cromolyn or nedocromil. Finally, clinical trials have established the efficacy of treatment for

asthma with a humanized monoclonal antibody, omalizumab, which is specifically targeted against IgE, the antibody responsible for allergic sensitization.

The distinction between "short-term relievers" and "long-term controllers" has become blurred. Theophylline, regarded as a bronchodilator, inhibits some lymphocyte functions and modestly reduces airway mucosal inflammation. Inhaled corticosteroids, regarded as long-term controllers, produce modest immediate bronchodilation. Two recently released long-acting β-adrenoceptor stimulants, salmeterol and formoterol, appear to be effective in improving asthma control when added to inhaled corticosteroid treatment.

This chapter presents the basic pharmacology of the methylxanthines, cromolyn, leukotriene pathway inhibitors, and monoclonal anti-IgE antibody—agents whose medical use is almost exclusively for pulmonary disease. The other classes of drugs listed above are discussed in relation to the therapy of asthma.

PATHOGENESIS OF ASTHMA

The classic immunologic model of asthma presents it as a disease mediated by reaginic immune globulin (IgE). Foreign materials that provoke IgE production are described as "allergens"; the most common are proteins from house dust mite, cockroach, cat dander, molds, and pollens. The tendency to produce IgE antibodies is genetically determined; asthma and other allergic diseases cluster in families. Once produced, IgE antibodies bind to mast cells in the airway mucosa (Figure 20–1). On reexposure to a specific allergen, antigen-antibody interaction on the surface of the mast cells triggers both the release of mediators stored in the cells' granules and the synthesis and release of other mediators. The histamine, tryptase, leukotrienes C_4 and D_4, and prostaglandin D_2, when released, diffuse through the airway mucosa triggering the muscle contraction and vascular leakage responsible for the acute bronchoconstriction of the "early asthmatic response." This response is often followed in 4–6 hours by a second, more sustained phase of bronchoconstriction, the "late asthmatic response," which is associated with an influx of inflammatory cells into the bronchial mucosa and with an increase in bronchial responsiveness that may last for several weeks after a single inhalation of allergen. The mediators responsible for this late

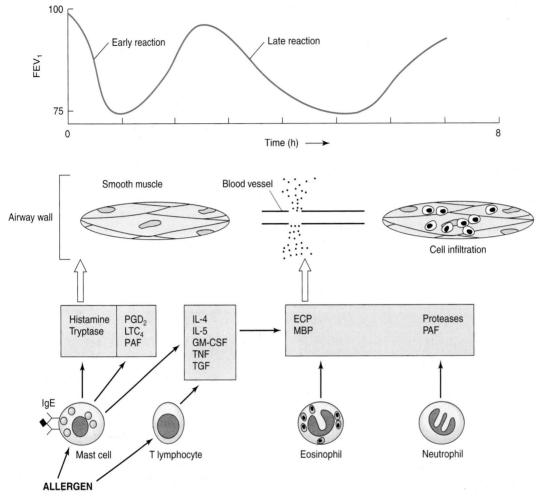

Figure 20–1. Conceptual model for the immunopathogenesis of asthma. Exposure to allergen causes synthesis of IgE, which binds to mast cells in the airway mucosa. On reexposure to allergen, antigen-antibody interaction on mast cell surfaces triggers release of mediators of anaphylaxis: histamine, tryptase, prostaglandin D₂ (PGD₂), leukotriene C₄, and platelet-activating factor (PAF). These agents provoke contraction of airway smooth muscle, causing the immediate fall in FEV_1. Reexposure to allergen also causes the synthesis and release of a variety of cytokines: interleukins 4 and 5, granulocyte-macrophage colony stimulating factor (GM-CSF), tumor necrosis factor (TNF), and tissue growth factor (TGF) from T cells and mast cells. These cytokines in turn attract and activate eosinophils and neutrophils, whose products include eosinophil cationic protein (ECP), major basic protein (MBP), proteases, and platelet-activating factor. These mediators cause the edema, mucus hypersecretion, smooth muscle contraction, and increase in bronchial reactivity associated with the late asthmatic response, indicated by a fall in FEV_1 2–8 hours after the exposure.

response are thought to be cytokines characteristically produced by TH2 lymphocytes, especially interleukins 5, 9, and 13. The cytokines are thought to attract and activate eosinophils, stimulate IgE production by B lymphocytes, and directly stimulate mucus production by bronchial epithelial cells. It is not clear whether lymphocytes or mast cells in the airway mucosa are the primary source of the mediators responsible for the late inflammatory response, but the

benefits of corticosteroid therapy are attributed to their inhibition of cytokine production in the airways.

The allergen challenge model does not reproduce all the features of asthma. Most asthma attacks are not triggered by inhalation of allergens. They are triggered by viral respiratory infection. Some adults with asthma have no evidence of allergic sensitivity to allergens, and even in people with allergic sensitivity, the severity of symptoms

Figure 20–2. Mechanisms of response to inhaled irritants. The airway is represented microscopically by a cross-section of the wall with branching vagal sensory endings lying adjacent to the lumen. Afferent pathways in the vagus nerves travel to the central nervous system; efferent pathways from the central nervous system travel to efferent ganglia. Postganglionic fibers release acetylcholine (ACh), which binds to muscarinic receptors on airway smooth muscle. Inhaled materials may provoke bronchoconstriction by several possible mechanisms. First, they may trigger the release of chemical mediators from mast cells. Second, they may stimulate afferent receptors to initiate reflex bronchoconstriction or to release tachykinins (eg, substance P) that directly stimulate smooth muscle contraction.

correlates poorly with levels of allergen in the atmosphere. Moreover, bronchospasm can be provoked by nonallergenic stimuli such as distilled water, exercise, cold air, sulfur dioxide, and rapid respiratory maneuvers.

This tendency to develop bronchospasm on encountering stimuli that do not affect healthy nonasthmatic airways is characteristic of asthma and is sometimes called "nonspecific bronchial hyperreactivity" to distinguish it from bronchial responsiveness to specific antigens. Bronchial reactivity is assessed by measuring the fall in forced expiratory volume in 1 second (FEV_1) provoked by inhaling serially increasing concentrations of aerosolized methacholine. The exaggerated reactivity of the airways appears to be fundamental to asthma's pathogenesis, because it is nearly ubiquitous in patients with asthma and its degree correlates with the clinical severity of the disease.

The mechanisms underlying bronchial hyperreactivity are somehow related to inflammation of the airway mucosa. The agents that increase bronchial reactivity, such as ozone exposure, allergen inhalation, and infection with respiratory viruses, also cause airway inflammation. The increase in reactivity due to allergen inhalation is associated with an increase in both eosinophils and polymorphonuclear leukocytes in bronchial lavage fluid. The increase in reactivity that is associated with the late asthmatic response to allergen inhalation (Figure 20–1) is sustained and, because it is prevented by treatment with an inhaled corticosteroid, is thought to be caused by airway inflammation.

Whatever the mechanisms responsible for bronchial hyperreactivity, bronchoconstriction itself seems to result not simply from the direct effect of the released mediators but also from their activation of neural or humoral pathways. Evidence for the importance of neural pathways stems largely from studies of laboratory animals. The bronchospasm provoked in dogs by inhalation of histamine is reduced by pretreatment with an inhaled topical anesthetic agent, by transection of the vagus nerves, and by pretreatment with atropine. Studies of asthmatic humans, however, have shown that treatment with atropine causes only a reduction in—not abolition of—the bronchospastic responses to antigens and to nonantigenic stimuli. It is possible that activity in another neural pathway, such as the nonadrenergic, noncholinergic system, contributes to bronchomotor responses stimuli (Figure 20–2).

The hypothesis suggested by these studies—that asthmatic bronchospasm results from a combination of release of mediators and an exaggeration of responsiveness to their effects—predicts that asthma may be effectively treated by drugs with different modes of action. Asthmatic bronchospasm might be reversed or prevented, for example, by drugs that reduce the amount of IgE bound to mast cells (anti-IgE antibody), prevent mast cell degranulation (cromolyn or nedocromil, sympathomimetic agents, calcium channel blockers), block the action of the products released (antihistamines and leukotriene receptor antagonists), inhibit the effect of acetylcholine released from vagal motor nerves (muscarinic antagonists), or directly relax airway smooth muscle (sympathomimetic agents, theophylline).

The second approach to the treatment of asthma is aimed not only at preventing or reversing acute bronchospasm but at reducing the level of bronchial responsiveness. Because increased responsiveness appears to be linked to airway inflammation and because airway inflammation is a feature of late asthmatic responses, this strategy is implemented both by reducing exposure to the allergens that provoke inflammation and by prolonged therapy with anti-inflammatory agents, especially inhaled corticosteroids.

■ I. BASIC PHARMACOLOGY OF AGENTS USED IN THE TREATMENT OF ASTHMA

The drugs most used for management of asthma are adrenoceptor agonists, or sympathomimetic agents (used as "relievers" or bronchodilators) and inhaled corticosteroids (used as "controllers" or anti-inflammatory agents). Their basic pharmacology is presented elsewhere (see Chapters 9 and 39). In this chapter, we review their pharmacology relevant to asthma.

SYMPATHOMIMETIC AGENTS

The adrenoceptor agonists have several pharmacologic actions that are important in the treatment of asthma. They relax airway smooth muscle and inhibit release of bronchoconstricting mediators from mast cells. They may also inhibit microvascular leakage and increase mucociliary transport by increasing ciliary activity. As in other tissues, the β agonists stimulate adenylyl cyclase and increase the formation of intracellular cAMP (Figure 20–3).

The best-characterized action of the adrenoceptor agonists in the airways is relaxation of airway smooth muscle. Although there is no evidence for significant sympathetic innervation of human airway smooth muscle, ample evidence exists for the presence of adrenoceptors on airway smooth muscle. In general, stimulation of β_2 receptors relaxes airway smooth muscle, inhibits mediator release, and causes tachycardia and skeletal muscle tremor as side effects.

The sympathomimetic agents that have been widely used in the treatment of asthma include epinephrine, ephedrine, isoproterenol, and albuterol and other β_2-selective agents (Figure 20–4). Because epinephrine and isoproterenol increase the rate and force of cardiac contraction (mediated mainly by β_1 receptors), they are reserved for special situations (see below).

In general, adrenoceptor agonists are best delivered by inhalation because this results in the greatest local effect on airway smooth muscle with the least systemic toxicity. Aerosol deposition depends on the particle size, the pattern of breathing (tidal volume and rate of airflow), and the geometry of the airways. Even with particles in the optimal size range of 2–5 mm, 80–90% of the total dose of aerosol is deposited in the mouth or

Figure 20–3. Bronchodilation is promoted by cAMP. Intracellular levels of cAMP can be increased by β-adrenoceptor agonists, which increase the rate of its synthesis by adenylyl cyclase (AC); or by phosphodiesterase (PDE) inhibitors such as theophylline, which slow the rate of its degradation. Bronchoconstriction can be inhibited by muscarinic antagonists and possibly by adenosine antagonists.

Figure 20–4. Structures of isoproterenol and several β_2-selective analogs.

pharynx. Particles under 1–2 µm remain suspended and may be exhaled. Deposition can be increased by holding the breath in inspiration.

Epinephrine is an effective, rapidly acting bronchodilator when injected subcutaneously (0.4 mL of 1:1000 solution) or inhaled as a microaerosol from a pressurized canister (320 mcg per puff). Maximal bronchodilation is achieved 15 minutes after inhalation and lasts 60–90 minutes. Because epinephrine stimulates α and β_1 as well as β_2 receptors, tachycardia, arrhythmias, and worsening of angina pectoris are troublesome adverse effects. The cardiovascular effects of epinephrine are of value for treating the acute vasodilation and shock as well as the bronchospasm of anaphylaxis, but its use in asthma has been displaced by other, more β_2-selective agents.

Ephedrine was used in China for more than 2000 years before its introduction into Western medicine in 1924. Compared with epinephrine, ephedrine has a longer duration, oral activity, more pronounced central effects, and much lower potency. Because of the development of more efficacious and β_2-selective agonists, ephedrine is now used infrequently in treating asthma.

Isoproterenol is a potent bronchodilator; when inhaled as a microaerosol from a pressurized canister, 80–120 mcg isoproterenol causes maximal bronchodilation within 5 minutes. Isoproterenol has a 60- to 90-minute duration of action. An increase in the asthma mortality rate that occurred in the United Kingdom in the mid 1960s was attributed to cardiac arrhythmias resulting from the use of high doses of inhaled isoproterenol. It is now rarely used for asthma.

Beta2-Selective Drugs

The β_2-selective adrenoceptor agonist drugs are the most widely used sympathomimetics for the treatment of asthma at present (Figure 20–4). These agents differ structurally from epinephrine in having a larger substitution on the amino group and in the position of the hydroxyl groups on the aromatic ring. They are effective after inhaled or oral administration and have a long duration of action.

Albuterol, terbutaline, metaproterenol, and **pirbuterol** are available as metered-dose inhalers. Given by inhalation, these agents cause bronchodilation equivalent to that produced by isoproterenol. Bronchodilation is maximal within 15–30 minutes and persists for 3–4 hours. All can be diluted in saline for administration from a hand-held nebulizer. Because the particles generated by a nebulizer are much larger than those from a metered-dose inhaler, much higher doses must be given (2.5–5.0 mg vs 100–400 mcg) but are no more effective. Nebulized therapy should thus be reserved for patients unable to coordinate inhalation from a metered-dose inhaler.

Albuterol and terbutaline are also available in tablet form. One tablet two or three times daily is the usual regimen; the principal adverse effects of skeletal muscle tremor, nervousness, and occasional weakness may be reduced by starting the patient on half-strength tablets for the first 2 weeks of therapy, but this route of administration presents no advantage over inhaled treatment.

Of these agents, only terbutaline is available for subcutaneous injection (0.25 mg). The indications for this route are similar to those for subcutaneous epinephrine—severe asthma requiring emergency treatment when aerosolized therapy is not available or has been ineffective—but it should be remembered that terbutaline's longer duration of action means that cumulative effects may be seen after repeated injections.

A new generation of long-acting β_2-selective agonists includes **salmeterol** and **formoterol.** Both drugs are potent selective β_2 agonists that achieve their long duration of action (12 hours or more) as a result of high lipid solubility. This permits them to dissolve in the smooth muscle cell membrane in high concentrations or, possibly, attach to "mooring" molecules in the vicinity of the adrenoceptor. These drugs appear to interact with inhaled corticosteroids to improve asthma control. They are not recommended as the sole therapy for asthma.

Toxicities

The use of sympathomimetic agents by inhalation at first raised fears about possible cardiac arrhythmias and about hypoxemia acutely and tachyphylaxis or tolerance when given repeatedly. It is true that the vasodilating action of β_2-agonist treatment may increase perfusion of poorly ventilated lung units, transiently decreasing arterial oxygen tension (PaO_2). This effect is usually small, however, and may occur with any bronchodilator

drug; the significance of such an effect depends on the initial PaO_2 of the patient. Administration of supplemental oxygen, routine in treatment of an acute severe attack of asthma, eliminates any concern over this effect. The other concern, that β-agonist treatment may cause lethal cardiac arrhythmias appears unsubstantiated. In patients presenting for emergency treatment of severe asthma, irregularities in cardiac rhythm *improve* with the improvements in gas exchange effected by bronchodilator treatment.

The concept that β-agonist drugs cause worsening of clinical asthma by inducing tachyphylaxis to their own action remains unestablished. Most studies have shown only a small change in the bronchodilator response to β stimulation after prolonged treatment with β-agonist drugs, but some studies have shown a loss in the ability of β-agonist treatment to inhibit the response to subsequent challenge with exercise, methacholine, or antigen challenge (referred to as a loss of bronchoprotective action).

Fears that heavy use of β-agonist inhalers could actually increase morbidity and mortality have not been borne out by careful epidemiologic investigations. Heavy use most often indicates that the patient should be receiving more effective prophylactic therapy with corticosteroids.

Although it is true that β_2-adrenoceptor agonists appear to be safe and effective bronchodilators for most patients, there is some evidence that the risk of adverse effects from chronic treatment with long-acting β agonists may be greater for some individuals, possibly as a function of genetic variants for the β receptor. Two retrospective and one prospective study have shown differences between patients homozygous for glycine versus arginine at the B-16 locus of the β receptor. Among patients homozygous for arginine, a genotype found in 16% of the Caucasian population in the USA, but more commonly in African Americans, asthma control deteriorated with regular use of albuterol or salmeterol, whereas asthma control improved with this treatment among those homozygous for glycine at the same locus. These findings need to be replicated in larger studies, but it is tempting to speculate that a genetic variant may underlie the report of an increase in asthma mortality from regular use of a long-acting β agonist in studies involving very large numbers of patients.

METHYLXANTHINE DRUGS

The three important methylxanthines are **theophylline, theobromine,** and **caffeine.** Their major source is beverages (tea, cocoa, and coffee, respectively). The importance of theophylline as a therapeutic agent in the treatment of asthma has waned as the greater effectiveness of inhaled adrenoceptor agents for acute asthma and of inhaled anti-inflammatory agents for chronic asthma has been established, but theophylline's very low cost is an important advantage for economically disadvantaged patients in societies in which health care resources are limited.

Chemistry

As shown below, theophylline is 1,3-dimethylxanthine; theobromine is 3,7-dimethylxanthine; and caffeine is 1,3,7-trimethylxanthine. A theophylline preparation commonly used for therapeutic purposes is **aminophylline,** a theophylline-ethylenediamine complex. The pharmacokinetics of theophylline are discussed below (see Clinical Use of Methylxanthines). The metabolic products, partially demethylated xanthines (not uric acid), are excreted in the urine.

Xanthine

Theobromine

Caffeine

Theophylline

Mechanism of Action

Several mechanisms have been proposed for the actions of methylxanthines, but none has been firmly established. At high concentrations, they can be shown in vitro to inhibit several members of the phosphodiesterase (PDE) enzyme family (Figure 20–3). Because the phosphodiesterases hydrolyze cyclic nucleotides, this inhibition results in higher concentrations of intracellular cAMP and, in some tissues, cGMP. Cyclic AMP is responsible for a myriad of cellular functions including, but not limited to, stimulation of cardiac function, relaxation of smooth muscle, and reduction in the immune and inflammatory activity of specific cells.

Of the various isoforms of phosphodiesterase that have been identified, PDE4 appears to be the most directly involved in actions of methylxanthines on airway smooth muscle and on inflammatory cells. The inhibition of PDE4 in inflammatory cells reduces their release of cytokines and chemokines, which in turn results in a decrease in immune cell migration and activation.

In an effort to reduce toxicity while maintaining therapeutic efficacy, more selective inhibitors of different isoforms of PDE4 have been developed, particularly for the treatment of chronic obstructive pulmonary disease (COPD). Several are now in advanced stages of clinical development, (eg, **roflumilast, cilomilast, tofimilast**), but at the time of writing, none has been approved for clinical use by the FDA. Although several appear promising, none is entirely free of the major adverse effect of this class of drugs, nausea and vomiting.

Another proposed mechanism is inhibition of cell surface receptors for adenosine. These receptors modulate adenylyl cyclase activity, and adenosine has been shown to provoke contraction of isolated airway smooth muscle and histamine release from airway mast cells. It has been shown, however, that xanthine derivatives devoid of adenosine antagonism (eg, enprofylline) may be potent in inhibiting bronchoconstriction in asthmatic subjects.

Pharmacodynamics of Methylxanthines

The methylxanthines have effects on the central nervous system, kidney, and cardiac and skeletal muscle as well as smooth muscle. Of the three agents, theophylline is most selective in its smooth muscle effects, whereas caffeine has the most marked central nervous system effects.

A. CENTRAL NERVOUS SYSTEM EFFECTS

In low and moderate doses, the methylxanthines—especially caffeine—cause mild cortical arousal with increased alertness and deferral of fatigue. The caffeine contained in beverages—eg, 100 mg in a cup of coffee—is sufficient to cause nervousness and insomnia in sensitive individuals and slight bronchodilation in patients with asthma. The larger doses necessary for more effective bronchodilation commonly cause nervousness and tremor in some patients. Very high doses, from accidental or suicidal overdose, cause medullary stimulation and convulsions and may lead to death.

B. CARDIOVASCULAR EFFECTS

The methylxanthines have positive chronotropic and inotropic effects. At low concentrations, these effects appear to result from inhibition of presynaptic adenosine receptors in sympathetic nerves increasing catecholamine release at nerve endings. The higher concentrations (> 10 µmol/L, 2 mg/L) associated with inhibition of phosphodiesterase and increases in cAMP may result in increased influx of calcium. At much higher concentrations (> 100 µmol/L), sequestration of calcium by the sarcoplasmic reticulum is impaired.

The clinical expression of these effects on cardiovascular function varies among individuals. Ordinary consumption of coffee and other methylxanthine-containing beverages usually produces slight tachycardia, an increase in cardiac output, and an increase in peripheral resistance, raising blood pressure slightly. In sensitive individuals, consumption of a few cups of coffee may result in arrhythmias. In large doses, these agents also relax vascular smooth muscle except in cerebral blood vessels, where they cause contraction.

Methylxanthines decrease blood viscosity and may improve blood flow under certain conditions. The mechanism of this action is not well defined, but the effect is exploited in the treatment of intermittent claudication with **pentoxifylline,** a dimethylxanthine agent. However, no evidence suggests that this therapy is superior to other approaches.

C. EFFECTS ON GASTROINTESTINAL TRACT

The methylxanthines stimulate secretion of both gastric acid and digestive enzymes. However, even decaffeinated coffee has a potent stimulant effect on secretion, which means that the primary secretagogue in coffee is not caffeine.

D. EFFECTS ON KIDNEY

The methylxanthines—especially theophylline—are weak diuretics. This effect may involve both increased glomerular filtration and reduced tubular sodium reabsorption. The diuresis is not of sufficient magnitude to be therapeutically useful.

E. EFFECTS ON SMOOTH MUSCLE

The bronchodilation produced by the methylxanthines is the major therapeutic action in asthma. Tolerance does not develop, but adverse effects, especially in the central nervous system, may limit the dose (see below). In addition to their effect on airway smooth muscle, these agents—in sufficient concentration—inhibit antigen-induced release of histamine from lung tissue; their effect on mucociliary transport is unknown.

F. EFFECTS ON SKELETAL MUSCLE

The respiratory actions of the methylxanthines may not be confined to the airways, for they also strengthen the contractions of isolated skeletal muscle in vitro and improve contractility and reverse fatigue of the diaphragm in patients with COPD. This effect on diaphragmatic performance—rather than an effect on the respiratory center—may account for theophylline's ability to improve the ventilatory response to hypoxia and to diminish dyspnea even in patients with irreversible airflow obstruction.

Clinical Use of Methylxanthines

Of the xanthines, theophylline is the most effective bronchodilator, and it has been shown repeatedly both to relieve airflow obstruction in acute asthma and to reduce the severity of symptoms and time lost from work or school in patients with chronic asthma. Theophylline base is only slightly soluble in water, so it has been administered as several salts containing varying amounts of theophylline base. Most preparations are well absorbed from the gastrointestinal tract, but absorption of rectal suppositories is unreliable.

Improvements in theophylline preparations have come from alterations in the physical state of the drugs rather than from new chemical formulations. For example, the increased surface area of anhydrous theophylline in a microcrystalline form facilitates solubilization for complete and rapid absorption after oral administration. Numerous sustained-release preparations (see Preparations Available) are available and can produce therapeutic blood levels for 12 hours or more. These preparations offer the advantages of less frequent drug administration, less fluctuation of theophylline blood levels, and, in many cases, more effective treatment of nocturnal bronchospasm.

Theophylline should be used only where methods to measure theophylline blood levels are available because it has a narrow therapeutic window, and its therapeutic and toxic effects are related to its blood level. Improvement in pulmonary function is correlated with plasma concentration in the range of 5–20 mg/L. Anorexia, nausea, vomiting, abdominal discomfort, headache, and anxiety occur at concentrations of 15 mg/L in some patients and become common at concentrations greater than 20 mg/L. Higher levels (> 40 mg/L) may cause seizures or arrhythmias; these may not be preceded by gastrointestinal or neurologic warning symptoms.

The plasma clearance of theophylline varies widely. Theophylline is metabolized by the liver, so usual doses may lead to toxic concentrations of the drug in patients with liver disease. Conversely, clearance may be increased through the induction of hepatic enzymes by cigarette smoking or by changes in diet. In normal adults, the mean plasma clearance is 0.69 mL/kg/min. Children clear theophylline faster than adults (1–1.5 mL/kg/min). Neonates and young infants have the slowest clearance (see Chapter 60). Even when maintenance doses are altered to correct for the above factors, plasma concentrations vary widely.

Theophylline improves long-term control of asthma when taken as the sole maintenance treatment or when added to inhaled corticosteroids. It is inexpensive, and it can be taken orally. Its use, however, also requires occasional measurement of plasma levels; it often causes unpleasant minor side effects (especially insomnia); and accidental or intentional overdose can result in severe toxicity or death. For oral therapy with the prompt-release formulation, the usual dose is 3–4 mg/kg of theophylline every 6 hours. Changes in dosage result in a new steady-state concentration of theophylline in 1–2 days, so the dosage may be increased at intervals of 2–3 days until therapeutic plasma concentrations are achieved (10–20 mg/L) or until adverse effects develop.

ANTIMUSCARINIC AGENTS

Observation of the use of leaves from *Datura stramonium* for asthma treatment in India led to the discovery of atropine, a potent competitive inhibitor of acetylcholine at postganglionic "muscarinic" receptors, as a bronchodilator. Interest in the potential value of antimuscarinic agents increased with demonstration of the importance of the vagus nerves in bronchospastic responses of laboratory animals and by the development of a potent atropine analog that is poorly absorbed after aerosol administration and that is therefore relatively free of systemic atropine-like effects.

Mechanism of Action

Muscarinic antagonists competitively inhibit the effect of acetylcholine at muscarinic receptors (see Chapter 8). In the airways, acetylcholine is released from efferent endings of the vagus nerves, and muscarinic antagonists block the contraction of airway smooth muscle and the increase in secretion of mucus that occurs in response to vagal activity (Figure 20–2). Very high concentrations—well above those achieved even with maximal therapy—are required to inhibit the response of airway smooth muscle to nonmuscarinic stimulation. This selectivity of muscarinic antagonists accounts for their usefulness as investigative tools in examining the role of parasympathetic pathways in bronchomotor responses but limits their usefulness in preventing bronchospasm. In the doses given, antimuscarinic agents inhibit only that portion of the response mediated by muscarinic receptors, which varies by stimulus, and which further appears to vary among individuals in responses to the same stimulus.

Clinical Use of Muscarinic Antagonists

Antimuscarinic agents are effective bronchodilators. When given intravenously, atropine, the prototypical muscarinic antagonist, causes bronchodilation at a lower dose than that needed to cause an increase in heart rate. The selectivity of atropine's effect can be increased further by administering the drug by inhalation or by use of a more selective quaternary ammonium derivative of atropine, **ipratropium bromide.** Ipratropium can be delivered in high doses by this route because it is poorly absorbed into the circulation and does not readily enter the central nervous system. Studies with this agent have shown that the degree of involvement of parasympathetic pathways in broncho-

motor responses varies among subjects. In some, bronchoconstriction is inhibited effectively; in others, only modestly. The failure of higher doses of the muscarinic antagonist to further inhibit the response in these individuals indicates that mechanisms other than parasympathetic reflex pathways must be involved.

Even in the subjects least protected by this antimuscarinic agent, however, the bronchodilation and partial inhibition of provoked bronchoconstriction are of potential clinical value, and antimuscarinic agents are valuable for patients intolerant of inhaled β-agonist agents. Although antimuscarinic drugs appear to be slightly less effective than β-agonist agents in reversing asthmatic bronchospasm, the addition of ipratropium enhances the bronchodilation produced by nebulized albuterol in acute severe asthma.

Ipratropium appears to be at least as effective in patients with COPD that includes a partially reversible component. A longer-acting, selective antimuscarinic agent, **tiotropium,** is approved as a treatment for COPD. This drug is also taken by inhalation, and a single dose of 18 mcg has 24-hour duration of action. Daily inhalation of tiotropium has been shown not only to improve functional capacity of patients with COPD, but also to reduce the frequency of exacerbations of their condition.

CORTICOSTEROIDS

Mechanism of Action

Corticosteroids have been used to treat asthma since 1950 and are presumed to act by their broad anti-inflammatory efficacy, mediated in part by inhibition of production of inflammatory cytokines (see Chapter 39). They do not relax airway smooth muscle directly but reduce bronchial reactivity and reduce the frequency of asthma exacerbations if taken regularly. Their effect on airway obstruction may be due in part to their contraction of engorged vessels in the bronchial mucosa and their potentiation of the effects of β-receptor agonists, but their most important action is inhibition of the lymphocytic, eosinophilic mucosal inflammation of asthmatic airways.

Clinical Use of Corticosteroids

Clinical studies of corticosteroids consistently show them to be effective in improving all indices of asthma control—severity of symptoms, tests of airway caliber and bronchial reactivity, frequency of exacerbations, and quality of life. Because of severe adverse effects when given chronically, oral and parenteral corticosteroids are reserved for patients who require urgent treatment, ie, those who have not improved adequately with bronchodilators or who experience worsening symptoms despite maintenance therapy. Regular or "controller" therapy is maintained with aerosol corticosteroids.

Urgent treatment is often begun with an oral dose of 30–60 mg prednisone per day or an intravenous dose of 1 mg/kg methylprednisolone every 6 hours; the daily dose is decreased after airway obstruction has improved. In most patients, systemic corticosteroid therapy can be discontinued in a week or 10 days, but in other patients symptoms may worsen as the dose is decreased to lower levels. Because adrenal suppression by corticosteroids is related to dose and because secretion of endogenous corticosteroids has a diurnal variation, it is customary to administer corticosteroids early in the morning after endogenous ACTH secretion has peaked. For prevention of nocturnal asthma, however, oral or inhaled corticosteroids are most effective when given in the late afternoon.

Aerosol treatment is the most effective way to avoid the systemic adverse effects of corticosteroid therapy. The introduction of corticosteroids such as **beclomethasone, budesonide, flunisolide, fluticasone, mometasone,** and **triamcinolone** has made it possible to deliver corticosteroids to the airways with minimal systemic absorption. An average daily dose of four puffs twice daily of beclomethasone (400 mcg/d) is equivalent to about 10–15 mg/d of oral prednisone for the control of asthma, with far fewer systemic effects. Indeed, one of the cautions in switching patients from oral to inhaled corticosteroid therapy is to taper oral therapy slowly to avoid precipitation of adrenal insufficiency. In patients requiring continued prednisone treatment despite inhalation of standard doses of an aerosol corticosteroid, higher doses appear to be more effective; inhaled dosages up to 2000 mcg/d of fluticasone are effective in weaning patients from chronic prednisone therapy. Although these high doses of inhaled steroids may cause adrenal suppression, the risks of systemic toxicity from chronic use appear negligible compared with those of the oral corticosteroid therapy they replace.

A special problem caused by inhaled topical corticosteroids is the occurrence of oropharyngeal candidiasis. The risk of this complication can be reduced by having patients gargle water and spit after each inhaled treatment. Hoarseness can also result from a direct local effect of inhaled corticosteroids on the vocal cords. These agents are remarkably free of other short-term complications in adults but may increase the risks of osteoporosis and cataracts over the long term. In children, inhaled corticosteroid therapy has been shown to slow the rate of growth, but this effect appears to be transient: Asthma itself delays puberty, and there is no evidence that inhaled corticosteroid therapy in childhood influences adult height.

A novel approach to minimizing the risk of toxicity from systemic absorption of an inhaled corticosteroid underlay the development of **ciclesonide.** This investigational corticosteroid is inhaled as a prodrug activated by cleavage by esterases in bronchial epithelial cells. When absorbed into the circulation, the active product is tightly bound to serum proteins, and so has little access to glucocorticoid receptors in skin, eye, and bone, minimizing its risk of causing cutaneous thinning, cataracts, osteoporosis, or temporary slowing of growth.

Chronic use of inhaled corticosteroids effectively reduces symptoms and improves pulmonary function in patients with mild asthma. Such use also reduces or eliminates the need for oral corticosteroids in patients with more severe disease. In contrast to β-stimulant agents and theophylline, chronic use of inhaled corticosteroids reduces bronchial reactivity. Because of the efficacy and safety of inhaled corticosteroids, they are now routinely prescribed for patients who require more than occasional inhalations of a β agonist for relief of symptoms. This therapy is continued for 10–12 weeks and then withdrawn to determine whether more prolonged therapy is needed. Inhaled corticosteroids are not curative. In most patients, the manifestations of asthma return within a few weeks after stopping therapy even if they have been taken in high doses for 2 years or longer.

CROMOLYN & NEDOCROMIL

Cromolyn sodium (disodium cromoglycate) and nedocromil sodium are stable but extremely insoluble salts (see structures below). When used as aerosols (by nebulizer or metered-dose inhaler), they effectively inhibit both antigen- and exercise-induced asthma, and chronic use (four times daily) slightly reduces the overall level of bronchial reactivity. However, these drugs have no effect on airway smooth muscle tone and are ineffective in reversing asthmatic bronchospasm; they are only of value when taken prophylactically.

Cromolyn sodium

Nedocromil sodium

Cromolyn is poorly absorbed from the gastrointestinal tract and must be inhaled as a microfine powder or aerosolized solution. Nedocromil also has a very low bioavailability and is available only in metered-dose aerosol form.

Mechanism of Action

Cromolyn and nedocromil differ structurally but are thought to share a common mechanism of action: an alteration in the function of delayed chloride channels in the cell membrane, inhibiting cell activation. This action on airway nerves is thought to be responsible for nedocromil's inhibition of cough; on mast cells, for inhibition of the early response to antigen challenge; and on eosinophils, for inhibition of the inflammatory response to inhalation of allergens. The inhibitory effect on mast cells appears to be specific for cell type, since cromolyn has little inhibitory effect on mediator release from human basophils. It may also be specific for different organs, since cromolyn inhibits mast cell degranulation in human and primate lung but not in skin. This in turn may reflect known differences in mast cells found in different sites, as in their neutral protease content.

Until recently, the idea that cromolyn inhibits mast cell degranulation was so well accepted that the inhibition of a response by cromolyn was thought to indicate the involvement of mast cells in the response. This simplistic idea has been overturned in part by the finding that cromolyn and nedocromil inhibit the function of cells other than mast cells and in part by the finding that nedocromil inhibits appearance of the late response even when given after the early response to antigen challenge, ie, after mast cell degranulation has occurred.

Clinical Use of Cromolyn & Nedocromil

In short-term clinical trials, pretreatment with cromolyn or nedocromil blocks the bronchoconstriction caused by allergen inhalation, by exercise, by sulfur dioxide, and by a variety of causes of occupational asthma. This acute protective effect of a single treatment makes cromolyn useful for administration shortly before exercise or before unavoidable exposure to an allergen.

When taken regularly (two to four puffs two to four times daily) by patients with perennial (nonseasonal) asthma, both agents modestly but significantly reduce symptomatic severity and the need for bronchodilator medications. These drugs are neither as potent nor as predictably effective as inhaled corticosteroids. In general, young patients with extrinsic asthma are most likely to respond favorably. At present, the only way of determining whether a patient will respond is by a therapeutic trial for 4 weeks. The addition of nedocromil to a standard dose of an inhaled corticosteroid appears to improve asthma control.

Cromolyn solution is also useful in reducing symptoms of **allergic rhinoconjunctivitis.** Applying the solution by nasal spray or eye drops several times a day is effective in about 75% of patients, even during the peak pollen season.

Because the drugs are so poorly absorbed, adverse effects of cromolyn and nedocromil are minor and are localized to the sites of deposition. These include such minor symptoms as throat irritation, cough, and mouth dryness, and, rarely, chest tightness, and wheezing. Some of these symptoms can be prevented by inhaling a β_2-adrenoceptor agonist before cromolyn or nedocromil treatment. Serious adverse effects are rare. Reversible dermatitis, myositis, or gastroenteritis occurs in less than 2% of patients, and a very few cases of pulmonary infiltration with eosinophilia and anaphylaxis have been reported. This lack of toxicity accounts for cromolyn's widespread use in children, especially those at ages of rapid growth. For children who have difficulty coordinating the use of the inhaler device, cromolyn may be given by aerosol of a 1% solution.

LEUKOTRIENE PATHWAY INHIBITORS

Because of the evidence of leukotriene involvement in many inflammatory diseases (see Chapter 18) and in anaphylaxis, considerable effort has been expended on the development of drugs that block the synthesis of these arachidonic acid derivatives or their receptors. Leukotrienes result from the action of 5-lipoxygenase on arachidonic acid and are synthesized by a variety of inflammatory cells in the airways, including eosinophils, mast cells, macrophages, and basophils. Leukotriene B_4 (LTB_4) is a potent neutrophil chemoattractant, and LTC_4 and LTD_4 exert many effects known to occur in asthma, including bronchoconstriction, increased bronchial reactivity, mucosal edema, and mucus hypersecretion. Early studies established that antigen challenge of sensitized human lung tissue results in the generation of leukotrienes, whereas other studies of human subjects have shown that inhalation of leukotrienes causes not only bronchoconstriction but also an increase in bronchial reactivity to histamine that persists for several days.

Two approaches to interrupting the leukotriene pathway have been pursued: inhibition of 5-lipoxygenase, thereby preventing leukotriene synthesis; and inhibition of the binding of LTD_4 to its receptor on target tissues, thereby preventing its action. Efficacy in blocking airway responses to exercise and to antigen challenge has been shown for drugs in both categories: **zileuton,** a 5-lipoxygenase inhibitor, and **zafirlukast** and **montelukast,** LTD_4-receptor antagonists. All have been shown to improve asthma control and to reduce the frequency of asthma exacerbations in outpatient clinical trials. Their effects on symptoms, airway caliber, bronchial reactivity, and airway inflammation are less marked than the effects of inhaled corticosteroids, but they are more nearly equal in reducing the frequency of exacerbations. Their principal advantage is that they are taken orally; some patients—especially children—comply poorly with inhaled therapies. Montelukast is approved for children as young as 6 years of age.

Zafirlukast

Montelukast

Zileuton

Some patients appear to have particularly favorable responses, but no clinical features allow identification of "responders" before a trial of therapy. In the USA, zileuton is approved for use in an oral dosage of 400–800 mg for administration 2–4 times daily; zafirlukast, 20 mg twice daily; and montelukast, 10 mg (for adults) or 4 mg (for children) once daily.

Trials with leukotriene inhibitors have demonstrated an important role for leukotrienes in aspirin-induced asthma. It has long been known that 5–10% of asthmatics are exquisitely sensitive to aspirin, so that ingestion of even a very small dose causes profound bronchoconstriction and symptoms of systemic release of histamine, such as flushing and abdominal cramping. Because this reaction to aspirin is not associated with any evidence of allergic sensitization to aspirin or its metabolites and because it is produced by any of the nonsteroidal anti-inflammatory agents, it is thought to result from inhibition of prostaglandin synthetase (cyclooxygenase), shifting arachidonic acid metabolism from the prostaglandin to the leukotriene pathway. Support for this idea was provided by the demonstra-

tion that leukotriene pathway inhibitors impressively reduce the response to aspirin challenge and improve overall control of asthma on a day-to-day basis.

Of these agents, zileuton is the least prescribed because of the former requirement of four-times-daily dosing (a formulation for twice-daily use has recently been developed) and because of occasional liver toxicity. The receptor antagonists appear to be safe to use. Reports of Churg-Strauss syndrome (a systemic vasculitis accompanied by worsening asthma, pulmonary infiltrates, and eosinophilia) appear to have been coincidental, with the syndrome unmasked by the reduction in prednisone dosage made possible by the addition of zafirlukast or montelukast.

OTHER DRUGS IN THE TREATMENT OF ASTHMA

Anti-IgE Monoclonal Antibodies

An entirely new approach to the treatment of asthma exploits advances in molecular biology to target IgE antibody. From a collection of monoclonal antibodies raised in mice against IgE antibody itself, a monoclonal antibody was selected that appeared to be targeted against the portion of IgE that binds to its receptors (FCe-R1 and FCe-R2 receptors) on mast cells and other inflammatory cells. **Omalizumab** (an anti-IgE monoclonal antibody) inhibits the binding of IgE to mast cells but does not activate IgE already bound to these cells and thus does not provoke mast cell degranulation. It may also inhibit IgE synthesis by B lymphocytes. The murine antibody has been genetically humanized by replacing all but a small fraction of its amino acids with those found in human proteins, and it does not appear to cause sensitization when given to human subjects.

Studies of omalizumab in asthmatic volunteers showed that its administration over 10 weeks lowered plasma IgE to undetectable levels and significantly reduced the magnitude of both the early and the late bronchospastic responses to antigen challenge. Clinical trials have shown that repeated intravenous or subcutaneous injection of anti-IgE MAb lessens asthma severity and reduces the corticosteroid requirement in patients with moderate to severe disease, especially those with a clear environmental antigen precipitating factor, and improves nasal and conjunctival symptoms in patients with perennial or seasonal allergic rhinitis. Omalizumab's most important effect is reduction of the frequency and severity of asthma exacerbations, even while enabling a reduction in corticosteroid requirements. Combined analysis of several clinical trials has shown that the patients most likely to respond are, fortunately, those with the greatest need, ie, patients with a history of repeated exacerbations, a high requirement for corticosteroid treatment, and poor pulmonary function.

Similarly, the exacerbations most prevented are the ones most important to prevent: Omalizumab treatment reduced exacerbations requiring hospitalization by 88%. These benefits justify the high cost of this treatment in selected individuals with severe disease characterized by frequent exacerbations.

Possible Future Therapies

The rapid advance in the scientific description of the immunopathogenesis of asthma has spurred the development of many new therapies targeting different sites in the immune cascade. These include monoclonal antibodies directed against cytokines (IL-4, IL-5, IL-13), antagonists of cell adhesion molecules, protease inhibitors, and immunomodulators aimed at shifting CD4 lymphocytes from the TH2 to the TH1 phenotype or at selective inhibition of the subset of TH2 lymphocytes directed against particular antigens. There is evidence that asthma may be aggravated—or even caused—by chronic airway infection with *Chlamydia pneumoniae* or *Mycoplasma pneumoniae*. This may explain the reports of benefit from treatment with macrolide antibiotics and, if confirmed, would stimulate the development of new diagnostic methods and antimicrobial therapies.

■ II. CLINICAL PHARMACOLOGY OF DRUGS USED IN THE TREATMENT OF ASTHMA

Asthma is best thought of as a disease in two time domains. In the present domain, it is important for the distress it causes—cough, nocturnal awakenings, and shortness of breath that interferes with the ability to exercise or to pursue desired activities. For mild asthma, occasional inhalation of a bronchodilator may be all that is needed. For more severe asthma, treatment with a long-term controller, like an inhaled corticosteroid, is necessary to relieve symptoms and restore function. The second domain of asthma is the risk it presents of future events, such as exacerbations, or of progressive loss of pulmonary function. A patient's satisfaction with his or her ability to control symptoms and maintain function by frequent use of an inhaled β_2 agonist does not mean that the risk of future events is also controlled. In fact, use of two or more canisters of an inhaled β agonist per month is a marker of increased risk of asthma fatality.

The challenges of assessing severity and adjusting therapy for these two domains of asthma are different. For relief of distress in the present domain, the key information can be obtained by asking specific questions about the frequency and severity of symptoms, the frequency of use of an inhaled β_2 agonist for relief of symptoms, the frequency of nocturnal awakenings, and the ability to exercise. Estimating the risk for future exacerbations is more difficult. In general, patients with poorly controlled symptoms in the present have a heightened risk of exacerbations in the future, but some patients seem unaware of the severity of their underlying airflow obstruction (sometimes described as "poor perceivers") and can be identified only by measurement of pulmonary function, as by spirometry. Reductions in the FEV_1 correlate with heightened risk of attacks of asthma in the future. Other possible markers of heightened risk are unstable pulmonary function (large variations in FEV_1 from visit to visit, large change with bronchodilator treatment), extreme bronchial reactivity, or high numbers of eosinophils in sputum or of nitric oxide in exhaled air. Assessment of these features may identify patients who need increases in therapy for protection against exacerbations.

BRONCHODILATORS

Bronchodilators, such as inhaled albuterol, are rapidly effective, safe, and inexpensive. Patients with only occasional symptoms of asthma require no more than an inhaled β_2-receptor agonist taken on an as-needed basis. If symptoms require this "rescue" therapy more than twice a week, if nocturnal symptoms occur more than twice a month, or if the FEV_1 is less than 80% predicted, additional treatment is needed. The treatment first recommended is a low dose of an inhaled corticosteroid, although treatment with a leukotriene receptor antagonist or with cromolyn may be used. Theophylline is now largely reserved for patients in whom symptoms remain poorly controlled despite the combination of regular treatment with an inhaled anti-inflammatory agent and as-needed use of a β_2 agonist. If the addition of theophylline fails to improve symptoms or if adverse effects become bothersome, it is important to check the plasma level of theophylline to be sure it is in the therapeutic range (10–20 mg/L).

An important caveat for patients with mild asthma is that although the risk of a severe, life-threatening attack is lower than in patients with severe asthma, it is not zero. All patients with asthma should be instructed in a simple action plan for severe, frightening attacks: to take up to four puffs of albuterol every 20 minutes over 1 hour. If they do not note clear improvement after the first four puffs, they should take the additional treatments while on their way to an Emergency Department or some other higher level of care.

MUSCARINIC ANTAGONISTS

Inhaled muscarinic antagonists have so far earned a limited place in the treatment of asthma. When adequate doses are given, their effect on baseline airway resistance is nearly as great as that of the sympathomimetic drugs. The airway effects of antimuscarinic and sympathomimetic drugs given in full doses have been shown to be additive only in patients with severe airflow obstruction who present for emergency care. Antimuscarinic agents appear to be of greater value in COPD—perhaps more so than in asthma. They are also useful as alternative therapies for patients intolerant of β_2-adrenoceptor agonists.

Although it was predicted that muscarinic antagonists would dry airway secretions and interfere with mucociliary clearance, direct measurements of fluid volume secretion from single airway submucosal glands in animals show that atropine decreases baseline secretory rates only slightly. The drugs do, however, inhibit the increase in mucus secretion caused by vagal stimulation. No cases of inspissation of mucus have been reported following administration of these drugs.

CORTICOSTEROIDS

If asthmatic symptoms occur frequently or if significant airflow obstruction persists despite bronchodilator therapy, inhaled corticosteroids should be started. For patients with severe symptoms or severe airflow obstruction (eg, $FEV_1 < 50\%$ predicted), initial treatment with a combination of inhaled and oral corticosteroid (eg, 30 mg/d of prednisone for 3 weeks) treatment is appropriate. Once clinical improvement is noted, usually after 7–10 days, the oral dose should be discontinued or reduced to the minimum necessary to control symptoms.

An issue for inhaled corticosteroid treatment is patient compliance. Analysis of prescription renewals shows that corticosteroids are taken regularly by a minority of patients. This may be a function of a general "steroid phobia" fostered by emphasis in the lay press over the hazards of long-term oral corticosteroid therapy and by ignorance over the difference between corticosteroids and anabolic steroids, taken to enhance muscle strength by now-infamous athletes. This fear of corticosteroid toxicity makes it hard to persuade patients whose symptoms have improved after starting the treatment that they should continue it for protection against attacks. This context accounts for the interest in a recent report that instructing patients with mild but persistent asthma to initiate inhaled corticosteroid therapy only when their symptoms worsened was as effective in maintaining pulmonary function and preventing attacks as taking it twice each day.

In patients with more severe asthma, whose symptoms are inadequately controlled by a standard dose of an inhaled corticosteroid, two options may be considered: to double the dose of inhaled corticosteroid or to add a *long-acting* inhaled β_2-receptor agonist (salmeterol or formoterol). Many studies have shown this combination therapy to be more effective than doubling the dose of the inhaled corticosteroid, but the FDA has issued a warning that the use of a long-acting β agonist is associated with a very small but statistically significant increase in the risk of death or near death from an asthma attack, especially in African Americans. This warning has not so far had much effect on prescriptions for a fixed-dose combination of inhaled fluticasone (a corticosteroid) and salmeterol (a long-acting β agonist), probably because their combination in a single inhaler offers several advantages. Combination inhalers are convenient; they ensure that the long-acting β agonist will not be taken as monotherapy (known not to protect against attacks); and they produce prompt, sustained improvements in clinical symptoms and pulmonary function and reduce the frequency of exacerbations requiring oral corticosteroid treatment. In patients prescribed such combination treatment, it is important to provide explicit instructions that a standard, short-acting inhaled β_2 agonist, such as albuterol, be used as needed for relief of acute symptoms.

CROMOLYN & NEDOCROMIL; LEUKOTRIENE ANTAGONISTS

Cromolyn or nedocromil by inhalation, or a leukotriene-receptor antagonist as an oral tablet, may be considered as alternatives to inhaled corticosteroid treatment in patients with symptoms occurring more than twice a week or who are wakened from sleep by asthma more than twice a month. Neither treatment is as effective as even a low dose of an inhaled corticosteroid, but both prevent the issue of "steroid phobia" described above.

Cromolyn and nedocromil may also be useful in patients whose symptoms occur seasonally or after clear-cut inciting stimuli such as exercise or exposure to animal danders or irritants. In patients whose symptoms are continuous or occur without an obvious inciting stimulus, the value of these drugs can be established only with a therapeutic trial of inhaled drug four times a day for 4 weeks. If the patient responds to this therapy, the dose can then be optimized.

Treatment with a leukotriene-receptor antagonist, particularly montelukast, is widely prescribed, especially by primary care providers. Taken orally, leukotriene-receptor antagonists are easy to use and appear to be taken more regularly than inhaled corticosteroids. They are rarely associated with troublesome side effects. Maintenance therapy with a leukotriene antagonist or with cromolyn or nedocromil appears to be roughly as effective as maintenance therapy with theophylline. Because of concerns over the possible long-term toxicity of systemic absorption of inhaled corticosteroids, this maintenance therapy has become widely used for treating children in the USA.

ANTI-IgE MONOCLONAL ANTIBODY

Treatment with omalizumab, the monoclonal humanized anti-IgE antibody, is reserved for patients with chronic severe asthma inadequately controlled by high-dose inhaled corticosteroid plus long-acting β-agonist combination treatment (eg, fluticasone 500 mcg plus salmeterol 50 mcg inhaled twice daily). This treatment reduces lymphocytic, eosinophilic bronchial inflammation and effectively reduces the frequency and severity of exacerbations. It is reserved for patients with demonstrated IgE-mediated sensitivity (by positive skin test or radioallergosorbent test [RAST] to common allergens) and an IgE level within a range that can be reduced sufficiently by twice weekly subcutaneous injection.

OTHER ANTI-INFLAMMATORY THERAPIES

Some reports suggest that agents commonly used to treat rheumatoid arthritis may also be used to treat patients with chronic steroid-dependent asthma. The development of an alternative treatment is important, because chronic treatment with oral corticosteroids may cause osteoporosis, cataracts, glucose intolerance, worsening of hypertension, and cushingoid changes in appearance. Initial studies suggested that oral methotrexate or gold salt injections were beneficial in prednisone-dependent asthmatics, but subsequent studies did not confirm this promise. In contrast, the benefit from treatment with cyclosporine seems real. However, this drug's great toxicity makes this finding only a source of hope that other immunomodulatory therapies will ultimately be developed for the small proportion of patients whose asthma can be managed only with high oral doses of prednisone. An immunomodulatory therapy recently reported to improve asthma is injection of etanercept, a TNF-α antagonist used for treatment of ankylosing spondylitis and severe rheumatoid arthritis.

MANAGEMENT OF ACUTE ASTHMA

The treatment of acute attacks of asthma in patients reporting to the hospital requires close, continuous clinical assessment and repeated objective measurement of lung function. For patients with mild attacks, inhalation of a β$_2$-receptor agonist is as effective as subcutaneous injection of epinephrine. Both of these treatments are more effective than intravenous administration of aminophylline (a soluble salt of theophylline). Severe attacks require treatment with oxygen, frequent or continuous administration of aerosolized albuterol, and systemic treatment with prednisone or methylprednisolone (0.5 mg/kg every 6 hours). Even this aggressive treatment is not invariably effective, and patients must be watched closely for signs of deterioration. General anesthesia, intubation, and mechanical ventilation of asthmatic patients cannot be undertaken lightly but may be lifesaving if respiratory failure supervenes.

PROSPECTS FOR PREVENTION

The high prevalence of asthma in the developed world and its rapid increases in the developing world call for a strategy for primary prevention. Strict antigen avoidance during infancy, once thought to be sensible, has now been shown to be ineffective. In fact, growing up in a household where cats and dogs are kept as pets may *protect* against developing asthma. The best hope seems to lie in understanding the importance of microbial exposures during infancy in shaping a balanced immune response, and one study showing that feeding *Lactobacillus caseii* to infants born to allergic parents reduced the rate of allergic dermatitis at age 2 years offers reason for hope.

Chapter continues on next page.

PREPARATIONS AVAILABLE

Sympathomimetics Used in Asthma

Albuterol (generic, Proventil, Ventolin)
Inhalant: 90 mcg/puff aerosol; 0.083, 0.5, 0.63% solution for nebulization
Oral: 2, 4 mg tablets; 2 mg/5 mL syrup
Oral sustained-release: 4, 8 mg tablets

Albuterol/Ipratropium (Combivent, DuoNeb)
Inhalant: 103 mcg albuterol + 18 mcg ipratropium/ puff; 3 mg albuterol + 0.5 mg ipratropium/3 mL solution for nebulization

Bitolterol (Tornalate)
Inhalant: 0.2% solution for nebulization

Ephedrine (generic)
Oral: 25 mg capsules
Parenteral: 50 mg/mL for injection

Epinephrine (generic, Adrenalin)
Inhalant: 1, 10 mg/mL for nebulization; 0.22 mg/spray epinephrine base aerosol
Parenteral: 1:10,000 (0.1 mg/mL), 1:1000 (1 mg/mL)

Formoterol (Foradil)
Inhalant: 12 mcg/unit inhalant powder

Isoetharine (generic)
Inhalant: 1% solution for nebulization

Isoproterenol (generic, Isuprel)
Inhalant: 0.5, 1% for nebulization; 80, 131 mcg/puff aerosols
Parenteral: 0.02, 0.2 mg/mL for injection

Levalbuterol (Xenopex)
Inhalant: 0.31, 0.63, 1.25 mg/3 mL solution

Metaproterenol (Alupent, generic)
Inhalant: 0.65 mg/puff aerosol in 7, 14 g containers; 0.4, 0.6, 5% for nebulization

Pirbuterol (Maxair)
Inhalant: 0.2 mg/puff aerosol in 80 and 300 dose containers

Salmeterol (Serevent)
Inhalant aerosol: 25 mcg salmeterol base/puff in 60 and 120 dose containers
Inhalant powder: 50 mcg/unit

Salmeterol/Fluticasone (Advair Diskus)
Inhalant: 100, 250, 500 mcg fluticasone + 50 mcg salmeterol/unit

Terbutaline (generic, Brethine)
Oral: 2.5, 5 mg tablets
Parenteral: 1 mg/mL for injection

Aerosol Corticosteroids (see also Chapter 39.)

Beclomethasone (QVAR)
Aerosol: 40, 80 mcg/puff in 100 dose containers

Budesonide (Pulmicort)
Aerosol powder (Turbuhaler): 160 mcg/activation
Inhalation suspension (Respules): 0.25, 0.5 mg/2 mL

Flunisolide (AeroBid, Aerospan)
Aerosol: 80, 250 mcg/puff in 80, 100, and 120 dose containers

Fluticasone (Flovent)
Aerosol: 44, 110, and 220 mcg/puff in 120 dose container; powder, 50, 100, 250 mcg/activation

Fluticasone/Salmeterol (Advair Diskus)
Inhalant: 100, 250, 500 mcg fluticasone + 50 mcg salmeterol/unit

Mometasone (Asmanex Twisthaler)
Inhalant: 220 mcg/actuation in 14, 30, 60, 120 dose units

Triamcinolone (Azmacort)
Aerosol: 100 mcg/puff in 240 dose container

Leukotriene Inhibitors

Montelukast (Singulair)
Oral: 10 mg tablets; 4, 5 mg chewable tablets; 4 mg/packet granules

Zafirlukast (Accolate)
Oral: 10, 20 mg tablets

Zileuton (Zyflo)
Oral: 600 mg tablets

Cromolyn Sodium & Nedocromil Sodium

Cromolyn sodium
Pulmonary aerosol (generic, Intal): 800 mcg/puff in 200 dose container; 20 mg/2 mL for nebulization (for asthma)
Nasal aerosol (Nasalcrom): 5.2 mg/puff (for hay fever)
Oral (Gastrocrom): 100 mg/5 mL concentrate (for gastrointestinal allergy)

Nedocromil sodium (Tilade)
Pulmonary aerosol: 1.75 mg/puff in 104 metered-dose container

Methylxanthines: Theophylline & Derivatives

Aminophylline (theophylline ethylenediamine, 79% theophylline) (generic)
Oral: 105 mg/5 mL liquid; 100, 200 mg tablets
Rectal: 250, 500 mg suppositories
Parenteral: 250 mg/10 mL for injection

(continued)

Theophylline (generic, Elixophyllin, Slo-Phyllin, Uniphyl, Theo-Dur, Theo-24, others)
Oral: 100, 125, 200, 250, 300 mg tablets; 100, 200 mg capsules; 26.7, 50 mg/5 mL elixirs, syrups, and solutions
Oral sustained-release, 8–12 hours: 50, 60, 75, 100, 125, 200, 250, 300 mg capsules
Oral sustained-release, 8–24 hours: 100, 200, 300, 450 mg tablets
Oral timed-release, 12 hours: 125, 130, 250, 260, 300 mg capsules
Oral timed-release, 12–24 hours: 100, 200, 300 tablets
Oral timed-release, 24 hours: 100, 200, 300 mg tablets and capsules; 400, 600 mg tablets
Parenteral: 200, 400, 800 mg/container, theophylline and 5% dextrose for injection

OTHER METHYLXANTHINES
Dyphylline (generic)
Oral: 200, 400 mg tablets; 33.3 mg/5 mL elixir

Oxtriphylline (generic, Choledyl)
Oral: equivalent to 64, 127, 254, 382 mg theophylline tablets; 32, 64 mg/5 mL syrup
Pentoxifylline (generic, Trental)
Oral: 400 mg tablets and controlled-release tablets
Note: Pentoxifylline is labeled for use in intermittent claudication only.

ANTIMUSCARINIC DRUGS USED IN ASTHMA
Ipratropium (generic, Atrovent)
Aerosol: 17 (freon-free), 18 mcg/puff in 200 metered-dose inhaler; 0.02% (500 mcg/vial) for nebulization
Nasal spray: 21, 42 mcg/spray
Tiotropium (Spiriva)
Aerosol: 18 mcg/puff in 6 packs

ANTIBODY
Omalizumab (Xolair)
Powder for SC injection, 202.5 mg

REFERENCES

Pathophysiology of Airway Disease

Mazzone SB, Canning BJ: Central nervous system control of the airways: Pharmacological implications. Curr Opin Pharmacol 2002;2:220.

Spina D, Page CP: Pharmacology of airway irritability. Curr Opin Pharmacol 2002;2:264.

Methylxanthines

Nakano J et al: Aminophilline suppresses the release of chemical mediators in treatment of acute asthma. Respir Med 2006;100:542.

Page CP: Recent advances in our understanding of the use of theophylline in the treatment of asthma. J Clin Pharmacol 1999;39:237.

Cromolyn & Nedocromil

Guevara J et al: Inhaled corticosteroids versus sodium cromoglycate in children and adults with asthma. Cochrane Database Syst Rev 2006;2:CD003558.

Yoshihara S et al: Effects of early intervention with inhaled sodium cromoglycate in childhood asthma. Lung 2006;184:63.

Corticosteroids

Boushey HA et al: Daily versus as-needed corticosteroids for mild persistent asthma. N Engl J Med 2005;352:1519.

Suissa S et al: Low-dose inhaled corticosteroids and the prevention of death from asthma. N Engl J Med 2000;343:332.

Wilson AM et al: Anti-inflammatory effects of once daily low dose inhaled ciclesonide in mild to moderate asthmatic patients. Allergy 2006;61:537.

Beta Agonists

Kelly HW, Harkins MS, Boushey H: The role of inhaled long-acting beta-2 agonists in the management of asthma. J Natl Med Assoc 2006;98:8.

Maneechotesuwan K et al: Formoterol attenuates neutrophilic airway inflammation in asthma. Chest 2005;128:1936.

Antimuscarinic Drugs

Lee AM, Jacoby DB, Fryer AD: Selective muscarinic receptor antagonists for airway diseases. Curr Opin Pharmacol 2001;1:223.

Leukotriene Pathway Inhibitors

Biernacki WA et al: Effect of montelukast on exhaled leukotrienes and quality of life in asthmatic patients. Chest 2005;128:1958.

Calhoun WJ: Anti-leukotrienes for asthma. Curr Opin Pharmacol 2001;1:230.

Krawiec ME, Wenzel SE: Leukotriene inhibitors and non-steroidal therapies in the treatment of asthma. Exp Opin Invest Drugs 2001;2:47.

Other Drugs For Asthma

Barnes J: Novel signal transduction modulators for the treatment of airway diseases. Pharmacol Ther 2006;109:238.

Bryan SA et al: Novel therapy for asthma. Exp Opin Invest Drugs 2000;9:25.

Leckie MJ et al: Effects of an interleukin-5 blocking monoclonal antibody on eosinophils, airway hyper-responsiveness, and the late asthmatic response. Lancet 2000;456:2144.

Lock SH et al: Double-blind, placebo-controlled study of cyclosporin A as a corticosteroid-sparing agent in corticosteroid-dependent asthma. Am J Respir Crit Care Med 1996;153:509.

Patacchini R, Maggi CA: Peripheral tachykinin receptors as targets for new drugs. Eur J Pharmacol 2001;429:13.

Walker S et al: Anti-IgE for chronic asthma in adults and children. Cochrane Database Syst Rev 2006;2:CD003559.

Clinical Management Of Airway Disease

Barnes PJ: Drugs for asthma. Br J Pharmacol 2006;147(Suppl 1):S297.

Tattersfield AE et al: Asthma. Lancet 2002;360:1313.

SECTION V
Drugs That Act in the Central Nervous System

Introduction to the Pharmacology of CNS Drugs

Roger A. Nicoll, MD

Drugs acting in the central nervous system (CNS) were among the first to be discovered by primitive humans and are still the most widely used group of pharmacologic agents. In addition to their use in therapy, many drugs acting on the CNS are used without prescription to increase one's sense of well-being.

The mechanisms by which various drugs act in the CNS have not always been clearly understood. In the last three decades, however, dramatic advances have been made in the methodology of CNS pharmacology. It is now possible to study the action of a drug on individual cells and even single ion channels within synapses. The information obtained from such studies is the basis for several major developments in studies of the CNS.

First, it is clear that nearly all drugs with CNS effects act on specific receptors that modulate synaptic transmission. A very few agents such as general anesthetics and alcohol may have nonspecific actions on membranes (although these exceptions are not fully accepted), but even these nonreceptor-mediated actions result in demonstrable alterations in synaptic transmission.

Second, drugs are among the most important tools for studying all aspects of CNS physiology, from the mechanism of convulsions to the laying down of long-term memory. As described below, agonists that mimic natural transmitters (and in many cases are more selective than the endogenous substances) and antagonists are extremely useful in such studies. The Box, Natural Toxins: Tools for Characterizing Ion Channels, describes a few of these substances.

Third, unraveling the actions of drugs with known clinical efficacy has led to some of the most fruitful hypotheses regarding the mechanisms of disease. For example, information on the action of antipsychotic drugs on dopamine receptors has provided the basis for important hypotheses regarding the pathophysiology of schizophrenia. Studies of the effects of a variety of agonists and antagonists on γ-aminobutyric acid (GABA) receptors has resulted in new concepts pertaining to the pathophysiology of several diseases, including anxiety and epilepsy.

This chapter provides an introduction to the functional organization of the CNS and its synaptic transmitters as a basis for understanding the actions of the drugs described in the following chapters.

NATURAL TOXINS: TOOLS FOR CHARACTERIZING ION CHANNELS

Evolution is tireless in the development of natural toxins. A vast number of variations are possible with even a small number of amino acids in peptides, and peptides make up only one of a broad array of toxic compounds. For example, the predatory marine snail genus *Conus* is estimated to include at least 500 different species. Each species kills or paralyzes its prey with a venom that contains 50–200 different peptides or proteins. Furthermore, there is little duplication of peptides among *Conus* species. Other animals with useful toxins include snakes, frogs, spiders, bees, wasps, and scorpions. Plant species with toxic (or therapeutic) substances are too numerous to mention here; they are referred to in many chapters of this book.

Since many toxins act on ion channels, they provide a wealth of chemical tools for studying the function of these channels. In fact, much of our current understanding of the properties of ion channels comes from studies utilizing only a small percentage of the highly potent and selective toxins that are now available. The toxins typically target voltage-sensitive ion channels, but a number of very useful toxins block ionotropic neurotransmitter receptors. Table 21–1 lists some of the toxins most commonly used in research, their mode of action, and their source.

Methods for the Study of CNS Pharmacology

Like many areas of science, major progress in the study of CNS drugs has depended on the development of new experimental techniques. The first detailed description of synaptic transmission was made possible by the invention of glass microelectrodes, which permit intracellular recording. The development of the brain slice technique permitted an analysis of the physiology and pharmacology of synapses. Detailed electrophysiologic studies of the action of drugs on both voltage- and transmitter-operated channels were further facilitated by the introduction of the patch clamp technique, which permits the recording of current through single channels. Histochemical, immunologic, and radioisotopic methods have made it possible to map the distribution of specific transmitters, their associated enzyme systems, and their receptors. Molecular cloning has had a major impact on our understanding of CNS receptors. These techniques make it possible to determine the precise molecular structure of the receptors and their associated channels. Finally, mice with mutated genes for specific receptors or enzymes (knockout mice) can provide important information regarding the physiologic and pharmacologic roles of these components.

ION CHANNELS & NEUROTRANSMITTER RECEPTORS

The membranes of nerve cells contain two types of channels defined on the basis of the mechanisms controlling their gating (opening and closing): **voltage-gated** and **ligand-gated** channels (Figure 21–1A and B). Voltage-gated channels respond to changes in the membrane potential of the cell. The voltage-gated sodium channel described in Chapter 14 for the heart is an example of the first type of channel. In nerve cells, these channels are concentrated on the initial segment and the axon and are responsible for the fast action potential, which transmits the signal from cell body to nerve terminal. There are many types of voltage-sensitive calcium and potassium channels on the cell body, dendrites, and initial segment, which act on a much slower time scale and modulate the rate at which the neuron discharges. For example, some types of potassium channels opened by depolarization of the cell result in slowing of further depolarization and act as a brake to limit further action potential discharge.

Ligand-gated channels, also called **ionotropic receptors,** are opened by the binding of neurotransmitters to the channel. The receptor is formed of subunits, and the channel is an integral part of the receptor complex (see Figures 22–6 and 27–1). These channels are insensitive or only weakly sensitive to membrane potential. Activation of these channels typically results in a brief (a few milliseconds to tens of milliseconds) opening of the channel. Ligand-gated channels are responsible for fast synaptic transmission typical of hierarchical pathways in the CNS (see below).

It is now well established that the traditional view of completely separate voltage-gated and ligand-gated channels requires substantial modifications. As discussed in Chapter 2, most neurotransmitters, in addition to binding to ionotropic receptors, also bind to G protein-coupled receptors, often referred to as **metabotropic receptors.** Metabotropic receptors, via G proteins, modulate voltage-gated channels. This interaction can occur entirely within the membrane and is then referred to as a **membrane delimited** pathway (Figure 21–1C). In this case, the G protein (often the $\beta\gamma$ subunit) interacts directly with the voltage-gated ion channel. In general, two types of voltage-gated ion channels are the targets of this type of signaling: calcium channels and potassium channels. When G proteins interact with calcium channels, they

Figure 21–1. Types of ion channels and neurotransmitter receptors in the CNS. **A** shows a voltage-gated channel in which a voltage sensor component of the protein controls the gating (broken arrow) of the channel. **B** shows a ligand-gated channel in which the binding of the neurotransmitter to the ionotropic channel receptor controls the gating (broken arrow) of the channel. **C** shows a G protein-coupled (metabotropic) receptor, which when bound, activates a G protein that then interacts directly with an ion channel. **D** shows a G protein-coupled receptor, which when bound, activates a G protein that then activates an enzyme. The activated enzyme generates a diffusible second messenger, eg, cAMP, which interacts with an ion channel.

inhibit channel function. This mechanism accounts for the presynaptic inhibition that occurs when presynaptic metabotropic receptors are activated. In contrast, when these receptors are postsynaptic, they activate (cause the opening of) potassium channels, resulting in a slow postsynaptic inhibition. Metabotropic receptors can also modulate voltage-gated channels less directly by the generation of **diffusible second messengers** (Figure 21–1D). A classic example of this type of action is pro-

vided by the β adrenoceptor, which generates cAMP via the activation of adenylyl cyclase (see Chapter 2). Whereas membrane-delimited actions occur within microdomains in the membrane, second messenger-mediated effects can occur over considerable distances. Finally, an important consequence of the involvement of G proteins in receptor signaling is that, in contrast to the brief effect of ionotropic receptors, the effects of metabotropic receptor activation can last tens of seconds

Table 21–1. Some toxins used to characterize ion channels.

Channel Types	Mode of Toxin Action	Source
Voltage-gated		
Sodium channels		
Tetrodotoxin (TTX)	Blocks channel from outside	Puffer fish
Batrachotoxin (BTX)	Slows inactivation, shifts activation	Colombian frog
Potassium channels		
Apamin	Blocks "small Ca-activated" K channel	Honeybee
Charybdotoxin	Blocks "big Ca-activated" K channel	Scorpion
Calcium channels		
Omega conotoxin (ω-CTX-GVIA)	Blocks N-type channel	Pacific cone snail
Agatoxin (ω-AGA-IVA)	Blocks P-type channel	Funnel web spider
Ligand-gated		
Nicotinic ACh receptor		
α-Bungarotoxin	Irreversible antagonist	Marine snake
GABA$_A$ receptor		
Picrotoxin	Blocks channel	South Pacific plant
Glycine receptor		
Strychnine	Competitive antagonist	Indian plant
AMPA receptor		
Philanthotoxin	Blocks channel	Wasp

to minutes. Metabotropic receptors predominate in the diffuse neuronal systems in the CNS (see below).

THE SYNAPSE & SYNAPTIC POTENTIALS

The communication between neurons in the CNS occurs through chemical synapses in the vast majority of cases. (A few instances of electrical coupling between neurons have been documented, and such coupling may play a role in synchronizing neuronal discharge. However, it is unlikely that these electrical synapses are an important site of drug action.) The events involved in synaptic transmission can be summarized as follows.

An action potential in the presynaptic fiber propagates into the synaptic terminal and activates voltage-sensitive calcium channels in the membrane of the terminal (see Figure 6–3). The calcium channels responsible for the release of transmitter are generally resistant to the calcium channel-blocking agents discussed in Chapter 12 (verapamil, etc) but are sensitive to blockade by certain marine toxins and metal ions (see Tables 12–4 and 21–1). Calcium flows into the terminal, and the increase in intraterminal calcium concentration promotes the fusion of synaptic vesicles with the presynaptic membrane. The transmitter contained in the vesicles is released into the synaptic cleft and diffuses to the

receptors on the postsynaptic membrane. Binding of the transmitter to its receptor causes a brief change in membrane conductance (permeability to ions) of the postsynaptic cell. The time delay from the arrival of the presynaptic action potential to the onset of the postsynaptic response is approximately 0.5 ms. Most of this delay is consumed by the release process, particularly the time required for calcium channels to open.

The first systematic analysis of synaptic potentials in the CNS was in the early 1950s by Eccles and associates, who recorded intracellularly from spinal motoneurons. When a microelectrode enters a cell, there is a sudden change in the potential recorded by the electrode, which is typically about -70 mV (Figure 21–2). This is the resting membrane potential of the neuron. Two types of pathways—excitatory and inhibitory—impinge on the motoneuron.

When an excitatory pathway is stimulated, a small depolarization or **excitatory postsynaptic potential (EPSP)** is recorded. This potential is due to the excitatory transmitter acting on an ionotropic receptor, causing an increase in sodium and potassium permeability. Changing the stimulus intensity to the pathway and, therefore, the number of presynaptic fibers activated, results in a graded change in the size of the depolarization. When a sufficient number of excitatory fibers are activated, the EPSP depolarizes the postsynaptic cell to threshold, and an all-or-none action potential is generated.

Figure 21–2. Excitatory synaptic potentials and spike generation. The figure shows entry of a microelectrode into a postsynaptic cell and subsequent recording of a resting membrane potential of -70 mV. Stimulation of an excitatory pathway (E) generates transient depolarization. Increasing the stimulus strength (second E) increases the size of the depolarization, so that the threshold for spike generation is reached.

When an inhibitory pathway is stimulated, the postsynaptic membrane is hyperpolarized owing to the selective opening of Cl⁻ channels, producing an **inhibitory postsynaptic potential (IPSP)** (Figure 21–3). However, because the equilibrium potential for Cl⁻ is only slightly more negative than the resting potential (~ –65 mV), the hyperpolarization is small and contributes only modestly to the inhibitory action. The opening of the Cl⁻ channel during the IPSP makes the neuron "leaky" so that changes in membrane potential are more difficult to achieve. This shunting effect decreases the change in membrane potential during the excitatory postsynaptic potential (EPSP). As a result an EPSP that evoked an action potential under resting conditions fails to evoke an action potential during the IPSP (Figure 21–3). A second type of inhibition is termed **presynaptic inhibition.** It was first described for sensory fibers entering the spinal cord, where excitatory synaptic terminals receive synapses called axoaxonic synapses (described later). When activated, axoaxonic synapses reduce the amount of transmitter released from the terminals of sensory fibers. It is interesting that presynaptic inhibitory receptors are present on virtually all presynaptic terminals in the brain even though axoaxonic synapses appear to be restricted to the spinal cord. In the brain, transmitter spills over to neighboring synapses to activate the presynaptic receptors.

SITES OF DRUG ACTION

Virtually all of the drugs that act in the CNS produce their effects by modifying some step in chemical synaptic transmission. Figure 21–4 illustrates some of the steps that can be altered. These transmitter-dependent actions can be divided into presynaptic and postsynaptic categories.

Drugs acting on the synthesis, storage, metabolism, and release of neurotransmitters fall into the presynaptic category. Synaptic transmission can be depressed by blockade of transmitter synthesis or storage. For example, reserpine depletes monoamine synapses of transmitter by interfering with intracellular storage. Blockade of transmitter catabolism inside the nerve terminal can increase transmitter concentrations and has been reported to increase the amount of transmitter released per impulse. Drugs can also alter the release of transmitter. The stimulant amphetamine induces the release of catecholamines from adrenergic synapses (Chapters 6 and 32). Capsaicin causes the release of the peptide substance P from sensory neurons, and tetanus toxin blocks the release of transmitters. After a transmitter has been released into the synaptic cleft, its action is terminated either by uptake or by degradation. For most neurotransmitters, there are uptake mechanisms into the synaptic terminal and also into surrounding neuroglia. Cocaine, for example, blocks the uptake of catecholamines at adrenergic synapses and thus potentiates the action of these amines. However, acetylcholine is inactivated by enzymatic degradation, not reuptake. Anticholinesterases block the degradation of acetylcholine and thereby prolong its action. No uptake mechanism has been found for any of the numerous CNS peptides, and it has yet to be demonstrated whether specific enzymatic degradation terminates the action of peptide transmitters.

In the postsynaptic region, the transmitter receptor provides the primary site of drug action. Drugs can act either as neurotransmitter agonists, such as the opioids, which mimic the action of enkephalin, or they can block receptor function. Receptor antagonism is a common mechanism of action for CNS drugs. An example is strychnine's block-

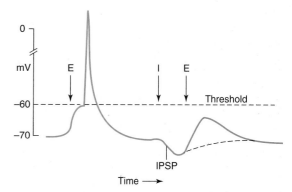

Figure 21–3. Interaction of excitatory and inhibitory synapses. On the left, a suprathreshold stimulus is given to an excitatory pathway (E) and an action potential is evoked. On the right, this same stimulus is given shortly after activating an inhibitory pathway (I), which results in an inhibitory postsynaptic potential (IPSP) that prevents the excitatory potential from reaching threshold.

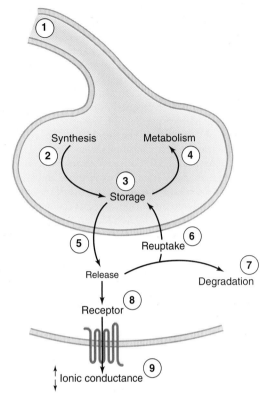

Figure 21–4. Sites of drug action. Schematic drawing of steps at which drugs can alter synaptic transmission. (1) Action potential in presynaptic fiber; (2) synthesis of transmitter; (3) storage; (4) metabolism; (5) release; (6) reuptake; (7) degradation; (8) receptor for the transmitter; (9) receptor-induced increase or decrease in ionic conductance.

ade of the receptor for the inhibitory transmitter glycine. This block, which underlies strychnine's convulsant action, illustrates how the blockade of inhibitory processes results in excitation. Drugs can also act directly on the ion channel of ionotropic receptors. For example, barbiturates can enter and block the channel of many excitatory ionotropic receptors. In the case of metabotropic receptors, drugs can act at any of the steps downstream of the receptor. Perhaps the best example is provided by the methylxanthines, which can modify neurotransmitter responses mediated through the second-messenger cAMP. At high concentrations, the methylxanthines elevate the level of cAMP by blocking its metabolism and thereby prolong its action.

The selectivity of CNS drug action is based almost entirely on the fact that different transmitters are used by different groups of neurons. Furthermore, these transmitters are often segregated into neuronal systems that subserve broadly different CNS functions. Without such segregation, it would be impossible to selectively modify CNS function even if one had a drug that operated on a single neurotransmitter system. That such segregation does occur has provided neuroscientists with a powerful pharmacologic approach for analyzing CNS function and treating pathologic conditions.

IDENTIFICATION OF CENTRAL NEUROTRANSMITTERS

Because drug selectivity is based on the fact that different pathways utilize different transmitters, a primary goal of neuropharmacologists is to identify the transmitters in CNS pathways. Establishing that a chemical substance is a transmitter has been far more difficult for central synapses than for peripheral synapses. The following criteria have been established for transmitter identification.

Localization

Approaches that have been used to prove that a suspected transmitter resides in the presynaptic terminal of the pathway under study include biochemical analysis of regional concentrations of suspected transmitters and immunocytochemical techniques for enzymes and peptides.

Release

To determine whether the substance is released from a particular region, local collection (in vivo) of the extracellular fluid can sometimes be accomplished. In addition, slices of brain tissue can be electrically or chemically stimulated in vitro and the released substances measured. To determine whether the release is relevant to synaptic transmission, it is important to establish that the release is calcium-dependent.

Synaptic Mimicry

Finally, application of the suspected substance should produce a response that mimics the action of the transmitter released by nerve stimulation. Furthermore, application of a selective antagonist should block the response. Microiontophoresis, which permits highly localized drug administration, has been a valuable technique in assessing the action of suspected transmitters. Because of the complexity of the CNS, specific pharmacologic antagonism of a synaptic response provides a particularly powerful technique for transmitter identification.

CELLULAR ORGANIZATION OF THE BRAIN

Most of the neuronal systems in the CNS can be divided into two broad categories: **hierarchical** systems and **nonspecific** or **diffuse** neuronal systems.

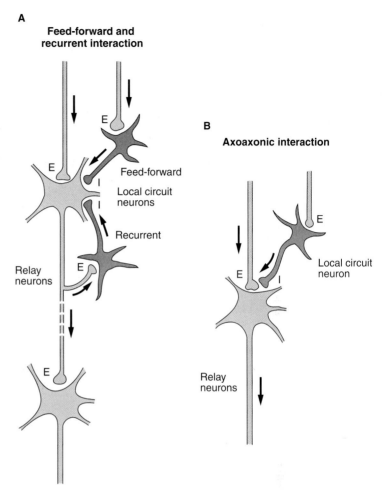

A

Feed-forward and recurrent interaction

Feed-forward

Local circuit neurons

Recurrent

Relay neurons

B

Axoaxonic interaction

Local circuit neuron

Relay neurons

Figure 21–5. Pathways in the central nervous system. **A** shows parts of three relay neurons (color) and two types of inhibitory pathways, recurrent and feed-forward. The inhibitory neurons are shown in gray. **B** shows the pathway responsible for presynaptic inhibition in which the axon of an inhibitory neuron (gray) synapses on the axon terminal of an excitatory fiber (color).

Hierarchical Systems

Hierarchical systems include all the pathways directly involved in sensory perception and motor control. The pathways are generally clearly delineated, being composed of large myelinated fibers that can often conduct action potentials at a rate in excess of 50 m/s. The information is typically phasic and occurs in bursts of action potentials. In sensory systems, the information is processed sequentially by successive integrations at each relay nucleus on its way to the cortex. A lesion at any link will incapacitate the system. Within each nucleus and in the cortex, there are two types of cells: **relay** or **projection neurons** and **local circuit neurons** (Figure 21–5A). The projection neurons that form the interconnecting pathways transmit signals over long distances. The cell bodies are relatively large, and their axons emit collaterals that arborize extensively in the vicinity of the neuron. These neurons are excitatory, and their synaptic influences, which involve ionotropic receptors, are very short-lived.

The excitatory transmitter released from these cells is, in most instances, **glutamate.** Local circuit neurons are typically smaller than projection neurons, and their axons arborize in the immediate vicinity of the cell body. The majority of these neurons are inhibitory, and they release either **GABA** or **glycine.** They synapse primarily on the cell body of the projection neurons but can also synapse on the dendrites of projection neurons as well as with each other. Two common types of pathways for these neurons (Figure 21–5A) include recurrent feedback pathways and feed-forward pathways. A special class of local circuit neurons in the spinal cord forms axoaxonic synapses on the terminals of sensory axons (Figure 21–5B). In some sensory pathways such as the retina and olfactory bulb, local circuit neurons may actually lack an axon and release neurotransmitter from dendritic synapses in a graded fashion in the absence of action potentials.

Although there is a great variety of synaptic connections in these hierarchical systems, the fact that a limited number of transmitters are utilized by these neurons indicates that any major pharmacologic manipulation of this system will have a profound effect on the overall excitability of the CNS. For instance, selectively blocking $GABA_A$ receptors with a drug such as picrotoxin results in generalized convulsions. Thus, although the mechanism of action of picrotoxin is specific in blocking the effects of GABA, the overall functional effect appears to be quite nonspecific, because GABA-mediated synaptic inhibition is so widely utilized in the brain.

Nonspecific or Diffuse Neuronal Systems

Neuronal systems that contain one of the monoamines—norepinephrine, dopamine, or 5-hydroxytryptamine (serotonin)—provide examples in this category. Certain other pathways emanating from the reticular formation and possibly some peptide-containing pathways also fall into this category. These systems differ in fundamental ways from the hierarchical systems, and the noradrenergic systems serve to illustrate the differences.

Noradrenergic cell bodies are found primarily in a compact cell group called the locus ceruleus located in the caudal pontine central gray matter. The number of neurons in this cell group is small, approximately 1500 on each side of the brain in the rat.

Because these axons are fine and unmyelinated, they conduct very slowly, at about 0.5 m/s. The axons branch repeatedly and are extraordinarily divergent. Branches from the same neuron can innervate several functionally different parts of the CNS. In the neocortex, these fibers have a tangential organization and therefore can monosynaptically influence large areas of cortex. The pattern of innervation by noradrenergic fibers in the cortex and nuclei of the hierarchical systems is diffuse, and these fibers form a very small percentage of the total number in the area. In addition, the axons are studded with periodic enlargements called varicosities, which contain large numbers of vesicles. In some instances, these varicosities do not form synaptic contacts, suggesting that norepinephrine may be released in a rather diffuse manner, as occurs with the noradrenergic autonomic innervation of smooth muscle. This indicates that the cellular targets of these systems are determined largely by the location of the receptors rather than by the location of the release sites. Finally, most neurotransmitters utilized by diffuse neuronal systems, including norepinephrine, act—perhaps exclusively—on metabotropic receptors and therefore initiate long-lasting synaptic effects. Based on these observations, it is clear that the monoamine systems cannot be conveying topographically specific types of information; rather, vast areas of the CNS must be affected simultaneously and in a rather uniform way. It is not surprising, then, that these systems have been implicated in such global functions as sleeping and waking, attention, appetite, and emotional states.

CENTRAL NEUROTRANSMITTERS

A vast number of small molecules have been isolated from the brain, and studies using a variety of approaches suggest that the agents listed in Table 21–2 are neurotransmitters. A brief summary of the evidence for some of these compounds follows.

Amino Acids

The amino acids of primary interest to the pharmacologist fall into two categories: the acidic amino acid **glutamate** and the neutral amino acids **glycine** and **GABA.** All of these compounds are present in high concentrations in the CNS and are extremely potent modifiers of neuronal excitability.

A. GLUTAMATE

Excitatory synaptic transmission is mediated by glutamate, which is present in very high concentrations in excitatory synaptic vesicles (~ 100 mM). Glutamate is released into the synaptic cleft by Ca^{2+}-dependent exocytosis (Figure 21–6). The released glutamate acts on postsynaptic glutamate receptors and is cleared by glutamate transporters present on surrounding glia. In glia, glutamate is converted to glutamine by glutamine synthetase, released from the glia, taken up by the nerve terminal, and converted back to glutamate by the enzyme glutaminase. The high concentration of glutamate in synaptic vesicles is achieved by the **vesicular glutamate transporter (VGLUT).**

Virtually all neurons that have been tested are strongly excited by glutamate. This excitation is caused by the activation of both ionotropic and metabotropic receptors, which have been extensively characterized by molecular cloning. The ionotropic receptors can be further divided into three subtypes based on the action of selective agonists: α-amino-3-hydroxy-5-methylisoxazole-4-propionic acid **(AMPA),** kainic acid **(KA)** and N-methyl-D-aspartate **(NMDA).** All of the ionotropic receptors are composed of four subunits. AMPA receptors, which are present on all neurons, are heterotetramers assembled from four subunits (GluR1-GluR4). The majority of AMPA receptors contain the GluR2 subunit and are permeable to Na^+ and K^+, but not to Ca^{2+}. Some AMPA receptors, typically present on inhibitory interneurons, lack the GluR2 subunit and are also permeable to Ca^{2+}.

Kainate receptors are not as uniformly distributed as AMPA receptors, being expressed at high levels in the hippocampus, cerebellum, and spinal cord. They are formed from a number of subunit combinations (GluR5-GluR7, and KA1 and KA2). Although KA1 and KA2 are unable to form channels on their own, their presence in the receptor changes the receptor's affinity and kinetics. Similar to AMPA receptors, kainate receptors are permeable to Na^+ and K^+ and in some subunit combinations can also be permeable to Ca^{2+}.

Table 21–2. Summary of neurotransmitter pharmacology in the central nervous system. (Many other central transmitters have been identified [see text].)

Transmitter	Anatomy	Receptor Subtypes and Preferred Agonists	Receptor Antagonists	Mechanisms
Acetylcholine	Cell bodies at all levels; long and short connections	Muscarinic (M_1): muscarine	Pirenzepine, atropine	Excitatory: $\downarrow$ in K^+ conductance; $\uparrow IP_3$, DAG
		Muscarinic (M_2): muscarine, bethanechol	Atropine, methoctramine	Inhibitory: $\uparrow K^+$ conductance; $\downarrow$ cAMP
	Motoneuron-Renshaw cell synapse	Nicotinic: nicotine	Dihydro-β-erythroidine, α-bungarotoxin	Excitatory: $\uparrow$ cation conductance
Dopamine	Cell bodies at all levels; short, medium, and long connections	D_1	Phenothiazines	Inhibitory (?): $\uparrow$ cAMP
		D_2: bromocriptine	Phenothiazines, butyrophenones	Inhibitory (presynaptic): $\downarrow Ca^{2+}$; Inhibitory (postsynaptic): $\uparrow$ in K^+ conductance, $\downarrow$ cAMP
GABA	Supraspinal and spinal interneurons involved in pre- and postsynaptic inhibition	$GABA_A$: muscimol	Bicuculline, picrotoxin	Inhibitory: $\uparrow Cl^-$ conductance
		$GABA_B$: baclofen	2-OH saclofen	Inhibitory (presynaptic): $\downarrow Ca^{2+}$ conductance Inhibitory (postsynaptic): $\uparrow K^+$ conductance
Glutamate	Relay neurons at all levels and some interneurons	N-Methyl-D-aspartate (NMDA): NMDA	2-Amino-5-phosphonovalerate, dizocilpine	Excitatory: $\uparrow$ cation conductance, particularly Ca^{2+}
		AMPA: AMPA	CNQX	Excitatory: $\uparrow$ cation conductance
		Kainate: kainic acid, domoic acid		
		Metabotropic: ACPD, quisqualate	MCPG	Inhibitory (presynaptic): $\downarrow Ca^{2+}$ conductance; $\downarrow$ cAMP Excitatory: $\downarrow K^+$ conductance, $\uparrow IP_3$, DAG
Glycine	Spinal interneurons and some brain stem interneurons	Taurine, β-alanine	Strychnine	Inhibitory: $\uparrow Cl^-$ conductance
5-Hydroxytryptamine (serotonin)	Cell bodies in midbrain and pons project to all levels	$5\text{-}HT_{1A}$: LSD	Metergoline, spiperone	Inhibitory: $\uparrow K^+$ conductance, $\downarrow$ cAMP
		$5\text{-}HT_{2A}$: LSD	Ketanserin	Excitatory: $\downarrow K^+$ conductance, $\uparrow IP_3$, DAG
		$5\text{-}HT_3$: 2-methyl-5-HT	Ondansetron	Excitatory: $\uparrow$ cation conductance
		$5\text{-}HT_4$		Excitatory: $\downarrow K^+$ conductance

(continued)

Table 21–2. Summary of neurotransmitter pharmacology in the central nervous system. (Many other central transmitters have been identified [see text].) (continued)

Transmitter	Anatomy	Receptor Subtypes and Preferred Agonists	Receptor Antagonists	Mechanisms
Norepinephrine	Cell bodies in pons and brain stem project to all levels	α_1: phenylephrine	Prazosin	Excitatory: ↓ K$^+$ conductance, ↑ IP$_3$, DAG
		α_2: clonidine	Yohimbine	Inhibitory (presynaptic): ↓ Ca^{2+} conductance Inhibitory: ↑ K$^+$ conductance, ↓ cAMP
		β_1: isoproterenol, dobutamine	Atenolol, practolol	Excitatory: ↓ K$^+$ conductance, ↑ cAMP
		β_2: albuterol	Butoxamine	Inhibitory: may involve ↑ in electrogenic sodium pump; ↑ cAMP
Histamine	Cells in ventral posterior hypothalamus	H$_1$: 2(m-fluorophenyl)-histamine	Mepyramine	Excitatory: ↓ K$^+$ conductance, ↑ IP$_3$, DAG
		H$_2$: dimaprit	Ranitidine	Excitatory: ↓ K$^+$ conductance, ↑ cAMP
		H$_3$: R-α-methyl-histamine	Thioperamide	Inhibitory autoreceptors
Opioid peptides	Cell bodies at all levels; long and short connections	Mu: bendorphin	Naloxone	Inhibitory (presynaptic): ↓ Ca^{2+} conductance, ↓ cAMP
		Delta: enkephalin	Naloxone	Inhibitory (postsynaptic): ↑ K$^+$ conductance, ↓ cAMP
		Kappa: dynorphin	Naloxone	
Tachykinins	Primary sensory neurons, cell bodies at all levels; long and short connections	NK1: Substance P methylester		Excitatory: ↓ K$^+$ conductance, ↑ IP$_3$, DAG
		NK2		
		NK3		
Endocannabinoids	Widely distributed	CB1: Anandamide, 2-arachidonylglyerol	Rimonabant	Inhibitory (presynaptic): ↓ Ca^{2+} conductance, ↓ cAMP

ACPD, trans-1-amino-cyclopentyl-1,3-dicarboxylate; AMPA, DL-α-amino-3-hydroxy-5-methylisoxazole-4-propionate; cAMP, cyclic adenosine monophosphate; CQNX, 6-cyano-7-nitroquinoxaline-2,3-dione; DAG, diacylglycerol; IP$_3$, inositol trisphosphate; LSD, lysergic acid diethylamide; MCPG, α-methyl-4-carboxyphenylglycine.

NMDA receptors are as ubiquitous as AMPA receptors, being present on essentially all neurons in the CNS. All NMDA receptors require the presence of the subunit NR1. The channel also contains one or two NR2 subunits (NR2A-D). Unlike AMPA and kainate receptors, all NMDA receptors are highly permeable to Ca^{2+} as well as to Na$^+$ and K$^+$. NMDA receptor function is controlled in a number of intriguing ways. In addition to glutamate binding, the channel also requires the binding of glycine to a separate site. The physiologic role for glycine binding is unclear because the glycine site appears to be saturated at normal ambient levels of glycine. Another key difference between AMPA and kainate receptors on the one hand, and NMDA receptors on the other, is that AMPA and kainate receptor activation results in channel opening at resting membrane potential, whereas NMDA

Figure 21–6. Schematic diagram of a glutamate synapse. Glutamine is imported into the glutamatergic neuron **(A)** and converted into glutamate by glutaminase. The glutamate is then concentrated in vesicles by the vesicular glutamate transporter (VGLUT). Upon release into the synapse, glutamate can interact with AMPA and NMDA ionotropic receptor channels (AMPAR, NMDAR) in the postsynaptic density (PSD) and with metabotropic receptors (MGluR) on the postsynaptic cell **(B)**. Synaptic transmission is terminated by active transport of the glutamate into a neighboring glial cell **(C)** by a glutamate transporter. It is synthesized into glutamine by glutamine synthetase and exported into the glutamatergic axon. **(D)** shows a model NMDA receptor channel complex consisting of a tetrameric protein that becomes permeable to Na^+ and Ca^{2+} when it binds a glutamate molecule.

receptor activation does not. This is due to the voltage-dependent block of the NMDA pore by extracellular Mg^{2+}. When the neuron is strongly depolarized, as occurs with intense activation of the synapse or by activation of neighboring synapses, the Mg^{2+} ion is expelled and the channel opens. Thus, there are two requirements for NMDA receptor channel opening: Glutamate must bind the receptor and the membrane must be depolarized. The rise in intracellular Ca^{2+} that accompanies channel opening results in a long-lasting enhancement in synaptic strength that is referred to as **long-term potentiation (LTP).** The change can last for many hours or even days and is generally accepted as an important cellular mechanism underlying learning and memory.

The metabotropic glutamate receptors are G protein-coupled receptors that act indirectly on ion channels via G proteins. Metabotropic receptors (mGluR1-mGluR8) have been divided into three groups (I, II, and III). A variety of agonists and antagonists have been developed that interact selectively with the different groups. Group I receptors are typically located postsynaptically and are thought to cause neuronal excitation by activating a non-selective cation channel. These receptors also activate phospholipase C, leading to IP_3-mediated intracellular Ca^{2+} release. In contrast, group II and group III receptors are typically located on presynaptic nerve terminals and act as inhibitory autoreceptors. Activation of these receptors causes the inhibition of Ca^{2+} channels resulting in inhibition of transmitter release. These receptors are activated only when the concentration of glutamate rises to high levels during repetitive stimulation of the synapse. Activation of these receptors causes the inhibition of adenylyl cyclase and decreases cAMP generation.

The postsynaptic membrane at excitatory synapses is thickened and referred to as the **postsynaptic density** (PSD; Figure 21–6). This is a highly complex structure containing glutamate receptors, signaling proteins, scaffolding proteins, and cytoskeletal proteins. A typical excitatory synapse contains AMPA receptors, which tend to be located toward the periphery, and NMDA receptors, which are concentrated in the center. Kainate receptors are present at a subset of excitatory synapses, but their exact location is unknown. Metabotropic glutamate receptors (group I), which are localized just outside the PSD, are also present at some excitatory synapses.

B. GABA AND GLYCINE

Both GABA and glycine are inhibitory neurotransmitters, which are typically released from local interneurons. Interneurons that release glycine are restricted to the spinal cord and brain stem, whereas interneurons releasing GABA are present throughout the CNS, including the spinal cord. It is interesting that some interneurons in the spinal cord can release both GABA and glycine. Glycine receptors are pentameric structures that are selectively permeable to Cl^-. Strychnine, which is a potent spinal cord convulsant and has been used in some rat poisons, selectively blocks glycine receptors.

GABA receptors are divided into two main types: $GABA_A$ and $GABA_B$. IPSPs in many areas of the brain have a fast and slow component. The fast component is mediated by $GABA_A$ receptors and the slow component by $GABA_B$ receptors. The difference in kinetics stems from the differences in coupling of the receptors to ion channels. $GABA_A$ receptors are inotropic receptors and, like glycine receptors, are pentameric structures that are selectively permeable to Cl^-. These receptors are selectively inhibited by picrotoxin and bicuculline, both of which cause generalized convulsions. A great many subunits for $GABA_A$ receptors have been cloned; this accounts for the large diversity in the pharmacology of $GABA_A$ receptors, making them key targets for clinically useful agents (see Chapter 22). $GABA_B$ receptors are metabotropic receptors that are selectively activated by the antispastic drug baclofen. These receptors are coupled to G proteins that, depending on their cellular location, either inhibit Ca^{2+} channels or activate K^+ channels. The $GABA_B$ component of the IPSP is due to a selective increase in K^+ conductance. This IPSP is long-lasting and slow because the coupling of receptor activation to K^+ channel opening is indirect and delayed. $GABA_B$ receptors are localized to the perisynaptic region and thus require the spillover of GABA from the synaptic cleft. $GABA_B$ receptors are also present on the axon terminals of many excitatory and inhibitory synapses. In this case, GABA spills over onto these presynaptic $GABA_B$ receptors, inhibiting transmitter release by inhibiting Ca^{2+} channels. In addition to their coupling to ion channels, $GABA_B$ receptors also inhibit adenylyl cyclase and decrease cAMP generation.

Acetylcholine

Acetylcholine was the first compound to be identified pharmacologically as a transmitter in the CNS. Eccles showed in the early 1950s that excitation of Renshaw cells by motor axon collaterals in the spinal cord was blocked by nicotinic antagonists. Furthermore, Renshaw cells were extremely sensitive to nicotinic agonists. These experiments were remarkable for two reasons. First, this early success at identifying a transmitter for a central synapse was followed by disappointment because it remained the sole central synapse for which the transmitter was known until the late 1960s, when comparable data became available for GABA and glycine. Second, the motor axon collateral synapse remains one of the best-documented examples of a cholinergic nicotinic synapse in the mammalian CNS, despite the rather widespread distribution of nicotinic receptors as defined by in situ hybridization studies. Most CNS responses to acetylcholine are mediated by a large family of G protein-coupled muscarinic receptors. At a few sites, acetylcholine causes slow inhibition of the neuron by activating the M_2 subtype of receptor, which opens potassium channels. A far more widespread muscarinic action in response to acetylcholine is a slow excitation that in some cases is mediated by M_1 receptors. These muscarinic effects are much slower than either nicotinic effects on Renshaw cells or the effect of amino acids. Furthermore, this M_1 muscarinic excitation is unusual in that acetylcholine produces it by *decreasing* the membrane permeability to potassium, ie, the opposite of conventional transmitter action.

A number of pathways contain acetylcholine, including neurons in the neostriatum, the medial septal nucleus, and the reticular formation. Cholinergic pathways appear to play an important role in cognitive functions, especially memory. Presenile dementia of the Alzheimer type is reportedly associated with a profound loss of cholinergic neurons. However, the specificity of this loss has been questioned because the levels of other putative transmitters, eg, somatostatin, are also decreased.

Monoamines

Monoamines include the catecholamines (dopamine and norepinephrine) and 5-hydroxytryptamine. Although these compounds are present in very small amounts in the CNS, they can be localized using extremely sensitive histochemical methods. These pathways are the site of action of many drugs; for example, the CNS stimulants cocaine and amphetamine appear to act primarily at catecholamine synapses. Cocaine blocks the reuptake of dopamine and norepinephrine, whereas amphetamines cause presynaptic terminals to release these transmitters.

A. DOPAMINE

The major pathways containing dopamine are the projection linking the substantia nigra to the neostriatum and the projection linking the ventral tegmental region to limbic structures, particularly the limbic cortex. The therapeutic action of the antiparkinsonism drug levodopa is associated with the former area (Chapter 28), whereas the therapeutic action of the antipsychotic drugs is thought to be associated with the latter (Chapter 29). Dopamine-containing neurons in the tuberobasal ventral hypothalamus play an important role in regulating hypothalamohypophysial function. Five dopamine receptors have been identified, and they fall into two categories: D_1-like (D_1 and D_5) and D_2-like (D_2, D_3, D_4). All dopamine receptors are metabotropic. Dopamine generally exerts a slow inhibitory action on CNS neurons. This action has been best characterized on dopamine-containing substantia nigra neurons, where D_2-receptor activation opens potassium channels via the G_i coupling protein.

B. NOREPINEPHRINE

Most noradrenergic neurons are located in the locus ceruleus or the lateral tegmental area of the reticular formation. Although the density of fibers innervating various sites differs considerably, most regions of the CNS receive diffuse noradrenergic input. All noradrenergic receptor subtypes are metabotropic. When applied to neurons, norepinephrine can hyperpolarize them by increasing potassium conductance. This effect is mediated by α_2 receptors and has been characterized most thoroughly on locus ceruleus neurons. In many regions of the CNS, norepinephrine actually enhances excitatory inputs by both indirect and direct mechanisms. The indirect mechanism involves disinhibition; that is, inhibitory local circuit neurons are inhibited. The direct mechanism involves blockade of potassium conductances that slow neuronal discharge. Depending on the type of neuron, this effect is mediated by either α_1 or β receptors. Facilitation of excitatory synaptic transmission is in accordance with many of the behavioral processes thought to involve noradrenergic pathways, eg, attention and arousal.

C. 5-HYDROXYTRYPTAMINE

Most 5-hydroxytryptamine (5-HT, serotonin) pathways originate from neurons in the raphe or midline regions of the pons and upper brain stem. 5-HT is contained in unmyelinated fibers that diffusely innervate most regions of the CNS, but the density of the innervation varies. 5-HT acts on more than a dozen receptor subtypes. Except for the 5-HT_3 receptor, all of these receptors are metabo-

tropic. The ionotropic 5-HT_3 receptor exerts a rapid excitatory action at a very limited number of sites in the CNS. In most areas of the CNS, 5-HT has a strong inhibitory action. This action is mediated by 5-HT_{1A} receptors and is associated with membrane hyperpolarization caused by an increase in potassium conductance. It has been found that 5-HT_{1A} receptors and $GABA_B$ receptors share the same potassium channels. Some cell types are slowly excited by 5-HT owing to its blockade of potassium channels via 5-HT_2 or 5-HT_4 receptors. Both excitatory and inhibitory actions can occur on the same neuron. It has often been speculated that 5-HT pathways may be involved in the hallucinations induced by LSD, since this compound can antagonize the peripheral actions of 5-HT. However, LSD does not appear to be a 5-HT antagonist in the CNS, and typical LSD-induced behavior is still seen in animals after raphe nuclei are destroyed. Other proposed regulatory functions of 5-HT-containing neurons include sleep, temperature, appetite, and neuroendocrine control.

Peptides

A great many CNS peptides have been discovered that produce dramatic effects both on animal behavior and on the activity of individual neurons. Many of the peptides have been mapped with immunohistochemical techniques and include opioid peptides (eg, enkephalins, endorphins), neurotensin, substance P, somatostatin, cholecystokinin, vasoactive intestinal polypeptide, neuropeptide Y, and thyrotropin-releasing hormone. As in the peripheral autonomic nervous system, peptides often coexist with a conventional nonpeptide transmitter in the same neuron. A good example of the approaches used to define the role of these peptides in the CNS comes from studies on substance P and its association with sensory fibers. Substance P is contained in and released from small unmyelinated primary sensory neurons in the spinal cord and brain stem and causes a slow EPSP in target neurons. These sensory fibers are known to transmit noxious stimuli, and it is therefore surprising that—although substance P receptor antagonists can modify responses to certain types of pain—they do not block the response. Glutamate, which is released with substance P from these synapses, presumably plays an important role in transmitting pain stimuli. Substance P is certainly involved in many other functions, because it is found in many areas of the CNS that are unrelated to pain pathways.

Many of these peptides are also found in peripheral structures, including peripheral synapses. They are described in Chapters 6 and 17.

Nitric Oxide

The CNS contains a substantial amount of nitric oxide synthase (NOS), which is found within certain classes of neurons. This neuronal NOS is an enzyme activated by calcium-calmodulin, and activation of NMDA receptors, which increases intracellular calcium, results in the generation of nitric oxide. Although a physiologic role for nitric oxide has been clearly established for vascular smooth muscle, its role in synaptic transmission and synaptic plasticity remains controversial.

Endocannabinoids

The primary psychoactive ingredient in cannabis, Δ^9-tetrahydrocannabinol (Δ^9-THC), affects the brain mainly by activating a specific cannabinoid receptor, CB1. CB1 is expressed at high levels in many brain regions, and several endogenous brain lipids, including anandamide and 2-arachidonylglycerol, have been identified as CB1 ligands. These ligands are not stored, as are classic neurotransmitters, but instead are rapidly synthesized by neurons in response to depolarization and consequent calcium influx. In further contradistinction to classic neurotransmitters, endogenous cannabinoids can function as retrograde synaptic messengers: They are released from postsynaptic neurons and travel backward across synapses, activating CB1 receptors on presynaptic neurons and suppressing transmitter release. Cannabinoids may affect memory, cognition, and pain perception by this mechanism.

REFERENCES

Aizenman CD et al: Use-dependent changes in synaptic strength at the Purkinje cell to deep nuclear synapse. Prog Brain Res 2000;124:257.

Bredt DS, Nicoll RA: AMPA receptor trafficking at excitatory synapses. Neuron 2003;40:361.

Catterall WA et al: Compendium of voltage-gated ion channels: Calcium channels. Pharmacol Rev 2003;55:579.

Catterall WA, Goldin AL, Waxman SG: Compendium of voltage-gated ion channels: Sodium channels. Pharmacol Rev 2003; 55:575.

Clapham DE et al: Compendium of voltage-gated ion channels: Transient receptor potential channels. Pharmacol Rev 2003; 55:591.

Fremeau RT, Jr et al: VGLUTs define subsets of excitatory neurons and suggest novel roles for glutamate. Trends Neurosci 2004; 27:98.

Freund TF, Katona I, Piomelli D: Role of endogenous cannabinoids in synaptic signaling. Physiol Rev 2003;83:1017.

Gouaux E, MacKinnon R: Principles of selective ion transport in channels and pumps. Science 2005;310:1461.

Hall ZW: In: *An Introduction to Molecular Neurobiology.* Sinauer, 1992.

Hille B: *Ionic Channels of Excitable Membranes,* 3rd ed. Sinauer, 2001.

Julius D, Basbaum AI: Molecular mechanisms of nociception. Nature 2001;413:203.

Koles L, Furst S, Illes P: P2X and P2Y receptors as possible targets of therapeutic manipulations in CNS illnesses. Drug News Perspect 2005;18:85.

Malenka RC, Nicoll RA: Long-term potentiation—A decade of progress? Science 1999;285:1870.

Mody I, Pearce RA: Diversity of inhibitory neurotransmission through GABA(A) receptors. Trends Neurosci 2004;27:569.

Moran MM, Xu H, Clapham DE: TRP ion channels in the nervous system. Curr Opin Neurobiol 2004;14:362.

Nestler EJ, Hyman SE, Malenka RC: *Molecular Neuropharmacology.* McGraw-Hill, 2001.

Rudolph U, Mohler H: Analysis of GABAA receptor function and dissection of the pharmacology of benzodiazepines and general anesthetics through mouse genetics. Annu Rev Pharmacol Toxicol 2004;44:475.

Sudhof TC: The synaptic vesicle cycle. Annu Rev Neurosci 2004; 27:509.

Wilson RI, Nicoll RA: Endocannabinoid signaling in the brain. Science 2002;296:678.

Sedative-Hypnotic Drugs

22

Anthony J. Trevor, PhD, & Walter L. Way, MD

Assignment of a drug to the sedative-hypnotic class indicates that it is able to cause sedation (with concomitant relief of anxiety) or to encourage sleep. Because there is considerable chemical variation within the group, this drug classification is based on clinical uses rather than on similarities in chemical structure. Anxiety states and sleep disorders are common problems, and sedative-hypnotics are widely prescribed drugs worldwide.

■ I. BASIC PHARMACOLOGY OF SEDATIVE-HYPNOTICS

An effective **sedative** (anxiolytic) agent should reduce anxiety and exert a calming effect. The degree of central nervous system depression caused by a sedative should be the minimum consistent with therapeutic efficacy. A **hypnotic** drug should produce drowsiness and encourage the onset and maintenance of a state of sleep. Hypnotic effects involve more pronounced depression of the central nervous system than sedation, and this can be achieved with many drugs in this class simply by increasing the dose. Graded dose-dependent depression of central nervous system function is a characteristic of most sedative-hypnotics. However, individual drugs differ in the relationship between the dose and the degree of central nervous system depression. Two examples of such dose-response relationships are shown in Figure 22–1. The linear slope for drug A is typical of many of the older sedative-hypnotics, including the barbiturates and alcohols. With such drugs, an increase in dose higher than that needed for hypnosis may lead to a state of general anesthesia. At still higher doses, these sedative-hypnotics may depress respiratory and vasomotor centers in the medulla, leading to coma and death. Deviations from a linear dose-response relationship, as shown for drug B, require proportionately greater dosage increments to achieve central nervous system depression more profound than hypnosis. This appears to be the case for benzodiazepines and for certain newer hypnotics that have a similar mechanism of action.

CHEMICAL CLASSIFICATION

The benzodiazepines are widely used sedative-hypnotics. All of the structures shown in Figure 22–2 are 1,4-benzodiazepines, and most contain a carboxamide group in the 7-membered heterocyclic ring structure. A substituent in the 7 position, such as a halogen or a nitro group, is required for sedative-hypnotic activity. The structures of triazolam and alprazolam include the addition of a triazole ring at the 1,2-position.

The chemical structures of some older and less commonly used sedative-hypnotics, including several barbiturates, are shown in Figure 22–3. Glutethimide and meprobamate are of distinctive chemical structure but are practically equivalent to barbiturates in their pharmacologic effects. Their clinical use is rapidly declining. The sedative-hypnotic class also includes compounds of simpler chemical structure, including ethanol (see Chapter 23) and chloral hydrate.

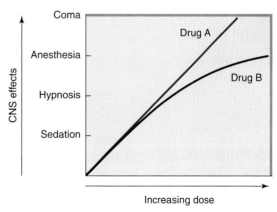

Figure 22–1. Dose-response curves for two hypothetical sedative-hypnotics.

Several drugs with novel chemical structures have been introduced more recently for use in sleep disorders. Zolpidem, an imidazopyridine, zaleplon, a pyrazolopyrimidine, and eszopiclone, a cyclopyrrolone (Figure 22–4), although structurally unrelated to benzodiazepines, share a similar mechanism of action, as described below. Eszopiclone is the *(S)*-enantiomer of zopiclone, a hypnotic drug that has been available outside the United States since 1989. Ramelteon, a melatonin receptor agonist, is a new hypnotic drug (see Box: Ramelteon). Buspirone is a slow-onset anxiolytic agent whose actions are quite different from

those of conventional sedative-hypnotics (see Box: Buspirone).

Other classes of drugs that exert sedative effects include antipsychotics (Chapter 29), and many antidepressant drugs (Chapter 30). The latter are currently used widely in management of chronic anxiety disorders. Certain antihistaminic agents including hydroxyzine and promethazine (Chapter 16) are also sedating. These agents commonly also exert marked effects on the peripheral autonomic nervous system. Certain antihistaminics with sedative effects are available in over-the-counter sleep aids.

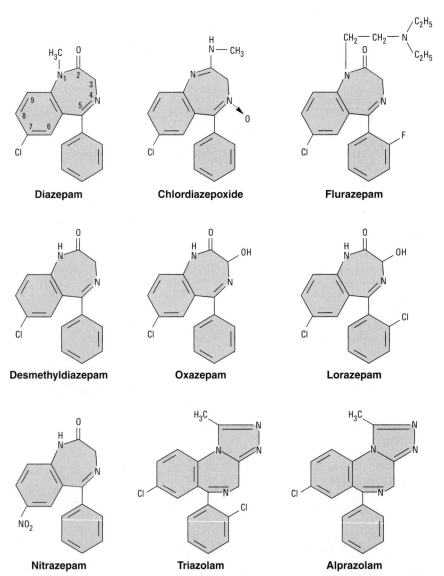

Figure 22–2. Chemical structures of benzodiazepines.

Figure 22–3. Chemical structures of barbiturates and other sedative-hypnotics.

Pharmacokinetics

A. ABSORPTION AND DISTRIBUTION

The rates of oral absorption of sedative-hypnotics differ depending on a number of factors, including lipophilicity. For example, the absorption of triazolam is extremely rapid, and that of diazepam and the active metabolite of clorazepate is more rapid than other commonly used benzodiazepines. Clorazepate, a prodrug, is converted to its active form, desmethyldiazepam (nordiazepam), by acid hydrolysis in the stomach. Most of the barbiturates and other older sedative-hypnotics, as well as the newer hypnotics (eszopiclone, zaleplon, zolpidem), are absorbed rapidly into the blood following oral administration.

Lipid solubility plays a major role in determining the rate at which a particular sedative-hypnotic enters the central nervous system. This property is responsible for the rapid onset of central nervous system effects of triazolam, thiopental (Chapter 25), and the newer hypnotics.

All sedative-hypnotics cross the placental barrier during pregnancy. If sedative-hypnotics are given during the predelivery period, they may contribute to the depression of neonatal vital functions. Sedative-hypnotics are also detectable in breast milk and may exert depressant effects in the nursing infant.

B. BIOTRANSFORMATION

Metabolic transformation to more water-soluble metabolites is necessary for clearance of sedative-hypnotics from the body. The microsomal drug-metabolizing enzyme systems of the liver are most important in this regard. Few sedative-hypnotics are excreted from the body in unchanged form, so elimination half-life depends mainly on the rate of metabolic transformation.

Figure 22–4. Chemical structures of newer hypnotics.

RAMELTEON

Melatonin receptors are thought to be involved in maintaining circadian rhythms underlying the sleep-wake cycle (Chapter 16). Ramelteon, a novel hypnotic drug prescribed specifically for patients who have difficulty in falling asleep, is an agonist at MT_1 and MT_2 melatonin receptors located in the suprachiasmatic nuclei of the brain. The drug has no direct effects on GABAergic neurotransmission in the central nervous system. In polysomnography studies of patients with chronic insomnia, ramelteon reportedly reduced the latency to persistent sleep with no rebound insomnia or withdrawal symptoms. The drug is rapidly ab-

sorbed after oral administration and undergoes extensive first-pass metabolism, forming an active metabolite with longer half-life (2–5 hours) than the parent drug. The CYP1A2 isoform of cytochrome P450 is mainly responsible for the metabolism of ramelteon; the drug should not be used with fluvoxamine (an inhibitor of CYP1A2) and should be used with caution in patients with liver dysfunction. Adverse effects of ramelteon include dizziness, somnolence, fatigue, and endocrine changes as well as decreases in testosterone and increases in prolactin. Ramelteon is not a controlled substance.

---

1. Benzodiazepines—Hepatic metabolism accounts for the clearance of all benzodiazepines. The patterns and rates of metabolism depend on the individual drugs. Most benzodiazepines undergo microsomal oxidation (phase I reactions), including *N*-dealkylation and aliphatic hydroxylation catalyzed by cytochrome P450 isozymes, especially CYP3A4. The metabolites are subsequently conjugated (phase II reactions) to form glucuronides that are excreted in the urine. However, many phase I metabolites of benzodiazepines are pharmacologi-

cally active, some with long half-lives (Figure 22–5). For example, desmethyldiazepam, which has an elimination half-life of more than 40 hours, is an active metabolite of chlordiazepoxide, diazepam, prazepam, and clorazepate. Alprazolam and triazolam undergo α-hydroxylation, and the resulting metabolites appear to exert short-lived pharmacologic effects because they are rapidly conjugated to form inactive glucuronides. The short elimination half-life of triazolam (2–3 hours) favors its use as a hypnotic rather than as a sedative drug.

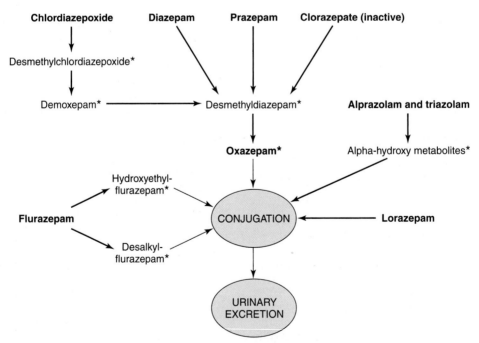

Figure 22–5. Biotransformation of benzodiazepines. (Boldface, drugs available for clinical use in various countries; *, active metabolite.)

BUSPIRONE

Buspirone has selective anxiolytic effects, and its pharmacologic characteristics are different from those of other drugs described in this chapter. Buspirone relieves anxiety without causing marked sedative, hypnotic, or euphoric effects. Unlike benzodiazepines, the drug has no anticonvulsant or muscle relaxant properties. Buspirone does not interact directly with GABAergic systems. It may exert its anxiolytic effects by acting as a partial agonist at brain 5-HT$_{1A}$ receptors, but it also has affinity for brain dopamine D$_2$ receptors. Buspirone-treated patients show no rebound anxiety or withdrawal signs on abrupt discontinuance. The drug is not effective in blocking the acute withdrawal syndrome resulting from abrupt cessation of use of benzodiazepines or other sedative-hypnotics. Buspirone has minimal abuse liability. In marked contrast to the benzodiazepines, the anxiolytic effects of buspirone may take more than a week to become established, making the drug unsuitable for management of acute anxiety states. The drug is used in generalized anxiety states but is less effective in panic disorders.

Buspirone is rapidly absorbed orally but undergoes extensive first-pass metabolism via hydroxylation and dealkylation reactions to form several active metabolites. The major metabolite is 1-(2-pyrimidyl)-piperazine (1-PP), which has α$_2$-adrenoceptor-blocking actions and which enters the central nervous system to reach higher levels than the parent drug. It is not known what role (if any) 1-PP plays in the central actions of buspirone. The elimination half-life of buspirone is 2–4 hours, and liver dysfunction may slow its clearance. Rifampin, an inducer of cytochrome P450, decreases the half-life of buspirone; inhibitors of CYP3A4 (eg, erythromycin, ketoconazole) increase its plasma levels.

Buspirone causes less psychomotor impairment than benzodiazepines and does not affect driving skills. The drug does not potentiate effects of conventional sedative-hypnotic drugs, ethanol, or tricyclic antidepressants, and elderly patients do not appear to be more sensitive to its actions. Tachycardia, palpitations, nervousness, gastrointestinal distress, and paresthesias and a dose-dependent pupillary constriction may occur. Blood pressure may be elevated in patients receiving MAO inhibitors.

The formation of active metabolites has complicated studies on the pharmacokinetics of the benzodiazepines in humans because the elimination half-life of the parent drug may have little relation to the time course of pharmacologic effects. Benzodiazepines for which the parent drug or active metabolites have long half-lives are more likely to cause cumulative effects with multiple doses. Cumulative and residual effects such as excessive drowsiness appear to be less of a problem with such drugs as estazolam, oxazepam, and lorazepam, which have relatively short half-lives and are metabolized directly to inactive glucuronides. Some pharmacokinetic properties of selected benzodiazepines are listed in Table 22–1. The metabolism of several commonly used benzodiazepines including diazepam, midazolam, and triazolam is affected by inhibitors and inducers of hepatic P450 isozymes (see Chapter 4).

2. Barbiturates—With the exception of phenobarbital, only insignificant quantities of the barbiturates are excreted unchanged. The major metabolic pathways involve oxidation by hepatic enzymes to form alcohols, acids, and ketones, which appear in the urine as glucuronide conjugates. The overall rate of hepatic metabolism in humans depends on the individual drug but (with the exception of the thiobarbiturates) is usually slow. The elimination half-lives of secobarbital and pentobarbital range from 18 to 48 hours in different individuals. The elimination half-life of phenobarbital in humans is 4–5 days. Multiple dosing with these agents can lead to cumulative effects.

3. Newer hypnotics—After oral administration of the standard formulation, zolpidem reaches peak plasma levels in 1.6 hours. A biphasic release formulation extends plasma levels by approximately 2 hours. Zolpidem is rapidly metabolized to inactive metabolites via oxidation and hydroxylation by hepatic cytochromes P450 including the CYP3A4 isozyme. The elimination half-life of the drug is 1.5–3.5 hours, with clearance decreased in elderly patients. Zaleplon is metabolized to inactive metabolites mainly by hepatic aldehyde oxidase and partly by the cytochrome P450 isoform CYP3A4. The half-life of the drug is about 1 hour. Dosage should be reduced in patients with hepatic impairment and in the elderly. Cimetidine, which inhibits both aldehyde dehydrogenase and CYP3A4, markedly increases the peak plasma level of zaleplon. Eszopiclone is metabolized by hepatic cytochromes P450 (especially CYP3A4) to form the inactive N-oxide derivative and weakly active desmethyleszopiclone. The elimination half-life of eszopiclone is approximately 6 hours and is prolonged in the

Table 22–1. Pharmacokinetic properties of some benzodiazepines and newer hypnotics in humans.

Drug	Peak Blood Level (hours)	Elimination Half-Life[1] (hours)	Comments
Alprazolam	1–2	12–15	Rapid oral absorption
Chlordiazepoxide	2–4	15–40	Active metabolites; erratic bioavailability from IM injection
Clorazepate	1–2 (nordiazepam)	50–100	Prodrug; hydrolyzed to active form in stomach
Diazepam	1–2	20–80	Active metabolites; erratic bioavailability from IM injection
Eszopiclone	1	6	Minor active metabolites
Flurazepam	1–2	40–100	Active metabolites with long half-lives
Lorazepam	1–6	10–20	No active metabolites
Oxazepam	2–4	10–20	No active metabolites
Temazepam	2–3	10–40	Slow oral absorption
Triazolam	1	2–3	Rapid onset; short duration of action
Zaleplon	<1	1–2	Metabolized via aldehyde dehydrogenase
Zolpidem	1–3	1.5–3.5	No active metabolites

[1]Includes half-lives of major metabolites.

elderly and in the presence of inhibitors of CYP3A4 (eg, ketoconazole). Inducers of CYP3A4 (eg, rifampin) increase the hepatic metabolism of eszopiclone.

C. Excretion

The water-soluble metabolites of sedative-hypnotics, mostly formed via the conjugation of phase I metabolites, are excreted mainly via the kidney. In most cases, changes in renal function do not have a marked effect on the elimination of parent drugs. Phenobarbital is excreted unchanged in the urine to a certain extent (20–30% in humans), and its elimination rate can be increased significantly by alkalinization of the urine. This is partly due to increased ionization at alkaline pH, since phenobarbital is a weak acid with a pK_a of 7.4.

D. Factors Affecting Biodisposition

The biodisposition of sedative-hypnotics can be influenced by several factors, particularly alterations in hepatic function resulting from disease or drug-induced increases or decreases in microsomal enzyme activities (see Chapter 4).

In very old patients and in patients with severe liver disease, the elimination half-lives of these drugs are often increased significantly. In such cases, multiple normal doses of these sedative-hypnotics can result in excessive central nervous system effects.

The activity of hepatic microsomal drug-metabolizing enzymes may be increased in patients exposed to certain older sedative-hypnotics on a long-term basis (enzyme induction; see Chapter 4). Barbiturates (especially phenobarbital) and meprobamate are most likely to cause this effect, which may result in an increase in their hepatic metabolism as well as that of other drugs. Increased biotransformation of other pharmacologic agents as a result of enzyme induction by barbiturates is a potential mechanism underlying drug interactions (Appendix II). In contrast, benzodiazepines and the newer hypnotics do not change hepatic drug-metabolizing enzyme activity with continuous use.

Pharmacodynamics of Benzodiazepines, Barbiturates, & Newer Hypnotics

A. Molecular Pharmacology of the GABA_A Receptor

The benzodiazepines, the barbiturates, zolpidem, zaleplon, eszopiclone, and many other drugs bind to molecular components of the $GABA_A$ receptor in neuronal membranes in the central nervous system. This receptor, which functions as a chloride ion channel, is activated by the inhibitory neurotransmitter GABA (see Chapter 21).

The GABA$_A$ receptor has a pentameric structure assembled from five subunits (each with four transmembrane-spanning domains) selected from multiple polypeptide classes (α, β, γ, δ, ε, π, ρ, etc). Multiple subunits of several of these classes have been characterized, eg, six different α, four β, and three γ. A model of the hypothetical GABA$_A$ receptor-chloride ion channel macromolecular complex is shown in Figure 22–6.

A major isoform of the GABA$_A$ receptor that is found in many regions of the brain consists of two α_1 and two β_2 subunits and one γ_2 subunit. In this isoform, the binding sites for GABA are located between adjacent α_1 and β_2 subunits, and the binding pocket for benzodiazepines

Figure 22–6. A model of the GABA$_A$ receptor-chloride ion channel macromolecular complex (others could be proposed). A heterooligomeric glycoprotein, the complex consists of five or more membrane-spanning subunits. Multiple forms of α, β, and γ subunits are arranged in different pentameric combinations so that GABA$_A$ receptors exhibit molecular heterogeneity. GABA appears to interact with α or β subunits triggering chloride channel opening with resulting membrane hyperpolarization. Binding of benzodiazepines to γ subunits or to an area of the α unit influenced by the γ unit facilitates the process of channel opening but does not directly initiate chloride current. (Modified and reproduced, with permission, from Zorumski CF, Isenberg KE: Insights into the structure and function of GABA receptors: Ion channels and psychiatry. Am J Psychiatry 1991;148:162.)

(the **BZ site** of the GABA$_A$ receptor) is between an α_1 and the γ_2 subunit. However, GABA$_A$ receptors in different areas of the central nervous system consist of various combinations of the essential subunits, and the benzodiazepines bind to many of these, including receptor isoforms containing α_2, α_3, and α_5 subunits. Barbiturates also bind to multiple isoforms of the GABA$_A$ receptor but at different sites from those with which benzodiazepines interact. In contrast to benzodiazepines, zolpidem, zaleplon, and eszopiclone bind more selectively because these drugs interact only with GABA$_A$-receptor isoforms that contain α_1 subunits. The heterogeneity of GABA$_A$ receptors may constitute the molecular basis for the varied pharmacologic actions of benzodiazepines and related drugs (see Box: GABA Receptor Heterogeneity & Pharmacologic Selectivity).

In contrast to GABA itself, benzodiazepines and other sedative-hypnotics have a low affinity for GABA$_B$ receptors, which are activated by the spasmolytic drug baclofen (see Chapters 21 and 27).

B. NEUROPHARMACOLOGY

GABA (gamma-aminobutyric acid) is the major inhibitory neurotransmitter in the central nervous system (Chapter 21). Electrophysiologic studies have shown that benzodiazepines potentiate GABAergic inhibition at all levels of the neuraxis, including the spinal cord, hypothalamus, hippocampus, substantia nigra, cerebellar cortex, and cerebral cortex. Benzodiazepines appear to increase the efficiency of GABAergic synaptic inhibition. The benzodiazepines do not substitute for GABA but appear to enhance GABA's effects allosterically without directly activating GABA$_A$ receptors or opening the associated chloride channels. The enhancement in chloride ion conductance induced by the interaction of benzodiazepines with GABA takes the form of an increase in the *frequency* of channel-opening events.

Barbiturates also facilitate the actions of GABA at multiple sites in the central nervous system, but—in contrast to benzodiazepines—they appear to increase the *duration* of the GABA-gated chloride channel openings. At high concentrations, the barbiturates may also be GABA-mimetic, directly activating chloride channels. These effects involve a binding site or sites distinct from the benzodiazepine binding sites. Barbiturates are less selective in their actions than benzodiazepines, because they also depress the actions of excitatory neurotransmitters (eg, glutamic acid) and exert nonsynaptic membrane effects in parallel with their effects on GABA neurotransmission. This multiplicity of sites of action of barbiturates may be the basis for their ability to induce full surgical anesthesia (see Chapter 25) and for their more pronounced central depressant effects (which result in their low margin of safety) compared with benzodiazepines and the newer hypnotics.

GABA RECEPTOR HETEROGENEITY & PHARMACOLOGIC SELECTIVITY

Studies involving genetically engineered mice have demonstrated that the specific pharmacologic actions elicited by benzodiazepines and other drugs that modulate GABA actions are influenced by the composition of the subunits assembled to form the $GABA_A$ receptor. Benzodiazepines interact only with brain $GABA_A$ receptors in which the α subunits (1,2,3, and 5) have a conserved histidine residue in the N-terminal domain. Strains of mice, in which a point mutation has been inserted converting histidine to arginine in the α_1 subunit, show resistance to both the sedative and amnestic effects of benzodiazepines, but anxiolytic and muscle-relaxing effects are largely unchanged. These animals are also unresponsive to the hypnotic actions of zolpidem and zaleplon, drugs that bind selectively to $GABA_A$

receptors containing α_1 subunits. In contrast, mice with selective histidine-arginine mutations in the α_2 subunit of $GABA_A$ receptors show selective resistance to the antianxiety effects of benzodiazepines. Based on studies of this type, it has been suggested that α_1 subunits in $GABA_A$ receptors mediate sedation, amnesia, and possibly antiseizure effects of benzodiazepines, whereas α_2 subunits are involved in their anxiolytic and muscle-relaxing actions. Other mutation studies have led to suggestions that an α_5 subtype is involved in at least some of the memory impairment caused by benzodiazepines. It should be noted that these studies involving genetic manipulations of the $GABA_A$ receptor utilize rodent models of the anxiolytic and amnestic actions of drugs.

C. Benzodiazepine Binding Site Ligands

The components of the $GABA_A$ receptor-chloride ion channel macromolecule that function as benzodiazepine binding sites exhibit heterogeneity (see Box: The Versatility of the Chloride Channel GABA Receptor Complex). Three types of ligand-benzodia-zepine receptor interactions have been reported: (1) **Agonists** facilitate GABA actions, and this occurs at multiple BZ binding sites in the case of the benzodiazepines. As noted above, the nonbenzodiazepines zolpidem, zaleplon, and eszopiclone are selective agonists at the BZ sites that contain an α_1 subunit. Endogenous agonist ligands for the BZ binding sites have been proposed, because benzodiazepine-like chemicals have been isolated from brain tissue of animals never exposed to these drugs. Nonbenzodiazepine molecules that have affinity for BZ sites on the $GABA_A$ receptor have also been detected in human brain. (2) **Antagonists** are typified by the synthetic benzodiazepine derivative **flumazenil,** which blocks the actions of benzodiazepines, eszopiclone, zaleplon, and zolpidem but does not antagonize the actions of barbiturates, meprobamate, or ethanol. Certain endogenous neuropeptides are also capable of blocking the interaction of benzodiazepines with BZ binding sites. (3) **Inverse agonists** act as negative allosteric modulators of GABA-receptor function. Their interaction with BZ sites on the $GABA_A$ receptor can *produce* anxiety and seizures, an action that has been demonstrated for several compounds, especially the β-carbolines, eg, *n*-butyl-β-carboline-3-carboxylate (β-CCB). In addition to their direct actions, these molecules can block the effects of benzodiazepines.

The physiologic significance of endogenous modulators of the functions of GABA in the central nervous system remains unclear. To date, it has not been established that the putative endogenous ligands of BZ binding sites play a role in the control of states of anxiety, sleep patterns, or any other characteristic behavioral expression of central nervous system function.

D. Organ Level Effects

1. Sedation—Benzodiazepines, barbiturates, and most older sedative-hypnotic drugs exert calming effects with concomitant reduction of anxiety at relatively low doses. In most cases, however, the anxiolytic actions of sedative-hypnotics are accompanied by some depressant effects on psychomotor and cognitive functions. In experimental animal models, benzodiazepines and older sedative-hypnotic drugs are able to disinhibit punishment-suppressed behavior. This disinhibition has been equated with antianxiety effects of sedative-hypnotics, and it is not a characteristic of all drugs that have sedative effects, eg, the tricyclic antidepressants and antihistamines. However, the disinhibition of previously suppressed behavior may be more related to behavioral disinhibitory effects of sedative-hypnotics, including euphoria, impaired judgment, and loss of self-control, which can occur at dosages in the range of those used for management of anxiety. The benzodiazepines also exert dose-dependent anterograde amnesic effects (inability to remember events occurring during the drug's duration of action).

2. Hypnosis—By definition, all of the sedative-hypnotics induce sleep if high enough doses are given. The effects of sedative-hypnotics on the stages of sleep depend on several factors, including the specific drug, the dose, and the frequency of its administration. The general effects of benzodiazepines and older sedative-hypnotics on patterns of normal sleep are as follows: (1) the latency of sleep onset is decreased (time to fall asleep); (2) the duration of stage 2 NREM sleep is increased; (3) the duration of REM sleep is decreased; and (4) the duration of stage 4 NREM slow-wave sleep is decreased. The newer hypnotics all decrease the latency to persistent sleep. Zolpidem decreases REM sleep but has minimal effect on slow-wave sleep. Zaleplon decreases the latency of sleep onset with little effect on total sleep time, NREM, or REM sleep. Eszopiclone increases total sleep time, mainly via increases in stage 2 NREM sleep, and at low doses has little effect on sleep patterns. At the highest recommended dose, eszopiclone decreases REM sleep.

More rapid onset of sleep and prolongation of stage 2 are presumably clinically useful effects. However, the significance of sedative-hypnotic drug effects on REM and slow-wave sleep is not clear. Deliberate interruption of REM sleep causes anxiety and irritability followed by a rebound increase in REM sleep at the end of the experiment. A similar pattern of "REM rebound" can be detected following abrupt cessation of drug treatment with older sedative-hypnotics, especially when drugs with short durations of action (eg, triazolam) are used at high doses. With respect to zolpidem and the other newer hypnotics, there is little evidence of REM rebound when these drugs are discontinued after use of recommended doses. However, rebound insomnia occurs with both zolpidem and zaleplon if used at higher doses. Despite possible reductions in slow-wave sleep, there are no reports of disturbances in the secretion of pituitary or adrenal hormones when either barbiturates or benzodiazepines are used as hypnotics. The use of sedative-hypnotics for more than 1–2 weeks leads to some tolerance to their effects on sleep patterns.

3. Anesthesia—As shown in Figure 22–1, high doses of certain sedative-hypnotics depress the central nervous system to the point known as stage III of general anesthesia (see Chapter 25). However, the suitability of a particular agent as an adjunct in anesthesia depends mainly on the physicochemical properties that determine its rapidity of onset and duration of effect. Among the barbiturates, thiopental and methohexital are very lipid-soluble, penetrating brain tissue rapidly following intravenous administration, a characteristic favoring their use for the induction of anesthesia. Rapid tissue redistribution (not rapid elimination) accounts for the short duration of action of these drugs, a feature useful in recovery from anesthesia.

Benzodiazepines—including diazepam, lorazepam, and midazolam—are used intravenously in anesthesia (see Chapter 25), often in combination with other agents. Not surprisingly, benzodiazepines given in large doses as adjuncts to general anesthetics may contribute to a persistent postanesthetic respiratory depression. This is probably related to their relatively long half-lives and the formation of active metabolites. However, such depressant actions of the benzodiazepines are usually reversible with flumazenil.

4. Anticonvulsant effects—Many sedative-hypnotics are capable of inhibiting the development and spread of epileptiform electrical activity in the central nervous system. Some selectivity exists in that some members of the group can exert anticonvulsant effects without marked central nervous system depression (although psychomotor function may be impaired). Several benzodiazepines—including clonazepam, nitrazepam, lorazepam, and diazepam—are sufficiently selective to be clinically useful in the management of seizures (see Chapter 24). Of the barbiturates, phenobarbital and metharbital (converted to phenobarbital in the body) are effective in the treatment of generalized tonic-clonic seizures. Zolpidem, zaleplon, and eszopiclone lack anticonvulsant activity, presumably because of their more selective binding than that of benzodiazepines to $GABA_A$ receptor isoforms.

THE VERSATILITY OF THE CHLORIDE CHANNEL GABA RECEPTOR COMPLEX

The $GABA_A$-chloride channel macromolecular complex is one of the most versatile drug-responsive machines in the body. In addition to the benzodiazepines, barbiturates, and the newer hypnotics (eg, zolpidem), many other drugs with central nervous system effects can modify the function of this important ionotropic receptor. These include alcohol; alphaxolone, etomidate, and propofol (intravenous anesthetics); volatile anesthetics (eg, halothane); several anticonvulsants (eg, gabapentin, vigabatrin); and ivermectin (an anthelmintic agent). Most of these agents facilitate or mimic the action of GABA. (It has not been shown that these drugs act exclusively or even primarily by this mechanism.) Central nervous system excitatory agents that act on the chloride channel include picrotoxin and bicuculline. These convulsant drugs block the channel directly (picrotoxin) or interfere with GABA binding (bicuculline).

5. Muscle relaxation—Some sedative-hypnotics, particularly members of the carbamate (eg, meprobamate) and benzodiazepine groups, exert inhibitory effects on polysynaptic reflexes and internuncial transmission and at high doses may also depress transmission at the skeletal neuromuscular junction. Somewhat selective actions of this type that lead to muscle relaxation can be readily demonstrated in animals and have led to claims of usefulness for relaxing contracted voluntary muscle in muscle spasm (see Clinical Pharmacology). Muscle relaxation is not a characteristic action of zolpidem, zaleplon, and eszopiclone.

6. Effects on respiration and cardiovascular function—At hypnotic doses in healthy patients, the effects of sedative-hypnotics on respiration are comparable to changes during natural sleep. However, even at therapeutic doses, sedative-hypnotics can produce significant respiratory depression in patients with pulmonary disease. Effects on respiration are dose-related, and depression of the medullary respiratory center is the usual cause of death due to overdose of sedative-hypnotics.

At doses up to those causing hypnosis, no significant effects on the cardiovascular system are observed in healthy patients. However, in hypovolemic states, heart failure, and other diseases that impair cardiovascular function, normal doses of sedative-hypnotics may cause cardiovascular depression, probably as a result of actions on the medullary vasomotor centers. At toxic doses, myocardial contractility and vascular tone may both be depressed by central and peripheral effects, leading to circulatory collapse. Respiratory and cardiovascular effects are more marked when sedative-hypnotics are given intravenously.

Tolerance; Psychologic & Physiologic Dependence

Tolerance—decreased responsiveness to a drug following repeated exposure—is a common feature of sedative-hypnotic use. It may result in the need for an increase in the dose required to maintain symptomatic improvement or to promote sleep. It is important to recognize that partial cross-tolerance occurs between the sedative-hypnotics described here and also with ethanol (Chapter 23)—a feature of some clinical importance, as explained below. The mechanisms responsible for tolerance to sedative-hypnotics are not well understood. An increase in the rate of drug metabolism (metabolic tolerance) may be partly responsible in the case of chronic administration of barbiturates, but changes in responsiveness of the central nervous system (pharmacodynamic tolerance) are of greater importance for most sedative-hypnotics. In the case of benzodiazepines, the development of tolerance in animals has been associated with down-regulation of brain benzodiazepine receptors. Tolerance has been reported to occur with the extended use of zolpidem. Minimal tolerance was observed with the use of zaleplon over a 5-week period and eszopiclone over a 6-month period.

The perceived desirable properties of relief of anxiety, euphoria, disinhibition, and promotion of sleep have led to the compulsive misuse of virtually all sedative-hypnotics. (See Chapter 32 for a detailed discussion.) For this reason, most sedative-hypnotic drugs are classified as Schedule III or Schedule IV drugs for prescribing purposes. The consequences of abuse of these agents can be defined in both psychologic and physiologic terms. The psychologic component may initially parallel simple neurotic behavior patterns difficult to differentiate from those of the inveterate coffee drinker or cigarette smoker. When the pattern of sedative-hypnotic use becomes compulsive, more serious complications develop, including physiologic dependence and tolerance.

Physiologic dependence can be described as an altered physiologic state that requires continuous drug administration to prevent an abstinence or withdrawal syndrome. In the case of sedative-hypnotics, this syndrome is characterized by states of increased anxiety, insomnia, and central nervous system excitability that may progress to convulsions. Most sedative-hypnotics—including benzodiazepines—are capable of causing physiologic dependence when used on a long-term basis. However, the severity of withdrawal symptoms differs among individual drugs and depends also on the magnitude of the dose used immediately before cessation of use. When higher doses of sedative-hypnotics are used, abrupt withdrawal leads to more serious withdrawal signs. Differences in the severity of withdrawal symptoms resulting from individual sedative-hypnotics relate in part to half-life, since drugs with long half-lives are eliminated slowly enough to accomplish gradual withdrawal with few physical symptoms. The use of drugs with very short half-lives for hypnotic effects may lead to signs of withdrawal even between doses. For example, triazolam, a benzodiazepine with a half-life of about 4 hours, has been reported to cause daytime anxiety when used to treat sleep disorders. The abrupt cessation of zolpidem, zaleplon, or eszopiclone may also result in withdrawal symptoms, though usually of less intensity than those seen with benzodiazepines.

BENZODIAZEPINE ANTAGONISTS: FLUMAZENIL

Flumazenil is one of several 1,4-benzodiazepine derivatives with a high affinity for the benzodiazepine binding site on the $GABA_A$ receptor that act as competitive antagonists. It blocks many of the actions of benzodiazepines, zolpidem, zaleplon, and eszopiclone, but does not antagonize the central nervous system effects of other sedative-hypnotics, ethanol, opioids, or general anesthetics. Flumazenil is approved for use in reversing the central nervous system depressant effects of benzodiazepine overdose and to hasten recovery following use of these drugs in anesthetic and diagnostic procedures. Although the drug reverses the sedative effects of benzodiazepines, antagonism of benzodiazepine-induced respiratory depression is less predictable. When given intravenously, flumazenil acts rapidly but has a short half-life (0.7–1.3 hours) due to rapid hepatic clearance. Because all benzodiazepines have a longer duration of action than flumazenil, sedation commonly recurs, requiring repeated administration of the antagonist.

Adverse effects of flumazenil include agitation, confusion, dizziness, and nausea. Flumazenil may cause a severe precipitated abstinence syndrome in patients who have developed physiologic benzodiazepine dependence. In patients who have ingested benzodiazepines with tricyclic antidepressants, seizures and cardiac arrhythmias may follow flumazenil administration.

■ II. CLINICAL PHARMACOLOGY OF SEDATIVE-HYPNOTICS

TREATMENT OF ANXIETY STATES

The psychologic, behavioral, and physiologic responses that characterize anxiety can take many forms. Typically, the psychic awareness of anxiety is accompanied by enhanced vigilance, motor tension, and autonomic hyperactivity. Anxiety is often secondary to organic disease states—acute myocardial infarction, angina pectoris, gastrointestinal ulcers, etc—which themselves require specific therapy. Another class of secondary anxiety states (situational anxiety) results from circumstances that may have to be dealt with only once or a few times, including anticipation of frightening medical or dental procedures and family illness or other stressful event. Even though situational anxiety tends to be self-limiting, the short-term use of sedative-hypnotics may be appropriate for the treatment of this and certain disease-associated anxiety states. Similarly, the use of a sedative-hypnotic as premedication prior to surgery or some unpleasant medical procedure is rational and proper (Table 22–2).

Excessive or unreasonable anxiety about life circumstances (generalized anxiety disorder, GAD), panic disorders, and agoraphobia are also amenable to drug therapy, sometimes in conjunction with psychotherapy. The benzodiazepines continue to be widely used for the management of acute anxiety states and for rapid control of panic attacks. They are also used in the long-

Table 22–2. Clinical uses of sedative-hypnotics.

For relief of anxiety
For insomnia
For sedation and amnesia before and during medical and surgical procedures
For treatment of epilepsy and seizure states
 As a component of balanced anesthesia (intravenous administration)
For control of ethanol or other sedative-hypnotic withdrawal states
For muscle relaxation in specific neuromuscular disorders
As diagnostic aids or for treatment in psychiatry

term management of GAD and panic disorders. Anxiety symptoms may be relieved by many benzodiazepines, but it is not always easy to demonstrate the superiority of one drug over another. However, alprazolam is particularly effective in the treatment of panic disorders and agoraphobia and appears to be more selective in these conditions than other benzodiazepines. The choice of benzodiazepines for anxiety is based on several sound pharmacologic principles: (1) a relatively high therapeutic index (see drug B in Figure 22–1), plus availability of flumazenil for treatment of overdose; (2) a low risk of drug interactions based on liver enzyme induction; (3) minimal effects on cardiovascular or autonomic functions.

Disadvantages of the benzodiazepines include the risk of dependence, depression of central nervous system functions, and amnestic effects. In addition, the benzodiazepines exert additive central nervous system depression when administered with other drugs, including ethanol. The patient should be warned of this possibility to avoid impairment of performance of any task requiring mental alertness and motor coordination. In the treatment of generalized anxiety disorders and certain phobias, newer antidepressants, including selective serotonin reuptake inhibitors, are now considered by many authorities to be drugs of first choice (see Chapter 30). However, these agents have minimal effectiveness in acute anxiety states.

Sedative-hypnotics should be used with appropriate caution so as to minimize adverse effects. A dose should be prescribed that does not impair mentation or motor functions during waking hours. Some patients may tolerate the drug better if most of the daily dose is given at bedtime, with smaller doses during the day. Prescriptions should be written for short periods, since there is little justification for long-term therapy (defined as use of therapeutic doses for 2 months or longer). The physician should make an effort to assess the efficacy of therapy from the patient's subjective responses. Combinations of antianxiety agents should be avoided, and people taking sedatives should be cautioned about the consumption of alcohol and the concurrent use of over-the-counter medications containing antihistaminic or anticholinergic drugs (see Chapter 64).

TREATMENT OF SLEEP PROBLEMS

Sleep disorders are common and often result from inadequate treatment of underlying medical conditions or psychiatric illness. True primary insomnia is rare. Nonpharmacologic therapies that are useful for sleep problems include proper diet and exercise, avoiding stimulants before retiring, ensuring a comfortable sleeping environment, and retiring at a regular time each night. In some cases, however, the patient will need and should be given a sedative-hypnotic for a limited period. It should be noted that the abrupt discontinuance of many drugs in this class can lead to rebound insomnia.

Benzodiazepines can cause a dose-dependent decrease in both REM and slow-wave sleep, though to a lesser extent than the barbiturates. The newer hypnotics zolpidem, zaleplon, and eszopiclone are less likely than the benzodiazepines to change sleep patterns. However, so little is known about the clinical impact of these effects that statements about the desirability of a particular drug based on its effects on sleep architecture have more theoretical than practical significance. Clinical criteria of efficacy in alleviating a particular sleeping problem are more useful. The drug selected should be one that provides sleep of fairly rapid onset (decreased sleep latency) and sufficient duration, with minimal "hangover" effects such as drowsiness, dysphoria, and

mental or motor depression the following day. Older drugs such as chloral hydrate, secobarbital, and pentobarbital continue to be used, but benzodiazepines, zolpidem, zaleplon, or eszopiclone are generally preferred. Daytime sedation is more common with benzodiazepines that have slow elimination rates (eg, lorazepam) and those that are biotransformed to active metabolites (eg, flurazepam, quazepam). If benzodiazepines are used nightly, tolerance can occur, which may lead to dose increases by the patient to produce the desired effect. Anterograde amnesia occurs to some degree with all benzodiazepines used for hypnosis.

Eszopiclone, zaleplon, and zolpidem have efficacies similar to those of the hypnotic benzodiazepines in the management of sleep disorders. Favorable clinical features of zolpidem and the other newer hypnotics include rapid onset of activity and modest day-after psychomotor depression with few amnestic effects. Zolpidem, currently the most frequently prescribed hypnotic drug in the United States, is available in a biphasic release formulation that provides sustained drug levels for sleep maintenance. Zaleplon acts rapidly, and because of its short half-life, the drug appears to have value in the management of patients who awaken early in the sleep cycle. At recommended doses, zaleplon and eszopiclone (despite its relatively long half-life) appear to cause less amnesia or day-after somnolence than zolpidem or benzodiazepines. The drugs commonly used for sedation and hypnosis are listed in Table 22–3 together with recommended doses. *Note:* Long-term use of hypnotics is an irrational and dangerous medical practice.

Table 22–3. Dosages of drugs used commonly for sedation and hypnosis.

Sedation		Hypnosis	
Drug	**Dosage**	**Drug**	**Dosage (at Bedtime)**
Alprazolam (Xanax)	0.25–0.5 mg 2–3 times daily	Chloral hydrate	500–1000 mg
Buspirone (BuSpar)	5–10 mg 2–3 times daily	Estazolam (ProSom)	0.5–2 mg
Chlordiazepoxide (Librium)	10–20 mg 2–3 times daily	Eszopiclone (Lunesta)	1–3 mg
Clorazepate (Tranxene)	5–7.5 mg twice daily	Lorazepam (Ativan)	2–4 mg
Diazepam (Valium)	5 mg twice daily	Quazepam (Doral)	7.5–15 mg
Halazepam (Paxipam)	20–40 mg 3–4 times daily	Secobarbital	100–200 mg
Lorazepam (Ativan)	1–2 mg once or twice daily	Temazepam (Restoril)	7.5–30 mg
Oxazepam	15–30 mg 3–4 times daily	Triazolam (Halcion)	0.125–0.5 mg
Phenobarbital	15–30 mg 2–3 times daily	Zaleplon (Sonata)	5–20 mg
		Zolpidem (Ambien)	5–10 mg

OTHER THERAPEUTIC USES

Table 22–2 summarizes several other important clinical uses of drugs in the sedative-hypnotic class. Drugs used in the management of seizure disorders and as intravenous agents in anesthesia are discussed in Chapters 24 and 25.

For sedative and possible amnestic effects during medical or surgical procedures such as endoscopy and bronchoscopy—as well as for premedication prior to anesthesia—oral formulations of shorter-acting drugs are preferred.

Long-acting drugs such as chlordiazepoxide and diazepam and, to a lesser extent, phenobarbital are administered in progressively decreasing doses to patients during withdrawal from physiologic dependence on ethanol or other sedative-hypnotics. Parenteral lorazepam is used to suppress the symptoms of delirium tremens.

Meprobamate and, more recently, the benzodiazepines have frequently been used as central muscle relaxants, though evidence for general efficacy without accompanying sedation is lacking. A possible exception is diazepam, which has useful relaxant effects in skeletal muscle spasticity of central origin (see Chapter 27).

Psychiatric uses of benzodiazepines other than treatment of anxiety states include the initial management of mania, the control of drug-induced hyperexcitability states (eg, phencyclidine intoxication), and possibly the treatment of major depressive disorders with alprazolam. Sedative-hypnotics are also used occasionally as diagnostic aids in neurology and psychiatry.

CLINICAL TOXICOLOGY OF SEDATIVE-HYPNOTICS

Direct Toxic Actions

Many of the common adverse effects of sedative-hypnotics result from dose-related depression of the central nervous system. Relatively low doses may lead to drowsiness, impaired judgment, and diminished motor skills, sometimes with a significant impact on driving ability, job performance, and personal relationships. Benzodiazepines may cause a significant dose-related anterograde amnesia; they can significantly impair ability to learn new information, particularly that involving effortful cognitive processes, while leaving the retrieval of previously learned information intact. This effect is utilized for uncomfortable clinical procedures, eg, endoscopy, because the patient is able to cooperate during the procedure but amnesic regarding it afterward. The criminal use of benzodiazepines in cases of "date rape" is based on their dose-dependent amnestic effects. Hangover effects are not uncommon following use of hypnotic drugs with long elimination half-lives. Because elderly patients are more sensitive to the effects of sedative-hypnotics, doses approximately half of those used in younger adults are safer and usually as effective. The most common reversible cause of confusional states in the elderly is overuse of sedative-hypnotics. At higher doses, toxicity may present as lethargy or a state of exhaustion or, alternatively, as gross symptoms equivalent to those of ethanol intoxication. The physician should be aware of variability among patients in terms of doses causing adverse effects. An increased sensitivity to sedative-hypnotics is more common in patients with cardiovascular disease, respiratory disease, or hepatic impairment and in older patients. Sedative-hypnotics can exacerbate breathing problems in patients with chronic pulmonary disease and in those with symptomatic sleep apnea.

Sedative-hypnotics are the drugs most frequently involved in deliberate overdoses, in part because of their general availability as very commonly prescribed pharmacologic agents. The benzodiazepines are considered to be safer drugs in this respect, since they have flatter dose-response curves. Epidemiologic studies on the incidence of drug-related deaths support this general assumption—eg, 0.3 deaths per million tablets of diazepam prescribed versus 11.6 deaths per million capsules of secobarbital in one study. Alprazolam is purportedly more toxic in overdose than other benzodiazepines. Of course, many factors other than the specific sedative-hypnotic could influence such data—particularly the presence of other central nervous system depressants, including ethanol. In fact, most serious cases of drug overdosage, intentional or accidental, do involve polypharmacy; and when combinations of agents are taken, the practical safety of benzodiazepines may be less than the foregoing would imply.

The lethal dose of any sedative-hypnotic varies with the patient and the circumstances (see Chapter 59). If discovery of the ingestion is made early and a conservative treatment regimen is started, the outcome is rarely fatal, even following very high doses. On the other hand, for most sedative-hypnotics—with the exception of benzodiazepines and possibly the newer hypnotic drugs that have a similar mechanism of action—a dose as low as ten times the hypnotic dose may be fatal if the patient is not discovered or does not seek help in time. With severe toxicity, the respiratory depression from central actions of the drug may be complicated by aspiration of gastric contents in the unattended patient—an even more likely occurrence if ethanol is present. Cardiovascular depression further complicates successful resuscitation. In such patients, treatment consists of ensuring a patent airway, with mechanical ventilation if needed, and maintenance of plasma volume, renal output, and cardiac function. Use of a positive inotropic drug such as dopamine, which preserves renal blood flow, is sometimes indicated. Hemodialysis or hemoperfusion may be used to hasten elimination of some of these drugs.

Flumazenil reverses the sedative actions of benzodiazepines, and probably those of eszopiclone, zaleplon, and zolpidem, although experience with its use in overdose of the newer hypnotics is limited. However, its duration of action is short, its antagonism of respiratory depression is unpredictable, and there is a risk of precipitation of withdrawal symptoms in long-term users of benzodiazpines (see below). Consequently, the use of flumazenil in benzodiazepine overdose remains controversial and *must* be accompanied by adequate monitoring and support of respiratory function. The extensive clinical use of triazolam has led to reports of serious central nervous system effects including behavioral disinhibition, delirium, aggression, and violence. Although behavioral disinhibition may occur with sedative-hypnotic drugs, it does not appear to be more prevalent with triazolam than with other benzodiazepines. Disinhibitory reactions during benzodiazepine treatment are more clearly associated with the use of very high doses and the pretreatment level of patient hostility.

Adverse effects of the sedative-hypnotics that are not referable to their central nervous system actions occur infrequently. Hypersensitivity reactions, including skin rashes, occur only occasionally with most drugs of this class. Reports of teratogenicity leading to fetal deformation following use of piperidinediones and certain benzodiazepines justify caution in the use of these drugs during pregnancy. Because barbiturates enhance porphyrin synthesis, they are *absolutely contraindicated* in patients with a history of acute intermittent porphyria, variegate porphyria, hereditary coproporphyria, or symptomatic porphyria.

Alterations in Drug Response

Depending on the dosage and the duration of use, tolerance occurs in varying degrees to many of the pharmacologic effects of sedative-hypnotics. However, it should not be assumed that the degree of tolerance achieved is identical for all pharmacologic effects. There is evidence that the lethal dose range is not altered significantly by the long-term use of sedative-hypnotics. Cross-tolerance between the different sedative-hypnotics, including ethanol, can lead to an unsatisfactory therapeutic response when standard doses of a drug are used in a patient with a recent history of excessive use of

these agents. However, there have been very few reports of tolerance development when eszopiclone, zolpidem, or zaleplon was used for less than 4 weeks.

With the long-term use of sedative-hypnotics, especially if doses are increased, a state of physiologic dependence can occur. This may develop to a degree unparalleled by any other drug group, *including the opioids.* Withdrawal from a sedative-hypnotic can have severe and life-threatening manifestations. Withdrawal symptoms range from restlessness, anxiety, weakness, and orthostatic hypotension to hyperactive reflexes and generalized seizures. Symptoms of withdrawal are usually more severe following discontinuance of sedative-hypnotics with shorter half-lives. However, eszopiclone, zolpidem, and zaleplon appear to be exceptions to this, because withdrawal symptoms are minimal following abrupt discontinuance of these newer short-acting agents. Symptoms are less pronounced with longer-acting drugs, which may partly accomplish their own "tapered" withdrawal by virtue of their slow elimination. Cross-dependence, defined as the ability of one drug to suppress abstinence symptoms from discontinuance of another drug, is quite marked among sedative-hypnotics. This provides the rationale for therapeutic regimens in the management of withdrawal states: Longer-acting drugs such as chlordiazepoxide, diazepam, and phenobarbital can be used to alleviate withdrawal symptoms of shorter-acting drugs, including ethanol.

Drug Interactions

The most common drug interactions involving sedative-hypnotics are interactions with other central nervous system depressant drugs, leading to additive effects. These interactions have some therapeutic usefulness when these drugs are used as adjuvants in anesthesia practice. However, if not anticipated, such interactions can lead to serious consequences, including enhanced depression with concomitant use of many other drugs. Additive effects can be predicted with concomitant use of alcoholic beverages, opioid analgesics, anticonvulsants, and phenothiazines. Less obvious but just as important is enhanced central nervous system depression with a variety of antihistamines, antihypertensive agents, and antidepressant drugs of the tricyclic class.

Interactions involving changes in the activity of hepatic drug-metabolizing enzyme systems have been discussed (see also Chapter 4 and Appendix II).

PREPARATIONS AVAILABLE

BENZODIAZEPINES

Alprazolam (generic, Xanax)
Oral: 0.25, 0.5, 1, 2 mg tablets, extended-release tablets, and orally disintegrating tablets; 1.0 mg/mL solution

Chlordiazepoxide (generic, Librium)
Oral: 5, 10, 25 mg capsules
Parenteral: 100 mg powder for injection

Clorazepate (generic, Tranxene)
Oral: 3.75, 7.5, 15 mg tablets and capsules
Oral sustained-release: 11.25, 22.5 mg tablets

Clonazepam (generic, Klonopin)
Oral: 0.5, 1, 2 mg tablets; 0.125, 0.25, 0.5, 1, 2 mg orally disintegrating tablets

Diazepam (generic, Valium)
Oral: 2, 5, 10 mg tablets; 1, 5 mg/mL solutions
Parenteral: 5 mg/mL for injection

Estazolam (generic, ProSom)
Oral: 1, 2 mg tablets

Flurazepam (generic, Dalmane)
Oral: 15, 30 mg capsules

Lorazepam (generic, Ativan)
Oral: 0.5, 1, 2 mg tablets; 2 mg/mL solution
Parenteral: 2, 4 mg/mL for injection

Midazolam (Versed)
Oral: 2 mg/mL syrup
Parenteral: 1, 5 mg/mL in 1, 2, 5, 10 mL vials for injection

Oxazepam (generic)
Oral: 10, 15, 30 mg capsules

Quazepam (Doral)
Oral: 7.5, 15 mg tablets

Temazepam (generic, Restoril)
Oral: 7.5, 15, 22.5, 30 mg capsules

Triazolam (generic, Halcion)
Oral: 0.125, 0.25 mg tablets

BENZODIAZEPINE ANTAGONIST

Flumazenil (Romazicon)
Parenteral: 0.1 mg/mL for IV injection

BARBITURATES

Amobarbital (Amytal)
Parenteral: powder in 250, 500 mg vials to reconstitute for injection

Mephobarbital (Mebaral)
Oral: 32, 50, 100 mg tablets

Pentobarbital (generic, Nembutal Sodium)
Oral: 50, 100 mg capsules; 4 mg/mL elixir
Rectal: 30, 60, 120, 200 mg suppositories
Parenteral: 50 mg/mL for injection

Phenobarbital (generic, Luminal Sodium)
Oral: 15, 16, 30, 60, 90, 100 mg tablets; 16 mg capsules; 15, 20 mg/5 mL elixirs
Parenteral: 30, 60, 65, 130 mg/mL for injection

Secobarbital (generic, Seconal)
Oral: 100 mg capsules

MISCELLANEOUS DRUGS

Buspirone (generic, BuSpar)
Oral: 5, 7.5, 10, 15, 30 mg tablets

Chloral hydrate (generic, Aquachloral Supprettes)
Oral: 500 mg capsules; 250, 500 mg/5 mL syrups
Rectal: 324, 648 mg suppositories

Eszopiclone (Lunesta)
Oral: 1, 2, 3 mg tablets

Hydroxyzine (generic, Atarax, Vistaril)
Oral: 10, 25, 50, 100 mg tablets; 25, 50, 100 mg capsules; 10 mg/5 mL syrup; 25 mg/5 mL suspension
Parenteral: 25, 50 mg/mL for injection

Meprobamate (generic, Equanil, Miltown)
Oral: 200, 400 mg tablets

Paraldehyde (generic)
Oral, rectal liquids: 1 g/mL

Ramelteon (Rozerem)
Oral: 8 mg tablets

Zaleplon (Sonata)
Oral: 5, 10 mg capsules

Zolpidem (Ambien, Ambien-CR)
Oral: 5, 10 mg tablets; 6.25, 12.5 mg extended-release tablets

REFERENCES

Ancoli-Israel S et al: Long-term use of sedative hypnotics in older patients with insomnia. Sleep Med 2005;6:107.

Bateson AN: The benzodiazepine site of the GABA A receptor: An old target with new potential? Sleep Med 2004;5(Suppl 1):S9.

Blednov YA et al: Deletion of the alpha$_1$ or beta$_2$ subunit of GABA$_A$ receptors reduces actions of alcohol and other drugs. J Pharmacol Exp Ther 2003;304:30.

Crestani F et al: Molecular targets for the myorelaxant action of diazepam. Mol Pharmacol 2001;59:442.

Drover DR: Comparative pharmacokinetics and pharmacodynamics of short-acting hypnosedatives: Zaleplon, zolpidem and zopiclone. Clin Pharmacokinet 2004;43:227.

Fricchione G: Generalized anxiety disorder. N Engl J Med 2004; 351:675.

Gottesmann C: GABA mechanisms and sleep. Neuroscience 2002; 111:231.

Hesse LM et al: Clinically important drug interactions with zopiclone, zolpidem and zaleplon. CNS Drugs 2003;17:513.

Israel AG, Kramer JA: Safety of zaleplon in the treatment of insomnia. Ann Pharmacother 2002;36:852.

Kato K et al: Neurochemical properties of ramelteon, a selective MT1/MT2 receptor agonist. Neuropharmacology 2005; 48:301.

Kralic JE et al: GABA(A) receptor alpha-1 subunit deletion alters receptor subtype assembly, pharmacological and behavioral responses to benzodiazepines and zolpidem. Neuropharmacology 2002;43:685.

Krystal AD: The changing perspective of chronic insomnia management. J Clin Psychiatry 2004;65(suppl 8):20.

Mahmood I, Sahalwalla C: Clinical pharmacokinetics and pharmacodynamics of buspirone, an anxiolytic drug. Clin Pharmacokinet 1999;36:277.

McKernan RM et al: Anxiolytic-like action of diazepam: Which GABA(A) receptor subtype is involved? Trends Pharmacol Sci 2001;22:402.

Mintzer MZ, Griffiths RR: Triazolam and zolpidem: Effects on human memory and attentional processes. Psychopharmacology (Berl) 1999;144:8.

Mohler H, Fritschy JM, Rudolph U: A new benzodiazepine pharmacology. J Pharmacol Exp Ther 2002;300:2.

Patat A, Paty I, Hindmarch I: Pharmacodynamic profile of Zaleplon, a new non-benzodiazepine hypnotic agent. Hum Psychopharmacol 2001;16:369.

Rickels K, Rynn M: Pharmacotherapy of generalized anxiety disorder. J Clin Psychiatry 2002;63(Suppl 14):9.

Rosenberg R et al: An assessment of the efficacy and safety of eszopiclone in the treatment of transient insomnia in healthy adults. Sleep Med 2005;6:15.

Silber MH: Chronic insomnia. N Engl J Med 2005;353:803.

Turek FW, Gillette MU: Melatonin, sleep and circadian rhythms: Rationale for development of specific melatonin agonists. Sleep Med 2004;5:523.

Verster JC et al: Residual effects of sleep medication on driving ability. Sleep Med Rev 2004;8:309.

The Alcohols

23

Susan B. Masters, PhD

Alcohol, primarily in the form of ethyl alcohol (ethanol), has occupied an important place in the history of humankind for at least 8000 years. In Western society, beer and wine were a main staple of daily life until the 19th century. These relatively dilute alcoholic beverages were preferred over water, which was known to be associated with acute and chronic illness. They provided important calories and nutrients and served as a main source of daily liquid intake. As systems for improved sanitation and water purification were introduced in the 1800s, beer and wine became less important components of the human diet, and the consumption of alcoholic beverages, including distilled preparations with higher concentrations of alcohol, shifted toward their present-day role, in many societies, as a socially acceptable form of recreation.

Today, alcohol is widely consumed. Like other sedative-hypnotic drugs, alcohol in low to moderate amounts relieves anxiety and fosters a feeling of well-being or even euphoria. However, alcohol is also the most commonly abused drug in the world, and a cause of vast medical and societal costs. In the United States, approximately 75% of the adult population drinks alcohol regularly. The majority of this drinking population are able to enjoy the pleasurable effects of alcohol without allowing their alcohol consumption to become a health risk. However, about 10% of the general population in the United States are unable to limit their ethanol consumption, a condition known as **alcohol abuse.** People who continue to drink alcohol in spite of adverse medical or social consequences related directly to their alcohol consumption suffer from **alcoholism,** a complex disorder that appears to have genetic as well as environmental determinants.

The societal and medical costs of alcohol abuse are staggering. It is estimated that about 30% of all people admitted to hospitals have coexisting alcohol problems. Once in the hospital, people with chronic alcoholism generally have poorer outcomes. In addition, each year thousands of children are born in the USA with morphologic and functional defects resulting from prenatal exposure to ethanol. Despite the investment of many resources and much basic research, alcoholism remains a common chronic disease that is difficult to treat.

Ethanol and many other alcohols with potentially toxic effects are used in industry, some in enormous quantities. In addition to ethanol, methanol and ethylene glycol toxicity occur with sufficient frequency to warrant discussion in this chapter.

■ I. BASIC PHARMACOLOGY OF ETHANOL

Pharmacokinetics

Ethanol is a small water-soluble molecule that is absorbed rapidly from the gastrointestinal tract. After ingestion of alcohol in the fasting state, peak blood alcohol concentrations are reached within 30 minutes. The presence of food in the gut delays absorption by slowing gastric emptying. Distribution is rapid, with tissue levels approximating the concentration in blood. The volume of distribution for ethanol approximates total body water (0.5–0.7 L/kg). For an equivalent oral dose of alcohol, women have a higher peak concentration than men, in part because women have a lower total body water content. In the central nervous system, the concentration of ethanol rises quickly since the brain receives a large proportion of total blood flow and ethanol readily crosses biologic membranes.

Over 90% of alcohol consumed is oxidized in the liver; much of the remainder is excreted through the lungs and in the urine. The excretion of a small but consistent proportion of alcohol by the lungs is utilized for breath alcohol tests that serve as a basis for a legal definition of "driving under the influence" in many countries. At levels of ethanol usually achieved in blood, the rate of oxidation follows zero-order kinetics; that is, it is independent of time and concentration of the drug. The typical adult can metabolize 7–10 g (150–220 mmol) of alcohol per hour, the equivalent of approximately one "drink" (10 oz of beer, 3.5 oz of wine, or 1 oz of distilled 80 proof spirits).

Two major pathways of alcohol metabolism to acetaldehyde have been identified (Figure 23–1). Acetaldehyde is then oxidized by a third metabolic process.

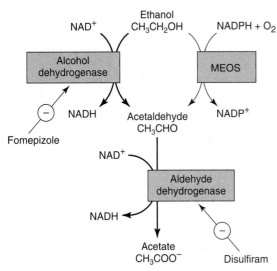

Figure 23–1. Metabolism of ethanol by alcohol dehydrogenase and the microsomal ethanol-oxidizing system (MEOS). Alcohol dehydrogenase and aldehyde dehydrogenase are inhibited by fomepizole and disulfiram, respectively.

A. ALCOHOL DEHYDROGENASE PATHWAY

The primary pathway for alcohol metabolism involves alcohol dehydrogenase (ADH), a cytosolic enzyme that catalyzes the conversion of alcohol to acetaldehyde (Figure 23–1, left). This enzyme is located mainly in the liver, but it is also found in other organs such as the brain and stomach. In some Asian populations with polymorphisms in ADH that affect enzyme activity, a form of ADH with reduced activity is associated with an increased risk of alcoholism.

A significant amount of ethanol metabolism by gastric ADH occurs in the stomach in men, but a smaller amount occurs in women, who appear to have lower levels of the gastric enzyme. This difference in gastric metabolism of alcohol in women probably contributes to the sex-related differences in blood alcohol concentrations noted above.

During conversion of ethanol to acetaldehyde, hydrogen ion is transferred from alcohol to the cofactor nicotinamide adenine dinucleotide (NAD$^+$) to form NADH. As a net result, alcohol oxidation generates an excess of reducing equivalents in the liver, chiefly as NADH. The excess NADH production appears to contribute to a number of metabolic disorders that accompany chronic alcoholism.

B. MICROSOMAL ETHANOL OXIDIZING SYSTEM (MEOS)

This enzyme system, also known as the mixed function oxidase system, uses NADPH as a cofactor in the metabolism of ethanol (Figure 23–1, right) and consists primarily of cytochrome P450 2E1, 1A2, and 3A4 (see Chapter 4).

At blood concentrations below 100 mg/dL (22 mmol/L), the MEOS system, which has a relatively high K_m for alcohol, contributes little to the metabolism of ethanol. However, when large amounts of ethanol are consumed, the alcohol dehydrogenase system becomes saturated owing to depletion of the required cofactor, NAD$^+$. As the concentration of ethanol increases above 100 mg/dL, there is increased contribution from the MEOS system, which does not rely upon NAD$^+$ as a cofactor.

During chronic alcohol consumption, MEOS activity is induced. As a result, chronic alcohol consumption results in significant increases not only in ethanol metabolism but also in the clearance of other drugs eliminated by the cytochrome P450s that constitute the MEOS system and the generation of the toxic byproducts of cytochrome P450 reactions (toxins, free radicals, H_2O_2).

C. ACETALDEHYDE METABOLISM

Much of the acetaldehyde formed from alcohol appears to be oxidized in the liver in a reaction catalyzed by mitochondrial NAD-dependent aldehyde dehydrogenase (ALDH). The product of this reaction is acetate (Figure 23–1), which can be further metabolized to CO_2 and water.

Oxidation of acetaldehyde is inhibited by disulfiram, a drug that has been used to deter drinking by alcohol-dependent patients undergoing treatment. When ethanol is consumed in the presence of disulfiram, acetaldehyde accumulates and causes an unpleasant reaction of facial flushing, nausea, vomiting, dizziness, and headache. Several other drugs (eg, metronidazole, cefotetan, trimethoprim) inhibit ALDH and can cause a disulfiram-like reaction if combined with ethanol.

Some people, primarily of Asian descent, have a genetic deficiency in the activity of the mitochondrial form of ALDH. When these individuals drink alcohol, they develop high blood acetaldehyde concentrations and experience a flushing reaction similar to that seen with the combination of disulfiram and ethanol. Although the presence of the form of ALDH with reduced activity appears to protect against alcoholism, its presence in alcoholics is associated with increased risk of severe liver disease, presumably owing to the toxic effects of aldehyde.

Pharmacodynamics of Acute Ethanol Consumption

A. CENTRAL NERVOUS SYSTEM

The central nervous system (CNS) is markedly affected by acute alcohol consumption. Alcohol causes sedation and relief of anxiety and, at higher concentrations, slurred speech, ataxia, impaired judgment, and disin-

Table 23–1. Blood alcohol concentration (BAC) and clinical effects in nontolerant individuals.

BAC (mg/dL)[1]	Clinical Effect
50–100	Sedation, subjective "high," slower reaction times
100–200	Impaired motor function, slurred speech, ataxia
200–300	Emesis, stupor
300–400	Coma
> 500	Respiratory depression, death

[1]In many parts of the USA, a blood level above 80–100 mg/dL for adults or 10 mg/dL for persons under 21 is sufficient for conviction of driving while "under the influence."

hibited behavior, a condition usually called intoxication or drunkenness (Table 23–1). These CNS effects are most marked as the blood level is rising, because acute tolerance to the effects of alcohol occurs after a few hours of drinking. For chronic drinkers who are tolerant to the effects of alcohol, much higher concentrations are needed to elicit these central nervous system effects. For example, a chronic alcoholic may appear sober or only slightly intoxicated with a blood alcohol concentration of 300–400 mg/dL, whereas this level is associated with marked intoxication or even coma in a nontolerant individual. The propensity of moderate doses of alcohol to inhibit the attention and information-processing skills as well as the motor skills required for operation of motor vehicles has profound effects. Approximately half of all traffic accidents resulting in a fatality in the United States involve at least one person with blood alcohol near or above the legal level of intoxication, and drunken driving is a leading cause of death in young adults.

Like other sedative-hypnotic drugs, alcohol is a central nervous system depressant. At high blood concentrations, it induces coma, respiratory depression, and death.

Ethanol affects a large number of membrane proteins that participate in signaling pathways, including neurotransmitter receptors for amines, amino acids, and opioids; enzymes such as Na^+/K^+ ATPase, adenylyl cyclase, phosphoinositide-specific phospholipase C, and ion channels. Much attention has focused on alcohol's effects on neurotransmission by glutamate and GABA, the main excitatory and inhibitory neurotransmitters in the CNS. Acute ethanol exposure enhances the action of GABA at $GABA_A$ receptors, which is consistent with the ability of GABA-mimetics to intensify many of the acute effects of alcohol and of $GABA_A$ antagonists to attenuate some of the actions of ethanol. Ethanol inhibits the abil-

ity of glutamate to open the cation channel associated with the N-methyl-D-aspartate (NMDA) subtype of glutamate receptors. The NMDA receptor is implicated in many aspects of cognitive function, including learning and memory. "Blackouts"—periods of memory loss that occur with high levels of alcohol—may result from inhibition of NMDA receptor activation. Experiments that use modern genetic approaches eventually will yield a more precise definition of ethanol's direct and indirect targets. In recent years, experiments with mutant strains of worms and flies have focused attention on several key genes, including a calcium-regulated and voltage-gated potassium channel that may be one of ethanol's direct targets (see Box: What Can Drunken Worms, Flies, And Mice Tell Us About Alcohol?).

B. HEART

Significant depression of myocardial contractility has been observed in individuals who acutely consume moderate amounts of alcohol, ie, at a blood concentration above 100 mg/dL.

C. SMOOTH MUSCLE

Ethanol is a vasodilator, probably as a result of both central nervous system effects (depression of the vasomotor center) and direct smooth muscle relaxation caused by its metabolite, acetaldehyde. In cases of severe overdose, hypothermia—caused by vasodilation—may be marked in cold environments. Ethanol also relaxes the uterus and—before the introduction of more effective and safer uterine relaxants (eg, calcium blockers, magnesium ion, and β_2-adrenoceptor stimulants)—was used intravenously for the suppression of premature labor.

Consequences of Chronic Alcohol Consumption

Chronic alcohol consumption profoundly affects the function of several vital organs—particularly the liver and skeletal muscle—and the nervous, gastrointestinal, cardiovascular, and immune systems. Since ethanol has low potency, it requires concentrations thousands of times higher than other misused drugs (eg, cocaine, opiates, amphetamines) to produce its intoxicating effects. As a result, ethanol is consumed in quantities that are unusually large for a pharmacologically active drug. The tissue damage caused by chronic alcohol ingestion results from a combination of the direct effects of ethanol and the metabolic consequences of processing a heavy load of a metabolically active substance. Specific mechanisms implicated in tissue damage include increased oxidative stress coupled with depletion of glutathione, damage to mitochondria, growth factor dysregulation, and potentiation of cytokine-induced injury.

WHAT CAN DRUNKEN WORMS, FLIES, AND MICE TELL US ABOUT ALCOHOL?

For a drug like ethanol, which exhibits low potency and specificity and modifies complex behaviors, the identification of direct molecular targets is difficult and has thus far proved elusive. Increasingly, ethanol researchers are employing genetic approaches to complement standard neurobiologic experimentation. Three experimental animal systems for which powerful genetic techniques exist—mice, flies, and worms—have yielded intriguing results.

Strains of mice with abnormal sensitivity to ethanol were identified many years ago by breeding and selection programs. Using sophisticated genetic mapping and sequencing techniques, researchers have made progress in identifying the genes that confer these traits. A more targeted approach is the use of transgenic mice to test hypotheses about specific genes. For example, after earlier experiments suggested a link between brain neuropeptide Y (NPY) and ethanol, researchers used two transgenic mouse models to further investigate the link. They found that a strain of mice that lacks the gene for NPY—NPY knockout mice—consume more ethanol than control mice and are less sensitive to ethanol's sedative effects. As would be expected if increased concentrations of NPY in the brain make mice more sensitive to ethanol, a strain of mice that overexpresses NPY drinks less alcohol than the controls even though their total consumption of food and liquid is normal. Work with other transgenic knockout mice have also implicated the dopamine D_2 and D_4 receptors and a subtype of protein kinase C with altered sensitivity to ethanol.

It is easy to imagine mice having measurable behavioral responses to alcohol but drunken worms and fruit flies are harder to imagine. Actually, both invertebrates respond to ethanol in ways that parallel mammalian responses. *Drosophila melanogaster* fruit flies that are exposed to ethanol vapor show increased locomotion at low concentrations but at higher concentrations, become poorly coordinated, sedated, and finally immobile. The behaviors can be monitored by sophisticated laser or video tracking methods or with an ingenious "chromatography" column that separates relatively insensitive flies from inebriated flies that drop to the bottom of the column. The worm *Caenorhabditis elegans* similarly exhibits increased locomotion at low ethanol concentrations and, at higher concentrations, reduced locomotion, sedation, and—something that can be turned into an effective screen for mutant worms that are resistant to ethanol—impaired egg laying. The advantage of using flies and worms as genetic models for ethanol research is their relatively simple neuroanatomy, well-established techniques for genetic manipulation, an extensive library of well-characterized mutants, and completely or nearly completely solved genetic code. Already, much information has accumulated about candidate proteins involved with the effects of ethanol in flies. In an elegant study on *C elegans*, researchers found evidence that a calcium-activated, voltage-gated BK potassium channel is a direct target of ethanol. This channel, which is activated by ethanol, has close homologs in flies and vertebrates, and evidence is accumulating that ethanol has similar effects in these homologs. Genetic experiments in these model systems should provide information that will help narrow and focus research into the complex and important effects of ethanol in humans.

Chronic consumption of large amounts of alcohol is associated with an increased risk of death. Deaths linked to alcohol consumption are caused by liver disease, cancer, accidents, and suicide.

A. Liver and Gastrointestinal Tract

Liver disease is the most common medical complication of alcohol abuse; an estimated 15–30% of chronic heavy drinkers eventually develop severe liver disease. Alcoholic fatty liver, a reversible condition, may progress to alcoholic hepatitis and finally to cirrhosis and liver failure. In the USA, chronic alcohol abuse is the leading cause of liver cirrhosis and of the need for liver transplantation. The risk of developing liver disease is related both to the average amount of daily consumption and to the duration of alcohol abuse. Women appear to be more susceptible to alcohol hepatotoxicity than men. Concurrent infection with hepatitis B or C virus increases the risk of severe liver disease.

The pathogenesis of alcoholic liver disease is a multifactorial process involving metabolic repercussions of ethanol oxidation in the liver, dysregulation of fatty acid oxidation and synthesis, and activation of the innate immune system by a combination of direct effects of ethanol and its metabolites and by bacterial endotoxins that access the liver as a result of ethanol-induced changes in the intestinal tract. Tumor necrosis factor-α, a pro-inflammatory cytokine that is consistently elevated in animal models of alcoholic liver disease and in patients with alcoholic liver disease, appears to play a pivotal role the progression of alcoholic liver disease and may be a fruitful therapeutic target.

Other portions of the gastrointestinal tract can also be injured. Chronic alcohol ingestion is by far the most common cause of chronic pancreatitis in the Western world. In addition to its direct toxic effect on pancreatic acinar cells, alcohol alters pancreatic epithelial permeability and promotes the formation of protein plugs and calcium carbonate-containing stones.

Chronic alcoholics are prone to gastritis and have increased susceptibility to blood and plasma protein loss during drinking, which may contribute to anemia and protein malnutrition. Alcohol also reversibly injures the small intestine, leading to diarrhea, weight loss, and multiple vitamin deficiencies.

Malnutrition from dietary deficiency and vitamin deficiencies due to malabsorption are common in alcoholic individuals. Malabsorption of water-soluble vitamins is especially severe.

B. NERVOUS SYSTEM

1. Tolerance and physical dependence—The consumption of alcohol in high doses over a long period results in tolerance and in physical and psychologic dependence. Tolerance to the intoxicating effects of alcohol is a complex process involving poorly understood changes in the nervous system as well as the metabolic changes described earlier. As with other sedative-hypnotic drugs, there is a limit to tolerance, so that only a relatively small increase in the lethal dose occurs with increasing alcohol use.

Chronic alcohol drinkers, when forced to reduce or discontinue alcohol, experience a withdrawal syndrome, which indicates the existence of physical dependence. Alcohol withdrawal symptoms classically consist of hyperexcitability in mild cases and seizures, toxic psychosis, and **delirium tremens** in severe ones. The dose, rate, and duration of alcohol consumption determine the intensity of the withdrawal syndrome. When consumption has been very high, merely reducing the rate of consumption may lead to signs of withdrawal.

Psychologic dependence upon alcohol is characterized by a compulsive desire to experience the rewarding effects of alcohol and, for current drinkers, a desire to avoid the negative consequences of withdrawal. People who have recovered from alcoholism and become abstinent still experience periods of intense craving for alcohol that can be set off by environmental cues associated in the past with drinking, such as familiar places, groups of people, or events.

The molecular basis of alcohol tolerance and dependence is not known, nor is it known if the two phenomena reflect opposing effects upon a shared molecular pathway. Tolerance may result from ethanol-induced up-regulation of a pathway in response to the continuous presence of ethanol. Dependence may result from overactivity of that same pathway after the ethanol effect dissipates and before the system has time to return to a normal ethanol-free state. Chronic exposure of animals or cultured cells to alcohol elicits a multitude of adaptive responses involving neurotransmitters and their receptors, ion channels, and enzymes that participate in signal transduction pathways. Up-regulation of the NMDA subtype of glutamate receptors and voltage-sensitive Ca^{2+} channels may underlie the seizures that accompany the alcohol withdrawal syndrome. Based on the ability of sedative-hypnotic drugs that enhance GABAergic neurotransmission to substitute for alcohol during alcohol withdrawal and evidence of down-regulation of $GABA_A$-mediated responses with chronic alcohol exposure, changes in GABA neurotransmission are believed to play a central role in tolerance and withdrawal.

Neurotransmission events involved in the sensation of reward are also important. Alcohol affects local concentrations of serotonin, opioids, and dopamine—neurotransmitters involved in brain reward circuits (see Chapter 32). Alcohol also has complex effects on the expression of receptors for these neurotransmitters and their signaling pathways. The discovery that naltrexone, a nonselective opioid receptor antagonist, helps patients who are recovering from alcoholism abstain from drinking supports the idea that a common neurochemical reward system is shared by very different drugs associated with physical and psychological dependence.

2. Neurotoxicity—Consumption of large amounts of alcohol over extended periods (usually years) often leads to neurologic deficits. The most common neurologic abnormality in chronic alcoholism is generalized symmetric peripheral nerve injury, which begins with distal paresthesias of the hands and feet. Chronic alcoholics may also exhibit gait disturbances and ataxia that are due to degenerative changes in the central nervous system. Other neurologic disturbances associated with alcoholism include dementia and, rarely, demyelinating disease.

Wernicke-Korsakoff syndrome is a relatively uncommon but important entity characterized by paralysis of the external eye muscles, ataxia, and a confused state that can progress to coma and death. It is associated with thiamin deficiency but is rarely seen in the absence of alcoholism. Because of the importance of thiamin in this pathologic condition and the absence of toxicity associated with thiamine administration, all patients suspected of having Wernicke-Korsakoff syndrome (including virtually all patients who present to the emergency department with altered consciousness, seizures, or both) should receive thiamine therapy. Often, the ocular signs, ataxia, and confusion improve promptly upon administration of thiamine. However, most patients are left with a chronic disabling memory disorder known as Korsakoff's psychosis.

Alcohol may also impair visual acuity, with painless blurring that occurs over several weeks of heavy alcohol consumption. Changes are usually bilateral and symmetric and may be followed by optic nerve degeneration. Ingestion of ethanol substitutes such as methanol (see III. Pharmacology of Other Alcohols) causes severe visual disturbances.

C. CARDIOVASCULAR SYSTEM

1. Cardiomyopathy and heart failure—Alcohol has complex effects on the cardiovascular system. Heavy alcohol consumption of long duration is associated with a dilated cardiomyopathy with ventricular hypertrophy and fibrosis. In animals and humans, alcohol induces a number of changes in heart cells that may contribute to cardiomyopathy. They include membrane disruption, depressed function of mitochondria and sarcoplasmic reticulum, intracellular accumulation of phospholipids and fatty acids, and up-regulation of voltage-dependent calcium channels. There is evidence that patients with alcohol-induced dilated cardiomyopathy do significantly worse than patients with idiopathic dilated cardiomyopathy, even though cessation of drinking is associated with a reduction in cardiac size and improved function. The poorer prognosis for patients who continue to drink appears to be due in part to interference by ethanol with the beneficial effects of β blockers and ACE inhibitors.

2. Arrhythmias—Heavy drinking—and especially "binge" drinking—are associated with both atrial and ventricular arrhythmias. Patients undergoing alcohol withdrawal syndrome can develop severe arrhythmias that may reflect abnormalities of potassium or magnesium metabolism as well as enhanced release of catecholamines. Seizures, syncope, and sudden death during alcohol withdrawal may be due to these arrhythmias.

3. Hypertension—A link between heavier alcohol consumption (more than three drinks per day) and hypertension has been firmly established in epidemiologic studies. Alcohol is estimated to be responsible for approximately 5% of cases of hypertension, making it one of the most common causes of reversible hypertension. This association is independent of obesity, salt intake, coffee drinking, and cigarette smoking. A reduction in alcohol intake appears to be effective in lowering blood pressure in hypertensives who are also heavy drinkers; the hypertension seen in this population is also responsive to standard blood pressure medications.

4. Coronary heart disease—Although the deleterious effects of excessive alcohol use on the cardiovascular system are well established, there is controversy over the effects of moderate drinking (one to three drinks per day) on the incidence of coronary heart disease (CHD). A number of observational studies concluded that moderate alcohol consumption actually prevents CHD and even reduces mortality. This type of relationship between mortality and the dose of a drug is called a "J-shaped" relationship. Results of these clinical studies are supported by ethanol's ability to raise serum levels of high-density lipoprotein (HDL) cholesterol (the form of cholesterol that appears to protect against atherosclerosis; see Chapter 35), its ability to inhibit some of the inflammatory processes that underlie atherosclerosis, and the presence in alcoholic beverages (especially red wine) of antioxidants and other substances that may protect against atherosclerosis. More recently, the relationship between moderate drinking and CHD has been called into question based on further investigation of confounders that affected the outcome of earlier epidemiologic studies. For example, moderate drinkers, especially wine drinkers, come from a higher socioeconomic level and may have healthier dietary habits; consumption tends to decrease with age; abstinence often is associated with ill health; and documenting precise amounts of consumption is difficult. Therefore, definitive conclusions regarding a cardioprotective effect of alcohol must await better clinical evidence.

D. BLOOD

Alcohol indirectly affects hematopoiesis through metabolic and nutritional effects and may also directly inhibit the proliferation of all cellular elements in bone marrow. The most common hematologic disorder seen in chronic drinkers is mild anemia resulting from alcohol-related folic acid deficiency. Iron deficiency anemia may result from gastrointestinal bleeding. Alcohol has also been implicated as a cause of several hemolytic syndromes, some of which are associated with hyperlipidemia and severe liver disease.

E. ENDOCRINE SYSTEM AND ELECTROLYTE BALANCE

Chronic alcohol use has important effects on the endocrine system and on fluid and electrolyte balance. Clinical reports of gynecomastia and testicular atrophy in alcoholics with or without cirrhosis suggest a derangement in steroid hormone balance.

Alcoholics with chronic liver disease may have disorders of fluid and electrolyte balance, including ascites, edema, and effusions. Alterations of whole body potassium induced by vomiting and diarrhea, as well as severe secondary aldosteronism, may contribute to muscle weakness and can be worsened by diuretic therapy. Some alcoholic patients develop hypoglycemia, probably as a result of impaired hepatic gluconeogenesis. Some alcoholics also develop ketosis, caused by excessive lipolytic factors, especially increased cortisol and growth hormone.

F. FETAL ALCOHOL SYNDROME

Chronic maternal alcohol abuse during pregnancy is associated with teratogenic effects, and alcohol appears to be a leading cause of mental retardation and congenital malformation. The abnormalities that have been characterized as fetal alcohol syndrome include (1) intrauterine growth retardation, (2) microcephaly, (3) poor coordination, (4) underdevelopment of midfacial region (appearing as a flattened face), and (5) minor joint anomalies. More severe cases may include congenital heart defects and mental retardation. While the level of alcohol intake required for causing serious neurologic deficits appears quite high, the threshold for causing more subtle neurologic deficits is uncertain.

The mechanisms that underlie ethanol's teratogenic effects are unknown. Ethanol rapidly crosses the placenta and reaches concentrations in the fetus that are similar to those in maternal blood. The fetal liver has little or no alcohol dehydrogenase activity, so the fetus must rely on maternal and placental enzymes for elimination of alcohol.

The neuropathologic abnormalities seen in humans and in animal models of fetal alcohol syndrome indicate that ethanol triggers apoptotic neurodegeneration and also causes aberrant neuronal and glial migration in the developing nervous system. In tissue culture systems, ethanol causes a striking reduction in neurite outgrowth.

G. IMMUNE SYSTEM

The effects of alcohol on the immune system are complex; immune function in some tissues is inhibited (eg, the lung), whereas pathologic, hyperactive immune function in other tissues is triggered (eg, liver, pancreas). In addition, acute and chronic exposure to alcohol have widely different effects on immune function. The types of immunologic changes reported for the lung include suppression of the function of alveolar macrophages, inhibition of chemotaxis of granulocytes, and reduced number and function of T cells. In the liver, there is enhanced function of key cells of the innate immune system (eg, Kupffer cells, hepatic stellate cells) and increased cytokine production. In addition to the inflammatory damage that chronic heavy alcohol use precipitates in the liver and pancreas, it predisposes to the development of infections, especially of the lung, and worsens the morbidity and increases the mortality risk of patients with pneumonia.

H. INCREASED RISK OF CANCER

Chronic alcohol use increases the risk for cancer of the mouth, pharynx, larynx, esophagus, and liver. Evidence also points to a small increase in the risk of breast cancer in women. Much more information is required before a threshold level for alcohol consumption as it relates to cancer can be established. Alcohol itself does not appear to be a carcinogen in most test systems. However, its primary metabolite, acetaldehyde, can damage DNA, as can the reactive oxygen species produced by increased cytochrome P450 activity. Other factors implicated in the link between alcohol and cancer include changes in folate metabolism and the growth-promoting effects of chronic inflammation.

Alcohol-Drug Interactions

Interactions between ethanol and other drugs can have important clinical effects that result from alterations in the pharmacokinetics or pharmacodynamics of the second drug.

The most frequent pharmacokinetic alcohol-drug interactions occur as a result of alcohol-induced increases of drug-metabolizing enzymes, as described in Chapter 4. Thus, prolonged intake of alcohol without damage to the liver may enhance the metabolic biotransformation of other drugs. Ethanol-mediated induction of hepatic cytochrome P450 enzymes is particularly important with regard to acetaminophen. Chronic consumption at the level of three or more drinks per day increases the risk of hepatotoxicity due to toxic or even high therapeutic levels of acetaminophen. This is probably due to increased P450-mediated conversion of acetaminophen to reactive hepatotoxic metabolites (see Figure 4–4). In 1998, the FDA announced that all OTC products containing acetaminophen must carry a warning about the relationship between chronic ethanol consumption and acetaminophen-induced hepatotoxicity.

In contrast, *acute* alcohol use may inhibit metabolism of other drugs. This inhibition may be due to decreased enzyme activity or decreased liver blood flow. Phenothiazines, tricyclic antidepressants, and sedative-hypnotic drugs are the most important drugs that may interact with alcohol by this pharmacokinetic mechanism.

Pharmacodynamic alcohol interactions are also of great clinical significance. Additive central nervous system depression with other central nervous system depressants, particularly sedative-hypnotics, is most important. Alcohol also potentiates the pharmacologic effects of many nonsedative drugs, including vasodilators and oral hypoglycemic agents.

■ II. CLINICAL PHARMACOLOGY OF ETHANOL

Ethanol is the cause of more preventable morbidity and mortality than all other drugs combined with the exception of tobacco. The search for specific etiologic factors or the identification of significant predisposing variables for alcohol abuse has generally led to disappointing results. Personality type, severe life stresses, psychiatric disorders, and parental role models are not reliable predictors of alcohol abuse. Although environmental factors clearly play a role, evidence suggests that there is a large genetic contribution to the development of alcoholism. Not surprisingly, polymorphisms in alcohol dehydrogenase and aldehyde dehydrogenase that lead to increased aldehyde accumulation (and therefore more severe hangover symptoms) appear to protect against alcoholism. Much attention in genetic mapping experiments has focused on membrane-signaling proteins known to be affected by ethanol and on protein constituents of reward pathways in the brain. Early reports of an association of an allele of the dopamine D_2 receptor with alcohol dependence have not been confirmed. Other candidate genes for susceptibility to alcoholism identified in genome-wide screens in humans include the dopamine D_4 receptor, the β_1 subunit of the $GABA_A$ receptor, and tyrosine hydroxylase, an enzyme involved in the synthesis of dopamine, norepinephrine, and epinephrine (see Chapter 6).

MANAGEMENT OF ACUTE ALCOHOL INTOXICATION

Nontolerant individuals who consume alcohol in large quantities develop typical effects of acute sedative-hypnotic drug overdose along with the cardiovascular effects described above (vasodilation, tachycardia) and gastrointestinal irritation. Since tolerance is not absolute, even chronic alcoholics may become severely intoxicated if sufficient alcohol is consumed.

The most important goals in the treatment of acute alcohol intoxication are to prevent severe respiratory depression and to prevent aspiration of vomitus. Even with very high blood ethanol levels, survival is probable as long as the respiratory and cardiovascular systems can be supported. The average blood alcohol concentration in fatal cases is above 400 mg/dL; however, the lethal dose of alcohol varies because of varying degrees of tolerance.

Metabolic alterations may require treatment of hypoglycemia and ketosis by administration of glucose. **Thiamine** is given to protect against the Wernicke-Korsakoff syndrome. Alcoholic patients who are dehydrated and vomiting should also receive electrolyte solutions. If vomiting is severe, large amounts of potassium may be required as long as renal function is normal. Especially important is recognition of decreased serum concentrations of phosphate, which may be aggravated by glucose administration.

MANAGEMENT OF ALCOHOL WITHDRAWAL SYNDROME

Abrupt alcohol withdrawal leads to a characteristic syndrome of motor agitation, anxiety, insomnia, and reduction of seizure threshold. The severity of the syndrome is usually proportionate to the degree and duration of alcohol abuse. However, this can be greatly modified by the use of other sedatives as well as by associated factors (eg, diabetes, injury). In its mildest form, the alcohol with-

drawal syndrome of tremor, anxiety, and insomnia occurs 6–8 hours after alcohol consumption is stopped. These effects usually abate in 1–2 days. In some patients, more severe withdrawal reactions occur in which visual hallucinations, total disorientation, and marked abnormalities of vital signs occur. Alcohol withdrawal is one of the most common causes of seizures in adults.

The major objective of drug therapy in the alcohol withdrawal period is prevention of seizures, delirium, and arrhythmias. Potassium, magnesium, and phosphate balance should be restored as rapidly as is consistent with renal function. Thiamine therapy is initiated in all cases. Persons in mild alcohol withdrawal do not need any other pharmacologic assistance.

Specific drug treatment for detoxification in severe cases involves two basic principles: substituting a long-acting sedative-hypnotic drug for alcohol and then gradually reducing ("tapering") the dose of the long-acting drug. Because of their wide margin of safety, benzodiazepines are preferred, though barbiturates such as phenobarbital were used in the past. Since any benzodiazepine will prevent symptoms of alcohol withdrawal, the choice of a specific agent in this class is generally based on pharmacokinetic or economic considerations. Long-acting benzodiazepines, including chlordiazepoxide, clorazepate, and diazepam, have the advantage of requiring less frequent dosing. Since their pharmacologically active metabolites are eliminated slowly, the long-acting drugs provide a built-in tapering effect. A disadvantage of the long-acting drugs is that they and their pharmacologically active metabolites may accumulate, especially in patients with compromised liver function. Short-acting drugs such as lorazepam and oxazepam are rapidly converted to inactive water-soluble metabolites that will not accumulate, and for this reason the short-acting drugs are especially useful in alcoholic patients with liver disease. Benzodiazepines can be administered orally in mild or moderate cases, or parenterally for patients with more severe withdrawal reactions.

After the alcohol withdrawal syndrome has been treated acutely, sedative-hypnotic medications must be tapered slowly over several weeks. Complete detoxification is not achieved with just a few days of alcohol abstinence. Several months may be required for restoration of normal nervous system function, especially sleep.

TREATMENT OF ALCOHOLISM

Following detoxification, psychosocial therapy either in intensive inpatient or in outpatient rehabilitation programs serves as the primary treatment for alcohol dependence. Other psychiatric problems, most commonly depressive or anxiety disorders, often coexist with alcoholism and, if untreated, can contribute to the tendency of detoxified alcoholics to relapse. Treatment of these associated disorders with counseling and drugs can help decrease the rate of relapse for alcoholic patients.

Three drugs—disulfiram, naltrexone, and acamprosate—have FDA approval for adjunctive treatment of alcohol dependence.

Naltrexone

Naltrexone is an orally active opioid receptor antagonist that blocks the effects at μ opioid receptors of exogenous and endogenous opioids (see Chapter 31). Studies in experimental animals first suggested a link between alcohol consumption and opioids. Injection of small amounts of opioids was followed by an increase in alcohol drinking, whereas administration of opioid antagonists inhibited self-administration of alcohol.

Naltrexone, a relatively long-acting oral opioid antagonist, has been shown in a number of short–term (12-week) placebo-controlled trials to reduce craving for alcohol and to reduce the rate of relapse to either drinking or alcohol dependence. Longer trials (6–12 months) have failed to show evidence to support long-term treatment. Naltrexone was approved in 1994 by the FDA for treatment of alcohol dependence.

Naltrexone is taken once a day in a dose of 50 mg for treatment of alcoholism. The drug should be used with caution in alcoholic patients with evidence of mild abnormalities in serum aminotransferase activity. The combination of naltrexone plus disulfiram should be avoided since both drugs are potential hepatotoxins. Administration of naltrexone to patients who are physically dependent on opioids will precipitate an acute withdrawal syndrome, so patients must be opioid-free before initiating naltrexone therapy. Naltrexone also blocks the therapeutic effects of usual doses of opioids.

Acamprosate

Acamprosate has been used in Europe for a number of years to treat alcohol dependence and was approved for this use by the FDA in 2004. Like ethanol itself, acamprosate has many molecular effects including effects on GABA, glutamate, serotonergic, noradrenergic, and dopaminergic effects. Probably its best characterized actions are as a weak NMDA-receptor antagonist and a $GABA_A$-receptor activator. In clinical trials, acamprosate reduces short-term and long-term (more than 6 months) relapse rates when combined with psychotherapy.

Acamprosate is administered as 1–2 enteric-coated 333-mg tablets three times per day. It is poorly absorbed, and food reduces its absorption even further. Acamprosate is widely distributed and is eliminated renally. It does not participate in drug-drug interactions. The most common adverse effects are gastrointestinal (nausea, vomiting, diarrhea) and rash. It is contraindicated in patients with severe renal impairment.

Disulfiram

Disulfiram causes extreme discomfort in patients who drink alcoholic beverages. Disulfiram given by itself to nondrinkers has little effect; however, flushing, throbbing headache, nausea, vomiting, sweating, hypotension, and confusion occur within a few minutes after drinking alcohol. The effect may last 30 minutes in mild cases or several hours in severe ones. Disulfiram acts by inhibiting aldehyde dehydrogenase. Thus, alcohol is metabolized as usual, but acetaldehyde accumulates.

Disulfiram is rapidly and completely absorbed from the gastrointestinal tract; however, a period of 12 hours is required for its full action. Its elimination rate is slow, so that its action may persist for several days after the last dose. The drug inhibits the metabolism of many other therapeutic agents, including phenytoin, oral anticoagulants, and isoniazid. It should not be administered with medications that contain alcohol, including nonprescription medications such as those listed in Table 64–3. Disulfiram can cause small increases in liver function tests. Its safety in pregnancy has not been demonstrated.

Because compliance with disulfiram therapy is low and because the evidence from clinical trials for its effectiveness is weak, disulfiram is no longer commonly used.

Other Drugs

There is some evidence that topiramate, a drug used for partial and generalized tonic-clonic seizures (Chapter 24), and ondansetron, a serotonin 5-HT$_3$-receptor antagonist (Chapters 16, 63), are effective in reducing craving in chronic alcoholics.

■ III. PHARMACOLOGY OF OTHER ALCOHOLS

Other alcohols related to ethanol have wide applications as industrial solvents and occasionally cause severe poisoning. Of these, **methanol** and **ethylene glycol** are two of the most common causes of intoxication.

Methanol

Methanol (methyl alcohol, wood alcohol) is widely used in the industrial production of synthetic organic compounds and as a constituent of many commercial solvents. In the home, methanol is most frequently found in the form of "canned heat" or in windshield-washing products. Poisonings occur from accidental ingestion of methanol-containing products or when it is used by alcoholics as an ethanol substitute.

Methanol can be absorbed through the skin or from the respiratory or gastrointestinal tract and is then distributed in body water. The primary mechanism of elimination of methanol in humans is by oxidation to formaldehyde, formic acid, and CO_2:

$$\underset{\text{Methanol}}{CH_3OH} \xrightarrow{\boxed{\substack{\text{Alcohol} \\ \text{dehydrogenase}}}} \underset{\text{Formaldehyde}}{H_2CO} \longrightarrow \underset{\text{Formate}}{HCOO^-} \longrightarrow CO_2 + H_2O$$

Animal species show great variability in mean lethal doses of methanol. The special susceptibility of humans to methanol toxicity is probably due to folate-dependent production of formate and not to methanol itself or to formaldehyde, the intermediate metabolite.

The most characteristic symptom in methanol poisoning is a visual disturbance, frequently described as "like being in a snowstorm." A complaint of blurred vision with a relatively clear sensorium should strongly suggest the diagnosis of methanol poisoning. Since much of the toxicity is due to metabolites of methanol, there is often a delay of up to 30 hours before development of visual disturbances and other signs of severe intoxication.

Physical findings in methanol poisoning are generally nonspecific. In severe cases, the odor of formaldehyde may be present on the breath or in the urine. Changes in the retina may sometimes be detected on examination, but these are usually late. The development of bradycardia, prolonged coma, seizures, and resistant acidosis all imply a poor prognosis. The cause of death in fatal cases is sudden cessation of respiration.

It is critical that the blood methanol level be determined as soon as possible if the diagnosis is suspected. Methanol concentrations higher than 50 mg/dL are thought to be an absolute indication for hemodialysis and ethanol treatment, though formate blood levels are a better indication of clinical pathology. Additional laboratory evidence includes metabolic acidosis with an elevated anion gap and osmolar gap (see Chapter 59). A decrease in serum bicarbonate is a uniform feature of severe methanol poisoning.

The first treatment for methanol poisoning, as in all critical poisoning situations, is support of respiration. There are three specific modalities of treatment for severe methanol poisoning: suppression of metabolism by alcohol dehydrogenase to toxic products, hemodialysis to enhance removal of methanol and its toxic products, and alkalinization to counteract metabolic acidosis.

The enzyme chiefly responsible for methanol oxidation in the liver is alcohol dehydrogenase. Ethanol has a higher affinity than methanol for alcohol dehydrogenase; thus, saturation of the enzyme with ethanol reduces formate production. Ethanol is often used intravenously as treatment for methanol poisoning. The dose-dependent characteristics of ethanol metabolism and the variability of ethanol metabolism require frequent monitoring of blood ethanol levels to ensure appropriate alcohol concentration. **Fomepizole,** an alcohol dehydrogenase inhibitor, is approved for the treatment of ethylene glycol poisoning (see next section) and methanol poisoning.

Hemodialysis rapidly eliminates both methanol and formate. However, ethanol is also eliminated in the dialysate, requiring alterations in the dose of ethanol. Hemodialysis is discussed in Chapter 59.

Two other measures are commonly taken. Because of profound metabolic acidosis in methanol poisoning, treatment with bicarbonate often is necessary. Since folate-dependent systems are responsible for the oxidation of formic acid to CO_2 in humans, it is probably useful to administer folic acid to patients poisoned with methanol, though this has never been fully tested in clinical studies.

Ethylene Glycol

Polyhydric alcohols such as ethylene glycol (CH_2OH-CH_2OH) are used as heat exchangers, in antifreeze formulations, and as industrial solvents. Young children and animals are sometimes attracted by the sweet taste of ethylene glycol and, rarely, it is ingested intentionally as an ethanol substitute or in attempted suicide. While ethylene glycol itself is relatively harmless and eliminated by the kidney, it is metabolized to toxic aldehydes and oxalate.

Three stages of ethylene glycol overdose occur. Within the first few hours after ingestion, there is transient excitation followed by central nervous system depression. After a delay of 4–12 hours, severe metabolic acidosis develops from accumulation of acid metabolites and lactate. Finally, delayed renal insufficiency follows deposition of oxalate in renal tubules. The key to the diagnosis of ethylene glycol poisoning is recognition of anion gap acidosis, osmolar gap, and oxalate crystals in the urine in a patient without visual symptoms.

As with methanol poisoning, early ethanol infusion and hemodialysis are standard treatments for ethylene glycol poisoning. Fomepizole, an inhibitor of alcohol dehydrogenase, has FDA approval for treatment of ethylene glycol poisoning in adults based on its ability to decrease concentrations of toxic metabolites in blood and urine and to prevent renal injury. Intravenous treatment with fomepizole is initiated immediately and continued until the patient's serum ethylene glycol concentration drops below a toxic threshold (20 mg/dL). Adverse effects associated with fomepizole are not severe. Headache, nausea, and dizziness are most frequently reported, and a few patients experience minor allergic reactions. Fomepizole is classified as an orphan drug (see Chapter 5) because ethylene glycol poisoning is relatively uncommon. Its cost—estimated to be $4000 per patient—is much higher than the cost of infusible ethanol, but fomepizole offers some advantages over ethanol as an antidote for this potentially fatal poisoning.

PREPARATIONS AVAILABLE

DRUGS FOR THE TREATMENT OF ACUTE ALCOHOL WITHDRAWAL SYNDROME

Diazepam (generic, Valium, others)
Oral: 2, 3, 10 mg tablets; 5 mg/5 mL solutions (see also Chapter 22)
Parenteral: 5 mg/mL for injection

Lorazepam (generic, Alzapam, Ativan)
Oral: 0.5, 1, 2 mg tablets
Parenteral: 2, 4 mg/mL for injection

Oxazepam (generic, Serax)
Oral: 10, 15, 30 mg capsules, 15 mg tablets

Thiamine (generic)
Parenteral: 100 mg/mL for IV injection

DRUGS FOR THE PREVENTION OF ALCOHOL ABUSE

Acamprosate (Campral)
Oral: 333 mg delayed-release tablets

Disulfiram (Antabuse)
Oral: 250 mg tablets

Naltrexone (generic, ReVia)
Oral: 50 mg tablets
Parenteral (Vivitrol): 380 mg for IM injection once per month

DRUGS FOR THE TREATMENT OF ACUTE METHANOL OR ETHYLENE GLYCOL POISONING

Ethanol (generic)
Parenteral: 5% or 10% ethanol and 5% dextrose in water for IV infusion

Fomepizole (Antizol)
Parenteral: 1 g/mL for IV injection

REFERENCES

Brent J et al: Fomepizole for the treatment of ethylene glycol poisoning. Methylpyrazole for Toxic Alcohols Study Group. N Engl J Med 1999;340:832.

CDC Fetal Alcohol Syndrome Website: http://www.cdc.gov/ncbddd/fas/

Corrao G et al: Alcohol and coronary heart disease: A meta-analysis. Addiction 2000;95:1505.

Crabbe JC et al: Identifying genes for alcohol and drug sensitivity: Recent progress and future directions. Trends Neurosci 1999; 22:173.

Davies AG et al: A central role of the BK potassium channel in behavioral responses to ethanol in *C. elegans*. Cell 2003; 115:655.

Hoffman PL et al: Transgenic and gene "knockout" models in alcohol research. Alcohol Clin Exp Res 2001;25(Suppl):606.

Jacobsen D: New treatment for ethylene glycol poisoning. N Engl J Med 1999;340:879.

Johnson BA et al: Ondansetron for reduction of drinking among biologically predisposed alcoholic patients: A randomized controlled trial. JAMA 2000;284:963.

Key TJ et al: The effect of diet on risk of cancer. Lancet 2002; 360:861.

Li TK: Pharmacogenetics of responses to alcohol and genes that influence alcohol drinking. J Stud Alcohol 2000;61:5.

Lieber CS: Medical disorders of alcoholism. N Engl J Med 1995; 333:1058.

Littleton J: Receptor regulation as a unitary mechanism for drug tolerance and physical dependence-not quite as simple as it seemed. Addiction 2001;96:87.

National Institute on Alcohol Abuse and Alcoholism Website: http://www.niaaa.nih.gov/

Nelson S, Knolls JK: Alcohol, host defense and society. Nat Rev Immunology 2002;2:205.

Srisurapanont M, Jarusuraisin N: Opioid antagonists for alcohol dependence. Cochrane Database Syst Rev 2005;(1):CD001867.

Williams SH: Medications for treating alcohol dependence. Am Fam Physician 2005;72:1755.

Wolf FW, Heberlein U: Invertebrate models of drug abuse. J Neurobiol 2003;54:161.

You M, Crabb DW: Recent advances in alcoholic liver disease II. Minireview: Molecular mechanisms of alcoholic fatty liver. Am J Physiol Gastrointest Liver Physiol 2004;287:G1.

Antiseizure Drugs

Roger J. Porter, MD, & Brian S. Meldrum, MB, PhD

Approximately 1% of the world's population has epilepsy, the second most common neurologic disorder after stroke. Although standard therapy permits control of seizures in 80% of these patients, millions (500,000 people in the USA alone) have uncontrolled epilepsy. Epilepsy is a heterogeneous symptom complex—a chronic disorder characterized by recurrent seizures. Seizures are finite episodes of brain dysfunction resulting from abnormal discharge of cerebral neurons. The causes of seizures are many and include the full range of neurologic diseases—from infection to neoplasm and head injury. In some subgroups, heredity has proved to be a predominant factor.

The antiseizure drugs described in this chapter are also used in patients with febrile seizures or with seizures occurring as part of an acute illness such as meningitis. The term "epilepsy" is not usually applied to such patients unless chronic seizures develop later. Seizures are occasionally caused by an acute underlying toxic or metabolic disorder, in which case appropriate therapy should be directed toward the specific abnormality, eg, hypocalcemia. In most cases of epilepsy, however, the choice of medication depends on the empiric seizure classification.

Drug Development for Epilepsy

For a long time it was assumed that a single drug could be developed for the treatment of all forms of epilepsy, but the causes of epilepsy are extremely diverse, encompassing genetic and developmental defects and infective, traumatic, neoplastic, and degenerative disease processes. Drug therapy to date shows little evidence of etiologic specificity. There is, however, some specificity according to seizure type (Table 24–1). This is most clearly seen with generalized seizures of the absence type. These are typically seen with 2–3 Hz spike-and-wave discharges on the electroencephalogram, which respond to ethosuximide and valproate but can be exacerbated by phenytoin and carbamazepine. Drugs acting selectively on absence seizures can be identified by animal screens, using either threshold pentylenetetrazol clonic seizures in mice or rats or mutant mice showing absence-like episodes (so-called lethargic, stargazer, or tottering mutants). In contrast, the maximal electroshock (MES) test, with suppression of the tonic extensor phase, identifies drugs such as phenytoin, carbamazepine, and lamotrigine that are active against generalized tonic-clonic seizures and complex partial seizures. Use of the maximal electroshock test as the major initial screen for new drugs has probably led to the identification of drugs with a common mechanism of action involving prolonged inactivation of the voltage-sensitive sodium channel. Limbic seizures induced in rats by the process of electrical kindling (involving repeated episodes of focal electrical stimulation) probably provide a better screen for predicting efficacy in complex partial seizures.

Existing antiseizure drugs provide adequate seizure control in about two thirds of patients. A fraction of the epileptic population is resistant to all available drugs, and this may be due to increased expression of the multidrug transporter P-glycoprotein 170, a product of the *ABCB1* gene. In children, some severe seizure syndromes associated with progressive brain damage are very difficult to treat. In adults, some focal seizures are refractory to medications. Some, particularly in the temporal lobe, are amenable to surgical resection. Some of the drug-resistant population may respond to vagus-nerve stimulation (VNS), a nonpharmacologic treatment for epilepsy now widely approved for treatment of patients with partial seizures. VNS is indicated for refractory cases or for patients in whom antiseizure drugs are poorly tolerated. Stimulating electrodes are implanted in the left vagus nerve, and the pacemaker is implanted in the chest wall or axilla. Use of this device may permit seizure control with lower doses of drugs.

New antiseizure drugs are being sought not only by the screening tests noted above but also by more rational approaches. Compounds are sought that act by one of three mechanisms: (1) enhancement of GABAergic (inhibitory) transmission, (2) diminution of excitatory (usually glutamatergic) transmission, or (3) modification of ionic conductances.

■ I. BASIC PHARMACOLOGY OF ANTISEIZURE DRUGS

Chemistry

Until 1990, approximately 16 antiseizure drugs were available, and 13 of them can be classified into five very similar chemical groups: barbiturates, hydantoins, oxa-

Table 24–1. Classification of seizure types.

Partial seizures
    Simple partial seizures
    Complex partial seizures
    Partial seizures secondarily generalized
Generalized seizures
    Generalized tonic-clonic (grand mal) seizures
    Absence (petit mal) seizures
    Tonic seizures
    Atonic seizures
    Clonic and myoclonic seizures
    Infantile spasms[1]

[1]An epileptic syndrome rather than a specific seizure type; drugs useful in infantile spasms will be reviewed separately.

zolidinediones, succinimides, and acetylureas. These groups have in common a similar heterocyclic ring structure with a variety of substituents (Figure 24–1). For drugs with this basic structure, the substituents on the heterocyclic ring determine the pharmacologic class, either anti-MES or antipentylenetetrazol. Very small changes in structure can dramatically alter the mechanism of action and clinical properties of the compound. The remaining drugs—carbamazepine, valproic acid, and the benzodiazepines—are structurally dissimilar, as are the newer compounds marketed since 1990, ie, felbamate, gabapentin, lamotrigine, levetiracetam, oxcarbazepine, pregabalin, tiagabine, topiramate, vigabatrin, and zonisamide.

Pharmacokinetics

The antiseizure drugs exhibit many similar pharmacokinetic properties—even those whose structural and chemical properties are quite diverse—because most have been selected for oral activity and all must enter the central nervous system. Although many of these compounds are only slightly soluble, absorption is usually good, with 80–100% of the dose reaching the circulation. Most antiseizure drugs are not highly bound to plasma proteins.

Figure 24–1. Antiseizure heterocyclic ring structure. The "X" varies as follows: hydantoin derivatives, –N–; barbiturates, –C–N–; oxazolidinediones, –O–; succinimides, –C–; acetylureas, –NH$_2$ (N connected to C$_2$). R$_1$, R$_2$, and R$_3$ vary within each subgroup.

Antiseizure drugs are cleared chiefly by hepatic mechanisms, although they have low extraction ratios (see Chapter 3). Many are converted to active metabolites that are also cleared by the liver. These drugs are predominantly distributed into total body water. Plasma clearance is relatively slow; many anticonvulsants are therefore considered to be medium- to long-acting. Some have half-lives longer than 12 hours. Many of the older antiseizure drugs are potent inducers of hepatic microsomal enzyme activity.

DRUGS USED IN PARTIAL SEIZURES & GENERALIZED TONIC-CLONIC SEIZURES

The classic major drugs for partial and generalized tonic-clonic seizures are phenytoin (and congeners), carbamazepine, valproate, and the barbiturates. However, the availability of newer drugs—lamotrigine, levetiracetam, gabapentin, oxcarbazepine, pregabalin, topiramate, vigabatrin, and zonisamide is altering clinical practice in countries where these compounds are available.

PHENYTOIN

Phenytoin is the oldest nonsedative antiseizure drug, introduced in 1938, after a systematic evaluation of compounds such as phenobarbital that altered electrically induced seizures in laboratory animals. It was known for decades as **diphenylhydantoin.**

Chemistry

Phenytoin is a diphenyl-substituted hydantoin with the structure shown below. It has much lower sedative properties than compounds with alkyl substituents at the 5 position. A more soluble prodrug of phenytoin, **fosphenytoin,** is available for parenteral use; this phosphate ester compound is rapidly converted to phenytoin in the plasma.

Phenytoin

Mechanism of Action

Phenytoin has major effects on several physiologic systems. It alters Na$^+$, K$^+$, and Ca^{2+} conductance, mem-

Figure 24–2. Effects of three antiseizure drugs on sustained high-frequency firing of action potentials by cultured neurons. Intracellular recordings were made from neurons while depolarizing current pulses, approximately 0.75 s in duration, were applied (on-off step changes indicated by arrows). In the absence of drug, a series of high-frequency repetitive action potentials filled the entire duration of the current pulse. Phenytoin, carbamazepine, and sodium valproate all markedly reduced the number of action potentials elicited by the current pulses. (Modified and reproduced, with permission, from Macdonald RL, Meldrum BS: Principles of antiepileptic drug action. In: Levy RH, et al [editors]: *Antiepileptic Drugs*, 4th ed. Raven Press, 1995.)

brane potentials, and the concentrations of amino acids and the neurotransmitters norepinephrine, acetylcholine, and γ-aminobutyric acid (GABA). Studies with neurons in cell culture show that phenytoin blocks sustained high-frequency repetitive firing of action potentials (Figure 24–2). This effect is seen at therapeutically relevant concentrations. It is a use-dependent effect (see Chapter 14) on Na$^+$ conductance, arising from preferential binding to—and prolongation of—the inactivated state of the Na$^+$ channel. This effect is also seen with therapeutically relevant concentrations of carbamazepine, lamotrigine, and valproate and probably contributes to their antiseizure action in the electroshock model and in partial seizures.

In addition, phenytoin paradoxically causes excitation in some cerebral neurons. A reduction of calcium permeability, with inhibition of calcium influx across the cell membrane, may explain the ability of phenytoin to inhibit a variety of calcium-induced secretory processes, including release of hormones and neurotransmitters. Recording of excitatory and inhibitory postsynaptic potentials show that phenytoin decreases the synaptic release of glutamate and enhances the release of GABA. The mechanism of phenytoin's action probably involves a combination of actions at several levels. At therapeutic concentrations, the major action of phenytoin is to block sodium channels and inhibit the generation of rapidly repetitive action potentials. Presynaptic actions on glutamate and GABA release probably arise from actions other than those on voltage-gated Na$^+$ channels.

Clinical Use

Phenytoin is effective against partial seizures and generalized tonic-clonic seizures. In the latter, it appears to be effective against attacks that are either primary or secondary to another seizure type.

Pharmacokinetics

Absorption of phenytoin is highly dependent on the formulation of the dosage form. Particle size and pharmaceutical additives affect both the rate and the extent of absorption. Absorption of phenytoin sodium from the gastrointestinal tract is nearly complete in most patients, although the time to peak may range from 3 hours to 12 hours. Absorption after intramuscular injection is unpredictable, and some drug precipitation in the muscle occurs; this route of administration is not recommended for phenytoin. In contrast, fosphenytoin, a more soluble phosphate prodrug of phenytoin, is well absorbed after intramuscular administration.

Phenytoin is highly bound to plasma proteins. The total plasma level decreases when the percentage that is bound decreases, as in uremia or hypoalbuminemia, but correlation of free levels with clinical states remains uncertain. Drug concentration in cerebrospinal fluid is proportionate to the free plasma level. Phenytoin accumulates in brain, liver, muscle, and fat.

Phenytoin is metabolized to inactive metabolites that are excreted in the urine. Only a very small proportion of phenytoin is excreted unchanged.

The elimination of phenytoin is dose-dependent. At very low blood levels, phenytoin metabolism follows first-order kinetics. However, as blood levels rise within the therapeutic range, the maximum capacity of the liver to metabolize phenytoin is approached (Figure 24–3). Further increases in dosage, even though relatively small, may produce very large changes in phenytoin concentrations. In such cases, the half-life of the drug increases markedly, steady state is not achieved in routine fashion

Figure 24–3. Nonlinear relationship of phenytoin dosage and plasma concentrations. Five different patients (identified by different symbols) received increasing dosages of phenytoin by mouth, and the steady-state serum concentration was measured at each dosage. The curves are not linear, since, as the dosage increases, the metabolism is saturable. Note also the marked variation among patients in the serum levels achieved at any dosage. (Modified, with permission, from Jusko WJ: Bioavailability and disposition kinetics of phenytoin in man. In: Kellaway P, Peterson I [editors]: *Quantitative Analytic Studies in Epilepsy.* Raven Press, 1977.)

(since the plasma level continues to rise), and patients quickly develop symptoms of toxicity.

The half-life of phenytoin varies from 12 hours to 36 hours, with an average of 24 hours for most patients in the low to mid therapeutic range. Much longer half-lives are observed at higher concentrations. At low blood levels, it takes 5–7 days to reach steady-state blood levels after every dosage change; at higher levels, it may be 4–6 weeks before blood levels are stable.

Therapeutic Levels & Dosage

The therapeutic plasma level of phenytoin for most patients is between 10 and 20 mcg/mL. A loading dose can be given either orally or intravenously; the latter, using fosphenytoin, is the method of choice for convulsive status epilepticus (discussed later). When oral therapy is started, it is common to begin adults at a dosage of 300 mg/d, regardless of body weight. This may be acceptable in some patients, but it frequently yields steady-state blood levels below 10 mcg/mL, which is the minimum therapeutic level for most patients. If seizures continue, higher doses are usually necessary to achieve plasma levels in the upper therapeutic range. Because of its dose-dependent kinetics, some toxicity

may occur with only small increments in dosage. The phenytoin dosage should be increased each time by only 25–30 mg in adults, and ample time should be allowed for the new steady state to be achieved before further increasing the dosage. A common clinical error is to increase the dosage directly from 300 mg/d to 400 mg/d; toxicity frequently occurs at a variable time thereafter. In children, a dosage of 5 mg/kg/d should be followed by readjustment after steady-state plasma levels are obtained.

Two types of oral phenytoin sodium are currently available in the USA, differing in their respective rates of dissolution; one is absorbed rapidly and one more slowly. Only the slow-release extended-action formulation can be given in a single daily dosage, and care must be used when changing brands (see Preparations Available). Although a few patients being given phenytoin on a long-term basis have been proved to have low blood levels from poor absorption or rapid metabolism, the most common cause of low levels is poor compliance. Fosphenytoin sodium is available for intravenous or intramuscular use and replaces intravenous phenytoin sodium, a much less soluble form of the drug.

Drug Interactions & Interference with Laboratory Tests

Drug interactions involving phenytoin are primarily related to protein binding or to metabolism. Since phenytoin is 90% bound to plasma proteins, other highly bound drugs, such as phenylbutazone and sulfonamides, can displace phenytoin from its binding site. In theory, such displacement may cause a transient increase in free drug. A decrease in protein binding—eg, from hypoalbuminemia—results in a decrease in the total plasma concentration of drug but not the free concentration. Intoxication may occur if efforts are made to maintain total drug levels in the therapeutic range by increasing the dose. The protein binding of phenytoin is decreased in the presence of renal disease. The drug has an affinity for thyroid-binding globulin, which confuses some tests of thyroid function; the most reliable screening test of thyroid function in patients taking phenytoin appears to be measurement of thyroid-stimulating hormone (TSH).

Phenytoin has been shown to induce microsomal enzymes responsible for the metabolism of a number of drugs. Autostimulation of its own metabolism, however, appears to be insignificant. Other drugs, notably phenobarbital and carbamazepine, cause decreases in phenytoin steady-state concentrations through induction of hepatic microsomal enzymes. On the other hand, isoniazid inhibits the metabolism of phenytoin, resulting in increased steady-state concentrations when the two drugs are given together.

Toxicity

Dose-related adverse effects caused by phenytoin are unfortunately similar to other antiseizure drugs in this group, making differentiation difficult in patients receiving multiple drugs. Nystagmus occurs early, as does loss of smooth extraocular pursuit movements, but neither is an indication for decreasing the dose. Diplopia and ataxia are the most common dose-related adverse effects requiring dosage adjustment; sedation usually occurs only at considerably higher levels. Gingival hyperplasia and hirsutism occur to some degree in most patients; the latter can be especially unpleasant in women. Long-term use is associated in some patients with coarsening of facial features and with mild peripheral neuropathy, usually manifested by diminished deep tendon reflexes in the lower extremities. Long-term use may also result in abnormalities of vitamin D metabolism, leading to osteomalacia. Low folate levels and megaloblastic anemia have been reported, but the clinical importance of this observation is unknown.

Idiosyncratic reactions to phenytoin are relatively rare. A skin rash may indicate hypersensitivity of the patient to the drug. Fever may also occur, and in rare cases the skin lesions may be severe and exfoliative. Lymphadenopathy may be difficult to distinguish from malignant lymphoma, and although some studies suggest a causal relationship between phenytoin and Hodgkin's disease, the data are far from conclusive. Hematologic complications are exceedingly rare, although agranulocytosis has been reported in combination with fever and rash.

MEPHENYTOIN, ETHOTOIN, & PHENACEMIDE

Many congeners of phenytoin have been synthesized, but only three have been marketed recently in the USA, and one of these (phenacemide) has been withdrawn from the market. The other two congeners, mephenytoin and ethotoin, like phenytoin, appear to be most effective against generalized tonic-clonic seizures and partial seizures. No well-controlled clinical trials have documented their effectiveness. The incidence of severe reactions such as dermatitis, agranulocytosis, or hepatitis is higher for mephenytoin than for phenytoin.

Ethotoin may be recommended for patients hypersensitive to phenytoin, but larger doses are required. The adverse effects and toxicity are generally less severe than those associated with phenytoin, but the drug appears to be less effective.

Both ethotoin and mephenytoin share with phenytoin the property of saturable metabolism within the therapeutic dosage range. Careful monitoring of the patient during dosage alterations with either drug is essential. Mephenytoin is metabolized to 5,5-ethylphenylhydantoin via demethylation. This metabolite, **nirvanol**, contributes most of the antiseizure activity of mephenytoin. Both mephenytoin and nirvanol are hydroxylated and undergo subsequent conjugation and excretion. Therapeutic levels for mephenytoin range from 5 mcg/mL to 16 mcg/mL, and levels above 20 mcg/mL are considered toxic.

Therapeutic blood levels of nirvanol are between 25 and 40 mcg/mL. A therapeutic range for ethotoin has not been established.

CARBAMAZEPINE

Closely related to imipramine and other antidepressants, carbamazepine is a tricyclic compound effective in treatment of bipolar depression. It was initially marketed for the treatment of trigeminal neuralgia but has proved useful for epilepsy as well.

Carbamazepine

Chemistry

Although not obvious from a two-dimensional representation of its structure, carbamazepine has many similarities to phenytoin. The ureide moiety ($-N-CO-NH_2$) present in the heterocyclic ring of most antiseizure drugs is also present in carbamazepine. Three-dimensional structural studies indicate that its spatial conformation is similar to that of phenytoin.

Mechanism of Action

The mechanism of action of carbamazepine appears to be similar to that of phenytoin. Like phenytoin, carbamazepine shows activity against maximal electroshock seizures. Carbamazepine, like phenytoin, blocks sodium channels at therapeutic concentrations and inhibits high-frequency repetitive firing in neurons in culture (Figure 24–2). It also acts presynaptically to decrease synaptic transmission. These effects probably account for the anticonvulsant action of carbamazepine. Binding studies show that carbamazepine interacts with adenosine receptors, but the functional significance of this observation is not known.

Clinical Use

Although carbamazepine has long been considered a drug of choice for both partial seizures and generalized tonic-clonic seizures, some of the newer antiseizure drugs are beginning to displace it from this role. Carbamazepine is not sedative in its usual therapeutic range. The drug is also very effective in some patients with trigeminal neuralgia, although older patients may tolerate higher doses poorly, with ataxia and unsteadiness. Carbamazepine is also useful in some patients with mania (bipolar disorder).

Pharmacokinetics

The rate of absorption of carbamazepine varies widely among patients, although almost complete absorption apparently occurs in all. Peak levels are usually achieved 6–8 hours after administration. Slowing absorption by giving the drug after meals helps the patient tolerate larger total daily doses.

Distribution is slow, and the volume of distribution is roughly 1 L/kg. The drug is only 70% bound to plasma proteins; no displacement of other drugs from protein binding sites has been observed.

Carbamazepine has a very low systemic clearance of approximately 1 L/kg/d at the start of therapy. The drug has a notable ability to induce microsomal enzymes. Typically, the half-life of 36 hours observed in subjects following an initial single dose decreases to as short as 8–12 hours in subjects receiving continuous therapy. Considerable dosage adjustments are thus to be expected during the first weeks of therapy. Carbamazepine also alters the clearance of other drugs (see below).

Carbamazepine is completely metabolized in humans to several derivatives. One of these, carbamazepine-10,11-epoxide, has been shown to have anticonvulsant activity. The contribution of this and other metabolites to the clinical activity of carbamazepine is unknown.

Therapeutic Levels & Dosage

Carbamazepine is available only in oral form. The drug is effective in children, in whom a dosage of 15–25 mg/kg/d is appropriate. In adults, daily doses of 1 g or even 2 g are tolerated. Higher dosage is achieved by giving multiple divided doses daily. Extended-release preparations permit twice-daily dosing for most patients. In patients in whom the blood is drawn just before the morning dose (trough level), the therapeutic level is usually 4–8 mcg/mL. Although many patients complain of diplopia at drug levels above 7 mcg/mL, others can tolerate levels above 10 mcg/mL, especially with monotherapy.

Drug Interactions

Drug interactions involving carbamazepine are almost exclusively related to the drug's enzyme-inducing properties. As noted previously, the increased metabolic capacity of the hepatic enzymes may cause a reduction in steady-state carbamazepine concentrations and an increased rate of metabolism of other drugs, eg, primidone, phenytoin, ethosuximide, valproic acid, and clonazepam. Other drugs such as propoxyphene, troleandomycin, and valproic acid may inhibit carbamazepine clearance and increase steady-state carbamazepine blood levels. Other anticonvulsants, however, such as phenytoin and phenobarbital, may decrease steady-state concentrations of carbamazepine through enzyme induction. No clinically significant protein-binding interactions have been reported.

Toxicity

The most common dose-related adverse effects of carbamazepine are diplopia and ataxia. The diplopia often occurs first and may last less than an hour during a particular time of day. Rearrangement of the divided daily dose can often remedy this complaint. Other dose-related complaints include mild gastrointestinal upsets, unsteadiness, and, at much higher doses, drowsiness. Hyponatremia and water intoxication have occasionally occurred and may be dose-related.

Considerable concern exists regarding the occurrence of idiosyncratic blood dyscrasias with carbamazepine, including fatal cases of aplastic anemia and agranulocytosis. Most of these have been in elderly patients with trigeminal neuralgia, and most have occurred within the first 4 months of treatment. The mild and persistent leukopenia seen in some patients is not necessarily an indication to stop treatment but requires careful monitoring. The most common idiosyncratic reaction is an erythematous skin rash; other responses such as hepatic dysfunction are unusual.

OXCARBAZEPINE

Oxcarbazepine is closely related to carbamazepine and useful in the same seizure types, but it may have an improved toxicity profile. Oxcarbazepine has a half-life of only 1–2 hours. Its activity, therefore, resides almost exclusively in the 10-hydroxy metabolite, to which it is rapidly converted and which has a half-life similar to that of carbamazepine, ie, 8–12 hours. The drug is mostly excreted as the glucuronide of the 10-hydroxy metabolite. Oxcarbazepine is less potent than carbamazepine, both in animal models of epilepsy and in epileptic patients; clinical doses of oxcarbazepine may need to be 50% higher than those of carbamazepine to obtain equivalent seizure control. Some studies report fewer hypersensitivity reactions to oxcarbazepine, and cross-reactivity with carbamazepine does not always occur. Furthermore, the drug appears to induce hepatic enzymes to a lesser extent than carbamazepine, minimizing drug interactions. Although hyponatremia may occur more commonly with oxcarbazepine than with carbamazepine, most adverse effects that occur with oxcarbazepine are similar in character to reactions reported with carbamazepine.

Oxcarbazepine

PHENOBARBITAL

Aside from the bromides, phenobarbital is the oldest of the currently available antiseizure drugs. Although it has long been considered one of the safest of the antiseizure agents, the use of other medications with lesser sedative effects has been urged. Many consider the barbiturates the drugs of choice for seizures only in infants.

Chemistry

The four derivatives of barbituric acid clinically useful as antiseizure drugs are phenobarbital, mephobarbital, metharbital, and primidone. The first three are so similar that they are considered together. Metharbital is methylated barbital, and mephobarbital is methylated phenobarbital; both are demethylated in vivo. The pKas of these three weak acid compounds range from 7.3 to 7.9. Slight changes in the normal acid-base balance, therefore, can cause significant fluctuation in the ratio of the ionized to the un-ionized species. This is particularly important for phenobarbital, the most commonly used barbiturate, whose pKa is similar to the plasma pH of 7.4.

The three-dimensional conformations of phenobarbital and *N*-methylphenobarbital are similar to that of phenytoin. Both compounds possess a phenyl ring and are active against partial seizures.

Mechanism of Action

The exact mechanism of action of phenobarbital is unknown, but enhancement of inhibitory processes and diminution of excitatory transmission probably contribute significantly. Recent data indicate that phenobarbital may selectively suppress abnormal neurons, inhibiting the spread and suppressing firing from the foci. Like phenytoin, phenobarbital suppresses high-frequency repetitive firing in neurons in culture through an action on Na^+ conductance, but only at high concentrations. Also at high concentrations, barbiturates block some Ca^{2+} currents (L-type and N-type). Phenobarbital binds to an allosteric regulatory site on the $GABA_A$ receptor, and it enhances the GABA receptor-mediated current by prolonging the openings of the chloride channels.

Phenobarbital also blocks excitatory responses induced by glutamate, principally those mediated by activation of the AMPA receptor (see Chapter 21). Both the enhancement of GABA-mediated inhibition and the reduction of glutamate-mediated excitation are seen with therapeutically relevant concentrations of phenobarbital.

Clinical Use

Phenobarbital is useful in the treatment of partial seizures and generalized tonic-clonic seizures, although the drug is often tried for virtually every seizure type, especially when attacks are difficult to control. There is little evidence for its effectiveness in generalized seizures such as absence, atonic attacks, and infantile spasms; it may worsen certain patients with these seizure types.

Some physicians prefer either metharbital or mephobarbital—especially the latter—to phenobarbital because of supposed decreased adverse effects. Only anecdotal data are available to support such comparisons.

Pharmacokinetics

See Chapter 22.

Therapeutic Levels & Dosage

The therapeutic levels of phenobarbital in most patients range from 10 mcg/mL to 40 mcg/mL. Documentation of effectiveness is best in febrile seizures, and levels below 15 mcg/mL appear ineffective for prevention of febrile seizure recurrence. The upper end of the therapeutic range is more difficult to define, because many patients appear to tolerate chronic levels above 40 mcg/mL.

Drug Interactions & Toxicity

See Chapter 22.

PRIMIDONE

Primidone, or 2-desoxyphenobarbital (Figure 24–4), was first marketed in the early 1950s. It was later reported that primidone was metabolized to phenobarbital and phenylethylmalonamide (PEMA). All three compounds are active anticonvulsants.

Mechanism of Action

Although primidone is converted to phenobarbital, the mechanism of action of primidone itself may be more like that of phenytoin.

Clinical Use

Primidone, like its metabolites, is effective against partial seizures and generalized tonic-clonic seizures and may be

Figure 24–4. Primidone and its active metabolites.

more effective than phenobarbital. It was previously considered to be the drug of choice for complex partial seizures, but the latest studies of partial seizures in adults strongly suggest that carbamazepine and phenytoin are superior to primidone. Attempts to determine the relative potencies of the parent drug and its two metabolites have been conducted in newborn infants, in whom drug-metabolizing enzyme systems are very immature and in whom primidone is only slowly metabolized. Primidone has been shown to be effective in controlling seizures in this group and in older patients beginning treatment with primidone; older patients show seizure control before phenobarbital concentrations reach the therapeutic range. Finally, studies of maximal electroshock seizures in animals suggest that primidone has an anticonvulsant action independent of its conversion to phenobarbital and PEMA (the latter is relatively weak).

Pharmacokinetics

Primidone is completely absorbed, usually reaching peak concentrations about 3 hours after oral administration, although considerable variation has been reported. Primidone is generally confined to total body water, with a volume of distribution of 0.6 L/kg. It is not highly bound to plasma proteins; approximately 70% circulates as unbound drug.

Primidone is metabolized by oxidation to phenobarbital, which accumulates very slowly, and by scission of the heterocyclic ring to form PEMA (Figure 24–4). Both primidone and phenobarbital also undergo subsequent conjugation and excretion.

Primidone has a larger clearance than most other antiseizure drugs (2 L/kg/d), corresponding to a half-life of 6–8 hours. PEMA clearance is approximately half that of primidone, but phenobarbital has a very low clearance. The appearance of phenobarbital corresponds to the disappearance of primidone. Phenobarbital therefore accumulates very slowly but eventually reaches therapeutic concentrations in most patients when therapeutic doses of primidone are administered. During chronic therapy, phenobarbital levels derived from primidone are usually two to three times higher than primidone levels. PEMA, which probably makes a minimal contribution to the efficacy of primidone, has a half-life of 8–12 hours and therefore reaches steady state more rapidly than phenobarbital.

Therapeutic Levels & Dosage

Primidone is most efficacious when plasma levels are in the range of 8–12 mcg/mL. Concomitant levels of its metabolite, phenobarbital, at steady state usually vary from 15 mcg/mL to 30 mcg/mL. Dosages of 10–20 mg/kg/d are necessary to obtain these levels. It is very important, however, to start primidone at low doses and gradually increase over days to a few weeks to avoid prominent sedation and gastrointestinal complaints. When adjusting doses of the drug, it is important to remember that the parent drug reaches steady state rapidly (30–40 hours), but the active metabolites phenobarbital (20 days) and PEMA (3–4 days) reach steady state much more slowly.

Toxicity

The dose-related adverse effects of primidone are similar to those of its metabolite, phenobarbital, except that drowsiness occurs early in treatment and may be prominent if the initial dose is too large. Gradual increments are indicated when starting the drug in either children or adults.

VIGABATRIN

Current investigations that seek drugs to enhance the effects of GABA include efforts to find GABA agonists and prodrugs, GABA transaminase inhibitors, and GABA uptake inhibitors. Vigabatrin (γ-vinyl-GABA) is one of these drugs and has been registered in Canada, Europe, and South America.

Vigabatrin

Mechanism of Action

Vigabatrin is an irreversible inhibitor of GABA aminotransferase (GABA-T), the enzyme responsible for the degradation of GABA. It apparently acts by increasing the amount of GABA released at synaptic sites, thereby enhancing inhibitory effects. A decrease in brain glutamine synthetase activity is probably secondary to the increased GABA concentrations. It is effective in a wide range of seizure models. Vigabatrin is marketed as a racemate; the $S(+)$ enantiomer is active and the $R(-)$ enantiomer appears to be inactive.

Clinical Use

Vigabatrin is useful in the treatment of partial seizures and West's syndrome. The half-life is approximately 6–8 hours, but considerable evidence suggests that the pharmacodynamic activity of the drug is more prolonged and not well correlated with the plasma half-life. In adults, vigabatrin should be started at an oral dosage of 500 mg twice daily; a total of 2–3 g (rarely more) daily may be required for full effectiveness. Typical toxicities include drowsiness, dizziness, and weight gain. Less common but more troublesome adverse reactions are agitation, confusion, and psychosis; preexisting mental illness is a relative contraindication. The drug was delayed in its worldwide introduction by the appearance in rats and dogs of a reversible intramyelinic edema; this phenomenon has not been observed in any patient to date. More recently, unfortunately, long-term therapy with vigabatrin has been associated with development of visual field defects in up to one third of patients. This adverse effect may not be reversible, and vigabatrin may therefore be relegated to use in patients—such as those with infantile spasms—who are refractory to other treatments.

LAMOTRIGINE

Lamotrigine was developed when some investigators thought that the antifolate effects of certain antiseizure drugs (eg, phenytoin) may contribute to their effectiveness. Several phenyltriazines were developed, and although their antifolate properties were weak, some were active in seizure screening tests.

Lamotrigine

Mechanism of Action

Lamotrigine, like phenytoin, suppresses sustained rapid firing of neurons and produces a voltage- and use-

dependent inactivation of sodium channels. This action probably explains lamotrigine's efficacy in focal epilepsy. It appears likely that lamotrigine has another mechanism of action to account for its efficacy in primary generalized seizures in childhood, including absence attacks; this mechanism may involve actions on voltage-activated Ca^{2+} channels. Lamotrigine also decreases the synaptic release of glutamate.

Clinical Use

Although most controlled studies have evaluated lamotrigine as add-on therapy, some suggest that the drug is effective as monotherapy for partial seizures, and the drug is now widely prescribed for this indication. Some authorities feel that the drug is also active against absence and myoclonic seizures in children. Adverse effects include dizziness, headache, diplopia, nausea, somnolence, and skin rash. The rash is considered a typical hypersensitivity reaction. Although the risk of rash may be diminished by introducing the drug slowly, pediatric patients are at high risk; some studies suggest that a potentially life-threatening dermatitis will develop in 1–2% of pediatric patients.

Pharmacokinetics & Dosage

Lamotrigine is almost completely absorbed and has a volume of distribution in the range of 1–1.4 L/kg. Protein binding is only about 55%. The drug has linear kinetics and is metabolized primarily by glucuronidation to the 2-N-glucuronide, which is excreted in the urine. Lamotrigine has a half-life of approximately 24 hours in normal volunteers; this decreases to 13–15 hours in patients taking enzyme-inducing drugs. Lamotrigine is effective against partial seizures in adults, with dosages typically between 100 and 300 mg/d and with a therapeutic blood level near 3 mcg/mL. Valproate causes a twofold increase in the drug's half-life; in patients receiving valproate, the initial dosage of lamotrigine must be reduced to 25 mg every other day.

FELBAMATE

Felbamate has been approved and marketed in the USA and in some European countries. Although it is effective in some patients with partial seizures, the drug causes aplastic anemia and severe hepatitis at unexpectedly high rates and has been relegated to the status of a third-line drug for refractory cases.

Felbamate appears to have multiple mechanisms of action. It produces a use-dependent block of the NMDA receptor, with selectivity for the NR1-2B subtype. It also potentiates $GABA_A$ receptor responses. Felbamate has a half-life of 20 hours (somewhat shorter when administered with either phenytoin or carbamazepine) and is metabolized by hydroxylation and conjugation; a significant percentage of the drug is excreted unchanged in the urine. When added to treatment with other antiseizure drugs, felbamate increases plasma phenytoin and valproic acid levels but decreases levels of carbamazepine.

Felbamate

In spite of the seriousness of the adverse effects, thousands of patients worldwide remain on the medication. Usual dosages are 2000–4000 mg/d in adults, and effective plasma levels range from 30 mcg/mL to 100 mcg/mL. In addition to its usefulness in partial seizures, felbamate has proved effective against the seizures that occur in Lennox-Gastaut syndrome.

GABAPENTIN & PREGABALIN

Gabapentin is an amino acid, an analog of GABA, that is effective against partial seizures. Originally planned as a spasmolytic, it was found to be more effective as an antiseizure drug. Pregabalin is another GABA analog, closely related to gabapentin. This drug was recently approved in the USA for both antiseizure activity and for its analgesic properties.

Gabapentin   **Pregabalin**

Mechanism of Action

In spite of their close structural resemblance to GABA, gabapentin and pregabalin do not act directly on GABA receptors. They may, however, modify the synaptic or nonsynaptic release of GABA. An increase in brain GABA concentration is observed in patients receiving gabapentin. Gabapentin is transported into the brain by the L-amino acid transporter. Gabapentin and pregabalin bind avidly to the $\alpha 2\delta$ subunit of voltage-gated Ca^{2+} channels. Gabapentin and pregabalin also act presynap-

tically to decrease the release of glutamate; this effect is probably dependent on reduced presynaptic entry of Ca^{2+} via voltage-activated channels.

Clinical Use & Dosage

Gabapentin is effective as an adjunct against partial seizures and generalized tonic-clonic seizures at dosages that range up to 2400 mg/d in controlled clinical trials. Open follow-on studies permitted dosages up to 4800 mg/d, but data are inconclusive on the effectiveness or tolerability of such doses. Monotherapy studies also document some efficacy. Some clinicians have found that very high dosages are needed to achieve improvement in seizure control. Effectiveness in other seizure types has not been well demonstrated. Gabapentin has also been found effective in the treatment of neuropathic pain and is now indicated for postherpetic neuralgia in adults at doses of 1800 mg and above. The most common adverse effects are somnolence, dizziness, ataxia, headache, and tremor.

Pregabalin is approved (as an adjunct) for the treatment of partial seizures, with or without secondary generalization; controlled clinical trials have documented its effectiveness. It is available only in oral form, and the daily dose ranges from 150 mg/d to 600 mg/d, usually in two or three divided administrations. Pregabalin is also approved for use in neuropathic pain, including painful diabetic peripheral neuropathy and postherpetic neuralgia.

Pharmacokinetics

Gabapentin is not metabolized and does not induce hepatic enzymes. Absorption is nonlinear and dose-dependent at very high doses, but otherwise the elimination kinetics are linear. The drug is not bound to plasma proteins. Drug-drug interactions are negligible. Elimination is via renal mechanisms; the drug is excreted unchanged. The half-life is short, ranging from 5 hours to 8 hours; the drug is typically administered two or three times per day.

Pregabalin, like gabapentin, is not metabolized and is almost entirely excreted unchanged in the urine. It is not bound to plasma proteins and has virtually no drug-drug interactions, again resembling the characteristics of gabapentin. Likewise, other drugs do not affect the pharmacokinetics of pregabalin. The half-life of pregabalin ranges from about 4.5 hours to 7.0 hours, thus requiring more than once-per-day dosing in most patients.

LEVETIRACETAM

Levetiracetam is a piracetam analog that is ineffective against seizures induced by maximum electroshock or pentylenetetrazol but has prominent activity in the kindling model.

Levetiracetam

Levetiracetam binds selectively to a synaptic vesicular protein SV2A. The function of this protein is not understood but it is likely that levetiracetam modifies the synaptic release of glutamate and GABA through an action on vesicular function.

The drug is marketed for the treatment of partial seizures. Oral absorption is nearly complete; it is rapid and unaffected by food, with peak plasma concentrations in 1.3 hours. Kinetics are linear. Protein binding is less than 10%. The plasma half-life is 6–8 hours and may be longer in the elderly. Two thirds of the drug is excreted unchanged in the urine. Drug interactions are minimal; levetiracetam is not metabolized by cytochrome P450. Dosing can begin with 500 mg orally twice daily; some patients require up to 3000 mg/d. Adverse effects include somnolence, asthenia, and dizziness. Idiosyncratic reactions are rare.

TIAGABINE

Tiagabine is a derivative of nipecotic acid and was "rationally designed" as an inhibitor of GABA uptake (as opposed to discovery through random screening).

Tiagabine

Mechanism of Action

Tiagabine is an inhibitor of GABA uptake in both neurons and glia. It preferentially inhibits the transporter isoform 1 (GAT-1) rather than GAT-2 or GAT-3 and increases extracellular GABA levels in the forebrain and hippocampus. It prolongs the inhibitory action of synaptically released GABA. In rodents, it is potent against kindled seizures but weak against the maximum electroshock model.

Clinical Use

Tiagabine is indicated for the adjunctive treatment of partial seizures and is effective in doses ranging from 16 mg/d to 56 mg/d. Divided doses as often as four times per day are sometimes required. Some patients appear to do well with tiagabine monotherapy, which is generally well tolerated. Minor adverse events are dose-related and include nervousness, dizziness, tremor, difficulty in concentrating, and depression. Excessive confusion, somnolence, or ataxia may require discontinuation. Psychosis occurs rarely. Rash is an uncommon idiosyncratic adverse effect. Laboratory studies are usually normal.

Pharmacokinetics

Tiagabine is 90–100% bioavailable, has linear kinetics, and is highly protein-bound. The half-life is 5–8 hours and decreases in the presence of enzyme-inducing drugs. Food decreases the peak plasma concentration but not the area under the concentration curve (see Chapter 3). Hepatic impairment causes a slight decrease in clearance (and may necessitate a lower dose), but the drug does not cause inhibition or induction of hepatic enzymes. The drug is oxidized in the liver by CYP3A. Elimination is primarily in the feces (60–65%) and urine (25%).

TOPIRAMATE

Topiramate is a substituted monosaccharide that is structurally different from all other antiseizure drugs.

Topiramate

Mechanism of Action

Topiramate blocks repetitive firing of cultured spinal cord neurons, as do phenytoin and carbamazepine. Its mechanism of action, therefore, is likely to involve blocking of voltage-gated sodium channels. Topiramate also appears to potentiate the inhibitory effect of GABA, acting at a site different from the benzodiazepine or barbiturate sites. Topiramate also depresses the excitatory action of kainate on glutamate receptors. It is possible that all three of these actions contribute to topiramate's anticonvulsant effect.

Clinical Use

Clinical trials of topiramate demonstrated a dose-response relationship, and monotherapy trials showed the drug to be effective against partial and generalized tonic-clonic seizures. Good evidence suggests that the drug has a broader spectrum, with effectiveness against Lennox-Gestaut syndrome, West's syndrome, and even absence seizures. Topiramate is also approved for the treatment of migraine headaches. Dosages typically range from 200 mg/d to 600 mg/d, with a few patients tolerating dosages higher than 1000 mg/d. Most clinicians begin at a low dose (50 mg/d) and increase slowly to avoid adverse effects. Although no idiosyncratic reactions have been noted, dose-related adverse effects occur most frequently in the first 4 weeks and include somnolence, fatigue, dizziness, cognitive slowing, paresthesias, nervousness, and confusion. Acute myopia and glaucoma may require prompt drug withdrawal. Urolithiasis has also been reported. However, the discontinuation rate is apparently only about 15%. The drug is teratogenic in animal models, and hypospadias has been reported in male infants exposed in utero to topiramate; however, no causal relationship could be established.

Pharmacokinetics

Topiramate is rapidly absorbed (about 2 hours) and is 80% bioavailable. There is no food effect on absorption, minimal (15%) plasma protein binding, and only moderate (20–50%) metabolism; no active metabolites are formed. The drug is primarily excreted unchanged in the urine. The half-life is 20–30 hours. Although increased levels are seen with renal failure and hepatic impairment, there is no age or gender effect, no autoinduction, no inhibition of metabolism, and kinetics are linear. Drug interactions do occur and can be complex, but the major effect is on topiramate levels rather than on the levels of other antiseizure drugs. Birth control pills may be less effective in the presence of topiramate, and higher estrogen doses may be required.

ZONISAMIDE

Zonisamide is a sulfonamide derivative. Its primary site of action appears to be the sodium channel; it may also act on voltage-gated calcium channels. The drug is effective against partial and generalized tonic-clonic seizures and may also be useful against infantile spasms and certain myoclonias. It has good bioavailability, linear kinetics, low protein-binding, renal excretion, and a half-life of 1–3 days. Doses range from 100 mg/d to 600 mg/d in adults and from 4 mg/d to 12 mg/d in children. Adverse effects include drowsiness, cognitive impairment, and potentially serious skin rashes. Zonisamide does not interact with other antiseizure drugs.

Zonisamide

DRUGS USED IN GENERALIZED SEIZURES

ETHOSUXIMIDE

Ethosuximide was introduced in 1960 as the third of three marketed succinimides in the USA. Ethosuximide has very little activity against maximal electroshock but considerable efficacy against pentylenetetrazol seizures, and it was introduced as a "pure petit mal" drug. Its continued popularity is based on its safety and efficacy, and its role as the first choice anti-absence drug remains undiminished—in part because of the idiosyncratic hepatotoxicity of the alternative drug, valproic acid.

Chemistry

Ethosuximide is the last antiseizure drug to be marketed whose origin is in the cyclic ureide structure. The three antiseizure succinimides marketed in the USA are ethosuximide, phensuximide, and methsuximide. Methsuximide and phensuximide have phenyl substituents, whereas ethosuximide is 2-ethyl-2-methylsuccinimide.

Ethosuximide

Mechanism of Action

Ethosuximide has an important effect on Ca^{2+} currents, reducing the low-threshold (T-type) current. This effect is seen at therapeutically relevant concentrations in thalamic neurons. The T-type calcium currents are thought to provide a pacemaker current in thalamic neurons responsible for generating the rhythmic cortical discharge of an absence attack. Inhibition of this current could therefore account for the specific therapeutic action of ethosuximide.

Clinical Use

As predicted from its activity in laboratory models, ethosuximide is particularly effective against absence seizures, but has a very narrow spectrum of clinical activity. Documentation of its effectiveness in human absence seizures was achieved with long-term electroencephalographic recording techniques.

Pharmacokinetics

Absorption is complete following administration of the oral dosage forms. Peak levels are observed 3–7 hours after oral administration of the capsules. Ethosuximide is not protein-bound.

Ethosuximide is completely metabolized, principally by hydroxylation, to inactive metabolites. The drug has a very low total body clearance (0.25 L/kg/d). This corresponds to a half-life of approximately 40 hours, although values from 18 to 72 hours have been reported.

Therapeutic Levels & Dosage

Therapeutic levels of 60–100 mcg/mL can be achieved in adults with dosages of 750–1500 mg/d, although lower or higher dosages and blood levels may be necessary and tolerated (up to 125 mcg/mL) in some patients. Ethosuximide has a linear relationship between dose and steady-state plasma levels. The drug might be administered as a single daily dose were it not for its adverse gastrointestinal effects; twice-a-day dosage is common.

Drug Interactions

Administration of ethosuximide with valproic acid results in a decrease in ethosuximide clearance and higher steady-state concentrations owing to inhibition of metabolism. No other important drug interactions have been reported for the succinimides.

Toxicity

The most common dose-related adverse effect of ethosuximide is gastric distress, including pain, nausea, and vomiting. When an adverse effect does occur, temporary dosage reductions may allow adaptation. Ethosuximide is a highly efficacious and safe drug for absence seizures; the appearance of relatively mild, dose-related adverse effects should not immediately call for its abandonment. Other dose-related adverse effects include transient lethargy or fatigue and, much less commonly, headache, dizziness, hiccup, and euphoria. Behavioral changes are usually in the direction of improvement.

Non-dose-related or idiosyncratic adverse effects of ethosuximide are extremely uncommon. Skin rashes have been reported, including at least one case of Stevens-Johnson syndrome. The development of systemic lupus erythematosus has also been reported, but other drugs may have been involved.

PHENSUXIMIDE & METHSUXIMIDE

Phensuximide and methsuximide are phenylsuccinimides that were developed and marketed before ethosuximide. They are used primarily as anti-absence drugs. Methsuximide is generally considered more toxic, and phensuximide less effective, than ethosuximide. Unlike ethosuximide, these two compounds have some activity against maximal electroshock seizures, and methsuximide has been used for partial seizures by some investigators. The desmethyl metabolite of methsuximide has a half-life of 25 hours or more and exerts the major anti-seizure effect. The toxicity and reduced effectiveness of phensuximide when compared with methsuximide has been investigated, and the failure of the desmethyl metabolite to accumulate in the former probably explains its relatively weak effect.

VALPROIC ACID & SODIUM VALPROATE

Sodium valproate, also used as the free acid, valproic acid, was found to have antiseizure properties when it was used as a solvent in the search for other drugs effective against seizures. It was marketed in France in 1969 but was not licensed in the USA until 1978. Valproic acid is fully ionized at body pH, and for that reason the active form of the drug may be assumed to be the valproate ion regardless of whether valproic acid or a salt of the acid is administered.

Chemistry

Valproic acid is one of a series of fatty carboxylic acids that have antiseizure activity; this activity appears to be greatest for carbon chain lengths of five to eight atoms. The amides and esters of valproic acid are also active antiseizure agents.

$$CH_3-CH_2-CH_2 \atop CH_3-CH_2-CH_2 \Big\rangle CH-COOH$$

Valproic acid

Mechanism of Action

The time course of valproate's anticonvulsant activity appears to be poorly correlated with blood or tissue levels of the parent drug, an observation giving rise to considerable speculation regarding both the active species and the mechanism of action of valproic acid. Valproate is active against both pentylenetetrazol and maximal electroshock seizures. Like phenytoin and carbamazepine, valproate blocks sustained high-frequency repetitive firing of neurons in culture at therapeutically relevant concentrations. Its action against partial seizures may be a consequence of this effect on Na^+ currents. Blockade of NMDA receptor-mediated excitation may also be important. Much attention has been paid to the effects of valproate on GABA. Several studies have shown increased levels of GABA in the brain after administration of valproate, although the mechanism for this increase remains unclear. An effect of valproate to facilitate glutamic acid decarboxylase (GAD), the enzyme responsible for GABA synthesis, has been described. An inhibitory effect on the GABA transporter GAT-1 may contribute. At very high concentrations, valproate inhibits GABA transaminase in the brain, thus blocking degradation of GABA. However, at the relatively low doses of valproate needed to abolish pentylenetetrazol seizures, brain GABA levels may remain unchanged. Valproate produces a reduction in the aspartate content of rodent brain, but the relevance of this effect to its anticonvulsant action is not known.

Valproic acid is a potent inhibitor of histone deacetylase and through this mechanism changes the transcription of many genes. A similar effect, but to a lesser degree, is shown by some other antiseizure drugs (topiramate, carbamazepine, and a metabolite of levetiracetam).

Clinical Use

Valproate is very effective against absence seizures. Although ethosuximide is the drug of choice when absence seizures occur alone, valproate is preferred when the patient has concomitant generalized tonic-clonic attacks. The reason for preferring ethosuximide for uncomplicated absence seizures is valproate's idiosyncratic hepatotoxicity, described below. Valproate is unique in its ability to control certain types of myoclonic seizures; in some cases the effect is very dramatic. The drug is effective in generalized tonic-clonic seizures, especially those which are primarily generalized. A few patients with atonic attacks may also respond, and some evidence suggests that the drug is effective in partial seizures.

Other uses of valproate include management of bipolar disorder and migraine prophylaxis.

Pharmacokinetics

Valproate is well absorbed following an oral dose, with bioavailability greater than 80%. Peak blood levels are observed within 2 hours. Food may delay absorption, and decreased toxicity may result if the drug is given after meals.

Valproic acid is 90% bound to plasma proteins, although the fraction bound is somewhat reduced at blood levels greater than 150 mcg/mL. Since valproate is both highly ionized and highly protein-bound, its distribution is essentially confined to extracellular water, with a volume of distribution of approximately 0.15 L/kg.

Clearance for valproate is low; its half-life varies from 9 hours to 18 hours. Approximately 20% of the drug is excreted as a direct conjugate of valproate.

The sodium salt of valproate is marketed in Europe as a tablet and is quite hygroscopic. In Central and South America, the magnesium salt is available, which is considerably less hygroscopic. The free acid of valproate was first marketed in the USA in a capsule containing corn oil; the sodium salt is also available in syrup, primarily for pediatric use. An enteric-coated tablet of divalproex sodium is also marketed in the USA. This improved product, a 1:1 coordination compound of valproic acid and sodium valproate, is as bioavailable as the capsule but is absorbed much more slowly and is preferred by many patients. Peak concentrations following administration of the enteric-coated tablets are seen in 3–4 hours.

Therapeutic Levels & Dosage

Dosages of 25–30 mg/kg/d may be adequate in some patients, but others may require 60 mg/kg/d or even more. Therapeutic levels of valproate range from 50 mcg/mL to 100 mcg/mL.

Drug Interactions

The clearance of valproate is dose-dependent, caused by changes in both the intrinsic clearance and protein binding. At higher doses, there is an increased free fraction of valproate, resulting in lower total drug levels than expected. It may be clinically useful, therefore, to measure both total and free drug levels. Valproate also displaces phenytoin from plasma proteins. In addition to binding interactions, valproate inhibits the metabolism of several drugs, including phenobarbital, phenytoin, and carbamazepine, leading to higher steady-state concentrations of these agents. The inhibition of phenobarbital metabolism, for example, may cause levels of the barbiturate to rise steeply, causing stupor or coma.

Toxicity

The most common dose-related adverse effects of valproate are nausea, vomiting, and other gastrointestinal complaints such as abdominal pain and heartburn. The drug should be started gradually to avoid these symptoms. Sedation is uncommon with valproate alone but may be striking when valproate is added to phenobarbital. A fine tremor is frequently seen at higher levels. Other reversible adverse effects, seen in a small number of patients, include weight gain, increased appetite, and hair loss.

The idiosyncratic toxicity of valproate is largely limited to hepatotoxicity, but this may be severe; there seems little doubt that the hepatotoxicity of valproate has been responsible for more than 50 fatalities in the USA alone. The risk is greatest for patients under the age of 2 years and for those taking multiple medications. Initial aspartate aminotransferase values may not be elevated in susceptible patients, although these levels do eventually become abnormal. Most fatalities have occurred within 4 months after initiation of therapy. Some clinicians recommend treatment with oral or intravenous L-carnitine as soon as severe hepatotoxicity is suspected. Careful monitoring of liver function is recommended when starting the drug; the hepatotoxicity is reversible in some cases if the drug is withdrawn. The other observed idiosyncratic response with valproate is thrombocytopenia, although documented cases of abnormal bleeding are lacking. It should be noted that valproate is an effective and popular antiseizure drug and that only a very small number of patients have had severe toxic effects from its use.

Several epidemiologic studies of valproate have confirmed an increased incidence of spina bifida in the offspring of women who took valproate during pregnancy. In addition, an increased incidence of cardiovascular, orofacial, and digital abnormalities has been reported. These observations must be strongly considered in the choice of drugs during pregnancy.

OXAZOLIDINEDIONES

Trimethadione, the first oxazolidinedione, was introduced as an antiseizure drug in 1945 and remained the drug of choice for absence seizures until the introduction of succinimides in the 1950s. The use of the oxazolidinediones (trimethadione, paramethadione, and dimethadione) is now very limited.

The oxazolidinediones contain an oxazolidine heterocyclic ring (Figure 24–1) and are similar in structure to other antiseizure drugs introduced before 1960. The structure includes only short-chain alkyl substituents on the heterocyclic ring, with no attached phenyl group.

$$H_3C \quad \overset{O}{\diagdown} \quad C=O$$
$$H_3C \diagup \overset{|}{\underset{5}{C}} \qquad |$$
$$\overset{|}{\underset{\parallel}{C}} \text{——} N\text{——}CH_3$$
$$O$$

Trimethadione

These compounds are active against pentylenetetrazol-induced seizures. Trimethadione raises the threshold for seizure discharges following repetitive thalamic stimulation. It—or, more notably, its active metabolite dimethadione—has the same effect on thalamic Ca^{2+} currents as ethosuximide (reducing the T-type calcium current). Thus, suppression of absence seizures is likely to depend on inhibiting the pacemaker action of thalamic neurons.

Trimethadione is rapidly absorbed, with peak levels reached within an hour after drug administration. It is not bound to plasma proteins. Trimethadione is completely metabolized in the liver by demethylation to dimethadione, which may exert the major antiseizure activity. Dimethadione has an extremely long half-life (240 hours).

The therapeutic plasma level range for trimethadione has never been established, although trimethadione blood levels above 20 mcg/mL and dimethadione levels above 700 mcg/mL have been suggested. A dosage of 30 mg/kg/d of trimethadione is necessary to achieve these levels in adults.

The most common and bothersome dose-related adverse effect of the oxazolidinediones is sedation. Trimethadione has been associated with many other toxic adverse effects, some of which are severe. These drugs should not be used during pregnancy.

OTHER DRUGS USED IN MANAGEMENT OF EPILEPSY

Some drugs not classifiable by application to seizure type are discussed in this section.

BENZODIAZEPINES

Six benzodiazepines play prominent roles in the therapy of epilepsy (see also Chapter 22). Although many benzodiazepines are similar chemically, subtle structural alterations result in differences in activity. They have two different mechanisms of antiseizure action, which are shown to different degrees by the six compounds. This is evident from the fact that diazepam is relatively more potent against electroshock and clonazepam against pentylenetetrazol (the latter effect correlating with an action at the GABA-benzodiazepine allosteric receptor sites). Possible mechanisms of action are discussed in Chapter 22.

Diazepam given intravenously or rectally is highly effective for stopping continuous seizure activity, especially generalized tonic-clonic status epilepticus (see below). The drug is occasionally given orally on a long-term basis, although it is not considered very effective in this application, probably because of the rapid development of tolerance. A rectal gel is available for refractory patients who need acute control of bouts of seizure activity. **Lorazepam** appears in some studies to be more effective and longer-acting than diazepam in the treatment of status epilepticus and is preferred by some experts.

Clonazepam is a long-acting drug with documented efficacy against absence seizures; on a milligram basis, it is one of the most potent antiseizure agents known. It is also effective in some cases of myoclonic seizures and has been tried in infantile spasms. Sedation is prominent, especially on initiation of therapy; starting doses should be small. Maximal tolerated doses are usually in the range of 0.1–0.2 mg/kg, but many weeks of gradually increasing daily doses may be needed to achieve these dosages in some patients. **Nitrazepam** is not marketed in the USA but is used in many other countries, especially for infantile spasms and myoclonic seizures.

It is less potent than clonazepam, and its clinical advantages over that drug have not been documented.

Clorazepate dipotassium is approved in the USA as an adjunct to treatment of complex partial seizures in adults. Drowsiness and lethargy are common adverse effects, but as long as the drug is increased gradually, dosages as high as 45 mg/d can be given.

Clobazam is not available in the USA but is marketed in most countries and is widely used in a variety of seizure types. It is a 1,5-benzodiazepine (other marketed benzodiazepines are 1,4-benzodiazepines) and reportedly has less sedative potential than benzodiazepines marketed in the USA. Whether the drug has significant clinical advantages is not clear. It has a half-life of 18 hours and is effective at dosages of 0.5–1 mg/kg/d. It does interact with some other antiseizure drugs and causes adverse effects typical of the benzodiazepines; efficacy, in some patients, is limited by the development of tolerance.

Pharmacokinetics

The pharmacokinetic properties of the benzodiazepines in part determine their clinical use. In general, the drugs are well absorbed, widely distributed, and extensively metabolized, with many active metabolites. The rate of distribution of benzodiazepines within the body is different from that of other antiseizure drugs. Diazepam and lorazepam in particular are rapidly and extensively distributed to the tissues, with volumes of distribution between 1 L/kg and 3 L/kg. The onset of action is very rapid. Total body clearances of the parent drug and its metabolites are low, corresponding to half-lives of 20–40 hours.

Limitations

Two prominent aspects of benzodiazepines limit their usefulness. The first is their pronounced sedative effect, which is unfortunate both in the treatment of status epilepticus and in chronic therapy. Children may manifest a paradoxical hyperactivity, as with barbiturates. The second problem is tolerance, in which seizures may respond initially but recur within a few months. The remarkable antiseizure potency of these compounds often cannot be realized because of these limiting factors.

ACETAZOLAMIDE

Acetazolamide is a diuretic whose main action is the inhibition of carbonic anhydrase (see Chapter 15). Mild acidosis in the brain may be the mechanism by which the drug exerts its antiseizure activity; alternatively, the depolarizing action of bicarbonate ions moving out of neurons via GABA receptor ion channels may be diminished by carbonic anhydrase inhibition. Acetazolamide has been used for all types of seizures but

is severely limited by the rapid development of tolerance, with return of seizures usually within a few weeks. The drug may have a special role in epileptic women who experience seizure exacerbations at the time of menses; seizure control may be improved and tolerance may not develop because the drug is not administered continuously. The usual dosage is approximately 10 mg/kg/d to a maximum of 1000 mg/d.

Another carbonic anhydrase inhibitor, **sulthiame,** was not found to be effective as an anticonvulsant in clinical trials in the USA. It is marketed in some other countries.

■ II. CLINICAL PHARMACOLOGY OF ANTISEIZURE DRUGS

SEIZURE CLASSIFICATION

The type of medication utilized for epilepsy depends on the empiric nature of the seizure. For this reason, considerable effort has been expended to classify seizures so that clinicians will be able to make a "seizure diagnosis" and on that basis prescribe appropriate therapy. Errors in seizure diagnosis cause use of the wrong drugs, and an unpleasant cycle ensues in which poor seizure control is followed by increasing drug doses and medication toxicity. As noted above, seizures are divided into two groups: partial and generalized. Drugs used for partial seizures are more or less the same for the entire group, but drugs used for generalized seizures are determined by the individual seizure type. A summary of the international classification of epileptic seizures is presented in Table 24–1.

Partial Seizures

Partial seizures are those in which a localized onset of the attack can be ascertained, either by clinical observation or by electroencephalographic recording; the attack begins in a specific locus in the brain. There are three types of partial seizures, determined to some extent by the degree of brain involvement by the abnormal discharge.

The least complicated partial seizure is the **simple partial seizure,** characterized by minimal spread of the abnormal discharge such that normal consciousness and awareness are preserved. For example, the patient may have a sudden onset of clonic jerking of an extremity lasting 60–90 seconds; residual weakness may last for 15–30 minutes after the attack. The patient is completely aware of the attack and can describe it in detail. The electroencephalogram may show an abnormal discharge highly localized to the involved portion of the brain.

The **complex partial seizure** also has a localized onset, but the discharge becomes more widespread (usually bilateral) and almost always involves the limbic system. Most complex partial seizures arise from one of the temporal lobes, possibly because of the susceptibility of this area of the brain to insults such as hypoxia or infection. Clinically, the patient may have a brief warning followed by an alteration of consciousness during which some patients stare and others stagger or even fall. Most, however, demonstrate fragments of integrated motor behavior called **automatisms** for which the patient has no memory. Typical automatisms are lip smacking, swallowing, fumbling, scratching, or even walking about. After 30–120 seconds, the patient makes a gradual recovery to normal consciousness but may feel tired or ill for several hours after the attack.

The last type of partial seizure is the **secondarily generalized attack,** in which a partial seizure immediately precedes a generalized tonic-clonic (grand mal) seizure. This seizure type is described in the text that follows.

Generalized Seizures

Generalized seizures are those in which there is no evidence of localized onset. The group is quite heterogeneous.

Generalized tonic-clonic (grand mal) seizures are the most dramatic of all epileptic seizures and are characterized by tonic rigidity of all extremities, followed in 15–30 seconds by a tremor that is actually an interruption of the tonus by relaxation. As the relaxation phases become longer, the attack enters the clonic phase, with massive jerking of the body. The clonic jerking slows over 60–120 seconds, and the patient is usually left in a stuporous state. The tongue or cheek may be bitten, and urinary incontinence is common. Primary generalized tonic-clonic seizures begin without evidence of localized onset, whereas secondary generalized tonic-clonic seizures are preceded by another seizure type, usually a partial seizure. The medical treatment of both primary and secondary generalized tonic-clonic seizures is the same and uses drugs appropriate for *partial* seizures.

The **absence (petit mal) seizure** is characterized by both sudden onset and abrupt cessation. Its duration is usually less than 10 seconds and rarely more than 45 seconds. Consciousness is altered; the attack may also be associated with mild clonic jerking of the eyelids or extremities, with postural tone changes, autonomic phenomena, and automatisms. The occurrence of automatisms can complicate the clinical differentiation from complex partial seizures in some patients. Absence attacks begin in childhood or adolescence and may occur up to hundreds of times a day. The electroencephalogram during the seizure shows a highly characteristic 2.5–3.5 Hz spike-and-wave pattern. Atypical absence patients have seizures with postural changes that are more abrupt, and such patients are often mentally retarded; the electroencephalogram may show a slower spike-and-wave discharge, and the seizures may be more refractory to therapy.

Myoclonic jerking is seen, to a greater or lesser extent, in a wide variety of seizures, including generalized tonic-clonic seizures, partial seizures, absence seizures, and infantile spasms. Treatment of seizures that include myoclonic jerking should be directed at the primary seizure type rather than at the myoclonus. Some patients, however, have myoclonic jerking as the major seizure type, and some have frequent myoclonic jerking and occasional generalized tonic-clonic seizures without overt signs of neurologic deficit. Many kinds of myoclonus exist, and much effort has gone into attempts to classify this entity.

Atonic seizures are those in which the patient has sudden loss of postural tone. If standing, the patient falls suddenly to the floor and may be injured. If seated, the head and torso may suddenly drop forward. Although most often seen in children, this seizure type is not unusual in adults. Many patients with atonic seizures wear helmets to prevent head injury.

Infantile spasms are an epileptic syndrome and not a seizure type. The attacks, although sometimes fragmentary, are most often bilateral and are included for pragmatic purposes with the generalized seizures. These attacks are most often characterized clinically by brief, recurrent myoclonic jerks of the body with sudden flexion or extension of the body and limbs; the forms of infantile spasms are, however, quite heterogeneous. Ninety percent of affected patients have their first attack before the age of 1 year. Most patients are mentally retarded, presumably from the same cause as the spasms. The cause is unknown in many patients, but such widely disparate disorders as infection, kernicterus, tuberous sclerosis, and hypoglycemia have been implicated. In some cases, the electroencephalogram is characteristic. Drugs used to treat infantile spasms are effective only in some patients; there is little evidence that the mental retardation is alleviated by therapy, even when the attacks disappear.

THERAPEUTIC STRATEGY

For most of the older antiseizure drugs, relationships between blood levels and therapeutic effects have been characterized to a high degree. The same is true for the pharmacokinetics of these drugs. These relationships provide significant advantages in the development of therapeutic strategies for the treatment of epilepsy. The therapeutic index for most antiseizure drugs is low, and toxicity is not uncommon. Thus, effective treatment of seizures often requires an awareness of the therapeutic levels and pharmacokinetic properties as well as the characteristic toxicities of each agent. Measurements of antiseizure drug plasma levels can be very useful when combined with clinical observations and pharmacoki-

Table 24–2. Effective plasma levels of six antiseizure drugs.

Drug	Effective Level (mcg/mL)	High Effective Level[1] (mcg/mL)	Toxic Level (mcg/mL)
Carbamazepine	4–12	7	> 8
Primidone	5–15	10	< 12
Phenytoin	10–20	18	> 20
Phenobarbital	10–40	35	> 40
Ethosuximide	50–100	80	> 100
Valproate	50–100	80	> 100

[1]Level that should be achieved, if possible, in patients with refractory seizures, assuming that the blood samples are drawn before administration of the morning medication. Higher levels are often possible—without toxicity—when the drugs are used alone, ie, as monotherapy.
Reprinted, with permission, from Porter RJ: *Epilepsy: 100 Elementary Principles,* 2nd ed. Saunders, 1989.

netic data (Table 24–2). The relationship between seizure control and plasma drug levels is variable and often less clear for the drugs marketed since 1990.

MANAGEMENT OF EPILEPSY

PARTIAL SEIZURES & GENERALIZED TONIC-CLONIC SEIZURES

Until the last 15 years, the choice of drugs for partial and tonic-clonic seizures was usually limited to phenytoin, carbamazepine, or barbiturates. There has been a strong tendency in the past few decades to limit the use of sedative antiseizure drugs such as barbiturates and benzodiazepines to patients who cannot tolerate other medications. Thus, in the 1980s, the trend was to increase the use of carbamazepine. Although carbamazepine and phenytoin are still very widely used, all of the newer drugs (marketed after 1990) have shown effectiveness against these same seizure types. An effort has been made to define the role for these new drugs (French et al, 2004). With the older drugs, the efficacy and the long-term adverse effects are well established; this creates a "confidence level" in spite of questionable tolerability. For the newer drugs, most have a broader spectrum of activity, and most are well tolerated, but the same "confidence level" is not yet present. These issues (plus the issues of drug cost) are the determining factors in choosing a drug for these seizure types.

GENERALIZED SEIZURES

The issues (described above) related to choosing between old and new drugs apply to the generalized group of seizures as well.

The drugs used for generalized tonic-clonic seizures are the same as for partial seizures; in addition, valproate is clearly useful.

At least three drugs are effective against absence seizures. Two are nonsedating and therefore preferred: ethosuximide and valproate. Clonazepam is also highly effective but has disadvantages of dose-related adverse effects and development of tolerance. Lamotrigine and topiramate may also be useful.

Specific myoclonic syndromes are usually treated with valproate; an intravenous formulation can be used acutely as needed. It is nonsedating and can be dramatically effective. Other patients respond to clonazepam, nitrazepam, or other benzodiazepines, although high doses may be necessary, with accompanying drowsiness. Zonisamide and levetiracetam may be useful. Another specific myoclonic syndrome, juvenile myoclonic epilepsy, can be aggravated by phenytoin or carbamazepine; valproate is the drug of choice followed by lamotrigine and topiramate.

Atonic seizures are often refractory to all available medications, although some reports suggest that valproate may be beneficial, as may lamotrigine. Benzodiazepines have been reported to improve seizure control in some of these patients but may worsen the attacks in others. Felbamate has been demonstrated to be effective in some patients, although the drug's idiosyncratic toxicity limits its use. If the loss of tone appears to be part of another seizure type (such as absence or complex partial seizures), every effort should be made to treat the other seizure type vigorously, hoping for simultaneous alleviation of the atonic component of the seizure. The ketogenic diet may also be useful.

DRUGS USED IN INFANTILE SPASMS

The treatment of infantile spasms is unfortunately limited to improvement of control of the seizures rather than other features of the disorder, such as retardation. Most patients receive a course of intramuscular corticotropin, although some clinicians note that prednisone may be equally effective and can be given orally. Clinical trials have been unable to settle the matter. In either case, therapy must often be discontinued because of adverse effects. If seizures recur, repeat courses of corticotropin or corticosteroids can be given, or other drugs may be tried. Other drugs widely used are the benzodiazepines such as clonazepam or nitrazepam; their efficacy in this heterogeneous syndrome may be nearly as good as that of corticosteroids. Vigabatrin may also be effective. The mechanism of action of corticosteroids or corticotropin in the treatment of infantile spasms is unknown. Further details may be sought in more specialized texts.

STATUS EPILEPTICUS

There are many forms of status epilepticus. The most common, generalized tonic-clonic status epilepticus, is a life-threatening emergency, requiring immediate cardiovascular, respiratory, and metabolic management as well as pharmacologic therapy. The latter virtually always requires intravenous administration of antiseizure medications. Diazepam is the most effective drug in most patients for stopping the attacks and is given directly by intravenous push to a maximum total dose of 20–30 mg in adults. Intravenous diazepam may depress respiration (less frequently, cardiovascular function), and facilities for resuscitation must be immediately at hand during its administration. The effect of diazepam is not lasting, but the 30- to 40-minute seizure-free interval allows more definitive therapy to be initiated. Some physicians prefer lorazepam, which is equivalent to diazepam in effect and perhaps somewhat longer-acting. For patients who are not actually in the throes of a seizure, diazepam therapy can be omitted and the patient treated at once with a long-acting drug such as phenytoin.

Until the introduction of fosphenytoin, the mainstay of continuing therapy for status epilepticus was intravenous phenytoin, which is effective and nonsedating. It can be given as a loading dose of 13–18 mg/kg in adults; the usual error is to give too little. Administration should be at a maximum rate of 50 mg/min. It is safest to give the drug directly by intravenous push, but it can also be diluted in saline; it precipitates rapidly in the presence of glucose. Careful monitoring of cardiac rhythm and blood pressure is necessary, especially in elderly people. At least part of the cardiotoxicity is from the propylene glycol in which the phenytoin is dissolved. Fosphenytoin, which is freely soluble in intravenous solutions without the need for propylene glycol or other solubilizing agents, is a safer parenteral agent. Because of its greater molecular weight, this prodrug is two thirds to three quarters as potent as phenytoin on a milligram basis.

In previously treated epileptic patients, the administration of a large loading dose of phenytoin may cause some dose-related toxicity such as ataxia. This is usually a relatively minor problem during the acute status episode and is easily alleviated by later adjustment of plasma levels.

For patients who do not respond to phenytoin, phenobarbital can be given in large doses: 100–200 mg intravenously to a total of 400–800 mg. Respiratory depression is a common complication, especially if benzodiazepines have already been given, and there should be no hesitation in instituting intubation and ventilation.

Although other drugs such as lidocaine have been recommended for the treatment of generalized tonic-clonic status epilepticus, general anesthesia is usually necessary in highly resistant cases.

For patients in absence status, benzodiazepines are still drugs of first choice. Rarely, intravenous valproate may be required.

SPECIAL ASPECTS OF THE TOXICOLOGY OF ANTISEIZURE DRUGS

TERATOGENICITY

The potential teratogenicity of antiseizure drugs is controversial and important. It is important because teratogenicity resulting from long-term drug treatment of millions of people throughout the world may have a profound effect even if the effect occurs in only a small percentage of cases. It is controversial because both epilepsy and antiseizure drugs are heterogeneous, and few epileptic patients are available for study who are not receiving these drugs. Furthermore, patients with severe epilepsy, in whom genetic factors rather than drug factors may be of greater importance in the occurrence of fetal malformations, are often receiving multiple antiseizure drugs in high doses.

In spite of these limitations, it appears—from whatever cause—that children born to mothers taking antiseizure drugs have an increased risk, perhaps twofold, of congenital malformations. Phenytoin has been implicated in a specific syndrome called **fetal hydantoin syndrome,** although not all investigators are convinced of its existence and a similar syndrome has been attributed both to phenobarbital and to carbamazepine. Valproate, as noted above, has also been implicated in a specific malformation, spina bifida. It is estimated that a pregnant woman taking valproic acid or sodium valproate has a 1–2% risk of having a child with spina bifida. Topiramate has shown some teratogenicity in animal testing and, as noted earlier, in the human male fetus.

In dealing with the clinical problem of a pregnant woman with epilepsy, most epileptologists agree that although it is important to minimize exposure to antiseizure drugs, both in numbers and dosages, it is also important not to allow maternal seizures to go unchecked.

WITHDRAWAL

Withdrawal of antiseizure drugs, whether by accident or by design, can cause increased seizure frequency and severity. The two factors to consider are the effects of the withdrawal itself and the need for continued drug suppression of seizures in the individual patient. In many patients, both factors must be considered. It is important to note, however, that the abrupt discontinuance of antiseizure drugs ordinarily does not cause seizures in nonepileptic patients, provided that the drug levels are not above the usual therapeutic range when the drug is stopped.

Some drugs are more easily withdrawn than others. In general, withdrawal of anti-absence drugs is easier than withdrawal of drugs needed for partial or generalized tonic-clonic seizures. Barbiturates and benzodiazepines are the most difficult to discontinue; weeks or months may be required, with very gradual dosage decrements, to accomplish their complete outpatient removal.

Because of the heterogeneity of epilepsy, complete discontinuance of antiseizure drug administration is an especially difficult problem. If a patient is seizure-free for 3 or 4 years, a trial of gradual discontinuance is often warranted.

OVERDOSE

Antiseizure drugs are central nervous system depressants but are rarely lethal. Very high blood levels are usually necessary before overdoses can be considered life-threatening. The most dangerous effect of antiseizure drugs after large overdoses is respiratory depression, which may be potentiated by other agents, such as alcohol. Treatment of antiseizure drug overdose is supportive; stimulants should not be used. Efforts to hasten removal of antiseizure drugs, such as alkalinization of the urine (phenytoin is a weak acid), are usually ineffective.

PREPARATIONS AVAILABLE

Carbamazepine (generic, Tegretol)
Oral: 200 mg tablets; 100 mg chewable tablets; 100 mg/5 mL suspension
Oral extended-release: 100, 200, 400 mg tablets; 200, 300 mg capsules
Clonazepam (generic, Klonopin)
Oral: 0.5, 1, 2 mg tablets
Clorazepate dipotassium (generic, Tranxene)
Oral: 3.75, 7.5, 15 mg tablets, capsules
Oral sustained-release (Tranxene-SD): 11.25, 22.5 mg tablets
Diazepam (generic, Valium, others)
Oral: 2, 5, 10 mg tablets; 5 mg/5 mL, 5 mg/mL solutions
Parenteral: 5 mg/mL for IV injection
Rectal: 2.5, 5, 10, 15, 20 mg viscous rectal solution
Ethosuximide (generic, Zarontin)
Oral: 250 mg capsules; 250 mg/5 mL syrup
Ethotoin (Peganone)
Oral: 250, 500 mg tablets
Felbamate (Felbatol)
Oral: 400, 600 mg tablets; 600 mg/5 mL suspension
Fosphenytoin (Cerebyx)
Parenteral: 75 mg/mL for IV or IM injection
Gabapentin (Neurontin)
Oral: 100, 300, 400 mg capsules; 600, 800 mg filmtabs; 50 mg/mL solution
Lamotrigine (Lamictal)
Oral: 25, 100, 150, 200 mg tablets; 2, 5, 25 mg chewable tablets
Levetiracetam (Keppra)
Oral: 250, 500, 750 mg tablets
Lorazepam (generic, Ativan)
Oral: 0.5, 1, 2 mg tablets; 2 mg/mL solution
Parenteral: 2, 4 mg/mL for IV or IM injection

Mephenytoin (Mesantoin)
Oral: 100 mg tablets
Mephobarbital (Mebaral)
Oral: 32, 50, 100 mg tablets
Oxcarbazepine (Trileptal)
Oral: 100, 300, 600 mg tablets; 60 mg/mL suspension
Pentobarbital sodium (generic, Nembutal)
Parenteral: 50 mg/mL for IV or IM injection
Phenobarbital (generic, Luminal Sodium, others)
Oral: 15, 16, 30, 60, 90, 100 mg tablets; 16 mg capsules; 15, 20 mg/5 mL elixirs
Parenteral: 30, 60, 65, 130 mg/mL for IV or IM injection
Phenytoin (generic, Dilantin, others)
Oral (prompt-release): 100 mg capsules; 50 mg chewable tablets; 30, 125 mg/5 mL suspension
Oral extended-action: 30, 100 mg capsules
Oral slow-release (Phenytek): 200, 300 mg capsules
Parenteral: 50 mg/mL for IV injection
Pregabalin (Lyrica)
Oral: 75, 150, 300 mg capsules
Primidone (generic, Mysoline)
Oral: 50, 250 mg tablets; 250 mg/5 mL suspension
Tiagabine (Gabitril)
Oral: 4, 12, 16, 20 mg tablets
Topiramate (Topamax)
Oral: 25, 100, 200 mg tablets; 15, 25 mg sprinkle capsules
Trimethadione (Tridione)
Oral: 150 mg chewable tablets; 300 mg capsules; 40 mg/mL solution

(continued)

Valproic acid (generic, Depakene)
Oral: 250 mg capsules; 250 mg/5 mL syrup (sodium valproate)
Oral sustained-release (Depakote): 125, 250, 500 mg tablets (as divalproex sodium)

Parenteral (Depacon): 100 mg/mL in 5 mL vial for IV injection
Zonisamide (Zonegran)
Oral: 25, 50, 100 mg tablets

REFERENCES

Backonja MM: Use of anticonvulsants for treatment of neuropathic pain. Neurology 2002;59(5 Suppl 2):S14.

Ben-Menachem E: Vagus-nerve stimulation for the treatment of epilepsy. The Lancet-Neurology 2002;1:477.

Beydoun A, Kutluay E: Oxcarbazepine. Expert Opin Pharmacother 2002;3:59.

Bialer M et al: Progress report on new antiepileptic drugs: A summary of the Fifth Eiliat Conference. Epilepsy Res 2001;43:11.

Cunningham MO et al: Dual effects of gabapentin and pregabalin on glutamate release at rat entorhinal synapses in vitro. Euro J Neurosci 2004;20:1566.

Delgado-Escueta AV et al: *Jasper's Basic Mechanisms of the Epilepsies,* Lippincott Williams & Wilkins, 1999.

Duncan JS: The promise of new antiepileptic drugs. Br J Clin Pharmacol 2002;53:123.

Elterman RD et al: Randomized trial of vigabatrin in patients with infantile spasms. Neurology 2001;57:1416.

Eyal S et al: The activity of antiepileptic drugs as histone deacetylase inhibitors. Epilepsia 2004;45:737.

Faught E et al: Randomized controlled trial of zonisamide for the treatment of refractory partial-onset seizures. Neurology 2001;57:1774.

Fisher RS et al: Rapid initiation of gabapentin: A randomized controlled trial. Neurology 2001;56:743.

French, JA et al: Efficacy and tolerability of the new antiepileptic drugs I: Treatment of new onset epilepsy. Report of the Therapeutics and Technology Assessment Subcommittee and Quality Standards Subcommittee of the American Academy of Neurology and the American Epilepsy Society. Neurology 2004;62(8):1252.

Hachad H et al: New antiepileptic drugs: Review on drug interactions. Ther Drug Monit 2002;24:91.

Levy RH et al: *Antiepileptic Drugs,* 5th ed. Lippincott Williams & Wilkins, 2002.

Löscher W: Basic pharmacology of valproate: A review after 35 years of clinical use for the treatment of epilepsy. CNS Drugs 2002;16:669.

Lynch BA et al: The synaptic vesicle protein SV2A is the binding site for the antiepileptic drug levetiracetam. Proc Natl Acad Sci U S A 2004;101:9861.

Marson AG et al: Levetiracetam, oxcarbazepine, remacemide and zonisamide for drug resistant localization-related epilepsy: A systematic review. Epilepsy Res 2001;46:259.

McAuley JW, Anderson GD: Treatment of epilepsy in women of reproductive age: Pharmacokinetic considerations. Clin Pharmacokinet 2002;41:559.

Privitera M: Efficacy of levetiracetam: A review of three pivotal trials. Epilepsia 2001;42(Suppl 4):31.

Pryor FM et al: Fosphenytoin: Pharmacokinetics and tolerance of intramuscular loading. Epilepsia 2001;42;245.

Siddiqui A et al: Association of multidrug resistance in epilepsy with a polymorphism in the drug-transporter gene *ABCB1.* N Engl J Med 2002;348:15.

Treiman DM et al: A comparison of four treatments for generalized convulsive status epilepticus. N Engl J Med 1998;339:792.

Wallace SJ: Newer antiepileptic drugs: Advantages and disadvantages. Brain Dev 2001;23:277.

Willmore LJ: Lamotrigine. Expert Review of Neurotherapeutics 2001;1:33.

General Anesthetics

Anthony J. Trevor, PhD, & Paul F. White, PhD, MD

The physiologic state induced by general anesthetics typically includes analgesia, amnesia, loss of consciousness, inhibition of sensory and autonomic reflexes, and skeletal muscle relaxation. The extent to which any individual anesthetic agent can exert these effects varies depending on the drug, the dosage, and the clinical situation.

An ideal anesthetic drug would induce loss of consciousness smoothly and rapidly, while allowing for prompt recovery of cognitive function after its administration is discontinued. The drug would also possess a wide margin of safety and be devoid of adverse effects. No single anesthetic agent is capable of achieving all of these desirable effects without some disadvantages when used alone. The modern practice of anesthesiology most commonly involves the use of combinations of intravenous and inhaled drugs, taking advantage of their individual favorable properties while minimizing their adverse reactions.

The anesthetic technique will vary according to the proposed type of diagnostic, therapeutic, or surgical intervention. For minor procedures, oral or parenteral sedatives may be used in conjunction with local anesthetics (see Chapter 26). These techniques provide profound analgesia, but with retention of the patient's ability to maintain a patent airway and to respond to verbal commands. For more extensive surgical procedures, anesthesia frequently includes preoperative benzodiazepines, induction of anesthesia with an intravenous anesthetic (eg, thiopental or propofol), and maintenance of anesthesia with a combination of inhaled (eg, volatile agents, nitrous oxide) and intravenous (eg, propofol, opioid analgesics) drugs.

TYPES OF GENERAL ANESTHESIA

General anesthetics are usually administered by intravenous injection or by inhalation. For many years, inhalation anesthesia was used for all major procedures. Recently, intravenous anesthesia has become the more commonly used technique.

Intravenous Anesthetics

Several drugs are administered intravenously, alone or in combination with other anesthetic drugs, to achieve an anesthetic state or to sedate patients in intensive care units (ICUs) who must be mechanically ventilated. These drugs include the following: (1) barbiturates (eg, thiopental, methohexital); (2) benzodiazepines (eg, midazolam, diazepam); (3) propofol (4) ketamine; (5) opioid analgesics (morphine, fentanyl, sufentanil, alfentanil, remifentanil); and (6) miscellaneous sedative-hypnotics (eg, etomidate, dexmedetomidine). Figure 25–1 shows the structures of some commonly used intravenous anesthetics.

Inhaled Anesthetics

The chemical structures of the currently available inhaled anesthetics are shown in Figure 25–2. The most commonly used inhaled anesthetics are isoflurane, desflurane, and sevoflurane. These compounds are volatile liquids. Nitrous oxide, a gas at ambient temperature and pressure, continues to be an important adjuvant to the volatile agents.

Balanced Anesthesia

Although general anesthesia can be produced using only intravenous or only inhaled anesthetic drugs, modern anesthesia typically involves a combination of intravenous (eg, for induction of anesthesia) and inhaled (eg, for maintenance of anesthesia) drugs. Muscle relaxants are commonly used to facilitate tracheal intubation and optimize surgical conditions (see Chapter 27). Local anesthetics are often administered by tissue infiltration and peripheral nerve blocks to provide perioperative analgesia (see Chapter 26). In addition, potent opioid analgesics and cardiovascular drugs (eg, β blockers, α_2 agonists, calcium channel blockers) are used to control autonomic responses to noxious (painful) surgical stimuli.

STAGES OF ANESTHESIA

The traditional description of the stages of anesthesia (the so-called Guedel's signs) were derived from observations of the effects of diethyl ether, which has a slow onset of central action owing to its high solubility in blood. Using these signs, anesthetic drug effects can be

Figure 25-1. Intravenous anesthetics.

divided into four stages of increasing depth of central nervous system depression:

I. Stage of analgesia: The patient initially experiences analgesia without amnesia. Later in Stage I, both analgesia and amnesia are produced.
II. Stage of excitement: During this stage, the patient often appears to be delirious and may vocalize but is definitely amnesic. Respiration is irregular both in volume and rate, and retching and vomiting may occur if the patient is stimulated. For these reasons, efforts are made to limit the duration and severity of this stage, which ends with the reestablishment of regular breathing.
III. Stage of surgical anesthesia: This stage begins with the recurrence of regular respiration and extends to complete cessation of spontaneous respiration (apnea). Four planes of stage III have been described in terms of changes in ocular movements, eye reflexes, and pupil size, which under specified conditions may represent signs of increasing depth of anesthesia.
IV. Stage of medullary depression: This deep stage of anesthesia includes severe depression of the vasomotor center in the medulla, as well as the respiratory center. Without circulatory and respiratory support, death rapidly ensues.

In current anesthesia practice, the distinctive signs of each of the four stages described above are usually obscured because of the more rapid onset of action of modern intravenous and inhaled anesthetics (compared with ether), and the fact that ventilation is often controlled mechanically. In addition, the practice of administering other pharmacologic agents preoperatively (eg, preanesthetic medication) or intraoperatively (eg, opioid analgesics, cardiovascular drugs) can also alter the clinical signs of anesthesia. The anticholinergic drugs, atropine and glycopyrrolate, are used to decrease secretions and to treat bradycardia; however, they also dilate the pupils. Muscle relaxants reduce muscle tone and prevent purposeful movements, whereas the opioid analgesics exert depressant effects on both the respiratory and heart rates. The most reliable indication that stage III (surgical anesthesia) has been achieved is loss of responsiveness to noxious stimuli (eg, trapezius muscle squeeze) and reestablishment of a regular respiratory pattern. The adequacy of the depth of anesthesia for a specific surgical stimulus is assessed by monitoring changes in respiratory and cardiovascular responses to the surgical stimulation, as well as electroencephalographic (EEG-based) cerebral indices.

Although vital sign monitoring remains the most common method of assessing depth of anesthesia during sur-

Figure 25–2. Inhaled anesthetics.

gery, techniques involving computer-assisted monitoring of cerebral function using EEG activity appear to offer some advantages. Automated techniques use processed variables derived from established effects of anesthetics on EEG activity and include the bispectral index (BIS), the physical state index (PSI), and the cerebral state index (CSI). The application of cerebral monitoring techniques has been shown to reduce the anesthetic requirement, contributing to a more rapid recovery from general anesthesia.

■ INHALED ANESTHETICS

PHARMACOKINETICS

Ensuring an adequate depth of anesthesia depends on achieving a therapeutic concentration of the anesthetic

in the central nervous system. The rate at which an effective brain concentration is achieved (ie, time to induction of general anesthesia) depends on multiple pharmacokinetic factors that influence the brain uptake and tissue distribution of the anesthetic agent. The pharmacokinetic properties of the intravenous anesthetics (Table 25–1) and the physicochemical properties of the inhaled agents (Table 25–2) directly influence the pharmacodynamic effects of these drugs. These factors also influence the rate of recovery when the anesthetic is discontinued.

Uptake & Distribution of Inhaled Anesthetics

The concentration of an inhaled anesthetic in a mixture of gases is proportional to its **partial pressure** (or **tension**). These terms are often used interchangeably in discussing the various transfer processes involving anesthetic gases in the body. Achievement of a brain concentration of an inhaled anesthetic to provide adequate anesthesia requires transfer of the anesthetic from the alveolar air to the blood and from the blood to the brain. The rate at which a therapeutic concentration of the anesthetic is achieved in the brain depends on the solubility properties of the anesthetic, its concentration in the inspired air, the volume of pulmonary ventilation, the pulmonary blood flow, and the partial pressure gradient between arterial and mixed venous blood anesthetic concentrations.

A. SOLUBILITY

One of the most important factors influencing the transfer of an anesthetic from the lungs to the arterial blood is its solubility characteristics (Table 25–2). The blood:gas partition coefficient is a useful index of solubility and defines the relative affinity of an anesthetic for the blood compared with that of inspired gas. The partition coefficients for desflurane and nitrous oxide, which are relatively insoluble in blood, are extremely low. When an anesthetic with low blood solubility diffuses from the lung into the arterial blood, relatively few molecules are required to raise its partial pressure, and therefore the arterial tension rises rapidly (Figure 25–3, top, nitrous oxide). Conversely, for anesthetics with moderate-to-high solubility (eg, halothane, isoflurane), more molecules dissolve before partial pressure changes significantly, and arterial tension of the gas increases less rapidly (Figure 25–3, bottom, halothane). This inverse relationship between the blood solubility of an anesthetic and the rate of rise of its tension in arterial blood is illustrated in Figure 25–4. Nitrous oxide, with low solubility in blood, reaches high arterial tensions rapidly, which in turn results in rapid equilibration with the brain and fast onset of action. A rapid onset of anesthetic action is also characteristic of desflu-

Table 25–1. Characteristics of intravenous anesthetics.

Drug	Induction and Recovery	Comments
Etomidate	Rapid onset and moderately fast recovery	Cardiovascular stability; decreased steroidogenesis; involuntary muscle movements
Ketamine	Moderately rapid onset and recovery	Cardiovascular stimulation; increased cerebral blood flow; emergence reactions impair recovery
Midazolam	Slow onset and recovery; flumazenil reversal available	Used in balanced anesthesia and conscious sedation; cardiovascular stability; marked amnesia
Propofol	Rapid onset and rapid recovery	Used in induction and for maintenance; hypotension; useful antiemetic action
Thiopental	Rapid onset and rapid recovery (bolus dose)— slow recovery following infusion	Standard induction agent; cardiovascular depression; avoid in porphyrias
Fentanyl	Slow onset and recovery; naloxone reversal available	Used in balanced anesthesia and conscious sedation; marked analgesia

rane and, to a lesser extent, sevoflurane, volatile anesthetics that have low blood:gas partition coefficients.

B. ANESTHETIC CONCENTRATION IN THE INSPIRED AIR

The concentration of an inhaled anesthetic in the inspired gas mixture has direct effects on both the maximum tension that can be achieved in the alveoli and the rate of increase in its tension in arterial blood. Increases in the inspired anesthetic concentration increase the rate of induction of anesthesia by increasing the rate of trans-

fer into the blood according to Fick's law (see Chapter 1). Advantage is taken of this effect in anesthetic practice with inhaled anesthetics that possess moderate blood solubility (eg, enflurane, isoflurane, and halothane). For example, a 1.5% concentration of isoflurane may be administered initially to increase the rate of induction; this is reduced to 0.75–1% for maintenance when adequate anesthesia is achieved. In addition, moderately soluble anesthetics are often administered in combination with a less soluble agent (eg, nitrous oxide) to reduce the

Table 25–2. Properties of inhaled anesthetics.

Anesthetic	Blood:Gas Partition Coefficient[1]	Brain:Blood Partition Coefficient[1]	Minimal Alveolar Conc (MAC) (%)[2]	Metabolism	Comments
Nitrous oxide	0.47	1.1	> 100	None	Incomplete anesthetic; rapid onset and recovery
Desflurane	0.42	1.3	6–7	< 0.05%	Low volatility; poor induction agent; rapid recovery
Sevoflurane	0.69	1.7	2.0	2–5% (fluoride)	Rapid onset and recovery; unstable in soda-lime
Isoflurane	1.40	2.6	1.40	< 2%	Medium rate of onset and recovery
Enflurane	1.80	1.4	1.7	8%	Medium rate of onset and recovery
Halothane	2.30	2.9	0.75	> 40%	Medium rate of onset and recovery
Methoxyflurane	12	2.0	0.16	> 70% (fluoride)	Very slow onset and recovery

[1]Partition coefficients (at 37 °C) are from multiple literature sources.
[2]MAC is the anesthetic concentration that produces immobility in 50% of patients exposed to a noxious stimulus.

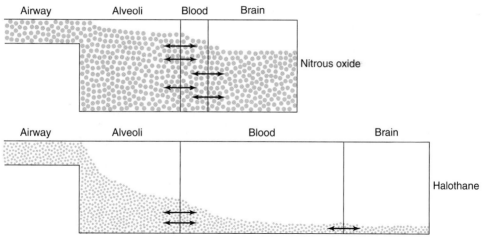

Figure 25–3. Why induction of anesthesia is slower with more soluble anesthetic gases. In this schematic diagram, solubility in blood is represented by the relative size of the blood compartment (the more soluble, the larger the compartment). Relative partial pressures of the agents in the compartments are indicated by the degree of filling of each compartment. For a given concentration or partial pressure of the two anesthetic gases in the inspired air, it will take much longer for the blood partial pressure of the more soluble gas (halothane) to rise to the same partial pressure as in the alveoli. Since the concentration of the anesthetic agent in the brain can rise no faster than the concentration in the blood, the onset of anesthesia will be slower with halothane than with nitrous oxide.

Figure 25–4. Tensions of three anesthetic gases in arterial blood as a function of time after beginning inhalation. Nitrous oxide is relatively insoluble (blood:gas partition coefficient = 0.47); methoxyflurane is much more soluble (coefficient = 12); and halothane is intermediate (2.3).

time required for loss of consciousness and achievement of a surgical depth of anesthesia.

C. PULMONARY VENTILATION

The rate of rise of anesthetic gas tension in arterial blood is directly dependent on both the rate and depth of ventilation (ie, minute ventilation). The magnitude of the effect varies according to the blood:gas partition coefficient. An increase in pulmonary ventilation is accompanied by only a slight increase in arterial tension of an anesthetic with low blood solubility or low coefficient but can significantly increase tension of agents with moderate-to-high blood solubility (Figure 25–5). For example, a fourfold increase in ventilation rate almost doubles the arterial tension of halothane during the first 10 minutes of anesthesia but increases the arterial tension of nitrous oxide by only 15%. Therefore, hyperventilation increases the speed of induction of anesthesia with inhaled anesthetics that would normally have a slow onset. Depression of respiration by opioid analgesics slows the onset of anesthesia of inhaled anesthetics if ventilation is not manually or mechanically assisted.

D. PULMONARY BLOOD FLOW

Changes in blood flow to and from the lungs influence transfer processes of the anesthetic gases. An increase in

Figure 25–5. Ventilation rate and arterial anesthetic tensions. Increased ventilation (8 versus 2 L/min) has a much greater effect on equilibration of halothane than nitrous oxide.

During the induction phase of anesthesia, the tissues that exert greatest influence on the arteriovenous anesthetic concentration gradient are those which are highly perfused (eg, brain, heart, liver, kidneys, and splanchnic bed). These tissues receive over 75% of the resting cardiac output. In the case of anesthetics with relatively high solubility in highly perfused tissues, venous blood concentration will initially be very low, and equilibrium with arterial blood is achieved slowly.

During maintenance of anesthesia with inhaled anesthetics, the drug continues to be transferred between various tissues at rates dependent on solubility and blood flow. Although muscle and skin constitute 50% of the total body mass, anesthetics accumulate more slowly in them than in highly perfused tissues (eg, brain) because they receive only one-fifth of the resting cardiac output. Although most anesthetic gases are highly soluble in adipose tissues, low blood perfusion to these tissues delays accumulation, and equilibrium is unlikely to occur with most anesthetics during an operation.

Elimination

The time to recovery from inhalation anesthesia depends on the rate of elimination of anesthetics from the brain. Many of the processes of anesthetic transfer during recovery are simply the reverse of those that occur during induction of anesthesia. One of the most important factors governing rate of recovery is the blood:gas partition coefficient of the anesthetic agent. Other factors controlling rate of recovery include the pulmonary blood flow, the magnitude of ventilation, and the tissue solubility of the anesthetic. Two features of recovery, however, are different from what happens during induction of anesthesia. First, although transfer of an anesthetic from the lungs to blood can be enhanced by increasing its concentration in inspired air, the reverse transfer process cannot be enhanced, because the concentration in the lungs cannot be reduced below zero. Second, at the beginning of recovery, the anesthetic gas tension in different tissues may be quite variable, depending on the specific agent and the duration of anesthesia. In contrast, with induction of anesthesia the initial anesthetic tension is zero in all tissues.

Inhaled anesthetics that are relatively insoluble in blood (ie, low blood:gas partition coefficient) and brain are eliminated at faster rates than more soluble anesthetics. The washout of nitrous oxide, desflurane, and sevoflurane occurs at a rapid rate, which leads to a more rapid recovery from their anesthetic effects compared with halothane and isoflurane. Halothane is approximately twice as soluble in brain tissue and five times more soluble in blood than nitrous oxide and desflurane; its elimination therefore takes place more slowly, and recovery from halothane anesthesia is predictably less rapid.

pulmonary blood flow (ie, increased cardiac output) slows the rate of rise in arterial tension, particularly for those anesthetics with moderate-to-high blood solubility. Increased pulmonary blood flow exposes a larger volume of blood to the anesthetic; thus, blood "capacity" increases and the anesthetic tension rises slowly. A decrease in pulmonary blood flow has the opposite effect, increasing the rate of rise of arterial tension of inhaled anesthetics. In patients with circulatory shock, the combined effects of decreased cardiac output (resulting in decreased pulmonary flow) and increased ventilation will accelerate induction of anesthesia with halothane and isoflurane. However, this is not likely to occur with less soluble agents such as nitrous oxide and desflurane.

E. ARTERIOVENOUS CONCENTRATION GRADIENT

The anesthetic concentration gradient between arterial and mixed venous blood is dependent mainly on uptake of the anesthetic by the tissues, including nonneural tissues. Depending on the rate and extent of tissue uptake, venous blood returning to the lungs may contain significantly less anesthetic than arterial blood. The greater this difference in anesthetic gas tensions, the more time it will take to achieve equilibrium with brain tissue. Anesthetic entry into tissues is influenced by factors similar to those that determine transfer from lung to blood, including tissue:blood partition coefficients, rates of blood flow to the tissues, and concentration gradients.

DO WE NEED ANOTHER INHALED ANESTHETIC?

After its introduction in 1956, halothane was the standard of comparison for inhaled anesthetics. However, the onset and recovery from its anesthetic action were slow compared with the commonly used intravenous agents (eg, thiopental). In addition, its hepatic metabolism can result in a reactive compound that may lead to halothane-associated hepatitis.

The newer volatile anesthetics, desflurane and sevoflurane, have physicochemical characteristics (ie, low blood:gas partition coefficients) that are favorable to a more rapid onset and shorter duration of anesthetic actions compared with isoflurane and halothane. However, both of these newer agents also have certain limitations. The low volatility of desflurane necessitates the use of a specialized heated vaporizer, and the pungency of the drug leads to a high incidence of coughing and sympath-

omimetic side effects that make it less than ideally suited for induction of anesthesia.

Anesthesia is achieved rapidly and smoothly with sevoflurane, and recovery is more rapid than with isoflurane. However, sevoflurane is chemically unstable when exposed to carbon dioxide absorbents in anesthesia machines, degrading to an olefinic compound (fluoromethyl-2,2-difluoro-1-[trifluoromethyl]vinyl ether, also known as compound A) that is potentially nephrotoxic. In addition, sevoflurane is metabolized by the liver to release fluoride ions, raising concerns about potential renal damage.

Sevoflurane comes close to having the characteristics of an ideal inhaled anesthetic; however, a more insoluble compound that lacks the pungency of desflurane and has greater chemical stability than sevoflurane could be a useful alternative to the currently available inhaled agents.

The duration of exposure to the anesthetic can also have a marked effect on recovery time, especially in the case of more soluble anesthetics (eg, isoflurane). Accumulation of anesthetics in muscle, skin, and fat increases with prolonged inhalation (especially in obese patients), and blood tension may decline slowly during recovery as the anesthetic is gradually eliminated from these tissues. Thus, if exposure to the anesthetic is short, recovery may be rapid even with the more soluble agents. However, after prolonged administration, recovery can be delayed even with anesthetics of moderate solubility (eg, isoflurane).

Clearance of inhaled anesthetics via the lungs is the major route of elimination from the body. However, hepatic metabolism may also contribute to the elimination of some volatile anesthetics. For example, the elimination of halothane during recovery is more rapid than that of enflurane, which would not be predicted from their respective tissue solubilities. However, over 40% of inspired halothane is metabolized during an average anesthetic procedure, whereas less than 10% of enflurane is metabolized over the same period. Oxidative metabolism of halothane results in the formation of trifluoroacetic acid and release of bromide and chloride ions. Under conditions of low oxygen tension, halothane is metabolized to the chlorotrifluoroethyl free radical, which is capable of reacting with hepatic membrane components and on rare occasions producing halothane hepatitis. Isoflurane and desflurane are the least metabolized of the fluorinated anesthetics; only traces of trifluoroacetic acid appear in the urine even after prolonged administration.

The metabolism of enflurane and sevoflurane results in the formation of fluoride ion; however, in contrast to the rarely used volatile anesthetic methoxyflurane, renal fluoride levels do not reach toxic levels under normal circumstances. In addition, sevoflurane is degraded by contact with the carbon dioxide absorbent in anesthesia machines, yielding a vinyl ether called "compound A," which can cause renal damage if high concentrations are absorbed. (See Box: Do We Need Another Inhaled Anesthetic?) Seventy percent of the absorbed methoxyflurane is metabolized by the liver, and released fluoride ions can very readily produce nephrotoxicity. In terms of the extent of hepatic metabolism, the rank order for the inhaled anesthetics is methoxyflurane > halothane > enflurane > sevoflurane > isoflurane > desflurane > nitrous oxide (Table 25–2). Nitrous oxide is not metabolized by human tissues. However, bacteria in the gastrointestinal tract may be able to break down the nitrous oxide molecule.

PHARMACODYNAMICS

Mechanism of Action

Both the inhaled and the intravenous anesthetics can depress spontaneous and evoked activity of neurons in many regions of the brain. Older concepts of the mechanism of anesthesia evoked nonspecific interactions of these agents with the lipid matrix of the nerve membrane (the Meyer-Overton principle)—interactions that were thought to lead to secondary changes in ion flux. More recently, evidence has accumulated suggesting that the modification of ion currents by anesthetics results from more direct interactions with specific nerve membrane components. The ionic mechanisms involved for different anesthetics may vary, but at clinically relevant concentrations they appear to involve interactions with members of the ligand-gated ion channel family.

In the past decade, considerable evidence has accumulated that a primary molecular target of general anesthetics is the **GABA_A receptor-chloride channel,** a major mediator of inhibitory synaptic transmission. Inhaled anesthetics, barbiturates, benzodiazepines, etomidate, and propofol facilitate GABA-mediated inhibition at GABA_A receptor sites. These receptors are sensitive to clinically relevant concentrations of the anesthetic agents and exhibit the appropriate stereospecific effects in the case of enantiomeric drugs. The GABA_A receptor-chloride channel is a pentameric assembly of five proteins derived from several polypeptide subclasses (see Chapter 22). Combinations of three major subunits—α, β, and γ—are necessary for normal physiologic and pharmacologic functions. GABA_A receptors in different areas of the central nervous system contain different subunit combinations, conferring different pharmacologic properties on each receptor subtype. Both inhaled and intravenous anesthetics with sedative-hypnotic properties directly activate GABA_A receptors, but at low concentrations they can also facilitate the action of GABA to increase chloride ion flux. In contrast, sedative benzodiazepines that lack general anesthetic properties (eg, diazepam, lorazepam) facilitate GABA action but have no direct actions on GABA_A receptors even at high concentrations in the absence of GABA.

Reconstitution studies with transfected cells utilizing chimeric and mutated GABA_A receptors reveal that anesthetic molecules do not interact directly with the GABA binding site but with specific sites in the transmembrane domains of both α and β subunits. Two specific amino acid residues in transmembrane segments 2 and 3 of the GABA_A receptor α_2 subunit, Ser270 and Ala291, are critical for the enhancement of GABA_A receptor function by inhaled anesthetics. One consequence of the interaction of isoflurane with this domain is an alteration in the gating of the chloride ion channel. However, differences occur in the precise binding sites of individual anesthetics. For example, a specific aspartate residue within transmembrane segment 2 of the GABA_A receptor α_2 subunit is required for etomidate activity but is not essential for the activity of barbiturates or propofol.

Ketamine does not produce its effects via facilitation of GABA_A receptor functions, but it may function via antagonism of the action of the excitatory neurotransmitter glutamic acid on the ***N*-methyl-D-aspartate** (NMDA) receptor. This receptor may also be a target for nitrous oxide.

In addition to their action on GABA_A chloride channels, certain general anesthetics have been reported to cause membrane hyperpolarization (ie, an inhibitory action) via their activation of potassium channels. These channels are ubiquitous in the central nervous system and some are linked to neurotransmitters, including acetylcholine, dopamine, norepinephrine, and serotonin. Electrophysiologic analyses of membrane ion flux in cultured cells have shown that inhaled anesthetics decrease the duration of opening of nicotinic receptor-activated cation channels—an action that decreases the excitatory effects of acetylcholine at cholinergic synapses. Most inhaled anesthetics inhibit nicotinic acetylcholine receptor isoforms, particularly those containing the α_4 subunit, though such actions do not appear to be involved in their immobilizing actions. The strychnine-sensitive **glycine receptor** is another ligand-gated ion channel that may function as a target for inhaled anesthetics, which can elicit channel opening directly and independently of their facilitatory effects on neurotransmitter binding.

The neuropharmacologic basis for the effects that characterize the stages of anesthesia appears to be differential sensitivity of specific neurons or neuronal pathways to the anesthetic drugs. Neurons in the substantia gelatinosa of the dorsal horn of the spinal cord are very sensitive to relatively low anesthetic concentrations. Interaction with neurons in this region interrupts sensory transmission in the spinothalamic tract, including transmission of nociceptive (pain) stimuli. These effects contribute to stage I analgesia and conscious sedation. The disinhibitory effects of general anesthetics (stage II), which occur at higher brain concentrations, result from complex neuronal actions, including blockade of many small inhibitory neurons such as Golgi type II cells, together with a paradoxical facilitation of excitatory neurotransmitters. A progressive depression of ascending pathways in the reticular activating system occurs during stage III of anesthesia; also occurring is suppression of spinal reflex activity, which contributes to muscle relaxation. Neurons in the respiratory and vasomotor centers of the medulla are relatively insensitive to the effects of general anesthetics, but at high concentrations their activity is depressed, leading to cardiorespiratory collapse (stage IV). It remains to be determined whether regional variation in anesthetic actions corresponds to the regional variation in the subtypes of GABA_A receptors. The differential sensitivity of specific neurons or neuronal pathways to anesthetics could reflect their interactions with other molecules in the fast ligand-gated ion channel family or could represent the existence of other molecular targets that have yet to be characterized.

Dose-Response Characteristics: The Concept of Minimum Alveolar Anesthetic Concentration

Inhaled anesthetics are delivered to the lungs in gas mixtures in which concentrations and flow rates are easy to measure and control. However, dose-response characteristics of gaseous anesthetics are difficult to measure. Although achievement of an anesthetic state depends on the concentration of the anesthetic in the brain (ie, effect site), concentrations in the brain tissue are obviously impossible to measure under clinical conditions. Furthermore, neither the lower nor the upper ends of the graded dose-response curve defining the effect on the central nervous system can be ethically determined because at very low gas concentrations awareness of pain may occur. Moreover, at high concentrations there is a high risk of severe cardiovascular and respiratory depression. Nevertheless, a useful estimate of anesthetic potency can be obtained using quantal dose-response principles.

During general anesthesia, the partial pressure of an inhaled anesthetic in the brain equals that in the lung when steady state is reached. Therefore, at a given level of anesthesia, measurements of the steady-state alveolar concentrations of different anesthetics provide a comparison of their relative potencies. The volatile anesthetic concentration is the percentage of the alveolar gas mixture, or partial pressure of the anesthetic as a percentage of 760 mm Hg (atmospheric pressure at sea level). The minimum alveolar anesthetic concentration (MAC) is defined as the *median concentration that results in immobility in 50% of patients when exposed to a noxious stimulus* (eg, surgical incision). Therefore, the MAC represents one point (the ED_{50}) on a conventional quantal dose-response curve (see Figure 2–16). Table 25–2 shows MAC values of the inhaled anesthetics, permitting comparison of their relative anesthetic potencies. The MAC value greater than 100% for nitrous oxide demonstrates that it is the least potent inhaled anesthetic. At normal barometric pressure, even 760 mm Hg partial pressure of nitrous oxide (100% of the inspired gas) is still less than 1 MAC, so it must be supplemented with other agents to achieve full surgical anesthesia (see below).

The dose of anesthetic gas that is being administered can be stated in multiples of MAC. A dose of 1 MAC of any anesthetic prevents movement in response to surgical incision in 50% of patients; however, individual patients may require 0.5–1.5 MAC. Unfortunately, MAC gives no information about the slope of the dose-response curve. In general, however, the dose-response relationship for inhaled anesthetics is very steep. Therefore, over 95% of patients may fail to respond to a noxious stimulus at 1.1 MAC.

The measurement of MAC values under controlled conditions has permitted quantitation of the effects of a number of variables on anesthetic requirements. For example, MAC values decrease in elderly patients and with hypothermia, but are not affected greatly by sex, height, and weight. Of particular importance is the presence of adjuvant drugs, which can change anesthetic requirement significantly. When intravenous drugs (eg, opioid analgesics, sympatholytics, or sedative-hypnotics) are administered as adjuvants to the volatile anesthetics, MAC is decreased in a dose-related fashion. The inspired concentration of anesthetic should be decreased in these situations.

MAC values of the inhaled anesthetics are additive. For example, nitrous oxide (60–70%) can be used as a "carrier" gas producing 40% of a MAC, thereby decreasing the anesthetic requirement of inhaled volatile and intravenous anesthetics. The addition of nitrous oxide (60% tension, 40% MAC) to 70% of a volatile agent's MAC would yield a total of 110% of a MAC, a value sufficient for surgical anesthesia in most patients.

Organ System Effects of Inhaled Anesthetics

A. EFFECTS ON THE CARDIOVASCULAR SYSTEM

Halothane, desflurane, enflurane, sevoflurane, and isoflurane all decrease mean arterial pressure in direct proportion to their alveolar concentration. With halothane and enflurane, the reduced arterial pressure appears to be caused by a reduction in cardiac output because there is little change in systemic vascular resistance despite marked changes in individual vascular beds (eg, an increase in cerebral blood flow). In contrast, isoflurane, desflurane, and sevoflurane have a depressant effect on arterial pressure as a result of a decrease in systemic vascular resistance with minimal effect on cardiac output.

Inhaled anesthetics change heart rate either directly by altering the rate of sinus node depolarization or indirectly by shifting the balance of autonomic nervous system activity. Bradycardia can be seen with halothane, probably because of direct vagal stimulation. In contrast, enflurane and sevoflurane have little effect, and both desflurane and isoflurane increase heart rate. In the case of desflurane, transient sympathetic activation with elevations in catecholamine levels can lead to marked increases in heart rate and blood pressure when high inspired gas concentrations are administered.

All inhaled anesthetics tend to increase right atrial pressure in a dose-related fashion, which reflects depression of myocardial function. In general, enflurane and halothane have greater myocardial depressant effects than isoflurane and the newer, less soluble halogenated anesthetics. Inhaled anesthetics reduce myocardial oxygen consumption, primarily by decreasing the variables that control oxygen demand, such as arterial blood pressure and contractile force (see Chapter 12). Although it produces less depression than the volatile anesthetics, nitrous oxide has also been found to depress the myocardium in a dose-dependent manner. However, administration of nitrous oxide in combination with the more potent inhaled (volatile) anesthetics can minimize cardiac depressant effects owing to its anesthetic-sparing effect.

Several factors influence the cardiovascular effects of inhaled anesthetics. Surgical stimulation, intravascular volume status, ventilatory status, and duration of anesthesia alter the cardiovascular depressant effects of these drugs. Hypercapnia releases catecholamines, which attenuate the decrease in blood pressure. As a result, the blood pressure decrease after 5 hours of anesthesia is less than it is after 1 hour; however, concomitant use of β blockers reduces this adaptive effect. Halothane and, to a lesser extent, isoflurane sensitize the myocardium to circulating catecholamines. Ventricular arrhythmias may occur in patients with cardiac disease who are given sympathomimetic drugs or have high circulating levels of endogenous catecholamines (eg, anxious patients, those given epinephrine-containing local anesthetics, and those with pheochromocytoma). However, the less soluble inhaled anesthetics appear to be less arrhythmogenic.

B. Effects on the Respiratory System

With the exception of nitrous oxide, all inhaled anesthetics in current use cause a dose-dependent decrease in tidal volume and an increase in respiratory rate. However, the increase in rate is insufficient to compensate for the decrease in volume, resulting in a decrease in minute ventilation. All volatile anesthetics are respiratory depressants, as indicated by a reduced response to increased levels of carbon dioxide. The degree of ventilatory depression varies among the volatile agents, with isoflurane and enflurane being the most depressant. All volatile anesthetics in current use increase the resting level of $PaCO_2$ (the partial pressure of carbon dioxide in arterial blood).

Volatile anesthetics increase the apneic threshold ($PaCO_2$ level below which apnea occurs through lack of CO_2-driven respiratory stimulation) and decrease the ventilatory response to hypoxia. The latter effect is especially important because subanesthetic concentrations during the early recovery period can depress the normal compensatory increase in ventilation that occurs during hypoxic states. The respiratory depressant effects of anesthetics are overcome by assisting (or controlling) ventilation mechanically. Furthermore, the ventilatory depressant effects of inhaled anesthetics are counteracted by surgical stimulation.

Inhaled anesthetics also depress mucociliary function in the airway. Thus, prolonged anesthesia may lead to pooling of mucus and then result in atelectasis and postoperative respiratory infections. However, volatile anesthetics possess varying degrees of bronchodilating properties), an effect of value in the treatment of active wheezing and status asthmaticus. The bronchodilating action of halothane and sevoflurane makes them the induction agents of choice in patients with underlying airway problems (eg, asthma, bronchitis, chronic obstructive pulmonary disease). Airway irritation, which may provoke coughing or breath-holding, is rarely a problem with halothane and sevoflurane. However, the pungency of desflurane make this agent less suitable for induction of anesthesia despite its low blood:gas partition coefficient.

C. Effects on the Brain

Inhaled anesthetics decrease the metabolic rate of the brain. Nevertheless, the more soluble volatile agents increase cerebral blood flow because they decrease cerebral vascular resistance. The increase in cerebral blood flow is clinically undesirable in patients who have increased intracranial pressure because of a brain tumor or head injury. Volatile anesthetic-induced increases in cerebral blood flow increase cerebral blood volume and further increase intracranial pressure.

Of the inhaled anesthetics, nitrous oxide is the least likely to increase cerebral blood flow. At low concentrations, all of the halogenated agents have similar effects on cerebral blood flow. However, at higher concentrations, the increase in cerebral blood flow is less with the more insoluble agents such as desflurane and sevoflurane. If the patient is hyperventilated before the volatile agent is started, the increase in intracranial pressure can be minimized.

Halothane, isoflurane, and enflurane have similar depressant effects on the EEG up to doses of 1–1.5 MAC. At higher doses, the cerebral irritant effects of enflurane may lead to development of a spike-and-wave pattern and mild generalized muscle twitching (ie, myoclonic activity). However, this seizure-like activity has not been found to have any adverse clinical consequences. Seizure-like EEG activity has also been described after sevoflurane, but not desflurane. Although nitrous oxide has a very low anesthetic potency, it does possess both analgesic and amnesic properties when used alone or in combination with other agents as part of a balanced anesthesia technique.

D. Effects on the Kidney

Depending on the concentration, volatile anesthetics decrease the glomerular filtration rate and renal blood flow, and increase the filtration fraction. Since renal blood flow decreases during general anesthesia in spite of well-maintained or even increased perfusion pressures (due to increased renal vascular resistance), autoregulation of renal flow may be impaired.

E. EFFECTS ON THE LIVER

Volatile anesthetics cause a concentration-dependent decrease in hepatic blood flow ranging from 15% to 45% below the preinduction (baseline) value. Despite transient intraoperative changes in liver function tests, permanent changes in liver enzyme function are rare.

F. EFFECTS ON UTERINE SMOOTH MUSCLE

Nitrous oxide appears to have little effect on uterine musculature. However, the halogenated anesthetics are potent uterine muscle relaxants and produce this effect in a concentration-dependent fashion. This pharmacologic effect can be used to advantage when profound uterine relaxation is required for an intrauterine fetal manipulation or manual extraction of a retained placenta during delivery.

Toxicity

A. HEPATOTOXICITY (HALOTHANE)

Postoperative hepatic dysfunction is typically associated with factors such as blood transfusions, hypovolemic shock, and other surgical stresses rather than volatile anesthetic toxicity. However, a small subset of individuals who have been previously exposed to halothane may develop potentially life-threatening hepatitis. The incidence of severe hepatotoxicity following exposure to halothane is in the range of one in 20,000–35,000. Obese patients who have had more than one exposure to halothane during a short time interval may be the most susceptible. There is no specific treatment for halothane hepatitis, and therefore liver transplantation may ultimately be required.

The mechanisms underlying hepatotoxicity from halothane remain unclear, but studies in animals have implicated the formation of reactive metabolites that either cause direct hepatocellular damage (eg, free radicals) or initiate immune-mediated responses. With regard to the latter mechanism, serum from patients with halothane hepatitis contains a variety of autoantibodies against hepatic proteins. Trifluoroacetylated (TFA) proteins in the liver could be formed in the hepatocyte during the biotransformation of halothane by liver drug-metabolizing enzymes. It is interesting that TFA proteins have also been identified in the sera of patients who did not develop hepatitis after halothane anesthesia.

B. NEPHROTOXICITY

Metabolism of methoxyflurane, enflurane, and sevoflurane leads to the formation of fluoride ions, and this has raised questions concerning the nephrotoxicity of these three volatile anesthetics. Changes in renal concentrating ability have been observed with prolonged exposure to both methoxyflurane and enflurane but not sevoflurane. Differences between the agents may be related to the fact that methoxyflurane and enflurane (but not sevoflurane) are metabolized in part by renal enzymes (eg, β-lyase), generating fluoride ions intrarenally. Sevoflurane degradation by carbon dioxide absorbents in anesthesia machines leads to formation of a haloalkene, compound A, which is metabolized by renal β-lyase to form thioacylhalide and causes a proximal tubular necrosis when administered to rats. However, there have been no reports of renal injury in humans receiving sevoflurane anesthesia. Moreover, the anesthetic does not appear to change standard markers of renal function. Renal dysfunction following methoxyflurane is caused by inorganic fluoride released during the extensive metabolism of this anesthetic by hepatic and renal enzymes. As a result, methoxyflurane, though still available, is no longer used in clinical practice.

C. MALIGNANT HYPERTHERMIA

Malignant hyperthermia is an autosomal dominant genetic disorder of skeletal muscle that occurs in susceptible individuals undergoing general anesthesia with volatile agents and muscle relaxants (eg, succinylcholine). The malignant hyperthermia syndrome consists of the rapid onset of tachycardia and hypertension, severe muscle rigidity, hyperthermia, hyperkalemia, and acid-base imbalance with acidosis that follows exposure to a triggering agent (see Table 16–4). Malignant hyperthermia is a rare but important cause of anesthetic morbidity and mortality. The specific biochemical abnormality is an increase in free calcium concentration in skeletal muscle cells. Treatment includes administration of dantrolene (to reduce calcium release from the sarcoplasmic reticulum) and appropriate measures to reduce body temperature and restore electrolyte and acid-base balance.

Malignant hyperthermia susceptibility is characterized by genetic heterogeneity, and several predisposing clinical myopathies have been identified. It has been associated with mutations in the gene loci corresponding to the skeletal muscle ryanodine receptor (RyRl), the calcium release channel on the sarcoplasmic reticulum. Mutations in the *RyR1* gene are inherited as mendelian dominant characteristics. Other chromosomal loci for malignant hyperthermia susceptibility include mutant alleles of the gene encoding the α_1 subunit of the human skeletal muscle dihydropyridine-sensitive L-type voltage-dependent calcium channel. However, the genetic loci identified to date account for no more than 50% of malignant hyperthermia-susceptible individuals. Given the degree of genetic heterogeneity, it is premature to use genetic testing methods for malignant hyperthermia susceptibility. Currently, the most reliable test to establish such susceptibility is the in vitro caffeine-halothane contracture test using skeletal muscle biopsy tissue.

D. CHRONIC TOXICITY

1. Mutagenicity—Under normal conditions, inhaled anesthetics (including nitrous oxide) are neither mutagens nor carcinogens in patients.

2. Carcinogenicity—Epidemiologic studies suggested an increase in the cancer rate in operating room personnel who were exposed to trace concentrations of anesthetic agents. However, no study has demonstrated the existence of a causal relationship between anesthetics and cancer. Many other factors might account for the questionably positive results seen after a careful review of epidemiologic data. Most operating rooms now use scavenging systems to remove trace concentrations of anesthetics released from anesthetic machines.

3. Effects on reproductive organs—The most consistent finding reported in surveys conducted to determine the reproductive success of female operating room personnel has been a questionably higher than expected incidence of miscarriages. However, there are several problems in interpreting these studies.

The association of obstetrical problems with surgery and anesthesia in pregnant patients is also an important consideration. In the USA, at least 50,000 pregnant women each year undergo anesthesia and surgery for indications unrelated to pregnancy. The risk of abortion is clearly higher following this experience. It is not obvious, however, whether the underlying disease, surgery, anesthesia, or a combination of these factors is the cause of the increased risk.

4. Hematotoxicity—Prolonged exposure to nitrous oxide decreases methionine synthase activity and theoretically can cause megaloblastic anemia, a potential occupational hazard for staff working in inadequately ventilated dental operating suites.

Clinical Use of Inhaled Anesthetics

Volatile anesthetics are rarely used as the sole agents for both induction and maintenance of anesthesia. Most commonly, they are combined with intravenous agents as part of a balanced anesthesia technique. Of the inhaled anesthetics, nitrous oxide, desflurane, sevoflurane, and isoflurane are the most commonly used in the USA. Use of less soluble volatile anesthetics (especially desflurane and sevoflurane) has increased during the last decade as more surgical procedures are performed on an ambulatory ("short-stay") basis. The low blood:gas coefficients of desflurane and sevoflurane afford a more rapid recovery and fewer postoperative adverse effects than halothane, enflurane, and isoflurane. Although halothane is still used in pediatric anesthesia, sevoflurane is rapidly replacing halothane in this setting. As indicated previously, nitrous oxide lacks sufficient potency to produce surgical anesthesia

by itself and therefore is used with volatile or intravenous anesthetics to produce a state of balanced general anesthesia. Despite the obvious advantages of the less soluble inhaled anesthetics, there is reason to believe that better ones might be developed (see Box: Do We Need Another Inhaled Anesthetic?).

■ INTRAVENOUS ANESTHETICS

In the last two decades there has been increasing use of intravenous anesthetics in anesthesia, both as adjuncts to inhaled anesthetics and as part of techniques that do not include any inhaled anesthetics (eg, total intravenous anesthesia). The properties of some of the commonly used intravenous anesthetics are summarized in Table 25–1. Unlike inhaled anesthetics, intravenous agents do not require specialized vaporizer equipment for their delivery or facilities for the disposal of exhaled gases. Intravenous drugs such as thiopental, methohexital, etomidate, ketamine, and propofol have an onset of anesthetic action faster than the most rapid inhaled agents (eg, desflurane and sevoflurane). Therefore, intravenous agents are commonly used for induction of general anesthesia.

Recovery is sufficiently rapid with most intravenous drugs to permit their use for short ambulatory (outpatient) surgical procedures. In the case of propofol, recovery times are similar to those seen with sevoflurane and desflurane. The anesthetic potency of intravenous anesthetics is adequate to permit their use as the sole anesthetic in short surgical procedures when combined with nitrous oxide. Adjunctive use of potent opioids (eg, fentanyl and sufentanil; see Chapter 31) contributes cardiovascular stability, enhanced sedation, and profound perioperative analgesia. Benzodiazepines (eg, midazolam, diazepam) have a slower onset and slower recovery than the barbiturates or propofol and are rarely used for induction of anesthesia. However, preanesthetic administration of benzodiazepines (eg, midazolam) can be used to provide anxiolysis, sedation, and amnesia when used in conjunction with other anesthetic agents.

BARBITURATES

The general pharmacology of the barbiturates is discussed in Chapter 22. Thiopental is a barbiturate commonly used for induction of anesthesia. Thiamylal is structurally almost identical to thiopental and has the same pharmacokinetic and pharmacodynamic profile.

After an intravenous bolus injection, thiopental rapidly crosses the blood-brain barrier and, if given in suf-

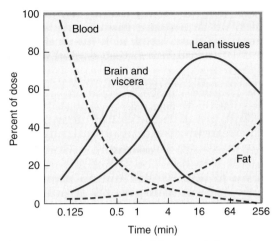

Figure 25–6. Redistribution of thiopental after an intravenous bolus administration. Note that the time axis is not linear.

ficient dosage, produces loss of consciousness (hypnosis) in one circulation time. Similar effects occur with the shorter-acting barbiturate, methohexital. With both of these barbiturates, plasma:brain equilibrium occurs rapidly (< 1 minute) because of their high lipid solubility. Thiopental rapidly diffuses out of the brain and other highly vascular tissues and is redistributed to muscle and fat (Figure 25–6). Because of this rapid removal from brain tissue, a single dose of thiopental produces only a brief period of unconsciousness. Thiopental is metabolized at the rate of only 12–16% per hour in humans following a single dose and less than 1% of the administered dose of thiopental is excreted unchanged by the kidney.

With large doses (or a continuous infusion), thiopental produces dose-dependent decreases in arterial blood pressure, stroke volume, and cardiac output. These hemodynamic effects are due primarily to a myocardial depressant effect and increased venous capacitance; there is little change in total peripheral resistance. Thiopental is also a potent respiratory depressant, producing transient apnea and lowering the sensitivity of the medullary respiratory center to carbon dioxide.

Cerebral metabolism and oxygen utilization are decreased after barbiturate administration in proportion to the degree of cerebral depression. Cerebral blood flow is also decreased, but less than oxygen consumption. Because intracranial pressure and blood volume are not increased (in contrast to the volatile anesthetics), thiopental is a desirable drug for patients with cerebral swelling (eg, head trauma, brain tumors). Methohexital can cause central excitatory activity (eg, myoclonus)

and has been useful for neurosurgical procedures involving ablation of seizure foci. However, it also has antiseizure activity and is the drug of choice for providing anesthesia in patients undergoing electroconvulsive therapy (ECT). Given its more rapid elimination, methohexital is also preferred over thiopental for short ambulatory procedures.

Barbiturates reduce hepatic blood flow and glomerular filtration rate, but these drugs produce no adverse effects on hepatic or renal function. Barbiturates can exacerbate acute intermittent porphyria by inducing the production of hepatic α-aminolevulinic acid (ALA) synthase (see Chapter 22). On rare occasions, thiopental has precipitated porphyric crisis when used as an induction agent in susceptible patients.

BENZODIAZEPINES

Diazepam, lorazepam, and midazolam are used in anesthetic procedures. The primary indication is for premedication because of their sedative, anxiolytic, and amnestic properties, and to control acute agitation. (The basic pharmacology of benzodiazepines is discussed in Chapter 22.) Diazepam and lorazepam are not water-soluble, and their intravenous use necessitates nonaqueous vehicles, which cause pain and local irritation. Midazolam is water-soluble and is the benzodiazepine of choice for parenteral administration. It is important that the drug becomes lipid-soluble at physiologic pH and can readily cross the blood-brain barrier to produce its central effects.

Compared with the intravenous barbiturates, benzodiazepines produce a slower onset of central nervous system depressant effects which reach a plateau at a depth of sedation that is inadequate for surgical anesthesia. Using large doses of benzodiazepines to achieve deep sedation prolongs the postanesthetic recovery period and can produce a high incidence of anterograde amnesia. Because it possesses sedative-anxiolytic properties and causes a high incidence of amnesia (> 50%), midazolam is frequently administered intravenously before patients enter the operating room. Midazolam has a more rapid onset, a shorter elimination half-life (2–4 hours), and a steeper dose-response curve than do the other available benzodiazepines.

The benzodiazepine antagonist flumazenil can be used to accelerate recovery when excessive doses of intravenous benzodiazepines are administered (especially in elderly patients). However, reversal of benzodiazepine-induced respiratory depression is less predictable. The short duration of action (< 90 minutes) of flumazenil may necessitate multiple doses to prevent recurrence of the central nervous system depressant effects of the longer-acting benzodiazepines (eg, lorazepam, diazepam).

CONSCIOUS & DEEP SEDATION

Many diagnostic and minor therapeutic surgical procedures can be performed without general anesthesia. In this setting, regional or local anesthesia supplemented with midazolam or propofol and opioid analgesics (or ketamine) may be a more appropriate and safer approach than general anesthesia.

Another approach has led to the development of **conscious sedation** or drug-induced alleviation of anxiety and pain in combination with an altered level of consciousness associated with minimal sedation and retention of the ability of the patient to maintain a patent airway and to respond to verbal commands. A wide variety of intravenous anesthetic agents have proved to be useful drugs in conscious sedation techniques (eg, diazepam, midazolam, propofol). For example, intravenous midazolam, propofol, and a potent opioid analgesic can provide amnestic, sedative, and analgesic effects without loss of consciousness as part of a monitored anesthesia care (MAC) technique. Use of benzodiazepines and opioid analgesics in conscious sedation protocols has the advantage of being reversible by the specific

receptor antagonist drugs (flumazenil and naloxone, respectively).

A specialized form of conscious sedation is occasionally required in the ICU, when patients are under severe stress and require mechanical ventilation for prolonged periods. In this situation, sedative-hypnotic drugs or low doses of intravenous anesthetics, neuromuscular blocking drugs, and dexmedetomidine may be combined. Dexmedetomidine is an α_2 agonist with sedative and analgesic effects. It has a half-life of 2–3 hours and is metabolized in the liver and excreted mainly as inactive urinary metabolites.

Deep sedation is similar to a light state of general anesthesia involving decreased consciousness from which the patient is not easily aroused. Because deep sedation is often accompanied by a loss of protective reflexes, an inability to maintain a patent airway, and lack of verbal responsiveness to surgical stimuli, this state may be indistinguishable from general anesthesia. Intravenous agents used in deep sedation protocols include thiopental, methohexital, ketamine, propofol, and the potent opioid analgesics.

OPIOID ANALGESICS

Large doses of opioid analgesics have been used in combination with large doses of benzodiazepines to achieve a general anesthetic state, particularly in patients undergoing cardiac surgery or other major surgery when the patient's circulatory reserve is limited. Although intravenous morphine, 1–3 mg/kg, was used many years ago, the high-potency opioids fentanyl, 100–150 mcg/kg, and sufentanil, 0.25–0.5 mcg/kg IV, have been used more recently in such patients. More recently also, remifentanil, a potent and extremely short-acting opioid, has been used to minimize residual ventilatory depression.

Despite the use of high doses of potent opioids (see Table 31–2), awareness during anesthesia and unpleasant postoperative recall can occur. Furthermore, high doses of opioids during surgery can cause chest wall (and laryngeal) rigidity, thereby acutely impairing ventilation, as well as increasing postoperative opioid requirements owing to the development of acute tolerance. Therefore, lower doses of fentanyl and sufentanil have been used as premedication and as an adjunct to both intravenous and inhaled anesthetics to provide perioperative analgesia. The shorter-acting alfentanil and remifentanil have been used as co-induction agents with intravenous sedative-hypnotic anesthetics because they have a rapid onset of action. Remifentanil is rapidly metabolized by esterases in the blood (not plasma cholinesterase) and muscle tissues, contributing to an extremely rapid recovery from its opioid

effects. The metabolism of remifentanil is not subject to genetic variability, and the drug does not interfere with the clearance of other compounds metabolized by plasma cholinesterase (eg, esmolol, mivacurium, or succinylcholine). Opioid analgesics can also be administered in very low doses by the epidural and subarachnoid (spinal) routes of administration to produce excellent postoperative analgesia. Fentanyl and droperidol (a butyrophenone related to haloperidol) administered together produce analgesia and amnesia and combined with nitrous oxide provide a state referred to as **neuroleptanesthesia.**

PROPOFOL

Propofol (2,6-diisopropylphenol) has become the most popular intravenous anesthetic. Its rate of onset of action is similar to that of the intravenous barbiturates but recovery is more rapid and patients are able to ambulate earlier after general anesthesia. Furthermore, patients subjectively "feel better" in the immediate postoperative period because of the reduction in postoperative nausea and vomiting. Propofol is used for both induction and maintenance of anesthesia as part of total intravenous or balanced anesthesia techniques and is the agent of choice for ambulatory surgery. The drug is also effective in producing prolonged sedation in patients in critical care settings (see Box: Conscious & Deep Sedation). When administered by prolonged infusion for sedation or ventilatory management in the intensive care unit, cumulative effects can lead to delayed arousal. In addition, prolonged administration of conventional emulsion formulations can elevate serum lipid levels. Use of propofol for the sedation of critically ill young children has led to severe acidosis in the presence of respiratory infections and to possible neurologic sequelae upon withdrawal.

After intravenous administration of propofol, the distribution half-life is 2–8 minutes, and the redistribution half-life is approximately 30–60 minutes. The drug is rapidly metabolized in the liver at a rate ten times faster than thiopental. Propofol is excreted in the urine as glucuronide and sulfate conjugates, with less than 1% of the parent drug excreted unchanged. Total body clearance of the anesthetic is greater than hepatic blood flow, suggesting that its elimination includes extrahepatic mechanisms in addition to metabolism by liver enzymes. This property can be useful in patients with impaired ability to metabolize other sedative-anesthetic drugs.

Effects on respiratory function are similar to those of thiopental at usual anesthetic doses and include dose-related depression of central ventilatory drive and apnea. However, propofol causes a marked decrease in blood pressure during induction of anesthesia through decreased peripheral arterial resistance and venodilation. In addition, propofol has greater direct negative inotropic effects than other intravenous anesthetics. Pain at the site of injection is the most common adverse effect of bolus administration. Muscle movements, hypotonus, and (rarely) tremors have also been reported after prolonged use. Clinical infections due to bacterial contamination of the propofol emulsion have led to the addition of antimicrobial adjuvants (eg, ethylenediaminetetraacetic acid [EDTA] and metabisulfite). Newer formulations of propofol have been developed that contain less lipid for prolonged administration (eg, Ampofol). However, pain on injection is increased when the lipid content is reduced. Admixture or pretreatment with lidocaine (20–50 mg) is the most effective approach to minimizing the pain on injection of propofol.

ETOMIDATE

Etomidate is a carboxylated imidazole that can be used for induction of anesthesia in patients with limited cardiovascular reserve. Its major advantage over other intravenous anesthetics is that it causes minimal cardiovascular and respiratory depression. Etomidate produces a rapid loss of consciousness, with minimal hypotension even in elderly patients with poor cardiovascular reserve. The heart rate is usually unchanged, and the incidence of apnea is low. The drug has no analgesic effects, and coadministration of opioids may be required to decrease cardiac responses during tracheal intubation and to lessen spontaneous muscle movements. Following an induction dose, initial recovery with etomidate is less rapid (< 10 minutes) compared with recovery with propofol.

Distribution of etomidate is rapid, with a biphasic plasma concentration curve showing initial and intermediate distribution half-lives of 3 and 29 minutes, respectively. Redistribution of the drug from brain to highly perfused tissues appears to be responsible for the relatively short duration of its anesthetic effects. Etomidate is extensively metabolized in the liver and plasma to inactive metabolites, with only 2% of the drug excreted unchanged in the urine.

Etomidate causes a high incidence of pain on injection, myoclonic activity, and postoperative nausea and vomiting. The involuntary muscle movements are not associated with electroencephalographic epileptiform activity. Etomidate may also cause adrenocortical suppression via inhibitory effects on steroidogenesis, with decreased plasma levels of cortisol after a single dose. Prolonged infusion of etomidate in critically ill patients may result in hypotension, electrolyte imbalance, and oliguria because of its adrenal suppressive effects.

KETAMINE

Ketamine is a racemic mixture of two optical isomers, $S(+)$ and $R(-)$ ketamine. The drug produces a **dissociative anesthetic state** characterized by catatonia, amnesia, and analgesia, with or without loss of consciousness (hypnosis). The drug is an arylcyclohexylamine chemically related to phencyclidine (PCP), a drug with a high abuse potential owing to its psychoactive properties. The mechanism of action of ketamine may involve blockade of the membrane effects of the excitatory neurotransmitter glutamic acid at the **NMDA receptor** subtype (see Chapter 21). Ketamine is a highly lipophilic drug and is rapidly distributed into well-perfused organs, including the brain, liver, and kidney. Subsequently ketamine is redistributed to less well perfused tissues with concurrent hepatic metabolism followed by both urinary and biliary excretion.

Ketamine is the only intravenous anesthetic that possesses both analgesic properties and the ability to produce dose-related cardiovascular stimulation. Heart rate, arterial blood pressure, and cardiac output can be significantly increased above baseline values. These variables reach a peak 2–4 minutes after an intravenous bolus injection, then slowly decline to normal values over the next 10–20 minutes. Ketamine produces its cardiovascular effects by stimulating the central sympathetic nervous system and, to a lesser extent, by inhibiting the reuptake of norepinephrine at sympathetic nerve terminals. Increases in plasma epinephrine and norepinephrine levels occur as early as 2 minutes after an intravenous bolus of ketamine and return to baseline levels in less than 15 minutes.

Ketamine markedly increases cerebral blood flow, oxygen consumption, and intracranial pressure. Similar to the volatile anesthetics, ketamine is a potentially dangerous drug when intracranial pressure is elevated. Although ketamine decreases the respiratory rate, upper airway muscle tone is well maintained and airway reflexes are usually preserved.

Use of ketamine has been associated with postoperative disorientation, sensory and perceptual illusions, and vivid dreams (so-called emergence phenomena). Diazepam, 0.2–0.3 mg/kg, or midazolam, 0.025–0.05 mg intravenously, given before the administration of ketamine reduce the incidence of these adverse effects. Because of the high incidence of postoperative psychic phenomena associated with its use, ketamine fell into disfavor. However, use of low doses of ketamine in combi- nation with other intravenous and inhaled anesthetics has become an increasingly popular alternative to opioid analgesics to minimize ventilatory depression. In addition, ketamine is very useful for poor-risk geriatric patients and high-risk patients in cardiogenic or septic shock because of its cardiostimulatory properties. It is also used in low doses for outpatient anesthesia in combination with propofol and in children undergoing painful procedures (eg, dressing changes for burns). In an effort to enhance ketamine's efficacy and reduce its side-effect profile, investigators separated the isomers and demonstrated that the $S(+)$ ketamine possessed greater anesthetic and analgesic potency. However, even the $S(+)$ isomer of ketamine possesses psychotomimetic side effects.

PREPARATIONS AVAILABLE*

Desflurane (Suprane)
   Liquid: 240 mL for inhalation
Dexmedetomidine (Precedex)
   Parenteral: 100 mcg/mL for IV infusion
Diazepam (generic, Valium)
   Oral: 2, 5, 10 mg tablets; 1 mg/mL and 5 mg/ mL solution
   Oral sustained-release: 15 mg capsules
   Rectal: 2.5, 5, 15, 19, 20 mg gel
   Parenteral: 5 mg/mL for injection
Droperidol (generic, Inapsine)
   Parenteral: 2.5 mg/mL for IV or IM injection
Enflurane (Enflurane, Ethrane)
   Liquid: 125, 250 mL for inhalation
Etomidate (Amidate)
   Parenteral: 2 mg/mL for injection
Halothane (generic, Fluothane)
   Liquid: 125, 250 mL for inhalation

Isoflurane (Isoflurane, Forane)
   Liquid: 100 mL for inhalation
Ketamine (generic, Ketalar)
   Parenteral: 10, 50, 100 mg/mL for injection
Lorazepam (generic, Ativan)
   Parenteral: 2, 4 mg/mL for injection
Methohexital (Brevital)
   Parenteral: 0.5, 2.5, 5 g powder to reconstitute for injection
Methoxyflurane (Penthrane)
   Liquid: 15, 125 mL for inhalation
Midazolam (generic, Versed)
   Parenteral: 1, 5 mg/mL for injection in 1, 2, 5, 10 mL vials
   Oral: 2 mg/mL syrup for children
Nitrous oxide (gas, supplied in blue cylinders)
Propofol (generic, Diprivan)
   Parenteral: 10 mg/mL for IV injection
Sevoflurane (Ultane)
   Liquid: 250 mL for inhalation
Thiopental (generic, Pentothal)
   Parenteral: powder to reconstitute 20, 25 mg/ mL for IV injection

---

*See Chapter 31 for formulations of opioid agents used in anesthesia.

REFERENCES

Angelini G, Ketzler JT, Coursin DB: Use of propofol and other nonbenzodiazepine sedatives in the intensive care unit. Crit Care Clin 2001;17:863.

Banoub M, Tetzlaff JE, Schubert A: Pharmacologic and physiologic influences affecting sensory evoked potentials: Implications for perioperative monitoring. Anesthesiology 2003;99:716.

Campagna JA, Miller KW, Forman SA: Mechanisms of actions of inhaled anesthetics. N Engl J Med 2003;348:2110.

Delgado-Herrera L, Ostroff RD, Rogers SA: Sevoflurane: approaching the ideal inhalational anesthetic. A pharmacologic, pharmacoeconomic, and clinical review. CNS Drug Rev 2001;7:48.

Dickinson R: Selective synaptic actions of thiopental and its enantiomers. Anesthesiology 2002;96:884.

Dilger JP: The effects of general anaesthetics on ligand-gated ion channels. Br J Anaesth 2002;89:41.

Ding Z, White PF: Anesthesia for electroconvulsive therapy. Anesth Analg 2002;94:1351.

Eger EI II et al: Clinical and economic factors important to anaesthetic choice for day-case surgery. Pharmacoeconomics 2000; 17:245.

Eger EI II, Saidman LJ, Brandstater B: Minimum alveolar anesthetic concentration: A standard of anesthetic potency. Anesthesiology 1965;26:756.

Eger EI II: Uptake and distribution. In: Miller RD (editor): *Anesthesia*, 4th ed. Churchill Livingstone, 1994.

Gupta A et al: Comparison of recovery profile after ambulatory anesthesia with propofol, isoflurane, sevoflurane and desflurane: A systematic review. Anesth Analg 2004;98:632.

Hemmings HC et al: Emerging molecular mechanisms of general anesthetic action. Trends Pharmacol Sci 2005;26:503.

Jurd R et al: General anesthetic actions in vivo strongly attenuated by a point mutation in the GABA$_A$ receptor beta$_3$ subunit. FASEB J 2003;17:250.

Kang TM: Propofol infusion syndrome in critically ill patients. Ann Pharmacother 2002;36:1453.

Kharasch ED et al: Compound A uptake and metabolism to mercapturic acids and 3,3,3-trifluoro-2-fluoromethoxypropanoic acid during low-flow sevoflurane anesthesia: Biomarkers for exposure, risk assessment, and interspecies comparison. Anesthesiology 1999;91:1267.

Krasowski MD, Harrison NL: General anaesthetic actions on ligand-gated ion channels. Cell Mol Life Sci 1999;55:1278.

Monk TG et al: Anesthetic management and one-year mortality after noncardiac surgery. Anesth Analg 2005;100:4.

Nelson LE et al: The sedative component of anesthesia is mediated by GABA$_A$ receptors in an endogenous sleep pathway. Nat Neurosci 2002;5:979.

Nishikawa K et al: Volatile anesthetic actions on the GABA$_A$ receptors: Contrasting effects of alpha 1(S270) and beta 2(N265) point mutations. Neuropharmacology 2002;42:337.

Park KW: Cardiovascular effects of inhalational anesthetics. Int Anesthesiol Clin 2002;40:1.

Patel S: Cardiovascular effects of intravenous anesthetics. Int Anesthesiol Clin 2002;40:15.

Siegwart R, Jurd R, Rudolph U: Molecular determinants for the action of general anesthetics at recombinant alpha(2)beta(3)gamma(2)gamma-aminobutyric acid(A) receptors. J Neurochem 2002;80:140.

Topf N et al: Effects of isoflurane on gamma-aminobutyric acid type A receptors activated by full and partial agonists. Anesthesiology 2003;98:306.

Trapani G et al: Propofol in anesthesia. Mechanism of action, structure-activity relationships, and drug delivery. Curr Med Chem 2000;7:249.

White PF et al: Does the use of electroencephalographic bispectral index or auditory evoked potential index monitoring facilitate recovery after desflurane anesthesia in the ambulatory setting? Anesthesiology 2004;100: 811.

White PF, Way WL, Trevor AJ: Ketamine—its pharmacology and therapeutic uses. Anesthesiology 1982;56:119.

White PF (editor): *Textbook of Intravenous Anesthesia*. Williams & Wilkins, 1997.

Local Anesthetics

26

Paul F. White, PhD, MD, & Bertram G. Katzung, MD, PhD

Local anesthetics reversibly block impulse conduction along nerve axons and other excitable membranes that utilize sodium channels as the primary means of action potential generation. Clinically, local anesthetics are used to block pain sensation from—or sympathetic vasoconstrictor impulses to—specific areas of the body. The first local anesthetic introduced into medical practice, cocaine, was isolated by Niemann in 1860 and introduced into practice by Koller in 1884 as an ophthalmic anesthetic. Despite the fact that its chronic use was associated with psychological dependence (addiction), cocaine was used clinically because it was the only local anesthetic drug available for 30 years. In an attempt to improve upon the clinical properties of cocaine, Einhorn in 1905 synthesized procaine, which became the dominant local anesthetic for the next 50 years. Subsequently, newer local anesthetics were introduced with the goal of reducing local tissue irritation, minimizing systemic cardiac and central nervous system (CNS) toxicity, and achieving a faster onset and longer duration of action. Lidocaine, which is still the most widely used local anesthetic, was synthesized in 1943 by Löfgren.

The development of newer agents continues because it is relatively easy to synthesize chemicals with local anesthetic properties. Unfortunately, it is difficult to reduce the toxicity of these compounds because the common side effects of local anesthetics represent extensions of their therapeutic effects. New research into the mechanisms of local anesthetic-induced cardiac and spinal toxicity and identification of alternative drug targets for spinal analgesia (eg, opioid receptors, α_2 adrenoceptors, NMDA receptors, N-type calcium channels, and adenosine receptors) suggest that it may be possible to develop safer drugs in the future. To extend the duration of the local anesthetic action, a variety of novel delivery systems are in development (eg, polymers, suspensions). Transdermal local anesthetic delivery systems have also been successfully introduced into clinical practice for providing topical analgesia.

■ I. BASIC PHARMACOLOGY OF LOCAL ANESTHETICS

Chemistry

Most local anesthetic agents consist of a lipophilic group (eg, an aromatic ring) connected by an intermediate chain via an ester or amide to an ionizable group (eg, a tertiary amine) (Figure 26–1; Table 26–1). In addition to the general physical properties of the molecules, specific stereochemical configurations are associated with differences in the potency of stereoisomers (eg, bupivacaine, ropivacaine). Because ester links are more prone to hydrolysis than amide links, esters usually have a shorter duration of action.

Local anesthetics are weak bases and are usually made available clinically as salts to increase solubility and stability. In the body, they exist either as the uncharged base or as a cation. The relative proportions of these two forms is governed by their pK_a and the pH of the body fluids according to the Henderson-Hasselbalch equation:

$$\log \frac{\text{Cationic form}}{\text{Uncharged form}} = pK_a - pH$$

Because the pK_a of most local anesthetics is in the range of 8.0–9.0, the larger percentage in body fluids at physiologic pH will be the charged, cationic form. The cationic form is the most active form at the receptor site because it cannot readily exit from closed channels. However, the uncharged form is important for rapid penetration of biologic membranes and producing a clinical effect, since the local anesthetic receptor is not readily accessible from the external side of the cell membrane. Therefore, local anesthetics are much less effective when they are injected into infected tissues because a smaller percentage of the local anesthetic is nonionized and available for diffusion across the membrane in an environment with a low extracellular pH.

Figure 26-1. Structures of two prototypical local anesthetics, the aminoester procaine and the aminoamide lidocaine. In both drugs, a lipophilic aromatic group is joined to a more hydrophilic tertiary amine base, by an intermediate amide or ester bond.

Pharmacokinetics

The pharmacokinetic properties of the commonly used amide local anesthetics are summarized in Table 26–2. The pharmacokinetics of the ester-based local anesthetics have not been extensively studied owing to their rapid breakdown in plasma (elimination half-life < 1 minute). Local anesthetics are usually administered by injection into dermis and soft tissues located in the area of nerves. Thus, absorption and distribution are not as important in controlling the onset of effect as in determining the rate of offset of local analgesia, and the likelihood of CNS and cardiac toxicity. Topical application of local anesthetics (eg, transmucosal or transdermal) requires drug diffusion for both onset and offset of anesthetic effect.

A. ABSORPTION

Systemic absorption of injected local anesthetic from the site of administration is determined by several factors, including dosage, site of injection, drug-tissue binding, local blood flow, use of vasoconstrictors (eg, epinephrine), and the physicochemical properties of the drug itself. Application of a local anesthetic to a highly vascular area such as the tracheal mucosa or the tissue surrounding intercostal nerves results in more rapid absorption and thus higher blood levels than if the local anesthetic had been injected into a poorly perfused tissue such as tendon, dermis, or subcutaneous fat. For regional anesthesia involving block of large nerves, maximum blood levels of local anesthetic decrease according to the site of administration in the following order: intercostal (highest) > caudal > epidural > brachial plexus > sciatic nerve (lowest).

Vasoconstrictor substances such as epinephrine reduce systemic absorption of local anesthetics from the injection site by decreasing blood flow in these areas. This is important for drugs with intermediate or short durations of action such as procaine, lidocaine, and mepivacaine (but not prilocaine).

Since blood levels are lowered up to 30% when vasoconstrictors are added to local anesthetics, localized neuronal uptake is enhanced because of higher local tissue concentrations in the region of drug administration, and the systemic toxic effects are reduced. Furthermore, when used in spinal anesthesia, epinephrine acts directly on the cord to both enhance and prolong local anesthetic-induced spinal anesthesia by acting on α_2 adrenoceptors, which inhibit release of substance P (neurokinin-1) and reduce sensory neuron firing. The recognition of this fact has led to the use of clonidine and dexmedetomidine to augment local anesthetic effect in the subarachnoid space and on peripheral nerves. The combination of reduced systemic absorption, enhanced local neuronal anesthetic uptake, and α_2 activation by epinephrine in the CNS is responsible for prolonging the local anesthetic effect by up to 50%. Vasoconstrictors are less effective in prolonging anesthetic action of the more lipid-soluble, long-acting drugs (eg, bupivacaine and ropivacaine), possibly

Table 26-1. Structure and properties of some ester and amide local anesthetics.[1]

	Lipophilic Group	Intermediate Chain	Amine Substituents	Potency (Procaine = 1)	Duration of Action
Esters					
Cocaine				2	Medium
Procaine (Novocain)				1	Short
Tetracaine (Pontocaine)				16	Long
Benzocaine				Surface use only	
Amides					
Lidocaine (Xylocaine)				4	Medium
Mepivacaine (Carbocaine, Isocaine)				2	Medium
Bupivicaine (Marcaine), levobupivacaine (Chirocaine)				16	Long
Prilocaine (Citanest)				3	Medium
Ropivacaine (Naropin)				16	Long

[1]Other chemical types are available including ethers (pramoxine), ketones (dyclonine), and phenetidin derivatives (phenacaine).

Table 26–2. Pharmacokinetic properties of several amide local anesthetics.

Agent	Half-Time of Distribution (min)	$t_{1/2}$ Elimination (h)	V_{dss} (L)	CL (L/min)
Bupivacaine	28	3.5	72	0.47
Lidocaine	10	1.6	91	0.95
Mepivacaine	7	1.9	84	0.78
Prilocaine	5	1.5	261	2.84
Ropivacaine	23	4.2	47	0.44

CL, clearance; V_{dss}, volume of distribution at steady state.

because these molecules are highly tissue-bound. Finally, cocaine is unique owing to its intrinsic sympathomimetic properties.

B. DISTRIBUTION

The amide local anesthetics are widely distributed after intravenous bolus administration. There is also evidence that sequestration can occur in lipophilic storage sites (eg, fat). After an initial rapid distribution phase, which consists of uptake into highly perfused organs such as the brain, liver, kidney, and heart, a slower distribution phase occurs with uptake into moderately well-perfused tissues, such as muscle and the gastrointestinal tract. As a result of the extremely short plasma half-lives of the ester type agents, their tissue distribution has not been extensively studied.

C. METABOLISM AND EXCRETION

The local anesthetics are converted in the liver (amide type) or in plasma (ester type) to more water-soluble metabolites and then excreted in the urine. Since local anesthetics in the uncharged form diffuse readily through lipid membranes, little or no urinary excretion of the neutral form occurs. Acidification of urine promotes ionization of the tertiary amine base to the more water-soluble charged form, which is more readily excreted.

Ester-type local anesthetics are hydrolyzed very rapidly in the blood by circulating butyrylcholinesterase (pseudocholinesterase) to inactive metabolites. Therefore, procaine and chloroprocaine have very short plasma half-lives (< 1 minute).

The amide linkage of amide local anesthetics is hydrolyzed by liver microsomal cytochrome P450 isozymes. There is considerable variation in the rate of liver metabolism of individual amide compounds, the approximate order being prilocaine (fastest) > lidocaine > mepivacaine > ropivacaine > bupivacaine and levobupivacaine (slowest). As a result, toxicity from amide-type

local anesthetics is more likely to occur in patients with hepatic disease. For example, the average elimination half-life of lidocaine may be increased from 1.6 hours in normal patients ($t_{1/2}$, Table 26–2) to more than 6 hours in patients with severe liver disease. Many other drugs used in anesthesia are metabolized by the same P450 isozymes, and concomitant use of these competing drugs may slow the hepatic metabolism of the local anesthetics.

Decreased hepatic elimination of local anesthetics would also be anticipated in patients with reduced hepatic blood flow. For example, the hepatic elimination of lidocaine in patients anesthetized with volatile anesthetics (which reduce liver blood flow) is slower than in patients anesthetized with intravenous anesthetics.

Pharmacodynamics

A. MECHANISM OF ACTION

The primary mechanism of action of local anesthetics is **blockade of voltage-gated sodium channels** (Figure 26–2). The excitable membrane of nerve axons, like the membrane of cardiac muscle (see Chapter 14) and neuronal cell bodies (see Chapter 21), maintains a resting transmembrane potential of –90 to –60 mV. During excitation, the sodium channels open, and a fast inward sodium current quickly depolarizes the membrane toward the sodium equilibrium potential (+40 mV). As a result of depolarization, the sodium channels close (inactivate) and potassium channels open. The outward flow of potassium repolarizes the membrane toward the potassium equilibrium potential (about –95 mV); repolarization returns the sodium channels to the rested state. The transmembrane ionic gradients are maintained by the sodium pump. These ionic fluxes are similar to those in heart muscle, and local anesthetics have similar effects in both tissues.

The function of sodium channels can be disrupted in several ways. Biologic toxins such as **batrachotoxin,**

Figure 26-2. Functional and structural features of the Na⁺ channel that determine local anesthetic (LA) interactions. **A:** Cartoon of the sodium channel in an axonal membrane in the resting (h gate open), activated (h gate open), and inactivated states (h gate closed). Recovery from the inactivated, refractory state requires opening of the h gate. Local anesthetics bind to a receptor (R) within the channel and access it via the membrane phase or from the cytoplasm. **B:** Molecular arrangement of the 6 membrane-spanning peptides, four of which combine to form the channel around a central pore. The S4 segments (marked with "+" signs) are thought to constitute the voltage-sensing "m" gates of the channel. The linker peptide connecting the III and IV hexamers acts as the inactivation "h" gate. Ions travel through an open channel along a pore defined at its narrowest dimension by partial membrane penetration of the four extracellular loops of protein connecting S5 and S6 in each domain. Local anesthetic binding occurs on S6 segments and at other regions of the channel. **C:** Three-dimensional cartoon showing the configuration of the four hexamers around the central pore in the membrane.

aconitine, veratridine, and some **scorpion venoms** bind to receptors within the channel and prevent inactivation. This results in prolonged influx of sodium through the channel and depolarization of the resting potential. The marine toxins **tetrodotoxin (TTX)** and **saxitoxin** block sodium channels by binding to channel receptors near the extracellular surface. Their clinical effects superficially resemble those of local anesthetics (ie, block of conduction without a change in the resting potential) even though their receptor site is quite different. Spinal neurons can be differentiated on the basis of tetrodotoxin effect into TTX-sensitive and TTX-resistant neurons. Some evidence suggests that the TTX-resistant neurons are responsible for pain transmission and are the primary targets for local anesthetics in producing spinal anesthesia. Local anesthetics bind to receptors near the intracellular end of the sodium channel and block the channel in a time- and voltage-dependent fashion (see below). The sodium channel has been cloned, its primary structure has been characterized, and mutational analysis has allowed identification of parts of the local anesthetic binding site.

When progressively increasing concentrations of a local anesthetic are applied to a nerve fiber, the threshold for excitation increases, impulse conduction slows, the rate of rise of the action potential declines, the action potential amplitude decreases, and, finally, the ability to generate an action potential is completely abolished. These progressive effects result from binding of the local anesthetic to more and more sodium channels. If the sodium current is blocked over a critical length of the nerve, propagation across the blocked area is no longer possible. In myelinated nerves, the critical length is 2 to 3 nodes of Ranvier. At the minimum dose required to block propagation, the resting potential is not significantly altered.

The blockade of sodium channels by most local anesthetics is both *voltage-* and *time-dependent:* Channels in the rested state, which predominate at more negative membrane potentials, have a much lower affinity for local anesthetics than activated (open state) and inactivated channels, which predominate at more positive membrane potentials (see Figure 14–8). Thus, the effect of a given drug concentration is more marked in rapidly firing axons than in resting fibers (Figure 26–3).

Between successive action potentials, a portion of the sodium channels will recover from the local anesthetic block (see Figure 14–8). The recovery from drug-induced block is 10 to 1000 times slower than the recovery of channels from normal inactivation (as shown for the cardiac membrane in Figure 14–4). As a result, the refractory period is lengthened and the nerve conducts fewer impulses.

Elevated extracellular calcium partially antagonizes the action of local anesthetics owing to the calcium-

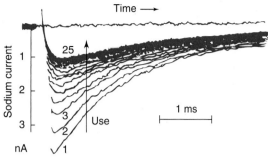

Figure 26–3. Effect of repetitive activity on the block of sodium current produced by a local anesthetic in a myelinated axon. A series of 25 pulses was applied, and the resulting sodium currents (downward deflections) are superimposed. Note that the current produced by the pulses rapidly decreased from the first to the 25th pulse. A long rest period following the train resulted in recovery from block, but the block could be reinstated by a subsequent train. (nA, nanoamperes.) (Modified and reproduced, with permission, from Courtney KR: Mechanism of frequency-dependent inhibition of sodium currents in frog myelinated nerve by the lidocaine derivative GEA. J Pharmacol Exp Ther 1975;195:225.)

induced increase in the surface potential on the membrane (which favors the low-affinity rested state). Conversely, increases in extracellular potassium depolarize the membrane potential and favor the inactivated state, enhancing the effect of local anesthetics.

Local anesthetics can be shown to block a variety of other ion channels, including nicotinic acetylcholine channels in the spinal cord. However, there is no convincing evidence that this mechanism is important in the clinical effects of these drugs. High concentrations of local anesthetics can interfere with intra-axonal transport and calcium homeostasis in the nerve terminal, contributing to potential spinal toxicity.

B. STRUCTURE-ACTIVITY CHARACTERISTICS OF LOCAL ANESTHETICS

The smaller and more lipophilic the local anesthetic, the faster the rate of interaction with the sodium channel receptor. Potency is also positively correlated with lipid solubility as long as the agent retains sufficient water solubility to diffuse to the site of action on the neuronal membrane. Lidocaine, procaine, and mepivacaine are more water-soluble than tetracaine, bupivacaine, and ropivacaine. The latter agents are more potent and have longer durations of local anesthetic action. These long-acting local anesthetics also bind more extensively to proteins and can be displaced from

Table 26–3. Relative size and susceptibility of different types of nerve fibers to local anesthetics.

Fiber Type	Function	Diameter (μm)	Myelination	Conduction Velocity (m/s)	Sensitivity to Block
Type A					
Alpha	Proprioception, motor	12–20	Heavy	70–120	+
Beta	Touch, pressure	5–12	Heavy	30–70	++
Gamma	Muscle spindles	3–6	Heavy	15–30	++
Delta	Pain, temperature	2–5	Heavy	12–30	+++
Type B	Preganglionic autonomic	< 3	Light	3–15	++++
Type C					
Dorsal root	Pain	0.4–1.2	None	0.5–2.3	++++
Sympathetic	Postganglionic	0.3–1.3	None	0.7–2.3	++++

these binding sites by other protein-bound drugs. In the case of optically active agents (eg, bupivacaine), the $S(+)$isomer can usually be shown to be moderately more potent than the $R(-)$ isomer.

C. OTHER ACTIONS ON NERVES

Since local anesthetics are capable of blocking all nerves, their actions are not limited to the desired loss of sensation from sites of noxious (painful) stimuli. Although motor paralysis can be desirable during surgery, it may also limit the ability of the patient to cooperate during obstetric delivery or ambulate after outpatient surgery. During spinal anesthesia, motor paralysis may impair respiratory activity and autonomic nerve blockade can lead to hypotension upon ambulation. Residual autonomic blockade interferes with bladder function resulting in urinary retention and the need for catheterization.

Nerve fibers differ significantly in their susceptibility to local anesthetic blockade on the basis of differences in size and degree of myelination (Table 26–3). Upon direct application of a local anesthetic to a nerve root, the smaller B and C fibers are blocked first, followed by other sensations, and motor function is the last to be blocked.

1. Effect of fiber diameter—Local anesthetics preferentially block small fibers because the distance over which such fibers can passively propagate an electrical impulse is shorter. During the onset of local anesthesia, when short sections of the nerve are blocked, the small-diameter fibers are the first to fail to conduct. For myelinated nerves, at least two and preferably three successive nodes of Ranvier must be blocked by the local anesthetic to halt impulse propagation. With larger and thicker nerve fibers (eg, motor neurons), the nodes are farther apart, creating greater resistance to blockade. Myelinated nerves tend to become blocked before unmyelinated

nerves of the same diameter. For this reason, the preganglionic B fibers are blocked before the smaller unmyelinated C fibers involved in pain transmission.

2. Effect of firing frequency—Another important reason for preferential blockade of sensory fibers follows directly from the state- and use-dependent mechanism of action of local anesthetics. Blockade by these drugs is more marked at higher frequencies of depolarization. Sensory (pain) fibers have a high firing rate and a relatively long action potential duration. Motor fibers fire at a slower rate and have a shorter action potential duration. Type A delta and C fibers are smaller-diameter fibers that participate in high-frequency pain transmission. Therefore, these fibers are blocked earlier with lower concentrations of local anesthetics than are the large A alpha fibers.

3. Effect of fiber position in the nerve bundle—An anatomic circumstance that sometimes creates exceptions to the above rules for differential nerve block is the location of the fibers in the peripheral nerve bundle. In large nerve trunks, motor nerves are usually located circumferentially, and for that reason they are the first to be exposed to the local anesthetic when it is administered into the tissue surrounding the nerve. Therefore, it is not uncommon for motor nerve block to occur before sensory block in large mixed nerves. In the extremities, proximal sensory fibers are located in the outer portion of the nerve trunk, whereas the distal sensory innervation is in the core of the nerve. Thus, during infiltration block of a large nerve, sensory analgesia first develops proximally and then spreads distally as the drug penetrates into the core of the nerve.

D. EFFECTS ON OTHER EXCITABLE MEMBRANES

Local anesthetics have weak neuromuscular blocking effects that are of little clinical importance. However, their effects on cardiac cell membranes are of major clinical significance, and some local anesthetics are useful antiarrhythmic agents (see Chapter 14) at concentrations lower than those required to produce nerve block. Others (eg, bupivacaine, ropivacaine) can *cause* lethal arrhythmias in high concentrations.

■ II. CLINICAL PHARMACOLOGY OF LOCAL ANESTHETICS

Local anesthetics can provide highly effective analgesia in well-defined regions of the body. The usual routes of administration include topical application (eg, nasal mucosa, wound margins), injection in the vicinity of peripheral nerve endings (infiltration) and major nerve trunks (blocks), and injection into the epidural or subarachnoid spaces surrounding the spinal cord (Figure 26–4). Intravenous regional anesthesia (so-called Bier block) is used for short surgical procedures (< 60 minutes) involving the upper and lower extremities. This is accomplished by intravenous injection of the anesthetic agent into a distal vein while the circulation of the limb is isolated with a proximally placed tourniquet. Finally, an infiltration block of autonomic sympathetic fibers can be used to evaluate the role of sympathetic tone in patients with peripheral vasospastic disorders.

The choice of local anesthetic for infiltration, peripheral nerve blocks, and central neuraxis blockade is usually based on the duration of action required. Procaine and chloroprocaine are short-acting; lidocaine, mepivacaine, and prilocaine have an intermediate duration of action; and tetracaine, bupivacaine, levobupivacaine, and ropivacaine are long-acting local anesthetics (Table 26–1).

The anesthetic effect of the agents with short and intermediate durations of action can be prolonged by increasing the dose or adding a vasoconstrictor agent (eg, epinephrine or phenylephrine). The vasoconstrictor slows the removal of the local anesthetic from the injection site. In addition, it decreases the blood level and the probability of CNS toxicity.

The onset of local anesthesia can be accelerated by the addition of sodium bicarbonate (1–2 mL) to the local anesthetic solution. This maximizes the amount of drug in the more lipid-soluble form.

Repeated injections of local anesthetics can result in loss of effectiveness (ie, tachyphylaxis) due to extracellular acidosis. Local anesthetics are commonly marketed as hydrochloride salts (pH 4.0–6.0). After injection, the salts are buffered in the tissue to physiologic pH, thereby providing sufficient free base concentration for diffusion through the axonal membrane. However, repeated injections of the local anesthetic can deplete the buffering capacity of the local tissues. The ensuing acidosis increases the extracellular cationic form, which diffuses poorly and results in tachyphylaxis. Tachyphylaxis to local anesthetics is common in areas with a limited buffer capacity (eg, the cerebrospinal fluid).

Pregnancy appears to increase susceptibility to local anesthetic toxicity, with reductions in the median doses required for neural blockade and to induce toxicity. Cardiac arrest leading to death following the epidural administration of 0.75% bupivacaine to women in labor resulted in the temporary withdrawal of the high concentration of this widely used long-acting local anesthetic. The subsequent introduction of purportedly less cardiotoxic alternatives to bupivacaine (ie, ropivacaine and levobupivacaine) has led to controversy because the evidence supporting enhanced safety is based on animal models. It is not clear whether the increased sensitivity to bupivacaine during pregnancy is due to elevated levels of estrogen, progesterone, or some other unrecognized factor.

Topical local anesthesia is often used for eye, ear, nose, and throat procedures and for cosmetic surgery. Satisfactory topical local anesthesia requires an agent capable of rapid penetration across the skin or mucosa, and with limited tendency to diffuse away from the site of application. Cocaine, because of its excellent penetration and local vasoconstrictor effects, has been used extensively for ear, nose and throat (ENT) procedures. Cocaine is somewhat irritating and therefore is less popular for ophthalmic procedures. Recent concern about its potential cardiotoxicity when combined with epinephrine has led most otolaryngologists and plastic surgeons to switch to a combination containing lidocaine and epinephrine. Other drugs used for topical anesthesia include tetracaine, pramoxine, dibucaine, benzocaine, and dyclonine.

Since local anesthetics have membrane-stabilizing effects, both parenteral (eg, intravenous lidocaine) and oral (eg, mexiletine, tocainide) formulations of local anesthetics have been used to treat patients with neuropathic pain syndromes because these syndromes are thought to involve uncontrolled, rapid, sensory fiber firing. Systemic local anesthetic drugs are commonly used as adjuvants to the combination of a tricyclic antidepressant (eg, amitriptyline) and an anticonvulsant (eg, carbamazepine) in patients who fail to respond to the combination of antidepressant and anticonvulsant. A period of 1–3 weeks may be required to observe a therapeutic effect after introduction of the local anesthetic in patients with neuropathic pain.

Toxicity

The two major forms of local anesthetic toxicity are: (1) systemic effects following absorption of the local anesthetic from their site of administration and (2) direct neurotoxicity from the local effects of these drugs when administered in close proximity to the spinal cord and other major nerve trunks. When blood levels

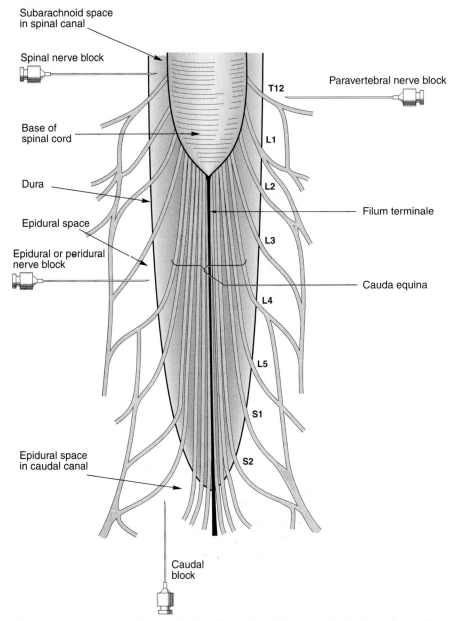

Subarachnoid space in spinal canal

Spinal nerve block

Base of spinal cord

Dura

Epidural space

Epidural or peridural nerve block

Epidural space in caudal canal

Caudal block

Paravertebral nerve block

T12

L1

L2

L3

L4

L5

S1

S2

Filum terminale

Cauda equina

Figure 26–4. Schematic diagram of sites of injection of local anesthetics in and near the spinal canal.

of local anesthetics rise rapidly, adverse effects on several major organ systems may be observed.

A. CENTRAL NERVOUS SYSTEM

1. All local anesthetics—At low concentrations, all local anesthetics have the ability to produce sleepiness, light-headedness, visual and auditory disturbances, and restlessness. An early symptom of local anesthetic toxicity is circumoral and tongue numbness and a metallic taste. At higher concentrations, nystagmus and muscular twitching occur, followed by overt tonic-clonic convulsions. Local anesthetics apparently cause depression of cortical inhibitory pathways, thereby allowing unopposed activity of excitatory neuronal pathways. This transitional stage of unbalanced excitation (ie, seizure activity) is then followed by generalized CNS depression.

Convulsions due to excessive blood levels can usually be prevented by administering the smallest effective dose of the local anesthetic required for adequate surgical analgesia and by avoiding inadvertent intravascular injection, or injection into highly perfused tissues. When large doses of a local anesthetic are required (eg, for major peripheral nerve block), premedication with a parenteral benzodiazepine (eg, diazepam or midazolam) provides significant prophylaxis against local anesthetic-induced CNS toxicity by raising the seizure threshold.

If seizures do occur, it is important to prevent hypoxemia and acidosis. Although administration of oxygen does not prevent seizure activity, hyperoxemia may be beneficial after onset of seizures. Hypercapnia and acidosis may lower the seizure threshold, and so hyperventilation is recommended during treatment of seizures. In addition, hyperventilation increases blood pH, which in turn lowers extracellular potassium. This action hyperpolarizes the transmembrane potential of axons, which favors the rested (or low-affinity) state of the sodium channels, resulting in decreased local anesthetic toxicity.

Seizures induced by local anesthetics can also be treated with intravenous anesthetic drugs (eg, thiopental 1–2 mg/kg, propofol 0.5–1 mg/kg, midazolam 0.03–0.06 mg/kg, or diazepam 0.1–0.2 mg/kg). The muscular manifestations of a seizure can be blocked using a short-acting neuromuscular relaxant drug (eg, succinylcholine, 0.5–1 mg/kg IV). It should be emphasized that succinylcholine does not obliterate CNS manifestations of seizure activity. Rapid tracheal intubation and mechanical ventilation can prevent pulmonary aspiration of gastric contents and facilitate hyperventilation.

2. Cocaine—Since prehistoric times, the natives of Peru and Bolivia have chewed the leaves of the indigenous plant *Erythroxylon coca,* the source of cocaine, to obtain a feeling of well-being and reduce fatigue. Intense CNS effects can be achieved by sniffing cocaine powder and smoking cocaine base ("free basing"). Cocaine has become one of the most widely abused drugs (see Chapter 32). High doses of inhaled and injected cocaine have all of the toxicities described for other local anesthetics. In addition, cocaine can produce severe cardiovascular toxicity, including hypertension, arrhythmias, and myocardial failure.

B. Neurotoxicity

When applied at excessively high concentrations, all local anesthetics can produce direct neural toxicity. Chloroprocaine and lidocaine appear to be more neurotoxic than other local anesthetics when used for spinal anesthesia, with high local concentrations producing so-called transient radicular irritation (or transient neuropathic symptoms). It has been suggested that this toxicity results

from pooling of high concentrations of the local anesthetic in the cauda equina (Figure 26–4). Although the precise mechanism of this neurotoxic action has not been established, both interference with axonal transport and disruption of calcium homeostasis have been implicated. Spinal neurotoxicity does not result from excessive sodium channel blockade.

C. Cardiovascular System

The cardiovascular effects of local anesthetics result partly from direct effects on the cardiac and smooth muscle membranes and partly from indirect effects on the autonomic nervous system. As described in Chapter 14, local anesthetics block cardiac sodium channels and thus depress abnormal cardiac pacemaker activity, excitability, and conduction. At extremely high concentrations, local anesthetics can also block calcium channels. With the notable exception of cocaine, local anesthetics also depress the strength of cardiac contraction and cause arteriolar dilation, leading to systemic hypotension. Cardiovascular collapse is rare, but has been reported after large doses of bupivacaine and ropivacaine.

Cocaine differs from the other local anesthetics with respect to its cardiovascular effects. Cocaine's blockade of norepinephrine reuptake results in vasoconstriction and hypertension, as well as cardiac arrhythmias. The vasoconstriction produced by cocaine can lead to local ischemia and, in chronic abusers who use the nasal route, ulceration of the mucous membrane and damage to the nasal septum have been reported. The vasoconstrictor properties of cocaine can be used clinically to decrease bleeding from mucosal damage in the nasopharynx.

It has been suggested that bupivacaine may be more cardiotoxic than other long-acting local anesthetics. This reflects the fact that bupivacaine-induced blockade of sodium channels is potentiated by the long action potential duration of cardiac cells compared with nerve fibers. The most common electrocardiographic finding in patients with bupivacaine intoxication is a slow idioventricular rhythm with broad QRS complexes and eventually electromechanical dissociation.

Resuscitation from bupivacaine cardiovascular toxicity is extremely difficult even for experienced clinicians. The *(S)*-isomer, levobupivacaine, appears to have a lower propensity for cardiovascular toxicity than the racemic mixture or the *(R)*-isomer and has been approved for clinical use. Ropivacaine has clinical (pharmacodynamic) effects similar to those of bupivacaine, but is allegedly associated with a lower potential for cardiovascular toxicity. Ropivacaine is available only as the *(S)*-stereoisomer, which has inherently less affinity for the cardiac sodium channel. However, both cardiac toxicity and CNS toxicity have been reported when ropivacaine was used for peripheral nerve blocks.

D. HEMATOLOGIC EFFECTS

The administration of large doses (> 10 mg/kg) of prilocaine during regional anesthesia may lead to accumulation of the metabolite *o*-toluidine, an oxidizing agent capable of converting hemoglobin to methemoglobin. When sufficient methemoglobin is present (3–5 mg/dL), the patient may appear cyanotic and the blood "chocolate-colored." Although moderate levels of methemoglobinemia are well tolerated by healthy individuals, elevated methemoglobinemia may cause decompensation in patients with preexisting cardiac or pulmonary disease. The treatment of methemoglobinemia involves the intravenous administration of a reducing agent (eg, methylene blue or ascorbic acid), which rapidly converts methemoglobin to hemoglobin.

E. ALLERGIC REACTIONS

The ester-type local anesthetics are metabolized to *p*-aminobenzoic acid derivatives. These metabolites are responsible for allergic reactions in a small percentage of the patient population. Amides are not metabolized to *p*-aminobenzoic acid, and allergic reactions to amide local anesthetics are extremely rare.

PREPARATIONS AVAILABLE

Articaine (Septocaine)
   Parenteral: 4% with 1:100,000 epinephrine
Benzocaine (generic)
   Topical: 5, 6% creams; 15, 20% gels; 5, 20% ointments; 0.8% lotion; 20% liquid; 20% spray
Bupivacaine (generic, Marcaine, Sensorcaine)
   Parenteral: 0.25, 0.5, 0.75% for injection; 0.25, 0.5, 0.75% with 1:200,000 epinephrine
Butamben picrate (Butesin Picrate)
   Topical: 1% ointment
Chloroprocaine (generic, Nesacaine)
   Parenteral: 1, 2, 3% for injection
Cocaine (generic)
   Topical: 40, 100 mg/mL regular and viscous solutions; 5, 25 g powder
Dibucaine (generic, Nupercainal)
   Topical: 0.5% cream; 1% ointment
Dyclonine (Dyclone)
   Topical: 0.5, 1% solution
Levobupivacaine (Chirocaine)
   Parenteral: 2.5, 5, 7.5 mg/mL
Lidocaine (generic, Xylocaine)
   Parenteral: 0.5, 1, 1.5, 2, 4% for injection; 0.5, 1, 1.5, 2% with 1:200,000 epinephrine; 1, 2% with 1:100,000 epinephrine, 2% with 1:50,000 epinephrine

   Topical: 2.5, 5% ointments; 0.5, 4% cream; 0.5, 2.5% gel; 2, 2.5, 4% solutions; 23, 46 mg/2 cm^2 patch
Lidocaine and bupivacaine mixture (Duocaine)
   Parenteral: 10 mg/mL lidocaine plus 3.75 mg/mL bupivacaine for injection
Lidocaine and prilocaine eutectic mixture (EMLA cream)
   Topical: lidocaine 2.5% plus prilocaine 2.5%
Mepivacaine (generic, Carbocaine)
   Parenteral: 1, 1.5, 2, 3% for injection; 2% with 1:20,000 levonordefrin
Pramoxine (generic, Tronothane)
   Topical: 1% cream, lotion, spray, and gel
Procaine (generic, Novocain)
   Parenteral: 1, 2, 10% for injection
Proparacaine (generic, Alcain, others)
   0.5% solution for ophthalmic use
Ropivacaine (Naropin)
   Parenteral: 0.2, 0.5, 0.75, 1.0 % solution for injection
Tetracaine (generic, Pontocaine)
   Parenteral: 1% for injection; 0.2, 0.3% with 6% dextrose for spinal anesthesia
   Topical: 1% ointment; 0.5% solution (ophthalmic); 1, 2% cream; 2% solution for nose and throat; 2% gel

REFERENCES

Brau ME et al: Effect of drugs used for neuropathic pain management on tetrodotoxin-resistant Na⁺ currents in rat sensory neurons. Anesthesiology 2001;94:137.

Davies PS, Galer BS: Review of lidocaine patch 5% studies in the treatment of postherpetic neuralgia. Drugs 2004;64:937.

Ferreira S et al: Effects of cocaine and its major metabolites on the HERG-encoded potassium channel. J Pharmacol Exp Ther 2001;299:220.

Hille B: Local anesthetics: Hydrophilic and hydrophobic pathways for the drug-receptor reactions. J Gen Physiol 1977;69:497.

Johnson ME et al: Effect of local anesthetic on neuronal cytoplasmic calcium and plasma membrane lysis (necrosis) in a cell culture model. Anesthesiology 2002;97:1466.

Kanai Y, Katsuki H, Takasaki M: Comparisons of the anesthetic potency and intracellular concentrations of S(-) and R(+) bupivacaine and ropivacaine in crayfish giant axon in vitro. Anesth Analg 2000;90:415.

Kanai Y, Katsuki H, Takasaki M: Lidocaine disrupts axonal membrane of rat sciatic nerve in vitro. Anesth Analg 2000;91:944.

Miyamoto Y et al: Direct inhibition of microtubule-based kinesin motility by local anesthetics. Biophys J 2000;78:940.

Oda A et al: Characteristics of ropivacaine block of Na⁺ channels in rat dorsal root ganglion neurons. Anesth Analg 2000; 91:1213.

Scholtz A: Mechanisms of (local) anaesthetics on voltage-gated sodium and other ion channels. Br J Anaesth 2002;89:52.

Sinnott CJ et al: On the mechanism by which epinephrine potentiates lidocaine's peripheral nerve block. Anesthesiology 2003; 98:181.

White JL, Durieux ME: Clinical pharmacology of local anesthetics. Anesthesiol Clin North Am 2005;23:73.

White PF: The changing role of non-opioid analgesic techniques in the management of postoperative pain. Anesth Analg 2005; 101:S5.

Zapata-Sudo G et al: Is comparative cardiotoxicity of S(-) and R(+) bupivacaine related to enantiomer-selective inhibition of L-type Ca²⁺ channels? Anesth Analg 2001;92:496.

Zhou W et al: Mechanism underlying bupivacaine inhibition of G protein-gated inwardly rectifying K⁺ channels. Proc Natl Acad Sci USA 2001;98:6482.

Skeletal Muscle Relaxants

27

Paul F. White, PhD, MD, & Bertram G. Katzung, MD, PhD

Drugs that affect skeletal muscle function as two very different therapeutic groups: those used during surgical procedures and in intensive care units to produce muscle paralysis for patients requiring ventilatory assistance (ie, **neuromuscular blockers**) and those used to reduce spasticity in a variety of neurologic conditions (ie, **spasmolytics**). Neuromuscular blocking drugs interfere with transmission at the neuromuscular end plate and lack central nervous system activity. These compounds are used primarily as adjuncts during general anesthesia to facilitate tracheal intubation and optimize surgical conditions while ensuring adequate ventilation. Drugs in the spasmolytic group have traditionally been called "centrally acting" muscle relaxants and are used primarily to treat chronic back pain and fibromyalgic conditions. Dantrolene, a spasmolytic agent that has no significant central effects and is used primarily to treat malignant hyperthermia, is also discussed in this chapter.

NEUROMUSCULAR BLOCKING DRUGS

History

During the 16th century, European explorers found that natives in the Amazon Basin of South America used curare, an arrow poison, to produce death by skeletal muscle paralysis. The active compound, *d*-tubocurarine, and its modern synthetic derivatives have had a significant influence on the practice of anesthesia and surgery and have proved useful in defining normal neuromuscular physiologic mechanisms.

Normal Neuromuscular Function

The mechanism of neuromuscular transmission at the motor end plate is similar to that described for preganglionic cholinergic nerves in Chapter 6. With the arrival of an electrical impulse at the motor nerve terminal, there is an influx of calcium and release of acetylcholine. Acetylcholine then diffuses across the synaptic cleft to the nicotinic receptor located on the motor end plate. As noted in Chapter 7, the adult N_M receptor is composed of five peptides: two alpha peptides, one beta, one gamma, and one delta peptide (Figure 27–1). The binding of two ace-

tylcholine molecules to receptors on the α-β and δ-α subunits causes opening of the channel. The subsequent movement of sodium and potassium is associated with a graded depolarization of the end plate membrane (Figure 27–2). This change in voltage is termed the motor end plate potential. The magnitude of the end plate potential is directly related to the amount of acetylcholine released. If the potential is small, the permeability and the end plate potential return to normal without an impulse being propagated from the end plate region to the rest of the muscle membrane. However, if the end plate potential is large, the adjacent muscle membrane is depolarized, and an action potential will be propagated along the entire muscle fiber. Muscle contraction is then initiated by excitation-contraction coupling. The released acetylcholine is quickly removed from the end plate region by diffusion and enzymatic destruction by the local acetylcholinesterase enzyme.

At least two additional types of acetylcholine receptors are associated with the neuromuscular apparatus. One type is located on the presynaptic motor axon terminal, and activation of these receptors mobilizes additional transmitter for subsequent release by moving more acetylcholine vesicles toward the synaptic membrane. The second type of receptor is found on perijunctional cells and is not normally involved in neuromuscular transmission. However, under certain conditions (eg, prolonged immobilization, thermal burns), these receptors may proliferate sufficiently to affect subsequent neuromuscular transmission.

Skeletal muscle relaxation and paralysis can occur from interruption of function at several sites along the pathway from the central nervous system to myelinated somatic nerves, unmyelinated motor nerve terminals, nicotinic acetylcholine receptors, the motor end plate, the muscle membrane, and the intracellular contractile apparatus itself.

In practice, blockade of end plate function is accomplished by two basic mechanisms. Pharmacologic blockade of the physiologic agonist acetylcholine is characteristic of the *antagonist* neuromuscular blocking drugs. These drugs prevent access of the transmitter to its receptor and thereby prevent depolarization. The prototype of this *nondepolarizing* subgroup is **d-tubocurarine.** The second mechanism of blockade can be produced by an

424

A

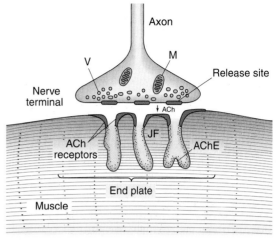

Figure 27–2. Schematic representation of the neuromuscular junction. (ACh, acetylcholine; AChE, acetylcholinesterase; JF, junctional folds; M, mitochondrion; V, transmitter vesicle.) (Reproduced, with permission, from Drachman DB: Myasthenia gravis. N Engl J Med 1978;298:135.)

B

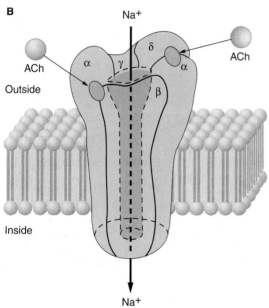

Figure 27–1. The adult nicotinic acetylcholine receptor (nAChR) is an intrinsic membrane protein with five distinct subunits ($\alpha_2\beta\delta\gamma$). **A:** Cartoon of the one of five subunits of the AChR in the end plate surface of adult mammalian muscle. Each subunit contains four helical domains labeled M1 to M4. The M2 domains line the channel pore. **B:** Cartoon of the full AChR. The N termini of two subunits cooperate to form two distinct binding pockets for acetylcholine (ACh). These pockets occur at the α-β and the δ-α subunit interfaces.

excess of a depolarizing *agonist,* such as acetylcholine. This paradoxical effect of acetylcholine also occurs at the ganglionic nicotinic acetylcholine receptor. The prototypical *depolarizing* blocking drug is **succinylcholine.** A similar depolarizing block can be produced by acetylcholine itself when high local concentrations are achieved in the synaptic cleft (eg, by cholinesterase inhibitor intoxication) and by nicotine and other nicotinic agonists. However, the neuromuscular block produced by these depolarizing drugs (other than succinylcholine) cannot be precisely controlled and is of no clinical value.

■ I. BASIC PHARMACOLOGY OF NEUROMUSCULAR BLOCKING DRUGS

Chemistry

All of the available neuromuscular blocking drugs bear a structural resemblance to acetylcholine. For example, succinylcholine is two acetylcholine molecules linked end-to-end (Figure 27–3). In contrast to the single linear structure of succinylcholine and other depolarizing drugs, the nondepolarizing agents (eg, pancuronium) conceal the "double-acetylcholine" structure in one of two types of bulky, semi-rigid ring systems (Figure 27–3). The two major families of nondepolarizing

Acetylcholine

Succinylcholine

Pancuronium

Figure 27–3. Structural relationship of succinylcholine, a depolarizing agent, and pancuronium, a nondepolarizing agent, to acetylcholine, the neuromuscular transmitter. Succinylcholine, originally called diacetylcholine, is simply two molecules of acetylcholine linked through the acetate methyl groups. Pancuronium may be viewed as two acetylcholine-like fragments (outlined in color) oriented on a steroid nucleus.

blocking drugs—the isoquinoline and steroid derivatives—are shown in Figures 27–4 and 27–5. Another feature common to all currently used neuromuscular blockers is the presence of one or two quaternary nitrogens, which makes them poorly lipid-soluble and limits entry into the central nervous system.

Pharmacokinetics of Neuromuscular Blocking Drugs

All of the neuromuscular blocking drugs are highly polar and inactive orally and must be administered parenterally.

A. NONDEPOLARIZING RELAXANT DRUGS

The rate of disappearance of a nondepolarizing neuromuscular blocking drug from the blood is characterized by a rapid initial distribution phase followed by a slower elimination phase. Neuromuscular blocking drugs are highly ionized and do not readily cross cell membranes. Therefore, their volume of distribution is only slightly larger than the blood volume (80–140 mL/kg).

The elimination half-life strongly correlates with the duration of action of nondepolarizing relaxants. Drugs that are excreted by the kidney typically have longer half-lives, leading to longer durations of action (> 60 minutes). Drugs eliminated by the liver tend to have shorter half-lives and durations of action (Table 27–1). All steroidal muscle relaxants are metabolized to their 3-hydroxy, 17-hydroxy, or 3,17-dihydroxy products in the liver. The 3-hydroxy metabolites are usually 40–80% as potent as the parent drug. Under normal circumstances, metabolites are not formed in sufficient quantities to produce a significant degree of neuromuscular blockade during or after anesthesia. However, if the parent compound is administered for several days in the intensive care setting, the 3-hydroxy metabolite may accumulate and cause prolonged paralysis because it has a longer half-life than the parent compound. The remaining metabolites possess minimal neuromuscular blocking properties.

The intermediate-acting steroid muscle relaxants (eg, vecuronium and rocuronium) tend to be more dependent on biliary excretion or hepatic metabolism for their elimination. These muscle relaxants are more commonly used clinically than the long-acting steroid-based drugs (eg, pancuronium, pipecuronium).

Atracurium (Figure 27–4) is an intermediate-acting isoquinoline nondepolarizing muscle relaxant. In addition to hepatic metabolism, atracurium is inactivated by a form of spontaneous breakdown known as Hofmann elimination. The main breakdown products are laudanosine and a related quaternary acid, neither of which possesses neuromuscular blocking properties. Laudanosine is slowly metabolized by the liver and has a long elimination half-life (ie, 150 minutes). It readily crosses the blood-brain barrier, and high blood concentrations may cause seizures and an increase in the volatile anesthetic requirement. During surgical anesthesia, blood levels of laudanosine range from 0.2 to 1 mcg/mL. However, with prolonged infusions of atracurium in the intensive care unit, laudanosine blood levels may exceed 5 mcg/mL.

Atracurium has several stereoisomers, and one of the more potent isomers, **cisatracurium,** has been approved for clinical use. It resembles atracurium but has even less dependence on hepatic inactivation, forms less laudanosine, and is less likely to release histamine.

Tubocurarine

Atracurium

Doxacurium

Figure 27–4. Structures of some isoquinoline neuromuscular blocking drugs. These agents are all nondepolarizing muscle relaxants.

From the clinical perspective, cisatracurium has all the advantages of atracurium with fewer side effects. Therefore, cisatracurium has largely replaced atracurium in clinical practice.

Mivacurium, another isoquinoline compound, has the shortest duration of action of all nondepolarizing muscle relaxants (Table 27–1). However, its onset of action is significantly slower than that of succinylcholine. In addition, the use of a larger dose to speed the onset can be associated with profound histamine release leading to hypotension, flushing, and bronchospasm. Clearance of mivacurium by plasma cholinesterase is rapid and independent of the liver or kidney (Table 27–1). However, because patients with renal failure often have decreased levels of plasma cholinesterase, the short duration of action of mivacurium may be prolonged in patients with impaired renal function.

B. DEPOLARIZING RELAXANT DRUGS

The extremely short duration of action of succinylcholine (5–10 minutes) is due to its rapid hydrolysis by cholinesterases (eg, butyrylcholinesterase and pseudocholinesterase) in the liver and plasma. Plasma cholinesterase metabolizes succinylcholine more rapidly than mivacurium, and consequently the duration of action of succinylcholine is shorter than that of mivacurium (Table

Pancuronium

Vecuronium

Pipecuronium

Rocuronium

Figure 27–5. Structures of steroid neuromuscular blocking drugs. These agents are all nondepolarizing muscle relaxants.

27–1). The primary metabolite, succinylmonocholine, is rapidly broken down to succinic acid and choline. Because plasma cholinesterase has an enormous capacity to hydrolyze succinylcholine, only a small percentage of the original intravenous dose ever reaches the neuromus-

cular junction. There is little if any plasma cholinesterase at the motor end plate, and a succinylcholine-induced blockade is terminated by its diffusion away from the end plate into extracellular fluid. Therefore, circulating levels of plasma cholinesterase influence the duration of

Table 27–1. Some properties of neuromuscular blocking drugs.

Drug	Elimination	Clearance (mL/kg/min)	Approximate Duration of Action (minutes)	Approximate Potency Relative to Tubocurarine
Isoquinoline derivatives				
Atracurium	Spontaneous[1]	6.6	20–35	1.5
Cisatracurium	Mostly spontaneous	5–6	25–44	1.5
Doxacurium	Kidney	2.7	> 35	6
Metocurine	Kidney (40%)	1.2	> 35	4
Mivacurium	Plasma ChE[2]	70–95	10–20	4
Tubocurarine	Kidney (40%)	2.3–2.4	> 35	1
Steroid derivatives				
Pancuronium	Kidney (80%)	1.7–1.8	> 35	6
Pipecuronium	Kidney (60%) and liver	2.5–3.0	> 35	6
Rocuronium	Liver (75–90%) and kidney	2.9	20–35	0.8
Vecuronium	Liver (75–90%) and kidney	3–5.3	20–35	6
Depolarizing agent				
Succinylcholine	Plasma ChE[2] (100%)	>100	< 8	0.4

[1]Nonenzymatic and enzymatic hydrolysis of ester bonds.
[2]Butyrylcholinesterase (pseudocholinesterase).

action of succinylcholine by determining the amount of the drug that reaches the motor end plate.

Neuromuscular blockade produced by succinylcholine and mivacurium can be prolonged in patients with a genetically abnormal variant of plasma cholinesterase. The *dibucaine number* is a measure of the ability of a patient to metabolize succinylcholine and can be used to identify at-risk patients. Under standardized test conditions, dibucaine inhibits the normal enzyme by 80% and the abnormal enzyme by only 20%. Many genetic variants of plasma cholinesterase have been identified, though the dibucaine-related variants are the most important. Given the rarity of these genetic variants, plasma cholinesterase testing is not a routine clinical procedure.

Mechanism of Action

The interactions of drugs with the acetylcholine receptor-end plate channel have been described at the molecular level. Several modes of action of drugs on the receptor are illustrated in Figure 27–6.

A. NONDEPOLARIZING RELAXANT DRUGS

All the neuromuscular blocking drugs in use in the USA except succinylcholine are classified as nondepolarizing agents. **Tubocurarine** is considered the prototype neuromuscular blocker. When small doses of nondepolarizing muscle relaxants are administered, they act predominantly at the nicotinic receptor site by competing with acetylcholine. The least potent nondepolarizing relaxants (eg, rocuronium) have the fastest onset and the shortest duration of action. In larger doses, nondepolarizing drugs can enter the pore of the ion channel (Figure 27–1) to cause a more intense motor blockade. This action further weakens neuromuscular transmission and diminishes the ability of acetylcholinesterase inhibitors (eg, neostigmine, edrophonium, pyridostigmine) to antagonize the effect of nondepolarizing muscle relaxants.

Nondepolarizing relaxants can also block prejunctional sodium channels. As a result of this action, muscle relaxants interfere with the mobilization of acetylcholine at the nerve ending. One consequence of the surmountable nature of the postsynaptic blockade produced by nondepolarizing muscle relaxants is the fact that tetanic stimulation, by releasing a large quantity of acetylcholine, is followed by transient posttetanic facilitation (ie, relief of blockade) of the twitch strength. An important clinical consequence of the same principle is the reversal of residual blockade by cholinesterase inhibitors. The characteristics of a nondepolarizing

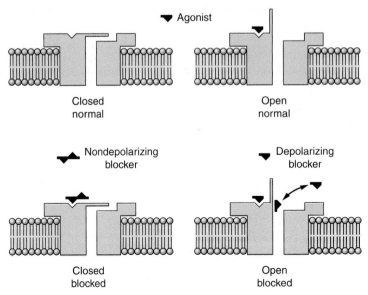

Figure 27–6. Schematic diagram of the interactions of drugs with the acetylcholine receptor on the end plate channel (structures are purely symbolic). **Top:** The action of the normal agonist, acetylcholine, in opening the channel. **Bottom, left:** A nondepolarizing blocker, eg, rocuronium, is shown as preventing the opening of the channel when it binds to the receptor. **Right:** A depolarizing blocker, eg, succinylcholine, both occupying the receptor and blocking the channel. Normal closure of the channel gate is prevented and the blocker may move rapidly in and out of the pore. Depolarizing blockers may desensitize the end plate by occupying the receptor and causing persistent depolarization. An additional effect of drugs on the end plate channel may occur through changes in the lipid environment surrounding the channel (not shown). General anesthetics and alcohols may impair neuromuscular transmission by this mechanism.

neuromuscular blockade are summarized in Table 27–2 and Figure 27–7).

B. DEPOLARIZING RELAXANT DRUGS

1. Phase I block (depolarizing)—Succinylcholine is the only clinically useful depolarizing blocking drug. Its neuromuscular effects are like those of acetylcholine except that succinylcholine produces a longer effect at the myoneural junction. Succinylcholine reacts with the nicotinic receptor to open the channel and cause depolarization of the motor end plate, and this in turn spreads to the adjacent membranes, causing contractions of muscle motor units. Data from single-channel recordings indicate that depolarizing blockers can enter the channel to produce a prolonged "flickering" of the ion conductance (Figure 27–8). Because succinylcholine is not metabolized effectively at the synapse, the depolarized membranes remain depolarized and unresponsive to subsequent impulses (ie, in a state of depolarizing block). Furthermore, because excitation-contraction coupling requires end plate repolarization ("repriming") and repetitive firing to maintain muscle tension, a flaccid paralysis results. This so-called phase I (depolarizing) block is thus augmented, not reversed, by cholinesterase inhibitors.

The characteristics of a depolarizing neuromuscular blockade are summarized in Table 27–2 and Figure 27–7.

2. Phase II block (desensitizing)—With continued exposure to succinylcholine, the initial end plate depolarization decreases and the membrane becomes repolarized. Despite this repolarization, the membrane cannot easily be depolarized again because it is *desensitized*. The mechanism for this desensitizing phase is unclear, but some evidence indicates that channel block may become more important than agonist action at the receptor in

Table 27–2. Comparison of a typical nondepolarizing muscle relaxant (rocuronium) and a depolarizing muscle relaxant (succinylcholine).

	Rocuronium	Succinylcholine Phase I	Succinylcholine Phase II
Administration of tubocurarine	Additive	Antagonistic	Augmented[1]
Administration of succinylcholine	Antagonistic	Additive	Augmented[1]
Effect of neostigmine	Antagonistic	Augmented[1]	Antagonistic
Initial excitatory effect on skeletal muscle	None	Fasciculations	None
Response to a tetanic stimulus	Unsustained (fade)	Sustained[2] (no fade)	Unsustained (fade)
Posttetanic facilitation	Yes	No	Yes
Rate of recovery	30–60 min[3]	4–8 min	> 20 min[3]

[1]It is not known whether this interaction is additive or synergistic (superadditive).
[2]The amplitude is decreased, but the response is sustained.
[3]The rate depends on the dose and on the completeness of neuromuscular blockade.

phase II of succinylcholine's neuromuscular blocking action. Regardless of the mechanism, the channels behave as if they are in a prolonged closed state (Figure 27–7). Later in phase II, the characteristics of the blockade are nearly identical to those of a nondepolarizing block (ie, a nonsustained twitch response to a tetanic stimulus) (Figure 27–7), with reversal by acetylcholinesterase inhibitors.

Figure 27–7. Muscle responses to different patterns of nerve stimulation used in monitoring skeletal muscle relaxation. The alterations produced by a nondepolarizing blocker and depolarizing and desensitizing blockade by succinylcholine are shown. In the train of four (TOF) pattern, four stimuli are applied at 2 Hz. The TOF ratio (TOF-R) is calculated from the strength of the fourth contraction divided by that of the first. In the double burst pattern, three stimuli are applied at 50 Hz, followed by a 700 ms rest period and then repeated. In the posttetanic potentiation pattern, several seconds of 50 Hz stimulation are applied, followed by several seconds of rest and then by single stimuli at a slow rate (eg, 0.5 Hz). The number of detectable posttetanic twitches is the posttetanic count (PTC). (*, first posttetanic contraction.)

Figure 27–8. Action of succinylcholine on single-channel end plate receptor currents in frog muscle. Currents through a single AchR channel were recorded using the patch clamp technique. The upper trace was recorded in the presence of a low concentration of succinylcholine; the downward deflections represent two openings of the channel and passage of inward (depolarizing) current. The lower trace was recorded in the presence of a much higher concentration of succinylcholine and shows prolonged "flickering" of the channel as it repetitively opens and closes or is "plugged" by the drug. (Reproduced, with permission, from Marshall CG, Ogden DC, Colquhoun D: The actions of suxamethonium (succinyldicholine) as an agonist and channel blocker at the nicotinic receptor of frog muscle. J Physiol [Lond] 1990;428:155.)

■ II. CLINICAL PHARMACOLOGY OF NEUROMUSCULAR BLOCKING DRUGS

Skeletal Muscle Paralysis

Before the introduction of neuromuscular blocking drugs, profound skeletal muscle relaxation for intracavitary operations could be achieved only by producing deep levels of anesthesia that are accompanied by profound depressant effects on the cardiovascular and respiratory systems. The adjunctive use of neuromuscular blocking drugs makes it possible to achieve adequate muscle relaxation for all types of surgical procedures without the cardiorespiratory depressant effects produced by deep anesthesia.

Assessment of Neuromuscular Transmission

Monitoring the effect of muscle relaxants during surgery (and recovery following the administration of cholinesterase inhibitors) typically involves the use of a device that produces transdermal electrical stimulation of one of the peripheral nerves to the hand (or face) and recording of the evoked contractions (ie, twitches). The motor responses to different patterns of peripheral nerve stimulation are measured (Figure 27–7). The three most commonly used patterns include (1) single-twitch stimulation, (2) train-of-four (TOF) stimulation, and (3) tetanic stimulation. Two newer modalities are also available to monitor neuromuscular transmission: double-burst stimulation and posttetanic count.

With single-twitch stimulation, a single supramaximal electrical stimulus is applied to a peripheral nerve at frequencies from 0.1 Hz to 1.0 Hz. The higher frequency is often used during induction and reversal to more accurately determine the peak (maximal) drug effect. TOF stimulation involves four successive supramaximal stimuli given at intervals of 0.5 second (2 Hz). Each stimulus in the TOF causes the muscle to contract, and the relative magnitude of the response of the fourth twitch compared with the first twitch is the TOF ratio. With a depolarizing block, all four twitches are reduced in a dose-related fashion. With a nondepolarizing block, the TOF ratio decreases ("fades") and is inversely proportional to the degree of blockade. During recovery from nondepolarizing block, the amount of fade decreases and the TOF ratio approaches 1.0. Fade in the TOF response after administration of succinylcholine signifies the development of a phase II block.

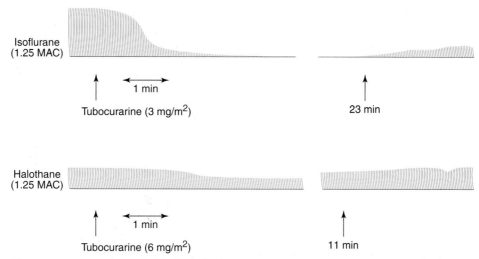

Figure 27–9. Neuromuscular blockade from tubocurarine during equivalent levels of isoflurane and halothane anesthesia in patients. Note that isoflurane augments the block far more than does halothane.

Tetanic stimulation consists of very rapid (30–100 Hz) delivery of electrical stimuli for several seconds. During a nondepolarizing block (and a phase II block after succinylcholine), the response is not sustained and fade is observed. Fade in response to tetanic stimulation is normally considered a presynaptic event. However, the degree of fade depends primarily on the degree of neuromuscular blockade. During a partial nondepolarizing blockade, tetanic nerve stimulation is followed by an increase in the posttetanic twitch response, so-called posttetanic facilitation of neuromuscular transmission. During intense neuromuscular blockade, there is no response to either tetanic or posttetanic stimulation. As the intensity of the block diminishes, the response to posttetanic twitch stimulation reappears. The time to reappearance of the first response to TOF stimulation is related to the posttetanic count.

The double-burst stimulation pattern is a newer mode of electrical nerve stimulation developed with the goal of allowing for manual detection of residual neuromuscular blockade when it is not possible to record the responses to single-twitch, TOF, or tetanic stimulation. In this pattern, three nerve stimuli are delivered at 50 Hz followed by a 700 ms rest period and then, by two or three additional stimuli at 50 Hz. It is easier to detect fade in the responses to double-burst stimulation than to TOF stimulation. The absence of fade in response to double-burst stimulation implies that clinically significant residual neuromuscular blockade does not exist.

A. NONDEPOLARIZING RELAXANT DRUGS

During anesthesia, administration of tubocurarine, 0.1–0.4 mg/kg IV, initially causes motor weakness, followed by the skeletal muscles becoming flaccid and inexcitable to electrical stimulation (Figure 27–9). In general, larger muscles (eg, abdominal, trunk, paraspinous, diaphragm) are more resistant to blockade and recover more rapidly than smaller muscles (eg, facial, foot, hand). The diaphragm is usually the last muscle to be paralyzed. Assuming that ventilation is adequately maintained, no adverse effects occur. When administration of muscle relaxants is discontinued, recovery of muscles usually occurs in reverse order, with the diaphragm regaining function first. The pharmacologic effect of tubocurarine, 0.3 mg/kg IV, usually lasts 45–60 minutes. However, subtle evidence of residual muscle paralysis detected using a neuromuscular monitor may last for another hour.

Potency and duration of action of the other nondepolarizing drugs are shown in Table 27–1. In addition to the duration of action, the most important property distinguishing the nondepolarizing relaxants is the time to onset of effect, which determines how rapidly the patient's trachea can be intubated. Of the currently available nondepolarizing drugs, rocuronium (60–120 seconds) is the most rapid.

B. DEPOLARIZING RELAXANT DRUGS

Following the administration of succinylcholine, 0.75–1.5 mg/kg IV, transient muscle fasciculations occur over the chest and abdomen within 30 seconds, although general anesthesia tends to attenuate them. As paralysis develops rapidly (< 90 seconds), the arm, neck, and leg muscles are initially relaxed followed by the respiratory muscles. As a result of succinylcholine's rapid hydrolysis by cholinesterase in the plasma

Table 27–3. Effects of neuromuscular blocking drugs on other tissues.

Drug	Effect on Autonomic Ganglia	Effect on Cardiac Muscarinic Receptors	Tendency to Cause Histamine Release
Isoquinoline derivatives			
Atracurium	None	None	Slight
Cisatracurium	None	None	None
Doxacurium	None	None	None
Metocurine	Weak block	None	Slight
Mivacurium	None	None	Moderate
Tubocurarine	Weak block	None	Moderate
Steroid derivatives			
Pancuronium	None	Moderate block	None
Pipecuronium	None	None	None
Rocuronium[1]	None	Slight	None
Vecuronium	None	None	None
Other agents			
Gallamine	None	Strong block	None
Succinylcholine	Stimulation	Stimulation	Slight

[1]Allergic reactions have been reported.

and liver, the duration of neuromuscular block typically lasts less than 10 minutes (Table 27–1).

Cardiovascular Effects

Vecuronium, pipecuronium, doxacurium, cisatracurium, and rocuronium all have minimal, if any, cardiovascular effects. The other nondepolarizing muscle relaxants (ie, pancuronium, atracurium, mivacurium) produce cardiovascular effects that are mediated by either autonomic or histamine receptors (Table 27–3). Tubocurarine and, to a lesser extent, metocurine, mivacurium, and atracurium can produce hypotension as a result of systemic histamine release, and with larger doses ganglionic blockade may occur with tubocurarine and metocurine. Premedication with an antihistaminic compound attenuates tubocurarine- and mivacurium-induced hypotension. Pancuronium causes a moderate increase in heart rate and a smaller increase in cardiac output, with little or no change in systemic vascular resistance. Although pancuronium-induced tachycardia is primarily due to a vagolytic action, release of norepinephrine from adrenergic nerve endings and blockade of neuronal uptake of norepinephrine may be secondary mechanisms. Although bronchospasm may be produced by neuromuscular blockers that release histamine (eg, mivacurium), insertion of a tracheal tube is the most common reason for bronchospasm after induction of general anesthesia.

Succinylcholine can cause cardiac arrhythmias when administered during halothane anesthesia. The drug stimulates autonomic cholinoceptors, including the nicotinic receptors at both sympathetic and parasympathetic ganglia and muscarinic receptors in the heart (eg, sinus node). The negative inotropic and chronotropic responses to succinylcholine can be attenuated by administration of an anticholinergic drug (eg, glycopyrrolate, atropine). With large doses of succinylcholine, positive inotropic and chronotropic effects may be observed. On the other hand, bradycardia has been repeatedly observed when a second dose of succinylcholine is given less than 5 minutes after the initial dose. This transient bradycardia can be prevented by thiopental, atropine, ganglionic-blocking drugs, and even nondepolarizing muscle relaxants (eg, pancuronium). Direct myocardial effects, increased muscarinic stimulation, and ganglionic stimulation contribute to this bradycardic response.

Other Adverse Effects of Depolarizing Blockade

A. HYPERKALEMIA

Patients with burns, nerve damage or neuromuscular disease, closed head injury, and other trauma can respond to succinylcholine by releasing potassium into the blood, which, on rare occasions, results in cardiac arrest.

B. Increased Intraocular Pressure

Administration of succinylcholine may be associated with the rapid onset of an increase in intraocular pressure (< 60 seconds), peaking at 2–4 minutes, and declining after 5 minutes. The mechanism may involve tonic contraction of myofibrils or transient dilation of ocular choroidal blood vessels. Despite the increase in intraocular pressure, the use of succinylcholine for ophthalmologic operations is not contraindicated unless the anterior chamber is open ("open globe") due to trauma.

C. Increased Intragastric Pressure

In heavily muscled patients, the fasciculations associated with succinylcholine may cause an increase in intragastric pressure ranging from 5 to 40 cm H_2O, increasing the risk for regurgitation and aspiration of gastric contents. This complication is more likely to occur in patients with delayed gastric emptying (eg, those with diabetes), traumatic injury, esophageal dysfunction, and morbid obesity.

D. Muscle Pain

Myalgias are a common postoperative complaint of heavily muscled patients and those who receive large doses of succinylcholine. The true incidence of myalgias related to muscle fasciculations is difficult to establish because of confounding factors, including the type of surgery and positioning during the operation. However, the incidence of myalgias has been reported to vary from less than 1% to 20%. It occurs more frequently in ambulatory than in bedridden patients. The pain is thought to be secondary to the unsynchronized contractions of adjacent muscle fibers just before the onset of paralysis. However, there is controversy over whether the incidence of muscle pain following succinylcholine is actually higher than with nondepolarizing muscle relaxants when other potentially confounding factors are taken into consideration.

Interactions with Other Drugs

A. Anesthetics

Inhaled (volatile) anesthetics potentiate the neuromuscular blockade produced by nondepolarizing muscle relaxants in a dose-dependent fashion. Of the general anesthetics that have been studied, volatile anesthetics augment the effects of muscle relaxants in the following order: isoflurane (most); sevoflurane, desflurane, enflurane, and halothane; and nitrous oxide (least) (Figure 27–9). The most important factors involved in this interaction are the following: (1) nervous system depression at sites proximal to the neuromuscular junction (ie, central nervous system); (2) increased muscle blood flow (ie, due to peripheral vasodilation produced by volatile anesthetics), which allows a larger fraction of the injected muscle relaxant to reach the neuromuscular junction; and (3) decreased sensitivity of the postjunctional membrane to depolarization.

A rare interatction of succinylcholine with volatile anesthetics results in malignant hyperthermia, a condition caused by abnormal release of calcium from stores in skeletal muscle. This condition is treated with dantrolcne and is discussed below under Spasmolytic Drugs and in Chapter 16.

B. Antibiotics

Numerous reports have described enhancement of neuromuscular blockade by antibiotics (eg, aminoglycosides). Many of the antibiotics have been shown to cause a depression of evoked release of acetylcholine similar to that caused by magnesium. The mechanism of this prejunctional effect appears to be blockade of specific P-type calcium channels.

C. Local Anesthetics and Antiarrhythmic Drugs

In small doses, local anesthetics depress posttetanic potentiation via a prejunctional neural effect. In large doses, local anesthetics can block neuromuscular transmission. With higher doses, local anesthetics block acetylcholine-induced muscle contractions as a result of blockade of the nicotinic receptor ion channels. Experimentally, similar effects can be demonstrated with sodium channel-blocking antiarrhythmic drugs such as quinidine. However, at the doses used for cardiac arrhythmias, this interaction is of little or no clinical significance. Higher concentrations of bupivacaine (0.75%) have been associated with cardiac arrhythmias independent of the muscle relaxant used.

D. Other Neuromuscular Blocking Drugs

The end plate-depolarizing effect of succinylcholine can be antagonized by administering a small dose of a nondepolarizing blocker. To prevent the fasciculations associated with succinylcholine administration, a small nonparalyzing dose of a nondepolarizing drug can be given before succinylcholine (eg, d-tubocurarine 2 mg IV or pancuronium 0.5 mg IV). Although this dose usually reduces fasciculations and postoperative myalgias, it can increase the amount of succinylcholine required for relaxation by 50–90% and can produce a feeling of weakness in awake patients. Therefore, "pre-curarization" before succinylcholine is no longer widely practiced.

Effects of Diseases & Aging on the Neuromuscular Response

Several diseases can diminish or augment the neuromuscular blockade produced by nondepolarizing muscle relaxants. Myasthenia gravis enhances the neuromuscular blockade produced by these drugs. Advanced age is associated with a prolonged duration of action from nondepolarizing relaxants as a result of decreased clearance of the drugs by the liver and kidneys. As a result, the dosage of neuromuscular blocking drugs should be reduced in elderly patients (> 70 years).

Conversely, patients with severe burns and those with upper motor neuron disease are resistant to nondepolarizing muscle relaxants. This desensitization is probably caused by proliferation of extrajunctional receptors, which results in an increased dose requirement for the nondepolarizing relaxant to block a sufficient number of receptors.

Reversal of Nondepolarizing Neuromuscular Blockade

The cholinesterase inhibitors effectively antagonize the neuromuscular blockade caused by nondepolarizing drugs. Their general pharmacology is discussed in Chapter 7. **Neostigmine** and **pyridostigmine** antagonize nondepolarizing neuromuscular blockade by increasing the availability of acetylcholine at the motor end plate, mainly by inhibition of acetylcholinesterase. To a lesser extent, these cholinesterase inhibitors also increase release of transmitter from the motor nerve terminal. In contrast, edrophonium antagonizes neuromuscular blockade purely by inhibiting acetylcholinesterase. Edrophonium may be less effective than neostigmine in reversing the effects of nondepolarizing blockers in the presence of a profound degree of neuromuscular blockade. These differences are important in determining recovery from *residual block*, the neuromuscular blockade remaining after completion of surgery and movement of the patient to the recovery room. Unsuspected residual block may result in hypoventilation, leading to hypoxia and even apnea, especially if patients receive central depressant medications during the early recovery period.

Since mivacurium is metabolized by plasma cholinesterase, the interaction with the reversal drugs is less predictable. On the one hand, the neuromuscular blockade is antagonized because of increased acetylcholine concentrations in the synapse. On the other hand, mivacurium concentration may be higher because of decreased plasma cholinesterase breakdown of the muscle relaxant.

A novel cyclodextrin reversal drug, **sugammadex,** has been recently introduced. It can rapidly inactivate steroidal neuromuscular blocking drugs by forming an inactive complex, which is excreted in the urine. This chelation process allows the practitioner to rapidly reverse even profound degrees of neuromuscular blockade at the end of surgery.

Uses of Neuromuscular Blocking Drugs

A. Surgical Relaxation

By far the most important application of the neuromuscular blockers is in facilitating intracavitary surgery. This is especially important in intra-abdominal and intrathoracic procedures.

B. Tracheal Intubation

By relaxing the pharyngeal and laryngeal muscles, neuromuscular blocking drugs facilitate laryngoscopy and placement of the tracheal tube. Placement of a tracheal tube ensures an adequate airway and minimizes the risk of pulmonary aspiration during general anesthesia.

C. Control of Ventilation

In critically ill patients who have ventilatory failure from various causes (eg, severe bronchospasm, pneumonia, chronic obstructive airway disease), it may be necessary to control ventilation to provide adequate gas exchange and to prevent atelectasis. Muscle paralysis is produced by neuromuscular blocking drugs to reduce chest wall resistance (ie, improve thoracic compliance) and ineffective spontaneous ventilation.

D. Treatment of Convulsions

Neuromuscular blocking drugs are occasionally used to attenuate the peripheral manifestations of convulsions associated with status epilepticus or local anesthetic toxicity. Although this approach is effective in eliminating the muscular manifestations of the seizures, it has no effect on the central processes because neuromuscular blocking drugs do not cross the blood-brain barrier.

SPASMOLYTIC DRUGS

Spasticity is characterized by an increase in tonic stretch reflexes and flexor muscle spasms (ie, increased basal muscle tone) together with muscle weakness. It is often associated with cerebral palsy, multiple sclerosis, and stroke. These conditions often involve abnormal function of the bowel and bladder as well as skeletal muscle. The mechanisms underlying clinical spasticity appear to involve not only the stretch reflex arc itself but also higher centers in the central nervous system (ie, upper motor neuron lesion), with damage to descending pathways in the spinal cord resulting in hyperexcitability of the alpha motoneurons in the cord. Pharmacologic therapy may ameliorate some of the symptoms of spasticity by modifying the stretch reflex arc or by interfering directly with skeletal muscle (ie, excitation-contraction coupling). The important components involved in these processes are shown in Figure 27–10.

Drugs that modify this reflex arc may modulate excitatory or inhibitory synapses (see Chapter 21). Thus, to reduce the hyperactive stretch reflex, it is desirable to reduce the activity of the Ia fibers that excite the primary motoneuron or to enhance the activity of the inhibitory internuncial neurons. These structures are shown in greater detail in Figure 27–11.

A variety of pharmacologic agents described as depressants of the spinal "polysynaptic" reflex arc (eg, barbiturates [phenobarbital] and glycerol ethers [mephenesin]) have been used to treat these conditions of excess skeletal muscle tone. However, as illustrated in Figure 27–11, nonspecific depression of syn-

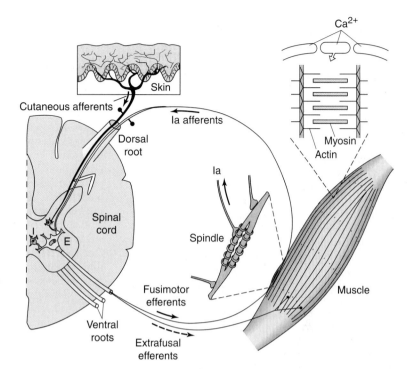

Figure 27–10. Diagram of the structures involved in the stretch reflex arc. *I* is an inhibitory interneuron; *E* indicates an excitatory presynaptic terminal; *Ia* is a primary intrafusal afferent fiber; Ca^{2+} denotes activator calcium stored in the sarcoplasmic reticulum of skeletal muscle. (Reproduced, with permission, from Young RR, Delwaide PJ: Drug therapy: Spasticity. N Engl J Med 1981;304:28.)

apses involved in the stretch reflex could reduce the desired inhibitory activity, as well as the excitatory transmission. Currently available drugs can provide significant relief from painful muscle spasms, but they are less effective in improving meaningful function (eg, mobility and return to work).

DIAZEPAM

As described in Chapter 22, benzodiazepines facilitate the action of γ-aminobutyric acid (GABA) in the central nervous system. Diazepam acts at $GABA_A$ synapses, and its action in reducing spasticity is at least partly mediated in the spinal cord because it is somewhat effective in patients with cord transection. Although diazepam can be used in patients with muscle spasm of almost any origin (including local muscle trauma), it produces sedation at the doses required to reduce muscle tone. The initial dosage is 4 mg/d, and it is gradually increased to a maximum of 60 mg/d. Other benzodiazepines have been used as spasmolytics (eg, midazolam), but clinical experience with them is limited.

BACLOFEN

Baclofen (*p*-chlorophenyl-GABA) was designed to be an orally active GABA-mimetic agent.

Baclofen exerts its spasmolytic activity at $GABA_B$ receptors. Activation of these receptors by baclofen results in hyperpolarization, probably by increased K^+ conductance. It has been suggested that hyperpolarization causes presynaptic inhibition by reducing calcium influx (Figure 27–11) and reduces the release of excitatory transmitters in both the brain and the spinal cord. Baclofen may also reduce pain in patients with spasticity, perhaps by inhibiting the release of substance P (neurokinin-1) in the spinal cord.

Baclofen

Baclofen is at least as effective as diazepam in reducing spasticity while producing less sedation. In addition, baclofen does not reduce overall muscle strength as much as dantrolene. It is rapidly and completely absorbed after oral administration and has a plasma half-life of 3–4 hours. Dosage is started at 15 mg twice daily, increasing as tolerated to 100 mg daily. Adverse effects of this drug include drowsiness; however, patients become tolerant to the sedative effect with chronic administration. Increased seizure activity has been reported in epileptic patients. Therefore, withdrawal from baclofen must be done very slowly.

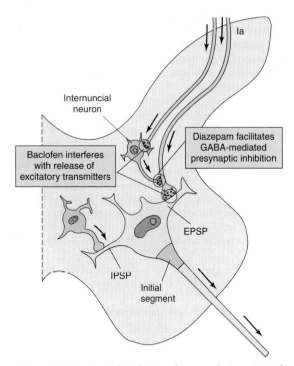

Figure 27–11. Postulated sites of spasmolytic action of diazepam and baclofen in the spinal cord. (Reproduced, with permission, from Young RR, Delwaide PJ: Drug therapy: Spasticity. N Engl J Med 1981;304:28.)

Studies have confirmed that intrathecal administration of baclofen can control severe spasticity and muscle pain that is not responsive to medication by other routes of administration. Owing to the poor egress of baclofen from the spinal cord, peripheral symptoms are rare. Therefore, higher central concentrations of the drug may be tolerated. Partial tolerance to the effect of the drug may occur after several months of therapy, but can be overcome by upward dosage adjustments to maintain the beneficial effect. Excessive somnolence, respiratory depression, and even coma have been described. Although a major disadvantage of this therapeutic approach is the difficulty of maintaining the drug delivery catheter in the subarachnoid space, long-term intrathecal baclofen therapy can improve the quality of life for patients with severe spastic disorders.

Oral baclofen has been studied in several other medical conditions. Preliminary studies suggest that it may be effective in reducing "craving" in recovering alcoholics (see Chapter 32). It has also been found to be effective in preventing migraine headaches in some patients.

TIZANIDINE

As noted in Chapter 11, α agonists such as clonidine and other imidazoline compounds have a variety of effects on the central nervous system that are not fully understood. Among these effects is the ability to reduce muscle spasm. Tizanidine is a congener of clonidine that has been studied for its spasmolytic actions. Tizanidine has significant α_2-adrenoceptor agonist effects, but it reduces spasticity in experimental models at doses that cause fewer cardiovascular effects than clonidine. Neurophysiologic studies in animals and humans suggest that tizanidine reinforces both presynaptic and postsynaptic inhibition in the cord. It also inhibits nociceptive transmission in the spinal dorsal horn.

Clinical trials with oral tizanidine report comparable efficacy in relieving muscle spasm to diazepam, baclofen, and dantrolene. However, tizanidine produces a different spectrum of adverse effects, including drowsiness, hypotension, dry mouth, and asthenia. The dosage requirements vary markedly among patients, suggesting that individual dosage titration is necessary to achieve an optimal clinical effect.

OTHER CENTRALLY ACTING SPASMOLYTIC DRUGS

Gabapentin is an antiepileptic drug (see Chapter 24) that has shown considerable promise as a spasmolytic agent in several studies involving patients with multiple sclerosis. Pregabalin is a new analog of gabapentin that may also prove useful. **Progabide** and **glycine** have also been found in preliminary studies to reduce spasticity. Progabide is a GABA$_A$ and GABA$_B$ agonist and has active metabolites, including GABA itself. **Glycine** is another inhibitory amino acid neurotransmitter (see Chapter 21). It appears to possess pharmacologic activity when given orally and readily passes the blood-brain barrier. **Idrocilamide** and **riluzole** are newer drugs for the treatment of amyotrophic lateral sclerosis that appear to have spasm-reducing effects, possibly through inhibition of glutamatergic transmission in the central nervous system.

DANTROLENE

Dantrolene is a hydantoin derivative related to phenytoin that has a unique mechanism of spasmolytic activity. In contrast to the centrally acting drugs, dantrolene reduces skeletal muscle strength by interfering with excitation-contraction coupling in the muscle fibers. The normal contractile response involves release of calcium from its stores in the sarcoplasmic reticulum (see Figures 13–2 and 27–10). This activator calcium brings about the tension-generating interaction of actin with myosin. Calcium is released from the sarcoplasmic reticulum via a calcium channel, called the **ryanodine** receptor (RyR) channel because the plant alkaloid ryanodine combines with a receptor on the channel protein. In the case of the skeletal muscle RyR channel, ryanodine facilitates the open configuration.

Dantrolene

Dantrolene interferes with the release of activator calcium through this sarcoplasmic reticulum calcium channel by binding to the RyR and blocking the opening of the channel. Motor units that contract rapidly are more sensitive to the drug's effects than are slower-responding units. Cardiac muscle and smooth muscle are minimally depressed because the release of calcium from their sarcoplasmic reticulum involves a different RyR channel.

Treatment with dantrolene is usually initiated with 25 mg daily as a single dose, increasing to a maximum of 100 mg four times daily as tolerated. Only about one third of an oral dose of dantrolene is absorbed, and the elimination half-life of the drug is approximately 8 hours. Major adverse effects are generalized muscle weakness, sedation, and occasionally hepatitis.

A special application of dantrolene is in the treatment of **malignant hyperthermia**, a rare heritable disorder that can be triggered by a variety of stimuli, including general anesthetics (eg, volatile anesthetics) and neuromuscular blocking drugs (eg, succinylcholine; see also Chapter 16). Patients at risk for this condition have a hereditary impairment in the ability of the sarcoplasmic reticulum to sequester calcium (Figure 27–10). After administration of one of the triggering agents, there is a sudden and prolonged release of calcium, with massive muscle contraction, lactic acid production, and increased body temperature. Prompt treatment is essential to control acidosis and body temperature and to reduce calcium release. The latter is accomplished with intravenous dantrolene, starting with a dose of 1 mg/kg IV, and repeating as necessary to a maximum dose of 10 mg/kg.

BOTULINUM TOXIN

The therapeutic use of botulinum toxin for ophthalmic purposes and for local muscle spasm was mentioned in Chapter 6. Local facial injections of botulinum toxin are widely used for the short-term treatment (1–3 months per treatment) of wrinkles around the eyes and mouth. Local injection of botulinum toxin has also become a useful treatment for generalized spastic disorders (eg, cerebral palsy). Most clinical studies to date have involved administration in one or two limbs, and the benefits appear to persist for weeks to several months after a single treatment. Most studies have used type A botulinum toxin, but type B is also available.

DRUGS USED TO TREAT ACUTE LOCAL MUSCLE SPASM

A large number of drugs (eg, **carisoprodol, chlorphenesin, chlorzoxazone, cyclobenzaprine, metaxalone, methocarbamol,** and **orphenadrine**) are promoted for the relief of acute muscle spasm caused by local tissue trauma or muscle strains. It has been suggested that these drugs act primarily at the level of the brainstem. Cyclobenzaprine may be regarded as the prototype of the group. Cyclobenzaprine is structurally related to the tricyclic antidepressants and possesses antimuscarinic effects. It is ineffective in treating muscle spasm due to cerebral palsy or spinal cord injury. The drug has strong antimuscarinic actions and may cause significant sedation, as well as confusion and transient visual hallucinations. The dosage of cyclobenzaprine for acute injury-related muscle spasm is 20–40 mg/d in divided doses.

Chapter continues on next page.

PREPARATIONS AVAILABLE

Neuromuscular Blocking Drugs

Atracurium (Tracrium)
Parenteral: 10 mg/mL for injection
Cisatracurium (Nimbex)
Parenteral: 2, 10 mg/mL for IV injection
Doxacurium (Nuromax)
Parenteral: 1 mg/mL for IV injection
Metocurine (generic, Metubine Iodide)
Parenteral: 2 mg/mL for injection
Mivacurium (Mivacron)
Parenteral: 0.5, 2 mg/mL for injection
Pancuronium (generic)
Parenteral: 1, 2 mg/mL for injection
Pipecuronium (Arduan)
Parenteral: powder for 1 mg/mL for IV injection
Rocuronium (Zemuron)
Parenteral: 10 mg/mL for IV injection
Succinylcholine (generic, Anectine)
Parenteral: 20, 50, 100 mg/mL for injection; 500, 1000 mg per vial powders to reconstitute for injection
Tubocurarine (generic)
Parenteral: 3 mg (20 units)/mL for injection
Vecuronium (generic, Norcuron)
Parenteral: 10, 20 mg powder to reconstitute for injection

Muscle Relaxants (Spasmolytics)

Baclofen (generic, Lioresal)
Oral: 10, 20 mg tablets
Intrathecal: 0.05, 0.5, 2 mg/mL
Botulinum toxin type A (Botox)
Parenteral: Powder for solution, 100 units/vial
Botulinum toxin type B (Myobloc)
Parenteral: 5000 units/mL for injection

Carisoprodol (generic, Soma)
Oral: 350 mg tablets
Chlorphenesin (Maolate)
Oral: 400 mg tablets
Chlorzoxazone (generic, Paraflex)
Oral: 250, 500 mg tablets, caplets
Cyclobenzaprine (generic, Flexeril)
Oral: 10 mg tablets
Dantrolene (Dantrium)
Oral: 25, 50, 100 mg capsules
Parenteral: 20 mg per vial powder to reconstitute for injection
Diazepam (generic, Valium)
Oral: 2, 5, 10 mg tablets; 5 mg/5 mL, 5 mg/mL solutions
Parenteral: 5 mg/mL for injection
Gabapentin (Neurontin)
Oral: 100, 300, 400 mg capsules; 600, 800 mg tablets; 50 mg/mL oral solution
Note: This drug is labeled for use only in epilepsy and postherpetic neuralgia
Metaxalone (Skelaxin)
Oral: 400 mg tablets
Methocarbamol (generic, Robaxin)
Oral: 500, 750 mg tablets
Parenteral: 100 mg/mL for IM, IV injection
Orphenadrine (generic, Norflex)
Oral: 100 mg tablets; 100 mg sustained-release tablets
Parenteral: 30 mg/mL for IM, IV injection
Riluzole (Rilutek)
Oral: 50 mg tablets
Note: This drug is labeled only for use in amyotrophic lateral sclerosis.
Tizanidine (Zanaflex)
Oral: 2, 4 mg tablets, capsules; 6 mg capsules

REFERENCES

Neuromuscular Blockers

Adt M, Baumert JH, Reimann HJ: The role of histamine in the cardiovascular effects of atracurium. Br J Anaesth 1992; 68:155.

Atherton DP, Hunter JM: Clinical pharmacokinetics of the newer neuromuscular blocking drugs. Clin Pharmacokinet 1999; 36:169.

Gibb AJ, Marshall IG: Pre- and postjunctional effects of tubocurarine and other nicotinic antagonists during repetitive stimulation in the rat. J Physiol 1984;351:275.

Jooste E et al: A mechanism for rapacuronium-induced bronchospasm. M2 muscarinic receptor antagonism. Anesthesiology 2003;98:906.

Kampe S et al: Muscle relaxants. Best Prac Res Clin Anesthesiol 2003;17:137.

Kaplan RF et al: The potency (ED$_{50}$) and cardiovascular effects of rapacuronium (ORG 9487) during narcotic-nitrous oxide-propofol anesthesia in neonates, infants, and children. Anesth Analg 1999;89:1172.

Kisor DF, Schmith VD: Clinical pharmacokinetics of cisatracurium besilate. Clin Pharmacokinet 1999;36:27.

Krause T et al: Dantrolene—a review of its pharmacology, therapeutic use and new developments. Anaesthesia 2004;59:364.

Lee C: Structure, conformation, and action of neuromuscular blocking drugs. Br J Anaesth 2001;87:755.

Marshall CG, Ogden DC, Colquhoun D: The actions of suxamethonium (succinyldicholine) as an agonist and channel blocker at the nicotinic receptor of frog muscle. J Physiol (Lond) 1990;428:155.

Meakin GH: Recent advances in myorelaxant therapy. Paed Anaesthesia 2001;11:523.

Moore EW, Hunter JM: The new neuromuscular blocking agents: Do they offer any advantages? Br J Anaesth 2001;87:912.

Naguib M et al: Advances in neurobiology of the neuromuscular junction: Implications for the anesthesiologist. Anesthesiology 2002;96:202.

Savarese JJ et al: Pharmacology of muscle relaxants and their antagonists. In: Miller RD (editor): *Anesthesia,* 5th ed. Churchill Livingstone, 2000.

Shields M et al: Org 25969 (sugammadex), a selective relaxant binding agent for antagonism of prolonged rocuronium-induced neuromuscular block. Br J Anaesth 2006;96:36.

Viby-Mogensen J: Neuromuscular monitoring. In: Miller RD (editor): *Anesthesia,* 5th ed. Churchill Livingstone, 2000.

White PF: Rapacuronium: Why did it fail as a replacement for succinylcholine? Br J Anaesth 2002;88:163.

Spasmolytics

Addolorato G et al: Ability of baclofen in reducing alcohol craving and intake: II. Preliminary clinical evidence. Alcohol Clin Exp Res 2000;24:67.

Albright AL, Cervi A, Singletary J: Intrathecal baclofen for spasticity in cerebral palsy. JAMA 1991;265:1418.

Cutter NC et al: Gabapentin effect on spasticity in multiple sclerosis: A placebo-controlled, randomized trial. Arch Phys Med Rehabil 2000;81:164.

Davidoff RA: Antispasticity drugs: Mechanisms of action. Ann Neurol 1985;17:107.

Groves L, Shellenberger MK, Davis CS: Tizanidine treatment of spasticity: A meta-analysis of controlled, double-blind, comparative studies with baclofen and diazepam. Adv Ther 1998;15:241.

Lopez JR et al: Effects of dantrolene on myoplasmic free [Ca^{2+}] measured in vivo in patients susceptible to malignant hyperthermia. Anesthesiology 1992;76:711.

Nolan KW, Cole LL, Liptak GS: Use of botulinum toxin type A in children with cerebral palsy. Phys Ther 2006;86:573.

Verrotti A et al: Pharmacotherapy of spasticity in children with cerebral palsy. Pediatr Neurol 2006;34:1.

Pharmacologic Management of Parkinsonism & Other Movement Disorders

Michael J. Aminoff, MD, DSc, FRCP

Several types of abnormal movement are recognized. **Tremor** consists of a rhythmic oscillatory movement around a joint and is best characterized by its relation to activity. Tremor at rest is characteristic of parkinsonism, when it is often associated with rigidity and an impairment of voluntary activity. Tremor may occur during maintenance of sustained posture (postural tremor) or during movement (intention tremor). A conspicuous postural tremor is the cardinal feature of benign essential or familial tremor. Intention tremor occurs in patients with a lesion of the brainstem or cerebellum, especially when the superior cerebellar peduncle is involved, and may also occur as a manifestation of toxicity from alcohol or certain other drugs.

Chorea consists of irregular, unpredictable, involuntary muscle jerks that occur in different parts of the body and impair voluntary activity. In some instances, the proximal muscles of the limbs are most severely affected, and because the abnormal movements are then particularly violent, the term *ballismus* has been used to describe them. Chorea may be hereditary or may occur as a complication of a number of general medical disorders and of therapy with certain drugs.

Abnormal movements may be slow and writhing in character **(athetosis)** and in some instances are so sustained that they are more properly regarded as abnormal postures **(dystonia).** Athetosis or dystonia may occur with perinatal brain damage, with focal or generalized cerebral lesions, as an acute complication of certain drugs, as an accompaniment of diverse neurologic disorders, or as an isolated inherited phenomenon of uncertain cause known as idiopathic torsion dystonia or dystonia musculorum deformans. Its physiologic basis is uncertain, and treatment is unsatisfactory.

Tics are sudden coordinated abnormal movements that tend to occur repetitively, particularly about the face and head, especially in children, and can be suppressed voluntarily for short periods of time. Common tics include repetitive sniffing or shoulder shrugging. Tics may be single or multiple and transient or chronic.

Gilles de la Tourette's syndrome is characterized by chronic multiple tics; its pharmacologic management is discussed at the end of this chapter.

Many of the movement disorders have been attributed to disturbances of the basal ganglia, but the precise function of these anatomic structures is not yet fully understood, and it is not possible to relate individual symptoms to involvement at specific sites.

■ PARKINSONISM (PARALYSIS AGITANS)

Parkinsonism is characterized by a combination of rigidity, bradykinesia, tremor, and postural instability that can occur for a variety of reasons but is usually idiopathic. The pathophysiologic basis of the idiopathic disorder may relate to exposure to some unrecognized neurotoxin or to the occurrence of oxidation reactions with the generation of free radicals. Studies in twins suggest that genetic factors may also be important, especially when the disease occurs in patients under age 50. Parkinson's disease is generally progressive, leading to increasing disability unless effective treatment is provided.

The normally high concentration of dopamine in the basal ganglia of the brain is reduced in parkinsonism, and pharmacologic attempts to restore dopaminergic activity with levodopa and dopamine agonists have been successful in alleviating many of the clinical features of the disorder. An alternative but complementary approach has been to restore the normal balance of cholinergic and dopaminergic influences on the basal ganglia with antimuscarinic drugs. The pathophysiologic basis for these therapies is that in idiopathic parkinsonism, dopaminergic neurons in the substantia nigra that normally inhibit the output of GABAergic cells in the corpus striatum are lost (Figure 28–1). (In

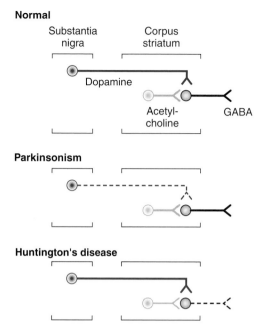

Figure 28–1. Schematic representation of the sequence of neurons involved in parkinsonism and Huntington's chorea. **Top:** Dopaminergic neurons (color) originating in the substantia nigra normally inhibit the GABAergic output from the striatum, whereas cholinergic neurons (gray) exert an excitatory effect. **Middle:** In parkinsonism, there is a selective loss of dopaminergic neurons (dashed, color). **Bottom:** In Huntington's chorea, some cholinergic neurons may be lost (gray), but even more GABAergic neurons (black) degenerate.

contrast, **Huntington's chorea** involves the loss of some cholinergic neurons and an even greater loss of the GABAergic cells that exit the corpus striatum.) Drugs that induce parkinsonian syndromes either are dopamine receptor antagonists (eg, antipsychotic agents; see Chapter 29) or lead to the destruction of the dopaminergic nigrostriatal neurons (eg, 1-methyl-4-phenyl-1,2,3,6-tetrahydropyridine [MPTP]; see below).

LEVODOPA

Dopamine does not cross the blood-brain barrier and if given into the peripheral circulation has no therapeutic effect in parkinsonism. However, (−)-3-(3,4-dihydroxyphenyl)-l-alanine (levodopa), the immediate metabolic precursor of dopamine, does enter the brain (via an L-amino acid transporter, LAT), where it is decarboxylated to dopamine (see Figure 6–5). Several noncatecholamine dopamine receptor agonists have also been developed and may lead to clinical benefit, as discussed below.

Dopamine receptors are discussed in detail in Chapters 21 and 29. Dopamine receptors of the D_1 type are located in the zona compacta of the substantia nigra and presynaptically on striatal axons coming from cortical neurons and from dopaminergic cells in the substantia nigra. The D_2 receptors are located postsynaptically on striatal neurons and presynaptically on axons in the substantia nigra belonging to neurons in the basal ganglia. The benefits of dopaminergic antiparkinsonism drugs appear to depend mostly on stimulation of the D_2 receptors, but D_1-receptor stimulation may also be required for maximal benefit and one of the newer drugs is D_3-selective. Dopamine agonist or partial agonist ergot derivatives such as lergotrile and bromocriptine that are powerful stimulators of the D_2 receptors have antiparkinsonism properties, whereas certain dopamine blockers that are selective D_2 antagonists can induce parkinsonism.

Chemistry

As discussed in Chapter 6, dopa is the amino acid precursor of dopamine and norepinephrine. Its structure is shown in Figure 28–2. Levodopa is the levorotatory stereoisomer of dopa.

Pharmacokinetics

Levodopa is rapidly absorbed from the small intestine, but its absorption depends on the rate of gastric emptying and the pH of the gastric contents. Ingestion of food delays the appearance of levodopa in the plasma. Moreover, certain amino acids from ingested food can compete with the drug for absorption from the gut and for transport from the blood to the brain. Plasma concentrations usually peak between 1 and 2 hours after an oral dose, and the plasma half-life is usually between 1 and 3 hours, although it varies considerably among individuals. About two thirds of the dose appears in the urine as metabolites within 8 hours of an oral dose, the main metabolic products being 3-methoxy-4-hydroxyphenyl acetic acid (homovanillic acid, HVA) and dihydroxyphenylacetic acid (DOPAC). Unfortunately, only about 1–3% of administered levodopa actually enters the brain unaltered; the remainder is metabolized extracerebrally, predominantly by decarboxylation to dopamine, which does not penetrate the blood-brain barrier. This means that levodopa must be given in large amounts when it is used alone. However, when it is given in combination with a dopa decarboxylase inhibitor that does not penetrate the blood-brain barrier, the peripheral metabolism of levodopa is reduced, plasma levels of levodopa are higher, plasma half-life is longer, and more dopa is available for entry into the brain (Figure 28–3). Indeed, concomitant administration of a peripheral dopa decarboxylase inhibitor such as carbi-

HO—

CH_2—CH—$COOH$
|
NH_2

**Dihydroxyphenylalanine
(dopa)**

CH_3
|
CH_2—C—$COOH$
|
NH—NH_2

Carbidopa

CH_3
|
CH_2—CH—N—CH_2—$C \equiv CH$
|
CH_3

Selegiline

$C \equiv N$
|
O_2N— $CH = C$—C—N
$\parallel$ CH_2CH_3
O CH_2CH_3

HO

OH

Entacapone

Figure 28–2. Some drugs used in the treatment of parkinsonism.

dopa may reduce the daily requirements of levodopa by approximately 75%.

Clinical Use

The best results of levodopa treatment are obtained in the first few years of treatment. This is sometimes because the daily dose of levodopa must be reduced over time to avoid side effects at doses that were well tolerated at the outset. Some patients also become less responsive to levodopa, so that previously effective doses eventually fail to produce any therapeutic benefit. Responsiveness to levodopa may ultimately be lost completely, perhaps because of the disappearance of dopaminergic nigrostriatal nerve terminals or some pathologic process directly involving the striatal dopamine receptors. For such reasons, the benefits of levo-

dopa treatment often begin to diminish after about 3 or 4 years of therapy regardless of the initial therapeutic response. Although levodopa therapy does not stop the progression of parkinsonism, its early initiation lowers the mortality rate. However, long-term therapy may lead to a number of problems in management such as the on-off phenomenon discussed below. The most appropriate time to introduce levodopa therapy must therefore be determined individually.

When levodopa is used, it is generally given in combination with carbidopa (Figure 28–2), a peripheral dopa decarboxylase inhibitor, which reduces peripheral conversion to dopamine. **Sinemet** treatment is started with a small dose, eg, Sinemet-25/100 (carbidopa 25 mg, levodopa 100 mg) three times daily, and gradually increased. It should be taken 30–60 minutes before meals. Most patients ultimately require Sinemet-25/250 (carbidopa 25 mg, levodopa 250 mg) three or four times daily. It is generally preferable to keep treatment with this agent at a low level (eg, Sinemet-25/100 three times daily) and to increase dopaminergic therapy by the addition of a dopamine agonist, if necessary, to reduce the risk of development of response fluctuations. A controlled-release formulation of Sinemet is available and may be helpful in patients with established response fluctuations or as a means of reducing dosing frequency. A commercially available combination (Stalevo) of levodopa, carbidopa, and a catechol-*O*-methyltransferase (COMT) inhibitor (entacapone) is discussed in a later section.

Levodopa can ameliorate all of the clinical features of parkinsonism, but it is particularly effective in relieving bradykinesia and any disabilities resulting from it. When it is first introduced, about one third of patients respond very well and one third less well. Most of the remainder either are unable to tolerate the medication or simply do not respond at all.

Adverse Effects

A. GASTROINTESTINAL EFFECTS

When levodopa is given without a peripheral decarboxylase inhibitor, anorexia and nausea and vomiting occur in about 80% of patients. These adverse effects can be minimized by taking the drug in divided doses, with or immediately after meals, and by increasing the total daily dose very slowly; antacids taken 30–60 minutes before levodopa may also be beneficial. The vomiting has been attributed to stimulation of the chemoreceptor trigger zone located in the brainstem but outside the blood-brain barrier. Fortunately, tolerance to this emetic effect develops in many patients. Antiemetics such as phenothiazines should be avoided because they reduce the antiparkinsonism effects of levodopa and may exacerbate the disease.

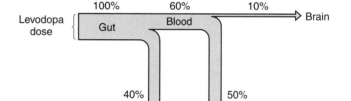

Figure 28–3. Fate of orally administered levodopa and the effect of carbidopa, estimated from animal data. The width of each pathway indicates the absolute amount of the drug at each site, whereas the percentages shown denote the relative proportion of the administered dose. The benefits of coadministration of carbidopa include reduction of the amount of levodopa diverted to peripheral tissues and an increase in the fraction of the dose that reaches the brain. (GI, gastrointestinal.) (Data from Nutt JG, Fellman JH: Pharmacokinetics of levodopa. Clin Neuropharmacol 1984;7:35.)

When levodopa is given in combination with carbidopa, adverse gastrointestinal effects are much less frequent and troublesome, occurring in less than 20% of cases, so that patients can tolerate proportionately higher doses.

B. CARDIOVASCULAR EFFECTS

A variety of cardiac arrhythmias have been described in patients receiving levodopa, including tachycardia, ventricular extrasystoles and, rarely, atrial fibrillation. This effect has been attributed to increased catecholamine formation peripherally. The incidence of such arrhythmias is low, even in the presence of established cardiac disease, and may be reduced still further if the levodopa is taken in combination with a peripheral decarboxylase inhibitor.

Postural hypotension is common, but often asymptomatic, and tends to diminish with continuing treatment. Hypertension may also occur, especially in the presence of nonselective monoamine oxidase inhibitors or sympathomimetics or when massive doses of levodopa are being taken.

C. DYSKINESIAS

Dyskinesias occur in up to 80% of patients receiving levodopa therapy for long periods. The form and nature of dopa dyskinesias vary widely among patients but tend to remain constant in character in individual patients. Choreoathetosis of the face and distal extremities is the most common presentation. The development of dyskinesias is dose-related, but there is considerable individual variation in the dose required to produce them.

D. BEHAVIORAL EFFECTS

A wide variety of adverse mental effects have been reported, including depression, anxiety, agitation, insomnia, somnolence, confusion, delusions, hallucinations, nightmares, euphoria, and other changes in mood or personality. Such adverse effects are more common in patients taking levodopa in combination with a decarboxylase inhibitor rather than levodopa alone, presumably because higher levels are reached in the brain. They may be precipitated by intercurrent illness or operation. It may be necessary to reduce or withdraw the medication. Several atypical antipsychotic agents (clozapine, olanzapine, quetiapine, and risperidone; see Chapter 29) are now available and may be particularly helpful in counteracting the behavioral complications of levodopa.

E. FLUCTUATIONS IN RESPONSE

Certain fluctuations in clinical response to levodopa occur with increasing frequency as treatment continues. In some patients, these fluctuations relate to the timing of levodopa intake, and they are then referred to as wearing-off reactions or end-of-dose akinesia. In other instances, fluctuations in clinical state are unrelated to the timing of doses (**on-off phenomenon**). In the on-off phenomenon, off-periods of marked akinesia alternate over the course of a few hours with on-periods of improved mobility but often marked dyskinesia. The phenomenon is most likely to occur in patients who responded well to treatment initially. The exact mechanism is unknown. For patients with severe off-periods who are unresponsive to other measures, subcutaneously injected apomorphine may provide temporary benefit.

F. MISCELLANEOUS ADVERSE EFFECTS

Mydriasis may occur and may precipitate an attack of acute glaucoma in some patients. Other reported but rare adverse effects include various blood dyscrasias; a positive Coombs test with evidence of hemolysis; hot flushes; aggravation or precipitation of gout; abnormalities of smell or taste; brownish discoloration of saliva, urine, or vaginal secretions; priapism; and mild—usually transient—elevations of blood urea nitrogen and of serum transaminases, alkaline phosphatase, and bilirubin.

Drug Holidays

A drug holiday (discontinuance of the drug for 3–21 days) may temporarily improve responsiveness to levodopa and alleviate some of its adverse effects but is usually of little help in the management of the on-off phenomenon. Furthermore, a drug holiday carries the risks of aspiration pneumonia, venous thrombosis, pulmonary embolism, and depression resulting from the immobility accompanying severe parkinsonism. For these reasons and because of the tempo-

rary nature of any benefit, drug holidays are no longer recommended.

Drug Interactions

Pharmacologic doses of pyridoxine (vitamin B_6) enhance the extracerebral metabolism of levodopa and may therefore prevent its therapeutic effect unless a peripheral decarboxylase inhibitor is also taken. Levodopa should not be given to patients taking monoamine oxidase A inhibitors or within 2 weeks of their discontinuance, because such a combination can lead to hypertensive crises.

Contraindications

Levodopa should not be given to psychotic patients because it may exacerbate the mental disturbance. It is also contraindicated in patients with angle-closure glaucoma, but those with chronic open-angle glaucoma may be given levodopa if intraocular pressure is well controlled and can be monitored. It is best given combined with carbidopa to patients with cardiac disease; even so, the risk of cardiac dysrhythmia is slight. Patients with active peptic ulcer must also be managed carefully, since gastrointestinal bleeding has occasionally occurred with levodopa. Because levodopa is a precursor of skin melanin and conceivably may activate malignant melanoma, its use should be avoided in patients with a history of melanoma or with suspicious undiagnosed skin lesions.

DOPAMINE RECEPTOR AGONISTS

Drugs acting directly on dopamine receptors may have a beneficial effect in addition to that of levodopa. Unlike levodopa, they do not require enzymatic conversion to an active metabolite, have no potentially toxic metabolites, and do not compete with other substances for active transport into the blood and across the blood-brain barrier. Moreover, drugs selectively affecting certain (but not all) dopamine receptors may have more limited adverse effects than levodopa. A number of dopamine agonists have antiparkinsonism activity. The older dopamine agonists (bromocriptine and pergolide) are ergot (ergoline) derivatives (see Chapter 16), and their side effects are of more concern than those of the newer agents (pramipexole and ropinirole). There is no evidence that one agonist is superior to another; individual patients, however, may respond to one but not another of these agents. Apomorphine is a potent dopamine agonist but is discussed separately in a later section in this chapter because it is used primarily as a rescue drug for patients with disabling response fluctuations to levodopa.

Dopamine agonists have an important role as first-line therapy for Parkinson's disease, and their use is associated with a lower incidence of the response fluctuations and dyskinesias that occur with long-term levodopa therapy. In consequence, dopaminergic therapy may best be initiated with a dopamine agonist. Alternatively, a low dose of carbidopa plus levodopa (eg, Sinemet-25/100 three times daily) is introduced and a dopamine agonist is then added. In either case, the dose of the dopamine agonist is built up gradually depending on response and tolerance. Dopamine agonists may also be given to patients with parkinsonism who are taking levodopa and who have end-of-dose akinesia or on-off phenomenon or are becoming resistant to treatment with levodopa. In such circumstances, it is generally necessary to lower the dose of levodopa to prevent intolerable adverse effects. The response to a dopamine agonist is generally disappointing in patients who have never responded to levodopa.

Bromocriptine

Bromocriptine is a D_2 agonist; its structure is shown in Table 16–4. This drug has been widely used to treat Parkinson's disease and has also been used to treat certain endocrinologic disorders, especially hyperprolactinemia (see Chapter 37), but in lower doses than for parkinsonism. Bromocriptine is absorbed to a variable extent from the gastrointestinal tract; peak plasma levels are reached within 1–2 hours after an oral dose. It is excreted in the bile and feces. The usual daily dose of bromocriptine in the treatment of parkinsonism is between 7.5 and 30 mg, depending on response and tolerance. To minimize adverse effects, the dose is built up slowly over 2 or 3 months from a starting level of 1.25 mg twice daily after meals; the daily dose is then increased by 2.5 mg every 2 weeks depending on the response or the development of adverse reactions.

Pergolide

Pergolide, another ergot derivative, directly stimulates both D_1 and D_2 receptors. It too has been widely used for parkinsonism, and comparative studies suggest that it is more effective than bromocriptine in relieving the symptoms and signs of the disease, increasing "on-time" among response fluctuators, and permitting the levodopa dose to be reduced. Because the use of pergolide has recently been associated with clinical or subclinical valvular heart disease in about one third of patients, one of the newer non-ergot agents is preferred when a dopamine agonist is required.

Pramipexole

Pramipexole, which is not an ergot derivative, has preferential affinity for the D_3 family of receptors. It is effective when used as monotherapy for mild parkinsonism. It is also helpful in patients with advanced disease, permitting the dose of levodopa to be reduced and smoothing out response fluctuations. It may ameliorate affective symptoms. A possible neuroprotective effect has been suggested by its ability to scavenge hydrogen peroxide and enhance neurotrophic activity in mesencephalic dopaminergic cell cultures.

Pramipexole

Pramipexole is rapidly absorbed after oral administration, reaching peak plasma concentrations in approximately 2 hours, and is excreted largely unchanged in the urine. It is started at a dosage of 0.125 mg three times daily, doubled after 1 week, and again after another week. Further increments in the daily dose are by 0.75 mg at weekly intervals, depending on response and tolerance. Most patients require between 0.5 and 1.5 mg three times daily. Renal insufficiency may necessitate dosage adjustment.

Ropinirole

Another nonergoline derivative, ropinirole is a relatively pure D_2 receptor agonist that is effective as monotherapy in patients with mild disease and as a means of smoothing the response to levodopa in patients with more advanced disease and response fluctuations. It is introduced at 0.25 mg three times daily, and the total daily dose is then increased by 0.75 mg at weekly intervals until the fourth week and by 1.5 mg thereafter. In most instances, a dose of between 2 and 8 mg three times daily is necessary. Ropinirole is metabolized by CYP1A2; other drugs metabolized by this isoform may significantly reduce its clearance.

Ropinirole

Adverse Effects of Dopamine Agonists

A. GASTROINTESTINAL EFFECTS

Anorexia and nausea and vomiting may occur when a dopamine agonist is introduced and can be minimized by taking the medication with meals. Constipation, dyspepsia, and symptoms of reflux esophagitis may also occur. Bleeding from peptic ulceration has been reported.

B. Cardiovascular Effects

Postural hypotension may occur, particularly at the initiation of therapy. Painless digital vasospasm is a dose-related complication of long-term treatment with the ergot derivatives (bromocriptine or pergolide). When cardiac arrhythmias occur, they are an indication for discontinuing treatment. Peripheral edema is sometimes problematic. Cardiac valvulopathy may occur with pergolide.

C. Dyskinesias

Abnormal movements similar to those introduced by levodopa may occur and are reversed by reducing the total dose of dopaminergic drugs being taken.

D. Mental Disturbances

Confusion, hallucinations, delusions, and other psychiatric reactions are other complications of dopaminergic treatment and are more common and severe with dopamine receptor agonists than with levodopa. They clear on withdrawal of the offending medication.

E. Miscellaneous

Headache, nasal congestion, increased arousal, pulmonary infiltrates, pleural and retroperitoneal fibrosis, and erythromelalgia are other reported side effects of the ergot-derived dopamine agonists. Erythromelalgia consists of red, tender, painful, swollen feet and, occasionally, hands, at times associated with arthralgia; symptoms and signs clear within a few days of withdrawal of the causal drug. In rare instances, an uncontrollable tendency to fall asleep at inappropriate times has occurred, particularly in patients receiving pramipexole or ropinirole, requiring the discontinuation of medication.

Contraindications

Dopamine agonists are contraindicated in patients with a history of psychotic illness or recent myocardial infarction, or with active peptic ulceration. The ergot-derived agonists are best avoided in patients with peripheral vascular disease.

MONOAMINE OXIDASE INHIBITORS

Two types of monoamine oxidase have been distinguished in the nervous system. Monoamine oxidase A metabolizes norepinephrine and serotonin; monoamine oxidase B metabolizes dopamine. **Selegiline**

(deprenyl) (Figure 28–2), a selective irreversible inhibitor of monoamine oxidase B at normal doses (at higher doses it inhibits MAO-A as well), retards the breakdown of dopamine; in consequence, it enhances and prolongs the antiparkinsonism effect of levodopa (thereby allowing the dose of levodopa to be reduced) and may reduce mild on-off or wearing-off phenomena. It is therefore used as adjunctive therapy for patients with a declining or fluctuating response to levodopa. The standard dose of selegiline is 5 mg with breakfast and 5 mg with lunch. Selegiline may cause insomnia when taken later during the day. It should not be taken by patients receiving meperidine, tricyclic antidepressants, or serotonin reuptake inhibitors because of the risk of acute toxic interactions of the serotonin syndrome type (see Chapter 16). The adverse effects of levodopa may be increased by selegiline.

Selegiline has only a minor therapeutic effect on parkinsonism when given alone, but studies in animals suggest that it may reduce disease progression. Such an effect of antioxidative therapy on disease progression may be expected if Parkinson's disease is associated with the oxidative generation of free radicals. However, any neuroprotective effect of selegiline may relate to its metabolite, desmethylselegiline, and involve antiapoptotic mechanisms. Studies to test the effect of selegiline on the progression of parkinsonism in humans have yielded ambiguous results. The findings in a large multicenter study have been taken to suggest a beneficial effect in slowing disease progression but may simply have reflected a symptomatic response.

Rasagiline, another monoamine oxidase B inhibitor, is more potent than selegiline in preventing MPTP-induced parkinsonism and is being used as a neuroprotective agent and for early symptomatic treatment. The standard dose is 0.5 mg/d.

The combined administration of levodopa and an inhibitor of both forms of monoamine oxidase must be avoided, because it may lead to hypertensive crises, probably because of the peripheral accumulation of norepinephrine.

CATECHOL-O-METHYLTRANSFERASE INHIBITORS

Inhibition of dopa decarboxylase is associated with compensatory activation of other pathways of levodopa metabolism, especially catechol-O-methyltransferase (COMT), and this increases plasma levels of 3-O-methyldopa (3OMD). Elevated levels of 3OMD have been associated with a poor therapeutic response to levodopa, perhaps in part because 3OMD competes with levodopa for an active carrier mechanism that governs its transport across the intestinal mucosa and the blood-brain barrier. Selective COMT inhibitors such as **tolcapone** and **entacapone** also prolong the action of levodopa by diminishing its peripheral metabolism. Levodopa clearance is decreased, and relative bioavailability of levodopa is thus increased. Neither the time to reach peak concentration nor the maximal concentration of levodopa is increased. These agents may be helpful in patients receiving levodopa who have developed response fluctuations—leading to a smoother response, more prolonged "on-time," and the option of reducing total daily levodopa dose. Tolcapone and entacapone are both widely available, but entacapone is generally preferred because it has not been associated with hepatotoxicity.

The pharmacologic effects of tolcapone and entacapone are similar, and both are rapidly absorbed, bound to plasma proteins, and metabolized prior to excretion. However, tolcapone has both central and peripheral effects, whereas the effect of entacapone is peripheral. The half-life of both drugs is approximately 2 hours, but tolcapone is slightly more potent and has a longer duration of action. Tolcapone is taken in a standard dosage of 100 mg three times daily; some patients require a daily dose of twice that amount. By contrast, entacapone (200 mg) needs to be taken with each dose of levodopa, up to five times daily.

Adverse effects of the COMT inhibitors relate in part to increased levodopa exposure and include dyskinesias, nausea, and confusion. It is often necessary to lower the daily dose of levodopa by about 30% in the first 48 hours to avoid or reverse such complications. Other side effects include diarrhea, abdominal pain, orthostatic hypotension, sleep disturbances, and an orange discoloration of the urine. Tolcapone may cause an increase in liver enzyme levels and has been rarely associated with death from acute hepatic failure; accordingly, its use in the USA requires signed patient consent (as provided in the product labeling) plus monitoring of liver function tests every 2 weeks during the first year and less frequently thereafter. No such toxicity has been reported with entacapone.

A commercial preparation named **Stalevo** consists of a combination of levodopa with both carbidopa and entacapone. Use of this preparation simplifies the drug regimen and requires the consumption of a lesser number of tablets than otherwise; Stalevo is priced at or below the price of its individual components.

APOMORPHINE

Subcutaneous injection of apomorphine hydrochloride (Apokyn), a potent dopamine agonist, is effective for the temporary relief of off-periods of akinesia in patients on dopaminergic therapy. It is rapidly taken up in the blood and then the brain, leading to clinical benefit that begins within about 10 minutes of injection and persists for up to 2 hours. The optimal dose is identified by administering increasing test doses until adequate benefit is achieved or a maximum of 10 mg is reached. Most patients require a dose of 3–6 mg, and this should be given no more than about three times daily.

Nausea is often troublesome, especially at the initiation of apomorphine treatment; accordingly, pretreatment with the antiemetic trimethobenzamide (300 mg three times daily) for 3 days is recommended before apomorphine is introduced and is then continued for at least 1 month, if not indefinitely. Other adverse effects include dyskinesias, drowsiness, sweating, hypotension, and bruising at the injection site.

AMANTADINE

Amantadine, an antiviral agent, was by chance found to have antiparkinsonism properties. Its mode of action in parkinsonism is unclear, but it may potentiate dopaminergic function by influencing the synthesis, release, or reuptake of dopamine. Release of catecholamines from peripheral stores has been documented.

Pharmacokinetics

Peak plasma concentrations of amantadine are reached 1–4 hours after an oral dose. The plasma half-life is between 2 and 4 hours, most of the drug being excreted unchanged in the urine.

Clinical Use

Amantadine is less potent than levodopa, and its benefits may be short-lived, often disappearing after only a few weeks of treatment. Nevertheless, during that time it may favorably influence the bradykinesia, rigidity, and tremor of parkinsonism. The standard dosage is 100 mg orally twice or three times daily. Amantadine may also help in reducing iatrogenic dyskinesias in patients with advanced disease.

Adverse Effects

Amantadine has a number of undesirable central nervous system effects, all of which can be reversed by stopping the drug. These include restlessness, depression, irritability, insomnia, agitation, excitement, hallucinations, and confusion. Overdosage may produce an acute toxic psychosis. With doses several times higher than recommended, convulsions have occurred.

Livedo reticularis sometimes occurs in patients taking amantadine and usually clears within a month after the drug is withdrawn. Other dermatologic reactions have also been described. Peripheral edema, another well-recognized complication, is not accompanied by signs of cardiac, hepatic, or renal disease and responds

Table 28–1. Some drugs with antimuscarinic properties used in parkinsonism.

Drug	Usual Daily Dose (mg)
Benztropine mesylate	1–6
Biperiden	2–12
Orphenadrine	150–400
Procyclidine	7.5–30
Trihexyphenidyl	6–20

to diuretics. Other adverse reactions include headache, heart failure, postural hypotension, urinary retention, and gastrointestinal disturbances (eg, anorexia, nausea, constipation, and dry mouth).

Amantadine should be used with caution in patients with a history of seizures or heart failure.

ACETYLCHOLINE-BLOCKING DRUGS

A number of centrally acting antimuscarinic preparations are available that differ in their potency and in their efficacy in different patients. Some of these drugs were discussed in Chapter 8. These agents may improve the tremor and rigidity of parkinsonism but have little effect on bradykinesia. Some of the more commonly used drugs are listed in Table 28–1.

Clinical Use

Treatment is started with a low dose of one of the drugs in this category, the level of medication gradually being increased until benefit occurs or adverse effects limit further increments. If patients do not respond to one drug, a trial with another member of the drug class is warranted and may be successful.

Adverse Effects

Antimuscarinic drugs have a number of undesirable central nervous system and peripheral effects (see Chapter 8). Dyskinesias occur in rare cases. Acute suppurative parotitis sometimes occurs as a complication of dryness of the mouth.

If medication is to be withdrawn, this should be accomplished gradually rather than abruptly to prevent acute exacerbation of parkinsonism. For contraindications to their use, see Chapter 8.

SURGICAL PROCEDURES

In patients with advanced disease that is poorly responsive to pharmacotherapy, worthwhile benefit may fol-

low thalamotomy (for conspicuous tremor) or postero-ventral pallidotomy. Ablative surgical procedures, however, are being replaced by functional, reversible lesions induced by high-frequency deep-brain stimulation, which has a lower morbidity.

Thalamic stimulation by an implanted electrode and stimulator is very effective for the relief of tremor, and stimulation of the subthalamic nucleus or globus pallidus internus has yielded good results for management of the clinical fluctuation occurring in advanced parkinsonism. The anatomic substrate for such therapy is indicated in Figure 28–4. Such procedures are contraindicated in patients with secondary or atypical parkinsonism.

Transplantation of dopaminergic tissue (fetal substantia nigra tissue) has been reported to confer benefit in some parkinsonism patients, but the results are conflicting. In one controlled trial, symptomatic benefit occurred in younger (less than 60 years old) but not older patients. In another trial, benefits were inconsequential. Further-

Figure 28–4. Functional circuitry between the cortex, basal ganglia, and thalamus. The involved neurotransmitters are indicated. In Parkinson's disease, there is degeneration of the pars compacta of the substantia nigra, leading to overactivity in the indirect pathway (color) and increased glutamatergic activity by the subthalamic nucleus.

more, uncontrollable dyskinesias occurred in some patients in both studies. This was attributed to a relative excess of dopamine from continued fiber outgrowth from the transplant. Further basic studies are required before other trials of cellular therapies are undertaken, and such approaches therefore remain investigational.

NEUROPROTECTIVE THERAPY

A number of different compounds are under investigation as potential neuroprotective agents that may slow disease progression. These compounds include antioxidants, antiapoptotic agents, glutamate antagonists, intraparenchymally administered glial-derived neurotrophic factor, coenzyme Q10, creatine, and anti-inflammatory drugs. The role of these agents remains to be established, however, and their use for therapeutic purposes is not indicated at this time.

GENERAL COMMENTS ON DRUG MANAGEMENT OF PATIENTS WITH PARKINSONISM

Parkinson's disease generally follows a progressive course. Moreover, the benefits of levodopa therapy often diminish with time, and serious adverse effects may complicate long-term levodopa treatment. Nevertheless, dopaminergic therapy at a relatively early stage may be most effective in alleviating symptoms of parkinsonism and may also favorably affect the mortality rate due to the disease. Symptomatic treatment of mild parkinsonism is probably best avoided until there is some degree of disability or until symptoms begin to have a significant impact on the patient's lifestyle. When treatment becomes necessary, a trial of amantadine or an antimuscarinic drug (or both) may be worthwhile. With disease progression, dopaminergic therapy becomes necessary. This can conveniently be initiated with a dopamine agonist, either alone or in combination with low-dose Sinemet therapy. Physical therapy is helpful in improving mobility. In patients with severe parkinsonism and long-term complications of levodopa therapy such as the on-off phenomenon, a trial of treatment with a COMT inhibitor may be worthwhile. Regulation of dietary protein intake may also improve response fluctuations. Deep-brain stimulation may be helpful in patients who fail to respond adequately to these measures. Treating patients who are young or have mild parkinsonism with selegiline or rasagiline may delay disease progression and merits consideration.

DRUG-INDUCED PARKINSONISM

Reserpine and the related drug tetrabenazine deplete biogenic monoamines from their storage sites, whereas haloperidol and the phenothiazines block dopamine receptors. These drugs may therefore produce a parkinsonian syndrome, usually within 3 months after introduction. This is related to high dosage and clears over a few weeks or months after withdrawal. If treatment is necessary, antimuscarinic agents are preferred. Levodopa is of no help if neuroleptic drugs are continued and may in fact aggravate the mental disorder for which antipsychotic drugs were prescribed originally.

In 1983, a drug-induced form of parkinsonism was discovered in individuals who attempted to synthesize and use a narcotic drug related to meperidine but actually synthesized and self-administered MPTP, as discussed in the Box: MPTP & Parkinsonism.

MPTP & PARKINSONISM

Reports in the early 1980s of a rapidly progressive form of parkinsonism in young persons opened a new area of research in the etiology and treatment of parkinsonism. The initial report described apparently healthy young people who attempted to support their opioid habit with a meperidine analog synthesized by an amateur chemist. They unwittingly self-administered 1-methyl-4-phenyl-1,2,3,6-tetrahydropyridine (MPTP) and subsequently developed a very severe form of parkinsonism.

MPTP is a protoxin that is converted by monoamine oxidase B to N-methyl-4-phenylpyridinium (MPP+). MPP+ is selectively taken up by cells in the substantia nigra through an active mechanism normally responsible for dopamine reuptake. MPP+ inhibits mitochondrial complex I, thereby inhibiting oxidative phosphorylation. The interaction of MPP+ with complex I probably leads to cell death and thus to striatal dopamine depletion and parkinsonism.

Recognition of the effects of MPTP suggested that spontaneously occurring Parkinson's disease may result from exposure to an environmental toxin that is similarly selective in its target. However, no such toxin has yet been identified. It also suggested a successful means of producing an experimental model of Parkinson's disease in animals, especially nonhuman primates. This model is assisting in the development of new antiparkinsonism drugs. Pretreatment of exposed animals with a monoamine oxidase B inhibitor such as selegiline prevents the conversion of MPTP to MPP+ and thus protects against the occurrence of parkinsonism. This observation has provided one reason to believe that selegiline or rasagiline may retard the progression of Parkinson's disease in humans.

■ OTHER MOVEMENT DISORDERS

Tremor

Tremor consists of rhythmic oscillatory movements. Physiologic postural tremor, which is a normal phenomenon, is enhanced in amplitude by anxiety, fatigue, thyrotoxicosis, and intravenous epinephrine or isoproterenol. Propranolol reduces its amplitude and, if administered intra-arterially, prevents the response to isoproterenol in the perfused limb, presumably through some peripheral action. Certain drugs—especially the bronchodilators, valproate, tricyclic antidepressants, and lithium—may produce a dose-dependent exaggeration of the normal physiologic tremor that is reversed by discontinuing the drug. Although the tremor produced by sympathomimetics such as terbutaline (a bronchodilator) is blocked by propranolol, which antagonizes both β_1 and β_2 receptors, it is not blocked by metoprolol, a β_1-selective antagonist; this suggests that such tremor is mediated mainly by the β_2 receptors.

Essential tremor is a postural tremor, sometimes familial, which is clinically similar to physiologic tremor. Dysfunction of β_1 receptors has been implicated in some instances, since the tremor may respond dramatically to standard doses of metoprolol as well as to propranolol. The most useful approach is with propranolol, but whether the response depends on a central or peripheral action is unclear. The pharmacokinetics, pharmacologic effects, and adverse reactions of propranolol are discussed in Chapter 10. Daily doses of propranolol on the order of 120 mg (range, 60–240 mg) are usually required, and reported adverse effects have been few. Propranolol should be used with caution in patients with heart failure, heart block, asthma, and hypoglycemia. Patients can be instructed to take their own pulse and call the physician if significant bradycardia develops. Metoprolol is sometimes useful in treating tremor when patients have concomitant pulmonary disease that contraindicates use of propranolol. Primidone (an antiepileptic drug; see Chapter 24), in gradually increasing doses up to 250 mg three times daily, is also effective in providing symptomatic control in some cases. Patients with tremor are very sensitive to primidone and often cannot tolerate the doses used to treat seizures; they should be started on 50 mg once daily and the daily dose increased by 50 mg every 2 weeks depending on response. Topiramate, another antiepileptic drug, may also be helpful in a dose of 400 mg daily, built up gradually. Small quantities of alcohol may suppress essential tremor but only for a short time and by an unknown mechanism. Alprazolam (in doses up to 3 mg daily) is

helpful in some patients. Others are helped by intramuscular injections of botulinum toxin. Thalamic stimulation (discussed earlier) is often worthwhile in advanced cases refractory to pharmacotherapy. Diazepam, chlordiazepoxide, mephenesin, and antiparkinsonism agents have been advocated in the past but are generally worthless. Anecdotal reports of benefit from mirtazapine were not confirmed in a double-blind study, which found no effect on the tremor in most patients.

Intention tremor is present during movement but not at rest; sometimes it occurs as a toxic manifestation of alcohol or drugs such as phenytoin. Withdrawal or reduction in dosage provides dramatic relief. There is no satisfactory pharmacologic treatment for intention tremor due to other neurologic disorders.

Rest tremor is usually due to parkinsonism.

Huntington's Disease

Huntington's disease is an autosomal dominant inherited disorder caused by an abnormality in chromosome 4. It is characterized by progressive chorea and dementia that usually begin in adulthood. The development of chorea seems to be related to an imbalance of dopamine, acetylcholine, GABA, and perhaps other neurotransmitters in the basal ganglia (Figure 28–1). Pharmacologic studies indicate that chorea results from functional overactivity in dopaminergic nigrostriatal pathways, perhaps because of increased responsiveness of postsynaptic dopamine receptors or deficiency of a neurotransmitter that normally antagonizes dopamine. Drugs that impair dopaminergic neurotransmission, either by depleting central monoamines (eg, reserpine, tetrabenazine) or by blocking dopamine receptors (eg, phenothiazines, butyrophenones), often alleviate chorea, whereas dopamine-like drugs such as levodopa tend to exacerbate it.

Both GABA and the enzyme (glutamic acid decarboxylase) concerned with its synthesis are markedly reduced in the basal ganglia of patients with Huntington's disease, and GABA receptors are usually implicated in inhibitory pathways. There is also a significant decline in concentration of choline acetyltransferase, the enzyme responsible for synthesizing acetylcholine, in the basal ganglia of these patients. These findings may be of pathophysiologic significance and have led to attempts to alleviate chorea by enhancing central GABA or acetylcholine activity. Unfortunately, such pharmacologic manipulations have been disappointing, yielding no consistently beneficial response. As a consequence, the most commonly used drugs for controlling dyskinesia in patients with Huntington's disease are still those that interfere with dopamine activity. With all the latter drugs, however, reduction of abnormal movements may be associated with iatrogenic parkinsonism.

Reserpine depletes cerebral dopamine by preventing intraneuronal storage (see Chapter 6); it is introduced in low doses (eg, 0.25 mg daily), and the daily dose is then built up gradually (eg, by 0.25 mg every week) until benefit occurs or adverse effects become troublesome. A daily dose of 2–5 mg is often effective in suppressing abnormal movements, but adverse effects may include hypotension, depression, sedation, diarrhea, and nasal congestion. **Tetrabenazine** resembles reserpine in depleting cerebral dopamine and has less troublesome adverse effects, but it is not available in the USA. Treatment with postsynaptic dopamine receptor blockers such as phenothiazines and butyrophenones may also be helpful. Haloperidol is started in a small dose, eg, 1 mg twice daily, and increased every 4 days depending on the response. If haloperidol is not helpful, treatment with increasing doses of perphenazine up to a total of about 20 mg daily sometimes helps. Several recent reports suggest that olanzapine may also be useful; the dose varies with the patient, but 10 mg daily is often sufficient although doses as high as 30 mg daily are sometimes required. The pharmacokinetics and clinical properties of these drugs are considered in greater detail elsewhere in this book.

Other Forms of Chorea

Treatment is directed at the underlying cause when chorea occurs as a complication of general medical disorders such as thyrotoxicosis, polycythemia vera rubra, systemic lupus erythematosus, hypocalcemia, and hepatic cirrhosis. Drug-induced chorea is managed by withdrawal of the offending substance, which may be levodopa, an antimuscarinic drug, amphetamine, lithium, phenytoin, or an oral contraceptive. Neuroleptic drugs may also produce an acute or tardive dyskinesia (discussed below). Sydenham's chorea is temporary and usually so mild that pharmacologic management of the dyskinesia is unnecessary, but dopamine-blocking drugs are effective in suppressing it.

Ballismus

The biochemical basis of ballismus is unknown, but the pharmacologic approach to management is the same as for chorea. Treatment with haloperidol, perphenazine, or other dopamine-blocking drugs may be helpful.

Athetosis & Dystonia

The pharmacologic basis of these disorders is unknown, and there is no satisfactory medical treatment for them. Occasional patients with dystonia may respond to diazepam, amantadine, antimuscarinic drugs (in high dosage), levodopa, carbamazepine, baclofen, haloperidol, or phenothiazines. A trial of these pharmacologic approaches is worthwhile even though often not successful. Patients with focal dystonias such as blepharospasm or torticollis may benefit from injection of botulinum toxin into the overactive muscles.

Tics

The pathophysiologic basis of tics is unknown. Chronic multiple tics (**Gilles de la Tourette's syndrome**) may require symptomatic treatment if the disorder is severe or is having a significant impact on the patient's life. The most effective pharmacologic approach is with **haloperidol,** and patients are better able to tolerate this drug if treatment is started with a small dosage (eg, 0.25 or 0.5 mg daily) and then increased very gradually over the following weeks. Most patients ultimately require a total daily dose of 3–8 mg. Adverse effects include extrapyramidal movement disorders, sedation, dryness of the mouth, blurred vision, and gastrointestinal disturbances. Pimozide, another dopamine-receptor antagonist, may be helpful in patients who are either unresponsive to or intolerant of haloperidol. Treatment is started at 1 mg/d, and the dosage is increased by 1 mg every 5 days; most patients require 7–16 mg/d.

If these measures fail, fluphenazine, clonazepam, clonidine, or carbamazepine should be tried. The pharmacologic properties of these drugs are discussed elsewhere in this book. Clonidine reduces motor or vocal tics in about 50% of children so treated. It may act by reducing activity in noradrenergic neurons in the locus caeruleus. It is introduced in a dose of 2–3 mcg/kg/d, increasing after 2 weeks to 4 mcg/kg/d and then, if required, to 5 mcg/kg/d. It may cause an initial transient fall in blood pressure. The most common side effect is sedation; other side effects include reduced or excessive salivation and diarrhea. Phenothiazines such as fluphenazine sometimes help the tics, as do dopamine agonists. The role of the newer atypical antipsychotic agents, such as risperidone, is unclear.

Injection of botulinum toxin A at the site of problematic tics is sometimes helpful. Treatment of any associated attention deficit disorder or obsessive-compulsive disorder may be required. Bilateral thalamic stimulation is sometimes worthwhile in otherwise intractable cases.

Drug-Induced Dyskinesias

The pharmacologic basis of the acute dyskinesia or dystonia sometimes precipitated by the first few doses of a phenothiazine is not clear. In most instances, parenteral administration of an antimuscarinic drug such as benztropine (2 mg intravenously), diphenhydramine (50 mg intravenously), or biperiden (2–5 mg intravenously or intramuscularly) is helpful, whereas in other instances diazepam (10 mg intravenously) alleviates the abnormal movements.

Tardive dyskinesia, a disorder characterized by a variety of abnormal movements, is a common complication of long-term neuroleptic drug treatment (see Chapter 29). Unfortunately, its precise pharmacologic basis is unclear. A reduction in dose of the offending medication, a dopamine receptor blocker, commonly worsens the dyskinesia, whereas an increase in dose may suppress it. The drugs most likely to provide immediate symptomatic benefit are those interfering with dopaminergic function, either by depletion (eg, reserpine, tetrabenazine) or receptor blockade (eg, phenothiazines, butyrophenones). Paradoxically, the receptor-blocking drugs are the very ones that also cause the dyskinesia.

Because tardive dyskinesia that develops in adults is often irreversible and has no satisfactory treatment, care must be taken to reduce the likelihood of its occurrence. Antipsychotic medication should be prescribed only when necessary and should be withheld periodically to assess the need for continued treatment and to unmask incipient dyskinesia. Thioridazine, a phenothiazine with a piperidine side chain, is an effective antipsychotic that seems less likely than most to cause extrapyramidal reactions, perhaps because it has little effect on dopamine receptors in the striatal system. Finally, antimuscarinic drugs should not be prescribed routinely in patients receiving neuroleptics, because the combination may increase the likelihood of dyskinesia.

Restless Legs Syndrome

Restless legs syndrome is characterized by an unpleasant creeping discomfort that seems to arise deep within the legs and occasionally the arms. Symptoms occur particularly when patients are relaxed, especially when they are lying down or sitting, and they lead to an urge to move about. Such symptoms may delay the onset of sleep. A sleep disorder associated with periodic movements during sleep may also occur. The cause is unknown, but the disorder is especially common among pregnant women and also among uremic or diabetic patients with neuropathy. In most patients, no obvious predisposing cause is found.

Symptoms may resolve with correction of coexisting iron-deficiency anemia and often respond to dopamine agonists, levodopa, diazepam, clonazepam, or opiates. Dopaminergic therapy is the preferred treatment for restless legs syndrome and should be initiated with long-acting dopamine agonists to avoid the complications associated with levodopa. **Ropinirole** has recently been approved for this condition. When opiates are required, those with long half-lives or low addictive potential should be used.

Wilson's Disease

A recessively inherited disorder of copper metabolism, Wilson's disease is characterized biochemically by reduced serum copper and ceruloplasmin concentrations, pathologically by markedly increased concentration of copper in the brain and viscera, and clinically by signs of hepatic and neurologic dysfunction. Neurologic signs include tremor, choreiform movements, rigidity, hypokinesia, and dysarthria and dysphagia. Treatment involves the removal of excess copper, followed by maintenance of copper balance. A commonly used agent for this purpose is **penicillamine** (dimethylcysteine), a chelating agent that forms a ring complex with copper. It is readily absorbed from the gastrointestinal tract and rapidly excreted in the urine. A common starting dose in adults is 500 mg three or four times daily. After remission occurs, it may be possible to lower the maintenance dose, generally to not less than 1 g daily, which must thereafter be continued indefinitely. Adverse effects include nausea and vomiting, nephrotic syndrome, a lupus-like syndrome, pemphigus, myasthenia, arthropathy, optic neuropathy, and various blood dyscrasias. Treatment should be monitored by frequent urinalysis and complete blood counts. Dietary copper should also be kept below 2 mg daily. **Potassium disulfide,** 20 mg three times daily with meals, reduces the intestinal absorption of copper and should also be prescribed.

For those patients who are unable to tolerate penicillamine, **trientine,** another chelating agent, may be used in a daily dose of 1–1.5 g. Trientine appears to have few adverse effects other than mild anemia due to iron deficiency in a few patients. **Zinc acetate** administered orally increases the fecal excretion of copper and is sometimes used for maintenance therapy. The dose is 50 mg three times a day. **Zinc sulfate** (200 mg/d orally) has also been used to decrease copper absorption. Zinc blocks copper absorption from the gastrointestinal tract by induction of intestinal cell metallothionein. Its main advantage is its low toxicity compared with that of other anticopper agents, although it may cause gastric irritation when introduced.

PREPARATIONS AVAILABLE

Amantadine (Symmetrel, others)
Oral: 100 mg capsules; 10 mg/mL syrup
Apomorphine (Apokyn)
Subcutaneous injection titration kit, 10 mg/mL
Benztropine (Cogentin, others)
Oral: 0.5, 1, 2 mg tablets
Parenteral: 1 mg/mL for injection
Biperiden (Akineton)
Oral: 2 mg tablets
Parenteral: 5 mg/mL for injection
Bromocriptine (Parlodel)
Oral: 2.5 mg tablets; 5 mg capsules
Carbidopa (Lodosyn)
Oral: 25 mg tablets
Carbidopa/levodopa (Sinemet, others)
Oral: 10 mg carbidopa and 100 mg levodopa, 25 mg carbidopa and 100 mg levodopa, 25 mg carbidopa and 250 mg levodopa tablets
Oral sustained-release (Sinemet CR): 25 mg carbidopa and 100 mg levodopa; 50 mg carbidopa and 200 mg levodopa
Carbidopa/levodopa/entacapone (Stalevo)
Oral: 12.5 mg carbidopa, 200 mg entacapone and 50 mg levodopa; 25 mg carbidopa, 200 mg entacapone, and 100 mg levodopa; 37.5 mg carbidopa, 200 mg entacapone, and 150 mg levodopa
Entacapone (Comtan)
Oral: 200 mg tablets

Levodopa (Dopar, Larodopa)
Oral: 100, 250, 500 mg tablets, capsules
Orphenadrine (various)
Oral: 100 mg tablets
Oral sustained-release: 100 mg tablets
Parenteral: 30 mg/mL for injection
Penicillamine (Cuprimine, Depen)
Oral: 125, 250 mg capsules; 250 mg tablets
Pergolide (Permax, other)
Oral: 0.05, 0.25, 1 mg tablets
Pramipexole (Mirapex)
Oral: 0.125, 0.25, 1, 1.5 mg tablets
Procyclidine (Kemadrin)
Oral: 5 mg tablets
Rasagiline (Azilect)
Oral: 0.5, 1 mg tablets
Ropinirole (Requip)
Oral: 0.25, 0.5, 1, 2, 5 mg tablets
Selegiline (deprenyl) (generic, Eldepryl)
Oral: 5 mg tablets, capsules
Tolcapone (Tasmar)
Oral: 100, 200 mg tablets
Trientine (Syprine)
Oral: 250 mg capsules
Trihexyphenidyl (Artane, others)
Oral: 2, 5 mg tablets; 2 mg/5 mL elixir
Oral sustained-release (Artane Sequels): 5 mg capsules

REFERENCES

Ahlskog JE: Slowing Parkinson's disease progression: Recent dopamine agonist trials. Neurology 2003;60:381.

Aminoff MJ: Neuroprotective treatment for Parkinson's disease. Expert Rev Neurotherapeutics 2003;3:797.

Anonymous: Apomorphine (Apokyn) for advanced Parkinson's disease. Med Lett Drugs Ther 2005;47:7.

Beal MF, Hantraye P: Novel therapies in the search for a cure for Huntington's disease. Proc Natl Acad Sci USA 2001;98:3.

Biglan KM, Holloway RG: A review of pramipexole and its clinical utility in Parkinson's disease. Expert Opin Pharmacother 2002;3:197.

Bonelli RM et al: High-dose olanzapine in Huntington's disease. Int Clin Psychopharmacol 2002;17:91.

Bonuccelli U et al: Pergolide in the treatment of patients with early and advanced Parkinson's disease. Clin Neuropharmacol 2002;25:1.

Brewer GJ: Zinc acetate for the treatment of Wilson's disease. Expert Opin Pharmacother 2001;2:1473.

Clarke CE, Guttman M: Dopamine agonist monotherapy in Parkinson's disease. Lancet 2002;360:1767.

Dawson TM, Dawson VL: Neuroprotective and neurorestorative strategies for Parkinson's disease. Nat Neurosci 2002;5(Suppl):1058.

Deleu D et al: Clinical pharmacokinetic and pharmacodynamic properties of drugs used in the treatment of Parkinson's disease. Clin Pharmacokinet 2002;41:261.

Deleu D et al: Subcutaneous apomorphine: An evidence-based review of its use in Parkinson's disease. Drugs Aging 2004; 21:687.

El-Youssef M: Wilson's disease. Mayo Clin Proc 2003;78:1126.

Etminan M et al: Increased risk of somnolence with the new dopamine agonists in patients with Parkinson's disease: A meta-analysis of randomised controlled trials. Drug Saf 2001;24:863.

Freed CR et al: Transplantation of embryonic dopamine neurons for severe Parkinson's disease. N Engl J Med 2001;344:710.

Koller WC, Tolosa E (editors): Current and emerging drug therapies in the management of Parkinson's disease. Neurology 1998;50:Suppl 6. [Entire issue.]

Lavenstein BL: Treatment approaches for children with Tourette's syndrome. Curr Neurol Neurosci Rep 2003;3:143.

Le WD, Jankovic J: Are dopamine receptor agonists neuroprotective in Parkinson's disease? Drugs Aging 2001;18:389.

Leckman JF: Tourette's syndrome. Lancet 2002;360:1577.

McMurray CT: Huntington's disease: New hope for therapeutics. Trends Neurosci 2001;24(Suppl):S32.

Miyasaki JM et al: Practice parameter: Initiation of treatment for Parkinson's disease: An evidence-based review. Neurology 2002;58:11.

Muller-Vahl KR: The treatment of Tourette's syndrome: Current opinions. Expert Opin Pharmacother 2002;3:899.

Murray KF et al: Current and future therapy in haemochromatosis and Wilson's disease. Expert Opin Pharmacother 2003;4:2239.

Pahwa R, Lyons KE: Essential tremor: Differential diagnosis and current therapy. Am J Med 2003;115:134.

Paleacu D et al: Olanzapine in Huntington's disease. Acta Neurol Scand 2002;105:441.

Parkinson Study Group: A controlled trial of rasagiline in early Parkinson disease: The TEMPO study. Arch Neurol 2002; 59:1937.

Schapira AH: Restless legs syndrome: An update on treatment options. Drugs 2004;64:149.

Schilsky ML: Diagnosis and treatment of Wilson's disease. Pediatr Transplant 2002;6:15.

Schwartz M, Hocherman S: Antipsychotic-induced rabbit syndrome: epidemiology, management and pathophysiology. CNS Drugs 2004;18:213.

Shapiro AK et al: Pimozide treatment of tic and Tourette disorders. Pediatrics 1987;79:6.

Silber MH et al: Pramipexole in the management of restless legs syndrome: An extended study. Sleep 2003;26:819.

Soares-Weiser KV, Joy C: Miscellaneous treatments for neuroleptic-induced tardive dyskinesia. Cochrane Database Syst Rev 2003;(2):CD000208.

Sydow O et al: Multicentre European study of thalamic stimulation in essential tremor: A six year follow up. J Neurol Neurosurg Psychiatry 2003;74:1387.

Tuite P, Ebbitt B: Dopamine agonists. Semin Neurol 2001;21:9.

Visser-Vandewalle V et al: Chronic bilateral thalamic stimulation: A new therapeutic approach in intractable Tourette syndrome. Report of three cases. J Neurosurg 2003;99:1094.

Whone AL et al: Slower progression of Parkinson's disease with ropinirole versus L-dopa: the REAL-PET study. Ann Neurol 2003;54:93.

Antipsychotic Agents & Lithium

29

William Z. Potter, MD, PhD, & Leo E. Hollister, MD*

■ I. ANTIPSYCHOTIC AGENTS

The terms **antipsychotic** and **neuroleptic** have been used interchangeably to denote a group of drugs that have been used mainly for treating schizophrenia but are also effective in some other psychoses and agitated states.

History

Antipsychotic drugs have been used in Western medicine for more than 50 years. Reserpine and chlorpromazine were the first drugs found to be useful in schizophrenia. Although chlorpromazine is still sometimes used for the treatment of psychoses, these forerunner drugs have been superseded by many newer agents. Their impact on psychiatry, however—especially on the treatment of schizophrenia—has been enormous: The number of patients hospitalized in mental institutions has markedly decreased, and schizophrenia is now recognized as a biologic illness.

Nature of Psychosis & Schizophrenia

The term "psychosis" denotes a variety of mental disorders. Schizophrenia is a particular kind of psychosis characterized mainly by a clear sensorium but a marked thinking disturbance.

The pathogenesis of schizophrenia is unknown. Largely as a result of research stimulated by the discovery of antipsychotic drugs, a genetic predisposition has been proposed as a necessary but not always sufficient condition underlying psychotic disorder. This assumption has been supported by the observed familial incidence of schizophrenia. At least one gene—that encoding neuregulin 1—is associated with schizophrenia in Icelandic and northern European populations. Additional genes associated with schizophrenia continue to be identified that may contribute to understanding the molecular basis for schizophrenia. Based on the efficacy of antipsychotic drugs, efforts continue to link the disorder with abnormalities of amine neurotransmitter function, especially that of dopamine (see Box: The Dopamine Hypothesis

of Schizophrenia). The defects of this hypothesis are significant, and it is now appreciated that schizophrenia is far more complex than originally supposed.

BASIC PHARMACOLOGY OF ANTIPSYCHOTIC AGENTS

Chemical Types

A number of chemical structures have been associated with antipsychotic properties. The drugs can be classified into several groups as shown in Figures 29–1 and 29–2.

A. PHENOTHIAZINE DERIVATIVES

Three subfamilies of phenothiazines, based primarily on the side chain of the molecule, were once the most widely used of the antipsychotics. Aliphatic derivatives (eg, **chlorpromazine**) and piperidine derivatives (eg, **thioridazine**) are the least potent. Piperazine derivatives are more potent (effective in lower doses) but not necessarily more efficacious. The piperazine derivatives are also more selective in their pharmacologic effects (Table 29–1).

B. THIOXANTHENE DERIVATIVES

This group of drugs is exemplified primarily by **thiothixene**. In general, these compounds are slightly less potent than their phenothiazine analogs.

C. BUTYROPHENONE DERIVATIVES

This group, of which **haloperidol** is the most widely used, has a very different structure from those of the two preceding groups. Diphenylbutylpiperidines are closely related compounds. The butyrophenones and congeners tend to be more potent and to have fewer autonomic effects but greater extrapyramidal effects (Table 29–1).

D. MISCELLANEOUS STRUCTURES

The newer drugs, not all of which are available in the USA, have a variety of structures and include **pimozide, molindone, loxapine, clozapine, olanzapine, quetiapine, risperidone, ziprasidone**, and **aripiprazole** (Figure 29–2).

---

*Deceased

THE DOPAMINE HYPOTHESIS OF SCHIZOPHRENIA

The dopamine hypothesis for schizophrenia is the most fully developed of several hypotheses and is the basis for much of the rationale for drug therapy. Several lines of circumstantial evidence suggest that excessive dopaminergic activity plays a role in the disorder: (1) many antipsychotic drugs strongly block postsynaptic D_2 receptors in the central nervous system, especially in the mesolimbic-frontal system; (2) drugs that increase dopaminergic activity, such as levodopa (a precursor), amphetamines (releasers of dopamine), and apomorphine (a direct dopamine receptor agonist), either aggravate schizophrenia or produce psychosis de novo in some patients; (3) dopamine receptor density has been found postmortem to be increased in the brains of schizophrenics who have not been treated with antipsychotic drugs; (4) positron emission tomography (PET) has shown increased dopamine receptor density in both treated and untreated schizophrenics when compared with such scans of nonschizophrenic persons; and (5) successful treatment of schizophrenic patients has been reported to change the amount of homovanillic acid (HVA), a metabolite of dopamine, in the cerebrospinal fluid, plasma, and urine.

The dopamine hypothesis is far from complete, however. If an abnormality of dopamine physiology were completely responsible for the pathogenesis of schizophrenia, antipsychotic drugs would do a much better job of treating patients—but they are only partially effective for most and ineffective for some patients. Moreover, it appears that antagonists of the NMDA receptor such as phencyclidine, when administered to nonpsychotic subjects, produce much more "schizophrenia-like" symptoms than do dopamine agonists. The cloning and characterization of multiple dopamine receptor types may permit more direct testing of the dopamine hypothesis if drugs can be developed that act more selectively on each receptor type. The traditional antipsychotics bind D_2 50 times more avidly than D_1 or D_3 receptors. Until recently, the main thrust in drug development was to find agents that were more potent and more selective in blocking D_2 receptors. The fact that several of the atypical antipsychotic drugs have much less effect on D_2 receptors and yet are effective in schizophrenia has redirected attention to the role of other dopamine receptors and to nondopamine receptors, especially serotonin receptor subtypes that may mediate synergistic effects or protect against the extrapyramidal consequences of D_2 antagonism. As a result of these considerations, the direction of research has changed to a greater focus on compounds that may act on several transmitter-receptor systems. The great hope is to produce drugs with greater efficacy and fewer adverse effects, especially extrapyramidal toxicity.

Pharmacokinetics

A. ABSORPTION AND DISTRIBUTION

Most antipsychotic drugs are readily but incompletely absorbed. Furthermore, many of these drugs undergo significant first-pass metabolism. Thus, oral doses of chlorpromazine and thioridazine have systemic availability of 25% to 35%, whereas haloperidol, which is less likely to be metabolized, has an average systemic availability of about 65%.

Most antipsychotic drugs are highly lipid-soluble and protein-bound (92–99%). They tend to have large volumes of distribution (usually > 7 L/kg). Probably because these drugs are sequestered in lipid compartments of the body and have a very high affinity for selected neurotransmitter receptors in the central nervous system, they generally have a much longer clinical duration of action than would be estimated from their plasma half-lives. This is paralleled by prolonged occupancy of dopamine D_2 receptors in brain. Metabolites of chlorpromazine may be excreted in the urine weeks after the last dose of chronically administered drug. Similarly, full relapse may not occur until 6 weeks or more after discontinuation of many antipsychotic drugs.

B. METABOLISM

Most antipsychotic drugs are almost completely metabolized by a variety of processes. Although some metabolites retain activity, eg, 7-hydroxychlorpromazine and reduced haloperidol, metabolites are not considered to be highly important to the action of these drugs. The sole exception is mesoridazine, the major metabolite of thioridazine, which is more potent than the parent compound and accounts for most of the effect. This compound has been marketed as a separate entity. Very little of these antipsychotic drugs is excreted unchanged, because they are almost completely metabolized to more polar substances.

Pharmacologic Effects

The first phenothiazine antipsychotic drugs, with chlorpromazine as the prototype, proved to have a wide variety of central nervous system, autonomic, and endocrine effects. These actions were traced to blocking

Figure 29–1. Structural formulas of some older antipsychotic drugs: phenothiazines, thioxanthenes, and butyrophenones. Only representative members of each type are shown.

effects at a wide range of receptors, including dopamine and α adrenoceptor, muscarinic, H_1 histaminic, and serotonin (5-HT_2) receptors. Dopamine receptor effects quickly became the major focus of interest.

A. DOPAMINERGIC SYSTEMS

Five important dopaminergic systems or pathways are now recognized in the brain. The first pathway—the one most closely related to behavior—is the **mesolimbic-mesocortical** pathway, which projects from cell bodies near the substantia nigra to the limbic system and neocortex. The second system—the **nigrostriatal** pathway—consists of neurons that project from the substantia nigra to the caudate and putamen; it is involved in the coordination of voluntary movement. The third pathway—the **tuberoinfundibular** system—connects arcuate nuclei and periventricular neurons to the hypothalamus and posterior pituitary. Dopamine released by these neurons physiologically inhibits prolactin secretion. The fourth dopaminergic system—the **medullary-periventricular** pathway—consists of neurons in the motor nucleus of the vagus whose projections are not well defined. This system may be involved in eating behavior. The fifth pathway—the **incertohypothalamic** pathway—forms connections from the medial zona incerta to the hypothalamus and the amygdala. It

appears to regulate the anticipatory motivational phase of copulatory behavior in rats.

After dopamine was recognized as a neurotransmitter in 1959, investigators showed that its effects on electrical activity in central synapses and on production of cAMP by adenylyl cyclase could be blocked by most antipsychotic drugs. This evidence led to the conclusion in the early 1960s that these drugs should be considered **dopamine antagonists.** The antipsychotic action is now thought to be produced (at least in part) by their ability to block dopamine in the mesolimbic and mesocortical systems. Furthermore, the antagonism of dopamine in the nigrostriatal system explains the unwanted effect of parkinsonism produced by these drugs. The hyperprolactinemia that follows treatment with antipsychotics is caused by blockade of dopamine's tonic inhibitory effect on prolactin release from the pituitary. Thus, the same pharmacodynamic action may have distinct psychiatric, neurologic, and endocrinologic consequences.

B. DOPAMINE RECEPTORS AND THEIR EFFECTS

At present, five dopamine receptors have been described, consisting of two separate families, the D_1-like and D_2-like receptor groups. The D_1 receptor is coded by a gene on chromosome 5, increases cAMP by G_s-cou-

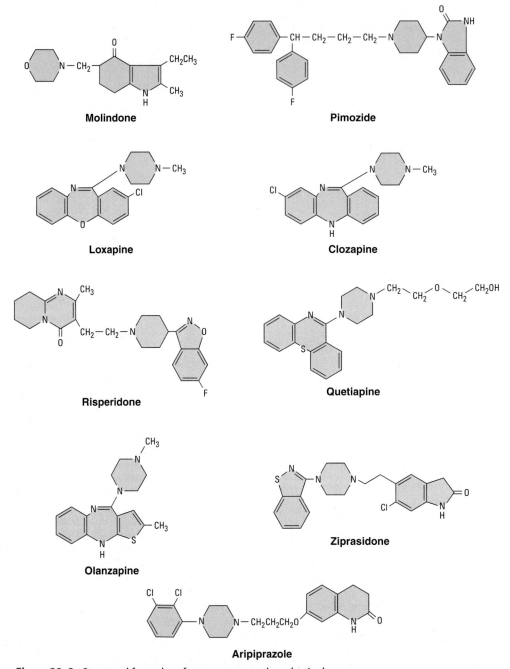

Figure 29–2. Structural formulas of some newer antipsychotic drugs.

pled activation of adenylyl cyclase, and is located mainly in the putamen, nucleus accumbens, and olfactory tubercle. The second member of this family, D_5, is coded by a gene on chromosome 4, also increases cAMP, and is found in the hippocampus and hypothal-amus. The therapeutic potency of antipsychotic drugs does not correlate with their affinity for binding the D_1 receptor (Figure 29–3, top) but for most, correlates strongly with D_2 affinity. The D_2 receptor is coded on chromosome 11, decreases cAMP (by G_i-coupled inhi-

Table 29–1. Antipsychotic drugs: Relation of chemical structure to potency and toxicities.

Chemical Class	Drug	D_2/5-HT$_{2A}$ Ratio[1]	Clinical Potency	Extrapyramidal Toxicity	Sedative Action	Hypotensive Actions
Phenothiazines						
Aliphatic	Chlorpromazine	High	Low	Medium	High	High
Piperazine	Fluphenazine	High	High	High	Low	Very low
Thioxanthene	Thiothixene	Very high	High	Medium	Medium	Medium
Butyrophenone	Haloperidol	Medium	High	Very high	Low	Very low
Dibenzodiazepine	Clozapine	Very low	Medium	Very low	Low	Medium
Benzisoxazole	Risperidone	Very low	High	Low[2]	Low	Low
Thienobenzodiazepine	Olanzapine	Low	High	Very low	Medium	Low
Dibenzothiazepine	Quetiapine	Low	Low	Very low	Medium	Low to medium
Dihydroindolone	Ziprasidone	Low	Medium	Very low	Low	Very low
Dihydrocarbostyril	Aripiprazole	Medium	High	Very low	Very low	Low

[1]Ratio of affinity for D_2 receptors to affinity for 5-HT$_{2A}$ receptors.
[2]At dosages below 8 mg/d.

bition of adenylyl cyclase), and inhibits calcium channels but opens potassium channels. It is found both pre- and postsynaptically on neurons in the caudate-putamen, nucleus accumbens, and olfactory tubercle. A second member of this family, the D_3 receptor, also coded by a gene on chromosome 11, is thought to decrease cAMP and is located in the frontal cortex, medulla, and midbrain. D_4 receptors also decrease cAMP.

The activation of D_2 receptors by a variety of direct or indirect agonists (eg, amphetamines, levodopa, apomorphine) causes increased motor activity and stereotyped behavior in rats, a model that has been extensively used for antipsychotic drug screening. When given to humans, the same drugs aggravate schizophrenia. The antipsychotic agents block D_2 receptors stereoselectively for the most part, and their binding affinity is very strongly correlated with clinical antipsychotic and extrapyramidal potency (Figure 29–3, bottom). Continuous treatment with antipsychotic drugs has been reported in some studies to produce a transient increase in levels of a dopamine metabolite, homovanillic acid (HVA), in the cerebrospinal fluid, plasma, and urine.

These findings have been incorporated into the dopamine hypothesis of schizophrenia. However, many questions have not been satisfactorily answered, and many observations have not been fully confirmed. For example, dopamine receptors exist in both high- and low-affinity forms, and it is not known whether schizophrenia or the antipsychotic drugs alter the proportions

of receptors in these two forms. With the introduction of aripiprazole, which in preclinical studies shows partial agonism at D_2 and 5-HT$_{1A}$ receptors, the relevance of the proportion of receptors in various affinity states may prove especially important for understanding the degree of response to this agent.

Furthermore, the drug-induced progression of extrapyramidal changes—from diminished function (resembling parkinsonism) to increased activity (manifested by dyskinesias)—often occurs over a period of months to years. This time scale is much longer than that described for other drug-induced changes in receptor function. Of most importance, newer drugs—clozapine, olanzapine, quetiapine, and aripiprazole—do not have very high affinity for the D_2 receptor, which suggests that additional actions are critical to their antipsychotic effects.

It has not been convincingly demonstrated that antagonism of any dopamine receptor other than the D_2 receptor plays a role in the action of antipsychotic drugs. Selective D_3-receptor antagonists may prove therapeutic but are not yet available. Most of the newer "atypical" antipsychotic agents and some of the traditional ones have significant affinity for the 5-HT$_{2A}$ receptor (Table 29–1), suggesting an important role for the serotonin system. Participation of glutamate, GABA, and acetylcholine receptors in the pathophysiology of schizophrenia has also been proposed. Agents targeted at glutamatergic and cholinergic systems are just beginning to be evaluated in schizophrenia.

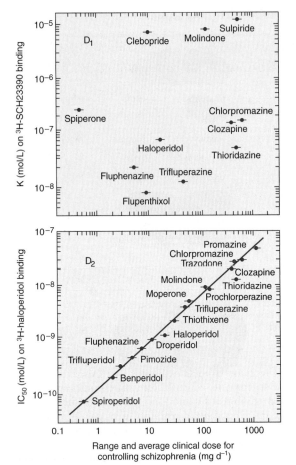

Figure 29–3. Correlations between the therapeutic potency of antipsychotic drugs and their affinity for binding to dopamine D_1 *(top)* or D_2 receptors *(bottom)*. Potency is indicated on the horizontal axes; it decreases to the right. Binding affinity for D_1 receptors was measured by displacing the selective D_1 ligand SCH 23390; affinity for D_2 receptors was similarly measured by displacing the selective D_2 ligand haloperidol. Binding affinity decreases upward. (Modified and reproduced, with permission, from Seeman P: Dopamine receptors and the dopamine hypothesis of schizophrenia. Synapse 1987;1:133.)

C. Differences Among Antipsychotic Drugs

Although all effective antipsychotic drugs block D_2 receptors, the degree of this blockade in relation to other actions on receptors varies considerably between drugs. Vast numbers of ligand-receptor binding experiments have been performed in an effort to discover a single receptor action that would best predict antipsychotic efficacy. A summary of the relative receptor-binding affinities of several key agents

in such comparisons illustrates the difficulty in drawing simple conclusions from such experiments:

Chlorpromazine: $\alpha_1 = 5\text{-HT}_{2A} > D_2 > D_1$
Haloperidol: $D_2 > \alpha_1 > D_4 > 5\text{-HT}_{2A} > D_1 > H_1$
Clozapine: $D_4 = \alpha_1 > 5\text{-HT}_{2A} > D_2 = D_1$
Olanzapine: $5\text{-HT}_{2A} > H_1 > D_4 > D_2 > \alpha_1 > D_1$
Aripiprazole: $D_2 = 5\text{-HT}_{2A} > D_4 > \alpha_1 = H_1 \gg D_1$
Quetiapine: $H_1 > \alpha_1 > M_{1,3} > D_2 > 5\text{-HT}_{2A}$

Thus, most of the atypical antipsychotic agents are at least as potent in inhibiting 5-HT_2 receptors as they are in inhibiting D_2 receptors. The newest, aripiprazole, appears to be a partial agonist of D_2 receptors. Varying degrees of antagonism of α_2 adrenoceptors are also seen with risperidone, clozapine, olanzapine, quetiapine, and aripiprazole. The clinical relevance of these actions remains to be ascertained.

Current research is directed toward discovering atypical antipsychotic compounds that are either more selective for the mesolimbic system (to reduce their effects on the extrapyramidal system) or have effects on central neurotransmitter receptors—such as those for acetylcholine and excitatory amino acids—that have been proposed as new targets for antipsychotic action.

In contrast to the search for *efficacy,* such differences in the receptor effects of various antipsychotics do explain many of their *toxicities* (Tables 29–1 and 29–2). In particular, extrapyramidal toxicity appears to be associated with high D_2 potency.

D. Psychological Effects

Most antipsychotic drugs cause unpleasant subjective effects in nonpsychotic individuals; the combination of sleepiness, restlessness, and autonomic effects creates experiences unlike those associated with more familiar sedatives or hypnotics. Nonpsychotic persons also experience impaired performance as judged by a number of psychomotor and psychometric tests. Psychotic individuals, however, may actually show improvement in their performance as the psychosis is alleviated.

E. Electroencephalographic Effects

Antipsychotic drugs produce shifts in the pattern of electroencephalographic frequencies, usually slowing them and increasing their synchronization. The slowing (hypersynchrony) is sometimes focal or unilateral, which may lead to erroneous diagnostic interpretations. Both the frequency and the amplitude changes induced by psychotropic drugs are readily apparent and can be quantitated by sophisticated electrophysiologic techniques. Some of the neuroleptic agents lower the seizure threshold and induce EEG patterns typical of seizure disorders; however, with careful dosage titration, most can be used safely in epileptic patients.

Table 29–2. Adverse pharmacologic effects of antipsychotic drugs.

Type	Manifestations	Mechanism
Autonomic nervous system	Loss of accommodation, dry mouth, difficulty urinating, constipation	Muscarinic cholinoceptor blockade
	Orthostatic hypotension, impotence, failure to ejaculate	Alpha adrenoceptor blockade
Central nervous system	Parkinson's syndrome, akathisia, dystonias	Dopamine receptor blockade
	Tardive dyskinesia	Supersensitivity of dopamine receptors
	Toxic-confusional state	Muscarinic blockade
Endocrine system	Amenorrhea-galactorrhea, infertility, impotence	Dopamine receptor blockade resulting in hyperprolactinemia
Other	Weight gain	Possibly combined H_1 and 5-HT_2 blockade

F. Endocrine Effects

Older antipsychotic drugs produce striking adverse effects on the reproductive system. Amenorrhea-galactorrhea, false-positive pregnancy tests, and increased libido have been reported in women, whereas men have experienced decreased libido and gynecomastia. Some of these effects are secondary to blockade of dopamine's tonic inhibition of prolactin secretion; others may be due to increased peripheral conversion of androgens to estrogens. Absent or minimal increases of prolactin after some of the newer antipsychotics such as olanzapine, quetiapine, and aripiprazole may be a marker of diminished D_2 antagonism and hence reduced risks of extrapyramidal system dysfunction and tardive dyskinesia as well as endocrine dysfunction.

G. Cardiovascular Effects

Orthostatic hypotension and high resting heart rates frequently result from use of the low-potency phenothiazines. Mean arterial pressure, peripheral resistance, and stroke volume are decreased, and heart rate is increased. These effects are predictable from the autonomic actions of these agents (Table 29–2). Abnormal ECGs have been recorded, especially with thioridazine. Changes include prolongation of QT interval and abnormal configurations of the ST segment and T waves. These changes are readily reversed by withdrawing the drug.

Among the newest antipsychotics, prolongation of the QT or QT_c interval—with increased risk of dangerous arrhythmias—has been of such concern that the atypical drug sertindole was withdrawn shortly after being marketed. Ziprasidone carries a warning about the risk of significant QT_c prolongation.

H. Animal Screening Tests

Inhibition of conditioned (but not unconditioned) avoidance behavior is one of the most predictive tests of anti-

psychotic action. Another is the inhibition of amphetamine- or apomorphine-induced stereotyped behavior. This inhibition is undoubtedly related to the D_2 receptor-blocking action of the drugs, countering these two dopamine agonists. Other tests that may predict antipsychotic action are reduction of exploratory behavior without undue sedation, induction of a cataleptic state, inhibition of intracranial self-stimulation of reward areas, and prevention of apomorphine-induced vomiting. Most of these tests are difficult to relate to any model of clinical psychosis.

The psychosis produced by phencyclidine (PCP) has been used as a model for schizophrenia. Because this drug is an antagonist of the NMDA glutamate receptor, attempts have been made to develop antipsychotics that work as NMDA agonists. Sigma opioid and cholecystokinin type b (CCK_b) antagonism have also been suggested as potential targets. Thus far, NMDA receptor-based models have pointed to agents that modulate glutamate release as potential antipsychotics.

CLINICAL PHARMACOLOGY OF ANTIPSYCHOTIC AGENTS

Indications

A. Psychiatric Indications

Schizophrenia is the primary indication for antipsychotic agents, which remain the mainstay of treatment for this condition. Unfortunately, many patients show little response and virtually none show a complete response.

Antipsychotics are also indicated for schizoaffective disorders, which share characteristics of both schizophrenia and affective disorders. The psychotic aspects of the illness require treatment with antipsychotic drugs, which may be used with other drugs such as antidepressants, lithium, or valproic acid. The manic phase in bipolar affective disorder often requires treatment with antipsychotic agents, though lithium or valproic acid supplemented with high-potency benzodiazepines (eg, lorazepam or clonazepam) may suffice in milder cases. Recent controlled trials support the efficacy of monotherapy with atypical antipsychotics in the acute phase (up to 4 weeks) of mania, and olanzapine has been approved for this indication.

As mania subsides, the antipsychotic drug may be withdrawn, although maintenance treatment with atypical antipsychotics has become more common. Nonmanic excited states may also be managed by antipsychotics, often in combination with benzodiazepines.

Other indications for the use of antipsychotics include Tourette's syndrome, disturbed behavior in patients with Alzheimer's disease, and, with antidepressants, psychotic depression. Antipsychotics are not indicated for the treatment of various withdrawal syndromes, eg, opioid withdrawal. In small doses antipsychotics have been promoted (wrongly) for the relief of anxiety associated with minor emotional disorders. The antianxiety sedatives (see Chapter 22) are preferred in terms of both safety and acceptability to patients.

B. NONPSYCHIATRIC INDICATIONS

Most older antipsychotic drugs, with the exception of thioridazine, have a strong antiemetic effect. This action is due to dopamine receptor blockade, both centrally (in the chemoreceptor trigger zone of the medulla) and peripherally (on receptors in the stomach). Some drugs, such as prochlorperazine and benzquinamide, are promoted solely as antiemetics.

Phenothiazines with shorter side chains have considerable H_1-receptor-blocking action and have been used for relief of pruritus or, in the case of promethazine, as preoperative sedatives. The butyrophenone droperidol is used in combination with an opioid, fentanyl, in neuroleptanesthesia. The use of these drugs in anesthesia practice is described in Chapter 25.

Drug Choice

Choice among antipsychotic drugs is based mainly on differences in adverse effects and possible differences in efficacy. Since use of the older drugs is still widespread, especially for patients treated in the public sector, knowledge of such agents as chlorpromazine and haloperidol remains relevant. Thus, one should be familiar with one member of each of the three subfamilies of phenothiazines, a member of the thioxanthine and butyrophenone group, and all of the newer compounds—clozapine, risperidone, olanzapine, quetiapine, ziprasidone, and aripiprazole. Each may have special benefits for selected patients. A representative group of antipsychotic drugs is presented in Table 29–3.

New antipsychotic drugs have been shown in some trials to be more effective than older ones for treating negative symptoms (emotional blunting, social withdrawal, lack of motivation). The floridly psychotic form of the illness accompanied by uncontrollable behavior probably responds equally well to all potent antipsychotics but is still frequently treated with older drugs that offer intramuscular formulations for acute and chronic treatment. Moreover, the low cost of the older drugs contributes to their widespread use despite their clear disadvantages in terms of extrapyramidal side effects and hyperprolactinemia. Several of the newer antipsychotics, including clozapine, risperidone, and olanzapine, show superiority over haloperidol in terms of overall response in some controlled trials. More comparative studies with aripiprazole are needed to evaluate its relative efficacy. Moreover, the superior side-effect profile of the newer agents and low to absent risk of tardive dyskinesia suggest that these should provide the first line of treatment.

It is not necessary for practitioners to know all the drugs intimately, but they should be familiar with the effects—including the adverse effects—of one or two drugs in each class. The best guide for selecting a drug for an individual patient is the patient's past responses to drugs. Within the older group, the trend has been away from low-potency agents such as chlorpromazine and thioridazine toward the high-potency drugs such as haloperidol. At present, clozapine is limited to those patients who have failed to respond to substantial doses of conventional antipsychotic drugs. The agranulocytosis and seizures associated with this drug prevent more widespread use. Risperidone's superior side-effect profile (compared with haloperidol) at dosages of 6 mg/d or less and the lower risk of tardive dyskinesia have contributed to its widespread use. Olanzapine and quetiapine may have even lower risk and have achieved widespread use. Whether any of the other recently introduced antipsychotic drugs can substitute for clozapine remains to be established.

Dosage

The range of effective dosages among various antipsychotics is quite broad. Therapeutic margins are substantial. Assuming that dosages are appropriate, antipsychotics, with the exception of clozapine and perhaps olanzapine, are of equal efficacy in broadly selected groups of patients. However, some patients who fail to respond to one drug may respond to another; for this reason, several drugs may have to be tried to find the one most effective for an individual patient. This phenomenon might be due to the differing profiles of receptor actions of the various drugs. Patients who have become refractory to two or three antipsychotic agents given in substantial doses now become candidates for

Table 29–3. Some representative antipsychotic drugs.

Drug Class	Drug	Advantages	Disadvantages
Phenothiazines			
Aliphatic	Chlorpromazine[1]	Generic, inexpensive	Many adverse effects, especially autonomic
Piperidine	Thioridazine[2]	Slight extrapyramidal syndrome; generic	800 mg/d limit; no parenteral form; cardiotoxicity
Piperazine	Fluphenazine[3]	Depot form also available (enanthate, decanoate)	(?) Increased tardive dyskinesia
Thioxanthene	Thiothixene	Parenteral form also available; (?) decreased tardive dyskinesia	Uncertain
Butyrophenone	Haloperidol	Parenteral form also available; generic	Severe extrapyramidal syndrome
Dibenzoxazepine	Loxapine	(?) No weight gain	Uncertain
Dibenzodiazepine	Clozapine	May benefit treatment-resistant patients; little extrapyramidal toxicity	May cause agranulocytosis in up to 2% of patients; dose-related lowering of seizure threshold
Benzisoxazole	Risperidone	Broad efficacy; little or no extrapyramidal system dysfunction at low doses	Extrapyramidal system dysfunction and hypotension with higher doses
Thienobenzodiazepine	Olanzapine	Effective against negative as well as positive symptoms; little or no extrapyramidal system dysfunction	Weight gain; dose-related lowering of seizure threshold
Dibenzothiazepine	Quetiapine	Similar to olanzapine; perhaps less weight gain	May require high doses if there is associated hypotension; short $t_{1/2}$ and twice-daily dosing
Dihydroindolone	Ziprasidone	Perhaps less weight gain than clozapine, parenteral form available	QT_c prolongation
Dihydrocarbostyril	Aripiprazole	Lower weight gain liability, long half-life, novel mechanism potential	Uncertain, novel toxicities possible

[1]Other aliphatic phenothiazines: promazine, triflupromazine.
[2]Other piperidine phenothiazines: piperacetazine, mesoridazine.
[3]Other piperazine phenothiazines: acetophenazine, perphenazine, carphenazine, prochlorperazine, trifluoperazine.

treatment with clozapine. This drug, in dosages up to 900 mg/d, salvages about 30–50% of patients previously refractory to 60 mg/d of haloperidol. In such cases, the increased risk of clozapine can well be justified. Risperidone does not appear to substitute for clozapine, although reports are mixed. Whether other antipsychotics will show efficacy similar to that of clozapine remains to be determined.

Some dosage relationships between various antipsychotic drugs, as well as possible therapeutic ranges, are shown in Table 29–4.

Parenteral Preparations

Well-tolerated parenteral forms of the high-potency older drugs are available for rapid initiation of treatment as well as for maintenance treatment in noncompliant patients. Since the parenterally administered drugs may have much greater bioavailability than the oral forms, doses should be only a fraction of what might be given orally, and the manufacturer's literature should be consulted. Fluphenazine decanoate and haloperidol decanoate are suitable for long-term parenteral maintenance therapy in patients who cannot or will not take oral medication.

Dosage Schedules

Antipsychotic drugs are often given in divided daily doses, titrating to an effective dosage. After an effective daily dosage has been defined for an individual patient, doses can be given less frequently. Once-daily doses, usually given at night, are feasible for many patients

Table 29–4. Dose relationships of antipsychotics.

	Minimum Effective Therapeutic Dose (mg)	Usual Range of Daily Doses (mg)
Chlorpromazine (Thorazine)	100	100–1000
Thioridazine (Mellaril)	100	100–800
Trifluoperazine (Stelazine)	5	5–60
Perphenazine (Trilafon)	10	8–64
Fluphenazine (Permitil, Prolixin)	2	2–60
Thiothixene (Navane)	2	2–120
Haloperidol (Haldol)	2	2–60
Loxapine (Loxitane)	10	20–160
Molindone (Lidone, Moban)	10	20–200
Clozapine (Clozaril)	50	300–600
Olanzapine (Zyprexa)	5	10–30
Quetiapine (Seroquel)	150	150–800
Risperidone (Risperdal)	4	4–16
Ziprasidone (Zeldox)	40	80–160
Aripiprazole (Abilify)	10	10–30

during chronic maintenance treatment. Simplification of dosage schedules leads to better compliance.

Maintenance Treatment

A very small minority of schizophrenic patients may recover from an acute episode and require no further drug therapy for prolonged periods. In most cases, the choice is between "as needed" increased doses or addition of other drugs for exacerbations versus continual maintenance treatment with full therapeutic doses. The choice depends on social factors such as the availability of family or friends familiar with the symptoms of early relapse and ready access to care.

Drug Combinations

Combining antipsychotic drugs confounds evaluation of the efficacy of the drugs being used. Use of combinations, however, is widespread, with more emerging experimental data supporting such practices. Tricyclic antidepressants or, more often, selective serotonin reuptake inhibitors may be used with antipsychotics for clear symptoms of depression complicating schizophrenia. Lithium or valproic acid is sometimes added to antipsychotic agents with benefit to patients who do

not respond to the latter drugs alone. It is uncertain whether such instances represent misdiagnosed cases of mania or schizoaffective disorder. Sedative drugs may be added for relief of anxiety or insomnia not controlled by antipsychotics.

Adverse Reactions

Most of the unwanted effects of antipsychotics are extensions of their known pharmacologic actions (Tables 29–1 and 29–2), but a few effects are allergic and some are idiosyncratic.

A. BEHAVIORAL EFFECTS

The older typical antipsychotic drugs are unpleasant to take. Many patients stop taking these drugs because of the adverse effects, which may be mitigated by giving small doses during the day and the major portion at bedtime. A "pseudodepression" that may be due to drug-induced akinesia usually responds to treatment with antiparkinsonism drugs. Other pseudodepressions may be due to higher doses than needed in a partially remitted patient, in which case decreasing the dose may relieve the symptoms. Toxic-confusional states may occur with very high doses of drugs that have prominent antimuscarinic actions.

B. NEUROLOGIC EFFECTS

Extrapyramidal reactions occurring early during treatment with older agents include typical **Parkinson's syndrome, akathisia** (uncontrollable restlessness), and **acute dystonic reactions** (spastic retrocollis or torticollis). Parkinsonism can be treated, when necessary, with conventional antiparkinsonism drugs of the antimuscarinic type or, in rare cases, with amantadine. (Levodopa should never be used in these patients.) Parkinsonism may be self-limiting, so that an attempt to withdraw antiparkinsonism drugs should be made every 3–4 months. Akathisia and dystonic reactions also respond to such treatment, but many prefer to use a sedative antihistamine with anticholinergic properties, eg, diphenhydramine, which can be given either parenterally or orally.

Tardive dyskinesia, as the name implies, is a late-occurring syndrome of abnormal choreoathetoid movements. It is the most important unwanted effect of antipsychotic drugs. It has been proposed that it is caused by a relative cholinergic deficiency secondary to supersensitivity of dopamine receptors in the caudate-putamen. The prevalence varies enormously, but tardive dyskinesia is estimated to have occurred in 20–40% of chronically treated patients prior to the introduction of the newer atypical antipsycotics. Early recognition is important, since advanced cases may be difficult to reverse. Many treatments have been proposed, but their evaluation is confounded by the fact that the course of the disorder is variable and sometimes self-limited. Most authorities agree that the first step would be to try to discontinue or reduce the dose of the current antipsychotic or switch to one of the newer atypical agents. A logical second step would be to eliminate all drugs with central anticholinergic action, particularly antiparkinsonism drugs and tricyclic antidepressants. These two steps are often enough to bring about improvement. If they fail, the addition of diazepam in doses as high as 30–40 mg/d may add to the improvement by enhancing GABAergic activity.

Seizures, though recognized as a complication of chlorpromazine treatment, were so rare with the high-potency older drugs as to merit little consideration. However, de novo seizures may occur in 2–5% of patients treated with clozapine.

C. AUTONOMIC NERVOUS SYSTEM EFFECTS

Most patients are able to tolerate the antimuscarinic adverse effects of antipsychotic drugs. Those who are made too uncomfortable or who develop urinary retention or other severe symptoms can be switched to an agent without significant antimuscarinic action. Orthostatic hypotension or impaired ejaculation—common complications of therapy with chlorpromazine or mesoridazine—should be managed by switching to drugs with less marked adrenoceptor-blocking actions.

D. METABOLIC AND ENDOCRINE EFFECTS

Weight gain is very common, especially with clozapine and olanzapine, and requires monitoring of food intake, especially carbohydrates. Hyperglycemia may develop, but whether secondary to weight gain-associated insulin resistance or due to other potential mechanisms remains to be clarified. Hyperprolactinemia in women results in the amenorrhea-galactorrhea syndrome and infertility; in men, loss of libido, impotence, and infertility may result.

E. TOXIC OR ALLERGIC REACTIONS

Agranulocytosis, cholestatic jaundice, and skin eruptions occur rarely with the high-potency antipsychotic drugs currently used.

In contrast to other antipsychotic agents, clozapine causes agranulocytosis in a small but significant number of patients—approximately 1–2% of those treated. This serious, potentially fatal effect can develop rapidly, usually between the 6th and 18th weeks of therapy. It is not known whether it represents an immune reaction, but it appears to be reversible upon discontinuance of the drug. *Because of the risk of agranulocytosis, patients receiving clozapine must have weekly blood counts for the first 6 months of treatment and every 3 weeks thereafter.*

F. OCULAR COMPLICATIONS

Deposits in the anterior portions of the eye (cornea and lens) are a common complication of chlorpromazine therapy. They may accentuate the normal processes of aging of the lens. Thioridazine is the only antipsychotic drug that causes retinal deposits, which in advanced cases may resemble retinitis pigmentosa. The deposits are usually associated with "browning" of vision. The maximum daily dose of thioridazine has been limited to 800 mg/d to reduce the possibility of this complication.

G. CARDIAC TOXICITY

Thioridazine in doses exceeding 300 mg daily is almost always associated with minor abnormalities of T waves that are easily reversible. Overdoses of thioridazine are associated with major ventricular arrhythmias, cardiac conduction block, and sudden death; it is not certain whether thioridazine can cause these same disorders when used in therapeutic doses. In view of possible additive antimuscarinic and quinidine-like actions with various tricyclic antidepressants, thioridazine should be combined with the latter drugs only with great care. Among the atypical agents, ziprasidone carries the greatest risk of QT prolongation and therefore should not be combined with other drugs that prolong the QT interval, including thioridazine, pimozide, and quinidine.

H. USE IN PREGNANCY; DYSMORPHOGENESIS

Although the antipsychotic drugs appear to be relatively safe in pregnancy, a small increase in teratogenic risk could be missed. Questions about whether to use these drugs during pregnancy and whether to abort a pregnancy in which the fetus has already been exposed must be decided individually.

I. NEUROLEPTIC MALIGNANT SYNDROME

This life-threatening disorder occurs in patients who are extremely sensitive to the extrapyramidal effects of antipsychotic agents (see also Chapter 16). The initial symptom is marked muscle rigidity. If sweating is impaired, as it often is during treatment with anticholinergic drugs, fever may ensue, often reaching dangerous levels. The stress leukocytosis and high fever associated with this syndrome may erroneously suggest an infectious process. Autonomic instability, with altered blood pressure and pulse rate, is often present. Creatine kinase isozymes are usually elevated, reflecting muscle damage. This syndrome is believed to result from an excessively rapid blockade of postsynaptic dopamine receptors. A severe form of extrapyramidal syndrome follows. Early in the course, vigorous treatment of the extrapyramidal syndrome with antiparkinsonism drugs is worthwhile. Muscle relaxants, particularly diazepam, are often useful. Other muscle relaxants, such as dantrolene, or dopamine agonists, such as bromocriptine, have been reported to be helpful. If fever is present, cooling by physical measures should be tried. Various minor forms of this syndrome are now recognized.

Drug Interactions

Antipsychotics produce more important pharmacodynamic than pharmacokinetic interactions because of their multiple effects. Additive effects may occur when these drugs are combined with others that have sedative effects, α-adrenoceptor-blocking action, anticholinergic effects, and—for thioridazine and ziprasidone—quinidine-like action.

A variety of pharmacokinetic interactions have been reported, but none are of major clinical significance.

Overdoses

Poisonings with antipsychotics (unlike tricyclic antidepressants) are rarely fatal, with the exception of those due to mesoridazine and thioridazine. In general, drowsiness proceeds to coma, with an intervening period of agitation. Neuromuscular excitability may be increased and proceed to convulsions. Pupils are miotic, and deep tendon reflexes are decreased. Hypotension and hypothermia are the rule, though fever may be present later in the course. The lethal effects of mesoridazine and thioridazine are related to induction of ventricular tachyarrhythmias. Patients should be given the usual "ABCD" treatment for poisonings (see Chapter 59) and treated supportively. Management of overdoses of thioridazine and mesoridazine, which are complicated by cardiac arrhythmias, is similar to that for tricyclic antidepressants (see Chapter 30).

Benefits & Limitations of Drug Treatment

As noted at the beginning of this chapter, antipsychotics have had a major impact on psychiatric treatment. First, they have shifted the care of patients from mental institutions to the community. For many patients, this shift has provided a better life under more humane circumstances and in many cases has made possible life without frequent use of physical restraints. For others, the tragedy of an aimless existence is now being played out in the streets of our communities rather than in mental institutions.

Second, these drugs have markedly shifted psychiatric thinking to a more biologic orientation. Partly because of research stimulated by the effects of these drugs on schizophrenia, we now know much more about central nervous system physiology and pharmacology than we did before the introduction of these agents. However, despite a great amount of research, schizophrenia remains a scientific mystery and a personal disaster for the patient. Although most schizophrenic patients obtain some degree of benefit from these drugs—in some cases substantial benefit—none are made well by them.

■ II. LITHIUM & OTHER MOOD-STABILIZING DRUGS

Lithium carbonate is often referred to as an "antimanic" drug, but in many parts of the world it is considered a "mood-stabilizing" agent because of its primary action of preventing mood swings in patients with bipolar affective (manic-depressive) disorder. Carbamazepine has also been recognized as effective in some groups of manic-depressive patients despite not being formally approved for such use. Valproate has recently been approved for the treatment of mania and is being evaluated as a mood stabilizer. Atypical antipsychotics, beginning with olanzapine, are being investigated and approved as antimanic agents and potential mood stabilizers.

Nature of Bipolar Affective Disorder

Bipolar affective (manic-depressive) disorder is a frequently diagnosed and very serious psychiatric disorder. Patients with cyclic attacks of mania have many symptoms of paranoid schizophrenia (grandiosity, bellicosity, paranoid thoughts, and overactivity). The ability to treat bipolar disorder effectively has made such diagnostic distinctions important.

The cause of the mood swings characteristic of bipolar affective disorder is unknown, although a preponderance of catecholamine-related activity may be present. Drugs that increase this activity tend to exacerbate mania, whereas those that reduce activity of dopamine or norepinephrine relieve mania. Acetylcholine or glutamate may also be involved. The nature of the abrupt switch from mania to depression experienced by some patients is uncertain. Bipolar disorder has a strong familial component. Genetic studies have identified at least three possible linkages to different chromosomes.

BASIC PHARMACOLOGY OF LITHIUM

Pharmacokinetics

Lithium is a small monovalent cation. Its pharmacokinetics are summarized in Table 29–5.

Pharmacodynamics

Despite considerable investigation, the mode of action of lithium remains unclear. The major possibilities being investigated include (1) effects on electrolytes and ion transport; (2) effects on neurotransmitters and their release; and (3) effects on second messengers and intracellular enzymes that mediate transmitter action. The last of these three approaches appears to be the most promising.

A. EFFECTS ON ELECTROLYTES AND ION TRANSPORT

Lithium is closely related to sodium in its properties. It can substitute for sodium in generating action potentials and in Na^+-Na^+ exchange across the membrane. It inhibits the latter process, ie, Li^+-Na^+ exchange is grad-

Table 29–5. Pharmacokinetics of lithium.

Absorption	Virtually complete within 6–8 hours; peak plasma levels in 30 minutes to 2 hours
Distribution	In total body water; slow entry into intracellular compartment. Initial volume of distribution is 0.5 L/kg, rising to 0.7–0.9 L/kg; some sequestration in bone. No protein binding.
Metabolism	None
Excretion	Virtually entirely in urine. Lithium clearance about 20% of creatinine. Plasma half-life about 20 hours.
Target plasma concentration	0.6–1.4 mEq/L
Dosage	0.5 mEq/kg/d in divided doses

Table 29–6. Enzymes affected by lithium at therapeutic concentrations.

Enzyme	Enzyme Function; Action of Lithium
Inositol monophosphatase	The rate-limiting enzyme in inositol recycling; inhibited by lithium, resulting in depletion of substrate for IP_3 production (see Figure 29–4)
Inositol polyphosphate 1-phosphatase	Another enzyme in inositol recycling; inhibited by lithium, resulting in depletion of substrate for IP_3 production (see Figure 29–4)
Bisphosphate nucleotidase	Involved in AMP production; inhibited by lithium; may be target that results in lithium-induced nephrogenic diabetes insipidus
Fructose 1,6-biphosphatase	Involved in gluconeogenesis; inhibition by lithium of unknown relevance
Phosphoglucomutase	Involved in glycogenolysis; inhibition by lithium of unknown relevance
Glycogen synthase kinase-3	Constitutively active enzyme that appears to limit neurotrophic and neuroprotective processes; lithium inhibits

AMP, adenosine monophosphate; IP_3, inositol 1,4,5-trisphosphate

ually slowed after lithium is introduced into the body. At therapeutic concentrations (around 1 mmol/L), it does not significantly affect the Na^+/Ca^{2+} exchange process or the Na^+/K^+ ATPase sodium pump.

B. EFFECTS ON NEUROTRANSMITTERS

Lithium appears to enhance some of the actions of serotonin, though findings have been contradictory. Its effects on norepinephrine are variable. The drug may decrease norepinephrine and dopamine turnover, and these effects, if confirmed, might be relevant to its antimanic action. Lithium also appears to block the development of dopamine receptor supersensitivity that may accompany chronic therapy with antipsychotic agents. Finally, lithium may augment the synthesis of acetylcholine, perhaps by increasing choline uptake into nerve terminals.

C. EFFECTS ON SECOND MESSENGERS

Some of the enzymes affected by lithium are listed in Table 29–6. One of the best-defined effects of lithium is its action on inositol phosphates. Early studies of lithium demonstrated changes in brain inositol phosphate levels, but the significance of these changes was not appreciated until the second-messenger roles of inositol-1,4,5-trisphosphate (IP_3) and diacylglycerol (DAG) were discovered. As described in Chapter 2, IP_3 and DAG are important second messengers for both α-adrenergic and muscarinic transmission. Lithium inhibits several important enzymes in the normal recycling of membrane phosphoinositides, including conversion of IP_2 to IP_1 (inositol monophosphate) and the conversion of IP_1 to inositol (Figure 29–4). This block leads to a depletion of phosphatidylinositol-4,5-bisphosphate (PIP_2), the membrane precursor of IP_3 and DAG. Over time, the effects of transmitters on the cell diminish in proportion to the amount of activity in the PIP_2-dependent pathways. Before therapy, such activity might be greatly increased in mania; thus, lithium could cause a selective depression of the overactive circuits.

Studies of noradrenergic effects in isolated brain tissue indicate that lithium can inhibit norepinephrine-sensitive adenylyl cyclase. Such an effect could relate to both its antidepressant and its antimanic effects. The relationship of these effects to lithium's actions on IP_3 mechanisms is currently unknown.

Because lithium affects second-messenger systems involving both activation of adenylyl cyclase and phosphoinositol turnover, it is not surprising that G proteins are also found to be affected. Several studies suggest that lithium may uncouple receptors from their G proteins; indeed, two of lithium's most common side effects, polyuria and subclinical hypothyroidism, may be due to uncoupling of the vasopressin and thyroid-stimulating hormone (TSH) receptors from their G proteins.

Figure 29–4. Effect of lithium on the IP_3 and DAG second-messenger system. The schematic diagram shows the synaptic membrane of a neuron. (PIP_2, phosphatidylinositol-4,5-bisphosphate; PLC, phospholipase-C; G, coupling protein; EFFECTS, activation of protein kinase C, mobilization of intracellular Ca^{2+}, etc.). Lithium, by inhibiting the recycling of inositol substrates, may cause depletion of the second-messenger source PIP_2 and therefore reduce the release of IP_3 and DAG. Lithium may also act by other mechanisms.

The major current working hypothesis for lithium's therapeutic mechanism of action supposes that its effects on phosphoinositol turnover, leading to an early relative reduction of myoinositol in human brain, are part of an initiating cascade of intracellular changes. Effects on specific isoforms of protein kinase C may be most relevant. Alterations of protein kinase C-mediated signaling alter gene expression and the production of proteins implicated in long-term neuroplastic events that could underlie long-term mood stabilization.

CLINICAL PHARMACOLOGY OF LITHIUM

Bipolar Affective Disorder

Until recently, lithium carbonate was the universally preferred treatment for bipolar disorder, especially in the manic phase. With the approval of valproate, olanzapine, and other newer antipsychotics for this indication, a smaller percentage of bipolar patients now receive lithium. This trend is reinforced by the slow onset of action of lithium, which has often been supplemented with concurrent use of antipsychotic drugs or potent benzodiazepines in severely manic patients. The overall success rate for achieving remission from the manic phase of bipolar disorder can be as high as 80%. However, among patients who require hospitalization, success rates are considerably lower. A similar situation applies to maintenance treatment, which is about 60% effective overall but less in severely ill patients. These considerations have led to increased use of combined treatment in severe cases. After mania is controlled, the antipsychotic drug may be stopped, then the benzodiazepine and lithium continued as maintenance therapy.

The depressive phase of manic-depressive disorder often requires concurrent use of an antidepressant drug (see Chapter 30). Tricyclic antidepressant agents have been linked to precipitation of mania, with more rapid cycling of mood swings, although most patients do not show this effect. Selective serotonin reuptake inhibitors are less likely to induce mania but may have limited efficacy. Bupropion has shown some promising effects but—like tricyclic antidepressants—may induce mania at higher doses. As shown in recent controlled trials, the anticonvulsant lamotrigine is effective for many patients with bipolar depression. For some patients, however, one of the older monoamine oxidase inhibitors may be the antidepressant of choice.

Unlike antipsychotic or antidepressant drugs, which exert several actions on the central or autonomic nervous system, lithium ion at therapeutic concentrations is devoid of autonomic blocking effects and of activating or sedating effects, though it can produce nausea and tremor. Most important is that the prophylactic use of lithium can prevent both mania and depression. Many experts believe that the aggressive marketing of newer drugs has inappropriately produced a shift to drugs that are less effective than lithium for substantial numbers of patients.

Other Applications

Recurrent endogenous depression with a cyclic pattern is controlled by either lithium or imipramine, both of which are superior to a placebo.

Schizoaffective disorder, another condition with an affective component characterized by a mixture of schizophrenic symptoms and depression or excitement, is treated with antipsychotic drugs alone or combined with lithium. Various antidepressants are added if depression is present.

Lithium alone is rarely successful in treating schizophrenia, but adding it to an antipsychotic may salvage an otherwise treatment-resistant patient. Carbamazepine may work equally well when added to an antipsychotic.

An interesting application of lithium that is relatively well supported by controlled studies is as an adjunct to tricyclic antidepressants and selective serotonin reuptake inhibitors in patients with unipolar depression who do not respond fully to monotherapy with the antidepressant. For this application, concentrations of lithium at the lower end of the recommended range for manic depressive illness appear to be adequate.

Monitoring Treatment

Clinicians rely on measurements of serum lithium concentrations for assessing both the dosage required for treatment of acute mania and for prophylactic maintenance. These measurements are customarily taken 10–12 hours after the last dose, so all data in the literature pertaining to these concentrations reflect this interval.

An initial determination of serum lithium concentration should be obtained about 5 days after the start of treatment, at which time steady-state conditions should have been attained. If the clinical response suggests a change in dosage, simple arithmetic (new dose equals present dose times desired blood level divided by present blood level) should produce the desired level. The serum concentration attained with the adjusted dosage can be checked in another 5 days. Once the desired concentration has been achieved, levels can be measured at increasing intervals unless the schedule is influenced by intercurrent illness or the introduction of a new drug into the treatment program.

Maintenance Treatment

The decision to use lithium as *prophylactic* treatment depends on many factors: the frequency and severity of previous episodes, a crescendo pattern of appearance, and the degree to which the patient is willing to follow a program of indefinite maintenance therapy. If the present attack was the patient's first or if the patient is unreliable, one might prefer to terminate treatment after the episode

has subsided. Patients who have one or more episodes of illness per year are candidates for maintenance treatment. Although some patients can be maintained with serum levels as low as 0.6 mEq/L, the best results have been obtained with higher levels, such as 0.9 mEq/L.

Drug Interactions

Renal clearance of lithium is reduced about 25% by diuretics (eg, thiazides), and doses may need to be reduced by a similar amount. A similar reduction in lithium clearance has been noted with several of the newer nonsteroidal anti-inflammatory drugs that block synthesis of prostaglandins. This interaction has not been reported for either aspirin or acetaminophen. All neuroleptics tested to date, with the possible exception of clozapine and the newer antipsychotics, may produce more severe extrapyramidal syndromes when combined with lithium.

Adverse Effects & Complications

Many adverse effects associated with lithium treatment occur at varying times after treatment is started. Some are harmless, but it is important to be alert to adverse effects that may signify impending serious toxic reactions.

A. NEUROLOGIC AND PSYCHIATRIC ADVERSE EFFECTS

Tremor is one of the most common adverse effects of lithium treatment, and it occurs with therapeutic doses. Propranolol and atenolol, which have been reported to be effective in essential tremor, also alleviate lithium-induced tremor. Other reported neurologic abnormalities include choreoathetosis, motor hyperactivity, ataxia, dysarthria, and aphasia. Psychiatric disturbances at toxic concentrations are generally marked by mental confusion and withdrawal. Appearance of any new neurologic or psychiatric symptoms or signs is a clear indication for temporarily stopping treatment with lithium and close monitoring of serum levels.

B. DECREASED THYROID FUNCTION

Lithium probably decreases thyroid function in most patients exposed to the drug, but the effect is reversible or nonprogressive. Few patients develop frank thyroid enlargement, and fewer still show symptoms of hypothyroidism. Although initial thyroid testing followed by regular monitoring of thyroid function has been proposed, such procedures are not cost-effective. Obtaining a serum TSH concentration every 6–12 months, however, is prudent.

C. NEPHROGENIC DIABETES INSIPIDUS AND OTHER RENAL ADVERSE EFFECTS

Polydipsia and polyuria are common but reversible concomitants of lithium treatment, occurring at therapeutic serum concentrations. The principal physiologic lesion involved is loss of responsiveness to antidiuretic hormone (nephrogenic diabetes insipidus). Lithium-induced diabetes insipidus is resistant to vasopressin but responds to amiloride.

An extensive literature has accumulated concerning other forms of renal dysfunction during long-term lithium therapy, including chronic interstitial nephritis and minimal-change glomerulopathy with nephrotic syndrome. Some instances of decreased glomerular filtration rate have been encountered but no instances of marked azotemia or renal failure.

Patients receiving lithium should avoid dehydration and the associated increased concentration of lithium in urine. Periodic tests of renal concentrating ability should be performed to detect changes.

D. EDEMA

Edema is a common adverse effect of lithium treatment and may be related to some effect of lithium on sodium retention. Although weight gain may be expected in patients who become edematous, water retention does not account for the weight gain observed in up to 30% of patients taking lithium.

E. CARDIAC ADVERSE EFFECTS

The bradycardia-tachycardia ("sick sinus") syndrome is a definite contraindication to the use of lithium because the ion further depresses the sinus node. T-wave flattening is often observed on ECG but is of questionable significance.

F. USE DURING PREGNANCY

Renal clearance of lithium increases during pregnancy and reverts to lower levels immediately after delivery. A patient whose serum lithium concentration is in a good therapeutic range during pregnancy may develop toxic levels following delivery. Special care in monitoring lithium levels is needed at these times. Lithium is transferred to nursing infants through breast milk, in which it has a concentration about one-third to one-half that of serum. Lithium toxicity in newborns is manifested by lethargy, cyanosis, poor suck and Moro reflexes, and perhaps hepatomegaly.

The issue of dysmorphogenesis is not settled. An earlier report suggested an increase in the frequency of cardiac anomalies, especially Ebstein's anomaly, in lithium babies, and it is listed as such in Table 60–1 in this book. However, more recent data suggest that lithium carries a relatively low risk of teratogenic effects. Further research is needed in this important area.

G. MISCELLANEOUS ADVERSE EFFECTS

Transient acneiform eruptions have been noted early in lithium treatment. Some of them subside with temporary discontinuance of treatment and do not recur with its resumption. Folliculitis is less dramatic and probably occurs more frequently. Leukocytosis is always present during lithium treatment, probably reflecting a direct effect on leukopoiesis rather than mobilization from the marginal pool. This adverse effect has now become a therapeutic effect in patients with low leukocyte counts.

Overdoses

Therapeutic overdoses of lithium are more common than those due to deliberate or accidental ingestion of the drug. Therapeutic overdoses are usually due to accumulation of lithium resulting from some change in the patient's status, such as diminished serum sodium, use of diuretics, or fluctuating renal function. Since the tissues will have already equilibrated with the blood, the plasma concentrations of lithium may not be excessively high in proportion to the degree of toxicity; any value over 2 mEq/L must be considered as indicating likely toxicity. Because lithium is a small ion, it is dialyzed readily. Both peritoneal dialysis and hemodialysis are effective, though the latter is preferred. Dialysis should be continued until the plasma concentration falls below the usual therapeutic range.

VALPROIC ACID

Valproic acid (valproate), discussed in detail in Chapter 24 as an antiepileptic, has been demonstrated to have antimanic effects and is now being widely used for this indication in the USA. Gabapentin is not effective, leaving the mechanism of action of valproate unclear. Overall, it shows efficacy equivalent to that of lithium during the early weeks of treatment. It is significant that valproic acid has been effective in some patients who have failed to respond to lithium. Moreover, its side-effect profile is such that one can rapidly increase the dosage over a few days to produce blood levels in the apparent therapeutic range, with nausea being the only limiting factor in some patients. The starting dosage is 750 mg/d, increasing rapidly to the 1500–2000 mg range with a recommended maximum dosage of 60 mg/kg/d.

Combinations of valproic acid with other psychotropic medications likely to be used in the management of either phase of bipolar illness are generally well tolerated. Valproic acid is becoming recognized as an appropriate first-line treatment for mania, although it is not clear that it will be as effective as lithium as a maintenance treatment in all subsets of patients. Many clinicians argue for combining valproic acid and lithium in patients who do not fully respond to either agent alone.

CARBAMAZEPINE

Carbamazepine has been considered to be a reasonable alternative to lithium when the latter is less than optimally efficacious. The mode of action of carbamazepine is unclear, and oxcarbazepine is not effective. Carbamazepine may be used to treat acute mania and also for prophylactic therapy. Adverse effects (discussed in Chapter 24) are generally no greater and sometimes less than those associated with lithium. Carbamazepine may be used alone or, in refractory patients, in combination with lithium or, rarely, valproate.

The use of carbamazepine as a mood stabilizer is similar to its use as an anticonvulsant (see Chapter 24). Dosage usually begins with 200 mg twice daily, with increases as needed. Maintenance dosage is similar to that used for treating epilepsy, ie, 800–1200 mg/d. Plasma concentrations between 3 and 14 mg/L are considered desirable, although no therapeutic range

has been established. Blood dyscrasias have figured prominently in the adverse effects of carbamazepine when it is used as an anticonvulsant, but they have not been a major problem with its use as a mood stabilizer. Overdoses of carbamazepine are a major emergency and should generally be managed like overdoses of tricyclic antidepressants.

OTHER DRUGS

Lamotrigine has been reported to be useful in preventing the depression that often follows the manic phase of bipolar disorder.

PREPARATIONS AVAILABLE

ANTIPSYCHOTIC AGENTS

Aripiprazole (Abilify)
Oral: 5, 10, 15, 20, 30 mg tablets; 1 mg/mL solution

Chlorpromazine (generic, Thorazine)
Oral: 10, 25, 50, 100, 200 mg tablets; 100 mg/mL concentrate
Rectal: 100 mg suppositories
Parenteral: 25 mg/mL for IM injection

Clozapine (generic, Clozaril)
Oral: 12.5, 25, 100 mg tablets; 25, 100 mg orally disintegrating tablets

Fluphenazine (generic, Prolixin)
Oral: 1, 2.5, 5, 10 mg tablets; 2.5 mg/5 mL elixir
Parenteral: (fluphenazine HCl): 2.5 mg/mL for IM injection

Fluphenazine decanoate (generic, Prolixin)
Parenteral: 25 mg/mL for IM or SC injection

Haloperidol (generic, Haldol)
Oral: 0.5, 1, 2, 5, 10, 20 mg tablets; 2 mg/mL concentrate
Parenteral: 5 mg/mL for IM injection

Haloperidol ester (Haldol Decanoate)
Parenteral: 50, 100 mg/mL for IM injection

Loxapine (generic, Loxitane)
Oral: 5, 10, 25, 50 mg capsules

Molindone (Moban)
Oral: 5, 10, 25, 50 mg tablets

Olanzapine (Zyprexa)
Oral: 2.5, 5, 7.5, 10, 15, 20 mg tablets; 5, 10, 15, 20 mg orally disintegrating tablets
Parenteral: 10 mg powder for injection

Perphenazine (generic)
Oral: 2, 4, 8, 16 mg tablets; 16 mg/5 mL concentrate

Pimozide (Orap)
Oral: 1, 2 mg tablets

Prochlorperazine (generic, Compazine)
Oral: 5, 10 mg tablets; 5 mg/5 mL syrup
Oral sustained-release: 10, 15 mg capsules
Rectal: 2.5, 5, 25 mg suppositories
Parenteral: 5 mg/mL for IM injection

Quetiapine (Seroquel)
Oral: 25, 100, 200, 300 mg tablets

Risperidone (Risperdal)
Oral: 0.25, 0.5, 1, 2, 3, 4 mg tablets; 0.5, 1, 2 mg orally disintegrating tablets; 1 mg/mL oral solution
Parenteral: 25, 37.5, 50 mg powder for injection

Thioridazine (generic, Mellaril)
Oral: 10, 15, 25, 50, 100, 150, 200 mg tablets; 30 mg/mL concentrate

Thiothixene (generic, Navane)
Oral: 1, 2, 5, 10, 20 mg capsules

Trifluoperazine (generic)
Oral: 1, 2, 5, 10 mg tablets

Ziprasidone (Geodon)
Oral: 20, 40, 60, 80 mg capsules
Parenteral: 20 mg powder for IM injection

MOOD STABILIZERS

Carbamazepine (generic, Tegretol)
Oral: 200, 300, 400 mg tablets, 100 mg chewable tablets; 100 mg/5 mL oral suspension
Oral extended-release: 100, 200, 400 mg tablets; 200, 300 mg capsules

Divalproex (Depakote)
Oral: 125, 250, 500 mg delayed-release tablets

Lithium carbonate (generic, Eskalith) (*Note*: 300 mg lithium carbonate = 8.12 mEq Li⁺.)
Oral: 150, 300, 600 mg capsules; 300 mg tablets; 8 mEq/5 mL syrup
Oral sustained-release: 300, 450 mg tablets

Valproic acid (generic, Depakene)
Oral: 250 mg capsules; 250 mg/5 mL syrup

REFERENCES

Antipsychotics

Bilder RM et al: Neurocognitive effects of clozapine, olanzapine, risperidone, and haloperidol in patients with chronic schizophrenia or schizoaffective disorder. Am J Psychiatry 2002;159:1018.

Breier A, Berg PH: The psychosis of schizophrenia: Prevalence, response to atypical antipsychotics, and prediction of outcome. Biol Psychiatry 1999;46:361.

Carlsson A, Waters N, Carlsson ML: Neurotransmitter interactions in schizophrenia—therapeutic implications. Biol Psychiatry 1999;46:1388.

Farde L et al: Central D_2-dopamine receptor occupancy in schizophrenic patients treated with antipsychotic drugs. Arch Gen Psychiatry 1987;45:71.

Freudenreich O, Goff DC: Antipsychotic combination therapy in schizophrenia. A review of efficacy and risks of current combinations. Acta Psychiatr Scand 2002;106:323.

Haddad PM, Anderson IM: Antipsychotic-related QT_c prolongation, torsade de pointes and sudden death. Drugs 2002;62:1649.

Jacobsen E: The early history of psychotherapeutic drugs. Psychopharmacology 1986;89:138.

Lieberman JA et al: Effectiveness of antipsychotic drugs in patients with chronic schizophrenia. N Engl J Med 2005;353:1209

McGavin JK, Goa KL: Aripiprazole. CNS Drugs 2002;16:779.

Meltzer HY: Treatment of schizophrenia and spectrum disorders: Pharmacotherapy, psychosocial treatments, and neurotransmitter interactions. Biol Psychiatry 1999;46:1321.

Seeman P: Dopamine receptors and the dopamine hypothesis of schizophrenia. Synapse 1987;1:133.

Stefansson H et al: Neuregulin 1 and susceptibility to schizophrenia. Am J Hum Genet 2002;71:877.

Tauscher J et al: Significant dissociation of brain and plasma kinetics with antipsychotics. Mol Psychiatry 2002;7:317.

Mood Stabilizers

Baraban JM, Worley PF, Snyder SH: Second messenger systems and psychoactive drug action: Focus on the phosphoinositide system and lithium. Am J Psychiatry 1989; 146:1251.

Bowden CL: Valproate in mania. In: Manji HK, Bowden CL, Belmaker RH (editors): *Bipolar Medications: Mechanisms of Action.* American Psychiatric Press, 2000.

Cowan WM et al: The human genome project and its impact on psychiatry. Annu Rev Neurosci 2002;25:1.

Jope RS: Anti-bipolar therapy: Mechanism of action of lithium. Mol Psychiatry 1999;4:117.

Manji HK, Chen G: PKC, MAP kinases and the bcl-2 family of proteins as long-term targets for mood stabilizers. Mol Psychiatry 2002;(7 Suppl 1):S46.

Quiroz JA et al: Emerging experimental therapeutics for bipolar disorder: Clues from the molecular pathophysiology. Mol Psychiatry 2004;9:756.

Schou M: Lithium treatment at 52. J Affect Disord 2001;67:21.

Sklar P: Linkage analysis in psychiatric disorders: The emerging picture. Ann Rev Genomics Hum Genet 2002;3:371.

Antidepressant Agents

30

William Z. Potter, MD, PhD, & Leo E. Hollister, MD*

Major depression is one of the most common psychiatric disorders. At any given moment, about 3–5% of the population is depressed (point prevalence), and an estimated 10% of people may become depressed during their lives (lifetime prevalence). The symptoms of depression are often subtle and unrecognized both by patients and by physicians. Patients with vague complaints that resist explanation as manifestations of somatic disorders and those who might be simplistically described as "neurotic" should be suspected of being depressed.

Depression is a heterogeneous disorder that has been characterized and classified in a variety of ways. According to the American Psychiatric Association's modified fourth edition (2000) of the *Diagnostic and Statistical Manual of Mental Disorders (DSM-IV-TR)*, several diagnoses of affective disorders are possible. Major depression and dysthymia (minor) are pure depressive syndromes, whereas bipolar disorder and cyclothymic disorder signify depression in association with mania. A simplified classification based on presumed origin is as follows: (1) brief reactive or secondary depression (most common), occurring in response to real stimuli such as grief, illness, etc; (2) melancholic and recurrent depression, a genetically determined biochemical disorder manifested by an inability to experience ordinary pleasure or to cope with ordinary life events; and (3) depression associated with bipolar affective (manic-depressive) disorder. Because safe antidepressants are now available, almost any individual with several symptoms of depression that persist beyond a few weeks is a candidate for pharmacologic treatment. Intensive efforts to formalize guidelines for the treatment of depression have been pursued for more than a decade, resulting in guidelines from the American Psychiatric Association, the Agency for Health Care Policy and Research, and the World Federation of Societies of Biological Psychiatry. Pharmacologic treatment is emphasized, although a continuing role for electroconvulsive therapy for delusional or severe forms of life-threatening depression is also noted.

---

*Deceased.

The Pathogenesis of Major Depression: The Amine Hypothesis and Subsequent Developments

Soon after the introduction of reserpine in the early 1950s, it became apparent that the drug could induce depression. Studies revealed that the principal mechanism of action of reserpine was to inhibit the neuronal storage of amine neurotransmitters such as serotonin and norepinephrine. Reserpine induced depression and depleted stores of amine neurotransmitters; therefore, it was reasoned, depression must be associated with decreased functional amine-dependent synaptic transmission. This idea provided the basis for what became known as the amine hypothesis of depression. By extension, drugs that increased amine function in appropriate synaptic areas would relieve depression. A major puzzle in applying this hypothesis was the fact that although the pharmacologic actions of both tricyclic and monoamine oxidase (MAO) inhibitor classes of antidepressants are prompt, the clinical effects require weeks to become manifest. Attempts have been made to explain this observation by invoking slow compensatory responses to the initial blockade of amine reuptake or MAO inhibition (see below).

Current brain imaging and biochemical studies in patients do not support a single biologic abnormality as common to most depressions. Rather, prevailing hypotheses emphasize an underlying role for several brain circuits that have a propensity to become dysfunctional, especially following certain stressors, in individuals with a range of genetic predispositions. It is likely that several pathophysiologic processes will ultimately be identified to account for the presentation of what is now termed *major depression*.

Nevertheless, the amine hypothesis has provided the major experimental models for the discovery of new antidepressant drugs. As a result, all currently available antidepressants, except bupropion, are classified as having their primary actions on the metabolism, reuptake, or selective receptor antagonism of serotonin, norepinephrine, or both.

$R_1: -(CH_2)_3N(CH_3)_2$
$R_2: H$

Imipramine

$R_1: = CH(CH_2)_2N(CH_3)_2$

Amitriptyline

$R_1: = CH(CH_2)_2N(CH_3)_2$

Doxepin

$R_1: -(CH_2)_3NHCH_3$
$R_2: H$

Desipramine

$R_1: = CH(CH_2)_2NHCH_3$

Nortriptyline

$R_1: -(CH_2)_3N(CH_3)_2$
$R_2: - Cl$

Clomipramine

$R_1: - (CH_2)_3NHCH_3$

Protriptyline

$R_1: - CH_2CH(CH_3)CH_2N(CH_3)_2$
$R_2: H$

Trimipramine

Figure 30–1. Structural relationships between various tricyclic antidepressants (TCAs).

■ I. BASIC PHARMACOLOGY OF ANTIDEPRESSANTS

Chemistry

A variety of chemical structures have been found to have antidepressant activity. With the exception of bupropion, however, the core antidepressant action of even the newest agents derives from mechanisms proposed for antidepressants that were introduced four decades ago.

A. TRICYCLIC ANTIDEPRESSANTS (TCAs)

Tricyclic antidepressants—so called because of the characteristic three-ring nucleus (Figure 30–1)—have been used clinically for four decades. They closely resemble the phenothiazines chemically and, to a lesser extent, pharmacologically. Like the phenothiazines, tricyclics were first thought to be useful as antihistamines with sedative properties. The discovery of their antidepressant properties was a fortuitous clinical observation. **Imipramine** and **amitriptyline** are the prototypical drugs of the class as mixed norepinephrine and seroto-

nin uptake inhibitors, although they also have several other effects.

B. SECOND-GENERATION AND SUBSEQUENT AGENTS

Between 1980 and 2005, thirteen structurally unique antidepressants and one isomeric variation were introduced. The agents classified as second generation and available for clinical use in the USA are shown in Figure 30–2. **Amoxapine** and **maprotiline** resemble the structure of the tricyclic agents, whereas **trazodone** and **bupropion** are distinctive. Newer, third generation drugs include **venlafaxine, mirtazapine, nefazodone,** and **duloxetine.** The structures of these compounds are shown in Figure 30–3. Six additional agents that work mainly through serotonin uptake inhibition are classified together in the following section.

C. SELECTIVE SEROTONIN REUPTAKE INHIBITORS (SSRIs)

Search for molecules with greater selectivity for the serotonin transporter led to the introduction of **fluoxetine**—an effective and more selective antidepressant with minimal autonomic toxicity. Since that time, four more SSRIs have been introduced as well as the active enantiomeric form of one, *(S)*-citalopram. All are structurally distinct from the tricyclic molecules (Figure 30–4).

Figure 30–2. Second-generation antidepressants.

Figure 30–3. Newer (third-generation) antidepressants.

Fluoxetine

Paroxetine

Sertraline

Fluvoxamine

Citalopram

Figure 30–4. Selective serotonin reuptake inhibitors (SSRIs).

These drugs have fewer adverse effects than the tricyclics and have become very popular.

D. MONOAMINE OXIDASE (MAO) INHIBITORS

MAO inhibitors may be classified as hydrazides, exemplified by the C–N–N moiety, as is the case with **phenelzine** and **isocarboxazid** (no longer marketed); or nonhydrazides, which lack such a moiety, as with **tranylcypromine** (Figure 30–5).

Tranylcypromine closely resembles dextroamphetamine, which is itself a weak inhibitor of MAO. Tranylcypromine retains some of the sympathomimetic characteristics of the amphetamines. The hydrazides appear to combine irreversibly with the enzyme, whereas tranylcypromine has a prolonged duration of effect even though it is not bound irreversibly. These older MAO inhibitors are nonselective inhibitors of both MAO-A and MAO-B. Selegiline, an MAO inhibitor used in Parkinson's disease that is selective for MAO-B at low doses but less selective at higher doses, has been approved for the treatment of major depression.

Phenelzine

Tranylcypromine

Figure 30–5. Some monoamine oxidase inhibitors. Phenelzine is the hydrazide of phenylethylamine (see Figure 9–3), whereas tranylcypromine has a cyclopropyl amine side chain and closely resembles dextroamphetamine (see Figure 9–4). These agents are unselective and produce an extremely long-lasting inhibition of the enzyme. Selegiline, which is partially selective for MAO-B, is shown in Figure 28–2.

Table 30–1. Pharmacokinetic parameters of various antidepressants.

Drug	Bioavail-ability (percent)	Protein Binding (percent)	Plasma $t_{1/2}$ (hours)	Active Metabolites	Volume of Distribution (L/kg)	Therapeutic Plasma Concentrations (ng/mL)[1]
Amitriptyline	31–61	82–96	31–46	Nortriptyline	5–10	80–200 total
Amoxapine	nd[2]	nd	8	7-,8-Hydroxy	nd	nd
Bupropion	60–80	85	11–14	Hydroxy, threohydro, erythreohydro	20–30	25–100
Citalopram	51–93	70–80	23–75	Desmethyl	12–16	nd
Clomipramine	nd	nd	22–84	Desmethyl	7–20	240–700
Desipramine	60–70	73–90	14–62	Hydroxy	22–59	> 125
Doxepin	13–45	nd	8–24	Desmethyl	9–33	30–150
Escitalopram	80	56	27–59	Desmethyl	12	nd
Fluoxetine	70	94	24–96	Norfluoxetine	12–97	nd
Fluvoxamine	> 90	77	7–63	None	> 5	nd
Imipramine	29–77	76–95	9–24	Desipramine	15–30	> 180 total
Maprotiline	66–75	88	21–52	Desmethyl	15–28	200–300
Mirtazapine	nd	nd	20–40	Desmethyl	nd	nd
Nefazodone	15–23	98	2–4	Hydroxy, *m*-chlorophenyl piperazine	nd	nd
Nortriptyline	32–79	93–95	18–93	10-Hydroxy	21–57	50–150
Paroxetine	50	95	24	None	28–31	nd
Protriptyline	77–93	90–95	54–198	nd	19–57	70–170
Sertraline	nd	98	22–35	Desmethyl	20	nd
Trazodone	nd	nd	4–9	*m*-Chloro-phe-nyl-piperazine	nd	nd
Venlafaxine	nd	27–30	4–10	*O*-Desmethyl	nd	nd

[1]Range includes active metabolites.
[2]nd = no data found.

Pharmacokinetics

A. TRICYCLIC ANTIDEPRESSANTS

Most tricyclics are incompletely absorbed and undergo significant first-pass metabolism. As a result of high tissue protein binding and relatively high lipid solubility, volumes of distribution tend to be very large. Tricyclics are metabolized by two major routes: transformation of the tricyclic nucleus and alteration of the aliphatic side chain. Monodemethylation of tertiary amines leads to active metabolites such as desipramine and nortrip-tyline (which are themselves available as drugs; Figure 30–1). The pharmacokinetic parameters of various antidepressants are summarized in Table 30–1.

B. SECOND-GENERATION AND SUBSEQUENT ANTIDEPRESSANTS

The pharmacokinetics of these drugs are similar to those of the TCAs (Table 30–1). Some have active metabolites. Trazodone and venlafaxine have short plasma half-lives, which mandates divided doses during the day when beginning treatment, although once-a-day dosing may be possible later. Extended-release forms of bupropion and venlafaxine allow for once-a-day dosing in some patients from the outset.

C. Selective Serotonin Reuptake Inhibitors

The pharmacokinetic parameters of these drugs are summarized in Table 30–1. Fluoxetine is notable for the long half-life of its active metabolite, norfluoxetine (7–9 days at steady state). This long $t_{1/2}$ has allowed the introduction of a formulation for once-weekly dosing. Sertraline and paroxetine have pharmacokinetic parameters similar to those of tricyclics. Citalopram and fluvoxamine resemble fluoxetine.

D. MAO Inhibitors

The monoamine oxidase inhibitors (MAOIs) are readily absorbed from the gastrointestinal tract. The hydrazide inhibitor phenelzine is acetylated in the liver and manifests differences in elimination, depending on the acetylation phenotype of the individual (see Chapter 4). However, inhibition of MAO persists even after these drugs (including selegiline) are no longer detectable in plasma. Therefore, conventional pharmacokinetic parameters (half-life, etc) are not very helpful in governing dosage. It is prudent to assume that the drug effect will persist for 7 days (tranylcypromine) to 2 or 3 weeks (phenelzine, selegiline) after discontinuance of the drug.

Pharmacodynamics

A. Actions of Antidepressants on Amine Neurotransmitters

The amine hypothesis was buttressed by studies on the mechanism of action of various types of antidepressant drugs. Tricyclics block the amine transporters (uptake pumps; Figure 30–6) known as the norepinephrine and serotonin transporters, NET and SERT, respectively. These transporters terminate amine neurotransmission (see Table 30–2 and Chapter 6). Blockade of these transporters presumably permits a longer sojourn of neurotransmitter in the intrasynaptic space at the receptor site. MAO inhibitors block a major intraneuronal degradative pathway for the amine neurotransmitters, which permits more amines to accumulate in presynaptic stores (Figure 30–6) and more to be released. Some of the second-generation antidepressants have similar strong effects on amine transporters, whereas others have only moderate or minimal effects on reuptake or metabolism. Countering this simple model of increased synaptic activity is increasing evidence of alterations in presynaptic regulation of neurotransmitter release. Presynaptic autoreceptors respond to increased synaptic transmitter by down-regulating transmitter synthesis and release. Furthermore, some (but not all) of these regulatory receptors may themselves be down-regulated. These changes occur on a slower time scale more in keeping with the clinically observed effects.

Trazodone, nefazodone, and mirtazapine stand out as agents in which antagonism of subtypes of serotonin receptors (5-HT$_{2A}$ or 5-HT$_{2C}$) may be important in their action. Mirtazapine is unique in including antagonism of α_2 norepinephrine receptors as presumably contributing to its therapeutic effects. Bupropion has been found to alter the output of norepinephrine in humans following chronic administration through some as yet unidentified primary mechanism as well as occupying about 25% of dopamine uptake transporters (DAT) in the brain as revealed by positron emission tomography. (Since it has been shown that effective doses of SSRIs occupy 80% of serotonin uptake sites, the clinical relevance of 25% DAT occupancy is uncertain.) Thus, even the newest antidepressants can still be categorized as possibly working through serotonergic and noradrenergic effects with the additional possibility of a role for dopamine. Increased synaptic dopamine has often been invoked as relevant to the efficacy of MAOIs.

B. Receptor and Postreceptor Effects

Considerable attention has been paid to the long-term postsynaptic effects of increased neurotransmitters in the synapses. In tests of postsynaptic effects, especially of the tricyclics, cAMP concentrations have consistently *decreased* rather than increased. In addition, the number of receptors for the neurotransmitters can decrease over the same time course as clinical improvement in patients. Thus, the initial increase in neurotransmitter seen with some antidepressants appears to produce, over time, a compensatory decrease in receptor activity, ie, down-regulation of certain postsynaptic as well as presynaptic receptors.

It has long been thought that enhanced serotonergic transmission, albeit mediated through diverse mechanisms, might be a common effect of antidepressants even without an increase in synaptic serotonin. Moreover, selective antagonism of either norepinephrine or serotonin receptors as opposed to that of the 5-HT transporter may lead to enhanced extracellular serotonin due to the complex manner in which these neurotransmitters are regulated.

Most recently, long-term intracellular changes involving phosphorylation of various regulatory elements, including those within the nucleus, have been implicated as relevant to antidepressant action. It is possible that effects on certain neurotrophic factors—factors critical to sustained survival and function of neurons in the adult nervous system—may be central to the actions of antidepressants.

Clinical studies have indirectly tested the relevance of findings from animals for norepinephrine or serotonin function. The approach has been to reduce the amino acid precursor of serotonin, tryptophan, in the diet and, by implication, the amount of available neurotransmitter in the brain, since tryptophan availability can be rate-limiting in the formation of serotonin. Severely tryptophan-depleted diets reduce plasma tryptophan and acutely reverse antidepressant responses to SSRIs but not

Figure 30–6. Schematic diagram showing some of the potential sites of action of antidepressant drugs. The primary neuron is shown as releasing a transmitter amine (NT). A modulating neuron may release a second transmitter (NT_x), regulating the activity of the primary neuron. The most consistent observed effect of the antidepressants (other than MAO inhibitors) is inhibition of the reuptake transporters (T) for norepinephrine or serotonin. The MAO inhibitors increase the vesicular stores of both NE and 5-HT. Other direct or indirect effects include initial increase in activation of pre- and postsynaptic receptors and subsequent desensitization or down-regulation of transmitter synthesis from an amino acid (AA), receptor numbers, or postreceptor mechanisms. Desensitization resulting from antidepressant use has been reported for α_2, β, and 5-HT_{1A} systems (color). VAT denotes a vesicle-associated transporter.

to NET inhibitors. Similarly, depletion of the norepinephrine amino acid precursor tyrosine can reverse antidepressant effects of the relatively selective NET inhibitor, desipramine. These findings support the hypothesis that enhanced serotonin and norepinephrine throughput is necessary for the antidepressant actions of the respective transporter inhibitors. However, tryptophan depletion does not consistently worsen the condition of unmedicated depressed patients. Thus, there is still no clear relationship between serotonin and depression or antidepressant mechanisms in general.

C. EFFECTS OF SPECIFIC ANTIDEPRESSANTS

1. Tricyclics—The first-generation antidepressants demonstrate varying degrees of selectivity for the reuptake

pumps for norepinephrine and serotonin (Table 30–2) but selectivity is much lower than for the SSRIs. They also have numerous autonomic actions, as described below under Adverse Effects.

2. Second-generation agents—Amoxapine is a metabolite of the antipsychotic drug loxapine and retains some of its antipsychotic action and dopamine receptor antagonism (see Chapter 29). A combination of antidepressant and antipsychotic actions might make it a suitable drug for depression in psychotic patients. However, the dopamine antagonism may cause akathisia, parkinsonism, amenorrhea-galactorrhea syndrome, and perhaps tardive dyskinesia.

Maprotiline (a tetracyclic drug) is most like desipramine in terms of its potent norepinephrine uptake inhibition.

Table 30–2. Pharmacologic differences among several antidepressants.[1]

Drug	Sedative Action	Antimuscarinic Action	Block of Amine Pump for:		
			Serotonin	Norepinephrine	Dopamine
Amitriptyline	+++	+++	+++	++	0
Amoxapine	++	++	+	++	+
Bupropion	0	0	0	+, 0	+
Citalopram, escitalopram	0	0	+++	0	0
Clomipramine	+++	++	+++	+++	0
Desipramine	+	+	0, +	+++	0
Doxepin	+++	+++	++	+	0
Duloxetine	0	0	+++	++	0
Fluoxetine	+	+	+++	0, +	0, +
Fluvoxamine	0	0	+++	0	0
Imipramine	++	++	+++	++	0
Maprotiline	++	++	0	+++	0
Mirtazapine [2]	+++	0	0	0	0
Nefazodone	++	+++	+, 0	0	0
Nortriptyline	++	++	+++	++	0
Paroxetine	+	0	+++	0	0
Protriptyline	0	++	?	+++	?
Sertraline	+	0	+++	0	0
Trazodone	+++	0	0, +	0	0
Venlafaxine	0	0	+++	++	0, +

[1] 0 = none; + = slight; ++ = moderate; +++ = high; ? = uncertain.
[2] Significant α_2-adrenoceptor antagonism.

Like desipramine, it has fewer sedative and antimuscarinic actions than the older tricyclics.

Clinical experience with trazodone has indicated unpredictable efficacy for depression, although it has proved very useful as a hypnotic, sometimes being combined with MAOIs, which disturb sleep.

3. Subsequent non-SSRI agents—Four antidepressants—nefazodone, venlafaxine, duloxetine, and mirtazapine—are all related to earlier agents in either structure or mechanism of action. Nefazodone is closely related to trazodone but is less sedating. It produces fewer adverse sexual effects than the SSRIs (see below) but is a potent inhibitor of CYP3A4. (Fluvoxamine causes the same inhibition of CYP3A4.)

Venlafaxine is a potent inhibitor of serotonin transport and a weaker inhibitor of norepinephrine transport.

At lower therapeutic doses, venlafaxine behaves like an SSRI. At high doses (more than 225 mg/d), it produces mild to moderate increases of heart rate and blood pressure attributable to norepinephrine transporter inhibition. Doses in the range of 225 mg/d or more may confer broader therapeutic effects than SSRIs, but titration up to these doses is needed to control adverse effects.

Mirtazapine is a potent antihistaminic with greater sedating effects than the other second- and third-generation antidepressants. Its use is also more likely to be associated with weight gain. The hypothesized mechanism of action of mirtazapine combines 5-HT$_2$ receptor and α-adrenoceptor antagonism and, if established in humans, would be unique among available drugs. Thus, mirtazapine may prove beneficial in patients who can tolerate its sedative effects and do not respond well to SSRIs or cannot tolerate their sexual adverse effects.

4. Selective serotonin reuptake inhibitors—These drugs achieve high ratios of SERT versus NET inhibition of 300 to 7000 (Table 30–2). Fluoxetine was the first SSRI to reach general clinical use. Paroxetine and sertraline differ mainly in having shorter half-lives and different potencies as inhibitors of specific P450 isoenzymes. Racemic citalopram and (S)-citalopram (escitalopram), the most selective SSRIs of all, have achieved very widespread use. Although the SSRIs have not been shown to be more effective overall than prior drugs, they lack many of the toxicities of the tricyclic and heterocyclic antidepressants. Thus, patient acceptance has been high despite their own adverse effects.

5. MAO inhibitors—MAO-A (isoform A) is the amine oxidase primarily responsible for norepinephrine, serotonin, and tyramine metabolism. MAO-B is more selective for dopamine. The irreversible inhibitors available in the USA are nonselective and at the doses used block both forms of the enzyme. Irreversible block of MAO, characteristic of the older MAO inhibitors, allows significant accumulation of tyramine and loss of the first-pass metabolism that protects against tyramine in foods (see Adverse Effects). Because they result in replacement of the normal transmitter (norepinephrine) stored in noradrenergic nerve terminal vesicles with a false transmitter (octopamine), they may cause significant hypotension.

■ II. CLINICAL PHARMACOLOGY OF ANTIDEPRESSANTS

Clinical Indications

The major indication for antidepressant drugs is to treat depression, but a number of other uses have been established by clinical experience and controlled trials.

A. Depression

This indication has been kept broad deliberately, even though evidence from clinical studies strongly suggests that the drugs are specifically useful only in major depressive episodes. Major depressive episodes are diagnosed primarily on the basis of the persistent degree and quality of depressed mood or loss of interest and pleasure in most activities, usually accompanied by disturbances of sleep, appetite, sexual drive, activity, or ability to concentrate. The diagnosis of major depression may be uncertain in individual patients, so that on balance this condition is underdiagnosed and undertreated. The depressed phase of bipolar illness definitely requires pharmacologic treatment given the high rate of suicide in persons with this disorder. Standard antidepressants are usually added to lithium or another antimanic agent; SSRIs are less likely to induce mania than the older

tricyclic agents. There are, however, few controlled studies on their relative efficacy or proper duration of use. Finally, recent controlled studies support the additional labeling of the anticonvulsant lamotrigine for maintenance and prophylaxis of the depressed phase of bipolar illness.

B. Anxiety Disorders: Panic, Generalized Anxiety, and Social Phobia

Imipramine was first shown in 1962 to have a beneficial effect in the acute episodes of anxiety that have come to be known as panic attacks. It has also been demonstrated that SSRIs, venlafaxine, and duloxetine are effective in panic, generalized anxiety disorder (GAD), and social phobia, but they require 6–8 weeks of treatment. Since there is considerable comorbidity between depression and anxiety disorders, it is advantageous for many patients to use a treatment that is helpful for both conditions. In some instances, because they are well tolerated and their clinical effects become evident promptly, benzodiazepines remain the preferred drugs for anxiety disorders despite the physiologic dependence associated with long-term use.

C. Obsessive-Compulsive Disorders

Potent SSRIs are uniquely effective for treating these disorders. Recent studies have focused on fluoxetine and other SSRIs, although clomipramine, the most potent mixed serotonin and norepinephrine transporter inhibitor, may be especially effective. Fluvoxamine is marketed exclusively for this disorder in the United States.

D. Enuresis

Enuresis is an established indication for tricyclics. Proof of efficacy for this indication is substantial, but drug therapy is not the preferred approach, especially given the risks of cardiovascular effects and the dangers from overdoses.

E. Chronic Pain

Clinicians in pain clinics have found tricyclics to be useful for treating a variety of chronically painful states that often cannot be definitively diagnosed. It is likely that tricyclics and other combined serotonin-norepinephrine transporter inhibitors work directly on pain pathways and do not work simply on depressive equivalents secondary to chronic pain.

In addition to TCAs, controlled studies of higher doses of venlafaxine show efficacy in pain. **Duloxetine** has similar effects at doses closer to standard antidepressant doses. SSRIs, however, are not effective for chronic pain.

F. Other Indications

Certain antidepressants have been shown to be effective for eating disorders, especially bulimia (fluoxetine), premenstrual dysphoric disorder (fluoxetine), and attention deficit hyperkinetic disorder (imipramine, desipramine). **Atomoxetine** was recently introduced for the treatment of attention deficit hyperactivity disorder (ADHD). This

CHAPTER 30

selective NET inhibitor does not appear to have the abuse liability of the standard drugs for this condition (methylphenidate and amphetamine; see Chapter 9).

Drug Choice

Controlled comparisons of the available antidepressants have usually led to the conclusion that they are roughly equivalent in efficacy. Although this may be true for groups of patients, individual patients may respond better to one drug than to another. European studies show that patients depressed enough to be hospitalized respond better to classic tricyclics than to monotherapy with SSRIs. Meta-analyses of outpatient studies also show a greater efficacy of tricyclics over SSRIs in patients who complete trials. The greater tolerability of the SSRIs, however, makes them the preferred agent for most patients. At high doses (> 225 mg), venlafaxine also shows greater efficacy than the SSRIs. Thus, finding the right drug and the right dose for the individual patient must be accomplished empirically. The history of the patient's drug experience is the most valuable guide.

Tricyclics and the second- and third-generation agents differ mainly in the degree of sedation they produce (greatest with amitriptyline, doxepin, trazodone, and mirtazapine) and their antimuscarinic effects (greatest with amitriptyline and doxepin; Table 30–2). SSRIs are generally free of sedative effects and safe in overdose. Combined with their mild adverse effects, these qualities account for the popularity of SSRIs as the most widely prescribed antidepressants.

In contrast, amoxapine and maprotiline seem to have as many sedative and autonomic actions as most tricyclics; more recently introduced antidepressants such as bupropion, venlafaxine, and duloxetine are, like SSRIs, mostly free of such effects, whereas nefazodone and mirtazapine are very sedating. Amoxapine and maprotiline are at least as dangerous as the tricyclics when taken in overdose; the other newer agents seem to be safer.

No special indications for particular types of depression have been found for SSRIs or other newer antidepressants. The popularity of these drugs, despite their higher cost, is due principally to their greater acceptance by patients. A provocative clinical report that fluoxetine use increased suicidal or aggressive ideation was not supported by subsequent analyses of massive databases. In 2004, however, because of an apparent increase in suicidal thoughts and behaviors in children on SSRIs, the FDA issued a general warning about increased risk of suicide with newer antidepressants. Studies of concurrent epidemiologic data involving much larger numbers than the trials cited by the FDA came to the opposite conclusion—any increase in suicide risk is seen only with older antidepressants (primarily tricyclics).

Clinical reports, prescription databases, and a few trials support the use of SSRIs in combination with the older tricyclics, especially desipramine; with bupropion; and, most recently, with mirtazapine in patients who do not show an adequate response to a single agent.

Table 30–3. Usual daily doses of antidepressant drugs.

Drug	Dose (mg)
Tricyclics	
Amitriptyline	75–200
Clomipramine	75–300
Desipramine	75–200
Doxepin	75–300
Imipramine	75–200
Nortriptyline	75–150
Protriptyline	20–40
Trimipramine	75–200
Second- and third-generation agents	
Amoxapine	150–300
Bupropion	200–400
Duloxetine	40–120
Maprotiline	75–300
Mirtazapine	15–60
Nefazodone	200–600
Trazodone	50–600
Venlafaxine	75–225
Monoamine oxidase inhibitors	
Phenelzine	45–75
Tranylcypromine	10–30
Selective serotonin reuptake inhibitors	
Citalopram	20–60
Fluoxetine	10–60
Fluvoxamine	100–300
Paroxetine	20–50
Sertraline	50–200

MAO inhibitors remain helpful despite their adverse effects but are reserved for patients who have failed to respond to at least two courses of monotherapy or combination treatment with different classes of antidepressants.

Lithium, a mood stabilizer (see Chapter 29), in combination with an antidepressant may achieve a favorable response not obtained by the antidepressant alone.

Dosages

The usual daily dose ranges of antidepressants are shown in Table 30–3. Doses are almost always determined empirically; the patient's acceptance of adverse effects is the usual limiting factor. Tolerance to some of the objectionable effects may develop, so that the usual pattern of treatment has been to start with small doses, increasing either to a predetermined daily dose, or to one that produces relief of depression, or to the maximum tolerated dose (except in the case of nortriptyline, which loses efficacy at plasma concentrations over 150 ng/mL).

MAO inhibitors, bupropion, fluoxetine, sertraline, paroxetine, citalopram, and venlafaxine are customarily given early in the day when initiating treatment, because they can be somewhat stimulating and may cause insomnia if given late. After a few weeks on the drug, however, any such effects should disappear, and time of day administered is rarely important. Virtually all the other antidepressants have varying degrees of sedative effects and are best given near bedtime. Autonomic adverse effects also tend to be less troublesome if the dose is given late.

Maintenance Treatment

Whether or not to undertake long-term maintenance treatment of a depressed patient depends entirely on the actual history of the disorder in that individual. If the depressive episode was the patient's first and if the patient responded quickly and satisfactorily to drug therapy, it is reasonable to gradually withdraw treatment over a period of a few weeks after treating for 6–9 months. If relapse does not occur, drug treatment can be stopped until another episode occurs, which is unpredictable but highly probable. Pooled data from randomized trials covering 6–36 months reveal a more than 50% reduction in relapses or recurrences if patients are maintained on an antidepressant. Thus, a patient who has had previous episodes of depression—especially if each succeeding one was more severe and more difficult to treat—is a candidate for maintenance therapy. Maintenance therapy requires the full dosage used to obtain the initial response. The duration of treatment varies, though many patients require maintenance treatment indefinitely.

Unresponsive Patients

One third or more of patients do not respond (defined as 50% or more improvement) to treatment, and almost two thirds fail to achieve or maintain full remission on any single regimen. In evaluating any patient's limited response to a treatment, one should consider the five D's: diagnosis, drug, dose, duration of treatment, and different treatment.

Diagnosis might be reassessed if the patient shows little response over a period of 2–3 weeks of adequate dosage or plasma concentrations. Whether or not the patient is bipolar, lithium might be added (see Chapter 29); if psychotic, treatment might be augmented with an antipsychotic agent. Combination of an SSRI with desipramine, bupropion, or mirtazapine is safe and effective for some patients. There is no good pharmacologic rationale for combining venlafaxine or duloxetine with SSRIs because they are full serotonin reuptake inhibitors at doses that inhibit norepinephrine uptake; rather, they might be combined with bupropion or mirtazapine. At least 6–8 weeks should be tried before giving up on a drug or combination as long as there is some evidence of improvement by 3–4 weeks.

One strategy is to begin treatment with an SSRI in mild to moderate outpatient depression and then augment by adding a drug of a different class for more impaired patients. Otherwise, switch to a drug of a different class. Most experts would move through various antidepressant drug classes in the search for the right drug rather than through various drugs within a class.

Dose and duration of treatment for depression must be considered. Many treatment failures are due to inadequate dosage, which should be pushed to the limits of the patient's tolerance in refractory cases. Duration of treatment is even more important. In over 50% of patients, full response does not occur until there has been at least 8 weeks of treatment.

Finally, some patients may need a completely different type of treatment, such as electroconvulsive therapy (ECT). ECT is often viewed as a treatment of last resort, but it should not be withheld from patients with depression who cannot be helped by drug therapy. For patients with psychotic depression, ECT may be a treatment of first choice.

Noncompliance is an important cause of lack of response to drugs. Patients should be warned also that noticeable improvement may be slow, with the first clear signs taking perhaps 3 weeks or more. Inability to tolerate adverse effects and discouragement with treatment are two major causes for noncompliance and for failure of antidepressants to show efficacy.

Adverse Effects

Adverse effects of various antidepressants are summarized in Table 30–4. Most common unwanted effects are minor, but they may seriously affect patient compliance. Seriously depressed patients, however, can tolerate unwanted effects, perhaps because they are too depressed to care. In healthy volunteers, even moderate doses of the tricyclics—amitriptyline, imipramine, clomipramine, and doxepin—are poorly tolerated. With the SSRIs, transient nausea is the most frequent complaint, and decreased libido and sexual dysfunction create the greatest concerns in patients during maintenance treatment. Concerns about teratogenic potential recently led to revised labeling of paroxetine.

Among the major drawbacks of most first-generation antidepressants are their many "irrelevant" pharmacologic actions, a trait inherited from the phenothiazine antipsychotic agents. It appears that the antimuscarinic, antihistaminic, and α-adrenoceptor-blocking actions of tricyclic antidepressants contribute only to the undesirable effects of these agents. Blurred vision, dry mouth, urinary hesitancy or retention, and constipation represent the most common antimuscarinic complaints. Postural hypotension is a significant and potentially dangerous manifestation of the α-blocking action, especially in the elderly.

Drug Interactions

A. PHARMACODYNAMIC INTERACTIONS

The pharmacodynamic interactions of antidepressants with other drugs depend on their class. Those with sedative effects may be additive with other sedatives, especially alcohol. Patients taking tricyclics or mirtazapine should be

Table 30–4. Adverse effects of antidepressants.

Tricyclics	
Sedation	Sleepiness, additive effects with other sedative drugs
Sympathomimetic	Tremor, insomnia
Antimuscarinic	Blurred vision, constipation, urinary hesitancy, confusion
Cardiovascular	Orthostatic hypotension, conduction defects, arrhythmias
Psychiatric	Aggravation of psychosis, withdrawal syndrome
Neurologic	Seizures
Metabolic-endocrine	Weight gain, sexual disturbances
Monoamine oxidase inhibitors	Headache, drowsiness, dry mouth, weight gain, postural hypotension, sexual disturbances, interactions[1]
Amoxapine	Similar to the tricyclics with the addition of some effects associated with the antipsychotics (Chapter 29)
Maprotiline	Similar to tricyclics; seizures are dose-related
Mirtazapine	Somnolence, increased appetite, weight gain, dizziness
Trazodone, nefazadone	Drowsiness, dizziness, insomnia, nausea, agitation
Venlafaxine	Nausea, somnolence, sweating, dizziness, anxiety, sexual disturbances, hypertension
Duloxetine	Nausea, dry mouth, decreased appetite, insomnia, dizziness, sweating
Bupropion	Dizziness, dry mouth, sweating, tremor, aggravation of psychosis, potential for seizures at high doses
Fluoxetine and other serotonin reuptake inhibitors	Anxiety, insomnia, gastrointestinal symptoms, decreased libido, sexual dysfunction, teratogenic potential with paroxetine

[1]Interactions with tyramine-containing foods; interactions that cause serotonin syndrome (see Chapter 16).

warned that use of alcohol may lead to greater than expected impairment of driving ability. MAO inhibitors, by increasing stores of catecholamines, sensitize the patient to indirectly acting sympathomimetics such as tyramine, which is found in some fermented foods and beverages, and to sympathomimetic drugs such as diethylpropion, phenylpropanolamine, or botanicals containing ephedrine. Such sensitization can result in dangerous and—rarely—fatal hypertensive reactions. A pharmacodynamic interaction may occur when fluoxetine or another SSRI is used in the presence of an MAO inhibitor. The combination of increased stores of 5-HT plus inhibition of reuptake after release is thought to result in a marked increase of serotonin in the synapses, leading to a **serotonin syndrome.** This sometimes fatal syndrome includes hyperthermia, muscle rigidity, myoclonus, and rapid changes in mental status and vital signs (see Chapter 16).

B. PHARMACOKINETIC INTERACTIONS

The most likely pharmacokinetic interactions are between the potent inhibitors of P450 2D6, paroxetine and fluoxetine, and those drugs highly dependent on this pathway for clearance (eg, desipramine, nortriptyline, flecainide; see also Chapter 4). Actual instances of clinically significant interactions are extremely rare, and there are only a

handful of case reports after cumulative exposure of more than 50 million patients to these SSRI drugs. Inhibition of P450 3A4 could possibly occur at high concentrations of nefazodone and fluvoxamine and block the metabolism of the many substrates of this isoform.

Overdoses

A. TRICYCLICS

Tricyclics are extremely dangerous when taken in overdose quantities, and depressed patients are more likely than others to be suicidal. Prescriptions should therefore be limited to amounts less than 1.25 g, or 50 dose units of 25 mg, on a "no refill" basis. If suicide is a serious possibility, the tablets should be entrusted to a family member. The drugs must be kept away from children. Both accidental and deliberate overdoses continue to occur and are serious medical emergencies. Major effects and management of overdosage are discussed in Chapter 59.

B. SECOND- AND THIRD-GENERATION DRUGS

Overdoses of amoxapine are characterized by severe neurotoxicity, with seizures that are difficult to control. Overdoses of maprotiline also have a tendency to cause seizures as well as cardiotoxicity. Overdoses of the other heterocyclic drugs appear to create only minor problems and can usually be managed with purely supportive measures.

C. MAO INHIBITORS

Intoxication with MAO inhibitors is unusual. Agitation, delirium, and neuromuscular excitability are followed by obtunded consciousness, seizures, shock, and hyperthermia. Supportive treatment is usually all that is required, though sedative phenothiazines with α-adrenoceptor-blocking action, such as chlorpromazine, may be useful.

D. SELECTIVE SEROTONIN REUPTAKE INHIBITORS

A few deaths have occurred during overdosage of SSRIs when other drugs were also being taken. The likelihood of fatalities from SSRI overdoses is extremely low. In case of overdose, only supportive treatment can be offered, since the high volume of distribution, as with other antidepressants, rules out removal of drug by dialysis. As much as 2.6 g of sertraline has been taken with survival. Overdoses of paroxetine are relatively benign: Up to 850 mg has been taken with no evidence of cardiotoxicity.

PREPARATIONS AVAILABLE

TRICYCLICS

Amitriptyline (generic, Elavil)
Oral: 10, 25, 50, 75, 100, 150 mg tablets
Parenteral: 10 mg/mL for IM injection
Amoxapine (generic)
Oral: 25, 50, 100, 150 mg tablets
Clomipramine (generic, Anafranil; labeled only for obsessive-compulsive disorder)
Oral: 25, 50, 75 mg capsules
Desipramine (generic, Norpramin)
Oral: 10, 25, 50, 75, 100, 150 mg tablets
Doxepin (generic, Sinequan)
Oral: 10, 25, 50, 75, 100, 150 mg capsules; 10 mg/mL concentrate
Imipramine (generic, Tofranil)
Oral: 10, 25, 50 mg tablets (as hydrochloride); 75, 100, 125, 150 mg capsules (as pamoate)
Nortriptyline (generic, Aventyl, Pamelor)
Oral: 10, 25, 50, 75 mg capsules; 10 mg/5 mL solution
Protriptyline (generic, Vivactil)
Oral: 5, 10 mg tablets
Trimipramine (Surmontil)
Oral: 25, 50, 100 mg capsules

SECOND-GENERATION & SUBSEQUENT DRUGS

Amoxapine (generic, Asendin)
Oral: 25, 50, 100, 150 mg tablets
Bupropion (generic, Wellbutrin)
Oral: 75, 100 mg tablets; 100, 150, 200 mg 12-hour sustained-release tablets; 150, 300 mg 24-hour sustained-release tablets
Duloxetine (Cymbalta)
Oral: 20, 30, 50 mg capsules
Maprotiline (generic)
Oral: 25, 50, 75 mg tablets
Mirtazapine (generic, Remeron)
Oral: 7.5, 15, 30, 45 mg tablets; 15, 30, 45 mg disintegrating tablets

Nefazodone (Serzone)
Oral: 50, 100, 150, 200, 250 mg tablets
Trazodone (generic, Desyrel)
Oral: 50, 100, 150, 300 mg tablets
Venlafaxine (Effexor)
Oral: 25, 37.5, 50, 75, 100 mg tablets; 37.5, 75, 150 mg extended-release capsules

SELECTIVE SEROTONIN REUPTAKE INHIBITORS

Citalopram (generic, Celexa)
Oral: 10, 20, 40 mg tablets; 10 mg/5 mL solution
Escitalopram (Lexapro)
Oral: 5, 10, 20 mg tablets; 5 mg/5 mL solution
Fluoxetine (generic, Prozac)
Oral: 10, 20, 40 mg capsules; 10, 20 mg tablets; 20 mg/5 mL liquid
Oral delayed-release (Prozac Weekly): 90 mg capsules
Fluvoxamine (generic, labeled only for obsessive-compulsive disorder)
Oral: 25, 50, 100 mg tablets
Paroxetine (generic, Paxil)
Oral: 10, 20, 30, 40 mg tablets; 10 mg/5 mL suspension; 12.5, 25, 37.5 mg controlled-release tablets
Sertraline (Zoloft)
Oral: 25, 50, 100 mg tablets; 20 mg/mL oral concentrate

MONOAMINE OXIDASE INHIBITORS

Phenelzine (Nardil)
Oral: 15 mg tablets
Tranylcypromine (Parnate)
Oral: 10 mg tablets

OTHER

Atomoxetine (Strattera)
Oral: 10, 18, 25, 40, 60 mg capsules

REFERENCES

American Psychiatric Association: DSM-IV-TR (*Diagnostic and Statistical Manual of Mental Disorders,* 4th ed). American Psychiatric Association, 1994, modified 2000.

American Psychiatric Association: APA practice guideline for major depressive disorder in adults (revision). Am J Psychiatry 2000;157:1.

Anderson IM, Tomenson BM: Selective serotonin reuptake inhibitors versus tricyclic antidepressants: A meta-analysis of efficacy and tolerability. J Affect Disord 2000;58:19.

Berton O, Nestler EJ: New approaches to antidepressant drug discovery: Beyond monoamines. Nat Rev Neurosci 2006;7:137.

Bradberry SM et al: Management of the cardiovascular complications of tricyclic antidepressant poisoning: Role of sodium bicarbonate. Toxicol Rev 2005;24:195.

Briley M: New hope in the treatment of painful symptoms in depression. Curr Opin Investig Drugs 2003;4:42.

Duman RS, Heninger G, Nestler E: A molecular and cellular theory of depression. Arch Gen Psychiatry 1997;54:597.

Ernst CL, Goldberg JF: Antidepressant properties of anticonvulsant drugs for bipolar disorder. J Clin Psychopharmacol 2003; 23:182.

Esposito E: Serotonin-dopamine interaction as a focus of novel antidepressant drugs. Curr Drug Targets 2006;7:177.

Geddes JR et al: Relapse prevention with antidepressant drug treatment in depressive disorders: A systematic review. Lancet 2003;361:653.

Harvey AT et al: Evidence of the dual mechanisms of action of venlafaxine. Arch Gen Psychiatry 2000;57:503.

Merikangas KR et al: Workgroup Reports: NIMH Strategic Plan for Mood Disorders Research, Future of Genetics of Mood Disorders Research. Biol Psychiatry 2002;52:457.

Meyer JH et al: Occupancy of serotonin transporters by paroxetine and citalopram during treatment of depression: A [(11)C]DASB PET imaging study. Am J Psychiatry 2001;158:1843.

Mottram P, Wilson K, Strobl J: Antidepressants for depressed elderly. Cochrane Database Syst Rev 2006;CD003491.

Nestler EJ et al: Preclinical models: Status of basic research in depression. Biol Psychiatry 2002;52:503.

Potter WZ: Adrenoceptors and serotonin receptor function: Relevance to antidepressant mechanisms of action. J Clin Psychiatry 1996;57(Suppl 4):4.

Rush JA, Ryan ND: Current and emerging therapeutics for depression. In: Davis KL et al (editors): *Neuropsychopharmacology: The Fifth Generation of Progress.* Lippincott Williams & Wilkins, 2002.

Schatzberg I et al: Molecular and cellular mechanisms in depression. In: Davis KL et al (editors): *Neuropsychopharmacology. The Fifth Generation of Progress.* Lippincott Williams & Wilkins, 2002.

Opioid Analgesics & Antagonists

31

Mark A. Schumacher, PhD, MD, Allan I. Basbaum, PhD, & Walter L. Way, MD

Morphine, the prototypical opioid agonist, has long been known to relieve severe pain with remarkable efficacy. The opium poppy is the source of crude opium from which Sertürner in 1803 isolated morphine, the pure alkaloid and named it after Morpheus, the Greek god of dreams. It remains the standard against which all drugs that have strong analgesic action are compared. These drugs are collectively known as opioid analgesics and include not only the natural and semisynthetic alkaloid derivatives from opium but also include synthetic surrogates, other opioid-like drugs whose actions are blocked by the nonselective antagonist naloxone, plus several endogenous peptides that interact with the several subtypes of opioid receptors.

■ I. BASIC PHARMACOLOGY OF THE OPIOID ANALGESICS

Source

Opium, the source of morphine, is obtained from the poppy, *Papaver somniferum* and *P album*. After incision, the poppy seed pod exudes a white substance that turns into a brown gum that is crude opium. Opium contains many alkaloids, the principle one being morphine, which is present in a concentration of about 10%. Codeine is synthesized commercially from morphine.

Classification & Chemistry

Opioid drugs include full agonists, partial agonists, and antagonists (see Chapter 2 for definitions). Morphine is a full agonist at the µ (mu) opioid receptor, the major analgesic opioid receptor (Table 31–1). In contrast, codeine functions as a partial (or "weak") µ-receptor agonist. Simple substitution of an allyl group on the nitrogen of the full *agonist* morphine plus addition of a single hydroxyl group results in naloxone, a strong µ-receptor *antagonist*. The structures of some of these compounds are shown later in this chapter. Some opioids, eg, nalbuphine, are capable of producing an agonist (or partial agonist) effect at one opioid receptor

subtype and an antagonist effect at another. Not only can the activating properties of opioid analgesics be manipulated by pharmaceutical chemistry, certain opioid analgesics are modified in the liver, resulting in compounds with greater analgesic action (see Pharmacokinetics, Metabolism).

Endogenous Opioid Peptides

Opioid alkaloids (eg, morphine) produce analgesia through actions at regions in the central nervous system (CNS) that contain peptides with opioid-like pharmacologic properties. The general term currently used for these endogenous substances is **endogenous opioid peptides.**

Three families of endogenous opioid peptides have been described in detail: the **endorphins,** the pentapeptides methionine-enkephalin (**met-enkephalin**) and leucine-enkephalin (**leu-enkephalin),** and the **dynorphins.** The three families of opioid receptors have overlapping affinities for these endogenous peptides (Table 31–1).

The endogenous opioid peptides are derived from three precursor proteins: prepro-opiomelanocortin (POMC), preproenkephalin (proenkephalin A), and prepro-dynorphin (proenkephalin B). POMC contains the met-enkephalin sequence, β-endorphin, and several nonopioid peptides, including adrenocorticotropic hormone (ACTH), β-lipotropin, and melanocyte-stimulating hormone. Preproenkephalin contains six copies of met-enkephalin and one copy of leu-enkephalin. Leu- and met-enkephalin have slightly higher affinity for the δ (delta) than for the µ opioid receptor (Table 31–1). Preprodynorphin yields several active opioid peptides that contain the leu-enkephalin sequence. These are **dynorphin A, dynorphin B,** and α and β **neoendorphins.** More recently, the endogenous peptides **endomorphin-1** and **endomorphin-2** have been found to possess many of the properties of opioid peptides, notably analgesia and high-affinity binding to the µ-receptor. Research is focused on whether endomorphins selectively activate µ-receptor subtypes and much remains unknown, including the identity of their gene. Both the endogenous opioid precursor molecules and the endomorphins are present at CNS sites that have been implicated in pain

Table 31–1. Opioid receptor subtypes, their functions, and their endogenous peptide affinities.

Receptor Subtype	Functions	Endogenous Opioid Peptide Affinity
μ (mu)	Supraspinal and spinal analgesia; sedation; inhibition of respiration; slowed GI transit; modulation of hormone and neurotransmitter release	Endorphins > enkephalins > dynorphins
δ (delta)	Supraspinal and spinal analgesia; modulation of hormone and neurotransmitter release	Enkephalins > endorphins and dynorphins
κ (kappa)	Supraspinal and spinal analgesia; psychotomimetic effects; slowed GI transit	Dynorphins > > endorphins and enkephalins

GI, gastrointestinal.

modulation. Evidence suggests that they can be released during stressful conditions such as pain or the anticipation of pain to diminish the sensation of noxious stimuli.

In contrast to the analgesic role of leu- and met-enkephalin, an analgesic action of dynorphin A—through its binding to κ (kappa) opioid receptors—remains controversial. Dynorphin A is also found in the dorsal horn of the spinal cord, where it plays a critical role in the *sensitization* of nociceptive neurotransmission. Increased levels of dynorphin can be found in the dorsal horn after tissue injury and inflammation. This elevated dynorphin level is believed to increase pain and induce a state of long-lasting hyperalgesia. The pronociceptive action of dynorphin in the spinal cord appears to be independent of the opioid receptor system. Rather, dynorphin A can bind and activate the *N*-methyl-D-aspartate (NMDA) receptor complex, a site of action that is the focus of intense therapeutic development.

Recently, a novel receptor-ligand system homologous to the opioid peptides has been found. The principle receptor for this system is the G protein-coupled **orphanin opioid-receptor-like subtype 1 (ORL1).** Its endogenous ligand has been termed **nociceptin** by one group of investigators and **orphanin FQ** by another group. This ligand-receptor system is currently known as the **N/OFQ** system. Nociceptin is structurally similar to dynorphin except for the absence of an N-terminal tyrosine; it acts only at the ORL1 receptor. Although widely expressed in the CNS and periphery, this system has a diverse pharmacology, capable of opposing classic μ receptor–mediated analgesia as well as modulating drug reward, reinforcement, learning, and memory processes.

Pharmacokinetics

Some properties of clinically important opioids are summarized in Table 31–2.

A. Absorption

Most opioid analgesics are well absorbed when given by subcutaneous, intramuscular, and oral routes. However, because of the first-pass effect, the oral dose of the opioid (eg, morphine) may need to be much higher than the parenteral dose to elicit a therapeutic effect. Considerable interpatient variability exists in first-pass opioid metabolism, making prediction of an effective oral dose difficult. Certain analgesics such as codeine and oxycodone are effective orally because they have reduced first-pass metabolism. Nasal insufflation of certain opioids can result in rapid therapeutic blood levels by avoiding first-pass metabolism. Other routes of opioid administration include oral mucosa via lozenges, and transdermal via transdermal patches. The latter can provide delivery of potent analgesics over days.

B. Distribution

The uptake of opioids by various organs and tissues is a function of both physiologic and chemical factors. Although all opioids bind to plasma proteins with varying affinity, the drugs rapidly leave the blood compartment and localize in highest concentrations in tissues that are highly perfused such as the brain, lungs, liver, kidneys, and spleen. Drug concentrations in skeletal muscle may be much lower, but this tissue serves as the main reservoir because of its greater bulk. Even though blood flow to fatty tissue is much lower than to the highly perfused tissues, accumulation can be very important, particularly after frequent high-dose administration or continuous infusion of highly lipophilic opioids that are slowly metabolized, eg, fentanyl.

C. Metabolism

The opioids are converted in large part to polar metabolites (mostly glucuronides), which are then readily excreted by the kidneys. For example, morphine, which contains free hydroxyl groups, is primarily conjugated to morphine-3-glucuronide (M3G), a compound with neuroexcitatory

Table 31–2. Common opioid analgesics.

Generic Name	Trade Name	Approximately Equivalent Dose (mg)	Oral:Parenteral Potency Ratio	Duration of Analgesia (hours)	Maximum Efficacy
Morphine[1]		10	Low	4–5	High
Hydromorphone	Dilaudid	1.5	Low	4–5	High
Oxymorphone	Numorphan	1.5	Low	3–4	High
Methadone	Dolophine	10	High	4–6	High
Meperidine	Demerol	60–100	Medium	2–4	High
Fentanyl	Sublimaze	0.1	Low	1–1.5	High
Sufentanyl	Sufenta	0.02	Parenteral only	1–1.5	High
Alfentanil	Alfenta	Titrated	Parenteral only	0.25–0.75	High
Remifentanyl	Ultiva	Titrated[2]	Parenteral only	0.05[3]	High
Levorphanol	Levo-Dromoran	2–3	High	4–5	High
Codeine		30–60[4]	High	3–4	Low
Hydrocodone[4]		5–10	Medium	4–6	Moderate
Oxycodone[1,5]	Percodan	4.5[6]	Medium	3–4	Moderate
Propoxyphene	Darvon	60–120[6]	Oral only	4–5	Very low
Pentazocine	Talwin	30–50[6]	Medium	3–4	Moderate
Nalbuphine	Nubain	10	Parenteral only	3–6	High
Buprenorphine	Buprenex	0.3	Low	4–8	High
Butorphanol	Stadol	2	Parenteral only	3–4	High

[1]Available in sustained-release forms, morphine (MSContin); oxycodone (OxyContin).
[2]Administered as an infusion at 0.025-0.2 mcg/kg/min.
[3]Duration is dependent on a context-sensitive half-time of 3–4 minutes.
[4]Available in tablets containing acetaminophen (Norco, Vicodin, Lortab, others).
[5]Available in tablets containing acetaminophen (Percocet); aspirin (Percodan).
[6]Analgesic efficacy at this dose not equivalent to 10 mg of morphine. See text for explanation.

properties. The neuroexcitatory effects of M3G do not appear to be mediated by μ receptors but rather by the GABA/glycinergic system. In contrast, approximately 10% of morphine is metabolized to morphine-6-glucuronide (M6G), an active metabolite with analgesic potency four to six times that of its parent compound. However, these relatively polar metabolites have limited ability to cross the blood-brain barrier and probably do not contribute significantly to the usual CNS effects of morphine given acutely. Nevertheless, accumulation of these metabolites may produce unexpected adverse effects in patients with renal failure or when exceptionally large doses of morphine are administered or high doses are administered over long periods. This can result in M3G-induced CNS excitation (seizures) or enhanced and prolonged opioid action produced by M6G. CNS uptake of M3G and, to a lesser extent, M6G can be

enhanced by coadministration with probenecid or with drugs that inhibit the P-glycoprotein drug transporter. Like morphine, hydromorphone is metabolized by conjugation, yielding hydromorphone-3-glucuronide (H3G), which has CNS excitatory properties. However, hydromorphone has not been shown to form significant amounts of a 6-glucuronide metabolite.

The effects of these active metabolites should be considered before the administration of morphine or hydromorphone, especially when given at high doses.

Esters (eg, heroin, remifentanil) are rapidly hydrolyzed by common tissue esterases. Heroin (diacetylmorphine) is hydrolyzed to monoacetylmorphine and finally to morphine, which is then conjugated with glucuronic acid.

Hepatic oxidative metabolism is the primary route of degradation of the phenylpiperidine opioids (meperidine, fentanyl, alfentanil, sufentanil) and eventually leaves only small quantities of the parent compound unchanged for excretion. However, accumulation of a demethylated metabolite of meperidine, normeperidine, may occur in patients with decreased renal function and in those receiving multiple high doses of the drug. In high concentrations, normeperidine may cause seizures. In contrast, no active metabolites of fentanyl have been reported. The P450 isozyme CYP3A4 metabolizes fentanyl by N-dealkylation in the liver. CYP3A4 is also present in the mucosa of the small intestine and contributes to the first-pass metabolism of fentanyl when it is taken orally. Codeine, oxycodone, and hydrocodone undergo metabolism in the liver by P450 isozyme CYP2D6, resulting in the production of metabolites of greater potency. For example, codeine is demethylated to morphine. Genetic polymorphism of CYP2D6 has been documented and linked to the variation in analgesic response seen among patients. Nevertheless, the metabolites of oxycodone and hydrocodone may be of minor consequence because the parent compounds are currently believed to be directly responsible for the majority of their analgesic actions. In the case of codeine, conversion to morphine may be of greater importance because codeine itself has relatively low affinity for opioid receptors.

D. EXCRETION

Polar metabolites, including glucuronide conjugates of opioid analgesics, are excreted mainly in the urine. Small amounts of unchanged drug may also be found in the urine. In addition, glucuronide conjugates are found in the bile, but enterohepatic circulation represents only a small portion of the excretory process.

Pharmacodynamics

A. MECHANISM OF ACTION

Opioid agonists produce analgesia by binding to specific G protein-coupled receptors that are located in brain and spinal cord regions involved in the transmission and modulation of pain.

1. Receptor types—As noted, three major classes of opioid receptors (μ, δ, and κ) have been identified in various nervous system sites and in other tissues (Table 31–1). Each of the three major receptors has now been cloned. All are members of the G protein-coupled family of receptors and show significant amino acid sequence homologies. Multiple receptor subtypes have been proposed based on pharmacologic criteria, including μ_1, μ_2; δ_1, δ_2; and κ_1, κ_2, and κ_3. However, genes encoding only one subtype from each of the μ, δ, and κ receptor families have been isolated and characterized thus far. One plausible explanation is that μ-receptor subtypes

arise from alternate splice variants of a common gene. Since an opioid drug may function with different potencies as an agonist, partial agonist, or antagonist at more than one receptor class or subtype, it is not surprising that these agents are capable of diverse pharmacologic effects. The N/OFQ-ORL1 receptor has not been as extensively studied.

2. Cellular actions—At the molecular level, opioid receptors form a family of proteins that physically couple to G proteins and through this interaction affect ion channel gating, modulate intracellular Ca^{2+} disposition, and alter protein phosphorylation (see Chapter 2). The opioids have two well-established direct G protein-coupled actions on neurons: (1) they close voltage-gated Ca^{2+} channels on presynaptic nerve terminals and thereby reduce transmitter release, and (2) they hyperpolarize and thus inhibit postsynaptic neurons by opening K^+ channels. Figure 31–1 schematically illustrates the presynaptic action at all three receptor types and the postsynaptic effect at μ receptors on nociceptive afferents in the spinal cord. The presynaptic action—depressed transmitter release—has been demonstrated for release of a large number of neurotransmitters including glutamate, the principle excitatory amino acid released from nociceptive nerve terminals, as well as acetylcholine, norepinephrine, serotonin, and substance P.

3. Relation of physiologic effects to receptor type—The majority of currently available opioid analgesics act primarily at the μ opioid receptor. Analgesia, as well as the euphoriant, respiratory depressant, and physical dependence properties of morphine result principally from actions at μ receptors. In fact, the μ receptor was originally defined using the relative potencies for clinical analgesia of a series of opioid alkaloids. However, opioid analgesic effects are complex and include interaction with δ and κ receptors. This is supported by the study of genetic knockouts of the μ, δ, and κ genes in mice. Delta-receptor agonists retain analgesic properties in μ receptor knockout mice. The development of δ-receptor-selective agonists could be clinically useful if their side-effect profiles (respiratory depression, risk of dependence) were more favorable than those found with current μ-receptor agonists, such as morphine. Although morphine does act at κ and δ receptor sites, it is unclear to what extent this contributes to its analgesic action. The endogenous opioid peptides differ from most of the alkaloids in their affinity for the δ and κ receptors (Table 31–1).

In an effort to develop opioid analgesics with a reduced incidence of respiratory depression or propensity for addiction and dependence, compounds that show preference for κ opioid receptors have been developed. Butorphanol and nalbuphine have shown some clinical success as analgesics, but they can cause dys-

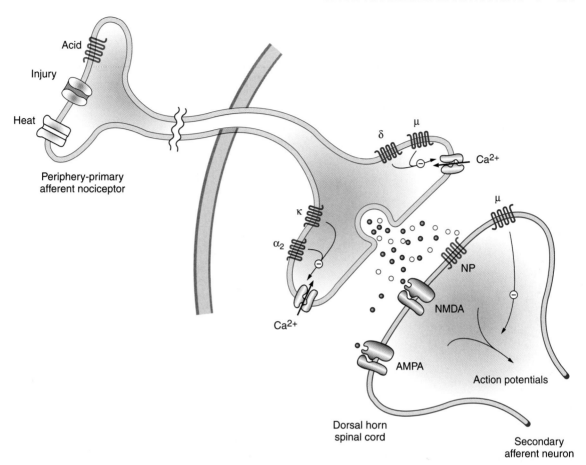

Figure 31–1. Spinal sites of action of opioids and some other analgesic agents. Mu (μ), delta (δ), and kappa (κ) agonists reduce transmitter release (often glutamate and excitatory neuropeptides) from presynaptic terminals of nociceptive primary afferents (cell body omitted). Mu agonists also hyperpolarize second-order pain transmission neurons by increasing K$^+$ conductance, evoking an inhibitory postsynaptic potential. Alpha$_2$ agonists appear to act on adrenoceptors on the presynaptic terminal of the primary afferent neuron and ziconotide may act by blocking the calcium channels on this structure (see text).

phoric reactions and have limited potency. It is interesting that butorphanol has also been shown to cause significantly greater analgesia in women than in men. The reason for this difference is not known.

4. Receptor distribution and neural mechanisms of analgesia—Opioid receptor binding sites have been localized autoradiographically with high-affinity radioligands and with antibodies to unique peptide sequences in each receptor subtype. All three major receptors are present in high concentrations in the dorsal horn of the spinal cord. Receptors are present both on spinal cord pain transmission neurons and on the primary afferents that relay the pain message to them (Figure 31–2, sites A and B). Opioid agonists inhibit the release of excita-

tory transmitters from these primary afferents, and they directly inhibit the dorsal horn pain transmission neuron. Thus, opioids exert a powerful analgesic effect directly on the spinal cord. This **spinal action** has been exploited clinically by direct application of opioid agonists to the spinal cord, which provides a regional analgesic effect while reducing the unwanted respiratory depression, nausea and vomiting, and sedation that may occur from the **supraspinal actions** of systemically administered opioids.

Under most circumstances, opioids are given systemically and so act simultaneously at multiple sites. These include not only the ascending pathways of pain transmission beginning with specialized peripheral sensory terminals that transduce painful stimuli (Figure

Transmission

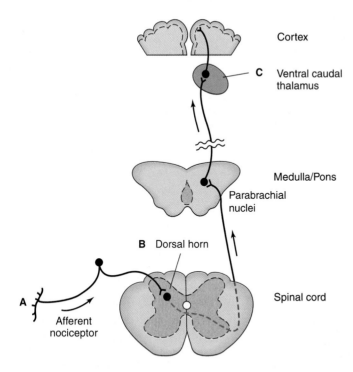

Figure 31–2. Putative sites of action of opioid analgesics. Sites of action on the afferent pain transmission pathway from the periphery to the higher centers are shown. **A:** Direct action of opioids on inflamed or damaged peripheral tissues (see Figure 31–1 for detail). **B:** Inhibition also occurs in the spinal cord. **C:** Possible sites of action in the thalamus.

31–2) but also descending (modulatory) pathways (Figure 31–3). At these sites as at others, opioids directly inhibit neurons; yet this action results in the *activation* of descending inhibitory neurons that send processes to the spinal cord and inhibit pain transmission neurons. This activation has been shown to result from the inhibition of inhibitory neurons in several locations (Figure 31–4). Taken together, interactions at these sites increase the overall analgesic effect of opioid agonists.

When pain-relieving opioid drugs are given systemically, they presumably act upon brain circuits normally regulated by endogenous opioid peptides. Part of the pain-relieving action of exogenous opioids involves the release of endogenous opioid peptides. An exogenous opioid agonist (eg, morphine) may act primarily and directly at the μ receptor, but this action may evoke the release of endogenous opioids that additionally act at δ and κ receptors. Thus, even a receptor-selective ligand can initiate a complex sequence of events involving multiple synapses, transmitters, and receptor types.

Animal and human clinical studies demonstrate that both endogenous and exogenous opioids can also produce opioid-mediated analgesia at sites *outside* the CNS. Pain associated with inflammation seems especially sensitive to these peripheral opioid actions. The identification of functional μ receptors on the peripheral terminals of sensory neurons supports this hypothesis. Furthermore, activation of peripheral μ receptors results in a decrease in sensory neuron activity and transmitter release. Peripheral administration of opioids, eg, into the knees of patients following arthroscopic knee surgery, has shown clinical benefit up to 24 hours after administration. If they can be developed, opioids selective for a peripheral site would be useful adjuncts in the treatment of inflammatory pain (see Box: Ion Channels & Novel Analgesic Targets). Moreover, new peripherally acting dynorphins may provide a novel means to treat visceral pain. Such compounds could have the additional benefit of reducing unwanted effects such as constipation.

5. Tolerance and physical dependence—With frequently repeated therapeutic doses of morphine or its surrogates, there is a gradual loss in effectiveness, ie, tolerance. To reproduce the original response, a larger dose must be administered. Along with tolerance, physical dependence develops. Physical dependence is defined as a characteristic **withdrawal** or **abstinence syndrome** when a drug is stopped or an antagonist is administered (see also Chapter 32).

The mechanism of development of tolerance and physical dependence is poorly understood, but persistent activation of μ receptors such as occurs with the treatment of severe chronic pain appears to play a primary role in its induction and maintenance. Current concepts

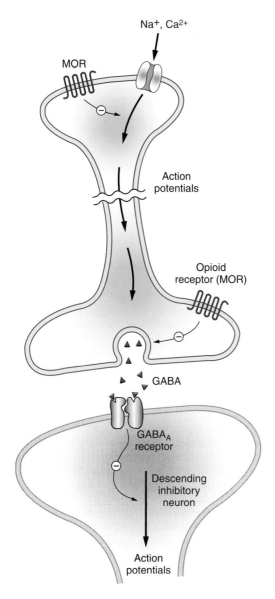

Figure 31–3. Brainstem local circuitry underlying the modulating effect of descending pathways by μ opioid receptor (MOR)–mediated analgesia. The pain inhibitory neuron is indirectly activated by opioids (exogenous or endogenous) that inhibit an inhibitory (GABAergic) interneuron. This results in enhanced inhibition of nociceptive processing in the dorsal horn of the spinal cord.

have shifted away from tolerance being driven by a simple up-regulation of the cyclic adenosine monophosphate (cAMP) system. Although this process is associated with tolerance, it is not sufficient to explain it. A second hypothesis for tolerance was based on the proposal that

repeated exposure to agonist caused μ receptors to be down-regulated by endocytosis. However, emerging research now implicates the *failure* of morphine to induce endocytosis of the μ opioid receptor as an important component of tolerance development. This suggests that maintenance of normal sensitivity of μ receptors requires reactivation by endocytosis and recycling (see Chapter 2). Another area of research suggests that the δ opioid receptor functions as an independent component in the maintenance of tolerance. In addition, the concept of **receptor uncoupling** has gained prominence. Under this hypothesis, tolerance is due to a dysfunction of structural interactions between the μ receptor and G proteins, second-messenger systems, and their target ion channels. Moreover, a particular ion channel complex, the NMDA receptor, has been shown to play a critical role in tolerance development and maintenance because NMDA-receptor antagonists such as ketamine can block tolerance development. The development of novel NMDA-receptor antagonists or other strategies to recouple μ receptors to their target ion channels provides hope for achieving a clinically effective means to prevent or reverse opioid analgesic tolerance.

In addition to the development of tolerance, persistent administration of opioid analgesics has been observed to *increase* the sensation of pain leading to a state of hyperalgesia. This phenomenon has been observed with several opioid analgesics, including morphine, fentanyl, and remifentanil. Spinal dynorphin has emerged as one important candidate for the mediation of opioid-induced pain and hyperalgesia.

B. Organ System Effects of Morphine and Its Surrogates

The actions described below for morphine, the prototypic opioid agonist, can also be observed with other opioid agonists, partial agonists, and those with mixed receptor effects. Characteristics of specific members of these groups are discussed below.

1. Central nervous system effects—The principal effects of opioid analgesics with affinity for μ receptors are on the CNS; the more important ones include analgesia, euphoria, sedation, and respiratory depression. With repeated use, a high degree of tolerance occurs to all of these effects (Table 31–3).

a. Analgesia—Pain consists of both sensory and affective (emotional) components. Opioid analgesics are unique in that they can reduce both aspects of the pain experience, especially the affective aspect.

b. Euphoria—Typically, patients or intravenous drug users who receive intravenous morphine experience a pleasant floating sensation with lessened anxiety and distress. However, dysphoria, an unpleasant state characterized by restlessness and malaise, may sometimes occur.

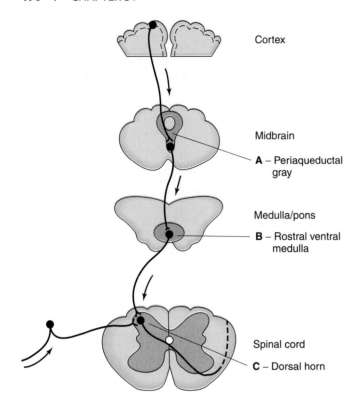

Cortex

Midbrain

A – Periaqueductal gray

Medulla/pons

B – Rostral ventral medulla

Spinal cord

C – Dorsal horn

Figure 31–4. Opioid analgesic action on the descending inhibitory pathway. Sites of action of opioids on pain-modulating neurons in the midbrain and medulla including the midbrain periaqueductal gray area **(A)**, rostral ventral medulla **(B)**, and the locus caeruleus indirectly control pain transmission pathways by enhancing descending inhibition to the dorsal horn **(C)**.

c. Sedation—Drowsiness and clouding of mentation are common concomitants of opioid action. There is little or no amnesia. Sleep is induced by opioids more frequently in the elderly than in young, healthy individuals. Ordinarily, the patient can be easily aroused from this sleep. However, the combination of morphine with other central depressant drugs such as the sedative-hypnotics may result in very deep sleep. Marked sedation occurs more frequently with compounds closely related to the phenanthrene derivatives and less frequently with the synthetic agents such as meperidine and fentanyl. In standard analgesic doses, morphine (a phenanthrene) disrupts normal REM and non-REM sleep patterns. This disrupting effect is probably characteristic of all opioids. In contrast to humans, a number of species (cats, horses, cows, pigs) may manifest excitation rather than sedation when given opioids. These paradoxic effects are at least partially dose-dependent.

d. Respiratory depression—All of the opioid analgesics can produce significant respiratory depression by inhibiting brainstem respiratory mechanisms. Alveolar PCO_2 may increase, but the most reliable indicator of this depression is a depressed response to a carbon dioxide challenge. The respiratory depression is dose-related and is influenced significantly by the degree of sensory input occurring at the time. For example, it is possible to par-

tially overcome opioid-induced respiratory depression by stimulation of various sorts. When strongly painful stimuli that have prevented the depressant action of a large dose of an opioid are relieved, respiratory depression may suddenly become marked. A small to moderate decrease in respiratory function, as measured by $PaCO_2$ elevation, may be well tolerated in the patient without prior respiratory impairment. However, in individuals with increased intracranial pressure, asthma, chronic obstructive pulmonary disease, or cor pulmonale, this decrease in respiratory function may not be tolerated. Opioid-induced respiratory depression remains one of the most difficult clinical challenges in the treatment of severe pain. Research is ongoing to understand and develop analgesic agents and adjuncts that avoid this effect. Research to overcome this problem is focused on δ receptor pharmacology and serotonin signaling pathways in the brainstem respiratory control centers.

e. Cough suppression—Suppression of the cough reflex is a well-recognized action of opioids. Codeine in particular has been used to advantage in persons suffering from pathologic cough and in patients in whom it is necessary to maintain ventilation via an endotracheal tube. However, cough suppression by opioids may allow accumulation of secretions and thus lead to airway obstruction and atelectasis.

ION CHANNELS & NOVEL ANALGESIA TARGETS

Even the most severe *acute* pain (lasting hours to days) can usually be well controlled—with significant but tolerable adverse effects—with currently available analgesics, especially the opioids. *Chronic* pain (lasting weeks to months), however, is not very satisfactorily managed with opioids. It is now known that in chronic pain, presynaptic receptors on sensory nerve terminals in the periphery contribute to increased excitability of sensory nerve endings (peripheral sensitization). The hyperexcitable sensory neuron bombards the spinal cord, leading to increased excitability and synaptic alterations in the dorsal horn (central sensitization). Such changes appear to be important in chronic inflammatory and neuropathic pain states.

In the effort to discover better analgesic drugs for chronic pain, renewed attention is being paid to synaptic transmission in nociception and peripheral sensory transduction. Potentially important ion channels associated with these processes in the periphery include members of the transient receptor potential family such as the capsaicin receptor, TRPV1 (which is activated by multiple noxious stimuli such as heat, mechanical injury, protons, and products of inflammation) as well as P2X receptors (which are responsive to purines released from tissue damage). A special type of tetrodotoxin-resistant voltage-gated sodium channel (Nav1.8), also known as the PN3/SNS channel, is apparently uniquely associated with nociceptive neurons in dorsal root ganglia. **Lidocaine** and **mexiletine,** which are useful in some chronic pain states, may act by blocking this channel. Given the importance of their peripheral sites of action, therapeutic strategies that deliver agents that block peripheral pain transduction or transmission have been introduced in the form of transdermal patches and balms. Such products that specifically target peripheral capsaicin receptors and sodium channel function are becoming available.

Ziconotide, a blocker of voltage-gated N-type calcium channels, has recently been approved for intrathecal analgesia in patients with refractory chronic pain. It is a synthetic peptide related to the marine snail toxin ω-conotoxin, which selectively blocks these calcium channels. **Gabapentin,** an anticonvulsant analog of GABA (see Chapter 24), is an effective treatment for neuropathic (nerve injury) pain. It has recently been shown to block the pain and hyperalgesia associated with inflammation. Potential sites of action of gabapentin include the $\alpha_2\delta$ family of calcium channels.

N-methyl-D-aspartate (NMDA) receptors appear to play a very important role in central sensitization at both spinal and supraspinal levels. Although certain NMDA antagonists have demonstrated analgesic activity (eg, **ketamine**), it has been difficult to find agents with an acceptably low profile of adverse effects or neurotoxicity. However, ketamine at very small doses appears to improve analgesia and reduce opioid requirements under conditions of opioid tolerance. GABA and acetylcholine (through nicotinic receptors) appear to control the central synaptic release of several transmitters involved in nociception. **Nicotine** itself and certain nicotine analogs cause analgesia, and their use for postoperative analgesia is under investigation. Finally, work on cannabinoids and vanilloids and their receptors suggest that Δ^9-**tetrahydrocannabinol,** which acts primarily on CB1 cannabinoid receptors, can interact with the TRPV1 capsaicin receptor to produce analgesia under certain circumstances.

As our understanding of peripheral and central pain transduction improves, additional therapeutic targets and strategies will become available. Combined with our present knowledge of opioid analgesics, a "multimodal" approach to pain therapy is emerging, which allows the use of complementary compounds resulting in improved analgesia with fewer adverse effects.

f. Miosis—Constriction of the pupils is seen with virtually all opioid agonists. Miosis is a pharmacologic action to which little or no tolerance develops (Table 31–3); thus, it is valuable in the diagnosis of opioid overdose. Even in highly tolerant addicts, miosis is seen. This action, which can be blocked by opioid antagonists, is mediated by parasympathetic pathways, which, in turn, can be blocked by atropine.

g. Truncal rigidity—An intensification of tone in the large trunk muscles has been noted with a number of opioids. It was originally believed that truncal rigidity involved a spinal cord action of these drugs, but there is now evidence that it results from an action at supraspinal levels. Truncal rigidity reduces thoracic compliance and thus interferes with ventilation. The effect is most apparent when high doses of the highly lipid-soluble opioids (eg, fentanyl, sufentanil, alfentanil, remifentanil) are rapidly administered intravenously. Truncal rigidity may be overcome by administration of an opioid antagonist, which of course will also antagonize the analgesic action of the opioid. Preventing truncal rigidity while preserving analgesia requires the concomitant use of neuromuscular blocking agents.

Table 31–3. Degrees of tolerance that may develop to some of the effects of the opioids.

High	Moderate	Minimal or None
Analgesia	Bradycardia	Miosis
Euphoria, dysphoria		Constipation
Mental clouding		Convulsions
Sedation		
Respiratory depression		
Antidiuresis		
Nausea and vomiting		
Cough suppression		

h. Nausea and vomiting—The opioid analgesics can activate the brainstem chemoreceptor trigger zone to produce nausea and vomiting. There may also be a vestibular component in this effect because ambulation seems to increase the incidence of nausea and vomiting.

i. Temperature—Homeostatic regulation of body temperature is mediated in part by the action of endogenous opioid peptides in the brain. This has been supported by experiments demonstrating that μ opioid receptor agonists such as morphine administered to the anterior hypothalamus produces hyperthermia, whereas administration of κ agonists induce hypothermia.

2. Peripheral effects—
a. Cardiovascular system—Most opioids have no significant *direct* effects on the heart and, other than bradycardia, no major effects on cardiac rhythm. Meperidine is an exception to this generalization because its antimuscarinic action can result in tachycardia. Blood pressure is usually well maintained in subjects receiving opioids unless the cardiovascular system is stressed, in which case hypotension may occur. This hypotensive effect is probably due to peripheral arterial and venous dilation, which has been attributed to a number of mechanisms including central depression of vasomotor-stabilizing mechanisms and release of histamine. No consistent effect on cardiac output is seen, and the electrocardiogram is not significantly affected. However, caution should be exercised in patients with decreased blood volume, because the above mechanisms make these patients susceptible to hypotension. Opioid analgesics affect cerebral circulation minimally except when PCO_2 rises as a consequence of respiratory depression. Increased PCO_2 leads to cerebral vasodilation associated with a decrease in cerebral vascular resistance, an increase in cerebral blood flow, and an increase in intracranial pressure.

b. Gastrointestinal tract—Constipation has long been recognized as an effect of opioids, an effect that does not diminish with continued use; that is, tolerance does not develop to opioid-induced constipation (Table 31–3). Opioid receptors exist in high density in the gastrointestinal tract, and the constipating effects of the opioids are mediated through an action on the enteric nervous system (see Chapter 6) as well as the CNS. In the stomach, motility (rhythmic contraction and relaxation) may decrease but tone (persistent contraction) may increase—particularly in the central portion; gastric secretion of hydrochloric acid is decreased. Small intestine resting tone is increased, with periodic spasms, but the amplitude of nonpropulsive contractions is markedly decreased. In the large intestine, propulsive peristaltic waves are diminished and tone is increased; this delays passage of the fecal mass and allows increased absorption of water, which leads to constipation. The large bowel actions are the basis for the use of opioids in the management of diarrhea.

c. Biliary tract—The opioids contract biliary smooth muscle, which can result in biliary colic. The sphincter of Oddi may constrict, resulting in reflux of biliary and pancreatic secretions and elevated plasma amylase and lipase levels.

d. Renal—Renal function is depressed by opioids. It is believed that in humans this is chiefly due to decreased renal plasma flow. In addition, μ opioids have been found to have an antidiuretic effect in humans. Mechanisms may involve both the CNS and peripheral sites. Opioids also enhance renal tubular sodium reabsorption. The role of opioid-induced changes in antidiuretic hormone (ADH) release is controversial. Ureteral and bladder tone are increased by therapeutic doses of the opioid analgesics. Increased sphincter tone may precipitate urinary retention, especially in postoperative patients. Occasionally, ureteral colic caused by a renal calculus is made worse by opioid-induced increase in ureteral tone.

e. Uterus—The opioid analgesics may prolong labor. The mechanism for this action is unclear, but both peripheral and central actions of the opioids can reduce uterine tone.

f. Neuroendocrine—Opioid analgesics stimulate the release of ADH, prolactin, and somatotropin but inhibit the release of luteinizing hormone. These effects suggest that endogenous opioid peptides, through effects in the hypothalamus, regulate these systems (Table 31–1).

g. Pruritus—Therapeutic doses of the opioid analgesics produce flushing and warming of the skin accompanied sometimes by sweating and itching; CNS effects and peripheral histamine release may be responsible for these reactions. Opioid-induced pruritus and occasionally urticaria appear more frequently when opioid analgesics are administered parenterally. In addition, when opioids such as morphine are administered to the neuraxis by the spinal or epidural route, their usefulness may be limited by intense pruritus over the lips and torso.

h. Miscellaneous—The opioids modulate the immune system by effects on lymphocyte proliferation, antibody production, and chemotaxis. Natural killer cell cytolytic activity and lymphocyte proliferative responses to mitogens are usually inhibited by opioids. Although the mechanisms involved are complex, activation of central opioid receptors could mediate a significant component of the changes observed in peripheral immune function. In general, these effects are mediated by the sympathetic nervous system in the case of acute administration and by the hypothalamic-pituitary-adrenal system in the case of prolonged administration of opioids.

C. EFFECTS OF OPIOIDS WITH BOTH AGONIST AND ANTAGONIST ACTIONS

Buprenorphine is an opioid agonist that displays high binding affinity but low intrinsic activity at the μ receptor. Its slow rate of dissociation from the μ receptor has also made it an attractive alternative to methadone for the management of opioid withdrawal. It functions as an *antagonist* at the δ and κ receptors and for this reason is referred to as a "mixed agonist-antagonist." Although buprenorphine is used as an analgesic, it can antagonize the action of more potent μ agonists such as morphine. Buprenorphine also binds to ORL1, the orphanin receptor. Whether this property also participates in opposing μ receptor function is under study. Pentazocine and nalbuphine are other examples of opioid analgesics with mixed agonist-antagonist properties. Psychotomimetic effects, with hallucinations, nightmares, and anxiety, have been reported after use of drugs with mixed agonist-antagonist actions.

■ II. CLINICAL PHARMACOLOGY OF THE OPIOID ANALGESICS

Successful treatment of pain is a challenging task that begins with careful attempts to assess the source and magnitude of the pain. The amount of pain experienced by the patient is often measured by means of a numeric visual analog scale (VAS) with word descriptors ranging from no pain (0) to excruciating pain (10). A similar scale can be used with children and with patients who cannot speak; this scale depicts five faces ranging from smiling (no pain) to crying (maximum pain).

For a patient in severe pain, the administration of an opioid analgesic is usually considered a primary part of the overall management plan. Determining the route of administration (oral, parenteral, neuraxial), duration of

drug action, ceiling effect (maximal intrinsic activity), duration of therapy, potential for adverse effects, and the patient's past experience with opioids all should be addressed. One of the principal errors made by physicians in this setting is failure to adequately assess a patient's pain and to match its severity with an appropriate level of therapy. Just as important is the principle that following delivery of the therapeutic plan, its effectiveness must be reevaluated and the plan modified, if necessary, if the response was excessive or inadequate.

Use of opioid drugs in acute situations may be contrasted with their use in chronic pain management, in which a multitude of other factors must be considered, including the development of tolerance to and physical dependence on opioid analgesics.

Clinical Use of Opioid Analgesics

A. ANALGESIA

Severe, *constant* pain is usually relieved with opioid analgesics with high intrinsic activity (see Table 31–2); whereas sharp, intermittent pain does not appear to be as effectively controlled.

The pain associated with cancer and other terminal illnesses must be treated aggressively and often requires a multidisciplinary approach for effective management. Such conditions may require continuous use of potent opioid analgesics and are associated with some degree of tolerance and dependence. However, this should not be used as a barrier to providing patients with the best possible care and quality of life. Research in the hospice movement has demonstrated that fixed-interval administration of opioid medication (ie, a regular dose at a scheduled time) is more effective in achieving pain relief than dosing on demand. New dosage forms of opioids that allow slower release of the drug are now available, eg, sustained-release forms of morphine (MSContin) and oxycodone (OxyContin). Their purported advantage is a longer and more stable level of analgesia.

If disturbances of gastrointestinal function prevent the use of oral sustained-release morphine, the fentanyl transdermal system (fentanyl patch) can be used over long periods. Furthermore, buccal transmucosal fentanyl can be used for episodes of breakthrough pain (see G. Alternative Routes of Administration). Administration of strong opioids by nasal insufflation has been shown to be efficacious, and nasal preparations are now available in some countries. Approval of such formulations in the USA is growing. In addition, stimulant drugs such as the amphetamines have been shown to enhance the analgesic actions of the opioids and thus may be very useful adjuncts in the patient with chronic pain.

Opioid analgesics are often used during obstetric labor. Because opioids cross the placental barrier and reach the fetus, care must be taken to minimize neonatal depression. If it occurs, immediate injection of the antagonist naloxone will reverse the depression. The phenylpiperidine drugs (eg, meperidine) appear to produce less depression, particularly respiratory depression, in newborn infants than does morphine; this may justify their use in obstetric practice.

The acute, severe pain of renal and biliary colic often requires a strong agonist opioid for adequate relief. However, the drug-induced increase in smooth muscle tone may cause a paradoxical *increase* in pain secondary to increased spasm. An increase in the dose of opioid is usually successful in providing adequate analgesia.

B. ACUTE PULMONARY EDEMA

The relief produced by intravenous morphine in dyspnea from pulmonary edema associated with left ventricular failure is remarkable. Proposed mechanisms include reduced anxiety (*perception* of shortness of breath), and reduced cardiac preload (reduced venous tone) and afterload (decreased peripheral resistance). Morphine can be particularly useful when treating painful myocardial ischemia with pulmonary edema.

C. COUGH

Suppression of cough can be obtained at doses lower than those needed for analgesia. However, in recent years the use of opioid analgesics to allay cough has diminished largely because a number of effective synthetic compounds have been developed that are neither analgesic nor addictive. These agents are discussed below.

D. DIARRHEA

Diarrhea from almost any cause can be controlled with the opioid analgesics, but if diarrhea is associated with infection such use must not substitute for appropriate chemotherapy. Crude opium preparations (eg, paregoric) were used in the past to control diarrhea, but now synthetic surrogates with more selective gastrointestinal effects and few or no CNS effects, eg, diphenoxylate, are used. Several preparations are available specifically for this purpose (Chapter 63).

E. SHIVERING

Although all opioid agonists have some propensity to reduce shivering, meperidine is reported to have the most pronounced anti-shivering properties. It is interesting that meperidine apparently blocks shivering through its action on subtypes of the α_2 adrenoceptor.

F. APPLICATIONS IN ANESTHESIA

The opioids are frequently used as premedicant drugs before anesthesia and surgery because of their sedative, anxiolytic, and analgesic properties. They are also used

intraoperatively both as adjuncts to other anesthetic agents and, in high doses (eg, 0.02–0.075 mg/kg of fentanyl), as a primary component of the anesthetic regimen (see Chapter 25). Opioids are most commonly used in cardiovascular surgery and other types of high-risk surgery in which a primary goal is to minimize cardiovascular depression. In such situations, mechanical respiratory assistance must be provided.

Because of their direct action on the superficial neurons of the spinal cord dorsal horn, opioids can also be used as regional analgesics by administration into the epidural or subarachnoid spaces of the spinal column. A number of studies have demonstrated that long-lasting analgesia with minimal adverse effects can be achieved by epidural administration of 3–5 mg of morphine, followed by slow infusion through a catheter placed in the epidural space. It was initially assumed that the epidural application of opioids might selectively produce analgesia without impairment of motor, autonomic, or sensory functions other than pain. However, respiratory depression can occur after the drug is injected into the epidural space and may require reversal with naloxone. Effects such as pruritus and nausea and vomiting are common after epidural and subarachnoid administration of opioids and may also be reversed with naloxone if necessary. Currently, the epidural route is favored because adverse effects are less common. Morphine is the most frequently used agent, but the use of low doses of local anesthetics in combination with fentanyl infused through a thoracic epidural catheter has also become an accepted method of pain control in patients recovering from major upper abdominal surgery. In rare cases, chronic pain management specialists may elect to surgically implant a programmable infusion pump connected to a spinal catheter for continuous infusion of opioids or other analgesic compounds.

G. ALTERNATIVE ROUTES OF ADMINISTRATION

Rectal suppositories of morphine and hydromorphone have long been used when oral and parenteral routes are undesirable. The **transdermal patch** provides stable blood levels of drug and better pain control while avoiding the need for repeated parenteral injections. Fentanyl has been the most successful opioid in transdermal application and finds great use in patients experiencing chronic pain. The **intranasal** route avoids repeated parenteral drug injections and the first-pass metabolism of orally administered drugs. Butorphanol is the only opioid currently available in the USA in a nasal formulation, but more are expected. Another alternative to parenteral administration is the **buccal transmucosal** route, which uses a fentanyl citrate lozenge or a "lollipop" mounted on a stick.

Another type of pain control called **patient-controlled analgesia (PCA)** is now in widespread use for the management of breakthrough pain. With PCA, the patient controls a parenteral (usually intravenous) infusion device by depressing a button to deliver a preprogrammed dose of the desired opioid analgesic. Claims of better pain control using less opioid are supported by well-designed clinical trials, making this approach very useful in postoperative pain control. However, health care personnel must be very familiar with the use of PCAs to avoid overdosage secondary to misuse or improper programming. There is a proven risk of respiratory depression with hypoxia that requires careful monitoring of vital signs and sedation level.

Toxicity & Undesired Effects

Direct toxic effects of the opioid analgesics that are extensions of their acute pharmacologic actions include respiratory depression, nausea, vomiting, and constipation (Table 31–4). In addition, tolerance and dependence, diagnosis and treatment of overdosage, as well as contraindications must be considered.

A. TOLERANCE AND DEPENDENCE

Drug dependence of the opioid type is marked by a relatively specific withdrawal or abstinence syndrome. Just as there are pharmacologic differences between the various opioids, there are also differences in psychologic dependence and the severity of withdrawal effects. For example, withdrawal from dependence on a strong agonist is associated with more severe withdrawal signs and symptoms than withdrawal from a mild or moderate agonist. Administration of an opioid *antagonist* to an opioid-dependent person is followed by brief but severe withdrawal symptoms (see antagonist-precipitated withdrawal, below). The potential for physical and psychologic dependence of the partial agonist-antagonist opioids appears to be less than that of the agonist drugs.

1. Tolerance—Although development of tolerance begins with the first dose of an opioid, tolerance generally does

Table 31–4. Adverse effects of the opioid analgesics.

Behavioral restlessness, tremulousness, hyperactivity (in dysphoric reactions)
Respiratory depression
Nausea and vomiting
Increased intracranial pressure
Postural hypotension accentuated by hypovolemia
Constipation
Urinary retention
Itching around nose, urticaria (more frequent with parenteral and spinal administration)

not become clinically manifest until after 2–3 weeks of frequent exposure to ordinary therapeutic doses. Tolerance develops most readily when large doses are given at short intervals and is minimized by giving small amounts of drug with longer intervals between doses.

Depending on the compound and the effect measured, the degree of tolerance may be as great as 35-fold. Marked tolerance may develop to the analgesic, sedating, and respiratory depressant effects. It is possible to produce respiratory arrest in a nontolerant person with a dose of 60 mg of morphine, whereas in addicts maximally tolerant to opioids as much as 2000 mg of morphine taken over a 2- or 3-hour period may not produce significant respiratory depression. Tolerance also develops to the antidiuretic, emetic, and hypotensive effects but not to the miotic, convulsant, and constipating actions (Table 31–3).

Tolerance to the sedating and respiratory effects of the opioids dissipates within a few days after the drugs are discontinued. Tolerance to the emetic effects may persist for several months after withdrawal of the drug. The rates at which tolerance appears and disappears, as well as the degree of tolerance, may also differ considerably among the different opioid analgesics and among individuals using the same drug. For instance, tolerance to methadone develops more slowly and to a lesser degree than to morphine.

Tolerance also develops to analgesics with mixed receptor effects but to a lesser extent than to the agonists. Such effects as hallucinations, sedation, hypothermia, and respiratory depression are reduced after repeated administration of the mixed receptor drugs. However, tolerance to the latter agents does not generally include cross-tolerance to the agonist opioids. It is also important to note that tolerance does not develop to the antagonist actions of the mixed agents or to those of the pure antagonists.

Cross-tolerance is an extremely important characteristic of the opioids, ie, patients tolerant to morphine show a reduction in analgesic response to other agonist opioids. This is particularly true of those agents with primarily μ-receptor agonist activity. Morphine and its congeners exhibit cross-tolerance not only with respect to their analgesic actions but also to their euphoriant, sedative, and respiratory effects. However, the cross-tolerance existing among the μ-receptor agonists can often be partial or incomplete. This clinical observation has led to the concept of "opioid rotation," which has been used in the treatment of cancer pain for many years. A patient who is experiencing decreasing effectiveness of one opioid analgesic regimen is "rotated" to a different opioid analgesic (eg, morphine to hydromorphone; hydromorphone to methadone) and typically experiences significantly improved analgesia at a reduced overall equivalent dosage. Another approach is to "recouple" opioid receptor function through the use of adjunctive nonopioid agents. NMDA-receptor antagonists (eg, ketamine) have shown promise in preventing or reversing opioid-induced tolerance in animals and humans. Use of these agents, especially ketamine, is increasing because well-controlled studies have shown clinical effectiveness in reducing postoperative pain and opioid requirements in opioid-tolerant patients.

The novel use of δ-receptor antagonists with μ-receptor agonists is also emerging as a strategy to avoid the development of tolerance. This idea has developed around the observation that mice lacking the δ opioid receptor fail to develop tolerance to morphine.

2. Physical dependence—The development of physical dependence is an invariable accompaniment of tolerance to repeated administration of an opioid of the μ type. Failure to continue administering the drug results in a characteristic withdrawal or abstinence syndrome that reflects an exaggerated rebound from the acute pharmacologic effects of the opioid.

The signs and symptoms of withdrawal include rhinorrhea, lacrimation, yawning, chills, gooseflesh (piloerection), hyperventilation, hyperthermia, mydriasis, muscular aches, vomiting, diarrhea, anxiety, and hostility (see Chapter 32). The number and intensity of the signs and symptoms are largely dependent on the degree of physical dependence that has developed. Administration of an opioid at this time suppresses abstinence signs and symptoms almost immediately.

The time of onset, intensity, and duration of abstinence syndrome depend on the drug previously used and may be related to its biologic half-life. With morphine or heroin, withdrawal signs usually start within 6–10 hours after the last dose. Peak effects are seen at 36–48 hours, after which most of the signs and symptoms gradually subside. By 5 days, most of the effects have disappeared, but some may persist for months. In the case of meperidine, the withdrawal syndrome largely subsides within 24 hours, whereas with methadone several days are required to reach the peak of the abstinence syndrome, and it may last as long as 2 weeks. The slower subsidence of methadone effects is associated with a less intense immediate syndrome, and this is the basis for its use in the detoxification of heroin addicts. After the abstinence syndrome subsides, tolerance also disappears, as evidenced by a restoration in sensitivity to the opioid agonist. However, despite the loss of physical dependence on the opioid, craving for it may persist for many months.

A transient, explosive abstinence syndrome—**antagonist-precipitated withdrawal**—can be induced in a subject physically dependent on opioids by administering naloxone or another antagonist. Within 3 minutes after injection of the antagonist, signs and symptoms similar to those seen after abrupt discontinuance appear, peaking in 10–20 minutes and largely subsiding after 1 hour. Even in the case of methadone, withdrawal of which results in a relatively mild abstinence syndrome, the antagonist-precipitated abstinence syndrome may be very severe.

In the case of agents with mixed effects, withdrawal signs and symptoms can be induced after repeated administration followed by abrupt discontinuance of pentazocine, cyclazocine, or nalorphine, but the syndrome appears to be somewhat different from that produced by morphine and other agonists. Anxiety, loss of appetite and body weight, tachycardia, chills, increase in body temperature, and abdominal cramps have been noted.

3. Psychologic dependence—The euphoria, indifference to stimuli, and sedation usually caused by the opioid analgesics, especially when injected intravenously, tend to promote their compulsive use. In addition, the addict experiences abdominal effects that have been likened to an intense sexual orgasm. These factors constitute the primary reasons for opioid abuse liability and are strongly reinforced by the development of physical dependence.

Obviously, the risk of causing dependence is an important consideration in the therapeutic use of these drugs. *Despite that risk, under no circumstances should adequate pain relief ever be withheld simply because an opioid exhibits potential for abuse or because legislative controls complicate the process of prescribing narcotics.* Furthermore, certain principles can be observed by the clinician to minimize problems presented by tolerance and dependence when using opioid analgesics:

Establish therapeutic goals before starting opioid therapy. This tends to limit the potential for physical dependence. The patient and his or her family should be included in this process.

Once a therapeutic dose is established, attempt to limit dosage to this level. This goal is facilitated by use of a written treatment contract which specifically prohibits early refills and having multiple prescribing physicians.

Instead of opioid analgesics—especially in chronic management—consider using other types of analgesics or compounds exhibiting less pronounced withdrawal symptoms on discontinuance.

Frequently evaluate continuing analgesic therapy and the patient's need for opioids.

B. DIAGNOSIS AND TREATMENT OF OPIOID OVERDOSAGE

Intravenous injection of naloxone dramatically reverses coma due to opioid overdose but not that due to other CNS depressants. Use of the antagonist should not, of course, delay the institution of other therapeutic measures, especially respiratory support.

See also the Antagonists section below and Chapter 59.

C. CONTRAINDICATIONS AND CAUTIONS IN THERAPY

1. Use of pure agonists with weak partial agonists—When a weak partial agonist such as pentazocine is given to a patient also receiving a full agonist (eg, morphine), there is a risk of diminishing analgesia or even inducing a state of withdrawal; combining full agonist with partial agonist opioids should be avoided.

2. Use in patients with head injuries—Carbon dioxide retention caused by respiratory depression results in cerebral vasodilation. In patients with elevated intracranial pressure, this may lead to lethal alterations in brain function.

3. Use during pregnancy—In pregnant women who are chronically using opioids, the fetus may become physically dependent in utero and manifest withdrawal symptoms in the early postpartum period. A daily dose as small as 6 mg of heroin (or equivalent) taken by the mother can result in a mild withdrawal syndrome in the infant, and twice that much may result in severe signs and symptoms, including irritability, shrill crying, diarrhea, or even seizures. Recognition of the problem is aided by a careful history and physical examination. When withdrawal symptoms are judged to be relatively mild, treatment is aimed at control of these symptoms with such drugs as diazepam; with more severe withdrawal, camphorated tincture of opium (paregoric; 0.4 mg of morphine/mL) in an oral dose of 0.12–0.24 mL/kg is used. Oral doses of methadone (0.1–0.5 mg/kg) have also been used.

4. Use in patients with impaired pulmonary function—In patients with borderline respiratory reserve, the depressant properties of the opioid analgesics may lead to acute respiratory failure.

5. Use in patients with impaired hepatic or renal function—Because morphine and its congeners are metabolized primarily in the liver, their use in patients in prehepatic coma may be questioned. Half-life is prolonged in patients with impaired renal function, and morphine and its active glucuronide metabolite may accumulate; dosage can often be reduced in such patients.

6. Use in patients with endocrine disease—Patients with adrenal insufficiency (Addison's disease) and those with hypothyroidism (myxedema) may have prolonged and exaggerated responses to opioids.

Drug Interactions

Because seriously ill or hospitalized patients may require a large number of drugs, there is always a possibility of drug interactions when the opioid analgesics are administered. Table 31–5 lists some of these drug interactions and the reasons for not combining the named drugs with opioids.

Table 31–5. Opioid drug interactions.

Drug Group	Interaction with Opioids
Sedative-hypnotics	Increased central nervous system depression, particularly respiratory depression.
Antipsychotic tranquilizers	Increased sedation. Variable effects on respiratory depression. Accentuation of cardiovascular effects (antimuscarinic and α-blocking actions).
MAO inhibitors	Relative contraindication to all opioid analgesics because of the high incidence of hyperpyrexic coma; hypertension has also been reported.

MAO, monoamine oxidase.

SPECIFIC AGENTS

The following section describes the most important and widely used opioid analgesics, along with features peculiar to specific agents. Data about doses approximately equivalent to 10 mg of intramuscular morphine, oral versus parenteral efficacy, duration of analgesia, and intrinsic activity (maximum efficacy) are presented in Table 31–2.

STRONG AGONISTS

1. Phenanthrenes

Morphine, hydromorphone, and **oxymorphone** are strong agonists useful in treating severe pain. These prototypic agents have been described in detail above.

Morphine

Heroin (diamorphine, diacetylmorphine) is potent and fast-acting, but its use is prohibited in the USA and Canada. In recent years, there has been considerable agitation to revive its use. However, double-blind studies have not supported the claim that heroin is more effective than morphine in relieving severe chronic pain, at least when given by the intramuscular route.

2. Phenylheptylamines

Methadone has undergone a dramatic revival as a potent and clinically useful analgesic. It can be administered by the oral, intravenous, subcutaneous, spinal, and rectal routes. It is well absorbed from the gastrointestinal tract and its bioavailability far exceeds that of oral morphine.

Methadone

Methadone is not only a potent μ-receptor agonist but its racemic mixture of D- and L-methadone isomers can also block both NMDA receptors and monoaminergic reuptake transporters. These nonopioid receptor properties may help explain its ability to relieve difficult-to-treat pain (neuropathic, cancer pain), especially when a previous trial of morphine has failed. In this regard, when analgesic tolerance or intolerable side effects have developed with the use of increasing doses of morphine or hydromorphone, "opioid rotation" to methadone has provided superior analgesia at 10–20% of the morphine-equivalent daily dose. In contrast to its use in suppressing symptoms of opioid withdrawal, use of methadone as an analgesic typically requires administration at intervals of no more than 8 hours. However, given methadone's highly variable pharmacokinetics and long half-life (25–52 hours), initial administration should be closely monitored to avoid potentially harmful adverse effects, especially respiratory depression.

Methadone is widely known for its use in the treatment of opioid abuse. Tolerance and physical dependence develop more slowly with methadone than with morphine. The withdrawal signs and symptoms occurring after abrupt discontinuance of methadone are milder, although more prolonged, than those of morphine. These properties make methadone a useful drug for detoxification and for maintenance of the chronic relapsing heroin addict.

For detoxification of a heroin-dependent addict, low doses of methadone (5–10 mg orally) are given two or three times daily for 2 or 3 days. Upon discontinuing methadone, the addict experiences a mild but endurable withdrawal syndrome.

For maintenance therapy of the opioid recidivist, tolerance to 50–100 mg/d of oral methadone may be deliberately produced; in this state, the addict experiences cross-tolerance to heroin, which prevents most of the addiction-reinforcing effects of heroin. One rationale of maintenance programs is that blocking the reinforcement obtained from abuse of illicit opioids removes the drive to obtain them, thereby reducing criminal activity and making the addict more amenable to psychiatric and rehabilitative therapy. The pharmacologic basis for the use of methadone in maintenance programs is sound and the sociologic basis is rational, but some methadone programs fail because nonpharmacologic management is inadequate.

The concurrent administration of methadone to heroin addicts known to be recidivists has been questioned because of the increased risk of overdose death secondary to respiratory arrest. Buprenorphine, a partial μ-receptor agonist with long-acting properties, has been found to be effective in opioid detoxification and maintenance programs and is presumably associated with a lower risk of such overdose fatalities.

3. Phenylpiperidines

Fentanyl is one of the most widely used agents in this family of synthetic opioids. The fentanyl subgroup now includes **sufentanil, alfentanil,** and **remifentanil** in addition to the parent compound, fentanyl.

Fentanyl

These opioids differ mainly in their potency and biodisposition. Sufentanil is five to seven times more potent than fentanyl. Alfentanil is considerably less potent than fentanyl, but acts more rapidly and has a markedly shorter duration of action. Remifentanil is metabolized very rapidly by blood and nonspecific tissue esterases, making its pharmacokinetic and pharmacodynamic half-lives extremely short. Such properties are useful when these compounds are used in anesthesia practice. Although fentanyl is now the predominant analgesic in the phenylpiperidine class, **meperidine** continues to be widely used. This older opioid has significant antimuscarinic effects, which may be a contraindication if tachycardia would be a problem. Meperidine is also reported to have a negative inotropic action on the heart. In addition, it has the potential for producing seizures secondary to accumulation of its metabolite, normeperidine, in patients receiving high doses or with concurrent renal failure.

4. Morphinans

Levorphanol is a synthetic opioid analgesic closely resembling morphine in its action.

MILD TO MODERATE AGONISTS

1. Phenanthrenes

Codeine, oxycodone, dihydrocodeine, and **hydrocodone** are all somewhat less efficacious than morphine (they are partial agonists) or have adverse effects that limit the maximum tolerated dose when one attempts to achieve analgesia comparable to that of morphine.

Codeine

These compounds are rarely used alone but are combined in formulations containing aspirin or acetaminophen and other drugs.

2. Phenylheptylamines

Propoxyphene is chemically related to methadone but has low analgesic activity. Various studies have reported its potency at levels ranging from no better than placebo to half as potent as codeine; that is, 120 mg propoxyphene = 60 mg codeine. Its true potency probably lies somewhere between these extremes, and its analgesic effect is additive to that of an optimal dose of aspirin. However, its low efficacy makes it unsuitable, even in combination with aspirin, for severe pain. Although propoxyphene has a low abuse liability, the increasing incidence of deaths associated with its misuse has caused it to be scheduled as a controlled substance with low potential for abuse.

3. Phenylpiperidines

Diphenoxylate and its metabolite, **difenoxin,** are not used for analgesia but for the treatment of diarrhea. They are scheduled for minimal control (difenoxin is schedule IV, diphenoxylate schedule V; see inside front cover) because the likelihood of their abuse is remote. The poor solubility of the compounds limits their use for parenteral injection. As antidiarrheal drugs, they are used in combination with atropine. The atropine is added in a concentration too low to have a significant antidiarrheal effect but is presumed to further reduce the likelihood of abuse.

Loperamide is a phenylpiperidine derivative used to control diarrhea. Its potential for abuse is considered very low because of its limited access to the brain. It is therefore available without a prescription.

The usual dose with all of these antidiarrheal agents is two tablets to start and then one tablet after each diarrheal stool.

OPIOIDS WITH MIXED RECEPTOR ACTIONS

Care should be taken not to administer any partial agonist or drug with mixed opioid receptor actions to patients receiving pure agonist drugs because of the unpredictability of both drugs' effects: reduction of analgesia or precipitation of an explosive abstinence syndrome may result.

1. Phenanthrenes

Nalbuphine is a strong κ receptor *agonist* and a μ receptor *antagonist;* it is given parenterally. At higher doses there seems to be a definite ceiling—not noted with morphine—to the respiratory depressant effect. Unfortunately, when respiratory depression does occur, it may be relatively resistant to naloxone reversal.

Buprenorphine is a potent and long-acting phenanthrene derivative that is a partial μ receptor agonist. When administered orally, the sublingual route is preferred to avoid significant first-pass effect. Its long duration of action is due to its slow dissociation from μ receptors. This property renders its effects resistant to naloxone reversal. Its clinical applications are much like those of nalbuphine. In addition, studies continue to suggest that buprenorphine is as effective as methadone in the detoxification and maintenance of heroin abusers. Buprenorphine was approved by the US Food and Drug Administration (FDA) in 2002 for the management of opioid dependence. In contrast to methadone, high-dose administration of buprenorphine results in a μ opioid *antagonist* action, limiting its properties of analgesia and respiratory depression. Moreover, buprenorphine is also available combined with a pure μ opioid antagonist to help prevent its diversion for illicit intravenous abuse.

2. Morphinans

Butorphanol produces analgesia equivalent to nalbuphine and buprenorphine but appears to produce more sedation at equianalgesic doses. Butorphanol is considered to be predominantly a κ agonist. However, it may also act as a partial agonist or antagonist at the μ-receptor.

3. Benzomorphans

Pentazocine is a κ agonist with weak μ antagonist or partial agonist properties. It is the oldest mixed agent available. It may be used orally or parenterally. However, because of its irritant properties, the injection of pentazocine subcutaneously is not recommended.

MISCELLANEOUS

Tramadol is a centrally acting analgesic whose mechanism of action is predominantly based on blockade of serotonin reuptake. Tramadol has also been found to inhibit norepinephrine transporter function. Because it is only partially antagonized by naloxone, it is believed to be only a weak μ-receptor agonist. The recommended dosage is 50–100 mg orally four times daily. Toxicity includes association with seizures; the drug is relatively contraindicated in patients with a history of epilepsy and for use with other drugs that lower the seizure threshold. Other side effects include nausea and dizziness, but these symptoms typically abate after several days of therapy. It is surprising that no clinically significant effects on respiration or the cardiovascular system have thus far been reported. Given the fact that the analgesic action of tramadol is largely independent of μ receptor action, tramadol may serve as an adjunct with pure opioid agonists in the treatment of chronic neuropathic pain.

ANTITUSSIVES

The opioid analgesics are among the most effective drugs available for the suppression of cough. This effect is often achieved at doses below those necessary to produce analgesia. The receptors involved in the antitussive effect appear to differ from those associated with the other actions of opioids. For example, the antitussive effect is also produced by stereoisomers of opioid molecules that are devoid of analgesic effects and addiction liability (see below).

The physiologic mechanism of cough is complex, and little is known about the specific mechanism of action of the opioid antitussive drugs. It is likely that both central and peripheral effects play a role.

The opioid derivatives most commonly used as antitussives are dextromethorphan, codeine, levopropoxyphene, and noscapine (levopropoxyphene and noscapine are not available in the USA). Although these agents (other than codeine) are largely free of the adverse effects associated with the opioids, they should be used with caution in patients taking monoamine oxide inhibitors (see Table 31–5). Antitussive preparations usually also contain expectorants to thin and liquefy respiratory secretions.

Dextromethorphan is the dextrorotatory stereoisomer of a methylated derivative of levorphanol. It is purported to be free of addictive properties and produces less constipation than codeine. The usual antitussive dose is 15–30 mg three or four times daily. It is available in many over-the-counter products. Dextromethorphan has also been found to enhance the analgesic action of morphine and presumably other μ-receptor agonists.

Codeine, as noted, has a useful antitussive action at doses lower than those required for analgesia. Thus, 15 mg are usually sufficient to relieve cough.

Levopropoxyphene is the stereoisomer of the weak opioid agonist dextropropoxyphene. It is devoid of opioid effects, although sedation has been described as a side effect. The usual antitussive dose is 50–100 mg every 4 hours.

THE OPIOID ANTAGONISTS

The pure opioid antagonist drugs **naloxone, naltrexone,** and **nalmefene** are morphine derivatives with bulkier substituents at the N_{17} position. These agents have a relatively high affinity for μ opioid binding sites. They have lower affinity for the other receptors but can also reverse agonists at δ and κ sites.

Naloxone

Pharmacokinetics

Naloxone is usually given by injection and has short duration of action (1–2 hours) when given by this route. Metabolic disposition is chiefly by glucuronide conjugation like that of the agonist opioids with free hydroxyl groups. Naltrexone is well absorbed after oral administration but may undergo rapid first-pass metabolism. It has a half-life of 10 hours, and a single oral dose of 100 mg blocks the effects of injected heroin for up to 48 hours. Nalmefene, the newest of these agents, is a derivative of naltrexone but is available only for intravenous administration. Like naloxone, nalmefene is used for opioid overdose but has a longer half-life (8–10 hours).

Pharmacodynamics

When given in the absence of an agonist drug, these antagonists are almost inert at doses that produce marked antagonism of agonist opioid effects.

When given intravenously to a morphine-treated subject, the antagonist completely and dramatically reverses the opioid effects within 1–3 minutes. In individuals who are acutely depressed by an overdose of an opioid, the antagonist effectively normalizes respiration, level of consciousness, pupil size, bowel activity, and awareness of pain. In dependent subjects who appear normal while taking opioids, naloxone or naltrexone almost instantaneously precipitates an abstinence syndrome.

There is no tolerance to the antagonistic action of these agents, nor does withdrawal after chronic administration precipitate an abstinence syndrome.

Clinical Use

Naloxone is a pure antagonist and is preferred over older weak agonist-antagonist agents that had been used primarily as antagonists, eg, nalorphine and levallorphan.

The major application of naloxone is in the treatment of acute opioid overdose (see also Chapter 59). *It is very important that the relatively short duration of action of naloxone be borne in mind, because a severely depressed patient may recover after a single dose of naloxone and appear normal, only to relapse into coma after 1–2 hours.*

The usual initial dose of naloxone is 0.1–0.4 mg intravenously for life-threatening respiratory and CNS depression. Maintenance is with the same drug, 0.4–0.8 mg given intravenously, and repeated whenever necessary. In using naloxone in the severely opioid-depressed newborn, it is important to start with doses of 5–10 mcg/kg and to consider a second dose of up to a total of 25 mcg/kg if no response is noted.

Low-dose naloxone (0.04 mg) has an increasing role in the treatment of adverse effects that are commonly associated with intravenous or epidural opioids. Careful titration of the naloxone dosage can often eliminate the itching, nausea, and vomiting while sparing the analgesia. Oral naloxone, and more recently developed nonabsorbable analogs of naloxone, have been shown to be efficacious in the treatment of opioid-induced ileus or constipation. The principal mechanism behind this selective therapeutic effect is believed to be local inhibition of μ receptors in the gut with minimal systemic absorption. Several of these compounds are in the final stages of evaluation by the FDA.

Because of its long duration of action, naltrexone has been proposed as a maintenance drug for addicts in treatment programs. A single dose given on alternate days blocks virtually all of the effects of a dose of heroin. It might be predicted that this approach to rehabilitation would not be popular with a large percentage of drug users unless they are motivated to become drug-free. There is evidence that naltrexone decreases the craving for alcohol in chronic alcoholics, and it has been approved by the FDA for this purpose (see Chapter 23).

Chapter continues on next page.

PREPARATIONS AVAILABLE[1]

ANALGESIC OPIOIDS

Alfentanil (Alfenta)
Parenteral: 0.5 mg/mL for injection

Buprenorphine (Buprenex, others)
Oral: 2, 8 mg sublingual tablets
Parenteral: 0.3 mg/mL for injection

Butorphanol (generic, Stadol)
Parenteral: 1, 2 mg/mL for injection
Nasal (generic, Stadol NS): 10 mg/mL nasal spray

Codeine (sulfate or phosphate) (generic)
Oral: 15, 30, 60 mg tablets, 15 mg/5 mL solution
Parenteral: 15, 30 mg/mL for injection

Fentanyl
Parenteral (generic, Sublimaze): 50 mg/mL for injection
Fentanyl Transdermal System (Duragesic): 12.5, 25, 50, 75, 100 mcg/h delivery
Fentanyl Oralet: 100, 200, 300, 400 mcg oral lozenge
Fentanyl Actiq: 200, 400, 600, 800, 1200, 1600 mcg lozenge on a stick

Hydromorphone (generic, Dilaudid)
Oral: 1, 2, 3, 4, 8 mg tablets; 1 mg/mL liquid
Parenteral: 1, 2, 4, 10 mg/mL for injection

Levomethadyl acetate (Orlaam)
Oral: 10 mg/mL solution. *Note:* Orphan drug approved only for the treatment of narcotic addiction.

Levorphanol (generic, Levo-Dromoran)
Oral: 2 mg tablets
Parenteral: 2 mg/mL for injection

Meperidine (generic, Demerol)
Oral: 50, 100 mg tablets; 50 mg/5 mL syrup
Parenteral: 25, 50, 75, 100 mg per dose for injection

Methadone (generic, Dolophine)
Oral: 5, 10 mg tablets; 40 mg dispersible tablets; 1, 2, 10 mg/mL solutions
Parenteral: 10 mg/mL for injection

Morphine sulfate (generic, others)
Oral: 15, 30 mg tablets; 15, 30 mg capsules; 10, 20, 100 mg/5 mL solution
Oral sustained-release tablets (MS-Contin, others): 15, 30, 60, 100, 200 mg tablets);
Oral sustained-release capsules (Avinza, Kadian): 20, 30, 50, 60, 90, 100, 120 mg capsules
Parenteral: 0.5, 1, 2, 4, 5, 8, 10, 15, 25, 50 mg/mL for injection
Rectal: 5, 10, 20, 30 mg suppositories

Nalbuphine (generic, Nubain)
Parenteral: 10, 20 mg/mL for injection

Oxycodone (generic)
Oral: 5 mg tablets, capsules; 1, 20 mg/mL solutions
Oral sustained-release (OxyContin): 10, 20, 40, 80 mg tablets

Oxymorphone (Numorphan)
Parenteral: 1, 1.5 mg/mL for injection
Rectal: 5 mg suppositories

Pentazocine (Talwin)
Oral: See combinations
Parenteral: 30 mg/mL for injection

Propoxyphene (generic, Darvon Pulvules, others)
Oral: 65 mg capsules, 100 mg tablets. *Note:* This product is not recommended.

Remifentanil (Ultiva)
Parenteral: 1, 2, 5 mg powder for reconstitution for injection

Sufentanil (generic, Sufenta)
Parenteral: 50 mcg /mL for injection

OTHER ANALGESICS

Tramadol (Ultram)
Oral: 50 mg tablets

Ziconotide (Prialt)
Intrathecal: 25, 100 mcg/mL for programmable pump

ANALGESIC COMBINATIONS[2]

Codeine/acetaminophen (generic, Tylenol w/ Codeine, others)
Oral: 15, 30, 60 mg codeine plus 300 or 325 mg acetaminophen tablets or capsules; 12 mg codeine plus 120 mg acetaminophen tablets

Codeine/aspirin (generic, Empirin Compound, others)
Oral: 30, 60 mg codeine plus 325 mg aspirin tablets

Hydrocodone/acetaminophen (generic, Norco, Vicodin, Lortab, others)
Oral: 2.5, 5, 7.5, 10 mg hydrocodone plus 500 or 650 mg acetaminophen tablets

(continued)

---

[1]Antidiarrheal opioid preparations are listed in Chapter 63.

[2]Dozens of combination products are available; only a few of the most commonly prescribed ones are listed here. Codeine combination products available in several strengths are usually denoted No. 2 (15 mg codeine), No. 3 (30 mg codeine), and No. 4 (60 mg codeine). Prescribers should be aware of the possible danger of renal damage with acetaminophen, aspirin, and nonsteroidal anti-inflammatory drugs contained in these analgesic combinations.

Hydrocodone/ibuprofen (Vicoprofen)
Oral: 7.5 mg hydrocodone plus 200 mg ibuprofen

Oxycodone/acetaminophen (generic, Percocet, Tylox, others). *Note:* High-dose acetaminophen has potential for hepatic toxicity with repeated use.
Oral: 5 mg oxycodone plus 325 or 500 mg acetaminophen tablets

Oxycodone/aspirin (generic, Percodan)
Oral: 4.9 mg oxycodone plus 325 mg aspirin

Propoxyphene/aspirin or **Propoxyphene/acetaminophen** (Darvon Compound-65, others)
Note: This product is not recommended.
Oral: 65 mg propoxyphene plus 389 mg aspirin plus 32.4 mg caffeine; 50, 65, 100 mg propoxyphene plus 325 or 650 mg acetaminophen

OPIOID ANTAGONISTS

Nalmefene (Revex)
Parenteral: 0.1, 1 mg/mL for injection

Naloxone (Narcan, various)
Parenteral: 0.4, 1 mg/mL; 0.02 mg/mL (for neonatal use) for injection

Naltrexone (ReVia, Depade)
Oral: 50 mg tablets

ANTITUSSIVES

Codeine (generic)
Oral: 15, 30, 60 mg tablets; constituent of many proprietary syrups[2]

Dextromethorphan (generic, Benylin DM, Delsym, others)
Oral: 5, 7.5 mg lozenges; 7.5, 10, 15, 30 mg/5 mL syrup; 30 mg sustained-action liquid; constituent of many proprietary syrups[2]

REFERENCES

Angst MS, Clark JD: Opioid-induced hyperalgesia. Anesthesiology 2006;104:570.

Basbaum AI, Woolf CJ: Pain. Curr Biol 1999;9:R429.

Basbaum AI, Jessel T: The perception of pain. In Kandel ER et al (editors): *Principles of Neural Science,* 4th ed, McGraw-Hill, 2000.

Benedetti C, Premuda L: The history of opium and its derivatives. In: Benedetti C et al (editors): *Advances in Pain Research and Therapy,* vol 14. Raven Press, 1990.

Bolan EA, Tallarida RJ, Pasternak GW: Synergy between mu opioid ligands: Evidence for functional interactions among mu opioid receptor subtypes. J Pharmacol Exp Ther 2002;303:557.

Bonci A, Williams JT: Increased probability of GABA release during withdrawal from morphine. J Neurosci 1997;17:796.

Daniels DJ et al: Opioid-induced tolerance and dependence in mice is modulated by the distance between pharmacophores in a bivalent ligand series. Proc Natl Acad Sci USA 2005; 102:19208.

Davis MP, Walsh D: Methadone for relief of cancer pain: A review of pharmacokinetics, pharmacodynamics, drug interactions and protocols of administration. Support Care Cancer 2001;9:73.

De Kock M, Lavand'homme P, Waterloos H: "Balanced analgesia" in the perioperative period: Is there a place for ketamine? Pain 2001;92:373.

Eilers HM et al: The reversal of fentanyl-induced tolerance by administration of "small-dose" ketamine. Anesth Analg 2001; 93:213.

Evans CJ et al: Cloning of a delta opioid receptor by functional expression. Science 1992;258:1952.

Ferner RE, Daniels AM: Office-based treatment of opioid-dependent patients. N Engl J Med 2003;348:81.

Ferrante FM: Principles of opioid pharmacotherapy: Practical implications of basic mechanisms. J Pain Symptom Manage 1996;11:265.

Fields HL, Basbaum AI: Central nervous system mechanisms of pain modulation. In: Wall PD, Melzack R (editors): *Textbook of Pain.* Churchill Livingstone, 1999.

Fields HL, Heinricher MM, Mason P: Neurotransmitters in nociceptive modulatory circuits. Annu Rev Neurosci 1991;14:219.

Fillingim RB, Gear RW: Sex differences in opioid analgesia: Clinical and experimental findings. Eur J Pain 2004;8:413.

Fischer BD, Carrigan KA, Dykstra LA: Effects of *N*-methyl-D-aspartate receptor antagonists on acute morphine-induced and L-methadone-induced antinociception in mice. J Pain 2005;6:425.

Goldman D, Barr CS: Restoring the addicted brain. N Engl J Med 2002;347:843.

Hill HF, Mather LE: Patient-controlled analgesia. Pharmacokinetic and therapeutic considerations. Clin Pharmacokinet 1993;24:124.

Irwin RS, Curley FJ, Bennett FM: Appropriate use of antitussives and protussives: A practical review. Drugs 1993;46:80.

Joly V et al: Remifentanil-induced postoperative hyperalgesia and its prevention with small-dose ketamine. Anesthesiology 2005; 103:147.

Julius D, Basbaum AI: Molecular mechanisms of nociception. Nature 2001;413:203.

Kalso E et al: No pain, no gain: Clinical excellence and scientific rigour—lessons learned from IA morphine. Pain 2002;98:269.

Kiefer BL: Opioids: First lessons from knockout mice. Trends Pharmacol Sci 1999;20:19.

King T et al: Role of NK-1 neurotransmission in opioid-induced hyperalgesia. Pain 2005;116:276.

Kirkwood LC et al: Characterization of the human cytochrome P450 enzymes involved in the metabolism of dihydrocodeine. Br J Clin Pharmacol 1997;44:549.

Kovelowski CJ et al: Supraspinal cholecystokinin may drive tonic descending facilitation mechanisms to maintain neuropathic pain in the rat. Pain 2000;87:265.

Kromer W: Endogenous and exogenous opioids in the control of gastrointestinal motility and secretion. Pharmacol Rev 1988; 40:121.

Laughlin TM, Larson AA, Wilcox GL: Mechanisms of induction of persistent nociception by dynorphin. J Pharmacol Exp Ther 2001;299:6.

Liu JG, Anand KJ: Protein kinases modulate the cellular adaptations associated with opioid tolerance and dependence. Brain Res Brain Res Rev 2001;38:1.

McGaraughty S, Heinricher MM: Microinjection of morphine into various amygdaloid nuclei differentially affects nociceptive responsiveness and RVM neuronal activity. Pain 2002;96:153.

Mercadante S: Opioid rotation for cancer pain: Rationale and clinical aspects. Cancer 1999;86:1856.

Mercadante S, Arcuri E: Opioids and renal function. J Pain 2004;5:2.

Meunier J, Mouledous L, Topham CM: The nociceptin (ORL1) receptor: Molecular cloning and functional architecture. Peptides 2000;21:893.

Mitchell JM, Basbaum AI, Fields HL: A locus and mechanism of action for associative morphine tolerance. Nat Neurosci 2000;3:47.

Pan YX et al: Generation of the mu opioid receptor (MOR-1) protein by three new splice variants of the Oprm gene. Proc Natl Acad Sci USA 2001;98;14084.

Paul D et al: Pharmacological characterization of morphine 6-β glucuronide, a very potent morphine metabolite. J Pharmacol Exp Ther 1989;251:477.

Quock RM et al: The delta-opioid receptor: Molecular pharmacology, signal transduction, and the determination of drug efficacy. Pharmacol Rev 1999;51:503.

Sindrup SH, Jensen TS: Efficacy of pharmacological treatments of neuropathic pain: An update and effect related to mechanism of drug action. Pain 1999;83:389.

Skarke C, Geisslinger G, Lotsch J: Is morphine-3-glucuronide of therapeutic relevance? Pain 2005;116:177.

Smith MT: Neuroexcitatory effects of morphine and hydromorphone: Evidence implicating the 3-glucuronide metabolites. Clin Exp Pharmacol Physiol 2000;27:524.

Stein C, Schafer M, Machelska H: Attacking pain at its source: New perspectives on opioids. Nat Med 2003;9:1003.

Vanderah TW et al: Mechanisms of opioid-induced pain and antinociceptive tolerance: Descending facilitation and spinal dynorphin. Pain 2001;92:5.

Von Dossow V et al: Thoracic epidural anesthesia combined with general anesthesia: The preferred anesthetic technique for thoracic surgery. Anesth Analg 2001;92:848.

Waldhoer M et al: A heterodimer-selective agonist shows in vivo relevance of G protein-coupled receptor dimers. Proc Natl Acad Sci USA 2005;102:9050.

Wang Z et al: Pronociceptive actions of dynorphin maintain chronic neuropathic pain. J Neurosci 2001;21:1779.

Williams JT, Christie MJ, Manzoni O: Cellular and synaptic adaptations mediating opioid dependence. Physiol Rev 2001; 81:299.

Woolf CJ, Salter MW: Neuronal plasticity: Increasing the gain in pain. Science 2000;288:1765.

Zhao GM et al: Profound spinal tolerance after repeated exposure to a highly selective mu-opioid peptide agonist: Role of delta-opioid receptors. J Pharmacol Exp Ther 2002; 302:188.

Zubieta JK et al: Regional mu opioid receptor regulation of sensory and affective dimensions of pain. Science 2001;293:311.

Drugs of Abuse

Christian Lüscher, MD

Drugs are abused (used in ways that are not medically approved) because they cause strong feelings of euphoria or alter perception. However, repetitive exposure induces widespread adaptive changes in the brain. As a consequence drug use may become compulsive—the hallmark of addiction.

■ I. BASIC NEUROBIOLOGY OF DRUG ABUSE

DEPENDENCE VERSUS ADDICTION

Recent neurobiologic research has led to the conceptual and mechanistic separation of "dependence" and "addiction." The older term "physical dependence" is now denoted **dependence,** while "psychological dependence" is more simply called **addiction.**

Every addictive drug causes its own characteristic spectrum of acute effects, but all have in common that they induce strong feelings of euphoria and reward. With repetitive exposure, addictive drugs induce adaptive changes such as tolerance (ie, escalation of dose to maintain effect). Once the abused drug is no longer available, signs of withdrawal become apparent. A combination of such signs, referred to as the withdrawal syndrome, defines *dependence.* Dependence is not always a correlate of drug abuse—it can also occur with many classes of nonpsychoactive drugs, eg, sympathomimetic vasoconstrictors and bronchodilators, and organic nitrate vasodilators. *Addiction,* on the other hand, consists of compulsive, relapsing drug use despite negative consequences, at times triggered by cravings that occur in response to contextual cues (see Box: Animal Models in Addiction Research). While dependence will invariably occur with chronic exposure, only a fraction of subjects will develop a habit, lose control, and become addicted. For example, very few patients who receive opioids as analgesics will desire the drug after withdrawal. And only one person out of six will become addicted within 10 years of first use of cocaine. Conversely, relapse is very common in addicts after a successful withdrawal when, by definition, they are no longer dependent.

ADDICTIVE DRUGS INCREASE THE LEVEL OF DOPAMINE: REINFORCEMENT

In order to understand the long-term changes induced by drugs of abuse, their initial molecular and cellular targets must be identified. A combination of approaches in animals and humans, including functional imaging, has revealed the mesolimbic dopamine system as the prime target of addictive drugs. This system originates in the ventral tegmental area (VTA), a tiny structure at the tip of the brainstem, which projects to the nucleus accumbens, the amygdala, and the prefrontal cortex (Figure 32–1). Most projection neurons of the VTA are dopamine-producing neurons. When the dopamine neurons of the VTA begin to fire in bursts, large quantities of dopamine are released in the nucleus accumbens and the prefrontal cortex. Early animal studies pairing electrical stimulation of the VTA with operant responses (eg, lever pressing) that result in strong reinforcement established the central role of the mesolimbic dopamine system in reward processing. Direct application of drugs into the VTA also acts as a strong reinforcer, and systemic administration of drugs of abuse causes release of dopamine. *As a general rule, all addictive drugs activate the mesolimbic dopamine system.* The behavioral significance of this increase of dopamine is still debated. An appealing hypothesis is that mesolimbic dopamine codes for the difference between expected and actual reward and thus constitutes a strong learning signal (see Box: The Dopamine Hypothesis of Addiction).

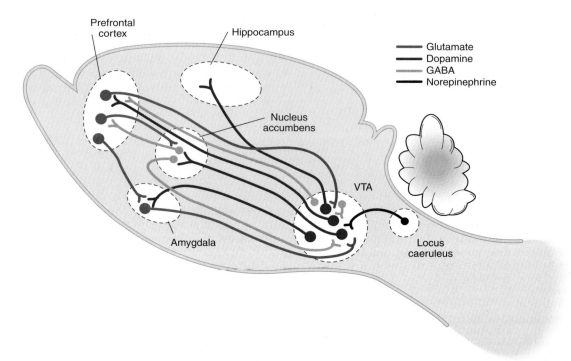

Figure 32–1. Major connections of the mesolimbic dopamine system in the rat brain. The dopamine projection originates in the ventral tegmental area (VTA). Main targets are the nucleus accumbens (NAc), prefrontal cortex (PFC), and amygdala. Excitatory inputs reach the VTA from the PFC and the amygdala. Inhibitory inputs onto dopamine neurons come from GABA neurons within the VTA (interneurons) or as a feedback loop from the NAc. The locus caeruleus releases norepinephrine onto the VTA. Transmitters used by the neurons are indicated by gray for glutamate, black for norepinephrine, dark color for dopamine, and light color for GABA.

ANIMAL MODELS IN ADDICTION RESEARCH

Many of the recent advances in addiction research have been made possible by the use of animal models. Since drugs of abuse are not only rewarding but also reinforcing, an animal will learn a behavior (eg, press a lever) when paired with drug administration. In such a self-administration paradigm, the number of times an animal is willing to press the lever in order to obtain a single dose reflects the strength of reinforcement and is therefore a measure of the rewarding properties of a drug. Observing withdrawal signs specific for rodents (eg, escape jumps or "wet-dog" shakes after abrupt termination of chronic morphine administration) allows the quantification of dependence. Behavioral tests for addiction in the rodent have proven difficult to develop and so far no test fully captures the complexity of the disease. However it is possible to model core components of addiction by monitoring behavioral sensitization and conditioned place preference. In the first test, an increase in locomotor activity is observed with intermittent drug exposure. The latter tests for the preference of a particular environment associated with drug exposure by measuring the time an animal spends in the compartment where a drug was received compared with the compartment where only saline was injected (conditioned place preference). Both tests have in common that they are sensitive to cue-conditioned effects of addictive drugs. Recent findings suggest that prolonged self-administration of cocaine leads to behaviors in rats that closely resemble human addiction. Such "addicted rats" are very strongly motivated to seek cocaine, continue looking for the drug even when no longer available, and self-administer cocaine in spite of negative consequences, such as an electric foot shock. These findings suggest that addiction is a disease that does not respect species boundaries.

THE DOPAMINE HYPOTHESIS OF ADDICTION

In the earliest version of the hypothesis described in this chapter, mesolimbic dopamine was believed to be the neurochemical correlate of pleasure and reward. However, during the past decade, experimental evidence has led to several revisions. Phasic dopamine release may actually code for the *prediction error* of reward rather than the reward itself. This distinction is based on pioneering observations in monkeys that dopamine neurons in the VTA are most efficiently activated by a reward (eg, a few drops of fruit juice) that is not anticipated. When the animal learns to predict the occurrence of a reward (eg, by pairing it with a stimulus such as a sound), dopamine neurons stop responding to the reward itself (juice), but increase their firing rate when the conditioned stimulus (sound) occurs. Finally, if reward is predicted but not delivered (sound but no juice), dopamine neurons are inhibited below their baseline activity and become completely silent. In other words, the mesolimbic system continuously scans the reward situation. It increases its activity when reward is larger than expected, and shuts down in the opposite case, thus coding for the prediction error of reward.

Under physiologic conditions the mesolimbic dopamine signal could represent a learning signal responsible for reinforcing constructive behavioral adaptation (eg, learning to press a lever for food). Addictive drugs, by directly increasing dopamine, would generate a strong but inappropriate learning signal, thus hijacking the reward system and leading to pathologic reinforcement, further drug consumption, and addiction.

This appealing hypothesis has been challenged based on the observation that some reward and drug-related learning is still possible in the absence of dopamine. Another intriguing observation is that mice genetically modified to lack the primary molecular target of cocaine, the dopamine transporter DAT, still self-administer the drug. Only when transporters of other biogenic amines are also knocked out does cocaine completely lose its rewarding properties. However, in DAT$^{-/-}$ mice, in which basal synaptic dopamine levels are high, cocaine still leads to increased dopamine release, presumably because other cocaine-sensitive amine transporters are able to clear some dopamine. When cocaine is given, these transporters (NET, SERT) are also inhibited and dopamine is again increased. This concept is supported by newer evidence showing that deletion of the cocaine binding site on DAT leaves basal dopamine levels unchanged but abolishes the rewarding effect of cocaine.

The dopamine hypothesis of addiction has also been challenged by the observation that salient stimuli that are not rewarding (they may actually even be aversive and therefore negative reinforcers) also activate the VTA. However, the neurons in the VTA that are activated by aversive stimuli do not release dopamine, and dopamine neurons are actually inhibited by aversive stimuli. These findings suggest that the controversy can be resolved in favor of dopamine reward theories.

Whatever the precise role of dopamine under physiologic conditions, all addictive drugs strongly increase its concentration in target structures of the mesolimbic projection. This suggests that high levels of dopamine may actually be at the origin of the adaptive changes that underlie dependence and addiction.

Since each addictive drug has a specific molecular target that engages distinct cellular mechanisms to activate the mesolimbic system, three classes can be distinguished: A first group binds to G_{io}-coupled receptors, a second group interacts with ionotropic receptors or ion channels, and a third group targets monoamine transporters (Table 32–1). G protein-coupled receptors (GPCRs) that are of the G_{io} family inhibit neurons through postsynaptic hyperpolarization and presynaptic regulation of transmitter release. In the VTA, the action of these drugs is preferentially on the γ-aminobutyric acid (GABA) neurons that act as local inhibitory interneurons. Addictive drugs that bind to ionotropic receptors and ion channels can have combined effects on dopamine neurons and GABA neurons, eventually leading to enhanced release of dopamine. Finally, addictive drugs that interfere with monoamine transporters block reuptake of or stimulate nonvesicular release of dopamine, causing an accumulation of extracellular dopamine in target structures. While drugs of this class also affect transporters of other monoamines (norepinephrine, serotonin), it is the action on the dopamine system that remains central for addiction. This is consistent with the observations that antidepressants that block serotonin and norepinephrine uptake, but not dopamine uptake, do not cause addiction even after prolonged use.

DEPENDENCE: TOLERANCE & WITHDRAWAL

With chronic exposure to addictive drugs, the brain shows signs of adaptation. For example, if morphine is used at short intervals, the dose has to be progressively increased over the course of several days to maintain rewarding or analgesic effects. This phenomenon is

Table 32–1. The mechanistic classification of drugs of abuse.[1]

Name	Main Molecular Target	Pharmacology	Effect on Dopamine (DA) Neurons	RR[2]
Drugs That Activate G Protein-Coupled Receptors				
Opioids	μ-OR (G_{io})	Agonist	Disinhibition	4
Cannabinoids	CB1R (G_{io})	Agonist	Disinhibition	2
γ-Hydroxybutyric acid (GHB)	$GABA_BR$ (G_{io})	Weak agonist	Disinhibition	?
LSD, mescaline, psilocybin	$5\text{-}HT_{2A}R$ (G_q)	Partial agonist	—	1
Drugs That Bind to Ionotropic Receptors and Ion Channels				
Nicotine	nAChR ($\alpha_2\beta_2$)	Agonist	Excitation, disinhibition (?)	4
Alcohol	$GABA_AR$, $5\text{-}HT_3R$, nAChR, NMDAR, Kir3 channels		Excitation, disinhibition (?)	3
Benzodiazepines	$GABA_AR$	Positive modulator	Disinhibition	3
Phencyclidine, ketamine	NMDAR	Antagonist	—	1
Drugs That Bind to Transporters of Biogenic Amines				
Cocaine	DAT, SERT, NET	Inhibitor	Blocks DA uptake	5
Amphetamine	DAT, NET, SERT, VMAT	Reverses transport	Blocks DA uptake, synaptic depletion	5
Ecstasy	SERT > DAT, NET	Reverses transport	Blocks DA uptake, synaptic depletion	?

5-HTxR, serotonin receptor; CB1R, cannabinoid-1; DAT, dopamine transporter; GABA, γ-aminobutyric acid; Kir3 channels, G protein-coupled inwardly rectifying potassium channels; LSD, lysergic acid diethylamide; μ-OR, μ-opioid receptor; nAChR, nicotinic acetylcholine receptor; NET, norepinephrine transporter; NMDAR, N-methyl-D-aspartate receptor; SERT, serotonin transporter; VMAT, vesicular monoamine transporter; ? indicates data not available.
[1]Drugs fall into one of three categories, targeting either G protein-coupled receptors, ionotropic receptors or ion channels, or biogenic amine transporters.
[2]RR, relative risk of addiction; 1 = nonaddictive; 5 = highly addictive.

called tolerance. It may become a serious problem because of increasing side-effects—eg, respiratory depression—that do not show much tolerance and may lead to fatalities associated with overdose.

Tolerance to opioids may be due to a reduction of the concentration of a drug or a shorter duration of action in a target system (pharmacokinetic tolerance). Alternatively, it may involve changes of μ opioid receptor function (pharmacodynamic tolerance). In fact, many μ opioid receptor agonists promote strong receptor phosphorylation that triggers the recruitment of the adaptor protein β-arrestin, causing G proteins to uncouple from the receptor and to internalize within minutes. Since this decreases signaling, it is tempting to explain tolerance by such a mechanism. However, morphine, which strongly induces tolerance, does not recruit β-arrestins and fails to promote receptor internalization. Conversely, other agonists that drive receptor internalization very efficiently induce only modest tolerance. Based on these observations it has been

hypothesized that desensitization and receptor internalization actually protect the cell from overstimulation. In this model, morphine, by failing to trigger receptor endocytosis, disproportionally stimulates adaptive processes, which eventually cause tolerance. Although the molecular identity of these processes is still under investigation, they may be similar to the ones involved in withdrawal (see below).

Adaptive changes become fully apparent once drug exposure is terminated. This state is called **withdrawal** and is observed to varying degrees following chronic exposure to most drugs of abuse. Withdrawal from opioids in humans is particularly strong and is described below. Studies in rodents have added significantly to our understanding of the neural and molecular mechanisms that underlie dependence. For example, dependence, as well as analgesia and reward, are abolished in knockout mice lacking the μ opioid receptor, but not in mice lacking other opioid receptors (δ, κ). While activation of the μ opioid receptor

Figure 32–2. CREB-mediated up-regulation of dynorphin during withdrawal from dependence. Supersensitization of adenylyl cyclase (AC) leads to an increase of cAMP concentration in medium spiny neurons of the accumbens. This activates the transcription factor CREB, which turns on several genes, including that for dynorphin. Dynorphin is then co-released with γ-aminobutyric acid (GABA), activating the κ-opioid receptor (KOR) located on dopamine neurons of the ventral tegmental area (VTA), and thereby leading to pre- and postsynaptic inhibition. (D_2R, dopamine D_2 receptor.)

initially strongly inhibits adenylyl cyclase, this inhibition becomes weaker after several days of repeated exposure. The waning of the inhibition of adenylyl cyclase is due to a counter adaptation of the enzyme system during exposure to the drug, which results in overproduction of cAMP during subsequent withdrawal. Several mechanisms exist for this adenylyl cyclase compensatory response, including up-regulation of transcription of the enzyme. Increased cAMP concentrations in turn strongly activate the transcription factor CREB, leading to the regulation of downstream genes. Of the few such genes identified to date, one of the most interesting is the gene for the endogenous κ opioid ligand dynorphin. During withdrawal, neurons of the nucleus accumbens produce high levels of dynorphin, which is then co-released with GABA onto the projection neurons of the VTA (Figure 32–2). These cells express κ opioid receptors on their synaptic terminals and on the dendrites. As a consequence, they are inhibited and dopamine release is reduced. This mechanism exemplifies the adaptive processes

engaged during dependence, and may underlie the intense dysphoria typically observed during withdrawal.

ADDICTION: A DISEASE OF MALADAPTIVE LEARNING

Addiction is characterized by a high motivation to obtain and use a drug despite negative consequences. With time, drug use becomes compulsive ("wanting without liking"). Addiction is a recalcitrant, chronic, and stubbornly relapsing disease that is very difficult to treat.

The central problem is that even after successful withdrawal and prolonged drug-free periods, addicted individuals are at high risk of relapsing. Relapse is typically triggered by one of the following three conditions: reexposure to the drug of abuse, stress, or a context that recalls prior drug use. It appears that when paired with drug use, a neutral stimulus may undergo a switch and motivate ("trigger") addiction-related behavior. This phenomenon may involve synaptic plasticity in the target nuclei of the mesolimbic projection (eg, nucleus accumbens). For example, cravings may recur at the presentation of contextual cues (eg, people, places, or drug paraphernalia), suggesting the involvement of learning and memory systems. If dopamine release codes for the prediction error of reward (see Box: The Dopamine Hypothesis of Addiction), the stimulation of the mesolimbic dopamine systems will generate an unusually strong learning signal. Unlike natural rewards, addictive drugs continue to increase dopamine even when reward is expected. Such overriding of the prediction error signal may eventually be responsible for the "usurping of memory processes" by addictive drugs. The involvement of learning and memory systems in addiction is also suggested by clinical studies. For example, the role of context in relapse is supported by the report that soldiers who became addicted to heroin during the Vietnam War had significantly better outcomes when treated after their return home, compared with addicts who remained in the environment where they had taken the drug. Current research therefore focuses on the effects of drugs on associative forms of synaptic plasticity, such as long-term potentiation (LTP), that underlie learning and memory (see Box: Synaptic Plasticity & Addiction).

Large individual differences exist in vulnerability to addiction. Whereas one person may become "hooked" after a few doses, others may be able to use a drug occasionally during their entire lives without ever having difficulty in stopping. Even when dependence is induced with chronic exposure, only a fraction of dependent users will go on to become addicted. The transition to addiction is determined by a combination of environmental and genetic factors. Heritability of addiction, as determined by comparing monozygotic with dizygotic twins, is relatively modest for cannabinoids but very

high for cocaine. It is of interest that the relative risk for addiction (addiction liability) of a drug (Table 32–1) correlates with its heritability, suggesting that the neurobiologic basis of addiction common to all drugs is what is being inherited. Further genomic analysis indicates that only a few alleles (or perhaps even a single recessive allele) need to function in combination to produce the phenotype. However, identification of the genes involved remains elusive. While some substance-specific candidate genes have been identified (eg, alcohol dehydrogenase), future research will also focus on genes implicated in the neurobiologic mechanisms common to all addictive drugs.

NONADDICTIVE DRUGS OF ABUSE

Some drugs of abuse do not lead to addiction. This is the case for substances that alter perception without causing sensations of reward and euphoria, such as the hallucinogens and the dissociative anesthetics (Table 32–1). These agents primarily target cortical and thalamic circuits unlike addictive drugs, which primarily target the mesolimbic dopamine system (see above). Lysergic acid diethylamide (LSD), for example, activates the serotonin 5-HT$_{2A}$ receptor in the prefrontal cortex, enhancing glutamatergic transmission onto pyramidal neurons. These excitatory afferents mainly come from the thalamus and carry sensory information of different modalities, which may constitute a link to enhanced perception. Phencyclidine (PCP) and ketamine produce a feeling of separation of mind and body (which is why they are called dissociative anesthetics) and, at higher doses, stupor and coma. The principal mechanism of action is a use-dependent inhibition of glutamate receptors of the NMDA type.

SYNAPTIC PLASTICITY & ADDICTION

Long-term potentiation (LTP) is a form of experience-dependent synaptic plasticity that is induced by activating glutamate receptors of the N-methyl-D-aspartate (NMDA) type. Since NMDA receptors are blocked by magnesium at negative potentials, their activation requires the concomitant release of glutamate (presynaptic activity) onto a receiving neuron that is depolarized (postsynaptic activity). Correlated pre- and postsynaptic activity durably enhances synaptic efficacy and triggers the formation of new connections. Because associativity is a critical component, LTP has become a leading candidate mechanism underlying learning and memory. LTP can be elicited at glutamatergic synapses of the mesolimbic reward system and is modulated by dopamine. Drugs of abuse could therefore interfere with LTP at sites of convergence of dopamine and glutamate projections (eg, nucleus accumbens or prefrontal cortex). Interestingly, exposure to an addictive drug triggers LTP at excitatory afferents and reduces GABA$_A$ receptor-mediated inhibition of the VTA, thus increasing the excitability of dopamine neurons. Genetic manipulations in mice that abolish LTP at this synapse also have effects on behavioral paradigms that model core components of addiction such as conditioned place preference, further supporting the idea that LTP is involved in context-dependent components of relapse. Similarly, interfering with transcriptional signaling implicated in the late phases of LTP affects conditioned place preference.

The classification of NMDA antagonists as nonaddictive drugs was based on early assessments, which, in the case of PCP, have recently been questioned. In fact, animal research shows that PCP can increase mesolimbic dopamine concentrations and has some reinforcing properties in rodents. Concurrent effects on both thalamocortical and mesolimbic systems also exist for other addictive drugs. Psychosis-like symptoms can be observed with cannabinoids, amphetamines, and cocaine, which may reflect their effects on thalamocortical structures. For example, cannabinoids, in addition to their documented effects on the mesolimbic dopamine system, also enhance excitation in cortical circuits through presynaptic inhibition of GABA release.

Hallucinogens and NMDA antagonists, even if they do not produce dependence or addiction, can still have long-term effects. Flashbacks of altered perception can occur years after LSD consumption. Moreover, chronic use of PCP may lead to an irreversible schizophrenia-like psychosis.

■ II. BASIC PHARMACOLOGY OF DRUGS OF ABUSE

Since all addictive drugs increase dopamine concentrations in target structures of the mesolimbic projections, we classify them on the basis of their molecular targets and the underlying mechanisms (Table 32–1). The first group contains the opioids, cannabinoids, γ-hydroxybutyric acid (GHB), and the hallucinogens, which all exert their action through G_{io} protein-coupled receptors. The second group includes nicotine, alcohol, the benzodiazepines, dissociative anesthetics, and some inhalants, which interact with ionotropic receptors or ion channels. The last group comprises cocaine, amphetamines, and ecstasy, which all bind to monoamine transporters. The nonaddictive drugs are classified using the same criteria.

DRUGS THAT ACTIVATE G_{io}-COUPLED RECEPTORS

OPIOIDS

Pharmacology & Clinical Aspects

As described in Chapter 31, the opioids comprise a large family of endogenous and exogenous agonists at three G protein-coupled receptors: the μ, κ, and δ opioid receptors. Although all three receptors couple to inhibitory G proteins (ie, they all inhibit adenylyl cyclase), they have distinct, sometimes even opposing

effects, mainly because of the cell type-specific expression throughout the brain. In the VTA, for example, μ opioid receptors are selectively expressed on GABA neurons (which they inhibit), while κ opioid receptors are expressed on and inhibit dopamine neurons. This may explain why μ opioid agonists cause euphoria while κ agonists induce dysphoria (see also Figure 32–3). In line with these observations, the rewarding effects of morphine are absent in knockout mice lacking μ receptors but persist when either of the other opioid receptors are ablated. In the VTA, μ opioids cause an inhibition of GABAergic inhibitory interneurons that leads eventually to a disinhibition of dopamine neurons (Figure 32–3).

The most commonly abused μ opioids include morphine, heroin (diacetylmorphine, which is rapidly metabolized to morphine), codeine, and oxycodone. Meperidine abuse is common among health professionals. All of these drugs induce strong tolerance and dependence. The withdrawal syndrome may be very severe (except for codeine) and includes intense dysphoria, nausea or vomiting, muscle aches, lacrimation, rhinorrhea, mydriasis, piloerection, sweating, diarrhea, yawning, and fever. Beyond the withdrawal syndrome, which usually lasts no longer than a few days, individuals who have received opioids as analgesics will only rarely develop addiction. In contrast, when taken for recreational purposes, opioids are highly addictive. The relative risk of addiction is 4 out of 5 on a widely used scale (Table 32–1).

Treatment

The opioid antagonist naloxone reverses the effects of a dose of morphine or heroin within minutes. This may be life-saving in the case of a massive overdose (see Chapters 31 and 59). Naloxone administration also provokes an acute withdrawal (precipitated abstinence) syndrome in a dependent person who has recently taken an opioid.

In the treatment of opioid addiction, a long-acting opioid (eg, methadone) is often substituted for the shorter-acting, more rewarding, opioid (eg, heroin). For substitution therapy, methadone is given orally once daily, facilitating supervised intake. The much longer half-life of methadone may also have some beneficial effects (eg, weaker drug sensitization, which typically requires intermittent exposures), but it is important to realize that abrupt termination of methadone administration invariably precipitates a withdrawal syndrome; that is, the subject on substitution therapy remains dependent. Some countries (eg, Switzerland, Netherlands) even allow substitution of heroin by heroin. A follow-up of a cohort of addicts who receive heroin injections in a controlled setting and have access to counseling indicates that addicts under heroin-substitution have an improved health status and are better integrated in society.

Figure 32–3. Disinhibition of dopamine (DA) neurons in the ventral tegmental area (VTA) through drugs that act via G_{io}-coupled receptors. ***Top:*** Opioids target μ opioid receptors (MORs) that in the VTA are located exclusively on γ-aminobutyric acid (GABA) neurons. MORs are expressed on the presynaptic terminal of these cells and the somatodendritic compartment of the postsynaptic cells. Each compartment has distinct effectors (*insets*). G protein-βγ-mediated inhibition of voltage-gated calcium channels (VGCC) is the major mechanism in the presynaptic terminal. Conversely, in dendrites MORs activate K channels. ***Middle:*** Δ⁹-tetrahydrocannabinol (THC) and other cannabinoids mainly act through presynaptic inhibition. ***Bottom:*** Gamma-hydroxybutyric acid (GHB) targets GABA$_B$ receptors, which are located on both cell types. However, GABA neurons are more sensitive to GHB than are DA neurons, leading to disinhibition at concentrations typically obtained with recreational use. (CB1R, cannabinoid receptors.)

CANNABINOIDS

Endogenous cannabinoids that act as neurotransmitters include 2-arachidonyl glycerol (2-AG) and anandamide, both of which bind to CB1 receptors. These very lipid-soluble compounds are released at the postsynaptic somatodendritic membrane, and diffuse through the extracellular space to bind at presynaptic CB1 receptors where they inhibit the release of either glutamate or GABA (Figure 32–3). Because of such backward signaling, endocannabinoids are called retrograde messengers. In the hippocampus, release of endocannabinoids from pyramidal neurons selectively affects inhibitory transmission and may contribute to the induction of synaptic plasticity during learning and memory formation.

Exogenous cannabinoids, eg in marijuana, comprise several pharmacologically active substances including Δ^9-tetrahydrocannabinol (THC), a powerful psychoactive substance. Like opioids, THC causes disinhibition of dopamine neurons, mainly by presynaptic inhibition of GABA neurons in the VTA. The half-life of THC is about 4 hours. The onset of effects of THC after smoking marijuana occurs within minutes and reaches a maximum after 1–2 hours. The most prominent effects are euphoria and relaxation. Users also report feelings of well-being, grandiosity, and altered perception of passage of time. Dose-dependent perceptual changes (eg, visual distortions), drowsiness, diminished coordination, and memory impairment may occur. Cannabinoids can also create a dysphoric state and in rare cases, following the use of very high doses, may result in visual hallucinations, depersonalization, and frank psychotic episodes. Additional effects of THC, eg, increased appetite, attenuation of nausea, decreased intraocular pressure, and relief of chronic pain, have led to the use of cannabinoids in medical therapeutics. The justification of medicinal use of marijuana was comprehensively examined by the Institute of Medicine (IOM) of the National Academy of Sciences in its 1999 report, *Marijuana & Medicine.* This continues to be a controversial issue, mainly because of the fear that cannabinoids may serve as a gateway to the consumption of "hard" drugs. Chronic exposure to marijuana leads to dependence, which is revealed by a distinctive, but mild and short-lived, withdrawal syndrome that includes restlessness, irritability, mild agitation, insomnia, nausea, and cramping. The relative risk for addiction is 2 (Table 32–1).

The synthetic Δ^9-THC analog **dronabinol** is the only Food and Drug Administration-approved cannabinoid agonist currently marketed in the USA and some European countries. **Nabilone,** an older commercial Δ^9-THC analog, may be reintroduced in the USA in the near future. The cannabinoid system is likely to emerge as an important drug target in the future because of its apparent involvement in several therapeutically desirable effects.

GAMMA-HYDROXYBUTYRIC ACID (GHB)

Gamma-hydroxybutyric acid is produced endogenously during the metabolism of GABA, but the function of this endogenous agent is unknown at present. The pharmacology of GHB is complex because there are two distinct binding sites. The protein that contains a high-affinity binding site (1 μM) for GHB has recently been cloned, but its involvement in the cellular effects of GHB at pharmacologic concentrations remains unclear. The low-affinity binding site (1 mM) has been identified as the $GABA_B$ receptor (Figure 32–3). In mice that lack $GABA_B$ receptors even very high doses of GHB have no effect, suggesting that $GABA_B$ receptors are the sole mediators of GHB's pharmacologic action.

Gamma-hydroxybutyric acid was first synthesized in 1960 and introduced as a general anesthetic. Because of its narrow safety margin and its addictive potential it is not available in the USA for this purpose at present. Before causing sedation and coma, GHB causes euphoria, enhanced sensory perceptions, a feeling of social closeness, and amnesia. These properties have made it a popular "club drug" that goes by colorful street names such as "liquid ecstasy," "grievous bodily harm," or "date rape drug." As the latter name suggests, GHB has been used in date rapes, because it is odorless and can be readily dissolved in beverages. It is rapidly absorbed after ingestion and reaches a maximal plasma concentration 20–30 minutes following ingestion of a 10–20 mg/kg dose. The elimination half-life is about 30 minutes.

Although $GABA_B$ receptors are expressed on all neurons of the VTA, GABA neurons are much more sensitive to GHB than dopamine neurons (the EC_{50} differs by about one order of magnitude). Because GHB is a weak agonist, only GABA neurons are inhibited at the concentrations typically obtained with recreational use. This feature may underlie the reinforcing effects of GHB and the basis for addiction to the drug. At higher doses, however, GHB also hyperpolarizes dopamine neurons, eventually completely inhibiting dopamine release. Such an inhibition of the VTA may in turn preclude its activation by other addictive drugs and may explain why GHB might have some utility as an "anticraving" compound.

LSD, MESCALINE, & PSILOCYBIN

These three drugs are commonly called hallucinogens because of their ability to alter consciousness such that the individual senses things that are not present. They induce, often in an unpredictable way, perceptual symptoms, including shape and color distortion. Psychosis-like manifestations (depersonalization, hallucinations, distorted time perception) have led some to classify these drugs as psychotomimetics. They also produce somatic symptoms (dizziness, nausea, paresthesias, and blurred vision). Some users have reported intense reexperiencing of perceptual effects (flashbacks) up to several years after the last drug exposure.

Hallucinogens differ from most other drugs described in this chapter in that they induce neither dependence nor addiction. However repetitive exposure still leads to rapid tolerance (also called tachyphylaxis). Animals will not self-administer hallucinogens, suggesting that they are not rewarding. Additional studies show that these drugs also fail to stimulate dopamine release, further supporting the idea that only drugs that activate the mesolimbic dopamine system are addictive. Instead, hallucinogens increase glutamate release in the cortex, presumably by enhancing excitatory afferent input from the thalamus.

The molecular target of hallucinogens is the 5-HT_{2A} receptor. This receptor couples to G proteins of the G_q type and generates inositol trisphosphate (IP_3), leading to a release of intracellular calcium. Although hallucinogens, and LSD in particular, have been proposed for several therapeutic indications, efficacy has never been demonstrated.

DRUGS THAT MEDIATE THEIR EFFECTS VIA IONOTROPIC RECEPTORS

NICOTINE

Pharmacology

In terms of numbers affected, addiction to nicotine exceeds all other forms of addiction, touching more than 50% of all adults in some countries. Nicotine exposure occurs primarily through smoking of tobacco, which causes associated diseases that are responsible for many preventable deaths. The chronic use of chewing tobacco and snuff tobacco is also addicting.

Nicotine is a selective agonist of the nicotinic acetylcholine receptor (nAChR) that is normally activated by acetylcholine (see Chapter 6). Based on nicotine's enhancement of cognitive performance and the association of Alzheimer's dementia with a loss of ACh-releasing neurons from the nucleus basalis of Meynert, nAChRs are believed to play an important role in many cognitive processes. The rewarding effect of nicotine requires involvement of the VTA, where nAChRs are expressed on dopamine neurons. When nicotine excites projection neurons, dopamine is released in the nucleus accumbens and the prefrontal cortex, thus fulfilling the dopamine requirement of addictive drugs. Recent work has identified $\alpha_4\beta_2$-containing channels in the VTA as the nAChRs that are required for the rewarding effects of nicotine. This statement is based on the observation that knockout mice deficient for the β_2 subunit lose interest in self-administering nicotine, and that in these mice, this behavior can be restored through an in-vivo transfection of the β_2 subunit

in neurons of the VTA. Electrophysiologic evidence suggests that homomeric nAChRs made exclusively of α_7 subunits also contribute to the reinforcing effects of nicotine. These receptors are mainly expressed on synaptic terminals of excitatory afferents projecting onto the dopamine neurons. They also contribute to nicotine-evoked dopamine release and the long-term changes induced by the drugs related to addiction (eg, long-term synaptic potentiation of excitatory inputs).

Nicotine withdrawal is mild compared with opioid withdrawal, and involves irritability and sleeplessness. However, nicotine is among the most addictive drugs (relative risk = 4, Table 32–1), and relapse after attempted cessation is very common.

Treatment

Treatment for nicotine addiction includes substituting nicotine that is chewed, inhaled, or transdermally delivered for the nicotine in cigarettes, thus slowing the pharmacokinetics and eliminating the many complications associated with the toxic substances found in tobacco smoke. At present, all available agents seem to be similarly effective in relieving craving, controlling the habit, and facilitating quitting. In addition, the antidepressant bupropion has been approved for nicotine cessation therapy. It is most effective when combined with behavioral therapies. Many countries have banned smoking in public places to create smoke-free environments. This important step not only reduces passive smoking and the hazards of secondhand smoke, but also the risk that ex-smokers will be exposed to smoke, which as a contextual cue, may trigger relapse.

BENZODIAZEPINES

Benzodiazepines are commonly prescribed as anxiolytics and sleep medications. They represent a moderate risk for abuse, which has to be weighed against their beneficial effects. Benzodiazepines are abused by some persons for their euphoriant effects, but most often abuse occurs concomitant with other drugs, eg, to attenuate anxiety during withdrawal from opioids.

Barbiturates, which preceded benzodiazepines as the most commonly abused sedative hypnotics (after ethanol), are now rarely prescribed to outpatients and therefore constitute a less common prescription drug problem than they did in the past. Street sales of barbiturates, however, continue. Management of barbiturate withdrawal and addiction is similar to that of benzodiazepines.

While benzodiazepine dependence is very common, cases that fulfill all the diagnostic criteria for addiction are rare. Withdrawal from benzodiazepines occurs within days of stopping the medication, and varies as a function of the half-life of elimination. Symptoms include irritability, insomnia, phono- and photophobia, depression, muscle cramps, and even seizures. Typically these symptoms taper off within 1–2 weeks.

Benzodiazepines are positive modulators of the $GABA_A$ receptor, increasing both single channel conductance and open-channel probability. $GABA_A$ receptors are pentameric structures consisting of α, β, and γ subunits (see Chapter 22). GABA receptors on dopamine neurons of the VTA lack α_1, a subunit that is typically present in GABA neurons. In addition, $GABA_A$ receptors are expressed in much higher density on interneurons, so that a disinhibition of the mesolimbic dopamine system may explain the rewarding effects of benzodiazepines. Receptors containing α_5 seem to be required for tolerance to the sedative effects of benzodiazepines, and studies in humans link $\alpha_2\gamma_3$-containing receptors to alcohol dependence (the $GABA_A$ receptor is also a target of alcohol, see below). Taken together, a picture is emerging linking $GABA_A$ receptors of specific subunit composition to their therapeutic effects and to dependence and addiction induced with chronic exposure.

ALCOHOL

Alcohol (ethanol, see Chapter 23) is regularly used by a majority of the population in many Western countries. Although only a minority becomes dependent and addicted, abuse is a very serious public health problem, because of the many diseases associated with alcoholism.

Pharmacology

The pharmacology of alcohol is complex and no single receptor mediates all of its effects. On the contrary, alcohol alters the function of several receptors and cellular functions, including $GABA_A$ receptors, Kir3/GIRK channels, adenosine reuptake (through the equilibrative nucleoside transporter, ENT1), glycine receptor, NMDA receptor, and $5-HT_3$ receptor. They are all, with the exception of ENT1, either ionotropic receptors or ion channels. It is not clear which of these targets is responsible for the increase of dopamine release from the mesolimbic reward system. The inhibition of ENT1 is probably not responsible for the rewarding effects (ENT1 knockout mice drink more than controls) but seems to be involved in alcohol dependence through an accumulation of adenosine, stimulation of adenosine A_2 receptors, and ensuing enhanced CREB signaling.

Dependence becomes apparent 6–12 hours after cessation of heavy drinking as a withdrawal syndrome that may include tremor (mainly of the hands), nausea and vomiting, excessive sweating, agitation, and anxiety. In some individuals this is followed by visual, tactile, and auditory hallucinations 12–24 hours after cessation. Generalized seizures may manifest after 24–48 hours. Finally, 48–72 hours after cessation, an alcohol withdrawal delirium (delirium tremens) may become apparent in which the person hallucinates, is disoriented, and shows evidence of autonomic instability. Delirium tremens is associated with 5–15% mortality.

Treatment

Treatment of ethanol withdrawal is supportive and relies on benzodiazepines, taking care to use compounds such as oxazepam and lorazepam, which are not as dependent on hepatic metabolism as most other benzodiazepines. In cases where monitoring is not reliable and liver function is adequate, a longer acting benzodiazepine such as chlordiazepoxide is preferred.

As in the treatment of all chronic drug abuse problems, heavy reliance is placed on psychosocial approaches to alcohol addiction. This is perhaps even more important for the alcoholic patient because of the ubiquitous presence of alcohol in many social contexts.

The pharmacologic treatment of alcohol addiction is limited although several compounds, with different goals, have been used. Disulfiram has been used as an adjunct to create aversion to drinking. Disulfiram inhibits acetaldehyde dehydrogenase, causing nausea, vomiting, and dysphoria with coincident alcohol use. Recently the efficacy of disulfiram has been questioned, and no large trials are available that conclusively demonstrate increased abstinence.

Naltrexone is an antagonist and partial agonist of the μ opioid receptor, which may decrease the craving for alcohol, resulting in fewer relapses. Although most, but not all, studies found that naltrexone decreases relapses, the effect is modest. Combining naltrexone therapy with cognitive behavioral therapy may enhance benefit.

The antiepileptic compound topiramate facilitates GABA function and antagonizes glutamate receptors (presumably the AMPA type), and may decrease mesocorticolimbic dopamine release after alcohol and reduce cravings. However, topiramate does not have FDA approval for this indication.

In Europe several trials have been carried out with acamprosate, an NMDA receptor antagonist. However, most patients returned to drinking while still using the drug. A direct comparison with naltrexone showed acamprosate to be less effective.

KETAMINE & PHENCYCLIDINE (PCP)

Ketamine and PCP were developed as general anesthetics (see Chapter 25), but only ketamine is still used for this application. Both drugs, along with others, are now classified as "club drugs" and sold under names such as "angel dust," "Hog," and "Special K." They owe their effects to their use-dependent, noncompetitive antagonism of the NMDA receptor. The effects of these substances became apparent when patients undergoing surgery reported unpleasant vivid dreams and hallucinations after anesthesia. Ketamine and PCP are white crystalline powders in their pure forms, but on the street they are also sold as a liquids, capsules, or pills, which can be snorted, ingested, injected, or smoked. Psychedelic effects last for about 1 hour and also include increased blood pressure, impaired memory function, and visual alterations. At high doses unpleasant out-of-body and near-death experiences have been reported. Although ketamine and phencyclidine do not cause dependence and addiction (relative risk = 1, Table 32–1), chronic exposure, particularly to PCP, may lead to long-lasting psychosis closely resembling schizophrenia, which may persist beyond drug exposure.

INHALANTS

Inhalant abuse is defined as recreational exposure to chemical vapors, such as nitrates, ketones, and aliphatic and aromatic hydrocarbons. These substances are present in a variety of household and industrial products that are inhaled by "sniffing," "huffing," or "bagging." Sniffing refers to inhalation from an open container, huffing to the soaking of a cloth in the volatile substance before inhalation, and bagging to breathing in and out of a paper or plastic bag filled with fumes. It is common for novices to start with sniffing and progress to huffing and bagging as addiction develops. Inhalant abuse is particularly prevalent in children and young adults.

The exact mechanism of action of most volatile substances remains unknown. Altered function of ionotropic receptors and ion channels throughout the central nervous system has been demonstrated for a few. Nitrous oxide, for example, binds to NMDA receptors and fuel additives enhance $GABA_A$ receptor function. Most inhalants produce euphoria; increased excitability of the VTA has been documented for toluene and may underlie its addiction risk. Other substances, such as amyl nitrite ("poppers"), primarily produce smooth muscle relaxation and enhance erection, but are not addictive. With chronic exposure to the aromatic hydrocarbons (eg, benzene, toluene) toxic effects can be observed in many organs, including white matter lesions in the central nervous system. Management of overdose remains supportive.

DRUGS THAT BIND TO TRANSPORTERS OF BIOGENIC AMINES

COCAINE

The prevalence of cocaine abuse has increased greatly over the past decade and now represents a major public health problem worldwide. Cocaine is highly addictive (relative risk = 5, Table 32–1), and its use is associated with a number of complications.

Cocaine is an alkaloid found in the leaves of *Erythroxylon coca*, a shrub indigenous to the Andes. For more than 100 years, it has been extracted and used in clinical medicine, mainly as a local anesthetic and to dilate pupils in ophthalmology. Sigmund Freud famously proposed its use to treat depression and alcohol dependence, but addiction quickly brought an end to this idea.

Cocaine hydrochloride is a water-soluble salt that can be injected or absorbed by any mucosal membrane (eg, nasal snorting). When heated in an alkaline solution it is transformed into the free base, "crack cocaine," which can then be smoked. Inhaled crack cocaine is rapidly absorbed in the lungs and penetrates swiftly into the brain, producing an almost instantaneous "rush."

In the peripheral nervous system, cocaine inhibits voltage-gated sodium channels, thus blocking initiation and conduction of action potentials (see Chapter 26). This effect, however, seems responsible for neither the acute rewarding nor the addictive effects. In the central nervous system, cocaine blocks the uptake of dopamine, noradrenaline, and serotonin through their respective transporters. The block of the dopamine transporter (DAT), by increasing dopamine concentrations in the nucleus accumbens, has been implicated in the rewarding effects of cocaine (Figure 32–4). In fact, rewarding effects of cocaine are abolished in mice with a cocaine-insensitive DAT. The activation of the sympathetic nervous system results mainly from the block of the norepinephrine transporter (NET) and leads to an acute increase in arterial pressure, tachycardia, and often, ventricular arrhythmias. Subjects typically lose appetite, are hyperactive, and sleep little. Cocaine exposure increases the risk for intracranial hemorrhage, ischemic stroke, myocardial infarction, and generalized or partial seizures. Cocaine overdose may lead to hyperthermia, coma, and death.

Susceptible individuals may become dependent and addicted after only a few exposures to cocaine. Although a withdrawal syndrome is reported, it is not as strong as the one observed with opioids. Tolerance may develop, but in some users a reverse tolerance is observed; that is, they become sensitized to small doses of cocaine. This behavioral sensitization is in part context-dependent. Cravings are very strong and underline the very high addiction liability of cocaine. To date, no specific antagonist is available and the management of intoxication remains supportive. Developing a pharmacologic treatment for cocaine addiction is a top priority.

AMPHETAMINES

Amphetamines are a group of synthetic, indirect-acting sympathomimetic drugs that cause the release of endogenous biogenic amines, such as dopamine and noradrenaline (see Chapters 6 and 9). Amphetamine, methamphet-

Figure 32–4. Mechanism of action of cocaine and amphetamine on synaptic terminal of dopamine (DA) neurons. **Left:** Cocaine inhibits the dopamine transporter (DAT), decreasing DA clearance from the synaptic cleft and causing an increase in extracellular DA concentration. **Right:** Since amphetamine (Amph) is a substrate of the DAT, it competitively inhibits DA transport. In addition, once in the cell, amphetamine interferes with the vesicular monoamine transporter (VMAT) and impedes the filling of synaptic vesicles. As a consequence, vesicles are depleted and cytoplasmic DA increases. This leads to a reversal of DAT direction, strongly increasing nonvesicular release of DA, and further increasing extracellular DA concentrations.

amine, and their many derivatives exert their effects by reversing the action of biogenic amine transporters at the plasma membrane. Amphetamines are substrates of these transporters and are taken up into the cell (Figure 32–4). Once in the cell, amphetamines interfere with the vesicular monoamine transporter (VMAT), depleting synaptic vesicles of their neurotransmitter content. As a consequence, levels of dopamine (or other transmitter amine) in the cytoplasm increase and quickly become sufficient to cause release into the synapse by reversal of the plasma membrane DAT. Normal vesicular release of dopamine consequently decreases (because synaptic vesicles contain less transmitter), while nonvesicular release increases. Similar mechanisms apply for other biogenic amines (serotonin and norepinephrine).

Together with GHB and ecstasy, amphetamines are often referred to as "club drugs," because they are increasingly popular in the club scene. They are often produced in small clandestine laboratories, which makes their precise chemical identification difficult. They differ from ecstasy chiefly in the context of use: intravenous administration and "hard core" addiction is far more common with amphetamines, especially methamphetamine. In general, amphetamines lead to elevated catecholamine levels that increase arousal and reduce sleep, while the effects on the dopamine system mediate euphoria but may also cause abnormal movements and precipitate psychotic episodes. Effects on

serotonin transmission may play a role in the hallucinogenic and anorexigenic functions as well as in the hyperthermia often caused by amphetamines.

Unlike many other abused drugs, amphetamines are neurotoxic. The exact mechanism is not known, but neurotoxicity depends on the NMDA receptor and affects mainly serotonin and dopamine neurons.

Amphetamines are typically taken initially in pill form by abusers, but can also be smoked or injected. Heavy users often progress rapidly to intravenous administration. Within hours after oral ingestion, amphetamines increase alertness, cause euphoria, agitation, and confusion. Bruxism (tooth grinding) and skin flushing may occur. Effects on heart rate may be minimal with some compounds (eg, methamphetamine), but with increasing dosage these agents often lead to tachycardia and dysrhythmias. Hypertensive crisis and vasoconstriction may lead to stroke. Spread of HIV and hepatitis infection in inner cities has been closely associated with needle sharing by intravenous users of methamphetamine.

With chronic use, tolerance may develop, leading to dose escalation. Withdrawal consists of dysphoria, drowsiness (in some cases, insomnia), and general irritability.

ECSTASY (MDMA)

Ecstasy is the name of a class of drugs that includes a large variety of derivatives of the amphetamine-related compound methylenedioxymethamphetamine (MDMA). MDMA was originally used in some forms of psychotherapy but no medically useful effects were documented. This is perhaps not surprising, because the main effect of ecstasy appears to be to foster feelings of intimacy and empathy without impairing intellectual capacities. Today, MDMA and its many derivatives are often produced in small quantities in ad hoc laboratories and distributed at parties or "raves" where it is taken orally. Ecstasy therefore is the prototypical designer drug and as such, increasingly popular.

Similar to the amphetamines, MDMA causes release of biogenic amines by reversing the action of their respective transporters. It has a preferential affinity for the serotonin transporter (SERT) and therefore most strongly increases the extracellular concentration of serotonin. This release is so profound that there is a marked intracellular depletion for 24 hours after a single dose. With repetitive administration, serotonin depletion may become permanent, which has triggered a debate on its neurotoxicity. Although direct proof from animal models for neurotoxicity remains weak, several studies report long-term cognitive impairment in heavy users of MDMA.

In contrast, there is a wide consensus that MDMA has several acute toxic effects, in particular hyperthermia, which along with dehydration (eg, caused by an all-night dance party) may be fatal. Other complications include serotonin syndrome (mental status change, autonomic hyperactivity, and neuromuscular abnormalities, see Chapter 16) and seizures. Following warnings about the dangers of MDMA, some users have attempted to compensate for hyperthermia by drinking excessive amounts of water, causing water intoxication involving severe hyponatremia, seizures, and even death.

Withdrawal is marked by a mood "offset" characterized by depression lasting up to several weeks. There have also been reports of increased aggression during periods of abstinence in chronic MDMA users.

Taken together, the evidence for irreversible damage to the brain, although not completely convincing, implies that even occasional recreational use of MDMA cannot be considered safe.

■ III. CLINICAL PHARMACOLOGY OF DEPENDENCE & ADDICTION

To date no single pharmacologic treatment (even in combination with behavioral interventions) efficiently eliminates addiction. This is not to say that addiction is irreversible. Pharmacologic interventions may in fact be useful at all stages of the disease. This is particularly true in the case of a massive overdose, in which reversal of drug action may be a life-saving measure. However, in this regard, FDA-approved antagonists are only available for opioids and benzodiazepines.

Pharmacologic interventions may also aim to alleviate the withdrawal syndrome, particularly after opioid exposure. On the assumption that withdrawal reflects at least in part a hyperactivity of central adrenergic systems, the α_2-adrenoceptor agonist clonidine (also used as a centrally active antihypertensive drug, see Chapter 11) has been used with some success to attenuate withdrawal. Today most clinicians prefer to manage opioid withdrawal by tapering very slowly the administration of long-acting opioids.

Another widely accepted treatment is substitution of a legally available agonist that acts at the same receptor as the abused drug. This approach has been approved for opioids and nicotine. For example, heroin addicts may receive methadone to replace heroin; smoking addicts may receive nicotine continuously via a transdermal patch system to replace smoking. In general, a rapidly acting substance is replaced with one that acts or is absorbed more slowly. Substitution treatments are largely justified by the benefits of reducing associated health risks, the reduction of drug-associated crime, and better social integration. While dependence persists, it may be possible, with the support of behavioral interventions, to motivate drug users to gradually reduce the dose and become abstinent.

The biggest challenge is the treatment of addiction itself. Several approaches have been taken, but all remain experimental. One approach is to pharmacologically reduce cravings. The μ opioid receptor antagonist and partial agonist naltrexone is FDA-approved for this indication in opioid and alcohol addiction. Its effect is modest and may involve a modulation of endogenous opioid systems.

Clinical trials are currently being conducted with a number of drugs, including the high-affinity $GABA_B$-receptor agonist baclofen, and initial results have shown a significant reduction of craving. This effect may be mediated by the inhibition of the dopamine neurons of the VTA, which is possible at baclofen concentrations obtained by oral administration because of its very high affinity for the $GABA_B$ receptor.

Rimonabant is a novel cannabinoid antagonist that should soon become available for the treatment of addiction. Initially developed for nicotine addiction, it may be useful in the treatment of abuse of cocaine, heroin, and alcohol. Although its cellular mechanism is unclear, data in rodents convincingly demonstrate that this compound can reduce self-administration in naïve as well as in drug-experienced animals.

REFERENCES

General

Goldman D, Oroszi G, Ducci F: The genetics of addictions: Uncovering the genes. Nat Rev Genet 2005;6:521.

Hyman SE: Addiction: A disease of learning and memory. Am J Psychiatry 2005;162:1414.

Kauer JA: Learning mechanisms in addiction: Synaptic plasticity in the ventral tegmental area as a result of exposure to drugs of abuse. Annu Rev Physiol 2004;66:447.

Lüscher C, Ungless MA: The mechanistic classification of addictive drugs. PLoS Med 2006;3:e437.

Robinson TE, Berridge KC: Addiction. Annu Rev Psychol 2003; 54:25.

Ungless MA: Dopamine: The salient issue. Trends Neurosci 2004; 27:702.

Wise RA: Dopamine, learning and motivation. Nat Rev Neurosci 2004;5:483.

Wolf ME: LTP may trigger addiction. Mol Interv 2003;3:248.

Pharmacology of Drugs of Abuse

Cruz HG et al: Bi-directional effects of GABA(B) receptor agonists on the mesolimbic dopamine system. Nat Neurosci 2004; 7:153.

Mansvelder HD, Keath JR, McGehee DS: Synaptic mechanisms underlie nicotine-induced excitability of brain reward areas. Neuron 2002;33:905.

Maskos U et al: Nicotine reinforcement and cognition restored by targeted expression of nicotinic receptors. Nature 2005; 436:103.

Morton J: Ecstasy: Pharmacology and neurotoxicity. Curr Opin Pharmacol 2005;5:79.

Nichols DE: Hallucinogens. Pharmacol Ther 2004;101:131.

Snead OC 3rd, Gibson KM: Gamma-hydroxybutyric acid. N Engl J Med 2005;352:2721.

Sulzer D et al: Mechanisms of neurotransmitter release by amphetamines: A review. Prog Neurobiol 2005;75:406.

Wilson RI, Nicoll RA: Endocannabinoid signaling in the brain. Science 2002;296:678.

SECTION VI
Drugs Used to Treat Diseases of the Blood, Inflammation, & Gout

Agents Used in Anemias; Hematopoietic Growth Factors

33

Susan B. Masters, PhD

Hematopoiesis, the production from undifferentiated stem cells of circulating erythrocytes, platelets, and leukocytes, is a remarkable process that produces over 200 billion new blood cells per day in the normal person and even greater numbers of cells in people with conditions that cause loss or destruction of blood cells. The hematopoietic machinery resides primarily in the bone marrow in adults and requires a constant supply of three essential nutrients—**iron, vitamin B_{12},** and **folic acid**—as well as the presence of **hematopoietic growth factors,** proteins that regulate the proliferation and differentiation of hematopoietic cells. Inadequate supplies of either the essential nutrients or the growth factors result in deficiency of functional blood cells. **Anemia,** a deficiency in oxygen-carrying erythrocytes, is the most common and easily treated of these conditions, but **thrombocytopenia** and **neutropenia** are not rare and some forms are amenable to drug therapy. In this chapter, we first consider treatment of anemia due to deficiency of iron, vitamin B_{12}, or folic acid and then turn to the medical use of hematopoietic growth factors to combat anemia, thrombocytopenia, and neutropenia, and to support stem cell transplantation.

■ AGENTS USED IN ANEMIAS

IRON

Basic Pharmacology

Iron deficiency is the most common cause of chronic anemia. Like other forms of chronic anemia, iron deficiency anemia leads to pallor, fatigue, dizziness, exertional dyspnea, and other generalized symptoms of tissue hypoxia. The cardiovascular adaptations to chronic anemia—tachycardia, increased cardiac output, vasodilation—can worsen the condition of patients with underlying cardiovascular disease.

Iron forms the nucleus of the iron-porphyrin heme ring, which together with globin chains forms hemoglobin. Hemoglobin reversibly binds oxygen and provides the critical mechanism for oxygen delivery from the lungs to other tissues. In the absence of adequate iron, small erythrocytes with insufficient hemoglobin are formed, giving rise to **microcytic hypochromic anemia.**

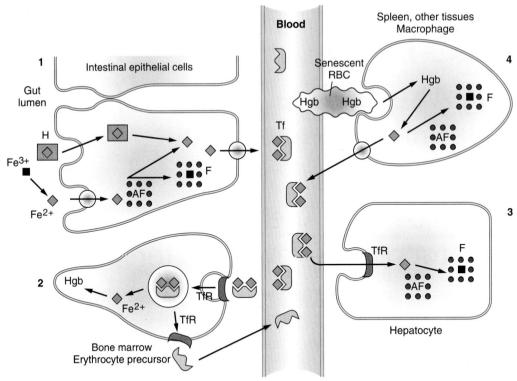

Figure 33–1. Absorption, transport, and storage of iron. Intestinal epithelial cells actively absorb inorganic iron and heme iron (H). Ferrous iron that is absorbed or released from absorbed heme iron in the intestine **(1)** is actively transported into the blood or complexed with apoferritin (AF) and stored as ferritin. In the blood, iron is transported by transferrin (Tf) to erythroid precursors in the bone marrow for synthesis of hemoglobin (Hgb) **(2)** or to hepatocytes for storage as ferritin **(3)**. The transferrin-iron complexes bind to transferrin receptors (TfR) in erythroid precursors and hepatocytes and are internalized. After release of the iron, the TfR-Tf complex is recycled to the plasma membrane and Tf is released. Macrophages that phagocytize senescent erythrocytes (RBC) reclaim the iron from the RBC hemoglobin and either export it or store it as ferritin **(4)**. Hepatocytes use several mechanisms to take up iron and store the iron as ferritin. See text.

Pharmacokinetics

Free inorganic iron is extremely toxic, but iron is required for essential proteins such as hemoglobin; therefore, evolution has provided an elaborate system for regulating iron absorption, transport, and storage (Figure 33–1). The system uses specialized transport and storage proteins whose concentrations are controlled by the body's demand for hemoglobin synthesis and adequate iron stores (Table 33–1). Nearly all of the iron used to support hematopoiesis is reclaimed from catalysis of the hemoglobin in senescent or damaged erythrocytes. Normally, only a small amount of iron is lost from the body each day, so dietary requirements are small and easily fulfilled by the iron available in a wide variety of foods. However, in special populations with either increased iron requirements

(eg, growing children, pregnant women) or increased losses of iron (eg, menstruating women), iron requirements can exceed normal dietary supplies and iron deficiency can develop.

A. ABSORPTION

The average diet in the USA contains 10–15 mg of elemental iron daily. A normal individual absorbs 5–10% of this iron, or about 0.5–1 mg daily. Iron is normally absorbed in the duodenum and proximal jejunum, although the more distal small intestine can absorb iron if necessary. Iron absorption increases in response to low iron stores or increased iron requirements. Total iron absorption increases to 1–2 mg/d in normal menstruating women and may be as high as 3–4 mg/d in pregnant women.

Table 33–1. Iron distribution in normal adults.[1]

	Iron Content (mg)	
	Men	Women
Hemoglobin	3050	1700
Myoglobin	430	300
Enzymes	10	8
Transport (transferrin)	8	6
Storage (ferritin and other forms)	750	300
Total	4248	2314

[1]Values are based on data from various sources and assume that "normal" men weigh 80 kg and have a hemoglobin of 16 g/dL and that "normal" women weigh 55 kg and have a hemoglobin of 14 g/dL.
Adapted, with permission, from Brown EB: Iron deficiency anemia. In: Wyngaarden JB, Smith LH (editors). *Cecil Textbook of Medicine*, 16th ed. Saunders, 1982.

Iron is available in a wide variety of foods but is especially abundant in meat. The iron in meat protein can be efficiently absorbed, because heme iron in meat hemoglobin and myoglobin can be absorbed intact without first having to be dissociated into elemental iron (Figure 33–1). Iron in other foods, especially vegetables and grains, is often tightly bound to organic compounds and is much less available for absorption. Nonheme iron in foods and iron in inorganic iron salts and complexes must be reduced to ferrous iron (Fe^{2+}) before it can be absorbed by intestinal mucosal cells.

Iron crosses the luminal membrane of the intestinal mucosal cell by two mechanisms: active transport of ferrous iron and absorption of iron complexed with heme (Figure 33–1). The divalent metal transporter, DMT1, efficiently transports ferrous iron across the luminal membrane of the intestinal enterocyte. The rate of iron uptake is regulated by mucosal cell iron stores such that more iron is transported when stores are low. Together with iron split from absorbed heme, the newly absorbed iron can be actively transported into the blood across the basolateral membrane, probably by the transporter IREG1, also known as ferroportin1. Other proteins are involved in this process, and some of them are regulated to control iron absorption and storage. Excess iron can be stored in the mucosal cell as ferritin, a water-soluble complex consisting of a core of ferric hydroxide covered by a shell of a specialized storage protein called apoferritin. In general, when total body iron stores are high and iron requirements by the body are low, newly absorbed iron is diverted into ferritin in the intestinal mucosal cells. When iron stores are low or iron requirements are high, newly absorbed iron is immediately transported from the mucosal cells to the bone marrow to support hemoglobin production.

B. TRANSPORT

Iron is transported in the plasma bound to **transferrin,** a β-globulin that specifically binds two molecules of ferrous iron (Figure 33–1). The transferrin-iron complex enters maturing erythroid cells by a specific receptor mechanism. Transferrin receptors—integral membrane glycoproteins present in large numbers on proliferating erythroid cells—bind and internalize the transferrin-iron complex through the process of receptor-mediated endocytosis. In endosomes, the iron is released and funneled into hemoglobin synthesis, whereas the transferrin-transferrin receptor complex is recycled to the plasma membrane, where the transferrin dissociates and returns to the plasma. This process provides an efficient mechanism for supplying the iron required by developing red blood cells.

Increased erythropoiesis is associated with an increase in the number of transferrin receptors on developing erythroid cells. Iron store depletion and iron deficiency anemia are associated with an increased concentration of serum transferrin.

C. STORAGE

In addition to the storage of iron in intestinal mucosal cells, iron is also stored, primarily as ferritin, in macrophages in the liver, spleen, and bone, and in parenchymal liver cells (Figure 33–1). Apoferritin synthesis is regulated by the levels of free iron. When these levels are low, apoferritin synthesis is inhibited and the balance of iron binding shifts toward transferrin. When free iron levels are high, more apoferritin is produced to sequester more iron and protect organs from the toxic effects of excess free iron.

Ferritin is detectable in serum. Since the ferritin present in serum is in equilibrium with storage ferritin in reticuloendothelial tissues, the serum ferritin level can be used to estimate total body iron stores.

D. ELIMINATION

There is no mechanism for excretion of iron. Small amounts are lost in the feces by exfoliation of intestinal mucosal cells, and trace amounts are excreted in bile, urine, and sweat. These losses account for no more than 1 mg of iron per day. Because the body's ability to excrete iron is so limited, regulation of iron balance must be achieved by changing intestinal absorption and storage of iron, in response to the body's needs. As noted below, impaired regulation of iron absorption leads to serious pathology.

Clinical Pharmacology

A. INDICATIONS FOR THE USE OF IRON

The only clinical indication for the use of iron preparations is the treatment or prevention of iron deficiency anemia. Iron deficiency is commonly seen in populations with increased iron requirements. These include infants, especially premature infants; children during rapid growth periods; pregnant and lactating women; and patients with chronic kidney disease who lose erythrocytes at a relatively high rate during hemodialysis and also form them at a high rate as a result of treatment with the erythrocyte growth factor erythropoietin (see below). Inadequate iron absorption can also cause iron deficiency. This is seen frequently after gastrectomy and in patients with severe small bowel disease that results in generalized malabsorption. Iron deficiency in these gastrointestinal conditions is due to inadequate iron absorption.

The most common cause of iron deficiency in adults is blood loss. Menstruating women lose about 30 mg of iron with each menstrual period; women with heavy menstrual bleeding may lose much more. Thus, many premenopausal women have low iron stores or even iron deficiency. In men and postmenopausal women, the most common site of blood loss is the gastrointestinal tract. Patients with unexplained iron deficiency anemia should be evaluated for occult gastrointestinal bleeding.

B. TREATMENT

Iron deficiency anemia is treated with oral or parenteral iron preparations. Oral iron corrects the anemia just as rapidly and completely as parenteral iron in most cases if iron absorption from the gastrointestinal tract is normal. An exception is the high requirement for iron of patients with advanced chronic kidney disease who are undergoing hemodialysis and treatment with erythropoietin; for these patients, parenteral iron administration is preferred.

1. Oral iron therapy—A wide variety of oral iron preparations are available. Because ferrous iron is most efficiently absorbed, only ferrous salts should be used. Ferrous sulfate, ferrous gluconate, and ferrous fumarate are all effective and inexpensive and are recommended for the treatment of most patients.

Different iron salts provide different amounts of elemental iron, as shown in Table 33–2. In an iron-deficient individual, about 50–100 mg of iron can be incorporated into hemoglobin daily, and about 25% of oral iron given as ferrous salt can be absorbed. Therefore, 200–400 mg of elemental iron should be given daily to correct iron deficiency most rapidly. Patients unable to tolerate such large doses of iron can be given lower daily doses of iron, which results in slower but still complete correction of iron deficiency. Treatment

with oral iron should be continued for 3–6 months after correction of the cause of the iron loss. This corrects the anemia and replenishes iron stores.

Common adverse effects of oral iron therapy include nausea, epigastric discomfort, abdominal cramps, constipation, and diarrhea. These effects are usually dose-related and can often be overcome by lowering the daily dose of iron or by taking the tablets immediately after or with meals. Some patients have less severe gastrointestinal adverse effects with one iron salt than another and benefit from changing preparations. Patients taking oral iron develop black stools; this has no clinical significance in itself but may obscure the diagnosis of continued gastrointestinal blood loss.

2. Parenteral iron therapy—Parenteral therapy should be reserved for patients with documented iron deficiency who are unable to tolerate or absorb oral iron and for patients with extensive chronic blood loss who cannot be maintained with oral iron alone. This includes patients with various postgastrectomy conditions and previous small bowel resection, inflammatory bowel disease involving the proximal small bowel, malabsorption syndromes, and advanced chronic renal disease including hemodialysis and treatment with erythropoietin.

Iron dextran is a stable complex of ferric hydroxide and low-molecular-weight dextran containing 50 mg of elemental iron per milliliter of solution. It can be given by deep intramuscular injection or by intravenous infusion, although the intravenous route is used most commonly. Intravenous administration eliminates the local pain and tissue staining that often occur with the intramuscular route and allows delivery of the entire dose of iron necessary to correct the iron deficiency at one time. Adverse effects of intravenous iron dextran therapy include headache, light-headedness, fever, arthralgias, nausea and vomiting, back pain, flushing, urticaria, bronchospasm, and,

Table 33–2. Some commonly used oral iron preparations.

Preparation	Tablet Size	Elemental Iron per Tablet	Usual Adult Dosage (Tablets per Day)
Ferrous sulfate, hydrated	325 mg	65 mg	3–4
Ferrous sulfate, desiccated	200 mg	65 mg	3–4
Ferrous gluconate	325 mg	36 mg	3–4
Ferrous fumarate	100 mg	33 mg	6–8
	325 mg	106 mg	2–3

rarely, anaphylaxis and death. Some of these effects represent a hypersensitivity reaction to the dextran component. Hypersensitivity reactions may be delayed for 48–72 hours after administration. Anaphylactic reactions to iron dextran, including fatal reactions, have been clearly documented. Owing to the risk of a hypersensitivity reaction, a small test dose of iron dextran should always be given before full intramuscular or intravenous doses are given. Patients with a strong history of allergy and patients who have previously received parenteral iron dextran are more likely to have hypersensitivity reactions after treatment with parenteral iron dextran.

Iron-sucrose complex and **iron sodium gluconate complex** are alternative preparations. These agents can be given only by the intravenous route. These preparations appear to be much less likely than iron dextran to cause hypersensitivity reactions.

For patients who are treated chronically with parenteral iron, it is important to periodically monitor iron storage levels to avoid the serious toxicity associated with iron overload. Unlike oral iron therapy, which is subject to the regulatory mechanism provided by the intestinal uptake system, parenteral administration, which bypasses this regulatory system, can deliver more iron than can be safely stored in intestinal cells and macrophages in the liver and tissues. Iron stores can be estimated on the basis of serum concentrations of ferritin and the transferrin saturation, which is the ratio of the total serum iron concentration to the total iron-binding capacity (TIBC).

Clinical Toxicity

A. ACUTE IRON TOXICITY

Acute iron toxicity is seen almost exclusively in young children who accidentally ingest iron tablets. Although adults are able to tolerate large doses of oral iron without serious consequences, as few as 10 tablets of any of the commonly available oral iron preparations can be lethal in young children. Adult patients taking oral iron preparations should be instructed to store tablets in child-proof containers out of the reach of children. Children who are poisoned with oral iron experience necrotizing gastroenteritis, with vomiting, abdominal pain, and bloody diarrhea followed by shock, lethargy, and dyspnea. Subsequently, improvement is often noted, but this may be followed by severe metabolic acidosis, coma, and death. Urgent treatment is necessary. **Whole bowel irrigation** (see Chapter 59) should be performed to flush out unabsorbed pills. **Deferoxamine,** a potent iron-chelating compound, can be given systemically to bind iron that has already been absorbed and to promote its excretion in urine and feces. Activated charcoal, a highly effective adsorbent for most toxins, **does not** bind iron and thus is ineffective. Appropriate supportive therapy for gastrointestinal bleeding, metabolic acidosis, and shock must also be provided.

B. CHRONIC IRON TOXICITY

Chronic iron toxicity (iron overload), also known as **hemochromatosis,** results when excess iron is deposited in the heart, liver, pancreas, and other organs. It can lead to organ failure and death. It most commonly occurs in patients with inherited hemochromatosis, a disorder characterized by excessive iron absorption, and in patients who receive many red cell transfusions over a long period of time (eg, patients with thalassemia major).

Chronic iron overload in the absence of anemia is most efficiently treated by intermittent phlebotomy. One unit of blood can be removed every week or so until all of the excess iron is removed. Iron chelation therapy using parenteral deferoxamine is much less efficient as well as more complicated, expensive, and hazardous, but it can be the only option for iron overload that cannot be managed by phlebotomy, such as the iron overload experienced by patients with thalassemia major.

Recently, an oral iron chelator **deferasirox** has been approved for treatment of iron overload. Deferasirox appears to be as effective as deferoxamine at reducing liver iron concentrations and is much more convenient. However, it is not clear whether deferasirox is as effective as deferoxamine at protecting the heart from iron overload.

VITAMIN B$_{12}$

Vitamin B$_{12}$ serves as a cofactor for several essential biochemical reactions in humans. Deficiency of vitamin B$_{12}$ leads to anemia, gastrointestinal symptoms, and neurologic abnormalities. Although deficiency of vitamin B$_{12}$ due to an inadequate supply in the diet is unusual, deficiency of B$_{12}$ in adults—especially older adults—due to inadequate absorption of dietary vitamin B$_{12}$ is a relatively common and easily treated disorder.

Chemistry

Vitamin B$_{12}$ consists of a porphyrin-like ring with a central cobalt atom attached to a nucleotide. Various organic groups may be covalently bound to the cobalt atom, forming different cobalamins. Deoxyadenosylcobalamin and methylcobalamin are the active forms of the vitamin in humans. **Cyanocobalamin** and **hydroxocobalamin** (both available for therapeutic use) and other cobalamins found in food sources are converted to the active forms. The ultimate source of vitamin B$_{12}$ is from microbial synthesis; the vitamin is not synthesized by animals or plants. The chief dietary source of vitamin B$_{12}$ is microbially derived vitamin B$_{12}$ in meat (especially liver), eggs, and dairy products. Vitamin B$_{12}$ is sometimes called **extrinsic factor** to differentiate it from **intrinsic factor,** a protein normally secreted by the stomach.

Pharmacokinetics

The average diet in the USA contains 5–30 mcg of vitamin B_{12} daily, 1–5 mcg of which is usually absorbed. The vitamin is avidly stored, primarily in the liver, with an average adult having a total vitamin B_{12} storage pool of 3000–5000 mcg. Only trace amounts of vitamin B_{12} are normally lost in urine and stool. Because the normal daily requirements of vitamin B_{12} are only about 2 mcg, it would take about 5 years for all of the stored vitamin B_{12} to be exhausted and for megaloblastic anemia to develop if B_{12} absorption stopped. Vitamin B_{12} in physiologic amounts is absorbed only after it complexes with intrinsic factor, a glycoprotein secreted by the parietal cells of the gastric mucosa. Intrinsic factor combines with the vitamin B_{12} that is liberated from dietary sources in the stomach and duodenum, and the intrinsic factor-vitamin B_{12} complex is subsequently absorbed in the distal ileum by a highly specific receptor-mediated transport system. Vitamin B_{12} deficiency in humans most often results from malabsorption of vitamin B_{12} due either to lack of intrinsic factor or to loss or malfunction of the specific absorptive mechanism in the distal ileum. Nutritional deficiency is rare but may be seen in strict vegetarians after many years without meat, eggs, or dairy products.

Once absorbed, vitamin B_{12} is transported to the various cells of the body bound to a plasma glycoprotein, transcobalamin II. Excess vitamin B_{12} is transported to the liver for storage.

Pharmacodynamics

Two essential enzymatic reactions in humans require vitamin B_{12} (Figure 33–2). In one, methylcobalamin serves as an intermediate in the transfer of a methyl group from N^5-methyltetrahydrofolate to homocysteine, forming methionine (Figure 33–2A; Figure 33–3, section 1). Without vitamin B_{12}, conversion of the major dietary and storage folate, N^5-methyltetrahydrofolate, to tetrahydrofolate, the precursor of folate cofactors, cannot occur. As a result, a deficiency of folate cofactors necessary for several biochemical reactions involving the transfer of one-carbon groups develops. In particular, the depletion of tetrahydrofolate prevents synthesis of adequate supplies of the deoxythymidylate (dTMP) and purines required for DNA synthesis in rapidly dividing cells, as shown in Figure 33–3, section 2. The accumulation of folate as N^5-methyltetrahydrofolate and the associated depletion of tetrahydrofolate cofactors in vitamin B_{12} deficiency have been referred to as the "methylfolate trap." This is the biochemical step whereby vitamin B_{12} and folic acid metabolism are linked, and it explains why the megaloblastic anemia of vitamin B_{12} deficiency can be partially corrected by ingestion of relatively large amounts of folic acid. Folic

A. Methyl transfer

B. Isomerization of L-Methylmalonyl-CoA

Figure 33–2. Enzymatic reactions that use vitamin B_{12}. See text for details.

acid can be reduced to dihydrofolate by the enzyme dihydrofolate reductase (Figure 33–3, reaction 3) and thus serve as a source of the tetrahydrofolate required for synthesis of the purines and dTMP that are needed for DNA synthesis.

The other enzymatic reaction that requires vitamin B_{12} is isomerization of methylmalonyl-CoA to succinyl-CoA by the enzyme methylmalonyl-CoA mutase (Figure 33–2B). In vitamin B_{12} deficiency, this conversion cannot take place, and the substrate, methylmalonyl-CoA, accumulates. In the past, it was thought that abnormal accumulation of methylmalonyl-CoA causes the neurologic manifestations of vitamin B_{12} deficiency. However, newer evidence instead implicates the disruption of the methionine synthesis pathway as the cause of neurologic problems. Whatever the biochemical explanation for neurologic damage, the important point is that administration of folic acid in the setting of vitamin B_{12} deficiency will not prevent *neurologic* manifestations even though it will largely correct the *anemia* caused by the vitamin B_{12} deficiency.

Clinical Pharmacology

Vitamin B_{12} is used to treat or prevent deficiency. There is no evidence that vitamin B_{12} injections have any benefit in persons who do not have vitamin B_{12} deficiency. The most characteristic clinical manifestation of vitamin B_{12} deficiency is **megaloblastic anemia.** The typical clinical findings in megaloblastic anemia are macrocytic anemia, often with associated mild or moderate leukopenia or thrombocytopenia (or both), and a characteristic hypercellular bone marrow with an accumulation of megaloblastic erythroid and

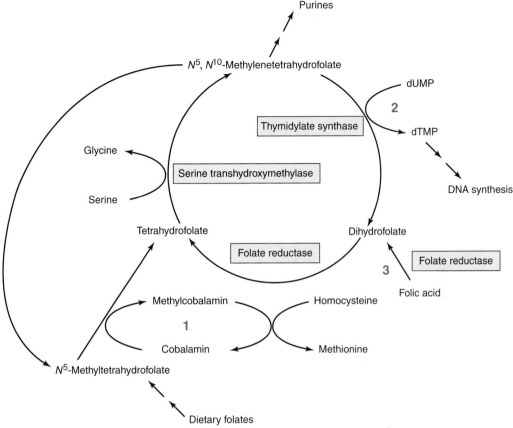

Figure 33–3. Enzymatic reactions that use folates. Section **1** shows the vitamin B_{12}-dependent reaction that allows most dietary folates to enter the tetrahydrofolate cofactor pool and becomes the "folate trap" in vitamin B_{12} deficiency. Section **2** shows the dTMP cycle. Section **3** shows the pathway by which folic acid enters the tetrahydrofolate cofactor pool. Double arrows indicate pathways with more than one intermediate step.

other precursor cells. The neurologic syndrome associated with vitamin B_{12} deficiency usually begins with paresthesias and weakness in peripheral nerves and progresses to spasticity, ataxia, and other central nervous system dysfunctions. Correction of vitamin B_{12} deficiency arrests the progression of neurologic disease, but it may not fully reverse neurologic symptoms that have been present for several months. Although most patients with neurologic abnormalities caused by vitamin B_{12} deficiency have megaloblastic anemia when first seen, occasional patients have few if any hematologic abnormalities.

Once a diagnosis of megaloblastic anemia is made, it must be determined whether vitamin B_{12} or folic acid deficiency is the cause. (Other causes of megaloblastic anemia are very rare.) This can usually be accomplished by measuring serum levels of the vitamins. The Schilling test, which measures absorption and urinary excretion of radioactively labeled vitamin B_{12}, can be used to further define the mechanism of vitamin B_{12} malabsorption when this is found to be the cause of the megaloblastic anemia.

The most common causes of vitamin B_{12} deficiency are pernicious anemia, partial or total gastrectomy, and conditions that affect the distal ileum, such as malabsorption syndromes, inflammatory bowel disease, or small bowel resection.

Pernicious anemia results from defective secretion of intrinsic factor by the gastric mucosal cells. Patients with pernicious anemia have gastric atrophy and fail to secrete intrinsic factor (as well as hydrochloric acid). The Schilling test shows diminished absorption of radioactively labeled vitamin B_{12}, which is corrected when intrinsic factor is administered with radioactive B_{12}, since the vitamin can then be normally absorbed.

Vitamin B_{12} deficiency also occurs when the region of the distal ileum that absorbs the vitamin B_{12}-intrinsic factor complex is damaged, as when the ileum is involved with inflammatory bowel disease or when the ileum is surgically resected. In these situations, radioactively labeled vitamin B_{12} is not absorbed in the Schilling test, even when intrinsic factor is added. Other rare causes of vitamin B_{12} deficiency include bacterial overgrowth of the small bowel, chronic pancreatitis, and thyroid disease. Rare cases of vitamin B_{12} deficiency in children have been found to be secondary to congenital deficiency of intrinsic factor and congenital selective vitamin B_{12} malabsorption due to defects of the receptor sites in the distal ileum.

Almost all cases of vitamin B_{12} deficiency are caused by malabsorption of the vitamin; therefore, parenteral injections of vitamin B_{12} are required for therapy. For patients with potentially reversible diseases, the underlying disease should be treated after initial treatment with parenteral vitamin B_{12}. Most patients, however, do not have curable deficiency syndromes and require lifelong treatment with vitamin B_{12}.

Vitamin B_{12} for parenteral injection is available as cyanocobalamin or hydroxocobalamin. Hydroxocobalamin is preferred because it is more highly protein-bound and therefore remains longer in the circulation. Initial therapy should consist of 100–1000 mcg of vitamin B_{12} intramuscularly daily or every other day for 1–2 weeks to replenish body stores. Maintenance therapy consists of 100–1000 mcg intramuscularly once a month for life. If neurologic abnormalities are present, maintenance therapy injections should be given every 1–2 weeks for 6 months before switching to monthly injections. Oral vitamin B_{12}-intrinsic factor mixtures and liver extracts should not be used to treat vitamin B_{12} deficiency; however, oral doses of 1000 mcg of vitamin B_{12} daily are usually sufficient to treat patients with pernicious anemia who refuse or cannot tolerate the injections. After pernicious anemia is in remission following parenteral vitamin B_{12} therapy, the vitamin can be administered intranasally as a spray or gel.

FOLIC ACID

Reduced forms of folic acid are required for essential biochemical reactions that provide precursors for the synthesis of amino acids, purines, and DNA. Folate deficiency is not uncommon, even though the deficiency is easily corrected by administration of folic acid. The consequences of folate deficiency go beyond the problem of anemia because folate deficiency is implicated as a cause of congenital malformations in newborns and may play a role in vascular disease (see Box: Folic Acid Supplementation: A Public Health Dilemma).

Chemistry

Folic acid (pteroylglutamic acid) is composed of a heterocycle (pteridine), p-aminobenzoic acid, and glutamic

Figure 33–4. The structure and numbering of atoms of folic acid. (Reproduced, with permission, from Murray RK et al: *Harper's Biochemistry,* 24th ed. McGraw-Hill, 1996.)

acid (Figure 33–4). Various numbers of glutamic acid moieties may be attached to the pteroyl portion of the molecule, resulting in monoglutamates, triglutamates, or polyglutamates. Folic acid can undergo reduction, catalyzed by the enzyme dihydrofolate reductase ("folate reductase"), to give dihydrofolic acid (Figure 33–3, section 3). Tetrahydrofolate can subsequently be transformed to folate cofactors possessing one-carbon units attached to the 5-nitrogen, to the 10-nitrogen, or to both positions (Figure 33–3). The folate cofactors are interconvertible by various enzymatic reactions and serve the important biochemical function of donating one-carbon units at various levels of oxidation. In most of these, tetrahydrofolate is regenerated and becomes available for reutilization.

Pharmacokinetics

The average diet in the USA contains 500–700 mcg of folates daily, 50–200 mcg of which is usually absorbed, depending on metabolic requirements. Pregnant women may absorb as much as 300–400 mcg of folic acid daily. Various forms of folic acid are present in a wide variety of plant and animal tissues; the richest sources are yeast, liver, kidney, and green vegetables. Normally, 5–20 mg of folates are stored in the liver and other tissues. Folates are excreted in the urine and stool and are also destroyed by catabolism, so serum levels fall within a few days when intake is diminished. Because body stores of folates are relatively low and daily requirements high, folic acid deficiency and megaloblastic anemia can develop within 1–6 months after the intake of folic acid stops, depending on the patient's nutritional status and the rate of folate utilization.

FOLIC ACID SUPPLEMENTATION: A PUBLIC HEALTH DILEMMA

Starting in January 1998, all products made from enriched grains in the USA were required to be supplemented with folic acid. This FDA ruling was issued to reduce the incidence of congenital neural tube defects. Epidemiologic studies show a strong correlation between maternal folic acid deficiency and the incidence of neural tube defects such as spina bifida and anencephaly. The FDA requirement for folic acid supplementation is a public health measure aimed at the significant number of women in the USA who do not receive prenatal care and are not aware of the importance of adequate folic acid ingestion for preventing birth defects in their babies.

There may be an added benefit for adults. N^5-Methyltetrahydrofolate is required for the conversion of homocysteine to methionine (Figure 33–2; Figure 33–3, reaction 1). Impaired synthesis of N^5-methyltetrahydrofolate results in elevated serum concentrations of homocysteine. Data from several sources suggest a positive correlation between elevated serum homocysteine and occlusive vascular diseases such as ischemic heart disease and stroke. Clinical data suggest that the folate supplementation program has improved the folate status and reduced the prevalence of hyperhomocysteinemia in a population of middle-aged and older adults who did not use vitamin supplements. It is possible, although the evidence thus far has been negative, that the increased ingestion of folic acid will also reduce the risk of vascular disease in this population.

Although the potential benefits of supplemental folic acid during pregnancy are compelling, the decision to require folic acid in grains was—and still is—controversial. As described in the text, ingestion of folic acid can partially or totally correct the anemia caused by vitamin B_{12} deficiency. However, folic acid supplementation *does not* prevent the potentially irreversible neurologic damage caused by vitamin B_{12} deficiency. People with pernicious anemia and other forms of vitamin B_{12} deficiency are usually identified because of signs and symptoms of anemia, which typically occur before neurologic symptoms. The opponents of folic acid supplementation are concerned that increased folic acid intake in the general population will mask vitamin B_{12} deficiency and increase the prevalence of neurologic disease in our elderly population. To put this in perspective, approximately 4000 pregnancies, including 2500 live births, in the USA each year are affected by neural tube defects. In contrast, it is estimated that over 10% of the elderly population in the USA, or several million people, are at risk for the neuropsychiatric complications of vitamin B_{12} deficiency. In acknowledgment of this controversy, the FDA has kept its requirements for folic acid supplementation at a somewhat low level.

Unaltered folic acid is readily and completely absorbed in the proximal jejunum. Dietary folates, however, consist primarily of polyglutamate forms of N^5-methyltetrahydrofolate. Before absorption, all but one of the glutamyl residues of the polyglutamates must be hydrolyzed by the enzyme α-1-glutamyl transferase ("conjugase") within the brush border of the intestinal mucosa. The monoglutamate N^5-methyltetrahydrofolate is subsequently transported into the bloodstream by both active and passive transport and is then widely distributed throughout the body. Inside cells, N^5-methyltetrahydrofolate is converted to tetrahydrofolate by the demethylation reaction that requires vitamin B_{12} (Figure 33–3, section 1).

Pharmacodynamics

Tetrahydrofolate cofactors participate in one-carbon transfer reactions. As described earlier in the discussion of vitamin B_{12}, one of these essential reactions produces the dTMP needed for DNA synthesis. In this reaction, the enzyme thymidylate synthase catalyzes the transfer of the one-carbon unit of N^5,N^{10}-methylenetetrahydrofolate to deoxyuridine monophosphate (dUMP) to form dTMP (Figure 33–3, section 2). Unlike all the other enzymatic reactions that use folate cofactors, in this reaction the cofactor is oxidized to dihydrofolate, and for each mole of dTMP produced, 1 mole of tetrahydrofolate is consumed. In rapidly proliferating tissues, considerable amounts of tetrahydrofolate are consumed in this reaction, and continued DNA synthesis requires continued regeneration of tetrahydrofolate by reduction of dihydrofolate, catalyzed by the enzyme dihydrofolate reductase. The tetrahydrofolate thus produced can then reform the cofactor N^5,N^{10}-methylenetetrahydrofolate by the action of serine transhydroxymethylase and thus allow for the continued synthesis of dTMP. The combined catalytic activities of dTMP synthase, dihydrofolate reductase, and serine transhydroxymethylase are often referred to as the *dTMP synthesis cycle*. Enzymes in the dTMP cycle are the targets of two anticancer drugs; methotrexate inhibits dihydrofolate reductase, and a metabolite of 5-fluorouracil inhibits thymidylate synthase (see Chapter 55).

Cofactors of tetrahydrofolate participate in several other essential reactions. N^5-Methylenetetrahydrofolate is required for the vitamin B_{12}-dependent reaction that generates methionine from homocysteine (Figure 33–2A; Figure 33–3, section 1). In addition, tetrahydrofolate cofactors donate one-carbon units during the de novo synthesis of essential purines. In these reactions, tetrahydrofolate is regenerated and can reenter the tetrahydrofolate cofactor pool.

Clinical Pharmacology

Folate deficiency results in a megaloblastic anemia that is microscopically indistinguishable from the anemia caused by vitamin B_{12} deficiency (see above). However, folate deficiency does not cause the characteristic neurologic syndrome seen in vitamin B_{12} deficiency. In patients with megaloblastic anemia, folate status is assessed with assays for serum folate or for red blood cell folate. Red blood cell folate levels are often of greater diagnostic value than serum levels, because serum folate levels tend to be labile and do not necessarily reflect tissue levels.

Folic acid deficiency, unlike vitamin B_{12} deficiency, is often caused by inadequate dietary intake of folates. Patients with alcohol dependence and patients with liver disease often develop folic acid deficiency because of poor diet and diminished hepatic storage of folates. Pregnant women and patients with hemolytic anemia have increased folate requirements and may become folic acid-deficient, especially if their diets are marginal. Evidence implicates maternal folic acid deficiency in the occurrence of fetal neural tube defects, eg, spina bifida. (See Box: Folic Acid Supplementation: A Public Health Dilemma.) Patients with malabsorption syndromes also frequently develop folic acid deficiency. Patients who require renal dialysis develop folic acid deficiency because folates are removed from the plasma during the dialysis procedure.

Folic acid deficiency can be caused by drugs. Methotrexate and, to a lesser extent, trimethoprim and pyrimethamine, inhibit dihydrofolate reductase and may result in a deficiency of folate cofactors and ultimately in megaloblastic anemia. Long-term therapy with phenytoin can also cause folate deficiency, but only rarely causes megaloblastic anemia.

Parenteral administration of folic acid is rarely necessary, since oral folic acid is well absorbed even in patients with malabsorption syndromes. A dose of 1 mg folic acid orally daily is sufficient to reverse megaloblastic anemia, restore normal serum folate levels, and replenish body stores of folates in almost all patients. Therapy should be continued until the underlying cause of the deficiency is removed or corrected. Therapy may be required indefinitely for patients with malabsorption or dietary inadequacy. Folic acid supplementation to prevent folic acid deficiency should be considered in high-risk patients, including pregnant women, patients with alcohol dependence, hemolytic anemia, liver disease, or certain skin diseases, and patients on renal dialysis.

■ HEMATOPOIETIC GROWTH FACTORS

The hematopoietic growth factors are glycoprotein hormones that regulate the proliferation and differentiation of hematopoietic progenitor cells in the bone marrow. The first growth factors to be identified were called colony-stimulating factors because they could stimulate the growth of colonies of various bone marrow progenitor cells in vitro. Many of these growth factors have been purified and cloned, and their effects on hematopoiesis have been extensively studied. Quantities of these growth factors sufficient for clinical use are produced by recombinant DNA technology.

Of the known hematopoietic growth factors, **erythropoietin (epoetin alfa), granulocyte colony-stimulating factor (G-CSF), granulocyte-macrophage colony-stimulating factor (GM-CSF),** and **interleukin-11 (IL-11)** are currently in clinical use. Thrombopoietin and other potentially useful hematopoietic factors are still in development.

The hematopoietic growth factors have complex effects on the function of a wide variety of cell types, including nonhematologic cells. Their usefulness in other areas of medicine, particularly as potential anticancer and anti-inflammatory drugs, is being investigated.

ERYTHROPOIETIN

Chemistry & Pharmacokinetics

Erythropoietin, a 34–39 kDa glycoprotein, was the first human hematopoietic growth factor to be isolated. It was originally purified from the urine of patients with severe anemia. Recombinant human erythropoietin (rHuEPO, epoetin alfa) is produced in a mammalian cell expression system. After intravenous administration, erythropoietin has a serum half-life of 4–13 hours in patients with chronic renal failure. It is not cleared by dialysis. It is measured in international units (IU). Darbepoetin alfa is a glycosylated form of erythropoietin and differs from it functionally only in having a twofold to threefold longer half-life.

Pharmacodynamics

Erythropoietin stimulates erythroid proliferation and differentiation by interacting with specific erythropoietin receptors on red cell progenitors. The erythropoietin

Table 33–3. Clinical uses of hematopoietic growth factors.

Hematopoietic Growth Factor	Clinical Condition Being Treated or Prevented	Recipients
Erythropoietin, darbepoetin alfa	Anemia	Patients with chronic renal failure HIV-infected patients treated with zidovudine Cancer patients treated with myelosuppressive cancer chemotherapy Patients scheduled to undergo elective, noncardiac, nonvascular surgery
Granulocyte colony-stimulating factor (G-CSF; filgrastim)	Neutropenia	Cancer patients treated with myelosuppressive cancer chemotherapy
Granulocyte-macrophage colony-stimulating factor (GM-CSF; sargramostim)		Patients with severe chronic neutropenia Patients with nonmyeloid malignancies with stem cell transplantation Mobilization of peripheral blood progenitor cells (PBPC)
	Stem cell transplantation	Patients with nonmyeloid malignancies
	Mobilization of peripheral blood progenitor cells (PBPC)	Donors of stem cells for allogeneic or autologous transplantation
Interleukin-11 (IL-11, oprelvekin)	Thrombocytopenia	Patients with nonmyeloid malignancies who receive myelosuppressive cancer chemotherapy

receptor is a member of the JAK/STAT superfamily of cytokine receptors that use protein phosphorylation and transcription factor activation to regulate cellular function (see Chapter 2). Erythropoietin also induces release of reticulocytes from the bone marrow. Endogenous erythropoietin is primarily produced in the kidney. In response to tissue hypoxia, more erythropoietin is produced through an increased rate of transcription of the erythropoietin gene. This results in correction of the anemia, provided that the bone marrow response is not impaired by red cell nutritional deficiency (especially iron deficiency), primary bone marrow disorders (see below), or bone marrow suppression from drugs or chronic diseases.

Normally, an inverse relationship exists between the hematocrit or hemoglobin level and the serum erythropoietin level. Nonanemic individuals have serum erythropoietin levels of less than 20 IU/L. As the hematocrit and hemoglobin levels fall and anemia becomes more severe, the serum erythropoietin level rises exponentially. Patients with moderately severe anemias usually have erythropoietin levels in the 100–500 IU/L range, and patients with severe anemias may have levels of thousands of IU/L. The most important exception to this inverse relationship is in the anemia of chronic renal failure. In patients with renal disease, erythropoietin levels are usually low because the kidneys cannot produce the growth factor. These are the patients most likely to respond to treatment with exogenous erythropoietin. In most primary bone marrow disorders (aplas-

tic anemia, leukemias, myeloproliferative and myelodysplastic disorders, etc) and most nutritional and secondary anemias, endogenous erythropoietin levels are high, so there is less likelihood of a response to exogenous erythropoietin (but see below).

Clinical Pharmacology

The availability of erythropoietin has had a significant positive impact for patients with anemia of **chronic renal failure** (Table 33–3). Erythropoietin consistently improves the hematocrit and hemoglobin level and usually eliminates the need for transfusions in these patients. An increase in reticulocyte count is usually observed in about 10 days and an increase in hematocrit and hemoglobin levels in 2–6 weeks. Most patients can maintain a hematocrit of about 35% with erythropoietin doses of 50–150 IU/kg intravenously or subcutaneously three times a week. Failure to respond to erythropoietin is most commonly due to concurrent iron deficiency, which can be corrected by giving oral or parenteral iron. Folate supplementation may also be necessary in some patients.

In selected patients, erythropoietin may also be useful for the treatment of anemia due to **primary bone marrow disorders** and **secondary anemias.** This includes patients with aplastic anemia and other bone marrow failure states, myeloproliferative and myelodysplastic disorders, multiple myeloma and perhaps other chronic bone marrow malignancies, and the anemias associated with chronic inflammation, AIDS, and cancer. Patients with these disorders who have disproportionately low serum erythropoietin levels for their degree of anemia are most likely to respond to treatment with this growth factor. Patients with endogenous erythropoietin levels of less than 100 IU/L have the best chance of response, although patients with erythropoietin levels between 100 and 500 IU/L respond occasionally. These patients generally require higher erythropoietin doses (150–300 IU/kg three times a week) to achieve a response, and responses are often incomplete.

Erythropoietin has been used successfully to offset the anemia produced by zidovudine treatment in patients with HIV infection and in the treatment of the anemia of prematurity. It can also be used to accelerate erythropoiesis after phlebotomies for autologous transfusion for elective surgery, or for treatment of iron overload (hemochromatosis).

Erythropoietin is one of the drugs banned by the International Olympic Committee. The use of erythropoietin by athletes is based on their hope that increased red blood cell concentration will increase oxygen delivery and improve performance.

Toxicity

The most common adverse effects of erythropoietin include hypertension and thrombotic complications. In March 2007, the FDA issued a warning that patients with chronic renal failure or cancer whose serum hemoglobin is raised to >12 g/dL with an erythropoiesis-stimulating agent face a greater risk of a thrombotic event or, in patients with advanced head and neck cancers, faster tumor growth. Allergic reactions have been infrequent and rare.

MYELOID GROWTH FACTORS

Chemistry & Pharmacokinetics

G-CSF and **GM-CSF,** the two myeloid growth factors currently available for clinical use, were originally purified from cultured human cell lines (Table 33–3). Recombinant human G-CSF (**rHuG-CSF; filgrastim**) is produced in a bacterial expression system. It is a nonglycosylated peptide of 175 amino acids, with a molecular weight of 18 kDa. Recombinant human GM-CSF (**rHuGM-CSF; sargramostim**) is produced in a yeast expression system. It is a partially glycosylated peptide of 127 amino acids, with three molecular species with molecular weights of 15,500; 15,800; and 19,500. These preparations have serum half-lives of 2–7 hours after intravenous or subcutaneous administration. **Pegfilgrastim,** a covalent conjugation product of filgrastim and a form of polyethylene glycol, has a much longer serum half-life than recombinant G-CSF, and so it can be injected once per myelosuppressive chemotherapy cycle instead of daily for several days.

Pharmacodynamics

The myeloid growth factors stimulate proliferation and differentiation by interacting with specific receptors found on various myeloid progenitor cells. Like the erythropoietin receptor, these receptors are members of the JAK/STAT superfamily (see Chapter 2). G-CSF stimulates proliferation and differentiation of progenitors already committed to the neutrophil lineage. It also activates the phagocytic activity of mature neutrophils and prolongs their survival in the circulation. G-CSF also has a remarkable ability to mobilize hematopoietic stem cells, ie, to increase their concentration in peripheral blood. This biologic effect underlies a major advance in transplantation—the use of **peripheral blood stem cells (PBSCs)** rather than bone marrow stem cells for autologous and allogeneic hematopoietic stem cell transplantation (see below).

GM-CSF has broader biologic actions than G-CSF. It is a multipotential hematopoietic growth factor that stimulates proliferation and differentiation of early and late granulocytic progenitor cells as well as erythroid and megakaryocyte progenitors. Like G-CSF, GM-CSF also stimulates the function of mature neutrophils. GM-CSF acts together with interleukin-2 to stimulate T-cell proliferation and appears to be a locally active factor at the site of inflammation. GM-CSF mobilizes peripheral blood stem cells, but it is significantly less efficacious than G-CSF in this regard.

Clinical Pharmacology

A. CANCER CHEMOTHERAPY-INDUCED NEUTROPENIA

Neutropenia is a common adverse effect of the cytotoxic drugs used to treat cancer and increases the risk of serious infection in patients receiving chemotherapy. Unlike the treatment of anemia and thrombocytopenia, transfusion of neutropenic patients with granulocytes collected from donors is performed rarely and with limited success. The introduction of G-CSF in 1991 represented a milestone in the treatment of chemotherapy-induced neutropenia. This growth factor dramatically accelerates the rate of neutrophil recovery after dose-intensive myelosuppressive chemotherapy (Figure 33–5). It reduces the duration of neutropenia and usually raises the nadir count, the lowest neutrophil count seen following a cycle of chemotherapy.

The ability of G-CSF to increase neutrophil counts after myelosuppressive chemotherapy is nearly universal, but its impact on clinical outcomes is more variable. Some clinical trials have shown that G-CSF reduces episodes of febrile neutropenia, requirements for broad-spectrum antibiotics, and days of hospitalization; however, other trials failed to find these favorable outcomes. To date, no

Figure 33–5. Effects of G-CSF (color) or placebo (black line) on absolute neutrophil count (ANC) after cytotoxic chemotherapy for lung cancer. Doses of chemotherapeutic drugs were administered on days 1 and 3. G-CSF or placebo injections were started on day 4 and continued daily through day 12 or 16. The first peak in ANC reflects the recruitment of mature cells by G-CSF. The second peak reflects a marked increase in new neutrophil production by the bone marrow under stimulation by G-CSF. (Normal ANC is 2.2–8.6 × 10⁹/L.) (Modified and reproduced, with permission, from Crawford et al: Reduction by granulocyte colony-stimulating factor of fever and neutropenia induced by chemotherapy in patients with small-cell lung cancer. N Engl J Med 1991;325:164.)

clinical trial has shown improved survival in cancer patients treated with G-CSF. Clinical guidelines for the use of G-CSF after cytotoxic chemotherapy recommend reserving G-CSF for patients with a prior episode of febrile neutropenia after cytotoxic chemotherapy, patients receiving dose-intensive chemotherapy, patients at high risk for febrile neutropenia, and patients who are unlikely to survive an episode of febrile neutropenia. Pegfilgrastim is an alternative to G-CSF for prevention of chemotherapy-induced febrile neutropenia. Pegfilgrastim can be administered less frequently, and it may shorten the period of severe neutropenia slightly more than G-CSF.

Like G-CSF and pegfilgrastim, GM-CSF also reduces the duration of neutropenia after cytotoxic chemotherapy. It has been more difficult to show that GM-CSF reduces the incidence of febrile neutropenia, probably because GM-CSF itself can induce fever. In the treatment of chemotherapy-induced neutropenia, G-CSF, 5 mcg/kg/d, or GM-CSF, 250 mcg/m²/d, is usually started within 24–72 hours after completing chemotherapy and is continued until the absolute neutrophil count is > 10,000 cells/μL. Pegfilgrastim is given as a single dose instead of daily injections.

The utility and safety of the myeloid growth factors in the postchemotherapy supportive care of patients with acute myeloid leukemia (AML) have been the subject of a number of clinical trials. Because leukemic cells arise from progenitors whose proliferation and differentiation are normally regulated by hematopoietic growth factors, including GM-CSF and G-CSF, there was concern that myeloid growth factors could stimulate leukemic cell growth and increase the rate of relapse. The results of randomized clinical trials suggest that both G-CSF and GM-CSF are safe following induction and consolidation treatment of myeloid and lymphoblastic leukemia. There has been no evidence that these growth factors reduce the rate of remission or increase relapse rate. On the contrary, the growth factors accelerate neutrophil recovery and reduce infection rates and days of hospitalization. Both G-CSF and GM-CSF have FDA approval for treatment of patients with AML.

B. OTHER APPLICATIONS

G-CSF and GM-CSF have also proved to be effective in treating the neutropenia associated with **congenital neutropenia, cyclic neutropenia, myelodysplasia,** and **aplastic anemia.** Many patients with these disorders respond with a prompt and sometimes dramatic increase in neutrophil count. In some cases, this results in a decrease in the frequency of infections. Because neither G-CSF nor GM-CSF stimulates the formation of erythrocytes and platelets, they are sometimes combined with other growth factors for treatment of pancytopenia.

The myeloid growth factors play an important role in **autologous stem cell transplantation** for patients undergoing high-dose chemotherapy. High-dose chemotherapy with autologous stem cell support is increasingly used to treat patients with tumors that are resistant to standard doses of chemotherapeutic drugs. The high-dose regimens produce extreme myelosuppression; the myelosuppression is then counteracted by reinfusion of the patient's own hematopoietic stem cells (which are collected prior to chemotherapy). The administration of G-CSF or GM-CSF early after autologous stem cell transplantation has been shown to reduce the time to engraftment and to recovery from neutropenia in patients receiving stem cells obtained either from bone marrow or from peripheral blood. These effects are seen in patients being treated for lymphoma or for solid tumors. G-CSF and GM-CSF are also used to support patients who have received allogeneic bone marrow transplantation for treatment of hematologic malignancies or bone marrow failure states. In this setting, the growth factors speed the recovery from neutropenia without increasing the incidence of acute graft-versus-host disease.

Perhaps the most important role of the myeloid growth factors in transplantation is for mobilization of peripheral blood stem cells (PBSCs). Stem cells collected from peripheral blood have nearly replaced bone marrow as the hematopoietic preparation used for autologous transplantation, and the use of PBSCs for allogeneic transplantation is also being investigated. The cells can be collected in an outpatient setting with a procedure that avoids much of the risk and discomfort of bone marrow collection, including the need for general anesthesia. In addition, there is evidence that PBSC transplantation results in more rapid engraftment of all hematopoietic cell lineages and in reduced rates of graft failure or delayed platelet recovery.

G-CSF is the cytokine most commonly used for PBSC mobilization because of its increased efficacy and reduced toxicity compared with GM-CSF. To mobilize stem cells, patients or donors are given 5–10 mcg/kg/d subcutaneously for 4 days. On the fifth day, they undergo leukapheresis. The success of PBSC transplantation depends on transfusion of adequate numbers of stem cells. CD34, an antigen present on early progenitor cells and absent from later, committed, cells, is used as a marker for the requisite stem cells. The goal is to reinfuse at least 5×10^6 CD34 cells/kg; this number of CD34 cells usually results in prompt and durable engraftment of all cell lineages. It can take several separate leukaphereses to collect enough CD34 cells, especially from older patients and patients who have been exposed to radiation therapy or chemotherapy.

Toxicity

Although the two growth factors have similar effects on neutrophil counts, G-CSF is used more frequently because it is better tolerated. G-CSF can cause bone pain, which clears when the drug is discontinued. GM-CSF can cause more severe side effects, particularly at higher doses. These include fever, malaise, arthralgias, myalgias, and a capillary leak syndrome characterized by peripheral edema and pleural or pericardial effusions. Allergic reactions may occur but are infrequent. Splenic rupture is a rare but serious complication of the use of G-CSF for PBSC.

MEGAKARYOCYTE GROWTH FACTORS

Chemistry & Pharmacokinetics

Interleukin-11 (IL-11) is a 65–85 kDa protein produced by fibroblasts and stromal cells in the bone marrow. **Oprelvekin,** the recombinant form of interleukin-11 approved for clinical use (Table 33–3), is produced by expression in *E coli.* The half-life of IL-11 is 7–8 hours when the drug is injected subcutaneously.

Thrombopoietin, a 65–85 kDa glycosylated protein, is constitutively expressed by a variety of organs and cell types. Hepatocytes appear to be the major source of human thrombopoietin, and patients with cirrhosis and thrombocytopenia have low serum thrombopoietin levels. Recombinant thrombopoietin is produced by expression in human cells; the recombinant product contains two intramolecular disulfide bonds and a number of carbohydrate side chains.

Pharmacodynamics

Interleukin-11 acts through a specific cell surface cytokine receptor to stimulate the growth of multiple lymphoid and myeloid cells. It acts synergistically with other growth factors to stimulate the growth of primitive megakaryocytic progenitors and, most importantly, increases the number of peripheral platelets and neutrophils.

Acting through its own cytokine receptor, thrombopoietin also independently stimulates the growth of primitive megakaryocytic progenitors. In addition, it stimulates mature megakaryocytes and even activates mature platelets to respond to aggregation-inducing stimuli. The critical in vivo role of thrombopoietin has been demonstrated in genetically engineered knockout mice who lack either thrombopoietin or its receptor. These mice have marked thrombocytopenia but do not display anemia or leukopenia.

Clinical Pharmacology

Patients with thrombocytopenia have a high risk of hemorrhage. Although platelet transfusion is commonly used to treat thrombocytopenia, this procedure can cause adverse reactions in the recipient; furthermore, a significant number of patients fail to exhibit the expected increase in platelet count.

Interleukin-11 is the first growth factor to gain FDA approval for treatment of thrombocytopenia. It is approved for the secondary prevention of thrombocytopenia in patients receiving cytotoxic chemotherapy for treatment of nonmyeloid cancers. Clinical trials show that it reduces the number of platelet transfusions required by patients who experience severe thrombocytopenia after a previous cycle of chemotherapy. Although IL-11 has broad stimulatory effects on hematopoietic cell lineages in vitro, it does not appear to have significant effects on the leukopenia caused by myelosuppressive chemotherapy. Interleukin-11 is given by subcutaneous injection at a dose of 50 mcg/kg/d. It is started 6–24 hours after completion of chemotherapy and continued for 14–21 days or until the platelet count passes the nadir and rises to > 50,000 cells/μL.

Recombinant thrombopoietin is still an investigational agent. The primary focus of current clinical trials is for the treatment of chemotherapy-induced thrombocytopenia and thrombocytopenia accompanying hematologic stem cell transplantation.

Toxicity

The most common adverse effects of interleukin-11 are fatigue, headache, dizziness, and cardiovascular effects. The cardiovascular effects include anemia (due to hemodilution), dyspnea (due to fluid accumulation in the lungs), and transient atrial arrhythmias. Hypokalemia has also been seen in some patients. All of these adverse effects appear to be reversible. In the limited clinical trial data available thus far, recombinant thrombopoietin appears to be well tolerated.

PREPARATIONS AVAILABLE

Darbepoetin alfa (Aranesp)
Parenteral: 25, 40, 60, 100, 200, 300, 500 mcg/mL for IV or SC injection
Deferasirox (Exjade)
Oral: 125, 250, 500 mg tablets
Deferoxamine (generic, Desferal)
Parenteral: 500, 2000 mg vials for IM, SC, or IV injection
Epoetin alfa (erythropoietin, EPO) (Epogen, Procrit)
Parenteral: 2000, 3000, 4000, 10000, 20000, 40000 IU/mL vials for IV or SC injection
Filgrastim (G-CSF) (Neupogen)
Parenteral: 300 mcg vials for IV or SC injection
Folic acid (folacin, pteroylglutamic acid) (generic)
Oral: 0.4, 0.8, 1 mg tablets
Parenteral: 5 mg/mL for injection
Iron (generic)
Oral: See Table 33–2.
Parenteral (Iron dextran) (InFeD, DexFerrum): 50 mg elemental iron/mL

Parenteral (Sodium ferric gluconate complex) (Ferrlecit): 12.5 mg elemental iron/mL
Parenteral (Iron sucrose)(Venofer): 20 mg elemental iron/mL
Oprelvekin (interleukin-11) (Neumega)
Parenteral: 5 mg vials for SC injection
Pegfilgrastim (Neulasta)
Parenteral: 10 mg/mL solution in single-dose syringe
Sargramostim (GM-CSF) (Leukine)
Parenteral: 250, 500 mcg vials for IV infusion
Vitamin B$_{12}$ (generic cyanocobalamin or hydroxocobalamin)
Oral (cyanocobalamin): 100, 500, 1000, 5000 mcg tablets, 100, 250, 500 mcg lozenges
Nasal (Nascobal): 5000 mcg/mL (500 mcg/spray)
Parenteral (cyanocobalamin): 100, 1000 mcg/mL for IM or SC injection
Parenteral (hydroxocobalamin): 1000 mcg/mL for IM injection only

REFERENCES

Anderson GJ et al: Mechanisms of haem and non-haem iron absorption: Lessons from inherited disorders of iron metabolism. Biometals 2005;18:339.

American Society of Clinical Oncology Supportive Care and Quality of Life Practice Guidelines Website: http://www.asco.org/portal/site/ASCO/menuitem.509189bfd2c2bf5ca7ffa807320041a0/?vgnextoid=04d61f886024a010VgnVCM100000ed730ad1RCRD

Crawford J et al: Reduction by granulocyte colony-stimulating factor of fever and neutropenia induced by chemotherapy in patients with small-cell lung cancer. N Engl J Med 1991;325:164.

Cook JD: Diagnosis and management of iron-deficiency anaemia. Best Pract Res Clin Haematol 2005;18:309.

Du X, Williams DA: Interleukin-11: Review of molecular, cell biology and clinical use. Blood 1997;89:3897.

Eschbach JW: Iron requirements in erythropoietin therapy. Best Pract Res Clin Haematol 2005;18:347.

Fetscher S, Mertelsmann R: Supportive care in hematological malignancies: Hematopoietic growth factors, infections, transfusion therapy. Curr Opin Hematol 1999;6:262.

Fisher JW: Erythropoietin: Physiology and pharmacology update. Exp Biol Med 2003;228:1.

Gazitt Y: Comparison between granulocyte colony-stimulating factor and granulocyte-macrophage colony stimulating factor in the mobilization of peripheral blood stem cells. Curr Opin Hematol 2002;9:190.

Green R, Miller JW: Folate deficiency beyond megaloblastic anemia: Hyperhomocysteinemia and other manifestations of dysfunctional folate status. Semin Hematol 1999;36:47.

Harker LA: Physiology and clinical applications of platelet growth factors. Curr Opin Hematol 1999;6:127.

Jacques PF et al: The effects of folic acid fortification on plasma folate and total homocysteine concentrations. N Engl J Med 1999;340:1449.

Kuter DJ, Begley CG: Recombinant human thrombopoietin: Basic biology and evaluation of clinical studies. Blood 2002; 100:3457.

Rothenberg SP: Increasing the dietary intake of folate: Pros and cons. Semin Hematol 1999;36:65.

Shpall EJ: The utilization of cytokines in stem cell mobilization strategies. Bone Marrow Transplant 1999;23(Suppl 2):S13.

Drugs Used in Disorders of Coagulation

34

James L. Zehnder, MD

Hemostasis refers to the finely regulated dynamic process of maintaining fluidity of the blood, repairing vascular injury, and limiting blood loss while avoiding vessel occlusion (thrombosis) and inadequate perfusion of vital organs. Either extreme—excessive bleeding or thrombosis—represents a breakdown of the hemostatic mechanism. Common causes of dysregulated hemostasis include hereditary or acquired defects in the clotting mechanism and secondary effects of infection or cancer. The drugs used to limit abnormal bleeding and to inhibit thrombosis are the subjects of this chapter.

MECHANISMS OF BLOOD COAGULATION

The vascular endothelial cell layer lining blood vessels has an anticoagulant phenotype, and circulating blood platelets and clotting factors do not normally adhere to it to an appreciable extent. In the setting of vascular injury, the endothelial cell layer rapidly undergoes a series of changes resulting in a more procoagulant phenotype. Injury exposes reactive subendothelial matrix proteins such as collagen and von Willebrand factor, which results in platelet adherence and activation, and secretion and synthesis of vasoconstrictors and platelet-recruiting and activating molecules. Thus, **thromboxane A_2 (TXA$_2$)** is synthesized from arachadonic acid within platelets and is a platelet activator and potent vasoconstrictor. Products secreted from platelet granules include **adenosine diphosphate (ADP),** a powerful inducer of platelet aggregation, and **serotonin (5-HT),** which stimulates aggregation and vasoconstriction. Activation of platelets results in a conformational change in the $\alpha_{IIb}\beta_{III}$ integrin (IIb/IIIa) receptor, enabling it to bind fibrinogen, which cross-links adjacent platelets, resulting in aggregation and formation of a platelet plug (Figure 34–1). Simultaneously, the coagulation system cascade is activated, resulting in thrombin generation and a fibrin clot, which stabilizes the platelet plug (see below). Knowledge of the hemostatic mechanism is important for diagnosis of bleeding disorders. Patients with defects in the formation of the primary platelet plug (defects in primary hemostasis, eg, platelet function defects, von Willebrand disease) typically bleed from mucosal sites (gingiva, skin, heavy menses) with injury. In contrast, patients with defects in the clotting mechanism (secondary hemostasis, eg, hemophilia A) tend to bleed into deep tissues (joints, muscle, retroperitoneum), often with no apparent inciting event, and bleeding may recur unpredictably.

The platelet is central to normal hemostasis and thromboembolic disease, and is the target of many therapies discussed in this chapter. Platelet-rich thrombi **(white thrombi)** form in the high flow rate and high shear force environment of arteries. Occlusive arterial thrombi cause serious disease by producing downstream ischemia of extremities or vital organs, and can result in limb amputation or organ failure. Venous clots tend to be more fibrin-rich, contain large numbers of trapped red blood cells, and are recognized pathologically as **red thrombi.** Venous thrombi can cause severe swelling and pain of the affected extremity, but the most feared consequence is pulmonary embolism. This occurs when part or all of the clot breaks off from its location in the deep venous system and travels as an embolus through the right side of the heart and into the pulmonary arterial circulation. Sudden occlusion of a large pulmonary artery can cause acute right heart failure and sudden death. In addition lung ischemia or infarction will occur distal to the occluded pulmonary arterial segment. Such emboli usually arise from the deep venous system of the proximal lower extremities or pelvis. Although all thrombi are mixed, the platelet nidus dominates the arterial thrombus and the fibrin tail dominates the venous thrombus.

BLOOD COAGULATION CASCADE

Blood coagulates by the transformation of soluble fibrinogen into insoluble fibrin. Several circulating proteins interact in a cascading series of limited proteolytic reactions (Figure 34–2). At each step, a clotting factor zymogen undergoes limited proteolysis and becomes an

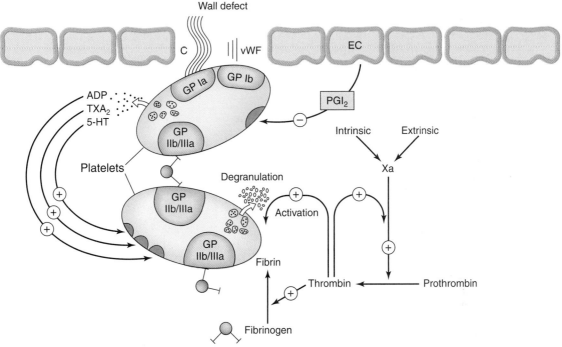

Figure 34–1. Thrombus formation at the site of the damaged vascular wall (EC, endothelial cell) and the role of platelets and clotting factors. Platelet membrane receptors include the glycoprotein (GP) Ia receptor, binding to collagen (C); GP Ib receptor binding von Willebrand factor (vWF), and GP IIb/IIIa, which binds fibrinogen and other macromolecules. Antiplatelet prostacyclin (PGI$_2$) is released from the endothelium. Aggregating substances released from the degranulating platelet include adenosine diphosphate (ADP), thromboxane A$_2$ (TXA$_2$), and serotonin (5-HT). Production of factor Xa is detailed in Figure 34–2. (Redrawn and reproduced, with permission, from Simoons ML, Decker JW: New directions in anticoagulant and antiplatelet treatment. [Editorial.] Br Heart J 1995;74:337.)

active protease (eg, factor VII is converted to factor VIIa). Each protease factor activates the next clotting factor in the sequence, culminating in the formation of thrombin (factor IIa). Several of these factors are targets for drug therapy (Table 34–1).

Thrombin has a central role in hemostasis and has many functions. In clotting, thrombin proteolytically cleaves small peptides from fibrinogen, allowing fibrinogen to polymerize and form a fibrin clot. Thrombin also activates many upstream clotting factors, leading to more thrombin generation, and activates factor XIII, a transaminase that cross-links the fibrin polymer and stabilizes the clot. Thrombin is a potent platelet activator and mitogen. Thrombin also exerts *anti*coagulant effects by activating the protein C pathway, which attenuates the clotting response (Figure 34–2). It should therefore be apparent that the response to vascular injury is a complex and precisely modulated process that ensures that under normal circumstances, repair of

vascular injury occurs without thrombosis and downstream ischemia; that is, the response is proportionate and reversible. Eventually vascular remodeling and repair occur with reversion to the quiescent resting anticoagulant endothelial cell phenotype.

Initiation of Clotting: The Tissue Factor-VIIa Complex

The main initiator of blood coagulation in vivo is the tissue factor (TF)-factor VIIa pathway (Figure 34–2). Tissue factor is a transmembrane protein ubiquitously expressed outside the vasculature, but not normally expressed in an active form within vessels. The exposure of TF on damaged endothelium or to blood that has extravasated into tissue binds TF to factor VIIa. This complex, in turn, activates factors X and IX. Factor Xa along with factor Va forms the prothrombinase complex on activated cell surfaces, which catalyzes the

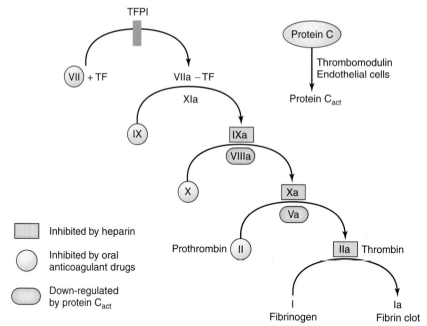

Figure 34–2. A model of blood coagulation. With tissue factor (TF), factor VII forms an activated complex (VIIa-TF) that catalyzes the activation of factor IX to factor IXa. Activated factor XIa also catalyzes this reaction. Tissue factor pathway inhibitor (TFPI) inhibits the catalytic action of the VIIa-TF complex. The cascade proceeds as shown, resulting ultimately in the conversion of fibrinogen to fibrin, an essential component of a functional clot. The two major anticoagulant drugs, heparin and warfarin (an oral anticoagulant), have very different actions. Heparin, acting in the blood, directly activates anticlotting factors, specifically antithrombin, which inactivates the factors enclosed in rectangles. Warfarin, acting in the liver, inhibits the synthesis of the factors enclosed in circles. Proteins C and S exert anticlotting effects by inactivating activated factors Va and VIIIa.

conversion of prothrombin (factor II) to thrombin (factor IIa). Thrombin, in turn, activates upstream clotting factors, primarily factors V, VIII, and XI, resulting in amplification of thrombin generation. The TF-factor VIIa-catalyzed activation of factor Xa is regulated by tissue factor pathway inhibitor (TFPI). Thus after initial activation of factor X to Xa by TF-VIIa, further propagation of the clot is by feedback amplification of thrombin through the intrinsic pathway factors VIII and IX (this provides an explanation of why patients with deficiency of factor VIII or IX—hemophilia A and hemophilia B, respectively—have a severe bleeding disorder).

It is also important to note that the coagulation mechanism in vivo does not occur in solution, but is localized to activated *cell surfaces* expressing anionic phospholipids such as phosphatidylserine, and is mediated by Ca^{2+} bridging between the anionic phospholip-

ids and γ-carboxyglutamic acid residues of the clotting factors. This is the basis for using calcium chelators such as ethylenediamine tetraacetic acid (EDTA) or citrate to prevent blood from clotting in a test tube.

Antithrombin (AT) is an endogenous anticoagulant and a member of the serine protease inhibitor (serpin) family; it inactivates the serine proteases IIa, IXa, Xa, XIa, and XIIa. The endogenous anticoagulants **protein C** and **protein S** attenuate the blood clotting cascade by proteolysis of the two cofactors Va and VIIIa. From an evolutionary standpoint, it is of interest that factors V and VIII have an identical overall domain structure and considerable homology, consistent with a common ancestor gene; likewise the serine proteases are descendents of a trypsin-like common ancestor. Thus, the TF-VIIa initiating complex, serine proteases, and cofactors each have their own lineage-specific attenuation mechanism (see Figure 34–2). Defects in natural anticoagu-

Table 34–1. Blood clotting factors and drugs that affect them.[1]

Component or Factor	Common Synonym	Target for the Action of:
I	Fibrinogen	
II	Prothrombin	Heparin (IIa); warfarin (synthesis)
III	Tissue thromboplastin	
IV	Calcium	
V	Proaccelerin	
VII	Proconvertin	Warfarin (synthesis)
VIII	Antihemophilic factor (AHF)	
IX	Christmas factor, plasma thromboplastin component (PTC)	Warfarin (synthesis)
X	Stuart-Prower factor	Heparin (Xa); warfarin (synthesis)
XI	Plasma thromboplastin antecedent (PTA)	
XII	Hageman factor	
XIII	Fibrin-stabilizing factor	
Proteins C and S		Warfarin (synthesis)
Plasminogen		Thrombolytic enzymes, aminocaproic acid

[1]See Figure 34–2 and text for additional details.

lants result in an increased risk of venous thrombosis. The most common defect in the natural anticoagulant system is a mutation in factor V (factor V Leiden), which results in resistance to inactivation by the protein C, protein S mechanism.

Fibrinolysis

Fibrinolysis refers to the process of fibrin digestion by the fibrin-specific protease, plasmin. The fibrinolytic system is similar to the coagulation system in that the precursor form of the serine protease plasmin circulates in an inactive form as plasminogen. In response to injury, endothelial cells synthesize and release tissue plasminogen activator (t-PA), which converts plasminogen to plasmin (Figure 34–3). Plasmin remodels the thrombus and limits its extension by proteolytic digestion of fibrin.

Both plasminogen and plasmin have specialized protein domains (kringles) that bind to exposed lysines on the fibrin clot and impart clot specificity to the fibrinolytic process. It should be noted that this clot specificity is only observed at *physiologic* levels of t-PA. At the *pharmacologic* levels of t-PA used in thrombolytic therapy, clot specificity is lost and a systemic lytic state is created, with attendant increase in bleeding risk. As in the coagulation cascade, there are negative regulators of fibrinolysis:

endothelial cells synthesize and release plasminogen activator inhibitor (PAI), which inhibits t-PA; in addition α_2 antiplasmin circulates in the blood at high concentrations and under physiologic conditions will rapidly inactivate any plasmin that is not clot-bound. However, this regulatory system is overwhelmed by therapeutic doses of plasminogen activators.

If the coagulation and fibrinolytic systems are pathologically activated, the hemostatic system may careen out of control, leading to generalized intravascular clotting and bleeding. This process is called **disseminated intravascular coagulation (DIC)** and may follow massive tissue injury, advanced cancers, obstetric emergencies such as abruptio placentae or retained products of conception, or bacterial sepsis. The treatment of DIC is to control the underlying disease process; if this is not possible, DIC is often fatal.

Regulation of the fibrinolytic system is useful in therapeutics. Increased fibrinolysis is effective therapy for thrombotic disease. **Tissue plasminogen activator, urokinase,** and **streptokinase** all activate the fibrinolytic system (Figure 34–3). Conversely, decreased fibrinolysis protects clots from lysis and reduces the bleeding of hemostatic failure. **Aminocaproic acid** is a clinically useful inhibitor of fibrinolysis. Heparin and the oral anticoagulant drugs do not affect the fibrinolytic mechanism.

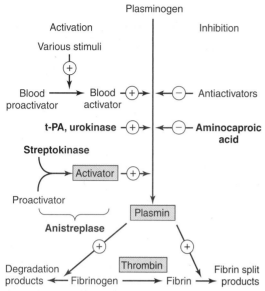

Plasminogen

Activation | Inhibition

Various stimuli

Blood proactivator → Blood activator ⊕ → ← ⊖ Antiactivators

t-PA, urokinase ⊕ → ← ⊖ **Aminocaproic acid**

Streptokinase

Activator ⊕ →

Proactivator

Anistreplase

Plasmin

⊕ ⊕

Degradation products ← Fibrinogen → Fibrin → Fibrin split products

Thrombin

Figure 34–3. Schematic representation of the fibrinolytic system. Plasmin is the active fibrinolytic enzyme. Several clinically useful activators are shown on the left in bold. Anistreplase is a combination of streptokinase and the proactivator plasminogen. Aminocaproic acid (right) inhibits the activation of plasminogen to plasmin and is useful in some bleeding disorders. (t-PA, tissue plasminogen activator.)

■ I. BASIC PHARMACOLOGY OF THE ANTICOAGULANT DRUGS

The ideal anticoagulant drug would prevent pathologic thrombosis and limit reperfusion injury, yet allow a normal response to vascular injury and limit bleeding. Theoretically this could be accomplished by preservation of the TF-VIIa initiation phase of the clotting mechanism with attenuation of the secondary intrinsic pathway propagation phase of clot development. At this time such a drug does not exist; all anticoagulants and fibrinolytic drugs have an increased bleeding risk as their principle toxicity.

INDIRECT THROMBIN INHIBITORS

The indirect thrombin inhibitors are so-named because their antithrombotic effect is exerted by their interaction with a separate protein, antithrombin. **Unfractionated heparin (UFH), low-molecular-weight heparin (LMWH),** and the synthetic pentasaccharide **fonda-** **parinux** bind to antithrombin and enhance its inactivation of factor Xa. Unfractionated heparin and to a lesser extent LMWH also enhance antithrombin's inactivation of thrombin.

HEPARIN

Chemistry & Mechanism of Action

Heparin is a heterogeneous mixture of sulfated mucopolysaccharides. It binds to endothelial cell surfaces and a variety of plasma proteins. Its biologic activity is dependent upon the endogenous anticoagulant **antithrombin.** Antithrombin inhibits clotting factor proteases, especially thrombin (IIa), IXa, and Xa, by forming equimolar stable complexes with them. In the absence of heparin, these reactions are slow; in the presence of heparin, they are accelerated 1000-fold. Only about a third of the molecules in commercial heparin preparations have an accelerating effect because the remainder lack the unique pentasaccharide sequence needed for high-affinity binding to antithrombin (Figure 34–4). The active heparin molecules bind tightly to antithrombin and cause a conformational change in this inhibitor. The conformational change of antithrombin exposes its active site for more rapid interaction with the proteases (the activated clotting factors). Heparin functions as a cofactor for the antithrombin-protease reaction without being consumed. Once the antithrombin-protease complex is formed, heparin is released intact for renewed binding to more antithrombin.

The antithrombin binding region of commercial unfractionated heparin consists of repeating sulfated disaccharide units composed of D-glucosamine-L-iduronic acid and D-glucosamine-D-glucuronic acid (Figure 34–4). High-molecular-weight fractions of heparin with high affinity for antithrombin markedly inhibit blood coagulation by inhibiting all three factors, especially thrombin and factor Xa. Unfractionated heparin has a molecular weight range of 5000–30,000. In contrast, the shorter-chain low-molecular-weight (LMW) fractions of heparin inhibit activated factor X but have less effect on thrombin than the HMW species. Nevertheless, numerous studies have demonstrated that LMW heparins such as **enoxaparin, dalteparin,** and **tinzaparin** are effective in several thromboembolic conditions. In fact, these LMW heparins—in comparison with UFH—have equal efficacy, increased bioavailability from the subcutaneous site of injection, and less frequent dosing requirements (once or twice daily is sufficient).

Because commercial heparin consists of a family of molecules of different molecular weights, the correlation between the concentration of a given heparin preparation and its effect on coagulation often is poor. Therefore, UFH is standardized by bioassay. Heparin sodium USP must contain at least 120 USP units per

Figure 34–4. Subunit structure of heparin. The small polymer section shown illustrates the repeating disaccharide units typical of heparin. The sequence shows the critical pentasaccharide portion required for binding to antithrombin. In addition to those shown, other saccharides occur. Heparin is a strongly acidic molecule because of its high content of anionic sulfate and carboxylic acid groups. (GlcN, glucosamine; IdUA, iduronic acid; GlcUA, glucuronic acid. The same five residues with the terminal groups shown in parentheses, constitute fondaparinux.)

milligram. Heparin is generally used as the sodium salt, but calcium heparin is equally effective. Lithium heparin is used in vitro as an anticoagulant for blood samples. Commercial heparin is extracted from porcine intestinal mucosa and bovine lung. Enoxaparin is obtained from the same sources as regular heparin, but doses are specified in milligrams. Dalteparin, tinzaparin and danaparoid (an LMW heparanoid containing heparan sulfate, dermatan sulfate, and chondroitin sulfate), on the other hand, are specified in anti-factor Xa units.

Monitoring of Heparin Effect

Close monitoring of the **activated partial thromboplastin time (aPTT)** is necessary in patients receiving UFH. Levels of UFH may also be determined by protamine titration (therapeutic levels 0.2–0.4 unit/mL) or anti-Xa units (therapeutic levels 0.3–0.7 unit/mL). Weight-based dosing of the LMW heparins results in predictable pharmacokinetics and plasma levels in patients with normal renal function. Therefore, LMW heparin levels are not generally measured except in the setting of renal insufficiency, obesity, and pregnancy. LMW heparin levels can be determined by anti-Xa units. Peak therapeutic levels should be 0.5–1 unit/mL for twice-daily dosing, determined 4 hours after administration, and approximately 1.5 units/mL for once-daily dosing.

Toxicity

A. BLEEDING

The major adverse effect of heparin is bleeding. This risk can be decreased by scrupulous patient selection, careful control of dosage, and close monitoring. Elderly women and patients with renal failure are more prone to hemorrhage. Heparin is of animal origin and should be used cautiously in patients with allergy. Increased

loss of hair and reversible alopecia have been reported. Long-term heparin therapy is associated with osteoporosis and spontaneous fractures. Heparin accelerates the clearing of postprandial lipemia by causing the release of lipoprotein lipase from tissues, and long-term use is associated with mineralocorticoid deficiency.

B. HEPARIN-INDUCED THROMBOCYTOPENIA

Heparin-induced thrombocytopenia (HIT) is a systemic hypercoagulable state that occurs in 1–4% of individuals treated with UFH for a minimum of 7 days. Surgical patients are at greatest risk. The reported incidence of HIT is lower in pediatric populations outside the critical care setting and is relatively rare in pregnant women. The risk of HIT may be higher in individuals treated with UFH of bovine origin compared with porcine heparin and is lower in those treated exclusively with LMWH.

Morbidity and mortality in HIT are related to thrombotic events. Venous thrombosis occurs most commonly, but occlusion of peripheral or central arteries is not infrequent. If an indwelling catheter is present, the risk of thrombosis is increased in that extremity. Skin necrosis has been described, particularly in individuals treated with warfarin in the absence of a direct thrombin inhibitor, presumably due to acute depletion of the vitamin K-dependent anticoagulant protein C occurring in the presence of high levels of procoagulant proteins and an active hypercoagulable state.

The following points should be considered in all patients receiving heparin: Platelet counts should be performed frequently; thrombocytopenia appearing in a time frame consistent with an immune response to heparin should be considered suspicious for HIT; and any new thrombus occuring in a patient receiving heparin therapy should raise suspicion of HIT. Patients who develop HIT are treated by discontinuance of heparin and administration of a direct thrombin inhibitor or fondaparinux (see below).

Contraindications

Heparin is contraindicated in patients with HIT, hypersensitivity to the drug, active bleeding, hemophilia, significant thrombocytopenia, purpura, severe hypertension, intracranial hemorrhage, infective endocarditis, active tuberculosis, ulcerative lesions of the gastrointestinal tract, threatened abortion, visceral carcinoma, or advanced hepatic or renal disease. Heparin should be avoided in patients who have recently had surgery of the brain, spinal cord, or eye, and in patients who are undergoing lumbar puncture or regional anesthetic block. Despite the apparent lack of placental transfer, heparin should be used in pregnant women only when clearly indicated.

Administration & Dosage

The indications for the use of heparin are described in the section on clinical pharmacology. A plasma concentration of heparin of 0.2–0.4 unit/mL (by protamine titration) or 0.3–0.7 unit/mL (anti-Xa units) usually prevents pulmonary emboli in patients with established venous thrombosis. This concentration of heparin will prolong the aPTT to 2–2.5 times that of the control value. This degree of anticoagulant effect should be maintained throughout the course of *continuous* intravenous heparin therapy. When *intermittent* heparin administration is used, the aPTT should be measured 6 hours after the administered dose to maintain prolongation of the aPTT to 2–2.5 times that of the control value.

Continuous intravenous administration of heparin is accomplished via an infusion pump. After an initial bolus injection of 80–100 units/kg, a continuous infusion of about 15–22 units/kg/h is required to maintain the aPTT at 2–2.5 times control. Patients with acute pulmonary emboli often require larger doses during the first few days because of binding to a variety of acute phase proteins, such as factor VIII and von Willebrand factor, and increased heparin clearance. Low-dose prophylaxis is achieved with subcutaneous administration of heparin, 5000 units every 8–12 hours. Because of the danger of hematoma formation at the injection site, heparin must never be administered intramuscularly.

Prophylactic enoxaparin is given subcutaneously in a dosage of 30 mg twice daily or 40 mg once daily. Full-dose enoxaparin therapy is 1 mg/kg subcutaneously every 12 hours. This corresponds to a therapeutic anti-factor Xa level of 0.5–1 unit/mL. Selected patients may be treated with enoxaparin 1.5 mg/kg once a day, with a target anti-Xa level of 1.5 units/mL. The prophylactic dose of dalteparin is 5000 units subcutaneously once a day; therapeutic dosing is 200 units/kg once a day for venous disease or 120 units/kg every 12 hours for acute coronary syndrome. Low-molecular-weight heparins should be used with caution in patients with renal insufficiency or body weight greater than 150 kg. Measurement of the anti-Xa level is useful to guide dosing in these individuals.

The synthetic pentasaccharide molecule fondaparinux (Figure 34–4) avidly binds antithrombin with high specific activity, resulting in efficient inactivation of factor Xa. Fondaparinux has a long half-life of 15 hours, allowing for once-daily dosing by subcutaneous administration. Fondaparinux is effective in the prevention and treatment of venous thromboembolism, and appears to not cross-react with pathologic HIT antibodies in most individuals. The use of fondaparinux as an alternative anticoagulant in HIT is currently being tested in clinical trials. Pharmaceutical companies have put much effort into developing an orally bioavailable anti-Xa inhibitor. The first of these have recently completed phase I clinical trials with promising results and are currently being evaluated for efficacy in prophylaxis and treatment of venous thromboembolism.

Reversal of Heparin Action

Excessive anticoagulant action of heparin is treated by discontinuance of the drug. If bleeding occurs, administration of a specific antagonist such as protamine sulfate is indicated. Protamine is a highly basic peptide that combines with heparin as an ion pair to form a stable complex devoid of anticoagulant activity. For every 100 units of heparin remaining in the patient, 1 mg of protamine sulfate is given intravenously; the rate of infusion should not exceed 50 mg in any 10-minute period. Excess protamine must be avoided; it also has an anticoagulant effect. Neutralization of LMW heparin by protamine is incomplete. Limited experience suggests that 1 mg of protamine sulfate may be used to partially neutralize 1 mg of enoxaparin. Protamine will not reverse the activity of fondaparinux. Excess danaparoid can be removed by plasmapheresis.

■ DIRECT THROMBIN INHIBITORS

The direct thrombin inhibitors (DTIs) exert their anticoagulant effect by directly binding to the active site of thrombin, thereby inhibiting thrombin's downstream effects. This is in contrast to indirect thrombin inhibitors such as heparin and LMWH (see above), which act through antithrombin. **Hirudin** and **bivalirudin** are bivalent DTIs in that they bind at both the catalytic or active site of thrombin as well as at a substrate recognition site. **Argatroban** and **melagatran** are small molecules that bind only at the thrombin active site.

Leeches have been used for bloodletting since the age of Hippocrates. More recently, surgeons have used medicinal leeches *(Hirudo medicinalis)* to prevent thrombosis in the fine vessels of reattached digits. **Hirudin** is a specific, irreversible thrombin inhibitor from leech saliva that is now available in recombinant form as **lepirudin.** Its action is independent of antithrombin, which means it can reach and inactivate fibrin-bound thrombin in thrombi. Lepirudin has little effect on platelets or the bleeding time. Like heparin, it must be administered parenterally and is monitored by the aPTT. Lepirudin is approved by the Food and Drug Administration for use in patients with thrombosis related to heparin-induced thrombocytopenia. Lepirudin is excreted by the kidney and should be used with great caution in patients with renal insufficiency as no antidote exists. Up to 40% of patients who receive long-term infusions develop an antibody directed against the thrombin-lepirudin complex. These antigen-antibody complexes are not cleared by the kidney and may result in an enhanced anticoagulant effect. Some patients re-exposed to the drug have developed life-threatening anaphylactic reactions.

Bivalirudin, another bivalent inhibitor of thrombin, is administered intravenously, with a rapid onset and offset of action. The drug has a short half-life with clearance that is 20% renal and the remainder metabolic. Bivalirudin also inhibits platelet activation and has been FDA-approved for use in percutaneous coronary angioplasty.

Argatroban is a small molecule thrombin inhibitor that is FDA-approved for use in patients with HIT with or without thrombosis and coronary angioplasty in patients with HIT. It, too, has a short half-life, is given by continuous intravenous infusion, and is monitored by aPTT. Its clearance is not affected by renal disease but is dependent on liver function; dose reduction is required in patients with liver disease. Patients on argatroban will demonstrate elevated international normalized ratios (INRs), rendering the transition to warfarin difficult (ie, the INR will reflect contributions from both warfarin and argatroban). (INR is discussed in detail in the discussion of warfarin administration.) A nomogram is supplied by the manufacturer to assist in this transition. No properly designed head-to-head trials have been performed to determine whether argatroban or lepirudin is superior in the treatment of HIT. However in practice, the choice of which DTI to use in a patient with HIT is usually dictated by the condition of the clearing organ. If the patient has severe renal insufficiency, then argatroban would be preferred. If there is severe hepatic insufficiency, then lepirudin would be a better choice.

Ximelagatran is an oral prodrug that is metabolized to the DTI melagatran. Potential advantages of ximelagatran include predictable pharmacokinetics and bioavailability. This allows for fixed dosing and predictable anticoagulant response; no need for routine coagulation monitoring; lack of interaction with P450-interacting drugs; and rapid onset and offset of action, which allow for immediate anticoagulation and thus no need for overlap with additional anticoagulant drugs. While clinical trials found that ximelagatran was as effective as other anticoagulants in venous thromboembolism and atrial fibrillation, hepatic toxicity was observed in 5–10% of individuals treated for more than one month. Thus while there is much enthusiasm for a nontoxic oral anticoagulant that might replace warfarin and not require routine monitoring, no such drug is currently FDA-approved.

WARFARIN & THE COUMARIN ANTICOAGULANTS

Chemistry & Pharmacokinetics

The clinical use of the coumarin anticoagulants began with the discovery of an anticoagulant substance formed in spoiled sweet clover silage which caused hemorrhagic disease in cattle. At the behest of local farmers, a chemist at the University of Wisconsin identified the toxic agent as bishydroxycoumarin. A synthesized derivative, dicumarol and its congeners, most notably warfarin (**W**isconsin **A**lumni **R**esearch **F**oundation, with "arin" from coumarin added; Figure 34–5), were initially used as rodenticides. In the 1950s warfarin (under the brand name Coumadin) was introduced as an antithrombotic agent in humans. Warfarin is one of the most commonly prescribed drugs, used by approximately 1.5 million individuals, and several studies have indicated that the drug is significantly underused in clinical situations where it has proven benefit.

Warfarin is generally administered as the sodium salt and has 100% bioavailability. Over 99% of racemic warfarin is bound to plasma albumin, which may contribute to its small volume of distribution (the albumin space), its long half-life in plasma (36 hours), and the lack of urinary excretion of unchanged drug. Warfarin used clinically is a racemic mixture composed of equal amounts of two enantiomorphs. The levorotatory *S*-warfarin is four times more potent than the dextrorotatory *R*-warfarin. This observation is useful in understanding the stereoselective nature of several drug interactions involving warfarin.

Mechanism of Action

Coumarin anticoagulants block the γ-carboxylation of several glutamate residues in prothrombin and factors VII, IX, and X as well as the endogenous anticoagulant

Dicumarol

Warfarin sodium

Phenindione

Phytonadione (vitamin K_1)

Figure 34–5. Structural formulas of several oral anticoagulant drugs and of vitamin K. The carbon atom of warfarin shown at the asterisk is an asymmetric center.

proteins C and S (See Figure 34–2, Table 34–1). The blockade results in incomplete coagulation factor molecules that are biologically inactive. The protein carboxylation reaction is coupled to the oxidation of vitamin K. The vitamin must then be reduced to reactivate it. Warfarin prevents reductive metabolism of the inactive vitamin K epoxide back to its active hydroquinone form (Figure 34–6). Mutational change of the responsible enzyme, vitamin K epoxide reductase, can give rise to genetic resistance to warfarin in humans and especially in rats.

There is an 8- to 12-hour delay in the action of warfarin. Its anticoagulant effect results from a balance between partially inhibited synthesis and unaltered degradation of the four vitamin K-dependent clotting factors. The resulting inhibition of coagulation is dependent on their degradation half-lives in the circulation. These half-lives are 6, 24, 40, and 60 hours for factors VII, IX, X, and II, respectively. Larger initial doses of warfarin—up to about 0.75 mg/kg—hasten the onset of the anticoagulant effect. Beyond this dosage, the speed of onset is independent of the dose size. The only effect of a larger loading dose is to prolong the time that the plasma concentration of drug remains above that required for suppression of clotting factor synthesis. The only difference among oral anticoagulants in producing and maintaining hypoprothrombinemia is the half-life of each drug.

Toxicity

Warfarin crosses the placenta readily and can cause a hemorrhagic disorder in the fetus. Furthermore, fetal proteins with γ-carboxyglutamate residues found in bone and blood may be affected by warfarin; the drug

Figure 34–6. Vitamin K cycle—metabolic interconversions of vitamin K associated with the synthesis of vitamin K–dependent clotting factors. Vitamin K_1 or K_2 is activated by reduction to the hydroquinone form (KH_2). Stepwise oxidation to vitamin K epoxide (KO) is coupled to prothrombin carboxylation by the enzyme carboxylase. The reactivation of vitamin K epoxide is the warfarin-sensitive step (warfarin). The *R* on the vitamin K molecule represents a 20-carbon phytyl side chain in vitamin K_1 and a 30- to 65-carbon polyprenyl side chain in vitamin K_2.

can cause a serious birth defect characterized by abnormal bone formation. Thus, warfarin should never be administered during pregnancy. Cutaneous necrosis with reduced activity of protein C sometimes occurs during the first weeks of therapy. Rarely, the same process causes frank infarction of the breast, fatty tissues, intestine, and extremities. The pathologic lesion associated with the hemorrhagic infarction is venous thrombosis, suggesting that it is caused by warfarin-induced depression of protein C synthesis.

Administration & Dosage

Treatment with warfarin should be initiated with standard doses of 5–10 mg rather than the large loading doses formerly used. The initial adjustment of the prothrombin time takes about 1 week, which usually results in a maintenance dose of 5–7 mg/d. The **prothrombin time (PT)** should be increased to a level representing a reduction of prothrombin activity to 25% of normal and maintained there for long-term therapy. When the activity is less than 20%, the warfarin dosage should be reduced or omitted until the activity rises above 20%.

The therapeutic range for oral anticoagulant therapy is defined in terms of an international normalized ratio (INR). The INR is the prothrombin time ratio (patient prothrombin time/mean of normal prothrombin time for lab)[ISI], where the ISI exponent refers to the International Sensitivity Index, and is dependent on the specific reagents and instruments used for the determination. The ISI serves to relate measured prothrombin times to a World Health Organization reference standard thromboplastin; thus the prothrombin times performed on different properly calibrated instruments with a variety of thromboplastin reagents should give the same INR results for a given sample. For most reagent and instrument combinations in current use, the ISI is close to 1, making the INR roughly the ratio of the patient prothrombin time to the mean normal prothrombin time. The recommended INR for prophylaxis and treatment of thrombotic disease is 2–3. Patients with some types of artificial heart valves (eg, tilting disk) or other medical conditions increasing thrombotic risk have a recommended range of 2.5–3.5.

Occasionally patients exhibit warfarin resistance, defined as progression or recurrence of a thrombotic event while in therapeutic range. These individuals may have their INR target raised (which is accompanied by an increase in bleeding risk) or be changed to an alternative form of anticoagulation (eg, daily injections of LMWH). Warfarin resistance is most commonly seen in patients with advanced cancers, typically of gastrointestinal origin (Trousseau's syndrome). A recent study has demonstrated the superiority of LMWH over warfarin in preventing recurrent venous thromboembolism in patients with cancer.

Drug Interactions

The oral anticoagulants often interact with other drugs and with disease states. These interactions can be broadly divided into pharmacokinetic and pharmacodynamic effects (Table 34–2). Pharmacokinetic mechanisms for drug interaction with oral anticoagulants are mainly enzyme induction, enzyme inhibition, and reduced plasma protein binding. Pharmacodynamic mechanisms for interactions with warfarin are synergism (impaired hemostasis, reduced clotting factor synthesis, as in hepatic disease), competitive antagonism (vitamin K), and an altered physiologic control loop for vitamin K (hereditary resistance to oral anticoagulants).

The most serious interactions with warfarin are those that increase the anticoagulant effect and the risk of bleed-

Table 34–2. Pharmacokinetic and pharmacodynamic drug and body interactions with oral anticoagulants.

Increased Prothrombin Time		Decreased Prothrombin Time	
Pharmacokinetic	Pharmacodynamic	Pharmacokinetic	Pharmacodynamic
Amiodarone	**Drugs**	Barbiturates	**Drugs**
Cimetidine	Aspirin (high doses)	Cholestyramine	Diuretics
Disulfiram	Cephalosporins, third-	Rifampin	Vitamin K
Metronidazole[1]	generation		**Body factors**
Fluconazole[1]	Heparin		Hereditary resistance
Phenylbutazone[1]	**Body factors**		Hypothyroidism
Sulfinpyrazone[1]	Hepatic disease		
Trimethoprim-	Hyperthyroidism		
sulfamethoxazole			

[1]Stereoselectively inhibits the oxidative metabolism of the (*S*)-warfarin enantiomorph of racemic warfarin.

ing. The most dangerous of these interactions are the pharmacokinetic interactions with the pyrazolones phenylbutazone and sulfinpyrazone. These drugs not only augment the hypoprothrombinemia but also inhibit platelet function and may induce peptic ulcer disease (see Chapter 36). The mechanisms for their hypoprothrombinemic interaction are a stereoselective inhibition of oxidative metabolic transformation of *S*-warfarin (the more potent isomer) and displacement of albumin-bound warfarin, increasing the free fraction. For this and other reasons, neither phenylbutazone nor sulfinpyrazone is in common use in the USA. Metronidazole, fluconazole, and trimethoprim-sulfamethoxazole also stereoselectively inhibit the metabolic transformation of *S*-warfarin, whereas amiodarone, disulfiram, and cimetidine inhibit metabolism of both enantiomorphs of warfarin. Aspirin, hepatic disease, and hyperthyroidism augment warfarin pharmacodynamically—aspirin by its effect on platelet function and the latter two by increasing the turnover rate of clotting factors. The third-generation cephalosporins eliminate the bacteria in the intestinal tract that produce vitamin K and, like warfarin, also directly inhibit vitamin K epoxide reductase.

Barbiturates and rifampin cause a marked *decrease* of the anticoagulant effect by induction of the hepatic enzymes that transform racemic warfarin. Cholestyramine binds warfarin in the intestine and reduces its absorption and bioavailability.

Pharmacodynamic reductions of anticoagulant effect occur with vitamin K (increased synthesis of clotting factors), the diuretics chlorthalidone and spironolactone (clotting factor concentration), hereditary resistance (mutation of vitamin K reactivation cycle molecules), and hypothyroidism (decreased turnover rate of clotting factors).

Drugs with *no* significant effect on anticoagulant therapy include ethanol, phenothiazines, benzodiazepines, acetaminophen, opioids, indomethacin, and most antibiotics.

Reversal of Warfarin Action

Excessive anticoagulant effect and bleeding from warfarin can be reversed by stopping the drug and administering oral or parenteral vitamin K_1 (phytonadione), fresh-frozen plasma, prothrombin complex concentrates such as Bebulin and Proplex T, and recombinant factor VIIa (rFVIIa). The disappearance of excessive effect is not correlated with plasma warfarin concentrations but rather with reestablishment of normal activity of the clotting factors. A modest excess of anticoagulant effect without bleeding may require no more than cessation of the drug. The warfarin effect can be rapidly reversed in the setting of severe bleeding with the administration of prothrombin complex or rFVIIa coupled with intravenous vitamin K. It is important to note that due to the long half life of warfarin, a single dose of vitamin K or rFVIIa may not be sufficient.

■ II. BASIC PHARMACOLOGY OF THE FIBRINOLYTIC DRUGS

Fibrinolytic drugs rapidly lyse thrombi by catalyzing the formation of the serine protease **plasmin** from its precursor zymogen, plasminogen (Figure 34–3). These drugs create a generalized lytic state when administered intravenously. Thus, both protective hemostatic thrombi and target thromboemboli are broken down. The Box: Thrombolytic Drugs for Acute Myocardial Infarction, describes the use of these drugs in one major application.

Pharmacology

Streptokinase is a protein (but not an enzyme in itself) synthesized by streptococci that combines with the proactivator plasminogen. This enzymatic complex catalyzes the conversion of inactive plasminogen to active plasmin. **Urokinase** is a human enzyme synthesized by the kidney that directly converts plasminogen to active plasmin. Plasmin itself cannot be used because naturally occurring inhibitors in plasma prevent its effects. However, the absence of inhibitors for urokinase and the streptokinase-proactivator complex permit their use clinically. Plasmin formed inside a thrombus by these activators is protected from plasma antiplasmins, which allows it to lyse the thrombus from within.

Anistreplase (anisoylated plasminogen streptokinase activator complex; APSAC) consists of a complex of purified human plasminogen and bacterial streptokinase that has been acylated to protect the enzyme's active site. When administered, the acyl group spontaneously hydrolyzes, freeing the activated streptokinase-proactivator complex. This product (recently discontinued in the USA) allows for rapid intravenous injection, greater clot selectivity (ie, more activity on plasminogen associated with clots than on free plasminogen in the blood), and more thrombolytic activity.

Plasminogen can also be activated endogenously by **tissue plasminogen activators (t-PAs).** These activators preferentially activate plasminogen that is bound to fibrin, which (in theory) confines fibrinolysis to the formed thrombus and avoids systemic activation. Human t-PA is manufactured as **alteplase** by means of recombinant DNA technology.

Reteplase is another recombinant human t-PA from which several amino acid sequences have been deleted. Reteplase is less expensive to produce than t-PA. Because it lacks the major fibrin-binding domain, reteplase is less fibrin-specific than t-PA. **Tenecteplase** is a mutant form of t-PA that has a longer half-life, and it can be given as an intravenous bolus. Tenecteplase is slightly more fibrin-specific than t-PA.

THROMBOLYTIC DRUGS FOR ACUTE MYOCARDIAL INFARCTION

The paradigm shift in 1980 on the causation of acute myocardial infarction to acute coronary occlusion by a thrombus created the rationale for thrombolytic therapy of this common lethal disease. At that time—and for the first time—intravenous thrombolytic therapy for acute myocardial infarction in the European Cooperative Study Group trial was found to reduce mortality significantly. Later studies, with thousands of patients in each trial, provided enough statistical power for the 20% reduction in mortality to be considered statistically significant. Although the standard of care in areas with adequate facilities and experience in percutaneous coronary intervention (PCI) now favors catheterization and placement of a stent, thrombolytic therapy is still very important where PCI is not readily available.

The proper selection of patients for thrombolytic therapy is critical. The diagnosis of acute myocardial infarction is made clinically and is confirmed by electrocardiography. Patients with ST-segment elevation and bundle branch block on electrocardiography have the best outcomes. All trials to date show the greatest benefit for thrombolytic therapy when it is given early, within 6 hours after symptomatic onset of acute myocardial infarction.

Thrombolytic drugs reduce the mortality of acute myocardial infarction. The early and appropriate use of any thrombolytic drug probably transcends possible advantages of a particular drug. Adjunctive drugs such as aspirin, heparin, β blockers, and angiotensin-converting enzyme (ACE) inhibitors reduce mortality even further. The principles of management are outlined in part 7 of the American Heart Association Guidelines, 2000.

Indications & Dosage

Administration of fibrinolytic drugs by the intravenous route is indicated in cases of **pulmonary embolism with hemodynamic instability,** severe **deep venous thrombosis** such as the superior vena caval syndrome, and **ascending thrombophlebitis** of the iliofemoral vein with severe lower extremity edema. These drugs are also given intra-arterially, especially for peripheral vascular disease.

Thrombolytic therapy in the management of **acute myocardial infarction** requires careful patient selection, the use of a specific thrombolytic agent, and the benefit of adjuvant therapy. Streptokinase is administered by intravenous infusion of a loading dose of 250,000 units, followed by 100,000 units/h for 24–72 hours. Patients with antistreptococcal antibodies can develop fever, allergic reactions, and therapeutic resistance. Urokinase requires a loading dose of 300,000 units given over 10 minutes and a maintenance dose of 300,000 units/h for 12 hours. Alteplase (t-PA) is given by intravenous infusion of 60 mg over the first hour and then 40 mg at a rate of 20 mg/h. Reteplase is given as two intravenous bolus injections of 10 units each, separated by 30 minutes. Tenecteplase is given as a single intravenous bolus of 0.5 mg/kg. Anistreplase (where available) is given as a single intravenous injection of 30 units over 3–5 minutes. A single course of fibrinolytic drugs is expensive: hundreds of dollars for streptokinase and thousands for urokinase and t-PA.

Recombinant t-PA has also been approved for use in acute ischmic stroke within 3 hours of symptom onset. In patients without hemorrhagic infarct or other contraindications, this therapy has been demonstrated to provide better outcomes in several randomized clinical trials. The recommended dose is 0.9 mg/kg, not to exceed 90 mg, with 10% given as a bolus and the remainder during a 1 hour infusion. Streptokinase has been associated with increased bleeding risk in acute ischemic stroke when given at a dose of 1.5 million units, and its use is not recommended in this setting.

■ III. BASIC PHARMACOLOGY OF ANTIPLATELET AGENTS

Platelet function is regulated by three categories of substances. The first group consists of agents generated outside the platelet that interact with platelet membrane receptors, eg, catecholamines, collagen, thrombin, and prostacyclin. The second category contains agents generated within the platelet that interact with membrane receptors, eg, ADP, prostaglandin D_2, prostaglandin E_2, and serotonin. The third group comprises agents generated within the platelet that act within the platelet, eg, prostaglandin endoperoxides and thromboxane A_2, the cyclic nucleotides cAMP and cGMP, and calcium ion. From this list of agents, several targets for platelet inhibitory drugs have been identified (see Figure 34–1): inhibition of prostaglandin synthesis (aspirin), inhibition of ADP-induced platelet aggregation (clopidogrel, ticlopidine), and blockade of glycoprotein IIb/IIIa receptors on platelets (abciximab, tirofiban, and eptifibatide). Dipyridamole and cilostazol are additional antiplatelet drugs.

ASPIRIN

The prostaglandin **thromboxane A_2** is an arachidonate product that causes platelets to change shape, release their granules, and aggregate (see Chapter 18). Drugs that antagonize this pathway interfere with platelet aggregation in vitro and prolong the bleeding time in vivo. Aspirin is the prototype of this class of drugs.

As described in Chapter 18, aspirin inhibits the synthesis of thromboxane A_2 by irreversible acetylation of the enzyme cyclooxygenase. Other salicylates and nonsteroidal anti-inflammatory drugs also inhibit cyclooxygenase but have a shorter duration of inhibitory action because they cannot acetylate cyclooxygenase; that is, their action is reversible.

The FDA has approved the use of 325 mg/d for *primary* prophylaxis of myocardial infarction but urges caution in this use of aspirin by the general population except when prescribed as an adjunct to risk factor management by smoking cessation and lowering of blood cholesterol and blood pressure. Meta-analysis of many published trials of aspirin and other antiplatelet agents confirms the value of this intervention in the *secondary* prevention of vascular events among patients with a history of vascular events.

CLOPIDOGREL & TICLOPIDINE

Clopidogrel and ticlopidine reduce platelet aggregation by inhibiting the ADP pathway of platelets. These drugs are thienopyridine derivatives that achieve their antiplatelet effects by irreversibly blocking the ADP receptor on platelets. Unlike aspirin, these drugs have no effect on prostaglandin metabolism. Randomized clinical trials with both drugs report efficacy in the prevention of vascular events among patients with transient ischemic attacks, completed strokes, and unstable angina pectoris. Use of clopidogrel or ticlopidine to prevent thrombosis is now considered standard practice in patients undergoing placement of a coronary stent.

Adverse effects of ticlopidine include nausea, dyspepsia, and diarrhea in up to 20% of patients, hemorrhage in 5%, and, most seriously, leukopenia in 1%. The leukopenia is detected by regular monitoring of the white blood cell count during the first 3 months of treatment. Development of thrombotic thrombocytopenic purpura has also been associated with the ingestion of ticlopidine. The dosage of ticlopidine is 250 mg twice daily. It is particularly useful in patients who cannot tolerate aspirin. Doses of ticlopidine less than 500 mg/d may be efficacious with fewer adverse effects.

Clopidogrel has fewer adverse effects than ticlopidine and is rarely associated with neutropenia. Thrombotic thrombocytopenic purpura associated with clopidogrel has been reported. Because of its superior side effect profile and dosing requirements, clopidogrel is preferred over ticlopidine. The antithrombotic effects of clopidogrel are dose-dependent; within 5 hours after an oral loading dose of 300 mg, 80% of platelet activity will be inhibited. The maintenance dose of clopidogrel is 75

mg/d, which achieves maximum platelet inhibition. The duration of the antiplatelet effect is 7–10 days.

Aspirin & Clopidogrel Resistance

The reported incidence of resistance to these drugs varies greatly, from less than 5% to 75%. In part this tremendous variation in incidence reflects the definition of resistance (recurrent thrombosis while on antiplatelet therapy vs in vitro testing), methods by which drug response is measured, and patient compliance. Several methods for testing aspirin and clopidogrel resistance in vitro are now FDA-approved; however, their utility outside of clinical trials remains controversial.

BLOCKADE OF PLATELET GLYCOPROTEIN IIB/IIIA RECEPTORS

The glycoprotein IIb/IIIa inhibitors are used in patients with acute coronary syndromes. These drugs target the platelet IIb/IIIa receptor complex (Figure 34–1). The IIb/IIIa complex functions as a receptor mainly for fibrinogen and vitronectin but also for fibronectin and von Willebrand factor. Activation of this receptor complex is the "final common pathway" for platelet aggregation. There are approximately 50,000 copies of this complex on the surface of each platelet. Persons lacking this receptor have a bleeding disorder called Glanzmann's thrombasthenia.

Abciximab, a chimeric monoclonal antibody directed against the IIb/IIIa complex including the vibronectin receptor, was the first agent approved in this class of drugs. It has been approved for use in percutaneous coronary intervention and in acute coronary syndromes. **Eptifibatide** is an analog of the sequence at the extreme carboxyl terminal of the delta chain of fibrinogen, which mediates the binding of fibrinogen to the receptor. **Tirofiban** is a smaller molecule with similar properties. Eptifibatide and tirofiban inhibit ligand binding to the IIb/IIIa receptor by their occupancy of the receptor but do not block the vibronectin receptor.

The three agents described above are administered parenterally. Oral formulations of IIb/IIIa antagonists have been developed and are in various stages of development.

ADDITIONAL ANTIPLATELET-DIRECTED DRUGS

Dipyridamole is a vasodilator that inhibits platelet function by inhibiting adenosine uptake and cyclic GMP phosphodiesterase activity. Dipyridamole by itself has little or no beneficial effect. Therefore, therapeutic use of this agent is primarily in combination with aspirin to prevent cerebrovascular ischemia. It may also be used in combination with warfarin for primary prophylaxis of thromboemboli in patients with prosthetic heart valves. A combination of dipyridamole complexed with

25 mg of aspirin is now available for secondary prophylaxis of cerebrovascular disease.

Cilostazol is a newer phosphodiesterase inhibitor that promotes vasodilation and inhibition of platelet aggregation. Cilostazol is used primarily to treat intermittent claudication.

■ IV. CLINICAL PHARMACOLOGY OF DRUGS USED TO PREVENT CLOTTING

VENOUS THROMBOSIS

Risk Factors

A. INHERITED DISORDERS

The inherited disorders characterized by a tendency to form thrombi (thrombophilia) derive from either quantitative or qualitative abnormalities of the natural anticoagulant system. Deficiencies (loss of function mutations) in the natural anticoagulants antithrombin, protein C, and protein S account for approximately 15% of selected patients with juvenile or recurrent thrombosis and 5–10% of unselected cases of acute venous thrombosis. Additional causes of thrombophilia include gain of function mutations such as the factor V Leiden mutation and the prothrombin 20210 mutation, elevated clotting factor and cofactor levels, and hyperhomocysteinemia that together account for the greater number of hypercoagulable patients. Although the loss of function mutations are less common, they are associated with the greatest thrombosis risk. Some patients have multiple inherited risk factors or combinations of inherited and acquired risk factors as discussed below. These individuals are at higher risk for recurrent thrombotic events and are often considered candidates for lifelong therapy.

B. ACQUIRED DISEASE

The increased risk of thromboembolism associated with atrial fibrillation and with the placement of mechanical heart valves has long been recognized. Similarly, prolonged bed rest, high-risk surgical procedures, and the presence of cancer are clearly associated with an increased incidence of deep venous thrombosis and embolism. Antiphospholipic antibody syndrome is another important acquired risk factor. Drugs may function as synergistic risk factors in concert with inherited risk factors. For example, women who have the factor V Leiden mutation and take oral contraceptives have a synergistic increase in risk.

Antithrombotic Management

A. PREVENTION

Primary prevention of venous thrombosis reduces the incidence of and mortality rate from pulmonary emboli. Heparin and warfarin may be used to prevent venous thrombosis. Subcutaneous administration of low-dose unfractionated heparin, low-molecular-weight heparin, or fondaparinux provides effective prophylaxis. Warfarin is also effective but requires laboratory monitoring of the prothrombin time.

B. TREATMENT OF ESTABLISHED DISEASE

Treatment for established venous thrombosis is initiated with unfractionated or low-molecular-weight heparin for the first 5–7 days, with an overlap with warfarin. Once therapeutic effects of warfarin have been established, therapy with warfarin is continued for a minimum of 3–6 months. Patients with recurrent disease or identifiable, nonreversible risk factors may be treated indefinitely. Small thrombi confined to the calf veins may be managed without anticoagulants if there is documentation over time that the thrombus is not extending.

Warfarin readily crosses the placenta. It can cause hemorrhage at any time during pregnancy as well as developmental defects when administered during the first trimester. Therefore, venous thromboembolic disease in pregnant women is generally treated with heparin, best administered by subcutaneous injection.

ARTERIAL THROMBOSIS

Activation of platelets is considered an essential process for arterial thrombosis. Thus, treatment with platelet-inhibiting drugs such as aspirin and clopidogrel or ticlopidine is indicated in patients with transient ischemic attacks and strokes or unstable angina and acute myocardial infarction. In angina and infarction, these drugs are often used in conjunction with β blockers, calcium channel blockers, and fibrinolytic drugs.

■ V. DRUGS USED IN BLEEDING DISORDERS

VITAMIN K

Vitamin K confers biologic activity upon prothrombin and factors VII, IX, and X by participating in their postribosomal modification. Vitamin K is a fat-soluble substance found primarily in leafy green vegetables. The dietary requirement is low, because the vitamin is additionally synthesized by bacteria that colonize the human intestine. Two natural forms exist: vitamins K_1 and K_2. Vitamin K_1 (phytonadione; Figure 34–5) is found in food. Vitamin K_2 (menaquinone) is found in human tissues and is synthesized by intestinal bacteria.

Vitamins K_1 and K_2 require bile salts for absorption from the intestinal tract. Vitamin K_1 is available clinically in oral and parenteral forms. Onset of effect is delayed for 6 hours but the effect is complete by 24 hours when treating depression of prothrombin activity by excess warfarin or vitamin K deficiency. Intravenous administration of vitamin K_1 should be slow, because rapid infusion can produce dyspnea, chest and back pain, and even death. Vitamin K repletion is best achieved with intravenous or oral administration, because its bioavailability after subcutaneous administration is erratic. Vitamin K_1 is currently administered to all newborns to prevent the hemorrhagic disease of vitamin K deficiency, which is especially common in premature infants. *The water-soluble salt of vitamin K_3 (menadione) should never be used in therapeutics.* It is particularly ineffective in the treatment of warfarin overdosage. Vitamin K deficiency frequently occurs in hospitalized patients in intensive care units because of poor diet, parenteral nutrition, recent surgery, multiple antibiotic therapy, and uremia. Severe hepatic failure results in diminished protein synthesis and a hemorrhagic diathesis that is unresponsive to vitamin K.

PLASMA FRACTIONS

Sources & Preparations

Deficiencies in plasma coagulation factors can cause bleeding (Table 34–3). Spontaneous bleeding occurs when factor activity is less than 5–10% of normal. Factor VIII deficiency (**classic hemophilia, or hemophilia A**) and factor IX deficiency (**Christmas disease,** or **hemophilia B**) account for most of the heritable coagulation defects. Concentrated plasma fractions are available for the treatment of these deficiencies. Administration of plasma-derived, heat- or detergent-treated factor concentrates and recombinant factor concentrates are the standard treatments for bleeding associated with hemophilia. Lyophilized factor VIII concentrates are prepared from large pools of plasma. Transmission of viral diseases such as hepatitis B and C and HIV is reduced or eliminated by pasteurization and by extraction of plasma with solvents and detergents. However, this treatment does not remove other potential causes of transmissable diseases such as prions. For this reason, recombinant clotting factor preparations are recommended whenever possible for factor replacement. The best use of these therapeutic materials requires diagnostic specificity of the deficient factor and quantitation of its activity in plasma. Intermediate purity factor VIII concentrates (as opposed to recombinant or high purity

concentrates) contain significant amounts of von Willebrand factor. Humate-P is a factor VIII concentrate that is approved by the FDA for the treatment of bleeding associated with von Willebrand disease.

Clinical Uses

An uncomplicated hemorrhage into a joint should be treated with sufficient factor VIII or factor IX replacement to maintain a level of at least 30–50% of the normal concentration for 24 hours. Soft tissue hematomas require a minimum of 100% activity for 7 days. Hematuria requires at least 10% activity for 3 days. Surgery and major trauma require a minimum of 100% activity for 10 days. The initial loading dose for factor VIII is 50 units/kg of body weight to achieve 100% activity of factor VIII from a baseline of $\leq$ 1%, assuming a normal hemoglobin. Each unit of factor VIII per kilogram of body weight raises its activity in plasma 2%. Replacement should be administered every 12 hours. Factor IX therapy requires twice the dose of factor VIII, but with an administration of about every 24 hours because of its longer half-life. Recombinant factor IX has only 80% recovery compared with plasma-derived factor IX products. Therefore, dosing with recombinant factor IX requires 120% of the dose used with the plasma-derived product.

Desmopressin acetate increases the factor VIII activity of patients with mild hemophilia A or von Willebrand disease. It can be used in preparation for minor surgery such as tooth extraction without any requirement for infusion of clotting factors if the patient has a documented adequate response. High-dose intranasal desmopressin (see Chapter 17) is available and has been shown to be efficacious and well tolerated by patients.

Freeze-dried concentrates of plasma containing prothrombin, factors IX and X, and varied amounts of factor VII (Proplex, etc) are commercially available for treating deficiencies of these factors (Table 34–3). Each unit of factor IX per kilogram of body weight raises its activity in plasma 1.5%. Heparin is often added to inhibit coagulation factors activated by the manufacturing process. However, addition of heparin does not eliminate all thromboembolic risk.

Some preparations of factor IX concentrate contain *activated* clotting factors, which has led to their use in treating patients with inhibitors or antibodies to factor VIII or factor IX. Two products are available expressly for this purpose: **Autoplex** (with factor VIII correctional activity) and **FEIBA** (**F**actor **E**ight **I**nhibitor **B**ypassing **A**ctivity). These products are not uniformly successful in arresting hemorrhage, and the factor IX inhibitor titers often rise after treatment with them. Acquired inhibitors of coagulation factors may also be treated with porcine factor VIII (for factor VIII inhibitors) and recombinant activated factor VII. Recombi-

Table 34–3. Therapeutic products for the treatment of coagulation disorders.

Factor	Deficiency State	Hemostatic Levels	Half-Life of Infused Factor	Replacement Source
I	Hypofibrinogenemia	1 g/dL	4 days	Cryoprecipitate FFP
II	Prothrombin deficiency	30–40%	3 days	Prothrombin complex concentrates (intermediate purity factor IX concentrates)
V	Factor V deficiency	20%	1 day	FFP
VII	Factor VII deficiency	30%	4–6 hours	FFP Prothrombin complex concentrates (intermediate purity factor IX concentrates) Recombinant factor VIIa
VIII	Hemophilia A	30–50% 100% for major bleeding or trauma	12 hours	Recombinant factor VIII products Plasma-derived high purity concentrates Cryoprecipitate[1] Some patients with mild deficiency will respond to DDAVP
IX	Hemophilia B Christmas disease	30–50% 100% for major bleeding or trauma	24 hours	Recombinant factor IX products Plasma-derived high purity concentrates
X	Stuart-Prower defect	25%	36 hours	FFP Prothrombin complex concentrates
XI	Hemophilia C	30–50%	3 days	FFP
XII	Hageman defect	Not required		Treatment not necessary
Von Willebrand	Von Willebrand disease	30%	Approximately 10 hours	Intermediate purity factor VIII concentrates that contain von Willebrand factor Some patients respond to DDAVP Cryoprecipitate[1]
XIII	Factor XIII deficiency	5%	6 days	FFP Cryoprecipitate

FFP, fresh frozen plasma; DDAVP, 1-deamino-8-D-arginine vasopressin.
Antithrombin and activated protein C concentrates are available for the appropriate indications that include thrombosis in the setting of antithrombin deficiency and sepsis respectively.
[1]Cryoprecipitate should be used to treat bleeding in the setting of factor VIII deficiency and von Willebrand disease only in an emergency in which pathogen-inactivated products are not available.

nant activated factor VII (**NovoSeven**) is being increasingly used to treat coagulopathy associated with liver disease and major blood loss in trauma and surgery. These recombinant and plasma-derived factor concentrates are very expensive, and the indications for them are very precise. Therefore, close consultation with a hematologist knowledgeable in this area is essential.

Cryoprecipitate is a plasma protein fraction obtainable from whole blood. It is used to treat deficiencies or qualitative abnormalities of fibrinogen, such as that which occurs with disseminated intravascular coagulation and liver disease. A single unit of cryoprecipitate contains 300 mg of fibrinogen.

Cryoprecipitate may also be used for patients with factor VIII deficiency and von Willebrand disease if desmopressin is not indicated and a pathogen-inactivated, recombinant, or plasma-derived product is not available. The concentration of factor VIII and von

Willebrand factor in cryoprecipitate is not as great as that found in the concentrated plasma fractions. Moreover, cryoprecipitate is not treated in any manner to decrease the risk of viral exposure. For infusion, the frozen cryoprecipitate unit is thawed and dissolved in a small volume of sterile citrate-saline solution and pooled with other units. Rh-negative women with potential for childbearing should receive only Rh-negative cryoprecipitate because of possible contamination of the product with Rh-positive blood cells.

FIBRINOLYTIC INHIBITORS: AMINOCAPROIC ACID

Aminocaproic acid (EACA), which is chemically similar to the amino acid lysine, is a synthetic inhibitor of fibrinolysis. It competitively inhibits plasminogen activation (Figure 34–3). It is rapidly absorbed orally and is cleared from the body by the kidney. The usual oral dosage of EACA is 6 g four times a day. When the drug is administered intravenously, a 5 g loading dose should be infused over 30 minutes to avoid hypotension. **Tranexamic acid** is an analog of aminocaproic acid and has the same properties. It is administered orally with a 15 mg/kg loading dose followed by 30 mg/kg every 6 hours, but the drug is not currently available in the USA.

Clinical uses of aminocaproic acid are as adjunctive therapy in hemophilia, as therapy for bleeding from fibrinolytic therapy, and as prophylaxis for rebleeding from intracranial aneurysms. Treatment success has also been reported in patients with postsurgical gastrointestinal bleeding and postprostatectomy bleeding and

bladder hemorrhage secondary to radiation- and drug-induced cystitis. Adverse effects of the drug include intravascular thrombosis from inhibition of plasminogen activator, hypotension, myopathy, abdominal discomfort, diarrhea, and nasal stuffiness. The drug should not be used in patients with disseminated intravascular coagulation or genitourinary bleeding of the upper tract, eg, kidney and ureters, because of the potential for excessive clotting.

SERINE PROTEASE INHIBITORS: APROTININ

Aprotinin is a serine protease inhibitor ("serpin") that inhibits fibrinolysis by free plasmin and may have other antihemorrhagic effects as well. It also inhibits the plasmin-streptokinase complex in patients who have received that thrombolytic agent. Aprotinin will reduce bleeding—by as much as 50%—from many types of surgery, especially that involving extracorporeal circulation for open heart procedures and liver transplantation. It is currently approved for use in patients undergoing coronary artery bypass grafting who are at high risk of excessive blood loss. In earlier placebo-controlled trials, adverse effects of aprotinin were little different from those reported in patients in the placebo group. A more recent study indicated an increased risk of myocardial infarction, stroke, and renal damage in aprotinin-treated patients. In larger studies, a possible association with anaphylaxis has been reported in < 0.5% of cases. Therefore, a small test dose is recommended before the full therapeutic dose is given.

PREPARATIONS AVAILABLE

Abciximab (ReoPro)
Parenteral: 2 mg/mL for IV injection
Alteplase recombinant [t-PA] (Activase*)
Parenteral: 50, 100 mg lyophilized powder to reconstitute for IV injection
Aminocaproic acid (generic, Amicar)
Oral: 500 mg tablets; 250 mg/mL syrup
Parenteral: 250 mg/mL for IV injection
Anisindione (Miradon)
Oral: 50 mg tablets
Antihemophilic factor [factor VIII, AHF] (Alphanate, Bioclate*, Helixate*, Hemofil M, Koate-HP, Kogenate*, Monoclate, Recombinate,* others)
Parenteral: in vials

Anti-inhibitor coagulant complex (Autoplex T, Feiba VH Immuno)
Parenteral: in vials
Antithrombin III (Thrombate III)
Parenteral: 500, 1000 IU powder to reconstitute for IV injection
Aprotinin (Trasylol)
Parenteral: 10,000 units/mL in 100 and 200 mL vials
Argatroban
Parenteral: 100 mg/mL in 2.5 mL vials
Bivalirudin (Angiomax)
Parenteral: 250 mg per vial
Cilostazol (Pletal)
Oral: 50, 100 mg tablets
Clopidogrel (Plavix)
Oral: 75 mg tablets

*Recombinant product.

(continued)

Coagulation factor VIIa recombinant (Novo-Seven*)
Parenteral: 1.2, 4.8 mg powder/vial for IV injection
Dalteparin (Fragmin)
Parenteral: 2500, 5000, 10,000 anti-factor Xa units/0.2 mL for SC injection only
Danaparoid (Orgaran)
Parenteral: 750 anti-Xa units/vial
Dipyridamole (Persantine)
Oral: 25, 50, 75 mg tablets
Oral combination product (Aggrenox): 200 mg extended-release dipyridamole plus 25 mg aspirin
Enoxaparin (low-molecular-weight heparin, Lovenox)
Parenteral: pre-filled, multiple-dose syringes for SC injection only
Eptifibatide (Integrilin)
Parenteral: 0.75, 2 mg/mL for IV infusion
Factor VIIa: see Coagulation factor VIIa recombinant
Factor VIII: see Antihemophilic factor
Factor IX complex, human (AlphaNine SD, Bebulin VH, BeneFix*, Konyne 80, Mononine, Profilnine SD, Proplex T, Proplex SX-T)
Parenteral: in vials
Fondaparinux (Arixtra)
Parenteral: 2.5 mg in 0.5 mL single-dose pre-filled syringes
Heparin sodium (generic, Liquaemin)
Parenteral: 1000, 2000, 2500, 5000, 10,000, 20,000, 40,000 units/mL for injection

Lepirudin (Refludan*)
Parenteral: 50 mg powder for IV injection
Phytonadione [K_1] (generic, Mephyton, Aqua-Mephyton)
Oral: 5 mg tablets
Parenteral: 2, 10 mg/mL aqueous colloidal solution or suspension for injection
Protamine (generic)
Parenteral: 10 mg/mL for injection
Reteplase (Retavase*)
Parenteral: 10.8 IU powder for injection
Streptokinase (Streptase)
Parenteral: 250,000, 750,000, 1,500,000 IU per vial powders to reconstitute for injection
Tenecteplase (TNKase*)
Parenteral: 50 mg powder for injection
Ticlopidine (Ticlid)
Oral: 250 mg tablets
Tinzaparin (Innohep)
Parenteral: 20,000 anti-Xa units/mL for subcutaneous injection only
Tirofiban (Aggrastat)
Parenteral: 50, 250 mcg/mL for IV infusion
Tranexamic acid (Cyklokapron)
Oral: 500 mg tablets
Parenteral: 100 mg/mL for IV infusion
Urokinase (Abbokinase)
Parenteral: 250,000 IU per vial for systemic use
Warfarin (generic, Coumadin)
Oral: 1, 2, 2.5, 3, 4, 5, 6, 7.5, 10 mg tablets

REFERENCES

Blood Coagulation & Bleeding Disorders

Dahlback B: Blood coagulation. Lancet 2000;355:1627.

Ginsburg D: Genetic risk factors for arterial thrombosis and inflammation. Hematology (Amer Soc Hematol Education Program) 2005;442.

Hayward CP: Diagnosis and management of mild bleeding disorders. Hematology (Amer Soc Hematol Educ Program) 2005;423.

Kessler CM: New perspectives in hemophilia treatment. Hematology (Amer Soc Hematol Educ Program) 2005;429.

Manno CS: Management of bleeding disorders in children. Hematology (Amer Soc Hematol Educ Program) 2005;416.

Rosendaal F: Venous thrombosis: The role of genes, environment and behavior. Hematology (Amer Soc Hematol Education Program) 2005;1.

Drugs Used in Bleeding Disorders

Hirsh J et al (editors): Seventh ACCP Consensus Conference on Antithrombotic Therapy. Chest 2004;126(Suppl):167S.

Mangano DT, Tudor IC, Dietzel C: The risk associated with aprotinin in cardiac surgery. N Engl J Med 2006;354:353.

Menon V et al: Thrombolysis and adjunctive therapy in acute myocardial infarction: The Seventh ACCP Conference on Antithrombotic and Thrombolytic Therapy. Chest 2004;126(Suppl):549S.

Weitz JI, Bates SM: New anticoagulants. J Thromb Haemost 2005;3:1843.

Agents Used in Hyperlipidemia

Mary J. Malloy, MD, & John P. Kane, MD, PhD

Plasma lipids are transported in complexes called **lipoproteins.** Metabolic disorders that involve elevations in any lipoprotein species are termed **hyperlipoproteinemias** or **hyperlipidemias. Hyperlipemia** denotes increased levels of triglycerides.

The two major clinical sequelae of hyperlipidemias are acute pancreatitis and atherosclerosis. The former occurs in patients with marked hyperlipemia. Control of triglycerides can prevent recurrent attacks of this life-threatening disease.

Atherosclerosis is the leading cause of death for both genders in the USA and other Western countries. Lipoproteins that contain **apolipoprotein (apo) B-100** convey lipids into the artery wall. These are **low-density (LDL), intermediate-density (IDL), very-low-density (VLDL),** and **lipoprotein(a) (Lp[a]).**

Cellular components in atherosclerotic plaques include foam cells, which are transformed macrophages and smooth muscle cells filled with **cholesteryl esters.** These cellular alterations result from endocytosis of modified lipoproteins via at least four species of **scavenger receptors.** Chemical modification of lipoproteins by free radicals creates ligands for these receptors. The atheroma grows with the accumulation of foam cells, collagen, fibrin, and frequently calcium. Whereas such lesions can slowly occlude coronary vessels, clinical symptoms are more frequently precipitated by rupture of unstable atheromatous plaques, leading to activation of platelets and formation of occlusive thrombi.

Although treatment of hyperlipidemia can cause slow physical regression of plaques, the well-documented reduction in acute coronary events that follows vigorous lipid-lowering treatment is attributable chiefly to mitigation of the inflammatory activity of macrophages and is evident within 2–3 months after starting therapy.

High-density lipoproteins (HDL) exert several *anti*atherogenic effects. They participate in retrieval of cholesterol from the artery wall and inhibit the oxidation of atherogenic lipoproteins. Low levels of HDL (hypoalphalipoproteinemia) are an independent risk factor for atherosclerotic disease and thus are a target for intervention.

ACRONYMS	
Apo	Apolipoprotein
CETP	Cholesteryl ester transfer protein
CK	Creatine kinase
HDL	High-density lipoproteins
HMG-CoA	3-Hydroxy-3-methylglutaryl-coenzyme A
IDL	Intermediate-density lipoproteins
LCAT	Lecithin:cholesterol acyltransferase
LDL	Low-density lipoproteins
Lp(a)	Lipoprotein(a)
LPL	Lipoprotein lipase
PPAR-α	Peroxisome proliferator-activated receptor-alpha
VLDL	Very-low-density lipoproteins

Cigarette smoking is a major risk factor for coronary disease. It is associated with reduced levels of HDL, impairment of cholesterol retrieval, cytotoxic effects on the endothelium, increased oxidation of lipoproteins, and stimulation of thrombogenesis. Diabetes, also a major risk factor, is another source of oxidative stress.

Normal coronary arteries can dilate in response to ischemia, increasing delivery of oxygen to the myocardium. This process is mediated by nitric oxide, acting upon smooth muscle cells of the arterial media. This function is impaired by atherogenic lipoproteins, thus aggravating ischemia. Reducing levels of atherogenic lipoproteins and inhibiting their oxidation restores endothelial function.

Because atherogenesis is multifactorial, therapy should be directed toward all modifiable risk factors. Atherogenesis is a dynamic process. Quantitative angiographic trials have demonstrated net regression of plaques during aggressive lipid-lowering therapy. Primary and secondary prevention trials have shown significant reduction in mortality from new coronary events and in all-cause mortality.

■ PATHOPHYSIOLOGY OF HYPERLIPOPROTEINEMIA

NORMAL LIPOPROTEIN METABOLISM

Structure

Lipoproteins have hydrophobic core regions containing cholesteryl esters and triglycerides surrounded by unesterified cholesterol, phospholipids, and apoproteins. Certain lipoproteins contain very high-molecular-weight B proteins that exist in two forms: **B-48,** formed in the intestine and found in chylomicrons and their remnants; and **B-100,** synthesized in liver and found in **VLDL, VLDL remnants (IDL), LDL** (formed from VLDL), and **Lp(a) lipoproteins.**

Synthesis & Catabolism

A. CHYLOMICRONS

Chylomicrons are formed in the intestine and carry **triglycerides** of dietary origin, **unesterified cholesterol,** and **cholesteryl esters.** They transit the thoracic duct to the bloodstream.

Triglycerides are removed in extrahepatic tissues through a pathway shared with VLDL that involves hydrolysis by the **lipoprotein lipase (LPL)** system. Decrease in particle diameter occurs as triglycerides are depleted. Surface lipids and small apoproteins are transferred to HDL. The resultant chylomicron remnants are taken up by receptor-mediated endocytosis into hepatocytes.

B. VERY-LOW-DENSITY LIPOPROTEINS

VLDL are secreted by liver and export triglycerides to peripheral tissues (Figure 35–1). VLDL triglycerides are hydrolyzed by LPL, yielding free fatty acids for storage in adipose tissue and for oxidation in tissues such as cardiac and skeletal muscle. Depletion of triglycerides produces remnants (IDL), some of which undergo endocytosis directly by liver. The remainder is converted to LDL by further removal of triglycerides mediated by hepatic lipase. This process explains the "beta shift" phenomenon, the increase of LDL (beta-lipoprotein) in serum as hypertriglyceridemia subsides. Increased levels of LDL can also result from increased secretion of VLDL and from decreased LDL catabolism.

C. LOW-DENSITY LIPOPROTEINS

LDL is catabolized chiefly in hepatocytes and other cells by receptor-mediated endocytosis. Cholesteryl esters from LDL are hydrolyzed, yielding free cholesterol for the synthesis of cell membranes. Cells also obtain cholesterol by synthesis via a pathway involving the formation of mevalonic acid by HMG-CoA reductase. Production of this enzyme and of LDL receptors is transcriptionally regulated by the content of cholesterol in the cell. Normally, about 70% of LDL is removed from plasma by hepatocytes. Even more cholesterol is delivered to the liver via IDL and chylomicrons. Unlike other cells, hepatocytes can eliminate cholesterol by secretion in bile and by conversion to bile acids.

D. LP(A) LIPOPROTEIN

Lp(a) lipoprotein is formed from LDL and the (a) protein, linked by a disulfide bridge. The (a) protein is highly homologous with plasminogen but is not activated by tissue plasminogen activator. It occurs in a number of isoforms of different molecular weights. Levels of Lp(a) vary from nil to over 500 mg/dL and are determined chiefly by genetic factors. Lp(a) can be found in atherosclerotic plaques and may also contribute to coronary disease by inhibiting thrombolysis. Levels are elevated in nephrosis.

E. HIGH-DENSITY LIPOPROTEINS

The apoproteins of HDL are secreted by the liver and intestine. Much of the lipid comes from the surface monolayers of chylomicrons and VLDL during lipolysis. HDL also acquires cholesterol from peripheral tissues, protecting the cholesterol homeostasis of cells. Free cholesterol is transported from the cell membrane by a transporter, ABCA1, acquired by a small particle termed prebeta-1 HDL, and then esterified by lecithin:cholesterol acyltransferase (LCAT), leading to the formation of larger HDL species. Cholesterol is also exported from macrophages by the ABCG1 transporter to large HDL particles. The cholesteryl esters are transferred to VLDL, IDL, LDL, and chylomicron remnants with the aid of cholesteryl ester transfer protein (CETP). Much of the cholesteryl ester thus transferred is ultimately delivered to the liver by endocytosis of the acceptor lipoproteins. HDL can also deliver cholesteryl esters directly to the liver via a docking receptor (scavenger receptor, SR-BI) that does not cause endocytosis of the lipoproteins.

■ LIPOPROTEIN DISORDERS

Lipoprotein disorders are detected by measuring lipids in serum after a 10-hour fast. Risk of heart disease increases with concentrations of the atherogenic lipoproteins, is inversely related to levels of HDL, and is modified by other risk factors (Table 35–1). Evidence from clinical trials suggests that LDL cholesterol levels

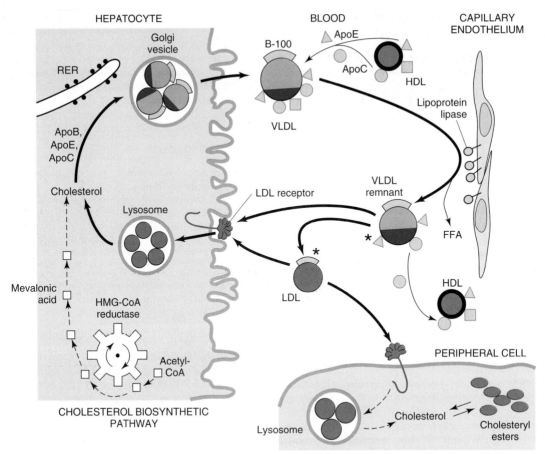

Figure 35–1. Metabolism of lipoproteins of hepatic origin. The heavy arrows show the primary pathways. Nascent VLDL are secreted via the Golgi apparatus. They acquire additional C apolipoproteins and apo E from HDL. VLDL are converted to VLDL remnants (IDL) by lipolysis via lipoprotein lipase in the vessels of peripheral tissues. In the process, C apolipoproteins and a portion of the apo E are given back to HDL. Some of the VLDL remnants are converted to LDL by further loss of triglycerides and loss of apo E. A major pathway for LDL degradation involves the endocytosis of LDL by LDL receptors in the liver and the peripheral tissues, for which apo B-100 is the ligand. (Dark color denotes cholesteryl esters; light color, triglycerides; the asterisk denotes a functional ligand for LDL receptors; triangles indicate apolipoprotein E; circles and squares represent C apolipoproteins; RER denotes rough endoplasmic reticulum.) (Modified and redrawn, with permission, from Kane J, Malloy M: Disorders of lipoproteins. In: Rosenberg RN et al (editors). *The Molecular and Genetic Basis of Neurological Disease.* Butterworth-Heinemann, 1993.)

of 60mg/dL may be optimal for patients with coronary disease. Ideally, triglycerides should be below 120 mg/dL. Differentiation of the disorders requires identification of the lipoproteins involved (Table 35–2). Diagnosis of a primary disorder usually requires further clinical and genetic data as well as ruling out secondary hyperlipidemias (Table 35–3).

Phenotypes of abnormal lipoprotein distribution are described in this section. Drugs mentioned for use in these conditions are described in the following section on basic and clinical pharmacology.

THE PRIMARY HYPERTRIGLYCERIDEMIAS

Hypertriglyceridemia is associated with increased risk of coronary disease. VLDL and IDL have been found in atherosclerotic plaques. These patients tend to have

Table 35–1. National Cholesterol Education Program: Adult Treatment Guidelines (2001).

	Desirable	Borderline to High[1]	High
Total cholesterol	< 200 (5.2)[2]	200–239[2] (5.2–6.2)	> 240 (6.2)[2]
LDL cholesterol	< 130 (3.4)[3]	130–159 (3.4–4.1)	> 160 (4.1)
HDL cholesterol Men Women	> 40 (1.04) > 50 (1.30)		> 60 (1.55)
Triglycerides	< 120 (1.4)	120–199 (1.4–2.3)	> 200 (2.3)

[1] Consider as high if coronary disease or more than 2 risk factors are present.
[2] mg/dL (mmol/L).
[3] Optimal level is < 100 (2.6).

cholesterol-rich VLDL of small particle diameter. Hypertriglyceridemic patients with coronary disease or risk equivalents should be treated aggressively. Patients with triglycerides above 700 mg/dL should be treated to prevent acute pancreatitis because the LPL clearance mechanism is saturated at about this level.

Primary Chylomicronemia

Chylomicrons are not present in the serum of normal individuals who have fasted 10 hours. The recessive traits of deficiency of lipoprotein lipase or its cofactor are usually associated with severe lipemia (2000–2500 mg/dL of triglycerides when the patient is consuming a typical American diet). These disorders might not be diagnosed until an attack of acute pancreatitis occurs. Patients may have eruptive xanthomas, hepatosplenomegaly, hypersplenism, and lipid-laden foam cells in bone marrow, liver, and spleen. The lipemia is aggravated by estrogens because they stimulate VLDL production, and pregnancy may cause marked increases in triglycerides despite

Table 35–2. The primary hyperlipoproteinemias and their drug treatment.

Disorder	Manifestations	Single Drug[1]	Drug Combination
Primary chylomicronemia (familial lipoprotein lipase or cofactor deficiency)	Chylomicrons, VLDL increased	Dietary management (niacin, fibrate)	Niacin plus fibrate
Familial hypertriglyceridemia Severe	VLDL, chylomicrons increased	Niacin, fibrate	Niacin plus fibrate
Moderate	VLDL increased; chylomicrons may be increased	Niacin, fibrate	
Familial combined hyperlipoproteinemia	VLDL increased	Niacin, fibrate	
	LDL increased	Niacin, reductase inhibitor, ezetimibe	Two or three of the individual drugs
	VLDL, LDL increased	Niacin, reductase inhibitor	Niacin or fibrate plus reductase inhibitor[2] or ezetimibe
Familial dysbetalipoproteinemia	VLDL remnants, chylomicron remnants increased	Fibrate, niacin	Fibrate plus niacin, or niacin plus reductase inhibitor
Familial hypercholesterolemia Heterozygous	LDL increased	Reductase inhibitor, resin, niacin, ezetimibe	Two or three of the individual drugs
Homozygous	LDL increased	Niacin, atorvastatin, ezetimibe, rosuvastatin	Niacin plus reductase inhibitor plus ezetimibe
Familial ligand-defective apo B	LDL increased	Niacin, reductase inhibitor, ezetimibe	Niacin plus reductase inhibitor or ezetimibe
Lp(a) hyperlipoproteinemia	Lp(a) increased	Niacin	

[1] Single-drug therapy should be evaluated before drug combinations are used.
[2] Select pharmacologically compatible reductase inhibitor (see text).

Table 35–3. Secondary causes of hyperlipoproteinemia.

Hypertriglyceridemia	Hypercholesterolemia
Diabetes mellitus	Hypothyroidism
Alcohol ingestion	Early nephrosis
Severe nephrosis	Resolving lipemia
Estrogens	Immunoglobulin-lipoprotein
Uremia	complex disorders
Corticosteroid excess	Anorexia nervosa
Myxedema	Cholestasis
Glycogen storage disease	Hypopituitarism
Hypopituitarism	Corticosteroid excess
Acromegaly	
Immunoglobulin-lipoprotein complex disorders	
Lipodystrophy	
Isotretinoin	
Protease inhibitors	

strict dietary control. Although these patients have a predominant chylomicronemia, they may also have moderately elevated VLDL, presenting with a pattern called mixed lipemia (fasting chylomicronemia and elevated VLDL). LPL deficiency is diagnosed by assay of lipolytic activity after intravenous injection of heparin. A presumptive diagnosis is made by demonstrating a pronounced decrease in triglycerides a few days after reduction of daily fat intake below 15 g. Marked restriction of total dietary fat is the basis of effective long-term treatment. Niacin or a fibrate may be of some benefit if VLDL levels are increased.

Familial Hypertriglyceridemia

A. SEVERE (USUALLY MIXED LIPEMIA)

Mixed lipemia usually results from impaired removal of triglyceride-rich lipoproteins. Factors that increase VLDL production aggravate the lipemia because VLDL and chylomicrons are competing substrates for LPL. The primary mixed lipemias probably reflect a variety of genetic determinants. Most patients have centripetal obesity with insulin resistance. Other factors that increase secretion of VLDL also worsen the lipemia. Eruptive xanthomas, lipemia retinalis, epigastric pain, and pancreatitis are variably present depending on the severity of the lipemia. Treatment is primarily dietary, with restriction of total fat, avoidance of alcohol and exogenous estrogens, weight reduction, and exercise. Most patients also require treatment with a fibrate or niacin.

B. MODERATE

Primary increases of VLDL also reflect a genetic predisposition and are worsened by factors that increase the rate of VLDL secretion from liver, ie, obesity, alcohol, diabetes, and estrogens. Treatment includes addressing these issues and the use of fibrates or niacin as needed. Marine omega-3 fatty acids are a valuable adjuvant.

Familial Combined Hyperlipoproteinemia

In this common disorder associated with an increased incidence of coronary disease, individuals may have elevated levels of VLDL, LDL, or both, and the pattern may change with time. Familial combined hyperlipoproteinemia involves an approximate doubling in VLDL secretion and appears to be transmitted as a semidominant trait. Triglycerides can be increased by the factors noted above. Elevations of cholesterol and triglycerides are generally moderate, and xanthomas are usually absent. Diet alone does not normalize lipid levels. A reductase inhibitor alone, or in combination with niacin or fenofibrate, is usually required to treat these patients. When fenofibrate is combined with a reductase inhibitor, pravastatin or rosuvastatin are recommended because they are not metabolized via CYP3A4.

Familial Dysbetalipoproteinemia

In this disorder, remnants of chylomicrons and VLDL accumulate and levels of LDL are decreased. Because remnants are rich in cholesteryl esters, the level of cholesterol may be as high as that of triglycerides. Diagnosis is confirmed by the absence of the E3 and E4 isoforms of apo E or the E2/E2 genotype. Patients often develop tuberous or tuberoeruptive xanthomas, or characteristic planar xanthomas of the palmar creases. They tend to be obese, and some have impaired glucose tolerance. These factors, as well as hypothyroidism, can aggravate the lipemia. Coronary and peripheral atherosclerosis occur with increased frequency. Weight loss, together with decreased fat, cholesterol, and alcohol consumption, may be sufficient, but a fibrate or niacin is usually needed to control the condition. These agents can be given together in more resistant cases, or a reductase inhibitor may be added.

THE PRIMARY HYPERCHOLESTEROLEMIAS

Familial Hypercholesterolemia

Familial hypercholesterolemia is an autosomal dominant trait. Although levels of LDL tend to increase throughout childhood, the diagnosis can often be made on the basis of elevated umbilical cord blood cholesterol. In most heterozygotes, cholesterol levels range from 260 to 500 mg/dL. Triglycerides are usually normal, tendon xanthomas are often present, and arcus corneae and xanthelasma may appear in the third

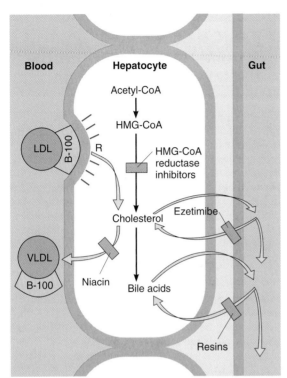

Figure 35–2. Sites of action of HMG-CoA reductase inhibitors, niacin, ezetimibe, and resins used in treating hyperlipidemias. LDL receptors (R) are increased by treatment with resins and HMG-CoA reductase inhibitors.

decade. Coronary disease tends to occur prematurely. In homozygous familial hypercholesterolemia, which can lead to coronary disease in childhood, levels of cholesterol often exceed 1000 mg/dL and early tuberous and tendinous xanthomas occur. These patients may also develop elevated plaque-like xanthomas of the aortic valve, digital webs, buttocks, and extremities.

Defects of LDL receptors underlie familial hypercholesterolemia. Some individuals have combined heterozygosity for alleles producing nonfunctional and kinetically impaired receptors. In heterozygous patients, LDL can be normalized with combined drug regimens (Figure 35–2). Homozygotes and those with combined heterozygosity whose receptors retain even minimal function may partially respond to niacin, ezetimibe, or reductase inhibitors.

Familial Ligand-Defective Apolipoprotein B

Defects in the domain of apo B-100 that binds to the LDL receptor impair the endocytosis of LDL, leading to hypercholesterolemia of moderate severity. Tendon xanthomas may occur. These disorders are as prevalent as familial

hypercholesterolemia. Response to reductase inhibitors is variable. Up-regulation of LDL receptors in liver increases endocytosis of LDL precursors but does not increase uptake of ligand-defective LDL particles. Niacin often has beneficial effects by reducing VLDL production.

Familial Combined Hyperlipoproteinemia

As described above, some persons with this disorder have only an elevation in LDL. Serum cholesterol is usually less than 350 mg/dL. Dietary and drug treatment, usually with a reductase inhibitor, is indicated. It may be necessary to add niacin or fenofibrate to normalize LDL or to reduce triglycerides.

Lp(a) Hyperlipoproteinemia

This familial disorder, which is associated with increased atherogenesis, is determined chiefly by alleles that dictate increased production of the (a) protein moiety. Niacin reduces levels of Lp(a) in many patients.

Other Disorders

Deficiency of cholesterol 7α-hydroxylase can increase LDL in the heterozygous state. Homozygotes can also have elevated triglycerides, resistance to reductase inhibitors, and increased risk of gallstones. Autosomal recessive hypercholesterolemia is due to mutations in a protein that normally assists in endocytosis of LDL. Mutations in the *PCSK9* gene also cause isolated elevations of LDL. Niacin, ezetimibe, and reductase inhibitors may be useful, variably, in these disorders.

HDL Deficiency

Rare genetic disorders, including Tangier disease and LCAT deficiency, are associated with extremely low levels of HDL. Familial hypoalphalipoproteinemia is a more common disorder with levels of HDL cholesterol usually below 35 mg/dL in men and 45 mg/dL in women. These patients tend to have premature atherosclerosis, and the low HDL may be the only identified risk factor. Management should include special attention to avoidance or treatment of other risk factors. Niacin increases HDL in many of these patients. Reductase inhibitors and fibric acid derivatives exert lesser effects.

In the presence of hypertriglyceridemia, HDL cholesterol is low because of exchange of cholesteryl esters from HDL into triglyceride-rich lipoproteins. Treatment of the hypertriglyceridemia may increase or normalize the HDL level.

SECONDARY HYPERLIPOPROTEINEMIA

Before primary disorders can be diagnosed, secondary causes of the phenotype must be considered. The more common conditions are summarized in Table 35–3. The lipoprotein abnormality usually resolves if the underlying disorder can be treated successfully.

DIETARY MANAGEMENT OF HYPERLIPOPROTEINEMIA

Dietary measures are initiated first—unless the patient has evident coronary or peripheral vascular disease—and may obviate the need for drugs. Patients with familial hypercholesterolemia or familial combined hyperlipidemia will always require drug therapy. Cholesterol and saturated and trans fats are the principal factors that increase LDL, whereas total fat, alcohol, and excess calories increase triglycerides.

Sucrose and other simple sugars raise VLDL in hypertriglyceridemic patients. Alcohol can cause significant hypertriglyceridemia by increasing hepatic secretion of VLDL. Synthesis and secretion of VLDL are increased by excess calories. During weight loss, LDL and VLDL levels may be much lower than can be maintained during neutral caloric balance. The conclusion that diet suffices for management can only be made after weight has stabilized for at least 1 month.

General recommendations include limiting total calories from fat to 20–25% of daily intake, saturated fats to less than 8%; and cholesterol to less than 200 mg/d. Reductions in serum cholesterol range from 10% to 20% on this regimen. Use of complex carbohydrates and fiber is recommended, and *cis*-monounsaturated fats should predominate. Weight reduction, caloric restriction, and avoidance of alcohol are especially important for patients with elevated VLDL and IDL.

The effect of dietary fats on hypertriglyceridemia is dependent upon the disposition of double bonds in the fatty acids. Omega-3 fatty acids found in fish oils, but not those from plant sources, can induce profound reduction of triglycerides in some patients with endogenous or mixed lipemia. In contrast, the omega-6 fatty acids present in vegetable oils may cause triglycerides to increase.

Patients with primary chylomicronemia and some with mixed lipemia must consume a diet severely restricted in total fat (10–15 g/d, of which 5 g should be vegetable oils rich in essential fatty acids), and fat-soluble vitamins should be given.

Homocysteine, which initiates proatherogenic changes in endothelium, can be reduced in many patients by restriction of total protein intake to the amount required for amino acid replacement. Supplementation with up to 2 mg of folic acid plus other B vitamins is also recommended.

BASIC & CLINICAL PHARMACOLOGY OF DRUGS USED IN HYPERLIPIDEMIA

The decision to use drug therapy is based on the specific metabolic defect and its potential for causing atherosclerosis or pancreatitis. Suggested regimens for the principal lipoprotein disorders are presented in Table 35–2. Diet should be continued to achieve the full potential of the drug regimen. Drugs should be avoided in pregnant and lactating women and those likely to become pregnant. All drugs that alter plasma lipoprotein concentrations may require adjustment of doses of warfarin and indandione anticoagulants. Children with heterozygous familial hypercholesterolemia may be treated with a resin or reductase inhibitor, usually after 7 or 8 years of age, when myelination of the central nervous system is essentially complete. The decision to treat a child should be based on the level of LDL, other risk factors, the family history, and the child's age. Drugs are rarely indicated before age 16.

COMPETITIVE INHIBITORS OF HMG-COA REDUCTASE (REDUCTASE INHIBITORS; "STATINS")

These compounds are structural analogs of HMG-CoA (3-hydroxy-3-methylglutaryl-coenzyme A, Figure 35–3). **Lovastatin, atorvastatin, fluvastatin, pravastatin, simvastatin,** and **rosuvastatin** belong to this class. They are most effective in reducing LDL. Other effects include decreased oxidative stress and vascular inflammation with increased stability of atherosclerotic lesions. It has become standard practice to initiate reductase inhibitor therapy immediately after acute coronary syndromes, irrespective of lipid levels.

Chemistry & Pharmacokinetics

Lovastatin and simvastatin are inactive lactone prodrugs that are hydrolyzed in the gastrointestinal tract to the active β-hydroxyl derivatives, whereas pravastatin has an open, active lactone ring. Atorvastatin, fluvastatin, and rosuvastatin are fluorine-containing congeners that are active as given. Absorption of the ingested doses of the reductase inhibitors varies from 40% to 75% with the exception of fluvastatin, which is almost completely absorbed. All have high first-pass extraction by the liver. Most of the absorbed dose is excreted in the bile; 5–20% is excreted in the urine. Plasma half-lives of these drugs range from 1 hour to 3 hours except for atorvastatin, which has a half-life of 14 hours, and rosuvastatin, 19 hours.

Figure 35–3. Inhibition of HMG-CoA reductase. **Top:** The HMG-CoA intermediate that is the immediate precursor of mevalonate, a critical compound in the synthesis of cholesterol. **Bottom:** The structure of lovastatin and its active form, showing the similarity to the normal HMG-CoA intermediate (shaded areas).

Mechanism of Action

HMG-CoA reductase mediates the first committed step in sterol biosynthesis. The active forms of the reductase inhibitors are structural analogs of the HMG-CoA intermediate (Figure 35–3) that is formed by HMG-CoA reductase in the synthesis of mevalonate. These analogs cause partial inhibition of the enzyme and thus may impair the synthesis of isoprenoids such as ubiquinone and dolichol and the prenylation of proteins. It is not known whether this has biologic significance. However, the reductase inhibitors clearly induce an increase in high-affinity LDL receptors. This effect increases both the fractional catabolic rate of LDL and the liver's extraction of LDL precursors (VLDL remnants) from the blood, thus reducing LDL (Figure 35–2). Because of marked first-pass hepatic extraction, the major effect is on liver. Preferential activity in liver of some congeners appears to be attributable to tissue-specific differences in uptake. Modest decreases in plasma triglycerides and small increases in HDL also occur.

Therapeutic Uses & Dosage

Reductase inhibitors are useful alone or with resins, niacin, or ezetimibe in reducing levels of LDL. Women who are pregnant, lactating, or likely to become pregnant should not be given these agents. Use in children is restricted to those with homozygous familial hypercholesterolemia and selected patients with heterozygous familial hypercholesterolemia.

Because cholesterol synthesis occurs predominantly at night, reductase inhibitors—except atorvastatin and rosuvastatin—should be given in the evening if a single daily dose is used. Absorption generally (with the exception of pravastatin) is enhanced by food. Daily doses of lovastatin vary from 10 mg to 80 mg. Pravastatin is nearly as potent on a mass basis as lovastatin up to the maximum recommended daily dose, 80 mg. Simvastatin is twice as potent and is given in doses of 5–80 mg daily. Fluvastatin appears to be about half as potent as lovastatin on a mass basis and is given in doses of 10–80 mg daily. Atorvastatin is given in doses of 10–80 mg/d, and rosuvastatin, the most efficacious agent for severe hypercholesterolemia, at 5–40 mg/d. The dose-response curves of pravastatin and especially of fluvastatin tend to level off in the upper part of the dosage range in patients with moderate to severe hypercholesterolemia. Those of lovastatin, simvastatin, and atorvastatin are somewhat more linear.

Toxicity

Elevations of serum aminotransferase activity (up to three times normal) occur in some patients. This is often intermittent and usually not associated with other evidence of hepatic toxicity. Therapy may be continued in such patients in the absence of symptoms if aminotransferase levels are monitored and stable. In some patients, who may have underlying liver disease or a history of alcohol abuse, levels may exceed three times normal. This finding portends more severe hepatic toxicity. These patients may present with malaise, anorexia, and precipitous decreases in LDL. Medication should be discontinued immediately in these patients and in asymptomatic patients whose aminotransferase activity is persistently elevated to more than three times the upper limit of normal. These agents should be used with caution and in reduced dosage in patients with hepatic parenchymal disease, Asians, and the elderly. In general, aminotransferase activity should be measured at baseline, at 1–2 months, and then every 6–12 months (if stable).

Minor increases in creatine kinase (CK) activity in plasma are observed in some patients receiving reductase inhibitors, frequently associated with heavy physical activity. Rarely, patients may have marked elevations in CK activity, often accompanied by generalized discomfort or weakness in skeletal muscles. If the drug is not discontinued, rhabdomyolysis may cause myoglobinuria, leading to renal injury. Myopathy may occur with monotherapy, but there is an increased incidence in patients receiving certain other drugs.

The catabolism of lovastatin, simvastatin, and atorvastatin proceeds chiefly through CYP3A4, whereas that of fluvastatin and rosuvastatin is mediated by CYP2C9. Pravastatin is catabolized through other pathways, including sulfation. The 3A4-dependent reductase inhibitors tend to accumulate in plasma in the presence of drugs that inhibit or compete for the 3A4 cytochrome. These include the macrolide antibiotics, cyclosporine, ketoconazole and its congeners, HIV protease inhibitors, tacrolimus, nefazodone, fibrates, and others (see Chapter 4). Concomitant use of reductase inhibitors with amiodarone or verapamil also causes an increased risk of myopathy. Conversely, drugs such as phenytoin, griseofulvin, barbiturates, rifampin, and thiazolidinediones increase expression of CYP3A4 and can reduce the plasma concentrations of the 3A4-dependent reductase inhibitors. Inhibitors of CYP2C9 such as ketoconazole and its congeners, metronidazole, sulfinpyrazone, amiodarone, and cimetidine may increase plasma levels of fluvastatin and rosuvastatin. Pravastatin appears to be the drug of choice for use with verapamil, the ketoconazole group of antifungal agents, macrolides, and cyclosporine. Plasma levels of lovastatin, simvastatin, and atorvastatin may be elevated in patients ingesting more than 1 liter of grapefruit juice daily.

Creatine kinase activity should be measured in patients receiving potentially interacting drug combinations. In all patients, CK should be measured at baseline. If muscle pain, tenderness, or weakness appears, CK should be measured immediately and the drug discontinued if activity is elevated significantly over baseline. The myopathy usually reverses promptly upon cessation of therapy. If the association is unclear, the patient can be rechallenged under close surveillance. Myopathy in the absence of elevated CK has been reported. Rarely, hypersensitivity syndromes have been reported that include a lupus-like disorder and peripheral neuropathy.

These drugs should be temporarily discontinued in the event of serious illness, trauma, or major surgery.

NIACIN (NICOTINIC ACID)

Niacin (but not niacinamide) decreases VLDL and LDL levels, and Lp(a) in most patients. It often increases HDL levels significantly.

Chemistry & Pharmacokinetics

Niacin (vitamin B_3) is converted in the body to the amide, which is incorporated into niacinamide adenine dinucleotide (NAD). It is excreted in the urine unmodified and as several metabolites.

Mechanism of Action

Niacin inhibits VLDL secretion, in turn decreasing production of LDL (Figure 35–2). Increased clearance of VLDL via the LPL pathway contributes to reduction of triglycerides. Niacin has no effect on bile acid production. Excretion of neutral sterols in the stool is increased acutely as cholesterol is mobilized from tissue pools and a new steady state is reached. The catabolic rate for HDL is decreased. Fibrinogen levels are reduced, and levels of tissue plasminogen activator appear to increase. Niacin inhibits the intracellular lipase of adipose tissue via receptor-mediated signaling, possibly reducing VLDL production by decreasing the flux of free fatty acids to the liver. Sustained inhibition of lipolysis has not been established, however.

Therapeutic Uses & Dosage

In combination with a resin or reductase inhibitor, niacin normalizes LDL in most patients with heterozygous familial hypercholesterolemia and other forms of hypercholesterolemia. These combinations are also indicated in some cases of nephrosis. In severe mixed lipemia that is incompletely responsive to diet, niacin often produces marked reduction of triglycerides, an effect enhanced by marine omega-3 fatty acids. It is useful in patients with combined hyperlipidemia and in those with dysbetalipoproteinemia. It is clearly the most effective agent for increasing HDL and the only agent that may reduce Lp(a).

For treatment of heterozygous familial hypercholesterolemia, most patients require 2–6 g of niacin daily; more than this should not be given. For other types of hypercholesterolemia and for hypertriglyceridemia, 1.5–3.5 g daily is often sufficient. Crystalline niacin should be given in divided doses with meals, starting with 100 mg two or three times daily and increasing gradually.

Toxicity

Most persons experience a harmless cutaneous vasodilation and sensation of warmth after each dose when the drug is started or the dose increased. Taking 81–325 mg of aspirin one half hour beforehand blunts this prostaglandin-mediated effect. Ibuprofen, once daily, also mitigates the flush. Tachyphylaxis to flushing usually occurs within a few days at doses above 1.5–3 g daily. Patients should be warned to expect the flush and understand that it is a harmless side effect. Pruritus, rashes, dry skin or mucous membranes, and acanthosis nigricans have been reported. The latter contraindicates use of niacin because of its association with insulin resistance. Some patients experience nausea and abdominal discomfort. Many can continue the drug at reduced dosage, with inhibitors of gastric acid secretion, or use of antacids not containing aluminum. Niacin should be avoided in most patients with severe peptic disease.

Reversible elevations in aminotransferases up to twice normal may occur, usually not associated with liver toxicity. However, liver function should be monitored at baseline and at appropriate intervals. Rarely, true hepatotoxicity may occur, and in these cases the drug should be discontinued. The association of severe hepatic dysfunction, including acute necrosis, with the use of over-the-counter sustained-release preparations of niacin has been reported. This effect has not been noted to date with one preparation, Niaspan, given at bedtime in doses of 2 g or less. Carbohydrate tolerance may be moderately impaired, but this is usually reversible except in some patients with latent diabetes. Niacin may be given to diabetics who are receiving insulin and to some receiving oral agents if insulin resistance is not increased. Hyperuricemia occurs in some patients and occasionally precipitates gout. Allopurinol can be given with niacin if needed. Rarely, niacin is associated with arrhythmias, mostly atrial, and a reversible toxic amblyopia. Patients should be instructed to report blurring of distance vision. Niacin may potentiate the action of antihypertensive agents, requiring adjustment of their dosages. Birth defects have been reported in animals given very high dosages.

FIBRIC ACID DERIVATIVES (FIBRATES)

Gemfibrozil and **fenofibrate** decrease levels of VLDL and, in some patients, LDL as well. Another fibrate, **bezafibrate,** is not yet available in the USA.

Chemistry & Pharmacokinetics

Gemfibrozil is absorbed quantitatively from the intestine and is tightly bound to plasma proteins. It undergoes enterohepatic circulation and readily passes the placenta. The plasma half-life is 1.5 hours. Seventy percent is eliminated through the kidneys, mostly unmodified. The liver modifies some of the drug to hydroxymethyl, carboxyl, or quinol derivatives. Fenofibrate is a methylethyl ester that is hydrolyzed completely in the intestine. Its plasma half-life is 20 hours. Sixty percent is excreted in the urine as the glucuronide, and about 25% in feces.

Gemfibrozil

Fenofibrate

Mechanism of Action

These agents function primarily as ligands for the nuclear transcription receptor, peroxisome proliferator-activated receptor-alpha (PPAR-α). They increase lipolysis of lipoprotein triglyceride via LPL. Intracellular lipolysis in adipose tissue is decreased. Levels of VLDL decrease, in part as a result of decreased secretion by the liver. Only modest reductions of LDL occur in most patients. In others, especially those with combined hyperlipidemia, LDL often increases as triglycerides are reduced. HDL cholesterol increases moderately. Part of this apparent increase is a consequence of decreasing triglycerides in plasma, with reduction in exchange of triglycerides into HDL in place of cholesteryl esters. Some increase in HDL protein has been reported.

Therapeutic Uses & Dosage

These drugs are useful in hypertriglyceridemias in which VLDL predominate and in dysbetalipoproteinemia. They also may be of benefit in treating the hypertriglyceridemia that results from treatment with viral protease inhibitors. The usual dose of gemfibrozil is 600 mg orally once or twice daily. The dosage of fenofibrate (as Tricor) is one to three 48 mg tablets (or a single 145 mg tablet) daily. Absorption of gemfibrozil is improved when the drug is taken with food.

Toxicity

Rare adverse effects include rashes, gastrointestinal symptoms, myopathy, arrhythmias, hypokalemia, and high blood levels of aminotransferases or alkaline phosphatase. A few patients show decreases in white blood count or hematocrit. Both agents potentiate the action of coumarin and indanedione anticoagulants, and doses of these agents should be adjusted. Rhabdomyolysis has occurred rarely. Risk of myopathy increases when fibrates are given with reductase inhibitors. The use of fenofibrate with rosuvastatin appears to minimize this risk. Fibrates should be avoided in patients with hepatic or renal dysfunction. There appears to be a modest increase in the risk of cholesterol gallstones, reflecting an increase in the cholesterol content of bile. Therefore, fibrates should be used with caution in patients with biliary tract disease or in those at high risk such as women, obese patients, and Native Americans.

BILE ACID–BINDING RESINS

Colestipol, cholestyramine, and **colesevelam** are useful only for isolated increases in LDL. In patients who also have hypertriglyceridemia, VLDL levels may be further increased during treatment with resins.

Chemistry & Pharmacokinetics

These agents are large polymeric cationic exchange resins that are insoluble in water. They bind bile acids in the intestinal lumen and prevent their reabsorption. The resin itself is not absorbed.

Mechanism of Action

The bile acids, metabolites of cholesterol, are normally efficiently reabsorbed in the jejunum and ileum (Figure 35–2). Excretion is increased up to tenfold when resins are given, resulting in enhanced conversion of cholesterol to bile acids in liver via 7α-hydroxylation, which is normally controlled by negative feedback by bile acids. Increased uptake of LDL and IDL from plasma results from up-regulation of LDL receptors, particularly in liver. Therefore, the resins are without effect in patients with homozygous familial hypercholesterolemia who have no functioning receptors but may be useful in patients with receptor-defective combined heterozygous states.

Therapeutic Uses & Dosage

The resins are used in treatment of patients with primary hypercholesterolemia, producing approximately 20% reduction in LDL cholesterol in maximal dosage. If resins are used to treat LDL elevations in persons with combined hyperlipidemia, they may cause an increase in VLDL requiring the addition of a second agent such as niacin. Resins are also used in combination with other drugs to achieve further hypocholesterolemic effect (see below). They may be helpful in relieving pruritus in patients who have cholestasis and bile salt accumulation. Because the resins bind digitalis glycosides, they may be useful in digitalis toxicity.

Colestipol and cholestyramine are available as granular preparations. A gradual increase of dosage of granules from 4 or 5 g/d to 20 g/d is recommended. Total dosages of 30–32 g/d may be needed for maximum effect. The usual dosage for a child is 10–20 g/d. Granular resins are mixed with juice or water and allowed to hydrate for 1 minute. Colestipol is also available in 1 g tablets that must be swallowed whole, with a maximum dose of 16 g daily. Colesevelam is available in 625 mg tablets. The maximum dose is six tablets daily. Resins should be taken in two or three doses with meals. They lack effect when taken between meals.

Toxicity

Common complaints are constipation and bloating, usually relieved by increasing dietary fiber or mixing psyllium seed with the resin. Resins should be avoided in patients with diverticulitis. Heartburn and diarrhea are occasionally reported. In patients who have preexisting bowel disease or cholestasis, steatorrhea may occur. Malabsorption of vitamin K occurs rarely, leading to hypoprothrombinemia. Prothrombin time should be measured frequently in patients who are taking resins and anticoagulants. Malabsorption of folic acid has been reported rarely. Increased formation of gallstones, particularly in obese persons, was an anticipated adverse effect but has rarely occurred in practice.

Absorption of certain drugs, including those with neutral or cationic charge as well as anions, may be impaired by the resins. These include digitalis glycosides, thiazides, warfarin, tetracycline, thyroxine, iron salts, pravastatin, fluvastatin, folic acid, phenylbutazone, aspirin, and ascorbic acid. Any additional medication (except niacin) should be given 1 hour before or at least 2 hours after the resin to ensure adequate absorption. Colesevelam does not bind digoxin, warfarin, or reductase inhibitors.

INHIBITORS OF INTESTINAL STEROL ABSORPTION

Ezetimibe is the first member of a group of drugs that inhibit intestinal absorption of phytosterols and cholesterol. Its primary clinical effect is reduction of LDL levels.

Chemistry & Pharmacokinetics

Ezetimibe is readily absorbed and conjugated in the intestine to an active glucuronide, reaching peak blood levels in 12–14 hours. It undergoes enterohepatic circulation and its half-life is 22 hours. Approximately 80% of the drug is excreted in feces. Plasma concentrations are substantially increased when it is administered with fibrates and reduced when it is given with cholestyramine. Other resins may also decrease its absorption. There are no significant interactions with warfarin or digoxin.

Ezetimibe

Mechanism of Action

Ezetimibe is a selective inhibitor of intestinal absorption of cholesterol and phytosterols. A transport protein, NPC1L1, appears to be the target of the drug. It is effective even in the absence of dietary cholesterol because it inhibits reabsorption of cholesterol excreted in the bile.

Therapeutic Uses & Dosage

The effect on cholesterol absorption is constant over the dosage range of 5–20 mg/d. Therefore, a single daily dose of 10 mg is used. Average reduction in LDL cholesterol with ezetimibe alone in patients with primary hypercholesterolemia is about 18%, with minimal increases in HDL cholesterol. It is also effective in patients with phytosterolemia. Ezetimibe is synergistic with reductase inhibitors, producing decrements as great as 25% in LDL cholesterol beyond that achieved with the reductase inhibitor alone.

Toxicity

Ezetimibe does not appear to be a substrate for cytochrome P450 enzymes. Experience to date reveals a low incidence of reversible impaired hepatic function with a small increase in incidence when given with a reductase inhibitor. Myositis has been reported rarely.

TREATMENT WITH DRUG COMBINATIONS

Combined drug therapy is useful (1) when VLDL levels are significantly increased during treatment of hypercholesterolemia with a resin; (2) when LDL and VLDL levels are both elevated initially; (3) when LDL or VLDL levels are not normalized with a single agent, or (4) when an elevated level of Lp(a) or an HDL deficiency coexists with other hyperlipidemias.

1. Fibric Acid Derivatives & Bile Acid–Binding Resins

This combination is sometimes useful in treating patients with familial combined hyperlipidemia who are intolerant of niacin or statins. However, it may increase the risk of cholelithiasis.

2. HMG-CoA Reductase Inhibitors & Bile Acid–Binding Resins

This synergistic combination is useful in the treatment of familial hypercholesterolemia but may not control levels of VLDL in some patients with familial combined hyperlipoproteinemia. Statins should be given at least 1 hour before or 4 hours after the resin to ensure their absorption.

3. Niacin & Bile Acid–Binding Resins

This combination effectively controls VLDL levels during resin therapy of familial combined hyperlipoproteinemia or other disorders involving both increased VLDL and LDL levels. When VLDL and LDL levels are both initially increased, doses of niacin as low as 1–3 g/d may be sufficient in combination with a resin. The niacin-resin combination is effective for treating heterozygous familial hypercholesterolemia.

The drugs may be taken together, because niacin does not bind to the resins. LDL levels in patients with heterozygous familial hypercholesterolemia require daily doses of up to 6 g of niacin with 24–30 g of resin.

4. Niacin & Reductase Inhibitors

This regimen is more effective than either agent alone in treating hypercholesterolemia. Experience indicates that it is an efficacious and practical combination for treatment of familial combined hyperlipoproteinemia.

5. Reductase Inhibitors & Ezetimibe

This combination is highly synergistic in treating primary hypercholesterolemia and has some use in the treatment of patients with homozygous familial hyper-cholesterolemia who have some receptor function.

6. Reductase Inhibitors & Fibrates

Fenofibrate appears to be complementary with rosuvastatin or pravastatin in the treatment of familial combined hyperlipoproteinemia and other conditions involving elevations of both LDL and VLDL. The combination of fenofibrate with rosuvastatin is particularly effective. Other statins may interact unfavorably due to effects on cytochrome P450 metabolism.

7. Ternary Combination of Resins, Ezetimibe, Niacin, & Reductase Inhibitors

These agents act in a complementary fashion to normalize cholesterol in patients with severe disorders involving elevated LDL. The effects are sustained, and little compound toxicity has been observed. Effective doses of the individual drugs may be lower than when each is used alone—eg, as little as 1–2 g of niacin may substantially increase the effects of the other agents.

PREPARATIONS AVAILABLE

Atorvastatin (Lipitor)
Oral: 10, 20, 40, 80 mg tablets

Cholestyramine (generic, Questran, Questran Light)
Oral: 4 g packets anhydrous granules cholestyramine resin; 210 g (Questran Light), 378 g (Questran) cans

Colesevelam (Welchol)
Oral: 625 mg tablets

Colestipol (Colestid)
Oral: 5 g packets granules; 300, 500 g bottles; 1 g tablets

Ezetimibe (Zetia)
Oral: 10 mg tablets

Fenofibrate
Oral (Tricor): 48, 145 mg tablets; (Antara): 43, 87, 130 mg capsules; (Lofibra): 67, 134, 200 mg capsules

Fluvastatin (Lescol)
Oral: 20, 40 mg capsules; extended release (Lescol XL): 80 mg capsules

Gemfibrozil (generic, Lopid)
Oral: 600 mg tablets

Lovastatin (generic, Mevacor)
Oral: 10, 20, 40 mg tablets; ; extended release (Altoprev): 10, 20, 40, 60 mg

Niacin, nicotinic acid, vitamin B$_3$ (generic, others)
Oral: 100, 250, 500, 1000 mg tablets; extended release (Niaspan): 500, 750, 1000 mg

Pravastatin (Pravachol)
Oral: 10, 20, 40, 80 mg tablets

Rosuvastatin (Crestor)
Oral: 5, 10, 20, 40 mg tablets

Simvastatin (Zocor)
Oral: 5, 10, 20, 40, 80 mg tablets

COMBINATION TABLETS

Advicor (sustained release niacin plus lovastatin)
Oral: 500 or 1000 mg niacin with 20 mg lovastatin tablets

Vytorin (ezetimibe plus simvastatin)
Oral: 10/10, 10/20, 10/40, 10/80 mg tablets

REFERENCES

Grundy SM et al: Diagnosis and management of the metabolic syndrome: An American Heart Association/National Heart, Lung, and Blood Institute scientific statement. Circulation 2005;112:2735.

Grundy SM et al, for the Coordinating Committee of the National Cholesterol Education Program: Implications of recent clinical trials for the National Cholesterol Education Adult Treatment Panel III guidelines. Circulation 2004;110:227.

Kromhout D et al: Prevention of coronary heart disease by diet and lifestyle. Circulation 2002;105:893.

Libby P, Ridker PM, Maseri A: Inflammation and atherosclerosis. Circulation 2002;105:1135.

Waters DD et al, for the TNT Steering Committee Members and Investigators: Treating to New Targets (TNT) Study; does lowering low density lipoprotein cholesterol levels below currently recommended guidelines yield incremental clinical benefit? Am J Cardiol 2004;93:154.

Nonsteroidal Anti-Inflammatory Drugs, Disease-Modifying Antirheumatic Drugs, Nonopioid Analgesics, & Drugs Used in Gout

36

Daniel E. Furst, MD, & Robert W. Ulrich, PharmD

THE IMMUNE RESPONSE

The immune response occurs when immunologically competent cells are activated in response to foreign organisms or antigenic substances liberated during the acute or chronic inflammatory response. The outcome of the immune response for the host may be beneficial, as when it causes invading organisms to be phagocytosed or neutralized. On the other hand, the outcome may be deleterious if it leads to chronic inflammation without resolution of the underlying injurious process (see Chapter 56). Chronic inflammation involves the release of a number of mediators that are not prominent in the acute response. One of the most important conditions involving these mediators is rheumatoid arthritis, in which chronic inflammation results in pain and destruction of bone and cartilage that can lead to severe disability and in which systemic changes occur that can result in shortening of life.

The cell damage associated with inflammation acts on cell membranes to cause leukocytes to release lysosomal enzymes; arachidonic acid is then liberated from precursor compounds, and various eicosanoids are synthesized. As discussed in Chapter 18, the cyclooxygenase (COX) pathway of arachidonate metabolism produces prostaglandins, which have a variety of effects on blood vessels, on nerve endings, and on cells involved in inflammation. The discovery of cyclooxygenase isoforms (COX-1 and COX-2) led to the concepts that the constitutive COX-1 isoform tends to be homeostatic in function, while COX-2 is induced during inflammation and tends to facilitate the inflammatory response. On this basis, highly selective COX-2 inhibitors have been developed and marketed on the assumption that such selective inhibitors would be safer than nonselective COX-1 inhibitors but without loss of efficacy. The lipoxygenase pathway of arachidonate metabolism yields leukotrienes, which have a powerful chemotactic effect on eosinophils, neutrophils, and macrophages and promote bronchoconstriction and alterations in vascular permeability.

Kinins, neuropeptides, and histamine are also released at the site of tissue injury, as are complement components, cytokines, and other products of leukocytes and platelets. Stimulation of the neutrophil membranes produces oxygen-derived free radicals. Superoxide anion is formed by the reduction of molecular oxygen, which may stimulate the production of other reactive molecules such as hydrogen peroxide and hydroxyl radicals. The interaction of these substances with arachidonic acid results in the generation of chemotactic substances, thus perpetuating the inflammatory process.

THERAPEUTIC STRATEGIES

The treatment of patients with inflammation involves two primary goals: first, the relief of pain, which is often the presenting symptom and the major continuing complaint of the patient; and second, the slowing or—in theory—arrest of the tissue-damaging process. In rheumatoid arthritis, response to therapy can be quantitated by means of the American College of Rheumatology scoring system values ACR20, ACR50, and ACR70, which denote the percentage of patients showing an improvement of 20%, 50%, or 70% in a global assessment of signs and symptoms.

Reduction of inflammation with **nonsteroidal anti-inflammatory drugs (NSAIDs)** often results in relief of pain for significant periods. Furthermore, most of the nonopioid analgesics (aspirin, etc) also have anti-inflammatory effects, so they are appropriate for the treatment of both acute and chronic inflammatory conditions.

The **glucocorticoids** also have powerful anti-inflammatory effects and when first introduced were considered to be the ultimate answer to the treatment of inflammatory arthritis. Although there are increasing data that low-dose corticosteroids have disease-modifying properties, the toxicity associated with chronic corticosteroid therapy usually limits their use except in the control of acute flare-ups of joint disease. The NSAIDs continue to have a significant role in the long-term treatment of arthritis.

Another important group of agents is characterized as **disease-modifying antirheumatic drugs (DMARDs).** They slow the bone damage associated with rheumatoid arthritis and are thought to affect more basic inflammatory mechanisms than do the NSAIDs. They may also be more toxic than the nonsteroidal anti-inflammatory agents.

■ I. NONSTEROIDAL ANTI-INFLAMMATORY DRUGS

Salicylates and other similar agents used to treat rheumatic disease share the capacity to suppress the signs and symptoms of inflammation. These drugs also exert antipyretic and analgesic effects, but it is their anti-inflammatory properties that make them most useful in the management of disorders in which pain is related to the intensity of the inflammatory process.

Although all NSAIDs are not approved by the Food and Drug Administration (FDA) for the whole range of rheumatic diseases, all are probably effective in rheumatoid arthritis, seronegative spondyloarthropathies (eg, psoriatic arthritis and arthritis associated with inflammatory bowel disease), osteoarthritis, localized musculoskeletal syndromes (eg, sprains and strains, low back pain), and gout (except tolmetin, which appears to be ineffective in gout). Since aspirin, the original NSAID, has a number of adverse effects, many other NSAIDs have been developed in attempts to improve upon aspirin's efficacy and decrease its toxicity.

Chemistry & Pharmacokinetics

The NSAIDs are grouped in several chemical classes, some of which are shown in Figure 36–1. This chemical diversity yields a broad range of pharmacokinetic characteristics (Table 36–1). Although there are many differences in the kinetics of NSAIDs, they have some general properties in common. All but one of the NSAIDs are weak organic acids as given; the exception, nabumetone, is a ketone prodrug that is metabolized to the acidic active drug. Most of these drugs are well absorbed, and food does not substantially change their bioavailability. Most of the NSAIDs are highly metabolized, some by phase I followed by phase II mechanisms and others by direct glucuronidation (phase II) alone. NSAID metabolism proceeds, in large part, by

way of the CYP3A or CYP2C families of P450 enzymes in the liver. While renal excretion is the most important route for final elimination, nearly all undergo varying degrees of biliary excretion and reabsorption (enterohepatic circulation). In fact, the degree of lower gastrointestinal tract irritation correlates with the amount of enterohepatic circulation. Most of the NSAIDs are highly protein-bound (~ 98%), usually to albumin. Some of the NSAIDs (eg, ibuprofen) are racemic mixtures, while one, naproxen, is provided as a single enantiomer and a few have no chiral center (eg, diclofenac).

All NSAIDs can be found in synovial fluid after repeated dosing. Drugs with short half-lives remain in the joints longer than would be predicted from their half-lives, while drugs with longer half-lives disappear from the synovial fluid at a rate proportionate to their half-lives.

Pharmacodynamics

The anti-inflammatory activity of the NSAIDs is mediated chiefly through inhibition of biosynthesis of prostaglandins. Various NSAIDs have additional possible mechanisms of action, including inhibition of chemotaxis, down-regulation of interleukin-1 production, decreased production of free radicals and superoxide, and interference with calcium-mediated intracellular events. Aspirin irreversibly acetylates and blocks platelet cyclooxygenase, while most non-COX-selective NSAIDs are reversible inhibitors.

Selectivity for COX-1 versus COX-2 is variable and incomplete for the older members, but the highly selective COX-2 inhibitor, celecoxib, is currently available and other highly selective coxibs are being developed. The highly selective COX-2 inhibitors do not affect platelet function at their usual doses. In testing using human whole blood, aspirin, indomethacin, piroxicam, and sulindac were somewhat more effective in inhibiting COX-1; ibuprofen and meclofenamate inhibited the two isozymes about equally. The efficacy of COX-2-selective drugs equals that of the older NSAIDs, while gastrointestinal safety may be improved. On the other hand, highly selective COX-2 inhibitors may increase the incidence of edema and hypertension. As of August 2006, celecoxib is the only COX-2 inhibitor marketed in the USA. Rofecoxib and valdecoxib, two previously marketed, highly selective COX-2 inhibitors, have been withdrawn from the market due to their association with increased cardiovascular thrombotic events. In early 2005 a joint meeting of the Arthritis Advisory Committee and the Drug Safety and Risk Management Advisory Committee conducted by the FDA convened to assess the risk and give recommendations concerning the COX-2 inhibitors and other NSAIDs. It was concluded that there was not sufficient evidence to withdraw the COX-2 inhibitors but "black box" warnings concerning the cardiovascular risks were added to the product label. Additionally, it was recommended that all

Figure 36–1. Chemical structures of some NSAIDs.

other NSAID product labels be revised to include cardiovascular risks. Presently, the future of the COX-2 inhibitors is unclear.

The NSAIDs decrease the sensitivity of vessels to bradykinin and histamine, affect lymphokine production from T lymphocytes, and reverse the vasodilation of inflammation. To varying degrees, all newer NSAIDs are analgesic, anti-inflammatory, and antipyretic, and all (except the COX-2-selective agents and the nonacetylated salicylates) inhibit platelet aggregation. NSAIDs are all gastric irritants as well, although as a group the newer agents tend to cause less gastric irritation than aspirin. Nephrotoxicity has been observed for all of the drugs for which extensive experience has been reported, and hepatotoxicity can also occur with any NSAID. Nephrotoxicity is due, in part, to interference with the autoregulation of renal blood flow, which is modulated by prostaglandins.

Although these drugs effectively inhibit inflammation, there is no evidence that—in contrast to drugs such as methotrexate and gold—they alter the course of an arthritic disorder.

Several NSAIDs (including aspirin) appear to reduce the incidence of colon cancer when taken chronically. Several large epidemiologic studies have shown a 50% reduction in relative risk when the drugs are taken for 5 years or longer. The mechanism for this protective effect is unclear.

ASPIRIN

Aspirin's long use and availability without prescription diminishes its glamour compared with that of the newer NSAIDs. Aspirin is now rarely used as an anti-inflammatory medication; it has been replaced by ibuprofen and naproxen, since they are effective, are also

Table 36–1. Properties of aspirin and some nonsteroidal anti-inflammatory drugs.

Drug	Half-Life (hours)	Urinary Excretion of Unchanged Drug	Recommended Anti-inflammatory Dosage
Aspirin	0.25	< 2%	1200–1500 mg tid
Salicylate[1]	2–19	2–30%	See footnote 2
Apazone	15	62%	600 mg bid
Celecoxib	11	27%[3]	100–200 mg bid
Diclofenac	1.1	< 1%	50–75 mg qid
Diflunisal	13	3–9%	500 mg bid
Etodolac	6.5	< 1%	200–300 mg qid
Fenoprofen	2.5	30%	600 mg qid
Flurbiprofen	3.8	< 1%	300 mg tid
Ibuprofen	2	< 1%	600 mg qid
Indomethacin	4–5	16%	50–70 mg tid
Ketoprofen	1.8	< 1%	70 mg tid
Ketorolac	4–10	58%	10 mg qid[4]
Meclofenamate	3	2–4%	100 mg qid
Meloxicam	20	Data not found	7.5–15 mg qd
Nabumetone[5]	26	1%	1000–2000 mg qd[6]
Naproxen	14	< 1%	375 mg bid
Oxaprozin	58	1–4%	1200–1800 mg qd[6]
Piroxicam	57	4–10%	20 mg qd[6]
Sulindac	8	7%	200 mg bid
Tolmetin	1	7%	400 mg qid
Valdecoxib	8–11	90%[3]	10 mg qd

[1]Major anti-inflammatory metabolite of aspirin.
[2]Salicylate is usually given in the form of aspirin.
[3]Total urinary excretion including metabolites.
[4]Recommended for treatment of acute (eg, surgical) pain only.
[5]Nabumetone is a prodrug; the half-life and urinary excretion are for its active metabolite.
[6]A single daily dose is sufficient because of the long half-life.

available over the counter, and have good to excellent safety records.

Pharmacokinetics

Salicylic acid is a simple organic acid with a pK_a of 3.0. Aspirin (acetylsalicylic acid; ASA) has a pK_a of 3.5 (see Table 1–1). Sodium salicylate and aspirin (Figure 36–2) are equally effective anti-inflammatory drugs, though aspirin may be more effective as an analgesic. The salicylates are rapidly absorbed from the stomach and upper small intestine, yielding a peak plasma salicylate level within 1–2 hours. Aspirin is absorbed as such and is rapidly hydrolyzed (serum half-life 15 minutes) to acetic acid and salicylate by esterases in tissue and blood. Salicylate is bound to albumin, but the binding and metabolism of salicylates are saturable so that the unbound fraction increases as total concentration increases. Beyond a total body load of 600 mg, increases in salicylate dosage increase salicylate concentration disproportionately. As doses of aspirin increase, salicylate elimination half-life increases from 3–5 hours (for 600 mg/d dosage) to 12–

Figure 36–2. Structure and metabolism of the salicylates. (Modified and reproduced, with permission, from Meyers FH, Jawetz E, Goldfien A: *Review of Medical Pharmacology,* 7th ed. McGraw-Hill, 1980.)

16 hours (dosage > 3.6 g/d). Alkalinization of the urine increases the rate of excretion of free salicylate and its water-soluble conjugates.

Mechanisms of Action

A. ANTI-INFLAMMATORY EFFECTS

Aspirin is a nonselective inhibitor of both COX iso-forms (Figure 36–3), but salicylate is much less effective in inhibiting either isoform. Nonacetylated salicylates may work as oxygen radical scavengers. Aspirin irreversibly inhibits COX and inhibits platelet aggregation, while nonacetylated salicylates do not.

B. ANALGESIC EFFECTS

Aspirin is most effective in reducing pain of mild to moderate intensity through its effects on inflammation and because it probably inhibits pain stimuli at a subcortical site.

C. ANTIPYRETIC EFFECTS

Aspirin's antipyretic effect is probably mediated by both COX inhibition in the central nervous system and inhibition of interleukin-1 (which is released from macrophages during episodes of inflammation).

D. ANTIPLATELET EFFECTS

Aspirin irreversibly inhibits platelet COX, so that aspirin's antiplatelet effect lasts 8–10 days (the life of the platelet).

Clinical Uses

A. ANALGESIA, ANTIPYRESIS, AND ANTI-INFLAMMATORY EFFECTS

Aspirin is employed for mild to moderate pain of varied origin but is not effective for severe visceral pain. Aspirin and other NSAIDs have been combined with opioid analgesics for treatment of cancer pain, where their anti-inflammatory effects act synergistically with the opioids to enhance analgesia. High-dose salicylates are effective for treatment of rheumatic fever, rheumatoid arthritis, and other inflammatory joint conditions.

B. OTHER EFFECTS

Aspirin decreases the incidence of transient ischemic attacks, unstable angina, coronary artery thrombosis with myocardial infarction, and thrombosis after coronary artery bypass grafting (see Chapter 34).

Epidemiologic studies suggest that long-term use of aspirin at low dosage is associated with a lower incidence of colon cancer, possibly related to its COX-inhibiting effects.

Dosage

The optimal analgesic or antipyretic dose of aspirin is less than the 0.6–0.65 g oral dose commonly used. The anti-inflammatory dose for children is 50–75 mg/kg/d in divided doses and the average starting anti-inflammatory dose for adults is 45 mg/kg/d in divided doses (Table 36–1).

Figure 36–3. Scheme for mediators derived from arachidonic acid and sites of drug action (dashed arrows). (LTB$_4$, LTC$_4$, leukotrienes B$_4$, C$_4$.)

Adverse Effects

At the usual dosage, aspirin's main adverse effects are gastric upset (intolerance) and gastric and duodenal ulcers; hepatotoxicity, asthma, rashes, and renal toxicity occur less frequently. A dose-related increase in fecal blood loss is routinely associated with aspirin administration, although some mucosal adaptation occurs in many patients, so that blood loss declines back to baseline over 4–6 weeks.

With higher doses, patients may experience *salicylism*—vomiting, tinnitus, decreased hearing, and vertigo—reversible by reducing the dosage. Still larger doses of salicylates cause hyperpnea through a direct effect on the medulla. At toxic salicylate levels, respiratory alkalosis followed by metabolic acidosis (salicylate accumulation), respiratory depression, and even cardiotoxicity and glucose intolerance can occur. Like other NSAIDs, aspirin can cause elevation of liver enzymes (a frequent but mild effect), hepatitis (rare), decreased renal function, bleeding, rashes, and asthma.

The antiplatelet action of aspirin contraindicates its use by patients with hemophilia. Although previously not recommended during pregnancy, aspirin may be valuable in treating preeclampsia-eclampsia.

Salicylate overdosage constitutes a medical emergency and requires hospitalization (see Chapter 59).

NONACETYLATED SALICYLATES

These drugs include magnesium choline salicylate, sodium salicylate, and salicylsalicylate. All nonacetylated salicylates are effective anti-inflammatory drugs, although they may be less effective analgesics than aspirin. Because they are much less effective than aspirin as COX inhibitors, they may be preferable when COX inhibition is undesirable, such as in patients with asthma, those with bleeding tendencies, and even (under close supervision) those with renal dysfunction.

The nonacetylated salicylates are administered in the same dosage as aspirin and can be monitored using serum salicylate measurements.

COX-2 Selective Inhibitors

COX-2 selective inhibitors, or coxibs, were developed in an attempt to inhibit prostaglandin synthesis by the COX-2 isoenzyme induced at sites of inflammation without affecting the action of the constitutively active "housekeeping" COX-1 isoenzyme found in the gastrointestinal tract, kidneys, and platelets. Coxibs selectively bind to and block the active site of the COX-2 enzyme much more effectively than that of COX-1. COX-2 inhibitors have analgesic, antipyretic, and anti-inflammatory effects similar to those of nonselective NSAIDs but with an approximate halving of gastrointestinal adverse effects. Likewise, COX-2 inhibitors at usual doses have been shown to have no impact on platelet aggregation, which is mediated by the COX-1 isoenzyme. As a result, COX-2 inhibitors do not offer the cardioprotective effects of traditional nonselective NSAIDs, which has resulted in some patients taking low-dose aspirin in addition to a coxib regimen to maintain this effect. Unfortunately, because COX-2 is constitutively active within the kidney, recommended doses of COX-2 inhibitors cause renal toxicities similar to those associated with traditional NSAIDs. Clinical data have suggested a higher incidence of cardiovascular thrombotic events associated with COX-2 inhibitors such as rofecoxib and valdecoxib, resulting in their withdrawal from the market.

1. Celecoxib

Celecoxib is a selective COX-2 inhibitor—about 10–20 times more selective for COX-2 than for COX-1. Pharmacokinetic and dosage considerations are given in Table 36–1.

Celecoxib

Celecoxib is as effective as other NSAIDs in the treatment of rheumatoid arthritis and osteoarthritis, and in trials it has caused fewer endoscopic ulcers than most other NSAIDs. Probably because it is a sulfonamide, celecoxib may cause rashes. It does not affect platelet aggregation at usual doses. It interacts occasionally with warfarin—as would be expected of a drug metabolized via CYP2C9.

Although celecoxib is associated with about half the gastrointestinal side effects of nonselective NSAIDs, the frequency of other adverse effects approximates that of other NSAIDs. Celecoxib causes no more edema or renal effects than other members of the NSAID group, but edema and hypertension have been documented.

2. Etoricoxib

Etoricoxib, a bipyridine derivative, is a second-generation COX-2-selective inhibitor with the highest selectivity ratio of any coxib for inhibition of COX-2 relative to COX-1. It is extensively metabolized by hepatic P450 enzymes followed by renal excretion and has an elimination half-life of 22 hours. Etoricoxib is approved in the United Kingdom for the treatment of the signs and symptoms of osteoarthritis (60 mg once daily) and rheumatoid arthritis (90 mg once daily), for treatment of acute gouty arthritis (120 mg once daily), and for relief of acute musculoskeletal pain (60 mg once daily). Approval in the USA is still pending. Ninety mg daily of etoricoxib has superior efficacy compared with 500 mg of naproxen twice daily in the treatment of rheumatoid arthritis over 12 weeks. Etoricoxib has similar efficacy to traditional NSAIDs for osteoarthritis, acute gouty arthritis, and primary dysmenorrhea and has a gastrointestinal safety profile similar to that of other coxibs. Since etoricoxib has structural similarities to diclofenac, it is appropriate to monitor hepatic function carefully in patients using this drug.

3. Meloxicam

Meloxicam is an enolcarboxamide related to piroxicam that has been shown to preferentially inhibit COX-2 over COX-1, particularly at its lowest therapeutic dose of 7.5 mg/d. It is not as selective as the other coxibs and may be considered "preferentially" selective rather than "highly" selective. The drug is popular in Europe and many other countries for most rheumatic diseases and has recently been approved for treatment of osteoarthritis in the USA. Its efficacy in this condition and rheumatoid arthritis is comparable to that of other NSAIDs. It is associated with fewer clinical gastrointestinal symptoms and complications than piroxicam, diclofenac, and naproxen. Similarly, while meloxicam is known to inhibit synthesis of thromboxane A_2, it appears that even at supratherapeutic doses its blockade of thromboxane A_2 does not reach levels that result in decreased in vivo platelet function. Other toxicities are similar to those of other NSAIDs.

4. Valdecoxib

Valdecoxib, a diaryl-substituted isoxazole, is a new highly selective COX-2 inhibitor. Pharmacokinetic characteristics and dosage in arthritis are set forth in

Table 36–1. The analgesic dose for valdecoxib is 20 mg twice daily. Gastrointestinal and other toxicities are similar to those of the other coxibs. Valdecoxib has no effect on platelet aggregation or bleeding time. Serious reactions have been reported in sulfonamide-sensitive individuals. Valdecoxib was withdrawn from the market in the USA in early 2005 in response to FDA concerns about cardiovascular risks and Stevens-Johnson syndrome, but the drug is still available in other countries.

Valdecoxib

NONSELECTIVE COX INHIBITORS

1. Diclofenac

Diclofenac is a phenylacetic acid derivative that is relatively nonselective as a COX inhibitor. Pharmacokinetic and dosage characteristics are set forth in Table 36–1.

Adverse effects occur in approximately 20% of patients and include gastrointestinal distress, occult gastrointestinal bleeding, and gastric ulceration, though ulceration may occur less frequently than with some other NSAIDs. A preparation combining diclofenac and misoprostol decreases upper gastrointestinal ulceration but may result in diarrhea. Another combination of diclofenac and omeprazole was also effective with respect to the prevention of recurrent bleeding, but renal adverse effects were common in high-risk patients. Diclofenac at a dosage of 150 mg/d appears to impair renal blood flow and glomerular filtration rate. Elevation of serum aminotransferases may occur more commonly with this drug than with other NSAIDs.

A 0.1% ophthalmic preparation is recommended for prevention of postoperative ophthalmic inflammation and can be used after intraocular lens implantation and strabismus surgery. A topical gel containing 3% diclofenac is effective for solar keratoses. Diclofenac in rectal suppository form can be considered a drug of choice for preemptive analgesia and postoperative nausea. In Europe, diclofenac is also available as an oral mouthwash and for intramuscular administration.

2. Diflunisal

Although diflunisal is derived from salicylic acid, it is not metabolized to salicylic acid or salicylate. It undergoes an enterohepatic cycle with reabsorption of its glucuronide metabolite followed by cleavage of the glucuronide to again release the active moiety. Diflunisal is subject to capacity-limited metabolism, with serum half-lives at various dosages approximating that of salicylates (Table 36–1). In rheumatoid arthritis the recommended dose is 500–1000 mg daily in two divided doses. It is claimed to be particularly effective for cancer pain with bone metastases and for pain control in dental (third molar) surgery. A 2% diflunisal oral ointment is a clinically useful analgesic for painful oral lesions.

Because its clearance depends on renal function as well as hepatic metabolism, diflunisal's dosage should be limited in patients with significant renal impairment. Its adverse event profile is similar to those of other NSAIDs; pseudoporphyria has also been reported.

3. Etodolac

Etodolac is a racemic acetic acid derivative with an intermediate half-life (Table 36–1). It is slightly more COX-2-selective than most other NSAIDs, with a COX-2:COX-1 activity ratio of about 10. Unlike many other racemic NSAIDs, etodolac does not undergo chiral inversion in the body. The dosage of etodolac is 200–400 mg three to four times daily. Etodolac provides good postoperative pain relief after coronary artery bypass operations, although transient impairment of renal function has been reported. There are no data to suggest that etodolac differs significantly from other NSAIDs except in its pharmacokinetic parameters, though it has been claimed to cause less gastric toxicity in terms of ulcer disease than other nonselective NSAIDs.

4. Fenoprofen

Fenoprofen, a propionic acid derivative, is the NSAID most closely associated with interstitial nephritis and is rarely used. Its other toxicities mirror those of other NSAIDs.

5. Flurbiprofen

Flurbiprofen is a propionic acid derivative with a possibly more complex mechanism of action than other NSAIDs. Its $(S)(-)$ enantiomer inhibits COX nonselectively, but it has been shown in rat tissue to also affect TNF-α and nitric oxide synthesis. Hepatic metabolism is extensive; its $(R)(+)$ and $(S)(-)$ enantiomers are metabolized differently, and it does not undergo chiral conversion. It does demonstrate enterohepatic circulation.

The efficacy of flurbiprofen at dosages of 200–400 mg/d is comparable to that of aspirin and other NSAIDs in clinical trials for patients with rheumatoid arthritis, ankylosing spondylitis, gout, and osteoarthritis. It is also available in a topical ophthalmic formulation for inhibition of intraoperative miosis. Flurbiprofen intravenously has been found to be effective for perioperative analgesia in minor ear, neck, and nose surgery and in lozenge form for sore throat.

Although its adverse effect profile is similar to that of other NSAIDs in most ways, flurbiprofen is also associated rarely with cogwheel rigidity, ataxia, tremor, and myoclonus.

6. Ibuprofen

Ibuprofen is a simple derivative of phenylpropionic acid. In doses of about 2400 mg daily, ibuprofen is equivalent to 4 g of aspirin in anti-inflammatory effect. Pharmacokinetic characteristics are given in Table 36–1.

Oral ibuprofen is often prescribed in lower doses (< 2400 mg/d), at which it has analgesic but not anti-inflammatory efficacy. It is available over the counter in low-dose forms under several trade names. A topical cream preparation appears to be absorbed into fascia and muscle; an *(S)(–)* formulation has been tested. Ibuprofen cream was more effective than placebo cream for the treatment of primary knee osteoarthritis. A liquid gel preparation of ibuprofen 400 mg provides prompt relief and good overall efficacy in postsurgical dental pain. In comparison with indomethacin, ibuprofen decreases urine output less and also causes less fluid retention than indomethacin. Ibuprofen is effective in closing patent ductus arteriosus in preterm infants, with much the same efficacy and safety as indomethacin. The oral and intravenous routes are equally effective for this indication.

Gastrointestinal irritation and bleeding occur, although less frequently than with aspirin. The use of ibuprofen concomitantly with aspirin may *decrease* the total anti-inflammatory effect. The drug is relatively contraindicated in individuals with nasal polyps, angioedema, and bronchospastic reactivity to aspirin. In addition to the gastrointestinal symptoms (which can be modified by ingestion with meals), rash, pruritus, tinnitus, dizziness, headache, aseptic meningitis (particularly in patients with systemic lupus erythematosus), and fluid retention have been reported. Interaction with anticoagulants is uncommon.

The concomitant administration of ibuprofen antagonizes the irreversible platelet inhibition induced by aspirin. Thus, treatment with ibuprofen in patients with increased cardiovascular risk may limit the cardioprotective effects of aspirin. Rare hematologic effects include agranulocytosis and aplastic anemia. Effects on the kidney (as with all NSAIDs) include acute renal failure, interstitial nephritis, and nephrotic syndrome, but these occur very rarely. Finally, hepatitis has been reported.

7. Indomethacin

Indomethacin, introduced in 1963, is an indole derivative (Figure 36–1). It is a potent nonselective COX inhibitor and may also inhibit phospholipase A and C, reduce neutrophil migration, and decrease T cell and B cell proliferation. Probenecid prolongs indomethacin's half-life by inhibiting both renal and biliary clearance. It differs somewhat from other NSAIDs in its indications and toxicities.

Indomethacin is indicated for use in rheumatic conditions and is particularly popular for gout and ankylosing spondylitis. In addition, it has been used to treat patent ductus arteriosus. Indomethacin has been tried in numerous small or uncontrolled trials for many other conditions, including Sweet's syndrome, juvenile rheumatoid arthritis, pleurisy, nephrotic syndrome, diabetes insipidus, urticarial vasculitis, postepisiotomy pain, and prophylaxis of heterotopic ossification in arthroplasty. An ophthalmic preparation seems to be efficacious for conjunctival inflammation and to reduce pain after traumatic corneal abrasion. Gingival inflammation is reduced after administration of indomethacin oral rinse. Epidural injections produce a degree of pain relief similar to that achieved with methylprednisolone in postlaminectomy syndrome.

At higher dosages, at least a third of patients have reactions to indomethacin requiring discontinuance. The gastrointestinal effects may include abdominal pain, diarrhea, gastrointestinal hemorrhage, and pancreatitis. Headache is experienced by 15–25% of patients and may be associated with dizziness, confusion, and depression. Rarely, psychosis with hallucinations has been reported. Hepatic abnormalities are rare. Serious hematologic reactions have been noted, including thrombocytopenia and aplastic anemia. Hyperkalemia has been reported and is related to inhibition of the synthesis of prostaglandins in the kidney. Renal papillary necrosis has also been observed. A number of interactions with other drugs have been reported (see Appendix II).

8. Ketoprofen

Ketoprofen is a propionic acid derivative that inhibits both COX (nonselectively) and lipoxygenase. Its pharmacokinetic characteristics are given in Table 36–1. Concurrent administration of probenecid elevates ketoprofen levels and prolongs its plasma half-life.

The effectiveness of ketoprofen at dosages of 100–300 mg/d is equivalent to that of other NSAIDs in the treatment of rheumatoid arthritis, osteoarthritis, gout, dysmenorrhea, and other painful conditions. In spite of its dual effect on prostaglandins and leukotrienes, ketoprofen is not superior to other NSAIDs. Its major adverse effects are on the gastrointestinal tract and the central nervous system.

9. Ketorolac

Ketorolac is an NSAID promoted for systemic use mainly as an analgesic, not as an anti-inflammatory drug (although it has typical NSAID properties). Pharmacokinetics are presented in Table 36–1. The drug is an effective analgesic and has been used successfully to replace morphine in some situations involving mild to moderate postsurgical pain. It is most often given intramuscularly or intravenously, but an oral dose formulation is available. When used with an opioid, it may decrease the opioid requirement by 25–50%. An ophthalmic preparation is available for ocular inflammatory conditions. Toxicities are similar to those of other NSAIDs, although renal toxicity may be more common with chronic use.

10. Meclofenamate & Mefenamic Acid

Meclofenamate and mefenamic acid (Table 36–1) inhibit both COX and phospholipase A_2. They are rarely used today.

11. Nabumetone

Nabumetone is the only nonacid NSAID in current use; it is converted to the active acetic acid derivative in the body. It is given as a ketone prodrug that resembles naproxen in structure (Figure 36–1). Its half-life of more than 24 hours (Table 36–1) permits once-daily dosing, and the drug does not appear to undergo enterohepatic circulation. Renal impairment results in a doubling of its half-life and a 30% increase in the area under the curve. Its properties are very similar to those of other NSAIDs, though it may be less damaging to the stomach than some other NSAIDs when given at a dosage of 1000 mg/d. Unfortunately, higher doses (eg, 1500–2000 mg/d) are often needed, and this is a very expensive NSAID. Like naproxen, nabumetone has been reported to cause pseudoporphyria and photosensitivity in some patients. Other adverse effects mirror those of other NSAIDs.

12. Naproxen

Naproxen is a naphthylpropionic acid derivative. It is the only NSAID presently marketed as a single enantiomer, and it is a nonselective COX inhibitor. Naproxen's free fraction is significantly higher in women than in men, although albumin binding is very high in both sexes (Table 36–1). Naproxen is effective for the usual rheumatologic indications and is available both in a slow-release formulation and as an oral suspension. A topical preparation and an ophthalmic solution are also available.

The incidence of upper gastrointestinal bleeding in over-the-counter use is low but still double that of over-the-counter ibuprofen (perhaps due to a dose effect). Rare cases of allergic pneumonitis, leukocytoclastic vasculitis, and pseudoporphyria as well as the more common NSAID-associated adverse effects have been noted.

13. Oxaprozin

Oxaprozin is another propionic acid derivative NSAID. As noted in Table 36–1, its major difference from the other members of this subgroup is a very long half-life (50–60 hours), although oxaprozin does not undergo enterohepatic circulation. The drug has the same benefits and risks that are associated with other NSAIDs. It is mildly uricosuric, making it potentially more useful in gout than some other NSAIDs.

14. Phenylbutazone

Phenylbutazone, a pyrazolone derivative, rapidly gained favor after its introduction in 1949 but, because of its toxicity, is rarely used today.

15. Piroxicam

Piroxicam, an oxicam (Figure 36–1), is a nonselective COX inhibitor that at high concentrations also inhibits polymorphonuclear leukocyte migration, decreases oxygen radical production, and inhibits lymphocyte function. Its long half-life (Table 36–1) permits once-daily dosing.

Piroxicam can be used for the usual rheumatic indications. Toxicity includes gastrointestinal symptoms (20% of patients), dizziness, tinnitus, headache, and rash. When piroxicam is used in dosages higher than 20 mg/d, an increased incidence of peptic ulcer and bleeding is encountered. Epidemiologic studies suggest that this risk is as much as 9.5 times higher with piroxicam than with other NSAIDs.

16. Sulindac

Sulindac is a sulfoxide prodrug. It is reversibly metabolized to the active sulfide metabolite, which is excreted in bile and then reabsorbed from the intestine. The enterohepatic cycling prolongs the duration of action to 12–16 hours.

The indications and adverse reactions of sulindac are similar to those of other NSAIDs. In addition to its rheumatic disease indications, sulindac suppresses familial intestinal polyposis; it may inhibit the development of colon, breast, and prostate cancer in humans. It appears to inhibit the occurrence of gastrointestinal cancer in rats. The latter effect may be caused by the sulfone rather than the sulfide.

Among the more severe adverse reactions, Stevens-Johnson epidermal necrolysis syndrome, thrombocytopenia, agranulocytosis, and nephrotic syndrome have all been observed. Like diclofenac, sulindac may have some propensity to cause elevation of serum aminotransferases; it is also sometimes associated with cholestatic liver damage, which disappears or becomes quiescent when the drug is stopped.

17. Tenoxicam

Tenoxicam is an oxicam similar to piroxicam and shares its nonselective COX inhibition, long half-life (72 hours), efficacy, and toxicity profile. It is available abroad but not in the USA.

18. Tiaprofen

Tiaprofen is a racemic propionic acid derivative but does not undergo stereoconversion. It has a short serum half-life (1–2 hours) with an increase to 2–4 hours in the elderly. This drug inhibits renal uric acid reabsorption and thus decreases serum uric acid slightly. It is available for oral and intramuscular administration. Its efficacy and adverse event profiles mirror those of other NSAIDs. Tiaprofen is not available in the USA.

19. Tolmetin

Tolmetin is a nonselective COX inhibitor with a short half-life (1–2 hours)and is not often used. Its efficacy and toxicity profiles are similar to those of other NSAIDs with the following exceptions: it is ineffective (for unknown reasons) in the treatment of gout, and it may cause (rarely) thrombocytopenic purpura.

20. Azapropazone & Carprofen

These drugs are available in many other countries but are not sold in the USA. Azapropazone (apazone), a pyrazolone derivative, is structurally related to phenylbutazone but appears less likely to cause agranulocytosis. Its half-life of 12–16 hours may be doubled in patients with decreased renal function. Carprofen is a propionic acid derivative with a half-life of 10–16 hours. The indications and adverse effects of azapropazone and carprofen are similar to those of other NSAIDs.

CLINICAL PHARMACOLOGY OF THE NSAIDS

All NSAIDs, including aspirin, are about equally efficacious with a few exceptions—tolmetin seems not to be effective for gout, and aspirin is less effective than other NSAIDs (eg, indomethacin) for ankylosing spondylitis. Thus, NSAIDs tend to be differentiated on the basis of toxicity and cost-effectiveness. For example, the gastrointestinal and renal side effects of ketorolac limit its use. Some surveys suggest that indomethacin, tolmetin, and meclofenamate are the NSAIDs associated with the greatest toxicity, while salsalate, aspirin, and ibuprofen are least toxic. The selective COX-2 inhibitors were not included in this analysis.

For patients with renal insufficiency, nonacetylated salicylates may be best. Fenoprofen is less often used because of its rare association with interstitial nephritis. Diclofenac and sulindac are associated with more liver function test abnormalities than other NSAIDs. The relatively expensive, selective COX-2 inhibitors are probably safest for patients at high risk for gastrointestinal bleeding but may have a higher risk of cardiovascular toxicity. Celecoxib or a nonselective NSAID plus omeprazole or misoprostol may be appropriate in patients at highest risk for gastrointestinal bleeding; in this subpopulation of patients, they are cost-effective despite their high acquisition costs.

The choice of an NSAID thus requires a balance of efficacy, cost-effectiveness, safety, and numerous personal factors (eg, other drugs also being used, concurrent illness, compliance, medical insurance coverage), so that there is no best NSAID for all patients. There may, however, be one or two best NSAIDs for a specific person.

■ II. DISEASE-MODIFYING ANTIRHEUMATIC DRUGS (DMARDS)

Careful clinical and epidemiologic studies have shown that rheumatoid arthritis is an immunologic disease that causes significant systemic effects which shorten life in addition to the joint disease that reduces mobility and quality of life. NSAIDs offer mainly symptomatic relief; they reduce inflammation and the pain it causes and often preserve function, but they have little effect on the progression of bone and cartilage destruction. Interest has therefore centered on finding treatments that might arrest—or at least slow—this progression by modifying the disease itself. The effects of disease-modifying therapies may take 6 weeks to 6 months to become evident; that is, they are slow-acting compared with NSAIDs. These therapies include methotrexate, azathioprine, penicillamine, hydroxychloroquine and chloroquine, organic gold compounds, sulfasalazine, several other immune-modulating agents, and immunoadsorption apheresis.

Considerable controversy surrounds the long-term efficacy of many of these therapies.

METHOTREXATE

Methotrexate is now considered the DMARD of first choice to treat rheumatoid arthritis and is used in up to 60% of patients. It is active in this condition at much lower doses than those needed in cancer chemotherapy (see Chapter 55).

Mechanism of Action

Methotrexate's principal mechanism of action at the low doses used in the rheumatic diseases probably relates to inhibition of aminoimidazolecarboxamide ribonucleotide (AICAR) transformylase and thymidylate synthetase, with secondary effects on polymorphonuclear chemotaxis. There is some effect on dihydrofolate reductase and this affects lymphocyte and macrophage function, but this is not its principal mechanism of action.

Pharmacokinetics

The drug is approximately 70% absorbed after oral administration (see Chapter 55). It is metabolized to a less active hydroxylated metabolite, and both the parent compound and the metabolite are polyglutamated within cells, where they stay for prolonged periods. Methotrexate's serum half-life is usually only 6–9 hours, although it may be as long as 24 hours in some individuals. Methotrexate's concentration is increased in the presence of hydroxychloroquine. This drug is excreted principally in the urine, but up to 30% may be excreted in bile.

Indications

Although the most common methotrexate dosing regimen for the treatment of rheumatoid arthritis is 15–25 mg weekly, there is an increased effect up to 30 or 35 mg weekly. The drug decreases the rate of appearance of new erosions. Evidence supports its use in juvenile chronic arthritis, and it has been used in psoriasis, psoriatic arthritis, ankylosing spondylitis, polymyositis, dermatomyositis, Wegener's granulomatosis, giant cell arteritis, systemic lupus erythematosus, and vasculitis.

Adverse Effects

Nausea and mucosal ulcers are the most common toxicities. Progressive dose-related hepatotoxicity in the form of enzyme elevation occurs frequently, but cirrhosis is rare (< 1%). Liver toxicity is not related to serum methotrexate concentrations, and liver biopsy follow-up is only recommended every 5 years. A rare "hypersensitivity" lung reaction with acute shortness of breath is documented, as are pseudolymphomatous reactions. The

incidence of gastrointestinal and liver function test abnormalities can be reduced by the use of leucovorin 24 hours after each weekly dose or by the use of daily folic acid. This drug is contraindicated in pregnancy.

CHLORAMBUCIL

Mechanism of Action & Pharmacokinetics

Chlorambucil, probably through its metabolite phenylacetic acid mustard, cross-links DNA, thereby preventing cell replication. Its bioavailability is about 70% and it is completely metabolized, with excretion completed within 24 hours.

Indications

One controlled, double-blind trial plus anecdotal evidence attest to the efficacy of chlorambucil in rheumatoid arthritis. Chlorambucil has also been used in Behçet's disease, systemic lupus erythematosus, vasculitis, and other autoimmune disorders.

Adverse Effects

The most common toxicity is dose-related bone marrow suppression. Infertility with azoospermia and amenorrhea also occurs. The risk of neoplasia is increased, with the relative risk of leukemia increased about tenfold compared with the general population, especially after more than 3 years of use.

CYCLOPHOSPHAMIDE

Mechanism of Action

Cyclophosphamide's major active metabolite is phosphoramide mustard, which cross-links DNA to prevent cell replication. It suppresses T cell and B cell function by 30–40%; T cell suppression correlates with clinical response in the rheumatic diseases.

Pharmacokinetics

See Chapter 55.

Indications

Cyclophosphamide is active against rheumatoid arthritis when given orally at dosages of 2 mg/kg/d but not when given intravenously. It is used regularly to treat systemic lupus erythematosus, vasculitis, Wegener's granulomatosis, and other severe rheumatic diseases.

Adverse Effects

Cyclophosphamide causes significant dose-related infertility in both men and women as well as bone marrow suppression, alopecia, hemorrhagic cystitis, and, rarely, bladder carcinoma (see Chapter 55).

CYCLOSPORINE

Mechanism of Action

Through regulation of gene transcription, cyclosporine inhibits interleukin-1 and interleukin-2 receptor production and secondarily inhibits macrophage-T cell interaction and T cell responsiveness (see Chapter 56). T cell-dependent B cell function is also affected.

Pharmacokinetics

Cyclosporine absorption is incomplete and somewhat erratic, although a new microemulsion formulation improves its consistency and provides 20–30% bioavailability. Grapefruit juice increases cyclosporine bioavailability by as much as 62%. Cyclosporine is metabolized by CYP3A and consequently is subject to a large number of drug interactions (see Chapter 56 and Appendix II).

Indications

Cyclosporine is approved for use in rheumatoid arthritis and retards the appearance of new bony erosions. Its usual dosage is 3–5 mg/kg/d divided into two doses. Anecdotal reports suggest that it may be useful in systemic lupus erythematosus, polymyositis and dermatomyositis, Wegener's granulomatosis, and juvenile chronic arthritis.

Adverse Effects

Cyclosporine has significant nephrotoxicity, and its toxicity can be increased by drug interactions with diltiazem, potassium-sparing diuretics, and other drugs inhibiting CYP3A. Serum creatinine should be closely monitored. Other toxicities include hypertension, hyperkalemia, hepatotoxicity, gingival hyperplasia, and hirsutism.

AZATHIOPRINE

Mechanism of Action

Azathioprine acts through its major metabolite, 6-thioguanine. 6-Thioguanine suppresses inosinic acid synthesis, B cell and T cell function, immunoglobulin production, and interleukin-2 secretion (see Chapter 56).

Pharmacokinetics

The metabolism of azathioprine is bimodal in the population, with rapid metabolizers clearing the drug four times more rapidly than slow metabolizers. Production of 6-thioguanine is dependent on thiopurine methyltransferase (TPMT), and patients with low or absent TPMT activity (0.3% of the population) are at particularly high risk of myelosuppression by excess concentrations of the parent drug if dosage is not adjusted.

Indications

Azathioprine is approved for use in rheumatoid arthritis and is used at a dosage of 2 mg/kg/d. Controlled trials show efficacy in psoriatic arthritis, reactive arthritis, polymyositis, systemic lupus erythematosus, and Behçet's disease.

Adverse Effects

Azathioprine's toxicity includes bone marrow suppression, gastrointestinal disturbances, and some increase in infection risk. As noted in Chapter 56, lymphomas may be increased with azathioprine use. Rarely, fever, rash, and hepatotoxicity signal acute allergic reactions.

MYCOPHENOLATE MOFETIL

Mechanism of Action

Mycophenolate mofetil (MMF) is converted to mycophenolic acid, the active form of the drug. The active product inhibits cytosine monophosphate dehydrogenase and, secondarily, inhibits T cell lymphocyte proliferation; downstream, it interferes with leukocyte adhesion to endothelial cells through inhibition of E-selectin, P-selectin, and intercellular adhesion molecule 1.

Pharmacokinetics

See Chapter 56.

Indications

MMF is effective for the treatment of renal disease due to systemic lupus erythematosus and may be useful in vasculitis and Wegener's granulomatosis. While occasionally used at a dosage of 2 g/d to treat rheumatoid arthritis, there are no well-controlled data regarding its efficacy in this disease.

Adverse Effects

Comparisons with azathioprine in the renal transplantation literature show that MMF and azathioprine have similar gastrointestinal, hematopoietic, and hepatic toxicity profiles, with a possibly decreased incidence of fungal infections among patients treated with MMF. Hepatic toxicities are infrequent but must be monitored.

CHLOROQUINE & HYDROXYCHLOROQUINE

Mechanism of Action

Chloroquine and hydroxychloroquine are used mainly in malaria (see Chapter 53) and in the rheumatic diseases. The mechanism of the anti-inflammatory action of these drugs in rheumatic diseases is unclear. The following mechanisms have been proposed: suppression of T lymphocyte responses to mitogens, decreased leukocyte chemotaxis, stabilization of lysosomal enzymes, inhibition of DNA and RNA synthesis, and the trapping of free radicals.

Pharmacokinetics

Antimalarials are rapidly absorbed but only 50% protein-bound in the plasma. They are very extensively tissue-bound, particularly in melanin-containing tissues such as the eyes. The drugs are deaminated in the liver and have blood elimination half-lives of up to 45 days.

Indications

Antimalarials are approved for rheumatoid arthritis, but they are not considered very efficacious DMARDs. Dose-response and serum concentration-response relationships have been documented for hydroxychloroquine and dose-loading may increase rate of response. While antimalarials improve symptoms, there is no evidence that these compounds alter bony damage in rheumatoid arthritis at their usual dosages (up to 6.4 mg/kg/d hydroxychloroquine or 200 mg/d chloroquine). It usually takes 3–6 months to obtain a response. Antimalarials are often used for the treatment of the skin manifestations, serositis, and joint pains of systemic lupus erythematosus, and they have been used in Sjögren's syndrome.

Adverse Effects

Although ocular toxicity (Chapter 53) may occur at dosages greater than 250 mg/d for chloroquine and greater than 6.4 mg/kg/d for hydroxychloroquine, it rarely occurs at lower doses. Nevertheless, ophthalmologic monitoring every 6–12 months is advised. Other toxicities include dyspepsia, nausea, vomiting, abdominal pain, rashes, and nightmares. These drugs appear to be relatively safe in pregnancy.

GOLD

Gold compounds were first proved to be effective in a large double-blind trial in 1960. Because of their toxicity, they are used infrequently today. Their intramuscular formulations (**aurothiomalate** and **aurothioglu-**

cose) contain 50% elemental gold. The oral formulation (**auranofin**) contains 29% elemental gold.

Mechanism of Action

Gold alters the morphology and functional capabilities of human macrophages—possibly its major mode of action. As a result, monocyte chemotactic factor-1, interleukin-8, interleukin-1β production, and vascular endothelial growth factor are all inhibited. Intramuscular gold compounds also alter lysosomal enzyme activity, reduce histamine release from mast cells, inactivate the first component of complement, and suppress the phagocytic activities of polymorphonuclear leukocytes. Oral gold (auranofin) also inhibits release of prostaglandin E_2 and leukotriene B_4.

Pharmacokinetics

These compounds have high bioavailability after intramuscular administration and tend to concentrate in synovial membranes, liver, kidney, spleen, lymph nodes, and bone marrow. One month after an intramuscular injection, 75–80% of the drug is eliminated from the serum, but intramuscular gold's total body half-life is approximately 1 year. Auranofin is only about 25% bioavailable. Gold compounds are excreted approximately 66% in the urine and 33% via the feces. No correlation has been found between serum gold concentration and either efficacy or toxicity.

Indications

Gold is effective for active rheumatoid arthritis and has been shown to slow radiologic progression of the disease. It has also been used in Sjögren's syndrome and juvenile rheumatoid arthritis, while use in psoriatic arthritis is controversial. In Japan, gold is used to treat asthma. The oral form of gold is effective in rheumatoid arthritis, but it appears less effective than the intramuscular formulation and is generally felt to have only modest effects.

Clinical Use

Intramuscular gold is given as a test dose of 5–25 mg and then as 50 mg intramuscular doses weekly for 20 weeks. Continued treatment, with maintained response, frequently allows lengthening of the dosing interval to 2, 3, or 4 weeks. Oral gold is generally given as 6 mg doses daily.

Adverse Effects

Pruritic skin rashes occur in 15–20% of patients, sometimes associated with eosinophilia. Stomatitis and a metallic taste in the mouth are common. Hematologic abnormalities, including thrombocytopenia, leukopenia, and even pancytopenia occur in 1–10% of patients. Aplastic anemia, while very rare, may be fatal. Eight to 10 percent of patients develop proteinuria that may progress to nephrotic syndrome. Rare toxicities include enterocolitis, cholestatic jaundice, peripheral neuropathy, and pulmonary infiltrates. Corneal gold deposition occurs but has little clinical import. Nitritoid reactions (sweating, flushing, and headaches) can occur, especially with gold thiomalate, and are presumably due to the vehicle rather than the gold salts. Adverse effects cause 30–40% of patients to discontinue gold therapy within a year.

PENICILLAMINE

Penicillamine, a metabolite of penicillin, is an analog of the amino acid cystine. The D isomer has been used in rheumatoid arthritis. Penicillamine is rarely used today because of toxicity.

SULFASALAZINE

Mechanism of Action

Sulfasalazine is metabolized to sulfapyridine and 5-aminosalicylic acid, and it is thought that the sulfapyridine is probably the active moiety when treating rheumatoid arthritis (unlike inflammatory bowel disease; see Chapter 63). Some authorities believe that the parent compound, sulfasalazine, also has an effect. In treated arthritis patients, IgA and IgM rheumatoid factor production are decreased. Suppression of T cell responses to concanavalin and inhibition of in vitro B cell proliferation have also been documented. It is not clear how these findings relate to the clinical efficacy of sulfasalazine in rheumatoid arthritis.

Pharmacokinetics

Only 10–20% of orally administered sulfasalazine is absorbed, although a fraction undergoes enterohepatic recirculation into the bowel, where sulfasalazine is reduced by intestinal bacteria to liberate sulfapyridine and 5-aminosalicylic acid. Sulfapyridine is well absorbed while 5-aminosalicylic acid remains unabsorbed. Some sulfasalazine is excreted unchanged in the urine whereas sulfapyridine is excreted after hepatic acetylation and hydroxylation. Sulfasalazine's half-life is 6–17 hours.

Indications

Sulfasalazine is effective in rheumatoid arthritis and reduces radiologic disease progression. It has been used in juvenile chronic arthritis and ankylosing spondylitis and its associated uveitis. The usual regimen is 2–3 g/d.

Adverse Effects

Approximately 30% of patients using sulfasalazine discontinue the drug because of toxicity. Common adverse effects include nausea, vomiting, headache, and rash. Hemolytic anemia and methemoglobinemia also occur, but rarely. Neutropenia occurs in 1.4–4.4% of patients, while thrombocytopenia is very rare. Pulmonary toxicity and positive double-stranded DNA are occasionally seen, but drug-induced lupus is rare. Reversible infertility occurs in men, but sulfasalazine does not affect fertility in women. The drug does not appear to be teratogenic.

TNF-α–BLOCKING AGENTS

Cytokines play a central role in the immune response (see Chapter 56) and in rheumatoid arthritis. Although a wide range of cytokines are expressed in the joints of rheumatoid arthritis patients, TNF-α appears to be at the heart of the inflammatory process.

TNF-α affects cellular function via activation of specific membrane-bound TNF receptors ($TNFR_1$, $TNFR_2$). Administered soluble TNF receptors, by combining with soluble TNF-α, can inhibit the effects of the endogenous cytokine. Monoclonal anti-TNF antibodies can, in theory, cross-link TNF receptors on the cell surface and inhibit T cell and macrophage function. Three drugs interfering with TNF-α have been approved for the treatment of rheumatoid arthritis and other rheumatic diseases.

1. Adalimumab

Mechanism of Action

Adalimumab is a fully human IgG_1 anti-TNF monoclonal antibody. This compound complexes with soluble TNF-α and prevents its interaction with p55 and p75 cell surface receptors. This results in down-regulation of macrophage and T cell function.

Pharmacokinetics

Adalimumab is given subcutaneously and has a half-life of 10–20 days. Its clearance is decreased by more than 40% in the presence of methotrexate, and the formation of human antimonoclonal antibody is decreased when methotrexate is given at the same time.

Indications

The compound is approved for the treatment of rheumatoid arthritis, ankylosing spondylitis, and psoriatic arthritis. It decreases the rate of formation of new erosions. It is effective both as monotherapy and in combination with methotrexate and other DMARDs. The usual dose is 40 mg every other week, although increased responses may be evident at higher dosages. Adalimumab is presently being tested in psoriasis, ankylosing spondylitis, Crohn's disease, and juvenile chronic arthritis.

Adverse Effects

In common with the other TNF-α blocking agents, the risk of macrophage-dependent infection (including tuberculosis and other opportunistic infections) is increased, although it remains very low. Patients should be screened for latent or active tuberculosis before starting adalimumab or other TNF-α blocking agents. There is no evidence of an increased incidence of solid malignancies. It is not clear if the incidence of lymphomas is increased by adalimumab. A low incidence of newly formed double-stranded DNA (dsDNA) antibodies and antinuclear antibodies (ANAs) has been documented when using adalimumab, but clinical lupus is extremely rare. Rare leukopenias and vasculitis, apparently associated with adalimumab, have been documented.

2. Infliximab

Mechanism of Action

Infliximab is a chimeric (25% mouse, 75% human) IgG$_1$ monoclonal antibody that binds with high affinity to soluble and possibly membrane-bound TNF-α. Its mechanism of action probably is the same as that of adalimumab.

Pharmacokinetics

Infliximab is given as an intravenous infusion at doses ranging from 3 mg/kg to 10 mg/kg, although the usual dose is 3–5 mg/kg every 8 weeks. There is a relationship between serum concentration and effect, although individual clearances vary markedly. The terminal half-life is 9–12 days without accumulation after repeated dosing at the recommended interval of 8 weeks. After intermittent therapy, infliximab elicits human antichimeric antibodies in up to 62% of patients. Concurrent therapy with methotrexate markedly decreases the prevalence of human antichimeric antibodies.

Indications

Infliximab is approved for use in rheumatoid arthritis, ankylosing spondylitis, Crohn's disease, and psoriatic arthritis. It is being used in other diseases, including psoriasis, ulcerative colitis, juvenile chronic arthritis, Wegener's granulomatosis, giant cell arteritis, and sarcoidosis. In rheumatoid arthritis, a regimen of infliximab plus methotrexate decreases the rate of formation of new erosions more than methotrexate alone over 52–104 weeks. While it is recommended that methotrexate be used in conjunction with infliximab, a number of other DMARDs,

including antimalarials, azathioprine, and cyclosporine, can be used as background therapy for this drug.

Adverse Effects

Upper respiratory tract infections, nausea, headache, sinusitis, rash, and cough are common when using infliximab, although their incidence does not appear to be very different from that of methotrexate. As a potent macrophage inhibitor, infliximab can be associated with activation of latent tuberculosis, and patients should be screened for latent or active tuberculosis before starting therapy. Other opportunistic infections have been documented, although rarely. There is no evidence for an increased incidence of solid malignancies and it is not clear if the incidence of lymphoma is increased with infliximab. Because rare demyelinating syndromes have been reported, patients with multiple sclerosis should not use infliximab. Rare cases of leukopenia, hepatitis, activation of hepatitis B, and vasculitis have been documented. The incidence of positive ANA and dsDNA antibodies is increased, although clinical lupus erythematosus remains an extremely rare occurrence and the presence of ANA and dsDNA does not contraindicate the use of infliximab. Infusion site reactions correlate with anti-infliximab antibodies. These reactions occur in approximately 3–11% of patients, and the combined use of antihistamines and H$_2$ blocking agents apparently prevents some of these reactions.

3. Etanercept

Mechanism of Action

Etanercept is a recombinant fusion protein consisting of two soluble TNF p75 receptor moieties linked to the Fc portion of human IgG$_1$; it binds TNF-α molecules and also inhibits lymphotoxin-α.

Pharmacokinetics

Etanercept is given subcutaneously in a dosage of 25 mg twice weekly or 50 mg weekly. The drug is slowly absorbed, with peak concentration 72 hours after drug administration. Etanercept has a mean serum elimination half-life of 4.5 days. Fifty milligrams given once weekly gives the same area under the curve and minimum serum concentrations as 25 mg twice weekly.

Indications

Etanercept is approved for the treatment of rheumatoid arthritis, juvenile chronic arthritis, psoriasis, psoriatic arthritis, and ankylosing spondylitis. It is used both as monotherapy and with methotrexate background; over 70% of patients taking etanercept are also using methotrexate. Etanercept decreases the rate of formation of new erosions relative to methotrexate alone. While etanercept is ineffective for treatment of Crohn's disease, it is being used in many rheumatic syndromes such as scleroderma, Wegener's granulomatosis, giant cell arteritis, and sarcoidosis.

Adverse Effects

The incidence of activation of latent tuberculosis in patients treated with etanercept is numerically but not statistically lower than other TNF-blocking agents and tuberculosis screening is appropriate before starting this medication. Similarly, opportunistic infections can rarely occur when using etanercept. The incidence of solid malignancies is not increased, but as with other TNF-blocking agents one must be alert for lymphomas (although their incidence may not be increased compared with other DMARDs or active rheumatoid arthritis itself). While positive ANAs and dsDNAs may be found in patients receiving this drug, these findings do not contraindicate continued use if clinical lupus symptoms do not occur. Injection site reactions occur in 20–40% of patients, although they rarely result in discontinuation of therapy. Antietanercept antibodies are present in up to 16% of treated patients, but they do not interfere with efficacy or predict toxicity.

ABATACEPT

Mechanism of Action

Abatacept is a costimulation modulator that inhibits the activation of T cells (see also Chapter 56). After a T cell has engaged an antigen-presenting cell (APC) a signal is produced by CD28 on the T cell that interacts with CD80 or CD86 on the APC, leading to activation. Abatacept (which contains the endogenous ligand CTLA-4) binds to CD80 and 86, thereby inhibiting the binding to CD28 and preventing the activation of T cells.

Pharmacokinetics

Abatacept is given as an intravenous infusion in three initial doses (day 0, week 2, and week 4), followed by monthly infusions. The dose is based on body weight, with patients weighing less than 60 kg receiving 500 mg, those 60–100 kg receiving 750 mg, and those more than 100 kg receiving 1000 mg. The terminal serum half-life is 13–16 days. Coadministration with methotrexate, NSAIDs, and corticosteroids does not influence abatacept clearance.

Indications

Abatacept can be used as monotherapy or in combination with other DMARDs in patients with moderate to severe rheumatoid arthritis who have had an inadequate response to DMARDs or TNF antagonists. It reduces the clinical signs and symptoms of rheumatoid arthritis, including slowing of radiographic progression.

Adverse Effects

There is an increased risk of infection, predominately of the upper respiratory tract. Concomitant use with TNF antagonists is not recommended due to the increased incidence of infection with this combination. Infusion-related reactions and hypersensitivity reactions, including anaphylaxis, have been reported but the incidence is rare. Antiabatacept antibody formation is low (< 5%) and has no effect on clinical outcomes. The incidence of malignancies is similar to placebo with the exception of a possible increase in lymphomas and lung cancer (not statistically significant). The role of abatacept in this increase is unknown.

RITUXIMAB

Rituximab is a chimeric monoclonal antibody that targets CD20 B lymphocytes (see Chapter 56). It has shown benefit in the treatment of rheumatoid arthritis refractory to antiTNF agents. Rituximab has been approved for the treatment of active rheumatoid arthritis when combined with methotrexate. It is given as two IV infusions 2 weeks apart.

LEFLUNOMIDE

Mechanism of Action

Leflunomide undergoes rapid conversion, both in the intestine and in the plasma, to its active metabolite, A77-1726. This metabolite inhibits dihydroorotate dehydrogenase, leading to a decrease in ribonucleotide synthesis and the arrest of stimulated cells in the G_1 phase of cell growth. Consequently, leflunomide inhibits T cell proliferation and production of autoantibodies by B cells. Secondary effects include increases of interleukin-10 receptor mRNA, decreased interleukin-8 receptor type A mRNA, and decreased TNF-α–dependent NF-κB activation.

Pharmacokinetics

Leflunomide is completely absorbed and has a mean plasma half-life of 19 days. A77-1726 is subject to enterohepatic recirculation and is efficiently reabsorbed. Cholestyramine can enhance leflunomide excretion and increases total clearance by approximately 50%.

Indications

Leflunomide is as effective as methotrexate in rheumatoid arthritis, including inhibition of bony damage. In one study, combined treatment with methotrexate and leflunomide resulted in a 46.2% ACR20 response compared with 19.5% in patients receiving methotrexate alone.

Adverse Effects

Diarrhea or loose bowels occur in approximately 25% of patients given leflunomide, although only about 3–5% discontinue the drug because of this effect. Elevation in liver enzymes also occurs. Both effects can be reduced by decreasing the dose of leflunomide. Other adverse effects associated with leflunomide are mild alopecia, weight gain, and increased blood pressure. Leukopenia and thrombocytopenia occur rarely. This drug is contraindicated in pregnancy.

COMBINATION THERAPY WITH DMARDS

In a 1998 study, approximately half of North American rheumatologists treated moderately aggressive rheumatoid arthritis with combination therapy, and the use of drug combinations is anticipated to be much higher now. Combinations of DMARDs can be designed rationally on the basis of complementary mechanisms of action, nonoverlapping pharmacokinetics, and nonoverlapping toxicity.

When added to methotrexate background therapy, cyclosporine, chloroquine, leflunomide, infliximab, adalimumab, rituximab, and etanercept have all shown improved efficacy. In contrast, azathioprine, auranofin, or sulfasalazine plus methotrexate results in no additional therapeutic benefit. Other combinations have occasionally been used, including the combination of intramuscular gold with hydroxychloroquine.

While it might be anticipated that combination therapy might result in more toxicity, this is often not the case. Combination therapy for patients not responding adequately to monotherapy is becoming the rule in the treatment of rheumatoid arthritis.

IMMUNOABSORPTION APHERESIS

Extracorporeal immunoabsorption of plasma over columns containing an inert silica matrix and covalently attached highly purified staphylococcal protein A (Prosorba column) involves apheresis of about 1200 mL plasma weekly for 3 months.

Mechanism of Action

Although this treatment has been available for idiopathic thrombocytopenic purpura for several years, its mechanism of action is not understood. Removal of IgG and IgG-containing immune complexes does not explain its effects in rheumatoid arthritis. The most recent hypothesis for this treatment's mechanism of action is down-regulation of B cell function through the release of small amounts of staphylococcal protein A complexed with immunoglobulins.

Indications

This treatment has been used in patients who have failed numerous other therapies, so its low efficacy in rheumatoid arthritis is better than it appears. The study establishing efficacy in rheumatoid arthritis showed a 41.7% ACR20 response among Prosorba-treated patients compared with 15.6% in the sham-treated group.

Adverse Effects

Common adverse events include joint pain, joint swelling, and hypotension. Central intravenous line usage may be associated with pulmonary emboli and sepsis. Other events, such as nausea, rash, pruritus, flushing, and fever, occurred in 1–6% of treatments in both sham and treatment groups in the double-blind trial. Rare leukocytoclastic vasculitis has been documented.

GLUCOCORTICOID DRUGS

The general pharmacology of corticosteroids, including mechanism of action, pharmacokinetics, and other applications, is discussed in Chapter 39.

Indications

Corticosteroids have been used in 60–70% of rheumatoid arthritis patients. Their effects are prompt and dramatic, and they are capable of slowing the appearance of new bone erosions. Corticosteroids may be administered for certain serious extra-articular manifestations of rheumatoid arthritis such as pericarditis or eye involvement or during periods of exacerbation. When prednisone is required for long-term therapy, the dosage should not exceed 7.5 mg daily, and gradual reduction of the dose should be encouraged. Alternate-day corticosteroid therapy is usually unsuccessful in rheumatoid arthritis.

Other rheumatic diseases in which the corticosteroids' potent anti-inflammatory effects may be useful include vasculitis, systemic lupus erythematosus, Wegener's granulomatosis, psoriatic arthritis, giant cell arteritis, sarcoidosis, and gout.

Intra-articular corticosteroids are often helpful to alleviate painful symptoms and, when successful, are preferable to increasing the dosage of systemic medication.

Adverse Effects

Prolonged use of these drugs leads to serious and disabling toxic effects as described in Chapter 39. There is controversy over whether many of these side effects occur at doses below 7.5 mg prednisone equivalent daily, although many experts believe that even 3–5 mg/d can cause these effects in susceptible individuals.

DIETARY MANIPULATION OF INFLAMMATION

Arachidonic acid is an eicosatetraenoic acid that is metabolized by the cyclooxygenase and lipoxygenase pathways, yielding several mediators (see Chapter 18). These mediators have potent effects on many systems, including the immune system. It has been demonstrated that dietary manipulation that substitutes unsaturated fatty acids (such as eicosapentaenoic acid, found in marine fish) causes the alternative fatty acids to be metabolized, changing the final prostaglandin and leukotriene products of the process. The products of eicosapentaenoic acid metabolism are less potent than the corresponding mediators derived from arachidonic acid (sometimes by several orders of magnitude), and they diminish the activities of the eicosatetraenoic mediators by competing with them for shared target-cell receptors.

The results of clinical studies suggest that therapy with dietary eicosapentaenoic acid decreases both morning stiffness and the number of tender joints in patients with rheumatoid arthritis and erythema associated with psoriasis. The efficacy of dietary eicosapentaenoic acid approximates that of the NSAIDs. These preliminary results and the near absence of significant adverse effects suggest that dietary alteration or supplementation to provide 2–4 g/d of eicosapentaenoic acid may be a beneficial addition to conventional treatment of rheumatoid arthritis.

■ III. OTHER ANALGESICS

Acetaminophen is one of the most important drugs used for the treatment of mild to moderate pain when an anti-inflammatory effect is not necessary. Phenacetin, a prodrug that is metabolized to acetaminophen, is more toxic than its active metabolite and has no rational indications.

ACETAMINOPHEN

Acetaminophen is the active metabolite of phenacetin and is responsible for its analgesic effect. It is a weak COX-1 and COX-2 inhibitor in peripheral tissues and possesses no significant anti-inflammatory effects. Recent evidence suggests that acetaminophen may inhibit a third enzyme, COX-3, in the central nervous system. COX-3 appears to be a splice variant product of the COX-1 gene.

**N-Acetyl-p-aminophenol
(acetaminophen)**

Pharmacokinetics

Acetaminophen is administered orally. Absorption is related to the rate of gastric emptying, and peak blood concentrations are usually reached in 30–60 minutes. Acetaminophen is slightly bound to plasma proteins and is partially metabolized by hepatic microsomal enzymes and converted to acetaminophen sulfate and glucuronide, which are pharmacologically inactive (see Figure 4–4). Less than 5% is excreted unchanged. A minor but highly active metabolite (N-acetyl-p-benzoquinone) is important in large doses because it is toxic to both liver and kidney. The half-life of acetaminophen is 2–3 hours and is relatively unaffected by renal function. With toxic doses or liver disease, the half-life may be increased twofold or more.

Indications

Although equivalent to aspirin as an effective analgesic and antipyretic agent, acetaminophen differs in that it lacks anti-inflammatory properties. It does not affect uric acid levels and lacks platelet-inhibiting properties. The drug is useful in mild to moderate pain such as headache, myalgia, postpartum pain, and other circumstances in which aspirin is an effective analgesic. Acetaminophen alone is inadequate therapy for inflammatory conditions such as rheumatoid arthritis, although it may be used as an analgesic adjunct to anti-inflammatory therapy. For mild analgesia, acetaminophen is the preferred drug in patients allergic to aspirin or when salicylates are poorly tolerated. It is preferable to aspirin in patients with hemophilia or a history of peptic ulcer and in those in whom bronchospasm is precipitated by aspirin. Unlike aspirin, acetaminophen does not antagonize the effects of uricosuric agents; it may be used concomitantly with probenecid in the treatment of gout. It is preferred to aspirin in children with viral infections.

Adverse Effects

In therapeutic doses, a mild increase in hepatic enzymes may occasionally occur in the absence of jaundice; this is reversible when the drug is withdrawn. With larger doses, dizziness, excitement, and disorientation are seen. Ingestion of 15 g of acetaminophen may be fatal, death being caused by severe hepatotoxicity with centrilobular necrosis, sometimes associated with acute renal tubular necrosis (see Chapters 4 and 59). Doses greater than 4 g/d are not recommended and a history of alcoholism contraindicates even this dose. Early symptoms of hepatic damage include nausea, vomiting, diarrhea, and abdominal pain. Cases of renal damage without hepatic damage have occurred, even after usual doses of acetaminophen. Therapy is much less satisfactory than for aspirin overdose. In addition to supportive therapy, the measure that has proved most useful is the provision of sulfhydryl groups in the form of acetylcysteine to neutralize the toxic metabolites (see Chapter 59).

Hemolytic anemia and methemoglobinemia are very rare. Interstitial nephritis and papillary necrosis—serious complications of phenacetin—have not occurred nor has gastrointestinal bleeding. Caution is necessary in patients with any type of liver disease.

Dosage

Acute pain and fever may be effectively treated with 325–500 mg four times daily and proportionately less for children.

PHENACETIN

Phenacetin is no longer prescribed in the USA and has been removed from many over-the-counter analgesic combinations. However, it is still present in several proprietary analgesics in this country and is in common use in many other parts of the world. The association between the excessive use of analgesic combinations—especially those that contain phenacetin—and the development of renal failure has been recognized for almost 30 years.

■ IV. DRUGS USED IN GOUT

Gout is a metabolic disease characterized by recurrent episodes of acute arthritis due to deposits of monosodium urate in joints and cartilage. Uric acid renal calculi, tophi, and interstitial nephritis may also occur. Gout is usually associated with high serum levels of uric acid, a poorly soluble substance that is the major end product of purine metabolism. In most mammals, uricase converts uric acid to the more soluble allantoin; this enzyme is absent in humans.

The treatment of gout aims to relieve acute gouty attacks and to prevent recurrent gouty episodes and urate lithiasis. Therapy for an attack of acute gouty arthritis is based on our current understanding of the pathophysiologic events that occur in this disease (Figure 36–4). Urate crystals are initially phagocytosed by synoviocytes, which then release prostaglandins, lysosomal enzymes, and interleukin-1. Attracted by these chemotactic media-

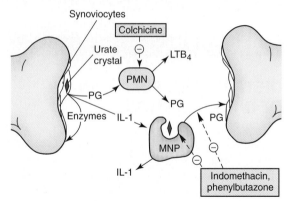

Figure 36–4. Pathophysiologic events in a gouty joint. Synoviocytes phagocytose urate crystals and then secrete inflammatory mediators, which attract and activate polymorphonuclear leukocytes (PMN) and mononuclear phagocytes (MNP) (macrophages). Drugs active in gout inhibit crystal phagocytosis and polymorphonuclear leukocyte and macrophage release of inflammatory mediators. (PG, prostaglandin; IL-1, interleukin-1; LTB$_4$, leukotriene B$_4$.)

tors, polymorphonuclear leukocytes migrate into the joint space and amplify the ongoing inflammatory process. In the later phases of the attack, increased numbers of mononuclear phagocytes (macrophages) appear, ingest the urate crystals, and release more inflammatory mediators. This sequence of events suggests that the most effective agents for the management of acute urate crystal-induced inflammation are those that suppress different phases of leukocyte activation.

Before starting chronic therapy for gout, patients in whom hyperuricemia is associated with gout and urate lithiasis must be clearly distinguished from those who have only hyperuricemia. In an asymptomatic person with hyperuricemia, the efficacy of long-term drug treatment is unproved. In some individuals, uric acid levels may be elevated up to 2 standard deviations above the mean for a lifetime without adverse consequences.

COLCHICINE

Although NSAIDs are now the first-line drugs for acute gout, colchicine was the primary treatment for many years. Colchicine is an alkaloid isolated from the autumn crocus, *Colchicum autumnale*. Its structure is shown in Figure 36–5.

Pharmacokinetics

Colchicine is absorbed readily after oral administration, reaches peak plasma levels within 2 hours, and is elimi-

Figure 36–5. Colchicine and uricosuric drugs.

nated with a serum half-life of 9 hours. Metabolites are excreted in the intestinal tract and urine.

Pharmacodynamics

Colchicine relieves the pain and inflammation of gouty arthritis in 12–24 hours without altering the metabolism or excretion of urates and without other analgesic effects. Colchicine produces its anti-inflammatory effects by binding to the intracellular protein tubulin, thereby preventing its polymerization into microtubules and leading to the inhibition of leukocyte migration and phagocytosis. It also inhibits the formation of leukotriene B_4. Several of colchicine's adverse effects are produced by its inhibition of tubulin polymerization and cell mitosis.

Indications

Although colchicine is more specific in gout than the NSAIDs, NSAIDs (eg, indomethacin and other NSAIDs [except aspirin]) have replaced it in the treatment of acute gout because of the troublesome diarrhea associated with colchicine therapy. Colchicine is now used for the prophylaxis of recurrent episodes of gouty arthritis, is effective in preventing attacks of acute Mediterranean fever, and may have a mild beneficial effect in sarcoid arthritis and in hepatic cirrhosis. Although it can be given intravenously, this route should be used cautiously because of increased bone marrow toxicity.

Adverse Effects

Colchicine often causes diarrhea and may occasionally cause nausea, vomiting, and abdominal pain. Colchicine may rarely cause hair loss and bone marrow depression as well as peripheral neuritis and myopathy.

Acute intoxication after overdoses is characterized by burning throat pain, bloody diarrhea, shock, hematuria, and oliguria. Fatal ascending central nervous system depression has been reported. Treatment is supportive.

Dosage

In prophylaxis (the most common use), the dose of colchicine is 0.6 mg one to three times daily. For terminating an attack of gout, the traditional initial dose of colchicine is usually 0.6 or 1.2 mg, followed by 0.6 mg every 2 hours until pain is relieved or nausea and diarrhea appear. The total dose can be given intravenously if necessary, but it should be remembered that as little as 8 mg in 24 hours may be fatal.

NSAIDS IN GOUT

In addition to inhibiting prostaglandin synthase, indomethacin and other NSAIDs also inhibit urate crystal phagocytosis. Indomethacin is commonly used as initial treatment of gout as the replacement for colchicine. For acute gout 50 mg three times daily is given; when a response occurs, the dosage is reduced to 25 mg three times daily for 5–7 days.

All other NSAIDs except aspirin, salicylates, and tolmetin have been successfully used to treat acute gouty episodes. Oxaprozin, which lowers serum uric acid, is theoretically a good choice although it should not be given to patients with uric acid stones because it increases uric acid excretion in the urine. These agents appear to be as effective and safe as the older drugs.

URICOSURIC AGENTS

Probenecid and sulfinpyrazone are uricosuric drugs employed to decrease the body pool of urate in patients with tophaceous gout or in those with increasingly frequent gouty attacks. In a patient who excretes large amounts of uric acid, the uricosuric agents should not be used.

Chemistry

Uricosuric drugs are organic acids (Figure 36–5) and, as such, act at the anionic transport sites of the renal tubule (see Chapter 15). Sulfinpyrazone is a metabolite of an analog of phenylbutazone.

Pharmacokinetics

Probenecid is completely reabsorbed by the renal tubules and is metabolized slowly with a terminal serum half-life of 5–8 hours. Sulfinpyrazone or its active hydroxylated derivative is rapidly excreted by the kidneys. Even so, the duration of its effect after oral administration is almost as long as that of probenecid, which is given once or twice daily.

Pharmacodynamics

Uric acid is freely filtered at the glomerulus. Like many other weak acids, it is also both reabsorbed and secreted in the middle segment (S_2) of the proximal tubule. Uricosuric drugs—probenecid, sulfinpyrazone, and large doses of aspirin—affect these active transport sites so that net reabsorption of uric acid in the proximal tubule is decreased. Because aspirin in doses of less than 2.6 g daily causes net *retention* of uric acid by inhibiting the secretory transporter, it should not be used for analgesia in patients with gout. The secretion of other weak acids (eg, penicillin) is also reduced by uricosuric agents. Probenecid was originally developed to prolong penicillin blood levels.

As the urinary excretion of uric acid increases, the size of the urate pool decreases, although the plasma concentration may not be greatly reduced. In patients who respond favorably, tophaceous deposits of urate are reabsorbed, with relief of arthritis and remineralization of bone. With the ensuing increase in uric acid excretion, a predisposition to the formation of renal stones is augmented rather than decreased; therefore, the urine volume should be maintained at a high level, and at least early in treatment the urine pH should be kept above 6.0 by the administration of alkali.

Indications

Uricosuric therapy should be initiated in gouty underexcretion of uric acid when allopurinol or febuxostat is contraindicated or when evidence of tophi appears. Therapy should not be started until 2–3 weeks after an acute attack.

Adverse Effects

Adverse effects do not provide a basis for preferring one or the other of the uricosuric agents. Both of these organic acids cause gastrointestinal irritation, but sulfin-pyrazone is more active in this regard. A rash may appear after the use of either compound. Nephrotic syndrome has occurred after the use of probenecid. Both sulfinpyrazone and probenecid may rarely cause aplastic anemia.

Contraindications & Cautions

It is essential to maintain a large urine volume to minimize the possibility of stone formation.

Dosage

Probenecid is usually started at a dosage of 0.5 g orally daily in divided doses, progressing to 1 g daily after 1 week. Sulfinpyrazone is started at a dosage of 200 mg orally daily, progressing to 400–800 mg daily. It should be given in divided doses with food to reduce adverse gastrointestinal effects.

ALLOPURINOL

The preferred and standard-of-care therapy for gout is allopurinol, which reduces total uric acid body burden by inhibiting xanthine oxidase.

Chemistry

The structure of allopurinol, an isomer of hypoxanthine, is shown in Figure 36–6.

Pharmacokinetics

Allopurinol is approximately 80% absorbed after oral administration and has a terminal serum half-life of 1–2 hours. Like uric acid, allopurinol is itself metabolized by xanthine oxidase, but the resulting compound, alloxanthine, retains the capacity to inhibit xanthine oxidase and has a long enough duration of action so that allopurinol is given only once a day.

Pharmacodynamics

Dietary purines are not an important source of uric acid. Quantitatively important amounts of purine are formed from amino acids, formate, and carbon dioxide in the body. Those purine ribonucleotides not incorporated into nucleic acids and derived from nucleic acid degradation are converted to xanthine or hypoxanthine and oxidized to uric acid (Figure 36–6). Allopurinol inhibits this last step, resulting in a fall in the plasma urate level and a decrease in the size of the urate pool. The more soluble xanthine and hypoxanthine are increased.

Indications

Treatment of gout with allopurinol, as with uricosuric agents, is begun with the expectation that it will be con-

Figure 36–6. Inhibition of uric acid synthesis by allopurinol. (Modified and reproduced, with permission, from Meyers FH, Jawetz E, Goldfien A: *Review of Medical Pharmacology,* 7th ed. McGraw-Hill, 1980.)

tinued for years if not for life. Allopurinol is often the first urate-lowering drug used. When starting allopurinol, colchicine should also be used until steady-state serum uric acid is normalized or decreased to less than 6 mg/dL. Thereafter colchicine can be stopped, while allopurinol is continued. Aside from gout, allopurinol is used as an antiprotozoal agent (see Chapter 52) and is indicated to prevent the massive uricosuria following therapy of blood dyscrasias that could otherwise lead to renal calculi.

Adverse Effects

See above for protection against an acute attack during the initial use of allopurinol. Gastrointestinal intolerance, including nausea, vomiting, and diarrhea, may occur. Peripheral neuritis and necrotizing vasculitis, depression of bone marrow elements, and, rarely, aplastic anemia may also occur. Hepatic toxicity and interstitial nephritis have been reported. An allergic skin reaction characterized by pruritic maculopapular lesions occurs in 3% of patients. Isolated cases of exfoliative dermatitis have been reported. In very rare cases, allopurinol has become bound to the lens, resulting in cataracts.

Interactions & Cautions

When chemotherapeutic mercaptopurines (eg, azathioprine) are given concomitantly with allopurinol, their dosage must be reduced by about 75%. Allopurinol may also increase the effect of cyclophosphamide. Allopurinol inhibits the metabolism of probenecid and oral anticoagulants and may increase hepatic iron concentration. Safety in children and during pregnancy has not been established.

Dosage

The initial dosage of allopurinol is 100 mg/d. It may be titrated upward until serum uric acid is below 6 mg/dL; this level is commonly achieved at 300 mg/d but is not restricted to this dose.

Colchicine or an NSAID should be given during the first weeks of allopurinol therapy to prevent the gouty arthritis episodes that sometimes occur.

FEBUXOSTAT

Febuxostat is the first nonpurine inhibitor of xanthine oxidase.

Pharmacokinetics

Febuxostat is more than 80% absorbed following oral administration. Maximum concentration is reached in approximately 1 hour. Febuxostat is extensively metabolized in the liver. All of the drug and its metabolites appear in the urine although less than 5% appears as unchanged drug. Because it is highly metabolized to inactive metabolites, no dosage adjustment is necessary for patients with renal impairment.

Pharmacodynamics

Febuxostat is a potent and selective inhibitor of xanthine oxidase, and thereby reduces the formation of xanthine and uric acid. No other enzymes involved in purine or pyrimidine metabolism are inhibited. Febuxostat at a daily dose of 80 mg or 120 mg was more effective than allopurinol at a standard 300 mg daily dose in lowering serum urate levels. The urate-lowering effect was comparable regardless of the pathogenic cause of hyperuricemia—overproduction or underexcretion.

Indications

Febuxostat is awaiting FDA approval at its 80 mg and 120 mg dose for the treatment of chronic gout. It is the first new drug for the treatment of gout in over 40 years.

Adverse Effects

As with allopurinol, prophylactic treatment with colchicine or NSAIDs should start at the beginning of treatment to avoid gout flares. The most frequent treatment-related adverse events are liver function abnormalities, diarrhea, headache, and nausea. Febuxostat appears to be well tolerated in patients with a history of allopurinol intolerance.

PREPARATIONS AVAILABLE

NSAIDs

Aspirin, acetylsalicylic acid (generic, Easprin, others)
Oral (regular, enteric-coated, buffered): 81, 165, 325, 500, 650, 800 mg tablets; 81, 650, 800 mg timed- or extended-release tablets
Rectal: 120, 200, 300, 600 mg suppositories
Bromfenac (Xibrom)
Ophthalmic: 0.09% solution
Celecoxib (Celebrex)
Oral: 100, 200 mg capsules
Choline salicylate (Arthropan)
Oral: 870 mg/5 mL liquid
Diclofenac (generic, Cataflam, Voltaren)
Oral: 50 mg tablets; 25, 50, 75 mg delayed-release tablets; 100 mg extended-release tablets
Ophthalmic: 0.1% solution
Diflunisal (generic, Dolobid)
Oral: 250, 500 mg tablets
Etodolac (generic, Lodine)
Oral: 200, 300 mg capsules; 400, 500 mg tablets; 400, 500, 600 mg extended-release tablets
Fenoprofen (generic, Nalfon)
Oral: 200, 300 mg capsules; 600 mg tablets
Flurbiprofen (generic, Ansaid)
Oral: 50, 100 mg tablets
Ophthalmic (generic, Ocufen): 0.03% solution
Ibuprofen (generic, Motrin, Rufen, Advil [otc], Nuprin [otc], others)
Oral: 100, 200, 400, 600, 800 mg tablets; 50, 100 mg chewable tablets; 200 mg capsules; 100 mg/2.5 mL suspension, 100 mg/5 mL suspension; 40 mg/mL drops
Indomethacin (generic, Indocin)
Oral: 25, 50 mg capsules; 75 mg sustained-release capsules; 25 mg/5 mL suspension
Rectal: 50 mg suppositories
Ketoprofen (generic, Orudis)
Oral: 12.5 mg tablets; 25, 50, 75 mg capsules; 100, 150, 200 mg extended-release capsules

Ketorolac tromethamine (generic, Toradol)
Oral: 10 mg tablets
Parenteral: 15, 30 mg/mL for IM injection
Ophthalmic: 0.4, 0.5% solution
Magnesium salicylate (Doan's Pills, Magan, MobidIn)
Oral: 545, 600 mg tablets; 467, 500, 580 mg caplets
Meclofenamate sodium (generic)
Oral: 50, 100 mg capsules
Mefenamic acid (Ponstel)
Oral: 250 mg capsules
Meloxicam (Mobic)
Oral: 7.5, 15 mg tablets; 7.5 mg/5 mL suspension
Nabumetone (generic, Relafen)
Oral: 500, 750 mg tablets
Naproxen (generic, Naprosyn, Anaprox, Aleve [otc])
Oral: 200, 220, 250, 375, 500 mg tablets; 375, 550 mg controlled-release tablets; 375, 500 mg delayed-release tablets; 125 mg/5 mL suspension
Oxaprozin (generic, Daypro)
Oral: 600 mg tablets
Piroxicam (generic, Feldene)
Oral: 10, 20 mg capsules
Salsalate, salicylsalicylic acid (generic, Disalcid)
Oral: 500, 750 mg tablets; 500 mg capsules
Sodium salicylate (generic)
Oral: 325, 650 mg enteric-coated tablets
Sodium thiosalicylate (generic, Rexolate)
Parenteral: 50 mg/mL for IM injection
Sulindac (generic, Clinoril)
Oral: 150, 200 mg tablets
Suprofen (Profenal)
Topical: 1% ophthalmic solution
Tolmetin (generic, Tolectin)
Oral: 200, 600 mg tablets; 400 mg capsules

(continued)

Valdecoxib (Bextra) (Not available in all countries)
Oral: 10, 20 mg tablets

DISEASE-MODIFYING ANTIRHEUMATIC DRUGS

Abatacept (Orencia)
Parenteral: 250 mg/vial lyophilized, for reconstitution for IV injection

Adalimumab (Humira)
Parenteral: 40 mg/0.8 mL for SC injection

Anakinra (Kineret)
Parenteral: 100 mg solution for SC injection

Auranofin (Ridaura)
Oral: 3 mg capsules

Aurothioglucose (Solganal)
Parenteral: 50 mg/mL suspension for injection

Etanercept (Enbrel)
Parenteral: 50 mg/mL, 25 mg powder for SC injection

Gold sodium thiomalate (generic, Aurolate)
Parenteral: 50 mg/mL for injection

Hydroxychloroquine (generic, Plaquenil)
Oral: 200 mg tablets

Infliximab (Remicade)
Parenteral: 100 mg powder for IV infusion

Leflunomide (Arava)
Oral: 10, 20, 100 mg tablets

Methotrexate (generic, Rheumatrex)
Oral: 2.5 mg tablet dose packs, 5, 7.5, 10, 15 mg tablets

Penicillamine (Cuprimine, Depen)
Oral: 125, 250 mg capsules; 250 mg tablets

Rituximab (Rituxan)
Parenteral: 10 mg/mL for IV infusion

Sulfasalazine (generic, Azulfidine)
Oral: 500 mg tablets; 500 mg delayed-release tablets

ACETAMINOPHEN

Acetaminophen (generic, Tylenol, Tempra, Panadol, Acephen, others)
Oral: 160, 325, 500, 650 mg tablets; 80 mg chewable tablets; 160, 500, 650 mg caplets; 325, 500 mg capsules; 80, 120, 160 mg/5 mL elixir; 500 mg/15 mL elixir; 80 mg/1.66 mL, 100 mg/mL solution
Rectal: 80, 120, 125, 300, 325, 650 mg suppositories

DRUGS USED IN GOUT

Allopurinol (generic, Zyloprim)
Oral: 100, 300 mg tablets

Colchicine (generic)
Oral: 0.6 mg tablets
Parenteral: 0.5 mg/mL for injection

Probenecid (generic)
Oral: 500 mg tablets

Sulfinpyrazone (generic, Anturane)
Oral: 100 mg tablets; 200 mg capsules

REFERENCES

General

Hellman DB, Stone JH: Arthritis and musculoskeletal disorders. In: McPhee ST, Papadakis MA (editors). *Current Medical Diagnosis & Treatment 2007.* McGraw-Hill, 2007.

Vane J, Botting R: Inflammation and the mechanism of action of anti-inflammatory drugs. FASEB J 1987;1:89.

NSAIDs

http://www.rheumatology.org/publications/hotline/0305NSAIDs.asp

Bensen W et al: Efficacy and safety of valdecoxib in treating the signs and symptoms of rheumatoid arthritis: A randomized, controlled comparison with placebo and naproxen. Rheumatology (Oxford) 2002;41:1008.

Bombardier C: An evidence-based evaluation of the gastrointestinal safety of coxibs. Am J Cardiol 2002;89(Suppl 6A):3D.

Bombardier C et al: Comparison of upper gastrointestinal toxicity of rofecoxib and naproxen in patients with rheumatoid arthritis. VIGOR Study Group. N Engl J Med 2000;343:1520.

Brix AE: Renal papillary necrosis. Toxicol Pathol 2002;30:672.

Chan FK et al: Celecoxib versus diclofenac and omeprazole in reducing the risk of recurrent ulcer bleeding in patients with arthritis. N Engl J Med 2002;347:2104.

Christmann V et al: Changes in cerebral, renal and mesenteric blood flow velocity during continuous and bolus infusion of indomethacin. Acta Paediatr 2002;91:440.

Deeks JJ, Smith LA, Bradley MD: Efficacy, tolerability, and upper gastrointestinal safety of celecoxib for treatment of osteoarthritis and rheumatoid arthritis: Systematic review of randomised controlled trials. BMJ 2002;325:619.

Furst DE et al: Dose response and safety study of meloxicam up to 22.5 mg daily in rheumatoid arthritis: A 12 week multicenter, double blind, dose response study versus placebo and diclofenac. J Rheumatol 2002;29:436.

Hanna MH et al: Comparative study of analgesic efficacy and morphine-sparing effect of intramuscular dexketoprofen trometamol with ketoprofen or placebo after major orthopaedic surgery. Br J Clin Pharmacol 2003;55:126.

Immer FF et al: Pain treatment with a COX-2 inhibitor after coronary artery bypass operation: A randomized trial. Ann Thorac Surg 2003;75:490.

Kivitz A et al: Randomized placebo-controlled trial comparing efficacy and safety of valdecoxib with naproxen in patients with osteoarthritis. J Fam Pract 2002;51:530.

Knijff-Dutmer EA et al: Platelet function is inhibited by non-selective non-steroidal anti-inflammatory drugs but not by cyclo-oxygenase-2-selective inhibitors in patients with rheumatoid arthritis. Rheumatology (Oxford) 2002;41:458.

Lago P et al: Safety and efficacy of ibuprofen versus indomethacin in preterm infants treated for patent ductus arteriosus: A randomized controlled trial. Eur J Pediatr 2002;161:202.

Laine L et al: Serious lower gastrointestinal clinical events with non-selective NSAID or coxib use. Gastroenterology 2003;124:288.

Makarowski W et al: Efficacy and safety of the COX-2 specific inhibitor valdecoxib in the management of osteoarthritis of the hip: A randomized, double-blind, placebo-controlled comparison with naproxen. Osteoarthritis Cartilage 2002;10:290.

Matsumoto AK et al: A randomized, controlled, clinical trial of etoricoxib in the treatment of rheumatoid arthritis. J Rheumatol 2002;29:1623.

Moran EM: Epidemiological and clinical aspects of nonsteroidal anti-inflammatory drugs and cancer risks. J Environ Pathol Toxicol Oncol 2002;21:193.

Niccoli L, Bellino S, Cantini F: Renal tolerability of three commonly employed non-steroidal anti-inflammatory drugs in elderly patients with osteoarthritis. Clin Exp Rheumatol 2002; 20:201.

Ray WA et al: COX-2 selective non-steroidal anti-inflammatory drugs and risk of serious coronary heart disease. Lancet 2002; 360:1071.

Reicin AS et al: Comparison of cardiovascular thrombotic events in patients with osteoarthritis treated with rofecoxib versus non-selective nonsteroidal anti-inflammatory drugs (ibuprofen, diclofenac, and nabumetone). Am J Cardiol 2002;89:204.

Rovensky J et al: Treatment of knee osteoarthritis with a topical non-steroidal anti-inflammatory drug. Results of a randomized, double-blind, placebo-controlled study on the efficacy and safety of a 5% ibuprofen cream. Drugs Exp Clin Res 2001;27:209.

Disease-Modifying Antirheumatic Drugs & Glucocorticoids

Caldwell J, Gendreau RM, Furst D: A pilot study using a staph protein A column (Prosorba) to treat refractory rheumatoid arthritis. J Rheumatol 1999;26:1657.

Charles P et al: Regulation of cytokines, cytokine inhibitors, and acute-phase proteins following anti-TNF-α therapy in rheumatoid arthritis. J Immunol 1999;163:1521.

Felson DT et al: The Prosorba column for treatment of refractory rheumatoid arthritis: A randomized, double-blind, sham-controlled trial. Arthritis Rheum 1999;42:2153.

Furst DE: Rational use of disease-modifying antirheumatic drugs. Drugs 1990;39:19.

Garrison L, McDonnell ND: Etanercept: Therapeutic use in patients with rheumatoid arthritis. Ann Rheum Dis 1999; 58(Suppl I):I165.

Genovese MC et al: Abatacept for rheumatoid arthritis refractory to tumor necrosis factor α inhibition. N Engl J Med 2005; 353:1114.

Jones RE, Moreland LW: Tumor necrosis factor inhibitors for rheumatoid arthritis. Bull Rheum Dis 1999;48:14.

Mease PJ et al: Adalimumab for the treatment of patients with moderately to severely active psoriatic arthritis. Arthritis Rheum 2005;52:3279.

Moreland LW et al: Etanercept therapy in rheumatoid arthritis. A randomized, controlled trial. Ann Intern Med 1999;130:478.

Teng GG, Turkiewicz AM, Moreland LW: Abatacept: A costimulatory inhibitor for treatment of rheumatoid arthritis. Expert Opin Biol Ther 2005;5:1245.

Other Analgesics

Chandrasekharan NV et al: COX-3, a cyclooxygenase-1 variant inhibited by acetaminophen and other analgesic/antipyretic drugs: Cloning, structure, and expression. Proc Natl Acad Sci U S A 2002;99:13926.

Linden CH, Rumack BH: Acetaminophen overdose. Emerg Med Clin North Am 1984;2:103.

Styrt B, Sugarman B: Antipyresis and fever. Arch Intern Med 1990; 150:1589.

Drugs Used in Gout

Becker MA et al: Febuxostat compared with allopurinol in patients with hyperuricemia and gout. N Engl J Med 2005;353:2450.

Emmerson BT: The management of gout. N Engl J Med 1996; 334:445.

Schumacher HR: Febuxostat: A non-purine, selective inhibitor of xanthine oxidase for the management of hyperuricaemia in patients with gout. Expert Opin Investig Drugs 2005;14:893.

SECTION VII
Endocrine Drugs

Hypothalamic & Pituitary Hormones

37

*Susan B. Masters, PhD**

The control of metabolism, growth, and reproduction is mediated by a combination of neural and endocrine systems located in the hypothalamus and pituitary gland. The pituitary weighs about 0.6 g and rests at the base of the brain in the bony sella turcica near the optic chiasm and the cavernous sinuses. The pituitary consists of an

---

ACRONYMS

ACTH	Adrenocorticotropic hormone
CRH	Corticotropin-releasing hormone
FSH	Follicle-stimulating hormone
GH	Growth hormone
GHRH	Growth hormone-releasing hormone
GnRH	Gonadotropin-releasing hormone
IGF	Insulin-like growth factor
LH	Luteinizing hormone
PRL	Prolactin
rhGH	Recombinant human growth hormone
SST	Somatostatin
TRH	Thyrotropin-releasing hormone
TSH	Thyroid-stimulating hormone (thyrotropin)

---

anterior lobe (adenohypophysis) and a posterior lobe (neurohypophysis) (Figure 37–1). It is connected to the overlying hypothalamus by a stalk of neurosecretory fibers and blood vessels, including a portal venous system that drains the hypothalamus and perfuses the anterior pituitary. The portal venous system carries small regulatory hormones (Figure 37–1, Table 37–1) from the hypothalamus to the anterior pituitary.

The posterior lobe hormones are synthesized in the hypothalamus and transported via the neurosecretory fibers in the stalk of the pituitary to the posterior lobe, from which they are released into the circulation.

Drugs that mimic or block the effects of hypothalamic and pituitary hormones have pharmacologic applications in three primary areas: (1) as replacement therapy for hormone deficiency states; (2) as antagonists for diseases that result from excess production of pituitary hormones; and (3) as diagnostic tools for identifying several endocrine abnormalities.

■ ANTERIOR PITUITARY HORMONES & THEIR HYPOTHALAMIC REGULATORS

All of the hormones produced by the anterior pituitary except prolactin (PRL) are key participants in hormonal

---

*The author acknowledges the contributions of the previous author, Dr. P. A. Fitzgerald.

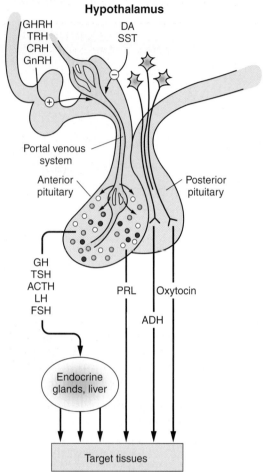

Hypothalamus

GHRH
TRH
CRH
GnRH

DA
SST

Portal venous
system

Anterior
pituitary

Posterior
pituitary

GH
TSH
ACTH
LH
FSH

PRL   Oxytocin

ADH

Endocrine
glands, liver

Target tissues

Figure 37–1. The hypothalamic-pituitary endocrine system. Except for prolactin, hormones released from the anterior pituitary stimulate the production of hormones by a peripheral endocrine gland or the liver. Prolactin and the hormones released from the posterior pituitary (vasopressin and oxytocin) act directly on target tissues. Hypothalamic factors regulate the release of anterior pituitary hormones. (ACTH, adrenocorticotropin; ADH, antidiuretic hormone [vasopressin]; CRH, corticotropin-releasing hormone; DA, dopamine; FSH, follicle-stimulating hormone; GH, growth hormone; GHRH, growth hormone-releasing hormone; GnRH, gonadotropin-releasing hormone; LH, luteinizing hormone; PRL, prolactin; SST, somatostatin; TRH, thyrotropin-releasing hormone; TSH, thyroid-stimulating hormone.)

systems in which they regulate the production by peripheral tissues of hormones that perform the ultimate regulatory functions. In these systems, the secretion of the pituitary hormone is under the control of a hypothalamic

hormone. Each hypothalamic-pituitary-endocrine gland system or axis provides multiple opportunities for complex neuroendocrine regulation of growth, development, and reproductive functions.

ANTERIOR PITUITARY & HYPOTHALAMIC HORMONE RECEPTORS

The anterior pituitary hormones can be classified according to hormone structure and the types of receptors that they activate. **Growth hormone** and **prolactin,** single-chain protein hormones with significant homology, form one group. Both hormones activate receptors of the JAK/STAT superfamily (see Chapter 2). Three pituitary hormones—**thyroid-stimulating hormone (TSH, thyrotropin), follicle-stimulating hormone (FSH),** and **luteinizing hormone (LH)**—are dimeric proteins that activate G protein-coupled receptors (Chapter 2). Thyroid-stimulating hormone, FSH, and LH share a common α chain. Their β chains, although somewhat similar to each other, differ enough to confer receptor specificity. Finally, **adrenocorticotropic hormone (ACTH),** a single peptide that is cleaved from a larger precursor that also contains the peptide β-endorphin (see Chapter 31), represents a third category. It does, however, like TSH, LH, and FSH, act through a G protein-coupled receptor.

Thyroid-stimulating hormone, FSH, LH, and ACTH share similarities in the regulation of their release from the pituitary. All are under the control of a hypothalamic peptide that stimulates their production by acting on G protein-coupled receptors (Table 37–1). Thyroid-stimulating hormone release is regulated by **thyrotropin-releasing hormone (TRH),** whereas the release of LH and FSH (known collectively as gonadotropins) is stimulated by pulses of **gonadotropin-releasing hormone (GnRH).** Adrenocorticotropin release is stimulated by **corticotropin-releasing hormone (CRH).** The final important regulatory feature shared by these three structurally related hormones is that they and their hypothalamic releasing factors are subject to feedback inhibitory regulation by the hormones whose production they control. Thyroid-stimulating hormone and TRH production is inhibited by the two key thyroid hormones, thyroxine and triiodothyronine (Chapter 38). Gonadotropin and GnRH production is inhibited in women by estrogen and progesterone, and in men by androgens such as testosterone. Production of ACTH is inhibited by cortisol. Feedback regulation is critical to the physiologic control of thyroid, adrenal cortical, and gonadal function and is also very important in pharmacologic treatments that affect these systems.

The hypothalamic hormonal control of GH and prolactin differs from the regulatory system for TSH, FSH,

Table 37–1. Links between hypothalamic, anterior pituitary, and target organ hormone or mediator.[1]

Anterior Pituitary Hormone	Hypothalamic Hormone	Target Organ	Primary Target Organ Hormone or Mediator
Growth hormone (GH, somatotropin)	Growth hormone-releasing hormone (GHRH) (+) Somatostatin (–)	Liver, muscle, bone, kidney, and others	Insulin-like growth factor-1 (IGF-1)
Thyroid-stimulating hormone (TSH)	Thyrotropin-releasing hormone (TRH) (+)	Thyroid	Thyroxine, triiodothyronine
Adrenocorticotropin (ACTH)	Corticotropin-releasing hormone (CRH) (+)	Adrenal cortex	Glucocorticoids, mineralocorticoids, androgens
Follicle-stimulating hormone (FSH) Luteinizing hormone (LH)	Gonadotropin-releasing hormone (GnRH) (+)[2]	Gonads	Estrogen, progesterone, testosterone
Prolactin (PRL)	Dopamine (–)	Breast	—

(+), stimulant; (–), inhibitor.
[1]All of these hormones act through G protein-coupled receptors except growth hormone and prolactin, which act through JAK/STAT receptors.
[2]Endogenous GnRH, which is released in pulses, stimulates LH and FSH release. When administered continuously as a drug, GnRH and its analogs inhibit LH and FSH release.

LH, and ACTH. The hypothalamus secretes two hormones that regulate GH; **growth hormone-releasing hormone (GHRH)** stimulates growth hormone production, whereas the peptide **somatostatin (SST)** inhibits growth hormone production. Growth hormone (GH) and its primary peripheral mediator, insulin-like growth factor-1 (IGF-1), also provide feedback to inhibit GH release. Prolactin production is inhibited by the catecholamine **dopamine** acting through the D$_2$ subtype of dopamine receptors. The hypothalamus does not produce a hormone that stimulates prolactin production.

Whereas all of the pituitary and hypothalamic hormones described above are available for use in humans, only a few are of major clinical importance. Because of the greater ease of administration of target endocrine gland hormones or their synthetic analogs, the related hypothalamic and pituitary hormones (TRH, TSH, CRH, ACTH, GHRH) are either not used clinically or are used rarely for specialized diagnostic testing. These agents are listed in Tables 37–2 and 37–3 and are not discussed further in this chapter. In contrast, GH, somatostatin, LH, FSH, GnRH, and dopamine or analogs of these hormones are commonly used and are described in the following text.

GROWTH HORMONE (SOMATOTROPIN)

Growth hormone, one of the peptide hormones produced by the anterior pituitary, is required during childhood and adolescence for attainment of normal adult size and has important effects throughout postnatal life on lipid and carbohydrate metabolism, and on lean body mass. Its effects are primarily mediated via **insulin-like growth factor 1 (IGF-1, somatomedin C)**

and to a lesser extent both directly and through **insulin-like growth factor 2 (IGF-2).** Individuals with congenital or acquired deficiency in GH during childhood or adolescence fail to reach their predicted adult

Table 37–2. Clinical uses of hypothalamic hormones and their analogs.

Hypothalamic Hormone	Clinical Uses
Growth hormone-releasing hormone (GHRH)	Used rarely as a diagnostic test for GH responsiveness
Thyrotropin-releasing hormone (TRH, protirelin)	Used rarely to diagnose hyper- or hypothyroidism
Corticotropin-releasing hormone (CRH)	Used rarely to distinguish Cushing's disease from ectopic ACTH secretion
Gonadotropin-releasing hormone (GnRH)	Used rarely in pulses to treat infertility caused by hypothalamic dysfunction
	Analogs used in long-acting formulations to inhibit gonadal function in men with prostate cancer and women undergoing assisted reproductive technology (ART) or women who require ovarian suppression for a gynecological disorder
Dopamine	Analogs used for treatment of hyperprolactinemia

Table 37–3. Diagnostic uses of thyroid-stimulating hormone and adrenocorticotropin.

Hormone	Diagnostic Use
Thyroid-stimulating hormone (TSH; thyrotropin)	In patients who have been treated surgically for thyroid carcinoma, to test for recurrence by assessing TSH-stimulated whole-body ^{131}I scans and serum thyroglobulin determinations
Adrenocorticotropin (ACTH)	In patients suspected of adrenal insufficiency, to test for a cortisol response.
	In patients suspected of congenital adrenal hyperplasia, to identify 21-hydroxylase deficiency, 11-hydroxylase deficiency, and 3β-hydroxy-Δ^5 steroid dehydrogenase deficiency, based on the steroids that accumulate in response to ACTH administration (see Figure 39-1 and Chapter 39)

height and have disproportionately increased body fat and decreased muscle mass. Adults with GH deficiency also have disproportionately small lean body mass.

Chemistry & Pharmacokinetics

A. STRUCTURE

Growth hormone (**somatotropin**) is a 191-amino-acid peptide with two sulfhydryl bridges. Its structure closely resembles that of prolactin. In the past, medicinal GH was isolated from the pituitaries of human cadavers. However, this form of GH was found to be contaminated with prions that could cause Creutzfeldt-Jakob disease. For this reason, it is no longer used.

Two types of recombinant human growth hormone (**rhGH**) are approved for clinical use. **Somatropin** has a 191-amino-acid sequence that is identical with the predominant native form of human growth hormone. **Somatrem** has 192 amino acids consisting of the 191 amino acids of GH plus an extra methionine residue at the amino terminal end. The two preparations appear to be equipotent.

B. ABSORPTION, METABOLISM, AND EXCRETION

Circulating endogenous GH has a half-life of 20–25 minutes and is predominantly cleared by the liver. Recombinant human GH is administered subcutaneously 3–6 times per week. Peak levels occur in 2–4 hours and active blood levels persist for approximately 36 hours.

Somatropin injectable suspension is a long-acting preparation of rhGH enclosed within microspheres. These microspheres degrade slowly after subcutaneous injection such that the rhGH is released over about 1 month.

Pharmacodynamics

Growth hormone mediates its effects via cell surface receptors of the JAK/STAT cytokine receptor superfamily. Dimerization of two GH receptors is stimulated by a single GH molecule and activates signaling cascades mediated by receptor-associated JAK tyrosine kinases and STATs (see Chapter 2). Growth hormone has complex effects on growth, body composition, and carbohydrate, protein, and lipid metabolism. The growth-promoting effects are mediated through an increase in the production of IGF-1. Much of the circulating IGF-1 is produced in the liver. Growth hormone also stimulates production of IGF-1 in bone, cartilage, muscle, and the kidney, where it plays autocrine or paracrine roles. Growth hormone stimulates longitudinal bone growth until the epiphyses close—near the end of puberty. In both children and adults, GH has anabolic effects in muscle and catabolic effects in lipid cells that shift the balance of body mass to an increase in muscle mass and a reduction in central adiposity. The effects of GH on carbohydrate metabolism are mixed, in part because GH and IGF-1 have opposite effects on insulin sensitivity. Growth hormone reduces insulin sensitivity, which results in mild hyperinsulinemia. In contrast, in patients who are unable to respond to endogenous GH because of mutated GH receptors, IGF-1 acting through its own IGF-1 receptors and through insulin receptors lowers serum glucose and reduces circulating insulin.

Clinical Pharmacology

A. GROWTH HORMONE DEFICIENCY

Growth hormone deficiency can have a genetic basis or can be acquired as a result of damage to the pituitary or hypothalamus by a tumor, infection, surgery, or radiation therapy. In childhood, GH deficiency presents as short stature and adiposity. (Neonates with isolated GH deficiency are of normal size at birth, presumably because fetal GH is not required for normal prenatal growth.) Another early sign of GH deficiency is hypoglycemia due to unopposed action of insulin, to which young children are especially sensitive. Criteria for diagnosis of GH deficiency usually include (1) a growth rate below 4 cm per year and (2) the absence of a serum GH response to two GH secretagogues. The incidence of congenital GH deficiency is approximately 1:4000 live births. Therapy with rhGH permits many children with short stature due to GH deficiency to achieve normal adult height.

In the past, it was believed that adults with GH deficiency did not exhibit a significant syndrome. However, more detailed studies suggest that adults with GH deficiency often have generalized obesity, reduced muscle

Table 37–4. Clinical uses of recombinant human growth hormone.

Primary Therapeutic Objective	Clinical Condition
Growth	Growth failure in pediatric patients associated with: Growth hormone deficiency Chronic renal failure Prader-Willi syndrome Turner syndrome
	Small for gestational age with failure to catch up by age 2
	Idiopathic short stature in pediatric patients
Improved metabolic state, increased lean body mass, sense of well-being	Growth hormone deficiency in adults
Increased lean body mass, weight, and physical endurance	Wasting in patients with AIDS
Improved gastrointestinal function	Short bowel syndrome in patients who are also receiving specialized nutritional support

mass, asthenia, and reduced cardiac output. GH-deficient adults who have been treated with GH have been shown to experience a reversal of many of these manifestations.

B. GROWTH HORMONE TREATMENT OF PEDIATRIC PATIENTS WITH SHORT STATURE

Although the greatest improvement in growth occurs in patients with GH deficiency, exogenous GH has some effect on height in children with short stature that is due to factors other than GH deficiency. Growth hormone has been approved for several conditions (Table 37–4) and has been used experimentally or off-label in many others. **Prader-Willi syndrome** is an autosomal dominant genetic disease that is associated with growth failure, obesity, and carbohydrate intolerance. In pediatric patients with Prader-Willi syndrome and growth failure, GH treatment decreases body fat and increases lean body mass, linear growth, and energy expenditure.

Growth hormone treatment has also been shown to have a strong beneficial effect on final height of girls with **Turner syndrome,** the syndrome associated with a 45,XO karyotype. In clinical trials, GH treatment has been shown to increase final height in girls with Turner syndrome by 10–15 cm (4–6 inches). Because girls with Turner syndrome also have either absent or rudimen-

tary ovaries, GH must be judiciously combined with gonadal steroids to achieve the maximal height effect.

Other conditions of growth failure for which GH treatment is approved include chronic renal failure in pediatric patients and small-for-gestational-age condition at birth in which the child has failed to catch up by age 2. In all of these pediatric patients as well as in patients with GH deficiency, it is critical to start GH treatment before the long bone epiphyses have closed.

The most controversial approved use of GH is for children with **idiopathic short stature,** also known as non-growth hormone-deficient short stature. This is a heterogeneous population that is defined clinically by a height that is 2.25 standard deviations or more below the national norm for children of the same age. Eligible children also have growth rates that are unlikely to result in an adult height in the normal range and the absence of a condition known to be associated with impaired growth. In this group of children, multiple years of GH therapy results in an average increase in adult height of 4–7 cm (1.57–2.76 inches) at an average cost of $35,000 per inch of height gained. The complex issues involved in the cost-risk-benefit relationship of this use of GH are important because an estimated 400,000 children in the USA fit the diagnostic criteria for idiopathic short stature.

Treatment of children with short stature should be carried out by specialists experienced in the use of GH. Treatment is begun with 0.025 mg/kg daily and may be increased to a maximum of 0.045 mg/kg daily. Somatropin injectable suspension is a long-acting preparation of rhGH that is administered subcutaneously in doses of 1.5 mg/kg monthly or 0.75 mg/kg twice monthly. Children must be observed closely for slowing of growth velocity, which could indicate a need to increase the dosage or the possibility of epiphyseal fusion or intercurrent problems such as hypothyroidism or malnutrition. Children with Turner syndrome or chronic renal insufficiency require somewhat higher doses.

Other Uses of Growth Hormone

Growth hormone affects many organ systems and also has a net anabolic effect. It has been tested in a number of conditions that are associated with a severe catabolic state and is approved for the treatment of wasting in patients with AIDS. In 2004, GH was approved for treatment of patients with short bowel syndrome who are dependent on total parenteral nutrition (TPN). After intestinal resection or bypass, the remaining functional intestine in many patients undergoes extensive adaptation that allows it to adequately absorb nutrients. However, other patients fail to adequately adapt and develop a malabsorption syndrome. Growth hormone has been shown in experimental animals to increase intestinal growth and improve its function. Results of GH treatment of patients with short bowel syndrome and dependence on total parenteral nutrition have been mixed in the clinical studies that have been published to date. Growth hormone is administered with glutamine, which also has trophic effects on the intestinal mucosa.

Growth hormone is a popular component of anti-aging programs. Serum levels of GH normally decline with aging; anti-aging programs claim that injection of GH or administration of drugs purported to increase GH release are effective anti-aging remedies. These claims are largely unsubstantiated. It is interesting that a number of studies in mice and the nematode *C elegans* have clearly demonstrated that analogs of human GH and IGF-1 consistently *shorten* lifespan and that loss-of-function mutations in the signaling pathways for the GH and IGF-1 analogs lengthen life-span. Another use of GH is by athletes for a purported increase in muscle mass and athletic performance. Growth hormone is one of the drugs banned by the Olympic Committee.

In 1993, the FDA approved the use of recombinant bovine growth hormone (rbGH) in dairy cattle to increase milk production. Although milk and meat from rbGH-treated cows appear to be safe, these cows have a higher incidence of mastitis, which could increase antibiotic use and result in greater antibiotic residues in milk and meat.

Toxicity & Contraindications

Children generally tolerate GH treatment well. A rarely reported side effect is intracranial hypertension, which may manifest as vision changes, headache, nausea, or vomiting. Some children develop scoliosis during rapid growth. Patients with Turner syndrome have an increased risk of otitis media while taking GH. Hypothyroidism is commonly discovered during GH treatment, so periodic assessment of thyroid function is indicated. Pancreatitis, gynecomastia, and nevus growth have occurred in patients receiving GH. Adults tend to have more adverse effects from GH therapy. Peripheral edema, myalgias, and arthralgias (especially in the hands and wrists) occur commonly but remit with dosage reduction. Carpal tunnel syndrome can occur. Growth hormone treatment increases the activity of cytochrome P450 isoforms, which could reduce the serum levels of drugs metabolized by that enzyme system (see Chapter 4). There has been no increased incidence of malignancy among patients receiving GH therapy, but GH treatment is contraindicated in a patient with a known malignancy. Proliferative retinopathy may rarely occur. Growth hormone treatment of critically ill patients appears to *increase* mortality.

Side effects of the long-acting somatropin injectable suspension have included injection-site nodules that persist for 5–7 days (96%), edema, arthralgias, transient fatigue (24%), mild-moderate nausea (24%), and headache (36%).

MECASERMIN

A small number of children with growth failure have severe IGF-1 deficiency that is not responsive to exogenous GH. Causes include mutations in the GH receptor and development of neutralizing antibodies to GH. In 2005, the FDA approved mecasermin for treatment of severe IGF-1 deficiency that is not responsive to GH. Mecasermin is a complex of recombinant human IGF-1 (rhIGF-1) and recombinant human insulin-like growth factor-binding protein-3 (rhIGFBP-3). The IGF-1 activates transmembrane receptors that, like insulin and EGF receptors, manifest tyrosine kinase activity at their intracellular domains (see Chapters 2 and 41). The binding protein rhIGFBP-3 is needed to maintain an adequate half-life of rhIGF-1. Normally, over 80% of the circulating IGF-1 is bound to IGFBP-3, which is produced by the liver under the control of GH. Patients with severe IGF-1 deficiency that is secondary to aberrant GH signaling also have deficiency of IGFBP-3, and so it is important to supply this with the IGF-1 replacement. Mecasermin is administered subcutaneously twice daily at a recommended starting dosage of 0.04–0.08 mg/kg and increased weekly up to a maximum twice-daily dosage of 0.12 mg/kg. The most important adverse effect observed with mecasermin is hypoglycemia. To avoid hypoglycemia, the prescribing instructions require consumption of a meal or snack 20 minutes before or after mecasermin administration. Several patients have experienced intracranial hypertension and asymptomatic elevation of liver enzymes.

GROWTH HORMONE ANTAGONISTS

The need for antagonists of GH stems from the tendency of GH-producing cells (somatotrophs) in the anterior pituitary to form secreting tumors. Pituitary adenomas occur most commonly in adults. In adults, GH-secreting adenomas cause **acromegaly,** which is characterized by abnormal growth of cartilage and bone tissue, and many organs including skin, muscle, heart, liver, and the gastrointestinal tract. Acromegaly adversely affects the skeletal, muscular, cardiovascular, respiratory, and metabolic systems. When a GH-secreting adenoma occurs before the long bone epiphyses close, it leads to the rare condition, **gigantism.** Small GH-secreting adenomas can be treated with GH antagonists. **Octreotide,** a somatostatin analog, and **bromocriptine,** a dopamine receptor agonist (described below) reduce the production of GH, whereas **pegvisomant** prevents GH from activating its receptor. Larger pituitary adenomas, which produce greater amounts of GH and also can impair visual and central nervous system function by encroaching on nearby brain structures, are treated with trans-sphenoidal surgery or radiation.

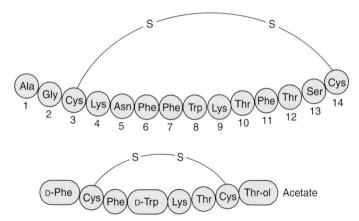

Figure 37–2. **Above:** Amino acid sequence of somatostatin. **Below:** Sequence of the synthetic analog, octreotide.

Somatostatin & Octreotide

Somatostatin, a 14-amino-acid peptide (Figure 37–2), is found in the hypothalamus, other parts of the central nervous system, the pancreas, and other sites in the gastrointestinal tract. It inhibits the release of GH, glucagon, insulin, and gastrin.

Exogenous somatostatin is rapidly cleared from the circulation, with an initial half-life of 1–3 minutes. The kidney appears to play an important role in its metabolism and excretion.

Somatostatin has limited therapeutic usefulness because of its short duration of action and its multiple effects in many secretory systems. **Octreotide,** an analog of somatostatin (Figure 37–2), is 45 times more potent than somatostatin in inhibiting GH release but only twice as potent in reducing insulin secretion. Because of this relatively reduced effect on pancreatic B cells, hyperglycemia rarely occurs during treatment. The plasma elimination half-life of octreotide is about 80 minutes, 30 times longer in humans than that of somatostatin.

Octreotide, 50–200 mcg given subcutaneously every 8 hours, reduces symptoms caused by a variety of hormone-secreting tumors: acromegaly; the carcinoid syndrome; gastrinoma; glucagonoma; nesidioblastosis; the watery diarrhea, hypokalemia, and achlorhydria (WDHA) syndrome; and diabetic diarrhea. Somatostatin receptor scintigraphy, using radiolabeled octreotide, is useful in localizing neuroendocrine tumors having somatostatin receptors and helps predict the response to octreotide therapy. Octreotide is also useful for the acute control of bleeding from esophageal varices.

Octreotide acetate injectable long-acting suspension is a slow-release microsphere formulation. It is instituted only after a brief course of shorter-acting octreotide has been demonstrated to be effective and tolerated. Injections into alternate gluteal muscles are repeated at 4-week intervals in doses of 20–40 mg. Octreotide is extremely costly.

Adverse effects of octreotide therapy include nausea, vomiting, abdominal cramps, flatulence, and steatorrhea with bulky bowel movements. Biliary sludge and gallstones may occur after 6 months of use in 20–30% of patients. However, the yearly incidence of symptomatic gallstones is about 1%. Cardiac effects include sinus bradycardia (25%) and conduction disturbances (10%). Pain at the site of injection is common, especially with the long-acting octreotide suspension. Vitamin B_{12} deficiency may occur with long-term use of octreotide.

Pegvisomant

Pegvisomant is a GH receptor antagonist that is useful for the treatment of acromegaly. Pegvisomant is the polyethylene glycol (PEG) derivative of a mutant GH, B2036, which has increased affinity for one site of the GH receptor but a reduced affinity at its second binding site. This allows dimerization of the receptor but blocks the conformational changes required for signal transduction. Pegvisomant is a less potent GH receptor antagonist than is B2036, but pegylation reduces its clearance and improves its overall clinical effectiveness. When pegvisomant was administered subcutaneously to 160 patients with acromegaly daily for 12 months or more, serum levels of IGF-1 fell into the normal range in 97%; two patients experienced growth of their GH-secreting pituitary tumors, and two patients developed increases in liver enzymes.

THE GONADOTROPINS— FOLLICLE-STIMULATING HORMONE & LUTEINIZING HORMONE—& HUMAN CHORIONIC GONADOTROPIN

The gonadotropins are produced by a single type of pituitary cell, the gonadotroph. These hormones serve complementary functions in the reproductive process.

In women, the principal function of FSH is to direct ovarian follicle development. Both FSH and LH are needed for ovarian steroidogenesis. In the ovary, LH stimulates androgen production by theca cells in the follicular stage of the menstrual cycle, whereas FSH stimulates the conversion by granulosa cells of androgens to estrogens. In the luteal phase of the menstrual cycle, estrogen and progesterone production is primarily under the control first of LH and then, if pregnancy occurs, under the control of human chorionic gonadotropin (hCG). Human chorionic gonadotropin is a placental protein nearly identical to LH; its actions are mediated through LH receptors.

In men, FSH is the primary regulator of spermatogenesis, whereas LH is the main stimulus for the production of testosterone by Leydig cells. FSH helps to maintain high local androgen concentrations in the vicinity of developing sperm by stimulating the production of androgen-binding protein by Sertoli cells. FSH also stimulates the conversion by Sertoli cells of testosterone to estrogen.

FSH, LH, and hCG are commercially available in several different forms. They are used in states of infertility to stimulate spermatogenesis in men and to induce ovulation in women. Their most common clinical use is for the controlled ovulation hyperstimulation that is the cornerstone of assisted reproductive technologies such as in vitro fertilization (IVF, see below).

Chemistry & Pharmacokinetics

All three hormones—FSH, LH, and hCG—are dimers that share an identical α chain in addition to a distinct β chain that confers receptor specificity. The β chains of hCG and LH are nearly identical, and these two hormones are used interchangeably. All of the gonadotropin preparations are administered by subcutaneous or intramuscular injection, usually on a daily basis. Half-lives vary by preparation and route of injection from 10 to 40 hours.

A. MENOTROPINS

The first commercial gonadotropin product was extracted from the urine of postmenopausal women, which contains a substance with FSH-like properties (but with 4% of the potency of FSH) and an LH-like substance. This purified extract of FSH and LH is known as **menotropins,** or human menopausal gonadotropins **(hMG).**

B. FOLLICLE-STIMULATING HORMONE

Three forms of purified FSH are available. **Urofollitropin,** also known as uFSH, is a purified preparation of human FSH that is extracted from the urine of postmenopausal women. Virtually all of the LH activity has

been removed through a form of immunoaffinity chromatography that uses anti-hCG antibodies. Two recombinant forms of FSH **(rFSH)** are also available: **follitropin alfa** and **follitropin beta.** The amino acid sequences of these two products are identical to that of human FSH. These preparations differ from each other and urofollitropin in the composition of the carbohydrate side chains. The rFSH preparations have a shorter half-life than preparations derived from human urine but stimulate estrogen secretion at least as efficiently and, in some studies, more efficiently. The rFSH preparations are considerably more expensive.

C. LUTEINIZING HORMONE

Lutropin, recombinant human LH (rLH), was introduced in the USA in 2004. When given by subcutaneous injection, it has a half-life of about 10 hours. Lutropin has only been approved for use in combination with follitropin alfa for stimulation of follicular development in infertile women with profound LH deficiency. It has not been approved for use with the other preparations of FSH nor for simulating the endogenous LH surge that is needed to complete follicular development and precipitate ovulation.

D. HUMAN CHORIONIC GONADOTROPIN

Human chorionic gonadotropin is produced by the human placenta and excreted into the urine, whence it can be extracted and purified. It is a glycoprotein consisting of a 92-amino-acid α chain virtually identical to that of FSH, LH, and TSH, and a β chain of 145 amino acids that resembles that of LH except for the presence of a carboxyl terminal sequence of 30 amino acids not present in LH. Choriogonadotropin alfa (rhCG) is a recombinant form of hCG. Because of its greater consistency in biologic activity, the rhCG is packaged and dosed on the basis of weight rather than units of activity. All of the other gonadotropins, including rFSH, are packaged and dosed on the basis of units of activity. The preparation of hCG that is purified from human urine is administered by intramuscular injection, whereas rhCG is administered by subcutaneous injection.

Pharmacodynamics

The gonadotropins and hCG exert their effects through G protein-coupled receptors. LH and FSH have complex effects on reproductive tissues in both sexes. In women, these effects change over the time course of a menstrual cycle as a result of a complex interplay between concentration-dependent effects of the gonadotropins, cross-talk between LH, FSH, and gonadal steroids, and the influence of other ovarian hormones. A coordinated pattern of FSH and LH secretion during the menstrual cycle (see Figure 40–1) is required for normal follicle development, ovulation, and pregnancy.

During the first 8 weeks of pregnancy, the progesterone and estrogen required to maintain pregnancy are produced by the ovarian corpus luteum. For the first few days after ovulation, the corpus luteum is maintained by maternal LH. However, as maternal LH concentrations fall owing to increasing concentrations of progesterone and estrogen, maintenance of the corpus luteum must be taken over by hCG produced by the placenta.

Clinical Pharmacology

A. Ovulation Induction

The gonadotropins are used to induce ovulation in women with anovulation due to hypogonadotropic hypogonadism, polycystic ovary syndrome, obesity, and other causes. Because of the high cost of gonadotropins and the need for close monitoring during their administration, gonadotropins are generally reserved for anovulatory women who fail to respond to other less complicated forms of treatment (eg, clomiphene, aromatase inhibitors, metformin; see Chapter 40). Gonadotropins are also used for controlled ovarian hyperstimulation in assisted reproductive technology procedures. A number of protocols make use of gonadotropins in ovulation induction and controlled ovulation hyperstimulation, and new ones are continually being developed to improve the rates of success and to decrease the two primary risks of ovulation induction: multiple pregnancies and the ovarian hyperstimulation syndrome (OHSS; see below). Although the details differ, all of these protocols are based on the complex physiology that underlies a normal menstrual cycle. Like a menstrual cycle, ovulation induction is discussed in relation to a cycle that begins on the first day of a menstrual bleed (Figure 37–3). Shortly after the first day (usually on day 3), daily injections with one of the FSH preparations (hMG, urofollitropin) are begun and are continued for approximately 7–12 days. In women with hypogonadotropic hypogonadism, follicle development requires treatment with a combination of FSH and LH because these women do not produce the basal level of LH that is required for adequate ovarian estrogen production and normal follicle development. The dose and duration of FSH treatment are based on the response as measured by the serum estradiol concentration and by ultrasound evaluation of ovarian follicle development and endometrial thickness. When exogenous gonadotropins are used to stimulate follicle development, there is risk of a premature endogenous surge in LH owing to the rapidly changing hormonal milieu. To prevent this, gonadotropins are almost always administered in conjunction with a drug that blocks the effects of endogenous GnRH—either continuous administration of a GnRH agonist, which down-regulates GnRH receptors, or a few days of treatment with a GnRH receptor antagonist (see below and Figure 37–3).

When appropriate follicular maturation has occurred, the FSH and GnRH agonist or GnRH antagonist injections are discontinued; the following day, hCG (5000–10,000 IU) is administered intramuscularly to induce final follicular maturation and, in ovulation induction protocols, ovulation. The hCG administration is followed by insemination in ovulation induction and by oocyte retrieval in assisted reproductive technology procedures. Because use of GnRH agonists or antagonists during the follicular phase of ovulation induction suppresses endogenous LH production, it is important to provide exogenous hormonal support of the luteal phase. In clinical trials, exogenous progesterone, hCG, or a combination of the two have been effective at providing adequate luteal support. However, progesterone is preferred because hCG for luteal support carries a higher risk of the ovarian hyperstimulation syndrome (see below).

B. Male Infertility

Most of the signs and symptoms of hypogonadism in males (eg, delayed puberty, maintenance of secondary sex characteristics after puberty) can be adequately treated with exogenous androgen; however, treatment of infertility in hypogonadal men requires the activity of both LH and FSH. For many years, conventional therapy has consisted of initial treatment for 8–12 weeks with injections of 1000–2500 IU hCG several times per week. After the initial phase, hMG is injected at a dose of 75–150 units three times per week. In men with hypogonadal hypogonadism, it takes an average of 4–6 months of such treatment for sperm to appear in the ejaculate. With the more recent availability of urofollitropin, rFSH, and rLH, a number of alternative protocols have been developed. An advance that has indirectly benefited gonadotropin treatment of male infertility is intracytoplasmic sperm injection (ICSI), in which a single sperm is injected directly into a mature oocyte that has been retrieved after controlled ovarian hyperstimulation of a female partner. With the advent of ICSI, the minimum threshold of spermatogenesis required for pregnancy is greatly lowered.

Toxicity & Contraindications

In women treated with gonadotropins and hCG, the two most serious complications are the **ovarian hyperstimulation syndrome** and **multiple pregnancies.** Overstimulation of the ovary during ovulation induction often leads to uncomplicated ovarian enlargement that usually resolves spontaneously. The ovarian hyperstimulation syndrome is a more serious complication that

Figure 37–3. Controlled ovarian hyperstimulation in preparation for an assisted reproductive technology such as in vitro fertilization. Follicular phase: Follicle development is stimulated with gonadotropin injections that begin about 3 days after menses begin. When the follicles are ready, as assessed by measurement of serum estrogen concentration and ultrasound measurement of follicle size, final oocyte maturation is induced by an injection of hCG. Luteal phase: Shortly thereafter oocytes are retrieved and fertilized in vitro. The recipient's luteal phase is supported with injections of progesterone. To prevent a premature luteinizing hormone surge, endogenous gonadotropin secretion is inhibited during the follicular phase with either a GnRH agonist or a GnRH antagonist. In most protocols, the GnRH agonist is started midway through the preceding luteal cycle.

occurs in 0.5–4% of patients. It is characterized by ovarian enlargement, ascites, hydrothorax, and hypovolemia, sometimes resulting in shock. Hemoperitoneum (from a ruptured ovarian cyst), fever, and arterial thromboembolism can occur.

The probability of multiple pregnancies is greatly increased when ovulation induction and assisted reproductive technologies are used. In ovulation induction, the risk of multiple pregnancy is estimated to be 15–20%, whereas the percentage of multiple pregnancies in the general population is closer to 1%. Multiple pregnancies carry an increased risk of complications, such as gestational diabetes, preeclampsia, and preterm labor. In IVF, the risk of multiple pregnancy is primarily determined by the number of embryos transferred to the recipient. A strong trend in recent years has been to transfer fewer embryos.

Other reported adverse effects of gonadotropin treatment are headache, depression, edema, precocious puberty, and (rarely) production of antibodies to hCG. In men treated with gonadotropins, the risk of gynecomastia is directly correlated with the level of testoste-

rone produced in response to treatment. An association between ovarian cancer and fertility drugs has been reported. However, it is not known which, if any, fertility drugs are causally related to cancer.

GONADOTROPIN-RELEASING HORMONE & ITS ANALOGS

Gonadotropin-releasing hormone is secreted by neurons in the hypothalamus. It travels through the hypothalamic-pituitary venous portal plexus to the anterior pituitary, where it binds to G protein-coupled receptors on the plasma membranes of gonadotroph cells. *Pulsatile* GnRH secretion is required to stimulate the gonadotroph cell to produce and release LH and FSH.

Sustained, *nonpulsatile* administration of GnRH or GnRH analogs *inhibits* the release of FSH and LH by the pituitary in both women and men, resulting in hypogonadism. GnRH agonists are used to produce gonadal suppression in men with prostate cancer. They are also used in women who are undergoing assisted reproductive technology procedures or have a gynecologic problem that is benefited by ovarian suppression.

Chemistry & Pharmacokinetics

A. STRUCTURE

GnRH is a decapeptide found in all mammals. **Gonadorelin** is an acetate salt of synthetic human GnRH. Synthetic analogs include **goserelin, histrelin, leuprolide, nafarelin,** and **triptorelin.** These analogs all have D-amino acids at position 6, and all but nafarelin have ethylamide substituted for glycine at position 10. Both modifications make them more potent and longer-lasting than native GnRH and gonadorelin.

B. PHARMACOKINETICS

Gonadorelin can be administered intravenously or subcutaneously. GnRH analogs can be administered subcutaneously, intramuscularly, via nasal spray (nafarelin), or as a subcutaneous implant. The half-life of intravenous gonadorelin is 4 minutes, and the half-lives of subcutaneous and intranasal GnRH analogs are approximately 3 hours. The duration of clinical uses of GnRH agonists varies from a few days for ovulation induction to a number of years for treatment of metastatic prostate cancer. Therefore, preparations have been developed with a range of durations of action from several hours (for daily administration) to 1, 4, 6, or 12 months (depot forms).

Pharmacodynamics

The pharmacodynamic actions of GnRH exhibit complex dose-response relationships that change dramatically from the fetal period through the end of puberty. This is not surprising in view of the complex physiologic role that GnRH plays in normal reproduction, particularly in female reproduction. Pulsatile GnRH release occurs and is responsible for stimulating LH and FSH production during the fetal and neonatal period. However, from the age of 2 years until the onset of puberty, GnRH secretion falls off and the pituitary simultaneously exhibits very low sensitivity to the GnRH that is produced. Just before puberty, an increase in the frequency and amplitude of GnRH release occurs. In early puberty, pituitary sensitivity to GnRH increases. This is due in part to the effect of increasing concentrations of gonadal steroids. In females, it usually takes several months to a year after the onset of puberty for the hypothalamic-pituitary system to produce an LH surge and ovulation. By the end of puberty, the system is well established so that menstrual cycles proceed at relatively constant intervals. The amplitude and frequency of GnRH pulses also vary in a regular pattern through the menstrual cycle with the highest amplitudes occurring during the luteal phase and the highest frequency occurring late in the follicular phase. Lower pulse frequencies favor FSH secretion, whereas higher pulse frequencies favor LH secretion. Gonadal steroids as well as the peptide hormones activin and inhibin have complex modulatory effects on the gonadotropin response to GnRH.

In the pharmacologic use of GnRH and its analogs, pulsatile intravenous administration of gonadorelin every 1–4 hours stimulates FSH and LH secretion. Continuous administration of gonadorelin or its longer-acting analogs produces a biphasic response. During the first 7–10 days, an agonist effect occurs that results in increased concentrations of gonadal hormones in males and females. This initial phase is referred to as a flare. After this period, the continued presence of GnRH results in an inhibitory action that manifests as a drop in the concentration of gonadotropins and gonadal steroids. The inhibitory action is due to a combination of receptor down-regulation and changes in the signaling pathways activated by GnRH.

Clinical Pharmacology

The GnRH agonists are occasionally used for stimulation of gonadotropin production. They are used far more commonly for suppression of gonadotropin release.

A. STIMULATION

1. Female infertility—In the current era of widespread availability of gonadotropins and assisted reproductive technology, the use of pulsatile GnRH administration to treat infertility has become less common. Although pulsatile GnRH is less likely than gonadotropins to cause multiple pregnancies and the ovarian hyperstimulation syndrome, the inconvenience and cost associated with continuous use of an intravenous pump and difficulties obtaining native GnRH (gonadorelin) are barriers to pulsatile GnRH. When this approach *is* used, a portable battery-powered programmable pump and intravenous tubing deliver pulses of gonadorelin every 90 minutes.

Gonadorelin or a GnRH agonist analog can be used to precipitate an LH surge and ovulation in women with infertility who are undergoing ovulation induction with gonadotropins. Traditionally, hCG has been used to precipitate ovulation in this situation. However, there is some evidence that gonadorelin or a GnRH agonist is less likely than hCG to cause multiple ova to be released and less likely to cause the ovarian hyperstimulation syndrome.

2. Male infertility—It is possible to use pulsatile gonadorelin for infertility in men with hypothalamic hypogonadotropic hypogonadism. A portable pump infuses gonadorelin intravenously every 90 minutes.

Serum testosterone levels and semen analyses must be done regularly. At least 3–6 months of pulsatile infusions are required before significant numbers of sperm are seen. The preferable alternative to intravenous gonadorelin treatment is the gonadotropin treatment described above.

3. Diagnosis of LH responsiveness—GnRH can be useful in determining whether delayed puberty in a hypogonadotropic adolescent is due to constitutional delay or to hypogonadotropic hypogonadism. The LH response (but not the FSH response) to a single dose of GnRH can distinguish between these two conditions. Serum LH levels are measured before and at various times after an intravenous or subcutaneous bolus of GnRH. An increase in serum LH with a peak that exceeds 15.6 mIU/mL is normal and suggests impending puberty. An impaired LH response suggests hypogonadotropic hypogonadism due to either pituitary or hypothalamic disease, but does not rule out constitutional delay of adolescence.

B. SUPPRESSION OF GONADOTROPIN PRODUCTION

1. Controlled ovarian hyperstimulation—In the controlled ovarian hyperstimulation that provides multiple mature oocytes for assisted reproductive technologies such as IVF, it is critical to suppress an endogenous LH surge that could prematurely trigger ovulation. This suppression is most commonly achieved by daily subcutaneous injections of leuprolide or daily nasal applications of nafarelin. For leuprolide, treatment is commonly initiated with 1.0 mg daily for about 10 days or until menstrual bleeding occurs. At that point, the dose is reduced to 0.5 mg daily until hCG is administered (Figure 37–3). For nafarelin, the beginning dosage is generally 400 mcg twice a day, which is decreased to 200 mcg when menstrual bleeding occurs. In women who respond poorly to the standard protocol, alternative protocols that use shorter courses and lower doses of GnRH agonists may improve the follicular response to gonadotropins.

2. Endometriosis—Endometriosis is a syndrome of cyclical abdominal pain in premenopausal women that is due to the presence of estrogen-sensitive endometrium-like tissue located outside the uterus. The pain of endometriosis is often reduced by abolishing exposure to the cyclical changes in the concentrations of estrogen and progesterone that are a normal part of the menstrual cycle. The ovarian suppression induced by continuous treatment with a GnRH agonist greatly reduces estrogen and progesterone concentrations and prevents cyclical changes. The recommended duration of treatment with a GnRH agonist is limited to 6 months because ovarian suppression beyond this period can result in decreased bone density. Leuprolide, goserelin, and nafarelin are approved for this indication. Leuprolide and goserelin are administered as depot preparations that provide 1 or 3 months of continuous GnRH agonist activity. Nafarelin is administered twice daily as a nasal spray at a dose of 0.2 mg per spray.

3. Uterine leiomyomata (uterine fibroids)—Uterine leiomyomata are benign, estrogen-sensitive, fibrous growths in the uterus that can cause menorrhagia, with associated anemia and pelvic pain. Treatment for 3–6 months with a GnRH agonist reduces fibroid size and, when combined with supplemental iron, improves anemia. Leuprolide, goserelin, and nafarelin are approved for this indication. The doses and routes of administration are similar to those described for treatment of endometriosis.

4. Prostate cancer—Antiandrogen therapy is the primary medical therapy for prostate cancer. Combined antiandrogen therapy with continuous GnRH agonist and an androgen receptor antagonist such as flutamide (see Chapter 40) is as effective as surgical castration in reducing serum testosterone concentrations. Leuprolide, goserelin, histrelin, and triptorelin are approved for this indication. The preferred formulation is one of the long-acting depot forms that provide 1, 3, 4, 6, or 12 months of active drug therapy. During the first 7–10 days of GnRH analog therapy, serum testosterone levels increase because of the agonist action of the drug; this can precipitate pain in patients with bone metastases, and tumor growth and neurologic symptoms in patients with vertebral metastases. It can also temporarily worsen symptoms of urinary obstruction. Such tumor flares can usually be avoided with the concomitant administration of bicalutamide or one of the other androgen receptor antagonists (see Chapter 40). Within about 2 weeks, serum testosterone levels fall to the hypogonadal range.

5. Central precocious puberty—Continuous administration of a GnRH agonist is indicated for treatment of central precocious puberty (onset of secondary sex characteristics before 8 years in girls or 9 years in boys). Before administering a GnRH agonist, one must confirm central precocious puberty by demonstrating a pubertal, not childhood, gonadotropin response to GnRH and a bone age at least 1 year beyond chronologic age. Pretreatment evaluation must also include gonadal steroid levels compatible with precocious puberty and not congenital adrenal hyperplasia; an hCG level that is low enough to exclude a chronic gonadotropin-secreting tumor; an MRI of the brain to exclude an intracranial tumor; and ultrasound examination of the adrenals and ovaries or testes to exclude a steroid-secreting tumor.

Treatment can be carried out with injections of leuprolide or nasal application of nafarelin. Leuprolide treatment is usually initiated at a dosage of 0.05 mg/kg body weight injected subcutaneously daily and then adjusted on the basis of the clinical response. Pediatric depot preparations of leuprolide are also available. The recommended initial dosage of nafarelin for central precocious puberty is 1.6 mg/d. This is achieved with two unit dose sprays (each spray contains 0.1 mL, 0.2 mg) into each nostril twice daily. Treatment with a GnRH agonist is generally continued to age 11 in females and age 12 in males.

6. Other—Other clinical uses for the gonadal suppression provided by continuous GnRH agonist treatment include advanced breast and ovarian cancer; thinning of the endometrial lining in preparation for an endometrial ablation procedure in women with dysfunctional uterine bleeding; and treatment of amenorrhea and infertility in women with polycystic ovary disease.

Toxicity

Gonadorelin can cause headache, light-headedness, nausea, and flushing. Local swelling often occurs at subcutaneous injection sites. Generalized hypersensitivity dermatitis has occurred after long-term subcutaneous administration. Rare acute hypersensitivity reactions include bronchospasm and anaphylaxis. Sudden pituitary apoplexy and blindness have been reported following administration of GnRH to a patient with a gonadotropin-secreting pituitary tumor.

Continuous treatment of women with a GnRH analog (leuprolide, nafarelin, goserelin) causes the typical symptoms of menopause, which include hot flushes, sweats, and headaches. Depression, diminished libido, generalized pain, vaginal dryness, and breast atrophy may also occur. Ovarian cysts may develop within the first 2 months of therapy and generally resolve after an additional 6 weeks; however, the cysts may persist and require discontinuation of therapy. Reduced bone density and osteoporosis may occur with prolonged use, so patients should be monitored with bone densitometry before repeated treatment courses. Depending on the condition being treated with the GnRH agonist, it may be possible to ameliorate the signs and symptoms of the hypoestrogenic state without losing clinical efficacy by adding back a small dose of a progestin and an estrogen. Contraindications to the use of GnRH agonists in women include pregnancy and breast-feeding.

In men treated with continuous GnRH agonist administration, adverse effects include hot flushes and sweats, edema, gynecomastia, decreased libido, decreased hematocrit, reduced bone density, asthenia, and injection site reactions. GnRH analog treatment of children is generally well tolerated. However, temporary exacerbation of precocious puberty may occur during the first few weeks of therapy. Nafarelin nasal spray may cause or aggravate sinusitis.

GNRH RECEPTOR ANTAGONISTS

Two synthetic decapeptides that function as competitive antagonists of GnRH receptors are available for clinical use. **Ganirelix** and **cetrorelix** inhibit the secretion of FSH and LH in a dose-dependent manner. Both are approved for use in controlled ovarian hyperstimulation as part of an assisted reproductive procedure such as IVF.

Pharmacokinetics

Ganirelix and cetrorelix are absorbed rapidly after subcutaneous injection. Administration of 0.25 mg daily maintains GnRH antagonism. Alternatively, a single 3.0-mg dose of cetrorelix suppresses LH secretion for 96 hours.

Clinical Pharmacology

GnRH antagonists are approved for preventing the LH surge during controlled ovarian hyperstimulation. They offer several advantages over continuous treatment with a GnRH agonist. Because they produce an immediate antagonist effect, their use can be delayed until day 6–8 of the IVF cycle (Figure 37–3) and thus the duration of administration is shorter. They also appear to have a less negative impact on the ovarian response to gonadotropin stimulation, which permits a decrease in the total duration and dose of gonadotropin. Finally, GnRH antagonists are associated with a lower risk of ovarian hyperstimulation syndrome, which can lead to cycle cancellation. On the other hand, because their antagonist effects reverse more quickly after their discontinuation, adherence to the treatment regimen is critical. The antagonists produce a more complete suppression of gonadotropin secretion than agonists. There is concern that the suppression of LH may inhibit ovarian steroidogenesis to an extent that impairs follicular development when recombinant or the purified form of FSH is used during the follicular phase of an IVF cycle. Clinical trials have shown a slightly lower rate of pregnancy in IVF cycles that used GnRH antagonist treatment compared with cycles that used GnRH agonist treatment.

Toxicity

The GnRH antagonists are well tolerated. The most common adverse effects are nausea and headache. When used for ovulation induction in combination with gonadotropins, the most serious toxicity is the ovarian hyperstimulation syndrome.

PROLACTIN

Prolactin is a 198-amino-acid peptide hormone produced in the anterior pituitary. Its structure resembles that of GH. Prolactin is the principal hormone responsible for lactation. Milk production is stimulated by prolactin when appropriate circulating levels of estrogens, progestins, corticosteroids, and insulin are present. A deficiency of prolactin—which can occur in rare states of pituitary deficiency—is manifested by failure to lactate or by a luteal phase defect. In rare cases of hypothalamic destruction, prolactin levels may be elevated as a result of impaired transport of dopamine (prolactin-inhibiting hormone) to the pituitary. Much more commonly, however, prolactin is elevated as a result of prolactin-secreting adenomas. Hyperprolactinemia produces a syndrome of amenorrhea and galactorrhea in women, and loss of libido and infertility in men. In the case of large tumors (macroadenomas), it can be associated with symptoms of a pituitary mass, including visual changes due to compression of the optic nerves. The hypogonadism and infertility associated with hyperprolactinemia result from inhibition of GnRH release.

No preparation of prolactin is available for use in prolactin-deficient patients. For patients with symptomatic hyperprolactinemia, inhibition of prolactin secretion can be achieved with dopamine agonists, which act in the pituitary to inhibit prolactin release.

DOPAMINE AGONISTS

Adenomas that secrete excess prolactin usually retain the sensitivity to inhibition by dopamine exhibited by the normal pituitary. **Bromocriptine, cabergoline,** and **pergolide** are ergot derivatives (see Chapters 16 and 28) with a high affinity for dopamine D_2 receptors. **Quinagolide,** a drug approved in Europe, is a nonergot agent with similarly high D_2 receptor affinity. The chemical structure and pharmacokinetic features of ergot alkaloids are presented in Chapter 16.

Dopamine agonists suppress prolactin release very effectively in patients with hyperprolactinemia. Growth hormone release is reduced in patients with acromegaly, although not as effectively. Cabergoline, bromocriptine, and pergolide are also used in Parkinson's disease to improve motor function and reduce levodopa requirements (see Chapter 28).

Pharmacokinetics

All available dopamine agonists are active as oral preparations, and all are eliminated by metabolism. They can also be absorbed systemically after vaginal insertion of tablets. Cabergoline, with a half-life of approximately 65 hours, has the longest duration of action. Pergolide and quinagolide have half-lives of about 20 hours, whereas the half-life of bromocriptine is about 7 hours. Following vaginal administration, serum levels peak more slowly.

Clinical Pharmacology

A. HYPERPROLACTINEMIA

A dopamine agonist is the standard medical treatment for hyperprolactinemia. These drugs shrink pituitary prolactin-secreting tumors, lower circulating prolactin levels, and restore ovulation in approximately 70% of women with microadenomas and 30% of women with macroadenomas (Figure 37–4). Cabergoline is initiated at 0.25 mg twice weekly orally or vaginally. It can be increased gradually, according to serum prolactin determinations, up to a maximum of 1 mg twice weekly. Bromocriptine is generally taken daily after the evening meal at the initial dose of 1.25 mg; the dose is then increased as tolerated. Most patients require 2.5–7.5 mg daily. Long-acting oral bromocriptine formulations (Parlodel SRO) and intramuscular formulations (Parlodel L.A.R.) are available outside the USA.

In doses of 0.15–0.6 mg/d orally, quinagolide suppresses prolactin and shrinks most prolactinomas. Quinagolide is sometimes better tolerated than ergot-derived dopamine agonists. It is not available in the USA.

B. PHYSIOLOGIC LACTATION

Dopamine agonists were used in the past to prevent breast engorgement when breast feeding was not desired. Their use for this purpose has been discouraged because of toxicity (see Toxicity & Contraindications).

C. ACROMEGALY

A dopamine agonist alone or in combination with pituitary surgery, radiation therapy, or octreotide administration can be used to treat acromegaly. The doses required are higher than those used to treat hyperprolactinemia. For example, patients with acromegaly require 20 to 30 mg/d of bromocriptine and seldom respond adequately to bromocriptine alone unless the pituitary tumor secretes prolactin as well as GH.

Toxicity & Contraindications

Dopamine agonists can cause nausea, headache, lightheadedness, orthostatic hypotension, and fatigue. Psychiatric manifestations occasionally occur, even at lower doses, and may take months to resolve. Erythromelalgia occurs rarely. High dosages of ergot-derived preparations can cause cold-induced peripheral digital vasospasm. Pulmonary infiltrates have occurred with chronic high-dosage therapy. Cabergoline appears to cause nausea less often than bromocriptine. Vaginal administration can reduce nausea, but may cause local irritation.

Dopamine agonist therapy during the early weeks of pregnancy has not been associated with an increased

Figure 37–4. Results from a clinical trial of cabergoline in women with hyperprolactinemia and anovulation. **A:** The dotted line indicates the upper limit of normal serum prolactin concentrations. **B:** Complete success was defined as pregnancy or at least two consecutive menses with evidence of ovulation at least once. Partial success was two menstrual cycles without evidence of ovulation or just one ovulatory cycle. The most common reasons for withdrawal from the trial were nausea, headache, dizziness, abdominal pain, and fatigue. (Modified and reproduced, with permission, from Webster J et al: A comparison of cabergoline and bromocriptine in the treatment of hyperprolactinemic amenorrhea. N Engl J Med 1994;331:904.)

risk of spontaneous abortion or congenital malformations. Although there has been a longer experience with the safety of bromocriptine during early pregnancy, there is growing evidence that cabergoline is also safe in women with macroadenomas who must continue a dopamine agonist during pregnancy. In patients with small pituitary adenomas, dopamine agonist therapy is discontinued upon conception because growth of microadenomas during pregnancy is rare. Patients with very large adenomas require vigilance for tumor progression and often require a dopamine agonist throughout pregnancy. There have been rare reports of stroke or coro-

nary thrombosis in postpartum women taking bromocriptine to suppress postpartum lactation.

■ POSTERIOR PITUITARY HORMONES

The two posterior pituitary hormones—vasopressin and oxytocin—are synthesized in neuronal cell bodies in the hypothalamus and then transported via their axons to the posterior pituitary, where they are stored and then released into the circulation. Each has limited but important clinical uses.

OXYTOCIN

Oxytocin is a peptide hormone secreted by the posterior pituitary that participates in labor and delivery and elicits milk ejection in lactating women. During the second half of pregnancy, uterine smooth muscle shows an increase in the expression of oxytocin receptors and becomes increasingly sensitive to the stimulant action of endogenous oxytocin. Pharmacologic concentrations of oxytocin powerfully stimulate uterine contraction.

Chemistry & Pharmacokinetics

A. STRUCTURE

Oxytocin is a 9-amino-acid peptide with an intrapeptide disulfide cross-link (Figure 37–5). Its amino acid sequence differs from that of vasopressin at positions 3 and 8. Vasotocin is similar to oxytocin and vasopressin and is found in nonmammalian vertebrates.

B. ABSORPTION, METABOLISM, AND EXCRETION

Oxytocin is administered intravenously for initiation and augmentation of labor. It also can be administered intramuscularly for control of postpartum bleeding. Oxytocin is not bound to plasma proteins and is eliminated by the kidneys and liver, with a circulating half-life of 5 minutes.

Pharmacodynamics

Oxytocin acts through G protein-coupled receptors and the phosphoinositide-calcium second-messenger system to contract uterine smooth muscle. Oxytocin also stimulates the release of prostaglandins and leukotrienes that augment uterine contraction. Oxytocin in small doses increases both the frequency and force of uterine contractions. At higher doses, it produces sustained contraction.

Figure 37–5. Posterior pituitary hormones and desmopressin. (Modified and reproduced, with permission, from Ganong WF: *Review of Medical Physiology*, 21st ed. McGraw-Hill, 2003.)

Oxytocin also causes contraction of myoepithelial cells surrounding mammary alveoli, which leads to milk ejection. Without oxytocin-induced contraction, normal lactation cannot occur. At high concentrations, oxytocin has weak antidiuretic and pressor activity due to activation of vasopressin receptors.

Clinical Pharmacology

Oxytocin is used to induce labor for conditions requiring early vaginal delivery such as Rh problems, maternal diabetes, preeclampsia, or ruptured membranes. It is also used to augment abnormal labor that is protracted or displays an arrest disorder. Oxytocin has several uses in the immediate postpartum period, including the control of uterine hemorrhage after vaginal or cesarean delivery. It is sometimes used during second-trimester abortions.

Before delivery, oxytocin is usually administered intravenously via an infusion pump with appropriate fetal and maternal monitoring. For induction of labor, an initial infusion rate of 0.5–2 mU/min is increased every 30–60 minutes until a physiologic contraction pattern is established. The maximum infusion rate is 20 mU/min. For postpartum uterine bleeding, 10–40 units are added to 1 L of 5% dextrose, and the infusion rate is titrated to control uterine atony. Alternatively, 10 units of oxytocin can be administered by intramuscular injection after delivery of the placenta.

During the antepartum period, oxytocin induces uterine contractions that transiently reduce placental blood flow to the fetus. The oxytocin challenge test measures the fetal heart rate response to a standardized oxytocin infusion and provides information about placental circulatory reserve. Oxytocin is infused at an initial rate of 0.5 mU/min, then doubled every 20 minutes until uterine contractions decrease the fetal blood supply. An abnormal response, seen as late decelerations in the fetal heart rate, indicates fetal hypoxia and may warrant immediate cesarean delivery.

Toxicity & Contraindications

When oxytocin is used judiciously, serious toxicity is rare. The toxicity that does occur is due either to excessive stimulation of uterine contractions or to inadvertent activation of vasopressin receptors. Excessive stimulation of uterine contractions before delivery can cause fetal distress, placental abruption, or uterine rupture. These complications can be detected early by means of standard fetal monitoring equipment. High concentrations of oxytocin with activation of vasopressin receptors can cause excessive fluid retention, or water intoxication, leading to hyponatremia, heart failure, seizures, and death. Bolus injections of oxytocin can cause hypotension. To avoid hypotension, oxytocin is administered intravenously as dilute solutions at a controlled rate.

Contraindications to oxytocin include fetal distress, prematurity, abnormal fetal presentation, cephalopelvic disproportion, and other predispositions for uterine rupture.

OXYTOCIN ANTAGONIST

Atosiban is an antagonist of the oxytocin receptor that has been approved outside the USA as a treatment for preterm labor (tocolysis). Atosiban is a modified form of oxytocin that is administered by IV infusion for 2–48 hours. In a small number of published clinical trials, atosiban appears to be as effective as β-adrenoceptor-agonist tocolytics and to produce fewer adverse effects. However, in one placebo-controlled trial, the subject group that received atosiban had more infant deaths than the placebo group. In 1998, the FDA decided not to approve atosiban based on concerns about efficacy and safety.

VASOPRESSIN (ANTIDIURETIC HORMONE, ADH)

Vasopressin is a peptide hormone released by the posterior pituitary in response to rising plasma tonicity or falling blood pressure. Vasopressin possesses antidiuretic and vasopressor properties. A deficiency of this hormone results in diabetes insipidus (see Chapters 15 and 17).

Chemistry & Pharmacokinetics

A. STRUCTURE

Vasopressin is a nonapeptide with a 6-amino-acid ring and a 3-amino-acid side chain. The residue at position 8 is arginine in humans and in most other mammals except pigs and related species, whose vasopressin contains lysine at position 8 (Figure 37–5). **Desmopressin** acetate (DDAVP, 1-desamino-8-D-arginine vasopressin) is a long-acting synthetic analog of vasopressin with minimal V_1 activity and an antidiuretic-to-pressor ratio 4000 times that of vasopressin. Desmopressin is modified at position 1 and contains a D-amino acid at position 8. Like vasopressin and oxytocin, desmopressin has a disulfide linkage between positions 1 and 6.

B. ABSORPTION, METABOLISM, AND EXCRETION

Vasopressin is administered by intravenous or intramuscular injection; oral administration is not effective because the peptide is inactivated by digestive enzymes. The half-life of circulating vasopressin is approximately 15 minutes, with renal and hepatic metabolism via reduction of the disulfide bond and peptide cleavage.

Desmopressin can be administered intravenously, subcutaneously, intranasally, or orally. The half-life of circulating desmopressin is 1.5–2.5 hours. Nasal desmopressin is available as a unit dose spray that delivers 0.1 mL per spray; it is also available with a calibrated nasal tube that can be used to deliver a more precise dose. Nasal bioavailability of desmopressin is 3–4%, whereas oral bioavailability is less than 1%.

Pharmacodynamics

Vasopressin activates two subtypes of G protein-coupled receptors (see Chapter 17). V_1 receptors are found on vascular smooth muscle cells and mediate vasoconstriction. V_2 receptors are found on renal tubule cells and reduce diuresis through increased water permeability and water resorption in the collecting tubules. Extrarenal V_2-like receptors regulate the release of coagulation factor VIII and von Willebrand factor.

Clinical Pharmacology

Vasopressin and desmopressin are treatments of choice for pituitary diabetes insipidus. The dosage of desmopressin is 10–40 mcg (0.1–0.4 mL) in two to three divided doses as a nasal spray or, as an oral tablet, 0.1–0.2 mg two to three times daily. The dosage by injection is 1–4 mcg (0.25–1 mL) every 12–24 hours as needed for polyuria, polydipsia, or hypernatremia. Bedtime desmopressin therapy, by intranasal or oral administration, ameliorates nocturnal enuresis by decreasing nocturnal urine production. Vasopressin infusion is effective in some cases of esophageal variceal bleeding and colonic diverticular bleeding.

Desmopressin is also used for the treatment of coagulopathy in hemophilia A and von Willebrand's disease (see Chapter 34).

Toxicity & Contraindications

Headache, nausea, abdominal cramps, agitation, and allergic reactions occur rarely. Therapy can result in hyponatremia and seizures.

Vasopressin (but not desmopressin) can cause vasoconstriction and should be used cautiously in patients with coronary artery disease. Nasal insufflation of desmopressin may be less effective when nasal congestion is present.

VASOPRESSIN ANTAGONISTS

A group of nonpeptide antagonists of vasopressin receptors is being investigated for use in patients with hyponatremia or acute heart failure which is often associated with elevated concentrations of vasopressin. **Conivaptan** has high affinity for both V_{1a} and V_2 receptors. **Tolvaptan** has 30-fold higher affinity for V_2 than for V_1 receptors. In several clinical trials, both agents relieved symptoms and reduced objective signs of hyponatremia and heart failure. Conivaptan has been approved by the FDA for intravenous administration in hyponatremia but not in congestive heart failure. Several other nonselective nonpeptide vasopressin receptor antagonists are being investigated for these conditions.

Chapter continues on next page.

PREPARATIONS AVAILABLE

GROWTH HORMONE AGONISTS & ANTAGONISTS

Mecasermin rinfabate (Iplex)
Parenteral: 36 mg per 0.6 mL for subcutaneous injection

Mecasermin (Increlex)
Parenteral: 36 mg/mL for subcutaneous injection

Octreotide (Sandostatin)
Parenteral: 0.05, 0.1, 0.2, 0.5, 1.0 mg/mL for subcutaneous or IV administration
Parenteral depot injection (Sandostatin LAR Depot): 10, 20, 30 mg for IM injection

Pegvisomant (Somavert)
Parenteral: 10, 15, 29 mg powder to reconstitute for subcutaneous injection

Sermorelin (Geref)
Parenteral: 0.5, 1.0 mg for subcutaneous injection; 50 mcg powder to reconstitute for intravenous injection

Somatrem (Protropin)
Parenteral: 5, 10 mg for subcutaneous or IM injection

Somatropin (Genotropin, Humatrope, Nutropin, Nutropin AQ, Norditropin, Saizen, Serostim, Tev-tropin)
Parenteral: 0.2, 0.4, 0.6, 0.8, 1.0, 1.2, 1.4, 1.6, 1.8, 2, 4, 5, 5.8, 6, 8, 8.8, 10, 12, 13.5, 13.8, 24 mg for subcutaneous or IM injection

GONADOTROPIN AGONISTS & ANTAGONISTS

Cetrorelix (Cetrotide)
Parenteral: 0.25, 3.0 mg in single-use vials for subcutaneous injection

Choriogonadotropin alfa [rhCG] (Ovidrel)
Parenteral: 250 mcg in single-dose prefilled syringes for subcutaneous injection

Chorionic gonadotropin [hCG] (generic, Profasi, Pregnyl, others)
Parenteral: powder to reconstitute 500, 1000, 2000 IU/mL for IM injection

Follitropin alfa [rFSH] (Gonal-f)
Parenteral: 82, 600, 1200 IU powder in single-dose vials or 415, 568, 1026 IU in prefilled pens with needles for subcutaneous injection

Follitropin beta [rFSH] (Follistim)
Parenteral: 37.5, 150 IU powder in sign-dose vials or 175, 350, 650, 975 IU in a solution of benzyl alcohol in cartridges for subcutaneous injection

Ganirelix (Antagon)
Parenteral: 500 mcg/mL in prefilled syringes for subcutaneous injection

Gonadorelin hydrochloride [GnRH] (Factrel)
Parenteral: 100, 500 mcg for subcutaneous or intravenous injection

Goserelin (Zoladex)
Parenteral: 3.6, 10.8 mg subcutaneous implant

Histrelin acetate (Vantas)
Parenteral: 50 mg subcutaneous implant

Leuprolide (generic, Eligard, Lupron)
Parenteral: 5 mg/mL in multiple-dose vials, or 7.5 mg powder in a single-use kit, or 30 mg (4-month depot), 45 mg (6-month depot) in a single-dose kit for subcutaneous injection
Parenteral depot polymeric delivery system (Eligard): 7.5, 22.5, 30, 45 mg in a single-dose kit for subcutaneous injection
Parenteral depot microspheres suspension (Lupron Depot, Depot-Ped, Depot-3, Depot-4): 3.75, 7.5, 11.25, 15, 22.5, 30 mg in a single-dose kit for IM injection
Parenteral implant: 72 mg for subcutaneous implant

Lutropin [rLH] (Luveris)
Parenteral: 82.5 IU powder for subcutaneous injection

Menotropins [hMG] (Menopur, Repronex)
Parenteral: 75 IU FSH and 75 IU LH activity, 150 IU FSH and 150 IU LH activity for subcutaneous or IM injection

Nafarelin (Synarel)
Nasal: 2 mg/mL (200 mcg/spray)

Urofollitropin (Bravelle)
Parenteral: 75 IU FSH for subcutaneous injection

PROLACTIN ANTAGONISTS (DOPAMINE AGONISTS)

Bromocriptine (generic, Parlodel)
Oral: 2.5 mg tablets, 5 mg capsules

Cabergoline (generic, Dostinex)
Oral: 0.5 mg scored tablets

Pergolide (generic, Permax)
Oral: 0.05, 0.25, 1.0 mg tablets

OXYTOCIN

Oxytocin (generic, Pitocin)
Parenteral: 10 units/mL for intravenous or IM injection

VASOPRESSIN AGONISTS AND ANTAGONISTS

Conivaptan (Vaprisol)
Parenteral: 5 mg/mL solution for IV injection

(continued)

Desmopressin (DDAVP, generic, Minirin, Stimate)
Nasal: 0.1, 1.5 mg/mL solution
Nasal: 0.1 mg/mL spray pump and rhinal tube delivery system
Parenteral: 4 mcg/mL solution for IV or subcutaneous injection
Oral: 0.1, 0.2 mg tablets
Vasopressin (generic, Pitressin)
Parenteral: 20 pressor IU/mL for IM or subcutaneous administration

OTHER
Corticorelin ovine (Acthrel)
Parenteral: 100 mcg for IV injection
Corticotropin (H.P. Acthar Gel)
Parenteral: 80 units/mL
Cosyntropin (Cortrosyn)
Parenteral: 0.25 mg/vial for IV or IM injection
Thyrotropin alpha (Thyrogen)
Parenteral: 1.1 mg (4 IU) for IM injection
Triptorelin (Trelstar)
Parenteral: 3.75, 11.25 mg microgranules for IM injection

REFERENCES

Attia AM, Al-Inany HG, Proctor ML: Gonadotropins for treatment of male factor subfertility. Cochrane Database Syst Rev 2006;1:CD005071.

Bankowski BJ, Zacur HA: Dopamine agonist therapy for hyperprolactinemia. Clin Obstet Gynecol 2003;46:349.

Barlier A, Jaquet P: Quinagolide—a valuable treatment option for hyperprolactinaemia. Eur J Endocrinol 2006;154:187.

Chandraharan E, Arulkumaran S: Acute tocolysis. Curr Opin Obstet Gynecol 2005;17:151.

Bevan JS et al: Primary medical therapy for acromegaly: An open, prospective, multicenter study of the effects of subcutaneous and intramuscular slow-release octreotide on growth hormone, insulin-like growth factor-I, and tumor size. J Clin Endocrinol Metab 2002;87:4554.

Blanks S, Thornton S: The role of oxytocin in parturition. Br J Obstet Gynecol 2003;110(Suppl 20):46.

Carter-Su C, Schwartz J, Smit LS: Molecular mechanism of growth hormone action. Annu Rev Physiol 1996;58:187.

Daya S: Updated meta-analysis of recombinant follicle-stimulating hormone (FSH) versus urinary FSH for ovarian stimulation in assisted reproduction. Fertil Steril 2002;77:711.

de Jong D et al: High dose gonadotropin-releasing hormone antagonist (ganirelix) may prevent ovarian hyperstimulation syndrome caused by ovarian stimulation for in-vitro fertilization. Hum Reprod 1998;13:573.

Demling R: Growth hormone therapy in critically ill patients. N Engl J Med 1999;341:837.

Devroey P et al: Reproductive biology and IVF: Ovarian stimulation and endometrial receptivity. Trends Endocrinol Metab 2004;15:84.

Ebling FJ: The neuroendocrine timing of puberty. Neuroendocrine 2005;129:675.

Gabe SG, Neibyl JR, Simpson JL: *Obstetrics: Normal and Problem Pregnancies*, 4th ed. Churchill Livingstone, 2002.

Gheorghiade M, Teerlink JR, Mebazaa A: Pharmacology of new agents for acute heart failure syndromes. Am J Cardiol 2005;96:68G.

Goffin V, Touraine P: Pegvisomant. Pharmacia. Curr Opin Investig Drugs 2002;3:752.

Hapgood JP et al: Regulation of expression of mammalian gonadotropin-releasing hormone receptor genes. J Neuroendocrinol 2005;17:619.

Larson PR et al: *Williams Textbook of Endocrinology*, 10th ed. Saunders, 2003.

Macklon NS et al: The science behind 25 years of ovulation stimulation for in vitro fertilization. Endocr Rev 2006;27:170.

Mammen AA, Ferrer FA: Nocturnal enuresis: Medical management. Urol Clin North Am 2004;31:491.

Maughan KL, Heim SW, Galazka SS: Preventing postpartum hemorrhage: Managing the third stage of labor. Am Fam Physician 2006;73:1025.

Melmed S et al: Consensus statement: Medical management of acromegaly. Eur J Endocrinol 2005;153:737.

Papatsonis D et al: Oxytocin receptor antagonists for inhibiting preterm labour. Cochrane Database Syst Rev 2005;20:CD004452.

Scolapio J: Short bowel syndrome: Recent clinical outcomes with growth hormone. Gastroenterology 2006;130:S122.

Speroff L, Fritz MA: *Clinical Gynecologic Endocrinology and Infertility*, 7th ed. Lippincott Williams & Wilkins, 2005.

van der Lely AJ et al: Long-term treatment of acromegaly with pegvisomant, a growth hormone receptor antagonist. Lancet 2001;358:1754.

Van Wely M et al: Human menopausal gonadotropin versus recombinant follicle stimulation hormone for ovarian stimulation in assisted reproductive cycles. Cochrane Database Syst Rev 2003;1:CD003973.

Webster J et al: A comparison of cabergoline and bromocriptine in the treatment of hyperprolactinemic amenorrhea. N Engl J Med 1994;331:904.

Zitzmann M, Nieschlag E: Hormone substitution in male hypogonadism. Mol Cell Endocrinol 2000;161:73.

Thyroid and Antithyroid Drugs

38

Francis S. Greenspan, MD, FACP, & Betty J. Dong, PharmD

THYROID PHYSIOLOGY

The normal thyroid gland secretes sufficient amounts of the thyroid hormones—**triiodothyronine (T_3)** and **tetraiodothyronine (T_4, thyroxine)**—to normalize growth and development, body temperature, and energy levels. These hormones contain 59% and 65% (respectively) of iodine as an essential part of the molecule. Calcitonin, the second type of thyroid hormone, is important in the regulation of calcium metabolism and is discussed in Chapter 42.

Iodide Metabolism

The recommended daily adult iodide (I^-)* intake is 150 mcg (200 mcg during pregnancy).

Iodide, ingested from food, water, or medication, is rapidly absorbed and enters an extracellular fluid pool. The thyroid gland removes about 75 mcg a day from this pool for hormone synthesis, and the balance is excreted in the urine. If iodide intake is increased, the fractional iodine uptake by the thyroid is diminished.

Biosynthesis of Thyroid Hormones

Once taken up by the thyroid gland, iodide undergoes a series of enzymatic reactions that convert it into active thyroid hormone (Figure 38–1). The first step is the transport of iodide into the thyroid gland by an intrinsic follicle cell basement membrane protein called the sodium/iodide symporter (NIS). This can be inhibited by such anions as thiocyanate (SCN^-), pertechnetate (TcO_4^-), and perchlorate (ClO_4^-). At the apical cell membrane a second I^- transport enzyme called pendrin controls the flow of iodide across the membrane. Pendrin is also found in the cochlea of the inner ear and if deficient or absent, a syndrome of deafness and goiter, called Pendred's syndrome, ensues. At the apical cell membrane, iodide is oxidized by thyroidal peroxidase to iodine, in which form it rapidly iodinates tyrosine residues within the thyroglobulin molecule to form monoiodotyrosine (MIT) and diiodotyrosine (DIT).

This process is called **iodide organification.** Thyroidal peroxidase is transiently blocked by high levels of intrathyroidal iodide and blocked more persistently by thioamide drugs.

Two molecules of DIT combine within the thyroglobulin molecule to form L-thyroxine (T_4). One molecule of MIT and one molecule of DIT combine to form T_3. In addition to thyroglobulin, other proteins within the gland may be iodinated, but these iodoproteins do not have hormonal activity. Thyroxine, T_3, MIT, and DIT are released from thyroglobulin by exocytosis and proteolysis of thyroglobulin at the apical colloid border. The MIT and DIT are deiodinated within the gland, and the iodine is reutilized. This process of proteolysis is also blocked by high levels of intrathyroidal iodide. The ratio of T_4 to T_3 within thyroglobulin is approximately 5:1, so that most of the hormone released is thyroxine. Most of the T_3 circulating in the blood is derived from peripheral metabolism of thyroxine (see below, Figure 38–2).

Transport of Thyroid Hormones

T_4 and T_3 in plasma are reversibly bound to protein, primarily thyroxine-binding globulin (TBG). Only about 0.04% of total T_4 and 0.4% of T_3 exist in the free form. Many physiologic and pathologic states and drugs affect T_4, T_3, and thyroid transport. However, the actual levels of free hormone generally remain normal, reflecting feedback control.

Peripheral Metabolism of Thyroid Hormones

The primary pathway for the peripheral metabolism of thyroxine is deiodination. Deiodination of T_4 may occur by monodeiodination of the outer ring, producing 3,5,3'-triiodothyronine (T_3), which is three to four times more potent than T_4. Alternatively, deiodination may occur in the inner ring, producing 3,3',5'-triiodothyronine (reverse T_3, or rT_3), which is metabolically inactive (Figure 38–2). Drugs such as amiodarone, iodinated contrast media, β blockers, and corticosteroids, and severe illness or starvation inhibit the 5'-deiodinase necessary for the conversion of T_4 to T_3, resulting in low T_3 and high rT_3 levels in the serum. The pharmacokinetics of thyroid hormones are

---

*In this chapter, the term "iodine" denotes all forms of the element; the term "iodide" denotes only the ionic form, I^-.

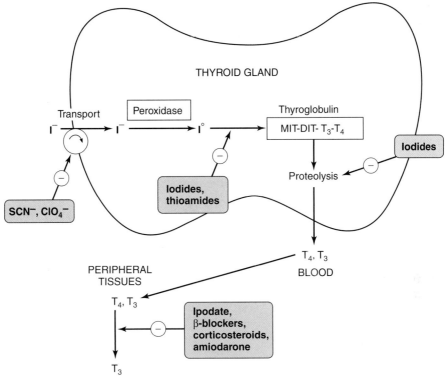

Figure 38–1. Biosynthesis of thyroid hormones. The sites of action of various drugs that interfere with thyroid hormone biosynthesis are shown.

Figure 38–2. Peripheral metabolism of thyroxine. (Modified from Greenspan FS: Thyroid gland. In: Greenspan FS, Gardner D [editors]: *Basic & Clinical Endocrinology,* 7th ed. McGraw-Hill, 2004.)

Table 38–1. Summary of thyroid hormone kinetics.

Variable	T$_4$	T$_3$
Volume of distribution	10 L	40 L
Extrathyroidal pool	800 mcg	54 mcg
Daily production	75 mcg	25 mcg
Fractional turnover per day	10%	60%
Metabolic clearance per day	1.1 L	24 L
Half-life (biologic)	7 days	1 day
Serum levels		
Total	5–12 mcg/dL (64–164 nmol/L)	70–132 ng/dL (1.1–2.0 nmol/L)
Free	0.7–1.86 ng/dL (9–24 pmol/L)	0.23–0.42 ng/dL (3.5–6.47 pmol/L)
Amount bound	99.96%	99.6%
Biologic potency	1	4
Oral absorption	80%	95%

listed in Table 38–1. The low serum levels of T$_3$ and rT$_3$ in normal individuals are due to the high metabolic clearances of these two compounds.

Evaluation of Thyroid Function

The tests used to evaluate thyroid function are listed in Table 38–2.

A. THYROID-PITUITARY RELATIONSHIPS

Control of thyroid function via thyroid-pituitary feedback is also discussed in Chapter 37. Briefly, hypothalamic cells secrete thyrotropin-releasing hormone (TRH) (Figure 38–3). TRH is secreted into capillaries of the pituitary portal venous system, and in the pituitary gland, TRH stimulates the synthesis and release of thyroid-stimulating hormone (TSH). TSH in turn stimulates an adenylyl cyclase–mediated mechanism in the thyroid cell to increase the synthesis and release of T$_4$ and T$_3$. These thyroid hormones act in a negative feedback fashion in the pituitary to block the action of TRH and in the hypothalamus to inhibit the synthesis and secretion of TRH. Other hormones or drugs may also affect the release of TRH or TSH.

B. AUTOREGULATION OF THE THYROID GLAND

The thyroid gland also regulates its uptake of iodide and thyroid hormone synthesis by intrathyroidal mechanisms that are independent of TSH. These mechanisms are primarily related to the level of iodine in the blood. Large doses of iodine inhibit iodide organification (Wolff-

Chaikoff block, see Figure 38–1). In certain disease states (eg, Hashimoto's thyroiditis), this can inhibit thyroid hormone synthesis and result in hypothyroidism. Hyperthyroidism can result from the loss of the Wolff-Chaikoff block in susceptible individuals (eg, multinodular goiter).

C. ABNORMAL THYROID STIMULATORS

In Graves' disease (see below), lymphocytes secrete a TSH receptor-stimulating antibody (TSH-R Ab [stim]), also known as thyroid-stimulating immunoglobulin (TSI). This immunoglobulin binds to the TSH receptor and turns on the gland in the same fashion as TSH itself. The duration of its effect, however, is much longer than that of TSH. TSH receptors are also found in orbital fibrocytes, which may be stimulated by high levels of TSH-R Ab [stim].

■ I. BASIC PHARMACOLOGY OF THYROID & ANTITHYROID DRUGS

THYROID HORMONES

Chemistry

The structural formulas of thyroxine and triiodothyronine as well as reverse triiodothyronine (rT$_3$) are shown

Table 38–2. Typical values for thyroid function tests.

Name of Test	Normal Value[1]	Results in Hypothyroidism	Results in Hyperthyroidism
Total thyroxine by RIA (T_4 [RIA])	5–12 mcg/dL (64–154 nmol/L)	Low	High
Total triiodothyronine by RIA (T_3 [RIA])	70–132 ng/dL (1.1–2.0 nmol/L)	Normal or low	High
Free T_4 (FT_4)	0.7–1.86 mg/dL (9–24 pmol/L)	Low	High
Free T_3 (FT_3)	0.2–0.42 ng/dL (3–6.5 pmol/L)	Low	High
Thyrotropic hormone (TSH)	0.5–5.0 μIU/mL (0.5–5.0 mIU/L)	High[2]	Low
[123]I uptake at 24 hours	5–35%	Low	High
Thyroglobulin autoantibodies (Tg-ab)	< 1 IU/mL	Often present	Usually present
Thyroid peroxidase antibodies (TPA)	< 1 IU/mL	Often present	Usually present
Isotope scan with ^{123}I or [99m]TcO_4	Normal pattern	Test not indicated	Diffusely enlarged gland
Fine-needle aspiration biopsy (FNA)	Normal pattern	Test not indicated	Test not indicated
Serum thyroglobulin	< 56 ng/mL	Test not indicated	Test not indicated
Serum calcitonin	Male: < 8 ng/L (< 2.3 pmol/L); female: < 4 ng/L (< 1.17 pmol/L)	Test not indicated	Test not indicated
TSH receptor-stimulating antibody (thyroid stimulating immunoglobulin)	< 125%	Test not indicated	Elevated in Graves' disease

[1]Results may vary with different laboratories.
[2]Exception is central hypothyroidism.

in Figure 38–2. All of these naturally occurring molecules are levo (L) isomers. The synthetic dextro (D) isomer of thyroxine, dextrothyroxine, has approximately 4% of the biologic activity of the L isomer as evidenced by its lesser ability to suppress TSH secretion and correct hypothyroidism.

Pharmacokinetics

Thyroxine is absorbed best in the duodenum and ileum; absorption is modified by intraluminal factors such as food, drugs, and intestinal flora. Oral bioavailability of current preparations of L-thyroxine averages 80% (Table 38–1). In contrast, T_3 is almost completely absorbed (95%). T_4 and T_3 absorption appears not to be affected by mild hypothyroidism but may be impaired in severe myxedema with ileus. These factors are important in switching from oral to parenteral therapy. For parenteral use, the intravenous route is preferred for both hormones.

In patients with hyperthyroidism, the metabolic clearances of T_4 and T_3 are increased and the half-lives decreased; the opposite is true in patients with hypothyroidism. Drugs that induce hepatic microsomal enzymes (eg, rifampin, phenobarbital, carbamazepine, phenytoin, imatinib, protease inhibitors) increase the metabolism of

both T_4 and T_3 (Table 38–3). Despite this change in clearance, the normal hormone concentration is maintained in euthyroid patients as a result of compensatory hyperfunction of the thyroid. However, patients receiving T_4 replacement medication may require increased dosages to maintain clinical effectiveness. A similar compensation occurs if binding sites are altered. If TBG sites are increased by pregnancy, estrogens, or oral contraceptives, there is an initial shift of hormone from the free to the bound state and a decrease in its rate of elimination until the normal hormone concentration is restored. Thus, the concentration of total and bound hormone will increase, but the concentration of free hormone and the steady-state elimination will remain normal. The reverse occurs when thyroid binding sites are decreased.

Mechanism of Action

A model of thyroid hormone action is depicted in Figure 38–4, which shows the free forms of thyroid hormones, T_4 and T_3, dissociated from thyroid-binding proteins, entering the cell by active transport. Within the cell, T_4 is converted to T_3 by 5′-deiodinase, and the T_3 enters the nucleus, where T_3 binds to a specific T_3 receptor protein, a member of the c-*erb* oncogene family. (This family also includes the steroid hormone

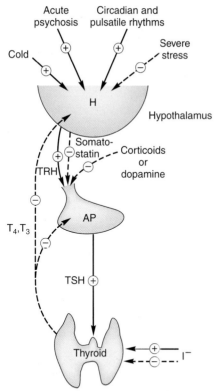

Figure 38–3. The hypothalamic-pituitary-thyroid axis. Acute psychosis or prolonged exposure to cold may activate the axis. Hypothalamic TRH stimulates pituitary TSH release, while somatostatin and dopamine inhibit it. TSH stimulates T_4 and T_3 synthesis and release from the thyroid, and they in turn inhibit both TRH and TSH synthesis and release. Small amounts of iodide are necessary for hormone production, but large amounts inhibit T_3 and T_4 production and release. (Solid arrows, stimulatory influence; dashed arrows, inhibitory influence. H, hypothalamus, AP, anterior pituitary.)

receptors and receptors for vitamins A and D.) The T_3 receptor exists in two forms, α and β. Differing concentrations of receptor forms in different tissues may account for variations in T_3 effect on different tissues.

Most of the effects of thyroid on metabolic processes appear to be mediated by activation of nuclear receptors that lead to increased formation of RNA and subsequent protein synthesis, eg, increased formation of Na^+/K^+ ATPase. This is consistent with the observation that the action of thyroid is manifested in vivo with a time lag of hours or days after its administration.

Large numbers of thyroid hormone receptors are found in the most hormone-responsive tissues (pituitary, liver, kidney, heart, skeletal muscle, lung, and intestine), while few receptor sites occur in hormone-unresponsive tissues (spleen, testes). The brain, which lacks an anabolic response to T_3, contains an intermediate number of receptors. In congruence with their biologic potencies, the affinity of the receptor site for T_4 is about ten times lower than that for T_3. The number of nuclear receptors may be altered to preserve body homeostasis. For example, starvation lowers both circulating T_3 hormone and cellular T_3 receptors.

Effects of Thyroid Hormones

The thyroid hormones are responsible for optimal growth, development, function, and maintenance of all body tissues. Excess or inadequate amounts result in the signs and symptoms of hyperthyroidism or hypothyroidism, respectively (Table 38–4). Since T_3 and T_4 are qualitatively similar, they may be considered as one hormone in the discussion that follows.

Thyroid hormone is critical for nervous, skeletal, and reproductive tissues. Its effects depend on protein synthesis as well as potentiation of the secretion and action of growth hormone. Thyroid deprivation in early life results in irreversible mental retardation and dwarfism—symptoms typical of congenital cretinism.

Effects on growth and calorigenesis are accompanied by a pervasive influence on metabolism of drugs as well as carbohydrates, fats, proteins, and vitamins. Many of these changes are dependent upon or modified by activity of other hormones. Conversely, the secretion and degradation rates of virtually all other hormones, including catecholamines, cortisol, estrogens, testosterone, and insulin, are affected by thyroid status.

Many of the manifestations of thyroid hyperactivity resemble sympathetic nervous system overactivity (especially in the cardiovascular system), although catecholamine levels are not increased. Changes in catecholamine-stimulated adenylyl cyclase activity as measured by cAMP are found with changes in thyroid activity. Possible explanations include increased numbers of β receptors or enhanced amplification of the β receptor signal. Other clinical symptoms reminiscent of excessive epinephrine activity (and partially alleviated by adrenoceptor antagonists) include lid lag and retraction, tremor, excessive sweating, anxiety, and nervousness. The opposite constellation of symptoms is seen in hypothyroidism (Table 38–4).

Thyroid Preparations

See the Preparations Available section at the end of this chapter for a list of available preparations. These preparations may be synthetic (levothyroxine, liothyronine, liotrix) or of animal origin (desiccated thyroid).

Thyroid hormones are not effective and can be detrimental in the management of obesity, abnormal vagi-

Table 38–3. Drug effects and thyroid function.

Drug Effect	Drugs
Change in thyroid hormone synthesis	
Inhibition of TRH or TSH secretion without induction of hypothyroidism or hyperthyroidism	Dopamine, levodopa, corticosteroids, somatostatin, metformin, bexarotene
Inhibition of thyroid hormone synthesis or release with the induction of hypothyroidism (or occasionally hyperthyroidism)	Iodides (including amiodarone), lithium, aminoglutethimide, thioamides, ethionamide
Alteration of thyroid hormone transport and serum total T_3 and T_4 levels, but usually no modification of FT_4 or TSH	
Increased TBG	Estrogens, tamoxifen, heroin, methadone, mitotane, fluorouracil
Decreased TBG	Androgens, glucocorticoids
Displacement of T_3 and T_4 from TBG with transient hyperthyroxinemia	Salicylates, fenclofenac, mefenamic acid, furosemide
Alteration of T_4 and T_3 metabolism with modified serum T_3 and T_4 levels but not FT_4 or TSH levels	
Induction of increased hepatic enzyme activity	Nicardipine, imatinib, protease inhibitors, phenytoin, carbamazepine, phenobarbital, rifampin, rifabutin
Inhibition of 5′-deiodinase with decreased T_3, increased rT_3	Iopanoic acid, ipodate, amiodarone, β blockers, corticosteroids, propylthiouracil, flavonoids
Other interactions	
Interference with T_4 absorption	Cholestyramine, colestipol, ciprofloxacin, aluminum hydroxide, sucralfate, sodium polystyrene sulfonate, raloxifene, ferrous sulfate, calcium carbonate, bran, soy
Induction of autoimmune thyroid disease with hypothyroidism or hyperthyroidism	Interferon-α, interleukin-2, interferon-β, lithium, amiodarone
Effect of thyroid function on drug effects	
Anticoagulation	Lower doses of warfarin required in hyperthyroidism, higher doses in hypothyroidism
Glucose control	Increased hepatic glucose production and glucose intolerance in hyperthyroidism; impaired insulin action and glucose disposal in hypothyroidism
Cardiac drugs	Higher doses of digoxin required in hyperthyroidism; lower doses in hypothyroidism
Sedatives; analgesics	Increased sedative and respiratory depressant effects from sedatives and opioids in hypothyroidsim; converse in hyperthyroidism

nal bleeding, or depression if thyroid hormone levels are normal. Anecdotal reports of a beneficial effect of T_3 administered with antidepressants have not been confirmed with a controlled study.

Synthetic levothyroxine is the preparation of choice for thyroid replacement and suppression therapy because of its stability, content uniformity, low cost, lack of allergenic foreign protein, easy laboratory measurement of serum levels, and long half-life (7 days), which permits once-daily administration. In addition, T_4 is converted to T_3 intracellularly; thus, administration of T_4 produces both hormones. Generic levothyroxine preparations provide comparable efficacy and are more cost-effective than branded preparations.

Although liothyronine (T_3) is three to four times more potent than levothyroxine, it is not recommended for routine replacement therapy because of its shorter half-life (24 hours), which requires multiple daily doses; its higher cost; and the greater difficulty of monitoring its adequacy of replacement by conventional laboratory tests. Furthermore, because of its greater hormone activity and consequent greater risk of cardiotoxicity,

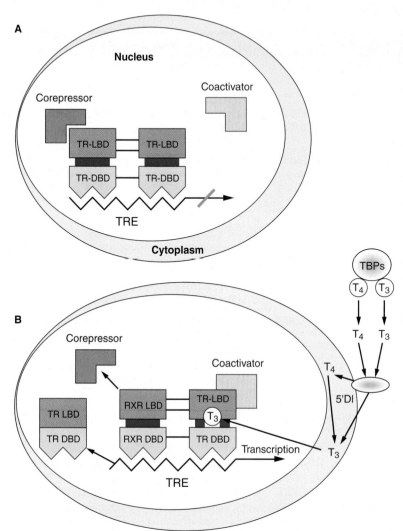

A

Nucleus

Corepressor

Coactivator

TR-LBD — TR-LBD

TR-DBD — TR-DBD

TRE

Cytoplasm

B

Corepressor

Coactivator

TR LBD

RXR LBD — TR-LBD

T₃

TR DBD

RXR DBD — TR DBD

Transcription

TRE

TBPs

T₄ T₃

T₄ T₃

T₄

5'DI

T₃

Figure 38–4. Model of the interaction of T_3 with the T_3 receptor. **A:** *Inactive phase*—the unliganded T_3 receptor dimer bound to the thyroid hormone response element (TRE) along with corepressors acts as a suppressor of gene transcription. **B:** *Active phase*—T_3 and T_4 circulate bound to thyroid-binding proteins (TBPs). The free hormones are transported into the cell by a specific transport system. Within the cytoplasm, T_4 is converted to T_3 by 5'-deiodinase; T_3 then moves into the nucleus. There it binds to the ligand-binding domain of the thyroid receptor (TR) monomer. This promotes disruption of the TR homodimer and heterodimerization with retinoid X receptor (RXR) on the TRE, displacement of corepressors, and binding of coactivators. The TR-coactivator complex activates gene transcription, which leads to alteration in protein synthesis and cellular phenotype. (TR-LBD, T_3 receptor ligand-binding domain; TR-DBD, T_3 receptor DNA-binding domain; RXR-LBD, retinoid X receptor ligand-binding domain; RXR-DBD, retinoid X receptor DNA-binding domain; T_3, triiodothyronine; T_4, tetraiodothyronine, L-thyroxine; 5'DI, 5'deiodinase. (Modified and reproduced, with permission, from Greenspan FS, Gardner DG [editors]: *Basic & Clinical Endocrinology,* 7th ed. McGraw-Hill, 2004.)

T_3 should be avoided in patients with cardiac disease. It is best used for short-term suppression of TSH. Because oral administration of T_3 is unnecessary, use of the more expensive mixture of thyroxine and liothyronine (liotrix) instead of levothyroxine is never required.

The use of desiccated thyroid rather than synthetic preparations is never justified, since the disadvantages of protein antigenicity, product instability, variable hormone concentrations, and difficulty in laboratory monitoring far outweigh the advantage of low cost. Significant amounts of T_3 found in some thyroid extracts and liotrix may produce significant elevations in T_3 levels and toxicity. Equivalent doses are 100 mg of desiccated thyroid, 100 mcg of levothyroxine, and 37.5 mcg of liothyronine.

The shelf life of synthetic hormone preparations is about 2 years, particularly if they are stored in dark bottles to minimize spontaneous deiodination. The shelf life of desiccated thyroid is not known with certainty, but its potency is better preserved if it is kept dry.

ANTITHYROID AGENTS

Reduction of thyroid activity and hormone effects can be accomplished by agents that interfere with the production of thyroid hormones, by agents that modify the tissue response to thyroid hormones, or by glandular destruction with radiation or surgery. *Goitrogens* are agents that suppress secretion of T_3 and T_4 to subnormal levels and thereby increase TSH, which in turn

Table 38–4. Manifestations of thyrotoxicosis and hypothyroidism.

System	Thyrotoxicosis	Hypothyroidism
Skin and appendages	Warm, moist skin; sweating; heat intolerance; fine, thin hair; Plummer's nails; pretibial dermopathy (Graves' disease)	Pale, cool, puffy skin; dry and brittle hair; brittle nails
Eyes, face	Retraction of upper lid with wide stare; periorbital edema; exophthalmos; diplopia (Graves' disease)	Drooping of eyelids; periorbital edema; loss of temporal aspects of eyebrows; puffy, nonpitting facies; large tongue
Cardiovascular system	Decreased peripheral vascular resistance, increased heart rate, stroke volume, cardiac output, pulse pressure; high-output heart failure; increased inotropic and chronotropic effects; arrhythmias; angina	Increased peripheral vascular resistance; decreased heart rate, stroke volume, cardiac output, pulse pressure; low-output heart failure; ECG: bradycardia, prolonged PR interval, flat T wave, low voltage; pericardial effusion
Respiratory system	Dyspnea; decreased vital capacity	Pleural effusions; hypoventilation and CO_2 retention
Gastrointestinal system	Increased appetite; increased frequency of bowel movements; hypoproteinemia	Decreased appetite; decreased frequency of bowel movements; ascites
Central nervous system	Nervousness; hyperkinesia; emotional lability	Lethargy; general slowing of mental processes; neuropathies
Musculoskeletal system	Weakness and muscle fatigue; increased deep tendon reflexes; hypercalcemia; osteoporosis	Stiffness and muscle fatigue; decreased deep tendon reflexes; increased alkaline phosphatase, LDH, AST
Renal system	Mild polyuria; increased renal blood flow; increased glomerular filtration rate	Impaired water excretion; decreased renal blood flow; decreased glomerular filtration rate
Hematopoietic system	Increased erythropoiesis; anemia[1]	Decreased erythropoiesis; anemia[1]
Reproductive system	Menstrual irregularities; decreased fertility; increased gonadal steroid metabolism	Hypermenorrhea; infertility; decreased libido; impotence; oligospermia; decreased gonadal steroid metabolism
Metabolic system	Increased basal metabolic rate; negative nitrogen balance; hyperglycemia; increased free fatty acids; decreased cholesterol and triglycerides; increased hormone degradation; increased requirements for fat- and water-soluble vitamins; increased drug metabolism	Decreased basal metabolic rate; slight positive nitrogen balance; delayed degradation of insulin, with increased sensitivity; increased cholesterol and triglycerides; decreased hormone degradation; decreased requirements for fat- and water-soluble vitamins; decreased drug metabolism

[1]The anemia of hyperthyroidism is usually normochromic and caused by increased red blood cell turnover. The anemia of hypothyroidism may be normochromic, hyperchromic, or hypochromic and may be due to decreased production rate, decreased iron absorption, decreased folic acid absorption, or to autoimmune pernicious anemia. (LDH, lactic dehydrogenase; AST, aspartate aminotransferase.)

produces glandular enlargement (goiter). The antithyroid compounds used clinically include the thioamides, iodides, and radioactive iodine.

1. Thioamides

The thioamides methimazole and propylthiouracil are major drugs for treatment of thyrotoxicosis. In the United Kingdom, carbimazole, which is converted to methimazole in vivo, is widely used. Methimazole is about ten times more potent than propylthiouracil.

The chemical structures of these compounds are shown in Figure 38–5. The thiocarbamide group is essential for antithyroid activity.

Pharmacokinetics

Propylthiouracil is rapidly absorbed, reaching peak serum levels after 1 hour. The bioavailability of 50–80% may be due to incomplete absorption or a large first-pass effect in the liver. The volume of distribution approximates total body water with accumulation in

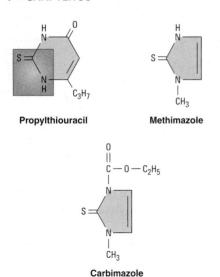

Figure 38–5. Structure of thioamides. The thiocarbamide moiety is shown in color.

the thyroid gland. Most of an ingested dose of propylthiouracil is excreted by the kidney as the inactive glucuronide within 24 hours.

In contrast, methimazole is completely absorbed but at variable rates. It is readily accumulated by the thyroid gland and has a volume of distribution similar to that of propylthiouracil. Excretion is slower than with propylthiouracil; 65–70% of a dose is recovered in the urine in 48 hours.

The short plasma half-life of these agents (1.5 hours for propylthiouracil and 6 hours for methimazole) has little influence on the duration of the antithyroid action or the dosing interval because both agents are accumulated by the thyroid gland. For propylthiouracil, giving the drug every 6–8 hours is reasonable since a single 100 mg dose can inhibit iodine organification by 60% for 7 hours. Since a single 30 mg dose of methimazole exerts an antithyroid effect for longer than 24 hours, a single daily dose is effective in the management of mild to moderate hyperthyroidism.

Both thioamides cross the placental barrier and are concentrated by the fetal thyroid, so that caution must be employed when using these drugs in pregnancy. Because of the risk of fetal hypothyroidism, both thioamides are classified as pregnancy category D (evidence of human fetal risk based on adverse reaction data from investigational or marketing experience). Of the two, propylthiouracil is preferable in pregnancy because it is more strongly protein-bound and, therefore, crosses the placenta less readily. In addition, methimazole has been, albeit rarely, associated with congenital malformations. Both thioamides are secreted in low concen-

trations in breast milk but are considered safe for the nursing infant.

Pharmacodynamics

The thioamides act by multiple mechanisms. The major action is to prevent hormone synthesis by inhibiting the thyroid peroxidase-catalyzed reactions and blocking iodine organification. In addition, they block coupling of the iodotyrosines. They do not block uptake of iodide by the gland. Propylthiouracil and (to a much lesser extent) methimazole inhibit the peripheral deiodination of T_4 and T_3 (Figure 38–1). Since the synthesis rather than the release of hormones is affected, the onset of these agents is slow, often requiring 3–4 weeks before stores of T_4 are depleted.

Toxicity

Adverse reactions to the thioamides occur in 3–12% of treated patients. Most reactions occur early, especially nausea and gastrointestinal distress. An altered sense of taste or smell may occur with methimazole. The most common adverse effect is a maculopapular pruritic rash (4–6%), at times accompanied by systemic signs such as fever. Rare adverse effects include an urticarial rash, vasculitis, a lupus-like reaction, lymphadenopathy, hypoprothrombinemia, exfoliative dermatitis, polyserositis, and acute arthralgia. Hepatitis (more common with propylthiouracil) and cholestatic jaundice (more common with methimazole) can be fatal; although asymptomatic elevations in transaminase levels also occur.

The most dangerous complication is agranulocytosis (granulocyte count < 500 cells/mm³), an infrequent but potentially fatal adverse reaction. It occurs in 0.1–0.5% of patients taking thioamides, but the risk may be increased in older patients and in those receiving high-dose methimazole therapy (> 40 mg/d). The reaction is usually rapidly reversible when the drug is discontinued, but broad-spectrum antibiotic therapy may be necessary for complicating infections. Colony-stimulating factors (eg, G-CSF; see Chapter 33) may hasten recovery of the granulocytes. The cross-sensitivity between propylthiouracil and methimazole is about 50%; therefore, switching drugs in patients with severe reactions is not recommended.

2. Anion Inhibitors

Monovalent anions such as perchlorate (ClO_4^-), pertechnetate (TcO_4^-), and thiocyanate (SCN^-) can block uptake of iodide by the gland through competitive inhibition of the iodide transport mechanism. Since these effects can be overcome by large doses of iodides, their effectiveness is somewhat unpredictable.

The major clinical use for potassium perchlorate is to block thyroidal reuptake of I^- in patients with iodide-induced hyperthyroidism (eg, amiodarone-induced hyperthyroidism). However, potassium perchlorate is rarely used clinically because it is associated with aplastic anemia.

3. Iodides

Prior to the introduction of the thioamides in the 1940s, iodides were the major antithyroid agents; today they are rarely used as sole therapy.

Pharmacodynamics

Iodides have several actions on the thyroid. They inhibit organification and hormone release and decrease the size and vascularity of the hyperplastic gland. In susceptible individuals, iodides can induce hyperthyroidism (*jodbasedow phenomenon*) or precipitate hypothyroidism.

In pharmacologic doses (> 6 mg/d), the major action of iodides is to inhibit hormone release, possibly through inhibition of thyroglobulin proteolysis. Improvement in thyrotoxic symptoms occurs rapidly—within 2–7 days—hence the value of iodide therapy in thyroid storm. In addition, iodides decrease the vascularity, size, and fragility of a hyperplastic gland, making the drugs valuable as preoperative preparation for surgery.

Clinical Use of Iodide

Disadvantages of iodide therapy include an increase in intraglandular stores of iodine, which may delay onset of thioamide therapy or prevent use of radioactive iodine therapy for several weeks. Thus, iodides should be initiated after onset of thioamide therapy and avoided if treatment with radioactive iodine seems likely. Iodide should not be used alone, because the gland will escape from the iodide block in 2–8 weeks, and its withdrawal may produce severe exacerbation of thyrotoxicosis in an iodine-enriched gland. Chronic use of iodides in pregnancy should be avoided, since they cross the placenta and can cause fetal goiter. In radiation emergencies, the thyroid-blocking effects of potassium iodide can protect the gland from subsequent damage if administered before radiation exposure.

Toxicity

Adverse reactions to iodine (iodism) are uncommon and in most cases reversible upon discontinuance. They include acneiform rash (similar to that of bromism), swollen salivary glands, mucous membrane ulcerations, conjunctivitis, rhinorrhea, drug fever, metallic taste, bleeding disorders and, rarely, anaphylactoid reactions.

4. Iodinated Contrast Media

The iodinated contrast agents—diatrizoate orally and iohexol orally or intravenously—are valuable in the treatment of hyperthyroidism, although they are not labeled for this indication. These drugs rapidly inhibit the conversion of T_4 to T_3 in the liver, kidney, pituitary gland, and brain. This accounts for the dramatic improvement in both subjective and objective parameters. For example, a decrease in heart rate is seen after only 3 days of administration of 0.5–1 g/d of oral contrast media. T_3 levels often return to normal during this time. The prolonged effect of suppressing T_4 as well as T_3 suggests that inhibition of hormone release due to the iodine released may be an additional mechanism of action. Fortunately, these agents are relatively nontoxic. They provide useful adjunctive therapy in the treatment of thyroid storm and offer valuable alternatives when iodides or thioamides are contraindicated. Surprisingly, these agents may not interfere with ^{131}I retention as much as iodides despite their large iodine content. Their toxicity is similar to that of the iodides, and their safety in pregnancy is undocumented.

5. Radioactive Iodine

^{131}I is the only isotope used for treatment of thyrotoxicosis (others are used in diagnosis). Administered orally in solution as sodium ^{131}I, it is rapidly absorbed, concentrated by the thyroid, and incorporated into storage follicles. Its therapeutic effect depends on emission of β rays with an effective half-life of 5 days and a penetration range of 400–2000 μm. Within a few weeks after administration, destruction of the thyroid parenchyma is evidenced by epithelial swelling and necrosis, follicular disruption, edema, and leukocyte infiltration. Advantages of radioiodine include easy administration, effectiveness, low expense, and absence of pain. Fears of radiation-induced genetic damage, leukemia, and neoplasia have not been realized after more than 50 years of clinical experience with radioiodine. Radioactive iodine should not be administered to pregnant women or nursing mothers, since it crosses the placenta to destroy the fetal thyroid gland and is excreted in breast milk.

6. Adrenoceptor-Blocking Agents

Beta blockers without intrinsic sympathomimetic activity (eg, metoprolol, propranolol, atenolol) are effective therapeutic adjuncts in the management of thyrotoxicosis since many of these symptoms mimic those associated with sympathetic stimulation. Propranolol has been the β blocker most widely studied and used in the therapy of thyrotoxicosis. Beta blockers cause clinical improvement of hyperthyroid symptoms but do not alter thyroid hormone levels.

■ II. CLINICAL PHARMACOLOGY OF THYROID & ANTITHYROID DRUGS

HYPOTHYROIDISM

Hypothyroidism is a syndrome resulting from deficiency of thyroid hormones and is manifested largely by a reversible slowing down of all body functions (Table 38–4). In infants and children, there is striking retardation of growth and development that results in dwarfism and irreversible mental retardation.

The etiology and pathogenesis of hypothyroidism are outlined in Table 38–5. Hypothyroidism can occur with or without thyroid enlargement (goiter). The laboratory diagnosis of hypothyroidism in the adult is easily made by the combination of a low free thyroxine and elevated serum TSH (Table 38–2).

The most common cause of hypothyroidism in the USA at this time is probably Hashimoto's thyroiditis, an immunologic disorder in genetically predisposed individuals. In this condition, there is evidence of humoral immunity in the presence of antithyroid antibodies and lymphocyte sensitization to thyroid antigens. Certain medications can also cause hypothyroidism (Table 38–5).

Management of Hypothyroidism

Except for hypothyroidism caused by drugs (Table 38–5), which can be treated in some cases by simply removing the depressant agent, the general strategy of replacement therapy is appropriate. The most satisfactory preparation is levothyroxine, administered as either a branded or generic preparation. Treatment with combination levothyroxine plus liothyronine has not been found to be superior to levothyroxine alone. Infants and children require more T_4 per kilogram of body weight than adults. The average dosage for an infant 1–6 months of age is 10–15 mcg/kg/d, whereas the average dosage for an adult is about 1.7 mcg/kg/d. Older adults (> 65 years of age) may require less thyroxine for replacement. There is some variability in the absorption of thyroxine, so this dosage will vary from patient to patient. Since interactions with certain foods (eg, bran, soy) and drugs (Table 38–3) can impair its absorption, thyroxine should be administered on an empty stomach (eg, 30 minutes before meals or 1 hour after meals). Its long half-life of 7 days permits once daily dosing. Children should be monitored for normal growth and development. Serum TSH and free thyroxine should be measured at regular intervals and TSH maintained within an optimal range of 0.5–2.5 mU/L. It takes 6–8 weeks after starting a given dose of thyroxine to reach steady-state levels in the bloodstream. Thus, dosage changes should be made slowly.

In long-standing hypothyroidism, in older patients, and in patients with underlying cardiac disease, it is imperative to start treatment with reduced dosages. In such adult patients, levothyroxine is given in a dosage of 12.5–25 mcg/d for 2 weeks, increasing the daily dose by 25 mcg every 2 weeks until euthyroidism or drug toxicity is observed. In older patients, the heart is very sensitive to the level of circulating thyroxine, and if angina pectoris or cardiac arrhythmia develops, it is essential to

Table 38–5. Etiology and pathogenesis of hypothyroidism.

Cause	Pathogenesis	Goiter	Degree of Hypothyroidism
Hashimoto's thyroiditis	Autoimmune destruction of thyroid	Present early, absent later	Mild to severe
Drug-induced[1]	Blocked hormone formation[2]	Present	Mild to moderate
Dyshormonogenesis	Impaired synthesis of T_4 due to enzyme deficiency	Present	Mild to severe
Radiation, ^{131}I, x-ray, thyroidectomy	Destruction or removal of gland	Absent	Severe
Congenital (cretinism)	Athyreosis or ectopic thyroid, iodine deficiency; TSH receptor-blocking antibodies	Absent or present	Severe
Secondary (TSH deficit)	Pituitary or hypothalamic disease	Absent	Mild

[1]Iodides, lithium, fluoride, thioamides, aminosalicylic acid, phenylbutazone, amiodarone, perchlorate, ethionamide, thiocyanate, cytokines (interferons, interleukins), bexarotene, etc.
[2]See Table 38–3 for specific pathogenesis.

stop or reduce the dose of thyroxine immediately. In younger patients or those with very mild disease, full replacement therapy may be started immediately.

The toxicity of thyroxine is directly related to the hormone level. In children, restlessness, insomnia, and accelerated bone maturation and growth may be signs of thyroxine toxicity. In adults, increased nervousness, heat intolerance, episodes of palpitation and tachycardia, or unexplained weight loss may be the presenting symptoms. If these symptoms are present, it is important to monitor serum TSH (Table 38–2), which will determine whether the symptoms are due to excess thyroxine blood levels. Chronic overtreatment with T_4, particularly in elderly patients, can increase the risk of atrial fibrillation and accelerated osteoporosis.

Special Problems in Management of Hypothyroidism

A. MYXEDEMA AND CORONARY ARTERY DISEASE

Since myxedema frequently occurs in older persons, it is often associated with underlying coronary artery disease. In this situation, the low levels of circulating thyroid hormone actually protect the heart against increasing demands that could result in angina pectoris or myocardial infarction. Correction of myxedema must be done cautiously to avoid provoking arrhythmia, angina, or acute myocardial infarction. If coronary artery surgery is indicated, it should be done first, prior to correction of the myxedema by thyroxine administration.

B. MYXEDEMA COMA

Myxedema coma is an end state of untreated hypothyroidism. It is associated with progressive weakness, stupor, hypothermia, hypoventilation, hypoglycemia, hyponatremia, water intoxication, shock, and death.

Management of myxedema coma is a medical emergency. The patient should be treated in the intensive care unit, since tracheal intubation and mechanical ventilation may be required. Associated illnesses such as infection or heart failure must be treated by appropriate therapy. It is important to give all preparations intravenously, because patients with myxedema coma absorb drugs poorly from other routes. Intravenous fluids should be administered with caution to avoid excessive water intake. These patients have large pools of empty T_3 and T_4 binding sites that must be filled before there is adequate free thyroxine to affect tissue metabolism. Accordingly, the treatment of choice in myxedema coma is to give a loading dose of levothyroxine intravenously—usually 300–400 mcg initially, followed by 50–100 mcg daily. Intravenous T_3 can also be used but may be more cardiotoxic and more difficult to monitor. Intravenous hydrocortisone is indicated if the patient has associated adrenal or pituitary insufficiency but is probably not necessary in most patients with primary myxedema. Opioids and sedatives must be used with extreme caution.

C. HYPOTHYROIDISM AND PREGNANCY

Hypothyroid women frequently have anovulatory cycles and are therefore relatively infertile until restoration of the euthyroid state. This has led to the widespread use of thyroid hormone for infertility, although there is no evidence for its usefulness in infertile euthyroid patients. In a pregnant hypothyroid patient receiving thyroxine, it is extremely important that the daily dose of thyroxine be adequate because early development of the fetal brain depends on maternal thyroxine. In many hypothyroid patients, an increase in the thyroxine dose (about 30–50%) is required to normalize the serum TSH level during pregnancy. Because of the elevated maternal TBG levels and, therefore, elevated total T_4 levels, adequate maternal thyroxine dosages warrant maintenance of TSH between 0.5 and 3.0 mU/L and the total T_4 at or above the upper range of normal.

D. SUBCLINICAL HYPOTHYROIDISM

Subclinical hypothyroidism, defined as an elevated TSH level and normal thyroid hormone levels, is found in 4–10% of the general population but increases to 20% in women older than age 50. The consensus of expert thyroid organizations concluded that thyroid hormone therapy should be considered for patients with TSH levels greater than 10 mU/L while close TSH monitoring is appropriate for those with lower TSH elevations.

E. DRUG-INDUCED HYPOTHYROIDISM

Drug-induced hypothyroidism (Table 38–3) can be satisfactorily managed with levothyroxine therapy if the offending agent cannot be stopped. In the case of amiodarone-induced hypothyroidism, levothyroxine therapy may be necessary even after discontinuance because of amiodarone's very long half-life.

HYPERTHYROIDISM

Hyperthyroidism (thyrotoxicosis) is the clinical syndrome that results when tissues are exposed to high levels of thyroid hormone (Table 38–4).

1. Graves' Disease

The most common form of hyperthyroidism is Graves' disease, or diffuse toxic goiter. The presenting signs and symptoms of Graves' disease are set forth in Table 38–4.

Pathophysiology

Graves' disease is considered to be an autoimmune disorder in which helper T lymphocytes stimulate B lymphocytes to synthesize antibodies to thyroidal antigens. The antibody described previously (TSH-R Ab [stim]) is directed against the TSH receptor site in the thyroid cell membrane and has the capacity to stimulate growth and biosynthetic activity of the thyroid cell. Spontaneous remission occurs but some patients require years of antithyroid therapy.

Laboratory Diagnosis

In most patients with hyperthyroidism, T_3, T_4, FT_4, and FT_3 are elevated and TSH is suppressed (Table 38–2). Radioiodine uptake is usually markedly elevated as well. Antithyroglobulin, thyroid peroxidase, and TSH-R Ab [stim] antibodies are usually present.

Management of Graves' Disease

The three primary methods for controlling hyperthyroidism are antithyroid drug therapy, surgical thyroidectomy, and destruction of the gland with radioactive iodine.

A. ANTITHYROID DRUG THERAPY

Drug therapy is most useful in young patients with small glands and mild disease. Methimazole or propylthiouracil is administered until the disease undergoes spontaneous remission. This is the only therapy that leaves an intact thyroid gland, but it does require a long period of treatment and observation (12–18 months), and there is a 50–68% incidence of relapse.

Methimazole is preferable to propylthiouracil (except in pregnancy) because it can be administered once daily, which may enhance adherence. Antithyroid drug therapy is usually begun with divided doses, shifting to maintenance therapy with single daily doses when the patient becomes clinically euthyroid. However, mild to moderately severe thyrotoxicosis can often be controlled with methimazole given in a single morning dose of 20–40 mg initially for 4–8 weeks to normalize hormone levels. Maintenance therapy requires 5–15 mg once daily. Alternatively, therapy is started with propylthiouracil, 100–150 mg every 6 or 8 hours until the patient is euthyroid, followed by gradual reduction of the dose to the maintenance level of 50–150 mg once daily. In addition to inhibiting iodine organification, propylthiouracil also inhibits the conversion of T_4 to T_3, so it brings the level of activated thyroid hormone down more quickly than does methimazole. The best clinical guide to remission is reduction in the size of the goiter. Laboratory tests most useful in monitoring the course of therapy are serum FT_3, FT_4, and TSH levels.

Reactivation of the autoimmune process may occur when the dosage of antithyroid drug is lowered during maintenance therapy and TSH begins to drive the gland. In some cases TSH release can be prevented by the daily administration of 50–150 mcg of levothyrox-ine with 5–15 mg of methimazole or 50–150 mg of propylthiouracil for the second year of therapy. The relapse rate with this program is probably comparable to the rate with antithyroid therapy alone, but the risk of hypothyroidism and overtreatment is avoided.

Reactions to antithyroid drugs have been described above. A minor rash can often be controlled by antihistamine therapy. Because the more severe reaction of agranulocytosis is often heralded by sore throat or high fever, patients receiving antithyroid drugs must be instructed to discontinue the drug and seek immediate medical attention if these symptoms develop. White cell and differential counts and a throat culture are indicated in such cases, followed by appropriate antibiotic therapy.

B. THYROIDECTOMY

A near-total thyroidectomy is the treatment of choice for patients with very large glands or multinodular goiters. Patients are treated with antithyroid drugs until euthyroid (about 6 weeks). In addition, for 10–14 days prior to surgery, they receive saturated solution of potassium iodide, 5 drops twice daily, to diminish vascularity of the gland and simplify surgery. About 80–90% of patients will require thyroid supplementation following near-total thyroidectomy.

C. RADIOACTIVE IODINE

Radioiodine therapy utilizing ^{131}I is the preferred treatment for most patients over 21 years of age. In patients without heart disease, the therapeutic dose may be given immediately in a range of 80–120 µCi/g of estimated thyroid weight corrected for uptake. In patients with underlying heart disease or severe thyrotoxicosis and in elderly patients, it is desirable to treat with antithyroid drugs (preferably methimazole) until the patient is euthyroid. The medication is then stopped for 5–7 days before the appropriate dose of ^{131}I is administered. Iodides should be avoided to ensure maximal ^{131}I uptake. Six to 12 weeks following the administration of radioiodine, the gland will shrink in size and the patient will usually become euthyroid or hypothyroid. A second dose may be required in some patients. Hypothyroidism occurs in about 80% of patients following radioiodine therapy. Serum FT_4 and TSH levels should be monitored regularly. When hypothyroidism develops, prompt replacement with oral levothyroxine, 50–150 mcg daily, should be instituted.

D. ADJUNCTS TO ANTITHYROID THERAPY

During the acute phase of thyrotoxicosis, β-adrenoceptor blocking agents without intrinsic sympathomimetic activity are extremely helpful. Propranolol, 20–40 mg orally every 6 hours, will control tachycardia, hypertension, and atrial fibrillation. Propranolol is gradually withdrawn as serum thyroxine levels return to normal. Diltiazem, 90–120 mg three or four times daily, can be used to control tachycardia in patients in whom β blockers are contraindicated, eg, those with asthma. Other calcium channel blockers may not be as effective as diltiazem. Adequate nutrition and vitamin supplements are essential. Barbiturates accelerate T_4 breakdown (by hepatic enzyme induction) and may be helpful both as sedatives and to lower T_4 levels.

2. Toxic Uninodular Goiter & Toxic Multinodular Goiter

These forms of hyperthyroidism occur often in older women with nodular goiters. FT_4 is moderately elevated or occasionally normal, but FT_3 or T_3 is strikingly elevated. Single toxic adenomas can be managed with either surgical excision of the adenoma or with radioiodine therapy. Toxic multinodular goiter is usually associated with a large goiter and is best treated by preparation with methimazole or propylthiouracil followed by subtotal thyroidectomy.

3. Subacute Thyroiditis

During the acute phase of a viral infection of the thyroid gland, there is destruction of thyroid parenchyma with transient release of stored thyroid hormones. A similar state may occur in patients with Hashimoto's thyroiditis. These episodes of transient thyrotoxicosis have been termed *spontaneously resolving hyperthyroidism*. Supportive therapy is usually all that is necessary, such as β-adrenoceptor blocking agents without intrinsic sympathomimetic activity (eg, propranolol) for tachycardia and aspirin or nonsteroidal anti-inflammatory drugs to control local pain and fever. Corticosteroids may be necessary in severe cases to control the inflammation.

4. Special Problems

Thyroid Storm

Thyroid storm, or thyrotoxic crisis, is sudden acute exacerbation of all of the symptoms of thyrotoxicosis, presenting as a life-threatening syndrome. Vigorous management is mandatory. Propranolol, 1–2 mg slowly intravenously or 40–80 mg orally every 6 hours, is helpful to control the severe cardiovascular manifestations. If propranolol is contraindicated by the presence of severe heart failure or asthma, hypertension and tachycardia may be controlled with diltiazem, 90–120 mg orally three or four times daily or 5–10 mg/h by intravenous infusion (asthmatic patients only). Release of thyroid hormones from the gland is retarded by the administration of saturated solution of potassium iodide, 10 drops orally daily, or iodinated contrast media, 1 g orally daily. The latter medication will also block peripheral conversion of T_4 to T_3. Hormone synthesis is blocked by the administration of propylthiouracil, 250 mg orally every 6 hours. If the patient is unable to take propylthiouracil by mouth, a rectal formulation* can be prepared and administered in a dosage of 400 mg every 6 hours as a retention enema. Methimazole may also be prepared for rectal administration in a dose of 60 mg daily. Hydrocortisone, 50 mg intravenously every 6 hours, will protect the patient against shock and will block the conversion of T_4 to T_3, rapidly bringing down the level of thyroactive material in the blood.

Supportive therapy is essential to control fever, heart failure, and any underlying disease process that may have precipitated the acute storm. In rare situations, where the above methods are not adequate to control the problem, plasmapheresis or peritoneal dialysis has been used to lower the levels of circulating thyroxine.

Ophthalmopathy

Although severe ophthalmopathy is rare, it is difficult to treat. Management requires effective treatment of the thyroid disease, usually by total surgical excision or ^{131}I ablation of the gland plus oral prednisone therapy (see below). In addition, local therapy may be necessary, eg, elevation of the head to diminish periorbital edema and artificial tears to relieve corneal drying. Smoking cessation should be advised to prevent progression of the ophthalmopathy. For the severe, acute inflammatory reaction, a short course of prednisone, 60–100 mg orally daily for about a week and then 60–100 mg every other day, tapering the dose over a period of 6–12 weeks, may be effective. If steroid therapy fails or is contraindicated, irradiation of the posterior orbit, using well-collimated high-energy x-ray therapy, will frequently result in marked improvement of the acute process. Threatened loss of vision is an indication for surgical decompression of the orbit. Eyelid or eye muscle surgery may be necessary to correct residual problems after the acute process has subsided.

Dermopathy

Dermopathy or pretibial myxedema will often respond to topical corticosteroids applied to the involved area and covered with an occlusive dressing.

Thyrotoxicosis during Pregnancy

Ideally, women in the childbearing period with severe disease should have definitive therapy with ^{131}I or subtotal thyroidectomy *prior* to pregnancy in order to avoid an acute exacerbation of the disease during pregnancy or following delivery. If thyrotoxicosis does develop during pregnancy, radioiodine is contraindicated because it crosses the placenta and may injure the fetal thyroid. In the first trimester, the patient can be

---

*To prepare a water suspension propylthiouracil enema, grind eight 50 mg tablets and suspend the powder in 90 mL of sterile water.

prepared with propylthiouracil and a subtotal thyroidectomy performed safely during the mid trimester. It is essential to give the patient a thyroid supplement during the balance of the pregnancy. However, most patients are treated with propylthiouracil during the pregnancy, and the decision regarding long-term management can be made after delivery. The dosage of propylthiouracil must be kept to the minimum necessary for control of the disease (ie, < 300 mg/d), because it may affect the function of the fetal thyroid gland. Methimazole is a potential alternative, although there is concern about a possible risk of fetal scalp defects.

Neonatal Graves' Disease

Graves' disease may occur in the newborn infant, either due to passage of maternal TSH-R Ab [stim] through the placenta, stimulating the thyroid gland of the neonate, or to genetic transmission of the trait to the fetus. Laboratory studies reveal an elevated free thyroxine, a markedly elevated T_3, and a low TSH—in contrast to the normal infant, in whom TSH is elevated at birth. TSH-R Ab [stim] is usually found in the serum of both the child and the mother.

If caused by maternal TSH-R Ab [stim], the disease is usually self-limited and subsides over a period of 4–12 weeks, coinciding with the fall in the infant's TSH-R Ab [stim] level. However, treatment is necessary because of the severe metabolic stress the infant experiences. Therapy includes propylthiouracil in a dose of 5–10 mg/kg/d in divided doses at 8-hour intervals; Lugol's solution (8 mg of iodide per drop), 1 drop every 8 hours; and propranolol, 2 mg/kg/d in divided doses. Careful supportive therapy is essential. If the infant is very ill, oral prednisone, 2 mg/kg/d in divided doses, will help block conversion of T_4 to T_3. These medications are gradually reduced as the clinical picture improves and can be discontinued by 6–12 weeks.

Subclinical Hyperthyroidism

Subclinical hyperthyroidism is defined as a suppressed TSH level (below the normal range) in conjunction with normal thyroid hormone levels. Cardiac toxicity (eg, atrial fibrillation), especially in older persons, is of greatest concern. The consensus of thyroid experts concluded that hyperthyroidism treatment is appropriate in those with TSH less than 0.1 mU/L, while close monitoring of the TSH level is appropriate for those with less TSH suppression.

Amiodarone-Induced Thyrotoxicosis

Approximately 3% of patients receiving amiodarone will develop hyperthyroidism. Two types of amiodarone-induced thyrotoxicosis have been reported: iodine-induced (type I), which often occurs in persons with underlying thyroid disease (eg, multinodular goiter); and an inflammatory thyroiditis (type II) that occurs in patients without thyroid disease due to leakage of thyroid hormone into the circulation. Treatment of type I requires thioamides while type II responds best to glucocorticoids. Since it is not always possible to differentiate between the two types, thioamides and glucocorticoids are often administered together. If possible, amiodarone should be discontinued; however, rapid improvement does not occur due to its long half-life.

NONTOXIC GOITER

Nontoxic goiter is a syndrome of thyroid enlargement without excessive thyroid hormone production. Enlargement of the thyroid gland is often due to TSH stimulation from inadequate thyroid hormone synthesis. The most common cause of nontoxic goiter worldwide is iodide deficiency, but in the USA, it is Hashimoto's thyroiditis. Other causes include germline or acquired mutations in genes involved in hormone synthesis, dietary goitrogens, and neoplasms (see below).

Goiter due to iodide deficiency is best managed by prophylactic administration of iodide. The optimal daily iodide intake is 150–200 mcg. Iodized salt and iodate used as preservatives in flour and bread are excellent sources of iodine in the diet. In areas where it is difficult to introduce iodized salt or iodate preservatives, a solution of iodized poppyseed oil has been administered intramuscularly to provide a long-term source of inorganic iodine.

Goiter due to ingestion of goitrogens in the diet is managed by elimination of the goitrogen or by adding sufficient thyroxine to shut off TSH stimulation. Similarly, in Hashimoto's thyroiditis and dyshormonogenesis, adequate thyroxine therapy—150–200 mcg/d orally—will suppress pituitary TSH and result in slow regression of the goiter as well as correction of hypothyroidism.

THYROID NEOPLASMS

Neoplasms of the thyroid gland may be benign (adenomas) or malignant. The primary diagnostic test is a fine needle aspiration biopsy and cytologic examination. Benign lesions may be monitored for growth or symptoms of local obstruction, which would mandate surgical excision. Management of thyroid carcinoma requires a total thyroidectomy, postoperative radioiodine therapy in selected instances, and lifetime replacement with levothyroxine. The evaluation for recurrence of some thyroid malignancies often involves withdrawal of thyroxine replacement for 4–6 weeks—accompanied by the development of hypothyroidism. Tumor recurrence is likely if there is a rise in serum thyroglobulin (ie, a tumor marker) or a positive ^{131}I scan when TSH is elevated. Alternatively, administration of recombinant human TSH (Thyrogen) can produce comparable TSH elevations without discontinuing thyroxine and avoiding hypothyroidism. Recombinant human TSH is administered intramuscularly once daily for 2 days. A rise in serum thyroglobulin or a positive ^{131}I scan will indicate a recurrence of the thyroid cancer.

PREPARATIONS AVAILABLE

Thyroid Agents

Levothyroxine [T₄] (generic, Levoxyl, Levo-T, Levothroid, Levolet, Novothyrox, Synthroid, Unithroid)
Oral: 0.025, 0.05, 0.075, 0.088, 0.1, 0.112, 0.125, 0.137, 0.15, 0.175, 0.2, 0.3 mg tablets
Parenteral: 200, 500 mcg per vial (100 mcg/mL when reconstituted) for injection

Liothyronine [T₃] (generic, Cytomel, Triostat)
Oral: 5, 25, 50 mcg tablets
Parenteral: 10 mcg/mL

Liotrix [a 4:1 ratio of T₄:T₃] (Thyrolar)
Oral: tablets containing 12.5, 25, 30, 50, 60, 100, 120, 150, 180 mcg T₄ and one fourth as much T₃

Thyroid desiccated [USP] (generic, Armour Thyroid, Thyroid Strong, Thyrar, S-P-T)
Oral: tablets containing 15, 30, 60, 90, 120, 180, 240, 300 mg; capsules (S-P-T) containing 120, 180, 300 mg

Antithyroid Agents

Diatrizoate sodium (Hypaque)
Parenteral: 25% (150 mg iodine/mL); 50% (300 mg iodine/mL) (unlabeled use); 250 g powder for reconstitution (oral use is unlabeled)

Iodide (¹³¹I) sodium (Iodotope, Sodium Iodide I 131 Therapeutic)
Oral: available as capsules and solution

Iohexol (Omnipaque)
Parenteral: 140, 180, 240, 300, 350 mg iodine/mL (unlabeled use)

Methimazole (Tapazole)
Oral: 5, 10 mg tablets

Potassium iodide
Oral solution (generic, SSKI): 1 g/mL
Oral solution (Lugol's solution): 100 mg/mL potassium iodide plus 50 mg/mL iodine
Oral syrup (Pima): 325 mg/5 mL
Oral controlled action tablets (Iodo-Niacin): 135 mg potassium iodide plus 25 mg niacinamide hydroiodide
Oral potassium iodide tablets (generic, IOSAT, RAD-Block, Thyro-Block): 65, 130 mg

Propylthiouracil [PTU] (generic)
Oral: 50 mg tablets

Thyrotropin; recombinant human TSH (Thyrogen)
Parenteral: 0.9 mg per vial

REFERENCES

General

Greenspan FS: Thyroid gland. In: Greenspan FS, Gardner DG (editors). *Basic & Clinical Endocrinology,* 7th ed. McGraw-Hill, 2004.

American Thyroid Association (http://thyroid.org/).

Guidelines

Anonymous: American Association of Clinical Endocrinologists medical guidelines for clinical practice for the evaluation and treatment of hyperthyroidism and hypothyroidism. Endocr Pract 2002;8:457.

Cooper DS et al: Management guidelines for patients with thyroid modules and differentiated thyroid cancer. Thyroid 2006;16:109.

Gharib H et al: Consensus statement #1: Subclinical thyroid dysfunction: A joint statement on management from the American Association of Clinical Endocrinologists, the American Thyroid Association, and The Endocrine Society. Thyroid. 2005;15:24.

Surks MI et al: Subclinical thyroid disease: Scientific review and guidelines for diagnosis and management. JAMA. 2004;291:228.

US Department of Health and Human Services: Potassium iodide as a thyroid blocking agent in radiation emergencies. December 2001 (http://www.fda.gov/cder/guidance/index.htm).

Hypothyroidism

Dong BJ et al: Bioequivalence of generic and brand-name levothyroxine products in the treatment of hypothyroidism. JAMA 1997;277:1205.

Escobar-Morreale HF et al: Treatment of hypothyroidism with combinations of levothyroxine plus liothyronine. J Clin Endocrinol Metab 2005;90:4946.

Gruters A et al: Long-term consequences of congenital hypothyroidism in the era of screening programs. Endocrinol Metab 2002;16:369.

Khouzam HR et al: Thyroid hormone therapy: A review of their effects in the treatment of psychiatric and medical conditions. Comp Ther 2004;30:148.

Toft A: Which thyroxine? Thyroid 2005;15:124.

Wartofsky L, Dickey RA: The evidence for a narrower thyrotropin reference range is compelling. J Clin Endocrinol Metab. 2005;90:5483.

Wiersinga QM: Thyroid hormone replacement therapy. Horm Res 2001;56(Suppl 1):74.

Hyperthyroidism

Abraham P et al: Antithyroid drug regimen for treating Graves' hyperthyroidism. Cochrane Database Syst Rev 2005;CD003420 (http://www.thecochranelibrary.com).

Abraham P et al: A systematic review of drug therapy for Graves' hyperthyroidism. Eur J Endocrinol 2005;153:489.

Braga M, Cooper DS: Oral cholecystographic agents and the thyroid. J Clin Endocrinol Metab 2001;86:1853.

Cooper DS: Antithyroid drugs. N Engl J Med 2005;352:905.

Cooper DS: Hyperthyroidism. Lancet 2003;362:459.

El-Kaissi S, Frauman AG, Wall JR: Thyroid-associated ophthalmopathy: A practical guide to classification, natural history and management. Intern Med J 2004;34:482.

Jongjaroenprasert W et al: Rectal administration of propylthiouracil in hyperthyroid patients: Comparison of suspension enema and suppository form. Thyroid 2002;12:627.

Mestman JH: Hyperthyroidism in pregnancy. Best Pract Res Clin Endocrinol Metab 2004;18:267.

Nontoxic Goiter, Nodules, & Cancer

Hegedus L: Clinical practice. The thyroid nodule. N Engl J Med 2004;351:1764.

Lawrence W Jr, Kaplan BJ: Diagnosis and management of patients with thyroid nodules. J Surg Oncol 2002;80:157.

The Effects of Drugs on Thyroid Function

Arafah BM: Increased need for thyroxine in women with hypothyroidism during estrogen therapy. N Engl J Med 2001; 344:1743.

Basaria S, Cooper DS: Amiodarone and the thyroid. Am J Med 2005;118:706.

Caraccop M et al: Long-term follow-up of 106 multiple sclerosis patients undergoing interferon-β 1a or 1b therapy: Predictive factors of thyroid disease development and duration. J Clin Endocrinol Metab 2005;90:4133.

Prummel MF, Laurberg P: Interferon-α and autoimmune thyroid disease. Thyroid 2003;13:547.

Adrenocorticosteroids & Adrenocortical Antagonists

39

George P. Chrousos, MD

The natural adrenocortical hormones are steroid molecules produced and released by the adrenal cortex. Both natural and synthetic corticosteroids are used for diagnosis and treatment of disorders of adrenal function. They are also used—more often and in much larger doses—for treatment of a variety of inflammatory and immunologic disorders.

Secretion of adrenocortical steroids is controlled by the pituitary release of corticotropin (ACTH). Secretion of the salt-retaining hormone aldosterone is primarily under the influence of angiotensin. Corticotropin has some actions that do not depend upon its effect on adrenocortical secretion. However, its pharmacologic value as an anti-inflammatory agent and its use in testing adrenal function depend on its secretory action. Its pharmacology is discussed in Chapter 37 and will be reviewed only briefly here.

Inhibitors of the synthesis or antagonists of the action of the adrenocortical steroids are important in the treatment of several conditions. These agents are described at the end of this chapter.

■ ADRENOCORTICOSTEROIDS

The adrenal cortex releases a large number of steroids into the circulation. Some have minimal biologic activity and function primarily as precursors, and there are some for which no function has been established. The hormonal steroids may be classified as those having important effects on intermediary metabolism and immune function (glucocorticoids), those having principally salt-retaining activity (mineralocorticoids), and those having androgenic or estrogenic activity (see Chapter 40). In humans, the major glucocorticoid is cortisol and the most important mineralocorticoid is aldosterone. Quantitatively, dehydroepiandrosterone (DHEA) in its sulfated form (DHEAS) is the major adrenal androgen, since about 20 mg is secreted daily. However, DHEA and two other adrenal androgens, androstenediol and androstenedione, are weak androgens or (by conversion) estrogens. Adrenal androgens constitute the major endogenous precursors of estrogen in women after menopause and in younger patients in whom ovarian function is deficient or absent.

THE NATURALLY OCCURRING GLUCOCORTICOIDS; CORTISOL (HYDROCORTISONE)

Pharmacokinetics

Cortisol (also called hydrocortisone, compound F) exerts a wide range of physiologic effects, including regulation of intermediary metabolism, cardiovascular function, growth, and immunity. Its synthesis and secretion are tightly regulated by the central nervous system, which is very sensitive to negative feedback by the circulating cortisol and exogenous (synthetic) glucocorticoids. Cortisol is synthesized from cholesterol (as shown in Figure 39–1). The mechanisms controlling its secretion are discussed in Chapter 37.

In the normal adult, in the absence of stress, 10–20 mg of cortisol is secreted daily. The rate of secretion follows a circadian rhythm governed by pulses of ACTH that peak in the early morning hours and after meals (Figure 39–2). In plasma, cortisol is bound to circulating proteins. Corticosteroid-binding globulin (CBG), an α_2 globulin synthesized by the liver, binds about 90% of the circulating hormone under normal circumstances. The remainder is free (about 5–10%) or loosely bound to albumin (about 5%) and is available to exert its effect on target cells. When plasma cortisol levels exceed 20–30 mcg/dL, CBG is saturated, and the concentration of free cortisol rises rapidly. CBG is increased in pregnancy and with estrogen administration and in hyperthyroidism. It is decreased by hypothyroidism, genetic defects in synthesis, and protein deficiency states. Albumin has a large capacity but low affinity for cortisol, and for practical purposes albumin-bound cortisol should be considered free. Synthetic corticosteroids such as dexamethasone are largely bound to albumin rather than CBG.

Figure 39–1. Outline of major pathways in adrenocortical hormone biosynthesis. The major secretory products are underlined. Pregnenolone is the major precursor of corticosterone and aldosterone, and 17-hydroxypregnenolone is the major precursor of cortisol. The enzymes and cofactors for the reactions progressing down each column are shown on the left and across columns at the top of the figure. When a particular enzyme is deficient, hormone production is blocked at the points indicated by the shaded bars. (Modified after Welikey et al; reproduced, with permission, from Ganong WF: *Review of Medical Physiology,* 17th ed. Originally published by Appleton & Lange. Copyright © 1995 by The McGraw-Hill Companies, Inc.)

The half-life of cortisol in the circulation is normally about 60–90 minutes; half-life may be increased when hydrocortisone (the pharmaceutical preparation of cortisol) is administered in large amounts or when stress, hypothyroidism, or liver disease is present. Only 1% of cortisol is excreted unchanged in the urine as free cortisol; about 20% of cortisol is converted to cortisone by 11-hydroxysteroid dehydrogenase in the kidney and other tissues with mineralocorticoid receptors (see below) before reaching the liver. Most cortisol is metabolized in the liver. About one third of the cortisol produced daily is excreted in the urine as dihydroxy ketone metabolites and is measured as 17-hydroxysteroids (see Figure 39–3 for carbon numbering). Many cortisol metabolites are conjugated with glucuronic acid or sulfate at the C_3 and C_{21} hydroxyls, respectively, in the liver; they are then excreted in the urine.

In some species (eg, the rat), corticosterone is the major glucocorticoid. It is less firmly bound to protein and therefore metabolized more rapidly. The pathways of its degradation are similar to those of cortisol.

Pharmacodynamics

A. MECHANISM OF ACTION

Most of the known effects of the glucocorticoids are mediated by widely distributed glucocorticoid recep-

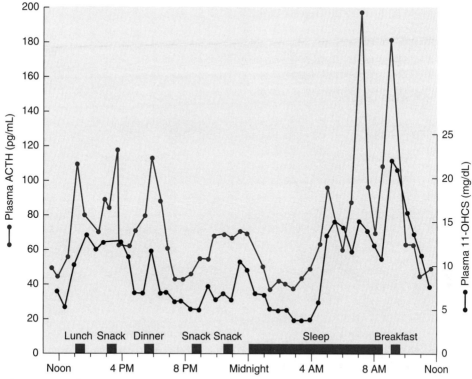

Figure 39–2. Fluctuations in plasma ACTH and glucocorticoids throughout the day in a normal girl (age 16). The ACTH was measured by immunoassay and the glucocorticoids as 11-oxysteroids (11-OHCS). Note the marked ACTH and glucocorticoid rises in the morning, before awakening from sleep. (Reproduced, with permission, from Krieger DT et al: Characterization of the normal temporal pattern of plasma corticosteroid levels. J Clin Endocrinol Metab 1971;32:266.)

tors. These proteins are members of the superfamily of nuclear receptors that includes steroid, sterol (vitamin D), thyroid, retinoic acid, and many other receptors with unknown or nonexistent ligands (orphan receptors). All these receptors interact with the promoters of—and regulate the transcription of—target genes (Figure 39–4). In the absence of the hormonal ligand, glucocorticoid receptors are primarily cytoplasmic, in oligomeric complexes with heat shock proteins (Hsp). The most important of these are two molecules of Hsp90, although other proteins are certainly involved. Free hormone from the plasma and interstitial fluid enters the cell and binds to the receptor, inducing conformational changes that allow it to dissociate from the heat shock proteins. The ligand-bound receptor complex then is actively transported into the nucleus, where it interacts with DNA and nuclear proteins. As a homodimer, it binds to glucocorticoid receptor elements (GRE) in the promoters of responsive genes. The GRE is composed of two palindromic sequences that bind to the hormone receptor dimer.

In addition to binding to GREs, the ligand-bound receptor also forms complexes with and influences the function of other transcription factors, such as AP1 and NF-κB, which act on non–GRE-containing promoters, to contribute to the regulation of transcription of their responsive genes. These transcription factors have broad actions on the regulation of growth factors, proinflammatory cytokines, etc, and to a great extent mediate the anti-growth, anti-inflammatory, and immunosuppressive effects of glucocorticoids.

Two genes for the corticoid receptor have been identified, one encoding the classic glucocorticoid receptor and the other the mineralocorticoid receptor. Alternative splicing of human glucocorticoid receptor pre-mRNA generates two highly homologous isoforms, termed hGR alpha and hGR beta. hGR alpha is the classic ligand-activated glucocorticoid receptor which, in the hormone-bound state, modulates the expression of glucocorticoid-responsive genes. In contrast, hGR beta does not bind glucocorticoids and is transcriptionally inactive. However, hGR beta is able to inhibit the effects of hormone-

Figure 39–3. Chemical structures of several glucocorticoids. The acetonide-substituted derivatives (eg, triamcinolone acetonide) have increased surface activity and are useful in dermatology. Dexamethasone is identical to betamethasone except for the configuration of the methyl group at C_{16}: in betamethasone it is beta (projecting *up* from the plane of the rings); in dexamethasone it is alpha.

activated hGR alpha on glucocorticoid-responsive genes, playing the role of a physiologically relevant endogenous inhibitor of glucocorticoid action.

The glucocorticoid receptor is composed of about 800 amino acids and can be divided into three functional domains (see Figure 2–6). The glucocorticoid-binding domain is located at the carboxyl terminal of the molecule and is the area where free glucocorticoids bind. The DNA-binding domain is located in the middle of the protein and contains nine cysteine residues. This region folds into a "two-finger" structure stabilized by zinc ions connected to cysteines to form two tetrahedrons. This part of the molecule binds to the GREs that regulate glucocorticoid action on glucocorticoid-regulated genes. The zinc-fingers represent the basic structure by which the DNA-binding domain recognizes specific nucleic acid sequences. The amino-terminal domain is involved in the transactivation activity of the receptor and increases its specificity.

The interaction of glucocorticoid receptors with GREs or other transcription factors is facilitated or inhibited by several families of proteins called steroid receptor *coregulators*, divided into *coactivators* and *corepressors*. The coregulators do this by serving as bridges between the receptors and other nuclear proteins and

by expressing enzymatic activities such as histone acetylase or deacetylase that alter the conformation of nucleosomes and the transcribability of genes.

Between 10% and 20% of expressed genes in a cell are regulated by glucocorticoids. The number and affinity of receptors for the hormone, the complement of transcription factors and coregulators, and posttranscription events determine the relative specificity of these hormones' actions in various cells. The effects of glucocorticoids are mainly due to proteins synthesized from mRNA transcribed by their target genes.

Some of the effects of glucocorticoids can be attributed to their binding to aldosterone receptors (ARs). Indeed, ARs bind aldosterone and cortisol with similar affinity. A mineralocorticoid effect of cortisol is avoided in some tissues by expression of 11β-hydroxysteroid dehydrogenase type 2, the enzyme responsible for biotransformation to its 11-keto derivative (cortisone), which has minimal affinity for aldosterone receptors.

Prompt effects such as initial feedback suppression of pituitary ACTH occur in minutes and are too rapid to be explained on the basis of gene transcription and protein synthesis. It is not known how these effects are mediated. Among the proposed mechanisms are direct effects on

Figure 39–4. A model of the interaction of a steroid, S (eg, cortisol), and its receptor, R, and the subsequent events in a target cell. The steroid is present in the blood in bound form on the corticosteroid-binding globulin (CBG) but enters the cell as the free molecule. The intracellular receptor is bound to stabilizing proteins, including two molecules of heat shock protein 90 (Hsp90) and several others, denoted as "X" in the figure. This receptor complex is incapable of activating transcription. When the complex binds a molecule of cortisol, an unstable complex is created and the Hsp90 and associated molecules are released. The steroid-receptor complex is able to enter the nucleus, bind to the glucocorticoid response element (GRE) on the gene, and regulate transcription by RNA polymerase II and associated transcription factors. A variety of regulatory factors (not shown) may participate in facilitating (coactivators) or inhibiting (corepressors) the steroid response. The resulting mRNA is edited and exported to the cytoplasm for the production of protein that brings about the final hormone response.

cell membrane receptors for the hormone or nongenomic effects of the classic hormone-bound glucocorticoid receptor. The putative membrane receptors might be entirely different from the known intracellular receptors.

B. PHYSIOLOGIC EFFECTS

The glucocorticoids have widespread effects because they influence the function of most cells in the body. The major metabolic consequences of glucocorticoid secretion or administration are due to direct actions of these hormones in the cell. However, some important effects are the result of homeostatic responses by insulin and glucagon. Although many of the effects of glucocorticoids are dose-related and become magnified when large amounts are administered for therapeutic purposes, there are also other effects—called *permissive* effects—in the absence of which many normal functions become deficient. For example, the response of vascular and bronchial smooth muscle to catecholamines is diminished in the absence of cortisol and restored by physiologic amounts of this glucocorticoid. Furthermore, the lipolytic responses of fat cells to catecholamines, ACTH, and growth hormone are attenuated in the absence of glucocorticoids.

C. METABOLIC EFFECTS

The glucocorticoids have important dose-related effects on carbohydrate, protein, and fat metabolism. The same effects are responsible for some of the serious adverse effects associated with their use in therapeutic doses. Glucocorticoids stimulate and are required for gluconeogenesis and glycogen synthesis in the fasting state. They stimulate phosphoenolpyruvate carboxykinase, glucose-6-phosphatase, and glycogen synthase and the release of amino acids in the course of muscle catabolism.

Glucocorticoids increase serum glucose levels and thus stimulate insulin release and inhibit the uptake of glucose by muscle cells, while they stimulate hormone-sensitive lipase and thus lipolysis. The increased insulin secretion stimulates lipogenesis and to a lesser degree inhibits lipolysis, leading to a net increase in fat deposition combined with increased release of fatty acids and glycerol into the circulation.

The net results of these actions are most apparent in the fasting state, when the supply of glucose from gluconeogenesis, the release of amino acids from muscle catabolism, the inhibition of peripheral glucose uptake, and the stimulation of lipolysis all contribute to maintenance of an adequate glucose supply to the brain.

D. CATABOLIC AND ANTIANABOLIC EFFECTS

Although glucocorticoids stimulate RNA and protein synthesis in the liver, they have catabolic and antianabolic effects in lymphoid and connective tissue, muscle, peripheral fat, and skin. Supraphysiologic amounts of glucocorticoids lead to decreased muscle mass and weakness and thinning of the skin. Catabolic and antianabolic effects on bone are the cause of osteoporosis in Cushing's syndrome and impose a major limitation in the long-term therapeutic use of glucocorticoids. In children, glucocorticoids reduce growth. This effect may be partially prevented by administration of growth hormone in high doses.

E. ANTI-INFLAMMATORY AND IMMUNOSUPPRESSIVE EFFECTS

Glucocorticoids dramatically reduce the manifestations of inflammation. This is due to their profound effects on the concentration, distribution, and function of peripheral leukocytes and to their suppressive effects on the inflammatory cytokines and chemokines and on other mediators of inflammation. Inflammation, regardless of its cause, is characterized by the extravasation and infiltration of leukocytes into the affected tissue. These events are mediated by a complex series of interactions of white cell adhesion molecules with those on endothelial cells and are inhibited by glucocorticoids. After a single dose of a short-acting glucocorticoid, the concentration of neutrophils in the circulation increases while the lymphocytes (T and B cells), monocytes, eosinophils, and basophils decrease. The changes are maximal at 6 hours and are dissipated in 24 hours. The increase in neutrophils is due both to the increased influx into the blood from the bone marrow and decreased migration from the blood vessels, leading to a reduction in the number of cells at the site of inflammation. The reduction in circulating lymphocytes, monocytes, eosinophils, and basophils is primarily the result of their movement from the vascular bed to lymphoid tissue.

Glucocorticoids also inhibit the functions of tissue macrophages and other antigen-presenting cells. The ability of these cells to respond to antigens and mitogens is reduced. The effect on macrophages is particularly marked and limits their ability to phagocytose and kill microorganisms and to produce tumor necrosis factor-α, interleukin-1, metalloproteinases, and plasminogen activator. Both macrophages and lymphocytes produce less interleukin-12 and interferon-γ, important inducers of TH1 cell activity, and cellular immunity.

In addition to their effects on leukocyte function, glucocorticoids influence the inflammatory response by reducing the prostaglandin, leukotriene, and platelet-activating factor synthesis that results from activation of phospholipase A_2. Finally, glucocorticoids reduce expression of cyclooxygenase-2, the inducible form of this enzyme, in inflammatory cells, thus reducing the amount of enzyme available to produce prostaglandins (see Chapters 18 and 36).

Glucocorticoids cause vasoconstriction when applied directly to the skin, possibly by suppressing mast cell degranulation. They also decrease capillary permeability by reducing the amount of histamine released by basophils and mast cells.

The anti-inflammatory and immunosuppressive effects of glucocorticoids are largely due to the actions described above. In humans, complement activation is unaltered, but its effects are inhibited. Antibody production can be reduced by large doses of steroids, though it is unaffected by moderate dosages (eg, 20 mg/d of prednisone).

The anti-inflammatory and immunosuppressive effects of these agents are widely useful therapeutically but are also responsible for some of their most serious adverse effects (see below).

F. OTHER EFFECTS

Glucocorticoids have important effects on the nervous system. Adrenal insufficiency causes marked slowing of the alpha rhythm of the electroencephalogram and is associated with depression. Increased amounts of glucocorticoids often produce behavioral disturbances in humans: initially insomnia and euphoria and subsequently depression. Large doses of glucocorticoids may increase intracranial pressure (pseudotumor cerebri).

Table 39–1. Some commonly used natural and synthetic corticosteroids for general use.

Agent	Activity[1]			Equivalent Oral Dose (mg)	Forms Available
	Anti-Inflammatory	Topical	Salt-Retaining		
Short- to medium-acting glucocorticoids					
Hydrocortisone (cortisol)	1	1	1	20	Oral, injectable, topical
Cortisone	0.8	0	0.8	25	Oral
Prednisone	4	0	0.3	5	Oral
Prednisolone	5	4	0.3	5	Oral, injectable
Methylprednisolone	5	5	0	4	Oral, injectable
Meprednisone[2]	5		0	4	Oral, injectable
Intermediate-acting glucocorticoids					
Triamcinolone	5	5[3]	0	4	Oral, injectable, topical
Paramethasone[2]	10		0	2	Oral, injectable
Fluprednisolone[2]	15	7	0	1.5	Oral
Long-acting glucocorticoids					
Betamethasone	25–40	10	0	0.6	Oral, injectable, topical
Dexamethasone	30	10	0	0.75	Oral, injectable, topical
Mineralocorticoids					
Fludrocortisone	10	0	250	2	Oral
Desoxycorticosterone acetate[2]	0	0	20		Injectable, pellets

[1]Potency relative to hydrocortisone.
[2]Outside USA.
[3]Acetonide: Up to 100.

Glucocorticoids given chronically suppress the pituitary release of ACTH, growth hormone, thyroid-stimulating hormone, and luteinizing hormone.

Large doses of glucocorticoids have been associated with the development of peptic ulcer, possibly by suppressing the local immune response against *Helicobacter pylori*. They also promote fat redistribution in the body, with increase of visceral, facial, nuchal, and supraclavicular fat, and they appear to antagonize the effect of vitamin D on calcium absorption. The glucocorticoids also have important effects on the hematopoietic system. In addition to their effects on leukocytes described above, they increase the number of platelets and red blood cells.

In the absence of physiologic amounts of cortisol, renal function (particularly glomerular filtration) is impaired, vasopressin secretion is augmented, and there is an inability to excrete a water load normally.

Glucocorticoids have important effects on the development of the fetal lungs. Indeed, the structural and functional changes in the lungs near term, including the pro-

duction of pulmonary surface-active material required for air breathing (surfactant), are stimulated by glucocorticoids.

SYNTHETIC CORTICOSTEROIDS

Glucocorticoids have become important agents for use in the treatment of many inflammatory, immunologic, hematologic, and other disorders. This has stimulated the development of many synthetic steroids with anti-inflammatory and immunosuppressive activity.

Pharmacokinetics

A. SOURCE

Pharmaceutical steroids are usually synthesized from cholic acid obtained from cattle or steroid sapogenins found in plants. Further modifications of these steroids have led to the marketing of a large group of synthetic steroids with special characteristics that are pharmacologically and therapeutically important (Table 39–1; Figure 39–3).

B. DISPOSITION

The metabolism of the naturally occurring adrenal steroids has been discussed above. The synthetic corticosteroids (Table 39–1) are in most cases rapidly and completely absorbed when given by mouth. Although they are transported and metabolized in a fashion similar to that of the endogenous steroids, important differences exist.

Alterations in the glucocorticoid molecule influence its affinity for glucocorticoid and mineralocorticoid receptors as well as its protein-binding affinity, side chain stability, rate of elimination, and metabolic products. Halogenation at the 9 position, unsaturation of the Δ1–2 bond of the A ring, and methylation at the 2 or 16 position prolong the half-life by more than 50%. The Δ1 compounds are excreted in the free form. In some cases, the agent given is a prodrug; for example, prednisone is rapidly converted to the active product prednisolone in the body.

Pharmacodynamics

The actions of the synthetic steroids are similar to those of cortisol (see above). They bind to the specific intracellular receptor proteins and produce the same effects but have different ratios of glucocorticoid to mineralocorticoid potency (Table 39–1).

Clinical Pharmacology

A. DIAGNOSIS AND TREATMENT OF DISTURBED ADRENAL FUNCTION

1. Adrenocortical insufficiency—
a. Chronic (Addison's disease)—Chronic adrenocortical insufficiency is characterized by weakness, fatigue, weight loss, hypotension, hyperpigmentation, and inability to maintain the blood glucose level during fasting. In such individuals, minor noxious, traumatic, or infectious stimuli may produce acute adrenal insufficiency with circulatory shock and even death.

In primary adrenal insufficiency, about 20–30 mg of hydrocortisone must be given daily, with increased amounts during periods of stress. Although hydrocortisone has some mineralocorticoid activity, this must be supplemented by an appropriate amount of a salt-retaining hormone such as fludrocortisone. Synthetic glucocorticoids that are long-acting and devoid of salt-retaining activity should not be administered to these patients.

b. Acute—When acute adrenocortical insufficiency is suspected, treatment must be instituted immediately. Therapy consists of correction of fluid and electrolyte abnormalities and treatment of precipitating factors in addition to large amounts of parenteral hydrocortisone. Hydrocortisone sodium succinate or phosphate in doses of 100 mg intravenously is given every 8 hours until the patient is stable. The dose is then gradually reduced, achieving maintenance dosage within 5 days.

The administration of salt-retaining hormone is resumed when the total hydrocortisone dosage has been reduced to 50 mg/d.

2. Adrenocortical hypo- and hyperfunction—
a. Congenital adrenal hyperplasia—This group of disorders is characterized by specific defects in the synthesis of cortisol. In pregnancies at high risk for congenital adrenal hyperplasia, fetuses can be protected from genital abnormalities by administration of dexamethasone to the mother. The most common defect is a decrease in or lack of P450c21 (21β-hydroxylase) activity.*

As can be seen in Figure 39–1, this would lead to a reduction in cortisol synthesis and thus produce a compensatory increase in ACTH release. The gland becomes hyperplastic and produces abnormally large amounts of precursors such as 17-hydroxyprogesterone that can be diverted to the androgen pathway, leading to virilization. Metabolism of this compound in the liver leads to pregnanetriol, which is characteristically excreted into the urine in large amounts in this disorder and can be used to make the diagnosis and to monitor efficacy of glucocorticoid substitution. However, the most reliable method of detecting this disorder is the increased response of plasma 17-hydroxyprogesterone to ACTH stimulation.

If the defect is in 11-hydroxylation, large amounts of deoxycorticosterone are produced, and because this steroid has mineralocorticoid activity, hypertension with or without hypokalemic alkalosis ensues. When 17-hydroxylation is defective in the adrenals and gonads, hypogonadism is also present. However, increased amounts of 11-deoxycorticosterone (DOC; see page 647) are formed, and the signs and symptoms associated with mineralocorticoid excess—such as hypertension and hypokalemia—are also observed.

When first seen, the infant with congenital adrenal hyperplasia may be in acute adrenal crisis and should be treated as described above, using appropriate electrolyte solutions and an intravenous preparation of hydrocortisone in stress doses.

Once the patient is stabilized, oral hydrocortisone, 12–18 mg/m²/d in two unequally divided doses (two thirds in the morning, one third in late afternoon) is begun. The dosage is adjusted to allow normal growth and bone maturation and to prevent androgen excess. Alternate-day therapy with prednisone has also been used to achieve greater ACTH suppression without increasing growth inhibition. Fludrocortisone, 0.05–0.2 mg/d, should also be administered by mouth, with added salt to maintain normal blood pressure, plasma renin activity, and electrolytes.

---

*Names for the adrenal steroid synthetic enzymes include the following:
P450c11 (11β-hydroxylase)
P450c17 (17α-hydroxylase)
P450c21 (21β-hydroxylase)

b. Cushing's syndrome—Cushing's syndrome is usually the result of bilateral adrenal hyperplasia secondary to an ACTH-secreting pituitary adenoma (Cushing's disease) but occasionally is due to tumors or nodular hyperplasia of the adrenal gland or ectopic production of ACTH by other tumors. The manifestations are those associated with the chronic presence of excessive glucocorticoids. When glucocorticoid hypersecretion is marked and prolonged, a rounded, plethoric face and trunk obesity are striking in appearance. The manifestations of protein loss are often found and include muscle wasting, thinning, purple striae, and easy bruising of the skin; poor wound healing; and osteoporosis. Other serious disturbances include mental disorders, hypertension, and diabetes. This disorder is treated by surgical removal of the tumor producing ACTH or cortisol, irradiation of the pituitary tumor, or resection of one or both adrenals. These patients must receive large doses of cortisol during and following the surgical procedure. Doses of up to 300 mg of soluble hydrocortisone may be given as a continuous intravenous infusion on the day of surgery. The dose must be reduced slowly to normal replacement levels, since rapid reduction in dose may produce withdrawal symptoms, including fever and joint pain. If adrenalectomy has been performed, long-term maintenance is similar to that outlined above for adrenal insufficiency.

c. Aldosteronism—Primary aldosteronism usually results from the excessive production of aldosterone by an adrenal adenoma. However, it may also result from abnormal secretion by hyperplastic glands or from a malignant tumor. The clinical findings of hypertension, weakness, and tetany are related to the continued renal loss of potassium, which leads to hypokalemia, alkalosis, and elevation of serum sodium concentrations. This syndrome can also be produced in disorders of adrenal steroid biosynthesis by excessive secretion of deoxycorticosterone, corticosterone, or 18-hydroxycorticosterone—all compounds with inherent mineralocorticoid activity.

In contrast to patients with secondary aldosteronism (see below), these patients have low (suppressed) levels of plasma renin activity and angiotensin II. When treated with fludrocortisone (0.2 mg twice daily orally for 3 days) or deoxycorticosterone acetate (20 mg/d intramuscularly for 3 days—but not available in the USA), they fail to retain sodium and their secretion of aldosterone is not significantly reduced. When the disorder is mild, it may escape detection when serum potassium levels are used for screening. However, it may be detected by an increased ratio of plasma aldosterone to renin. Patients generally improve when treated with spironolactone, and the response to this agent is of diagnostic and therapeutic value.

3. Use of glucocorticoids for diagnostic purposes—It is sometimes necessary to suppress the production of ACTH in order to identify the source of a particular hormone or to establish whether its production is influenced by the secretion of ACTH. In these circumstances, it is advantageous to employ a very potent substance such as dexamethasone because the use of small quantities reduces the possibility of confusion in the interpretation of hormone assays in blood or urine. For example, if complete suppression is achieved by the use of 50 mg of cortisol, the urinary 17-hydroxycorticosteroids will be 15–18 mg/24 h, since one third of the dose given will be recovered in urine as 17-hydroxycorticosteroid. If an equivalent dose of 1.5 mg of dexamethasone is employed, the urinary excretion will be only 0.5 mg/24 h and blood levels will be low.

The **dexamethasone suppression test** is used for the diagnosis of Cushing's syndrome and has also been used in the differential diagnosis of depressive psychiatric states. As a screening test, dexamethasone, 1 mg, is given orally at 11 PM, and a plasma sample is obtained the following morning. In normal individuals, the morning cortisol concentration is usually less than 3 mcg/dL, whereas in Cushing's syndrome the level is usually greater than 5 mcg/dL. The results are not reliable in the presence of depression, anxiety, concurrent illness, and other stressful conditions or if the patient receives a medication that enhances the catabolism of dexamethasone in the liver. To distinguish between hypercortisolism due to anxiety, depression, and alcoholism (pseudo-Cushing syndrome) and bona fide Cushing's syndrome, a combined test is carried out, consisting of dexamethasone (0.5 mg orally every 6 hours for 2 days) followed by a standard corticotropin-releasing hormone (CRH) test (1 mg/kg given as a bolus intravenous infusion 2 hours after the last dose of dexamethasone).

In patients in whom the diagnosis of Cushing's syndrome has been established clinically and confirmed by a finding of elevated free cortisol in the urine, suppression with large doses of dexamethasone will help to distinguish patients with Cushing's disease from those with steroid-producing tumors of the adrenal cortex or with the ectopic ACTH syndrome. Dexamethasone is given in a dosage of 0.5 mg orally every 6 hours for 2 days, followed by 2 mg orally every 6 hours for 2 days, and the urine is then assayed for cortisol or its metabolites (Liddle's test); or dexamethasone is given as a single dose of 8 mg at 11 PM and the plasma cortisol is measured at 8 AM the following day. In patients with Cushing's disease, the suppressant effect of dexamethasone will usually produce a 50% reduction in hormone levels. In patients in whom suppression does not occur, the ACTH level will be low in the presence of a cortisol-producing adrenal tumor and elevated in patients with an ectopic ACTH-producing tumor.

B. CORTICOSTEROIDS AND STIMULATION OF LUNG MATURATION IN THE FETUS

Lung maturation in the fetus is regulated by the fetal secretion of cortisol. Treatment of the mother with large

Table 39–2. Some therapeutic indications for the use of glucocorticoids in nonadrenal disorders.

Disorder	Examples
Allergic reactions	Angioneurotic edema, asthma, bee stings, contact dermatitis, drug reactions, allergic rhinitis, serum sickness, urticaria
Collagen-vascular disorders	Giant cell arteritis, lupus erythematosus, mixed connective tissue syndromes, polymyositis, polymyalgia rheumatica, rheumatoid arthritis, temporal arteritis
Eye diseases	Acute uveitis, allergic conjunctivitis, choroiditis, optic neuritis
Gastrointestinal diseases	Inflammatory bowel disease, nontropical sprue, subacute hepatic necrosis
Hematologic disorders	Acquired hemolytic anemia, acute allergic purpura, leukemia, autoimmune hemolytic anemia, idiopathic thrombocytopenic purpura, multiple myeloma
Systemic inflammation	Acute respiratory distress syndrome (sustained therapy with moderate dosage accelerates recovery and decreases mortality)
Infections	Acute respiratory distress syndrome, sepsis, systemic inflammatory syndrome
Inflammatory conditions of bones and joints	Arthritis, bursitis, tenosynovitis
Neurologic disorders	Cerebral edema (large doses of dexamethasone are given to patients following brain surgery to minimize cerebral edema in the postoperative period), multiple sclerosis
Organ transplants	Prevention and treatment of rejection (immunosuppression)
Pulmonary diseases	Aspiration pneumonia, bronchial asthma, prevention of infant respiratory distress syndrome, sarcoidosis
Renal disorders	Nephrotic syndrome
Skin diseases	Atopic dermatitis, dermatoses, lichen simplex chronicus (localized neurodermatitis), mycosis fungoides, pemphigus, seborrheic dermatitis, xerosis
Thyroid diseases	Malignant exophthalmos, subacute thyroiditis
Miscellaneous	Hypercalcemia, mountain sickness

doses of glucocorticoid reduces the incidence of respiratory distress syndrome in infants delivered prematurely. When delivery is anticipated before 34 weeks of gestation, intramuscular betamethasone, 12 mg, followed by an additional dose of 12 mg 18–24 hours later, is commonly used. Betamethasone is chosen because maternal protein binding and placental metabolism of this corticosteroid is less than that of cortisol, allowing increased transfer across the placenta to the fetus.

C. Corticosteroids and Nonadrenal Disorders

The synthetic analogs of cortisol are useful in the treatment of a diverse group of diseases unrelated to any known disturbance of adrenal function (Table 39–2). The usefulness of corticosteroids in these disorders is a function of their ability to suppress inflammatory and immune responses and to alter leukocyte function, as described above and in Chapter 56. In disorders in which host response is the cause of the major manifestations of the disease, these agents are useful. In instances where the inflammatory or immune response is impor-

tant in controlling the pathologic process, therapy with corticosteroids may be dangerous but justified to prevent irreparable damage from an inflammatory response—if used in conjunction with specific therapy for the disease process.

Since the corticosteroids are not usually curative, the pathologic process may progress while clinical manifestations are suppressed. Therefore, chronic therapy with these drugs should be undertaken with great care and only when the seriousness of the disorder warrants their use and less hazardous measures have been exhausted.

In general, attempts should be made to bring the disease process under control using medium- to intermediate-acting glucocorticoids such as prednisone and prednisolone (Table 39–1), as well as all ancillary measures possible to keep the dose low. Where possible, alternate-day therapy should be utilized (see below). Therapy should not be decreased or stopped abruptly. When prolonged therapy is anticipated, it is helpful to obtain chest x-rays and a tuberculin test, since glucocorticoid therapy can reactivate dormant disease. The presence of diabetes, peptic ulcer, osteoporosis, and psychologic disturbances should be taken into consideration, and cardiovascular function should be assessed.

Treatment of transplant rejection is a very important application of glucocorticoids. The efficacy of these agents is based on their ability to reduce antigen expression from the grafted tissue, delay revascularization, and interfere with the sensitization of cytotoxic T lymphocytes and the generation of primary antibody-forming cells.

Toxicity

The benefits obtained from use of the glucocorticoids vary considerably. Use of these drugs must be carefully weighed in each patient against their widespread effects on every part of the organism. The major undesirable effects of the glucocorticoids are the result of their hormonal actions (see above), which lead to the clinical picture of iatrogenic Cushing's syndrome (see below).

When the glucocorticoids are used for short periods (< 2 weeks), it is unusual to see serious adverse effects even with moderately large doses. However, insomnia, behavioral changes (primarily hypomania), and acute peptic ulcers are occasionally observed even after only a few days of treatment. Acute pancreatitis is a rare but serious acute adverse effect of high-dose glucocorticoids.

A. METABOLIC EFFECTS

Most patients who are given daily doses of 100 mg of hydrocortisone or more (or the equivalent amount of synthetic steroid) for longer than 2 weeks undergo a series of changes that have been termed iatrogenic Cushing's syndrome. The rate of development is a function of the dose and the genetic background of the patient. In the face, rounding, puffiness, fat deposition, and plethora usually appear (moon facies). Similarly, fat tends to be redistributed from the extremities to the trunk, the back of the neck, and the supraclavicular fossae. There is an increased growth of fine hair over the face, thighs and trunk. Steroid-induced punctate acne may appear, and insomnia and increased appetite are noted. In the treatment of dangerous or disabling disorders, these changes may not require cessation of therapy. However, the underlying metabolic changes accompanying them can be very serious by the time they become obvious. The continuing breakdown of protein and diversion of amino acids to glucose production increase the need for insulin and over a period of time result in weight gain; visceral fat deposition; myopathy and muscle wasting; thinning of the skin, with striae and bruising; hyperglycemia; and eventually the development of osteoporosis, diabetes, and aseptic necrosis of the hip. Wound healing is also impaired under these circumstances. When diabetes occurs, it is treated by diet and insulin. These patients are often resistant to insulin but rarely develop ketoacidosis. In general,

patients treated with corticosteroids should be on high-protein and potassium-enriched diets.

B. OTHER COMPLICATIONS

Other serious side effects include peptic ulcers and their consequences. The clinical findings associated with certain disorders, particularly bacterial and mycotic infections, may be masked by the corticosteroids, and patients must be carefully watched to avoid serious mishap when large doses are used. The frequency of severe myopathy is greater in patients treated with long-acting glucocorticoids. The administration of such compounds has been associated with nausea, dizziness, and weight loss in some patients. It is treated by changing drugs, reducing dosage, and increasing potassium and protein intake.

Hypomania or acute psychosis may occur, particularly in patients receiving very large doses of corticosteroids. Long-term therapy with intermediate- and long-acting steroids is associated with depression and the development of posterior subcapsular cataracts. Psychiatric follow-up and periodic slit lamp examination is indicated in such patients. Increased intraocular pressure is common, and glaucoma may be induced. Benign intracranial hypertension also occurs. In dosages of 45 $mg/m^2/d$ or more of hydrocortisone or its equivalent, growth retardation occurs in children. Medium-, intermediate-, and long-acting glucocorticoids have greater growth-suppressing potency than the natural steroid at equivalent doses.

When given in greater than physiologic amounts, steroids such as cortisone and hydrocortisone, which have mineralocorticoid effects in addition to glucocorticoid effects, cause some sodium and fluid retention and loss of potassium. In patients with normal cardiovascular and renal function, this leads to a hypokalemic, hypochloremic alkalosis and eventually a rise in blood pressure. In patients with hypoproteinemia, renal disease, or liver disease, edema may also occur. In patients with heart disease, even small degrees of sodium retention may lead to heart failure. These effects can be minimized by using synthetic non–salt-retaining steroids, sodium restriction, and judicious amounts of potassium supplements.

C. ADRENAL SUPPRESSION

When corticosteroids are administered for more than 2 weeks, adrenal suppression may occur. If treatment extends over weeks to months, the patient should be given appropriate supplementary therapy at times of minor stress (twofold dose increases for 24–48 hours) or severe stress (up to tenfold dose increases for 48–72 hours) such as accidental trauma or major surgery. If corticosteroid dosage is to be reduced, it should be tapered slowly. If therapy is to be stopped, the reduction process should be quite slow when the dose reaches replacement levels. It may take 2–12 months for the hypothalamic-pituitary-adrenal axis to function acceptably, and cortisol levels may not return to normal for another 6–9 months. The glucocorticoid-induced suppression is not a pituitary problem, and treatment with ACTH does not reduce the time required for the return of normal function.

If the dose is reduced too rapidly in patients receiving glucocorticoids for a certain disorder, the symptoms of the disorder may reappear or increase in intensity. However, patients without an underlying disorder (eg, patients cured surgically of Cushing's disease) will also develop symptoms with rapid reductions in corticosteroid levels. These symptoms include anorexia, nausea or vomiting, weight loss, lethargy, headache, fever, joint or muscle pain, and postural hypotension. Although many of these symptoms may reflect true glucocorticoid deficiency, they may also occur in the presence of normal or even elevated plasma cortisol levels, suggesting glucocorticoid dependence.

Contraindications & Cautions

A. SPECIAL PRECAUTIONS

Patients receiving these drugs must be monitored carefully for the development of hyperglycemia, glycosuria, sodium retention with edema or hypertension, hypokalemia, peptic ulcer, osteoporosis, and hidden infections.

The dosage should be kept as low as possible, and intermittent administration (eg, alternate-day) should be employed when satisfactory therapeutic results can be obtained on this schedule. Even patients maintained on relatively low doses of corticosteroids may require supplementary therapy at times of stress, such as when surgical procedures are performed or intercurrent illness or accidents occur.

B. CONTRAINDICATIONS

These agents must be used with great caution in patients with peptic ulcer, heart disease or hypertension with heart failure, certain infectious illnesses such as varicella and tuberculosis, psychoses, diabetes, osteoporosis, or glaucoma.

Selection of Drug & Dosage Schedule

Since these preparations differ with respect to relative anti-inflammatory and mineralocorticoid effect, duration of action, cost, and dosage forms available (Table 39–1), these factors should be taken into account in selecting the drug to be used.

A. ACTH VERSUS ADRENOCORTICAL STEROIDS

In patients with normal adrenals, ACTH was used to induce the endogenous production of cortisol to obtain similar effects. However, except when the increase in androgens is desirable, the use of ACTH as a therapeutic agent has been abandoned. Instances in which ACTH was claimed to be more effective than glucocorticoids were probably due to the administration of smaller amounts of corticosteroids than were produced by the dosage of ACTH.

B. DOSAGE

In determining the dosage regimen to be used, the physician must consider the seriousness of the disease, the amount of drug likely to be required to obtain the desired effect, and the duration of therapy. In some diseases, the amount required for maintenance of the desired therapeutic effect is less than the dose needed to obtain the initial effect, and the lowest possible dosage for the needed effect should be determined by gradually lowering the dose until a small increase in signs or symptoms is noted.

When it is necessary to maintain continuously elevated plasma corticosteroid levels in order to suppress ACTH, a slowly absorbed parenteral preparation or small oral doses at frequent intervals are required. The opposite situation exists with respect to the use of corticosteroids in the treatment of inflammatory and allergic disorders. The same total quantity given in a few doses may be more effective than when given in many smaller doses or in a slowly absorbed parenteral form.

Severe autoimmune conditions involving vital organs must be treated aggressively, and undertreatment is as dangerous as overtreatment. In order to minimize the deposition of immune complexes and the influx of leukocytes and macrophages, 1 mg/kg/d of prednisone in divided doses is required initially. This dose is maintained until the serious manifestations respond. The dose can then be gradually reduced.

When large doses are required for prolonged periods of time, alternate-day administration of the compound may be tried after control is achieved. When used in this manner, very large amounts (eg, 100 mg of prednisone) can sometimes be administered with less marked adverse effects because there is a recovery period between each dose. The transition to an alternate-day schedule can be made after the disease process is under control. It should be done gradually and with additional supportive measures between doses.

When selecting a drug for use in large doses, a medium- or intermediate-acting synthetic steroid with little mineralocorticoid effect is advisable. If possible, it should be given as a single morning dose.

C. SPECIAL DOSAGE FORMS

The use of local therapy, such as topical preparations for skin disease, ophthalmic forms for eye disease, intra-articular injections for joint disease, inhaled steroids for asthma, and hydrocortisone enemas for ulcerative colitis, provides a means of delivering large amounts of steroid to the diseased tissue with reduced systemic effects.

Beclomethasone dipropionate and several other glucocorticoids—primarily budesonide and flunisolide and mometasone furoate, administered as aerosols—have been found to be effective in the treatment of asthma (see Chapter 20).

Beclomethasone dipropionate, triamcinolone acetonide, budesonide, flunisolide, and mometasone furoate are available as nasal sprays for the topical treatment of allergic rhinitis. They are effective at doses (one or two sprays one, two, or three times daily) that in most patients result in plasma levels too low to influence adrenal function or have any other systemic effects.

Corticosteroids incorporated in ointments, creams, lotions, and sprays are used extensively in dermatology. These preparations are discussed in more detail in Chapter 62.

MINERALOCORTICOIDS (ALDOSTERONE, DEOXYCORTICOSTERONE, FLUDROCORTISONE)

The most important mineralocorticoid in humans is aldosterone. However, small amounts of deoxycorticosterone (DOC) are also formed and released. Although the amount is normally insignificant, DOC was of some importance therapeutically in the past. Its actions, effects, and metabolism are qualitatively similar to those described below for aldosterone.

Fludrocortisone, a synthetic corticosteroid, is the most commonly prescribed salt-retaining hormone.

1. Aldosterone

Aldosterone is synthesized mainly in the zona glomerulosa of the adrenal cortex. Its structure and synthesis are illustrated in Figure 39–1.

The rate of aldosterone secretion is subject to several influences. ACTH produces a moderate stimulation of its release, but this effect is not sustained for more than a few days in the normal individual. Although aldosterone is no less than one third as effective as cortisol in suppressing ACTH, the quantities of aldosterone produced by the adrenal cortex and its plasma concentrations are insufficient to participate in any significant feedback control of ACTH secretion.

In the absence of ACTH, aldosterone secretion falls to about half the normal rate, indicating that other factors, eg, angiotensin, are able to maintain and perhaps regulate its secretion (see Chapter 17). Independent variations between cortisol and aldosterone secretion can also be demonstrated by means of lesions in the nervous system such as decerebration, which decreases the secretion of cortisol while increasing the secretion of aldosterone.

Physiologic & Pharmacologic Effects

Aldosterone and other steroids with mineralocorticoid properties promote the reabsorption of sodium from the distal part of the distal convoluted tubule and from the cortical collecting renal tubules, loosely coupled to the excretion of potassium and hydrogen ion. Sodium reabsorption in the sweat and salivary glands, gastrointestinal mucosa, and across cell membranes in general is also increased. Excessive levels of aldosterone produced by tumors or overdosage with synthetic mineralocorticoids lead to hypokalemia, metabolic alkalosis, increased plasma volume, and hypertension.

Mineralocorticoids act by binding to the mineralocorticoid receptor in the cytoplasm of target cells, especially principal cells of the distal convoluted and collecting tubules of the kidney. The drug-receptor complex activates a series of events similar to those described above for the glucocorticoids and illustrated in Figure 39–4. It is of interest that this receptor has the same affinity for cortisol, which is present in much higher concentrations in the extracellular fluid. The specificity for mineralocorticoids at this site appears to be conferred, at least in part, by the presence of the enzyme 11β-hydroxysteroid dehydrogenase type 2, which converts cortisol to cortisone. The latter has low affinity for the receptor and is inactive as a mineralocorticoid or glucocorticoid. The major effect of activation of the aldosterone receptor is increased expression of Na^+/K^+ ATPase and the epithelial sodium channel (ENaC).

Metabolism

Aldosterone is secreted at the rate of 100–200 mcg/d in normal individuals with a moderate dietary salt intake. The plasma level in men (resting supine) is about 0.007 mcg/dL. The half-life of aldosterone injected in tracer quantities is 15–20 minutes, and it does not appear to be firmly bound to serum proteins.

The metabolism of aldosterone is similar to that of cortisol, about 50 mcg/24 h appearing in the urine as conjugated tetrahydroaldosterone. Approximately 5–15 mcg/24 h is excreted free or as the 3-oxo glucuronide.

2. Deoxycorticosterone (DOC)

DOC, which also serves as a precursor of aldosterone (Figure 39–1), is normally secreted in amounts of about 200 mcg/d. Its half-life when injected into the human circulation is about 70 minutes. Preliminary estimates of its concentration in plasma are approximately 0.03 mcg/dL. The control of its secretion differs from that of aldosterone in that the secretion of DOC is primarily under the control of ACTH. Although the response to ACTH is enhanced by dietary sodium restriction, a low-salt diet does not increase DOC secretion. The secretion of DOC may be markedly increased in abnormal conditions such as adrenocortical carcinoma and congenital adrenal hyperplasia with reduced P450c11 or P450c17 activity.

3. Fludrocortisone

This compound, a potent steroid with both glucocorticoid and mineralocorticoid activity, is the most widely used mineralocorticoid. Doses of 0.1 mg two to seven times weekly have potent salt-retaining activity and are used in the treatment of adrenocortical insufficiency associated with mineralocorticoid deficiency. These dosages are too small to have important anti-inflammatory or antigrowth effects.

ADRENAL ANDROGENS

The adrenal cortex secretes large amounts of DHEA and smaller amounts of androstenedione and testosterone. Although these androgens are thought to contribute to the normal maturation process, they do not stimulate or support major androgen-dependent pubertal changes in humans. Recent studies suggest that DHEA and its sulfate may have other important physiologic actions. If that is correct, these results are probably due to the peripheral conversion of DHEA to more potent androgens or to estrogens and interaction with androgen and estrogen receptors, respectively. Additional effects may be exerted through an interaction with the $GABA_A$ and glutamate receptors in the brain or with a nuclear receptor in several central and peripheral sites. The therapeutic use of DHEA in humans is being explored, but the substance has already been adopted with uncritical enthusiasm by members of the sports drug culture and the vitamin and food supplement culture. The results of a placebo-controlled trial of DHEA in patients with systemic lupus erythematosus were recently reported as well as those of a study of DHEA replacement in women with adrenal insufficiency. In both studies a small beneficial effect was seen, with significant improvement of the disease in the former and a clearly added sense of well-being in the latter. The androgenic or estrogenic actions of DHEA could explain the effects of the compound in both situations.

■ ANTAGONISTS OF ADRENOCORTICAL AGENTS

SYNTHESIS INHIBITORS & GLUCOCORTICOID ANTAGONISTS

1. Metyrapone

Metyrapone (Figure 39–5) is a relatively selective inhibitor of steroid synthesis. It inhibits 11-hydroxylation,

interfering with cortisol and corticosterone synthesis. In the presence of a normal pituitary gland, there is a compensatory increase in pituitary ACTH release and adrenal 11-deoxycortisol secretion. This response is a measure of the capacity of the anterior pituitary to produce ACTH and has been adapted for clinical use as a diagnostic test. Although the toxicity of metyrapone is much lower than that of mitotane (see below), the drug may produce transient dizziness and gastrointestinal disturbances. This agent has not been widely used for the treatment of Cushing's syndrome. However, in doses of 0.25 g twice daily to 1 g four times daily, metyrapone can reduce cortisol production to normal levels in some patients with endogenous Cushing's syndrome. Thus, it may be useful in the management of severe manifestations of cortisol excess while the cause of this condition is being determined or in conjunction with radiation or surgical treatment. It is the only adrenal-inhibiting medication that can be administered to pregnant women with Cushing's syndrome. The major adverse effects observed are salt and water retention and hirsutism resulting from diversion of the 11-deoxycortisol precursor to DOC and androgen synthesis.

Metyrapone is commonly used in tests of adrenal function. The blood levels of 11-deoxycortisol and the urinary excretion of 17-hydroxycorticoids are measured before and after administration of the compound. Normally, there is a twofold or greater increase in the urinary 17-hydroxycorticoid excretion. A dose of 300–500 mg every 4 hours for six doses is often used, and urine collections are made on the day before and the day after treatment. In patients with Cushing's syndrome, a normal response to metyrapone indicates that the cortisol excess is not the result of a cortisol-secreting adrenal carcinoma or adenoma, since secretion by such tumors produces suppression of ACTH and atrophy of normal adrenal cortex.

Pituitary function may also be tested by administering metyrapone, 2–3 g orally at midnight, and measuring the level of ACTH or 11-deoxycortisol in blood drawn at 8 AM, or by comparing the excretion of 17-hydroxycorticosteroids in the urine during the 24-hour periods preceding and following administration of the drug. In patients with suspected or known lesions of the pituitary, this procedure is a means of estimating the ability of the gland to produce ACTH. The drug has been withdrawn from the market in the USA but is available on a compassionate basis.

2. Aminoglutethimide

Aminoglutethimide (Figure 39–5) blocks the conversion of cholesterol to pregnenolone and causes a reduction in the synthesis of all hormonally active steroids (see Figure 39–1). It has been used in conjunction with dexamethasone or hydrocortisone to reduce or eliminate estrogen production in patients with carcinoma of

Figure 39–5. Some adrenocortical antagonists. Because of their toxicity, several of these compounds are no longer available in the USA.

the breast. In a dosage of 1 g/d it was well tolerated; however, with higher dosages, lethargy and skin rash was a common effect. The use of aminoglutethimide in breast cancer patients has now been supplanted by the use of tamoxifen or another class of drugs, the aromatase inhibitors (see Chapters 40 and 55). Aminoglutethimide can be used in conjunction with metyrapone or ketoconazole to reduce steroid secretion in patients with Cushing's syndrome due to adrenocortical cancer who do not respond to mitotane.

Aminoglutethimide also apparently increases the clearance of some steroids. It has been shown to enhance the metabolism of dexamethasone, reducing its half-life from 4–5 hours to 2 hours.

3. Ketoconazole

Ketoconazole, an antifungal imidazole derivative (see Chapter 48), is a potent and rather nonselective inhibitor of adrenal and gonadal steroid synthesis. This compound inhibits the cholesterol side chain cleavage, P450c17, C17,20-lyase, 3β-hydroxysteroid dehydrogenase, and P450c11 enzymes required for steroid hormone synthesis. The sensitivity of the P450 enzymes to this compound in mammalian tissues is much lower than that needed to treat fungal infections, so that its

inhibitory effects on steroid biosynthesis are seen only at high doses.

Ketoconazole has been used for the treatment of patients with Cushing's syndrome due to several causes. Dosages of 200–1200 mg/d have produced a reduction in hormone levels and impressive clinical improvement. This drug has some hepatotoxicity and should be started at 200 mg/d and slowly increased by 200 mg/d every 2–3 days up to a total daily dose of 1000 mg.

4. Mifepristone (RU 486)

The search for a glucocorticoid receptor antagonist finally succeeded in the early 1980s with the development of the 11β-aminophenyl-substituted 19-norsteroid called RU 486, later named mifepristone. This compound has strong antiprogestin activity and initially was proposed as a contraceptive-contragestive agent. High doses of mifepristone exert antiglucocorticoid activity by blocking the glucocorticoid receptor, since mifepristone binds to it with high affinity, causing (1) some stabilization of the Hsp-glucocorticoid receptor complex and inhibition of the dissociation of the RU 486-bound glucocorticoid receptor from the Hsp chaperone proteins; and (2) alteration of the interaction of the glucocorticoid receptor with coregulators, favoring the formation of a transcriptionally inactive complex in the cell nucleus. The result is inhibition of glucocorticoid receptor activation.

The mean half-life of mifepristone is 20 hours. This is longer than that of many natural and synthetic glucocorticoid agonists (dexamethasone has a half-life of 4–5 hours). Less than 1% of the daily dose is excreted in the urine, suggesting a minor role of kidneys in the clearance of the compound. The long plasma half-life of mifepristone results from extensive and strong binding to plasma proteins. Less than 5% of the compound is found in the free form when plasma is analyzed by equilibrium dialysis. Mifepristone can bind to albumin and α_1-acid glycoprotein, but it has no affinity for CBG.

In humans, mifepristone causes generalized glucocorticoid resistance. Given orally to several patients with Cushing's syndrome due to ectopic ACTH production or adrenal carcinoma, it was able to reverse the cushingoid phenotype, to eliminate carbohydrate intolerance, normalize blood pressure, correct thyroid and gonadal hormone suppression, and ameliorate the psychologic sequelae of hypercortisolism in these patients. At present, this use of mifepristone can only be recommended for inoperable patients with ectopic ACTH secretion or adrenal carcinoma who have failed to respond to other therapeutic manipulations. Its pharmacology and use in women as a progesterone antagonist are discussed in Chapter 40.

5. Mitotane

Mitotane (Figure 39–5) has adrenolytic properties in dogs and to a lesser extent in humans. This drug is administered orally in divided doses up to 12 g daily. About one third of patients with adrenal carcinoma show a reduction in tumor mass. In 80% of patients, the toxic effects are sufficiently severe to require dose reduction. These include diarrhea, nausea, vomiting, depression, somnolence, and skin rashes. The drug has been withdrawn from the market in the USA but is available on a compassionate basis.

6. Trilostane

Trilostane is a 3β-17 hydroxysteroid dehydrogenase inhibitor that interferes with the synthesis of adrenal and gonadal hormones and is comparable to aminoglutethimide. Its side effects are predominantly gastrointestinal; adverse effects occur in about 50% of patients with both agents. There is no cross-resistance or crossover of side effects between these compounds.

MINERALOCORTICOID ANTAGONISTS

In addition to agents that interfere with aldosterone synthesis (see above), there are steroids that compete with

aldosterone for its receptor and decrease its effect peripherally. Progesterone is mildly active in this respect.

Spironolactone is a 7α-acetylthiospironolactone. Its onset of action is slow, and the effects last for 2–3 days after the drug is discontinued. It is used in the treatment of primary aldosteronism in dosages of 50–100 mg/d. This agent reverses many of the manifestations of aldosteronism. It has been useful in establishing the diagnosis in some patients and in ameliorating the signs and symptoms when surgical removal of an adenoma is delayed. When used diagnostically for the detection of aldosteronism in hypokalemic patients with hypertension, dosages of 400–500 mg/d for 4–8 days—with an adequate intake of sodium and potassium—will restore potassium levels to or toward normal. This agent is also useful in preparing these patients for surgery. Dosages of 300–400 mg/d for 2 weeks are used for this purpose and may reduce the incidence of cardiac arrhythmias.

Spironolactone is also an androgen antagonist and as such is sometimes used in treatment of hirsutism in women. Dosages of 50–200 mg/d cause a reduction in the density, diameter, and rate of growth of facial hair in patients with idiopathic hirsutism or hirsutism secondary to androgen excess. The effect can usually be seen in 2 months and becomes maximal in about 6 months.

Spironolactone

The use of spironolactone as a diuretic is discussed in Chapter 15. The drug has benefits in heart failure greater than those predicted from its diuretic effects alone (see Chapter 13). Adverse effects reported for spironolactone include hyperkalemia, cardiac arrhythmia, menstrual abnormalities, gynecomastia, sedation, headache, gastrointestinal disturbances, and skin rashes.

Eplerenone, another aldosterone antagonist, is approved for the treatment of hypertension (see Chapters 11 and 15). This aldosterone receptor antagonist is somewhat more selective than spironolactone and has no reported effects on androgen receptors. The standard dosage in hypertension is 50–100 mg/d. The most common toxicity is hyperkalemia but this is usually mild.

Drospirenone, a progestin in an oral contraceptive, also antagonizes the effects of aldosterone.

PREPARATIONS AVAILABLE[1]

GLUCOCORTICOIDS FOR ORAL & PARENTERAL USE

Betamethasone (Celestone)
Oral: 0.6 mg tablets; 0.6 mg/5 mL syrup

Betamethasone sodium phosphate (Celestone Phosphate)
Parenteral: 4 mg/mL for IV, IM, intralesional, or intra-articular injection

Cortisone (Cortone Acetate)
Oral: 25 mg tablets

Dexamethasone (generic, Decadron)
Oral: 0.25, 0.5, 0.75, 1, 1.5, 2, 4, 6 mg tablets; 0.5 mg/5 mL elixir; 0.5 mg/5 mL, 1 mg/mL solution

Dexamethasone acetate (generic, Decadron-LA)
Parenteral: 8 mg/mL suspension for IM, intralesional, or intra-articular injection; 16 mg/mL suspension for intralesional injection

Dexamethasone sodium phosphate (generic, Decadron Phosphate)
Parenteral: 4, 10, 20 mg/mL for IV, IM, intralesional, or intra-articular injection; 24 mg/mL for IV use only

Hydrocortisone [cortisol] (generic, Cortef)
Oral: 5, 10, 20 mg tablets

Hydrocortisone acetate (generic)
Parenteral: 25, 50 mg/mL suspension for intralesional, soft tissue, or intra-articular injection

Hydrocortisone cypionate (Cortef)
Oral: 10 mg/5 mL suspension

Hydrocortisone sodium phosphate (Hydrocortone)
Parenteral: 50 mg/mL for IV, IM, or SC injection

Hydrocortisone sodium succinate (generic, SoluCortef)
Parenteral: 100, 250, 500, 1000 mg/vial for IV, IM injection

Methylprednisolone (generic, Medrol)
Oral: 2, 4, 8, 16, 24, 32 mg tablets

Methylprednisolone acetate (generic, DepoMedrol)
Parenteral: 20, 40, 80 mg/mL for IM, intralesional, or intra-articular injection

Methylprednisolone sodium succinate (generic, Solu-Medrol)
Parenteral: 40, 125, 500, 1000, 2000 mg/vial for injection

Prednisolone (generic, Delta-Cortef, Prelone)
Oral: 5 mg tablets; 5, 15 mg/5 mL syrup

Prednisolone acetate (generic)
Parenteral: 25, 50 mg/mL for soft tissue or intra-articular injection

Prednisolone sodium phosphate (generic, Hydeltrasol)
Oral: 5 mg/5 mL solution
Parenteral: 20 mg/mL for IV, IM, intra-articular, or intralesional injection

Prednisolone tebutate (generic)
Oral: 5 mg/5 mL liquid
Parenteral: 20 mg/mL for intra-articular or intralesional injection

Prednisone (generic, Meticorten)
Oral: 1, 2.5, 5, 10, 20, 50 mg tablets; 1, 5 mg/mL solution and syrup

Triamcinolone (generic, Aristocort, Kenacort)
Oral: 4, 8 mg tablets; 4 mg/5 mL syrup

Triamcinolone acetonide (generic, Kenalog)
Parenteral: 3, 10, 40 mg/mL for IM, intra-articular, or intralesional injection

Triamcinolone diacetate (generic)
Parenteral: 25, 40 mg/mL for IM, intra-articular, or intralesional injection

Triamcinolone hexacetonide (Aristospan)
Parenteral: 5, 20 mg/mL for intra-articular, intralesional, or sublesional injection

MINERALOCORTICOIDS

Fludrocortisone acetate (generic, Florinef Acetate)
Oral: 0.1 mg tablets

ADRENAL STEROID INHIBITORS

Aminoglutethimide (Cytadren)
Oral: 250 mg tablets

Ketoconazole (generic, Nizoral)
Oral: 200 mg tablets (unlabeled use)

Mifepristone (Mifeprex)
Oral: 200 mg tablets

Mitotane (Lysodren)
Oral: 500 mg tablets

---

[1]Glucocorticoids for Aerosol Use: See Chapter 20.
Glucocorticoids for Dermatologic Use: See Chapter 62.
Glucocorticoids for Gastrointestinal Use: See Chapter 63.

REFERENCES

Alesci S et al: Glucocorticoid-induced osteoporosis: From basic mechanisms to clinical aspects. Neuroimmunomodulation 2005;12:1.

Bamberger CM, Schulte HM, Chrousos GP: Molecular determinants of glucocorticoid receptor function and tissue sensitivity to glucocorticoids. Endocr Rev 1996;17:245.

Charmandari E, Tsigos C, Chrousos GP: Neuroendocrinology of stress. Ann Rev Physiol 2005;67:259.

Chrousos G: The glucocorticoid receptor gene, longevity, and the highly prevalent complex disorders of western societies. Am J Med 2004;117:204.

Elenkov IJ, Chrousos GP: Stress hormones, TH1/TH2 patterns, pro/anti-inflammatory cytokines and susceptibility to disease. Trends Endocrinol Metab 1999;10:359.

Elenkov IJ et al: Cytokine dysregulation, inflammation, and well-being. Neuroimmunomodulation 2005;12:255.

Franchimont D et al: Glucocorticoids and inflammation revisited: The state of the art. Neuroimmunomodulation 2002–03;10:247.

Graber AL et al: Natural history of pituitary-adrenal recovery following long-term suppression with corticosteroids. J Clin Endocrinol Metab 1965;25:11.

Hochberg Z, Pacak K, Chrousos GP: Endocrine withdrawal syndromes. Endocrine Rev 2003;24:523.

Kalantaridou S, Chrousos GP: Clinical review 148: Monogenic disorders of puberty. J Clin Endocrinol Metab 2002;87:2481.

Kino T, Charmandari E, Chrousos G (editors): Glucocorticoid action: Basic and clinical implications. Ann N Y Acad Sci 2004; 1024 (entire volume).

Kino T et al: The GTP-binding (G) protein β interacts with the activated glucocorticoid receptor and suppresses its transcriptional activity in the nucleus. J Cell Biol 2005;20:885.

Koch CA, Pacak K, Chrousos GP: The molecular pathogenesis of hereditary and sporadic adrenocortical and adrenomedullary tumors. J Clin Endocrinol Metab 2002;87:5367.

Mao J, Regelson W, Kalimi M: Molecular mechanism of RU 486 action: A review. Mol Cellular Biochem 1992;109:1.

Meduri GU, Chrousos GP: Effectiveness of prolonged glucocorticoid treatment in ARDS: The right drug the right way? Crit Care Med 2006;34:236.

Merke DP et al: Future directions in the study and management of congenital adrenal hyperplasia due to 21-hydroxylase deficiency. Ann Intern Med 2002;136:320.

Tsigos C, Chrousos GP: Differential diagnosis and management of Cushing's syndrome. Annu Rev Med 1996;47:443.

The Gonadal Hormones & Inhibitors | 40

George P. Chrousos, MD

■ I. THE OVARY (ESTROGENS, PROGESTINS, OTHER OVARIAN HORMONES, ORAL CONTRACEPTIVES, INHIBITORS & ANTAGONISTS, & OVULATION-INDUCING AGENTS)

The ovary has important gametogenic functions that are integrated with its hormonal activity. In the human female, the gonad is relatively quiescent during childhood, the period of rapid growth and maturation. At puberty, the ovary begins a 30- to 40-year period of cyclic function called the **menstrual cycle** because of the regular episodes of bleeding that are its most obvious manifestation. It then fails to respond to gonadotropins secreted by the anterior pituitary gland, and the cessation of cyclic bleeding that occurs is called the **menopause.**

The mechanism responsible for the onset of ovarian function at the time of puberty is thought to be neural in origin, because the immature gonad can be stimulated by gonadotropins already present in the pituitary and because the pituitary is responsive to exogenous hypothalamic gonadotropin-releasing hormone. The maturation of centers in the brain may withdraw a childhood-related inhibitory effect upon hypothalamic arcuate nucleus neurons, allowing them to produce **gonadotropin-releasing hormone (GnRH)** in pulses with the appropriate amplitude, which stimulates the release of **follicle-stimulating hormone (FSH)** and **luteinizing hormone (LH)** (see Chapter 37). At first, small amounts of the latter two hormones are released during the night, and the limited quantities of ovarian estrogen secreted in response start to cause breast development. Subsequently, FSH and LH are secreted throughout the day and night, causing secretion of higher amounts of estrogen and leading to further breast enlargement, alterations in fat distribution, and a growth spurt that culminates in epiphysial closure in the long bones. The beginning of ovarian function at puberty is called **gonadarche.**

A year or so after gonadarche, sufficient estrogen is produced to induce endometrial changes and periodic bleeding. After the first few irregular cycles, which may be anovulatory, normal cyclic function is established.

At the beginning of each cycle, a variable number of follicles (vesicular follicles), each containing an ovum, begin to enlarge in response to FSH. After 5 or 6 days, one follicle, called the dominant follicle, begins to develop more rapidly. The outer theca and inner granulosa cells of this follicle multiply and, under the influence of LH, synthesize and release estrogens at an increasing rate. The estrogens appear to inhibit FSH release and may lead to regression of the smaller, less mature follicles. The mature dominant ovarian follicle consists of an ovum surrounded by a fluid-filled antrum lined by granulosa and theca cells. The estrogen secretion reaches a peak just before midcycle, and the granulosa cells begin to secrete progesterone. These changes stimulate the brief surge in LH and FSH release that precedes and causes ovulation. When the follicle ruptures, the ovum is released into the abdominal cavity near the opening of the uterine tube.

Following the above events, the cavity of the ruptured follicle fills with blood (corpus hemorrhagicum), and the luteinized theca and granulosa cells proliferate and replace the blood to form the corpus luteum. The cells of this structure produce estrogens and progesterone for the remainder of the cycle, or longer if pregnancy occurs.

If pregnancy does not occur, the corpus luteum begins to degenerate and ceases hormone production, eventually becoming a corpus albicans. The endometrium, which proliferated during the follicular phase and developed its glandular function during the luteal phase, is shed in the process of menstruation. These events are summarized in Figure 40–1.

The ovary normally ceases its gametogenic and endocrine function with time. This change is accompanied by a cessation in uterine bleeding (menopause) and occurs at a mean age of 52 years in the USA. Although the ovary ceases to secrete estrogen, significant levels of estrogen persist in many women as a result of conversion of adrenal and ovarian steroids such as androstenedione to estrone and estradiol in adipose and possibly other nonendocrine tissues.

Disturbances in Ovarian Function

Disturbances of cyclic function are common even during the peak years of reproduction. A minority of these result from inflammatory or neoplastic processes that influence the functions of the uterus, ovaries, or pituitary. Many of the minor disturbances leading to periods of amenorrhea or anovulatory cycles are self-limited. They are often associated with emotional or physical stress and represent temporary alterations in the stress centers in the brain that control the secretion of GnRH. Anovulatory cycles are also associated with eating disorders (bulimia, anorexia nervosa) and with severe exercise such as distance running and swimming. Among the more common organic causes of persistent ovulatory disturbances are pituitary prolactinomas and syndromes and tumors characterized by excessive ovarian or adrenal androgen production. Normal ovarian function can be modified by androgens produced by the adrenal cortex or tumors arising from it. The ovary also gives rise to androgen-producing neoplasms such as arrhenoblastomas, as well as to estrogen-producing granulosa cell tumors.

THE ESTROGENS

Estrogenic activity is shared by a large number of chemical substances. In addition to the variety of steroidal estrogens derived from animal sources, numerous nonsteroidal estrogens have been synthesized. Many phenols are estrogenic, and estrogenic activity has been identified in such diverse forms of life as those found in ocean sediments. Estrogen-mimetic compounds (flavonoids) are found in many plants, including saw palmetto, and soybeans and other foods. Studies have shown that a diet rich in these plant products may produce slight estrogenic effects. Additionally, some com-

Figure 40–1. The menstrual cycle, showing plasma levels of pituitary and ovarian hormones and histologic changes.

pounds used in the manufacture of plastics (bisphenols, alkylphenols, phthalate phenols) have been found to be estrogenic. It has been proposed that these agents are associated with an increased breast cancer incidence in both women and men in the industrialized world.

Natural Estrogens

The major estrogens produced by women are **estradiol** (estradiol-17β, E_2), **estrone** (E_1), and **estriol** (E_3) (Figure 40–2). Estradiol is the major secretory product of the ovary. Although some estrone is produced in the ovary, most estrone and estriol are formed in the liver from estradiol or in peripheral tissues from androstenedione and other androgens (see Figure 39–1). As noted

FOLLICULAR PHASE

Pregnenolone

17α-Hydroxypregnenolone

Dehydroepiandrosterone

LUTEAL PHASE

Pregnenolone

Progesterone

17α-Hydroxyprogesterone

Androstenedione

Testosterone

AROMATASE

Estriol

16α-Hydroxyestrone

Estrone

17β-Estradiol

2-Hydroxyestrone
and other metabolites

2-Hydroxyestradiol
and other metabolites

Figure 40–2. Biosynthesis and metabolism of estrogens and testosterone.

above, during the first part of the menstrual cycle estrogens are produced in the ovarian follicle by the theca and granulosa cells. After ovulation, the estrogens as well as progesterone are synthesized by the luteinized granulosa and theca cells of the corpus luteum, and the pathways of biosynthesis are slightly different.

During pregnancy, a large amount of estrogen is synthesized by the fetoplacental unit—consisting of the fetal adrenal zone, secreting androgen precursor, and the placenta, which aromatizes it into estrogen. The estriol synthesized by the fetoplacental unit is released into the maternal circulation and excreted into the urine. Repeated assay of maternal urinary estriol excretion has been used in the assessment of fetal well-being.

One of the most prolific natural sources of estrogenic substances is the stallion, which liberates more of these hormones than the pregnant mare or pregnant woman. The equine estrogens—equilenin and equilin—and their congeners are unsaturated in the B as well as the A ring and are excreted in large quantities in urine, from which they can be recovered and used for medicinal purposes.

In normal women, estradiol is produced at a rate that varies during the menstrual cycle, resulting in plasma levels as low as 50 pg/mL in the early follicular phase to as high as 350–850 pg/mL at the time of the preovulatory peak (Figure 40–1).

Synthetic Estrogens

A variety of chemical alterations have been produced in the natural estrogens. The most important effect of these alterations has been to increase the oral effectiveness of

Figure 40–3. Compounds with estrogenic activity.

the estrogens. Some structures are shown in Figure 40–3. Those with therapeutic use are listed in Table 40–1.

In addition to the steroidal estrogens, a variety of nonsteroidal compounds with estrogenic activity have been synthesized and used clinically. These include dienestrol, diethylstilbestrol, benzestrol, hexestrol, methestrol, methallenestril, and chlorotrianisene (Figure 40–3).

Pharmacokinetics

When released into the circulation, estradiol binds strongly to an α_2 globulin (sex hormone-binding globulin [SHBG]) and with lower affinity to albumin. Bound estrogen is relatively unavailable for diffusion into cells, so it is the free fraction that is physiologically active. Estradiol is converted by the liver and other tissues to estrone and estriol (which have low affinity for the estrogen receptor, Figure 40–2) and

their 2-hydroxylated derivatives and conjugated metabolites (which are too insoluble in lipid to cross the cell membrane readily) and excreted in the bile. However, the conjugates may be hydrolyzed in the intestine to active, reabsorbable compounds. Estrogens are also excreted in small amounts in the breast milk of nursing mothers.

Because significant amounts of estrogens and their active metabolites are excreted in the bile and reabsorbed from the intestine, the resulting enterohepatic circulation ensures that orally administered estrogens will have a high ratio of hepatic to peripheral effects. As noted below, the hepatic effects are thought to be responsible for some undesirable actions such as synthesis of increased clotting factors and plasma renin substrate. The hepatic effects of estrogen can be minimized by routes that avoid first-pass liver exposure, ie, vaginal, transdermal, or by injection.

Table 40–1. Commonly used estrogens.

	Average Replacement Dosage
Ethinyl estradiol	0.005–0.02 mg/d
Micronized estradiol	1–2 mg/d
Estradiol cypionate	2–5 mg every 3–4 weeks
Estradiol valerate	2–20 mg every other week
Estropipate	1.25–2.5 mg/d
Conjugated, esterified, or mixed estrogenic substances:	
Oral	0.3–1.25 mg/d
Injectable	0.2–2 mg/d
Transdermal	Patch
Quinestrol	0.1–0.2 mg/week
Chlorotrianisene	12–25 mg/d
Methallenestril	3–9 mg/d

Physiologic Effects

A. MECHANISM

Plasma estrogens in the blood and interstitial fluid are bound to SHBG, from which they dissociate to enter the cell and bind to their receptor. Two genes code for two estrogen receptor isoforms, α and β, which are members of the superfamily of steroid, sterol, retinoic acid, and thyroid receptors. The estrogen receptors are found predominantly in the nucleus bound to heat shock proteins that stabilize them (see Figure 39–4).

Binding of the hormone to its receptor alters its conformation and releases it from the stabilizing proteins (predominantly Hsp90). The receptor-hormone complex forms homodimers that bind to a specific sequence of nucleotides called **estrogen response elements (EREs)** in the promoters of various genes and regulate their transcription. The ERE is composed of two half-sites arranged as a palindrome separated by a small group of nucleotides called the spacer. The interaction of a receptor dimer with the ERE also involves a number of nuclear proteins, the coregulators, as well as components of the transcription machinery. The receptor may also bind to other transcription factors to influence the effects of these factors on their responsive genes.

The relative concentrations and types of receptors, receptor coregulators, and transcription factors confer the cell specificity of the hormone's actions. The genomic effects of estrogens are mainly due to proteins synthesized by translation of RNA transcribed from a responsive gene. Some of the effects of estrogens are indirect, mediated by the autocrine and paracrine actions of autacoids such as growth factors, lipids, glycolipids, and cytokines produced by the target cells in response to estrogen.

Rapid estrogen-induced effects such as granulosa cell Ca^{2+} uptake and increased uterine blood flow do not require gene activation. These appear to be mediated by nongenomic effects of the classic estrogen receptor-estrogen complex, influencing several intracellular signaling pathways.

B. FEMALE MATURATION

Estrogens are required for the normal sexual maturation and growth of the female. They stimulate the development of the vagina, uterus, and uterine tubes as well as the secondary sex characteristics. They stimulate stromal development and ductal growth in the breast and are responsible for the accelerated growth phase and the closing of the epiphyses of the long bones that occur at puberty. They contribute to the growth of axillary and pubic hair and alter the distribution of body fat to produce typical female body contours. Larger quantities also stimulate development of pigmentation in the skin, most prominent in the region of the nipples and areolae and in the genital region.

C. ENDOMETRIAL EFFECTS

In addition to its growth effects on uterine muscle, estrogen also plays an important role in the development of the endometrial lining. When estrogen production is properly coordinated with the production of progesterone during the normal human menstrual cycle, regular periodic bleeding and shedding of the endometrial lining occur. Continuous exposure to estrogens for prolonged periods leads to hyperplasia of the endometrium that is usually associated with abnormal bleeding patterns.

D. METABOLIC AND CARDIOVASCULAR EFFECTS

Estrogens have a number of important metabolic and cardiovascular effects. They seem to be partially responsible for maintenance of the normal structure and function of the skin and blood vessels in women. Estrogens also decrease the rate of resorption of bone by promoting the apoptosis of osteoclasts and by antagonizing the osteoclastogenic and pro-osteoclastic effects of parathyroid hormone and interleukin-6. Estrogens also stimulate adipose tissue production of leptin and are in part responsible for the higher levels of this hormone in women than in men.

In addition to stimulating the synthesis of enzymes and growth factors leading to uterine and breast growth and differentiation, estrogens alter the production and activity of many other proteins in the body. Metabolic alterations in the liver are especially important, so that there is a higher circulating level of proteins such as transcortin (CBG), thyroxine-binding globulin (TBG), SHBG, transferrin, renin substrate, and fibrinogen. This leads to increased circulating levels of thyroxine, estrogen, testosterone, iron, copper, and other substances.

Alterations in the composition of the plasma lipids caused by estrogens are characterized by an increase in the high-density lipoproteins (HDL), a slight reduction in the low-density lipoproteins (LDL), and a reduction in total plasma cholesterol levels. Plasma triglyceride levels are increased. Estrogens decrease hepatic oxidation of adipose tissue lipid to ketones and increase synthesis of triglycerides.

E. Effects on Blood Coagulation

Estrogens enhance the coagulability of blood. Many changes in factors influencing coagulation have been reported, including increased circulating levels of factors II, VII, IX, and X and decreased antithrombin III, partially as a result of the hepatic effects mentioned above. Increased plasminogen levels and decreased platelet adhesiveness have also been found (see Hormonal Contraception, below).

F. Other Effects

Estrogens induce the synthesis of progesterone receptors. They are responsible for estrous behavior in animals and may influence behavior and libido in humans. Administration of estrogens stimulates central components of the stress system, including the production of corticotropin-releasing hormone and the activity of the sympathetic system, and promotes a sense of well-being when given to women who are estrogen-deficient. They also facilitate the loss of intravascular fluid into the extracellular space, producing edema. The resulting decrease in plasma volume causes a compensatory retention of sodium and water by the kidney. Estrogens also modulate sympathetic nervous system control of smooth muscle function.

Clinical Uses*

A. Primary Hypogonadism

Estrogens have been used extensively for replacement therapy in estrogen-deficient patients. The estrogen deficiency may be due to primary failure of development of the ovaries, premature menopause, castration, or menopause.

Treatment of primary hypogonadism is usually begun at 11–13 years of age in order to stimulate the development of secondary sex characteristics and menses, to stimulate optimal growth, to prevent osteoporosis and to avoid the psychologic consequences of delayed puberty and estrogen deficiency. Treatment attempts to mimic the physiology of puberty. It is initiated with small doses of estrogen (0.3 mg conjugated estrogens or 5–10 mcg ethinyl estradiol) on days 1–21 each

month and is slowly increased to adult doses and then maintained until the age of menopause (approximately 51 years of age). A progestin is added after the first uterine bleeding. When growth is completed, chronic therapy consists mainly of the administration of adult doses of both estrogens and progestins, as described below.

B. Postmenopausal Hormonal Therapy

In addition to the signs and symptoms that follow closely upon the cessation of normal ovarian function—such as loss of periods, vasomotor symptoms, sleep disturbances, and genital atrophy—there are longer-lasting changes that influence the health and well-being of postmenopausal women. These include an acceleration of bone loss, which in susceptible women may lead to vertebral, hip, and wrist fractures; and lipid changes, which may contribute to the acceleration of atherosclerotic cardiovascular disease noted in postmenopausal women. The effects of estrogens on bone have been extensively studied, and the effects of hormone withdrawal have been well-characterized. However, the role of estrogens and progestins in the cause and prevention of cardiovascular disease, which is responsible for 350,000 deaths per year, and breast cancer, which causes 35,000 deaths per year, is less well understood.

When normal ovulatory function ceases and the estrogen levels fall after menopause, oophorectomy, or premature ovarian failure, there is an accelerated rise in plasma cholesterol and LDL concentrations, while LDL receptors decline. HDL is not much affected, and levels remain higher than in men. Very-low-density lipoprotein and triglyceride levels are also relatively unaffected. Since cardiovascular disorders account for most deaths in this age group, the risk for these disorders constitutes a major consideration in deciding whether or not hormonal "replacement" therapy (HRT, also called HT) is indicated and influences the selection of hormones to be administered. Estrogen replacement therapy has a beneficial effect on circulating lipids and lipoproteins, and this was earlier thought to be accompanied by a reduction in myocardial infarction by about 50% and of fatal strokes by as much as 40%. These findings, however, have been recently disputed by the results of a large study from the Women's Health Initiative (WHI) project showing no cardiovascular benefit from estrogen plus progestin replacement therapy in perimenopausal or older postmenopausal patients. In fact, there may be a small increase in cardiovascular problems as well as breast cancer in women who received the replacement therapy. Interestingly, a small protective effect against colon cancer was observed. Although current clinical guidelines do not recommend routine hormone therapy in postmenopausal women, the validity of the WHI report has been questioned. Young women with premature menopause

---

*The use of estrogens in contraception is discussed below.

should definitely recieve HRT. In other recent studies, a protective effect of estrogen replacement therapy against Alzheimer's disease was observed.

Progestins antagonize estrogen's effects on LDL and HDL to a variable extent. However, one large study has shown that the addition of a progestin to estrogen replacement therapy does not influence the cardiovascular risk.

Optimal management of the postmenopausal patient requires careful assessment of her symptoms as well as consideration of her age and the presence of (or risks for) cardiovascular disease, osteoporosis, breast cancer, and endometrial cancer. Bearing in mind the effects of the gonadal hormones on each of these disorders, the goals of therapy can then be defined and the risks of therapy assessed and discussed with the patient.

If the main indication for therapy is hot flushes and sleep disturbances, therapy with the lowest dose of estrogen required for symptomatic relief is recommended. Treatment may be required for only a limited period of time and the possible increased risk for breast cancer avoided. In women who have undergone hysterectomy, estrogens alone can be given 5 days per week or continuously, since progestins are not required to reduce the risk for endometrial hyperplasia and cancer. Hot flushes, sweating, insomnia, and atrophic vaginitis are generally relieved by estrogens; many patients experience some increased sense of well-being; and climacteric depression and other psychopathologic states are improved.

The role of estrogens in the prevention and treatment of osteoporosis has been carefully studied (see Chapter 42). The amount of bone present in the body is maximal in the young active adult in the third decade of life and begins to decline more rapidly in middle age in both men and women. The development of osteoporosis also depends on the amount of bone present at the start of this process, on vitamin D and calcium intake, and on the degree of physical activity. The risk of osteoporosis is highest in smokers who are thin, Caucasian, and inactive and have a low calcium intake and a strong family history of osteoporosis. Depression also is a major risk factor for development of osteoporosis in women.

Estrogens should be used in the smallest dosage consistent with relief of symptoms. In women who have not undergone hysterectomy, it is most convenient to prescribe estrogen on the first 21–25 days of each month. The recommended dosages of estrogen are 0.3–1.25 mg/d of conjugated estrogen or 0.01–0.02 mg/d of ethinyl estradiol. Dosages in the middle of these ranges have been shown to be maximally effective in preventing the decrease in bone density occurring at menopause. From this point of view, it is important to begin therapy as soon as possible after the menopause for maximum effect. In these patients and others not taking estrogen, calcium supplements that bring the total daily calcium intake up to 1500 mg are useful.

Patients at low risk of developing osteoporosis who manifest only mild atrophic vaginitis can be treated with topical preparations. The vaginal route of application is also useful in the treatment of urinary tract symptoms in these patients. It is important to realize, however, that although locally administered estrogens escape the first-pass effect (so that some undesirable hepatic effects are reduced), they are almost completely absorbed into the circulation, and these preparations should be given cyclically.

As noted below, the administration of estrogen is associated with an increased risk of endometrial carcinoma. The administration of a progestational agent with the estrogen prevents endometrial hyperplasia and markedly reduces the risk of this cancer. When estrogen is given for the first 25 days of the month and the progestin medroxyprogesterone (10 mg/d) is added during the last 10–14 days, the risk is only half of that in women not receiving hormone replacement therapy. On this regimen, some women will experience a return of symptoms during the period off estrogen administration. In these patients, the estrogen can be given continuously. If the progestin produces sedation or other undesirable effects, its dose can be reduced to 2.5–5 mg for the last 10 days of the cycle with a slight increase in the risk for endometrial hyperplasia. These regimens are usually accompanied by bleeding at the end of each cycle. Some women experience migraine headaches during the last few days of the cycle. The use of a continuous estrogen regimen will often prevent their occurrence. Women who object to the cyclic bleeding associated with sequential therapy can also consider continuous therapy. Daily therapy with 0.625 mg of conjugated equine estrogens and 2.5–5 mg of medroxyprogesterone will eliminate cyclic bleeding, control vasomotor symptoms, prevent genital atrophy, maintain bone density, and show a favorable lipid profile with a small decrease in LDL and an increase in HDL concentrations. These women have endometrial atrophy on biopsy. About half of these patients experience breakthrough bleeding during the first few months of therapy. Seventy to 80 percent become amenorrheic after the first 4 months, and most remain so. The main disadvantage of continuous therapy is the need for uterine biopsy if bleeding occurs after the first few months.

As noted above, estrogens may also be administered vaginally or transdermally. When estrogens are given by these routes, the liver is bypassed on the first circulation, and the ratio of the liver effects to peripheral effects is reduced.

In patients in whom estrogen replacement therapy is contraindicated, such as those with estrogen-sensitive tumors, relief of vasomotor symptoms may be obtained by the use of clonidine.

C. OTHER USES

Estrogens combined with progestins can be used to suppress ovulation in patients with intractable dysmenorrhea or when suppression of ovarian function is used in the treatment of hirsutism and amenorrhea due to excessive secretion of androgens by the ovary. Under these circumstances, greater suppression may be needed, and oral contraceptives containing 50 mcg of estrogen or a combination of a low estrogen pill with GnRH suppression may be required.

Adverse Effects

Adverse effects of variable severity have been reported with the therapeutic use of estrogens. Many other effects reported in conjunction with hormonal contraceptives may be related to their estrogen content. These are discussed below.

A. UTERINE BLEEDING

Estrogen therapy is a major cause of postmenopausal uterine bleeding. Unfortunately, vaginal bleeding at this time of life may also be due to carcinoma of the endometrium. In order to avoid confusion, patients should be treated with the smallest amount of estrogen possible. It should be given cyclically so that bleeding, if it occurs, will be more likely to occur during the withdrawal period. As noted above, endometrial hyperplasia can be prevented by administration of a progestational agent with estrogen in each cycle.

B. CANCER

The relation of estrogen therapy to cancer continues to be the subject of active investigation. Although no adverse effect of short-term estrogen therapy on the incidence of breast cancer has been demonstrated, a small increase in the incidence of this tumor may occur with prolonged therapy. Although the risk factor is small (1.25), the impact may be great since this tumor occurs in 10% of women, and addition of progesterone does not confer a protective effect. Studies indicate that following unilateral excision of breast cancer, women receiving tamoxifen (an estrogen partial agonist, see below) show a 35% decrease in contralateral breast cancer compared with controls. These studies also demonstrate that tamoxifen is well tolerated by most patients, produces estrogen-like alterations in plasma lipid levels, and stabilizes bone mineral loss. Studies bearing on the possible efficacy of tamoxifen in postmenopausal women at high risk for breast cancer are under way. A recent study shows that postmenopausal hormone replacement therapy with estrogens plus progestins was associated with greater breast epithelial cell proliferation and breast epithelial cell density than estrogens alone or no replacement therapy. Furthermore, with estrogens plus progestins, breast proliferation was localized to the terminal duct-lobular unit of the breast, which is the main site of development of breast cancer. Thus, further studies are needed to conclusively assess the possible association between progestins and breast cancer risk.

Many studies show an increased risk of endometrial carcinoma in patients taking estrogens alone. The risk seems to vary with the dose and duration of treatment: 15 times greater in patients taking large doses of estrogen for 5 or more years, in contrast with two to four times greater in patients receiving lower doses for short periods. However, as noted above, the concomitant use of a progestin prevents this increased risk and may in fact reduce the incidence of endometrial cancer to less than that in the general population.

There have been a number of reports of adenocarcinoma of the vagina in young women whose mothers were treated with large doses of diethylstilbestrol early in pregnancy. These cancers are most common in young women (ages 14–44). The incidence is less than 1 per 1000 women exposed—too low to establish a cause-and-effect relationship with certainty. However, the risks for infertility, ectopic pregnancy, and premature delivery are also increased. It is now recognized that there is no indication for the use of diethylstilbestrol during pregnancy, and it should be avoided. It is not known whether other estrogens have a similar effect or whether the observed phenomena are peculiar to diethylstilbestrol. This agent should be used only in the treatment of cancer (eg, of the prostate) or as a "morning after" contraceptive (see below).

C. OTHER EFFECTS

Nausea and breast tenderness are common and can be minimized by using the smallest effective dose of estrogen. Hyperpigmentation also occurs. Estrogen therapy is associated with an increase in frequency of migraine headaches as well as cholestasis, gallbladder disease, and hypertension.

Contraindications

Estrogens should not be used in patients with estrogen-dependent neoplasms such as carcinoma of the endometrium or in those with—or at high risk for—carcinoma of the breast. They should be avoided in patients with undiagnosed genital bleeding, liver disease, or a history of thromboembolic disorder. In addition, the use of estrogens should be avoided by heavy smokers.

Preparations & Dosages

The dosages of commonly used natural and synthetic preparations are listed in Table 40–1. Although all of the estrogens produce almost the same hormonal effects, their potencies vary both between agents and depending on the route of administration. As noted above, estradiol is the most active endogenous estrogen, and it has the highest affinity for the estrogen receptor. However, its metabolites estrone and estriol have weak uterine effects.

For a given level of gonadotropin suppression, oral estrogen preparations have more effect on the circulating levels of CBG, SHBG, and a host of other liver proteins, including angiotensinogen, than do transdermal preparations. The oral route of administration allows greater concentrations of hormone to reach the liver, thus increasing the synthesis of these proteins. Transdermal preparations were developed to avoid this effect. When administered transdermally, 50–100 mcg of estradiol has effects similar to those of 0.625–1.25 mg of conjugated oral estrogens on gonadotropin concentrations, endometrium, and vaginal epithelium. Furthermore, the transdermal estrogen preparations do not significantly increase the concentrations of renin substrate, CBG, and TBG and do not produce the characteristic changes in serum lipids. Combined oral preparations containing 0.625 mg of conjugated estrogens and 2.5 mg of medroxyprogesterone acetate are available for menopausal replacement therapy. Tablets containing 0.625 of conjugated estrogens and 5 mg of medroxyprogesterone acetate are available to be used in conjunction with conjugated estrogens in a sequential fashion. Estrogens alone are taken on days 1–14 and the combination on days 15–28.

THE PROGESTINS

Natural Progestins: Progesterone

Progesterone is the most important progestin in humans. In addition to having important hormonal effects, it serves as a precursor to the estrogens, androgens, and adrenocortical steroids. It is synthesized in the ovary, testis, and adrenal from circulating cholesterol. Large amounts are also synthesized and released by the placenta during pregnancy.

In the ovary, progesterone is produced primarily by the corpus luteum. Normal males appear to secrete 1–5 mg of progesterone daily, resulting in plasma levels of about 0.03 mcg/dL. The level is only slightly higher in the female during the follicular phase of the cycle, when only a few milligrams per day of progesterone are secreted. During the luteal phase, plasma levels range from 0.5 mcg/dL to more than 2 mcg/dL (Figure 40–1). Plasma levels of progesterone are further elevated and reach their peak levels in the third trimester of pregnancy.

Synthetic Progestins

A variety of progestational compounds have been synthesized. Some are active when given by mouth. They are not a uniform group of compounds, and all of them differ from progesterone in one or more respects. Table 40–2 lists some of these compounds and their effects. In general, the 21-carbon compounds (hydroxyprogesterone, medroxyprogesterone, megestrol, and dimethisterone) are the most closely related, pharmacologically as well as chemically, to progesterone. A new group of third-generation synthetic progestins has been introduced, principally as components of oral contraceptives. These "19-nor, 13-ethyl" steroid compounds include desogestrel (Figure 40–4), gestodene, and norgestimate. They are claimed to have lower androgenic activity than older synthetic progestins.

Pharmacokinetics

Progesterone is rapidly absorbed following administration by any route. Its half-life in the plasma is approximately 5 minutes, and small amounts are stored temporarily in body fat. It is almost completely metabolized in one passage through the liver, and for that reason it is quite ineffective when the usual formulation is administered orally. However, high-dose oral micronized progesterone preparations have been developed that provide adequate progestational effect.

In the liver, progesterone is metabolized to pregnanediol and conjugated with glucuronic acid. It is excreted into the urine as pregnanediol glucuronide. The amount of pregnanediol in the urine has been used as an index of progesterone secretion. This measure has been very useful in spite of the fact that the proportion of secreted progesterone converted to this compound varies from day to day and from individual to individual. In addition to progesterone, 20α- and 20β-hydroxyprogesterone (20α- and 20β-hydroxy-4-pregnene-3-one) are also found. These compounds have about one fifth the progestational activity of progesterone in humans and other species. Little is known of their physiologic role, but 20α-hydroxyprogesterone is produced in large amounts in some species and may be of some importance biologically.

The usual routes of administration and durations of action of the synthetic progestins are listed in Table 40–2. Most of these agents are extensively metabolized to inactive products that are excreted mainly in the urine.

Physiologic Effects

A. MECHANISM

The mechanism of action of progesterone—described in more detail above—is similar to that of other steroid hormones. Progestins enter the cell and bind to progesterone receptors that are distributed between the nucleus and the cytoplasm. The ligand-receptor complex binds

Table 40–2. Properties of some progestational agents.

	Route	Duration of Action	Estro-genic	Andro-genic	Anties-trogenic	Antian-drogenic	Anabolic
Progesterone and derivatives							
Progesterone	IM	1 day	–	–	+	–	–
Hydroxyprogesterone caproate	IM	8–14 days	sl	sl	–	–	–
Medroxyprogesterone acetate	IM, PO	Tabs: 1–3 days; in-jection: 4–12 weeks	–	+	+	–	–
Megestrol acetate	PO	1–3 days	–	+	–	+	–
17-Ethinyl testosterone derivatives							
Dimethisterone	PO	1–3 days	–	–	sl	–	–
19-Nortestosterone derivatives							
Desogestrel	PO	1–3 days	–	–	–	–	–
Norethynodrel[2]	PO	1–3 days	+	–	–	–	–
Lynestrenol[3]	PO	1–3 days	+	+	–	–	+
Norethindrone[2]	PO	1–3 days	sl	+	+	–	+
Norethindrone acetate[2]	PO	1–3 days	sl	+	+	–	+
Ethynodiol diacetate[2]	PO	1–3 days	sl	+	+	–	–
L-Norgestrel[2]	PO	1–3 days	–	+	+	–	+

The "Activities[1]" header spans the columns: Estrogenic, Androgenic, Antiestrogenic, Antiandrogenic, Anabolic.

[1]**Interpretation:** + = active; – = inactive; sl = slightly active. Activities have been reported in various species using various end points and may not apply to humans.
[2]See Table 40–3.
[3]Not available in USA.

Figure 40–4. Progesterone and some progestational agents in clinical use.

to a progesterone response element (PRE) to activate gene transcription. The response element for progesterone appears to be similar to the corticosteroid response element, and the specificity of the response depends upon which receptor is present in the cell as well as upon other cell-specific receptor coregulators and interacting transcription factors. The progesterone-receptor complex forms a dimer before binding to DNA. Like the estrogen receptor, it can form heterodimers as well as homodimers between two isoforms: A and B. These isoforms are produced by alternative splicing of the same gene.

B. EFFECTS OF PROGESTERONE

Progesterone has little effect on protein metabolism. It stimulates lipoprotein lipase activity and seems to favor fat deposition. The effects on carbohydrate metabolism are more marked. Progesterone increases basal insulin levels and the insulin response to glucose. There is usually no manifest change in carbohydrate tolerance. In the liver, progesterone promotes glycogen storage, possibly by facilitating the effect of insulin. Progesterone also promotes ketogenesis.

Progesterone can compete with aldosterone for the mineralocorticoid receptor of the renal tubule, causing a decrease in Na^+ reabsorption. This leads to an increased secretion of aldosterone by the adrenal cortex (eg, in pregnancy). Progesterone increases body temperature in humans. The mechanism of this effect is not known, but an alteration of the temperature-regulating centers in the hypothalamus has been suggested. Progesterone also alters the function of the respiratory centers. The ventilatory response to CO_2 is increased (synthetic progestins with an ethinyl group do not have respiratory effects). This leads to a measurable reduction in arterial and alveolar P_{CO_2} during pregnancy and in the luteal phase of the menstrual cycle. Progesterone and related steroids also have depressant and hypnotic effects on the brain.

Progesterone is responsible for the alveolobular development of the secretory apparatus in the breast. It also participates in the preovulatory LH surge and causes the maturation and secretory changes in the endometrium that are seen following ovulation (Figure 40–1).

Progesterone decreases the plasma levels of many amino acids and leads to increased urinary nitrogen excretion. It induces changes in the structure and function of smooth endoplasmic reticulum in experimental animals.

Other effects of progesterone and its analogs are noted below in the section on Hormonal Contraception.

C. SYNTHETIC PROGESTINS

The 21-carbon progesterone analogs antagonize aldosterone-induced sodium retention (see above). The remaining compounds ("19-nortestosterone" third-generation agents) produce a decidual change in the endometrial stroma, do not support pregnancy in test animals, are more effective gonadotropin inhibitors, and may have minimal estrogenic and androgenic or anabolic activity (Table 40–2, Figure 40–4). They are sometimes referred to as "impeded androgens." Progestins without androgenic activity include desogestrel, norgestimate, and gestodene. The first two of these compounds are dispensed in combination with ethinyl estradiol for oral contraception (Table 40–3) in the USA. Oral contraceptives containing the progestins cyproterone acetate (also an antiandrogen) in combination with ethinyl estradiol are investigational in the USA.

Clinical Uses of Progestins

A. THERAPEUTIC APPLICATIONS

The major uses of progestational hormones are for hormone replacement therapy (see above) and hormonal contraception (see below). In addition, they are useful in producing long-term ovarian suppression for other purposes. When used alone in large doses parenterally (eg, medroxyprogesterone acetate, 150 mg intramuscularly every 90 days), prolonged anovulation and amenorrhea result. This therapy has been employed in the treatment of dysmenorrhea, endometriosis, and bleeding disorders when estrogens are contraindicated, and for contraception. The major problem with this regimen is the prolonged time required in some patients for ovulatory function to return after cessation of therapy. It should not be used for patients planning a pregnancy in the near future. Similar regimens will relieve hot flushes in some menopausal women and can be used if estrogen therapy is contraindicated.

Medroxyprogesterone acetate, 10–20 mg orally twice weekly—or intramuscularly in doses of 100 mg/m^2 every 1–2 weeks—will prevent menstruation, but it will not arrest accelerated bone maturation in children with precocious puberty.

Progestins do not appear to have any place in the therapy of threatened or habitual abortion. Early reports of the usefulness of these agents resulted from the unwarranted assumption that after several abortions the likelihood of repeated abortions was over 90%. When progestational agents were administered to patients with previous abortions, a salvage rate of 80% was achieved. It is now recognized that similar patients abort only 20% of the time even when untreated. On the other hand, progesterone was experimentally given recently to delay premature labor with encouraging results.

Progesterone and medroxyprogesterone have been used in the treatment of women who have difficulty in conceiving and who demonstrate a slow rise in basal body temperature. There is no convincing evidence that this treatment is effective.

Preparations of progesterone and medroxyprogesterone have been used to treat premenstrual syndrome. Controlled studies have not confirmed the effectiveness of such therapy except when doses sufficient to suppress ovulation have been used.

B. Diagnostic Uses

Progesterone can be used as a test of estrogen secretion. The administration of progesterone, 150 mg/d, or medroxyprogesterone, 10 mg/d, for 5–7 days, is followed by withdrawal bleeding in amenorrheic patients only when the endometrium has been stimulated by estrogens. A combination of estrogen and progestin can be given to test the responsiveness of the endometrium in patients with amenorrhea.

Contraindications, Cautions, & Adverse Effects

Studies of progestational compounds alone and with combination oral contraceptives indicate that the progestin in these agents may increase blood pressure in some patients. The more androgenic progestins also reduce plasma HDL levels in women. (See Hormonal Contraception, below.) Two recent studies suggest that combined progestin plus estrogen replacement therapy in postmenopausal women may increase breast cancer risk significantly compared with the risk in women taking estrogen alone. These findings require careful examination and if confirmed will lead to important changes in postmenopausal hormone replacement practice.

OTHER OVARIAN HORMONES

The normal ovary produces small amounts of **androgens,** including testosterone, androstenedione, and dehydroepiandrosterone. Of these, only testosterone has a significant amount of biologic activity, although androstenedione can be converted to testosterone or estrone in peripheral tissues. The normal woman produces less than 200 mcg of testosterone in 24 hours, and about one third of this is probably formed in the ovary directly. The physiologic significance of these small amounts of androgens is not established, but they may be partly responsible for normal hair growth at puberty, for stimulation of female libido, and, possibly, for metabolic effects. Androgen production by the ovary may be markedly increased in some abnormal states, usually in association with hirsutism and amenorrhea as noted above.

The ovary also produces **inhibin** and **activin.** These peptides consist of several combinations of α and β subunits and are described in greater detail later. The αβ dimer (inhibin) inhibits FSH secretion while the ββ dimer (activin) increases FSH secretion. Studies in primates indicate that inhibin has no direct effect on ovarian steroidogenesis but that activin modulates the response to LH and FSH. For example, simultaneous treatment with activin and human FSH enhances FSH stimulation of progesterone synthesis and aromatase activity in granulosa cells. When combined with LH, activin suppressed the LH-induced progesterone response by 50% but markedly enhanced basal and LH-stimulated aromatase activity. Activin may also act as a growth factor in other tissues. The physiologic roles of these modulators are not fully understood.

Relaxin is another peptide that can be extracted from the ovary. The three-dimensional structure of relaxin is related to that of growth-promoting peptides and is similar to that of insulin. Although the amino acid sequence differs from that of insulin, this hormone, like insulin, consists of two chains linked by disulfide bonds, cleaved from a prohormone. It is found in the ovary, placenta, uterus, and blood. Relaxin synthesis has been demonstrated in luteinized granulosa cells of the corpus luteum. It has been shown to increase glycogen synthesis and water uptake by the myometrium and decreases uterine contractility. In some species, it changes the mechanical properties of the cervix and pubic ligaments, facilitating delivery.

In women, relaxin has been measured by immunoassay. Levels were highest immediately after the LH surge and during menstruation. A physiologic role for this peptide has not been established.

Clinical trials with relaxin have been conducted in patients with dysmenorrhea. Relaxin has also been administered to patients in premature labor and during prolonged labor. When applied to the cervix of a woman at term, it facilitates dilation and shortens labor.

Several other nonsteroidal substances such as corticotropin-releasing hormone, follistatin, and prostaglandins are produced by the ovary. These probably have paracrine effects within the ovary.

HORMONAL CONTRACEPTION (ORAL, PARENTERAL, & IMPLANTED CONTRACEPTIVES)

A large number of oral contraceptives containing estrogens or progestins (or both) are now available for clinical use (Table 40–3). These preparations vary chemically and pharmacologically and have many properties in common as well as definite differences important for the correct selection of the optimum agent.

Two types of preparations are used for oral contraception: (1) combinations of estrogens and progestins and (2) continuous progestin therapy without concomitant administration of estrogens. The combination agents are further divided into **monophasic** forms (constant dosage

Table 40–3. Some oral and implantable contraceptive agents in use. The estrogen-containing compounds are arranged in order of increasing content of estrogen. (Ethinyl estradiol and mestranol have similar potencies.)

	Estrogen (mg)		Progestin (mg)	
Monophasic combination tablets				
Alesse, Aviane, Lessinea, Levlite	Ethinyl estradiol	0.02	L-Norgestrel	0.1
Levlen, Levora, Nordette, Portia	Ethinyl estradiol	0.03	L-Norgestrel	0.15
Crysella, Lo-Ovral, Low-Ogestrel	Ethinyl estradiol	0.03	Norgestrel	0.30
Yasmin	Ethinyl estradiol	0.03	Drospirenone	3.0
Brevicon, Modicon, Necon 0.5/35, Nortrel 0.5/35	Ethinyl estradiol	0.035	Norethindrone	0.5
Ortho-Cyclen, Sprintec	Ethinyl estradiol	0.035	Norgestimate	0.25
Necon 1/35, Norinyl 1+, Nortrel 1/35, Ortho-Novum 1/35	Ethinyl estradiol	0.035	Norethindrone	1.0
Ovcon-35	Ethinyl estradiol	0.035	Norethindrone	0.4
Demulen 1/50	Ethinyl estradiol	0.05	Ethynodiol diacetate	1.0
Ovcon 50	Ethinyl estradiol	0.05	Norethindrone	1.0
Ovral-28	Ethinyl estradiol	0.05	D,L-Norgestrel	0.5
Norinyl 1/50, Ortho-Novum 1/50	Mestranol	0.05	Norethindrone	1.0
Biphasic combination tablets				
Ortho-Novum 10/11, Necon 10/11				
Days 1–10	Ethinyl estradiol	0.035	Norethindrone	0.5
Days 11–21	Ethinyl estradiol	0.035	Norethindrone	1.0
Triphasic combination tablets				
Enpresse, Triphasil, Tri-Levlen, Trivora				
Days 1–6	Ethinyl estradiol	0.03	L-Norgestrel	0.05
Days 7–11	Ethinyl estradiol	0.04	L-Norgestrel	0.075
Days 12–21	Ethinyl estradiol	0.03	L-Norgestrel	0.125
Ortho-Novum 7/7/7, Necon 7/7/7				
Days 1–7	Ethinyl estradiol	0.035	Norethindrone	0.5
Days 8–14	Ethinyl estradiol	0.035	Norethindrone	0.75
Days 15–21	Ethinyl estradiol	0.035	Norethindrone	1.0
Ortho-Tri-Cyclen				
Days 1–7	Ethinyl estradiol	0.035	Norgestimate	0.18
Days 8–14	Ethinyl estradiol	0.035	Norgestimate	0.215
Days 15–21	Ethinyl estradiol	0.035	Norgestimate	0.25
Daily progestin tablets				
Micronor, Nor-QD, Ortho Micronor, Nor-QD, Camila, Errin			Norethindrone	0.35
Ovrette			D,L-Norgestrel	0.075
Implantable progestin preparation				
Norplant System	. . .		L-Norgestrel (six tubes of 36 mg each)	

of both components during the cycle) and **biphasic** or **triphasic** forms (dosage of one or both components is changed once or twice during the cycle). The preparations for oral use are all adequately absorbed, and in combination preparations the pharmacokinetics of neither drug is significantly altered by the other.

Few implantable contraceptive preparations are available at present in the USA. Norgestrel, also used in some oral contraceptives, is available in the subcutaneous implant form listed in Table 40–3, and has been available for several years. An implant containing etonogestrel, a newer progestin, is available overseas and will be marketed in the USA as Implanon. Several hormonal contraceptives are available as vaginal rings or intrauterine devices. Intramuscular injection of large doses of medroxyprogesterone also provides contraception of long duration.

Pharmacologic Effects

A. MECHANISM OF ACTION

The combinations of estrogens and progestins exert their contraceptive effect largely through selective inhibition of pituitary function that results in inhibition of ovulation. The combination agents also produce a change in the cervical mucus, in the uterine endometrium, and in motility and secretion in the uterine tubes, all of which decrease the likelihood of conception and implantation. The continuous use of progestins alone does not always inhibit ovulation. The other factors mentioned, therefore, play a major role in the prevention of pregnancy when these agents are used.

B. EFFECTS ON THE OVARY

Chronic use of combination agents depresses ovarian function. Follicular development is minimal, and corpora lutea, larger follicles, stromal edema, and other morphologic features normally seen in ovulating women are absent. The ovaries usually become smaller even when enlarged before therapy.

The great majority of patients return to normal menstrual patterns when these drugs are discontinued. About 75% will ovulate in the first posttreatment cycle and 97% by the third posttreatment cycle. About 2% of patients remain amenorrheic for periods of up to several years after administration is stopped.

The cytologic findings on vaginal smears vary depending on the preparation used. However, with almost all of the combined drugs, a low maturation index is found because of the presence of progestational agents.

C. EFFECTS ON THE UTERUS

After prolonged use, the cervix may show some hypertrophy and polyp formation. There are also important effects on the cervical mucus, making it more like postovulation mucus, ie, thicker and less copious.

Agents containing both estrogens and progestins produce further morphologic and biochemical changes of the endometrial stroma under the influence of the progestin, which also stimulates glandular secretion throughout the luteal phase. The agents containing "19-nor" progestins—particularly those with the smaller amounts of estrogen—tend to produce more glandular atrophy and usually less bleeding.

D. EFFECTS ON THE BREAST

Stimulation of the breasts occurs in most patients receiving estrogen-containing agents. Some enlargement is generally noted. The administration of estrogens and combinations of estrogens and progestins tends to suppress lactation. When the doses are small, the effects on breast feeding are not appreciable. Studies of the transport of the oral contraceptives into breast milk suggest that only small amounts of these compounds cross into the milk, and they have not been considered to be of importance.

E. OTHER EFFECTS OF ORAL CONTRACEPTIVES

1. Effects on the central nervous system—The central nervous system effects of the oral contraceptives have not been well studied in humans. A variety of effects of estrogen and progesterone have been noted in animals. Estrogens tend to increase excitability in the brain, whereas progesterone tends to decrease it. The thermogenic action of progesterone and some of the synthetic progestins is also thought to occur in the central nervous system.

It is very difficult to evaluate any behavioral or emotional effects of these compounds in humans. Although the incidence of pronounced changes in mood, affect, and behavior appears to be low, milder changes are commonly reported, and estrogens are being successfully employed in the therapy of premenstrual tension syndrome, postpartum depression, and climacteric depression.

2. Effects on endocrine function—The inhibition of pituitary gonadotropin secretion has been mentioned. Estrogens also alter adrenal structure and function. Estrogens given orally or at high doses increase the plasma concentration of the α_2 globulin that binds cortisol (corticosteroid-binding globulin). Plasma concentrations may be more than double the levels found in untreated individuals, and urinary excretion of free cortisol is elevated.

These preparations cause alterations in the renin-angiotensin-aldosterone system. Plasma renin activity has been found to increase, and there is an increase in aldosterone secretion.

Thyroxine-binding globulin is increased. As a result, total plasma thyroxine (T_4) levels are increased to those commonly seen during pregnancy. Since more of the thyroxine is bound, the free thyroxine level in these patients is normal. Estrogens also increase the plasma level of SHBG and decrease plasma levels of free androgens by increasing their binding; large amounts of estrogen may decrease androgens by gonadotropin suppression.

3. Effects on blood—Serious thromboembolic phenomena occurring in women taking oral contraceptives gave rise to a great many studies of the effects of these compounds on blood coagulation. A clear picture of such effects has not yet emerged. The oral contraceptives do not consistently alter bleeding or clotting times. The changes that have been observed are similar to those reported in pregnancy. There is an increase in factors VII, VIII, IX, and X and a decrease in antithrombin III. Increased amounts of coumarin anticoagulants may be required to prolong prothrombin time in patients taking oral contraceptives.

There is an increase in serum iron and total ironbinding capacity similar to that reported in patients with hepatitis.

Significant alterations in the cellular components of blood have not been reported with any consistency. A number of patients have been reported to develop folic acid deficiency anemias.

4. Effects on the liver—These hormones also have profound effects on the function of the liver. Some of these effects are deleterious and will be considered below in the section on adverse effects.

The effects on serum proteins result from the effects of the estrogens on the synthesis of the various α_2 globulins and fibrinogen. Serum haptoglobins produced in the liver are depressed rather than increased by estrogen.

Some of the effects on carbohydrate and lipid metabolism are probably influenced by changes in liver metabolism (see below).

Important alterations in hepatic drug excretion and metabolism also occur. Estrogens in the amounts seen during pregnancy or used in oral contraceptive agents delay the clearance of sulfobromophthalein and reduce the flow of bile. The proportion of cholic acid in bile acids is increased while the proportion of chenodeoxycholic acid is decreased. These changes may be responsible for the observed increase in cholelithiasis associated with the use of these agents.

5. Effects on lipid metabolism—As noted above, estrogens increase serum triglycerides and free and esterified cholesterol. Phospholipids are also increased, as are HDL; levels of LDL usually decrease. Although the effects are marked with doses of 100 mcg of mestranol or ethinyl estradiol, doses of 50 mcg or less have minimal effects. The progestins (particularly the "19-nortestosterone" derivatives) tend to antagonize these effects of estrogen. Preparations containing small amounts of estrogen and a progestin may slightly decrease triglycerides and HDL.

6. Effects on carbohydrate metabolism—The administration of oral contraceptives produces alterations in carbohydrate metabolism similar to those observed in pregnancy. There is a reduction in the rate of absorption of carbohydrates from the gastrointestinal tract. Progesterone increases the basal insulin level and the rise in insulin induced by carbohydrate ingestion. Preparations with more potent progestins such as norgestrel may cause progressive decreases in carbohydrate tolerance over several years. However, the changes in glucose tolerance are reversible on discontinuing medication.

7. Effects on the cardiovascular system—These agents cause small increases in cardiac output associated with higher systolic and diastolic blood pressure and heart rate. The pressure returns to normal when treatment is terminated. Although the magnitude of the pressure change is small in most patients, it is marked in a few. It is important that blood pressure be followed in each patient. An increase in blood pressure has been reported to occur in few postmenopausal women treated with estrogens alone.

8. Effects on the skin—The oral contraceptives have been noted to increase pigmentation of the skin (chloasma). This effect seems to be enhanced in women with dark complexions and by exposure to ultraviolet light. Some of the androgen-like progestins might increase the production of sebum, causing acne in some patients. However, since ovarian androgen is suppressed, many patients note decreased sebum production, acne, and terminal hair growth. The sequential oral contraceptive preparations as well as estrogens alone often decrease sebum production.

Clinical Uses

The most important use of combined estrogens and progestins is for oral contraception. A large number of preparations are available for this specific purpose, some of which are listed in Table 40–3. They are specially packaged for ease of administration. In general, they are very effective; when these agents are taken according to directions, the risk of conception is extremely small. The pregnancy rate with combination agents is estimated to be about 0.5–1 per 100 woman years at risk. Contraceptive failure has been observed in some patients when one or more doses are missed, if phenytoin is also being used (which may increase catabolism of the compounds), or if antibiotics are taken that alter enterohepatic cycling of metabolites.

Progestins and estrogens are also useful in the treatment of endometriosis. When severe dysmenorrhea is the major symptom, the suppression of ovulation with estrogen alone may be followed by painless periods. However, in most patients this approach to therapy is inadequate. The long-term administration of large doses of progestins or combinations of progestins and estrogens prevents the periodic breakdown of the endometrial tissue and in some cases will lead to endometrial fibrosis and prevent the reactivation of implants for prolonged periods.

As is true with most hormonal preparations, many of the undesired effects are physiologic or pharmacologic actions that are objectionable only because they are not pertinent to the situation for which they are being used. Therefore, the product containing the smallest effective amounts of hormones should be selected for use.

Adverse Effects

The incidence of serious known toxicities associated with the use of these drugs is low—far lower than the risks associated with pregnancy. There are a number of reversible changes in intermediary metabolism. Minor adverse effects are frequent, but most are mild and many are transient. Continuing problems may respond to simple changes in pill formulation. Although it is not often necessary to discontinue medication for these reasons, as many as one third of all patients started on oral contraception discontinue use for reasons other than a desire to become pregnant.

A. Mild Adverse Effects

1. Nausea, mastalgia, breakthrough bleeding, and edema are related to the amount of estrogen in the preparation. These effects can often be alleviated by a shift to a preparation containing smaller amounts of estrogen or to agents containing progestins with more androgenic effects.

2. Changes in serum proteins and other effects on endocrine function (see above) must be taken into account when thyroid, adrenal, or pituitary function is being evaluated. Increases in sedimentation rate are thought to be due to increased levels of fibrinogen.

3. Headache is mild and often transient. However, migraine is often made worse and has been reported to be associated with an increased frequency of cerebrovascular accidents. When this occurs or when migraine has its onset during therapy with these agents, treatment should be discontinued.

4. Withdrawal bleeding sometimes fails to occur—most often with combination preparations—and may cause confusion with regard to pregnancy. If this is disturbing to the patient, a different preparation may be tried or other methods of contraception used.

B. Moderate Adverse Effects

Any of the following may require discontinuance of oral contraceptives:

1. Breakthrough bleeding is the most common problem in using progestational agents alone for contraception. It occurs in as many as 25% of patients. It is

more frequently encountered in patients taking low-dose preparations than in those taking combination pills with higher levels of progestin and estrogen. The biphasic and triphasic oral contraceptives (Table 40–3) decrease breakthrough bleeding without increasing the total hormone content.

2. Weight gain is more common with the combination agents containing androgen-like progestins. It can usually be controlled by shifting to preparations with less progestin effect or by dieting.

3. Increased skin pigmentation may occur, especially in dark-skinned women. It tends to increase with time, the incidence being about 5% at the end of the first year and about 40% after 8 years. It is thought to be exacerbated by vitamin B deficiency. It is often reversible upon discontinuance of medication but may disappear very slowly.

4. Acne may be exacerbated by agents containing androgen-like progestins (Table 40–2), whereas agents containing large amounts of estrogen usually cause marked improvement in acne.

5. Hirsutism may also be aggravated by the "19-nortestosterone" derivatives, and combinations containing nonandrogenic progestins are preferred in these patients.

6. Ureteral dilation similar to that observed in pregnancy has been reported, and bacteriuria is more frequent.

7. Vaginal infections are more common and more difficult to treat in patients who are receiving oral contraceptives.

8. Amenorrhea occurs in some patients. Following cessation of administration of oral contraceptives, 95% of patients with normal menstrual histories resume normal periods and all but a few resume normal cycles during the next few months. However, some patients remain amenorrheic for several years. Many of these patients also have galactorrhea. Patients who have had menstrual irregularities before taking oral contraceptives are particularly susceptible to prolonged amenorrhea when the agents are discontinued. Prolactin levels should be measured in these patients, since many have prolactinomas.

C. Severe Adverse Effects

1. Vascular disorders—Thromboembolism was one of the earliest of the serious unanticipated effects to be reported and has been the most thoroughly studied.

a. Venous thromboembolic disease—Superficial or deep thromboembolic disease in women not taking oral contraceptives occurs in about one patient per 1000 woman years. The overall incidence of these disorders in patients taking low-dose oral contraceptives is about threefold higher. The risk for this disorder is increased during the first month of contraceptive use and remains constant for several years or more. The risk returns to normal within a month when use is discontinued. The risk of venous thrombosis or pulmonary embolism is increased among women with predisposing conditions such as stasis, altered clotting factors such as antithrombin III, increased levels of homocysteine, or injury. Genetic disorders, including mutations in the genes governing the production of protein C (factor V Leiden), protein S, hepatic cofactor II, and others, markedly increase the risk of venous thromboembolism. The incidence of these disorders is too low for cost-effective screening by current methods, but prior episodes or a family history may be helpful in identifying patients with increased risk.

The incidence of venous thromboembolism appears to be related to the estrogen but not the progestin content of oral contraceptives and is not related to age, parity, mild obesity, or cigarette smoking. Decreased venous blood flow, endothelial proliferation in veins and arteries, and increased coagulability of blood resulting from changes in platelet functions and fibrinolytic systems contribute to the increased incidence of thrombosis. The major plasma inhibitor of thrombin, antithrombin III, is substantially decreased during oral contraceptive use. This change occurs in the first month of treatment and lasts as long as treatment persists, reversing within a month thereafter.

b. Myocardial infarction—The use of oral contraceptives is associated with a slightly higher risk of myocardial infarction in women who are obese, have a history of preeclampsia or hypertension, or have hyperlipoproteinemia or diabetes. There is a much higher risk in women who smoke. The risk attributable to oral contraceptives in women 30–40 years of age who do not smoke is about 4 cases per 100,000 users per year, as compared with 185 cases per 100,000 among women 40–44 who smoke heavily. The association with myocardial infarction is thought to involve acceleration of atherogenesis because of decreased glucose tolerance, decreased levels of HDL, increased levels of LDL, and increased platelet aggregation. In addition, facilitation of coronary arterial spasm may play a role in some of these patients. The progestational component of oral contraceptives decreases HDL cholesterol levels, in proportion to the androgenic activity of the progestin. The net effect, therefore, will depend on the specific composition of the pill used and the patient's susceptibility to the particular effects. Recent studies suggest that risk of infarction is not increased in past users who have discontinued oral contraceptives.

c. Cerebrovascular disease—The risk of strokes is concentrated in women over age 35. It is increased in current users of oral contraceptives but not in past users. However, subarachnoid hemorrhages have been found to be increased among both current and past users and may increase with time. The risk of thrombotic or hemorrhagic stroke attributable to oral contraceptives (based on older, higher-dose preparations) has been estimated to about 37 cases per 100,000 users per year.

In summary, available data indicate that oral contraceptives increase the risk of various cardiovascular disorders at all ages and among both smokers and nonsmokers. However, this risk appears to be concentrated in women 35 years of age or older who are heavy smokers. It is clear that these risk factors must be considered in each individual patient for whom oral contraceptives are being considered. Some experts have suggested that screening for coagulopathy should be performed before starting oral contraception.

2. Gastrointestinal disorders—Many cases of cholestatic jaundice have been reported in patients taking progestin-containing drugs. The differences in incidence of these disorders from one population to another suggest that genetic factors may be involved. The jaundice caused by these agents is similar to that produced by other 17-alkyl-substituted steroids. It is most often observed in the first three cycles and is particularly common in women with a history of cholestatic jaundice during pregnancy. Jaundice and pruritus disappear 1–8 weeks after the drug is discontinued.

These agents have also been found to increase the incidence of symptomatic gallbladder disease, including cholecystitis and cholangitis. This is probably the result of the alterations responsible for jaundice and bile acid changes described above.

It also appears that the incidence of hepatic adenomas is increased in women taking oral contraceptives. Ischemic bowel disease secondary to thrombosis of the celiac and superior and inferior mesenteric arteries and veins has also been reported in women using these drugs.

3. Depression—Depression of sufficient degree to require cessation of therapy occurs in about 6% of patients treated with some preparations.

4. Cancer—The occurrence of malignant tumors in patients taking oral contraceptives has been studied extensively. It is now clear that these compounds *reduce* the risk of endometrial and ovarian cancer. The lifetime risk of breast cancer in the population as a whole does not seem to be affected by oral contraceptive use. Some studies have shown an increased risk in younger women, and it is possible that tumors that develop in younger women become clinically apparent sooner. The relation of risk of cervical cancer to oral contraceptive use is still controversial. It should be noted that a number of recent studies associate the use of oral contraceptives by women with cervical infection with the human papillomavirus to an increased risk of cervical cancer.

5. Other—In addition to the above effects, a number of other adverse reactions have been reported for which a causal relation has not been established. These include alopecia, erythema multiforme, erythema nodosum, and other skin disorders.

Contraindications & Cautions

These drugs are contraindicated in patients with thrombophlebitis, thromboembolic phenomena, and cardiovascular and cerebrovascular disorders or a past history of these conditions. They should not be used to treat vaginal bleeding when the cause is unknown. They should be avoided in patients with known or suspected tumors of the breast or other estrogen-dependent neoplasms. Since these preparations have caused aggravation of preexisting disorders, they should be avoided or used with caution in patients with liver disease, asthma, eczema, migraine, diabetes, hypertension, optic neuritis, retrobulbar neuritis, or convulsive disorders.

The oral contraceptives may produce edema, and for that reason they should be used with great caution in patients in heart failure or in whom edema is otherwise undesirable or dangerous.

Estrogens may increase the rate of growth of fibroids. Therefore, for women with these tumors, agents with the smallest amounts of estrogen and the most androgenic progestins should be selected. The use of progestational agents alone for contraception might be especially useful in such patients (see below).

These agents are contraindicated in adolescents in whom epiphysial closure has not yet been completed.

Women using oral contraceptives must be made aware of an important interaction that occurs with antimicrobial drugs. Because the normal gastrointestinal flora increases the enterohepatic cycling (and bioavailability) of estrogens, antimicrobial drugs that interfere with these organisms may reduce the efficacy of oral contraceptives. Additionally, coadministration with potent inducers of the hepatic microsomal metabolizing enzymes, such as rifampin, may increase liver catabolism of estrogens or progestins and diminish the efficacy of oral contraceptives.

Contraception with Progestins Alone

Small doses of progestins administered orally or by implantation under the skin can be used for contraception. They are particularly suited for use in patients for whom estrogen administration is undesirable. They are about as effective as intrauterine devices or combination pills containing 20–30 mcg of ethinyl estradiol. There is a high incidence of abnormal bleeding.

Effective contraception can also be achieved by injecting 150 mg of **depot medroxyprogesterone acetate (DMPA)** every 3 months. After a 150 mg dose, ovulation is inhibited for at least 14 weeks. Almost all users experience episodes of unpredictable spotting and bleeding, particularly during the first year of use. Spotting and bleeding decrease with time, and amenorrhea is common. This preparation is not desirable for women planning a pregnancy soon after cessation of therapy because ovulation suppression can sometimes persist for as long as 18 months

after the last injection. Long-term DMPA use reduces menstrual blood loss and is associated with a decreased risk of endometrial cancer. Suppression of endogenous estrogen secretion may be associated with a reversible reduction in bone density, and changes in plasma lipids are associated with an increased risk of atherosclerosis.

The progestin implant method utilizes the subcutaneous implantation of capsules containing a progestin. These capsules release one fifth to one third as much steroid as oral agents, are extremely effective, and last for 5–6 years (Norplant) or 2–4 years (Implanon). The low levels of hormone have little effect on lipoprotein and carbohydrate metabolism or blood pressure. The disadvantages include the need for surgical insertion and removal of capsules and some irregular bleeding rather than predictable menses. An association of intracranial hypertension with implanted norgestrel has been observed in a small number of women. Patients experiencing headache or visual disturbances should be checked for papilledema.

Contraception with progestins is useful in patients with hepatic disease, hypertension, psychosis or mental retardation, or prior thromboembolism. The side effects include headache, dizziness, bloating and weight gain of 1–2 kg, and a reversible reduction of glucose tolerance.

Postcoital Contraceptives

Pregnancy can be prevented following coitus by the administration of estrogens alone or in combination with progestins (**"morning after"** contraception). When treatment is begun within 72 hours, it is effective 99% of the time. Some effective schedules are shown in Table 40–4. The hormones are often administered with antiemetics, since 40% of the patients have nausea or vomiting. Other adverse effects include headache, dizziness, breast tenderness, and abdominal and leg cramps.

Mifepristone (RU 486), an antagonist at progesterone and glucocorticoid receptors, has a luteolytic effect and is effective as a postcoital contraceptive. When combined with a prostaglandin it is also an effective abortifacient.

Table 40–4. Schedules for use of postcoital contraceptives.

Conjugated estrogens: 10 mg three times daily for 5 days
Ethinyl estradiol: 2.5 mg twice daily for 5 days
Diethylstilbestrol: 50 mg daily for 5 days
Mifepristone, 600 mg once with misoprostol, 400 mcg once[1]
L-Norgestrel: 0.75 mg twice daily for 1 day (eg, Plan B[2])
Norgestrel, 0.5 mg, with ethinyl estradiol, 0.05 mg (eg, Ovral, Preven[2]): Two tablets and then two in 12 hours

[1]Mifepristone given on day 1, misoprostol on day 3.
[2]Sold as emergency contraceptive kits.

Beneficial Effects of Oral Contraceptives

It has become apparent that reduction in the dose of the constituents of oral contraceptives has markedly reduced mild and severe adverse effects, providing a relatively safe and convenient method of contraception for many young women. Treatment with oral contraceptives has also been shown to be associated with many benefits unrelated to contraception. These include a reduced risk of ovarian cysts, ovarian and endometrial cancer, and benign breast disease. There is a lower incidence of ectopic pregnancy. Iron deficiency and rheumatoid arthritis are less common, and premenstrual symptoms, dysmenorrhea, endometriosis, acne, and hirsutism may be ameliorated with their use.

ESTROGEN & PROGESTERONE INHIBITORS & ANTAGONISTS

TAMOXIFEN & RELATED PARTIAL AGONIST ESTROGENS

Tamoxifen, a competitive partial agonist inhibitor of estradiol at the estrogen receptor (Figure 40–5), was the first **selective estrogen receptor modulator (SERM)** to be introduced. It is extensively used in the palliative treatment of breast cancer in postmenopausal women and is approved for chemoprevention of breast cancer in high-risk women (see Chapter 55). It is a nonsteroidal agent (see structure below) that is given orally. Peak plasma levels are reached in a few hours. Tamoxifen has an initial half-life of 7–14 hours in the circulation and is predominantly excreted by the liver. It is used in doses of 10–20 mg twice daily. Hot flushes and nausea and vomiting occur in 25% of patients, and many other minor adverse effects are observed. Studies of patients treated with tamoxifen as adjuvant therapy for early breast cancer have shown a 35% decrease in contralateral breast cancer. However, adjuvant therapy extended beyond 5 years in patients with breast cancer has shown no further improvement in outcome. **Toremifene** is a structurally similar compound with very similar properties, indications, and toxicities.

Prevention of the expected loss of lumbar spine bone density and plasma lipid changes consistent with a reduction in the risk for atherosclerosis have also been reported in tamoxifen-treated patients following spon-

Figure 40–5. Control of ovarian secretion and the actions of its hormones. In the follicular phase the ovary produces mainly estrogens; in the luteal phase it produces estrogens and progesterone. (SERMs, selective estrogen receptor modulators. See text.)

Tamoxifen

taneous or surgical menopause. However, this agonist activity also affects the uterus and may increase the risk of endometrial cancer.

Raloxifene is another partial estrogen agonist-antagonist (SERM) at some but not all target tissues. It has similar effects on lipids and bone but appears not to stimulate the endometrium or breast. Although subject to a high first-pass effect, raloxifene has a very large volume of distribution and a long half-life (> 24 hours), so it can be taken once a day. Raloxifene has been approved in the USA for the prevention of postmenopausal osteoporosis.

Clomiphene is an older partial agonist, a weak estrogen that also acts as a competitive inhibitor of endogenous estrogens (Figure 40–5). It has found use as an ovulation-inducing agent (see below).

MIFEPRISTONE

Mifepristone (RU 486) is a "19-norsteroid" that binds strongly to the progesterone receptor and inhibits the activity of progesterone. The drug has luteolytic properties in 80% of women when given in the midluteal period. The mechanism of this effect is unknown, but it may provide the basis for using mifepristone as a contraceptive (as opposed to an abortifacient). However, because the compound has a long half-life, large doses may prolong the follicular phase of the subsequent cycle and so make it difficult to use continuously for this purpose. A single dose of 600 mg is an effective emergency postcoital contraceptive, though it may result in delayed ovulation in the following cycle. As noted in Chapter 39, the drug also binds to and acts as an antagonist at the glucocorticoid receptor. Limited clinical studies suggest that mifepristone or other analogs with similar properties may be useful in the treatment of endometriosis, Cushing's syndrome, breast cancer, and possibly other neoplasms such as meningiomas that contain glucocorticoid or progesterone receptors.

Mifepristone

Mifepristone's major use thus far has been to terminate early pregnancies. Doses of 400–600 mg/d for 4 days or 800 mg/d for 2 days successfully terminated pregnancy in over 85% of the women studied. The major adverse effect was prolonged bleeding that on most occasions did not require treatment. The combination of a single oral dose of 600 mg of mifepristone and a vaginal pessary containing 1 mg of prostaglandin E_1 or oral misoprostol has been found to effectively terminate pregnancy in over 95% of patients treated during the first 7 weeks after conception. The adverse effects of the medications included vomiting, diarrhea, and abdominal or pelvic pain. As many as 5% of patients have vaginal bleeding requiring intervention. Because of these adverse effects, RU 486 is administered only by physicians at family planning centers. In a very small number of cases, use of a vaginal tablet for the prostaglandin dose has been associated with sepsis, so it is recommended that *both* drugs be given by mouth in all patients.

ZK 98734 (lilopristone) is a potent experimental progesterone inhibitor and abortifacient in doses of 25 mg twice daily. Like mifepristone, it also appears to have antiglucocorticoid activity.

DANAZOL

Danazol, an isoxazole derivative of ethisterone (17α-ethinyltestosterone) with weak progestational, androgenic, and glucocorticoid activities, is used to suppress ovarian function. Danazol inhibits the midcycle surge of LH and FSH and can prevent the compensatory increase in LH and FSH following castration in animals, but it does not significantly lower or suppress basal LH or FSH levels in normal women (Figure 40–5). Danazol binds to androgen, progesterone, and glucocorticoid receptors and can translocate the androgen receptor into the nucleus to initiate androgen-specific RNA synthesis. It does not bind to intracellular estrogen receptors, but it does bind to sex hormone-binding and corticosteroid-binding globulins. It inhibits P450scc (the cholesterol side chain-cleaving enzyme), 3β-hydroxysteroid dehydrogenase, 17α-hydroxysteroid dehydrogenase, P450c17 (17α-hydroxylase), P450c11 (11β-hydroxylase), and P450c21 (21β-hydroxylase). However, it does not inhibit aromatase, the enzyme required for estrogen synthesis. It increases the mean clearance of progesterone, probably by competing with the hormone for binding proteins, and may have similar effects on other active steroid hormones. Ethisterone, a major metabolite of danazol, has both progestational and mild androgenic effects.

Danazol is slowly metabolized in humans, having a half-life of over 15 hours. This results in stable circulating levels when the drug is administered twice daily. It is highly concentrated in the liver, adrenals, and kidneys and is excreted in both feces and urine.

Danazol has been employed as an inhibitor of gonadal function and has found its major use in the treatment of endometriosis. For this purpose, it can be given in a dosage of 600 mg/d. The dosage is reduced to 400 mg/d after 1 month and to 200 mg/d in 2 months. About 85% of patients show marked improvement in 3–12 months.

Danazol has also been used in the treatment of fibrocystic disease of the breast and hematologic or allergic disorders, including hemophilia, Christmas disease, idiopathic thrombocytopenic purpura, and angioneurotic edema.

The major adverse effects are weight gain, edema, decreased breast size, acne and oily skin, increased hair growth, deepening of the voice, headache, hot flushes, changes in libido, and muscle cramps. Although mild adverse effects are very common, it is seldom necessary to discontinue the drug because of them. Occasionally, because of its inherent glucocorticoid activity, danazol may cause adrenal suppression.

Danazol should be used with great caution in patients with hepatic dysfunction, since it has been reported to produce mild to moderate hepatocellular damage in some patients, as evidenced by enzyme changes. It is also contraindicated during pregnancy and breast feeding, as it may produce urogenital abnormalities in the offspring.

OTHER INHIBITORS

Anastrozole, a selective nonsteroidal inhibitor of aromatase (the enzyme required for estrogen synthesis, Figures 40–2, 40–5), is effective in some women whose breast tumors have become resistant to tamoxifen (see Chapter 55). **Letrozole** is similar. **Exemestane,** a steroid molecule, is an irreversible inhibitor of aromatase. Like anastrazole and letrozole, it is approved for use in women with advanced breast cancer (see Chapter 55).

Several other aromatase inhibitors are undergoing clinical trials in patients with breast cancer. **Fadrozole** is a newer oral nonsteroidal (triazole) inhibitor of aromatase activity. These compounds appear to be as effective as tamoxifen. In addition to their use in breast cancer, aromatase inhibitors have been successfully employed as adjuncts to androgen antagonists in the treatment of precocious puberty and as primary treatment in the excessive aromatase syndrome.

Fulvestrant is a pure estrogen receptor antagonist that has been somewhat more effective than those with partial agonist effects in some patients who have become resistant to tamoxifen. ICI 164,384 is a newer antagonist; it inhibits dimerization of the occupied estrogen receptor and interferes with its binding to DNA. It has also been used experimentally in breast cancer patients who have become resistant to tamoxifen.

GnRH and its analogs (**nafarelin, buserelin,** etc) have become important in both stimulating and inhibiting ovarian function. They are discussed in Chapter 37.

OVULATION-INDUCING AGENTS

CLOMIPHENE

Clomiphene citrate, a partial estrogen agonist, is closely related to the estrogen chlorotrianisene (Figure 40–3). This compound is active when taken orally. Very little is known about its metabolism, but about half of the compound is excreted in the feces within 5 days after administration. It has been suggested that clomiphene is slowly excreted from an enterohepatic pool.

Pharmacologic Effects

A. MECHANISMS OF ACTION

Clomiphene is a partial agonist at estrogen receptors. The estrogenic agonist effects are best demonstrated in animals with marked gonadal deficiency. Clomiphene has also been shown to effectively inhibit the action of stronger estrogens. In humans it leads to an increase in the secretion of gonadotropins and estrogens by inhibiting estradiol's negative feedback effect on the gonadotropins (Figure 40–5).

B. EFFECTS

The pharmacologic importance of this compound rests on its ability to stimulate ovulation in women with oligomenorrhea or amenorrhea and ovulatory dysfunction. The majority of patients suffer from polycystic ovary syndrome, a common disorder affecting about 7% of women of reproductive age. The syndrome is characterized by gonadotropin-dependent ovarian hyperandrogenism associated with anovulation and infertility. The disorder is frequently accompanied by adrenal hyperandrogenism. Clomiphene probably blocks the feedback inhibitory influence of estrogens on the hypothalamus, causing a surge of gonadotropins, which leads to ovulation.

Clinical Use

Clomiphene is used in the treatment of disorders of ovulation in patients who wish to become pregnant. Usually, a single ovulation is induced by a single course of therapy, and the patient must be treated repeatedly until pregnancy is achieved, since normal ovulatory function does not usually resume. The compound is of no value in patients with ovarian or pituitary failure.

When clomiphene is administered in doses of 100 mg/d for 5 days, a rise in plasma LH and FSH is observed after several days. In patients who ovulate, the initial rise is followed by a second rise of gonadotropin levels just prior to ovulation.

Adverse Effects

The most common adverse effects in patients treated with this drug are hot flushes, which resemble those experienced by menopausal patients. They tend to be mild, and disappear when the drug is discontinued. There have been occasional reports of eye symptoms due to intensification and prolongation of afterimages. These are generally of short duration. Headache, constipation, allergic skin reactions, and reversible hair loss have been reported occasionally.

The effective use of clomiphene is associated with some stimulation of the ovaries and usually with ovarian enlargement. The degree of enlargement tends to be greater and its incidence higher in patients who have enlarged ovaries at the beginning of therapy.

A variety of other symptoms such as nausea and vomiting, increased nervous tension, depression, fatigue, breast soreness, weight gain, urinary frequency, and heavy menses have also been reported. However, these appear to result from the hormonal changes associated with an ovulatory menstrual cycle rather than from the medication. The incidence of multiple pregnancy is approximately 10%. Clomiphene has not been shown to have an adverse effect when inadvertently given to women who are already pregnant.

Contraindications & Cautions

Special precautions should be observed in patients with enlarged ovaries. These women are thought to be more sensitive to this drug and should receive small doses. Any patient who complains of abdominal symptoms should be examined carefully. Maximum ovarian enlargement occurs after the 5-day course has been completed, and many patients can be shown to have a palpable increase in ovarian size by the seventh to tenth days. Treatment with clomiphene for more than a year may be associated with an increased risk for low-grade ovarian cancer; however, the evidence for this effect is not conclusive.

Special precautions must also be taken in patients who have visual symptoms associated with clomiphene therapy, since these symptoms may make activities such as driving more hazardous.

OTHER DRUGS USED IN OVULATORY DISORDERS

In addition to clomiphene, a variety of other hormonal and nonhormonal agents are used in treating anovulatory disorders. They are discussed in Chapter 37.

■ II. THE TESTIS (ANDROGENS & ANABOLIC STEROIDS, ANTIANDROGENS, & MALE CONTRACEPTION)

The testis, like the ovary, has both gametogenic and endocrine functions. The onset of gametogenic function of the testes is controlled largely by the secretion of FSH by the pituitary. High concentrations of testosterone locally are also required for continuing sperm production in the seminiferous tubules. The Sertoli cells in the seminiferous tubules may be the source of the estradiol produced in the testes via aromatization of locally produced testosterone. With LH stimulation, testosterone is produced by the interstitial or Leydig cells found in the spaces between the seminiferous tubules.

The Sertoli cells in the testis synthesize and secrete a variety of active proteins, including müllerian duct inhibitory factor, inhibin, and activin. As in the ovary, inhibin and activin appear to be the product of three genes that produce a common α subunit and two β subunits, A and B. Activin is composed of the two β subunits ($\beta_A\beta_B$). There are two inhibins (A and B), which contain the α subunit and one of the β subunits. Activin stimulates pituitary FSH release and is structurally similar to transforming growth factor-β, which also increases FSH. The inhibins in conjunction with testosterone and dihydrotestosterone are responsible for the feedback inhibition of pituitary FSH secretion.

ANDROGENS & ANABOLIC STEROIDS

In humans, the most important androgen secreted by the testis is testosterone. The pathways of synthesis of testosterone in the testes are similar to those previously described for the adrenal and ovary (Figures 39–1 and 40–2).

In men, approximately 8 mg of testosterone is produced daily. About 95% is produced by the Leydig cells and only 5% by the adrenal. The testis also secretes small amounts of another potent androgen, dihydrotestosterone, as well as androstenedione and dehydroepiandrosterone, which are weak androgens. Pregnenolone and progesterone and their 17-hydroxylated derivatives are also released in small amounts. Plasma levels of testosterone in males are about 0.6 mcg/dL after puberty and appear to decline after age 50. Testosterone is also present in the plasma of women in concentrations of approximately 0.03 mcg/dL and is derived in approximately equal parts from the ovaries and adrenals and by the peripheral conversion of other hormones.

About 65% of circulating testosterone is bound to sex hormone-binding globulin. SHBG is increased in plasma by estrogen, by thyroid hormone, and in patients with cirrhosis of the liver. It is decreased by androgen and growth hormone and is lower in obese individuals. Most of the remaining testosterone is bound to albumin. Approximately 2% remains free and available to enter cells and bind to intracellular receptors.

Metabolism

In many target tissues, testosterone is converted to dihydrotestosterone by 5α-reductase. In these tissues, dihydrotestosterone is the major active androgen. The conversion of testosterone to estradiol by P450 aromatase also occurs in some tissues, including adipose tissue, liver, and the hypothalamus, where it may be of importance in regulating gonadal function.

The major pathway for the degradation of testosterone in humans occurs in the liver, with the reduction of the double bond and ketone in the A ring, as is seen in other steroids with a Δ^4-ketone configuration in the A ring. This leads to the production of inactive substances such as androsterone and etiocholanolone that are then conjugated and excreted in the urine.

Androstenedione, dehydroepiandrosterone (DHEA), and dehydroepiandrosterone sulfate (DHEAS) are also produced in significant amounts in humans, although largely in the adrenal rather than in the testes. They contribute slightly to the normal maturation process supporting other androgen-dependent pubertal changes in the human, primarily development of pubic and axillary hair and bone maturation. As noted in Chapter 39, some studies suggest that DHEA and DHEAS may have other central nervous system and metabolic effects and may prolong life in rabbits. In men they may improve the sense of well-being and inhibit atherosclerosis. In a recent placebo-controlled clinical trial in patients with systemic lupus erythematosus, DHEA demonstrated some beneficial effects (see Adrenal Androgens, Chapter 39). Adrenal androgens are to a large extent metabolized in the same fashion as testosterone. Both steroids—but particularly androstenedione—can be converted by peripheral tissues to estrone in very small amounts (1–5%). The P450 aromatase enzyme responsible for this conversion is also found in the brain and is thought to play an important role in development.

Physiologic Effects

In the normal male, testosterone or its active metabolite 5α-dihydrotestosterone is responsible for the many changes that occur in puberty. In addition to the general growth-promoting properties of androgens on body tissues, these hormones are responsible for penile and scrotal growth. Changes in the skin include the appearance of pubic, axillary, and beard hair. The sebaceous glands become more active, and the skin tends to become thicker and oilier. The larynx grows and the vocal cords become thicker, leading to a lower-pitched voice. Skeletal growth is stimulated and epiphysial closure accelerated. Other effects include growth of the prostate and seminal vesicles, darkening of the skin, and increased skin circulation. Androgens play an important role in stimulating and maintaining sexual function in men. Androgens increase lean body mass and stimulate body hair growth and sebum secretion. Metabolic effects include the reduction of hormone binding and other carrier proteins and increased liver synthesis of clotting factors, triglyceride lipase, α_1-antitrypsin, haptoglobin, and sialic acid. They also stimulate renal erythropoietin secretion and decrease HDL levels.

Synthetic Steroids with Androgenic & Anabolic Action

Testosterone, when administered by mouth, is rapidly absorbed. However, it is largely converted to inactive metabolites, and only about one sixth of the dose administered is available in active form. Testosterone can be administered parenterally, but it has a more prolonged absorption time and greater activity in the propionate, enanthate, undecanoate, or cypionate ester forms. These derivatives are hydrolyzed to release free testosterone at the site of injection. Testosterone derivatives alkylated at the 17 position, eg, methyltestosterone and fluoxymesterone, are active when given by mouth.

Testosterone and its derivatives have been used for their anabolic effects as well as in the treatment of testosterone deficiency. Although testosterone and other known active steroids can be isolated in pure form and measured by weight, biologic assays are still used in the investigation of new compounds. In some of these studies in animals, the anabolic effects of the compound as measured by trophic effects on muscles or the reduction of nitrogen excretion may be dissociated from the other androgenic effects. This has led to the marketing of compounds claimed to have anabolic activity associated with only weak androgenic effects. Unfortunately, this dissociation is less marked in humans than in the animals used for testing (Table 40–5), and all are potent androgens.

Pharmacologic Effects

A. MECHANISMS OF ACTION

Like other steroids, testosterone acts intracellularly in target cells. In skin, prostate, seminal vesicles, and epididymis, it is converted to 5α-dihydrotestosterone by 5α-reductase. In these tissues, dihydrotestosterone is the dominant androgen. The distribution of

Table 40–5. Androgens: Preparations available and relative androgenic: anabolic activity in animals.

	Androgenic: Anabolic Activity
Testosterone	1:1
Testosterone cypionate	1:1
Testosterone enanthate	1:1
Methyltestosterone	1:1
Fluoxymesterone	1:2
Oxymetholone	1:3
Oxandrolone	1:3–1:13
Nandrolone decanoate	1:2.5–1:4

this enzyme in the fetus is different and has important developmental implications.

Testosterone and dihydrotestosterone bind to the intracellular androgen receptor, initiating a series of events similar to those described above for estradiol and progesterone, leading to growth, differentiation, and synthesis of a variety of enzymes and other functional proteins.

B. EFFECTS

In the male at puberty, androgens cause development of the secondary sex characteristics (see above). In the adult male, large doses of testosterone—when given alone—or its derivatives suppress the secretion of gonadotropins and result in some atrophy of the interstitial tissue and the tubules of the testes. Since fairly large doses of androgens are required to suppress gonadotropin secretion, it has been postulated that inhibin, in combination with androgens, is responsible for the feedback control of secretion. In women, androgens are capable of producing changes similar to those observed in the prepubertal male. These include growth of facial and body hair, deepening of the voice, enlargement of the clitoris, frontal baldness, and prominent musculature. The natural androgens stimulate erythrocyte production.

The administration of androgens reduces the excretion of nitrogen into the urine, indicating an increase in protein synthesis or a decrease in protein breakdown within the body. This effect is much more pronounced in women and children than in normal men.

Clinical Uses

A. ANDROGEN REPLACEMENT THERAPY IN MEN

Androgens are used to replace or augment endogenous androgen secretion in hypogonadal men (Table 40–6).

Even in the presence of pituitary deficiency, androgens are used rather than gonadotropin except when normal spermatogenesis is to be achieved. In patients with hypopituitarism, androgens are not added to the treatment regimen until puberty, at which time they are instituted in gradually increasing doses to achieve the growth spurt and the development of secondary sex characteristics. In these patients, therapy should be started with long-acting agents such as testosterone enanthate or cypionate in doses of 50 mg intramuscularly, initially every 4, then every 3, and finally every 2 weeks, with each change taking place at 3-month intervals. The dose is then doubled to 100 mg every 2 weeks until maturation is complete. Finally, it is changed to the adult replacement dose of 200 mg at 2-week intervals. Testosterone propionate, though potent, has a short duration of action and is not practical for long-term use. Testosterone undecanoate can be given orally, administering large amounts of the steroid twice daily (eg, 40 mg/d); however, this is not recommended because oral testosterone administration has been associated with liver tumors. Testosterone can also be administered transdermally; skin patches or gels are available for scrotal or other skin area application. Two applications daily are usually required for replacement therapy. Implanted pellets and other longer-acting preparations are under study. The development of polycythemia or hypertension may require some reduction in dose.

B. GYNECOLOGIC DISORDERS

Androgens are used occasionally in the treatment of certain gynecologic disorders, but the undesirable effects in women are such that they must be used with great caution. Androgens have been used to reduce breast engorgement during the postpartum period, usually in conjunction with estrogens. The weak androgen danazol is used in the treatment of endometriosis (see above).

Table 40–6. Androgen preparations for replacement therapy.

	Route of Administration	Dosage
Methyltestosterone	Oral	25–50 mg/d
	Sublingual (buccal)	5–10 mg/d
Fluoxymesterone	Oral	2–10 mg/d
Testosterone enanthate	Intramuscular	See text
Testosterone cypionate	Intramuscular	See text
Testosterone	Transdermal	2.5–10 mg/d
	Topical gel (1%)	5–10 g gel/d

Androgens are sometimes given in combination with estrogens for replacement therapy in the postmenopausal period in an attempt to eliminate the endometrial bleeding that may occur when only estrogens are used and to enhance libido. They have been used for chemotherapy of breast tumors in premenopausal women.

C. Use as Protein Anabolic Agents

Androgens and anabolic steroids have been used in conjunction with dietary measures and exercises in an attempt to reverse protein loss after trauma, surgery, or prolonged immobilization and in patients with debilitating diseases.

D. Anemia

In the past, large doses of androgens were employed in the treatment of refractory anemias such as aplastic anemia, Fanconi's anemia, sickle cell anemia, myelofibrosis, and hemolytic anemias. Recombinant erythropoietin has largely replaced androgens for this purpose.

E. Osteoporosis

Androgens and anabolic agents have been used in the treatment of osteoporosis, either alone or in conjunction with estrogens. With the exception of substitution therapy in hypogonadism, bisphosphonates have largely replaced androgen use for this purpose.

F. Use as Growth Stimulators

These agents have been used to stimulate growth in boys with delayed puberty. If the drugs are used carefully, these children will probably achieve their expected adult height. If treatment is too vigorous, the patient may grow rapidly at first but will not achieve full predicted final stature because of the accelerated epiphysial closure that occurs. It is difficult to control this type of therapy adequately even with frequent x-ray examination of the epiphyses, since the action of the hormones on epiphysial centers may continue for many months after therapy is discontinued.

G. Anabolic Steroid and Androgen Abuse in Sports

The use of anabolic steroids by athletes has received worldwide attention. Many athletes and their coaches believe that anabolic steroids—in doses 10–200 times larger than the daily normal production—increase strength and aggressiveness, thereby improving competitive performance. Such effects have been unequivocally demonstrated only in women. Furthermore, the adverse effects of these drugs clearly make their use inadvisable.

H. Aging

Androgen production falls with age in men and may contribute to the decline in muscle mass, strength, and libido. Preliminary studies of androgen replacement in aging males with low androgen levels show an increase in lean body mass and hematocrit and a decrease in bone turnover. Longer studies will be required to assess the usefulness of this therapy.

Adverse Effects

The adverse effects of these compounds are due largely to their masculinizing actions and are most noticeable in women and prepubertal children. In women, the administration of more than 200–300 mg of testosterone per month is usually associated with hirsutism, acne, amenorrhea, clitoral enlargement, and deepening of the voice. These effects may occur with even smaller doses in some women. Some of the androgenic steroids exert progestational activity, leading to endometrial bleeding upon discontinuation. These hormones also alter serum lipids and could conceivably increase susceptibility to atherosclerotic disease in women.

Except under the most unusual circumstances, androgens should not be used in infants. Recent studies in animals suggest that administration of androgens in early life may have profound effects on maturation of central nervous system centers governing sexual development, particularly in the female. Administration of these drugs to pregnant women may lead to masculinization or undermasculinization of the external genitalia in the female and male fetus, respectively. Although the above-mentioned effects may be less marked with the anabolic agents, they do occur.

Sodium retention and edema are not common but must be carefully watched for in patients with heart and kidney disease.

Most of the synthetic androgens and anabolic agents are 17-alkyl-substituted steroids. Administration of drugs with this structure is often associated with evidence of hepatic dysfunction. Hepatic dysfunction usually occurs early in the course of treatment, and the degree is proportionate to the dose. Bilirubin levels occasionally increase until clinical jaundice is apparent. The cholestatic jaundice is reversible upon cessation of therapy, and permanent changes do not occur. In older males, prostatic hyperplasia may develop, causing urinary retention.

Replacement therapy in men may cause acne, sleep apnea, erythrocytosis, gynecomastia, and azoospermia. Supraphysiologic doses of androgens produce azoospermia and decrease in testicular size, both of which may take months to recover after cessation of therapy. The alkylated androgens in high doses can produce peliosis hepatica, cholestasis, and hepatic failure. They lower plasma HDL_2 and may increase LDL. Hepatic adenomas and carcinomas have also been reported. Behavioral effects include psychologic dependence, increased aggressiveness, and psychotic symptoms.

Contraindications & Cautions

The use of androgenic steroids is contraindicated in pregnant women or women who may become pregnant during the course of therapy.

Androgens should not be administered to male patients with carcinoma of the prostate or breast. Until more is known about the effects of these hormones on the central nervous system in developing children, they should be avoided in infants and young children.

Special caution is required in giving these drugs to children to produce a growth spurt. In most patients, the use of somatotropin is more appropriate (see Chapter 37).

Care should be exercised in the administration of these drugs to patients with renal or cardiac disease predisposed to edema. If sodium and water retention occurs, it will respond to diuretic therapy.

Methyltestosterone therapy is associated with creatinuria, but the significance of this finding is not known.

Caution: Several cases of hepatocellular carcinoma have been reported in patients with aplastic anemia treated with androgen anabolic therapy. Colony-stimulating factors (see Chapter 33) should be used instead.

ANDROGEN SUPPRESSION & ANTIANDROGENS

ANDROGEN SUPPRESSION

The treatment of advanced prostatic carcinoma often requires orchiectomy or large doses of estrogens to reduce available endogenous androgen. The psychologic effects of the former and gynecomastia produced by the latter make these approaches undesirable. As noted in Chapter 37, the GnRH analogs such as goserelin, nafarelin, buserelin, and leuprolide acetate produce gonadal suppression when blood levels are continuous rather than pulsatile (see Chapter 37 and Figure 40–6).

ANTIANDROGENS

The potential usefulness of antiandrogens in the treatment of patients producing excessive amounts of testosterone has led to the search for effective drugs that can be used for this purpose. Several approaches to the problem, especially inhibition of synthesis and receptor antagonism, have met with some success.

Steroid Synthesis Inhibitors

Ketoconazole, used primarily in the treatment of fungal disease, is an inhibitor of adrenal and gonadal steroid synthesis, as described in Chapter 39. It does not affect ovarian aromatase, but it reduces human placental aromatase activity. It displaces estradiol and dihy-

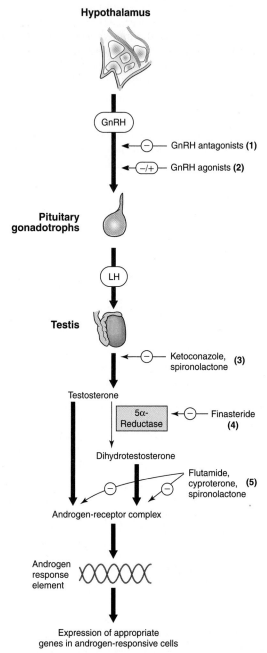

Figure 40–6. Control of androgen secretion and activity and some sites of action of antiandrogens. **(1),** competitive inhibition of GnRH receptors; **(2),** stimulation (+, pulsatile administration) or inhibition via desensitization of GnRH receptors (–, continuous administration); **(3),** decreased synthesis of testosterone in the testis; **(4),** decreased synthesis of dihydrotestosterone by inhibition of 5α-reductase; **(5),** competition for binding to cytosol androgen receptors.

drotestosterone from sex hormone–binding protein in vitro and increases the estradiol:testosterone ratio in plasma in vivo by a different mechanism. However, it does not appear to be clinically useful in women with increased androgens because of the toxicity associated with prolonged use of the 400–800 mg/d required. The drug has also been used experimentally to treat prostatic carcinoma, but the results have not been encouraging. Men treated with ketoconazole often develop reversible gynecomastia during therapy; this may be due to the demonstrated increase in the estradiol:testosterone ratio.

Conversion of Steroid Precursors to Androgens

Several compounds have been developed that inhibit the 17-hydroxylation of progesterone or pregnenolone, thereby preventing the action of the side chain-splitting enzyme and the further transformation of these steroid precursors to active androgens. A few of these compounds have been tested clinically but have been too toxic for prolonged use.

Since dihydrotestosterone—not testosterone—appears to be the essential androgen in the prostate, androgen effects in this and similar dihydrotestosterone-dependent tissues can be reduced by an inhibitor of 5α-reductase (Figure 40–6). **Finasteride,** a steroid-like inhibitor of this enzyme, is orally active and causes a reduction in dihydrotestosterone levels that begins within 8 hours after administration and lasts for about 24 hours. The half-life is about 8 hours (longer in elderly individuals). Forty to 50 percent of the dose is metabolized; more than half is excreted in the feces. Finasteride has been reported to be moderately effective in reducing prostate size in men with benign prostatic hyperplasia and is approved for this use in the USA. The dosage is 5 mg/d. Its use in advanced prostatic carcinoma is under study. The drug is not approved for use in women or children, although it has been used successfully in the treatment of hirsutism in women and early male pattern baldness in men (1 mg/d).

Finasteride

Receptor Inhibitors

Cyproterone and **cyproterone acetate** are effective antiandrogens that inhibit the action of androgens at the target organ. The acetate form has a marked progestational effect that suppresses the feedback enhancement of LH and FSH, leading to a more effective antiandrogen effect. These compounds have been used in women to treat hirsutism and in men to decrease excessive sexual drive and are being studied in other conditions in which the reduction of androgenic effects would be useful. Cyproterone acetate in a dosage of 2 mg/d administered concurrently with an estrogen is used in the treatment of hirsutism in women, doubling as a contraceptive pill; it has orphan drug status in the USA.

Flutamide, a substituted anilide, is a potent antiandrogen that has been used in the treatment of prostatic carcinoma. Although not a steroid, it behaves like a competitive antagonist at the androgen receptor. It is rapidly metabolized in humans. It frequently causes mild gynecomastia (probably by increasing testicular estrogen production) and occasionally causes mild reversible hepatic toxicity. Administration of this compound causes some improvement in most patients who have not had prior endocrine therapy. Preliminary studies indicate that flutamide is also useful in the management of excess androgen effect in women.

Flutamide

Bicalutamide and **nilutamide** are potent orally active antiandrogens that can be administered as a single daily dose and are used in patients with metastatic carcinoma of the prostate. Studies in patients with carcinoma of the prostate indicate that these agents are well tolerated. Bicalutamide is recommended for use in combination with a GnRH analog (to reduce tumor flare) and may have fewer gastrointestinal side effects than flutamide. A dosage of 150–200 mg/d (when used alone) is required to reduce prostate-specific antigen levels to those achieved by castration, but, in combination with a GnRH analog, 50 mg/d may be adequate. Nilutamide is approved for use following surgical castration in a dosage of 300 mg/d for 30 days followed by 150 mg/d.

Spironolactone, a competitive inhibitor of aldosterone (see Chapter 15), also competes with dihydrotestosterone for the androgen receptors in target tissues. It also reduces 17α-hydroxylase activity, lowering plasma levels of testosterone and androstenedione. It is used in dosages of 50–200 mg/d in the treatment of hirsutism in women and appears to be as effective as finasteride, flutamide, or cyproterone in this condition.

CHEMICAL CONTRACEPTION IN MEN

Although many studies have been conducted, an effective oral contraceptive for men has not yet been found. For example, various androgens, including testosterone and testosterone enanthate, in a dosage of 400 mg per month, produced azoospermia in less than half the men treated. Minor adverse reactions, including gynecomastia and acne, were encountered. Testosterone in combination with danazol was well tolerated but no more effective than testosterone alone. Androgens in combination with a progestin such as medroxyprogesterone acetate were no more effective. However, preliminary studies indicate that the intramuscular administration of 100 mg of testosterone enanthate weekly together with 500 mg of levonorgestrel daily orally can produce azoospermia in 94% of men.

Cyproterone acetate, a very potent progestin and antiandrogen, also produces oligospermia; however, it does not cause reliable contraception.

At present, pituitary hormones—and potent antagonist analogs of GnRH—are receiving increased attention. A GnRH antagonist in combination with testosterone has been shown to produce reversible azoospermia in nonhuman primates.

GOSSYPOL

Extensive trials of this cottonseed derivative have been conducted in China. This compound destroys elements of the seminiferous epithelium but does not significantly alter the endocrine function of the testis.

In Chinese studies, large numbers of men were treated with 20 mg/d of gossypol or gossypol acetic acid for 2 months, followed by a maintenance dosage of 60 mg/wk. On this regimen, 99% of men developed sperm counts below 4 million/mL. Preliminary data indicate that recovery (return of normal sperm count) following discontinuance of gossypol administration is more apt to occur in men whose counts do not fall to extremely low levels and when administration is not continued for more than 2 years. Hypokalemia is the major adverse effect and may lead to transient paralysis. The drug has also been tried as an intravaginal spermicide contraceptive.

PREPARATIONS AVAILABLE[1]

ESTROGENS

Conjugated estrogens (Premarin)
Oral: 0.3, 0.45, 0.625, 0.9, 1.25 mg tablets
Parenteral: 25 mg/5 mL for IM, IV injection
Vaginal: 0.625 mg/g cream base
Diethylstilbestrol diphosphate (Stilphostrol)
Oral: 50 mg tablets
Parenteral: 50 mg/mL injection
Estradiol cypionate in oil (Depo-Estradiol Cypionate)
Parenteral: 5 mg/mL for IM injection
Estradiol (generic, Estrace)
Oral: 0.45, 0.5, 0.9, 1, 1.5, 1.8, 2 mg tablets
Vaginal: 0.1 mg/g cream
Estradiol transdermal (Estraderm, others)
Transdermal patch: 0.014, 0.025, 0.0375, 0.05, 0.6, 0.075, 0.1 mg/d release rates
Topical: 2.5 mg/g emulsion (Estrasorb); 0.75 mg/1.25 g unit dose (Estrogel)
Estradiol valerate in oil (generic)
Parenteral: 10, 20, 40 mg/mL for IM injection
Estrone (Menest)
Oral: 0.3, 0.625, 1.25, 2.5 mg tablets

Estropipate (generic, Ogen)
Oral: 0.625, 1.25, 2.5, 5 mg tablets
Vaginal: 1.5 mg/g cream base

PROGESTINS

Hydroxyprogesterone caproate (generic, Hylutin)
Parenteral: 125, 250 mg/mL for IM injection
Levonorgestrel (Norplant)
Kit for subcutaneous implant: 6 capsules of 36 mg each
Intrauterine system: 52 mg
Medroxyprogesterone acetate (generic, Provera)
Oral: 2.5, 5, 10 mg tablets
Parenteral (Depo-Provera): 150, 400 mg/mL for IM injection
Megestrol acetate (generic, Megace)
Oral: 20, 40 mg tablets; 40 mg/mL suspension
Norethindrone acetate (generic, Aygestin)
Oral: 5 mg tablets
Norgestrel (Ovrette) (See also Table 40–3)
Oral: 0.075 mg tablets

---

[1]Oral contraceptives are listed in Table 40–3.

(continued)

Progesterone (generic)
  Oral: 100, 200 mg capsules
  Topical: 4, 8% vaginal gel
  Parenteral: 50 mg/mL in oil for IM injection
  Intrauterine contraceptive system: 38 mg in silicone

ANDROGENS & ANABOLIC STEROIDS

Fluoxymesterone (generic)
  Oral: 10 mg tablets
Methyltestosterone (generic)
  Oral: 10, 25 mg tablets; 10 mg capsules; 10 mg buccal tablets
  Parenteral: 200 mg/mL injection
Nandrolone decanoate (generic)
  Parenteral: 100, 200 mg/mL in oil for injection
Oxandrolone (Oxandrin)
  Oral: 2.5, 10 mg tablets
Oxymetholone (Androl-50)
  Oral: 50 mg tablets
Testosterone
  Buccal system: 30 mg
Testosterone cypionate in oil (Depo-testosterone)
  Parenteral: 100, 200 mg/mL for IM injection
Testosterone enanthate in oil (Deletestryl)
  Parenteral: 200 mg/mL for IM injection
Testosterone transdermal system
  Patch (Testoderm): 4, 6 mg/24 h release rate
  Patch (Androderm): 2.5, 5 mg/24 h release rate
  Gel (Androgel): 1%
Testosterone pellets (Testopel)
  Parenteral: 75 mg/pellet for parenteral injection (not IV)

ANTAGONISTS & INHIBITORS

(See also Chapter 37)
Anastrozole (Arimidex)
  Oral: 1 mg tablets
Bicalutamide (Casodex)
  Oral: 50 mg tablets
Clomiphene (generic, Clomid, Serophene, Milophene)
  Oral: 50 mg tablets
Danazol (generic, Danocrine)
  Oral: 50, 100, 200 mg capsules
Dutasteride (Avodart)
  Oral: 0.5 mg tablets
Exemestane (Aromasin)
  Oral: 25 mg tablets
Finasteride
  Oral: 1 mg tablets (Propecia); 5 mg tablets (Proscar)
Flutamide (Eulexin)
  Oral: 125 mg capsules
Fulvestrant (Faslodex)
  Parenteral: 50 mg/mL for IM injection
Letrozole (Femara)
  Oral: 2.5 mg tablets
Mifepristone (Mifeprex)
  Oral: 200 mg tablets
Nilutamide (Nilandron)
  Oral: 50, 150 mg tablets
Raloxifene (Evista)
  Oral: 60 mg tablets
Tamoxifen (generic, Nolvadex)
  Oral: 10, 20 mg tablets
Testolactone (Teslac)
  Oral: 50 mg tablets
Toremifene (Fareston)
  Oral: 60 mg tablets

REFERENCES

Anderson GL et al for the Women's Health Initiative Steering Committee: Effects of conjugated equine estrogen in postmenopausal women with hysterectomy. JAMA 2004;291:1701.

Bagatell CJ, Bremmer WJ: Androgens in men—uses and abuses. N Engl J Med 1996;334:707.

Bamberger CM, Schulte HM, Chrousos GP: Molecular determinants of glucocorticoid receptor function and tissue sensitivity. Endo Rev 1996;17:221.

Baulieu E-E: Contragestion and other clinical applications of RU 486, an antiprogesterone at the receptor. Science 1989;245:1351.

Burkman R, Schlesselman JJ, Zieman M: Safety concerns and health benefits associated with oral contraception. Am J Obstet Gynecol 2004;190(Suppl 4):S5.

Chrousos GP, Torpy DJ, Gold PW: Interactions between the hypothalamic-pituitary-adrenal axis and the female reproductive system: Clinical implications. Ann Intern Med 1998;129:229.

Giangrande PH, McDonnell DP: The A and B isoforms of the human progesterone receptor: Two functionally different transcription factors encoded by a single gene. Recent Prog Horm Res 1999;54:291.

Gomes MPV, Deitcher SR: Risk of venous thromboembolic disease associated with hormonal contraceptives and hormone replacement therapy: A clinical review. Arch Intern Med 2004;164:1965.

Hall JM, McDonnell DP, Korach KS: Allosteric regulation of estrogen receptor structure, function, and co-activator recruitment by different estrogen response elements. Mol Endocrinol 2002;16:469.

Harman SM et al: Longitudinal effects of aging on serum total and free testosterone levels in healthy men. Baltimore Longitudinal Study of Aging. J Clin Endocrinol Metab 2001; 86:724.

Kalantaridou S, Chrousos GP: Monogenic disorders of puberty. J Clin Endocrinol Metab 2002;87:2481.

Kalantaridon S et al: Premature ovarian failure, endothelial dysfunction, and estrogen-progesterone replacement. Trends Endocrinol Metab 2006;17:101.

Lacey JV Jr et al: Oral contraceptives as risk factors for cervical adenocarcinomas and squamous cell carcinomas. Cancer Epidemiol Biomarkers Prev 1999;8:1079.

Manson JE et al: Estrogen plus progestin and the risk of coronary heart disease. N Engl J Med 2003;349:523.

Merke DP et al: Future directions in the study and management of congenital adrenal hyperplasia due to 21-hydroxylase deficiency. Ann Intern Med 2002;136:320.

Mooradian AD, Morley JD, Korenman SG: Biological action of androgens. Endocr Rev 1987;8:1.

Price VH: Treatment of hair loss. N Engl J Med 1999;341:964.

Rossouw JE et al: Risks and benefits of estrogen plus progestin in healthy postmenopausal women: Principal results from the Women's Health Initiative randomized controlled trial. JAMA 2002;288:321.

Smith RE: A review of selective estrogen receptor modulators in national surgical adjuvant breast and bowel project clinical trials. Semin Oncol 2003;30(5 Suppl 16):4.

Snyder PJ et al: Effect of testosterone replacement in hypogonadal men. J Clin Endocrinol Metab 2000;85:2670.

US Preventive Services Task Force: Hormone therapy for the prevention of chronic conditions in postmenopausal women. Ann Intern Med 2005;142:855.

Wehrmacher WH, Messmore H: Women's health initiative is fundamentally flawed. Gend Med 2005;2:4.

Weisberg E: Interactions between oral contraceptives and antifungals/antibacterials. Is contraceptive failure the result? Clin Pharmacokinet 1999;36:309.

Young NR et al: Body composition and muscle strength in healthy men receiving T enanthate for contraception. J Clin Endocrinol Metab 1993;77:1028.

Zandi PP et al: Hormone replacement therapy and incidence of Alzheimer's disease in older women. JAMA 2002;288:2123.

Pancreatic Hormones & Antidiabetic Drugs

41

Martha S. Nolte, MD, & John H. Karam, MD*

■ THE ENDOCRINE PANCREAS

The endocrine pancreas in the adult human consists of approximately 1 million islets of Langerhans interspersed throughout the pancreatic gland. Within the islets, at least four hormone-producing cells are present (Table 41–1). Their hormone products include **insulin,** the storage and anabolic hormone of the body; **islet amyloid polypeptide (IAPP, or amylin),** which modulates appetite, gastric emptying, and glucagon and insulin secretion; **glucagon,** the hyperglycemic factor that mobilizes glycogen stores; **somatostatin,** a universal inhibitor of secretory cells; and **pancreatic peptide,** a small protein that facilitates digestive processes by a mechanism not yet clarified.

The elevated blood glucose associated with diabetes mellitus results from absent or inadequate pancreatic insulin secretion, with or without concurrent impairment of insulin action. The disease states underlying the diagnosis of diabetes mellitus are now classified into four categories: type 1, *insulin-dependent diabetes;* type 2, *noninsulin-dependent diabetes;* type 3, other; and type 4, *gestational diabetes mellitus* (Expert Committee, 2003).

Type 1 Diabetes Mellitus

The hallmark of type 1 diabetes is selective B-cell destruction and *severe* or *absolute* insulin deficiency. Administration of insulin is essential in patients with type 1 diabetes. Type 1 diabetes is further subdivided into immune and idiopathic causes. The immune form is the most common form of type 1 diabetes. Although most patients are younger than 30 years of age at the time of diagnosis, the onset can occur at any age. Type 1 diabetes is found in all ethnic groups, but the highest incidence is in people from northern Europe and from Sardinia. Susceptibility appears to involve a multifactorial genetic linkage but only 10–15% of patients have a positive family history.

Type 2 Diabetes Mellitus

Type 2 diabetes is characterized by tissue resistance to the action of insulin combined with a *relative* deficiency in insulin secretion. A given individual may have more resistance or more B-cell deficiency, and the abnormalities may be mild or severe. Although insulin is produced by the B cells in these patients, it is inadequate to overcome the resistance, and the blood glucose rises. The impaired insulin action also affects fat metabolism, resulting in increased free fatty acid flux and triglyceride levels and reciprocally low levels of high-density lipoprotein (HDL).

Individuals with type 2 diabetes may not require insulin to survive, but 30% or more will benefit from insulin therapy to control the blood glucose. It is likely that 10–20% of individuals in whom type 2 diabetes was initially diagnosed actually have both type 1 and type 2 or a slowly progressing type 1, and ultimately will require full insulin replacement. Although persons with type 2 diabetes ordinarily do not develop ketosis, ketoacidosis may occur as the result of stress such as infection or use of medication that enhances resistance, eg, corticosteroids. Dehydration in untreated and poorly controlled individuals with type 2 diabetes can lead to a life-threatening condition called *nonketotic hyperosmolar coma.* In this condition, the blood glucose may rise to 6–20 times the normal range and an altered mental state develops or the person loses consciousness. Urgent medical care and rehydration is required.

Type 3 Diabetes Mellitus

The type 3 designation refers to multiple *other* specific causes of an elevated blood glucose: nonpancreatic diseases, drug therapy, etc. For a detailed list the reader is referred to Expert Committee, 2003.

Type 4 Diabetes Mellitus

Gestational diabetes (GDM) is defined as any abnormality in glucose levels noted for the first time during

*Deceased.

683

Table 41–1. Pancreatic islet cells and their secretory products.

Cell Types	Approximate Percent of Islet Mass	Secretory Products
A cell (alpha)	20	Glucagon, proglucagon
B cell (beta)	75	Insulin, C-peptide, proinsulin, amylin
D cell (delta)	3–5	Somatostatin
F cell (PP cell)[1]	< 2	Pancreatic polypeptide (PP)

[1]Within pancreatic polypeptide-rich lobules of adult islets, located only in the posterior portion of the head of the human pancreas, glucagon cells are scarce (< 0.5%) and F cells make up as much as 80% of the cells.

pregnancy. Gestational diabetes is diagnosed in approximately 4% of all pregnancies in the USA. During pregnancy, the placenta and placental hormones create an insulin resistance that is most pronounced in the last trimester. Risk assessment for diabetes is suggested starting at the first prenatal visit. High-risk women should be screened immediately. Screening may be deferred in lower-risk women until the 24th to 28th week of gestation.

INSULIN

Chemistry

Insulin is a small protein with a molecular weight in humans of 5808. It contains 51 amino acids arranged in two chains (A and B) linked by disulfide bridges; there are species differences in the amino acids of both chains. Proinsulin, a long single-chain protein molecule, is processed within the Golgi apparatus and packaged into granules, where it is hydrolyzed into insulin and a residual connecting segment called C-peptide by removal of four amino acids (shown in dashed circles in Figure 41–1).

Insulin and C-peptide are secreted in equimolar amounts in response to all insulin secretagogues; a small quantity of unprocessed or partially hydrolyzed proinsulin is released as well. Although proinsulin may have some mild hypoglycemic action, C-peptide has no known physiologic function. Granules within the B cells store the insulin in the form of crystals consisting of two atoms of zinc and six molecules of insulin. The entire human pancreas contains up to 8 mg of insulin, representing approximately 200 biologic units. Originally, the unit was defined on the basis of the hypoglycemic activity of insulin in rabbits. With improved purification techniques, the unit is presently defined on the basis of weight, and present insulin standards used for assay purposes contain 28 units per milligram.

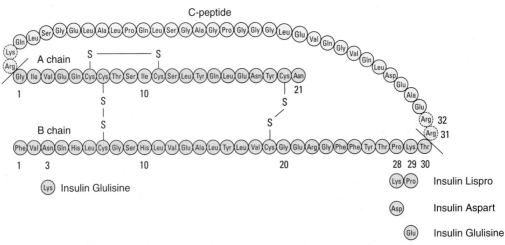

Figure 41–1. Structure of human proinsulin and some commercially available insulin analogs. Insulin is shown as the shaded (darker color) peptide chains, A and B. Differences in the A and B chains and amino acid modifications for insulin aspart, lispro, and glulisine are noted.

Figure 41–2. One model of control of insulin release from the pancreatic B cell by glucose and by sulfonylurea drugs. In the resting cell with normal (low) ATP levels, potassium diffuses down its concentration gradient through ATP-gated potassium channels, maintaining the intracellular potential at a fully polarized, negative level. Insulin release is minimal. If glucose concentration rises, ATP production increases, potassium channels close, and depolarization of the cell results. As in muscle and nerve, voltage-gated calcium channels open in response to depolarization, allowing more calcium to enter the cell. Increased intracellular calcium results in increased insulin secretion. Insulin secretagogues close the ATP-dependent potassium channel, thereby depolarizing the membrane and causing increased insulin release by the same mechanism. (Modified and reproduced, with permission, from *Basic & Clinical Endocrinology*, 4th ed. Greenspan F, Baxter JD [editors]: Originally published by Appleton & Lange. Copyright © 1994 by The McGraw-Hill Companies, Inc.)

Insulin Secretion

Insulin is released from pancreatic B cells at a low basal rate and at a much higher stimulated rate in response to a variety of stimuli, especially glucose. Other stimulants such as other sugars (eg, mannose), certain amino acids (eg, leucine, arginine), hormones such as glucagon-like polypeptide-1 and vagal activity are recognized. One mechanism of stimulated insulin release is diagrammed in Figure 41–2. As shown in the figure, hyperglycemia results in increased intracellular ATP levels, which close the ATP-dependent potassium channels. Decreased outward potassium efflux results in depolarization of the B cell and opening of voltage-gated calcium channels. The resulting increased intracellular calcium triggers secretion of the hormone. The insulin secretagogue drug group (sulfonylureas, meglitinides, and D-phenylalanine) exploits parts of this mechanism.

Insulin Degradation

The liver and kidney are the two main organs that remove insulin from the circulation. The liver normally clears the blood of approximately 60% of the insulin released from the pancreas by virtue of its location as the terminal site of portal vein blood flow, with the kidney removing 35–40% of the endogenous hormone. However, in insulin-treated diabetics receiving subcutaneous insulin injections, this ratio is reversed, with as much as 60% of exogenous insulin being cleared by the kidney and the liver removing no more than 30–40%. The half-life of circulating insulin is 3–5 minutes.

Circulating Insulin

Basal insulin values of 5–15 µU/mL (30–90 pmol/L) are found in normal humans, with a peak rise to 60–90 µU/mL (360–540 pmol/L) during meals.

The Insulin Receptor

After insulin has entered the circulation, it diffuses into tissues, where it is bound by specialized receptors that are found on the membranes of most tissues. The biologic responses promoted by these insulin-receptor complexes have been identified in the primary target tissues, ie, liver, muscle, and adipose tissue. The receptors bind insulin with high specificity and affinity in the picomolar range. The full insulin receptor consists of two covalently linked heterodimers, each containing an α subunit, which is entirely extracellular and constitutes the recognition site, and a β subunit that spans the membrane (Figure 41–3). The β subunit contains a tyrosine kinase. The binding of an insulin molecule to the α subunits at the outside surface of the cell activates the receptor and through a conformational change brings the catalytic loops of the opposing cytoplasmic β subunits into closer proximity. This facilitates mutual phosphorylation of tyrosine residues on the β subunits and tyrosine kinase activity directed at cytoplasmic proteins.

The first proteins to be phosphorylated by the activated receptor tyrosine kinases are the docking proteins, insulin receptor substrate-1 through -6 (IRS-1 to IRS-6). After tyrosine phosphorylation at several critical sites, the IRS molecules bind to and activate other kinases—most significantly phosphatidylinositol-3-kinase—which produce further phosphorylations or to an adaptor protein such as growth factor receptor-binding protein 2, which translates the insulin signal to a guanine nucleotide-releasing factor that ultimately activates the GTP binding protein ras, and the mitogen-activated protein kinase (MAPK) system. The particular IRS-phosphorylated tyrosine kinases have binding specificity with downstream molecules based on their surrounding 4–5 amino acid sequences or motifs that recognize specific Src homology 2 (SH2) domains on the other protein. This network of phosphorylations within the cell represents insulin's second message and results in multiple effects, including translocation of glucose transporters (especially GLUT 4, Table 41–2) to the cell membrane with a resultant increase in glucose uptake; increased glycogen synthase activity and increased glycogen formation; multiple effects on protein synthesis, lipolysis, and lipogenesis; and activation of transcription factors that enhance DNA synthesis and cell growth and division. The IRS-2 signaling pathway is associated with cellular proliferation and mitogenesis.

Various hormonal agents (eg, glucocorticoids) lower the affinity of insulin receptors for insulin; growth hormone in excess increases this affinity slightly. Aberrant serine and threonine phosphorylation of the insulin

Figure 41–3. Schematic diagram of the insulin receptor heterodimer in the activated state. IRS, insulin receptor substrate; P, phosphate; tyr, tyrosine.

receptor β subunits or IRS molecules may result in insulin resistance and functional receptor down-regulation.

Effects of Insulin on Its Targets

Insulin promotes the storage of fat as well as glucose (both sources of energy) within specialized target cells (Figure 41–4) and influences cell growth and the metabolic functions of a wide variety of tissues (Table 41–3).

Characteristics of Available Insulin Preparations

Commercial insulin preparations differ in a number of ways, such as differences in the recombinant DNA pro-

Table 41–2. Glucose transporters.

Transporter	Tissues	Glucose K_m (mmol/L)	Function
GLUT 1	All tissues, especially red cells, brain	1–2	Basal uptake of glucose; transport across the blood-brain barrier
GLUT 2	B cells of pancreas; liver, kidney; gut	15–20	Regulation of insulin release, other aspects of glucose homeostasis
GLUT 3	Brain, kidney, placenta, other tissues	< 1	Uptake into neurons, other tissues
GLUT 4	Muscle, adipose	≈ 5	Insulin-mediated uptake of glucose
GLUT 5	Gut, kidney	1–2	Absorption of fructose

Table 41–3. Endocrine effects of insulin.

Effect on liver:
  Reversal of catabolic features of insulin deficiency
    Inhibits glycogenolysis
    Inhibits conversion of fatty acids and amino acids to keto acids
    Inhibits conversion of amino acids to glucose
  Anabolic action
    Promotes glucose storage as glycogen (induces glucokinase and glycogen synthase, inhibits phosphorylase)
    Increases triglyceride synthesis and very-low-density lipoprotein formation

Effect on muscle:
  Increased protein synthesis
    Increases amino acid transport
    Increases ribosomal protein synthesis
  Increased glycogen synthesis
    Increases glucose transport
    Induces glycogen synthase and inhibits phosphorylase

Effect on adipose tissue:
  Increased triglyceride storage
    Lipoprotein lipase is induced and activated by insulin to hydrolyze triglycerides from lipoproteins
    Glucose transport into cell provides glycerol phosphate to permit esterification of fatty acids supplied by lipoprotein transport
    Intracellular lipase is inhibited by insulin

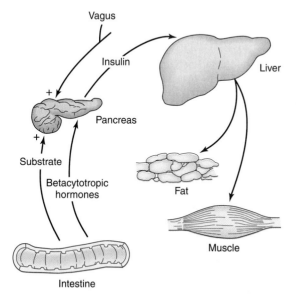

Figure 41–4. Insulin promotes synthesis (from circulating nutrients) and storage of glycogen, triglycerides, and protein in its major target tissues: liver, fat, and muscle. The release of insulin from the pancreas is stimulated by increased blood glucose, incretins, vagal nerve stimulation, and other factors (see text).

duction techniques, amino acid sequence, concentration, solubility, and the time of onset and duration of their biologic action. In 2006, 17 insulin formulations were available in the USA.

A. PRINCIPAL TYPES AND DURATION OF ACTION OF INSULIN PREPARATIONS

Four principal types of injected insulins are available: (1) rapid-acting, with very fast onset and short duration; (2) short-acting, with rapid onset of action; (3) intermediate-acting; and (4) long-acting, with slow onset of action (Figure 41–5, Table 41–4). An inhaled form of rapid-acting insulin also is marketed. Injected rapid-acting and short-acting insulins are dispensed as clear solutions at neutral pH and contain small amounts of zinc to improve their stability and shelf-life. Inhaled rapid-acting human insulin is available as a powder for alveolar absorption. Injected intermediate-acting NPH insulins have been modified to provide prolonged action and are dispensed as a turbid suspension at neutral pH with protamine in phosphate buffer (neutral protamine Hagedorn [NPH] insulin). Insulin glargine and insulin detemir are the soluble long-acting insulins. The goal of subcutaneous insulin therapy is to

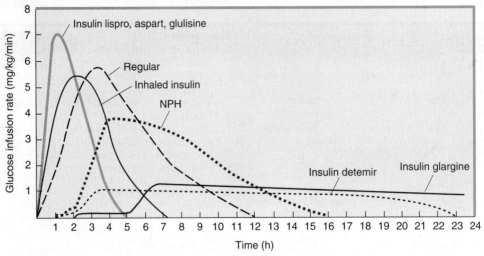

Figure 41–5. Extent and duration of action of various types of insulin as indicated by the glucose infusion rates (mg/kg/min) required to maintain a constant glucose concentration. The durations of action shown are typical of an average dose of 0.2–0.3 U/kg; with the exception of insulin lispro, aspart, and glulisine, duration increases considerably when dosage is increased.

replace the normal basal (overnight, fasting, and between meal) as well as bolus or prandial (mealtime) insulin. Current regimens generally use long-acting insulins to provide basal or background coverage, and rapid-acting insulin to meet the mealtime requirements. The latter insulins are given as supplemental doses to correct transient hyperglycemia. Intensive therapy ("tight control") attempts to restore near-normal glucose patterns throughout the day while minimizing the risk of hypoglycemia.

An exact reproduction of the normal glycemic profile is technically not possible because of the limitations inherent in subcutaneous administration of insulin. The most sophisticated insulin regimen delivers rapid-acting insulin through a continuous subcutaneous insulin infusion device; alternative intensive regimens referred to as multiple daily injections (MDI) use long-acting insulins with multiple boluses of rapid-acting insulin. Conventional therapy presently consists of split-dose injections of mixtures of rapid- or short-acting and intermediate-acting insulins.

1. Rapid-acting insulin—Three injected rapid-acting insulin analogs: **insulin lispro, insulin aspart,** and **insulin glulisine,** and one inhaled form of rapid-acting insulin, **human insulin recombinant inhaled,** are commercially available. The rapid-acting insulins permit more physiologic prandial insulin replacement because their rapid onset and early peak action more closely mimic normal endogenous prandial insulin secretion than does regular insulin, and

they have the additional benefit of allowing insulin to be taken immediately before the meal without sacrificing glucose control. Their duration of action is rarely more than 3–5 hours (with the exception of inhaled insulin, which may last 6–7 hours), which decreases the risk of late postmeal hypoglycemia. The injected rapid-acting insulins have the lowest variability of absorption (approximately 5%) of all available commercial insulins (compared to 25% for regular insulin and 25–50% for intermediate- and long-acting formulations). They are the preferred insulins for use in continuous subcutaneous insulin infusion devices.

Insulin lispro, the first monomeric insulin analog to be marketed, is produced by recombinant technology wherein two amino acids near the carboxyl terminal of the B chain have been reversed in position: Proline at position B28 has been moved to B29, and lysine at position B29 has been moved to B28 (Figure 41–1). Reversing these two amino acids does not interfere in any way with insulin lispro's binding to the insulin receptor, its circulating half-life, or its immunogenicity, which are similar to those of human regular insulin. However, the advantage of this analog is its very low propensity—in contrast to human insulin—to self-associate in antiparallel fashion and form dimers. To enhance the shelf-life of insulin in vials, insulin lispro is stabilized into hexamers by a cresol preservative. When injected subcutaneously, the drug quickly dissociates into monomers and is rapidly absorbed with onset of action

Table 41–4. Some insulin preparations available in the USA.[1]

Preparation	Species Source	Concentration
Rapid-acting insulins		
Insulin Lispro, Humalog (Lilly)	Human analog	U100
Insulin Aspart, Novolog (Novo Nordisk)	Human analog	U100
Insulin Glulisine, Apidra (Aventis)	Human analog	U100
Short-acting insulins		
Regular Novolin R (Novo Nordisk)	Human	U100
Regular Humulin R (Lilly)	Human	U100, U500
Velosulin BR (Novo Nordisk)[2]	Human	U100
Regular, Exubera (Pfizer)	Human	1, 3, 6 mg powder (inhaled)
Intermediate-acting insulins		
NPH Humulin N (Lilly)	Human	U100
NPH Novolin N (Novo Nordisk)	Human	U100
Premixed insulins (% NPH/ % regular)		
Novolin 70/30 (Novo Nordisk)	Human	U100
Humulin 70/30 and 50/50 (Lilly)	Human	U100
50/50 NPL, Lispro (Lilly)	Human analog	U100
75/25 NPL, Lispro (Lilly)	Human analog	U100
70/30 NPA, Aspart (Novo Nordisk)	Human analog	U100
Long-acting insulins		
Insulin detemir, Levemir (Novo Nordisk)	Human analog	U100
Insulin glargine, Lantus (Aventis/Hoechst Marion Roussel)	Human analog	U100

[1]All of these agents (except insulin lispro, insulin aspart, insulin detemir, insulin glulisine, inhaled insulin, and U500 regular Humulin) are available without a prescription. All insulins should be refrigerated and brought to room temperature just before injection.
[2]Velosulin contains phosphate buffer, which favors its use to prevent insulin aggregation in pump tubing but precludes its being mixed with lente insulin.

within 5–15 minutes and peak activity as early as 1 hour. The time to peak action is relatively constant, regardless of the dose.

Insulin aspart is created by the substitution of the B28 proline with a negatively charged aspartic acid (Figure 41–1). This modification reduces the normal ProB28 and GlyB23 monomer-monomer interaction, thereby inhibiting insulin self-aggregation. Its absorption and activity profile is similar to that of insulin lispro, and it is more reproducible than regular insulin, but has similar binding properties, activity, and mitogenicity characteristics to regular insulin and equivalent immunogenicity.

Insulin glulisine is formulated by substituting an asparagine for lysine at B3 and glutamic acid for lysine at B29. Its absorption, action, and immunologic characteristics are similar to the other injected rapid-acting insulins. After high-dose insulin glulisine-insulin receptor interaction, there may be downstream differences in IRS-2 pathway activation relative to human insulin. The clinical significance of such differences is unclear.

Inhaled human insulin is a powder form of rDNA human insulin that is administered through an inhaler device and is marketed for pre-prandial and blood sugar correction use in adults with type 1 and 2 diabetes. Because of concerns about lung safety, it is not approved for use in children, teenagers, or adults with asthma, bronchitis, emphysema, smokers, or those within 6 months of quitting smoking. Although this route of administration is well tolerated, studies have shown that less than 30% of users were able to achieve target blood glucoses after 6 months of therapy with inhaled human insulin.

2. Short-acting insulin—Regular insulin is a short-acting soluble crystalline zinc insulin made by recombinant DNA techniques to produce a molecule identical to human insulin. Its effect appears within 30 minutes and peaks between 2 and 3 hours after subcutaneous injection and generally lasts 5–8 hours. In high concentrations, eg, in the vial, regular insulin molecules self-aggregate in antiparallel fashion to form dimers that stabilize around zinc ions to create insulin hexamers. The hexameric nature of regular insulin causes a delayed onset and prolongs the time to peak action. After subcutaneous injection, the insulin hexamers are too large and bulky to be transported across the vascular endothelium into the bloodstream. As the insulin depot is diluted by interstitial fluid and the concentration begins to fall, the hexamers break down into dimers and finally monomers. This results in three rates of absorption of the injected insulin, with the final monomeric phase having the fastest uptake out of the injection site. The delayed absorption results in a mismatching of insulin availability with need.

Specifically, when regular insulin is administered at mealtime, the blood glucose rises faster than the insulin with resultant early postprandial hyperglycemia and an increased risk of late postprandial hypoglycemia. Regular insulin should be injected 30–45 or more minutes before the meal to minimize the mismatching. As with all older insulin formulations, the duration of action as well as the time of onset and the intensity of peak action increase with the size of the dose. Clinically, this is a critical issue because the pharmacokinetics and pharmacodynamics of small doses of regular and NPH insulins differ greatly from those of large doses. Short-acting soluble insulin is the only type that should be administered intravenously because the dilution causes the hexameric insulin to immediately dissociate into monomers. It is particularly useful for intravenous therapy in the management of diabetic ketoacidosis and when the insulin requirement is changing rapidly, such as after surgery or during acute infections.

3. Intermediate-acting and long-acting insulins—
  a. NPH (neutral protamine Hagedorn, or isophane) insulin—NPH insulin is an intermediate-acting insulin wherein absorption and the onset of action are delayed by combining appropriate amounts of insulin and protamine so that neither is present in an uncomplexed form ("isophane"). Protamine is a mixture of six major and some minor compounds of similar structure isolated from the sperm of rainbow trout. They appear to be basic, arginine-rich peptides with an average molecular weight of approximately 4400. To form an isophane complex (one in which neither component retains any free binding sites), approximately a 1:10 ratio by weight of protamine to insulin is required, representing approximately six molecules of insulin per

molecule of protamine. After subcutaneous injection, proteolytic tissue enzymes degrade the protamine to permit absorption of insulin. NPH insulin has an onset of approximately 2–5 hours and duration of 4–12 hours (Figure 41–5); it is usually mixed with regular, lispro, aspart, or glulisine insulin and given two to four times daily for insulin replacement in patients with type 1 diabetes. The dose regulates the action profile; specifically, small doses have lower, earlier peaks and a short duration of action with the converse true for large doses.

  b. Insulin glargine—Insulin glargine is a soluble, "peakless" (ie, having a broad plasma concentration plateau), ultra-long-acting insulin analog. This product was designed to provide reproducible, convenient, background insulin replacement. The attachment of two arginine molecules to the B chain carboxyl terminal and substitution of a glycine for asparagine at the A21 position created an analog that is soluble in an acidic solution but precipitates in the more neutral body pH after subcutaneous injection. Individual insulin molecules slowly dissolve away from the crystalline depot and provide a low, continuous level of circulating insulin. Insulin glargine has a slow onset of action (1–1.5 hours) and achieves a maximum effect after 4–6 hours. This maximum activity is maintained for 11–24 hours or longer. Glargine is usually given once daily, although some very insulin-sensitive individuals benefit from split (twice a day) dosing. To maintain solubility, the formulation is unusually acidic (pH 4.0) and insulin glargine should not be mixed with other insulins. Separate syringes must be used to minimize the risk of contamination and subsequent loss of efficacy. The absorption pattern of insulin glargine appears to be independent of the anatomic site of injection, and this drug is associated with less immunogenicity than human insulin in animal studies. Glargine's interaction with the insulin receptor is similar to that of native insulin and shows no increase in mitogenic activity in vitro. It has sixfold to sevenfold greater binding than native insulin to the insulin-like growth factor-1 (IGF-1) receptor, but the clinical significance of this is unclear.

  c. Insulin detemir—This insulin is the most recently developed long-acting insulin analog. The terminal threonine is dropped from the B30 position and myristic acid (a C-14 fatty acid chain) is attached to the terminal B29 lysine. These modifications prolong the availability of the injected analog by increasing both self-aggregation in subcutaneous tissue and reversible albumin binding. Insulin detemir has the most reproducible effect of the intermediate- and long-acting insulins, and its use is associated with less hypoglycemia than NPH insulin. Insulin detemir has a dose-dependent onset of action of 1–2 hours and duration of action of more than 24 hours. It is given twice daily to obtain a smooth background insulin level.

4. Mixtures of insulins—Because intermediate-acting NPH insulins require several hours to reach adequate therapeutic levels, their use in type 1 diabetic patients requires supplements of rapid- or short-acting insulin before meals. For convenience, these are often mixed together in the same syringe before injection. Insulin lispro, aspart, and glulisine can be *acutely* mixed (ie, just before injection) with NPH insulin without affecting their rapid absorption. However, *premixed* preparations have thus far been unstable. To remedy this, intermediate insulins composed of isophane complexes of protamine with insulin lispro and insulin aspart have been developed. These intermediate insulins have been designated as "NPL" (neutral protamine lispro) and "NPA" (neutral protamine aspart) and have the same duration of action as NPH insulin. They have the advantage of permitting formulation as premixed combinations of NPL and insulin lispro, and as NPA and insulin aspart, and they have been shown to be safe and effective in clinical trials. The FDA has approved 50%/50% and 75%/25% NPL/insulin lispro and 70%/30% NPA/insulin aspart premixed formulations. Additional ratios are available abroad. Insulin glargine and detemir must be given as separate injections. They are not miscible acutely or in a premixed preparation with any other insulin formulation.

B. Insulin Production

Human insulins—Mass production of human insulin and insulin analogs by recombinant DNA techniques is carried out by inserting the human or a modified proinsulin gene into *Escherichia coli* or yeast and treating the extracted proinsulin to form the insulin or insulin analog molecules.

C. Concentration

All insulins in the USA and Canada are currently available in a concentration of 100 U/mL (U100). A limited supply of U500 regular human insulin is available for use in rare cases of severe insulin resistance in which larger doses of insulin are required.

Insulin Delivery Systems

The standard mode of insulin therapy is subcutaneous injection using conventional disposable needles and syringes. During the last three decades, much effort has gone into exploration of other means of administration, and inhaled insulin is now available.

A. Portable Pen Injectors

To facilitate multiple subcutaneous injections of insulin, particularly during intensive insulin therapy, portable pen-sized injectors have been developed. These contain cartridges of insulin and replaceable needles.

Disposable insulin pens are also available for selected formulations. These are regular insulin, insulin lispro, insulin aspart, insulin glulisine, insulin glargine, insulin detemir, and several mixtures of NPH with regular, lispro, or aspart insulin (Table 41–4). They have been well accepted by patients because they eliminate the need to carry syringes and bottles of insulin to the workplace and while traveling.

B. Continuous Subcutaneous Insulin Infusion Devices (CSII, Insulin Pumps)

Continuous subcutaneous insulin infusion devices are external open-loop pumps for insulin delivery. The devices have a user-programmable pump that delivers individualized basal and bolus insulin replacement doses based on blood glucose self-monitoring results. Normally, the 24-hour background basal rates are relatively constant from day to day, although temporarily altered rates can be superimposed to adjust for a short-term change in requirement. For example, the basal delivery rate might need to be decreased for several hours because of the increased insulin sensitivity associated with strenuous activity. In contrast, the bolus amounts frequently vary and are used to correct high blood glucose levels and to cover mealtime insulin requirements based on the carbohydrate content of the food and concurrent activity. The pump—which contains an insulin reservoir, the program chip, the keypad, and the display screen—is about the size of a pager. It is usually placed on a belt or in a pocket, and the insulin is infused through thin plastic tubing that is connected to the subcutaneously inserted infusion set. The abdomen is the favored site for the infusion set, although flanks and thighs are also used. The insulin reservoir, tubing, and infusion set need to be changed using sterile techniques every 2 or 3 days. CSII delivery is regarded as the most physiologic method of insulin replacement.

The use of these continuous infusion devices is encouraged for individuals who are unable to obtain target control while on multiple injection regimens and in circumstances in which excellent glycemic control is desired, such as during pregnancy. Their optimal use requires responsible involvement and commitment by the patient. Velosulin (a regular insulin) and insulin aspart, lispro, and glulisine are all specifically approved for pump use. Insulins aspart, lispro, and glulisine are preferred pump insulins because their favorable pharmacokinetic attributes allow glycemic control without increasing the risk of hypoglycemia.

C. Inhaled Insulin

The FDA has approved an inhaled insulin preparation of finely powdered and aerosolized human insulin. Insulin is readily absorbed into the bloodstream through alveolar walls, but the challenge has been to create particles that are small enough to pass through the bronchial tree without being trapped and still enter the alveoli in sufficient amounts to have a clinical effect. Insulin delivered by the inhaled route has pharmacokinetic and pharmacodynamic characteristics of both rapid- and short-acting insulin. It has a rapid onset and peak insulin levels (by 30 minutes) similar to insulin lispro, aspart, and glulisine, and peak effect (2–2.5 hours) and duration of action (6–8 hours) similar to regular insulin. Inhaled insulin can be used to cover mealtime insulin requirements or to correct high glucose levels, but not to provide background or basal insulin coverage. Less than 10% of the inhaled insulin dose (which ranges from 1 mg to 6 mg) is absorbed. One milligram of inhaled insulin is equivalent to 2–3 units of regular human insulin injected subcutaneously. Safety concerns include possible pulmonary fibrosis or hypertension, reduced lung volume or oxygen diffusing capacity, and excessive insulin antibody formation.

Treatment with Insulin

The current classification of diabetes mellitus identifies a group of patients who have virtually no insulin secretion and whose survival depends on administration of exogenous insulin. This insulin-dependent group (type 1) represents 5–10% of the diabetic population in the USA. Most type 2 diabetics do not require exogenous insulin for survival, but many need exogenous supplementation of their endogenous secretion to achieve optimum health.

Benefit of Glycemic Control in Diabetes Mellitus

The consensus of the American Diabetes Association is that intensive glycemic control associated with comprehensive self-management training should become standard therapy in type 1 patients (see Box: Benefits of Tight Glycemic Control in Diabetes). Exceptions include patients with advanced renal disease and the elderly, since the risks of hypoglycemia outweigh the benefit of tight glycemic control in these groups. In children under the age of 7 years, the extreme susceptibility of the developing brain to damage from hypoglycemia contraindicates attempts at intensive glycemic control. A similar conclusion regarding the benefits of tight control in type 2 diabetes was reached as the result of a large study in the United Kingdom.

Complications of Insulin Therapy

A. Hypoglycemia

1. Mechanisms and diagnosis—Hypoglycemic reactions are the most common complication of insulin therapy. They may result from a delay in taking a meal, inadequate carbohydrate consumed, unusual physical exertion, or a dose of insulin that is too large for immediate needs.

Rapid development of hypoglycemia in individuals with intact hypoglycemic awareness causes signs of autonomic hyperactivity, both sympathetic (tachycardia, palpitations, sweating, tremulousness) and parasympathetic (nausea, hunger) and may progress to convulsions and coma if untreated.

In individuals exposed to frequent hypoglycemic episodes during tight glycemic control, autonomic warning signals of hypoglycemia are less common or even absent. This dangerous acquired condition is termed "hypoglycemic unawareness." When patients lack the early warning signs of low blood glucose, they may not take corrective measures in time. In patients with persistent, untreated hypoglycemia, the manifestations of insulin excess may develop—confusion, weakness, bizarre behavior, coma, seizures—at which point they may not be able to procure or safely swallow glucose-containing foods. Hypoglycemic awareness may be restored by preventing frequent hypoglycemic episodes. An identification bracelet, necklace, or card in the wallet or purse, as well as some form of rapidly absorbed glucose, should be carried by every diabetic who is receiving hypoglycemic drug therapy.

2. Treatment of hypoglycemia—All the manifestations of hypoglycemia are relieved by glucose administration. To expedite absorption, simple sugar or glucose should be given, preferably in a liquid form. To treat mild hypoglycemia in a patient who is conscious and able to swallow, dextrose tablets, glucose gel, or any sugar-containing beverage or food may be given. If more severe hypoglycemia has produced unconsciousness or stupor, the treatment of choice is to give 20–50 mL of 50% glucose solution by intravenous infusion over a period of 2–3 minutes. If intravenous therapy is not available, 1 mg of glucagon injected either subcutaneously or intramuscularly usually restores consciousness within 15 minutes to permit ingestion of sugar. If the patient is stuporous and glucagon is not available, small amounts of honey or syrup can be inserted into the buccal pouch. In general, however, oral feeding is contraindicated in unconscious patients. Emergency medical services should be called for all episodes of severely impaired consciousness.

B. Immunopathology of Insulin Therapy

At least five molecular classes of insulin antibodies may be produced in diabetics during the course of insulin therapy: IgA, IgD, IgE, IgG, and IgM. There are two major types of immune disorders in these patients:

1. Insulin allergy—Insulin allergy, an immediate type hypersensitivity, is a rare condition in which local or systemic urticaria results from histamine release from tissue mast cells sensitized by anti-insulin IgE antibodies. In severe cases, anaphylaxis results. Because sensitivity is often to noninsulin protein contaminants, the human and analog insulins have markedly reduced the incidence of insulin allergy, especially local reactions.

BENEFITS OF TIGHT GLYCEMIC CONTROL IN DIABETES

A long-term randomized prospective study involving 1441 type 1 patients in 29 medical centers reported in 1993 that "near normalization" of blood glucose resulted in a delay in onset and a major slowing of progression of microvascular and neuropathic complications of diabetes during follow-up periods of up to 10 years (Diabetes Control And Complications Trial [DCCT] Research Group, 1993). In the intensively treated group, a mean glycated hemoglobin HbA_{1c} of 7.2% (normal <6%) and a mean blood glucose of 155 mg/dL were achieved, whereas in the conventionally treated group, HbA_{1c} averaged 8.9% with an average blood glucose of 225 mg/dL. Over the study period, which averaged 7 years, approximately a 60% reduction in risk of diabetic retinopathy, nephropathy, and neuropathy was noted in the tight control group compared with the standard control group.

The DCCT study, in addition, has introduced the concept of *glycemic memory*, which comprises the long-term benefits of any significant period of glycemic control. During a 6-year follow-up period, both the intensively and the conventionally treated groups had similar levels of glycemic control, and both had progression of carotid intimal-medial thickness. However, the intensively treated cohort had significantly less progression of intimal thickness.

The United Kingdom Prospective Diabetes Study (UKPDS) was a very large randomized prospective study carried out to study the effects of intensive glycemic control with several types of therapies and the effects of blood pressure control in type 2 diabetic patients. A total of 3867 newly diagnosed type 2 diabetic patients were studied over 10 years. A significant fraction of these were overweight and hypertensive. Patients were given dietary treatment alone or intensive therapy with insulin, chlorpropamide, glyburide, or glipizide. Metformin was an option for patients with inadequate response to other therapies. Tight control of blood pressure was added as a variable, with an angiotensin-converting enzyme inhibitor, β-blocker or, in some cases, a calcium channel blocker available for this purpose.

Tight control of diabetes, with reduction of HbA_{1c} from 9.1% to 7%, was shown to reduce the risk of microvascular complications overall compared with that achieved with conventional therapy (mostly diet alone, which decreased HbA_{1c} to 7.9%). Cardiovascular complications were not noted for any particular therapy; metformin treatment alone reduced the risk of macrovascular disease (myocardial infarction, stroke).

Tight control of hypertension also had a surprisingly significant effect on microvascular disease (as well as more conventional hypertension-related sequelae) in these diabetic patients. These studies show that tight glycemic control benefits both type 1 and type 2 patients.

The STOP-NIDDM trial followed up 1429 patients with impaired glucose tolerance who were randomized to treatment with acarbose or placebo over 3 years. This trial demonstrated that normalization of glycemic control in subjects with impaired glucose tolerance significantly diminished cardiovascular risk. The acarbose-treated group had a significant reduction in the development of major cardiovascular events and hypertension. A prospective placebo-controlled subgroup analysis has shown a marked decrease in the progression of intimal-medial thickness.

---

2. Immune insulin resistance—A low titer of circulating IgG anti-insulin antibodies that neutralize the action of insulin to a negligible extent develops in most insulin-treated patients. Rarely, the titer of insulin antibodies leads to insulin resistance and may be associated with other systemic autoimmune processes such as lupus erythematosus.

C. LIPODYSTROPHY AT INJECTION SITES

Injection of older animal insulin preparations sometimes led to atrophy of subcutaneous fatty tissue at the site of injection. This type of immune complication is almost never seen since the development of human and analog insulin preparations of neutral pH. Injection of these newer preparations directly into the atrophic area often results in restoration of normal contours. Hypertrophy of subcutaneous fatty tissue remains a problem if injected repeatedly at the same site. However, this may be corrected by avoidance of that specific injection site or with liposuction.

■ ORAL ANTIDIABETIC AGENTS

Four categories of oral antidiabetic agents are now available in the USA: **insulin secretagogues** (sulfonylureas, meglitinides, D-phenylalanine derivatives), **biguanides, thiazolidinediones,** and **α-glucosidase inhibitors.** The sulfonylureas and biguanides have been available the longest and are the traditional initial treatment choice for type 2 diabetes. Novel classes of rapidly acting insulin secretagogues, the meglitinides and D-phenylalanine derivatives, are alternatives to the short-acting sulfonylurea, tolbutamide. The thiazolidinediones, under development since the early 1980s, are very effective agents that reduce insulin resistance. Alpha-glucosidase inhibitors have a relatively weak antidiabetic effect and significant adverse effects, and they are used primarily as adjunctive therapy in individuals who cannot achieve their glycemic goals with other medications.

INSULIN SECRETAGOGUES: SULFONYLUREAS

Mechanism of Action

The major action of sulfonylureas is to increase insulin release from the pancreas (Table 41–5). Two additional mechanisms of action have been proposed—a reduction of serum glucagon levels and closure of potassium channels in extrapancreatic tissues.

A. INSULIN RELEASE FROM PANCREATIC B CELLS

Sulfonylureas bind to a 140-kDa high-affinity sulfonylurea receptor (Figure 41–2) that is associated with a B-cell inward rectifier ATP-sensitive potassium channel. Binding of a sulfonylurea inhibits the efflux of potassium ions through the channel and results in depolarization. Depolarization opens a voltage-gated calcium channel and results in calcium influx and the release of preformed insulin.

B. REDUCTION OF SERUM GLUCAGON CONCENTRATIONS

Long-term administration of sulfonylureas to type 2 diabetics reduces serum glucagon levels, which may contribute to the hypoglycemic effect of the drugs. The mechanism for this suppressive effect of sulfonylureas on glucagon levels is unclear but appears to involve indirect inhibition due to enhanced release of both insulin and somatostatin, which inhibit A-cell secretion.

C. POTASSIUM CHANNEL CLOSURE IN EXTRAPANCREATIC TISSUES

Insulin secretagogues bind to sulfonylurea receptors in potassium channels in extrapancreatic tissues, but the binding affinity varies among the drug classes and is much less avid than for the B-cell receptors. The clinical significance of extrapancreatic binding is not known.

Efficacy & Safety of the Sulfonylureas

In 1970, the University Group Diabetes Program (UGDP) in the USA reported that the number of deaths due to cardiovascular disease in diabetic patients treated with tolbutamide was excessive compared with either insulin-treated patients or those receiving place-

Table 41–5. Regulation of insulin release in humans.

Stimulants of insulin release
Glucose, mannose
Leucine
Vagal stimulation
Sulfonylureas
Amplifiers of glucose-induced insulin release
Enteric hormones:
Glucagon-like peptide 1(7–37)
Gastrin inhibitory peptide
Cholecystokinin
Secretin, gastrin
Neural amplifiers:
β-Adrenoceptor stimulation
Amino acids:
Arginine
Inhibitors of insulin release
Neural: α-Sympathomimetic effect of catecholamines
Humoral: Somatostatin, amylin
Drugs: Diazoxide, phenytoin, vinblastine, colchicine

Modified and reproduced, with permission, from Greenspan FS, Strewler GJ (editors): Basic & Clinical Endocrinology, 5th ed. Originally published by Appleton & Lange. Copyright © 1997 by The McGraw-Hill Companies, Inc.

bos. Owing to design flaws, this study and its conclusions were not generally accepted. A study in the United Kingdom, the UKPDS, did not find an untoward cardiovascular effect of sulfonylurea usage in their large, long-term study.

The sulfonylureas continue to be widely prescribed, and six are available in the USA (Table 41–6). They are conventionally divided into first-generation and second-generation agents, which differ primarily in their potency and adverse effects. The first-generation sulfonylureas are increasingly difficult to procure, and as the second-generation agents become generic and less expensive, the older compounds probably will be discontinued.

1. First-Generation Sulfonylureas

Tolbutamide is well absorbed but rapidly metabolized in the liver. Its duration of effect is relatively short, with an elimination half-life of 4–5 hours, and it is best administered in divided doses. Because of its short half-life, it is the safest sulfonylurea for elderly diabetics. Prolonged hypoglycemia has been reported rarely, mostly in patients receiving certain drugs (eg, dicumarol, phenylbutazone, some sulfonamides) that inhibit the metabolism of tolbutamide.

Chlorpropamide has a half-life of 32 hours and is slowly metabolized in the liver to products that retain

Table 41–6. Sulfonylureas.

Sulfonylureas	Chemical Structure	Daily Dose	Duration of Action (hours)
Tolbutamide (Orinase)	H_3C—〈〉—SO_2—NH—C(=O)—NH—$(CH_2)_3$—CH_3	0.5–2 g in divided doses	6–12
Tolazamide (Tolinase)	H_3C—〈〉—SO_2—NH—C(=O)—NH—N〈ring〉	0.1–1 g as single dose or in divided doses	10–14
Chlorpropamide (Diabinese)	Cl—〈〉—SO_2—NH—C(=O)—NH—$(CH_2)_2$—CH_3	0.1–0.5 g as single dose	Up to 60
Glyburide (glibenclamide[1]) (Diaβeta, Micronase, Glynase PresTab)	Cl, OCH_3 substituted benzamide—C(=O)—NH—$(CH_2)_2$—〈〉—SO_2—NH—C(=O)—NH—〈cyclohexyl〉	0.00125–0.02 g	10–24
Glipizide (glydiazinamide[1]) (Glucotrol, Glucotrol XL)	H_3C, N, N pyrazine—C(=O)—NH—$(CH_2)_2$—〈〉—SO_2—NH—C(=O)—NH—〈cyclohexyl〉	0.005–0.03 g (0.02 g in Glucotrol XL)	10–24[2]
Glimepiride (Amaryl)	H_3C, H_5C_2, O pyrroline—N—$CONHCH_2CH_2$—〈〉—$SO_2NHCONH$—〈cyclohexyl〉—CH_3	0.001–0.004 g	12–24

[1]Outside USA.
[2]Elimination half-life considerably shorter (see text).

some biologic activity; approximately 20–30% is excreted unchanged in the urine. Chlorpropamide also interacts with the drugs mentioned above that depend on hepatic oxidative catabolism, and it is contraindicated in patients with hepatic or renal insufficiency. Dosages higher than 500 mg daily increase the risk of jaundice. The average maintenance dosage is 250 mg daily, given as a single dose in the morning. Prolonged hypoglycemic reactions are more common in elderly patients, and the drug is contraindicated in this group. Other side effects include a hyperemic flush after alcohol ingestion in genetically predisposed patients and dilutional hyponatremia. Hematologic toxicity (transient leukopenia, thrombocytopenia) occurs in less than 1% of patients.

Tolazamide is comparable to chlorpropamide in potency but has a shorter duration of action. Tolazamide is more slowly absorbed than the other sulfonylureas, and its effect on blood glucose does not appear for several hours. Its half-life is about 7 hours. Tolazamide is metabolized to several compounds that retain hypoglycemic effects. If more than 500 mg/d are required, the dose should be divided and given twice daily.

2. Second-Generation Sulfonylureas

The second-generation sulfonylureas are more frequently prescribed in the USA than the first-generation agents because they have fewer adverse effects and drug interactions. These potent sulfonylurea compounds—glyburide, glipizide, and glimepiride—should be used with caution in patients with cardiovascular disease or in elderly patients, in whom hypoglycemia would be especially dangerous.

Glyburide is metabolized in the liver into products with very low hypoglycemic activity. The usual starting dosage is 2.5 mg/d or less, and the average maintenance dosage is 5–10 mg/d given as a single morning dose; maintenance dosages higher than 20 mg/d are not recommended. A formulation of "micronized" glyburide (Glynase PresTab) is available in a variety of tablet sizes. However, there is some question as to its bioequivalence with nonmicronized formulations, and the FDA recommends careful monitoring to retitrate dosage when switching from standard glyburide doses or from other sulfonylurea drugs.

Glyburide has few adverse effects other than its potential for causing hypoglycemia. Flushing has rarely been reported after ethanol ingestion, and the compound slightly enhances free water clearance. Glyburide is contraindicated in the presence of hepatic impairment and in patients with renal insufficiency.

Glipizide has the shortest half-life (2–4 hours) of the more potent agents. For maximum effect in reducing postprandial hyperglycemia, this agent should be ingested 30 minutes before breakfast, because absorption is delayed when the drug is taken with food. The recommended starting dosage is 5 mg/d, with up to 15 mg/d given as a single dose. When higher daily dosages are required, they should be divided and given before meals. The maximum total daily dosage recommended by the manufacturer is 40 mg/d, although some studies indicate that the maximum therapeutic effect is achieved by 15–20 mg of the drug. An extended-release preparation (Glucotrol XL) provides 24-hour action after a once-daily morning dose (maximum of 20 mg/d). However, this formulation appears to have sacrificed its lower propensity for severe hypoglycemia compared with longer-acting glyburide without showing any demonstrable therapeutic advantages over the latter (which can be obtained as a generic drug).

Because of its shorter half-life, the regular formulation of glipizide is much less likely than glyburide to produce serious hypoglycemia. At least 90% of glipizide is metabolized in the liver to inactive products, and 10% is excreted unchanged in the urine. Glipizide therapy is therefore contraindicated in patients with significant hepatic or renal impairment, who would be at high risk for hypoglycemia.

Glimepiride is approved for once-daily use as monotherapy or in combination with insulin. Glimepiride achieves blood glucose lowering with the lowest dose of any sulfonylurea compound. A single daily dose of 1 mg has been shown to be effective, and the recommended maximal daily dose is 8 mg. It has a long duration of effect with a half-life of 5 hours, allowing once-daily dosing and thereby improving compliance. It is completely metabolized by the liver to inactive products.

Secondary Failure & Tachyphylaxis to Sulfonylureas

Secondary failure, ie, failure to maintain a good response to sulfonylurea therapy over the long term, remains a disconcerting problem in the management of type 2 diabetes. A progressive decrease in B-cell mass, reduction in physical activity, decline in lean body mass, or increase in ectopic fat deposition in chronic type 2 diabetes also may contribute to secondary failure.

INSULIN SECRETAGOGUES: MEGLITINIDES

The meglitinides are a relatively new class of insulin secretagogues. **Repaglinide,** the first member of the group, was approved for clinical use in 1998 (Table 41–7). These drugs modulate B-cell insulin release by regulating potassium efflux through the potassium channels previously discussed. There is overlap with the sulfonylureas in their molecular sites of action because the meglitinides have two binding sites in common with the sulfonylureas and one unique binding site.

Repaglinide has a very fast onset of action, with a peak concentration and peak effect within approximately 1 hour after ingestion, but the duration of action is 5–8 hours. It is hepatically cleared by CYP3A4 with a plasma half-life of 1 hour. Because of its rapid onset, repaglinide is indicated for use in controlling postprandial glucose excursions. The drug should be taken just before each meal in doses of 0.25–4 mg (maximum, 16 mg/d); hypoglycemia is a risk if the meal is delayed or skipped or contains inadequate carbohydrate. This drug should be used cautiously in individuals with renal and hepatic impairment. Repaglinide is approved as monotherapy or in combination with biguanides. There is no sulfur in its structure, so repaglinide may be used in type 2 diabetic individuals with sulfur or sulfonylurea allergy.

INSULIN SECRETAGOGUE: D-PHENYLALANINE DERIVATIVE

Nateglinide, a D-phenylalanine derivative, is the latest insulin secretagogue to become clinically available. Nateglinide stimulates very rapid and transient release of insulin from B cells through closure of the ATP-sensitive K^+ channel. It also partially restores initial insulin release in response to an intravenous glucose tolerance test. This may be a significant advantage of the drug because type 2 diabetes is associated with loss of this initial insulin response. The restoration of more normal insulin secretion may suppress glucagon release early in

Table 41–7. Meglitinides.

Drug	Chemical Structure	Oral Dose	$t_{1/2}$	Duration of Action (hours)
Repaglinide (Prandin)		0.25–4 mg before meals	1 hour	4–5
Nateglinide (Starlix)		60–120 mg before meals	1 hour	4

the meal and result in less endogenous or hepatic glucose production. Nateglinide may have a special role in the treatment of individuals with isolated postprandial hyperglycemia, but it has minimal effect on overnight or fasting glucose levels. Nateglinide is efficacious when given alone or in combination with nonsecretagogue oral agents (such as metformin). In contrast to other insulin secretagogues, dose titration is not required.

Nateglinide is ingested just before meals. It is absorbed within 20 minutes after oral administration with a time to peak concentration of less than 1 hour and is hepatically metabolized by CYP2C9 and CYP3A4 with a half-life of 1.5 hours. The overall duration of action is less than 4 hours.

Nateglinide amplifies the insulin secretory response to a glucose load but has a markedly diminished effect in the presence of normoglycemia. The incidence of hypoglycemia may be the lowest of all the secretagogues, and it has the advantage of being safe in individuals with very reduced renal function.

BIGUANIDES

The structure of metformin is shown below. Phenformin (an older biguanide) was discontinued in the USA because of its association with lactic acidosis and because there was no documentation of any long-term benefit from its use.

Metformin

Mechanisms of Action

A full explanation of the biguanides' mechanism of action remains elusive. Their blood glucose-lowering action does not depend on functioning pancreatic B cells. Patients with type 2 diabetes have considerably less fasting hyperglycemia as well as lower postprandial hyperglycemia after biguanides; however, hypoglycemia during biguanide therapy is essentially unknown. These agents are therefore more appropriately termed "euglycemic" agents. Currently proposed mechanisms of action include (1) reduced hepatic and renal gluconeogenesis; (2) slowing of glucose absorption from the gastrointestinal tract, with increased glucose to lactate conversion by enterocytes; (3) direct stimulation of glycolysis in tissues, with increased glucose removal from blood; and (4) reduction of plasma glucagon levels.

Metabolism & Excretion

Metformin has a half-life of 1.5–3 hours, is not bound to plasma proteins, is not metabolized, and is excreted by the kidneys as the active compound. As a consequence of metformin's blockade of gluconeogenesis, the drug may impair the hepatic metabolism of lactic acid. In patients with renal insufficiency, biguanides accumulate and thereby increase the risk of lactic acidosis, which appears to be a dose-related complication.

Clinical Use

Biguanides have been most often prescribed for patients whose hyperglycemia is due to ineffective insulin action, ie, insulin resistance syndrome. Because metformin is an insulin-sparing agent and does not increase weight or provoke hypoglycemia, it offers obvious advantages over insulin or sulfonylureas in treating hyperglycemia in such individuals. The UKPDS reported that metformin therapy decreases the risk of macrovascular as well as microvascular disease; this is in contrast to the other therapies, which only modified microvascular morbidity. Biguanides are also indicated for use in combination with insulin secretagogues or thiazolidinediones in type 2 diabetics in whom oral monotherapy is inadequate. Metformin is useful in the prevention of type 2 diabetes; the landmark Diabetes Prevention Program concluded that metformin is efficacious in preventing the new onset of type 2 diabetes in middle-aged, obese persons with impaired glucose tolerance and fasting hyperglycemia. It is interesting that metformin did not prevent diabetes in older, leaner prediabetics.

The dosage of metformin is from 500 mg to a maximum of 2.55 g daily, with the lowest effective dose being recommended. A common schedule would be to begin with a single 500-mg tablet given with breakfast for several days. If this is tolerated without gastrointestinal discomfort and if hyperglycemia persists, a second 500-mg tablet may be added with the evening meal. If further dose increases are required after 1 week, an additional 500-mg tablet can be added to be taken with the midday meal, or the larger (850-mg) tablet can be prescribed twice daily or even three times daily (the maximum recommended dosage) if needed. Dosage should always be divided because ingestion of more than 1000 mg at any one time usually provokes significant gastrointestinal side effects.

Toxicities

The most common toxic effects of metformin are gastrointestinal (anorexia, nausea, vomiting, abdominal discomfort, diarrhea) and occur in up to 20% of patients. They are dose-related, tend to occur at the onset of ther-

apy, and are often transient. However, metformin may have to be discontinued in 3–5% of patients because of persistent diarrhea. Absorption of vitamin B_{12} appears to be reduced during long-term metformin therapy, and annual screening of serum vitamin B_{12} levels and red blood cell parameters has been encouraged by the manufacturer to determine the need for vitamin B_{12} injections. In the absence of hypoxia or renal or hepatic insufficiency, lactic acidosis is less common with metformin therapy than with phenformin therapy.

Biguanides are contraindicated in patients with renal disease, alcoholism, hepatic disease, or conditions predisposing to tissue anoxia (eg, chronic cardiopulmonary dysfunction), because of an increased risk of lactic acidosis induced by biguanide drugs in the presence of these diseases.

THIAZOLIDINEDIONES

Thiazolidinediones (Tzds) act to decrease insulin resistance. Their primary action is the regulation of genes involved in glucose and lipid metabolism and adipocyte differentiation. Tzds are ligands of **peroxisome proliferator-activated receptor-gamma (PPAR-γ),** part of the steroid and thyroid superfamily of nuclear receptors. These PPAR receptors are found in muscle, fat, and liver. PPAR-γ receptors are complex and modulate the expression of the genes involved in lipid and glucose metabolism, insulin signal transduction, and adipocyte and other tissue differentiation. The available Tzds do not have identical clinical effects, and new drug development will focus on defining PPAR effects and designing ligands that have selective action—much like the selective estrogen receptor modulators (see Chapter 40).

In addition to targeting adipocytes, myocytes, and hepatocytes, Tzds also have significant effects on vascular endothelium, the immune system, the ovaries, and tumor cells. Some of these responses may be independent of the PPAR-γ pathway.

In persons with diabetes, a major site of Tzd action is adipose tissue, where the drug promotes glucose uptake and utilization and modulates synthesis of lipid hormones or cytokines and other proteins involved in energy regulation. Tzds also regulate adipocyte apoptosis and differentiation. Numerous other effects have been documented in animal studies but applicability to human tissues has yet to be determined.

Two thiazolidinediones are currently available: pioglitazone and rosiglitazone (Table 41–8). Their distinct side chains create differences in therapeutic action, metabolism, metabolite profile, and adverse effects. A third compound, troglitazone, was withdrawn from the market because of hepatic toxicity thought to be related to its side chain. **Pioglitazone** has PPAR-α as well as PPAR-γ activity. It is absorbed within 2 hours of inges-

Table 41–8. Thiazolidinediones.

Thiazolidinedione	Chemical Structure	Oral Dose
Pioglitazone (Actos)		15–45 mg once daily
Rosiglitazone (Avandia)		2–8 mg once daily

tion; although food may delay uptake, total bioavailability is not affected. Pioglitazone is metabolized by CYP2C8 and CYP3A4 to active metabolites. The bioavailability of numerous other drugs also degraded by these enzymes may be affected by pioglitazone therapy, including estrogen-containing oral contraceptives; additional methods of contraception are advised. Pioglitazone may be taken once daily; the usual starting dose is 15–30 mg. The triglyceride lowering effect is more significant than that observed with rosiglitazone, presumably because of its PPAR-α binding characteristics. Pioglitaxone therapy reduces mortality and macrovascular events (myocardial infarction and stroke). Pioglitazone is approved as a monotherapy and in combination with metformin, sulfonylureas, and insulin for the treatment of type 2 diabetes.

Rosiglitazone is rapidly absorbed and highly protein-bound. It is metabolized in the liver to minimally active metabolites, predominantly by CYP2C8 and to a lesser extent by CYP2C9. It is administered once or twice daily; 4–8 mg is the usual total dose. Rosiglitazone shares the common Tzd adverse effects but does not seem to have any significant drug interactions. The drug is approved for use in type 2 diabetes as monotherapy or in combination with a biguanide, sulfonylurea, in combination with a biguanide and sulfonylurea, and insulin.

Tzds are considered "euglycemics" and are efficacious in about 70% of new users. The overall response is similar to sulfonylurea and biguanide monotherapy. Individuals experiencing secondary failure to other oral agents should benefit from the addition (rather than substitution) of a Tzd. Because their mechanism of action involves gene regulation, the Tzds have a slow onset and

offset of activity over weeks or even months. Combination therapy with sulfonylureas and insulin can lead to hypoglycemia and may require dosage adjustment. Long-term therapy is associated with a drop in triglyceride levels and a slight rise in HDL and low-density lipoprotein (LDL) cholesterol values. An adverse effect common to both Tzds is fluid retention, which presents as a mild anemia and peripheral edema, especially when used in combination with insulin or insulin secretagogues. Some reports have suggested an increased risk of heart failure. Rarely, new or worsening macular edema has been reported in association with rosiglitazone treatment. Many users have a dose-related weight gain (average 1–3 kg), which may be fluid-related. These agents should not be used during pregnancy or in the presence of significant liver disease (ALT more than 2.5 × upper limit of normal), or if there is a concurrent diagnosis of heart failure. Anovulatory women may resume ovulation and should be counseled on the increased risk of pregnancy. Because of the hepatotoxicity observed with troglitazone, a discontinued Tzd, the FDA continues to require monitoring of liver function tests before initiation of Tzd therapy and periodically afterward. To date, hepatotoxicity has not been associated with rosiglitazone or pioglitazone.

Thiazolidinediones have an emerging benefit in the prevention of type 2 diabetes. The Diabetes Prevention Trial reported a 75% reduction in the diabetes incidence rate when troglitazone was administered to patients with prediabetes. Another study reported that troglitazone therapy significantly decreased the recurrence of diabetes mellitus in high-risk Hispanic women with a history of gestational diabetes. Other trials using clinically available Tzds are in progress.

ALPHA-GLUCOSIDASE INHIBITORS

Only monosaccharides, such as glucose and fructose, can be transported out of the intestinal lumen and into the bloodstream. Complex starches, oligosaccharides, and disaccharides must be broken down into individual monosaccharides before being absorbed in the duodenum and upper jejunum. This digestion is facilitated by enteric enzymes, including pancreatic α-amylase, and α-glucosidases that are attached to the brush border of the intestinal cells. **Acarbose** and **miglitol** are competitive inhibitors of the intestinal α-glucosidases and reduce the postprandial digestion and absorption of starch and disaccharides (Table 41–9). Miglitol differs structurally from acarbose and is six times more potent in inhibiting sucrase. Although the binding affinity of the two compounds differs, acarbose and miglitol both target the α-glucosidases: sucrase, maltase, glycoamylase, and dextranase. Miglitol alone has effects on isomaltase and on β-glucosidases, which split β-linked sugars such as lactose. Acarbose alone has a small effect on α-amylase. The consequence of enzyme inhibition is to minimize upper intestinal digestion and defer digestion (and thus absorption) of the ingested starch and disaccharides to the distal small intestine, thereby lowering postmeal glycemic excursions as much as 45–60 mg/dL and creating an insulin-sparing effect. Monotherapy with these drugs is associated with a modest drop (0.5–1%) in glycohemoglobin levels and a 20–25 mg/dL fall in fasting glucose levels. They are FDA-approved for persons with type 2 diabetes as monotherapy and in combination with sulfonylureas, in which the glycemic effect is additive. Both acarbose and miglitol are taken in doses of 25–100 mg just before ingesting the first portion of each meal; therapy should be initiated with the lowest dose and slowly titrated upward.

Prominent adverse effects include flatulence, diarrhea, and abdominal pain and result from the appearance of undigested carbohydrate in the colon that is then fermented into short-chain fatty acids, releasing gas. These side effects tend to diminish with ongoing use because chronic exposure to carbohydrate induces the expression of α-glucosidase in the jejunum and ileum, increasing distal small intestine glucose absorption and minimizing the passage of carbohydrate into the colon. Although not a problem with monotherapy or combination therapy with a biguanide, hypoglycemia may occur with concurrent sulfonylurea treatment. Hypoglycemia should be treated with glucose (dextrose) and not sucrose, whose breakdown may be blocked. These drugs are contraindicated in patients with inflammatory bowel disease or any intestinal condition that could be worsened by gas and distention. Because both miglitol and acarbose are excreted by the kidneys, these medications should not be prescribed in individuals with renal impairment. Acarbose has been associated with reversible hepatic enzyme elevation and should be used with caution in the presence of hepatic disease.

The STOP-NIDDM trial demonstrated that α-glucosidase therapy in prediabetic individuals successfully prevented a significant number of new cases of type 2 diabetes and helped restore B-cell function, in addition to reducing cardiovascular disease and hypertension. Intervention with acarbose also reduced cardiovascular events in individuals with diabetes. Diabetes and cardiovascular disease prevention may become a further indication for this class of medications.

PRAMLINTIDE

Pramlintide, a synthetic analog of amylin, is an injectable antihyperglycemic that modulates postprandial glucose levels and is approved for preprandial use in individuals with type 1 and type 2 diabetes. It is administered in addition to insulin in those individuals who are unable to achieve their target postprandial blood sugars. Pramlintide suppresses glucagon release via undetermined mechanisms, delays gastric emptying, and has central nervous system–mediated anorectic effects. It is rapidly absorbed after subcutaneous administration; levels peak within 20 minutes, and the duration of action is not more than 150 minutes.

Table 41–9. Alpha-glucosidase inhibitors.

Alpha-Glucosidase Inhibitor	Chemical Structure	Oral Dose
Acarbose (Precose)		25–100 mg before meals
Miglitol (Glyset)		25–100 mg before meals

Pramlintide is renally metabolized and excreted, but even at low creatinine clearance there is no significant change in bioavailability. It has not been evaluated in dialysis patients. The most reliable absorption is from the abdomen and thigh; arm administration is less reliable. Pramlintide should be injected immediately before eating; doses range from 15 mcg to 120 mcg subcutaneously. Therapy with this agent should be initiated with the lowest dose and titrated upward. Because of the risk of hypoglycemia, concurrent rapid- or short-acting mealtime insulin doses should be decreased by 50% or more. Pramlintide should always be injected by itself with a separate syringe; it cannot be mixed with insulin. The major side effects of pramlintide are hypoglycemia and gastrointestinal symptoms including nausea, vomiting, and anorexia.

EXENATIDE

As a synthetic analog of glucagon-like-polypeptide 1 (GLP-1), exenatide is the first incretin therapy to become available for the treatment of diabetes. Exenatide is approved as an injectable, adjunctive therapy in individuals with type 2 diabetes treated with metformin or sulfonylureas who still have suboptimal glycemic control. In clinical studies, exenatide therapy is shown to have multiple actions such as potentiation of glucose-mediated insulin secretion, suppression of postprandial glucagon release through as-yet unknown mechanisms, slowed gastric emptying and a central loss of appetite. The increased insulin secretion is speculated to be due in part to an increase in B-cell mass. It is not known whether the increased B-cell mass results from a decreased B-cell turnover, increased B-cell formation, or both.

Exenatide is absorbed equally from arm, abdomen, or thigh injection sites, reaching a peak concentration in approximately 2 hours with a duration of up to 10 hours. It undergoes glomerular filtration, and dosage adjustment is required only when the creatinine clearance is less than 30 mL/min. Exenatide is injected subcutaneously within 60 minutes before a meal; therapy is initiated at 5 mcg twice daily, with a maximum dosage of 10 mcg twice daily. When exenatide is added to preexisting sulfonylurea therapy, the oral hypoglycemic dosage may need to be decreased to prevent hypoglycemia. The major side effects are nausea (about 44% of users) and vomiting and diarrhea. The nausea decreases with ongoing exenatide usage.

SITAGLIPTIN

Sitagliptin is an inhibitor of dipeptidyl peptidase-4 (DPP-4), the enzyme that degrades incretin and other GLP-1-like molecules. This drug appears likely to be approved for use in type 2 diabetes. In phase 2 and 3 clinical trials, sitagliptin was reported to have a bioavailability of approximately 80% and a half-life of 8–14 hours. Control of hyperglycemia and reductions in HbA_{1c} were documented at doses of 100 mg orally once

daily. Dosage should be reduced in patients with renal impairment. Hypoglycemic episodes were rare and the drug facilitated weight loss. Sitagliptin therapy can be combined with metformin, Tzds, or sulfonylureas. The drug will be marketed as Januvia.

Combination Therapy with Oral Antidiabetic Agents & Injectable Medication

A. COMBINATION THERAPY IN TYPE 2 DIABETES MELLITUS

1. Combination therapy with exenatide—Exenatide is approved for use in individuals who fail to achieve desired glycemic control on biguanides, sulfonylureas, or both. Although the combination of exenatide and Tzds, D-phenylalanine derivatives, meglitinides, α-glucosidase inhibitors, and insulin has not been studied, these regimens are clinically prescribed. Hypoglycemia is a risk when exenatide is used with an insulin secretagogue or insulin. The doses of the latter drugs have to be reduced at the initiation of exenatide therapy and subsequently titrated.

2. Combination therapy with pramlintide—Pramlintide is approved for concurrent mealtime administration in individuals with type 2 diabetes treated with insulin, metformin, or a sulfonylurea who are unable to achieve their postmeal glucose targets. Combination therapy results in a significant reduction in early postprandial glucose excursions; mealtime insulin or sulfonylurea doses usually have to be reduced to prevent hypoglycemia.

3. Combination therapy with insulin—Bedtime insulin has been suggested as an adjunct to oral antidiabetic therapy in patients with type 2 diabetes patients who have not responded to maximal oral therapy. Clinical practice has evolved to include sulfonylureas, meglitinides, D-phenylalanine derivatives, biguanides, thiazolidinediones, or α-glucosidase inhibitors given in conjunction with insulin.

Individuals unable to achieve glycemic control with bedtime insulin as described above generally require full insulin replacement and multiple daily injections of insulin. Insulin secretagogues are redundant when an individual is receiving multiple daily insulin injections, but persons with severe insulin resistance may benefit from the addition of one of the biguanides, thiazolidinediones, or α-glucosidase inhibitors. In some cases, multiple oral agents have been required together with insulin. When oral agents are added to the regimen of a person already taking insulin, the blood glucose should be closely monitored and the insulin dosage decreased as needed to avoid hypoglycemia.

B. COMBINATION THERAPY IN TYPE 1 DIABETES MELLITUS

1. Combination therapy with pramlintide—Pramlintide is approved for concurrent mealtime administration in individuals with type 1 diabetes who have poor glucose control after eating despite optimal insulin therapy. The addition of pramlintide leads to a significant reduction in early postprandial glucose excursions; mealtime insulin doses usually have to be reduced to prevent hypoglycemia.

2. Combination therapy with oral medications— There is no indication for combining insulin with insulin secretagogues (sulfonylureas, meglitinides, or D-phenylalanine derivatives) in individuals with type 1 diabetes. Type 1 diabetics with diets very high in starch may benefit from the addition of α-glucosidase inhibitors, but this is not typically practiced in the USA. Although not approved for use in type 1 diabetes, Tzds have been prescribed for type 1 individuals with significant insulin resistance and a combined type 1, type 2 phenotype, or latent autoimmune diabetes mellitus of adulthood (LADA). The insulin dose has to be reduced with the addition of Tzd therapy to prevent hypoglycemia.

■ GLUCAGON

Chemistry & Metabolism

Glucagon is synthesized in the A cells of the pancreatic islets of Langerhans (see Table 41–1). Glucagon is a peptide—identical in all mammals—consisting of a single chain of 29 amino acids, with a molecular weight of 3485. Selective proteolytic cleavage converts a large precursor molecule of approximately 18,000 MW to glucagon. One of the precursor intermediates consists of a 69-amino-acid peptide called **glicentin,** which contains the glucagon sequence interposed between peptide extensions.

Glucagon is extensively degraded in the liver and kidney as well as in plasma and at its tissue receptor sites. Because of its rapid inactivation by plasma, chilling of the collecting tubes and addition of inhibitors of proteolytic enzymes are necessary when samples of blood are collected for immunoassay of circulating glucagon. Its half-life in plasma is between 3 and 6 minutes, which is similar to that of insulin.

"Gut Glucagon"

Glicentin immunoreactivity has been found in cells of the small intestine as well as in pancreatic A cells and in effluents of perfused pancreas. The intestinal cells secrete **enteroglucagon,** a family of glucagon-like peptides, of which glicentin is a member, along with glucagon-like peptides 1 and 2 (GLP-1 and GLP-2). Unlike the pancreatic A cell, these intestinal cells lack the enzymes to convert glucagon precursors to true glucagon by removing the carboxyl terminal extension from the molecule.

The function of the enteroglucagons has not been clarified, although smaller peptides can bind hepatic glucagon receptors where they exert partial activity. A derivative of the 37-amino-acid form of GLP-1 that lacks the first six amino acids (GLP-1[7–37]) is a potent stimulant of insulin release. It represents the predominant form of GLP in the human intestine and has been termed "insulinotropin." It has been considered as a potential therapeutic agent in type 2 diabetes. However, it requires continuous subcutaneous infusion to produce a sustained lowering of both fasting and postprandial hyperglycemia in type 2 diabetic patients; therefore, its clinical usefulness is limited. Exenatide (see above) is an analog of GLP-1.

Pharmacologic Effects of Glucagon

A. METABOLIC EFFECTS

The first six amino acids at the amino terminal of the glucagon molecule bind to specific receptors on liver cells. This leads to a G_s protein-coupled increase in adenylyl cyclase activity and the production of cAMP, which facilitates catabolism of stored glycogen and increases gluconeogenesis and ketogenesis. The immediate pharmacologic result of glucagon infusion is to raise blood glucose at the expense of stored hepatic glycogen. There is no effect on skeletal muscle glycogen, presumably because of the lack of glucagon receptors on skeletal muscle. Pharmacologic amounts of glucagon cause release of insulin from normal pancreatic B cells, catecholamines from pheochromocytoma, and calcitonin from medullary carcinoma cells.

B. CARDIAC EFFECTS

Glucagon has a potent inotropic and chronotropic effect on the heart, mediated by the cAMP mechanism described above. Thus, it produces an effect very similar to that of β-adrenoceptor agonists without requiring functioning β receptors.

C. EFFECTS ON SMOOTH MUSCLE

Large doses of glucagon produce profound relaxation of the intestine. In contrast to the above effects of the peptide, this action on the intestine may be due to mechanisms other than adenylyl cyclase activation.

Clinical Uses

A. SEVERE HYPOGLYCEMIA

The major use of glucagon is for emergency treatment of severe hypoglycemic reactions in patients with type 1 diabetes when unconsciousness precludes oral feedings and intravenous glucose is not possible. Recombinant glucagon is currently available in 1-mg vials for parenteral use (Glucagon Emergency Kit). Nasal sprays have been developed for this purpose but have not yet received FDA approval.

B. ENDOCRINE DIAGNOSIS

Several tests use glucagon to diagnose endocrine disorders. In patients with type 1 diabetes mellitus, a standard test of pancreatic B-cell secretory reserve uses 1 mg of glucagon administered as an intravenous bolus. Because insulin-treated patients develop circulating anti-insulin antibodies that interfere with radioimmunoassays of insulin, measurements of C-peptide are used to indicate B-cell secretion.

C. BETA-BLOCKER POISONING

Glucagon is sometimes useful for reversing the cardiac effects of an overdose of β-blocking agents because of its ability to increase cAMP production in the heart. However, it is not clinically useful in the treatment of cardiac failure.

D. RADIOLOGY OF THE BOWEL

Glucagon has been used extensively in radiology as an aid to x-ray visualization of the bowel because of its ability to relax the intestine.

Adverse Reactions

Transient nausea and occasional vomiting can result from glucagon administration. These are generally mild, and glucagon is relatively free of severe adverse reactions.

■ ISLET AMYLOID POLYPEPTIDE (IAPP, AMYLIN)

Amylin is a 37-amino-acid peptide originally derived from islet amyloid deposits in pancreas material from patients with long-standing type 2 diabetes or insulinomas. It is produced by pancreatic B cells, packaged within B-cell granules in a concentration 1–2% that of insulin and co-secreted with insulin in a pulsatile manner and in response to physiologic secretory stimuli. Approximately 1 molecule of amylin is released for every 10 molecules of insulin. It circulates in a glycated (active) and nonglycated (inactive) form with physiologic concentrations ranging from 4–25 pmol/L and is primarily renally excreted. Amylin appears to be a member of the superfamily of neuroregulatory peptides, with 46% homology with the calcitonin gene-related peptide CGRP (see Chapter 17). The physiologic effect of amylin may be to modulate insulin release by acting as a negative feed back on insulin secretion. At pharmacologic doses, amylin reduces glucagon secretion, slows gastric emptying by a vagally medicated mechanism, and centrally decreases appetite. An analog of amylin, **pramlintide** (see above), differs from amylin by the substitution of proline at positions 25, 28, and 29. These modifications make pramlintide soluble and non–self-aggregating.

Chapter continues on next page.

PREPARATIONS AVAILABLE*

SULFONYLUREAS
Chlorpropamide (generic, Diabinese)
Oral: 100, 250 mg tablets
Glimepiride (Amaryl)
Oral: 1, 2, 4 mg tablets
Glipizide (generic, Glucotrol, Glucotrol XL)
Oral: 5, 10 mg tablets; 5, 10 mg extended-release tablets
Glyburide (generic, Diaβeta, Micronase, Glynase PresTab)
Oral: 1.25, 2.5, 5 mg tablets; 1.5, 3, 4.5, 6 mg Glynase PresTab, micronized tablets
Tolazamide (generic, Tolinase)
Oral: 100, 250, 500 mg tablets
Tolbutamide (generic, Orinase)
Oral: 500 mg tablets

MEGLITINIDE & RELATED DRUGS
Repaglinide (Prandin)
Oral: 0.5, 1, 2 mg tablets
Nateglinide (Starlix)
Oral: 60, 120 mg tablets

BIGUANIDE
Metformin (generic, Glucophage, Glucophage XR)
Oral: 500, 850, 1000 mg tablets; extended-release (XR): 500 mg tablets; 500 mg/5 mL solution

METFORMIN COMBINATIONS
Glipizide plus metformin (Metaglip)
Oral: 2.5/250, 2.5/500, 5/500 mg tablets

Glyburide plus metformin (Glucovance)
Oral: 1.25/250, 2.5/500, 5/500 mg tablets
Rosiglitazone plus metformin (Avandamet)
Oral: 1/500, 2/500, 4/500; 2/1000, 4/1000 mg tablets

THIAZOLIDINEDIONE DERIVATIVES
Pioglitazone (Actos)
Oral: 15, 30, 45 mg tablets
Rosiglitazone (Avandia)
Oral: 2, 4, 8 mg tablets

THIAZOLIDINEDIONE COMBINATIONS
Rosiglitazone plus glimeperide (Avandaryl)
Oral: 4/1, 4/2, 4/4 mg rosiglitazone/mg glimeperide tablets

ALPHA-GLUCOSIDASE INHIBITORS
Acarbose (Precose)
Oral: 25, 50, 100 mg tablets
Miglitol (Glyset)
Oral: 25, 50, 100 mg tablets

AMYLIN ANALOGS
Pramlintide (Symlin)
Parenteral: vial: 0.6 mg/mL (2.5 units [15 mcg] to 20 units [120 mcg])

GLUCAGON-LIKE POLYPEPTIDE-1 ANALOGS
Exenatide (Byetta)
Parenteral: 5, 10 mcg/dose pen injectors

GLUCAGON
Glucagon (generic)
Parenteral: 1 mg lyophilized powder to reconstitute for injection

*See Table 41–4 for insulin preparations.

REFERENCES

Bloomgarden ZT: Gut-derived incretin hormones and new therapeutic approaches. Diabetes Care 2004;27:2554.

Buchanan TA: Protection from type 2 diabetes persists in the TRIPOD cohort eight months after stopping troglitazone. Diabetes 2001;50(Suppl 2):A81.

Chapman I et al: Effect of pramlintide on satiety and food intake in obese subjects and subjects with type 2 diabetes. Diabetologia 2005;48:838.

Chiasson JL et al: Acarbose for prevention of type 2 diabetes mellitus: The STOP-NIDDM randomized trial. Lancet 2002;359:2072.

Chaisson JL et al: Acarbose treatment and the risk of cardiovascular disease and hypertension in patients with impaired glucose tolerance: The STOP-NIDDM trial. JAMA 2003; 290:486.

Diabetes Control and Complications Trial Research Group: Epidemiology of severe hypoglycemia in the diabetes control and complications trial. Am J Med 1991;90:450.

Diabetes Control and Complications Trial Research Group: The effect of intensive treatment of diabetes on the development and progression of long-term complications in insulin-dependent diabetes mellitus. N Engl J Med 1993; 329:977.

Diabetes Control and Complications Trial/Epidemiology of Diabetes Interventions and Complications Research Group: Intensive Diabetes Therapy and Carotid Intima-Media Thickness in Type 1 Diabetes Mellitus. N Engl J Med 2003;348:2294.

Diabetes Prevention Program Research Group: Reduction in the incidence of type 2 diabetes with lifestyle intervention or metformin. N Engl J Med 2002;346:393.

Diabetes Prevention Program Research Group: Prevention of type 2 diabetes with troglitazone in the diabetes prevention program. Diabetes 2005;54:1150.

Dormandy JA et al: Secondary prevention of macrovascular events in patients with type 2 diabetes in the PROactive study (PROspective pioglitAzone Clinical Trial in macroVascular Events): A randomized controlled trial. Lancet 2005,366:1280.

Dunn CJ et al: Nateglinide. Drugs 2000;60:607.

Dunning BE et al: Alpha cell function in health and disease: Influence of glucagon-like peptide-1. Diabetologia 2005;48:1700.

Dupre J: Extendin-4 Normalized Postcibial Glycemic Excursions in Type 1 Diabetes. J Clin Endocrinol Metab 2004;89:3469.

Dupre J: Glycemic effects of incretins in Type 1 diabetes mellitus: A concise review, with emphasis on studies in humans. Regul Pept 2005;128:149.

Expert Committee on the Diagnosis and Classification of Diabetes Mellitus: Report of the expert committee on the diagnosis and classification of diabetes mellitus. Diabetes Care 2003,26(Suppl 1):S5.

Goldberg RB et al: A comparison of lipid and glycemic effects of pioglitazone and rosiglitazone in patients with type 2 diabetes and dyslipidemia. Diabetes Care 2005;28:1547.

Hanefeld M et al: Acarbose reduces the risk for myocardial infarction in type 2 diabetic patients: Meta-analysis of seven long term studies. Eur Heart J 2004;25:10.

Heinemann L et al: Time action profile of the long-acting insulin analog insulin glargine (HOE901) in comparison with those of NPH insulin and placebo. Diabetes Care 2000;23:644.

Heptulla RA et al: The role of amylin and glucagon in the dampening of glycemic excursions in children with type 1 diabetes. Diabetes 2005;54:1100.

Kolterman O et al: Pharmacokinetics, pharmacodynamics, and safety of exenatide in patients with type 2 diabetes mellitus. Am J Health-Syst Pharm 2005;62:173.

Lepore M et al: Pharmacokinetics and pharmacodynamics of subcutaneous injection of long-acting human insulin analog glargine, NPH insulin and ultralente human insulin and continuous subcutaneous infusion of insulin lispro. Diabetes 2000;49:2142.

Levien TL: Nateglinide therapy for type 2 diabetes mellitus. Ann Pharmacother 2001;35:1426.

Mudaliar S et al: New oral therapies for type 2 diabetes mellitus: The glitazones or insulin sensitizers. Annu Rev Med 2001;52:239.

Nauck MA et al: Glucagon-like peptide 1 and its derivatives in the treatment of diabetes. Regul Pept 2005;128:135.

Ottensmeyer FP et al: Mechanism of transmembrane signalling: Insulin binding and the insulin receptor. Biochemistry 2000; 39:12103.

Owens DR: Repaglinide: A new short-acting insulinotropic agent for the treatment of type 2 diabetes. Eur J Clin Invest 1999; 29(Suppl 2):30.

Plank J et al: A double-blind, randomized, dose-response study investigating the pharmacodynamic and pharmacokinetic properties of the long-acting insulin analog detemir. Diabetes Care 2005;28:1107.

Quattrin T et al: Efficacy and safety of inhaled insulin (Exubera) compared with subcutaneous insulin therapy in patients with type 1 diabetes. Diabetes Care 2004;27:2622.

Ratner RE et al: Amylin replacement with pramlintide as an adjunct to insulin therapy improves long term glycemic and weight control in type 1 diabetes mellitus: A 1-year randomized controlled trial. Diabetic Med 2004;21:1204.

Rave K et al: Time-action profile of inhaled insulin in comparison with subcutaneously injected insulin lispro and regular human insulin. Diabetes Care 2005;28:1077.

Schmitz O et al: Amylin agonists: A novel approach in the treatment of diabetes. Diabetes 2004;53(Suppl 3):S233.

Shepherd PR, Kahn BB: Glucose transporters and insulin action— implications for insulin resistance and diabetes mellitus. N Engl J Med 1999;341:248.

Skyler JS et al: Use of inhaled insulin in a basal/bolus insulin regimen in type 1 diabetic subjects. Diabetes Care 2005; 28:1630.

Toft-Nielsen MB, Madsbad S, Holst JJ: Continuous subcutaneous infusion of glucagon-like peptide 1 lowers plasma glucose and reduces appetite in type 2 diabetic patients. Diabetes Care 1999;22:1137.

United Kingdom Prospective Diabetes Study (UKPDS) Group: Effect of intensive blood-glucose control with metformin on complications in overweight patients with type 2 diabetes: UKPDS 34. Lancet 1998;352:854.

United Kingdom Prospective Diabetes Study (UKPDS) Group: Glycemic control with diet, sulfonylurea, metformin, or insulin in patients with type 2 diabetes mellitus: Progressive requirement for multiple therapies: UKPDS 49. JAMA 1999;281:2005.

United Kingdom Prospective Diabetes Study (UKPDS) Group: Intensive blood-glucose control with sulphonylureas or insulin compared with conventional treatment and risk of complications in patients with type 2 diabetes: UKPDS 33. Lancet 1998;352:837.

United Kingdom Prospective Diabetes Study (UKPDS) Group: Tight blood pressure control and risk of macrovascular and microvascular complications in type 2 diabetes: UKPDS 38. BMJ 1998;317:703.

Agents That Affect Bone Mineral Homeostasis

42

Daniel D. Bikle, MD, PhD

■ I. BASIC PHARMACOLOGY

Calcium and phosphate, the major mineral constituents of bone, are also two of the most important minerals for general cellular function. Accordingly, the body has evolved a complex set of mechanisms by which calcium and phosphate homeostasis are carefully maintained (Figure 42–1). Approximately 98% of the 1–2 kg of calcium and 85% of the 1 kg of phosphorus in the human adult are found in bone, the principal reservoir for these minerals. These functions are dynamic, with constant remodeling of bone and ready exchange of bone mineral with that in the extracellular fluid. Bone also serves as the principal structural support for the body and provides the space for hematopoiesis. Thus, abnormalities in bone mineral homeostasis can lead not only to a wide variety of cellular dysfunctions (eg, tetany, coma, muscle weakness) but also to disturbances in structural support of the body (eg, osteoporosis with fractures) and loss of hematopoietic capacity (eg, infantile osteopetrosis).

Calcium and phosphate enter the body from the intestine. The average American diet provides 600–1000 mg of calcium per day, of which approximately 100–250 mg is absorbed. This figure represents net absorption, because both absorption (principally in the duodenum and upper jejunum) and secretion (principally in the ileum) occur. The amount of phosphorus in the American diet is about the same as that of calcium. However, the efficiency of absorption (principally in the jejunum) is greater, ranging from 70% to 90%, depending on intake. In the steady state, renal excretion of calcium and phosphate balances intestinal absorption. In general, over 98% of filtered calcium and 85% of filtered phosphate is reabsorbed by the kidney. The movement of calcium and phosphate across the intestinal and renal epithelia is closely regulated. Intrinsic disease of the intestine (eg, nontropical sprue) or kidney (eg, chronic renal failure) disrupts bone mineral homeostasis.

Two hormones serve as the principal regulators of calcium and phosphate homeostasis: the peptide parathyroid hormone (PTH) and the steroid vitamin D (Figure 42–2). Vitamin D is a prohormone rather than a true hormone, because it must be further metabolized to gain biologic activity. PTH stimulates the production of the active metabolite of vitamin D, $1,25(OH)_2D$. $1,25(OH)_2D$, on the other hand, suppresses the production of PTH. $1,25(OH)_2D$ stimulates the intestinal absorption of calcium and phosphate. $1,25(OH)_2D$ and PTH promote both bone formation and resorption in part by stimulating the proliferation and differentiation of osteoblasts and osteoclasts. Both PTH and $1,25(OH)_2D$ enhance renal retention of calcium, but PTH promotes renal phosphate excretion. Fibroblast growth factor 23 (FGF23) is a newly discovered hormone that stimulates renal phosphate excretion and inhibits renal production of $1,25(OH)_2D$. Other hormones—calcitonin, prolactin, growth hormone, insulin, thyroid hormone, glucocorticoids, and sex steroids—influence calcium and phosphate homeostasis under certain physiologic circumstances and can be considered secondary regulators. Deficiency or excess of these secondary regulators within a physiologic range does not produce the disturbance of calcium and phosphate homeostasis that is observed in situations of deficiency or excess of PTH and vitamin D. However, certain of these secondary regulators—especially calcitonin, glucocorticoids, and estrogens—are useful therapeutically and are discussed in subsequent sections.

In addition to these hormonal regulators, calcium and phosphate themselves, other ions such as sodium and fluoride, and a variety of drugs (bisphosphonates, plicamycin, and diuretics) also alter calcium and phosphate homeostasis.

PRINCIPAL HORMONAL REGULATORS OF BONE MINERAL HOMEOSTASIS

PARATHYROID HORMONE

Parathyroid hormone (PTH) is a single-chain peptide hormone composed of 84 amino acids. It is produced

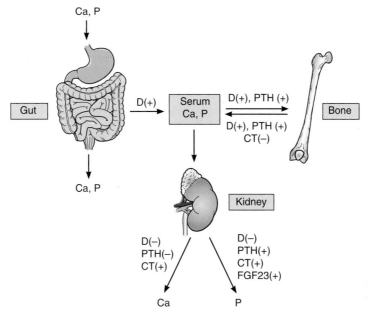

Ca, P

Gut → D(+) → **Serum Ca, P** → D(+), PTH (+) ⇌ D(+), PTH (+) CT(−) → **Bone**

Ca, P

Kidney

D(−) PTH(−) CT(+) / **Ca**

D(−) PTH(+) CT(+) FGF23(+) / **P**

Figure 42–1. Some mechanisms contributing to bone mineral homeostasis. Direct actions are shown and feedback may alter the net effect. Calcium and phosphorus concentrations in the serum are controlled principally by two hormones, 1,25(OH)$_2$D$_3$ *(D)* and parathyroid hormone *(PTH)*, through their action on absorption from the gut and from bone and on excretion in the urine. Both hormones increase input of calcium and phosphorus from bone into the serum; both hormones also stimulate bone formation; vitamin D also increases absorption from the gut. Vitamin D decreases urinary excretion of both calcium and phosphorus, whereas PTH reduces calcium but increases phosphorus excretion. Calcitonin *(CT)* is a less critical hormone for calcium homeostasis, but in pharmacologic concentrations CT can reduce serum calcium and phosphorus by inhibiting bone resorption and stimulating their renal excretion. FGF23 is a recently discovered hormone that stimulates renal excretion of phosphate. Feedback may alter the effects shown; for example, vitamin D usually increases urinary calcium excretion because of effects on calcium absorption from the gut and effects on PTH.

in the parathyroid gland in a precursor form of 115 amino acids, the remaining 31 amino terminal amino acids being cleaved off before secretion. Within the gland is a calcium-sensitive protease capable of cleaving the intact hormone into fragments. Biologic activity resides in the amino terminal region such that synthetic 1–34 PTH is fully active. Loss of the first two amino terminal amino acids eliminates most biologic activity.

The metabolic clearance of intact PTH is rapid, with a half-time of disappearance measured in minutes. Most of the clearance occurs in the liver and kidney. The biologically inactive carboxyl terminal fragments produced during metabolism of the intact hormone have a much lower clearance, especially in renal failure. This accounts in part for the very high PTH values often observed in the past in patients with renal failure when measured by radioimmunoassays directed against the carboxyl terminal region of the molecule. However, most PTH assays currently in use measure the intact hormone by a double antibody method, so that this circumstance is less frequently encountered in clinical practice. PTH regulates calcium and phosphate flux across cellular membranes in bone and kidney, resulting in increased serum calcium and decreased serum phosphate. In bone, PTH increases the activity and number of osteoclasts, the cells responsible for bone resorption. However, this stimulation of osteoclasts is not a direct effect. Rather,

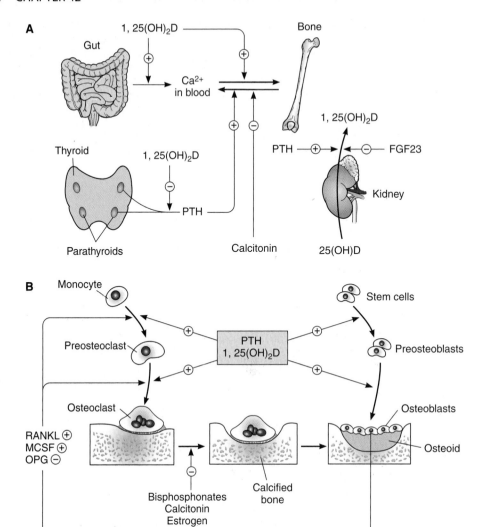

Figure 42–2. The hormonal interactions controlling bone mineral homeostasis. 1,25(OH)$_2$D is produced by the kidney under the control of PTH, which stimulates its production, and FGF23, which inhibits its production. 1,25(OH)$_2$D in turn inhibits the production of PTH by the parathyroid glands. 1,25(OH)$_2$D is the principal regulator of intestinal calcium and phosphate absorption. Both PTH and 1,25(OH)$_2$D regulate bone formation and resorption, each capable of stimulating both processes. This is accomplished by their stimulation of preosteoblast proliferation and differentiation into osteoblasts, the bone forming cell. PTH and 1,25(OH)$_2$D stimulate the expression of RANKL by the osteoblast, which, with MCSF, stimulates the differentiation and subsequent activation of osteoclasts, the bone resorbing cell. FGF23, fibroblast growth factor; MCSF, macrophage colony-stimulating factor; OPG, osteoprotegerin; RANK, receptor for activation of nuclear factor-κB.

PTH acts on the osteoblast (the bone-forming cell) to induce a membrane-bound protein called **RANK ligand (RANKL).** This factor acts on osteoclasts and osteoclast precursors to increase both the numbers and the activity of osteoclasts. This action increases bone turnover or bone remodeling, a specific sequence of cellular events initiated by osteoclastic bone resorption and followed by osteoblastic bone formation. Although both bone resorption and bone formation are enhanced by PTH, the net effect of excess PTH is to increase bone resorption. PTH in low and intermittent doses increases bone formation without first stimulating bone resorption. This action appears to be indirect, involving other growth factors such as IGF-1. This has led to the recent approval of recombinant PTH 1-34 **(teriparatide)** for the treatment of osteoporosis. In the kidney, PTH increases the ability of the nephron to reabsorb calcium and magnesium but reduces its ability to reabsorb phosphate, amino acids, bicarbonate, sodium, chloride, and sulfate. Another important action of PTH on the kidney is its stimulation of 1,25-dihydroxyvitamin D (1,25[OH]$_2$D) production.

VITAMIN D

Vitamin D is a secosteroid produced in the skin from 7-dehydrocholesterol under the influence of ultraviolet irradiation. Vitamin D is also found in certain foods and is used to supplement dairy products. Both the natural form (vitamin D$_3$, cholecalciferol) and the plant-derived form (vitamin D$_2$, ergocalciferol) are present in the diet. These forms differ in that ergocalciferol contains a double bond (C$_{22-23}$) and an additional methyl group in the side chain (Figure 42–3). In humans, this difference apparently is of limited physiologic consequence (although ergocalciferol is less potent), and the following comments apply equally well to both forms of vitamin D.

Vitamin D is a prohormone that serves as precursor to a number of biologically active metabolites (Figure 42–3). Vitamin D is first hydroxylated in the liver to form 25-hydroxyvitamin D (25[OH]D). This metabolite is further converted in the kidney to a number of other forms, the best-studied of which are 1,25-dihy-

Figure 42–3. Conversion of 7-dehydrocholesterol to vitamin D$_3$ and metabolism of D$_3$ to 1,25(OH)$_2$D$_3$ and 24,25(OH)$_2$D$_3$. Control of the latter step is exerted primarily at the level of the kidney, where low serum phosphorus, low serum calcium, and high parathyroid hormone favor the production of 1,25(OH)$_2$D$_3$. The inset shows the side chain for ergosterol. Ergosterol undergoes similar transformation to vitamin D$_2$ (ergocalciferol), which, in turn, is metabolized to 25(OH)D$_2$, 1,25(OH)$_2$D$_2$, and 24,25(OH)$_2$D$_2$. In humans, corresponding D$_2$ and D$_3$ derivatives have equivalent effects and potency. They are therefore referred to in the text without a subscript.

Table 42–1. VItamin D and its major metabolites and analogs.

Chemical and Generic Names	Abbreviation
Vitamin D₃; cholecalciferol	D_3
Vitamin D₂; ergocalciferol	D_2
25-Hydroxyvitamin D₃; calcifediol	$25(OH)D_3$
1,25-Dihydroxyvitamin D₃; calcitriol	$1,25(OH)_2D_3$
24,25-Dihydroxyvitamin D₃; secalcifediol	$24,25(OH)_2D_3$
Dihydrotachysterol	DHT
Calcipotriene (calcipotriol)	None
1α-Hydroxyvitamin D₂; doxercalciferol	$1\alpha(OH)D_2$
19-nor-1,25-Dihydroxyvitamin D₂; paricalcitol	$19\text{-nor-}1,25(OH)D_2$

droxyvitamin D (1,25[OH]₂D) and 24,25-dihydroxy-vitamin D (24,25[OH]₂D). Of the natural metabolites, only vitamin D and 1,25(OH)₂D (as **calcitriol**) are available for clinical use (Table 42–1). Moreover, a number of analogs of 1,25(OH)₂D are being synthesized to extend the usefulness of this metabolite to a variety of nonclassic conditions. **Calcipotriene** (calcipotriol), for example, is being used to treat psoriasis, a hyperproliferative skin disorder. **Doxercalciferol** and **paricalcitol** have recently been approved for the treatment of secondary hyperparathyroidism in patients with chronic kidney disease. Other analogs are being investigated for the treatment of various malignancies. The regulation of vitamin D metabolism is complex, involving calcium, phosphate, and a variety of hormones, the most important of which is PTH, which stimulates the production of 1,25(OH)₂D by the kidney.

Vitamin D and its metabolites circulate in plasma tightly bound to a carrier protein, the vitamin D-binding protein. This α-globulin binds 25(OH)D and 24,25(OH)₂D with comparable high affinity and vitamin D and 1,25(OH)₂D with lower affinity. In normal subjects, the terminal half-life of injected calcifediol is 23 days, whereas in anephric subjects it is 42 days. The half-life of 24,25(OH)₂D is probably similar. Tracer studies with vitamin D have shown a rapid clearance from the blood. The liver appears to be the principal organ for clearance. Excess vitamin D is stored in adipose tissue. The metabolic clearance of calcitriol in humans indicates a rapid turnover, with a terminal half-life measured in hours. Several of the 1,25(OH)₂D analogs are bound poorly by the vitamin D-binding protein. As a result, their clearance is very rapid, with a terminal half-life measured in minutes. Such analogs have little of the hypercalcemic, hypercalciuric effects of calcitriol, an

important aspect of their use for the management of conditions such as psoriasis and hyperparathyroidism.

The mechanism of action of the vitamin D metabolites remains under active investigation. However, calcitriol is well established as the most potent agent with respect to stimulation of intestinal calcium and phosphate transport and bone resorption. Calcitriol appears to act on the intestine both by induction of new protein synthesis (eg, calcium-binding protein) and by modulation of calcium flux across the brush border and basolateral membranes by a means that does not require new protein synthesis. The molecular action of calcitriol on bone has received less attention. However, like PTH, calcitriol can induce RANK ligand in osteoblasts and proteins such as osteocalcin, which may regulate the mineralization process. The metabolites 25(OH)D and 24,25(OH)₂D are far less potent stimulators of intestinal calcium and phosphate transport or bone resorption. However, 25(OH)D appears to be more potent than 1,25(OH)₂D in stimulating renal reabsorption of calcium and phosphate and may be the major metabolite regulating calcium flux and contractility in muscle. Specific receptors for 1,25(OH)₂D exist in target tissues. However, the role and even the existence of separate receptors for 25(OH)D and 24,25(OH)₂D remain controversial.

The receptor for 1,25(OH)₂D exists in a wide variety of tissues—not just bone, gut, and kidney. In these "nonclassic" tissues, 1,25(OH)₂D exerts a number of actions including regulation of parathyroid hormone secretion from the parathyroid gland, insulin secretion from the pancreas, cytokine production by macrophages and T cells, and proliferation and differentiation of a large number of cells, including cancer cells. Thus, the clinical utility of 1,25(OH)₂D analogs is likely to expand.

INTERACTION OF PTH & VITAMIN D

A summary of the principal actions of PTH and vitamin D on the three main target tissues—intestine, kidney, and bone—is presented in Table 42–2. The net effect of PTH is to raise serum calcium and reduce serum phosphate; the net effect of vitamin D is to raise both. Regulation of calcium and phosphate homeostasis is achieved through a variety of feedback loops. Calcium is the principal regulator of PTH secretion. It binds to a novel ion recognition site that is part of a G_q protein–coupled receptor called the calcium sensing receptor (CaR) and links changes in intracellular free calcium concentration to changes in extracellular calcium. As serum calcium levels rise and bind to this receptor, intracellular calcium levels increase and inhibit PTH secretion. Phosphate regulates PTH secretion directly and indirectly by forming complexes with calcium in the serum. Because it is the ionized free concentration of calcium that is detected by the parathyroid gland, increases in serum phosphate levels reduce the ionized calcium and

Table 42–2. Actions of parathyroid hormone (PTH) and vitamin D on gut, bone, and kidney.

	PTH	Vitamin D
Intestine	Increased calcium and phosphate absorption (by increased 1,25[OH]$_2$D production)	Increased calcium and phosphate absorption by 1,25 (OH)$_2$D
Kidney	Decreased calcium excretion, increased phosphate excretion	Calcium and phosphate excretion may be decreased by 25(OH)D and 1,25(OH)$_2$D[1]
Bone	Calcium and phosphate resorption increased by high doses. Low doses may increase bone formation.	Increased calcium and phosphate resorption by 1,25(OH)$_2$D; bone formation may be increased by 1,25 (OH)$_2$D and 24,25(OH)$_2$D
Net effect on serum levels	Serum calcium increased, serum phosphate decreased	Serum calcium and phosphate both increased

[1]Direct effect. Vitamin D often *increases* urine calcium owing to increased calcium absorption from the intestine and resulting decreased PTH.

lead to enhanced PTH secretion. Such feedback regulation is appropriate to the net effect of PTH to raise serum calcium and reduce serum phosphate levels. Likewise, both calcium and phosphate at high levels reduce the amount of 1,25(OH)$_2$D produced by the kidney and increase the amount of 24,25(OH)$_2$D produced. The high calcium works directly and indirectly by reducing PTH secretion. The high phosphate works directly and indirectly by increasing FGF23 levels. Since 1,25(OH)$_2$D raises serum calcium and phosphate, whereas 24,25(OH)$_2$D has less effect, such feedback regulation is again appropriate. 1,25(OH)$_2$D itself directly inhibits PTH secretion (independently of its effect on serum calcium) by a direct action on PTH gene transcription. This provides yet another negative feedback loop. The ability of 1,25(OH)$_2$D to inhibit PTH secretion directly is being exploited using calcitriol analogs that have less effect on serum calcium because of their lesser effect on intestinal calcium absorption. Such drugs are proving useful in the management of secondary hyperparathyroidism accompanying chronic kidney disease and may be useful in selected cases of primary hyperparathyroidism.

SECONDARY HORMONAL REGULATORS OF BONE MINERAL HOMEOSTASIS

A number of hormones modulate the actions of PTH and vitamin D in regulating bone mineral homeostasis. Compared with that of PTH and vitamin D, the physiologic impact of such secondary regulation on bone mineral homeostasis is minor. However, in pharmacologic amounts, a number of these hormones have actions on the bone mineral homeostatic mechanisms that can be exploited therapeutically.

CALCITONIN

The calcitonin secreted by the parafollicular cells of the mammalian thyroid is a single-chain peptide hormone with 32 amino acids and a molecular weight of 3600. A disulfide bond between positions 1 and 7 is essential for biologic activity. Calcitonin is produced from a precursor with MW 15,000. The circulating forms of calcitonin are multiple, ranging in size from the monomer (MW 3600) to forms with an apparent molecular weight of 60,000. Whether such heterogeneity includes precursor forms or covalently linked oligomers is not known. Because of its heterogeneity, calcitonin is standardized by bioassay in rats. Activity is compared to a standard maintained by the British Medical Research Council (MRC) and expressed as MRC units.

Human calcitonin monomer has a half-life of about 10 minutes with a metabolic clearance of 8–9 mL/kg/min. Salmon calcitonin has a longer half-life and a reduced metabolic clearance (3 mL/kg/min), making it more attractive as a therapeutic agent. Much of the clearance occurs in the kidney, although little intact calcitonin appears in the urine.

The principal effects of calcitonin are to lower serum calcium and phosphate by actions on bone and kidney. Calcitonin inhibits osteoclastic bone resorption. Although bone formation is not impaired at first after calcitonin administration, with time both formation and resorption of bone are reduced. In the kidney, calcitonin reduces both calcium and phosphate reabsorption as well as reabsorption of other ions, including sodium, potassium, and magnesium. Tissues other than bone and kidney are also affected by calcitonin. Calcitonin in pharmacologic amounts decreases gastrin secretion and reduces gastric acid output while increasing secretion of sodium, potassium, chloride, and water in the gut. Pentagastrin is a potent stimulator of calcitonin secretion (as is hypercalcemia), suggesting a possible physiologic relationship between gastrin and calcitonin. In the adult human, no readily demonstrable problem develops in cases of calcitonin deficiency (thyroidectomy) or excess (medullary carcinoma of the thyroid). However, the ability of calcitonin to block bone resorption and lower serum calcium makes it a useful drug for the treatment of Paget's disease, hypercalcemia, and osteoporosis.

GLUCOCORTICOIDS

Glucocorticoid hormones alter bone mineral homeostasis by antagonizing vitamin D-stimulated intestinal calcium transport, by stimulating renal calcium excretion, and by blocking bone formation. Although these observations underscore the negative impact of glucocorticoids on bone mineral homeostasis, these hormones have proved useful in reversing the hypercalcemia associated with lymphomas and granulomatous diseases such as sarcoidosis (in which production of $1,25[OH]_2D$ is increased) or in cases of vitamin D intoxication. Prolonged administration of glucocorticoids is a common cause of osteoporosis in adults and stunted skeletal development in children.

ESTROGENS

Estrogens can prevent accelerated bone loss during the immediate postmenopausal period and at least transiently increase bone in the postmenopausal woman.

The prevailing hypothesis advanced to explain these observations is that estrogens reduce the bone-resorbing action of PTH. Estrogen administration leads to an increased $1,25(OH)_2D$ level in blood, but estrogens have no direct effect on $1,25(OH)_2D$ production in vitro. The increased $1,25(OH)_2D$ levels in vivo following estrogen treatment may result from decreased serum calcium and phosphate and increased PTH. Estrogen receptors have been found in bone, and estrogen has direct effects on bone remodeling. Recent case reports of men who lack the estrogen receptor or who are unable to produce estrogen because of aromatase deficiency noted marked osteopenia and failure to close epiphyses. This further substantiates the role of estrogen in bone development, even in men. The principal therapeutic application for estrogen administration in disorders of bone mineral homeostasis is the treatment or prevention of postmenopausal osteoporosis. However, long-term use of estrogen is being discouraged because of its deleterious side effects. Rather, selective estrogen receptor modulators (SERMs) have been developed to retain the beneficial effects on bone while minimizing these deleterious side effects on breast, uterus, and the cardiovascular system (see Box: Newer Therapies for Osteoporosis).

NEWER THERAPIES FOR OSTEOPOROSIS

Bone undergoes a continuous remodeling process involving bone resorption and formation. Any process that disrupts this balance by increasing resorption relative to formation results in osteoporosis. Inadequate sex hormone production is a major cause of osteoporosis in men and women. Estrogen replacement therapy at menopause is a well-established means of preventing osteoporosis in the female, but many women fear its adverse effects, particularly the increased risk of breast cancer from continued estrogen use (the well-demonstrated increased risk of endometrial cancer is prevented by cycling with a progestin) and do not like the persistence of menstrual bleeding that often accompanies this form of therapy. Medical enthusiasm for this treatment has waned with the demonstration that it does not protect against heart disease. Raloxifene is the first of the selective estrogen receptor modulators (SERMs; see Chapter 40) to be approved for the prevention of osteoporosis. Raloxifene shares some of the beneficial effects of estrogen on bone without increasing the risk of breast or endometrial cancer (it may actually reduce the risk of breast cancer). Although not as effective as estrogen in increasing bone density, raloxifene has been shown to reduce vertebral fractures.

Nonhormonal forms of therapy for osteoporosis with proven efficacy in reducing fracture risk have also been developed. Bisphosphonates such as alendronate,

risedronate, and ibandronate have been conclusively shown to increase bone density and reduce fractures over at least 5 years when used continuously at a dosage of 10 mg/d or 70 mg/wk for alendronate and 5 mg/d or 35 mg/wk for risedronate, 2.5 mg/d or 150 mg/mo for ibandronate. Side-by-side trials between alendronate and calcitonin (another approved nonestrogen drug for osteoporosis) indicated a greater efficacy of alendronate. Bisphosphonates are poorly absorbed and must be given on an empty stomach or infused intravenously. At the higher oral doses used in the treatment of Paget's disease, alendronate causes gastric irritation, but this is not a significant problem at the doses recommended for osteoporosis when patients are instructed to take the drug with a glass of water and remain upright. The most recently approved drug for osteoporosis is teriparatide, the recombinant form of PTH_{1-34}. Unlike other approved drugs for osteoporosis, teriparatide stimulates bone formation rather than inhibiting bone resorption. However, teriparatide must be given daily by subcutaneous injection. Its efficacy in preventing fractures appears to be at least as great as that of the bisphosphonates. In all cases, adequate intake of calcium and vitamin D needs to be maintained.

Thus, we now have several well-validated, efficacious forms of treatment for this common debilitating disease.

NONHORMONAL AGENTS AFFECTING BONE MINERAL HOMEOSTASIS

BISPHOSPHONATES

The bisphosphonates are analogs of pyrophosphate in which the P-O-P bond has been replaced with a nonhydrolyzable P-C-P bond (Figure 42–4). **Etidronate, pamidronate,** and **alendronate** have now been joined by **risedronate, tiludronate, ibandronate,** and **zoledronate** for clinical use. The bisphosphonates owe at least part of their clinical usefulness and toxicity to their ability to retard formation and dissolution of hydroxyapatite crystals within and outside the skeletal system. They localize to regions of bone resorption and so exert their greatest effects on osteoclasts. However, the exact mechanism by which they selectively inhibit bone resorption is not clear.

The results from animal and clinical studies indicate that less than 10% of an oral dose of these drugs is absorbed. Food reduces absorption even further, necessitating their administration on an empty stomach. Because it causes gastric irritation, pamidronate is not available as an oral preparation. However, with the pos-sible exception of etidronate, all currently available bisphosphonates have this complication. Nearly half of the absorbed drug accumulates in bone; the remainder is excreted unchanged in the urine. Decreased renal function, esophageal motility disorders, and peptic ulcer disease are the main contraindications to the use of these drugs. The portion bound to bone is retained for months, depending on the turnover of bone itself.

Etidronate and the other bisphosphonates exert a variety of effects on bone mineral homeostasis. In particular, bisphosphonates are useful for the treatment of hypercalcemia associated with malignancy, for Paget's disease, and for osteoporosis (See Box: Newer Therapies for Osteoporosis). Contrary to expectations, alendronate appears to increase bone mineral density well beyond the 2-year period predicted for a drug whose effects are limited to blocking bone resorption. The bisphosphonates exert a variety of other cellular effects, including inhibition of $1,25(OH)_2D$ production, inhibition of intestinal calcium transport, metabolic changes in bone cells such as inhibition of glycolysis, inhibition of cell growth, and changes in acid and alkaline phosphatase.

Amino bisphosphonates such as alendronate have recently been found to block farnesyl pyrophosphate synthase, an enzyme in the mevalonate pathway that appears to be critical for osteoclast survival. Statins, which block mevalonate synthesis, stimulate bone formation at least in animal studies. Thus, the mevalonate pathway appears to be important in bone cell function and provides new targets for drug development. These effects vary depending on the bisphosphonate being studied (ie, only amino bisphosphonates have this property) and may account for some of the clinical differences observed in the effects of the various bisphosphonates on bone mineral homeostasis. However, with the exceptions of the induction of a mineralization defect by higher than approved doses of etidronate and gastric and esophageal irritation by pamidronate and by high doses of alendronate, these drugs have proved to be remarkably free of adverse effects when used at the doses recommended for the treatment of osteoporosis. Higher doses used in the treatment of hypercalcemia have been associated with renal deterioration and osteonecrosis of the jaw. Esophageal irritation can be minimized by taking the drug with a full glass of water and remaining upright for 30 minutes.

Figure 42–4. The structure of pyrophosphate and of the first three bisphosphonates—etidronate, pamidronate, and alendronate—that were approved for use in the USA.

CALCIMIMETICS

Cinacalcet is the first representative of a new class of drugs that activates the calcium sensing receptor (CaR). CaR is widely distributed but has its greatest concentration in the parathyroid gland. Cinacalcet blocks PTH secretion by this mechanism and is approved for the treatment of secondary hyperparathyroidism in chronic kidney disease and for the treatment of parathyroid carcinoma.

PLICAMYCIN (MITHRAMYCIN)

Plicamycin is a cytotoxic antibiotic (see Chapter 55) that has been used clinically for two disorders of bone mineral metabolism: Paget's disease and hypercalcemia. The cytotoxic properties of the drug appear to involve its binding to DNA and interruption of DNA-directed RNA synthesis. The reasons for its usefulness in the treatment of Paget's disease and hypercalcemia are unclear but may relate to the need for protein synthesis to sustain bone resorption. The doses required to treat Paget's disease and hypercalcemia are about one tenth the amounts required to achieve cytotoxic effects.

THIAZIDES

The chemistry and pharmacology of this family of drugs are covered in Chapter 15. The principal application of thiazides in the treatment of bone mineral disorders is in reducing renal calcium excretion. Thiazides may increase the effectiveness of parathyroid hormone in stimulating reabsorption of calcium by the renal tubules or may act on calcium reabsorption secondarily by increasing sodium reabsorption in the proximal tubule. In the distal tubule, thiazides block sodium reabsorption at the luminal surface, increasing the calcium-sodium exchange at the basolateral membrane and thus enhancing calcium reabsorption into the blood at this site. Thiazides have proved to be useful in reducing the hypercalciuria and incidence of stone formation in subjects with idiopathic hypercalciuria. Part of their efficacy in reducing stone formation may lie in their ability to decrease urine oxalate excretion and increase urine magnesium and zinc levels (both of which inhibit calcium oxalate stone formation).

FLUORIDE

Fluoride is well established as effective for the prophylaxis of dental caries and has been under investigation for the treatment of osteoporosis. Both therapeutic applications originated from epidemiologic observations that subjects living in areas with naturally fluoridated water (1–2 ppm) had less dental caries and fewer vertebral compression fractures than subjects living in nonfluoridated water areas. Fluoride is accumulated by bones and teeth, where it may stabilize the hydroxyapatite crystal. Such a mechanism may explain the effectiveness of fluoride in increasing the resistance of teeth to dental caries, but it does not explain new bone growth.

Fluoride in drinking water appears to be most effective in preventing dental caries if consumed before the eruption of the permanent teeth. The optimum concentration in drinking water supplies is 0.5–1 ppm. Topical application is most effective if done just as the teeth erupt. There is little further benefit to giving fluoride

after the permanent teeth are fully formed. Excess fluoride in drinking water leads to mottling of the enamel proportionate to the concentration above 1 ppm.

Because of the paucity of agents that stimulate new bone growth in patients with osteoporosis, fluoride for this disorder has been examined (see Osteoporosis, below). Results of earlier studies indicated that fluoride alone without adequate calcium supplementation produced osteomalacia. More recent studies, in which calcium supplementation has been adequate, have demonstrated an improvement in calcium balance, an increase in bone mineral, and an increase in trabecular bone volume. However, studies of the ability of fluoride to reduce fractures reach opposite conclusions. Adverse effects observed—at the doses used for testing fluoride's effect on bone—include nausea and vomiting, gastrointestinal blood loss, arthralgias, and arthritis in a substantial proportion of patients. Such effects are usually responsive to reduction of the dose or giving fluoride with meals (or both). At present, fluoride is not approved by the Food and Drug Administration for use in osteoporosis.

■ II. CLINICAL PHARMACOLOGY

Disorders of bone mineral homeostasis generally present with abnormalities in serum or urine calcium levels (or both), often accompanied by abnormal serum phosphate levels. These abnormal mineral concentrations may themselves cause symptoms requiring immediate treatment (eg, coma in malignant hypercalcemia, tetany in hypocalcemia). More commonly, they serve as clues to an underlying disorder in hormonal regulators (eg, primary hyperparathyroidism), target tissue response (eg, chronic kidney disease), or drug misuse (eg, vitamin D intoxication). In such cases, treatment of the underlying disorder is of prime importance.

Since bone and kidney play central roles in bone mineral homeostasis, conditions that alter bone mineral homeostasis usually affect one or both of these tissues secondarily. Effects on bone can result in osteoporosis (abnormal loss of bone; remaining bone histologically normal), osteomalacia (abnormal bone formation due to inadequate mineralization), or osteitis fibrosa (excessive bone resorption with fibrotic replacement of resorption cavities and marrow). Biochemical markers of skeletal involvement include changes in serum levels of the skeletal isoenzyme of alkaline phosphatase and osteocalcin (reflecting osteoblastic activity) and urine levels of hydroxyproline and pyridinoline cross-links (reflecting osteoclastic activity). The kidney becomes involved when the calcium × phosphate product in serum exceeds the point at which ectopic calcification occurs (nephrocalcinosis) or when the calcium × oxalate (or phosphate) product in urine exceeds saturation, leading to nephrolithiasis. Subtle early indicators of such renal involvement include polyuria, nocturia, and hyposthenuria. Radiologic evidence of nephrocalcinosis and stones is not generally observed until later. The degree of the ensuing renal failure is best followed by monitoring the decline in creatinine clearance. On the other hand, chronic kidney disease can be a primary cause of bone disease because of altered handling of calcium and phosphate, decreased $1,25(OH)_2D$ production, and secondary hyperparathyroidism.

ABNORMAL SERUM CALCIUM & PHOSPHATE LEVELS

HYPERCALCEMIA

Hypercalcemia causes central nervous system depression, including coma, and is potentially lethal. Its major causes (other than thiazide therapy) are hyperparathyroidism and cancer with or without bone metastases. Less common causes are hypervitaminosis D, sarcoidosis, thyrotoxicosis, milk-alkali syndrome, adrenal insufficiency, and immobilization. With the possible exception of hypervitaminosis D, the latter disorders seldom require emergency lowering of serum calcium. A number of approaches are used to manage the hypercalcemic crisis.

Saline Diuresis

In hypercalcemia of sufficient severity to produce symptoms, rapid reduction of serum calcium is required. The first steps include rehydration with saline and diuresis with furosemide. Most patients presenting with severe hypercalcemia have a substantial component of prerenal azotemia owing to dehydration, which prevents the kidney from compensating for the rise in serum calcium by excreting more calcium in the urine. Therefore, the initial infusion of 500–1000 mL/h of saline to reverse the dehydration and restore urine flow can by itself substantially lower serum calcium. The addition of a loop diuretic such as furosemide not only enhances urine flow but also inhibits calcium reabsorption in the ascending limb of the loop of Henle (see Chapter 15). Monitoring central venous pressure is important to forestall the development of heart failure and pulmonary edema in predisposed subjects. In many subjects, saline diuresis suffices to reduce serum calcium levels to a point at which more definitive diagnosis and treatment of the underlying condition can be achieved. If this is not the case or if more prolonged medical treatment of hypercalcemia is required, the following agents are available (discussed in order of preference).

Bisphosphonates

Pamidronate, 60–90 mg, infused over 2–4 hours, and zoledronate, 4 mg, infused over at least 15 minutes, have been approved for the treatment of hypercalcemia of malignancy and have largely replaced the less effective etidronate for this indication. The effects generally persist for weeks, but treatment can be repeated after a 7-day interval if necessary and if renal function is not impaired. Some patients experience a self-limited flu-like syndrome after the infusion. Repeated doses of these drugs have been linked to renal deterioration and osteonecrosis of the jaw, but this adverse effect is rare.

Calcitonin

Calcitonin has proved useful as ancillary treatment in a large number of patients. Calcitonin by itself seldom restores serum calcium to normal, and refractoriness frequently develops. However, its lack of toxicity permits frequent administration at high doses (200 MRC units or more). An effect on serum calcium is observed within 4–6 hours and lasts for 6–10 hours. Calcimar (salmon calcitonin) is available for parenteral and nasal administration.

Gallium Nitrate

Gallium nitrate is approved by the FDA for the management of hypercalcemia of malignancy and is undergoing trials for the treatment of advanced Paget's disease. This drug acts by inhibiting bone resorption. At a dosage of 200 mg/m^2 body surface area per day given as a continuous intravenous infusion in 5% dextrose for 5 days, gallium nitrate proved superior to calcitonin in reducing serum calcium in cancer patients. Because of potential nephrotoxicity, patients should be well hydrated and have good renal output before starting the infusion.

Plicamycin (Mithramycin)

Because of its toxicity, plicamycin (mithramycin) is not the drug of first choice for the treatment of hypercalcemia. However, when other forms of therapy fail, 25–50 mcg/kg given intravenously usually lowers serum calcium substantially within 24–48 hours. This effect can last for several days. This dose can be repeated as necessary. The most dangerous toxic effect is sudden thrombocytopenia followed by hemorrhage. Hepatic and renal toxicity can also occur. Hypocalcemia, nausea, and vomiting may limit therapy. Use of this drug must be accompanied by careful monitoring of platelet counts, liver and kidney function, and serum calcium levels.

Phosphate

Giving intravenous phosphate is probably the fastest and surest way to reduce serum calcium, but it is a hazardous procedure if not done properly. Intravenous phosphate should be used only after other methods of treatment (bisphosphonates, calcitonin, and saline diuresis with furosemide) have failed to control symptomatic hypercalcemia. Phosphate must be given slowly (50 mmol or 1.5 g elemental phosphorus over 6–8 hours) and the patient switched to oral phosphate (1–2 g/d elemental phosphorus, as one of the salts indicated below) as soon as symptoms of hypercalcemia have cleared. The risks of intravenous phosphate therapy include sudden hypocalcemia, ectopic calcification, acute renal failure, and hypotension. Oral phosphate can also lead to ectopic calcification and renal failure if serum calcium and phosphate levels are not carefully monitored, but the risk is less and the time of onset much longer. Phosphate is available in oral and intravenous forms as sodium or potassium salt. Amounts required to provide 1 g of elemental phosphorus are as follows:

> **Intravenous:**
> In-Phos: 40 mL
> Hyper-Phos-K: 15 mL
> **Oral:**
> Fleet Phospho-Soda: 6.2 mL
> Neutra-Phos: 300 mL
> K-Phos-Neutral: 4 tablets

Glucocorticoids

Glucocorticoids have no clear role in the acute treatment of hypercalcemia. However, the chronic hypercalcemia of sarcoidosis, vitamin D intoxication, and certain cancers may respond within several days to glucocorticoid therapy. Prednisone in oral doses of 30–60 mg daily is generally used, although equivalent doses of other glucocorticoids are effective. The rationale for the use of glucocorticoids in these diseases differs, however. The hypercalcemia of sarcoidosis is secondary to increased production of $1,25(OH)_2D$, possibly by the sarcoid tissue itself. Glucocorticoid therapy directed at the reduction of sarcoid tissue results in restoration of normal serum calcium and $1,25(OH)_2D$ levels. The treatment of hypervitaminosis D with glucocorticoids probably does not alter vitamin D metabolism significantly but is thought to reduce vitamin D-mediated intestinal calcium transport. An action of glucocorticoids to reduce vitamin D-mediated bone resorption has not been excluded, however. The effect of glucocorticoids on the hypercalcemia of cancer is probably twofold. The malignancies responding best to glucocorticoids (ie, multiple myeloma and related lymphoproliferative diseases) are sensitive to the lytic action of glucocorticoids. Therefore part of the effect may be related to decreased tumor mass and activity. Glucocorticoids have also been shown to inhibit the secretion or effectiveness of cytokines elaborated by mul-

tiple myeloma and related cancers that stimulate osteoclastic bone resorption. Other causes of hypercalcemia—particularly primary hyperparathyroidism—do not respond to glucocorticoid therapy.

HYPOCALCEMIA

The main features of hypocalcemia are neuromuscular—tetany, paresthesias, laryngospasm, muscle cramps, and convulsions. The major causes of hypocalcemia in the adult are hypoparathyroidism, vitamin D deficiency, chronic kidney disease, and malabsorption. Neonatal hypocalcemia is a common disorder that usually resolves without therapy. The roles of PTH, vitamin D, and calcitonin in the neonatal syndrome are under active investigation. Large infusions of citrated blood can produce hypocalcemia by the formation of citrate-calcium complexes. Calcium and vitamin D (or its metabolites) form the mainstay of treatment of hypocalcemia.

Calcium

A number of calcium preparations are available for intravenous, intramuscular, and oral use. Calcium gluceptate (0.9 mEq calcium/mL), calcium gluconate (0.45 mEq calcium/mL), and calcium chloride (0.68–1.36 mEq calcium/mL) are available for intravenous therapy. Calcium gluconate is the preferred form because it is less irritating to veins. Oral preparations include calcium carbonate (40% calcium), calcium lactate (13% calcium), calcium phosphate (25% calcium), and calcium citrate (21% calcium). Calcium carbonate is often the preparation of choice because of its high percentage of calcium, ready availability (eg, Tums), low cost, and antacid properties. In achlorhydric patients, calcium carbonate should be given with meals to increase absorption or the patient switched to calcium citrate, which is somewhat better absorbed. Combinations of vitamin D and calcium are available, but treatment must be tailored to the individual patient and individual disease, a flexibility lost by fixed-dosage combinations. Treatment of severe symptomatic hypocalcemia can be accomplished with slow infusion of 5–20 mL of 10% calcium gluconate. Rapid infusion can lead to cardiac arrhythmias. Less severe hypocalcemia is best treated with oral forms sufficient to provide approximately 400–1200 mg of elemental calcium (1–3 g calcium carbonate) per day. Dosage must be adjusted to avoid hypercalcemia and hypercalciuria.

Vitamin D

When rapidity of action is required, $1,25(OH)_2D_3$ (calcitriol), 0.25–1 mcg daily, is the vitamin D metabolite of choice, because it is capable of raising serum calcium within 24–48 hours. Calcitriol also raises serum phosphate, although this action is usually not observed early in treatment. The combined effects of calcitriol and all other vitamin D metabolites and analogs on both calcium and phosphate make careful monitoring of these mineral levels especially important to avoid ectopic calcification secondary to an abnormally high serum calcium × phosphate product. Since the choice of the appropriate vitamin D metabolite or analog for long-term treatment of hypocalcemia depends on the nature of the underlying disease, further discussion of vitamin D treatment is found under the headings of the specific diseases.

HYPERPHOSPHATEMIA

Hyperphosphatemia is a common complication of renal failure but is also found in all types of hypoparathyroidism (idiopathic, surgical, and pseudo-), vitamin D intoxication, and the rare syndrome of tumoral calcinosis. Emergency treatment of hyperphosphatemia is seldom necessary but can be achieved by dialysis or glucose and insulin infusions. In general, control of hyperphosphatemia involves restriction of dietary phosphate plus the use of phosphate-binding gels such as **sevelamer** and of calcium supplements. Because of their potential to induce aluminum-associated bone disease, aluminum-containing antacids should be used sparingly and only when other measures fail to control the hyperphosphatemia.

HYPOPHOSPHATEMIA

A variety of conditions are associated with hypophosphatemia, including primary hyperparathyroidism, vitamin D deficiency, idiopathic hypercalciuria, vitamin D-resistant rickets, various other forms of renal phosphate wasting (eg, Fanconi's syndrome), overzealous use of phosphate binders, and parenteral nutrition with inadequate phosphate content. Acute hypophosphatemia may lead to a reduction in the intracellular levels of high-energy organic phosphates (eg, ATP), interfere with normal hemoglobin-to-tissue oxygen transfer by decreasing red cell 2,3-diphosphoglycerate levels, and lead to rhabdomyolysis. However, clinically significant acute effects of hypophosphatemia are seldom seen, and emergency treatment is generally not indicated. The long-term effects of hypophosphatemia include proximal muscle weakness and abnormal bone mineralization (osteomalacia). Therefore, hypophosphatemia should be avoided during other forms of therapy and treated in conditions such as hypophosphatemic rickets, of which it is a cardinal feature. Oral forms of phosphate available for use are listed above in the section on hypercalcemia.

SPECIFIC DISORDERS INVOLVING THE BONE MINERAL-REGULATING HORMONES

PRIMARY HYPERPARATHYROIDISM

This rather common disease, if associated with symptoms and significant hypercalcemia, is best treated surgically. Oral phosphate and bisphosphonates have been tried but cannot be recommended. Asymptomatic patients with mild disease in general do not get worse and may be left untreated. The calcimimetic agent **cinacalcet,** the first representative of a new class of drugs that act through the calcium sensing receptor, has been approved for secondary hyperparathyroidism and is in clinical trials for the treatment of primary hyperparathyroidism. If such drugs prove efficacious, medical management of this disease will need to be reconsidered.

HYPOPARATHYROIDISM

In the absence of PTH (idiopathic or surgical hypoparathyroidism) or an abnormal target tissue response to PTH (pseudohypoparathyroidism), serum calcium falls and serum phosphate rises. In such patients, $1,25(OH)_2D$ levels are usually low, presumably reflecting the lack of stimulation by PTH of $1,25(OH)_2D$ production. The skeletons of patients with idiopathic or surgical hypoparathyroidism are normal except for a slow turnover rate. A number of patients with pseudohypoparathyroidism appear to have osteitis fibrosa, suggesting that the normal or high PTH levels found in such patients are capable of acting on bone but not on the kidney. The distinction between pseudohypoparathyroidism and idiopathic hypoparathyroidism is made on the basis of normal or high PTH levels but deficient renal response (ie, diminished excretion of cAMP or phosphate) in patients with pseudohypoparathyroidism.

The principal therapeutic concern is to restore normocalcemia and normophosphatemia. Under most circumstances, vitamin D (25,000–100,000 units three times per week) and dietary calcium supplements suffice. More rapid increments in serum calcium can be achieved with calcitriol, although it is not clear whether this metabolite offers a substantial advantage over vitamin D itself for long-term therapy. Many patients treated with vitamin D develop episodes of hypercalcemia. This complication is more rapidly reversible with cessation of therapy using calcitriol rather than vitamin D. This would be of importance to the patient in whom such hypercalcemic crises are common.

NUTRITIONAL VITAMIN D DEFICIENCY OR INSUFFICIENCY

Vitamin D *deficiency* (generally defined as 25(OH)D levels < 10 ng/mL), once thought to be rare in this country, is being recognized more often, especially in the pediatric and geriatric populations on vegetarian diets and with reduced sunlight exposure. Vitamin D *insufficiency*, generally defined as 25(OH)D levels between 10 ng/mL and 32 ng/mL, is very frequently found in most populations, and is associated with decreased bone mineral density and predisposition to falls and fractures in the elderly. This problem can be avoided by daily intake of 800–1200 units of vitamin D and treated by higher dosages (4000 units per day or 50,000 units per week for several weeks). No other metabolite is indicated. The diet should also contain adequate amounts of calcium and phosphate.

CHRONIC KIDNEY DISEASE

The major problems of chronic kidney disease that impact on bone mineral homeostasis are the loss of $1,25(OH)_2D$ production, the retention of phosphate that reduces ionized calcium levels, and the secondary hyperparathyroidism that results. With the loss of $1,25(OH)_2D$ production, less calcium is absorbed from the intestine and less bone is resorbed under the influence of PTH. As a result hypocalcemia usually develops, furthering the development of hyperparathyroidism. The bones show a mixture of osteomalacia and osteitis fibrosa.

In contrast to the hypocalcemia that is more often associated with chronic kidney disease, some patients may become hypercalcemic from two causes (in addition to overzealous treatment with calcium). The most common cause of hypercalcemia is the development of severe secondary (sometimes referred to as tertiary) hyperparathyroidism. In such cases, the PTH level in blood is very high. Serum alkaline phosphatase levels also tend to be high. Treatment often requires parathyroidectomy.

A less common circumstance leading to hypercalcemia is development of a form of bone disease characterized by a profound decrease in bone cell activity and loss of the calcium buffering action of bone (adynamic bone disease). In the absence of kidney function, any calcium absorbed from the intestine accumulates in the blood. Therefore, such patients are very sensitive to the hypercalcemic action of $1,25(OH)_2D$. These individuals generally have a high serum calcium but nearly normal alkaline phosphatase and PTH levels. The bone in such patients may have a high aluminum content, especially in the mineralization front, which blocks normal bone mineralization. These patients do not respond favorably to parathyroidectomy. Deferoxamine, an agent used to chelate iron (see Chapter 58), also binds aluminum and is being used as therapy for this disorder. However, with less use of aluminum-containing phosphate binders, most cases of adynamic bone disease are not associated with aluminum deposition but are attributed to overzealous suppression of PTH secretion.

Vitamin D Preparations

The choice of vitamin D preparation to be used in the setting of chronic kidney disease depends on the type and extent of bone disease and hyperparathyroidism. Individuals with vitamin D deficiency or insufficiency should first have their 25(OH)D levels restored to normal (above 32 ng/mL) with vitamin D. $1,25(OH)_2D_3$ (calcitriol) rapidly corrects hypocalcemia and at least partially reverses the secondary hyperparathyroidism and osteitis fibrosa. Many patients with muscle weakness and bone pain gain an improved sense of well-being.

Two analogs of calcitriol, doxercalciferol and paricalcitol, are approved for the treatment of secondary hyperparathyroidism of chronic kidney disease. Their principal advantage is that they are less likely than calcitriol to induce hypercalcemia for any given reduction in PTH. Their greatest impact is in patients in whom the use of calcitriol may lead to unacceptably high serum calcium levels.

Regardless of the drug used, careful attention to serum calcium and phosphate levels is required. A calcium × phosphate product (in mg/dL units) less than 55 is desired with both calcium and phosphate in the normal range. Calcium adjustments in the diet and dialysis bath and phosphate restriction (dietary and with oral ingestion of phosphate binders) should be used along with vitamin D metabolites. Monitoring serum PTH and alkaline phosphatase levels is useful in determining whether therapy is correcting or preventing secondary hyperparathyroidism. Although not generally available, percutaneous bone biopsies for quantitative histomorphometry may help in choosing appropriate therapy and following the effectiveness of such therapy, especially in cases suspected of having adynamic bone disease. Unlike the rapid changes in serum values, changes in bone morphology require months to years. Monitoring serum levels of the vitamin D metabolites is useful to determine compliance, absorption, and metabolism.

INTESTINAL OSTEODYSTROPHY

A number of gastrointestinal and hepatic diseases result in disordered calcium and phosphate homeostasis that ultimately leads to bone disease. The bones in such patients show a combination of osteoporosis and osteomalacia. Osteitis fibrosa does not occur, as in renal osteodystrophy. The common features that appear to be important in this group of diseases are malabsorption of calcium and malabsorption of vitamin D. Liver disease may, in addition, reduce the production of 25(OH)D from vitamin D, although its importance in all but patients with terminal liver failure remains in dispute. The malabsorption of vitamin D is probably not limited to exogenous vitamin D. The liver secretes into bile a

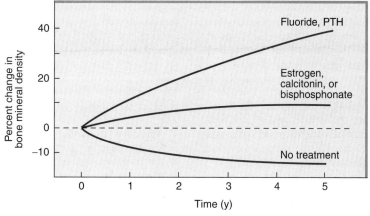

Figure 42–5. Typical changes in bone mineral density with time after the onset of menopause, with and without treatment. In the untreated condition, bone is lost during aging in both men and women. Fluoride and PTH promote new bone formation and can increase bone mineral density in subjects who respond to it throughout the period of treatment. In contrast, estrogen, calcitonin, and bisphosphonates block bone resorption. This leads to a transient increase in bone mineral density because bone formation is not initially decreased. However, with time, both bone formation and bone resorption are decreased and bone mineral density reaches a new plateau.

substantial number of vitamin D metabolites and conjugates that are reabsorbed in (presumably) the distal jejunum and ileum. Interference with this process could deplete the body of endogenous vitamin D metabolites as well as limit absorption of dietary vitamin D.

In mild forms of malabsorption, vitamin D (25,000–50,000 units three times per week) should suffice to raise serum levels of 25(OH)D into the normal range. Many patients with severe disease do not respond to vitamin D. Clinical experience with the other metabolites is limited, but both calcitriol and calcifediol have been used successfully in doses similar to those recommended for treatment of renal osteodystrophy. Theoretically, calcifediol should be the drug of choice under these conditions, because no impairment of the renal metabolism of 25(OH)D to 1,25(OH)$_2$D and 24,25(OH)$_2$D exists in these patients. Both calcitriol and 24,25(OH)$_2$D may be of importance in reversing the bone disease. However, calcifediol is no longer available. As in the other diseases discussed, treatment of intestinal osteodystrophy with vitamin D and its metabolites should be accompanied by appropriate dietary calcium supplementation and monitoring of serum calcium and phosphate levels.

OSTEOPOROSIS

Osteoporosis is defined as abnormal loss of bone predisposing to fractures. It is most common in postmenopausal women but also occurs in men. The annual cost of fractures in older women and men in the USA was estimated at $13.8 billion in 1996 and would be much higher today. It may occur as a side effect of long-term administration of glucocorticoids or other drugs; as a manifestation of endocrine disease such as thyrotoxicosis or hyperparathyroidism; as a feature of malabsorption syndrome; as a consequence of alcohol abuse and cigarette smoking; or without obvious cause (idiopathic). The ability of some agents to reverse the bone loss of osteoporosis is shown in Figure 42–5. The postmenopausal form of osteoporosis may be accompanied by lower 1,25(OH)$_2$D levels and reduced intestinal calcium transport. This form of osteoporosis is due to estrogen deficiency and can be treated with estrogen (cycled with a progestin in women with a uterus to prevent endometrial carcinoma). However, concern that estrogen increases the risk of breast cancer and fails to reduce the development of heart disease has reduced enthusiasm for this form of therapy.

As noted above, estrogen-like SERMs (selective estrogen receptor modulators, Chapter 40) have been developed that prevent the increased risk of breast and uterine cancer associated with estrogen while maintaining the benefit to bone. **Raloxifene** is such a drug approved for treatment of osteoporosis. Like tamoxifen, it appears to reduce the risk of breast cancer. Raloxifene protects against spine fractures but not hip fractures—unlike bisphosphonates and teriparatide, which protect against both. Raloxifene does not prevent hot flushes and imposes the same increased risk of thrombophlebitis as estrogen. To counter the reduced intestinal calcium transport associated with osteoporosis, vitamin D therapy is often used in addition to dietary calcium supplementation. There is no clear evidence that pharmacologic doses of vitamin D are of much additional benefit beyond cyclic estrogens and calcium supplementation. However, in several large studies, vitamin D supplementation (800 IU/d) has been shown to be useful. In addition, calcitriol and its analog $1\alpha(OH)D_3$ have been shown to increase bone mass and reduce fractures in several recent studies. Use of these agents for osteoporosis is not FDA-approved, although they are used in other countries.

Despite early promise that **fluoride** might be useful in the prevention or treatment of postmenopausal osteoporosis, this form of therapy remains controversial. A new formulation of fluoride (slow release, lower dose) appears to avoid much of the toxicity of earlier formulations and may reduce fracture rates. However, this formulation has not been approved by the FDA. **Teriparatide,** the recombinant form of PTH 1-34, has recently been approved for treatment of osteoporosis. Teriparatide is given in a dosage of 20 mcg subcutaneously daily. Like fluoride, teriparatide stimulates new bone formation, but unlike fluoride, this new bone appears structurally normal and is associated with a substantial reduction in the incidence of fractures.

Calcitonin is approved for use in the treatment of postmenopausal osteoporosis. It has been shown to increase bone mass and reduce fractures, but only in the spine. It does not appear to be as effective as bisphosphonates or teriparatide.

Bisphosphonates are potent inhibitors of bone resorption. They increase bone density and reduce the risk of fractures in the hip, spine, and other locations. **Alendronate, risedronate,** and **ibandronate** are approved for the treatment of osteoporosis, using either daily dosing schedules: alendronate 10 mg/d, risedronate 5 mg/d, ibandronate 2.5 mg/d; weekly schedules: alendronate 70 mg/wk, risedronate 35 mg/wk; or monthly schedules: ibandronate 150 mg/mo. These drugs are effective in men as well as women and for various causes of osteoporosis.

X-LINKED & AUTOSOMAL DOMINANT HYPOPHOSPHATEMIA

These disorders are manifested by the appearance of rickets and hypophosphatemia in children, although they may first present in adults. X-linked hypophosphatemia is caused by mutations in a gene encoding a protein called PHEX, which appears to be an endopeptidase. Mutations in the gene responsible for the autosomal dominant form target FGF23. The current concept is that FGF23 blocks the renal uptake of phosphate and blocks $1,25(OH)_2D_3$ production. Muta-

tions in PHEX inactivate it, and FGF23 levels increase. Similarly, mutations in FGF23 that resist hydrolysis, as seen in patients with the autosomal form of hypophosphatemic rickets, also have elevated FGF23 levels.

Initially, it was thought that FGF23 was a direct substrate for PHEX, but this no longer appears to be the case. In either disease, intact and biologically active FGF23 accumulates, leading to phosphate wasting in the urine and hypophosphatemia.

Phosphate is critical to normal bone mineralization; when phosphate stores are deficient, a clinical and pathologic picture resembling vitamin D–deficient rickets develops. However, such children fail to respond to the usual doses of vitamin D used in the treatment of nutritional rickets. A defect in $1,25(OH)_2D$ production by the kidney has also been noted, because the serum $1,25(OH)_2D$ levels tend to be low in comparison with the degree of hypophosphatemia observed. This combination of low serum phosphate and low or low-normal serum $1,25(OH)_2D$ provides the rationale for treating such patients with oral phosphate (1–3 g daily) and calcitriol (0.25–2 mcg daily). Reports of such combination therapy are encouraging in this otherwise debilitating disease.

VITAMIN D–DEPENDENT RICKETS TYPES I & II

These distinctly different autosomal recessive diseases present as childhood rickets that does not respond to conventional doses of vitamin D. Type I vitamin D–dependent rickets, now known as pseudovitamin D deficiency rickets, is due to an isolated deficiency of $1,25(OH)_2D$ production caused by mutations in $25(OH)D\text{-}1\alpha\text{-hydroxylase}$. This condition can be treated with vitamin D (4000 units daily) or calcitriol (0.25–0.5 mcg daily). Type II vitamin D–dependent rickets, now known as hereditary vitamin D resistant rickets, is caused by mutations in the gene for the vitamin D receptor, which disrupt the functions of this receptor and lead to this syndrome. The serum levels of $1,25(OH)_2D$ are very high in type II but not in type I vitamin D-dependent rickets. Treatment with large doses of calcitriol has been claimed to be effective in restoring normocalcemia in some patients, presumably those with a partially functional vitamin D receptor. Some patients are totally refractory to vitamin D. One recent report indicates a reversal of resistance to calcitriol when $24,25(OH)_2D$ was given. These diseases are rare.

NEPHROTIC SYNDROME

Patients with nephrotic syndrome can lose vitamin D metabolites in the urine, presumably by loss of the vitamin D-binding protein. Such patients may have very low 25(OH)D levels. Some of them develop bone disease. It is not yet clear what value vitamin D therapy has in such patients, because therapeutic trials with vitamin D (or any other vitamin D metabolite) have not yet been carried out. Because the problem is not related to vitamin D metabolism, one would not anticipate any advantage in using the more expensive vitamin D metabolites in place of vitamin D itself.

IDIOPATHIC HYPERCALCIURIA

People with idiopathic hypercalciuria, characterized by hypercalciuria and nephrolithiasis with normal serum calcium and PTH levels, have been subdivided into three groups: (1) hyperabsorbers, patients with increased intestinal absorption of calcium, resulting in high-normal serum calcium, low-normal PTH, and a secondary increase in urine calcium; (2) renal calcium leakers, patients with a primary decrease in renal reabsorption of filtered calcium, leading to low-normal serum calcium and high-normal serum PTH; and (3) renal phosphate leakers, patients with a primary decrease in renal reabsorption of phosphate, leading to stimulation of $1,25(OH)_2D$ production, increased intestinal calcium absorption, increased ionized serum calcium, low-normal PTH levels, and a secondary increase in urine calcium. There is some disagreement about this classification, and many patients are not readily categorized. Many such patients present with mild hypophosphatemia, and oral phosphate has been used with some success to reduce stone formation. However, a clear role for phosphate in the treatment of this disorder has not been established.

Therapy with hydrochlorothiazide, up to 50 mg twice daily, or chlorthalidone, 50–100 mg daily, is recommended. Loop diuretics such as furosemide and ethacrynic acid should not be used because they increase urinary calcium excretion. The major toxicity of thiazide diuretics, besides hypokalemia, hypomagnesemia, and hyperglycemia, is hypercalcemia. This is seldom more than a biochemical observation unless the patient has a disease such as hyperparathyroidism in which bone turnover is accelerated. Accordingly, one should screen patients for such disorders before starting thiazide therapy and monitor serum and urine calcium when therapy has begun.

An alternative to thiazides is allopurinol. Some studies indicate that hyperuricosuria is associated with idiopathic hypercalcemia and that a small nidus of urate crystals could lead to the calcium oxalate stone formation characteristic of idiopathic hypercalcemia. Allopurinol, 300 mg daily, may reduce stone formation by reducing uric acid excretion.

OTHER DISORDERS OF BONE MINERAL HOMEOSTASIS

PAGET'S DISEASE OF BONE

Paget's disease is a localized bone disease characterized by uncontrolled osteoclastic bone resorption with sec-

ondary increases in bone formation. This new bone is poorly organized, however. The cause of Paget's disease is obscure, although some studies suggest that a slow virus may be involved. The disease is fairly common, although symptomatic bone disease is less common. The biochemical parameters of elevated serum alkaline phosphatase and urinary hydroxyproline are useful for diagnosis. Along with the characteristic radiologic and bone scan findings, these biochemical determinations provide good markers by which to follow therapy.

The goal of treatment is to reduce bone pain and stabilize or prevent other problems such as progressive deformity, hearing loss, high-output cardiac failure, and immobilization hypercalcemia. Calcitonin and bisphosphonates are the first-line agents for this disease. Treatment failures may respond to plicamycin. Calcitonin is administered subcutaneously or intramuscularly in doses of 50–100 MRC units every day or every other day. Nasal inhalation at 200–400 units per day is also effective. Higher or more frequent doses have been advocated when this initial regimen is ineffective. Improvement in bone pain and reduction in serum alkaline phosphatase and urine hydroxyproline levels require weeks to months. Often a patient who responds well initially loses the response to calcitonin. This refractoriness is not correlated with the development of antibodies.

Alendronate, etidronate, pamidronate, risedronate, tiludronate, and zoledronic acid are the bisphosphonates currently approved for clinical use in this condition in the USA. The recommended dosages of bisphosphonates are alendronate, 40 mg/d; etidronate, 5 mg/kg/d; pamidronate, 30 mg/d IV for 3 days; risedronate, 30 mg/d; tiludronate, 400 mg/d; and zoledronic acid, 5 mg IV once. Long-term (months to years) remission may be expected in patients who respond to these agents. Treatment should not exceed 6 months per course but can be repeated after 6 months if necessary. The principal toxicity of etidronate is the development of osteomalacia and an increased incidence of fractures when the dosage is raised substantially above 5 mg/kg/d. The newer bisphosphonates such as risedronate and alendronate do not share this side effect. Some patients treated with etidronate develop bone pain similar in nature to the bone pain of osteomalacia. This subsides after stopping the drug. The principal side effect of alendronate and the newer bisphosphonates is gastric irritation when used at these high doses. This is reversible on cessation of the drug.

The use of a potentially lethal cytotoxic drug such as plicamycin in a generally benign disorder such as Paget's disease is recommended only when other less toxic agents (calcitonin, alendronate) have failed and the symptoms are debilitating. Insufficient clinical data on long-term use of plicamycin are available to determine its usefulness for extended therapy. However, short courses involving 15–25 mcg/kg/d intravenously for 5–10 days followed by 15 mcg/kg intravenously each week have been used to control the disease.

ENTERIC OXALURIA

Patients with short bowel syndromes associated with fat malabsorption can present with renal stones composed of calcium and oxalate. Such patients characteristically have normal or low urine calcium levels but elevated urine oxalate levels. The reasons for the development of oxaluria in such patients are thought to be twofold: first, in the intestinal lumen, calcium (which is now bound to fat) fails to bind oxalate and no longer prevents its absorption; second, enteric flora, acting on the increased supply of nutrients reaching the colon, produce larger amounts of oxalate. Although one would ordinarily avoid treating a patient with calcium oxalate stones with calcium supplementation, this is precisely what is done in patients with enteric oxaluria. The increased intestinal calcium binds the excess oxalate and prevents its absorption. One to 2 g of calcium carbonate can be given daily in divided doses, with careful monitoring of urinary calcium and oxalate to be certain that urinary oxalate falls without a dangerous increase in urinary calcium.

PREPARATIONS AVAILABLE

VITAMIN D, METABOLITES, AND ANALOGS

Calcitriol
Oral (generic, Rocaltrol): 0.25, 0.5 mcg capsules, 1 mcg/mL solution
Parenteral (generic, Calcijex): 1, 2 mcg/mL for injection

Cholecalciferol [D_3] (vitamin D_3, Delta-D)
Oral: 400, 1000 IU tablets

Doxercalciferol (Hectoral)
Oral: 2.5 mcg capsules

Ergocalciferol [D_2] (vitamin D_2, Calciferol, Drisdol)
Oral: 50,000 IU capsules; 8000 IU/mL drops
Parenteral: 500,000 IU/mL for injection

Paricalcitol (Zemplar)
Oral: 1, 2, 4 mcg capsules
Parenteral: 5 mcg/mL for injection

CALCIUM

Calcium acetate [25% calcium] (PhosLo)
Oral: 668 mg (167 mg calcium) tablets; 333.5 mg (84.5 mg calcium), 667 mg (169 mg calcium) capsules

Calcium carbonate [40% calcium] (generic, Tums, Cal-Sup, Os-Cal 500, others)
Oral: Numerous forms available containing 260–600 mg calcium per unit

Calcium chloride [27% calcium] (generic)
Parenteral: 10% solution for IV injection only

Calcium citrate [21% calcium] (generic, Citracal)
Oral: 950 mg (200 mg calcium), 2376 mg (500 mg calcium)

Calcium glubionate [6.5% calcium] (Calcionate, Calciquid)
Oral: 1.8 g (115 mg calcium)/5 mL syrup

Calcium gluceptate [8% calcium] (Calcium Gluceptate)

Parenteral: 1.1 g/5 mL solution for IM or IV injection

Calcium gluconate [9% calcium] (generic)
Oral: 500 mg (45 mg calcium), 650 mg (58.5 mg calcium), 975 mg (87.75 mg calcium), 1 g (90 mg calcium) tablets
Parenteral: 10% solution for IV or IM injection

Calcium lactate [13% calcium] (generic)
Oral: 650 mg (84.5 mg calcium), 770 mg (100 mg calcium) tablets

Tricalcium phosphate [39% calcium] (Posture)
Oral: 1565 mg (600 mg calcium) tablets (as phosphate)

PHOSPHATE AND PHOSPHATE BINDER

Phosphate
Oral (Fleet Phospho-soda): solution containing 2.5 g phosphate/5 mL (816 mg phosphorus/5 mL; 751 mg sodium/5 mL)
Oral (K-Phos-Neutral): tablets containing 250 mg phosphorus, 298 mg sodium
Oral (Neutra-Phos): For reconstitution in 75 mL water, packet containing 250 mg phosphorus; 164 mg sodium; 278 mg potassium
Oral (Neutra-Phos-K): For reconstitution in 75 mL water, packet containing 250 mg phosphorus; 556 mg potassium; 0 mg sodium
Parenteral (potassium or sodium phosphate): 3 mmol/mL

Sevelamer (Renagel)
Oral: 403 mg capsules

OTHER DRUGS

Alendronate (Fosamax)
Oral: 5, 10, 35, 40, 70 mg tablets; 70 mg/75 mL oral solution

(continued)

Calcitonin-Salmon
Nasal spray (Miacalcin): 200 IU/puff
Parenteral (Calcimar, Miacalcin, Salmonine): 200 IU/mL for injection

Cinacalcet (Sensipar)
Oral: 30, 60, 90 mg tablets

Etidronate (Didronel)
Oral: 200, 400 mg tablets
Parenteral: 300 mg/6 mL for IV injection

Gallium nitrate (Ganite)
Parenteral: 500 mg/20 mL vial

Ibandronate (Boniva)
Oral: 2.5, 150 mg tablets

Pamidronate (generic, Aredia)
Parenteral: 30, 60, 90 mg/vial

Plicamycin (mithramycin) (Mithracin)
Parenteral: 2.5 mg per vial powder to reconstitute for injection

Risedronate (Actonel)
Oral: 5, 30, 35 mg tablets

Sodium fluoride (generic)
Oral: 0.55 mg (0.25 mg F), 1.1 mg (0.5 mg F), 2.2 mg (1.0 mg F) tablets; drops

Teriparatide (Forteo)
Subcutaneous: 250 mcg/mL from prefilled pen (3 mL)

Tiludronate (Skelid)
Oral: 200 mg tablets (as tiludronic acid)

Zoledronic acid (Zometa)
Parenteral: 4 mg/vial

REFERENCES

Andress DL: Vitamin D treatment in chronic kidney disease. Semin Dial 2005;18:315.

Berenson JR et al: American Society of Clinical Oncology clinical practice guidelines: The role of bisphosphonates in multiple myeloma. J Clin Oncol 2002;20:3719.

Cho HY et al: A clinical and molecular genetic study of hypophosphatemic rickets in children. Pediatr Res 2005;58:329.

Clines GA, Guise TA: Mechansims and treatment for bone metastases. Clin Adv Hematol Oncol 2004;2:295.

Fowler VG et al: Daptomycin versus standard therapy for bacteremia and endocarditis caused by *Staphylococcus aureus*. N Engl J Med 2006;355:653.

Gaugris S et al: Vitamin D inadequacy among post-menopausal women: A systematic review. Quart J Med 2005;98:667.

Hodsman AB et al: Parathyroid hormone and teriparatide for the treatment of osteoporosis: A review of the evidence and suggested guidelines for use. Endocr Rev 2005;26:688.

Hutton E: Evaluation and management of hypercalcemia. JAAPA 2005;18:30.

Ishida M et al: Management of calcium, phosphorus, and bone metabolism in dialysis patients using sevalamer hydrochloride and vitamin D therapy. Ther Apher Dial 2005;9(Suppl 1):S16.

Liberman et al: Effect of oral alendronate on bone mineral density and the incidence of fractures in postmenopausal osteoporosis. N Engl J Med 1995;333:1437.

McClung MR et al: Effect of risedronate on the risk of hip fracture in elderly women. N Engl J Med 2001;344:333.

McIntyre CW et al: A prospective study of combination therapy for hyperphosphataemia with calcium-containing phosphate binders and sevelamer in hypercalcaemic haemodialysis patients. Nephrol Dial Transplant 2002;17:1643.

Merigo E et al: Jaw bone necrosis without previous dental extractions associated with the use of bisphosphonates (pamidronate and zoledronate): A four-case report. J Oral Pathol Med 2005;34:613.

Morony S et al: The inhibition of RANKL causes greater suppression of bone resorption and hypercalcemia compared with bisphosphonates in two models of humoral hypercalcemia and malignancy. Endocrinology 2005;146:3235.

Neer RM et al: Effect of parathyroid hormone (1-34) on fractures and bone mineral density in postmenopausal women with osteoporosis. N Engl J Med 2001;344:1434.

Orwoll E et al: Alendronate for the treatment of osteoporosis in men. N Engl J Med 2000;343:604.

Park S, Johnson MA: Living in low-latitude regions in the United States does not prevent poor vitamin D status. Nutr Rev 2005;63:203.

Pettifor JM: Rickets and vitamin D deficiency in children and adolescents. Endocrinol Metab Clin North Am 2005;34:537.

Quarles LD: Cinacalcet HCl: A novel treatment for secondary hyperparathyroidism in stage 5 chronic kidney disease. Kidney Int Suppl 2005;Jul(96):S24.

Rizzoli R: A new treatment for post-menopausal osteoporosis: strontium ranelate. J Endocrinol Invest 2005;28:50.

Rosen CJ: Clinical practice. Postmenopausal osteoporosis. N Engl J Med 2005;353:595.

Steddon SJ, Cunningham J: Calcimimetics and calcilytics—fooling the calcium receptor. Lancet 2005;365:2237.

Salusky IB: Are new vitamin D analogues in renal bone disease superior to calcitriol? Pediatr Nephrol 2005;20:393.

Stewart AF: Clinical practice. Hypercalcemia associated with cancer. N Engl J Med 2005;352:373.

Strewler GJ: FGF23, hypophosphatemia, and rickets: Has phosphatonin been found? Proc Natl Acad Sci U S A 2001;98:5945.

Tfelt-Hanson J, Brown EM: The calcium-sensing receptor in normal physiology and pathophysiology: A review. Crit Rev Clin Lab Sci 2005;42:35.

Wilkins CH, Birge SJ: Prevention of osteoporotic fractures in the elderly. Am J Med 2005;118:1190.

Zisman AL et al: Inhibition of parathyroid hormone: A dose equivalency study of paracalcitol and doxercalciferol. Am J Nephrol 2005;25:591.

SECTION VIII
Chemotherapeutic Drugs

INTRODUCTION TO ANTIMICROBIAL AGENTS

Antimicrobial agents are among the most dramatic examples of the advances of modern medicine. Many infectious diseases once considered incurable and lethal are now amenable to treatment with a few pills. The remarkably powerful and specific activity of antimicrobial drugs is due to their selectivity for targets that are either unique to microorganisms or much more important in them than in humans. Among these targets are bacterial and fungal cell wall-synthesizing enzymes (see Chapters 43 and 48), the bacterial ribosome (see Chapters 44 and 45), the enzymes required for nucleotide synthesis and DNA replication (see Chapter 46), and the machinery of viral replication (see Chapter 49). The special group of drugs used in mycobacterial infections is discussed in Chapter 47. The much older and less selective cytotoxic antiseptics and disinfectants are discussed in Chapter 50. The clinical uses of all these agents are presented in Chapter 51.

Microorganisms can adapt to environmental pressures in a variety of effective ways, and their response to antibiotic pressure is no exception. An inevitable consequence of antimicrobial usage is the selection of resistant microorganisms, perhaps the most obvious example of evolution in action. Overuse and inappropriate use of antibiotics has fueled a major increase in prevalence of multidrug-resistant pathogens, leading some to speculate that we are nearing the end of the antibiotic era. Unfortunately, as the need has grown in recent years, development of novel drugs has slowed. The most vulnerable molecular targets of antimicrobial drugs have been identified, and in many cases crystallized and characterized. Pending the identification of new targets and compounds, it seems likely that over the next decade we will have to rely on currently available families of drugs. In the face of continuing development of resistance, considerable effort will be required to maintain the effectiveness of these drug groups.

Beta-Lactam & Other Cell Wall- & Membrane-Active Antibiotics

43

Henry F. Chambers, MD

◼ BETA-LACTAM COMPOUNDS

PENICILLINS

The penicillins share features of chemistry, mechanism of action, pharmacology, and immunologic characteristics with cephalosporins, monobactams, carbapenems, and β-lactamase inhibitors. All are β-lactam compounds, so named because of their unique four-membered lactam ring.

Chemistry

All penicillins have the basic structure shown in Figure 43–1. A thiazolidine ring (A) is attached to a β-lactam ring (B) that carries a secondary amino group (RNH–). Substituents (R; examples shown in Figure 43–2) can be attached to the amino group. Structural integrity of the 6-aminopenicillanic acid nucleus is essential for the biologic activity of these compounds. Hydrolysis of the β-lactam ring by bacterial β-lactamases yields penicilloic acid, which lacks antibacterial activity.

A. CLASSIFICATION

Substituents of the 6-aminopenicillanic acid moiety determine the essential pharmacologic and antibacterial properties of the resulting molecules. Penicillins can be assigned to one of three groups (below). Within each of these groups are compounds that are relatively stable to gastric acid and suitable for oral administration, eg, penicillin V, dicloxacillin, and amoxicillin. The side chains of some representatives of each group are shown in Figure 43–2, with a few distinguishing characteristics.

1. Penicillins (eg, penicillin G)—These have greatest activity against gram-positive organisms, gram-negative cocci, and non-β-lactamase-producing anaerobes. However, they have little activity against gram-negative rods, and they are susceptible to hydrolysis by β-lactamases.

2. Antistaphylococcal penicillins (eg, nafcillin)—These penicillins are resistant to staphylococcal β-lactamases. They are active against staphylococci and strep-

tococci but not against enterococci, anaerobic bacteria, and gram-negative cocci and rods.

3. Extended-spectrum penicillins (ampicillin and the antipseudomonal penicillins)—These drugs retain the antibacterial spectrum of penicillin and have improved activity against gram-negative organisms. Like penicillin, however, they are relatively susceptible to hydrolysis by β-lactamases.

B. PENICILLIN UNITS AND FORMULATIONS

The activity of penicillin G was originally defined in units. Crystalline sodium penicillin G contains approximately 1600 units per mg (1 unit = 0.6 mcg; 1 million units of penicillin = 0.6 g). Semisynthetic penicillins are prescribed by weight rather than units. The **minimum inhibitory concentration (MIC)** of any penicillin (or other antimicrobial) is usually given in mcg /mL. Most penicillins are dispensed as the sodium or potassium salt of the free acid. Potassium penicillin G contains about 1.7 mEq of K^+ per million units of penicillin (2.8 mEq/g). Nafcillin contains Na^+, 2.8 mEq/g. Procaine salts and benzathine salts of penicillin G provide repository forms for intramuscular injection. In dry crystalline form, penicillin salts are stable for years at 4 °C. Solutions lose their activity rapidly (eg, 24 hours at 20 °C) and must be prepared fresh for administration.

Mechanism of Action

Penicillins, like all β-lactam antibiotics, inhibit bacterial growth by interfering with the transpeptidation reaction of bacterial cell wall synthesis. The cell wall is a rigid outer layer unique to bacterial species. It completely surrounds the cytoplasmic membrane (Figure 43–3), maintains cell shape and integrity, and prevents cell lysis from high osmotic pressure. The cell wall is composed of a complex cross-linked polymer of polysaccharides and polypeptides, peptidoglycan (murein, mucopeptide). The polysaccharide contains alternating amino sugars, *N*-acetylglucosamine and *N*-acetylmuramic acid (Figure 43–4). A five-amino-acid peptide is linked to the *N*-acetylmuramic acid sugar. This peptide terminates in D-

Figure 43–1. Core structures of four β-lactam antibiotic families. The ring marked B in each structure is the β-lactam ring. The penicillins are susceptible to bacterial metabolism and inactivation by amidases and lactamases at the points shown. Note that the carbapenems have a different stereochemical configuration in the lactam ring that apparently imparts resistance to β-lactamases. Substituents for the penicillin and cephalosporin families are shown in Figures 43–2 and 43–6, respectively.

alanyl-D-alanine. Penicillin-binding protein (PBP, an enzyme) removes the terminal alanine in the process of forming a cross-link with a nearby peptide. Cross-links give the cell wall its structural rigidity. β-Lactam antibiotics, structural analogs of the natural D-Ala-D-Ala substrate, covalently bind to the active site of PBPs. This inhibits the transpeptidation reaction (Figure 43–5), halting peptidoglycan synthesis, and the cell dies. The exact mechanism of cell death is not completely understood, but autolysins and disruption of cell wall morphogenesis are involved. Penicillins and cephalosporins kill bacterial cells only when they are actively growing and synthesizing cell wall.

Resistance

Resistance to penicillins and other β-lactams is due to one of four general mechanisms: (1) inactivation of antibiotic by β-lactamase, (2) modification of target PBPs, (3) impaired penetration of drug to target PBPs, and (4) efflux. β-Lactamase production is the most common mechanism of resistance. Many hundreds of different β-lactamases have been identified. Some, such as those produced by *Staphylococcus aureus, Haemophilus* sp, and *Escherichia coli,* are relatively narrow in substrate specificity, preferring penicillins to cephalosporins. Other β-lactamases, eg, AmpC β-lactamase produced by *Pseudomonas aeruginosa* and *Enterobacter* sp, and extended-spectrum β-lactamases (ESBLs), hydrolyze both cephalosporins and penicillins. Carbapenems are highly resistant to hydrolysis by penicillinases and cephalosporinases but they are hydrolyzed by metallo-β-lactamase and carbapenemases.

Altered target PBPs are the basis of methicillin resistance in staphylococci and of penicillin resistance in pneumococci and enterococci. These resistant organisms produce PBPs that have low affinity for binding β-lactam antibiotics, and consequently they are not inhibited except at relatively high, often clinically unachievable, drug concentrations.

Resistance due to impaired penetration of antibiotic to target PBPs occurs only in gram-negative species because of their impermeable outer cell wall membrane, which is absent in gram-positive bacteria. β-Lactam antibiotics cross the outer membrane and enter gram-negative organisms via outer membrane protein channels (porins). Absence of the proper channel or down-regulation of its production can greatly impair drug entry into the cell. Poor penetration alone is usually not sufficient to confer resistance, because enough antibiotic eventually enters the cell to inhibit growth. However, this barrier can become important in the presence of a β-lactamase, even a relatively inactive one, as long as it can hydrolyze drug faster than it enters the cell. Gram-negative organisms also may produce an efflux pump, which consists of cytoplasmic and periplasmic protein components that efficiently transport some β-lactam antibiotics from the periplasm back across the outer membrane.

Pharmacokinetics

Absorption of orally administered drug differs greatly for different penicillins, depending in part on their acid

6-Aminopenicillanic acid

The following structures can each be substituted at the R to produce a new penicillin.

Penicillin G (benzylpenicillin):
High activity against gram-positive bacteria. Low activity against gram-negative bacteria. Acid-labile. Destroyed by β-lactamase. 60% protein-bound.

Oxacillin (no Cl atoms); cloxacillin (one Cl in structure); dicloxacillin (2 Cls in structure); flucloxacillin (one Cl and one F in structure) (isoxazolyl penicillins):
Similar to methicillin in β-lactamase resistance, but acid-stable. Can be taken orally. Highly protein-bound (95–98%).

Nafcillin (ethoxynaphthamidopenicillin):
Similar to isoxazolyl penicillins. Less strongly protein-bound (90%). Resistant to staphylococcal β-lactamase.

Ampicillin (alpha-aminobenzylpenicillin):
Similar to Penicillin G (destroyed by β-lactamase) but acid-stable and more active against gram-negative bacteria. Carbenicillin has –COONa instead of NH₂ group.

Ticarcillin:
Similar to carbenicillin but gives higher blood levels. Piperacillin, azlocillin, and mezlocillin resemble ticarcillin in action against gram-negative aerobes.

Amoxicillin:
Similar to ampicillin but better absorbed, gives higher blood levels.

Figure 43–2. Side chains of some penicillins (R groups of Figure 43–1).

stability and protein binding. Gastrointestinal absorption of nafcillin is erratic, so it is not suitable for oral administration. Dicloxacillin, ampicillin, and amoxicillin are acid-stable and relatively well absorbed, producing serum concentrations in the range of 4–8 mcg/mL following a 500 mg oral dose. Absorption of most oral penicillins (amoxicillin being an exception) is impaired by food, and the drugs should be administered at least 1–2 hours before or after a meal.

After parenteral administration, absorption of most penicillins is complete and rapid. Intravenous administration is preferred to the intramuscular route because of irritation and local pain from intramuscular injection of large doses. Serum concentrations 30 minutes after an intravenous injection of 1 g of a penicillin (equivalent to approximately 1.6 million units of penicillin G) are 20–50 mcg/mL. Only a small amount of the total drug in serum is present as free drug, the concentration

Figure 43–3. A highly simplified diagram of the cell envelope of a gram-negative bacterium. The outer membrane, a lipid bilayer, is present in gram-negative but not gram-positive organisms. It is penetrated by porins, proteins that form channels providing hydrophilic access to the cytoplasmic membrane. The peptidoglycan layer is unique to bacteria and is much thicker in gram-positive organisms than in gram-negative ones. Together, the outer membrane and the peptidoglycan layer constitute the cell wall. Penicillin-binding proteins (PBPs) are membrane proteins that cross-link peptidoglycan. β-Lactamases, if present, reside in the periplasmic space or on the outer surface of the cytoplasmic membrane, where they may destroy β-lactam antibiotics that penetrate the outer membrane.

of which is determined by protein binding. Highly protein-bound penicillins (eg, nafcillin) generally achieve lower free-drug concentrations in serum than less protein-bound penicillins (eg, penicillin G, ampicillin). Protein binding becomes clinically relevant when the protein-bound percentage is approximately 95% or more. Penicillins are widely distributed in body fluids and tissues with a few exceptions. They are polar molecules, so intracellular concentrations are well below those found in extracellular fluids.

Benzathine and procaine penicillins are formulated to delay absorption, resulting in prolonged blood and tissue concentrations. A single intramuscular injection of 1.2 million units of benzathine penicillin maintains serum levels above 0.02 mcg/mL for 10 days, sufficient to treat β-hemolytic streptococcal infection. After 3 weeks, levels still exceed 0.003 mcg/mL, which is enough to prevent β-hemolytic streptococcal infection. A 600,000 unit dose of procaine penicillin yields peak concentrations of 1–2 mcg/mL and clinically useful concentrations for 12–24 hours after a single intramuscular injection.

Penicillin concentrations in most tissues are equal to those in serum. Penicillin is also excreted into sputum and milk to levels 3–15% of those present in the serum. Penetration into the eye, the prostate, and the central nervous system is poor. However, with active inflammation of the meninges, as in bacterial meningitis, penicillin concentrations of 1–5 mcg/mL can be achieved with a daily parenteral dose of 18–24 million units.

M

L-Ala

M

L-Ala
|
R

G

G

M

M

L-Ala

L-Ala

G

D-Glu

+

G

D-Glu

L-Lys — [Gly]₅

L-Lys — [Gly]₅*

D-Ala*

R

D-Ala

D-Ala

D-Ala

| Transpeptidase |

M

M

L-Ala

L-Ala
|
R

G

G

M

M

L-Ala

L-Ala

G

D-Glu

G

D-Glu

L-Lys — [Gly]₅ — D-Ala — L-Lys — [Gly]₅

D-Ala

D-Ala

+ D-Ala

These concentrations are sufficient to kill susceptible strains of pneumococci and meningococci.

Penicillin is rapidly excreted by the kidneys; small amounts are excreted by other routes. About 10% of renal excretion is by glomerular filtration and 90% by tubular secretion. The normal half-life of penicillin G is approximately 30 minutes; in renal failure, it may be as long as 10 hours. Ampicillin and the extended-spectrum penicillins are secreted more slowly than penicillin G and have half-lives of 1 hour. For penicillins that are cleared by the kidney, the dose must be adjusted according to renal function, with approximately one fourth to one third the normal dose being administered if creatinine clearance is 10 mL/min or less (Table 43–1).

Nafcillin is primarily cleared by biliary excretion. Oxacillin, dicloxacillin, and cloxacillin are eliminated by both the kidney and biliary excretion; no dosage adjustment is required for these drugs in renal failure. Because clearance of penicillins is less efficient in the newborn, doses adjusted for weight alone result in higher systemic concentrations for longer periods than in the adult.

Clinical Uses

Except for oral amoxicillin, penicillins should be given 1–2 hours before or after a meal; they should not be given with food to minimize binding to food proteins and acid inactivation. Blood levels of all penicillins can be raised by simultaneous administration of probenecid, 0.5 g (10 mg/kg in children) every 6 hours orally, which impairs renal tubular secretion of weak acids such as β-lactam compounds.

A. PENICILLIN

Penicillin G is a drug of choice for infections caused by streptococci, meningococci, enterococci, penicillin-susceptible pneumococci, non–β-lactamase-producing staphylococci, *Treponema pallidum* and many other spirochetes, clostridium species, actinomyces, and other

Figure 43–4. The transpeptidation reaction in *Staphylococcus aureus* that is inhibited by β-lactam antibiotics. The cell wall of gram-positive bacteria is made up of long peptidoglycan polymer chains consisting of the alternating aminohexoses N-acetylglucosamine (G) and N-acetylmuramic acid (M) with pentapeptide side chains linked (in *S aureus*) by pentaglycine bridges. The exact composition of the side chains varies among species. The diagram illustrates small segments of two such polymer chains and their amino acid side chains. These linear polymers must be cross-linked by transpeptidation of the side chains at the points indicated by the asterisk to achieve the strength necessary for cell viability.

Figure 43–5. The biosynthesis of cell wall peptidoglycan, showing the sites of action of five antibiotics (shaded bars; 1 = fosfomycin, 2 = cycloserine, 3 = bacitracin, 4 = vancomycin, 5 = β-lactam antibiotics). Bactoprenol (BP) is the lipid membrane carrier that transports building blocks across the cytoplasmic membrane; M = *N*-acetylmuramic acid; Glc = glucose; NAcGlc or G = *N*-acetylglucosamine.

gram-positive rods and non-β-lactamase-producing gram-negative anaerobic organisms. Depending on the organism, the site, and the severity of infection, effective doses range between 4 and 24 million units per day administered intravenously in four to six divided doses. High-dose penicillin G can also be given as a continuous intravenous infusion.

Penicillin V, the oral form of penicillin, is indicated only in minor infections because of its relatively poor bioavailability, the need for dosing four times a day, and its narrow antibacterial spectrum. Amoxicillin (see below) is often used instead.

Benzathine penicillin and procaine penicillin G for intramuscular injection yield low but prolonged drug levels. A single intramuscular injection of benzathine penicillin, 1.2 million units, is effective treatment for β-hemolytic streptococcal pharyngitis; given intramuscularly once every 3–4 weeks, it prevents reinfection. Benzathine penicillin G, 2.4 million units intramuscularly once a week for 1–3 weeks, is effective in the treatment of syphilis. Procaine penicillin G, formerly a work horse for treating uncomplicated pneumococcal pneumonia or gonorrhea, is rarely used nowadays because many strains are penicillin-resistant.

Table 43–1. Guidelines for dosing of some commonly used penicillins.

Antibiotic (Route of Administration)	Adult Dose	Pediatric Dose[1]	Neonatal Dose[2]	Adjusted Dose as a Percentage of Normal Dose for Renal Failure Based on Creatinine Clearance (Cl$_{cr}$)	
				Cl$_{cr}$ Approx 50 mL/min	Cl$_{cr}$ Approx 10 mL/min
Penicillins					
Penicillin G (IV)	1–4 mU q4–6h	25,000–400,000 units/kg/d in 4–6 doses	75,000–150,000 units/kg/d in 2 or 3 doses	50–75%	25%
Penicillin VK (PO)	0.25–0.5 g qid	25–50 mg/kg/d in 4 doses		None	None
Antistaphylococcal penicillins					
Cloxacillin, dicloxacillin (PO)	0.25–0.5 g qid	25–50 mg/kg/d in 4 doses		100%	100%
Nafcillin (IV)	1–2 g q4–6h	50–100 mg/kg/d in 4–6 doses	50–75 mg/kg/d in 2 or 3 doses	100%	100%
Oxacillin (IV)	1–2 g q4–6h	50–100 mg/kg/d in 4–6 doses	50–75 mg/kg/d in 2 or 3 doses	100%	100%
Extended-spectrum penicillins					
Amoxicillin (PO)	0.25–0.5 g tid	20–40 mg/kg/d in 3 doses		66%	33%
Amoxicillin/ potassium clavulanate (PO)	500/125 tid– 875/125 mg bid	20–40 mg/kg/d in 3 doses		66%	33%
Piperacillin (IV)	3–4 g q4–6h	300 mg/kg/d in 4–6 doses	150 mg/kg/d in 2 doses	50–75%	25–33%
Ticarcillin (IV)	3 g q4–6h	200–300 mg/kg/d in 4–6 doses	150–200 mg/kg/d in 2 or 3 doses	50–75%	25–33%

[1]The total dose should not exceed the adult dose.
[2]The dose shown is during the first week of life. The daily dose should be increased by approximately 33–50% after the first week of life. The lower dosage range should be used for neonates weighing less than 2 kg. After the first month of life, pediatric doses may be used.

B. Penicillins Resistant to Staphylococcal Beta-Lactamase (Methicillin, Nafcillin, and Isoxazolyl Penicillins)

These semisynthetic penicillins are indicated for infection by β-lactamase-producing staphylococci, although penicillin-susceptible strains of streptococci and pneumococci are also susceptible. Listeria, enterococci, and methicillin-resistant strains of staphylococci are resistant.

An isoxazolyl penicillin such as oxacillin, cloxacillin, or dicloxacillin, 0.25–0.5 g orally every 4–6 hours (15–25 mg/kg/d for children), is suitable for treatment of mild to moderate localized staphylococcal infections. All are relatively acid-stable and have reasonable bio-availability. However, food interferes with absorption, and the drugs should be administered 1 hour before or after meals.

For serious systemic staphylococcal infections, oxacillin or nafcillin, 8–12 g/d, is given by intermittent intravenous infusion of 1–2 g every 4–6 hours (50–100 mg/kg/d for children).

C. Extended-Spectrum Penicillins (Aminopenicillins, Carboxypenicillins, and Ureidopenicillins)

These drugs have greater activity than penicillin against gram-negative bacteria because of their enhanced ability to penetrate the gram-negative outer membrane. Like penicillin G, they are inactivated by many β-lactamases.

The aminopenicillins, ampicillin and amoxicillin, have identical spectrum and activity, but amoxicillin is better absorbed orally. Amoxicillin, 250–500 mg three times daily, is equivalent to the same amount of ampicillin given four times daily. These drugs are given orally to treat urinary tract infections, sinusitis, otitis, and lower respiratory tract infections. Ampicillin and amoxicillin are the most active of the oral β-lactam antibiotics against penicillin-resistant pneumococci and are the preferred β-lactam antibiotics for treating infections suspected to be caused by these resistant strains. Ampicillin (but not amoxicillin) is effective for shigellosis. Its use to treat uncomplicated salmonella gastroenteritis is controversial because it may prolong the carrier state.

Ampicillin, at dosages of 4–12 g/d intravenously, is useful for treating serious infections caused by penicillin-susceptible organisms, including anaerobes, enterococci, *Listeria monocytogenes,* and β-lactamase-negative strains of gram-negative cocci and bacilli such as *E coli,* and salmonella species. Non-β-lactamase-producing strains of *H influenzae* are generally susceptible, but strains that are resistant because of altered PBPs are emerging. Many gram-negative species produce β-lactamases and are resistant, precluding use of ampicillin for empirical therapy of urinary tract infections, meningitis, and typhoid fever. Ampicillin is not active against klebsiella, enterobacter, *Pseudomonas aeruginosa,* citrobacter, serratia, indole-positive proteus species, and other gram-negative aerobes that are commonly encountered in hospital-acquired infections.

Carbenicillin, the very first antipseudomonal carboxypenicillin, is obsolete. A derivative, carbenicillin indanyl sodium, can be given orally for urinary tract infections. There are more active, better tolerated alternatives. A carboxypenicillin with activity similar to that of carbenicillin is ticarcillin. It is less active than ampicillin against enterococci. The ureidopenicillins, piperacillin, mezlocillin, and azlocillin, are also active against selected gram-negative bacilli, such as *Klebsiella pneumoniae.* Although supportive clinical data are lacking for superiority of combination therapy over single-drug therapy, because of the propensity of *P aeruginosa* to develop resistance, an antipseudomonal penicillin is frequently used in combination with an aminoglycoside or fluoroquinolone for pseudomonal infections outside the urinary tract.

Ampicillin, amoxicillin, ticarcillin, and piperacillin are also available in combination with one of several β-lactamase inhibitors: clavulanic acid, sulbactam, or tazobactam. The addition of a β-lactamase inhibitor extends the activity of these penicillins to include β-lactamase-producing strains of *S aureus* as well as some β-lactamase-producing gram-negative bacteria (see below).

Adverse Reactions

The penicillins are remarkably nontoxic. Most of the serious adverse effects are due to hypersensitivity. All penicillins are cross-sensitizing and cross-reacting. The antigenic determinants are degradation products of penicillins, particularly penicilloic acid and products of alkaline hydrolysis bound to host protein. A history of a penicillin reaction is not reliable; about 5–8% of people claim such a history, but only a small number of these will have an allergic reaction when given penicillin. Less than 1% of persons who previously received penicillin without incident will have an allergic reaction when given penicillin. Because of the potential for anaphylaxis, however, penicillin should be administered with caution or a substitute drug given if there is a history of penicillin allergy. The incidence of allergic reactions in small children is negligible.

Allergic reactions include anaphylactic shock (very rare—0.05% of recipients); serum sickness-type reactions (now rare—urticaria, fever, joint swelling, angioneurotic edema, intense pruritus, and respiratory embarrassment occurring 7–12 days after exposure); and a variety of skin rashes. Oral lesions, fever, interstitial nephritis (an autoimmune reaction to a penicillin-protein complex), eosinophilia, hemolytic anemia and other hematologic disturbances, and vasculitis may also occur. Most patients allergic to penicillins can be treated with alternative drugs. However, if necessary (eg, treatment of enterococcal endocarditis or neurosyphilis in a highly penicillin-allergic patient), desensitization can be accomplished with gradually increasing doses of penicillin.

In patients with renal failure, penicillin in high doses can cause seizures. Nafcillin is associated with neutropenia; oxacillin can cause hepatitis; and methicillin causes interstitial nephritis (and is no longer used for this reason). Large doses of penicillins given orally may lead to gastrointestinal upset, particularly nausea, vomiting, and diarrhea. Ampicillin has been associated with pseudomembranous colitis. Secondary infections such as vaginal candidiasis may occur. Ampicillin and amoxicillin can cause skin rashes that are not allergic in nature.

■ CEPHALOSPORINS & CEPHAMYCINS

Cephalosporins are similar to penicillins, but more stable to many bacterial β-lactamases and therefore have a broader spectrum of activity. However, strains of *E coli* and *Klebsiella* species expressing extended-spectrum β-lactamases that can hydrolyze most cephalosporins are becoming a problem. Cephalosporins are not active against enterococci and *L monocytogenes.*

Chemistry

The nucleus of the cephalosporins, 7-aminocephalosporanic acid (Figure 43–6), bears a close resemblance to 6-aminopenicillanic acid (Figure 43–1). The intrinsic antimicrobial activity of natural cephalosporins is low, but the attachment of various R_1 and R_2 groups has yielded hundreds of potent compounds of low toxicity (Figure 43–6). Cephalosporins can be classified into four major groups or generations, depending mainly on the spectrum of antimicrobial activity.

FIRST-GENERATION CEPHALOSPORINS

First-generation cephalosporins include **cefadroxil, cefazolin, cephalexin, cephalothin, cephapirin,** and **cephradine.** These drugs are very active against gram-positive cocci, such as pneumococci, streptococci, and staphylococci. Cephalosporins are not active against methicillin-resistant strains of staphylococci. *E coli, K pneumoniae,* and *Proteus mirabilis* are often sensitive, but activity against *P aeruginosa,* indole-positive proteus, enterobacter, *Serratia marcescens,* citrobacter, and acinetobacter is poor. Anaerobic cocci (eg, peptococcus, peptostreptococcus) are usually sensitive, but *Bacteroides fragilis* is not.

Pharmacokinetics & Dosage

A. ORAL

Cephalexin, cephradine, and cefadroxil are absorbed from the gut to a variable extent. After oral doses of 500 mg, serum levels are 15–20 mcg/mL. Urine concentration is usually very high, but in most tissues levels are variable and generally lower than in serum. Cephalexin and cephradine are given orally in dosages of 0.25–0.5 g four times daily (15–30 mg/kg/d) and cefadroxil in dosages of 0.5–1 g twice daily. Excretion is mainly by glomerular filtration and tubular secretion into the urine. Drugs that block tubular secretion, eg, probenecid, may increase serum levels substantially. In patients with impaired renal function, dosage must be reduced (Table 43–2).

B. PARENTERAL

Cefazolin is the only first-generation parenteral cephalosporin still in general use. After an intravenous infusion of 1 g, the peak level of cefazolin is 90–120 mcg/mL. The usual intravenous dosage of cefazolin for adults is 0.5–2 g intravenously every 8 hours. Cefazolin can also be administered intramuscularly. Excretion is via the kidney, and dose adjustments must be made for impaired renal function.

Clinical Uses

Although the first-generation cephalosporins are broad spectrum and relatively nontoxic, they are rarely the drug of choice for any infection. Oral drugs may be used for the treatment of urinary tract infections, for staphylococcal, or for streptococcal infections including cellulitis or soft tissue abscess. However, oral cephalosporins should not be relied on in serious systemic infections.

Cefazolin penetrates well into most tissues. It is a drug of choice for surgical prophylaxis. Cefazolin may be a choice in infections for which it is the least toxic drug (eg, *K pneumoniae*) and in persons with staphylococcal or streptococcal infections who have a history of penicillin allergy other than immediate hypersensitivity. Cefazolin does not penetrate the central nervous system and cannot be used to treat meningitis. Cefazolin is an alternative to an antistaphylococcal penicillin for patients who are allergic to penicillin.

SECOND-GENERATION CEPHALOSPORINS

Members of the second-generation cephalosporins include **cefaclor, cefamandole, cefonicid, cefuroxime, cefprozil, loracarbef,** and **ceforanide** and the structurally related cephamycins **cefoxitin, cefmetazole,** and **cefotetan,** which have activity against anaerobes. This is a heterogeneous group of drugs with marked individual differences in activity, pharmacokinetics, and toxicity. In general, they are active against organisms inhibited by first-generation drugs, but in addition they have extended gram-negative coverage. Klebsiellae (including those resistant to cephalothin) are usually sensitive. Cefamandole, cefuroxime, cefonicid, ceforanide, and cefaclor are active against *H influenzae* but not against serratia or *B fragilis.* In contrast, cefoxitin, cefmetazole, and cefotetan are active against *B fragilis* and some serratia strains but are less active against *H influenzae.* As with first-generation agents, none is active against enterococci or *P aeruginosa.* Second-generation cephalosporins may exhibit in vitro activity against enterobacter species, but resistant mutants that constitutively express a chromosomal β-lactamase that hydrolyzes these compounds (and third-generation cephalosporins) are readily selected, and they should not be used to treat enterobacter infections.

Pharmacokinetics & Dosage

A. ORAL

Cefaclor, cefuroxime axetil, cefprozil, and loracarbef can be given orally. The usual dosage for adults is 10–15 mg/kg/d in two to four divided doses; children should be given 20–40 mg/kg/d up to a maximum of 1 g/d. Except for cefuroxime axetil, these drugs are not predictably active against penicillin-resistant pneumococci and should be used cautiously, if at all, to treat suspected or proved pneumococcal infections. Cefaclor is more susceptible to β-lactamase hydrolysis compared with the other agents, and its usefulness is correspondingly diminished.

7-Aminocephalosporanic acid nucleus. The following structures can each be substituted at R_1 and R_2 to produce the named derivatives.

Figure 43–6. Structures of some cephalosporins R_1 and R_2 structures are substituents on the 7-aminocephalosporanic acid nucleus pictured at the top. Other structures (cefoxitin and below) are complete in themselves.

Table 43–2. Guidelines for dosing of some commonly used cephalosporins and other cell-wall inhibitor antibiotics.

Antibiotic (Route of Administration)	Adult Dose	Pediatric Dose[1]	Neonatal Dose[2]	Adjusted Dose as a Percentage of Normal Dose for Renal Failure Based on Creatinine Clearance (Cl$_{cr}$)	
				Cl$_{cr}$ Approx 50 mL/min	Cl$_{cr}$ Approx 10 mL/min
First-generation cephalosporins					
Cefadroxil (PO)	0.5–1 g qd–bid	30 mg/kg/d in 2 doses		50%	25%
Cephalexin, cephradine (PO)	0.25–0.5 g qid	25–50 mg/kg/d in 4 doses		50%	25%
Cefazolin (IV)	0.5–2 g q8h	25–100 mg/kg/d in 3 or 4 doses		50%	25%
Second-generation cephalosporins					
Cefoxitin (IV)	1–2 g q6–8h	75–150 mg/kg/d in 3 or 4 doses		50–75%	25%
Cefotetan (IV)	1–2 g q12h			50%	25%
Cefuroxime (IV)	0.75–1.5 g q8h	50–100 mg/kg/d in 3 or 4 doses		66%	25–33%
Cefuroxime axetil (PO)	0.25–0.5 g bid	0.125–0.25 g bid		100%	25%
Third- and fourth-generation cephalosporins					
Cefotaxime (IV)	1–2 g q6–12h	50–200 mg/kg/d in 4–6 doses	100 mg/kg/d in 2 doses	50%	25%
Ceftazidime (IV)	1–2 g q8–12h	75–150 mg/kg/d in 3 doses	100–150 mg/kg/d in 2 or 3 doses	50%	25%
Ceftriaxone (IV)	1–4 g q24h	50–100 mg/kg/d in 1 or 2 doses	50 mg/kg/d once a day	None	None
Cefepime (IV)	0.5–2 g q12h	75–120 mg/kg/d in 2 or 3 divided doses		50%	25%
Carbapenems					
Ertapenem (IM or IV)	1 g			100%[3]	50%
Imipenem (IV)	0.25–0.5 g q6–8h			75%	50%
Meropenem (IV)	1 g q8h (2 g q8h for meningitis)	60–120 mg/kg/d in 3 doses (maximum of 2 g q8h)		66%	50%
Glycopeptides					
Vancomycin (IV)	30 mg/kg/d in 2–3 doses	40 mg/kg/d in 3 or 4 doses	15 mg/kg load, then 20 mg/kg/d in 2 doses	40%	10%

[1]The total dose should not exceed the adult dose.
[2]The dose shown is during the first week of life. The daily dose should be increased by approximately 33–50% after the first week of life. The lower dosage range should be used for neonates weighing less than 2 kg. After the first month of life, pediatric doses may be used.
[3]50% of dose for Cl$_{cr}$ < 30 mL/min.

B. PARENTERAL

After a 1-g intravenous infusion, serum levels are 75–125 mcg/mL for most second-generation cephalosporins. Intramuscular administration is painful and should be avoided. Doses and dosing intervals vary depending on the specific agent (Table 43–2). There are marked differences in half-life, protein binding, and interval between doses. All are renally cleared and require dosage adjustment in renal failure.

Clinical Uses

The oral second-generation cephalosporins are active against β-lactamase-producing *H influenzae* or *Moraxella catarrhalis* and have been primarily used to treat sinusitis, otitis, or lower respiratory tract infections, in which these organisms have an important role. Because of their activity against anaerobes (including *B fragilis*), cefoxitin, cefotetan, or cefmetazole can be used to treat mixed anaerobic infections such as peritonitis or diverticulitis. Cefuroxime is used to treat community-acquired pneumonia because it is active against β-lactamase-producing *H influenzae* or *K pneumoniae* and penicillin-resistant pneumococci. Although cefuroxime crosses the blood-brain barrier, it is less effective in treatment of meningitis than ceftriaxone or cefotaxime and should not be used.

THIRD-GENERATION CEPHALOSPORINS

Third-generation agents include **cefoperazone, cefotaxime, ceftazidime, ceftizoxime, ceftriaxone, cefixime, cefpodoxime proxetil, cefdinir, cefditoren pivoxil, ceftibuten,** and **moxalactam.**

Antimicrobial Activity

Compared with second-generation agents, these drugs have expanded gram-negative coverage, and some are able to cross the blood-brain barrier. Third-generation drugs are active against citrobacter, *S marcescens,* and providencia (though resistance can emerge during treatment of infections caused by these species due to selection of mutants that constitutively produce cephalosporinase). They are also effective against β-lactamase-producing strains of haemophilus and neisseria. Ceftazidime and cefoperazone are the only two drugs with useful activity against *P aeruginosa*. Like the second-generation drugs, third-generation cephalosporins are hydrolyzable by constitutively produced AmpC β-lactamase, and they are not reliably active against enterobacter species. Serratia, providencia, and citrobacter also produce a chromosomally encoded cephalosporinase that, when constitutively expressed, can confer resistance to third-generation cephalosporins. Ceftizoxime and moxalactam are active against *B fragilis*. Cefixime, cefdinir, ceftibuten, and cef-

podoxime proxetil are oral agents possessing similar activity except that cefixime and ceftibuten are much less active against pneumococci (and completely inactive against penicillin-resistant strains) and have poor activity against *S aureus*.

Pharmacokinetics & Dosage

Intravenous infusion of 1 g of a parenteral cephalosporin produces serum levels of 60–140 mcg/mL. Cephalosporins penetrate body fluids and tissues well and, with the exception of cefoperazone and all oral cephalosorins, achieve levels in the cerebrospinal fluid sufficient to inhibit most pathogens, including gram-negative rods, except pseudomonas.

The half-lives of these drugs and the necessary dosing intervals vary greatly: Ceftriaxone (half-life 7–8 hours) can be injected once every 24 hours at a dosage of 15–50 mg/kg/d. A single daily 1-g dose is sufficient for most serious infections, with 4 g once daily recommended for treatment of meningitis. Cefoperazone (half-life 2 hours) can be injected every 8–12 hours in a dosage of 25–100 mg/kg/d. The remaining drugs in the group (half-life 1–1.7 hours) can be injected every 6–8 hours in dosages between 2 and 12 g/d, depending on the severity of infection. Cefixime can be given orally (200 mg twice daily or 400 mg once daily) for respiratory or urinary tract infections. The adult dose for cefpodoxime proxetil or cefditoren pivoxil is 200–400 mg twice daily; for ceftibuten, 400 mg once daily; and for cefdinir, 300 mg/12 h. The excretion of cefoperazone and ceftriaxone is mainly through the biliary tract, and no dosage adjustment is required in renal insufficiency. The others are excreted by the kidney and therefore require dosage adjustment in renal insufficiency.

Clinical Uses

Third-generation cephalosporins are used to treat a wide variety of serious infections caused by organisms that are resistant to most other drugs. Strains expressing extended-spectrum β-lactamases, however, are not susceptible. Third-generation cephalosporins should be avoided in treatment of enterobacter infections—even if the clinical isolate appears susceptible in vitro—because of emergence of resistance. Ceftriaxone and cefotaxime are approved for treatment of meningitis, including meningitis caused by pneumococci, meningococci, *H influenzae,* and susceptible enteric gram-negative rods, but not by *L monocytogenes.* Ceftriaxone and cefotaxime are the most active cephalosporins against penicillin-resistant strains of pneumococci and are recommended for empirical therapy of serious infections that may be caused by these strains. Meningitis caused by highly penicillin-resistant strains of pneumococci (ie, those susceptible only to penicillin MICs > 1 mcg/mL) may not respond even to these agents, and addition of vancomycin is recommended. Other potential indications include empirical therapy of sepsis of unknown cause in both the immunocompetent and the immunocompromised patient and treatment of infections for which a cephalosporin is the least toxic drug available. In neutropenic, febrile immunocompromised patients, third-generation cephalosporins are often used in combination with an aminoglycoside.

FOURTH-GENERATION CEPHALOSPORINS

Cefepime is an example of a so-called fourth-generation cephalosporin. It is more resistant to hydrolysis by chromosomal β-lactamases (eg, those produced by enterobacter). It has good activity against *P aeruginosa,* Enterobacteriaceae, *S aureus,* and *S pneumoniae.* Cefepime is highly active against haemophilus and neisseria. It penetrates well into cerebrospinal fluid. It is cleared by the kidneys and has a half-life of 2 hours, and its pharmacokinetic properties are very similar to those of ceftazidime. Unlike ceftazidime, however, cefepime has good activity against most penicillin-resistant strains of streptococci, and it may be useful in treatment of enterobacter infections. Otherwise, its clinical role is similar to that of third-generation cephalosporins.

ADVERSE EFFECTS OF CEPHALOSPORINS

Allergy

Cephalosporins are sensitizing and may elicit a variety of hypersensitivity reactions that are identical to those of penicillins, including anaphylaxis, fever, skin rashes, nephritis, granulocytopenia, and hemolytic anemia. However, the chemical nucleus of cephalosporins is sufficiently different from that of penicillins so that some individuals with a history of penicillin allergy may tolerate cephalosporins. The frequency of cross-allergenicity between the two groups of drugs is uncertain but is probably around 5–10%. However, patients with a history of anaphylaxis to penicillins should not receive cephalosporins.

Toxicity

Local irritation can produce severe pain after intramuscular injection and thrombophlebitis after intravenous injection. Renal toxicity, including interstitial nephritis and even tubular necrosis, has been demonstrated and has caused the withdrawal of cephaloridine from clinical use.

Cephalosporins that contain a methylthiotetrazole group (eg, cefamandole, cefmetazole, cefotetan, cefoperazone) frequently cause hypoprothrombinemia and bleeding disorders. Administration of vitamin K$_1$, 10 mg twice weekly, can prevent this. Drugs with the methylthiotetrazole ring can also cause severe disulfiram-like reactions; consequently, alcohol and alcohol-containing medications must be avoided.

■ OTHER BETA-LACTAM DRUGS

MONOBACTAMS

Monobactams are drugs with a monocyclic β-lactam ring (Figure 43–1). They are relatively resistant to β-lactamases and active against gram-negative rods (including pseudomonas and serratia). They have no activity against gram-positive bacteria or anaerobes. Aztreonam is the only monobactam available in the USA. It resembles aminoglycosides (Chapter 45) in its spectrum of activity. Aztreonam is given intravenously every 8 hours in a dose of 1–2 g, providing peak serum levels of 100 mcg/mL. The half-life is 1–2 hours and is greatly prolonged in renal failure.

Penicillin-allergic patients tolerate aztreonam without reaction. Occasional skin rashes and elevations of serum aminotransferases occur during administration of aztreonam, but major toxicity has not yet been reported. The clinical usefulness of aztreonam has not been fully defined.

BETA-LACTAMASE INHIBITORS (CLAVULANIC ACID, SULBACTAM, & TAZOBACTAM)

These substances resemble β-lactam molecules (Figure 43–7) but they have very weak antibacterial action. They are potent inhibitors of many but not all bacterial β-lactamases and can protect hydrolyzable penicillins from inactivation by these enzymes. β-Lactamase inhibitors are most active against Ambler class A β-lactamases (plasmid-encoded transposable element [TEM] β-lactamases in particular), such as those produced by staphylococci, *H influenzae, N gonorrhoeae,* salmonella, shigella, *E coli,* and *K pneumoniae.* They are not good inhibitors of class C β-lactamases, which typically are chromosomally encoded and inducible, produced by enterobacter, citrobacter, serratia, and pseudomonas, but they do inhibit chromosomal β-lactamases of bacteroides and branhamella.

The three inhibitors differ slightly with respect to pharmacology, stability, potency, and activity, but these differences usually are of little therapeutic significance. β-Lactamase inhibitors are available only in fixed combinations with specific penicillins. The antibacterial spectrum of the combination is determined by the companion penicillin, not the β-lactamase inhibitor. (The fixed combinations available in the USA are listed in the Preparations Available section.) An inhibitor

Figure 43–7. β-lactamase inhibitors.

Clavulanic acid **Sulbactam** **Tazobactam**

extends the spectrum of a penicillin provided that the inactivity of the penicillin is due to destruction by β-lactamase and that the inhibitor is active against the β-lactamase that is produced. Thus, ampicillin-sulbactam is active against β-lactamase-producing *S aureus* and *H influenzae* but not serratia, which produces a β-lactamase that is not inhibited by sulbactam. Similarly, if a strain of *P aeruginosa* is resistant to piperacillin, it is also resistant to piperacillin-tazobactam, because tazobactam does not inhibit the chromosomal β-lactamase.

The indications for penicillin-β-lactamase inhibitor combinations are empirical therapy for infections caused by a wide range of potential pathogens in both immuno-compromised and immunocompetent patients and treatment of mixed aerobic and anaerobic infections, such as intra-abdominal infections. Doses are the same as those used for the single agents except that the recommended dosage of piperacillin in the piperacillin-tazobactam combination is 3 g every 6 hours. Adjustments for renal insufficiency are made based on the penicillin component.

CARBAPENEMS

The carbapenems are structurally related to β-lactam antibiotics (Figure 43–1). Ertapenem, imipenem, and meropenem are licensed for use in the USA. Imipenem has a wide spectrum with good activity against many gram-negative rods, including *P aeruginosa,* gram-positive organisms, and anaerobes. It is resistant to most β-lactamases but not metallo-β-lactamases. *Enterococcus faecium,* methicillin-resistant strains of staphylococci, *Clostridium difficile, Burkholderia cepacia,* and *Stenotrophomonas maltophilia* are resistant. Imipenem is inactivated by dehydropeptidases in renal tubules, resulting in low urinary concentrations. Consequently, it is administered together with an inhibitor of renal dehydropeptidase, cilastatin, for clinical use. Meropenem is similar to imipenem but has slightly greater activity against gram-negative aerobes and slightly less activity against gram-positives. It is not significantly degraded by renal dehydropeptidase and does not require an inhibitor. Ertapenem is less active than meropenem or imipenem against *P aeruginosa* and acinetobacter species. It is not degraded by renal dehydropeptidase.

Carbapenems penetrate body tissues and fluids well, including the cerebrospinal fluid. All are cleared renally,

and the dose must be reduced in patients with renal insufficiency. The usual dose of imipenem is 0.25–0.5 g given intravenously every 6–8 hours (half-life 1 hour). The usual adult dose of meropenem is 1 g intravenously every 8 hours. Ertapenem has the longest half-life (4 hours) and is administered as a once-daily dose of 1 g intravenously or intramuscularly. Intramuscular ertapenem is irritating, and for that reason the drug is formulated with 1% lidocaine for administration by this route.

A carbapenem is indicated for infections caused by susceptible organisms, eg, *P aeruginosa,* which are resistant to other available drugs and for treatment of mixed aerobic and anaerobic infections. Carbapenems are active against many highly penicillin-resistant strains of pneumococci. A carbapenem is the β-lactam antibiotic of choice for treatment of enterobacter infections because it is resistant to destruction by the β-lactamase produced by these organisms; it is also the treatment of choice for infections caused by ESBL-producing gram-negatives. Ertapenem is insufficiently active against *P aeruginosa* and should not be used to treat infections caused by that organism. Imipenem or meropenem with or without an aminoglycoside may be effective treatment for febrile neutropenic patients.

The most common adverse effects of carbapenems—which tend to be more common with imipenem—are nausea, vomiting, diarrhea, skin rashes, and reactions at the infusion sites. Excessive levels of imipenem in patients with renal failure may lead to seizures. Meropenem and ertapenem are less likely to cause seizures than imipenem. Patients allergic to penicillins may be allergic to carbapenems as well.

■ OTHER CELL WALL OR MEMBRANE-ACTIVE AGENTS

VANCOMYCIN

Vancomycin is an antibiotic produced by *Amycolatopsis orientalis.* With the single exception of flavobacterium, it is active only against gram-positive bacteria, particularly staphylococci. Vancomycin is a glycopeptide of molecular weight 1500. It is water-soluble and quite stable.

Mechanisms of Action & Basis of Resistance

Vancomycin inhibits cell wall synthesis by binding firmly to the D-Ala-D-Ala terminus of nascent peptidoglycan pentapeptide (Figure 43–5). This inhibits the transglycosylase, preventing further elongation of peptidoglycan and cross-linking. The peptidoglycan is thus weakened, and the cell becomes susceptible to lysis. The cell membrane is also damaged, which contributes to the antibacterial effect.

Resistance to vancomycin in enterococci is due to modification of the D-Ala-D-Ala binding site of the peptidoglycan building block in which the terminal D-Ala is replaced by D-lactate. This results in the loss of a critical hydrogen bond that facilitates high-affinity binding of vancomycin to its target and loss of activity. This mechanism is also present in vancomycin-resistant *S aureus* strains (MIC ≥ 32 mcg/mL), which have acquired the enterococcal resistance determinants. The mechanism for reduced vancomycin susceptibility of vancomycin-intermediate strains (MICs = 8–16 mcg/mL) is not known.

Antibacterial Activity

Vancomycin is bactericidal for gram-positive bacteria in concentrations of 0.5–10 mcg/mL. Most pathogenic staphylococci, including those producing β-lactamase and those resistant to nafcillin and methicillin, are killed by 2 mcg/mL or less. Vancomycin kills staphylococci relatively slowly and only if cells are actively dividing; the rate is less than that of the penicillins both in vitro and in vivo. Vancomycin is synergistic in vitro with gentamicin and streptomycin against *Enterococcus faecium* and *Enterococcus faecalis* strains that do not exhibit high levels of aminoglycoside resistance.

Pharmacokinetics

Vancomycin is poorly absorbed from the intestinal tract and is administered orally only for the treatment of antibiotic-associated enterocolitis caused by *C difficile*. Parenteral doses must be administered intravenously. A 1-hour intravenous infusion of 1 g produces blood levels of 15–30 mcg/mL for 1–2 hours. The drug is widely distributed in the body. Cerebrospinal fluid levels 7–30% of simultaneous serum concentrations are achieved if there is meningeal inflammation. Ninety percent of the drug is excreted by glomerular filtration. In the presence of renal insufficiency, striking accumulation may occur (Table 43–2). In functionally anephric patients, the half-life of vancomycin is 6–10 days. The drug is not removed by hemodialysis.

Clinical Uses

The main indication for parenteral vancomycin is sepsis or endocarditis caused by methicillin-resistant staphylococci.

However, vancomycin is not as effective as an antistaphylococcal penicillin for treatment of serious infections such as endocarditis caused by methicillin-susceptible strains. Vancomycin in combination with gentamicin is an alternative regimen for treatment of enterococcal endocarditis in a patient with serious penicillin allergy. Vancomycin (in combination with cefotaxime, ceftriaxone, or rifampin) is also recommended for treatment of meningitis suspected or known to be caused by a highly penicillin-resistant strain of pneumococcus (ie, MIC > 1 mcg/mL). The recommended dosage is 30 mg/kg/d in two or three divided doses. A typical dosing regimen for most infections in adults with normal renal function is 1 g every 12 hours. The dosage in children is 40 mg/kg/d in three or four divided doses. Clearance of vancomycin is directly proportional to creatinine clearance, and the dose is reduced accordingly in patients with renal insufficiency. For functionally anephric adult patients, a 1-g dose administered once a week is usually sufficient. Patients receiving a prolonged course of therapy should have serum concentrations checked. Recommended peak serum concentrations are 20–50 mcg/mL, and trough concentrations are 10–15 mcg/mL.

Oral vancomycin, 0.125–0.25 g every 6 hours, is used to treat antibiotic-associated enterocolitis caused by *C difficile*. However, because of the emergence of vancomycin-resistant enterococci and the strong selective pressure of oral vancomycin for these resistant organisms, metronidazole is strongly preferred as initial therapy and vancomycin should be reserved for treatment of refractory cases.

Adverse Reactions

Adverse reactions are encountered in about 10% of cases. Most reactions are minor. Vancomycin is irritating to tissue, resulting in phlebitis at the site of injection. Chills and fever may occur. Ototoxicity is rare and nephrotoxicity uncommon with current preparations. However, administration with another ototoxic or nephrotoxic drug, such as an aminoglycoside, increases the risk of these toxicities. Ototoxicity can be minimized by maintaining peak serum concentrations below 60 mcg/mL. Among the more common reactions is the so-called "red man" or "red neck" syndrome. This infusion-related flushing is caused by release of histamine. It can be largely prevented by prolonging the infusion period to 1–2 hours or increasing the dosing interval.

TEICOPLANIN

Teicoplanin is a glycopeptide antibiotic that is very similar to vancomycin in mechanism of action and antibacterial spectrum. Unlike vancomycin, it can be given intramuscularly as well as intravenously. Teicoplanin has a long half-life (45–70 hours), permitting once-daily dosing. This drug is available in Europe but has not been approved for use in the United States.

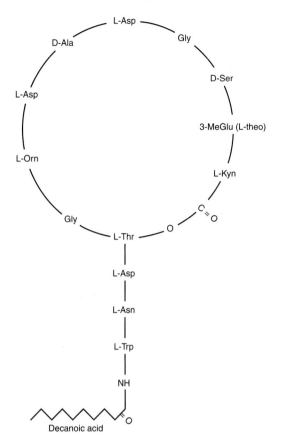

Figure 43–8. Structure of daptomycin.

DAPTOMYCIN

Daptomycin is a cyclic lipopeptide fermentation product of *Streptomyces roseosporus* (Figure 43–8). Its spectrum of activity is similar to that of vancomycin except that it is more rapidly bactericidal in vitro and it is active against vancomycin-resistant strains of enterococci and vancomycin-intermediate and -resistant strains of *S aureus*. The precise mechanism of action is not known, but it appears to bind to and depolarize the cell membrane, causing potassium efflux and rapid cell death. Daptomycin is cleared renally. The recommended doses are 4 mg/kg dose for treatment of skin and soft tissue infections and 6 mg/kg dose for treatment of bacteremia and endocarditis once daily in patients with normal renal function and every other day in patients with creatinine clearance of less than 30 mL/min. In clinical trials powered for noninferiority, daptomycin was equivalent in efficacy to vancomycin. It can cause myopathy, and creatine phosphokinase levels should be monitored. Pulmonary surfactant antagonizes daptomycin and it should not be used to treat pneumonia. Scattered cases of treatment failures have been reported in association with an increase in daptomycin MIC for clinical isolates obtained during therapy. The rela-

tion between an increase in MIC and treatment failure is unclear at this point. Daptomycin is an effective alternative to vancomycin, and its ultimate role continues to unfold.

FOSFOMYCIN

Fosfomycin trometamol, a stable salt of fosfomycin (phosphonomycin), inhibits a very early stage of bacterial cell wall synthesis (Figure 43–5). An analog of phosphoenolpyruvate, it is structurally unrelated to any other antimicrobial agent. It inhibits the cytoplasmic enzyme enolpyruvate transferase by covalently binding to the cysteine residue of the active site and blocking the addition of phosphoenolpyruvate to UDP-*N*-acetylglucosamine. This reaction is the first step in the formation of UDP-*N*-acetylmuramic acid, the precursor of *N*-acetylmuramic acid, which is found only in bacterial cell walls. The drug is transported into the bacterial cell by glycerophosphate or glucose 6-phosphate transport systems. Resistance is due to inadequate transport of drug into the cell.

Fosfomycin is active against both gram-positive and gram-negative organisms at concentrations ≤ 125 mcg/mL. Susceptibility tests should be performed in growth medium supplemented with glucose 6-phosphate to minimize false-positive indications of resistance. In vitro synergism occurs when fosfomycin is combined with β-lactam antibiotics, aminoglycosides, or fluoroquinolones.

Fosfomycin trometamol is available in both oral and parenteral formulations, although only the oral preparation is approved for use in the USA. Oral bioavailability is approximately 40%. Peak serum concentrations are 10 mcg/mL and 30 mcg/mL following a 2-g or 4-g oral dose, respectively. The half-life is approximately 4 hours. The active drug is excreted by the kidney, with urinary concentrations exceeding MICs for most urinary tract pathogens.

Fosfomycin is approved for use as a single 3-g dose for treatment of uncomplicated lower urinary tract infections in women. The drug appears to be safe for use in pregnancy.

BACITRACIN

Bacitracin is a cyclic peptide mixture first obtained from the Tracy strain of *Bacillus subtilis* in 1943. It is active against gram-positive microorganisms. Bacitracin inhibits cell wall formation by interfering with dephosphorylation in cycling of the lipid carrier that transfers peptidoglycan subunits to the growing cell wall (Figure 43–5). There is no cross-resistance between bacitracin and other antimicrobial drugs.

Bacitracin is highly nephrotoxic when administered systemically and is only used topically (Chapter 62). Bacitracin is poorly absorbed. Topical application results in local antibacterial activity without systemic toxicity. Bacitracin, 500 units/g in an ointment base (often combined with polymyxin or neomycin), is indicated for the suppression of mixed bacterial flora in surface lesions of the skin, in wounds, or on mucous membranes. Solutions of bacitracin containing 100–200 units/mL in saline can be used for irrigation of joints, wounds, or the pleural cavity.

CYCLOSERINE

Cycloserine is an antibiotic produced by *Streptomyces orchidaceus*. It is water-soluble and very unstable at acid pH. Cycloserine inhibits many gram-positive and gram-negative organisms, but it is used almost exclusively to treat tuberculosis caused by strains of *Mycobacterium tuberculosis* resistant to first-line agents. Cycloserine is a structural analog of D-alanine and inhibits the incorporation of D-alanine into peptidoglycan pentapeptide by inhibiting alanine racemase, which converts L-alanine to D-alanine, and D-alanyl-D-alanine ligase (Figure 43–5). After ingestion of 0.25 g of cycloserine blood levels reach 20–30 mcg/mL—sufficient to inhibit many strains of mycobacteria and gram-negative bacteria. The drug is widely distributed in tissues. Most of the drug is excreted in active form into the urine. The dosage for treating tuberculosis is 0.5 to 1 g/d in two or three divided doses.

Cycloserine causes serious dose-related central nervous system toxicity with headaches, tremors, acute psychosis, and convulsions. If oral dosages are maintained below 0.75 g/d, such effects can usually be avoided.

PREPARATIONS AVAILABLE

PENICILLINS

Amoxicillin (generic, Amoxil, others)
Oral: 125, 200, 250, 400 mg chewable tablets; 500, 875 mg tablets; 250, 500 mg capsules; powder to reconstitute for 50, 125, 200, 250, 400 mg/mL solution

Amoxicillin/potassium clavulanate (generic, Augmentin)[1]
Oral: 250, 500, 875 mg tablets; 125, 200, 250, 400 mg chewable tablets; 1000 mg extended-release tablet powder to reconstitute for 125, 200, 250 mg/5 mL suspension

Ampicillin (generic)
Oral: 250, 500 mg capsules; powder to reconstitute for 125, 250 mg suspensions
Parenteral: powder to reconstitute for injection (125, 250, 500 mg, 1, 2 g per vial)

Ampicillin/sulbactam sodium (generic, Unasyn)[2]
Parenteral: 1, 2 g ampicillin powder to reconstitute for IV or IM injection

Carbenicillin (Geocillin)
Oral: 382 mg tablets

Dicloxacillin (generic)
Oral: 250, 500 mg capsules

Mezlocillin (Mezlin)
Parenteral: powder to reconstitute for injection (in 1, 2, 3, 4 g vials)

Nafcillin (generic)
Oral: 250 mg capsules
Parenteral: 1, 2 g per IV piggyback units

Oxacillin (generic)
Oral: 250, 500 mg capsules; powder to reconstitute for 250 mg/5 mL solution

Parenteral: powder to reconstitute for injection (0.5, 1, 2, 10 g per vial)

Penicillin G (generic, Pentids, Pfizerpen)
Oral: 0.2, 0.25, 0.4, 0.5, 0.8 million unit tablets; powder to reconstitute 400,000 units/5mL suspension
Parenteral: powder to reconstitute for injection (1, 2, 3, 5, 10, 20 million units)

Penicillin G benzathine (Permapen, Bicillin)
Parenteral: 0.6, 1.2, 2.4 million units per dose

Penicillin G procaine (generic)
Parenteral: 0.6, 1.2 million units/mL for IM injection only

Penicillin V (generic, V-Cillin, Pen-Vee K, others)
Oral: 250, 500 mg tablets; powder to reconstitute for 125, 250 mg/5 mL solution

Piperacillin (Pipracil)
Parenteral: powder to reconstitute for injection (2, 3, 4 g per vial)

Piperacillin and tazobactam sodium (Zosyn)[3]
Parenteral: 2, 3, 4 g powder to reconstitute for IV injection

Ticarcillin (Ticar)
Parenteral: powder to reconstitute for injection (1, 3, 6 g per vial)

Ticarcillin/clavulanate potassium (Timentin)[4]
Parenteral: 3 g powder to reconstitute for injection

CEPHALOSPORINS & OTHER BETA-LACTAM DRUGS

Narrow-Spectrum (First-Generation) Cephalosporins
Cefadroxil (generic, Duricef)
Oral: 500 mg capsules; 1 g tablets; 125, 250, 500 mg/5 mL suspension

(continued)

---

[1]Clavulanate content varies with the formulation; see package insert.
[2]Sulbactam content is half the ampicillin content.

[3]Tazobactam content is 12.5% of the piperacillin content.
[4]Clavulanate content 0.1 g.

Cefazolin (generic, Ancef, Kefzol)
Parenteral: powder to reconstitute for injection (0.25, 0.5, 1 g per vial or IV piggyback unit)
Cephalexin (generic, Keflex, others)
Oral: 250, 500 mg capsules and tablets; 1 g tablets; 125, 250 mg/5 mL suspension
Cephalothin (generic, Keflin)[5]
Parenteral: powder to reconstitute for injection and solution for injection (1 g per vial or infusion pack)
Cephapirin (Cefadyl)
Parenteral: powder to reconstitute for injection (1 g per vial or IV piggyback unit)
Cephradine (generic, Velosef)
Oral: 250, 500 mg capsules; 125, 250 mg/5 mL suspension
Parenteral: powder to reconstitute for injection (0.25, 0.5, 1, 2 g per vial)

Intermediate-Spectrum (Second-Generation) Cephalosporins
Cefaclor (generic, Ceclor)
Oral: 250, 500 mg capsules; 375, 500 mg extended-release tablets; powder to reconstitute for 125, 187, 250, 375 mg/5 mL suspension
Cefamandole (Mandol)
Parenteral: 1, 2 g (in vials) for IM, IV injection
Cefmetazole (Zefazone)
Parenteral: 1, 2 g powder for IV injection
Cefonicid (Monocid)
Parenteral: powder to reconstitute for injection (1, 10 g per vial)
Cefotetan (Cefotan)
Parenteral: powder to reconstitute for injection (1, 2, 10 g per vial)
Cefoxitin (Mefoxin)
Parenteral: powder to reconstitute for injection (1, 2, 10 g per vial)
Cefprozil (Cefzil)
Oral: 250, 500 mg tablets; powder to reconstitute 125, 250 mg/5 mL suspension
Cefuroxime (generic, Ceftin, Kefurox, Zinacef)
Oral: 125, 250, 500 mg tablets; 125, 250 mg/5 mL suspension
Parenteral: powder to reconstitute for injection (0.75, 1.5, 7.5 g per vial or infusion pack)
Loracarbef (Lorabid)
Oral: 200, 400 mg capsules; powder for 100, 200 mg/5 mL suspension

Broad-Spectrum (Third- & Fourth-Generation) Cephalosporins
Cefdinir (Omnicef)
Oral: 300 mg capsules; 125 mg/5 mL suspension

Cefditoren (Spectracef)
Oral: 200 mg tablets
Cefepime (Maxipime)
Parenteral: powder for injection 0.5, 1, 2 g
Cefixime (Suprax)
Oral: 200, 400 mg tablets; powder for oral suspension, 100 mg/5 mL
Cefoperazone (Cefobid)
Parenteral: powder to reconstitute for injection (1, 2 g per vial, 10 g bulk)
Cefotaxime (Claforan)
Parenteral: powder to reconstitute for injection (0.5, 1, 2 g per vial)
Cefpodoxime proxetil (Vantin)
Oral: 100, 200 mg tablets; 50, 100 mg granules for suspension in 5 mL
Ceftazidime (generic, Fortaz, Tazidime)
Parenteral: powder to reconstitute for injection (0.5, 1, 2 g per vial)
Ceftibuten (Cedax)
Oral: 400 mg capsules; 90, 180 mg/5 mL powder for oral suspension
Ceftizoxime (Cefizox)
Parenteral: powder to reconstitute for injection and solution for injection (0.5, 1, 2 g per vial)
Ceftriaxone (Rocephin)
Parenteral: powder to reconstitute for injection (0.25, 0.5, 1, 2, 10 g per vial)

Carbapenems & Monobactam
Aztreonam (Azactam)
Parenteral: powder to reconstitute for injection (0.5, 1, 2 g)
Ertapenem (Invanz)
Parenteral: 1 g powder to reconstitute for intravenous (0.9% NaCl diluent) or intramuscular (1% lidocaine diluent) injection
Imipenem/cilastatin (Primaxin)
Parenteral: powder to reconstitute for injection (250, 500, 750 mg imipenem per vial)
Meropenem (Merrem IV)
Parenteral: powder for injection (0.5, 1 g per vial)

OTHER DRUGS DISCUSSED IN THIS CHAPTER
Cycloserine (Seromycin Pulvules)
Oral: 250 mg capsules
Daptomycin (Cubicin)
Parenteral: 0.25 or 0.5 g lyophilized powder to reconstitute for IV injection
Fosfomycin (Monurol)
Oral: 3 g packet
Vancomycin (generic, Vancocin, Vancoled)
Oral: 125, 250 mg pulvules; powder to reconstitute for 250 mg/5 mL, 500 mg/6 mL solution
Parenteral: 0.5, 1, 5, 10 g powder to reconstitute for IV injection

---

[5]Not available in the USA.

REFERENCES

Balbisi EA: Cefditoren, a new aminothiazolyl cephalosporin. Pharmacology 2002;22:1278.

Carpenter CF, Chambers HF: Daptomycin: Another novel agent for treating infections due to drug-resistant gram-positive pathogens. Clin Infect Dis 2004;38:994.

Centers for Disease Control and Prevention: Vancomycin resistant *Staphylococcus aureus*—Pennsylvania, 2002. JAMA 2002;288:2116.

Chow JW et al: *Enterobacter* bacteremia: Clinical features and emergence of antibiotic resistance during therapy. Ann Intern Med 1991;115:585.

Fowler VG et al: Daptomycin versus standard therapy for bacteremia and endocarditis caused by *Staphylococcus aureus.* N Engl J Med 2006;355:653.

Hiramatsu K et al: Methicillin resistant *Staphylococcus aureus* clinical strain with reduced vancomycin susceptibility. J Antimicrob Chemother 1997;40:135.

Jacoby GA, Munoz-Price LS: The new beta-lactamases. N Engl J Med 2005;352:380.

Keating GM, Perry CM: Ertapenem: A review of its use in the treatment of bacterial infections. Drugs 2005;65:2151.

Park MA, Li JT: Diagnosis and management of penicillin allergy. Mayo Clin Proc 2005;80:405.

Perry CM, Scott LJ: Cefdinir: A review of its use in the management of mild-to-moderate bacterial infections. Drugs 2004; 64:1433.

Wexler HM. In vitro activity of ertapenem: Review of recent studies. J Antimicrob Chemother 2004;53(Suppl 2):ii11.

Tetracyclines, Macrolides, Clindamycin, Chloramphenicol, & Streptogramins

44

Henry F. Chambers, MD

The drugs described in this chapter inhibit bacterial protein synthesis by binding to and interfering with ribosomes.

■ TETRACYCLINES

All of the tetracyclines have the basic structure shown below:

Tigecycline

	R_7	R_6	R_5	Renal Clearance (mL/min)
Chlortetracycline	— Cl	— CH_3	— H	35
Oxytetracycline	— H	— CH_3	— OH	90
Tetracycline	— H	— CH3	— H	65
Demeclocycline	— Cl	— H	— H	35
Methacycline	— H	$= CH_2$*	— OH	31
Doxycycline	— H	— CH_3*	— OH	16
Minocycline	— $N(CH_3)_2$	— H	— H	10

*There is no — OH at position 6 on methacycline and doxycycline.

Free tetracyclines are crystalline amphoteric substances of low solubility. They are available as hydrochlorides, which are more soluble. Such solutions are acid and, with the exception of chlortetracycline, fairly stable. Tetracyclines chelate divalent metal ions, which can interfere with their absorption and activity. A newly approved tetracycline analog, tigecycline, is a glycylcycline and a semisynthetic derivative of minocycline.

Antimicrobial Activity

Tetracyclines are broad-spectrum bacteriostatic antibiotics that inhibit protein synthesis. They are active against many gram-positive and gram-negative bacteria, including anaerobes, rickettsiae, chlamydiae, mycoplasmas, and L forms; and against some protozoa, eg, amebas. The antibacterial activities of most tetracyclines are similar except that tetracycline-resistant strains may be susceptible to doxycycline, minocycline, and tigecycline, all of which are poor substrates for the efflux pump that mediates resistance. Differences in clinical efficacy for susceptible organisms are minor and attributable largely to features of absorption, distribution, and excretion of individual drugs.

Tetracyclines enter microorganisms in part by passive diffusion and in part by an energy-dependent process of active transport. Susceptible cells concentrate the drug intracellularly. Once inside the cell, tetracyclines bind reversibly to the 30S subunit of the bacterial ribosome, blocking the binding of aminoacyl-tRNA to the acceptor site on the mRNA-ribosome complex (Figure 44–1). This prevents addition of amino acids to the growing peptide.

Resistance

Three mechanisms of resistance to tetracycline analogs have been described: (1) impaired influx or increased efflux by an active transport protein pump; (2) ribosome

Figure 44–1. Steps in bacterial protein synthesis and targets of several antibiotics. Amino acids are shown as numbered circles. The 70S ribosomal mRNA complex is shown with its 50S and 30S subunits. In step 1, the charged tRNA unit carrying amino acid 8 binds to the acceptor site A on the 70S ribosome. The peptidyl tRNA at the donor site, with amino acids 1 through 7, then binds the growing amino acid chain to amino acid 8 (transpeptidation, step 2). The uncharged tRNA left at the donor site is released (step 3), and the new 8-amino acid chain with its tRNA shifts to the peptidyl site (translocation, step 4). The antibiotic binding sites are shown schematically as triangles. Chloramphenicol (C) and macrolides (M) bind to the 50S subunit and block transpeptidation (step 2). The tetracyclines (T) bind to the 30S subunit and prevent binding of the incoming charged tRNA unit (step 1).

protection due to production of proteins that interfere with tetracycline binding to the ribosome; and (3) enzymatic inactivation. The most important of these are production of an efflux pump and ribosomal protection. Tet(AE) efflux pump-expressing gram-negative species are resistant to the older tetracyclines, doxycycline, and minocycline. They are susceptible, however, to tigecycline, which is not a substrate of these pumps. Similarly, the Tet(K) efflux pump of staphylococci confers resistance to tetracyclines, but not to doxycycline, minocycline, or tigecycline, none of which are pump substrates. The Tet(M) ribosomal protection protein expressed by gram-positives produces resistance to the tetracyclines, doxycycline, and minocycline, but not to tigecycline, which because of its bulky *t*-butylglycylamido substituent has a steric hindrance effect on Tet(M) binding to the ribosome. Tigecycline is a substrate of the chromosomally encoded multidrug efflux pumps of *Proteus* sp, and

Pseudomonas aeruginosa, accounting for their intrinsic resistance to all tetracyclines including tigecycline.

Pharmacokinetics

Tetracyclines mainly differ in their absorption after oral administration and their elimination. Absorption after oral administration is approximately 30% for chlortetracycline; 60–70% for tetracycline, oxytetracycline, demeclocycline, and methacycline; and 95–100% for doxycycline and minocycline. Tigecycline is poorly absorbed orally and must be administered intravenously. A portion of an orally administered dose of tetracycline remains in the gut lumen, modifies intestinal flora, and is excreted in the feces. Absorption occurs mainly in the upper small intestine and is impaired by food (except doxycycline and minocycline); by divalent cations (Ca^{2+}, Mg^{2+}, Fe^{2+}) or Al^{3+}; by dairy products and antacids, which contain multivalent cations; and by alkaline pH. Specially buffered tetracycline solutions are formulated for intravenous administration.

Tetracyclines are 40–80% bound by serum proteins. Oral dosages of 500 mg every 6 hours of tetracycline hydrochloride or oxytetracycline produce peak blood levels of 4–6 mcg/mL. Intravenously injected tetracyclines give somewhat higher levels, but only temporarily. Peak levels of 2–4 mcg/mL are achieved with a 200-mg dose of doxycycline or minocycline. Steady-state peak serum concentrations of tigecycline are 0.6 mcg/mL at the usual dosage. Tetracyclines are distributed widely to tissues and body fluids except for cerebrospinal fluid, where concentrations are 10–25% of those in serum. Minocycline reaches very high concentrations in tears and saliva, which makes it useful for eradication of the meningococcal carrier state. Tetracyclines cross the placenta to reach the fetus and are also excreted in milk. As a result of chelation with calcium, tetracyclines are bound to—and damage—growing bones and teeth. Carbamazepine, phenytoin, barbiturates, and chronic alcohol ingestion may shorten the half-life of doxycycline 50% by induction of hepatic enzymes that metabolize the drug.

Tetracyclines are excreted mainly in bile and urine. Concentrations in bile exceed those in serum tenfold. Some of the drug excreted in bile is reabsorbed from the intestine (enterohepatic circulation) and may contribute to maintenance of serum levels. Ten to 50 percent of various tetracyclines is excreted into the urine, mainly by glomerular filtration. Ten to 40 percent of the drug is excreted in feces. Doxycycline and tigecycline, in contrast to other tetracyclines, are eliminated by nonrenal mechanisms, do not accumulate significantly and require no dosage adjustment in renal failure.

Tetracyclines are classified as short-acting (chlortetracycline, tetracycline, oxytetracycline), intermediate-acting (demeclocycline and methacycline), or long-acting (doxycycline and minocycline) based on serum half-lives of 6–8 hours, 12 hours, and 16–18 hours, respectively. Tigecycline has a half-life of 36 hours. The almost complete absorption and slow excretion of doxycycline and minocycline allow for once-daily dosing.

Clinical Uses

A tetracycline is the drug of choice in infections with *Mycoplasma pneumoniae,* chlamydiae, rickettsiae, and some spirochetes. They are used in combination regimens to treat gastric and duodenal ulcer disease caused by *Helicobacter pylori.* They may be used in various gram-positive and gram-negative bacterial infections, including vibrio infections, provided the organism is not resistant. In cholera, tetracyclines rapidly stop the shedding of vibrios, but tetracycline resistance has appeared during epidemics. Tetracyclines remain effective in most chlamydial infections, including sexually transmitted diseases. Tetracyclines are no longer recommended for treatment of gonococcal disease because of resistance. A tetracycline—usually in combination with an aminoglycoside—is indicated for plague, tularemia, and brucellosis. Tetracyclines are sometimes used in the treatment of protozoal infections, eg, those due to *Entamoeba histolytica* or *Plasmodium falciparum* (see Chapter 53). Other uses include treatment of acne, exacerbations of bronchitis, community-acquired pneumonia, Lyme disease, relapsing fever, leptospirosis, and some nontuberculous mycobacterial infections (eg, *Mycobacterium marinum*). Tetracyclines formerly were used for a variety of common infections, including bacterial gastroenteritis, pneumonia (other than mycoplasmal or chlamydial pneumonia), and urinary tract infections. However, many strains of bacteria causing these infections now are resistant, and other agents have largely supplanted tetracyclines.

Minocycline, 200 mg orally daily for 5 days, can eradicate the meningococcal carrier state, but because of side effects and resistance of many meningococcal strains, rifampin is preferred. Demeclocycline inhibits the action of ADH in the renal tubule and has been used in the treatment of inappropriate secretion of ADH or similar peptides by certain tumors (see Chapter 15).

Tigecycline, the first glycylcycline to reach the clinic, has several unique features that warrant its consideration apart from the older tetracyclines. Many tetracycline-resistant strains are susceptible to tigecycline because the common resistance determinants have no activity against it. Its spectrum is very broad. Coagulase-negative staphylococci and *Staphylococcus aureus*, including methicillin-resistant, vancomycin-intermediate, and vancomycin-resistant strains; streptococci, penicillin-susceptible and -resistant; enterococci, including vancomycin-resistant strains; gram-positive rods; Enterobacteriaceae; multidrug-resistant strains of *Acinetobacter* sp; anaerobes, both gram-positive and gram-negative; atypical agents, rickettsiae, chlamydia, and legionella; and rapidly growing mycobacteria all are susceptible. *Proteus* and *P aeruginosa*, however, are intrinsically resistant.

Tigecycline, formulated for intravenous administration only, is given as a 100-mg loading dose; then 50 mg every 12 hours. As with all tetracyclines, tissue and intracellular penetration is excellent; consequently, the volume of distribution is quite large and peak serum concentrations are somewhat blunted. Elimination is primarily biliary, and no dosage adjustment is needed for patients with renal insufficiency. In addition to the tetracycline class effects, the chief adverse effect of tigecycline is nausea, which occurs in up to one third of patients, and occasionally vomiting. Neither nausea nor vomiting usually requires discontinuation of the drug.

Tigecycline is FDA-approved for treatment of skin and skin-structure infection and intraabdominal infections. Because active drug concentrations in the urine are relatively low, tigecycline may not be effective for urinary tract infections and has no indication for this use. Because it is active against a wide variety of multidrug-resistant nosocomial pathogens (eg, methicillin-resistant *S aureus*, extended-spectrum β-lactamase-producing gram-negatives, and acinetobacter sp.), tigecycline is a welcome addition to the antimicrobial drug group.

A. ORAL DOSAGE

The oral dosage for rapidly excreted tetracyclines, equivalent to tetracycline hydrochloride, is 0.25–0.5 g four times daily for adults and 20–40 mg/kg/d for children (8 years of age and older). For severe systemic infections, the higher dosage is indicated, at least for the first few days. The daily dose is 600 mg for demeclocycline or methacycline, 100 mg once or twice daily for doxycycline, and 100 mg twice daily for minocycline. Doxycycline is the oral tetracycline of choice because it can be given as a once-daily dose and its absorption is not significantly affected by food. All tetracyclines chelate with metals, and none should be orally administered with milk, antacids, or ferrous sulfate. To avoid deposition in growing bones or teeth, tetracyclines should be avoided in pregnant women and children under 8 years of age.

B. PARENTERAL DOSAGE

Several tetracyclines are available for intravenous injection in doses of 0.1–0.5 g every 6–12 hours (similar to oral doses) but doxycycline is the usual preferred agent, at a dosage of 100 mg every 12–24 hours. Intramuscular injection is not recommended because of pain and inflammation at the injection site.

Adverse Reactions

Hypersensitivity reactions (drug fever, skin rashes) to tetracyclines are uncommon. Most adverse effects are due to direct toxicity of the drug or to alteration of microbial flora.

A. GASTROINTESTINAL ADVERSE EFFECTS

Nausea, vomiting, and diarrhea are the most common reasons for discontinuing tetracycline medication. These effects are attributable to direct local irritation of the intestinal tract. Nausea, anorexia, and diarrhea can usually be controlled by administering the drug with food or carboxymethylcellulose, reducing drug dosage, or discontinuing the drug.

Tetracyclines modify the normal flora, with suppression of susceptible coliform organisms and overgrowth of pseudomonas, proteus, staphylococci, resistant coliforms, clostridia, and candida. This can result in intestinal functional disturbances, anal pruritus, vaginal or oral candidiasis, or enterocolitis with shock and death.

B. BONY STRUCTURES AND TEETH

Tetracyclines are readily bound to calcium deposited in newly formed bone or teeth in young children. When a tetracycline is given during pregnancy, it can be deposited in the fetal teeth, leading to fluorescence, discoloration, and enamel dysplasia; it can also be deposited in bone, where it may cause deformity or growth inhibition. If the drug is given for long periods to children under 8 years of age, similar changes can result.

C. LIVER TOXICITY

Tetracyclines can probably impair hepatic function, especially during pregnancy, in patients with preexisting hepatic insufficiency and when high doses are given intravenously. Hepatic necrosis has been reported with daily doses of 4 g or more intravenously.

D. KIDNEY TOXICITY

Renal tubular acidosis and other renal injury resulting in nitrogen retention have been attributed to the administration of outdated tetracycline preparations. Tetracyclines given along with diuretics may produce nitrogen retention. Tetracyclines other than doxycycline may accumulate to toxic levels in patients with impaired kidney function.

E. LOCAL TISSUE TOXICITY

Intravenous injection can lead to venous thrombosis. Intramuscular injection produces painful local irritation and should be avoided.

F. PHOTOSENSITIZATION

Systemically administered tetracycline, especially demeclocycline, can induce sensitivity to sunlight or ultraviolet light, particularly in fair-skinned persons.

G. VESTIBULAR REACTIONS

Dizziness, vertigo, nausea, and vomiting have been noted particularly with doxycycline at doses above 100 mg. With dosages of 200–400 mg/d of minocycline, 35–70% of patients will have these reactions.

■ MACROLIDES

The macrolides are a group of closely related compounds characterized by a macrocyclic lactone ring (usually containing 14 or 16 atoms) to which deoxy sugars are attached. The prototype drug, erythromycin, which consists of two sugar moieties attached to a 14-atom lactone ring, was obtained in 1952 from *Streptomyces erythreus*. Clarithromycin and azithromycin are semisynthetic derivatives of erythromycin.

Erythromycin ($R_1 = CH_3$, $R_2 = H$)
Clarithromycin (R_1, $R_2 = CH_3$)

ERYTHROMYCIN

Chemistry

The general structure of erythromycin is shown above with the macrolide ring and the sugars desosamine and cladinose. It is poorly soluble in water (0.1%) but dissolves readily in organic solvents. Solutions are fairly stable at 4 °C but lose activity rapidly at 20 °C and at acid pH. Erythromycins are usually dispensed as various esters and salts.

Antimicrobial Activity

Erythromycin is effective against gram-positive organisms, especially pneumococci, streptococci, staphylococci, and corynebacteria, in plasma concentrations of 0.02–2 mcg/mL. Mycoplasma, legionella, *Chlamydia trachomatis, C psittaci, C pneumoniae,* helicobacter, listeria, and certain mycobacteria *(Mycobacterium kansasii, M scrofulaceum)* are also susceptible. Gram-negative organisms such as *Neisseria* sp, *Bordetella pertussis, Bartonella henselae,* and *B quintana* (etiologic agents of cat-scratch disease and bacillary angiomatosis), some rickettsia sp, *Treponema pallidum,* and campylobacter sp are susceptible. *Haemophilus influenzae* is somewhat less susceptible.

The antibacterial action of erythromycin may be inhibitory or bactericidal, particularly at higher concentrations, for susceptible organisms. Activity is enhanced at alkaline pH. Inhibition of protein synthesis occurs via binding to the 50S ribosomal RNA, which blocks the aminoacyl translocation reaction and formation of initiation complexes (Figure 44–1).

Resistance

Resistance to erythromycin is usually plasmid-encoded. Three mechanisms have been identified: (1) reduced permeability of the cell membrane or active efflux; (2) production (by Enterobacteriaceae) of esterases that hydrolyze macrolides; and (3) modification of the ribosomal binding site (so-called ribosomal protection) by chromosomal mutation or by a macrolide-inducible or constitutive methylase. Efflux and methylase production are by far the most important resistance mechanisms in gram-positive organisms. Cross-resistance is complete between erythromycin and the other macrolides. Constitutive methylase production also confers resistance to structurally unrelated but mechanistically similar compounds such as clindamycin and streptogramin B (so-called macrolide-lincosamide-streptogramin, or MLS-type B, resistance), which share the same ribosomal binding site. Because nonmacrolides are poor inducers of the methylase, strains expressing an inducible methylase will appear susceptible in vitro. However, constitutive mutants that are resistant can be selected out and emerge during therapy with clindamycin.

Pharmacokinetics

Erythromycin base is destroyed by stomach acid and must be administered with enteric coating. Food interferes with absorption. Stearates and esters are fairly acid-resistant and somewhat better absorbed. The lauryl salt of the propionyl ester of erythromycin (erythromycin estolate) is the best-absorbed oral preparation. Oral dosage of 2 g/d results in serum erythromycin base and ester concentrations of approximately 2 mcg/mL. However, only the base is microbiologically active, and its concentration tends to be similar regardless of the formulation. A 500-mg intravenous dose of erythromycin lactobionate produces serum concentrations of 10 mcg/mL 1 hour after dosing. The serum half-life is approximately 1.5 hours normally and 5 hours in patients with anuria. Adjustment for renal failure is not necessary.

Erythromycin is not removed by dialysis. Large amounts of an administered dose are excreted in the bile and lost in feces, and only 5% is excreted in the urine. Absorbed drug is distributed widely except to the brain and cerebrospinal fluid. Erythromycin is taken up by polymorphonuclear leukocytes and macrophages. It traverses the placenta and reaches the fetus.

Clinical Uses

An erythromycin is a drug of choice in corynebacterial infections (diphtheria, corynebacterial sepsis, erythrasma); in respiratory, neonatal, ocular, or genital chlamydial infections; and in treatment of community-acquired pneumonia because its spectrum of activity includes pneumococcus, mycoplasma, and legionella. Erythromycin is also useful as a penicillin substitute in penicillin-allergic individuals with infections caused by staphylococci (assuming that the isolate is susceptible), streptococci, or pneumococci. Emergence of erythromycin resistance in strains of group A streptococci and pneumococci (penicillin-resistant pneumococci in particular) has made macrolides less attractive as first-line agents for treatment of pharyngitis, skin and soft tissue infections, and pneumonia. Erythromycin has been recommended as prophylaxis against endocarditis during dental procedures in individuals with valvular heart disease, although clindamycin, which is better tolerated, has largely replaced it. Although erythromycin estolate is the best-absorbed salt, it imposes the greatest risk of adverse reactions. Therefore, the stearate or succinate salt may be preferred.

The oral dosage of erythromycin base, stearate, or estolate is 0.25–0.5 g every 6 hours (for children, 40 mg/kg/d). The dosage of erythromycin ethylsuccinate is 0.4–0.6 g every 6 hours. Oral erythromycin base (1 g) is sometimes combined with oral neomycin or kanamycin for preoperative preparation of the colon. The intravenous dosage of erythromycin gluceptate or lactobionate is 0.5–1.0 g every 6 hours for adults and 20–40 mg/kg/d for children. The higher dosage is recommended when treating pneumonia caused by *Legionella* sp.

Adverse Reactions

A. GASTROINTESTINAL EFFECTS

Anorexia, nausea, vomiting, and diarrhea occasionally accompany oral administration. Gastrointestinal intolerance, which is due to a direct stimulation of gut motility, is the most common reason for discontinuing erythromycin and substituting another antibiotic.

B. LIVER TOXICITY

Erythromycins, particularly the estolate, can produce acute cholestatic hepatitis (fever, jaundice, impaired liver function), probably as a hypersensitivity reaction. Most patients recover from this, but hepatitis recurs if the drug is readministered. Other allergic reactions include fever, eosinophilia, and rashes.

C. DRUG INTERACTIONS

Erythromycin metabolites can inhibit cytochrome P450 enzymes and thus increase the serum concentrations of numerous drugs, including theophylline, oral anticoagulants, cyclosporine, and methylprednisolone. Erythromycin increases serum concentrations of oral digoxin by increasing its bioavailability.

CLARITHROMYCIN

Clarithromycin is derived from erythromycin by addition of a methyl group and has improved acid stability and oral absorption compared with erythromycin. Its mechanism of action is the same as that of erythromycin. Clarithromycin and erythromycin are virtually identical with respect to antibacterial activity except that clarithromycin is more active against *Mycobacterium avium* complex (see Chapter 47). Clarithromycin also has activity against *M leprae* and *Toxoplasma gondii*. Erythromycin-resistant streptococci and staphylococci are also resistant to clarithromycin.

A 500-mg dose of clarithromycin produces serum concentrations of 2–3 mcg/mL. The longer half-life of clarithromycin (6 hours) compared with erythromycin permits twice-daily dosing. The recommended dosage is 250–500 mg twice daily or 1000 mg of the extended release formulation once daily. Clarithromycin penetrates most tissues well, with concentrations equal to or exceeding serum concentrations.

Clarithromycin is metabolized in the liver. The major metabolite is 14-hydroxyclarithromycin, which also has antibacterial activity. A portion of active drug and this major metabolite is eliminated in the urine, and dosage reduction (eg, a 500-mg loading dose, then 250 mg once or twice daily) is recommended for patients with creatinine clearances less than 30 mL/min. Clarithromycin has drug interactions similar to those described for erythromycin.

The advantages of clarithromycin compared with erythromycin are lower incidence of gastrointestinal intolerance and less frequent dosing. Except for the specific organisms noted above, the two drugs are otherwise therapeutically very similar, and the choice of one over the other usually turns out to be cost and tolerability.

AZITHROMYCIN

Azithromycin, a 15-atom lactone macrolide ring compound, is derived from erythromycin by addition of a methylated nitrogen into the lactone ring. Its spectrum of activity and clinical uses are virtually identical to those of clarithromycin. Azithromycin is active against *M avium* complex and *T gondii*. Azithromycin is slightly less active than erythromycin and clarithromycin against staphylococci and streptococci and slightly more active against *H influenzae*. Azithromycin is highly active against chlamydia.

Azithromycin differs from erythromycin and clarithromycin mainly in pharmacokinetic properties. A 500-mg dose of azithromycin produces relatively low serum concentrations of approximately 0.4 mcg/mL. However, azithromycin penetrates into most tissues (except cerebrospinal fluid) and phagocytic cells extremely well, with tissue concentrations exceeding serum concentrations by 10- to 100-fold. The drug is slowly released from tissues (tissue half-life of 2–4 days) to produce an elimination half-life approaching 3 days. These unique properties permit once-daily dosing and shortening of the duration of treatment in many cases. For example, a single 1-g dose of azithromycin is as effective as a 7-day course of doxycycline for chlamydial cervicitis and urethritis. Community-acquired pneumonia can be treated with azithromycin given as a 500-mg loading dose, followed by a 250-mg single daily dose for the next 4 days.

Azithromycin is rapidly absorbed and well tolerated orally. It should be administered 1 hour before or 2 hours after meals. Aluminum and magnesium antacids do not alter bioavailability but delay absorption and reduce peak serum concentrations. Because it has a 15-member (not 14-member) lactone ring, azithromycin does not inactivate cytochrome P450 enzymes and therefore is free of the drug interactions that occur with erythromycin and clarithromycin.

KETOLIDES

Ketolides are semisynthetic 14-membered-ring macrolides, differing from erythromycin by substitution of a 3-keto group for the neutral sugar l-cladinose. **Telithromycin** is approved for clinical use. It is active in vitro against *Streptococcus pyogenes, S pneumoniae, S aureus, H influenzae, Moraxella catarrhalis,* mycoplasmas, *Legionella* sp, *chlamydia* sp, *H pylori, N gonorrhoeae, B fragilis, T gondii,* and nontuberculosis mycobacteria. Many macrolide-resistant strains are susceptible to ketolides because the structural modification of these compounds renders them poor substrates for efflux pump-mediated resistance and they bind to ribosomes of some bacterial species with higher affinity than macrolides.

Oral bioavailability of telithromycin is 57%, and tissue and intracellular penetration is generally good. Telithromycin is metabolized in the liver and eliminated by a combination of biliary and urinary routes of excretion. It is administered as a once-daily dose of 800 mg, which results in peak serum concentrations of approximately 2 mcg/mL. Telithromycin is indicated for treatment of respiratory tract infections, including community-acquired bacterial pneumonia, acute exacerbations of chronic bronchitis, sinusitis, and streptococcal pharyngitis. It is a reversible inhibitor of the CYP3A4 enzyme system and may slightly prolong the QT_c interval. Rare cases of hepatitis and liver failure have been reported.

■ CLINDAMYCIN

Clindamycin is a chlorine-substituted derivative of **lincomycin,** an antibiotic that is elaborated by *Streptomyces lincolnensis.*

Clindamycin

Antibacterial Activity

Streptococci, staphylococci, and pneumococci are inhibited by clindamycin, 0.5–5 mcg/mL. Enterococci and gram-negative aerobic organisms are resistant (in contrast to their susceptibility to erythromycin). Bacteroides sp and other anaerobes, both gram-positive and gram-negative, are usually susceptible. Clindamycin, like erythromycin, inhibits protein synthesis by interfering with the formation of initiation complexes and with aminoacyl translocation reactions. The binding site for clindamycin on the 50S subunit of the bacterial ribosome is identical with that for erythromycin. Resistance to clindamycin, which generally confers cross-resistance to macrolides, is due to (1) mutation of the ribosomal receptor site; (2) modification of the receptor by a constitutively expressed methylase (see section on erythromycin resistance, above); and (3) enzymatic inactivation of clindamycin. Gram-negative aerobic species are intrinsically resistant because of poor permeability of the outer membrane.

Pharmacokinetics

Oral dosages of clindamycin, 0.15–0.3 g every 8 hours (10–20 mg/kg/d for children), yield serum levels of 2–3 mcg/mL. When administered intravenously, 600 mg of clindamycin every 8 hours gives levels of 5–15 mcg/mL. The drug is about 90% protein-bound. Clindamycin penetrates well into most tissues, with brain and cerebrospinal fluid being important exceptions. It penetrates well into abscesses and is actively taken up and concentrated by phagocytic cells. Clindamycin is metabolized by the liver, and both active drug and active metabolites are excreted in bile and urine. The half-life is about 2.5 hours in normal individuals, increasing to 6 hours in patients with anuria. No dosage adjustment is required for renal failure.

Clinical Uses

Clindamycin is indicated for treatment of anaerobic infection caused by bacteroides and other anaerobes that often participate in mixed infections. Clindamycin, sometimes in combination with an aminoglycoside or cephalosporin, is used to treat penetrating wounds of the abdomen and the gut; infections originating in the female genital tract, eg, septic abortion and pelvic abscesses; and aspiration pneumonia. Clindamycin is now recommended rather than erythromycin for prophylaxis of endocarditis in patients with valvular heart disease who are undergoing certain dental procedures. Clindamycin plus primaquine is an effective alternative to trimethoprim-sulfamethoxazole for moderate to moderately severe *Pneumocystis jiroveci* pneumonia in AIDS patients. It is also used in combination with pyrimethamine for AIDS-related toxoplasmosis of the brain.

Adverse Effects

Common adverse effects are diarrhea, nausea, and skin rashes. Impaired liver function (with or without jaundice) and neutropenia sometimes occur. Severe diarrhea and enterocolitis have followed clindamycin administration. Administration of clindamycin is a risk factor for diarrhea and colitis due to *Clostridium difficile.*

■ CHLORAMPHENICOL

Crystalline chloramphenicol is a neutral, stable compound with the following structure:

Chloramphenicol

It is soluble in alcohol but poorly soluble in water. Chloramphenicol succinate, which is used for parenteral administration, is highly water-soluble. It is hydrolyzed in vivo with liberation of free chloramphenicol.

Antimicrobial Activity

Chloramphenicol is a potent inhibitor of microbial protein synthesis. It binds reversibly to the 50S subunit of the bacterial ribosome (Figure 44–1) and inhibits the peptidyl transferase step of protein synthesis. Chloramphenicol is a bacteriostatic broad-spectrum antibiotic that is active against both aerobic and anaerobic gram-positive and gram-negative organisms. It is active also against rickettsiae but not chlamydiae. Most gram-positive bacteria are inhibited at concentrations of 1–10 mcg/mL, and many gram-negative bacteria are inhibited by concentrations of 0.2–5 mcg/mL. *H influenzae, N meningitidis,* and some strains of bacteroides are highly susceptible, and for them chloramphenicol may be bactericidal.

Low-level resistance to chloramphenicol may emerge from large populations of chloramphenicol-susceptible cells by selection of mutants that are less permeable to the drug. Clinically significant resistance is due to production of chloramphenicol acetyltransferase, a plasmid-encoded enzyme that inactivates the drug.

Pharmacokinetics

The usual dosage of chloramphenicol is 50–100 mg/kg/d. After oral administration, crystalline chloramphenicol is rapidly and completely absorbed. A 1-g oral dose produces blood levels between 10 and 15 mcg/mL. Chloramphenicol palmitate is a prodrug that is hydrolyzed in the intestine to yield free chloramphenicol. The parenteral formulation is a prodrug, chloramphenicol succinate, which hydrolyzes to yield free chloramphenicol, giving blood levels somewhat lower than those achieved with orally administered drug. Chloramphenicol is widely distributed to virtually all tissues and body fluids, including the central nervous system and cerebrospinal fluid, such that the concentration of chloramphenicol in brain tissue may be equal to that in serum. The drug penetrates cell membranes readily.

Most of the drug is inactivated either by conjugation with glucuronic acid (principally in the liver) or by reduction to inactive aryl amines. Active chloramphenicol (about 10% of the total dose administered) and its inactive degradation products (about 90% of the total) are eliminated in the urine. A small amount of active drug is excreted into bile and feces. The systemic dosage of chloramphenicol need not be altered in renal insufficiency, but it must be reduced markedly in hepatic failure. Newborns less than a week old and premature infants also clear chloramphenicol less well, and the dosage should be reduced to 25 mg/kg/d.

Clinical Uses

Because of potential toxicity, bacterial resistance, and the availability of many other effective alternatives, chloramphenicol is rarely used. It may be considered for treatment of serious rickettsial infections such as typhus and Rocky Mountain spotted fever. It is an alternative to a β-lactam antibiotic for treatment of meningococcal meningitis occurring in patients who have major hypersensitivity reactions to penicillin or bacterial meningitis caused by penicillin-resistant strains of pneumococci. The dosage is 50–100 mg/kg/d in four divided doses.

Chloramphenicol is used topically in the treatment of eye infections because of its broad spectrum and its penetration of ocular tissues and the aqueous humor. It is ineffective for chlamydial infections.

Adverse Reactions

A. GASTROINTESTINAL DISTURBANCES

Adults occasionally develop nausea, vomiting, and diarrhea. This is rare in children. Oral or vaginal candidiasis may occur as a result of alteration of normal microbial flora.

B. BONE MARROW DISTURBANCES

Chloramphenicol commonly causes a dose-related reversible suppression of red cell production at dosages exceeding 50 mg/kg/d after 1–2 weeks. Aplastic anemia, a rare consequence (1 in 24,000 to 40,000 courses of therapy) of chloramphenicol administration by any route, is an idiosyncratic reaction unrelated to dose, although it occurs more frequently with prolonged use. It tends to be irreversible and can be fatal.

C. TOXICITY FOR NEWBORN INFANTS

Newborn infants lack an effective glucuronic acid conjugation mechanism for the degradation and detoxification of chloramphenicol. Consequently, when infants are given dosages above 50 mg/kg/d, the drug may accumulate, resulting in the **gray baby syndrome,** with vomiting, flaccidity, hypothermia, gray color, shock, and collapse. To avoid this toxic effect, chloramphenicol should be used with caution in infants and the dosage limited to 50 mg/kg/d or less (during the first week of life) in full-term infants more than 1 week old and 25 mg/kg/d in premature infants.

D. INTERACTION WITH OTHER DRUGS

Chloramphenicol inhibits hepatic microsomal enzymes that metabolize several drugs. Half-lives are prolonged, and the serum concentrations of phenytoin, tolbutamide, chlorpropamide, and warfarin are increased. Like other bacteriostatic inhibitors of microbial protein synthesis, chloramphenicol can antagonize bactericidal drugs such as penicillins or aminoglycosides.

STREPTOGRAMINS

Quinupristin-dalfopristin is a combination of two streptogramins—quinupristin, a streptogramin B, and dalfopristin, a streptogramin A—in a 30:70 ratio. It is rapidly bactericidal for most organisms except *Enterococcus faecium,* which is killed slowly. Quinupristin-dalfopristin is active against gram-positive cocci, including multidrug-resistant strains of streptococci, penicillin-resistant strains of *S pneumoniae,* methicillin-susceptible and -resistant strains of staphylococci, and *E faecium* (but not *E faecalis*). Resistance is due to modification of the quinupristin binding site (MLS-B type), enzymatic inactivation of dalfopristin, or efflux.

Quinupristin-dalfopristin is administered intravenously at a dosage of 7.5 mg/kg every 8–12 hours. Peak serum concentrations following an infusion of 7.5 mg/kg over 60 minutes are 3 mcg/mL for quinupristin and 7 mcg/mL for dalfopristin. Quinupristin and dalfopristin are rapidly metabolized, with half-lives of 0.85 and 0.7 hours, respectively. Elimination is principally by the fecal route. Dose adjustment is not necessary for renal failure, peritoneal dialysis, or hemodialysis. Patients with hepatic insufficiency may not tolerate the drug at usual doses, however, because of increased area under the concentration curve of both parent drugs and metabolites. This may necessitate a dose reduction to 7.5 mg/kg every 12 hours or 5 mg/kg every 8 hours. Quinupristin and dalfopristin significantly inhibit CYP3A4, which metabolizes warfarin, diazepam, astemizole, terfenadine, cisapride, nonnucleoside reverse transcriptase inhibitors, and cyclosporine, among others. Dosage reduction of cyclosporine may be necessary.

Quinupristin-dalfopristin is approved for treatment of infections caused by staphylococci or by vancomycin-resistant strains of *E faecium,* but not *E faecalis,* which is intrinsically resistant probably because of an efflux-type resistance mechanism. The principal toxicities are infusion-related events, such as pain at the infusion site, and an arthralgia-myalgia syndrome.

OXAZOLIDINONES

Linezolid is a member of the oxazolidinones, a new class of synthetic antimicrobials. It is active against gram-positive organisms including staphylococci, streptococci, enterococci, gram-positive anaerobic cocci, and gram-positive rods such as corynebacteria and *Listeria monocytogenes.* It is primarily a bacteriostatic agent except for streptococci, for which it is bactericidal. It is active in vitro against *Mycobacterium tuberculosis.*

Linezolid inhibits protein synthesis by preventing formation of the ribosome complex that initiates protein synthesis. Its unique binding site, located on 23S ribosomal RNA of the 50S subunit, results in no cross-resistance with other drug classes. Resistance is caused by mutation of the linezolid binding site on 23S ribosomal RNA.

The principal toxicity of linezolid is hematologic—reversible and generally mild. Thrombocytopenia is the most common manifestation (seen in approximately 3% of treatment courses), particularly when the drug is administered for longer than 2 weeks. Neutropenia may also occur, most commonly in patients with a predisposition to or underlying bone marrow suppression. Linezolid is 100% bioavailable after oral administration and has a half-life of 4–6 hours. It is metabolized by oxidative metabolism, yielding two inactive metabolites. It is neither an inducer nor an inhibitor of cytochrome P450 enzymes. Peak serum concentrations average 18 mcg/mL following a 600-mg oral dose. The recommended dosage for most indications is 600 mg twice daily, either orally or intravenously. Linezolid is approved for vancomycin-resistant *E faecium* infections; nosocomial pneumonia; community-acquired pneumonia; and skin infections, complicated or uncomplicated. It should be reserved for treatment of infections caused by multidrug-resistant gram-positive bacteria.

PREPARATIONS AVAILABLE

CHLORAMPHENICOL

Chloramphenicol (generic, Chloromycetin)
Oral: 250 mg capsules
Parenteral: 100 mg powder to reconstitute for injection

TETRACYCLINES

Demeclocycline (Declomycin)
Oral: 150, 300 mg tablets; 150 mg capsules
Doxycycline (generic, Vibramycin, others)
Oral: 50, 75, 100 mg tablets and capsules; powder to reconstitute for 25 mg/5 mL suspension; 50 mg/5 mL syrup
Parenteral: 100, 200 mg powder to reconstitute for injection
Methacycline (Rondomycin)
Oral: 150, 300 mg capsules
Minocycline (Minocin)
Oral: 50, 75, 100 mg tablets and capsules; 50 mg/5 mL suspension
Parenteral: 100 mg powder to reconstitute for injection
Oxytetracycline (Terramycin)
Parenteral: 50, 125 mg/mL for IM injection
Tetracycline (generic, others)
Oral: 250, 500 mg capsules; 125 mg/5 mL suspension
Tigecycline (Tygacil)
Parenteral: 50 mg powder to reconstitute for IV administration

MACROLIDES

Azithromycin (Zithromax)
Oral: 250, 500, 600 mg capsules; powder for 100, 200 mg/5 mL oral suspension
Parenteral: 500 mg powder for injection

Clarithromycin (Biaxin)
Oral: 250, 500 mg tablets, 500 mg extended-release tablets; granules for 125, 250 mg/5 mL oral suspension
Erythromycin (generic, others)
Oral (base): 250, 333, 500 mg enteric-coated tablets
Oral (base) delayed-release: 250 mg capsules, 500 mg tablets
Oral (estolate): 125, 250 mg/5 mL suspension
Oral (ethylsuccinate): 400 mg tablets; 200, 400 mg/5 mL suspension
Oral (stearate): 250, 500 mg film-coated tablets
Parenteral: lactobionate, 0.5, 1 g powder to reconstitute for IV injection

KETOLIDES

Telithromycin (Keteck)
Oral: 400 mg tablets

LINCOMYCINS

Clindamycin (generic, Cleocin)
Oral: 75, 150, 300 mg capsules; 75 mg/5 mL granules to reconstitute for solution
Parenteral: 150 mg/mL in 2, 4, 6, 60 mL vials for injection

STREPTOGRAMINS

Quinupristin and dalfopristin (Synercid)
Parenteral: 30:70 formulation in 500 mg vial for reconstitution for IV injection

OXAZOLIDINONES

Linezolid (Zyvox)
Oral: 400, 600 mg tablets; 100 mg powder for 5 mL suspension
Parenteral: 2 mg/mL for IV infusion

REFERENCES

Anonymous: Tigecycline (tygacil). Med Lett Drugs Ther 2005;47:73.

Fortun J et al: Linezolid for the treatment of multidrug-resistant tuberculosis. J Antimicrob Chemother 2005;56:180.

Gee T et al: Pharmacokinetics and tissue penetration of linezolid following multiple oral doses. Antimicrob Agents Chemother 2001;45:1843.

Hancock RE: Mechanisms of action of newer antibiotics for gram-positive pathogens. Lancet Infect Dis 2005;5:209.

Livermore DM. Tigecycline: What is it, and where should it be used? J Antimicrob Chemother 2005;56:611.

Noskin GA: Tigecycline: A new glycylcycline for treatment of serious infections. Clin Infect Dis 2005;41(Suppl 5):S303.

Schlossberg D: Azithromycin and clarithromycin. Med Clin North Am 1995;79:803.

Speer BS, Shoemaker MB, Salyers AA: Bacterial resistance to tetracycline: Mechanism, transfer, and clinical significance. Clin Microbiol Rev 1992;5:387.

Zhanel GG et al: The ketolides: A critical review. Drugs 2002; 62:1771.

Zuckerman JM: Macrolides and ketolides: Azithromycin, clarithromycin, telithromycin. Infect Dis Clin North Am 2004; 18:621.

Aminoglycosides & Spectinomycin

Henry F. Chambers, MD

The drugs described in this chapter are bactericidal inhibitors of protein synthesis that interfere with ribosomal function. These agents are useful mainly against aerobic gram-negative microorganisms.

■ AMINOGLYCOSIDES

The aminoglycosides include **streptomycin, neomycin, kanamycin, amikacin, gentamicin, tobramycin, sisomicin, netilmicin,** and others. They are used most widely against gram-negative enteric bacteria, especially in bacteremia and sepsis, in combination with vancomycin or a penicillin for endocarditis, and for treatment of tuberculosis.

General Properties of Aminoglycosides

A. PHYSICAL AND CHEMICAL PROPERTIES

Aminoglycosides have a hexose ring, either streptidine (in streptomycin) or 2-deoxystreptamine (other aminoglycosides), to which various amino sugars are attached by glycosidic linkages (Figures 45–1 and 45–2). They are water-soluble, stable in solution, and more active at alkaline than at acid pH.

B. MECHANISM OF ACTION

The mode of action of streptomycin has been studied far more closely than that of other aminoglycosides, but probably all act similarly. Aminoglycosides are irreversible inhibitors of protein synthesis, but the precise mechanism for bactericidal activity is not known. The initial event is passive diffusion via porin channels across the outer membrane. Drug is then actively transported across the cell membrane into the cytoplasm by an oxygen-dependent process. The transmembrane electrochemical gradient supplies the energy for this process, and transport is coupled to a proton pump. Low extracellular pH and anaerobic conditions inhibit transport by reducing the gradient. Transport may be enhanced by cell wall-active drugs such as penicillin or

vancomycin; this enhancement may be the basis of the synergism of these antibiotics with aminoglycosides.

Inside the cell, aminoglycosides bind to specific 30S-subunit ribosomal proteins (S12 in the case of streptomycin). Protein synthesis is inhibited by aminoglycosides in at least three ways (Figure 45–3): (1) interference with the initiation complex of peptide formation; (2) misreading of mRNA, which causes incorporation of incorrect amino acids into the peptide, resulting in a nonfunctional or toxic protein; and (3) breakup of polysomes into nonfunctional monosomes. These activities occur more or less simultaneously, and the overall effect is irreversible and lethal for the cell.

C. MECHANISMS OF RESISTANCE

Three principal mechanisms have been established: (1) production of a transferase enzyme or enzymes inactivates the aminoglycoside by adenylylation, acetylation, or phosphorylation. This is the principal type of resistance encountered clinically. (Specific transferase enzymes are discussed below.) (2) There is impaired entry of aminoglycoside into the cell. This may be genotypic, ie, resulting from mutation or deletion of a porin protein or proteins involved in transport and maintenance of the electrochemical gradient; or phenotypic, eg, resulting from growth conditions under which the oxygen-dependent transport process

Figure 45–1. Structure of streptomycin.

described above is not functional. (3) The receptor protein on the 30S ribosomal subunit may be deleted or altered as a result of a mutation.

D. PHARMACOKINETICS AND ONCE-DAILY DOSING

Aminoglycosides are absorbed very poorly from the intact gastrointestinal tract; almost the entire oral dose is excreted in feces after oral administration. However, the drugs may be absorbed if ulcerations are present. After intramuscular injection, aminoglycosides are well absorbed, giving peak concentrations in blood within 30–90 minutes. Aminoglycosides are usually administered intravenously as a 30- to 60-minute infusion; after a brief distribution phase, this results in serum concentrations that are identical to those following intramuscular injection.

Traditionally, aminoglycosides have been administered in two or three equally divided daily doses for patients with normal renal function. However, once-daily aminoglycoside dosing may be preferred in certain clinical situations. Aminoglycosides have **concentration-dependent killing;** that is, increasing concentrations kill an increasing proportion of bacteria and at a more rapid rate. They also have a significant **postantibiotic effect,** such that the antibacterial activity persists beyond the time during which measurable drug is present. The postantibiotic effect of aminoglycosides can reach several hours. Because of these properties, a given total amount of aminoglycoside may have better efficacy when administered as a single large dose than when administered as multiple smaller doses.

Aminoglycoside toxicity is both time- and concentration-dependent. Toxicity is unlikely to occur until a certain threshold concentration is achieved, but once that concentration is achieved the time above this threshold becomes critical. This threshold is not precisely defined, but a trough concentration above 2 mcg/mL is predictive of toxicity. At clinically relevant doses, the time above this threshold will be greater with multiple smaller doses of drug than with a single large dose.

Numerous clinical studies demonstrate that a single daily dose of aminoglycoside is just as effective—and no

Kanamycin R = H

Amikacin R = C — CH — CH$_2$ — CH$_2$ — NH$_2$ (with O double bond and OH shown)

Gentamicin, netilmicin

	Ring I			Ring II
	R_1	R_2	C4–C5 bond	R_3
Gentamicin C_1	CH$_3$	CH$_3$	Single	H
Gentamicin C_2	CH$_3$	H	Single	H
Gentamicin C_{1a}	H	H	Single	H
Netilmicin	H	H	Double	C_2H_5

Figure 45–2. Structures of several important aminoglycoside antibiotics. Ring II is 2-deoxystreptamine. The resemblance between kanamycin and amikacin and between gentamicin, netilmicin, and tobramycin can be seen. The circled numerals on the kanamycin molecule indicate points of attack of plasmid-mediated bacterial transferase enzymes that can inactivate this drug. ①, ②, and ③, acetyltransferase; ④, phosphotransferase; ⑤, adenylyltransferase. Amikacin is resistant to modification at ②, ③, ④, and ⑤.

Tobramycin

Figure 45–3. Putative mechanisms of action of the aminoglycosides. Normal protein synthesis is shown in the top panel. At least three aminoglycoside effects have been described, as shown in the bottom panel: block of formation of the initiation complex; miscoding of amino acids in the emerging peptide chain due to misreading of the mRNA; and block of translocation on mRNA. Block of movement of the ribosome may occur after the formation of a single initiation complex, resulting in an mRNA chain with only a single ribosome on it, a so-called monosome. (Reproduced, with permission, from Trevor AT, Katzung BG, Masters SB: *Pharmacology: Examination & Board Review,* 6th ed. McGraw-Hill, 2002.)

more (and often less) toxic—than multiple smaller doses. Therefore, many authorities now recommend that aminoglycosides be administered as a single daily dose in many clinical situations. The efficacy of once-daily aminoglycoside dosing in combination therapy of enterococcal, streptococcal, and staphylococcal endocarditis remains to be defined, and the standard low-dose, thrice-daily administration is still recommended. The role of once-daily dosing in pregnancy and in neonates also is not well-defined.

Once-daily dosing has potential practical advantages. For example, determination of serum concentrations is probably unnecessary unless aminoglycoside is given for more than 3 days. A drug administered once a day rather than three times a day saves time. And once-a-day dosing lends itself to outpatient therapy.

Once-daily dosing, however, does not eliminate responsibility for careful monitoring and dosage adjustment to minimize toxicity. Selection of the appropriate dose is particularly critical if renal function is impaired. Aminoglycosides are cleared by the kidney, and excretion is directly proportional to creatinine clearance. Rapidly changing renal function, which may occur with acute renal failure in the patient with septic shock, must be anticipated to avoid overdose. Provided these pitfalls are avoided, once-daily aminoglycoside dosing is safe and effective. If the creatinine clearance is 100 mL/min, gentamicin is given as a 5 mg/kg dose (15 mg/kg for amikacin) over 30–60 minutes. If the creatinine clearance is 80 mL/min, the dose is 4 mg/kg (12 mg/kg for

amikacin); if creatinine clearance is 50 mL/min, the dose is 3 mg/kg (9 mg/kg for amikacin). If the creatinine clearance is less than 50 mL/min, a 2 mg/kg gentamicin loading dose is given and subsequent doses are adjusted as would normally be done. Serum concentrations need not be routinely checked until the second or third day of therapy, depending on the stability of renal function and the anticipated duration of therapy. It is probably unnecessary to check peak concentrations, because they will be high. The goal is to administer drug so that concentrations of less than 1 mcg/mL are present between 18 and 24 hours after dosing. This provides a sufficient period of time for washout of drug to occur before the next dose is given. This is most easily determined either by measuring serum concentrations in samples obtained 2 hours and 12 hours after dosing and then adjusting the dose based on the actual clearance of drug or by measuring the concentration in a sample obtained 8 hours after a dose. If the 8-hour concentration is between 1.5 mcg and 6 mcg/mL, the target trough will be achieved at 18 hours.

Aminoglycosides are highly polar compounds that do not enter cells readily. They are largely excluded from the central nervous system and the eye. In the presence of active inflammation, however, cerebrospinal fluid levels reach 20% of plasma levels, and in neonatal meningitis the levels may be higher. Intrathecal or intraventricular injection is required for high levels in cerebrospinal fluid. Even after parenteral administration, concentrations of aminoglycosides are not high in most tissues except the renal cortex. Concentration in most secretions is also modest; in the bile, it may reach 30% of the blood level. With prolonged therapy, diffusion into pleural or synovial fluid may result in concentrations 50–90% of that of plasma.

The normal half-life of aminoglycosides in serum is 2–3 hours, increasing to 24–48 hours in patients with significant impairment of renal function. Aminoglycosides are only partially and irregularly removed by hemodialysis—eg, 40–60% for gentamicin—and even less effectively by peritoneal dialysis.

Dosage adjustments must be made to avoid accumulation of drug and toxicity in patients with renal insufficiency. Either the dose of drug is kept constant and the interval between doses is increased, or the interval is kept constant and the dose is reduced. Nomograms and formulas have been constructed relating serum creatinine levels to adjustments in treatment regimens. The simplest formula divides the dose (calculated on the basis of normal renal function) by the serum creatinine value (mg/dL). Thus, a 60-kg patient with normal renal function might receive 300 mg/d of gentamicin (maximum daily dose of 5 mg/kg), whereas a 60-kg patient with a serum creatinine of 3 mg/dL would receive 100 mg/d. However, this approach fails to take into account the age and gender of the patient, both of which significantly affect creatinine clearance without necessarily being reflected as a change in serum creatinine. Because aminoglycoside clearance is directly proportional to the creatinine clearance, a better method for determining the aminoglycoside dose is to estimate creatinine clearance using the Cockcroft-Gault formula described in Chapter 61.

The daily dosage of aminoglycoside is calculated by multiplying the maximum daily dose by the ratio of estimated creatinine clearance to normal creatinine clearance, ie, 120 mL/min, which is a typical value for a 70-kg young adult male. For a 60-year-old female weighing 60 kg with a serum creatinine of 3 mg/dL, the corrected dosage of gentamicin would be approximately 50 mg/d, half the dose calculated by the simplest formula. There is considerable individual variation in aminoglycoside serum levels among patients with similar estimated creatinine clearance values. Therefore, it is mandatory, especially when using higher dosages for more than a few days or when renal function is rapidly changing, to measure serum drug levels to avoid severe toxicity. For a traditional twice- or thrice-daily dosing regimen, peak serum concentrations should be determined from a blood sample obtained 30–60 minutes after a dose and trough concentrations from a sample obtained just before the next dose.

E. ADVERSE EFFECTS

All aminoglycosides are ototoxic and nephrotoxic. Ototoxicity and nephrotoxicity are more likely to be encoun-

tered when therapy is continued for more than 5 days, at higher doses, in the elderly, and in the setting of renal insufficiency. Concurrent use with loop diuretics (eg, furosemide, ethacrynic acid) or other nephrotoxic antimicrobial agents (eg, vancomycin or amphotericin) can potentiate nephrotoxicity and should be avoided if possible. Ototoxicity can manifest itself either as auditory damage, resulting in tinnitus and high-frequency hearing loss initially, or as vestibular damage, evident by vertigo, ataxia, and loss of balance. Nephrotoxicity results in rising serum creatinine levels or reduced creatinine clearance, although the earliest indication often is an increase in trough serum aminoglycoside concentrations. Neomycin, kanamycin, and amikacin are the most ototoxic agents. Streptomycin and gentamicin are the most vestibulotoxic. Neomycin, tobramycin, and gentamicin are the most nephrotoxic.

In very high doses, aminoglycosides can produce a curare-like effect with neuromuscular blockade that results in respiratory paralysis. This paralysis is usually reversible by calcium gluconate (given promptly) or neostigmine. Hypersensitivity occurs infrequently.

F. CLINICAL USES

Aminoglycosides are mostly used against gram-negative enteric bacteria, especially when the isolate may be drug-resistant and when there is suspicion of sepsis. They are almost always used in combination with a β-lactam antibiotic to extend coverage to include potential gram-positive pathogens and to take advantage of the synergism between these two classes of drugs. Penicillin-aminoglycoside combinations also are used to achieve bactericidal activity in treatment of enterococcal endocarditis and to shorten duration of therapy for viridans streptococcal and staphylococcal endocarditis. Which aminoglycoside and what dose should be used depend on the infection being treated and the susceptibility of the isolate.

STREPTOMYCIN

Streptomycin (Figure 45–1) was isolated from a strain of *Streptomyces griseus.* The antimicrobial activity of streptomycin is typical of that of other aminoglycosides, as are the mechanisms of resistance. Resistance has emerged in most species, severely limiting the current usefulness of streptomycin, with the exceptions listed below. Ribosomal resistance to streptomycin develops readily, limiting its role as a single agent.

Clinical Uses

A. MYCOBACTERIAL INFECTIONS

Streptomycin is mainly used as a second-line agent for treatment of tuberculosis. The dosage is 0.5–1 g/d

(7.5–15 mg/kg/d for children), which is given intramuscularly or intravenously. It should be used only in combination with other agents to prevent emergence of resistance. See Chapter 47 for additional information regarding the use of streptomycin in mycobacterial infections.

B. NONTUBERCULOUS INFECTIONS

In plague, tularemia, and sometimes brucellosis, streptomycin, 1 g/d (15 mg/kg/d for children), is given intramuscularly in combination with an oral tetracycline.

Penicillin plus streptomycin is effective for enterococcal endocarditis and 2-week therapy of viridans streptococcal endocarditis. Gentamicin has largely replaced streptomycin for these indications. Streptomycin remains a useful agent for treating enterococcal infections, however, because approximately 15% of enterococcal isolates that are resistant to gentamicin (and therefore to netilmicin, tobramycin, and amikacin) will be susceptible to streptomycin.

Adverse Reactions

Fever, skin rashes, and other allergic manifestations may result from hypersensitivity to streptomycin. This occurs most frequently with prolonged contact with the drug either in patients who receive a prolonged course of treatment (eg, for tuberculosis) or in medical personnel who handle the drug. Desensitization is occasionally successful.

Pain at the injection site is common but usually not severe. The most serious toxic effect with streptomycin is disturbance of vestibular function—vertigo and loss of balance. The frequency and severity of this disturbance are in proportion to the age of the patient, the blood levels of the drug, and the duration of administration. Vestibular dysfunction may follow a few weeks of unusually high blood levels (eg, in individuals with impaired renal function) or months of relatively low blood levels. Vestibular toxicity tends to be irreversible. Streptomycin given during pregnancy can cause deafness in the newborn and therefore is relatively contraindicated.

GENTAMICIN

Gentamicin is an aminoglycoside (Figure 45–2) isolated from *Micromonospora purpurea*. It is effective against both gram-positive and gram-negative organisms, and many of its properties resemble those of other aminoglycosides. **Sisomicin** is very similar to the C_{1a} component of gentamicin.

Antimicrobial Activity

Gentamicin sulfate, 2–10 mcg/mL, inhibits in vitro many strains of staphylococci and coliforms and other gram-negative bacteria. It is active alone, but also as a synergistic companion with β-lactam antibiotics, against pseudomonas, proteus, enterobacter, klebsiella, serratia, stenotrophomonas, and other gram-negative rods that may be resistant to multiple other antibiotics. Like all aminoglycosides, it has no activity against anaerobes.

Resistance

Streptococci and enterococci are relatively resistant to gentamicin owing to failure of the drug to penetrate into the cell. However, gentamicin in combination with vancomycin or a penicillin produces a potent bactericidal effect, which in part is due to enhanced uptake of drug that occurs with inhibition of cell wall synthesis. Resistance to gentamicin rapidly emerges in staphylococci owing to selection of permeability mutants. Ribosomal resistance is rare. Among gram-negative bacteria, resistance is most commonly due to plasmid-encoded aminoglycoside-modifying enzymes. Gram-negative bacteria that are gentamicin-resistant usually are susceptible to amikacin, which is much more resistant to modifying enzyme activity. The enterococcal enzyme that modifies gentamicin is a bifunctional enzyme that also inactivates amikacin, netilmicin, and tobramycin, but not streptomycin; the latter is modified by a different enzyme. This is why some gentamicin-resistant enterococci are susceptible to streptomycin.

Clinical Uses

A. INTRAMUSCULAR OR INTRAVENOUS ADMINISTRATION

Gentamicin is used mainly in severe infections (eg, sepsis and pneumonia) caused by gram-negative bacteria that are likely to be resistant to other drugs, especially pseudomonas, enterobacter, serratia, proteus, acinetobacter, and klebsiella. It usually is used in combination with a second agent, as an aminoglycoside alone may not be effective for infections outside the urinary tract. For example, gentamicin should not be used as a single agent to treat staphylococcal infections because resistance develops rapidly. Aminoglycosides should not be used for single-agent therapy of pneumonia because penetration of infected lung tissue is poor and local conditions of low pH and low oxygen tension contribute to poor activity. Gentamicin 5–6 mg/kg/d traditionally is given intravenously in three equal doses, but once-daily administration is just as effective for some organisms and less toxic.

Serum gentamicin concentrations and renal function should be monitored if gentamicin is administered for more than a few days or if renal function is changing (eg, in sepsis, which often is complicated by acute renal failure). For patients receiving dosing every 8 hours, target peak concentrations are 5–10 mcg/mL, and trough concentrations should be less than 1–2 mcg/mL. Trough concentrations above 2 mcg/mL indicate accumulation of drug and are associated with toxicity; in this case, the dose should be lowered or the interval extended to achieve the target range.

B. TOPICAL ADMINISTRATION

Creams, ointments, and solutions containing 0.1–0.3% gentamicin sulfate have been used for the treatment of infected burns, wounds, or skin lesions and the prevention of intravenous catheter infections. Topical gentamicin is partly inactivated by purulent exudates. Ten milligrams can be injected subconjunctivally for treatment of ocular infections.

C. INTRATHECAL ADMINISTRATION

Meningitis caused by gram-negative bacteria has been treated by the intrathecal injection of gentamicin sulfate, 1–10 mg/d. However, neither intrathecal nor intraventricular gentamicin was beneficial in neonates with meningitis, and intraventricular gentamicin was toxic, raising questions about the utility of this form of therapy. Moreover, the availability of third-generation cephalosporins for gram-negative meningitis has rendered this therapy obsolete in most cases.

Adverse Reactions

Nephrotoxicity is usually reversible and mild. It occurs in 5–25% of patients receiving gentamicin for longer than 3–5 days. Such toxicity requires, at the very least, adjustment of the dosing regimen and should prompt reconsideration of the need for the drug, particularly if there is a less toxic alternative agent. Measurement of gentamicin serum levels is essential. Ototoxicity, which tends to be irreversible, manifests itself mainly as vestibular dysfunction. Loss of hearing can also occur. The incidence of ototoxicity is in part genetically determined, having been linked to point mutations in mitochondrial DNA, and occurs in 1–5% for patients receiving gentamicin for more than 5 days. Hypersensitivity reactions to gentamicin are uncommon.

TOBRAMYCIN

This aminoglycoside (Figure 45–2) has an antibacterial spectrum similar to that of gentamicin. Although there is some cross-resistance between gentamicin and tobramycin, it is unpredictable in individual strains. Separate laboratory susceptibility tests are therefore necessary.

The pharmacokinetic properties of tobramycin are virtually identical to those of gentamicin. The daily dose of tobramycin is 5–6 mg/kg intramuscularly or intravenously, traditionally divided into three equal amounts and given every 8 hours. Monitoring blood levels in renal insufficiency is an essential guide to proper dosing.

Tobramycin has almost the same antibacterial spectrum as gentamicin with a few exceptions. Gentamicin is slightly more active against serratia, whereas tobramycin is slightly more active against pseudomonas; *Enterococcus faecalis* is susceptible to both gentamicin and tobramycin, but *E faecium* is resistant to tobramycin. Gentamicin and tobramycin are otherwise interchangeable clinically. Gentamicin is much less expensive, however, and is preferred for this reason.

Like other aminoglycosides, tobramycin is ototoxic and nephrotoxic. Nephrotoxicity of tobramycin may be slightly less than that of gentamicin, but the difference is clinically inconsequential.

Tobramycin is also formulated in solution (300 mg in 5 mL) for inhalation for treatment of *Pseudomonas aeruginosa* lower respiratory tract infections complicating cystic fibrosis. The drug is recommended as a 300-mg dose regardless of the patient's age or weight for administration twice daily in repeated cycles of 28 days on therapy followed by 28 days off therapy. Serum concentrations 1 hour after inhalation average 1 mcg/mL; consequently, nephrotoxicity and ototoxicity rarely occur. Caution should be used when administering the tobramycin to patients with preexisting renal, vestibular, or hearing disorders.

AMIKACIN

Amikacin is a semisynthetic derivative of kanamycin; it is less toxic than the parent molecule (Figure 45–2). It is resistant to many enzymes that inactivate gentamicin and tobramycin, and it therefore can be used against some microorganisms resistant to the latter drugs. Many gram-negative enteric bacteria, including many strains of proteus, pseudomonas, enterobacter, and serratia, are inhibited by 1–20 mcg/mL amikacin in vitro. After injection of 500 mg of amikacin every 12 hours (15 mg/kg/d) intramuscularly, peak levels in serum are 10–30 mcg/mL.

Strains of multidrug-resistant *Mycobacterium tuberculosis,* including streptomycin-resistant strains, are usually susceptible to amikacin. Kanamycin-resistant strains may be cross-resistant to amikacin. The dosage of amikacin for tuberculosis is 7.5–15 mg/kg/d as a once-daily or two to three times weekly injection and always in combination with other drugs to which the isolate is susceptible.

Like all aminoglycosides, amikacin is nephrotoxic and ototoxic (particularly for the auditory portion of the eighth nerve). Serum concentrations should be monitored. Target peak serum concentrations for an every-12-hours dosing regimen are 20–40 mcg/mL, and troughs should be maintained at less than 2 mcg/mL.

NETILMICIN

Netilmicin shares many characteristics with gentamicin and tobramycin. However, the addition of an ethyl group to the 1-amino position of the 2-deoxy-streptamine ring (ring II, Figure 45–2) sterically protects the netilmicin molecule from enzymatic degradation at the 3-amino (ring II) and 2-hydroxyl (ring III) positions. Consequently, netilmicin may be active against some gentamicin-resistant and tobramycin-resistant bacteria.

The dosage (5–7 mg/kg/d) and the routes of administration are the same as for gentamicin. It is completely therapeutically interchangeable with gentamicin or tobramycin and has similar toxicities.

NEOMYCIN & KANAMYCIN

Neomycin and kanamycin are closely related. **Paromomycin** is also a member of this group. All have similar properties.

Antimicrobial Activity & Resistance

Drugs of the neomycin group are active against gram-positive and gram-negative bacteria and some mycobacteria. Pseudomonas and streptococci are generally resistant. Mechanisms of antibacterial action and resistance are the same as with other aminoglycosides. The widespread use of these drugs in bowel preparation for elective surgery has resulted in the selection of resistant organisms and some outbreaks of enterocolitis in hospitals. Cross-resistance between kanamycin and neomycin is complete.

Pharmacokinetics

Drugs of the neomycin group are poorly absorbed from the gastrointestinal tract. After oral administration, the intestinal flora is suppressed or modified, and the drug is excreted in the feces. Excretion of any absorbed drug is mainly through glomerular filtration into the urine.

Clinical Uses

Neomycin and kanamycin are now limited to topical and oral use. Neomycin is too toxic for parenteral use. With the advent of more potent and less toxic aminoglycosides, parenteral administration of kanamycin has also been largely abandoned.

A. TOPICAL ADMINISTRATION

Solutions containing 1–5 mg/mL are used on infected surfaces or injected into joints, the pleural cavity, tissue spaces, or abscess cavities where infection is present. The total amount of drug given in this fashion must be limited to 15 mg/kg/d because at higher doses enough drug may be absorbed to produce systemic toxicity. Whether topical application for active infection adds anything to appropriate systemic therapy is question-able. Ointments, often formulated as a neomycin-polymyxin-bacitracin combination, can be applied to infected skin lesions or in the nares for suppression of staphylococci but they are largely ineffective.

B. ORAL ADMINISTRATION

In preparation for elective bowel surgery, 1 g of neomycin is given orally every 6–8 hours for 1–2 days, often combined with 1 g of erythromycin base. This reduces the aerobic bowel flora with little effect on anaerobes. In hepatic coma, coliform flora can be suppressed by giving 1 g every 6–8 hours together with reduced protein intake, thus reducing ammonia intoxication. Use of neomycin for hepatic coma has been almost entirely supplanted by lactulose, which is much less toxic. Paromomycin, 1 g every 6 hours orally for 2 weeks, has been effective in intestinal amebiasis (see Chapter 53).

Adverse Reactions

All members of the neomycin group have significant nephrotoxicity and ototoxicity. Auditory function is affected more than vestibular. Deafness has occurred, especially in adults with impaired renal function and prolonged elevation of drug levels.

The sudden absorption of postoperatively instilled kanamycin from the peritoneal cavity (3–5 g) has resulted in curare-like neuromuscular blockade and respiratory arrest. Calcium gluconate and neostigmine can act as antidotes.

Although hypersensitivity is not common, prolonged application of neomycin-containing ointments to skin and eyes has resulted in severe allergic reactions.

■ SPECTINOMYCIN

Spectinomycin is an aminocyclitol antibiotic that is structurally related to aminoglycosides. It lacks amino sugars and glycosidic bonds.

Spectinomycin

Spectinomycin is active in vitro against many gram-positive and gram-negative organisms, but it is used almost solely as an alternative treatment for drug-resistant gonorrhea or gonorrhea in penicillin-allergic patients. The majority of gonococcal isolates are inhibited by 6 mcg/mL of spectinomycin. Strains of gonococci may be resistant to spectinomycin, but there is no cross-resistance with other drugs used in gonorrhea. Spectinomycin is rapidly absorbed after intramuscular injection. A single dose of 40 mg/kg up to a maximum of 2 g is given. There is pain at the injection site and occasionally fever and nausea. Nephrotoxicity and anemia have been observed rarely.

 PREPARATIONS AVAILABLE

Amikacin (generic, Amikin)
   Parenteral: 50, 250 mg (in vials) for IM, IV injection
Gentamicin (generic, Garamycin)
   Parenteral: 10, 40 mg/mL vials for IM, IV injection
Kanamycin (Kantrex)
   Oral: 500 mg capsules
   Parenteral: 500, 1000 mg for IM, IV injection;
      75 mg for pediatric injection
Neomycin (generic, Mycifradin)
   Oral: 500 mg tablets; 125 mg/5 mL solution
Netilmicin (Netromycin)
   Parenteral: 100 mg/mL for IM, IV injection

Paromomycin (Humatin)
   Oral: 250 mg capsules
Spectinomycin (Trobicin)
   Parenteral: 2 g powder to reconstitute for 400 mg/mL IM injection
Streptomycin (generic)
   Parenteral: 400 mg/mL for IM injection
Tobramycin (generic, Nebcin)
   Parenteral: 10, 40 mg/mL for IM, IV injection; powder to reconstitute for injection
   Solution for inhalation (TOBI): 300 mg in 5 mL sodium chloride solution

---

REFERENCES

Busse H-J, Wöstmann C, Bakker EP: The bactericidal action of streptomycin: Membrane permeabilization caused by the insertion of mistranslated proteins into the cytoplasmic membrane of *Escherichia coli* and subsequent caging of the antibiotic inside the cells due to degradation of these proteins. J Gen Microbiol 1992;138:551.

Cheer SM, Waugh J, Noble S: Inhaled tobramycin (TOBI): A review of its use in the management of *Pseudomonas aeruginosa* infections in patients with cystic fibrosis. Drugs 2003;63:2501.

Contopoulos-Ioannidis DG et al: Extended-interval aminoglycoside administration for children: A meta-analysis. Pediatrics 2004;114:111.

Kaye D: Current use for old antibacterial agents: Polymyxins, rifampin, and aminoglycosides. Infect Dis Clin North Am 2004;18:669.

Le T, Bayer AS: Combination antibiotic therapy for infective endocarditis. Clin Infect Dis 2003;36:615.

Olsen KM et al: Effect of once-daily dosing vs. multiple daily dosing of tobramycin on enzyme markers of nephrotoxicity. Crit Care Med 2004;32:1678.

Pappas G et al: Brucellosis. N Engl J Med 2005;352:2325.

Paul M et al: Beta lactam monotherapy versus beta lactam-aminoglycoside combination therapy for sepsis in immunocompetent patients: Systematic review and meta-analysis of randomised trials. BMJ 2004;328:668.

Paul M, Soares-Weiser K, Leibovici L: Beta lactam monotherapy versus beta lactam-aminoglycoside combination therapy for fever with neutropenia: Systematic review and meta-analysis. BMJ 2003;326:1111.

Poole K: Aminoglycoside resistance in *Pseudomonas aeruginosa*. Antimicrob Agents Chemother 2005;49:479.

Sulfonamides, Trimethoprim, & Quinolones

Henry F. Chambers, MD

46

■ I. ANTIFOLATE DRUGS

SULFONAMIDES

Chemistry

The basic formula of the sulfonamides and their structural similarity to *p*-aminobenzoic acid (PABA) are shown in Figure 46–1. Sulfonamides with varying physical, chemical, pharmacologic, and antibacterial properties are produced by attaching substituents to the amido group ($-SO_2-NH-R$) or the amino group ($-NH_2$) of the sulfanilamide nucleus. Sulfonamides tend to be much more soluble at alkaline than at acid pH. Most can be prepared as sodium salts, which are used for intravenous administration.

Antimicrobial Activity

Sulfonamide-susceptible organisms, unlike mammals, cannot use exogenous folate but must synthesize it from PABA (Figure 46–2). This pathway is thus essential for production of purines and nucleic acid synthesis. Because sulfonamides are structural analogs of PABA, they inhibit dihydropteroate synthase and folate production. Sulfonamides inhibit both gram-positive and gram-negative bacteria, nocardia, *Chlamydia trachomatis*, and some protozoa. Some enteric bacteria, such as *E coli*, klebsiella, salmonella, shigella, and enterobacter, are also inhibited. It is interesting that rickettsiae are not inhibited by sulfonamides but are actually stimulated in their growth. Activity is poor against anaerobes.

Combination of a sulfonamide with an inhibitor of dihydrofolate reductase (trimethoprim or pyrimethamine) provides synergistic activity because of sequential inhibition of folate synthesis (Figure 46–2).

Resistance

Mammalian cells (and some bacteria) lack the enzymes required for folate synthesis from PABA and depend on exogenous sources of folate; therefore, they are not susceptible to sulfonamides. Sulfonamide resistance may occur as a result of mutations that (a) cause overproduction of PABA, (b) cause production of a folic acid-synthesizing enzyme that has low affinity for sulfonamides, or (c) impair permeability to the sulfonamide. Dihydropteroate synthase with low sulfonamide affinity is often encoded on a plasmid that is transmissible and can disseminate rapidly and widely. Sulfonamide-resistant dihydropteroate synthase mutants also can emerge under selective pressure.

Pharmacokinetics

Sulfonamides can be divided into three major groups: (1) oral, absorbable; (2) oral, nonabsorbable; and (3) topical. The oral, absorbable sulfonamides can be classified as short-, intermediate-, or long-acting on the basis of their half-lives (Table 46–1). They are absorbed from the stomach and small intestine and distributed widely to tissues and body fluids (including the central nervous system and cerebrospinal fluid), placenta, and fetus. Protein binding varies from 20% to over 90%. Therapeutic concentrations are in the range of 40–100 mcg/mL of blood. Blood levels generally peak 2–6 hours after oral administration.

A portion of absorbed drug is acetylated or glucuronidated in the liver. Sulfonamides and inactive metabolites are then excreted into the urine, mainly by glomerular filtration. In significant renal failure, the dosage of sulfonamide must be reduced.

Clinical Uses

Sulfonamides are infrequently used as single agents. Many strains of formerly susceptible species, including meningococci, pneumococci, streptococci, staphylococci, and gonococci, are now resistant. The fixed-drug combination of trimethoprim-sulfamethoxazole is the drug of choice for infections such as *Pneumocystis jiroveci* (formerly *P carinii*) pneumonia, toxoplasmosis, nocardiosis, and occasionally other bacterial infections.

Figure 46–1. Structures of some sulfonamides and *p*-aminobenzoic acid.

A. ORAL ABSORBABLE AGENTS

Sulfisoxazole and sulfamethoxazole are short- to medium-acting agents used almost exclusively to treat urinary tract infections. The usual adult dosage is 1 g of sulfisoxazole four times daily or 1 g of sulfamethoxazole two or three times daily.

Sulfadiazine in combination with pyrimethamine is first-line therapy for treatment of acute toxoplasmosis. The combination of sulfadiazine with pyrimethamine, a potent inhibitor of dihydrofolate reductase, is synergistic because these drugs block sequential steps in the folate synthetic pathway blockade (Figure 46–2). The dosage of sulfadiazine is 1 g four times daily, with pyrimethamine given as a 75-mg loading dose followed by a 25-mg once-daily dose. Folinic acid, 10 mg orally each day, should also be administered to minimize bone marrow suppression.

Sulfadoxine is the only long-acting sulfonamide currently available in the United States and only as a combi-nation formulation with pyrimethamine (Fansidar), a second-line agent in treatment for malaria (see Chapter 53).

B. ORAL NONABSORBABLE AGENTS

Sulfasalazine (salicylazosulfapyridine) is widely used in ulcerative colitis, enteritis, and other inflammatory bowel disease (see Chapter 63).

C. TOPICAL AGENTS

Sodium sulfacetamide ophthalmic solution or ointment is effective treatment for bacterial conjunctivitis and as adjunctive therapy for trachoma. Another sulfonamide, mafenide acetate, is used topically but can be absorbed from burn sites. The drug and its primary metabolite inhibit carbonic anhydrase and can cause metabolic acidosis, a side effect that limits its usefulness. Silver sulfadiazine is a much less toxic topical sulfonamide and is preferred to mafenide for prevention of infection of burn wounds.

Adverse Reactions

All sulfonamides, including antimicrobial sulfas, diuretics, diazoxide, and the sulfonylurea hypoglycemic agents, have been considered to be partially cross-allergenic. However, evidence for this is not extensive. The most common adverse effects are fever, skin rashes, exfoliative dermatitis, photosensitivity, urticaria, nausea, vomiting, diarrhea, and difficulties referable to the urinary tract (see below). Stevens-Johnson syndrome, although relatively uncommon (ie, less than 1% of treatment courses), is a particularly serious and potentially fatal type of skin and

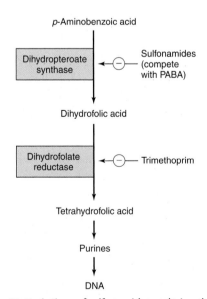

Figure 46–2. Actions of sulfonamides and trimethoprim.

Table 46–1. Pharmacokinetic properties of some sulfonamides and trimethoprim.

Drug	Half-Life	Oral Absorption
Sulfonamides		
Sulfacytine	Short	Prompt (peak levels in 1–4 hours)
Sulfisoxazole	Short (6 hours)	Prompt
Sulfamethizole	Short (9 hours)	Prompt
Sulfadiazine	Intermediate (10–17 hours)	Slow (peak levels in 4–8 hours)
Sulfamethoxazole	Intermediate (10–12 hours)	Slow
Sulfapyridine	Intermediate (17 hours)	Slow
Sulfadoxine	Long (7–9 days)	Intermediate
Pyrimidines		
Trimethoprim	Intermediate (11 hours)	Prompt

mucous membrane eruption associated with sulfonamide use. Other unwanted effects include stomatitis, conjunctivitis, arthritis, hematopoietic disturbances (see below), hepatitis, and, rarely, polyarteritis nodosa and psychosis.

A. URINARY TRACT DISTURBANCES

Sulfonamides may precipitate in urine, especially at neutral or acid pH, producing crystalluria, hematuria, or even obstruction. This is rarely a problem with the more soluble sulfonamides (eg, sulfisoxazole). Sulfadiazine when given in large doses, particularly if fluid intake is poor, can cause crystalluria. Crystalluria is treated by administration of sodium bicarbonate to alkalinize the urine and fluids to maintain adequate hydration. Sulfonamides have also been implicated in various types of nephrosis and in allergic nephritis.

B. HEMATOPOIETIC DISTURBANCES

Sulfonamides can cause hemolytic or aplastic anemia, granulocytopenia, thrombocytopenia, or leukemoid reactions. Sulfonamides may provoke hemolytic reactions in patients with glucose-6-phosphate dehydrogenase deficiency. Sulfonamides taken near the end of pregnancy increase the risk of kernicterus in newborns.

TRIMETHOPRIM & TRIMETHOPRIM-SULFAMETHOXAZOLE MIXTURES

Trimethoprim, a trimethoxybenzylpyrimidine, selectively inhibits bacterial dihydrofolic acid reductase, which con-

verts dihydrofolic acid to tetrahydrofolic acid, a step leading to the synthesis of purines and ultimately to DNA (Figure 46–2). Trimethoprim is about 50,000 times less efficient in inhibition of mammalian dihydrofolic acid reductase. Pyrimethamine, another benzylpyrimidine, selectively inhibits dihydrofolic acid reductase of protozoa compared with that of mammalian cells. As noted above, trimethoprim or pyrimethamine in combination with a sulfonamide blocks sequential steps in folate synthesis, resulting in marked enhancement (synergism) of the activity of both drugs. The combination often is bactericidal, compared with the bacteriostatic activity of a sulfonamide alone.

Trimethoprim

Pyrimethamine

Resistance

Resistance to trimethoprim can result from reduced cell permeability, overproduction of dihydrofolate reductase, or production of an altered reductase with reduced drug binding. Resistance can emerge by mutation, although more commonly it is due to plasmid-encoded trimethoprim-resistant dihydrofolate reductases. These resistant enzymes may be coded within transposons on conjugative plasmids that exhibit a broad host range, accounting for rapid and widespread dissemination of trimethoprim resistance among numerous bacterial species.

Pharmacokinetics

Trimethoprim is usually given orally, alone or in combination with sulfamethoxazole, which has a similar half-life. Trimethoprim-sulfamethoxazole can also be given intravenously. Trimethoprim is well absorbed from the gut and distributed widely in body fluids and tissues, including cerebrospinal fluid. Because trimethoprim is more lipid-soluble than sulfamethoxazole, it has a larger volume of distribution than the latter drug.

Therefore, when 1 part of trimethoprim is given with 5 parts of sulfamethoxazole (the ratio in the formulation), the peak plasma concentrations are in the ratio of 1:20, which is optimal for the combined effects of these drugs in vitro. About 30–50% of the sulfonamide and 50–60% of the trimethoprim (or their respective metabolites) are excreted in the urine within 24 hours. The dose should be reduced by half for patients with creatinine clearances of 15–30 mL/min.

Trimethoprim concentrates in prostatic fluid and in vaginal fluid, which are more acidic than plasma. Therefore, it has more antibacterial activity in prostatic and vaginal fluids than many other antimicrobial drugs.

Clinical Uses

A. Oral Trimethoprim

Trimethoprim can be given alone (100 mg twice daily) in acute urinary tract infections. Most community-acquired organisms tend to be susceptible to the high concentrations that are found in the urine (200–600 mcg/mL).

B. Oral Trimethoprim-Sulfamethoxazole (TMP-SMZ)

A combination of trimethoprim-sulfamethoxazole is effective treatment for a wide variety of infections including *P jiroveci* pneumonia, shigellosis, systemic salmonella infections, urinary tract infections, prostatitis, and some nontuberculous mycobacterial infections. It is active against most *S aureus* strains, both methicillin-susceptible and methicillin-resistant, and against respiratory tract pathogens such as the pneumococcus, *Haemophilus* species, *Moraxella catarrhalis*, and *Klebsiella pneumoniae* (but not *Mycoplasma pneumoniae*). However, the increasing prevalence of strains of *E coli* (up to 30% or more) and pneumococci that are resistant to trimethoprim-sulfamethoxazole must be considered before using this combination for empirical therapy of upper urinary tract infections or pneumonia.

One double-strength tablet (each tablet contains trimethoprim 160 mg plus sulfamethoxazole 800 mg) given every 12 hours is effective treatment for urinary tract infections and prostatitis. One half of the regular (single-strength) tablet given three times weekly for many months may serve as prophylaxis in recurrent urinary tract infections of some women. One double-strength tablet every 12 hours is effective treatment for infections caused by susceptible strains of shigella and salmonella. The dosage for children treated for shigellosis, urinary tract infection, or otitis media is 8 mg/kg trimethoprim and 40 mg/kg sulfamethoxazole every 12 hours.

Infections with *P jiroveci* and some other pathogens can be treated orally with high doses of the combination (dosed on the basis of the trimethoprim component at 15–20 mg/kg) or can be prevented in immunosuppressed patients by one double-strength tablet daily or three times weekly.

C. Intravenous Trimethoprim-Sulfamethoxazole

A solution of the mixture containing 80 mg trimethoprim plus 400 mg sulfamethoxazole per 5 mL diluted in 125 mL of 5% dextrose in water can be administered by intravenous infusion over 60–90 minutes. It is the agent of choice for moderately severe to severe pneumocystis pneumonia. It may be used for gram-negative bacterial sepsis, including that caused by some multidrug-resistant species such as enterobacter and serratia; shigellosis; typhoid fever; or urinary tract infection caused by a susceptible organism when the patient is unable to take the drug by mouth. The dosage is 10–20 mg/kg/d of the trimethoprim component.

D. Oral Pyrimethamine with Sulfonamide

Pyrimethamine and sulfadiazine have been used for treatment of leishmaniasis and toxoplasmosis. In falciparum malaria, the combination of pyrimethamine with sulfadoxine (Fansidar) has been used (see Chapter 53).

Adverse Effects

Trimethoprim produces the predictable adverse effects of an antifolate drug, especially megaloblastic anemia, leukopenia, and granulocytopenia. The combination trimethoprim-sulfamethoxazole may cause all of the untoward reactions associated with sulfonamides. Nausea and vomiting, drug fever, vasculitis, renal damage, and central nervous system disturbances occasionally occur also. Patients with AIDS and pneumocystis pneumonia have a particularly high frequency of untoward reactions to trimethoprim-sulfamethoxazole, especially fever, rashes, leukopenia, diarrhea, elevations of hepatic aminotransferases, hyperkalemia, and hyponatremia.

■ II. DNA GYRASE INHIBITORS

FLUOROQUINOLONES

The important quinolones are synthetic fluorinated analogs of nalidixic acid (Figure 46–3). They are active against a variety of gram-positive and gram-negative bacteria. Quinolones block bacterial DNA synthesis by inhibiting bacterial topoisomerase II (DNA gyrase) and topoisomerase IV. Inhibition of DNA gyrase prevents the relaxation of positively supercoiled DNA that is required for normal transcription and replication. Inhi-

Figure 46–3. Structures of nalidixic acid and some fluoroquinolones.

bition of topoisomerase IV interferes with separation of replicated chromosomal DNA into the respective daughter cells during cell division.

Earlier quinolones such as nalidixic acid did not achieve systemic antibacterial levels and were useful only for treatment of lower urinary tract infections. Fluorinated derivatives (ciprofloxacin, levofloxacin, and others; Figure 46–3 and Table 46–2) have greatly improved antibacterial activity compared with nalidixic acid and achieve bactericidal levels in blood and tissues.

Antibacterial Activity

Fluoroquinolones were originally developed because of their excellent activity against gram-negative aerobic bacteria; they had limited activity against gram-positive organisms. Several newer agents have improved activity against gram-positive cocci. This relative activity against gram-negative versus gram-positive species is useful for classification of these agents. Norfloxacin is the least active of the fluoroquinolones against both gram-negative and gram-positive organisms, with minimum inhibitory concentrations (MICs) fourfold to eightfold higher than those of ciprofloxacin. Ciprofloxacin, enoxacin, lomefloxacin, levofloxacin, ofloxacin, and pefloxacin make up a second group of similar agents possessing excellent gram-negative activity and moderate to good activity against gram-positive bacteria. MICs for gram-negative cocci and bacilli, including Enterobacteriaceae, pseudomonas, neisseria, haemophilus, and campylobacter, are 1–2 mcg/mL and often less. Methicillin-susceptible strains of *S aureus* are generally susceptible to these fluoroquinolones, but methicillin-resistant strains of staphylococci are often resistant. Streptococci and

Table 46–2. Pharmacokinetic properties of fluoroquinolones.

Drug	Half-Life (h)	Oral Bioavailability (%)	Peak Serum Concentration (μg/mL)	Oral Dose (mg)	Primary Route of Excretion
Ciprofloxacin	3–5	70	2.4	500	Renal
Gatifloxacin	8	98	3.4	400	Renal
Gemifloxacin	8	70	1.6	320	Renal & nonrenal
Levofloxacin	5–7	95	5.7	500	Renal
Lomefloxacin	8	95	2.8	400	Renal
Moxifloxacin	9–10	> 85	3.1	400	Nonrenal
Norfloxacin	3.5–5	80	1.5	400	Renal
Ofloxacin	5–7	95	2.9	400	Renal

enterococci tend to be less susceptible than staphylococci, and efficacy in infections caused by these organisms is limited. Ciprofloxacin is the most active agent of this group against gram-negatives, *P aeruginosa* in particular. Levofloxacin, the L-isomer of ofloxacin, has superior activity against gram-positive organisms, including *S pneumoniae.*

Gatifloxacin, gemifloxacin, and moxifloxacin make up a third group of fluoroquinolones with improved activity against gram-positive organisms, particularly *S pneumoniae* and some staphylococci. Gemifloxacin is active in vitro against ciprofloxacin-resistant strains of *S pneumoniae*, but in vivo efficacy is unproven. Although MICs of these agents for staphylococci are lower than those of ciprofloxacin (and the other compounds mentioned in the paragraph above) and may fall within the susceptible range, it is not known whether the enhanced activity is sufficient to permit use of these agents for treatment of infections caused by ciprofloxacin-resistant strains. In general, none of these agents is as active as ciprofloxacin against gram-negative organisms. Fluoroquinolones also are active against agents of atypical pneumonia (eg, mycoplasmas and chlamydiae) and against intracellular pathogens such as *Legionella* species and some mycobacteria, including *Mycobacterium tuberculosis* and *M avium* complex. Moxifloxacin also has good activity against anaerobic bacteria. Because of toxicity, gatifloxacin is no longer available in the USA.

Resistance

During fluoroquinolone therapy, resistant organisms emerge about once in 10^7–10^9, especially among staphylococci, pseudomonas, and serratia. Resistance is due to one or more point mutations in the quinolone binding region of the target enzyme or to a change in the permeability of the organism. Resistance to one fluoroquinolone, particularly if it is of high level, generally confers cross-resistance to all other members of this class.

Pharmacokinetics

After oral administration, the fluoroquinolones are well absorbed (bioavailability of 80–95%) and distributed widely in body fluids and tissues (Table 46–2). Serum half-lives range from 3 to 10 hours. The relatively long half-lives of levofloxacin, gemifloxacin gatifloxacin, and moxifloxacin permit once-daily dosing. Oral absorption is impaired by divalent cations, including those in antacids. Serum concentrations of intravenously administered drug are similar to those of orally administered drug. Most fluoroquinolones are eliminated by renal mechanisms, either tubular secretion or glomerular filtration (Table 46–2). Dose adjustment is required for patients with creatinine clearances less than 50 mL/min, the exact adjustment depending on the degree of renal impairment and the specific fluoroquinolone being used. Dose adjustment for renal failure is not necessary for moxifloxacin. Nonrenally cleared fluoroquinolones are relatively contraindicated in patients with hepatic failure.

Clinical Uses

Fluoroquinolones (other than moxifloxacin, which achieves relatively low urinary levels) are effective in urinary tract infections even when caused by multidrug-resistant bacteria, eg, pseudomonas. These agents are also effective for bacterial diarrhea caused by shigella, salmonella, toxigenic *E coli,* and campylobacter. Fluoroquinolones (except norfloxacin, which does not achieve adequate systemic concentrations) have been used in infections of soft tissues, bones, and joints and in intra-abdominal and respiratory tract infections, including those caused by multidrug-resistant organisms such as pseudomonas and enterobacter. Ciprofloxacin is a drug of choice for prophylaxis and treatment of anthrax, although the newer fluoroquinolones are active in vitro and very likely in vivo as well.

Ciprofloxacin and levofloxacin are effective for gonococcal infection, including disseminated disease and chlamydial urethritis or cervicitis. Ciprofloxacin, levofloxacin, or moxifloxacin is occasionally used for treatment of tuberculosis and atypical mycobacterial infections. They may be suitable for eradication of meningococci from carriers or for prophylaxis of infection in neutropenic patients.

Levofloxacin, gatifloxacin, gemifloxacin, and moxifloxacin, so-called respiratory fluoroquinolones, with their enhanced gram-positive activity and activity against atypical pneumonia agents (eg, chlamydia, mycoplasma, and legionella), are effective and used increasingly for treatment of upper and lower respiratory tract infections.

Adverse Effects

Fluoroquinolones are extremely well tolerated. The most common effects are nausea, vomiting, and diarrhea. Occasionally, headache, dizziness, insomnia, skin rash, or abnormal liver function tests develop. Photosensitivity has been reported with lomefloxacin and pcfloxacin. QT_c prolongation may occur with gatifloxacin, levofloxacin, gemifloxacin, and moxifloxacin. Ideally, these agents should be avoided or used with caution in patients with known QT_c interval prolongation or uncorrected hypokalemia; in those receiving class IA (eg, quinidine or procainamide) or class III antiarrhythmic agents (sotalol, ibutilide, amiodarone); and in patients receiving other agents known to increase the QT_c interval (eg, erythromycin, tricyclic antidepressants). Gatifloxacin has been associated with hyperglycemia in diabetic patients and with hypoglycemia in patients also receiving oral hypoglycemic agents. Because of these serious effects (including some fatalities), gatifloxacin was withdrawn from sales in the USA in 2006; it may be available elsewhere.

Fluoroquinolones may damage growing cartilage and cause an arthropathy. Thus, these drugs are not routinely recommended for patients under 18 years of age. However, the arthropathy is reversible, and there is a growing consensus that fluoroquinolones may be used in children in some cases (eg, for treatment of pseudomonal infections in patients with cystic fibrosis). Tendinitis, a rare complication that has been reported in adults, is potentially more serious because of the risk of tendon rupture. They should be avoided during pregnancy in the absence of specific data documenting their safety.

Chapter continues on next page.

PREPARATIONS AVAILABLE

GENERAL-PURPOSE SULFONAMIDES

Sulfadiazine (generic)
Oral: 500 mg tablets
Sulfamethizole (Thiosulfil Forte)
Oral: 500 mg tablets
Sulfamethoxazole (generic, Gantanol)
Oral: 500 mg tablets
Sulfanilamide (AVC)
Vaginal cream: 15%
Sulfisoxazole (generic)
Oral: 500 mg tablets; 500 mg/5 mL syrup
Ophthalmic: 4% solution

SULFONAMIDES FOR SPECIAL APPLICATIONS

Mafenide (Sulfamylon)
Topical: 85 mg/g cream; 5% solution
Silver sulfadiazine (generic, Silvadene)
Topical: 10 mg/g cream
Sulfacetamide sodium (generic)
Ophthalmic: 1, 10, 15, 30% solutions; 10%
ointment

TRIMETHOPRIM

Trimethoprim (generic, Proloprim, Trimpex)
Oral: 100, 200 mg tablets
Trimethoprim-sulfamethoxazole [co-trimox-azole, TMP-SMZ] (generic, Bactrim, Septra, others)
Oral: 80 mg trimethoprim + 400 mg sulfamethoxazole per single-strength tablet; 160 mg trimethoprim + 800 mg sulfamethoxazole per double-strength tablet; 40 mg trimethoprim + 200 mg sulfamethoxazole per 5 mL suspension
Parenteral: 80 mg trimethoprim + 400 mg sulfamethoxazole per 5 mL for infusion (in 5 mL ampules and 5, 10, 20 mL vials)

QUINOLONES & FLUOROQUINOLONES

Ciprofloxacin (generic, Cipro, Cipro I.V.)
Oral: 100, 250, 500, 750 mg tablets; 500 mg extended-release tablet; 50, 100 mg/mL suspension
Parenteral: 10 mg/mL for IV infusion
Ophthalmic (Ciloxan): 3 mg/mL solution; 3.3 mg/g ointment
Enoxacin (Penetrex)
Oral: 200, 400 mg tablets
Gatifloxacin (Tequin) (withdrawn from the market in the USA)
Oral: 200, 400 mg tablets; 200 mg/5 mL oral suspension
Parenteral: 200, 400 mg for IV injection
Gemifloxacin (Factive)
Oral: 320 mg tablet
Levofloxacin (Levaquin)
Oral: 250, 500, 750 mg tablets; 25 mg/mL solution
Parenteral: 5, 25 mg/mL for IV injection
Ophthalmic (Quixin): 5 mg/mL solution
Lomefloxacin (Maxaquin)
Oral: 400 mg tablets
Moxifloxacin (Avelox, Avelox I.V.)
Oral: 400 mg tablets
Parenteral: 400 mg in IV bag
Norfloxacin (Noroxin)
Oral: 400 mg tablets
Ofloxacin (Floxin)
Oral: 200, 300, 400 mg tablets
Parenteral: 200 mg in 50 mL 5% D/W for IV administration; 20, 40 mg/mL for IV injection
Ophthalmic (Ocuflox): 3 mg/mL solution
Otic (Floxin Otic): 0.3% solution

REFERENCES

Davidson R et al: Resistance to levofloxacin and failure of treatment of pneumococcal pneumonia. N Engl J Med 2002;346:747.

Ferrero L, Cameron B, Crouzet J: Analysis of *gyrA* and *grlA* mutations in stepwise-selected ciprofloxacin-resistant mutants of *Staphylococcus aureus*. Antimicrob Agents Chemother 1995;39:1554.

Frothingham R: Rates of torsades de pointes associated with ciprofloxacin, ofloxacin, levofloxacin, gatifloxacin, and moxifloxacin. Pharmacotherapy 2001;21:1468.

Keating GM, Scott LJ: Moxifloxacin: A review of its use in the management of bacterial infections. Drugs 2004;64:2347.

Mandell LA et al: Update of practice guidelines for the management of community-acquired pneumonia in immunocompetent adults. Clin Infect Dis 2003;37:1405.

Scheld WM: Maintaining fluoroquinolone class efficacy: Review of influencing factors. Emerg Infect Dis 2003;9:1.

Yoo BK et al: Gemifloxacin: A new fluoroquinolone approved for treatment of respiratory infections. Ann Pharmacother 2004; 38:1226.

Antimycobacterial Drugs

47

Henry F. Chambers, MD

Mycobacteria are intrinsically resistant to most antibiotics. Because they grow slowly compared with other bacteria, antibiotics that are most active against growing cells are relatively ineffective. Mycobacterial cells can also be dormant and thus completely resistant to many drugs or killed only very slowly. The lipid-rich mycobacterial cell wall is impermeable to many agents. Mycobacterial species are intracellular pathogens, and organisms residing within macrophages are inaccessible to drugs that penetrate these cells poorly. Finally, mycobacteria are notorious for their ability to develop resistance. Combinations of two or more drugs are required to overcome these obstacles and to prevent emergence of resistance during the course of therapy. The response of mycobacterial infections to chemotherapy is slow, and treatment must be administered for months to years, depending on which drugs are used. The drugs used to treat tuberculosis, atypical mycobacterial infections, and leprosy are described in this chapter.

■ DRUGS USED IN TUBERCULOSIS

Isoniazid (INH), rifampin (or other rifamycin), pyrazinamide, ethambutol, and **streptomycin** are the five first-line agents for treatment of tuberculosis (Table 47–1). Isoniazid and rifampin are the two most active drugs. An isoniazid-rifampin combination administered for 9 months will cure 95–98% of cases of tuberculosis caused by susceptible strains. The addition of pyrazinamide to an isoniazid-rifampin combination for the first 2 months allows the total duration of therapy to be reduced to 6 months without loss of efficacy (Table 47–2). In practice, therapy is initiated with a four-drug regimen of isoniazid, rifampin, pyrazinamide, and either ethambutol or streptomycin until susceptibility of the clinical isolate has been determined. Neither ethambutol nor streptomycin adds substantially to the overall activity of the regimen (ie, the duration of treatment cannot be further reduced if either drug is used), but they provide additional coverage if the isolate proves to be resistant to isoniazid, rifampin, or both. The prevalence of isoniazid resistance among US clinical isolates

is approximately 10%. Prevalence of resistance to both isoniazid and rifampin (ie, multiple drug resistance) is about 3%.

ISONIAZID (INH)

Isoniazid is the most active drug for the treatment of tuberculosis caused by susceptible strains. It is small (MW 137) and freely soluble in water. The structural similarity to pyridoxine is shown below.

Isoniazid

Pyridoxine

In vitro, isoniazid inhibits most tubercle bacilli in a concentration of 0.2 mcg/mL or less and is bactericidal for actively growing tubercle bacilli. It is less effective against atypical mycobacterial species. Isoniazid penetrates into macrophages and is active against both extracellular and intracellular organisms.

Mechanism of Action & Basis of Resistance

Isoniazid inhibits synthesis of mycolic acids, which are essential components of mycobacterial cell walls. Isoniazid is a prodrug that is activated by KatG, the mycobacterial catalase-peroxidase. The activated form of isoniazid forms a covalent complex with an acyl carrier protein (AcpM) and KasA, a beta-ketoacyl carrier protein synthetase, which blocks mycolic acid synthesis and kills the cell. Resistance to isoniazid is associated with mutations resulting in overexpression of *inhA,* which

Table 47–1. Antimicrobials used in the treatment of tuberculosis.

Drug	Typical Adult Dosage[1]
First-line agents (in approximate order of preference)	
Isoniazid	300 mg/d
Rifampin	600 mg/d
Pyrazinamide	25 mg/kg/d
Ethambutol	15–25 mg/kg/d
Streptomycin	15 mg/kg/d
Second-line agents	
Amikacin	15 mg/kg/d
Aminosalicylic acid	8–12 g/d
Capreomycin	15 mg/kg/d
Ciprofloxacin	1500 mg/d, divided
Clofazimine	200 mg/d
Cycloserine	500–1000 mg/d, divided
Ethionamide	500–750 mg/d
Levofloxacin	500 mg/d
Rifabutin	300 mg/d[2]
Rifapentine	600 mg once or twice weekly

[1] Assuming normal renal function.
[2] 150 mg/d if used concurrently with a protease inhibitor.

encodes an NADH-dependent acyl carrier protein reductase; mutation or deletion of the *katG* gene; promoter mutations resulting in overexpression of *ahpC*, a putative virulence gene involved in protection of the cell from oxidative stress; and mutations in *kasA*. Overproducers of *inhA* express low-level isoniazid resistance and cross-resistance to ethionamide. *KatG* mutants express high-level isoniazid resistance and often are not cross-resistant to ethionamide.

Drug-resistant mutants are normally present in susceptible mycobacterial populations at about 1 bacillus in 10^6. Since tuberculous lesions often contain more than 10^8 tubercle bacilli, resistant mutants are readily selected out if isoniazid or any other drug is given as a single agent. The use of two independently acting drugs in combination is much more effective. The probability that a bacillus is resistant to both drugs is approximately 1 in $10^6 \times 10^6$, or 1 in 10^{12}, several orders of magnitude greater than the number of infecting organisms. Thus, at least two (or more in certain cases) active agents should always be used to treat active tuberculosis to prevent emergence of resistance during therapy.

Pharmacokinetics

Isoniazid is readily absorbed from the gastrointestinal tract. A 300-mg oral dose (5 mg/kg in children) achieves peak plasma concentrations of 3–5 mcg/mL within 1–2 hours. Isoniazid diffuses readily into all body fluids and tissues. The concentration in the central nervous system and cerebrospinal fluid ranges between 20% and 100% of simultaneous serum concentrations.

Metabolism of isoniazid, especially acetylation by liver *N*-acetyltransferase, is genetically determined (see Chapter 4). The average plasma concentration of isoniazid in rapid acetylators is about one third to one half of that in slow acetylators, and average half-lives are less than 1 hour and 3 hours, respectively. More rapid clearance of isoniazid by rapid acetylators is usually of no therapeutic consequence when appropriate doses are administered daily, but subtherapeutic concentrations may occur if drug is administered as a once-weekly dose or if there is malabsorption.

Isoniazid metabolites and a small amount of unchanged drug are excreted mainly in the urine. The dose need not be adjusted in renal failure. Dose adjustment is not well defined in patients with severe preexisting hepatic insufficiency (isoniazid is contraindicated if it is the cause of the hepatitis) and should be guided by serum concentrations if a reduction in dose is contemplated.

Clinical Uses

The usual dosage of isoniazid is 5 mg/kg/d; a typical adult dose is 300 mg given once daily. Up to 10 mg/kg/d may be used for serious infections or if malabsorption is a problem. A 15 mg/kg dose, or 900 mg, may be used in a twice-weekly dosing regimen in combination with a second antituberculous agent (eg, rifampin 600 mg). Pyridoxine, 25–50 mg/d, is recommended for those with conditions predisposing to neuropathy, an adverse

Table 47–2. Recommended duration of therapy for tuberculosis.

Regimen (in Approximate Order of Preference)	Duration in Months
Isoniazid, rifampin, pyrazinamide	6
Isoniazid, rifampin	9
Rifampin, ethambutol, pyrazinamide	6
Rifampin, ethambutol	12
Isoniazid, ethambutol	18
All others	≥ 24

effect of isoniazid. Isoniazid is usually given by mouth but can be given parenterally in the same dosage.

Isoniazid as a single agent is also indicated for treatment of latent tuberculosis. The dosage is 300 mg/d (5 mg/kg/d) or 900 mg twice weekly for 9 months.

Adverse Reactions

The incidence and severity of untoward reactions to isoniazid are related to dosage and duration of administration.

A. IMMUNOLOGIC REACTIONS

Fever and skin rashes are occasionally seen. Drug-induced systemic lupus erythematosus has been reported.

B. DIRECT TOXICITY

Isoniazid-induced hepatitis is the most common major toxic effect. This is distinct from the minor increases in liver aminotransferases (up to three or four times normal), which do not require cessation of the drug and which are seen in 10–20% of patients, who usually are asymptomatic. Clinical hepatitis with loss of appetite, nausea, vomiting, jaundice, and right upper quadrant pain occurs in 1% of isoniazid recipients and can be fatal, particularly if the drug is not discontinued promptly. There is histologic evidence of hepatocellular damage and necrosis. The risk of hepatitis depends on age. It occurs rarely under age 20, in 0.3% of those aged 21–35, 1.2% of those aged 36–50, and 2.3% for those aged 50 and above. The risk of hepatitis is greater in alcoholics and possibly during pregnancy and the postpartum period. Development of isoniazid hepatitis contraindicates further use of the drug.

Peripheral neuropathy is observed in 10–20% of patients given dosages greater than 5 mg/kg/d but is infrequently seen with the standard 300 mg adult dose. It is more likely to occur in slow acetylators and patients with predisposing conditions such as malnutrition, alcoholism, diabetes, AIDS, and uremia. Neuropathy is due to a relative pyridoxine deficiency. Isoniazid promotes excretion of pyridoxine, and this toxicity is readily reversed by administration of pyridoxine in a dosage as low as 10 mg/d. Central nervous system toxicity, which is less common, includes memory loss, psychosis, and seizures. These may also respond to pyridoxine.

Miscellaneous other reactions include hematologic abnormalities, provocation of pyridoxine deficiency anemia, tinnitus, and gastrointestinal discomfort. Isoniazid can reduce the metabolism of phenytoin, increasing its blood level and toxicity.

RIFAMPIN

Rifampin is a semisynthetic derivative of rifamycin, an antibiotic produced by *Streptomyces mediterranei*. It is active in vitro against gram-positive and gram-negative cocci, some enteric bacteria, mycobacteria, and chlamydia. Susceptible organisms are inhibited by less than 1 mcg/mL. Resistant mutants are present in all microbial populations at approximately 1 in 10^6 and are rapidly selected out if rifampin is used as a single drug, especially if there is active infection. There is no cross-resistance to other classes of antimicrobial drugs, but there is cross-resistance to other rifamycin derivatives, eg, rifabutin and rifapentine.

Antimycobacterial Activity, Resistance, & Pharmacokinetics

Rifampin binds to the β subunit of bacterial DNA-dependent RNA polymerase and thereby inhibits RNA synthesis. Resistance results from any one of several possible point mutations in *rpoB,* the gene for the β subunit of RNA polymerase. These mutations result in reduced binding of rifampin to RNA polymerase. Human RNA polymerase does not bind rifampin and is not inhibited by it. Rifampin is bactericidal for mycobacteria. It readily penetrates most tissues and into phagocytic cells. It can kill organisms that are poorly accessible to many other drugs, such as intracellular organisms and those sequestered in abscesses and lung cavities.

Rifampin is well absorbed after oral administration and excreted mainly through the liver into bile. It then undergoes enterohepatic recirculation, with the bulk excreted as a deacylated metabolite in feces and a small amount in the urine. Dosage adjustment for renal or hepatic insufficiency is not necessary. Usual doses result in serum levels of 5–7 mcg/mL. Rifampin is distributed widely in body fluids and tissues. Rifampin is relatively highly protein-bound, and adequate cerebrospinal fluid concentrations are achieved only in the presence of meningeal inflammation.

Clinical Uses

A. MYCOBACTERIAL INFECTIONS

Rifampin, usually 600 mg/d (10 mg/kg/d) orally, must be administered with isoniazid or other antituberculous drugs to patients with active tuberculosis to prevent emergence of drug-resistant mycobacteria. In some short-course therapies, 600 mg of rifampin are given twice weekly. Rifampin 600 mg daily or twice weekly for 6 months also is effective in combination with other agents in some atypical mycobacterial infections and in leprosy. Rifampin, 600 mg daily for 4 months as a single drug, is an alternative to isoniazid prophylaxis for patients with latent tuberculosis only who are unable to take isoniazid or who have had exposure to a case of active tuberculosis caused by an isoniazid-resistant, rifampin-susceptible strain.

B. Other Indications

Rifampin has other uses. An oral dosage of 600 mg twice daily for 2 days can eliminate meningococcal carriage. Rifampin, 20 mg/kg/d for 4 days, is used as prophylaxis in contacts of children with *Haemophilus influenzae* type b disease. Rifampin combined with a second agent is used to eradicate staphylococcal carriage. Rifampin combination therapy is also indicated for treatment of serious staphylococcal infections such as osteomyelitis and prosthetic valve endocarditis.

Adverse Reactions

Rifampin imparts a harmless orange color to urine, sweat, tears, and contact lenses (soft lenses may be permanently stained). Occasional adverse effects include rashes, thrombocytopenia, and nephritis. It may cause cholestatic jaundice and occasionally hepatitis. Rifampin commonly causes light-chain proteinuria. If administered less often than twice weekly, rifampin causes a flu-like syndrome characterized by fever, chills, myalgias, anemia, and thrombocytopenia and sometimes is associated with acute tubular necrosis. Rifampin strongly induces most cytochrome P450 isoforms (CYPs 1A2, 2C9, 2C19, 2D6, and 3A4), which increases the elimination of numerous other drugs including methadone, anticoagulants, cyclosporine, some anticonvulsants, protease inhibitors, some nonnucleoside reverse transcriptase inhibitors, contraceptives, and a host of others. Administration of rifampin results in significantly lower serum levels of these drugs.

ETHAMBUTOL

Ethambutol is a synthetic, water-soluble, heat-stable compound, the dextro-isomer of the structure shown below, dispensed as the dihydrochloride salt.

$$CH_2OH \qquad\qquad C_2H_5$$
$$H-C-NH-(CH_2)_2-NH-C-H$$
$$C_2H_5 \qquad\qquad CH_2OH$$

Ethambutol

Susceptible strains of *Mycobacterium tuberculosis* and other mycobacteria are inhibited in vitro by ethambutol, 1–5 mcg/mL. Ethambutol inhibits mycobacterial arabinosyl transferases, which are encoded by the *embCAB* operon. Arabinosyl transferases are involved in the polymerization reaction of arabinoglycan, an essential component of the mycobacterial cell wall. Resistance to ethambutol is due to mutations resulting in overexpression of *emb* gene products or within the *embB* structural gene.

Ethambutol is well absorbed from the gut. After ingestion of 25 mg/kg, a blood level peak of 2–5 mcg/mL is reached in 2–4 hours. About 20% of the drug is excreted in feces and 50% in urine in unchanged form. Ethambutol accumulates in renal failure, and the dose should be reduced by half if creatinine clearance is less than 10 mL/min. Ethambutol crosses the blood-brain barrier only if the meninges are inflamed. Concentrations in cerebrospinal fluid are highly variable, ranging from 4% to 64% of serum levels in the setting of meningeal inflammation.

As with all antituberculous drugs, resistance to ethambutol emerges rapidly when the drug is used alone. Therefore, ethambutol is always given in combination with other antituberculous drugs.

Clinical Use

Ethambutol hydrochloride, 15–25 mg/kg, is usually given as a single daily dose in combination with isoniazid or rifampin. The higher dose is recommended for treatment of tuberculous meningitis. The dose of ethambutol is 50 mg/kg when a twice-weekly dosing schedule is used.

Adverse Reactions

Hypersensitivity to ethambutol is rare. The most common serious adverse event is retrobulbar neuritis, resulting in loss of visual acuity and red-green color blindness. This dose-related side effect is more likely to occur at doses of 25 mg/kg/d continued for several months. At 15 mg/kg/d or less, visual disturbances are very rare. Periodic visual acuity testing is desirable if the 25 mg/kg/d dosage is used. Ethambutol is relatively contraindicated in children too young to permit assessment of visual acuity and red-green color discrimination.

PYRAZINAMIDE

Pyrazinamide (PZA) is a relative of nicotinamide, stable, and slightly soluble in water. It is inactive at neutral pH, but at pH 5.5 it inhibits tubercle bacilli and some other mycobacteria at concentrations of approximately 20 mcg/mL. The drug is taken up by macrophages and exerts its activity against mycobacteria residing within the acidic environment of lysosomes.

Pyrazinamide is converted to pyrazinoic acid—the active form of the drug—by mycobacterial pyrazinamidase, which is encoded by *pncA*. The drug target and mechanism of action are unknown. Resistance may be due to impaired uptake of pyrazinamide or mutations in *pncA* that impair conversion of pyrazinamide to its active form.

Pyrazinamide (PZA)

Clinical Use

Serum concentrations of 30–50 mcg/mL at 1–2 hours after oral administration are achieved with dosages of 25 mg/kg/d. Pyrazinamide is well absorbed from the gastrointestinal tract and widely distributed in body tissues, including inflamed meninges. The half-life is 8–11 hours. The parent compound is metabolized by the liver, but metabolites are renally cleared; therefore, pyrazinamide should be administered at 25–35 mg/kg three times weekly (not daily) in hemodialysis patients and those in whom the creatinine clearance is less than 30 mL/min. In patients with normal renal function, a dose of 40–50 mg/kg is used for thrice-weekly or twice-weekly treatment regimens. Pyrazinamide is an important front-line drug used in conjunction with isoniazid and rifampin in short-course (ie, 6-month) regimens as a "sterilizing" agent active against residual intracellular organisms that may cause relapse. Tubercle bacilli develop resistance to pyrazinamide fairly readily, but there is no cross-resistance with isoniazid or other antimycobacterial drugs.

Adverse Reactions

Major adverse effects of pyrazinamide include hepatotoxicity (in 1–5% of patients), nausea, vomiting, drug fever, and hyperuricemia. The latter occurs uniformly and is not a reason to halt therapy. Hyperuricemia may provoke acute gouty arthritis.

STREPTOMYCIN

The mechanism of action and other pharmacologic features of streptomycin are discussed in Chapter 45. The typical adult dose is 1 g/d (15 mg/kg/d). If the creatinine clearance is less than 30 mL/min or the patient is on hemodialysis, the dose is 15 mg/kg two or three times a week. Most tubercle bacilli are inhibited by streptomycin, 1–10 mcg/mL, in vitro. Nontuberculosis species of mycobacteria other than *Mycobacterium avium* complex (MAC) and *Mycobacterium kansasii* are resistant. All large populations of tubercle bacilli contain some streptomycin-resistant mutants. On average, 1 in 10^8 tubercle bacilli can be expected to be resistant to streptomycin at levels of 10–100 mcg/mL. Resistance is due to a point mutation in either the *rpsL* gene encoding the S12 ribosomal protein gene or the *rrs* gene encoding 16S ribosomal rRNA, which alters the ribosomal binding site.

Streptomycin penetrates into cells poorly and is active mainly against extracellular tubercle bacilli. Streptomycin crosses the blood-brain barrier and achieves therapeutic concentrations with inflamed meninges.

Clinical Use in Tuberculosis

Streptomycin sulfate is used when an injectable drug is needed or desirable, principally in individuals with severe, possibly life-threatening forms of tuberculosis, eg, meningitis and disseminated disease, and in treatment of infections resistant to other drugs. The usual dosage is 15 mg/kg/d intramuscularly or intravenously daily for adults (20–40 mg/kg/d, not to exceed 1–1.5 g for children) for several weeks, followed by 1–1.5 g two or three times weekly for several months. Serum concentrations of approximately 40 mcg/mL are achieved 30–60 minutes after intramuscular injection of a 15 mg/kg dose. Other drugs are always given in combination to prevent emergence of resistance.

Adverse Reactions

Streptomycin is ototoxic and nephrotoxic. Vertigo and hearing loss are the most common side effects and may be permanent. Toxicity is dose-related, and the risk is increased in the elderly. As with all aminoglycosides, the dose must be adjusted according to renal function (see Chapter 45). Toxicity can be reduced by limiting therapy to no more than 6 months whenever possible.

ALTERNATIVE SECOND-LINE DRUGS FOR TUBERCULOSIS

The alternative drugs listed below are usually considered only (1) in case of resistance to first-line agents; (2) in case of failure of clinical response to conventional therapy; (3) in case of serious treatment-limiting adverse drug reactions; and (4) when expert guidance is available to deal with the toxic effects. For many of the second-line drugs listed in the following text, the dosage, emergence of resistance, and long-term toxicity have not been fully established.

Ethionamide

Ethionamide is chemically related to isoniazid and also blocks the synthesis of mycolic acids. It is poorly water-soluble and available only in oral form. It is metabolized by the liver.

Ethionamide

Most tubercle bacilli are inhibited in vitro by ethionamide, 2.5 mcg/mL or less. Some other species of mycobacteria also are inhibited by ethionamide, 10 mcg/mL. Serum concentrations in plasma and tissues of approximately 20 mcg/mL are achieved by a dosage of 1 g/d. Cerebrospinal fluid concentrations are equal to those in serum.

Ethionamide is administered at an initial dose of 250 mg once daily, which is increased in 250-mg increments to the recommended dosage of 1 g/d (or 15 mg/kg/d), if possible. The 1 g/d dosage, although theoretically desirable, is poorly tolerated because of the intense gastric irritation and neurologic symptoms that commonly occur, and one often must settle for a total daily dose of 500–750 mg. Ethionamide is also hepatotoxic. Neurologic symptoms may be alleviated by pyridoxine.

Resistance to ethionamide as a single agent develops rapidly in vitro and in vivo. There can be low-level cross-resistance between isoniazid and ethionamide.

Capreomycin

Capreomycin is a peptide protein synthesis inhibitor antibiotic obtained from *Streptomyces capreolus.* Daily injection of 1 g intramuscularly results in blood levels of 10 mcg/mL or more. Such concentrations in vitro are inhibitory for many mycobacteria, including multidrug-resistant strains of *M tuberculosis.*

Capreomycin (15 mg/kg/d) is an important injectable agent for treatment of drug-resistant tuberculosis. Strains of *M tuberculosis* that are resistant to streptomycin or amikacin (eg, the multidrug-resistant W strain) usually are susceptible to capreomycin. Resistance to capreomycin, when it occurs, may be due to an *rrs* mutation.

Capreomycin is nephrotoxic and ototoxic. Tinnitus, deafness, and vestibular disturbances occur. The injection causes significant local pain, and sterile abscesses may occur.

Dosing of capreomycin is the same as that of streptomycin. Toxicity is reduced if 1 g is given two or three times weekly after an initial response has been achieved with a daily dosing schedule.

Cycloserine

Cycloserine is an inhibitor of cell wall synthesis and is discussed in Chapter 43. Concentrations of 15–20 mcg/mL inhibit many strains of *M tuberculosis.* The dosage of cycloserine in tuberculosis is 0.5–1 g/d in two divided doses. Cycloserine is cleared renally, and the dose should be reduced by half if creatinine clearance is less than 50 mL/min.

The most serious toxic effects are peripheral neuropathy and central nervous system dysfunction, including depression and psychotic reactions. Pyridoxine 150 mg/d should be given with cycloserine because this ameliorates neurologic toxicity. Adverse effects, which are most common during the first 2 weeks of therapy, occur in 25% or more of patients, especially at higher doses. Side effects can be minimized by monitoring peak serum concentrations. The peak concentration is reached 2–4 hours after dosing. The recommended range of peak concentrations is 20–40 mcg/mL.

Aminosalicylic Acid (PAS)

Aminosalicylic acid is a folate synthesis antagonist that is active almost exclusively against *M tuberculosis.* It is structurally similar to *p*-aminobenzoic aid (PABA) and to the sulfonamides (see Chapter 46).

Aminosalicylic acid (PAS)

Tubercle bacilli are usually inhibited in vitro by aminosalicylic acid, 1–5 mcg/mL. Aminosalicylic acid is readily absorbed from the gastrointestinal tract. Serum levels are 50 mcg/mL or more after a 4-g oral dose. The dosage is 8–12 g/d orally for adults and 300 mg/kg/d for children. The drug is widely distributed in tissues and body fluids except the cerebrospinal fluid. Aminosalicylic acid is rapidly excreted in the urine, in part as active aminosalicylic acid and in part as the acetylated compound and other metabolic products. Very high concentrations of aminosalicylic acid are reached in the urine, which can result in crystalluria.

Aminosalicylic acid is used infrequently now because other oral drugs are better tolerated. Gastrointestinal symptoms are common and may be diminished by giving the drug with meals and with antacids. Peptic ulceration and hemorrhage may occur. Hypersensitivity reactions manifested by fever, joint pains, skin rashes, hepatosplenomegaly, hepatitis, adenopathy, and granulocytopenia often occur after 3–8 weeks of aminosalicylic acid therapy, making it necessary to stop aminosalicylic acid administration temporarily or permanently.

Kanamycin & Amikacin

The aminoglycoside antibiotics are discussed in Chapter 45. Kanamycin has been used for treatment of tuberculosis caused by streptomycin-resistant strains, but the availability of less toxic alternatives (eg, capreomycin and amikacin) has rendered it obsolete.

The role of amikacin in treatment of tuberculosis has increased with the increasing incidence and prevalence of multidrug-resistant tuberculosis. Prevalence of amikacin-resistant strains is low (less than 5%), and most multidrug-resistant strains remain amikacin-susceptible. *M tuberculosis* is inhibited at concentrations of 1 mcg/mL or less. Amikacin is also active against atypical mycobacteria. There is no cross-resistance between streptomycin and amikacin, but kanamycin resistance often indicates resistance to amikacin as well. Serum concentrations of 30–50 mcg/mL are achieved 30–60 minutes after a 15 mg/kg intravenous infusion. Amikacin is indicated for treatment of tuberculosis suspected or known to be caused by streptomycin-resistant or multidrug-resistant strains. Amikacin must be used in combination with at least one and preferably two or three other drugs to which the isolate is susceptible for treatment of drug-resistant cases. The recommended dosages are the same as that for streptomycin.

Fluoroquinolones

In addition to their activity against many gram-positive and gram-negative bacteria (discussed in Chapter 46), ciprofloxacin, levofloxacin, gatifloxacin, and moxifloxacin inhibit strains of *M tuberculosis* at concentrations less than 2 mcg/mL. They are also active against atypical mycobacteria. Moxifloxacin is the most active against *M tuberculosis* by weight in vitro. Levofloxacin tends to be slightly more active than ciprofloxacin against *M tuberculosis,* whereas ciprofloxacin is slightly more active against atypical mycobacteria.

Fluoroquinolones are an important addition to the drugs available for tuberculosis, especially for strains that are resistant to first-line agents. Resistance, which may result from any one of several single point mutations in the gyrase A subunit, develops rapidly if a fluoroquinolone is used as a single agent; thus, the drug must be used in combination with two or more other active agents. The standard dosage of ciprofloxacin is 750 mg orally twice a day. The dosage of levofloxacin is 500–750 mg once a day. The dosage of moxifloxacin is 400 mg once a day.

Linezolid

Linezolid (discussed in Chapter 44) inhibits strains of *M tuberculosis* in vitro at concentrations of 4 to 8 mcg/mL. It achieves good intracellular concentrations, and it is active in murine models of tuberculosis. Linezolid has been used in combination with other second- and third-line drugs to treat patients with tuberculosis caused by multidrug-resistant strains. Conversion of sputum cultures to negative was associated with linezolid use in these cases, and some may have been cured. Significant and at times treatment-limiting adverse effects, including bone marrow suppression and irreversible peripheral and optic neuropathy, have been reported with the prolonged courses of therapy that are necessary for treatment of tuberculosis. A 600-mg (adult) dose administered once a day (half of that used for treatment of other bacterial infections) seems to be sufficient and may limit the occurrence of these adverse effects. Although linezolid may eventually prove to be an important new agent for treatment of

tuberculosis, at this point it should be considered a drug of last resort for infection caused by multidrug-resistant strains that also are resistant to several other first- and second-line agents.

Rifabutin (Ansamycin)

Rifabutin is derived from rifamycin and is related to rifampin. It has significant activity against *M tuberculosis, M avium-intracellulare,* and *M fortuitum* (see below). Its activity is similar to that of rifampin, and cross-resistance with rifampin is virtually complete. Some rifampin-resistant strains may appear susceptible to rifabutin in vitro, but a clinical response is unlikely because the molecular basis of resistance, *rpoB* mutation, is the same. Rifabutin is both substrate and inducer of cytochrome P450 enzymes. Because it is a less potent inducer, rifabutin is indicated in place of rifampin for treatment of tuberculosis in HIV-infected patients who are receiving concurrent antiretroviral therapy with a protease inhibitor or nonnucleoside reverse transcriptase inhibitor (eg, efavirenz)—drugs that also are cytochrome P450 substrates.

The usual dose of rifabutin is 300 mg/d unless the patient is receiving a protease inhibitor, in which case the dose should be reduced to 150 mg/d. If efavirenz (also a P450 inducer) is used, the recommended dose of rifabutin is 450 mg/d.

Rifabutin is effective in prevention and treatment of disseminated atypical mycobacterial infection in AIDS patients with CD4 counts below 50/μL. It is also effective for preventive therapy of tuberculosis, either alone in a 3–4 month regimen or with pyrazinamide in a 2-month regimen.

Rifapentine

Rifapentine is an analog of rifampin. It is active against both *M tuberculosis* and *M avium.* As with all rifamycins, it is a bacterial RNA polymerase inhibitor, and cross-resistance between rifampin and rifapentine is complete. Like rifampin, rifapentine is a potent inducer of cytochrome P450 enzymes, and it has the same drug interaction profile. Toxicity is similar to that of rifampin. Rifapentine and its microbiologically active metabolite, 25-desacetylrifapentine, have an elimination half-life of 13 hours. Rifapentine 600 mg (10 mg/kg) once weekly is indicated for treatment of tuberculosis caused by rifampin-susceptible strains during the continuation phase only (ie, after the first 2 months of therapy and ideally after conversion of sputum cultures to negative). Rifapentine should not be used to treat HIV-infected patients because of an unacceptably high relapse rate with rifampin-resistant organisms.

Table 47–3. Clinical features and treatment options for infections with atypical mycobacteria.

Species	Clinical Features	Treatment Options
M kansasii	Resembles tuberculosis	Ciprofloxacin, clarithromycin, ethambutol, isoniazid, rifampin, trimethoprim-sulfamethoxazole
M marinum	Granulomatous cutaneous disease	Amikacin, clarithromycin, ethambutol, doxycycline, minocycline, rifampin, trimethoprim-sulfamethoxazole
M scrofulaceum	Cervical adenitis in children	Amikacin, erythromycin (or other macrolide), rifampin, streptomycin (Surgical excision is often curative and the treatment of choice.)
M avium complex	Pulmonary disease in patients with chronic lung disease; disseminated infection in AIDS	Amikacin, azithromycin, clarithromycin, ciprofloxacin, ethambutol, rifabutin
M chelonae	Abscess, sinus tract, ulcer; bone, joint, tendon infection	Amikacin, doxycycline, imipenem, macrolides, tobramycin
M fortuitum	Abscess, sinus tract, ulcer; bone, joint, tendon infection	Amikacin, cefoxitin, ciprofloxacin, doxycycline, ofloxacin, trimethoprim-sulfamethoxazole
M ulcerans	Skin ulcers	Isoniazid, streptomycin, rifampin, minocycline (Surgical excision may be effective.)

◼ DRUGS ACTIVE AGAINST ATYPICAL MYCOBACTERIA

About 10% of mycobacterial infections seen in clinical practice in the USA are caused not by *M tuberculosis* or *M tuberculosis* complex organisms, but by nontuberculous or so-called "atypical" mycobacteria. These organisms have distinctive laboratory characteristics, are present in the environment, and are not communicable from person to person. As a rule, these mycobacterial species are less susceptible than *M tuberculosis* to antituberculous drugs. On the other hand, agents such as erythromycin, sulfonamides, or tetracycline, which are not active against *M tuberculosis,* may be effective for infections caused by atypical strains. Emergence of resistance during therapy is also a problem with these mycobacterial species, and active infection should be treated with combinations of drugs. *M kansasii* is susceptible to rifampin and ethambutol, partially resistant to isoniazid, and completely resistant to pyrazinamide. A three-drug combination of isoniazid, rifampin, and ethambutol is the conventional treatment for *M kansasii* infection. A few representative pathogens, with the clinical presentation and the drugs to which they are often susceptible, are given in Table 47–3.

M avium complex, which includes both *M avium* and *M intracellulare,* is an important and common cause of disseminated disease in late stages of AIDS (CD4 counts < 50/μL). *M avium* complex is much less susceptible than *M tuberculosis* to most antituberculous drugs. Combinations of agents are required to suppress the disease. Azithromycin, 500 mg once daily, or clarithromycin, 500 mg twice daily, plus ethambutol, 15–25 mg/kg/d, is an effective and well-tolerated regimen for treatment of disseminated disease. Some authorities recommend use of a third agent, such as ciprofloxacin 750 mg twice daily or rifabutin, 300 mg once daily. Other agents that may be useful are listed in Table 47–3. Rifabutin in a single daily dose of 300 mg has been shown to reduce the incidence of *M avium* complex bacteremia in AIDS patients with CD4 less than 100/μL. Clarithromycin also effectively prevents MAC bacteremia in AIDS patients, but if breakthrough bacteremia occurs, the isolate often is resistant to both clarithromycin and azithromycin, precluding the use of the most effective drugs for treatment.

◼ DRUGS USED IN LEPROSY

Mycobacterium leprae has never been grown in vitro, but animal models, such as growth in injected mouse footpads, have permitted laboratory evaluation of drugs. Only those drugs that have the widest clinical use are presented here. Because of increasing reports of dapsone resistance, treatment of leprosy with combinations of the drugs listed below is recommended.

DAPSONE & OTHER SULFONES

Several drugs closely related to the sulfonamides have been used effectively in the long-term treatment of leprosy. The most widely used is dapsone (diaminodiphenylsulfone). Like the sulfonamides, it inhibits folate synthesis. Resistance can emerge in large populations of *M leprae*, eg, in lepromatous leprosy, if very low doses are given. Therefore, the combination of dapsone, rifampin, and clofazimine is recommended for initial therapy. Dapsone may also be used to prevent and treat *Pneumocystis jiroveci* pneumonia in AIDS patients.

Dapsone

Sulfones are well absorbed from the gut and widely distributed throughout body fluids and tissues. Dapsone's half-life is 1–2 days, and drug tends to be retained in skin, muscle, liver, and kidney. Skin heavily infected with *M leprae* may contain several times more drug than normal skin. Sulfones are excreted into bile and reabsorbed in the intestine. Excretion into urine is variable, and most excreted drug is acetylated. In renal failure, the dose may have to be adjusted. The usual adult dosage in leprosy is 100 mg daily. For children, the dose is proportionately less depending on weight.

Dapsone is usually well tolerated. Many patients develop some hemolysis, particularly if they have glucose-6-phosphate dehydrogenase deficiency. Methemoglobinemia is common, but usually is not a problem clinically. Gastrointestinal intolerance, fever, pruritus, and various rashes occur. During dapsone therapy of lepromatous leprosy, erythema nodosum leprosum often develops. It is sometimes difficult to distinguish reactions to dapsone from manifestations of the underlying illness. Erythema nodosum leprosum may be suppressed by **corticosteroids** or by **thalidomide.**

RIFAMPIN

Rifampin (see earlier discussion) in a dosage of 600 mg daily is highly effective in lepromatous leprosy. Because of the probable risk of emergence of rifampin-resistant *M leprae*, the drug is given in combination with dapsone or another antileprosy drug. A single monthly dose of 600 mg may be beneficial in combination therapy.

CLOFAZIMINE

Clofazimine is a phenazine dye that can be used as an alternative to dapsone. Its mechanism of action is unknown but may involve DNA binding.

Absorption of clofazimine from the gut is variable, and a major portion of the drug is excreted in feces. Clofazimine is stored widely in reticuloendothelial tissues and skin, and its crystals can be seen inside phagocytic reticuloendothelial cells. It is slowly released from these deposits, so that the serum half-life may be 2 months.

Clofazimine is given for sulfone-resistant leprosy or when patients are intolerant to sulfones. A common dosage is 100 mg/d orally. The most prominent untoward effect is skin discoloration ranging from red-brown to nearly black. Gastrointestinal intolerance occurs occasionally.

PREPARATIONS AVAILABLE

DRUGS USED IN TUBERCULOSIS

Aminosalicylate sodium (Paser)
  Oral: 4 g delayed-release granules
Capreomycin (Capastat Sulfate)
  Parenteral: 1 g powder to reconstitute for injection
Cycloserine (Seromycin Pulvules)
  Oral: 250 mg capsules
Ethambutol (Myambutol)
  Oral: 100, 400 mg tablets
Ethionamide (Trecator-SC)
  Oral: 250 mg tablets
Isoniazid (generic)
  Oral: 100, 300 mg tablets; syrup, 50 mg/5 mL
  Parenteral: 100 mg/mL for injection
Pyrazinamide (generic)
  Oral: 500 mg tablets

Rifabutin (Mycobutin)
  Oral: 150 mg capsules
Rifampin (generic, Rifadin, Rimactane)
  Oral: 150, 300 mg capsules
  Parenteral: 600 mg powder for IV injection
Rifapentine (Priftin)
  Oral: 150 mg tablets
Streptomycin (generic)
  Parenteral: 1 g lyophilized for IM injection

DRUGS USED IN LEPROSY

Clofazimine (Lamprene)
  Oral: 50 mg capsules
Dapsone (generic)
  Oral: 25, 100 mg tablets

REFERENCES

Anonymous: Update: Adverse event data and revised American Thoracic Society/CDC recommendations against the use of rifampin and pyrazinamide for treatment of latent tuberculosis infection–United States, 2003. MMWR Morb Mortal Wkly Rep. 2003;52:735.

Anonymous: Diagnosis and treatment of disease caused by nontuberculous mycobacteria. Am J Respir Crit Care Med 1997; 156(2 Part 2):S1.

Anonymous: Targeted tuberculin testing and treatment of latent tuberculosis infection. Am J Respir Crit Care Med 2000; 161(4 Part 2):S221.

Gillespie SH et al: Early bactericidal activity of a moxifloxacin and isoniazid combination in smear-positive pulmonary tuberculosis. J Antimicrob Chemother 2005;56:1169.

Jasmer RM, Nahid P, Hopewell PC: Latent tuberculosis infection. N Engl J Med 2002;347:1860.

Kinzig-Schippers M et al: Should we use *N*-acetyltransferase type 2 genotyping to personalize isoniazid doses? Antimicrob Agents Chemother 2005;49:1733.

Sulochana S, Rahman F, Paramasivan CN: In vitro activity of fluoroquinolones against *Mycobacterium tuberculosis*. J Chemother 2005;17:169.

von der Lippe B, Sandven P, Brubakk O: Efficacy and safety of linezolid in multidrug resistant tuberculosis (MDR-TB)—a report of ten cases. J Infect 2006;52:92.

Antifungal Agents

Don Sheppard, MD, & Harry W. Lampiris, MD

Human fungal infections have increased dramatically in incidence and severity in recent years, owing mainly to advances in surgery, cancer treatment, and critical care accompanied by increases in the use of broad-spectrum antimicrobials and the HIV epidemic. These changes have resulted in increased numbers of patients at risk for fungal infections.

Pharmacotherapy of fungal disease has been revolutionized by the introduction of the relatively nontoxic oral azole drugs and the echinocandins. Combination therapy is being reconsidered, and new formulations of old agents are becoming available. Unfortunately, the appearance of azole-resistant organisms, as well as the rise in the number of patients at risk for mycotic infections, has created new challenges.

The antifungal drugs presently available fall into several categories: systemic drugs (oral or parenteral) for systemic infections, oral drugs for mucocutaneous infections, and topical drugs for mucocutaneous infections.

■ SYSTEMIC ANTIFUNGAL DRUGS FOR SYSTEMIC INFECTIONS

AMPHOTERICIN B

Amphotericin A and B are antifungal antibiotics produced by *Streptomyces nodosus*. Amphotericin A is not in clinical use.

Chemistry

Amphotericin B is an amphoteric polyene macrolide (polyene = containing many double bonds; macrolide = containing a large lactone ring of 12 or more atoms). It is nearly insoluble in water and is therefore prepared as a colloidal suspension of amphotericin B and sodium desoxycholate for intravenous injection. Several new formulations have been developed in which amphotericin B is packaged in a lipid-associated delivery system (Table 48–1 and Box: Liposomal Amphotericin B).

Pharmacokinetics

Amphotericin B is poorly absorbed from the gastrointestinal tract. Oral amphotericin B is thus effective only on fungi within the lumen of the tract and cannot be used for treatment of systemic disease. The intravenous injection of 0.6 mg/kg/d of amphotericin B results in average blood levels of 0.3–1 mcg/mL; the drug is more than 90% bound by serum proteins. Although it is mostly metabolized, some amphotericin B is excreted slowly in the urine over a period of several days. The serum $t_{1/2}$ is approximately 15 days. Hepatic impairment, renal impairment, and dialysis have little impact on drug concentrations, and therefore no dose adjustment is required. The drug is widely distributed in most tissues, but only 2–3% of the blood level is reached in cerebrospinal fluid, thus occasionally necessitating intrathecal therapy for certain types of fungal meningitis.

Amphotericin B

LIPOSOMAL AMPHOTERICIN B

Therapy with amphotericin B is often limited by toxicity, especially drug-induced renal impairment. This has led to the development of lipid drug formulations on the assumption that lipid-packaged drug binds to the mammalian membrane less readily, permitting the use of effective doses of the drug with lower toxicity. Liposomal amphotericin preparations package the active drug in lipid delivery vehicles, in contrast to the colloidal suspensions, which were previously the only available forms. Amphotericin binds to the lipids in these vehicles with an affinity between that for fungal ergosterol and that for human cholesterol. The lipid vehicle then serves as an amphotericin reservoir, reducing nonspecific binding to human cell membranes. This preferential binding allows for a reduction of toxicity without sacrificing efficacy and permits use of larger doses. Furthermore, some fungi contain lipases that may liberate free amphotericin B directly at the site of infection.

Three such formulations are now available and have differing pharmacologic properties as summarized in Table 48–1. Although clinical trials have demonstrated different renal and infusion-related toxicities for these preparations compared with regular amphotericin B, there are no trials comparing the different formulations with each other. Limited studies have suggested at best a moderate improvement in the clinical efficacy of the lipid formulations compared with conventional amphotericin B. Because the lipid preparations are much more expensive, their use is usually restricted to patients intolerant to, or not responding to, conventional amphotericin treatment.

Mechanism of Action

Amphotericin B is selective in its fungicidal effect because it exploits the difference in lipid composition of fungal and mammalian cell membranes. **Ergosterol,** a cell membrane sterol, is found in the cell membrane of fungi, whereas the predominant sterol of bacteria and human cells is **cholesterol.** Amphotericin B binds to ergosterol and alters the permeability of the cell by forming amphotericin B-associated pores in the cell membrane. As suggested by its chemistry, amphotericin B combines avidly with lipids (ergosterol) along the double bond-rich side of its structure and associates with water molecules along the hydroxyl-rich side. This amphipathic characteristic facilitates pore formation by multiple amphotericin molecules, with the lipophilic portions around the outside of the pore and the hydrophilic regions lining the inside. The pore allows the leakage of intracellular ions and macromolecules, eventually leading to cell death. Some binding to human membrane sterols does occur, probably accounting for the drug's prominent toxicity.

Resistance to amphotericin B occurs if ergosterol binding is impaired, either by decreasing the membrane concentration of ergosterol or by modifying the sterol target molecule to reduce its affinity for the drug.

Antifungal Activity

Amphotericin B remains the antifungal agent with the broadest spectrum of action. It has activity against the clinically significant yeasts, including *Candida albicans* and *Cryptococcus neoformans;* the organisms causing endemic mycoses, including *Histoplasma capsulatum, Blastomyces dermatitidis,* and *Coccidioides immitis;* and the pathogenic molds, such as *Aspergillus fumigatus* and

---

Table 48–1. Properties of conventional amphotericin B and some lipid formulations.[1]

Drug	Physical Form	Dosing (mg/kg/d)	C_{max}	Clearance	Nephro-toxicity	Infusional Toxicity	Daily Cost
Conventional formulation							
Fungizone	Micelles	1	--	--	--	--	24
Lipid formulations							
AmBisome	Spheres	3–5	↑	↓	↓	↓	1300
Amphotec	Disks	5	↓	↑	↓	↑(?)	660
Abelcet	Ribbons	5	↓	↑	↓	↓(?)	570

[1]Changes in C_{max} (peak plasma concentration), clearance, nephrotoxicity, and infusional toxicity are relative to conventional amphotercin B.

mucor. Some fungal organisms such as *Candida lusitaniae* and *Pseudallescheria boydii* display intrinsic amphotericin B resistance.

Clinical Use

Owing to its broad spectrum of activity and fungicidal action, amphotericin B remains a useful agent for nearly all life-threatening mycotic infections, although newer less toxic agents have begun to replace amphotericin B for many conditions. It is often used as the initial induction regimen for serious fungal infections and is then replaced by one of the newer azole drugs (described below) for chronic therapy or prevention of relapse. Such induction therapy is especially important for immunosuppressed patients and those with severe fungal pneumonia, cryptococcal meningitis with altered mental status, or sepsis syndrome due to fungal infection. Once a clinical response has been elicited, these patients then often continue maintenance therapy with an azole; therapy may be lifelong in patients at high risk for disease relapse. Amphotericin has also been used as empiric therapy for selected patients in whom the risks of leaving a systemic fungal infection untreated are high. The most common such patient is the cancer patient with neutropenia who remains febrile on broad-spectrum antibiotics.

For treatment of systemic fungal disease, amphotericin B is given by slow intravenous infusion at a dosage of 0.5–1 mg/kg/d. It is usually continued to a defined total dose (eg, 1–2 g), rather than a defined time span, as used with other antimicrobial drugs.

Intrathecal therapy for fungal meningitis is poorly tolerated and fraught with difficulties related to maintaining cerebrospinal fluid access. Thus, intrathecal therapy with amphotericin B is being increasingly supplanted by other therapies but remains an option in cases of fungal central nervous system infections that have not responded to other agents.

Local administration of amphotericin B has been used with success. Mycotic corneal ulcers and keratitis can be cured with topical drops as well as by direct subconjunctival injection. Fungal arthritis has been treated with adjunctive local injection directly into the joint. Candiduria responds to bladder irrigation with amphotericin B, and this route has been shown to produce no significant systemic toxicity.

Adverse Effects

The toxicity of amphotericin B can be divided into two broad categories: immediate reactions, related to the infusion of the drug, and those occurring more slowly.

A. INFUSION-RELATED TOXICITY

These infusion-related reactions are nearly universal and consist of fever, chills, muscle spasms, vomiting, headache,

and hypotension. They can be ameliorated by slowing the infusion rate or decreasing the daily dose. Premedication with antipyretics, antihistamines, meperidine, or corticosteroids can be helpful. When starting therapy, many clinicians administer a test dose of 1 mg intravenously to gauge the severity of the reaction. This can serve as a guide to an initial dosing regimen and premedication strategy.

B. CUMULATIVE TOXICITY

Renal damage is the most significant toxic reaction. Renal impairment occurs in nearly all patients treated with clinically significant doses of amphotericin. The degree of azotemia is variable and often stabilizes during therapy, but it can be serious enough to necessitate dialysis. A reversible component is associated with decreased renal perfusion and represents a form of prerenal renal failure. An irreversible component results from renal tubular injury and subsequent dysfunction. The irreversible form of amphotericin nephrotoxicity usually occurs in the setting of prolonged administration (> 4 g cumulative dose). Renal toxicity commonly manifests as renal tubular acidosis and severe potassium and magnesium wasting. There is some evidence that the prerenal component can be attenuated with sodium loading, and it is common practice to administer normal saline infusions with the daily doses of amphotericin B.

Abnormalities of liver function tests are occasionally seen, as is a varying degree of anemia due to reduced erythropoietin production by damaged renal tubular cells. After intrathecal therapy with amphotericin, seizures and a chemical arachnoiditis may develop, often with serious neurologic sequelae.

FLUCYTOSINE

Flucytosine (5-FC) was discovered in 1957 during a search for novel antineoplastic agents. Though devoid of anticancer properties, it became apparent that it was a potent antifungal agent. Flucytosine is a water-soluble pyrimidine analog related to the chemotherapeutic agent fluorouracil (5-FU). Its spectrum of action is much narrower than that of amphotericin B.

Flucytosine

Pharmacokinetics

Flucytosine is currently available in North America only in an oral formulation. The dosage is 100–150 mg/kg/d in patients with normal renal function. It is well absorbed (> 90%), with serum concentrations peaking 1–2 hours after an oral dose. It is poorly protein-bound and penetrates well into all body fluid compartments, including the cerebrospinal fluid. It is eliminated by glomerular filtration with a half-life of 3–4 hours and is removed by hemodialysis. Levels rise rapidly with renal impairment and can lead to toxicity. Toxicity is more likely to occur in AIDS patients and those with renal insufficiency. Peak serum concentrations should be measured periodically in patients with renal insufficiency and maintained between 50 and 100 mcg/mL.

Mechanism of Action

Flucytosine is taken up by fungal cells via the enzyme cytosine permease. It is converted intracellularly first to 5-FU and then to 5-fluorodeoxyuridine monophosphate (FdUMP) and fluorouridine triphosphate (FUTP), which inhibit DNA and RNA synthesis, respectively. Human cells are unable to convert the parent drug to its active metabolites.

Synergy with amphotericin B has been demonstrated in vitro and in vivo. It may be related to enhanced penetration of the flucytosine through amphotericin-damaged fungal cell membranes. In vitro synergy with azole drugs has also been seen, although the mechanism is unclear.

Resistance is thought to be mediated through altered metabolism of flucytosine, and, though uncommon in primary isolates, it develops rapidly in the course of flucytosine monotherapy.

Clinical Use

The spectrum of activity of flucytosine is restricted to *Cryptococcus neoformans,* some candida species, and the dematiaceous molds that cause chromoblastomycosis. Flucytosine is not used as a single agent because of its demonstrated synergy with other agents and to avoid the development of secondary resistance. Clinical use at present is confined to combination therapy, either with amphotericin B for cryptococcal meningitis or with itraconazole for chromoblastomycosis.

Adverse Effects

The adverse effects of flucytosine result from metabolism (possibly by intestinal flora) to the toxic antineoplastic compound fluorouracil. Bone marrow toxicity with anemia, leukopenia, and thrombocytopenia are the most common adverse effects, with derangement of liver enzymes occurring less frequently. A form of toxic enterocolitis can occur. There seems to be a narrow therapeutic window, with an increased risk of toxicity at higher drug levels and resistance developing rapidly

at subtherapeutic concentrations. The use of drug concentration measurements may be helpful in reducing the incidence of toxic reactions, especially when flucytosine is combined with nephrotoxic agents such as amphotericin B.

AZOLES

Azoles are synthetic compounds that can be classified as either imidazoles or triazoles according to the number of nitrogen atoms in the five-membered azole ring as indicated below. The imidazoles consist of ketoconazole, miconazole, and clotrimazole (Figure 48–1). The latter two drugs are now used only in topical therapy. The triazoles include itraconazole, fluconazole, and voriconazole.

X = C, imidazole
X = N, triazole

Azole nucleus

Pharmacology

The pharmacology of each of the azoles is unique and accounts for some of the variations in clinical use. Table 48–2 summarizes the differences among four of the azoles.

Mechanism of Action

The antifungal activity of azole drugs results from the reduction of ergosterol synthesis by inhibition of fungal cytochrome P450 enzymes. The specificity of azole drugs results from their greater affinity for fungal than for human cytochrome P450 enzymes. Imidazoles exhibit a lesser degree of specificity than the triazoles, accounting for their higher incidence of drug interactions and side effects.

Resistance to azoles occurs via multiple mechanisms. Once rare, increasing numbers of resistant strains are being reported, suggesting that increasing use of these agents for prophylaxis and therapy may be selecting for clinical drug resistance in certain settings.

Clinical Use

The spectrum of action of azole medications is broad, ranging from many candida species, *Cryptococcus neoformans,* the endemic mycoses (blastomycosis, coccidioidomycosis, histoplasmosis), the dermatophytes, and, in the case of itraconazole and voriconazole, even aspergillus infections. They are also useful in the treatment of intrinsically amphotericin-resistant organisms such as *Pseudallescheria boydii.*

Clotrimazole

Miconazole

Voriconazole

Itraconazole

Ketoconazole

Fluconazole

Figure 48–1. Structural formulas of some antifungal azoles.

Adverse Effects

As a group, the azoles are relatively nontoxic. The most common adverse reaction is relatively minor gastrointestinal upset. All azoles have been reported to cause abnormalities in liver enzymes and, very rarely, clinical hepatitis. Adverse effects specific to individual agents are discussed below.

Drug Interactions

All azole drugs affect the mammalian cytochrome P450 system of enzymes to some extent, and consequently they are prone to drug interactions. The most significant reactions are indicated below.

1. Ketoconazole

Ketoconazole was the first oral azole introduced into clinical use. It is distinguished from triazoles by its greater propensity to inhibit mammalian cytochrome P450 enzymes; that is, it is less selective for fungal P450 than are the newer azoles. As a result, systemic ketoconazole has fallen out of clinical use in the USA and is not discussed in any detail here. Its dermatologic use is discussed in Chapter 62.

2. Itraconazole

Itraconazole is available in oral and intravenous formulations and is used at a dosage of 100–400 mg/d. Drug

Table 48–2. Pharmacologic properties of four systemic azole drugs.

	Water Solubility	Absorption	CSF:Serum Concentration Ratio	$t_{1/2}$ (Hours)	Elimination	Formulations
Ketoconazole	Low	Variable	< 0.1	7–10	Hepatic	Oral
Itraconazole	Low	Variable	< 0.01	24–42	Hepatic	Oral, IV
Fluconazole	High	High	> 0.7	22–31	Renal	Oral, IV
Voriconazole	High	High	...	6	Hepatic	Oral, IV

absorption is increased by food and by low gastric pH. Like other lipid-soluble azoles, it interacts with hepatic microsomal enzymes, though to a lesser degree than ketoconazole. An important drug interaction is reduced bioavailability of itraconazole when taken with rifamycins (rifampin, rifabutin, rifapentine). It does not affect mammalian steroid synthesis, and its effects on the metabolism of other hepatically cleared medications are much less than those of ketoconazole. While itraconazole displays potent antifungal activity, effectiveness can be limited by reduced bioavailability. Newer formulations, including an oral liquid and an intravenous preparation, have utilized cyclodextran as a carrier molecule to enhance solubility and bioavailability. Like ketoconazole, it penetrates poorly into the cerebrospinal fluid. Itraconazole is the azole of choice for treatment of disease due to the dimorphic fungi histoplasma, blastomyces, and sporothrix. Itraconazole has activity against aspergillus species, but it has been replaced by voriconazole as the azole of choice for aspergillosis. Itraconazole is used extensively in the treatment of dermatophytoses and onychomycosis.

3. Fluconazole

Fluconazole displays a high degree of water solubility and good cerebrospinal fluid penetration. Unlike ketoconazole and itraconazole, its oral bioavailability is high. Drug interactions are also less common because fluconazole has the least effect of all the azoles on hepatic microsomal enzymes. Because of fewer hepatic enzyme interactions and better gastrointestinal tolerance, fluconazole has the widest therapeutic index of the azoles, permitting more aggressive dosing in a variety of fungal infections. The drug is available in oral and intravenous formulations and is used at a dosage of 100–800 mg/d.

Fluconazole is the azole of choice in the treatment and secondary prophylaxis of cryptococcal meningitis. Intravenous fluconazole has been shown to be equivalent to amphotericin B in treatment of candidemia in ICU patients with normal white blood cell counts. Flu-

conazole is the agent most commonly used for the treatment of mucocutaneous candidiasis. Activity against the dimorphic fungi is limited to coccidioidal disease, and in particular for meningitis, where high doses of fluconazole often obviate the need for intrathecal amphotericin B. Fluconazole displays no activity against aspergillus or other filamentous fungi.

Prophylactic use of fluconazole has been demonstrated to reduce fungal disease in bone marrow transplant recipients and AIDS patients, but the emergence of fluconazole-resistant fungi has raised concerns about this indication.

4. Voriconazole

Voriconazole is the newest triazole to be licensed in the USA. It is available in intravenous and oral formulations. The recommended dosage is 400 mg/d. The drug is well absorbed orally, with a bioavailability exceeding 90%, and it exhibits less protein binding than itraconazole. Metabolism is predominantly hepatic, but the propensity for inhibition of mammalian P450 appears to be low. Observed toxicities include rash and elevated hepatic enzymes. Visual disturbances are common, occurring in up to 30% of patients receiving voriconazole, and include blurring and changes in color vision or brightness. These visual changes usually occur immediately after a dose of voriconazole and resolve within 30 minutes.

Voriconazole is similar to itraconazole in its spectrum of action, having excellent activity against candida species (including fluconazole-resistant species such as *C krusei*) and the dimorphic fungi. Voriconazole is less toxic than amphotericin B and is probably more effective in the treatment of invasive aspergillosis.

ECHINOCANDINS

Echinocandins are the newest class of antifungal agent to be developed. They are large cyclic peptides linked to a long-chain fatty acid. **Caspofungin, micafungin,** and **anidulafungin** are the only licensed agents in this category of antifungals, although other drugs are under active investigation. These agents are active against both candida and aspergillus, but not *Cryptococcus neoformans*.

Pharmacology

Echinocandins are available only in intravenous forms. Caspofungin is administered as a single loading dose of 70 mg, followed by a daily dose of 50 mg. Caspofungin is water-soluble and highly protein-bound. The half-life is 9–11 hours, and the metabolites are excreted by the kidneys and gastrointestinal tract. Dosage adjustments are required only in the presence of severe hepatic insufficiency. Micafungin displays similar properties with a half-life of 11–15 hours and is used at a dose of 150 mg/day for treatment and 50 mg/d for prophylaxis of fungal infections. Anidulafungin has a half-life of 24–48 hours. For esophageal candidiasis, it is administered intravenously at 100 mg on the first day and 50 mg/d thereafter for 14 days. For systemic candidemia, a loading dose of 200 mg is recommended with 100 mg/d thereafter for at least 14 days after the last positive blood culture.

Mechanism of Action

Echinocandins act at the level of the fungal cell wall by inhibiting the synthesis of $\beta(1–3)$ glucan. This results in disruption of the fungal cell wall and cell death.

Adverse Effects

Echinocandin agents are extremely well tolerated, with minor gastrointestinal side effects and flushing reported infrequently. Elevated liver enzymes have been noted in several patients receiving caspofungin in combination with cyclosporine, and this combination should be avoided. Micafungin has been shown to increase levels of nifedipine, cyclosporine, and sirolimus. Anidulafungin does not seem to have significant drug interactions, but histamine release may occur during IV infusion.

Clinical Use

Caspofungin is currently licensed for disseminated and mucocutaneous candida infections, as well as for empiric antifungal therapy during febrile neutropenia. Note that caspofungin is licensed for use in invasive aspergillosis only as salvage therapy in patients who have failed to respond to amphotericin B, and not as primary therapy. Micafungin is licensed only for mucocutaneous candidiasis and prophylaxis of candida infections in bone marrow transplant patients. Anidulafungin is approved for use in esophageal candidiasis and invasive candidiasis, including septicemia.

■ SYSTEMIC ANTIFUNGAL DRUGS FOR MUCOCUTANEOUS INFECTIONS

GRISEOFULVIN

Griseofulvin is a very insoluble fungistatic drug derived from a species of penicillium. Its only use is in the systemic treatment of dermatophytosis (see Chapter 62). It is administered in a microcrystalline form at a dosage of 1 g/d. Absorption is improved when it is given with fatty foods. Griseofulvin's mechanism of action at the cellular level is unclear, but it is deposited in newly forming skin where it binds to keratin, protecting the skin from new infection. Because its action is to prevent infection of these new skin structures, griseofulvin must be administered for 2–6 weeks for skin and hair infections to allow the replacement of infected keratin by the resistant structures. Nail infections may require therapy for months to allow regrowth of the new protected nail and is often followed by relapse. Adverse effects include an allergic syndrome much like serum sickness, hepatitis, and drug interactions with warfarin and phenobarbital. Griseofulvin has been largely replaced by newer antifungal medications such as itraconazole and terbinafine.

TERBINAFINE

Terbinafine is a synthetic allylamine that is available in an oral formulation and is used at a dosage of 250 mg/d. It is used in the treatment of dermatophytoses, especially onychomycosis (see Chapter 62). Like griseofulvin, terbinafine is a keratophilic medication, but unlike griseofulvin, it is fungicidal. Like the azole drugs, it interferes with ergosterol biosynthesis, but rather than interacting with the P450 system, terbinafine inhibits the fungal enzyme squalene epoxidase. This leads to the accumulation of the sterol squalene, which is toxic to the organism. One tablet given daily for 12 weeks achieves a cure rate of up to 90% for onychomycosis and is more effective than griseofulvin or itraconazole. Adverse effects are rare, consisting primarily of gastrointestinal upset and headache. Terbinafine does not seem to affect the P450 system and has demonstrated no significant drug interactions to date.

■ TOPICAL ANTIFUNGAL THERAPY

NYSTATIN

Nystatin is a polyene macrolide much like amphotericin B. It is too toxic for parenteral administration and is only used topically. Nystatin is currently available in creams, ointments, suppositories, and other forms for application to skin and mucous membranes. It is not absorbed to a significant degree from skin, mucous membranes, or the gastrointestinal tract. As a result, nystatin has little toxicity, although oral use is often limited by the unpleasant taste.

Nystatin is active against most candida species and is most commonly used for suppression of local candidal infections. Some common indications include oropharyngeal thrush, vaginal candidiasis, and intertriginous candidal infections.

TOPICAL AZOLES

The two azoles most commonly used topically are clotrimazole and miconazole; several others are available (see Preparations Available). Both are available over-the-counter and are often used for vulvovaginal candidiasis. Oral clotrimazole troches are available for treatment of oral thrush and are a pleasant-tasting alternative to nystatin. In cream form, both agents are useful for dermatophytic infections, including tinea corporis, tinea pedis, and tinea cruris. Absorption is negligible, and adverse effects are rare.

Topical and shampoo forms of ketoconazole are also available and useful in the treatment of seborrheic dermatitis and pityriasis versicolor. Several other azoles are available for topical use (see Preparations Available).

TOPICAL ALLYLAMINES

Terbinafine and naftifine are allylamines available as topical creams (see Chapter 62). Both are effective for treatment of tinea cruris and tinea corporis. These are prescription drugs in the USA.

PREPARATIONS AVAILABLE

Anidulafungin (Eraxis)
  Parenteral: 50 mg powder for injection
Amphotericin B
  Parenteral:
  Conventional formulation (Amphotericin B, Fungizone): 50 mg powder for injection
  Lipid formulations:
  (Abelcet): 100 mg/20 mL suspension for injection
  (AmBisome): 50 mg powder for injection
  (Amphotec): 50, 100 mg powder for injection
  Topical: 3% cream, lotion, ointment
Butaconazole (Gynazole-1, Mycelex-3)
  Topical: 2% vaginal cream
Butenafine (Lotrimin Ultra, Mentax)
  Topical: 1% cream
Caspofungin (Cancidas)
  Parenteral: 50, 70 mg powder for injection
Clotrimazole (generic, Lotrimin)
  Topical: 1% cream, solution, lotion; 100, 200 mg vaginal suppositories
Econazole (generic, Spectazole)
  Topical: 1% cream
Fluconazole (Diflucan)
  Oral: 50, 100, 150, 200 mg tablets; powder for 10, 40 mg/mL suspension
  Parenteral: 2 mg/mL in 100 and 200 mL vials
Flucytosine (Ancobon)
  Oral: 250, 500 mg capsules
Griseofulvin (Grifulvin, Grisactin, Fulvicin P/G)
  Oral microsize: 125, 250 mg tablets; 250 mg capsule, 125 mg/5 mL suspension

Oral ultramicrosize:* 125, 165, 250, 330 mg tablets
Itraconazole (Sporanox)
  Oral: 100 mg capsules; 10 mg/mL solution
  Parenteral: 10 mg/mL for IV infusion
Ketoconazole (generic, Nizoral)
  Oral: 200 mg tablets
  Topical: 2% cream, shampoo
Miconazole (generic, Micatin)
  Topical: 2% cream, powder, spray; 100, 200 mg vaginal suppositories
Micafungin (Mycamine)
  Parenteral: 50 mg powder for injection
Naftifine (Naftin)
  Topical: 1% cream, gel
Natamycin (Natacyn)
  Topical: 5% ophthalmic suspension
Nystatin (generic, Mycostatin)
  Oral: 500,000 unit tablets
  Topical: 100,000 units/g cream, ointment, powder; 100,000 units vaginal tablets
Oxiconazole (Oxistat)
  Topical: 1% cream, lotion
Sulconazole (Exelderm)
  Topical: 1% cream, solution

                                                   (continued)

---

*Ultramicrosize formulations of griseofulvin are approximately 1.5 times more potent, milligram for milligram, than the microsize preparations.

Terbinafine (Lamisil)
Oral: 250 mg tablets
Topical: 1% cream, gel
Terconazole (Terazol 3, Terazol 7)
Topical: 0.4%, 0.8% vaginal cream; 80 mg vaginal suppositories
Tioconazole (Vagistat-1, Monistat 1)
Topical: 6.5% vaginal ointment

Tolnaftate (generic, Aftate, Tinactin)
Topical: 1% cream, gel, solution, aerosol powder
Voriconazole (Vfend)
Oral: 50, 200 mg tablets; oral suspension 40 mg/mL
Parenteral: 200 mg vials, reconstituted to a 5 mg/mL solution

REFERENCES

Diekema DJ et al: Activities of caspofungin, itraconazole, posaconazole, ravuconazole, voriconazole, and amphotericin B against 448 recent clinical isolates of filamentous fungi. J Clin Microbiol 2003;41:3623.

Groll A, Piscitelli SC, Walsh TJ: Clinical pharmacology of systemic antifungal agents: A comprehensive review of agents in clinical use, current investigational compounds, and putative targets for antifungal drug development. Adv Pharmacol 1998; 44:343.

Herbrecht R et al: Voriconazole versus amphotericin B for primary therapy of invasive aspergillosis. N Engl J Med 2002; 347:408.

Sheehan DJ, Hitchcock CA, Sibley CM: Current and emerging azole antifungal agents. Clin Microbiol Rev 1999;12:40.

Wiederhold NP, Lewis RE: The echinocandin antifungals: An overview of the pharmacology, spectrum and clinical efficacy. Expert Opin Investig Drugs 2003;12:1313.

Wong-Beringer A, Jacobs RA, Guglielmo BJ: Lipid formulations of amphotericin B. Clinical efficacy and toxicities. Clin Infect Dis 1998;27:603.

Antiviral Agents

49

Sharon Safrin, MD

Viruses are obligate intracellular parasites; their replication depends primarily on synthetic processes of the host cell. Therefore, to be effective, antiviral agents must either block viral entry into or exit from the cell or be active inside the host cell. As a corollary, nonselective inhibitors of virus replication may interfere with host cell function and produce toxicity.

Progress in antiviral chemotherapy began in the early 1950s, when the search for anticancer drugs generated several new compounds capable of inhibiting viral DNA synthesis. The two first-generation antivirals, 5-iododeoxyuridine and trifluorothymidine, had poor specificity (ie, they inhibited host cell DNA as well as viral DNA) that rendered them too toxic for systemic use. However, both agents are effective when used topically for the treatment of herpes keratitis.

Recent research has focused on the identification of agents with greater selectivity, in vivo stability, and lack of toxicity. Selective antiretroviral agents that inhibit a critical HIV-1 enzyme such as reverse transcriptase or the protease required for final packaging of the virus particle have become available. However, because replication of the virus peaks at or before the manifestation of clinical symptoms in many viral infections, chemoprophylaxis or early initiation of therapy may be key. In chronic illnesses such as viral hepatitis or HIV infection, potent inhibition of viral replication is crucial in limiting the extent of systemic damage.

Viral replication consists of several steps (Figure 49–1): (1) attachment of the virus to the host cell; (2) entry of the virus through the host cell membrane; (3) uncoating of viral nucleic acid; (4) synthesis of early regulatory proteins, eg, nucleic acid polymerases; (5) synthesis of RNA or DNA; (6) synthesis of late, structural proteins; (7) assembly (maturation) of viral particles; and (8) release from the cell. Antiviral agents can potentially target any of these steps.

■ I. AGENTS TO TREAT HERPES SIMPLEX VIRUS (HSV) & VARICELLA-ZOSTER VIRUS (VZV) INFECTIONS

Three oral nucleoside analogs are licensed for the treatment of HSV and VZV infections: acyclovir, valacyclovir, and famciclovir. They have similar mechanisms of action and similar indications for clinical use; all are well tolerated. Acyclovir has been the most extensively studied; it was licensed first and is the only one of the three available for intravenous use in the United States. Comparative trials have demonstrated similar efficacies of these three agents for the treatment of HSV but modest superiority of famciclovir and valacyclovir over

---

ACRONYMS & OTHER NAMES

3TC	Lamivudine
AZT	Zidovudine (previously azido-thymidine)
CMV	Cytomegalovirus
CYP	Cytochrome P450
d4T	Stavudine
ddC	Zalcitabine
ddI	Didanosine
EBV	Epstein-Barr virus
FTC	Emtricitabine
HAART	Highly active antiretroviral therapy
HBV	Hepatitis B virus
HCV	Hepatitis C virus
HHV-6	Human herpesvirus-6
HIV	Human immunodeficiency virus
HPV	Human papillomavirus
HSV	Herpes simplex virus
IFN	Interferon
KSHV	Kaposi's sarcoma-associated herpesvirus
NNRTI	Nonnucleoside reverse transcriptase inhibitor
NRTI	Nucleoside reverse transcriptase inhibitor
PI	Protease inhibitor
RSV	Respiratory syncytial virus
SVR	Sustained antiviral response
VZV	Varicella-zoster virus

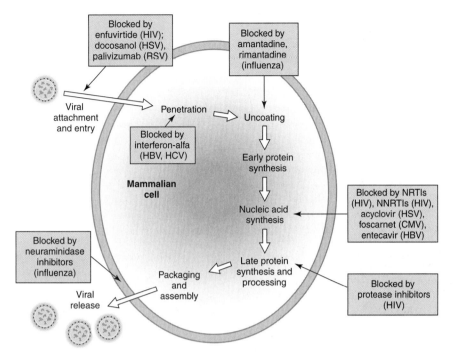

Figure 49–1. The major sites of antiviral drug action. Note: Interferon alfas are speculated to have multiple sites of action. (Modified and reproduced, with permission, from Trevor AT, Katzung BG, Masters SM: *Pharmacology: Examination & Board Review,* 6th ed. McGraw-Hill, 2002.)

acyclovir for the treatment of herpes zoster. Neither valacyclovir nor famciclovir have been fully evaluated in pediatric patients; thus, neither is indicated for the treatment of varicella infection.

ACYCLOVIR

Acyclovir (Figure 49–2) is an acyclic guanosine derivative with clinical activity against HSV-1, HSV-2, and VZV. In vitro activity against Epstein-Barr virus (EBV), cytomegalovirus (CMV), and human herpesvirus-6 (HHV-6) is present but comparatively weaker.

Acyclovir requires three phosphorylation steps for activation. It is converted first to the monophosphate derivative by the virus-specified thymidine kinase and then to the di- and triphosphate compounds by host cell enzymes (Figure 49–3). Because it requires the viral kinase for initial phosphorylation, acyclovir is selectively activated, and the active metabolite accumulates, only in infected cells. Acyclovir triphosphate inhibits viral DNA synthesis by two mechanisms: competition with deoxyGTP for the viral DNA polymerase, resulting in binding to the DNA template as an irreversible complex; and chain termination following incorporation into the viral DNA.

The bioavailability of oral acyclovir is 15–20% and is unaffected by food. An intravenous formulation is available. Topical formulations produce high concentrations in herpetic lesions, but systemic concentrations are undetectable by this route.

Acyclovir is cleared primarily by glomerular filtration and tubular secretion. The half-life is approximately 3 hours in patients with normal renal function and 20 hours in patients with anuria. Acyclovir is readily cleared by hemodialysis but not by peritoneal dialysis. Acyclovir diffuses readily into most tissues and body fluids. Cerebrospinal fluid concentrations are 50% of serum values.

Oral acyclovir has multiple uses. In first episodes of genital herpes, oral acyclovir shortens the duration of symptoms by approximately 2 days, the time to lesion healing by 4 days, and the duration of viral shedding by 7 days. In recurrent genital herpes, the time course is shortened by 1–2 days. Treatment of first-episode genital herpes does not alter the frequency or severity of recurrent outbreaks. Long-term suppression of genital herpes with oral acyclovir in patients with frequent recurrences decreases the frequency of symptomatic recurrences and of asymptomatic viral shedding, thus decreasing the rate of sexual transmission. However, outbreaks may resume

A. Antiherpes agents

Acyclovir

Valacyclovir (prodrug)

Ganciclovir

Foscarnet

Valganciclovir (prodrug)

Penciclovir

Famciclovir (prodrug)

Cidofovir

B. Anti-HIV NRTI agents

Zidovudine (AZT)

Stavudine (d4T)

Zalcitabine (ddC)

Lamivudine (3TC)

Didanosine (ddl)

Abacavir

Tenofovir disoproxil

Emtricitabine

C. Anti-HBV agents

Adefovir

Entecavir

Figure 49–2. Chemical structures of some antiviral nucleoside and nucleotide analogs.

upon discontinuation of suppressive acyclovir. Oral acyclovir is only modestly beneficial in recurrent herpes labialis. It significantly decreases the total number of lesions, duration of symptoms, and viral shedding in patients with varicella (if begun within 24 hours after the onset of rash) or cutaneous zoster (if begun within 72 hours). However, because VZV is less susceptible to acyclovir than HSV, higher doses are required (Table 49–1). When given prophylactically to patients undergoing organ transplantation, oral acyclovir (200 mg every 8 hours or 800 mg every 12 hours) or intravenous acyclovir (5 mg/kg every 8 hours) prevents reactivation of HSV infection.

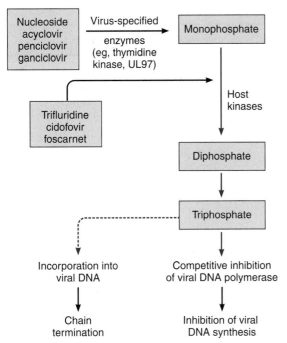

Figure 49–3. Mechanism of action of antiherpes agents.

Intravenous acyclovir is the treatment of choice for herpes simplex encephalitis, neonatal HSV infection, and serious HSV or VZV infections (Table 49–1). In immunocompromised patients with VZV infection, intravenous acyclovir reduces the incidence of cutaneous and visceral dissemination.

Topical acyclovir is substantially less effective than oral therapy for primary HSV infection. It is of no benefit in treating recurrent genital herpes.

Resistance to acyclovir can develop in HSV or VZV through alteration in either the viral thymidine kinase or the DNA polymerase, and clinically resistant infections have been reported in immunocompromised hosts. Most clinical isolates are resistant on the basis of deficient thymidine kinase activity and thus are cross-resistant to valacyclovir, famciclovir, and ganciclovir. Agents such as foscarnet, cidofovir, and trifluridine do not require activation by viral thymidine kinase and thus have preserved activity against the most prevalent acyclovir-resistant strains (Figure 49–3).

Acyclovir is generally well tolerated. Nausea, diarrhea, and headache have occasionally been reported. Intravenous infusion may be associated with reversible renal dysfunction (due to crystalline nephropathy) or neurologic toxicity (eg, tremors, delirium, seizures). However, these are uncommon with adequate hydration and avoidance of rapid infusion rates. High doses of acyclovir cause chromosomal damage and testicular atrophy in rats, but there has been no evidence of teratogenicity, reduction in sperm production, or cytogenetic alterations in peripheral blood lymphocytes in patients receiving chronic daily suppression of genital herpes for more than 10 years.

VALACYCLOVIR

Valacyclovir is the L-valyl ester of acyclovir (Figure 49–2). It is rapidly converted to acyclovir after oral administration via intestinal and hepatic first-pass metabolism, resulting in serum levels that are three to five times greater than those achieved with oral acyclovir and approximate those achieved with intravenous acyclovir administration. Oral bioavailability is 54%, and cerebrospinal fluid levels are 50% of those in serum. Elimination half-life is 2.5–3.3 hours.

Approved uses of valacyclovir include treatment of first or recurrent genital herpes, suppression of frequently recurring genital herpes, and as a 1-day treatment for orolabial herpes (Table 49–1). Once-daily dosing of valacyclovir (500 mg) for chronic suppression in persons with recurrent genital herpes has been shown to markedly decrease the risk of sexual transmission. In comparative trials with acyclovir for the treatment of patients with zoster, rates of cutaneous healing were similar, but valacyclovir was associated with a shorter duration of zoster-associated pain. Valacyclovir has also been shown to be effective in preventing cytomegalovirus disease after organ transplantation when compared with placebo.

Valacyclovir is generally well tolerated, although nausea, vomiting, or rash occasionally occur. Agitation, dizziness, headache, liver enzyme elevation, anemia, and neutropenia are rare. At high doses, confusion, hallucinations, and seizures have been reported. AIDS patients who received high-dosage valacyclovir chronically (ie, 8 g/d) had an increased incidence of gastrointestinal intolerance as well as thrombotic microangiopathies (thrombotic thrombocytopenic purpura and hemolytic-uremic syndrome).

FAMCICLOVIR

Famciclovir is the diacetyl ester prodrug of 6-deoxypenciclovir, an acyclic guanosine analog (Figure 49–2). After oral administration, famciclovir is rapidly converted by first-pass metabolism to penciclovir. It is active in vitro against HSV-1, HSV-2, VZV, EBV, and HBV. As with acyclovir, activation by phosphorylation is catalyzed by the virus-specified thymidine kinase in infected cells, followed by competitive inhibition of the viral DNA polymerase to block DNA synthesis. Unlike acyclovir, however, penciclovir does not cause chain termination. Penciclovir triphosphate has lower affinity for the viral DNA polymerase than acyclovir triphosphate, but it

Table 49–1. Agents to treat or prevent herpes simplex virus (HSV) and varicella-zoster virus (VZV) infections.

	Route of Administration	Use	Recommended Adult Dosage and Regimen
Acyclovir[1]	Oral	First episode genital herpes	400 mg tid or 200 mg 5 times daily × 7–10 days
		Recurrent genital herpes	400 mg tid or 200 mg 5 times daily or 800 mg bid × 3–5 days
		Genital herpes suppression	400 mg bid
		Herpes proctitis	400 mg 5 times daily until healed
		Orolabial herpes	400 mg 5 times daily × 5 days
		Mucocutaneous herpes in the immunocompromised host	400 mg 5 times daily × 7–10 days
		Varicella	20 mg/kg (maximum 800 mg) qid × 5 days
		Zoster	800 mg 5 times daily × 7–10 days
	Intravenous	Severe HSV infection	5 mg/kg q8h × 7–10 days
		Mucocutaneous herpes in the immunocompromised host	10 mg/kg q8h × 7–14 days
		Herpes encephalitis	10–15 mg/kg q8h × 14–21 days
		Neonatal HSV infection	10–20 mg/kg q8h × 14–21 days
		Varicella or zoster in the immunosuppressed host	10 mg/kg q8h × 7 days
	Topical	Herpes labialis	Thin film covering leasion 5 times daily × 4 days
Famciclovir[1]	Oral	First episode genital herpes	250 mg tid × 7–10 days
		Recurrent genital herpes	125 mg bid × 3–5 days or 1000 mg bid × 2 doses
		Genital herpes suppression	250 mg bid
		Orolabial herpes	500 mg bid × 7 days
		Orolabial or genital herpes in the immunosuppressed host	500 mg bid × 7–10 days
		Zoster	500 mg tid × 7 days
Valacyclovir[1]	Oral	First episode genital herpes	1 g bid × 7–10 days
		Recurrent genital herpes	500 mg bid × 3 days
		Genital herpes suppression	500–1000 mg daily
		Orolabial herpes	2 g bid × 2 doses
		Orolabial or genital herpes in the immunosuppressed host	1 g bid × 7–10 days
		Zoster	1 g tid × 7 days
Foscarnet[1]	Intravenous	Acyclovir-resistant HSV and VZV infections	40 mg/kg q8h until healed
Docosanol	Topical	Herpes labialis	Thin film covering lesion 5 times daily until healed
Penciclovir	Topical	Recurrent herpes labialis	Thin film covering lesion every 2 hours × 4 days
Trifluridine	Topical	Herpes keratitis	1 drop every 2 hours
		Acyclovir-resistant HSV infection	Thin film covering lesion 5 times daily until healed

[1]Dosage must be reduced in patients with renal insufficiency.

achieves higher intracellular concentrations and has a more prolonged intracellular effect in experimental systems. The most commonly encountered clinical mutants of HSV are thymidine kinase-deficient; these are cross-resistant to acyclovir and famciclovir.

The bioavailability of penciclovir from orally administered famciclovir is 70%. Penciclovir triphosphate has an intracellular half-life of 10 hours in HSV-1-infected cells, 20 hours in HSV-2-infected cells, and 7 hours in VZV-infected cells in vitro. Penciclovir is excreted primarily in the urine.

Oral famciclovir is effective for the treatment of first and recurrent genital herpes, for chronic daily suppression of genital herpes, and for the treatment of acute zoster (Table 49–1). One-day usage of famciclovir (1000 mg twice daily) significantly accelerates time to healing of recurrent genital herpes compared with placebo, by approximately 2 days. A single dose of 1500 mg or two 750 mg doses (BID) accelerates herpes labialis healing time. Comparison of famciclovir to valacyclovir for treatment of herpes zoster in immunocompetent patients showed similar rates of cutaneous healing and pain resolution, although both agents were associated with a shortened duration of zoster-associated pain compared with acyclovir.

Oral famciclovir is generally well tolerated, although headache, diarrhea, and nausea may occur. As with acyclovir, testicular toxicity has been demonstrated in animals receiving repeated doses. However, men receiving daily famciclovir (250 mg every 12 hours) for 18 weeks had no changes in sperm morphology or motility. The incidence of mammary adenocarcinoma was increased in female rats receiving famciclovir for 2 years.

PENCICLOVIR

The guanosine analog penciclovir, the active metabolite of famciclovir, is also available for topical use. One percent penciclovir cream is effective for the treatment of recurrent herpes labialis in immunocompetent adults (Table 49–1). When therapy was initiated within 1 hour after the onset of signs or symptoms and continued every 2 hours during waking hours for 4 days, treatment with topical penciclovir resulted in a shortening of the median time until healing by approximately 0.7 days compared with placebo. Side effects are uncommon.

DOCOSANOL

Docosanol is a saturated 22-carbon aliphatic alcohol that inhibits fusion between the plasma membrane and the HSV envelope, thereby preventing viral entry into cells and subsequent viral replication. Topical docosanol 10% cream is available without a prescription. When therapy is initiated within 12 hours of the onset of prodromal symptoms and applied five times daily, the healing time

is decreased by approximately 18 hours compared with placebo in recurrent orolabial herpes.

TRIFLURIDINE

Trifluridine (trifluorothymidine) is a fluorinated pyrimidine nucleoside that inhibits viral DNA synthesis in HSV-1, HSV-2, vaccinia, and some adenoviruses. It is phosphorylated intracellularly to its active form by host cell enzymes, and then competes with thymidine triphosphate for incorporation by the viral DNA polymerase (Figure 49–3). Incorporation of trifluridine triphosphate into both viral and host DNA prevents its systemic use. Application of a 1% solution is effective in treating keratoconjunctivitis and recurrent epithelial keratitis due to HSV-1 and HSV-2. Topical application of trifluridine solution, alone or in combination with interferon alfa, has been used successfully in the treatment of acyclovir-resistant HSV infections.

■ II. AGENTS TO TREAT CYTOMEGALOVIRUS (CMV) INFECTIONS

CMV infections occur primarily in the setting of advanced immunosuppression and are typically due to reactivation of latent infection. Dissemination of infection results in end-organ disease, including retinitis, colitis, esophagitis, central nervous system disease, and pneumonitis. Although the incidence in HIV-infected patients has markedly decreased with the advent of potent antiretroviral therapy, reactivation of CMV infection after organ transplantation is still clinically prevalent.

The availability of oral valganciclovir and the ganciclovir intraocular implant has decreased the usage of intravenous ganciclovir, intravenous foscarnet, and intravenous cidofovir for the treatment of end-organ CMV disease (Table 49–2). Oral valganciclovir has largely replaced oral ganciclovir because of its lower pill burden. The choice of therapy in patients with CMV retinitis must also take into account the location of the lesion and the extent of immediate visual impairment or threat.

GANCICLOVIR

Ganciclovir is an acyclic guanosine analog (Figure 49–2) that requires activation by triphosphorylation before inhibiting the viral DNA polymerase. Initial phosphorylation is catalyzed by the virus-specified protein kinase phosphotransferase UL97 in CMV-infected cells. The activated compound competitively inhibits viral DNA polymerase and causes termination of viral DNA elongation (Figure

Table 49–2. Agents to treat cytomegalovirus (CMV) infection.

Agent	Route of Administration	Use	Recommended Adult Dosage[1]
Valganciclovir	Oral	CMV retinitis treatment	Induction: 900 mg bid Maintenance: 900 mg daily
	Oral	CMV prophylaxis (transplant patients)	900 mg daily
Ganciclovir	Intravenous	CMV retinitis treatment	Induction: 5 mg/kg q12h Maintenance: 5 mg/kg/d or 6 mg/kg five times per week
	Oral	CMV prophylaxis	1 g tid
		CMV retinitis treatment	1 g tid
	Intraocular implant	CMV retinitis treatment	4.5 mg every 5–8 months
Foscarnet	Intravenous	CMV retinitis treatment	Induction: 60 mg/kg q8h or 90 mg/kg q12h Maintenance: 90–120 mg/kg/d
Cidofovir	Intravenous	CMV retinitis treatment	Induction: 5 mg/kg every 7 days Maintenance: 5 mg/kg every 14 days

[1]Dosage must be reduced in patients with renal insufficiency.

49–3). Ganciclovir has in vitro activity against CMV, HSV, VZV, EBV, HHV-6, and KSHV (Kaposi's sarcoma-associated herpesvirus). Its activity against CMV is up to 100 times greater than that of acyclovir.

Ganciclovir may be administered intravenously, orally, or via intraocular implant. Cerebrospinal fluid concentrations are approximately 50% of those in serum. The elimination half-life is 4 hours with normal renal function and the intracellular half-life is 18 hours. Clearance of the drug is linearly related to creatinine clearance. Ganciclovir is readily cleared by hemodialysis. The bioavailability of oral ganciclovir is poor. In patients with an intraocular implant, ganclovir is released into the vitreous cavity at a rate of approximately 1.4 mcg/h.

Intravenous ganciclovir has been shown to delay progression of CMV retinitis in patients with AIDS when compared with no treatment. Dual therapy with foscarnet and ganciclovir has been shown to be more effective in delaying progression of retinitis than either drug administered alone (see Foscarnet), although side effects are compounded. Intravenous ganciclovir is also used to treat CMV colitis and esophagitis. The risk of Kaposi's sarcoma is reduced in AIDS patients receiving long-term ganciclovir. Intravenous ganciclovir, followed by either oral ganciclovir or high-dose oral acyclovir, reduces the risk of CMV infection in transplant recipients. Intravenous ganciclovir for CMV pneumonitis in immunocompromised patients may be beneficial, particularly in combination with intravenous cytomegalovirus immunoglobulin. Oral ganciclovir is indicated for prevention of end-organ CMV disease in

AIDS patients and as maintenance therapy of CMV retinitis after induction. Although less effective than intravenous ganciclovir, the risk of myelosuppression and of catheter-related complications is diminished.

Ganciclovir may also be administered intraocularly to treat CMV retinitis, either by direct intravitreal administration or via an intraocular implant. The implant, which achieves high and prolonged intraocular levels of ganciclovir, has been shown to delay progression of retinitis to a greater degree than systemic therapy with ganciclovir. Surgical replacement is required at intervals of 5–8 months. Concurrent therapy with a systemic anti-CMV agent is recommended.

Resistance to ganciclovir increases with duration of usage. The more common mutation is in UL97, resulting in decreased levels of the triphosphorylated (ie, active) form of ganciclovir. The less common UL54 mutation in DNA polymerase results in higher levels of resistance and potential cross-resistance with cidofovir and foscarnet. Antiviral susceptibility testing is recommended in patients in whom resistance is suspected clinically, as is the substitution of alternative therapies and concomitant reduction in immunosuppressive therapies, if possible. The addition of CMV hyperimmune globulin may also be considered.

The most common adverse effect of systemic ganciclovir treatment, particularly after intravenous administration, is myelosuppression. Myelosuppression may be additive in patients receiving concurrent zidovudine, azathioprine, or mycophenolate mofetil. Other potential adverse effects are nausea, diarrhea, fever, rash, headache, insomnia, and peripheral neuropathy, as well as retinal detachment in patients with CMV retinitis. Central nervous system toxicity (confusion, seizures, psychiatric disturbance) and hepatotoxicity have been rarely reported. Ganciclovir is mitogenic in mammalian cells and carcinogenic and embryotoxic at high doses in animals and causes aspermatogenesis; the clinical significance of these preclinical data is unclear.

Levels of ganciclovir may rise in patients concurrently taking probenecid or trimethoprim. Concurrent use of ganciclovir with didanosine may result in increased levels of didanosine.

VALGANCICLOVIR

Valganciclovir is an L-valyl ester prodrug of ganciclovir that exists as a mixture of two diastereomers (Figure 49–2). After oral administration, both diastereomers are rapidly hydrolyzed to ganciclovir by intestinal and hepatic esterases.

Valganciclovir is well absorbed and rapidly metabolized in the intestinal wall and liver to ganciclovir; no other metabolites have been detected. The absolute bioavailability of oral valganciclovir is 60%; it is recommended that the drug be taken with food. The AUC_{0-24h} resulting from valganciclovir (900 mg once daily) is similar to that after 5 mg/kg once daily of intravenous ganciclovir, and approximately 1.65 times that of oral ganciclovir. Plasma protein binding is less than 2%. The major route of elimination is renal—through glomerular filtration and active tubular secretion. Plasma concentrations of valganciclovir are reduced approximately 50% by hemodialysis.

Valganciclovir is indicated for the treatment of CMV retinitis in patients with AIDS and for the prevention of CMV disease in high-risk kidney, heart, and kidney-pancreas transplant patients. Adverse effects, drug interactions, and resistance patterns are the same as those associated with ganciclovir.

FOSCARNET

Foscarnet (phosphonoformic acid) is an inorganic pyrophosphate compound (Figure 49–2) that inhibits viral DNA polymerase, RNA polymerase, and HIV reverse transcriptase directly without requiring activation by phosphorylation. It has in vitro activity against HSV, VZV, CMV, EBV, HHV-6, KSHV, and HIV-1.

Foscarnet is available in an intravenous formulation only; poor oral bioavailability and gastrointestinal intolerance preclude oral use. Cerebrospinal fluid concentrations are 43–67% of steady-state serum concentrations. Although the mean plasma half-life is 3–6.8 hours, up to 30% of foscarnet may be deposited in bone, with a half-life of several months. The clinical repercussions of this are unknown. Clearance of foscarnet is primarily by the kidney and is directly proportional to creatinine clearance. Serum drug concentrations are reduced approximately 50% by hemodialysis.

An effective treatment for CMV retinitis, foscarnet has an efficacy approximately equal to that of ganciclovir. Foscarnet is also used for treatment of CMV colitis, CMV esophagitis, acyclovir-resistant HSV infection, and acyclovir-resistant VZV infection. The dosage of foscarnet must be titrated according to the patient's calculated creatinine clearance before each infusion. Use of an infusion pump to control the rate of infusion is important to avoid toxicity, and relatively large volumes of fluid are required because of the drug's poor solubility. The combination of ganciclovir and foscarnet is synergistic in vitro against CMV and has been shown to be superior to either agent alone in delaying progression of retinitis; however, toxicity is also increased when both agents are administered concurrently. As with ganciclovir, a decrease in the incidence of Kaposi's sarcoma has been observed in patients who have received long-term foscarnet.

Foscarnet has been administered intravitreally for the treatment of CMV retinitis in patients with AIDS, but data regarding efficacy and safety are lacking.

Resistance to foscarnet in HSV and CMV isolates is due to point mutations in the DNA polymerase gene and is typically associated with prolonged or repeated exposure to the drug. Mutations in the HIV-1 reverse transcriptase gene have also been described. Although foscarnet-resistant CMV isolates are typically cross-resistant to ganciclovir, foscarnet activity is usually maintained against ganciclovir- and cidofovir-resistant isolates of CMV.

Potential adverse effects of foscarnet include renal impairment, hypo- or hypercalcemia, hypo- or hyperphosphatemia, hypokalemia, and hypomagnesemia. Saline preloading helps to prevent nephrotoxicity, as does avoidance of concomitant administration of drugs with nephrotoxic potential (eg, amphotericin B, pentamidine, aminoglycosides). The risk of severe hypocalcemia is increased with concomitant use of pentamidine. Penile ulcerations associated with foscarnet therapy may be due to high levels of ionized drug in the urine. Nausea, vomiting, anemia, elevation of liver enzymes, and fatigue have been reported; the risk of anemia may be additive in patients receiving concurrent zidovudine. Central nervous system toxicities include headache, hallucinations, and seizures; seizures may be increased with concurrent use of imipenem. Foscarnet caused chromosomal damage in preclinical studies.

CIDOFOVIR

Cidofovir (Figure 49–2) is a cytosine nucleotide analog with in vitro activity against CMV, HSV-1, HSV-2, VZV, EBV, HHV-6, KSHV, adenovirus, poxviruses, polyomaviruses, and human papillomavirus. In contrast to ganciclovir, phosphorylation of cidofovir to the active diphosphate is independent of viral enzymes (Figure 49–3). After phosphorylation, cidofovir acts both as a potent inhibitor of and as an alternative substrate for viral DNA polymerase, competitively inhibiting DNA synthesis and becoming incorporated into the viral DNA chain. Isolates with resistance to cidofovir have been selected in vitro; these isolates tend to be cross-resistant with ganciclovir but retain susceptibility to foscarnet. Clinical resistance to cidofovir has not been reported to date in patients.

Although the terminal half-life of cidofovir is about 2.6 hours, the active metabolite, cidofovir diphosphate, has a prolonged intracellular half-life of 17–65 hours, thus allowing widely spaced administration. A separate metabolite, cidofovir phosphocholine, has a half-life of at least 87 hours and may serve as an intracellular reservoir of active drug. Cerebrospinal fluid penetration is poor. Elimination involves active renal tubular secretion. High-flux hemodialysis has been shown to reduce the serum levels of cidofovir by approximately 75%.

Intravenous cidofovir is effective for the treatment of CMV retinitis and is used experimentally to treat adenovirus infections. Intravenous cidofovir must be administered with probenecid (2 g at 3 hours before the infusion and 1 g at 2 and 8 hours after), which blocks active tubular secretion and decreases nephrotoxicity. Cidofovir dosage must be adjusted for alterations in the calculated creatinine clearance or the presence of urine protein before each infusion, and aggressive adjunctive hydration is required. Initiation of cidofovir therapy is contraindicated in patients with existing renal insufficiency. Direct intravitreal administration of cidofovir is not recommended because of ocular toxicity.

The primary adverse effect of intravenous cidofovir is a dose-dependent nephrotoxicity, which may be reduced with prehydration using normal saline. Concurrent administration of other potentially nephrotoxic agents (eg, amphotericin B, aminoglycosides, nonsteroidal antiinflammatory drugs, pentamidine, foscarnet) should be avoided. Prior administration of foscarnet may increase the risk of nephrotoxicity. Other potential side effects include uveitis, ocular hypotony, neutropenia (15%), and metabolic acidosis. Gastrointestinal intolerance, fever, and rash due to probenecid may occur. The drug caused mammary adenocarcinomas in rats and is embryotoxic.

■ III. ANTIRETROVIRAL AGENTS

Substantial advances have been made in antiretroviral therapy since the introduction of the first agent, zidovudine, in 1987, and many antiretroviral agents are now available (Table 49–3). In addition, greater knowledge of viral dynamics through the use of viral load and resistance testing has made clear that combination therapy with maximally efficacious and potent agents will reduce viral replication to the lowest possible level and decrease the likelihood of emergence of resistance. Thus, administration of highly active antiretroviral therapy (HAART), typically comprising a combination of 3–4 antiretroviral agents, has become the standard of care. Such regimens may be composed of nucleoside reverse transcriptase inhibitors, nonnucleoside reverse transcriptase inhibitors, protease inhibitors, and a fusion inhibitor (see below). Viral susceptibility to specific agents varies among patients and may change with time, owing to development of resistance. Therefore, such combinations must be chosen with care and tailored to the individual, as must changes to a given regimen. In addition to potency and susceptibility, important factors in the selection of agents for any given patient are tolerability, convenience, and optimization of adherence (see Box: Treatment of HIV-Infected Individuals: Importance of Pharmacokinetic Knowledge).

Four classes of antiretroviral agents are available for use: nucleoside/nucleotide reverse transcriptase inhibitors (NRTIs), nonnucleoside reverse transcriptase inhibitors (NNRTIs), protease inhibitors (PIs), and fusion inhibitors. As new agents have become available, several older ones have had diminished usage, because of either suboptimal safety profile or inferior antiviral potency.

NUCLEOSIDE & NUCLEOTIDE REVERSE TRANSCRIPTASE INHIBITORS

The NRTIs act by competitive inhibition of HIV-1 reverse transcriptase and can also be incorporated into the growing viral DNA chain to cause termination (Figure 49–4). Each requires intracytoplasmic activation via phosphorylation by cellular enzymes to the triphosphate form. Most have activity against HIV-2 as well as HIV-1.

Nucleoside analogs may be associated with mitochondrial toxicity, probably owing to inhibition of mitochondrial DNA polymerase gamma, and they can increase the risk of lactic acidosis with hepatic steatosis, which may be fatal, as well as disorders of lipid metabolism. NRTI treatment should be suspended in the setting of rapidly rising aminotransferase levels, progressive hepatomegaly, or metabolic acidosis of unknown cause.

ABACAVIR

Abacavir is a guanosine analog (Figure 49–2) that is well absorbed following oral administration (83%) and unaffected by food. The elimination half-life is 1.5

Table 49–3. Currently available antiretroviral agents.

Agent	Class of Agent	Recommended Adult Dosage	Administration Recommendation	Characteristic Side Effects	Comments
Abacavir	NRTI[1]	300 mg bid or 600 mg daily		Rash, hypersensitivity reaction, nausea	Avoid alcohol.
Amprenavir	PI[2]	1400 mg bid (oral solution).[3] Adjust dose in hepatic insufficiency; avoid use in severe hepatic insufficiency.	Separate dosing from ddl or antacids by 1 hour. Avoid high-fat meals.	Nausea, vomiting, diarrhea, rash, headache, oral paresthesias, ↑ liver enzymes	See footnote 4 for contraindicated medications. Also avoid cimetidine, disulfiram, lopinavir, metronidazole, vitamin E, ritonavir oral solution, and alcohol.
Atazanavir	PI[2]	400 mg daily or 300 mg daily with ritonavir 100 daily. Adjust dose in hepatic insufficiency; avoid in severe hepatic insufficiency.	Take with food. Separate dosing from ddl or antacids by 1 hour. Separate dosing from cimetidine and other acid-reducing agents by 12 hours.	Nausea, vomiting, diarrhea, abdominal pain, headache, peripheral neuropathy, skin rash, indirect hyperbilirubinemia, prolonged PR and/or QT$_c$ interval	See footnote 4 for contraindicated medications. Also avoid indinavir, irinotecan, and omeprazole.
Darunavir	PI[2]	600 mg bid with ritonavir 100 mg bid	Take with food.	Diarrhea, headache, nausea, rash, hyperlipidemia, ↑ liver enzymes, ↑ serum amylase	Avoid in patients with sulfa allergy. See footnote 4 for contraindicated medications.
Delavirdine	NNRTI	400 mg tid	Separate dosing from ddl or antacids by 1 hour.	Rash, ↑ liver enzymes, headache	See footnote 4 for contraindicated medications. Also avoid amprenavir, fosamprenavir, and rifabutin. Teratogenic in rats.
Didanosine (ddl)	NRTI[1]	Capsules: 250–400 mg daily, depending on weight. Tablets or powder: 125–250 mg bid, depending on weight Adjust dose in renal insufficiency.	30 minutes before or 2 hours after meals	Peripheral neuropathy, pancreatitis, diarrhea, nausea, hyperuricemia	Avoid concurrent neuropathic drugs (eg, stavudine, zalcitabine, isoniazid), ribavirin, and alcohol.
Efavirenz	NNRTI	600 mg daily	Take on empty stomach. Bedtime dosing recommended initially to minimize central nervous system side effects.	Central nervous system effects, rash, ↑ liver enzymes	Avoid concurrent astemizole, carbamazepine, ergot derivative, indinavir, itraconazole, ketoconazole, methadone, phenobarbital, phenytoin, triazolam, voriconazole. Teratogenic in primates.
Emtricitabine	NRTI[1]	200 mg daily Adjust dose in renal insufficiency.	Oral solution should be refrigerated.	Headache, diarrhea, nausea, asthenia, skin hyperpigmentation	Do not administer concurrent lamivudine. Avoid disulfram and metronidazole with oral solution.
Enfuvirtide	Fusion inhibitor	90 mg subcutaneously bid	Store at room temperature as a powder; refrigerate once reconstituted.	Local injection site reactions, hypersensitivity reation	

(continued)

Table 49–3. Currently available antiretroviral agents. (continued)

Agent	Class of Agent	Recommended Adult Dosage	Administration Recommendation	Characteristic Side Effects	Comments
Fosampren-avir	PI[2]	1400 mg bid or 700 mg bid with ritonavir 100 bid or 1400 mg daily with ritonavir 200 mg daily Adjust dose in hepatic insufficiency; avoid use in severe hepatic insufficiency.	Separate dosing from antacids by 2 hours	See amprenavir.	See amprenavir.
Indinavir	PI[2]	800 mg tid or 800 mg bid with ritonavir 100 mg bid Adjust dose in hepatic insufficiency.	Take on empty stomach. Drink at least 48 oz of liquid daily. Separate dosing from ddI by 1 hour. Store in original container, which contains dessicant.	Nephrolithiasis, nausea, indirect hyperbilirubinemia, headache, asthenia, blurred vision	See footnote 4 for contraindicated medications. Also avoid efavirenz.
Lamivudine	NRTI[1]	150 mg bid or 300 mg daily, depending on weight Adjust dose in renal insufficiency.		Nausea, headache, fatigue	
Lopinavir/ ritonavir	PI/PI[2]	400 mg/l00 mg bid May need dose adjustment in hepatic insufficiency	Take with food. Separate dosing from ddI by 1 hour. Store capsules and solution in refrigerator.	Diarrhea, abdominal pain, nausea, headache, ↑ liver enzymes	See footnote 4 for contraindicated medications. Also avoid amprenavir, fosamprenavir. Avoid disulfiram and metronidazole with oral solution.
Nelfinavir	PI[2]	750 mg tid or 1250 mg bid	Take with food.	Diarrhea, nausea, flatulence	See footnote 4 for contraindicated medications.
Nevirapine	NNRTI	200 mg bid Adjust dose in hepatic insufficiency.	Dose-escalate from 200 mg daily over 14 days to decrease frequency of rash.	Rash, hepatitis (occasionally fulminant), nausea, headache	Avoid rifampin, ketoconazole, and St. John's wort.
Ritonavir	PI[2]	600 mg bid	Take with food. Separate dosing with ddI by 2 hours. Dose-escalate over 5 days to improve tolerance. Refrigerate capsules but not oral solution.	Nausea, diarrhea, paresthesias, hepatitis	See footnote 4 for contraindicated medications.
Saquinavir	PI[2]	Tablets and hard gel capsules: 600 mg tid or 1000 mg bid with ritonavir 100 mg bid Soft gel capsules: 1200 mg tid or 1800 mg bid or 1000 mg bid with ritonavir 100 mg bid	Take within 2 hours of a full meal. Refrigeration recomended.	Nausea, diarrhea, rhinitis, abdominal pain, dyspepsia, rash	See footnote 4 for contraindicated medications. Use sunscreen owing to an increase in photosensitivity.

(continued)

Table 49–3. Currently available antiretroviral agents. (continued)

Agent	Class of Agent	Recommended Adult Dosage	Administration Recommendation	Characteristic Side Effects	Comments
Stavudine	NRTI[1]	Immediate release: 30–40 mg bid, depending on weight Extended release: 75–100 mg daily, depending on weight Adjust dose in renal insufficiency.		Peripheral neuropathy, lipodystrophy, hyperlipidemia, rapidly progressive ascending neuromuscular weakness (rare), pancreatitis	Avoid concurrent zidovudine and neuropathic drugs (eg, ddl, zalcitabine, isoniazid).
Tenofovir	NRTI[1]	300 mg qd Adjust dose in renal insufficiency.	Take with food.	Asthenia, headache, diarrhea, nausea, vomiting, flatulence, renal insufficiency	Avoid concurrent atazanavir, probenecid.
Tipranavir	PI[2]	Must be taken with ritonavir to achieve effective levels: tipranavir 500 mg bid/ ritonavir 200 mg bid. Avoid use in hepatic insufficiency.	Take with food. Separate from ddl by at least 2 hours. Avoid antacids. Avoid in patients with sulfa allergy. Refrigeration required.	Diarrhea, nausea, vomiting, abdominal pain, rash, ↑ liver enzymes, hypercholesterolemia, hypertriglyceridemia	Avoid concurrent amprenavir, fosamprenavir, saquinavir.
Zalcitabine	NRTI[1]	0.75 mg tid Adjust dose in renal insufficiency.	Administer 1 hour before or 2 hours after an antacid.	Peripheral neuropathy; oral ulcerations, pancreatitis	Avoid concurrent cimetidine; avoid concurrent neuropathic drugs (eg, ddl, zalcitabine, isoniazid).
Zidovudine	NRTI[1]	200 mg tid or 300 mg bid Adjust dose in renal insufficiency.		Macrocytic anemia, neutropenia, nausea, headache, insomnia, asthenia	Avoid concurrent stavudine and myelosuppressive drugs (eg, ganciclovir, ribavirin).

NRTI, nucleoside reverse transcriptase inhibitor; NNRTI, nonnucleoside reverse transcriptase inhibitor; PI, protease inhibitor; RTI, reverse transcriptase inhibitor.

[1]All NRTI agents, as well as tenofovir, carry the risk of lactic acidosis with hepatic steatosis as a potential adverse event.

[2]All PI agents, with the possible exception of amprenavir, carry the risk of hyperlipidemia, fat maldistribution, hyperglycemia, and insulin resistance as a potential adverse event..

[3]Capsules are no longer available and have been replaced by fosamprenavir.

[4]Because of altered systemic exposures, contraindicated concurrent drugs generally include anti-arrhythmics (flecainide, propafenone), antihistamines (astemizole, terfenadine), sedative-hypnotics (alprazolam, diazepam, flurazepam, midazolam, triazolam, trazodone, clorazepate), neuroleptics (pimozide), ergot alkaloid derivatives, HMG CoA reductase inhibitors (atorvastatin, simvastatin, lovastatin), anticonvulsants (phenobarbital, phenytoin), oral contraceptives (ethinyl estradiol/norethidrone acetate), cisapride, rifampin, rifapentine, and St. John's wort. Drugs that should be used with caution owing to altered levels include amiodarone, bepridil, quinidine, lidocaine, nifedipine, nicardipine, sildenafil, vardenafil, warfarin, levodopa, tacrolimus, cyclosporine, rapamycin, voriconazole, itraconazole, ketoconazole, carbamazepine, desipramine, bupropion, dofetilide, atovaquone, dapsone, dexamethasone, methadone, omeprazole, and lansoprazole. The dosages of rifabutin and clarithromycin should be decreased when administered concurrently.

hours, and the intracellular half-life ranges from 12 to 26 hours. Cerebrospinal fluid levels are approximately one third those of plasma.

High-level resistance to abacavir appears to require at least two or three concomitant mutations (eg, M184V, L74V, D67N) and thus tends to develop slowly. The K65R mutation is associated with reduced susceptibility to lamivudine, abacavir, tenofovir, and emtricitabine.

Hypersensitivity reactions, occasionally fatal, have been reported in approximately 5% of patients receiving abacavir. Symptoms, which generally occur within the first 6 weeks of therapy, include fever, malaise, nausea, vomiting, diarrhea, and anorexia. Respiratory symptoms such as dyspnea, pharyngitis, and cough may also be present, and skin rash occurs in about 50% of patients. Laboratory abnormalities such as mildly elevated serum aminotransferase or creatine kinase levels may be present but are not specific for the hypersensitivity reaction. Although the syndrome tends to resolve quickly with discontinuation of medication, rechallenge with abacavir results in return of symptoms within hours and may be fatal. Other potential adverse events are rash, fever, nausea, vomiting, diarrhea, headache, dyspnea, fatigue, and pancreatitis (rare).

DIDANOSINE

Didanosine (ddI) is a synthetic analog of deoxyadenosine (Figure 49–2). Oral bioavailability is 30–40%; dosing on an empty stomach is required. Cerebrospinal fluid concentrations of the drug are approximately 20% of serum concentrations. The elimination half-life is 1.5 hours, but the intracellular half-life of the activated compound is as long as 20–24 hours. The drug is eliminated by glomerular filtration and tubular secretion. Dosage reduction is therefore required for low creatinine clearance and for low body weight (Table 49–3).

Buffered powder for oral solution and chewable tablets are taken twice daily; enteric-coated capsules can be taken once daily because of greater bioavailability. The buffer in the tablets and powder interferes with absorption of indinavir, delavirdine, dapsone, and itraconazole; therefore, concurrent administration is to be avoided. Because the tablets contain both phenylalanine (36.5 mg) and sodium (1380 mg), caution should be exercised in patients with phenylketonuria and those on sodium-restricted diets.

Resistance to didanosine is typically associated with the L74V mutation, although decreased susceptibility may also occur in the presence of K65R and multiple thymidine analog mutations (TAMs). These may partially restore susceptibility to zidovudine but may confer cross-resistance to abacavir, zalcitabine, and lamivudine. The M184V mutation is found in a significant proportion of isolates selected by didanosine and may confer resistance to lamivudine.

The major clinical toxicity associated with didanosine therapy is dose-dependent pancreatitis. Other risk factors for pancreatitis (eg, alcoholism, hypertriglyceridemia) are relative contraindications to administration of didanosine, and other drugs with the potential to cause pancreatitis, including zalcitabine and stavudine, should be avoided (Table 49–3). Other reported adverse effects include painful peripheral distal neuropathy, diarrhea (particularly with tablets and powder), hepatitis, esophageal ulceration, cardiomyopathy, and central nervous system toxicity (headache, irritability, insomnia). Asymptomatic hyperuricemia may precipitate attacks of gout in susceptible individuals. Reports of retinal changes and optic neuritis in patients receiving didanosine, particularly in adults receiving high doses and in children, mandate periodic retinal examinations.

TREATMENT OF HIV-INFECTED INDIVIDUALS: IMPORTANCE OF PHARMACOKINETIC KNOWLEDGE

Concurrent use of many medications is necessary in most HIV-infected patients. These medications include combinations of antiretroviral agents, prophylaxis or treatment for opportunistic infections, antiemetics, neuropsychiatric drugs, and opioid pain medications. Such extreme polypharmacy necessitates awareness of pharmacokinetic and pharmacodynamic interactions.

Perhaps the most important of the pharmacokinetic complications results from the metabolism of the NNRTI and PI agents by the CYP450 enzyme system, primarily the 3A4 isoform. Because many are inducers or inhibitors of CYP3A4 as well as substrates, drug-drug interactions may have marked clinical ramifications. However, variable effects on different CYP450 isoforms may make interactions somewhat unpredictable. For example, in the treatment of tuberculosis, the use of rifampin, a standard antimycobacterial agent but also one of the most potent 3A4 inducers, may either decrease efficacy (eg, atazanavir, lopinavir) or increase

toxicity (eg, saquinavir) of concurrent antiretroviral agents, owing to alteration of serum levels. Increased levels of rifabutin (associated with uveitis) or trazodone (causing hypotension, syncope), when co-administered with ritonavir, may markedly increase toxicity. Increased levels of clarithromycin used for treatment or prophylaxis of *Mycobacterium avium* infection or as an antibacterial agent, when co-administered with indinavir, ritonavir, and atazanavir, may increase the potential for QT interval prolongation. Conversely, decreased levels of clarithromycin with efavirenz may reduce antibacterial efficacy. Most recently, these types of interactions have been used to advantage in the form of dual protease inhibitor regimens (boosted regimens), based on resultant increased plasma concentrations of the substrate (eg, lopinavir, saquinavir) when co-administered with an inducer (most often ritonavir). Improved drug exposure, increased antiviral potency, more convenient dosing, and improved tolerability result, thus improving patient adherence.

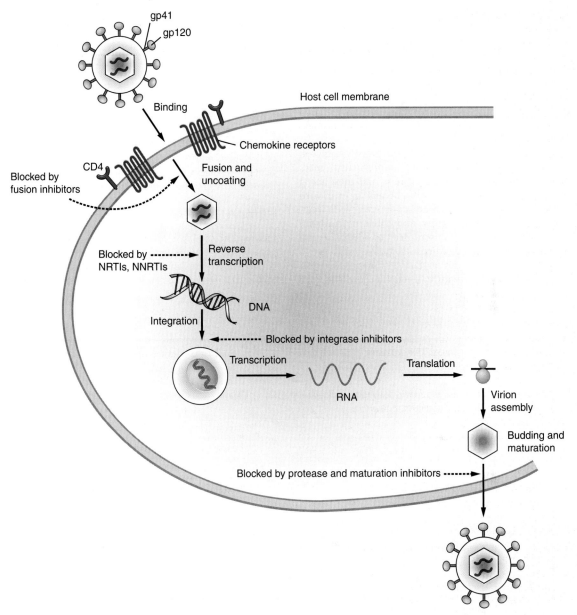

Figure 49–4. Life cycle of HIV. Binding of viral glycoproteins to host cell CD4 and chemokine receptors precedes fusion and entry into the cell. After uncoating, reverse transcription copies the single-stranded HIV RNA genome into double-stranded DNA, which is integrated into the host cell genome. Gene transcription by host cell enzymes produces messenger RNA, which is translated into proteins that assemble into immature noninfectious virions that bud from the host cell membrane. Maturation into fully infectious virions is through proteolytic cleavage.

Fluoroquinolones and tetracyclines should be administered at least 2 hours before or after didanosine to avoid decreased antibiotic plasma concentrations due to chelation. Serum levels of didanosine are increased when co-administered with tenofovir and ganciclovir, thus increasing the risk of toxicity; they are decreased by atazanavir, delavirdine, ritonavir, tipranavir, and methadone (Table 49–4).

EMTRICITABINE

Emtricitabine (formerly called FTC) is a fluorinated analog of lamivudine with a long intracellular half-life (> 39 hours), allowing for once-daily dosing (Figure 49–2). Oral bioavailability of the capsules is 93% and is unaffected by food, but penetration into the cerebrospinal fluid is low. Elimination is by both glomerular filtration and active tubular secretion. The mean plasma elimination half-life is 8–9 hours.

The oral solution, which contains propylene glycol, is contraindicated in young children, pregnant women, patients with renal or hepatic failure, and those using metronidazole or disulfiram. Also, because of its in vitro activity against HBV, patients co-infected with HIV and HBV should be closely monitored if treatment with emtricitabine is interrupted or discontinued, owing to the likelihood of hepatitis flares.

Like lamivudine, the M184V/I mutation is most frequently associated with emtricitabine use and may emerge rapidly in patients receiving HAART regimens that are not fully suppressive. There is cross-resistance to lamivudine but not to other NRTI agents. Isolates with the K65R mutation may have decreased susceptibility to emtricitabine. Because of their similar mechanisms of action and resistance profiles, the combination of lamivudine and emtricitabine is not recommended.

The most common adverse effects observed in patients receiving emtricitabine are headache, diarrhea, nausea, and asthenia. In addition, hyperpigmentation of the palms and/or soles may be observed (~ 3%), particularly in blacks (up to 13%). No drug-drug interactions of note have been reported to date.

LAMIVUDINE

Lamivudine (3TC) is a cytosine analog (Figure 49–2) with in vitro activity against HIV-1 that is synergistic with a variety of antiretroviral nucleoside analogs—including zidovudine and stavudine—against both

Table 49–4. Potential drug-drug interactions pertaining to two-drug antiretroviral combinations.

Agent	Drugs That Increase Its Serum Levels	Drugs That Decrease Its Serum Levels
Abacavir		Tipranavir
Amprenavir/fos-amprenavir	Abacavir, atazanavir, delavirdine, indinavir, lopinavir, ritonavir, tipranavir, zidovudine	Didanosine, efavirenz, nevirapine, saquinavir
Atazanavir	Ritonavir	Amprenavir, didanosine, efavirenz, stavudine, tenofovir
Darunavir	Indinavir	Lopinavir, ritonavir, saquinavir
Delavirdine		Amprenavir, didanosine, lopinavir, nelfinavir, ritonavir
Didanosine	Tenofovir, ganciclovir	Atazanavir, delavirdine, ritonavir, tipranavir
Efavirenz	Ritonavir	Lopinavir, nelfinavir, nevirapine
Enfuvirtide	Ritonavir	
Indinavir	Delavirdine, nelfinavir, ritonavir, zidovudine, darunavir	Amprenavir, didanosine, efavirenz, nevirapine
Lamivudine	Nelfinavir	Abacavir, tenofovir, tipranavir
Lopinavir	Delavirdine, indinavir, ritonavir, darunavir	Amprenavir, efavirenz, nelfinavir, nevirapine, tenofovir
Nelfinavir	Amprenavir, delavirdine, efavirenz, indinavir, ritonavir, saquinavir	
Nevirapine	Amprenavir, lopinavir	Tipranavir
Ritonavir	Amprenavir, delavirdine, efavirenz, indinavir	Didanosine, tenofovir, zidovudine
Saquinavir	Atazanavir, delavirdine, indinavir, lopinavir, nelfinavir, tenofovir, tipranavir	Efavirenz, nevirapine
Stavudine	Indinavir	Tipranavir
Tenofovir	Atazanavir, lopinavir, ritonavir	Tipranavir
Tipranavir	Didanosine, efavirenz	
Zidovudine	Amprenavir, indinavir, lamivudine	Didanosine, nelfinavir, ritonavir, tipranavir

zidovudine-sensitive and zidovudine-resistant HIV-1 strains. Activity against HBV is described below.

Oral bioavailability exceeds 80% and is not food-dependent. In children, the mean cerebrospinal fluid:plasma ratio of lamivudine was 0.2. Mean elimination half-life is 2.5 hours, whereas the intracellular half-life of the active 5'-triphosphate metabolite in HIV-1-infected cell lines is 10.5–15.5 hours. The majority of lamivudine is eliminated unchanged in the urine, and the dose should be reduced in patients with renal insufficiency or low body weight (Table 49–3).

Lamivudine therapy rapidly selects for the M184V mutation in regimens that are not fully suppressive; this mutation confers high-level resistance as well as a reduction in susceptibility to abacavir, didanosine, and zalcitabine. Conversely, the M184V mutation may restore phenotypic susceptibility to zidovudine, indicating that this two-drug combination regimen may be particularly beneficial. However, HIV-1 strains resistant to both lamivudine and zidovudine have been isolated. The K65R mutation is associated with reduced susceptibility to lamivudine, abacavir, tenofovir, and emtricitabine.

Potential adverse effects are headache, insomnia, fatigue, and gastrointestinal discomfort, although these are typically mild. Lamivudine's bioavailability increases when it is co-administered with trimethoprim-sulfamethoxazole. Lamivudine and zalcitabine may inhibit the intracellular phosphorylation of one another in vitro, thus decreasing potency; therefore, their concurrent use should be avoided if possible.

STAVUDINE

The thymidine analog stavudine (d4T) (Figure 49–2) has high oral bioavailability (86%) that is not food-dependent. The plasma half-life is 1.2 hours, the intracellular half-life is approximately 3.5 hours, and mean cerebrospinal fluid concentrations are 55% of those of plasma. Excretion is by active tubular secretion and glomerular filtration. The dosage of stavudine should be reduced in patients with renal insufficiency and low body weight (Table 49–3).

A number of mutations are associated with reduced susceptibility to stavudine; the predominant mutations are M41L, D67N, K70R, L210W, T215Y/F, and K219O.

The major dose-limiting toxicity is a dose-related peripheral sensory neuropathy. The incidence of neuropathy may be increased when stavudine is administered with other neuropathy-inducing drugs such as didanosine and zalcitabine. Symptoms typically resolve completely upon discontinuation of stavudine; in such cases, a reduced dosage may be cautiously restarted. Other potential adverse effects include pancreatitis, arthralgias, and elevation in serum aminotransferases. Lactic acidosis with hepatic steatosis, as well as fat atrophy, appears to occur more frequently in patients receiving stavudine than in those receiving other NRTI agents. Moreover, because the co-administration of stavudine and didanosine may increase the incidence of lactic acidosis and pancreatitis, concurrent use should be avoided, if possible. This combination has been implicated in several deaths in HIV-infected pregnant women. A rare side effect is a rapidly progressive ascending neuromuscular weakness. Since zidovudine may reduce the phosphorylation of stavudine, these two drugs should generally not be used together.

TENOFOVIR

Tenofovir is an acyclic nucleoside phosphonate (ie, nucleotide) analog of adenosine (Figure 49–2). Like the nucleoside analogs, tenofovir competitively inhibits HIV reverse transcriptase and causes chain termination after incorporation into DNA.

Tenofovir disopoxilfumarate is a water-soluble prodrug of active tenofovir. The oral bioavailability in fasted patients is approximately 25% and increases to 39% after a high-fat meal. Serum half-life is 17 hours and intracellular half-life is prolonged at more than 60 hours. Elimination occurs by a combination of glomerular filtration and active tubular secretion, and the dosage must be adjusted in patients with renal insufficiency.

The primary mutation associated with resistance to tenofovir is K65R, although varying degrees of decreased susceptibility to tenofovir may be conferred by zidovudine-associated mutations (eg, M41L, L210W), according to the number of specific mutations present.

Gastrointestinal complaints (eg, nausea, diarrhea, vomiting, flatulence) are the most common side effects but rarely require discontinuation of therapy. Other potential adverse effects include headache and asthenia. Preclinical studies in several animal species have demonstrated bone toxicity (eg, osteomalacia); however, to date there has been no evidence of bone toxicity in humans. Cases of renal impairment, including acute renal failure and Fanconi's syndrome, have been reported in patients receiving tenofovir. Tenofovir may compete with other drugs that are actively secreted by the kidneys, such as cidofovir, acyclovir, and ganciclovir. The combination of tenofovir with didanosine is associated with both decreased virologic efficacy and increased toxicity (due to increased didanosine levels) and therefore should be avoided.

ZALCITABINE

Zalcitabine (ddC) is a cytosine analog with high oral bioavailability (> 80%) and a relatively long intracellular half-life (10 hours) despite its elimination half-life of 1–2 hours (Figure 49–2). However, plasma levels decrease by 25–39% when the drug is administered with food or antacids. Cerebrospinal fluid concentrations are approximately 20% of those in the plasma.

Although a variety of mutations associated with in vitro resistance to zalcitabine have been described (eg,

T69D, K65R, M184V, L74V), phenotypic resistance appears to be rare, particularly in combination regimens.

Zalcitabine therapy is associated with a dose-dependent peripheral neuropathy that can be treatment-limiting in 10–20% of patients but appears to be slowly reversible if treatment is stopped promptly. The potential for causing peripheral neuropathy constitutes a relative contraindication to use with other drugs that may cause this toxicity, including stavudine, didanosine, and isoniazid. Decreased renal clearance caused by amphotericin B, foscarnet, and aminoglycosides may increase the risk of zalcitabine neuropathy. The other major reported toxicity is oral and esophageal ulcerations. Pancreatitis occurs less frequently than with didanosine administration, but co-administration of other drugs that cause pancreatitis may increase the frequency of this adverse effect. Headache, nausea, rash, and arthralgias may occur but tend to be mild or resolve during therapy. Cardiomyopathy has rarely been reported. Zalcitabine causes thymic lymphomas in rodents, but no clinical correlates have been observed in humans.

The AUC of zalcitabine increases when co-administered with probenecid or cimetidine, and bioavailability decreases with concurrent antacids or metoclopramide. Lamivudine inhibits the phosphorylation of zalcitabine in vitro, potentially interfering with its efficacy.

ZIDOVUDINE

Zidovudine (azidothymidine; AZT) is a deoxythymidine analog (Figure 49–2) that is well absorbed from the gut and distributed to most body tissues and fluids, including the cerebrospinal fluid, where drug levels are 60–65% of those in serum. The serum half-life averages 1 hour, and the intracellular half life of the phosphorylated compound is 3–7 hours. Zidovudine is eliminated primarily by renal excretion following glucuronidation in the liver. Clearance of zidovudine is reduced by approximately 50% in uremic patients, and toxicity may increase in patients with advanced hepatic insufficiency.

Zidovudine was the first antiretroviral agent to be approved and has been well studied. The drug has been shown to decrease the rate of clinical disease progression and prolong survival in HIV-infected individuals. Efficacy has also been demonstrated in the treatment of HIV-associated dementia and thrombocytopenia. In pregnancy (Table 49–5), a regimen of oral zidovudine beginning between 14 and 34 weeks of gestation (100 mg five times a day), intravenous zidovudine during labor (2 mg/kg over 1 hour, then 1 mg/kg/h by continuous infusion), and zidovudine syrup to the neonate from birth through 6 weeks of age (2 mg/kg every 6 hours) has been shown to reduce the rate of vertical (mother-to-newborn) transmission of HIV by up to 23%.

As with other NRTI agents, resistance may limit clinical efficacy. High-level zidovudine resistance is generally

Table 49–5. The use of antiretroviral agents in pregnancy.

Recommended Agents	Alternate Agents
Nucleoside/nucleotide reverse transcriptase inhibitors (NRTIs)	
Zidovudine, lamivudine	Didanosine, emtricitabine, stavudine, abacavir
Nonnucleoside reverse transcriptase inhibitors (NNRTIs)	
Nevirapine	
Protease inhibitors (PIs)	
Nelfinavir, saquinavir-S	Indinavir, lopinavir/ritonavir, ritonavir

seen in strains with three or more of the five most common mutations: M41L, D67N, K70R, T215F, and K219Q. However, the emergence of certain mutations that confer decreased susceptibility to one drug (eg, L74V for didanosine and M184V for lamivudine) seems to enhance zidovudine susceptibility in previously zidovudine-resistant strains. Withdrawal of zidovudine exposure may permit the reversion of zidovudine-resistant HIV-1 isolates to the susceptible wild-type phenotype.

The most common adverse effect of zidovudine is myelosuppression, resulting in macrocytic anemia (1–4%) or neutropenia (2–8%). Gastrointestinal intolerance, headaches, and insomnia may occur but tend to resolve during therapy. Less frequent toxicities include thrombocytopenia, hyperpigmentation of the nails, and myopathy. Very high doses can cause anxiety, confusion, and tremulousness. Zidovudine causes vaginal neoplasms in mice; however, no human cases of genital neoplasms have been reported to date.

Increased serum levels of zidovudine may occur with concomitant administration of probenecid, phenytoin, methadone, fluconazole, atovaquone, valproic acid, and lamivudine, either through inhibition of first-pass metabolism or through decreased clearance. Zidovudine may decrease phenytoin levels, and this warrants monitoring of serum phenytoin levels in epileptic patients taking both agents. Hematologic toxicity may be increased during co-administration of other myelosuppressive drugs such as ganciclovir, ribavirin, and cytotoxic agents. Combination regimens containing zidovudine and stavudine should be avoided; antagonism has been demonstrated in vitro.

NONNUCLEOSIDE REVERSE TRANSCRIPTASE INHIBITORS

The NNRTIs bind directly to HIV-1 reverse transcriptase (Figure 49–4), resulting in blockade of RNA- and DNA-dependent DNA polymerase. The binding site of NNRTIs is near to but distinct from that of NRTIs. Unlike the NRTI agents, NNRTIs neither compete with nucleoside triphosphates nor require phosphorylation to be active. NNRTI resistance occurs rapidly with monotherapy and can be due to a single mutation (eg, K103N). The K103N and Y181C mutations confer resistance across the entire class of NNRTIs, whereas L100I, Y188C, and G190A confer resistance to both nevirapine and efavirenz.

As a class, NNRTI agents tend to be associated with varying levels of gastrointestinal intolerance and skin rash, the latter of which may infrequently be serious (eg, Stevens-Johnson syndrome). A further limitation to use of NNRTI agents as a component of HAART is their metabolism by the CYP450 system, leading to innumerable potential drug-drug interactions (Tables 49–3 and 49–4). NNRTI agents are all substrates for CYP3A4 and can act as inducers (nevirapine), inhibitors (delavirdine), or mixed inducers and inhibitors (efavirenz). Given the large number of non-HIV medications that are also metabolized by this pathway (see Chapter 4); drug-drug interactions must be expected and looked for.

DELAVIRDINE

Delavirdine has an oral bioavailability of about 85%, but this is reduced by antacids or H_2-blockers. It is extensively bound (~ 98%) to plasma proteins and has correspondingly low cerebrospinal fluid levels.

Skin rash occurs in approximately 18% of patients receiving delavirdine; it typically occurs during the first 1–3 weeks of therapy and does not preclude rechallenge. However, severe rash such as erythema multiforme and Stevens-Johnson syndrome have rarely been reported. Other possible adverse effects are headache, fatigue, nausea, diarrhea, and increased serum aminotransferase levels. Delavirdine has been shown to be teratogenic in rats, causing ventricular septal defects and other malformations at dosages not unlike those achieved in humans. Thus, pregnancy should be avoided when taking delavirdine.

Delavirdine is extensively metabolized to inactive metabolites by the CYP3A and CYP2D6 enzymes and also inhibits CYP3A4 and 2C9. Therefore, there are numerous potential drug-drug interactions to consider (Tables 49–3 and 49–4). Because of this effect, however, co-administration with delavirdine may allow indinavir or saquinavir to be dosed twice daily rather than the usual three times a day. The concurrent use of delavirdine with amprenavir/fosamprenavir and rifabutin is not recommended because of decreased delavirdine levels.

EFAVIRENZ

Efavirenz can be given once daily because of its long half-life (40–55 hours). It is moderately well absorbed following oral administration (45%). Since toxicity

may increase owing to increased bioavailability after a high-fat meal, efavirenz should be taken on an empty stomach. Peak plasma concentrations occur 3–5 hours after administration of daily doses; steady-state plasma concentrations are reached in 6–10 days. Efavirenz is principally metabolized by CYP3A4 and CYP2B6 to inactive hydroxylated metabolites; the remainder is eliminated in the feces as unchanged drug. It is highly bound to albumin (~ 99%), and cerebrospinal fluid levels range from 0.3% to 1.2% of plasma levels.

The principal adverse effects of efavirenz involve the central nervous system (dizziness, drowsiness, insomnia, headache, confusion, amnesia, agitation, delusions, depression, nightmares, euphoria); these may occur in up to 50% of patients and may be severe. However, they tend to resolve after the first month of treatment. Skin rash has also been reported early in therapy in up to 28% of patients, is usually mild to moderate in severity, and typically resolves despite continuation. Other potential adverse reactions are nausea, vomiting, diarrhea, crystalluria, elevated liver enzymes, and an increase in total serum cholesterol by 10–20%. High rates of fetal abnormalities occurred in pregnant monkeys exposed to efavirenz in doses roughly equivalent to the human dosage; several cases of congenital anomalies have been reported in humans. Therefore, efanirenz should be avoided in pregnant women, particularly in the first trimester.

Efavirenz is both an inducer and an inhibitor of CYP3A4, thus inducing its own metabolism and interacting with the metabolism of many other drugs (Tables 49–3 and 49–4).

NEVIRAPINE

The oral bioavailability of nevirapine is excellent (~ 90%) and is not food-dependent. The drug is highly lipophilic and achieves cerebrospinal fluid levels that are 45% of those in plasma. Serum half-life is 25–30 hours. It is extensively metabolized by the CYP3A isoform to hydroxylated metabolites and then excreted, primarily in the urine.

In addition to its use as a component of a combination antiretroviral regimen, a single dose of nevirapine (200 mg) has been shown to be effective in the prevention of transmission of HIV from mother to newborn when administered to women at the onset of labor and followed by a 2-mg/kg oral dose to the neonate within 3 days after delivery. However, resistance has been documented after this single dose.

Rash occurs in approximately 17% of patients, most typically in the first 4–6 weeks of therapy, and is dose-limiting in about 7% of patients. When initiating therapy, gradual dose escalation over 14 days is recommended to decrease the incidence of rash. Women may have a greater propensity for rash. Severe and life-threatening skin rashes have been rarely reported, including Stevens-Johnson syndrome and toxic epidermal necrolysis. Nevirapine therapy should be immediately discontinued in patients with severe rash and in those with accompanying constitutional symptoms. Hepatotoxicity occurs in about 4% of patients and appears to occur more frequently in those with higher pre-therapy CD4 cell counts (ie, > 250 cells/mm^3 in women and > 400 cells/mm^3 in men), in women, and in those with hepatitis B or C co-infection. Fulminant hepatitis may rarely occur, typically within the first 18 weeks of therapy and can be fatal. Other adverse effects associated with nevirapine therapy are fever, nausea, headache, and somnolence.

Nevirapine is a moderate inducer of CYP3A metabolism, resulting in decreased levels of amprenavir, indinavir, lopinavir, saquinavir, efavirenz, and methadone if administered concurrently (Table 49–4). Drugs that induce the CYP3A system, such as tipranavir, rifampin, rifabutin, and St. John's wort, can decrease levels of nevirapine, whereas those that inhibit CYP3A activity, such as fluconazole, ketoconazole, and clarithromycin, can increase nevirapine levels.

PROTEASE INHIBITORS

During the later stages of the HIV growth cycle, the *Gag* and *Gag-Pol* gene products are translated into polyproteins, and these become immature budding particles. Protease is responsible for cleaving these precursor molecules to produce the final structural proteins of the mature virion core. By preventing cleavage of the Gag-Pol polyprotein, protease inhibitors (PIs) result in the production of immature, noninfectious viral particles (Figure 49–4). Unfortunately, specific genotypic alterations that confer phenotypic resistance are fairly common with these agents, thus contraindicating monotherapy. Some of the most common mutations conferring resistance to most if not all of the PI agents are L10I/R/V, M46I/L, I54V/M/L, V82A/F/T/S, and I84V.

A syndrome of redistribution and accumulation of body fat that results in central obesity, dorsocervical fat enlargement (buffalo hump), peripheral and facial wasting, breast enlargement, and a cushingoid appearance has been observed in patients receiving antiretroviral therapy. These abnormalities may be particularly associated with the use of PIs, although the recently licensed atazanavir appears to be an exception (see below). Concurrent increases in triglyceride and LDL levels, along with glucose intolerance and insulin resistance, have also been noted. The cause is not yet known.

Protease inhibitors have been associated with increased spontaneous bleeding in patients with hemophilia A or B.

All of the antiretroviral PIs are substrates and inhibitors of CYP3A4, with ritonavir having the most pro-

nounced inhibitory effect and saquinavir the least. Some PI agents such as amprenavir and ritonavir are also inducers of specific CYP isoforms. As a result, there is enormous potential for drug-drug interactions with other antiretroviral agents and other commonly used medications (Tables 49–3 and 49–4). It is noteworthy that the potent CYP3A4 inhibitory properties of ritonavir have been utilized to clinical advantage by having it "boost" the levels of other PI agents when given in combination.

AMPRENAVIR

Amprenavir is rapidly absorbed from the gastrointestinal tract and can be taken with or without food. However, high-fat meals decrease absorption and thus should be avoided. The plasma half-life is relatively long (7–10.6 hours). Amprenavir is metabolized in the liver by CYP3A4 and should be used with caution in the setting of hepatic insufficiency.

The key mutation conferring resistance to amprenavir appears to be I50V. Evidence to date suggests that cross-resistance to other members of the PI class of drugs may be less prevalent with amprenavir than with previously available compounds.

The most common adverse effects of amprenavir are nausea, diarrhea, vomiting, perioral paresthesias, depression, and rash. Up to 3% of patients in clinical trials to date have had rashes (including Stevens-Johnson syndrome) severe enough to warrant drug discontinuation.

Amprenavir is both an inducer and an inhibitor of CYP3A4 and is contraindicated with numerous other drugs (Tables 49–3 and 49–4). The oral solution, which contains propylene glycol, is contraindicated in young children, pregnant women, patients with renal or hepatic failure, and those using metronidazole or disulfiram. Also, the oral solutions of amprenavir and ritonavir should not be co-administered because the propylene glycol in one and the ethanol in the other may compete for the same metabolic pathway, leading to accumulation of either. Because the oral solution also contains vitamin E at several times the recommended daily dosage, supplemental vitamin E should be avoided. Amprenavir is contraindicated in patients with a history of sulfa allergy because it is itself a sulfonamide. Lopinavir/ritonavir should not be co-administered with amprenavir owing to decreased amprenavir and increased lopinavir exposures. An increased dosage of amprenavir is recommended when co-administered with efavirenz (with or without the addition of ritonavir to boost levels).

ATAZANAVIR

Atazanavir is a newer azapeptide PI with a pharmacokinetic profile that allows once-daily dosing. Its oral bioavailability is approximately 60–68%; the drug should be taken with food. Atazanavir requires an acidic medium for absorption and exhibits pH-dependent aqueous solubility; therefore, separation of ingestion from acid-reducing agents by at least 12 hours is recommended. Atazanavir is able to penetrate both the cerebrospinal and seminal fluids. The plasma half-life is 6–7 hours, which increases to approximately 11 hours when co-administered with ritonavir. The primary route of elimination is biliary; atazanavir should not be given to patients with severe hepatic insufficiency.

Resistance to atazanavir has been associated with various known PI mutations including the novel I50L substitution, which has been associated with *increased* susceptibility to other PIs.

The most common adverse effects in patients receiving atazanavir in clinical trials were nausea, vomiting, diarrhea, abdominal pain, headache, peripheral neuropathy, and skin rash. As with indinavir, indirect hyperbilirubinemia with overt jaundice may occur, in all likelihood owing to inhibition of the UGT1A1 enzyme. Although bilirubinemia is not regularly associated with hepatic injury, elevation of hepatic enzymes has also been observed, usually in patients with underlying hepatitis B or C infection. In contrast to the other PIs, atazanavir does not appear to be associated with dyslipidemias, fat redistribution, or the metabolic syndrome. Atazanavir may be associated with electrocardiographic PR interval prolongation, which is usually inconsequential but may be exacerbated by other causative agents such as calcium channel blockers. Also, a possible concentration-dependent increase in the QT_c interval may occur in patients receiving atazanavir in dosages greater than 400 mg/d or in conjunction with the CYP3A4 inhibitor clarithromycin.

As an inhibitor of CYP3A4 and CYP2C9, the potential for drug-drug interactions with atazanavir is great (see Tables 49–3 and 49–4). Atazanavir AUC is reduced by 76% on average when combined with omeprazole; thus, the combination is to be avoided. In addition, co-administration of atazanavir with other drugs that inhibit the glucuronidation enzyme UGT1A1, such as indinavir and irinotecan, is contraindicated because of enhanced toxicity. Tenofovir and efavirenz should not be co-administered with atazanavir unless ritonavir is added to boost levels.

FOSAMPRENAVIR

Fosamprenavir is a prodrug of amprenavir that is rapidly hydrolyzed by enzymes in the intestinal epithelium. Tablets may be taken with or without food. Because of its significantly lower daily pill burden, fosamprenavir tablets have replaced amprenavir capsules for adults. All pharmacokinetic and pharmacodynamic attributes are those of amprenavir (see above).

INDINAVIR

Indinavir must be consumed on an empty stomach for maximal absorption; however, if co-administered with ritonavir, it may be taken without regard to food. Oral bioavailability is about 65%, and the drug has a high level of cerebrospinal fluid penetration (up to 76% of serum levels). Serum half-life is 1.5–2 hours. Excretion is primarily fecal. An increase in AUC by 60% and in half-life to 2.8 hours in the setting of hepatic insufficiency necessitates dose reduction.

Resistance may be associated with multiple mutations, particularly at positions 46 and 82, and the number of codon alterations (typically substitutions) tends to predict the level of phenotypic resistance. Resistance to indinavir is associated with a loss of susceptibility to ritonavir.

The most common adverse effects are indirect hyperbilirubinemia and nephrolithiasis due to crystallization of the drug. Nephrolithiasis can occur within days after initiating therapy, with an estimated incidence of 10–20%, and it may be associated with renal failure. Consumption of at least 48 ounces of water daily is important to maintain adequate hydration and prevent nephrolithiasis. Thrombocytopenia, elevations of serum aminotransferase levels, nausea, diarrhea, and irritability have also been reported. Insulin resistance may be more common with indinavir than with the other PI agents, occurring in 3–5% of patients. There have also been rare cases of acute hemolytic anemia. In rats, high doses of indinavir are associated with development of thyroid adenomas.

Since indinavir is an inhibitor of CYP3A4, numerous and complex drug interactions can occur (Tables 49–3 and 49–4). Combination with ritonavir (boosting) allows for twice-daily rather than thrice-daily dosing and eliminates the food restriction associated with use of indinavir. However, there is potential for an increase in nephrolithiasis with this combination compared with indinavir alone; thus, a high fluid intake (1.5–2 L/d) is advised.

LOPINAVIR/RITONAVIR

Lopinavir 100/ritonavir 400 is a licensed combination in which subtherapeutic doses of ritonavir inhibit the CYP3A-mediated metabolism of lopinavir, thereby resulting in increased exposure to lopinavir. Trough levels of lopinavir are greater than the median HIV-1 wild-type 50% inhibitory concentration, thus maintaining potent viral suppression as well as providing a pharmacologic barrier to the emergence of resistance. In this combination, therefore, ritonavir is acting as a pharmacokinetic enhancer rather than an antiretroviral agent. In addition to improved patient compliance due to reduced pill burden, lopinavir/ritonavir is generally well tolerated.

Absorption of lopinavir is enhanced with food. The oral solution contains alcohol. Lopinavir is extensively metabolized by the CYP3A isozyme of the hepatic cytochrome P450 system, which is inhibited by ritonavir. Serum levels of lopinavir may be increased in patients with hepatic impairment.

The most common adverse effects of lopinavir are diarrhea, abdominal pain, nausea, vomiting, and asthenia. Potential drug-drug interactions are extensive (see ritonavir and Tables 49–3 and 49–4). Increased dosage of lopinavir/ritonavir is recommended when co-administered with efavirenz or nevirapine, which induce lopinavir metabolism. Concurrent use of fosamprenavir should be avoided owing to increased exposure to lopinavir with decreased levels of amprenavir.

NELFINAVIR

Nelfinavir has higher absorption in the fed state (increased AUC by two- to threefold), undergoes metabolism by CYP3A, and is excreted primarily in the feces. The plasma half-life in humans is 3.5–5 hours. The D30N mutation appears to be particularly closely linked with phenotypic resistance in isolates obtained from clinical trials.

The most common adverse effects associated with nelfinavir are diarrhea and flatulence. Diarrhea often responds to antidiarrheal medications but can be dose-limiting. Like other PIs, nelfinavir is an inhibitor of the CYP3A system, and multiple drug interactions may occur (Tables 49–3 and 49–4). An increased dosage of nelfinavir is recommended when co-administered with rifabutin (with a decreased dose of rifabutin), whereas a decrease in saquinavir dose is suggested with concurrent nelfinavir. Nelfinavir has a favorable safety and pharmacokinetic profile for pregnant women compared with that of other PIs (Table 49–5).

RITONAVIR

Ritonavir is an inhibitor of HIV-1 and HIV-2 proteases with high bioavailability (about 75%) that increases when the drug is given with food. Metabolism to an active metabolite occurs via the CYP3A and CYP2D6 isoforms; excretion is primarily in the feces. Caution is advised when administering the drug to persons with impaired hepatic function.

Resistance is associated with mutations at positions 84, 82, 71, 63, and 46, of which the I84V mutation appears to be the most critical.

The most common adverse effects of ritonavir are gastrointestinal disturbances, paresthesias (circumoral and peripheral), elevated serum aminotransferase levels, altered taste, and hypertriglyceridemia. Nausea, vomiting, and abdominal pain typically occur during the first few weeks of therapy. Slow dose escalation over

4–5 days is recommended to decrease the dose-limiting side effects. Liver adenomas and carcinomas have been induced in male mice receiving ritonavir; no similar effects have been observed to date in humans.

Ritonavir is a potent inhibitor of CYP3A4; as such, co-administration with agents heavily metabolized by CYP3A must be approached with caution (Tables 49–3 and 49–4). In addition, therapeutic levels of digoxin and theophylline should be monitored when co-administered with ritonavir owing to likely increase in their concentrations. However, the CYP3A4 inhibitory properties of ritonavir have been exploited to raise the trough concentration and prolong the half-life of more potent and less toxic PI agents. Thus, lower than therapeutic doses of ritonavir are commonly given in combination with agents such as lopinavir, indinavir, or amprenavir to reduce the risk of resistance by increasing the time of drug exposure. Moreover, the prolonged half-life allows for less frequent dosing of the other PI agent, thus enhancing adherence.

SAQUINAVIR

In its original formulation as a hard gel capsule (saquinavir-H; Invirase), oral saquinavir is poorly bioavailable (only about 4% after food). It was therefore largely replaced in clinical use by a soft gel capsule formulation (saquinavir-S; Fortovase) in which absorption was increased approximately threefold. However, reformulation of saquinavir-H for once-daily dosing in combination with low-dose ritonavir (see below) has both improved antiviral efficacy and decreased the gastrointestinal side effects typically associated with saquinavir-S. Moreover, co-administration of saquinavir-H with ritonavir results in blood levels of saquinavir similar to those associated with saquinavir-S, thus capitalizing on the pharmacokinetic interaction of the two agents. The manufacturer announced plans to discontinue the manufacture of saquinavir-S in early 2006.

The most common critical resistance mutations are L90M and G48V, conferring an approximately tenfold decrease in susceptibility to saquinavir.

Both formulations of saquinavir should be taken within 2 hours after a fatty meal for enhanced absorption. Saquinavir has a large volume of distribution, but penetration into the cerebrospinal fluid is negligible. The elimination half-life is 12 hours. Excretion is primarily in the feces. Reported adverse effects include gastrointestinal discomfort (nausea, diarrhea, abdominal discomfort, dyspepsia; these are more common with saquinavir-S) and rhinitis.

Saquinavir is subject to extensive first-pass metabolism by CYP3A4, and functions as a CYP3A4 inhibitor as well as a substrate; thus, it should be used with the same precautions regarding drug-drug interactions as are the other PIs (Table 49–4). Co-administration with the CYP3A4 inhibitor ritonavir has been adopted by clinicians because of the higher—and thus more efficacious—levels of saquinavir while enabling reduction in daily dose and frequency of saquinavir. A decreased dose of saquinavir is recommended when co-administered with nelfinavir. Liver function tests should be monitored if saquinavir is co-administered with delavirdine or rifampin.

TIPRANAVIR

Tipranavir is another newer PI. Bioavailability is poor but is increased when taken with a high-fat meal. The drug is metabolized by the liver microsomal system. Tipranavir must be taken in combination with ritonavir to achieve effective serum levels. It is contraindicated in patients with hepatic insufficiency. Tipranavir contains a sulfonamide moiety and should not be administered to patients with known sulfa allergy.

The most common adverse effects are diarrhea, nausea, vomiting, abdominal pain, and rash; the latter is more common in women. Liver toxicity, including life-threatening hepatic decompensation, has been observed and is more common in patients with chronic hepatitis B or C. In 2006 a black box warning was added noting a possible increase in intracranial hemorrhage in patients taking tipranavir. Other potential adverse effects include depression; elevations in total cholesterol, triglycerides, and amylase; and decreased white blood cell count.

Tipranavir both inhibits and induces the CYP3A4 system. When used in combination with ritonavir, its net effect is inhibition. Tipranavir also induces P-glycoprotein transporter and thus may alter the disposition of many other drugs (see Table 49–4). Concurrent administration of tipranavir with amprenavir or saquinavir should be avoided owing to decreased blood levels of the latter drugs.

FUSION INHIBITORS— ENFUVIRTIDE

Enfuvirtide (formerly called T-20) is the first representative of a new class of antiretroviral agents: It is a fusion inhibitor that blocks entry into the cell (Figure 49–4). Enfuvirtide, a synthetic 36-amino-acid peptide, binds to the gp41 subunit of the viral envelope glycoprotein, preventing the conformational changes required for the fusion of the viral and cellular membranes. Enfuvirtide must be administered by subcutaneous injection. Metabolism appears to be by proteolytic hydrolysis without involvement of the CYP450 system. Elimination half-life is 3.8 hours.

Resistance to enfuvirtide can occur, and the frequency and mechanisms of this phenomenon are being investigated. However, enfuvirtide lacks cross-resistance to the other currently approved antiretroviral drug classes.

The most common adverse effects associated with enfuvirtide therapy are local injection site reactions. Hypersensitivity reactions may rarely occur, are of varying severity, and may recur on rechallenge. Eosinophilia has also been noted. No interactions have been identified that would require the alteration of the dosage of other antiretroviral drugs.

INVESTIGATIONAL ANTIRETROVIRAL AGENTS

New therapies are being sought that offer convenient dosing, lower incidence of adverse effects, new viral targets, and activity against resistant viruses. Agents under evaluation or reformulation for once-daily dosing include stavudine and nevirapine. New agents currently in advanced stages of clinical development include the NRTI agent elvucitabine, the NNRTI agents TMC-125 and TMC-278, the PI agents TMC-114* and GSK-640385, and chemokine co-receptor inhibitors to block virus entry such as maraviroc. In addition, new drug classes such as maturation inhibitors and integrase inhibitors are under clinical investigation.

■ IV. ANTIHEPATITIS AGENTS

Several agents effective against hepatitis B virus (HBV) and hepatitis C virus (HCV) are now available (Table 49–6). Although treatment is suppressive rather than curative, the high prevalence of these infections worldwide, with their concomitant morbidity and mortality, reflect a critical need for improved therapeutics.

INTERFERON ALFA

Interferons are host cytokines that exert complex antiviral, immunomodulatory, and antiproliferative activities (see Chapter 56). Interferon (IFN)-alfa appears to function by induction of intracellular signals following binding to specific cell membrane receptors, resulting in inhibition of viral penetration, translation, transcription, protein processing, maturation, and release, as well as increased expression of major histocompatibility complex antigens, enhanced phagocytic activity of macrophages, and augmentation of the proliferation and survival of cytotoxic T cells.

Injectable preparations of interferon alfa are available for treatment of both HBV and HCV virus infections (Table 49–6). Interferon alfa-2a and interferon alfa-2b

---

*TMC-114 was licensed as **darunavir** in the USA in 2006, to be co-administered with ritonavir in treatment-experienced patients with resistance to other PIs (Table 49–3).

Table 49–6. Drugs used to treat viral hepatitis.

Agent	Indication	Recommended Adult Dosage	Route of Administration
Hepatitis B			
Lamivudine[1]	Chronic hepatitis B	100 mg once daily	Oral
Adefovir[1]	Chronic hepatitis B	10 mg once daily	Oral
Entecavir[1]	Chronic hepatitis B	0.5–1 mg once daily	Oral
Interferon alfa-2b	Chronic hepatitis B	5 million units once daily or 10 million units three times weekly	Subcutaneous or intramuscular
Hepatitis C			
Pegylated interferon alfa-2a[1]	Chronic hepatitis C	18 mcg once weekly with ribavirin or 180 mcg once weekly as monotherapy	Subcutaneous
Pegylated interferon alfa-2b[1]	Chronic hepatitis C	1.5 mcg/kg once weekly with ribavirin or 1.0 mcg/kg once weekly as monotherapy	Subcutaneous
Ribavirin[2]	Chronic hepatitis C	800–1200 mg daily, according to weight	Oral
Interferon alfa-2b[1]	Acute hepatitis C	5 million units once daily for 3–4 weeks, then 5 million units three times weekly	Subcutaneous or intramuscular
Interferon alfa-2a[1]	Chronic hepatitis C	3 million units three times weekly	Subcutaneous or intramuscular
Interferon alfa-2b[1]	Chronic hepatitis C	3 million units three times weekly	Subcutaneous or intramuscular
Interferon alfacon-1	Chronic hepatitis C	9–15 mcg three times weekly as monotherapy	Subcutaneous

[1]Dose must be reduced in patients with renal insufficiency.
[2]Not recommended as monotherapy.

may be administered subcutaneously or intramuscularly, whereas interferon alfacon-1 is administered subcutaneously. Elimination half-life is 2–5 hours for interferon alfa 2a and 2b, depending on the route of administration. The half-life of interferon alfacon-1 in patients with chronic hepatitis C ranges from 6 hours to 10 hours. Alfa interferons are filtered at the glomeruli and undergo rapid proteolytic degradation during tubular reabsorption, such that detection in the systemic circulation is negligible. Liver metabolism and subsequent biliary excretion are considered minor pathways.

Pegylated interferon alfa-2a and pegylated interferon alfa-2b have recently been introduced for the treatment of patients with HBV and HCV infections. Slower clearance of these agents results in substantially longer terminal half-lives and steadier drug concentrations, allowing for less frequent dosing. Renal elimination accounts for about 30% of clearance, and clearance is approximately halved in subjects with impaired renal function; dosage must therefore be adjusted.

In patients with chronic HBV infection, a recent meta-analysis of clinical trials showed that treatment with interferon alfa is associated with a higher incidence of hepatitis e antigen (HBeAg) seroconversion and undetectable HBV DNA levels than placebo. The addition of the pegylated moiety results in further increases in the proportion of patients with HBeAg seroconversion (~ 30%) and a decline by approximately 4 log copies/mL (99.99%) in HBV DNA after 1 year. Trials of the pegylated interferon alfas in chronic HCV infection are discussed below.

Typical side effects of interferon alfa include a flu-like syndrome (ie, headache, fevers, chills, myalgias, and malaise) that occurs within 6 hours after dosing in more than 30% of patients during the first week of therapy and tends to resolve upon continued administration. Transient hepatic enzyme elevations may occur in the first 8–12 weeks of therapy and appear to be more common in responders. Potential adverse effects during chronic therapy include neurotoxicities (mood disorders, depression, somnolence, confusion, seizures), myelosuppression, profound fatigue, weight loss, rash, cough, myalgia, alopecia, tinnitus, reversible hearing loss, retinopathy, pneumonitis, and possibly cardiotoxicity. Induction of autoantibodies may occur, causing exacerbation or unmasking of autoimmune or thyroid disease. The polyethylene glycol molecule is a nontoxic polymer that is readily excreted in the urine.

Contraindications to interferon alfa therapy include hepatic decompensation, autoimmune disease, and history of cardiac arrhythmia. Caution is advised in the setting of psychiatric disease, epilepsy, thyroid disease, ischemic cardiac disease, severe renal insufficiency, and cytopenia. Alfa interferons are abortifacient in primates and should not be administered in pregnancy. Potential drug-drug interactions include increased theophylline levels and increased methadone levels. Combination therapy with NRTI agents may cause hepatic failure; in particular, co-administration with didanosine is not recommended. Co-administration with zidovudine may exacerbate cytopenias.

TREATMENT OF HEPATITIS B VIRUS INFECTION

The most common efficacy end points in clinical trials of hepatitis B virus infection are seroconversion from HBeAg from positive to negative and suppression of HBV DNA to undetectable levels. These end points are correlated with improvement in necroinflammatory disease, a decreased risk of hepatocellular carcinoma and cirrhosis, and a decreased need for liver transplantation. However, because current therapies suppress HBV replication rather than eradicate the virus, initial responses may not be durable. The covalently closed circular (ccc) DNA exists in stable form indefinitely within the cell, serving as a reservoir for HBV throughout the life of the cell and resulting in the capacity to reactivate. Relapse is more common in patients co-infected with HBV and hepatitis D virus.

As of 2006 there were three oral nucleoside/nucleotide analogs and two injectable interferon drugs available in the United States for the treatment of chronic HBV infection. Although three of the current antiretroviral NRTIs (emtricitabine, lamivudine, and tenofovir) have potent activity against HBV, only lamivudine is approved for clinical treatment. Although not FDA-approved, tenofovir is recommended by recent consensus guidelines for the treatment of patients co-infected with HBV and HIV-1. The anti-herpes agent famciclovir also has anti-HBV activity, but it is relatively weak and requires thrice-daily dosing. Because NRTI agents may be used in patients co-infected with hepatitis B and HIV, it is important to note that acute exacerbation of hepatitis may occur upon discontinuation or interruption of these agents.

LAMIVUDINE

The pharmacokinetics of lamivudine are described earlier in this chapter (see page 804). The more prolonged intracellular half-life in HBV cell lines (17–19 hours) than in HIV-infected cell lines (10.5–15.5 hours) allows for lower doses and less frequent administration. Lamivudine can be safely administered to patients with decompensated liver disease.

Lamivudine inhibits HBV DNA polymerase and HIV reverse transcriptase by competing with deoxycyti-

dine triphosphate for incorporation into the viral DNA, resulting in chain termination. Lamivudine achieves 3–4 log decreases in viral replication in most patients and suppression of HBV DNA to undetectable levels in about 44% of patients. Seroconversion of HBeAg from positive to negative occurs in about 17% of patients and is durable at 3 years in about 70% of responders. Continuation of treatment for 4–8 months after seroconversion may improve the durability of response. Response in HBeAg-negative patients is initially high but less durable.

Chronic therapy with lamivudine in patients with hepatitis may ultimately be limited by the emergence of lamivudine-resistant HBV isolates (eg, with the YMDD mutation). Resistance has been associated with flares of hepatitis and progressive liver disease. Cross-resistance between lamivudine and either emtricitabine or entecavir may occur; however, cross-resistance between lamivudine and adefovir has not been reported.

In the doses used for HBV infection, lamivudine has an excellent safety profile. Headache, nausea, and dizziness are rare. Co-infection with HIV may increase the risk of pancreatitis. No evidence of mitochondrial toxicity has been reported.

ADEFOVIR DIPIVOXIL

Although initially and abortively developed for treatment of HIV infection, adefovir dipivoxil gained approval, at lower and less toxic doses, for treatment of HBV infection. Adefovir dipivoxil is the diester prodrug of adefovir, an acyclic phosphonated adenine nucleotide analog (Figure 49–2). It is phosphorylated by cellular kinases to the active diphosphate metabolite and then competitively inhibits HBV DNA polymerase to result in chain termination after incorporation into the viral DNA. Naturally occuring (ie, primary) adefovir-resistant rt233 HBV mutants have recently been described.

Oral bioavailability is about 59% and is unaffected by meals. The terminal elimination half-life is approximately 7.5 hours. Adefovir is excreted by a combination of glomerular filtration and active tubular secretion and thus may be administered to patients with decompensated liver disease.

Recent placebo-controlled trials showed that adefovir resulted in a mean of 3.5 logs reduction of HBV DNA copies/mL, normalization of aspartate aminotransferase in 48%–72% of patients, and improvement in liver histology and fibrosis in 53%–64% of patients at 48 weeks. More prolonged therapy results in higher rates of response, with anti-HBeAg seroconversion in 23% by 72 weeks and improved inflammation and fibrosis on liver biopsy at 5 years. Although emergence of resistance during therapy is rare (~ 4% after 3 years of use), specific mutations have been associated with viral rebound. There is no cross-resistance between adefovir and lamivudine.

Adefovir dipivoxil is well tolerated. A dose-dependent nephrotoxicity has been observed in clinical trials, manifested by increased serum creatinine with decreased serum phosphorous and more common in patients with baseline renal insufficiency. Other potential adverse effects are headache, diarrhea, asthenia, and abdominal pain. As with other NRTI agents, lactic acidosis and hepatic steatosis are considered a risk owing to mitochondrial dysfunction. Adefovir is embryotoxic in rats.

ENTECAVIR

Entecavir is an orally administered guanosine nucleoside analog (Figure 49–2) that competitively inhibits all three functions of HBV DNA polymerase, including base priming, reverse transcription of the negative strand, and synthesis of the positive strand of HBV DNA. Oral bioavailability approaches 100% but is decreased by food; therefore, entecavir should be taken on an empty stomach. The intracellular half-life of the active phosphorylated compound is 15 hours. It is excreted by the kidney, undergoing both glomerular filtration and net tubular secretion.

Comparison with lamivudine in patients with chronic HBV infection demonstrated similar rates of HBeAg seroconversion but significantly higher rates of HBV DNA viral suppression with entecavir, normalization of serum alanine aminotransferase levels, and histologic improvement in the liver. No primary resistance was observed to emerge after entecavir use for up to 48 weeks. However, decreased susceptibility to entecavir occurs in association with lamivudine resistance. Adefovir maintains activity against entecavir-resistant strains.

Entecavir is well tolerated. The most frequently reported adverse events are headache, fatigue, dizziness, and nausea. Lung adenomas and carcinomas in mice, hepatic adenomas and carcinomas in rats and mice, vascular tumors in mice, and brain gliomas and skin fibromas in rats have been observed at varying exposures. Co-administration of entecavir with drugs that reduce renal function or compete for active tubular secretion may increase serum concentrations of either entecavir or the co-administered drug.

INVESTIGATIONAL AGENTS

Compounds in advanced stages of clinical development for the treatment of patients with HBV infection include the nucleoside/nucleotide analogs clevudine, telbivudine, valtorcitabine, and alamifovir, as well as the immunologic modulator thymosin alpha-1, agents that facilitate uptake by the liver using conjugation to ligands, and RNA interference compounds.

TREATMENT OF HEPATITIS C INFECTION

The primary goal of treatment in patients with HCV infection is viral eradication. In clinical trials, the primary efficacy end point is typically achievement of sustained viral response (SVR), defined as the absence of detectable viremia for 6 months after completion of therapy. SVR is associated with improvement in liver histology and reduction in risk of hepatocellular carcinoma and occasionally with regression of cirrhosis as well. Late relapse occurs in fewer than 5% of patients who achieve SVR.

In acute hepatitis C, the rate of clearance of the virus without therapy is estimated to be 15–30%. In one (uncontrolled) study, treatment of acute infection with interferon alfa-2b, in doses higher than those used for chronic hepatitis C (Table 49–6), resulted in a sustained rate of clearance of 95% at 6 months. Therefore, if HCV RNA testing documents persistent viremia 12 weeks after initial seroconversion, antiviral therapy is recommended.

The current standard of treatment in patients with chronic HCV infection is once-weekly pegylated interferon alfa in combination with daily oral ribavirin. Pegylated interferon alfa-2a and -2b have replaced their unmodified interferon alfa counterparts because of superior efficacy in combination with ribavirin, regardless of genotype. It is also clear that combination therapy with oral ribavirin is more effective than monotherapy with either interferon or ribavirin alone. Therefore, monotherapy with pegylated interferon alfa is recommended only in patients who cannot tolerate ribavirin. Factors associated with a favorable response to therapy include HCV genotype 2 or 3, absence of cirrhosis on liver biopsy, and low pretreatment HCV RNA levels.

RIBAVIRIN

Ribavirin is a guanosine analog that is phosphorylated intracellularly by host cell enzymes. Although its mechanism of action has not been fully elucidated, it appears to interfere with the synthesis of guanosine triphosphate, to inhibit capping of viral messenger RNA, and to inhibit the viral RNA-dependent polymerase of certain viruses. Ribavirin triphosphate inhibits the replication of a wide range of DNA and RNA viruses, including influenza A and B, parainfluenza, respiratory syncytial virus, paramyxoviruses, HCV, and HIV-1.

The absolute oral bioavailability of ribavirin is about 64%, increases with high-fat meals, and decreases with co-administration of antacids. Ribavirin elimination is primarily through the urine; therefore, clearance is decreased in patients with creatinine clearances less than 30 mL/min.

Evidence suggests that both a higher dose (ie, > 10.6 mg/kg) and a longer duration of ribavirin therapy, in combination with one of the interferon alfas, may improve response. This must be balanced with an increased likelihood of toxicity. A dose-dependent hemolytic anemia occurs in 10–20% of patients. Other potential adverse effects are depression, fatigue, irritability, rash, cough, insomnia, nausea, and pruritus. Contraindications to ribavirin therapy include uncorrected anemia, end-stage renal failure, ischemic vascular disease, and pregnancy. Ribavirin is teratogenic and embryotoxic in animals as well as mutagenic in mammalian cells. Patients exposed to the drug should not conceive children for at least 6 months thereafter.

INVESTIGATIONAL AGENTS

Investigational agents for the treatment of HCV infection include inhibitors of the HCV RNA polymerase such as valopicitabine, the nucleoside analogs isatoribine and viramidine, monoclonal antibodies against the glycoprotein, several new types of interferons, congeners of ribavirin, PIs, and the immunomodulator thymosin alpha-1.

■ V. ANTI-INFLUENZA AGENTS

Influenza virus strains are classified by their core proteins (ie, A, B, or C), species of origin (eg, avian, swine), and geographic site of isolation. Influenza A, the only strain that causes pandemics, is classified into 16 H (hemagglutinin) and 9 N (neuraminidase) known subtypes based on surface proteins. Although influenza B viruses usually infect only people, influenza A viruses can infect a variety of animal hosts. Current influenza A subtypes that are circulating among people worldwide include H1N1, H1N2, and H3N2. Fifteen subtypes are known to infect birds, providing an extensive reservoir. Although avian influenza subtypes are typically highly species-specific, they have on rare occasions crossed the species barrier to infect humans and cats. Viruses of the H5 and H7 subtypes (eg, H5N1, H7N7, and H7N3) may rapidly mutate within poultry flocks from a low to high pathogenic form and have recently expanded their host range to cause both avian and human disease. Of particular concern is the H5N1 virus, which first caused human infection (including severe disease and death) in 1997 and has become endemic in Southeast Asia poultry since 2003. It is feared that the virus will become transmissible from person to person rather than solely from poultry to human, thus initiating the potential for a global outbreak (ie, pandemic).

Although both classes of antiviral drugs available for influenza have activity against influenza A, many or most of the circulating strains of avian H5N1, as well as the H1 and H3 strains causing seasonal influenza in the United States, are resistant to the adamantanamine agents.

AMANTADINE & RIMANTADINE

Amantadine (1-aminoadamantane hydrochloride) and its α-methyl derivative, rimantadine, are cyclic amines of the adamantine family that block the M2 proton ion channel of the virus particle and inhibit uncoating of the viral RNA within infected host cells, thus preventing its replication. They are active against influenza A only. Rimantadine is four to ten times more active than amantadine in vitro. Amantadine is excreted unchanged in the urine, whereas rimantadine undergoes extensive metabolism by hydroxylation, conjugation, and glucuronidation before urinary excretion. Dose reductions are required for both agents in the elderly and in patients with renal insufficiency and for rimantadine in patients with marked hepatic insufficiency.

In the absence of resistance, both amantadine and rimantadine, at 100 mg twice daily or 200 mg once daily, are 70–90% protective in the prevention of clinical illness when initiated before exposure. When begun within 1–2 days after the onset of illness, the duration of fever and systemic symptoms is reduced by 1–2 days.

The primary target for both agents is the M2 protein within the viral membrane, incurring both influenza A specificity and a mutation-prone site that results in the rapid development of resistance in up to 50% of treated individuals. Resistant isolates with single-point mutation are genetically stable, retain pathogenicity, can be transmitted to close contacts, and may be shed chronically by immunocompromised patients. The prevalence of resistance to both agents in clinical isolates in the United States increased from 2% in the 2003–2004 influenza season, to 12% in 2004–2005, to an alarming 91% in 2005–2006 (99% in H3N2, 1% in H1N1). Cross-resistance to zanamivir and oseltamivir does not occur.

The most common adverse effects are gastrointestinal (nausea, anorexia) and central nervous system (nervousness, difficulty in concentrating, insomnia, light-headedness). Central nervous system toxicity may be due to alteration of dopamine neurotransmission (see Chapter 28), is less frequent with rimantadine than with amantadine, tends to diminish after the first week of use, and may increase with concomitant antihistamines, anticholinergic drugs, hydrochlorothiazide, and trimethoprim-sulfamethoxazole. Serious neurotoxic reactions, occasionally fatal, may occur in association with high amantadine plasma concentrations and are more likely in the elderly or with renal insufficiency. Peripheral edema is another potential adverse effect. Both agents are teratogenic in rodents, and birth defects have been reported after exposure during pregnancy.

ZANAMIVIR & OSELTAMIVIR

The neuraminidase inhibitors zanamivir and oseltamivir, analogs of sialic acid, interfere with release of progeny influenza virus from infected to new host cells, thus halting the spread of infection within the respiratory tract.

Unlike amantadine and rimantadine, zanamivir and oseltamivir have activity against both influenza A and influenza B viruses. Early administration is crucial because replication of influenza virus peaks at 24–72 hours after the onset of illness. When a 5-day course of therapy is initiated within 36–48 hours after the onset of symptoms, the duration of illness is decreased by 1–2 days compared with those on placebo, severity is diminished, and the incidence of secondary complications in children and adults decreases. Once-daily prophylaxis is 70–90% effective in preventing disease after exposure. Oseltamivir is FDA-approved for patients 1 year and older, whereas zanamivir is approved in patients 7 years or older.

Zanamivir is delivered directly to the respiratory tract via inhalation. Ten to twenty percent of the active compound reaches the lungs, and the remainder is deposited in the oropharynx. The concentration of the drug in the respiratory tract is estimated to be more than 1000 times the 50% inhibitory concentration for neuraminidase. Five to fifteen percent of the total dose (10 mg twice daily for treatment and 10 mg once daily for prevention) is absorbed and excreted in the urine with minimal metabolism. Potential side effects include cough, bronchospasm (occasionally severe), reversible decrease in pulmonary function, and transient nasal and throat discomfort.

Oseltamivir is an orally administered prodrug that is activated by hepatic esterases and widely distributed throughout the body. The dosage is 75 mg twice daily for treatment and 75 mg once daily for prevention; dosage must be modified in patients with renal insufficiency. The half-life of oseltamivir is 6–10 hours, and excretion is primarily in the urine. Potential side effects include nausea, vomiting, and abdominal pain, which occur in 5–10% of patients early in therapy but tend to resolve spontaneously. Taking oseltamivir with food does not interfere with absorption and may decrease nausea and vomiting. Headache, fatigue, and diarrhea have also been reported and appear to be more common with prophylactic use.

In adults, resistance during therapy is rare but may cause fatal disease. It is unknown whether resistant mutants retain pathogenicity or are spread between people. Worldwide resistance is rare and has not been documented in any clinical isolate from the 2005–2006 influenza season to date in the USA. Avian influenza is expected to retain susceptibility to the neuraminidase inhibitors.

■ VI. OTHER ANTIVIRAL AGENTS

INTERFERONS

Interferons have been studied for numerous clinical indications. In addition to HBV and HCV infections

(see IV. Antihepatitis Agents), intralesional injection of interferon alfa-2b or alfa-n3 may be used for treatment of condylomata acuminata (see also Chapter 62).

RIBAVIRIN

In addition to oral administration for hepatitis C infection in combination with interferon alfa, aerosolized ribavirin is administered by nebulizer (20 mg/mL for 12–18 hours per day) to children and infants with severe respiratory syncytial virus (RSV) bronchiolitis or pneumonia to reduce the severity and duration of illness. Aerosolized ribavirin has also been used to treat influenza A and B infections but has not gained widespread use. Aerosolized ribavirin is generally well tolerated but may cause conjunctival or bronchial irritation. Health care workers should be protected against extended inhalation exposure.

Intravenous ribavirin decreases mortality in patients with Lassa fever and other viral hemorrhagic fevers if started early. High concentrations inhibit West Nile virus in vitro, but clinical data are lacking. Clinical benefit has been reported in cases of severe measles pneumonitis and certain encephalitides, and continuous infusion of ribavirin has decreased virus shedding in several patients with severe lower respiratory tract influenza or parainfluenza infections. At steady state, cerebrospinal fluid levels are about 70% of those in plasma.

PALIVIZUMAB

Palivizumab is a humanized monoclonal antibody directed against an epitope in the A antigen site on the F surface protein of RSV. It is licensed for the prevention of RSV infection in high risk infants and children such as premature infants and those with bronchopulmonary dysplasia or congenital heart disease. A placebo-controlled trial using once-monthly intramuscular injections (15 mg/kg) for 5 months beginning at the start of the RSV season demonstrated a 55% reduction in the risk of hospitalization for RSV in treated patients, as well as decreases in the need for supplemental oxygen, illness severity score, and need for intensive care. Although resistant strains have been isolated in the laboratory, no resistant clinical isolates have yet been identified. Potential adverse effects include upper respiratory tract infection, fever, rhinitis, rash, diarrhea, vomiting, cough, otitis media, and elevation in serum aminotransferase levels.

IMIQUIMOD

Imiquimod is an immune response modifier shown to be effective in the topical treatment of external genital and perianal warts (ie, condyloma acuminatum; see Chapter 62). The mechanism of action against these human papillomavirus (HPV)-induced lesions is unknown. The 5% cream is applied three times weekly and washed off 6–10 hours after each application. Recurrences appear to be less common than after ablative therapies. Imiquimod is also effective against actinic keratoses. Local skin reactions are the most common side effect; these resolve within weeks after therapy. However, pigmentary skin changes may persist. Systemic adverse effects such as fatigue and influenza-like syndrome have occasionally been reported.

PREPARATIONS AVAILABLE

Abacavir
Oral (Ziagen): 300 mg tablets; 20 mg/mL solution
Oral (Epzicom): 600 mg plus 300 mg lamivudine
Oral (Trizivir): 300 mg tablets in combination with 150 mg lamivudine and 300 mg zidovudine

Acyclovir (generic, Zovirax)
Oral: 200 mg capsules; 400, 800 mg tablets; 200 mg/5 mL suspension
Parenteral: 50 mg/mL; powder to reconstitute for injection (500, 1000 mg/vial)
Topical: 5% ointment

Adefovir (Hepsera)
Oral: 10 mg tablets

Amantadine (generic, Symmetrel)
Oral: 100 mg capsules, tablets; 50 mg/5 mL syrup

Amprenavir (Agenerase)
Oral: 50 mg capsules; 15 mg/mL solution

Atazanavir (Reyataz)
Oral: 100, 150, 200 mg capsules

Cidofovir (Vistide)
Parenteral: 375 mg/vial (75 mg/mL) for IV injection

Darunavir (Prezista)
Oral: 300 mg tablets (must be taken with ritonavir)

Delavirdine (Rescriptor)
Oral: 100, 200 mg tablets

Didanosine (dideoxyinosine, ddI)
Oral (Videx): 25, 50, 100, 150, 200 mg tablets; 100, 167, 250 mg powder for oral solution; 2, 4 g powder for pediatric solution
Oral (Videx-EC): 125, 200, 250, 400 mg delayed-release capsules

Docosanol (Abreva) (over-the-counter)
Topical: 10% cream

Efavirenz (Sustiva)
Oral: 50, 100, 200 mg capsules; 600 mg tablets

Emtricitabine
Oral (Emtriva): 200 mg tablets
Oral (Truvada): 200 mg plus 300 mg tenofovir tablets

Enfuvirtide (Fuzeon)
Parenteral: 90 mg/mL for injection

Entacavir (Baraclude)
Oral: 0.5, 1 mg tablets; 0.05 mg/mL oral solution

Famciclovir (Famvir)
Oral: 125, 250, 500 mg tablets

Fosamprenavir (Lexiva)
Oral: 700 mg tablets

Fomivirsen (Vitravene)
Intraocular injection: 6.6 mg/mL

Foscarnet (Foscavir)
Parenteral: 24 mg/mL for IV injection

Ganciclovir (Cytovene)
Oral: 250, 500 mg capsules
Parenteral: 500 mg/vial for IV injection
Intraocular implant (Vitrasert): 4.5 mg ganciclovir/implant

Idoxuridine (Herplex)
Ophthalmic: 0.1% solution

Imiquimod (Aldera)
Topical: 5% cream

Indinavir (Crixivan)
Oral: 100, 200, 333, 400 mg capsules

Interferon alfa-2a (Roferon-A)
Parenteral: 3, 6, 9, 36 million IU vials

Interferon alfa-2b (Intron A)
Parenteral: 3, 5, 10, 18, 25, and 50 million IU vials

Interferon alfa-2b (Rebetron)
Parenteral: 3 million IU vials (supplied with oral ribavirin, 200 mg capsules)

Interferon alfa-n3 (Alferon N)
Parenteral: 5 million IU/vial

Interferon alfacon-1 (Infergen)
Parenteral: 9 and 15 mcg vials

Lamivudine
Oral (Epivir): 150, 300 mg tablets; 10 mg/mL oral solution
Oral (Epivir-HBV): 100 mg tablets; 5 mg/mL solution
Oral (Combivir): 150 mg tablets in combination with 300 mg zidovudine
Oral (Trizivir): 150 mg tablets in combination with 300 mg abacavir and 300 mg zidovudine

(continued)

Lopinavir/ritonavir (Kaletra)
Oral: 133.3 mg/33.3 mg capsules; 80 mg/20 mg per mL solution
Nelfinavir (Viracept)
Oral: 250, 625 mg tablets; 50 mg/g powder
Nevirapine (Viramune)
Oral: 200 mg tablets; 50 mg/5 mL suspension
Oseltamivir (Tamiflu)
Oral: 75 mg capsules; powder to reconstitute as suspension (12 mg/mL)
Palivizumab (Synagis)
Parenteral: 50, 100 mg/vial
Peginterferon alfa-2a (pegylated interferon alfa-2a, Pegasys)
Parenteral: 180 mcg/mL
Peginterferon alfa-2b (pegylated interferon alfa-2b, PEG-Intron)
Parenteral: powder to reconstitute as 100, 160, 240, 300 mcg/mL injection
Penciclovir (Denavir)
Topical: 1% cream
Ribavirin
Aerosol (Virazole): powder to reconstitute for aerosol; 6 g/100 mL vial
Oral (Rebetol, generic): 200 mg capsules, tablets; 40 mg/mL oral solution
Oral (Rebetron): 200 mg in combination with 3 million units interferon alfa-2b (Intron-A)
Rimantadine (Flumadine)
Oral: 100 mg tablets; 50 mg/5 mL syrup
Ritonavir (Norvir)
Oral: 100 mg capsules; 80 mg/mL oral solution

Saquinavir
Oral (Invirase): 200 mg hard gel capsules, 500 mg tablets
Oral (Fortovase): 200 mg soft gel capsules
Stavudine
Oral (Zerit): 15, 20, 30, 40 mg capsules; powder for 1 mg/mL oral solution
Oral extended-release (Zerit XR): 37.5, 50, 75, 100 mg capsules
Tenofovir (Viread)
Oral: 300 mg tablets
Tipranavir (Aptivus)
Oral: 250 mg capsules
Trifluridine (Viroptic)
Topical: 1% ophthalmic solution
Valacyclovir (Valtrex)
Oral: 500, 1000 mg tablets
Valganciclovir (Valcyte)
Oral: 450 mg capsules
Vidarabine (Vira-A)
Topical: 3% ointment
Zalcitabine (dideoxycytidine, ddC) (Hivid)
Oral: 0.375, 0.75 mg tablets
Zanamivir (Relenza)
Inhalational: 5 mg/blister
Zidovudine (azidothymidine, AZT) (Retrovir)
Oral: 100 mg capsules, 300 mg tablets, 50 mg/5 mL syrup
Oral (Combivir): 300 mg tablets in combination with 150 mg lamivudine
Oral (Trizivir): 300 mg tablets in combination with 150 mg lamivudine and 300 mg zidovudine
Parenteral: 10 mg/mL

REFERENCES

Asmuth DM, Nguyen HH, Melcher GP et al: Treatments for hepatitis B. Clinical Infect Dis 2004;39:1353.

Drugs for non-HIV viral infections. Med Lett Drugs Ther 2005;23.

Gnann JW, Whitley RJ: Herpes zoster. N Engl J Med 2002;347:340.

Hammer SM et al: Treatment for Adult HIV Infection, 2006. Recommendations of the International AIDS Society-USA Panel. JAMA 2006;296:827.

Kimberlin DW, Rouse DJ: Genital herpes. N Engl J Med 2004;350:1970.

Moscona A: Neuraminidase inhibitors for influenza. N Engl J Med 2005;353:1363.

Panel on Clinical Practices for Treatment of HIV Infection convened by the Department of Health and Human Services (DHHS). Guidelines for the Use of Antiretroviral Agents in HIV-1-Infected Adults and Adolescents. April 7, 2005. Available at http://AIDSinfo.nih.gov

Piscitelli SC, Gallicano KD: Interactions among drugs for HIV and opportunistic infections. N Engl J Med 2001;344:984.

Public Health Service Task Force. Recommendations for Use of Antiretroviral Drugs in Pregnant HIV-1-Infected Women for Maternal Health and Interventions to Reduce Perinatal HIV-1 Transmission in the United States. February 24, 2005. Available at http://AIDSinfo.nih.gov

Thio CL, Sulkowski MS, Thomas DL: Treatment of chronic hepatitis B in HIV-infected persons: Thinking outside the black box. Clin Infect Dis 2005;41:1035.

RELEVANT WEB SITES

www.aidsinfo.nih.gov
www.hiv-druginteractions.org
www.hivinsite.com
http://hopkins-aids.edu [the pocket guide to adults HIV/AIDS treatment]
http://www.iasusa.org [treatment guidelines and listing of resistance mutations]

Miscellaneous Antimicrobial Agents; Disinfectants, Antiseptics, & Sterilants

50

Henry F. Chambers, MD

■ METRONIDAZOLE, MUPIROCIN, POLYMYXINS, & URINARY ANTISEPTICS

METRONIDAZOLE

Metronidazole is a nitroimidazole antiprotozoal drug (see Chapter 53) that also has potent antibacterial activity against anaerobes, including bacteroides and clostridium species. It is well absorbed after oral administration, is widely distributed in tissues, and reaches serum levels of 4–6 mcg/mL after a 250-mg oral dose. Metronidazole can also be given intravenously or by rectal suppository. The drug penetrates well into the cerebrospinal fluid and brain, reaching levels similar to those in serum. Metronidazole is metabolized in the liver and may accumulate in hepatic insufficiency.

Metronidazole is indicated for treatment of anaerobic or mixed intra-abdominal infections, vaginitis (trichomonas infection, bacterial vaginosis), *C difficile* colitis, and brain abscess. The typical dosage is 500 mg three times daily orally or intravenously (30 mg/kg/d). Vaginitis may respond to a single 2-g dose. A vaginal gel is available for topical use.

Adverse effects include nausea, diarrhea, stomatitis, and peripheral neuropathy with prolonged use. Metronidazole has a disulfiram-like effect, and patients should be instructed to avoid alcohol. Although teratogenic in some animals, metronidazole has not been associated with this effect in humans. Other properties of metronidazole are discussed in Chapter 53.

A structurally similar agent, tinidazole, is a once-daily drug approved for treatment of trichomonas infection, giardiasis, and amebiasis. It also is active against anaerobic bacteria, but is not FDA-approved for treatment of anaerobic infections.

MUPIROCIN

Mupirocin (pseudomonic acid) is a natural product produced by *Pseudomonas fluorescens*. It is rapidly inactivated after absorption, and systemic levels are undetectable. It is available as an ointment for topical application.

Mupirocin is active against gram-positive cocci, including methicillin-susceptible and methicillin-resistant strains of *Staphylococcus aureus*. Mupirocin inhibits staphylococcal isoleucyl tRNA synthetase. Low-level resistance, defined as a minimum inhibitory concentration (MIC) of up to 100 mcg/mL, is due to point mutation in the gene of the target enzyme. Low-level resistance has been observed after prolonged use. However, local concentrations achieved with topical application are well above this MIC, and this level of resistance appears not to result in clinical failure. High-level resistance, with MICs exceeding 1000 mcg/mL, is due to the presence of a second isoleucyl tRNA synthetase gene, which is plasmid-encoded. High-level resistance results in complete loss of activity. Strains with high-level resistance have caused nosocomial (hospital) outbreaks of staphylococcal infection and colonization. Although higher rates of resistance are encountered with intensive use of mupirocin, more than 95% of staphylococcal isolates are still susceptible.

Mupirocin is indicated for topical treatment of minor skin infections, such as impetigo (see Chapter 62). Topical application over large infected areas, such as decubitus ulcers or open surgical wounds, has been identified as an important factor leading to emergence of mupirocin-resistant strains and is not recommended. Mupirocin effectively eliminates *S aureus* nasal carriage by patients or health care workers, but results are mixed with respect to its ability to prevent subsequent staphylococcal infection.

POLYMYXINS

The polymyxins are a group of basic peptides active against gram-negative bacteria and include **polymyxin**

B and **polymyxin E (colistin)**. Polymyxins act like cationic detergents. They attach to and disrupt bacterial cell membranes. They also bind and inactivate endotoxin. Gram-positive organisms, proteus, and neisseria are resistant.

Owing to their significant toxicity with systemic administration, polymyxins have been largely restricted to topical use. Ointments containing polymyxin B, 0.5 mg/g, in mixtures with bacitracin or neomycin (or both) are commonly applied to infected superficial skin lesions. Emergence of strains of *Acinetobacter baumannii* and *Pseudomonas aeruginosa* that are resistant to all other agents has led to renewed interest in polymixins, eg, colistin as a parenteral agent for salvage therapy of infections caused by these organisms.

URINARY ANTISEPTICS

Urinary antiseptics are oral agents that exert antibacterial activity in the urine but have little or no systemic antibacterial effect. Their usefulness is limited to lower urinary tract infections. Prolonged suppression of bacteriuria by means of urinary antiseptics may be desirable in chronic urinary tract infections in which eradication of infection by short-term systemic therapy has not been possible.

1. Nitrofurantoin

Nitrofurantoin is bacteriostatic and bactericidal for many gram-positive and gram-negative bacteria but *P aeruginosa* and many strains of proteus are resistant. There is no cross-resistance between nitrofurantoin and other antimicrobial agents and resistance emerges slowly. As *Escherichia coli* resistant to trimethoprim-sulfamethoxazole and fluoroquinolones has become more common, nitrofurantoin has become an important alternative oral agent for treatment of uncomplicated urinary tract infection.

Nitrofurantoin is well absorbed after ingestion. It is metabolized and excreted so rapidly that no systemic antibacterial action is achieved. The drug is excreted into the urine by both glomerular filtration and tubular secretion. With average daily doses, concentrations of 200 mcg/mL are reached in urine. In renal failure, urine levels are insufficient for antibacterial action, but high blood levels may cause toxicity. Nitrofurantoin is contraindicated in patients with significant renal insufficiency.

The dose for urinary tract infection in adults is 100 mg orally taken four times daily. It should not be used to treat upper urinary tract infection. Oral nitrofurantoin can be given for months for the suppression of chronic urinary tract infection. It is desirable to keep urinary pH below 5.5, which greatly enhances drug activity. A single daily dose of nitrofurantoin, 100 mg, can prevent recurrent urinary tract infections in some women.

Anorexia, nausea, and vomiting are the principal side effects of nitrofurantoin. Neuropathies and hemolytic anemia occur in glucose-6-phosphate dehydrogenase deficiency. Nitrofurantoin antagonizes the action of nalidixic acid. Rashes, pulmonary infiltration and fibrosis, and other hypersensitivity reactions have been reported.

2. Methenamine Mandelate & Methenamine Hippurate

Methenamine mandelate is the salt of mandelic acid and methenamine and possesses properties of both of these urinary antiseptics. Methenamine hippurate is the salt of hippuric acid and methenamine. Below pH 5.5, methenamine releases formaldehyde, which is antibacterial. Mandelic acid or hippuric acid taken orally is excreted unchanged in the urine, in which these drugs are bactericidal for some gram-negative bacteria when pH is less than 5.5.

Methenamine mandelate, 1 g four times daily, or methenamine hippurate, 1 g twice daily by mouth (children, 50 mg/kg/d or 30 mg/kg/d, respectively), is used only as a urinary antiseptic to suppress, not treat, urinary tract infection. Acidifying agents (eg, ascorbic acid, 4–12 g/d) may be given to lower urinary pH below 5.5. Sulfonamides should not be given at the same time because they may form an insoluble compound with the formaldehyde released by methenamine. Persons taking methenamine mandelate may exhibit falsely elevated tests for catecholamine metabolites.

■ DISINFECTANTS, ANTISEPTICS, & STERILANTS

Disinfectants are strong chemical agents that inhibit or kill microorganisms (Table 50–1). Antiseptics are disinfecting agents with sufficiently low toxicity for host cells that they can be used directly on skin, mucous membranes, or wounds. Sterilants kill both vegetative cells and spores when applied to materials for appropriate times and temperatures. Some of the terms used in this context are defined in Table 50–2.

Disinfection prevents infection by reducing the number of potentially infective organisms by killing, removing, or diluting them. Disinfection can be accomplished by application of chemical agents or use of physical agents such as ionizing radiation, dry or moist heat, or superheated steam (autoclave, 120°C) to kill microorganisms. Often a combination of agents is used, eg, water and moderate heat over time (pasteurization); ethylene oxide and moist heat (a sterilant); or addition of disinfectant to a detergent. Prevention of infection

Table 50–1. Activities of disinfectants.

	Bacteria				Viruses		Other		
	Gram-positive	Gram-negative	Acid-Fast	Spores	Lipo-philic	Hydro-philic	Fungi	Amebic Cysts	Prions
Alcohols (isopropanol, ethanol)	HS	HS	S	R	S	V	—	—	R
Aldehydes (glutaraldehyde, formaldehyde)	HS	HS	MS	S (slow)	S	MS	S	—	R
Chlorhexidine gluconate	HS	MS	R	R	V	R	—	—	R
Sodium hypochlorite, chlorine dioxide	HS	HS	MS	S (pH 7.6)	S	S (at high conc)	MS	S	MS (at high conc)
Hexachlorophene	S (slow)	R	R	R	R	R	R	R	R
Povidone, iodine	HS	HS	S	S (at high conc)	S	R	S	S	R
Phenols, quaternary ammonium compounds	HS	HS	MS	R	S	R	—	—	R
Strong oxidizing agents, cresols	HS	MS to R	R	R	S	R	R	R	R

HS, highly susceptible; S, susceptible; MS, moderately susceptible; R, resistant; V, variable; —, no data.

also can be achieved by washing, which dilutes the potentially infectious organism, or by establishing a barrier, eg, gloves, condom, or respirator, which prevents the pathogen from entry into the host.

Handwashing is the most important means of preventing transmission of infectious agents from person to person or from regions of high microbial load, eg, mouth, nose, or gut, to potential sites of infection. Soap and warm water efficiently and effectively remove bacteria. Skin disinfectants along with detergent and water are usually used preoperatively as a surgical scrub for surgeons' hands and the patient's surgical incision.

Evaluation of effectiveness of antiseptics, disinfectants, and sterilants, although seemingly simple in principle, is very complex. Factors in any evaluation include the intrinsic resistance of the microorganism, the number of microorganisms present, mixed populations of organisms, amount of organic material present (eg, blood, feces, tissue), concentration and stability of disinfectant or sterilant, time and temperature of exposure, pH, and hydration and binding of the agent to surfaces. Specific, standardized assays of activity are defined for each use. Toxicity for humans also must be evaluated. The Environmental Protection Agency (EPA) regulates disinfectants and sterilants and the Food and Drug Administration regulates antiseptics.

Users of antiseptics, disinfectants, and sterilants need to consider their short-term and long-term toxicity because they may have general biocidal activity and may accumulate in the environment or in the body of the patient or caregiver using the agent. Disinfectants and antiseptics may also become contaminated by resistant microorganisms—eg, spores, *P aeruginosa,* or *Serratia marcescens*—and actually transmit infection. Most topical antiseptics interfere with wound healing to some degree. Simple cleansing with soap and water is less damaging than antiseptics to wounds. Topical antibiotics with a narrow spectrum of action and low toxicity (eg, bacitracin and mupirocin) can be used for temporary control of bacterial growth and are generally preferred to antiseptics. Methenamine mandelate releases formaldehyde in a low antibacterial concentration at acid pH and can be an effective urinary antiseptic for long-term control of urinary tract infections.

Some of the chemical classes of antiseptics, disinfectants, and sterilants are described briefly in the text that follows. The reader is referred to the general references for descriptions of physical disinfection and sterilization methods.

Table 50–2. Commonly used terms related to chemical and physical killing of microorganisms.

Antisepsis	Application of an agent to living tissue for the purpose of preventing infection
Decontamination	Destruction or marked reduction in number or activity of microorganisms
Disinfection	Chemical or physical treatment that destroys most vegetative microbes or viruses, but not spores, in or on inanimate surfaces
Sanitization	Reduction of microbial load on an inanimate surface to a level considered acceptable for public health purposes
Sterilization	A process intended to kill or remove all types of microorganisms, including spores, and usually including viruses with an acceptable low probability of survival
Pasteurization	A process that kills nonsporulating microorganisms by hot water or steam at 65–100°C

ALCOHOLS

The two alcohols most frequently used for antisepsis and disinfection are ethanol and isopropyl alcohol (isopropanol). They are rapidly active, killing vegetative bacteria, *Mycobacterium tuberculosis,* and many fungi and inactivating lipophilic viruses. The optimum bactericidal concentration is 60–90% by volume in water. They probably act by denaturation of proteins. They are not used as sterilants because they are not sporicidal, do not penetrate protein-containing organic material, may not be active against hydrophilic viruses, and lack residual action because they evaporate completely. The alcohols are useful in situations in which sinks with running water are not available for washing with soap and water. Their skin-drying effect can be partially alleviated by addition of emollients to the formulation. Use of alcohol-based hand rubs has been shown to reduce transmission of nosocomial bacterial pathogens and is recommended by the Centers for Disease Control and Prevention (CDC) as the preferred method of hand decontamination. Alcohol-based hand rubs are ineffective against spores of *Clostridium difficile* and assiduous handwashing with a disinfectant soap and water is still required for decontamination after caring for a patient with infection from this organism.

Alcohols are flammable and must be stored in cool, well-ventilated areas. They must be allowed to evaporate before cautery, electrosurgery, or laser surgery.

Alcohols may be damaging if applied directly to corneal tissue. Therefore, instruments such as tonometers that have been disinfected in alcohol should be rinsed with sterile water, or the alcohol should be allowed to evaporate before they are used.

CHLORHEXIDINE

Chlorhexidine is a cationic biguanide with very low water solubility. Water-soluble chlorhexidine digluconate is used in water-based formulations as an antiseptic. It is active against vegetative bacteria and mycobacteria and has moderate activity against fungi and viruses. It strongly adsorbs to bacterial membranes, causing leakage of small molecules and precipitation of cytoplasmic proteins. It is active at pH 5.5–7.0. Chlorhexidine gluconate is slower in its action than alcohols, but because of its persistence it has residual activity when used repeatedly, producing bactericidal action equivalent to alcohols. It is most effective against gram-positive cocci and less active against gram-positive and gram-negative rods. Spore germination is inhibited by chlorhexidine. Chlorhexidine digluconate is resistant to inhibition by blood and organic materials. However, anionic and nonionic agents in moisturizers, neutral soaps, and surfactants may neutralize its action. Chlorhexidine digluconate formulations of 4% concentration have slightly greater antibacterial activity than newer 2% formulations. Chlorhexidine 0.5% in 70% alcohol formulations are available in some countries. Chlorhexidine has a very low skin-sensitizing or irritating capacity. Oral toxicity is low because it is poorly absorbed from the alimentary tract. Chlorhexidine must not be used during surgery on the middle ear because it causes sensorineural deafness. Similar neural toxicity may be encountered during neurosurgery.

HALOGENS

1. Iodine

Iodine in a 1:20,000 solution is bactericidal in 1 minute and kills spores in 15 minutes. Tincture of iodine USP contains 2% iodine and 2.4% sodium iodide in alcohol. It is the most active antiseptic for intact skin. It is not commonly used because of serious hypersensitivity reactions that may occur and because of its staining of clothing and dressings.

2. Iodophors

Iodophors are complexes of iodine with a surface-active agent such as **polyvinyl pyrrolidone (PVP; povidone-iodine).** Iodophors retain the activity of iodine. They kill vegetative bacteria, mycobacteria, fungi, and lipid-containing viruses. They may be sporicidal upon prolonged exposure. Iodophors can be used as antiseptics or disinfectants, the latter containing more iodine. The amount of free iodine is low, but it is released as the solution is diluted. An iodophor solution must be diluted according to the manufacturer's directions to obtain full activity.

Iodophors are less irritating and less likely to produce skin hypersensitivity than tincture of iodine. They act as rapidly as chlorhexidine and have a broader spectrum of action, including sporicidal action, but they lack the persistent action of chlorhexidine.

3. Chlorine

Chlorine is a strong oxidizing agent and universal disinfectant that is most commonly provided as a 5.25% **sodium hypochlorite** solution, a typical formulation for **household bleach.** Because formulations may vary, the exact concentration should be verified on the label. A 1:10 dilution of household bleach provides 5000 ppm of available chlorine. The CDC recommends this concentration for disinfection of blood spills. Less than 5 ppm kills vegetative bacteria, whereas up to 5000 ppm is necessary to kill spores. A concentration of 1000–10,000 ppm is tuberculocidal. One hundred ppm kills vegetative fungal cells in 1 hour, but fungal spores require 500 ppm. Viruses are inactivated by 200–500 ppm. Dilutions of 5.25% sodium hypochlorite made up in pH 7.5–8.0 tap water retain their activity for months when kept in tightly closed, opaque containers. Frequent opening and closing of the container reduces the activity markedly.

Because chlorine is inactivated by blood, serum, feces, and protein-containing materials, surfaces should be cleaned before chlorine disinfectant is applied. Undissociated hypochlorous acid (HOCl) is the active biocidal agent. When pH is increased, the less active hypochlorite ion, OCl⁻ is formed. When hypochlorite solutions contact formaldehyde, the carcinogen *bis*-chloromethyl is formed. Rapid evolution of irritating chlorine gas occurs when hypochlorite solutions are mixed with acid and urine. Solutions are corrosive to aluminum, silver, and stainless steel.

Alternative chlorine-releasing compounds include **chlorine dioxide** and **chloramine T.** These agents retain chlorine longer and have a prolonged bactericidal action.

PHENOLICS

Phenol itself (perhaps the oldest of the surgical antiseptics) is no longer used even as a disinfectant because of its corrosive effect on tissues, its toxicity when absorbed, and its carcinogenic effect. These adverse actions are diminished by forming derivatives in which a functional group replaces a hydrogen atom in the aromatic ring. The phenolic agents most commonly used are **o-**

phenylphenol, *o*-benzyl-*p*-chlorophenol, and **p-tertiary amylphenol.** Mixtures of phenolic derivatives are often used. Some of these are derived from coal tar distillates, eg, cresols and xylenols. Skin absorption and skin irritation still occur with these derivatives, and appropriate care is necessary in their use. Detergents are often added to formulations to clean and remove organic material that may decrease the activity of a phenolic compound.

Phenolic compounds disrupt cell walls and membranes, precipitate proteins, and inactivate enzymes. They are bactericidal (including mycobacteria) and fungicidal and they are capable of inactivating lipophilic viruses. They are not sporicidal. Dilution and time of exposure recommendations of the manufacturer must be followed.

Phenolic disinfectants are used for hard surface decontamination in hospitals and laboratories, eg, floors, beds, and counter or bench tops. They are not recommended for use in nurseries and especially in bassinets, where their use has been associated with hyperbilirubinemia. Use of **hexachlorophene** as a skin disinfectant has caused cerebral edema and convulsions in premature infants and occasionally in adults.

QUATERNARY AMMONIUM COMPOUNDS

The quaternary ammonium compounds ("quats") are cationic surface-active detergents. The active cation has at least one long water-repellent hydrocarbon chain, which causes the molecules to concentrate as an oriented layer on the surface of solutions and colloidal or suspended particles. The charged nitrogen portion of the cation has high affinity for water and prevents separation out of solution. The bactericidal action of quaternary compounds has been attributed to inactivation of energy-producing enzymes, denaturation of proteins, and disruption of the cell membrane. These agents are bacteriostatic, fungistatic, and sporistatic and also inhibit algae. They are bactericidal for gram-positive bacteria and moderately active against gram-negative bacteria. Lipophilic viruses are inactivated. They are not tuberculocidal or sporicidal, and they do not inactivate hydrophilic viruses. Quaternary ammonium compounds bind to the surface of colloidal protein in blood, serum, and milk and to the fibers in cotton, mops, cloths, and paper towels used to apply them, which can cause inactivation of the agent by removing it from solution. They are inactivated by anionic detergents (soaps), by many nonionic detergents, and by calcium, magnesium, ferric, and aluminum ions.

Quaternary compounds are used for sanitation of noncritical surfaces (floors, bench tops, etc). Their low toxicity has led to their use as sanitizers in food production facilities. CDC recommends that quaternary ammonium compounds such as **benzalkonium chloride** *not* be used as antiseptics because several outbreaks of infections have occurred that were due to growth of pseudomonas and other gram-negative bacteria in quaternary ammonium antiseptic solutions.

ALDEHYDES

Formaldehyde and **glutaraldehyde** are used for disinfection or sterilization of instruments such as fiberoptic endoscopes, respiratory therapy equipment, hemodialyzers, and dental handpieces that cannot withstand exposure to the high temperatures of steam sterilization. They are not corrosive for metal, plastic, or rubber. These agents have a broad spectrum of activity against microorganisms and viruses. They act by alkylation of chemical groups in proteins and nucleic acids. Failures of disinfection or sterilization can occur as a result of dilution below the known effective concentration, the presence of organic material, and the failure of liquid to penetrate into small channels in the instruments. Automatic circulating baths are available that increase penetration of aldehyde solution into the instrument while decreasing exposure of the operator to irritating fumes.

Formaldehyde is available as a 40% w/v solution in water (100% **formalin**). An 8% formaldehyde solution in water has a broad spectrum of activity against bacteria, fungi, and viruses. Sporicidal activity may take as long as 18 hours. Its rapidity of action is increased by solution in 70% isopropanol. Formaldehyde solutions are used for high-level disinfection of hemodialyzers, preparation of vaccines, and preservation and embalming of tissues. The 4% formaldehyde (10% formalin) solutions used for fixation of tissues and embalming may not be mycobactericidal.

Glutaraldehyde is a dialdehyde (1,5-pentanedial). Solutions of 2% w/v glutaraldehyde are most commonly used. The solution must be alkalinized to pH 7.4–8.5 for activation. Activated solutions are bactericidal, sporicidal, fungicidal, and virucidal for both lipophilic and hydrophilic viruses. Glutaraldehyde has greater sporicidal activity than formaldehyde, but its tuberculocidal activity may be less. Lethal action against mycobacteria and spores may require prolonged exposure. Once activated, solutions have a shelf life of 14 days, after which polymerization reduces activity. Other means of activation and stabilization can increase the shelf life. Because glutaraldehyde solutions are frequently reused, the most common reason for loss of activity is dilution and exposure to organic material. Test strips to measure residual activity are recommended.

Formaldehyde has a characteristic pungent odor and is highly irritating to respiratory mucous membranes and eyes at concentrations of 2–5 ppm. OSHA has declared that formaldehyde is a potential carcinogen and has established an employee exposure standard that limits the 8-hour time-weighted average (TWA) exposure to 0.75 ppm. Protection of health care workers from exposure to glutaraldehyde concentrations greater than 0.2 ppm is advisable. Increased air exchange, enclosure in hoods with exhausts, tight-fitting lids on exposure devices, and use of protective personal equipment such as goggles, respirators, and gloves may be necessary to achieve these exposure limits.

Ortho-phthalaldehyde (OPA) is a phenolic dialdehyde chemical sterilant with a spectrum of activity comparable to glutaraldehyde, although it is several times more rapidly bactericidal. OPA solution typically contains 0.55% OPA. Its label claim is that high-level disinfection can be achieved at 12 minutes at room temperature compared with 45 minutes for 2.4% glutaraldehyde. Unlike glutaraldehyde, OPA requires no activation, is less irritating to mucous membranes, and does not require exposure monitoring. It has good materials compatibility and an acceptable environmental safety profile. OPA is useful for disinfection or sterilization of endoscopes, surgical instruments, and other medical devices.

SUPEROXIDIZED WATER

Electrolysis of saline yields a mixture of oxidants, primarily hypochlorous acid and chlorine, with potent disinfectant and sterilant properties. The solution generated by the process, which has been commercialized and marketed as Sterilox for disinfection of endoscopes and dental materials, is rapidly bactericidal, fungicidal, tuberculocidal, and sporicidal. High-level disinfection is achieved with a contact time of 10 minutes. The solution is nontoxic and nonirritating and requires no special disposal precautions.

PEROXYGEN COMPOUNDS

The peroxygen compounds, **hydrogen peroxide** and **peracetic acid,** have high killing activity and a broad spectrum against bacteria, spores, viruses, and fungi when used in appropriate concentration. They have the advantage that their decomposition products are not toxic and do not injure the environment. They are powerful oxidizers that are used primarily as disinfectants and sterilants.

Hydrogen peroxide is a very effective disinfectant when used for inanimate objects or materials with low organic content such as water. Organisms with the enzymes catalase and peroxidase rapidly degrade hydrogen peroxide. The innocuous degradation products are oxygen and water. Concentrated solutions containing 90% w/v H_2O_2 are prepared electrochemically. When diluted in high-quality deionized water to 6% and 3% and put into clean containers, they remain stable. Hydrogen peroxide has been proposed for disinfection of respirators, acrylic resin implants, plastic eating utensils, soft contact lenses, and cartons intended to contain milk or juice products. Concentrations of 10–25% hydrogen peroxide are sporicidal. Vapor phase hydrogen peroxide (VPHP) is a cold gaseous sterilant that has the potential to replace the toxic or carcinogenic gases ethylene oxide and formaldehyde. VPHP does not require a pressurized chamber and is active at temperatures as low as 4°C and concentrations as low as 4 mg/L. It is incompatible with liquids and cellulose products. It penetrates the surface of some plastics. Automated equipment using vaporized hydrogen peroxide (eg, Sterrad) or hydrogen peroxide mixed with formic acid (Endoclens) is available for sterilizing endoscopes.

Peracetic acid (CH_3COOOH) is prepared commercially from 90% hydrogen peroxide, acetic acid, and sulfuric acid as a catalyst. It is explosive in the pure form. It is usually used in dilute solution and transported in containers with vented caps to prevent increased pressure as oxygen is released. Peracetic acid is more active than hydrogen peroxide as a bactericidal and sporicidal agent. Concentrations of 250–500 ppm are effective against a broad range of bacteria in 5 minutes at pH 7.0 at 20°C. Bacterial spores are inactivated by 500–30,000 ppm peracetic acid. Only slightly increased concentrations are necessary in the presence of organic matter. Viruses require variable exposures. Enteroviruses require 2000 ppm for 15–30 minutes for inactivation.

An automated machine (Steris) that uses buffered peracetic acid liquid of 0.1–0.5% concentration has been developed for sterilization of medical, surgical, and dental instruments. Peracetic acid sterilization systems have also been adopted for hemodialyzers. The food processing and beverage industries use peracetic acid extensively because the breakdown products in high dilution do not produce objectionable odor, taste, or toxicity. Because rinsing is not necessary in this use, time and money are saved.

Peracetic acid is a potent tumor promoter but a weak carcinogen. It is not mutagenic in the Ames test.

HEAVY METALS

Heavy metals, principally mercury and silver, are now rarely used as disinfectants. Mercury is an environmental hazard, and some pathogenic bacteria have developed plasmid-mediated resistance to mercurials. Hypersensitivity to thimerosal is common, possibly in up to 40% of the population. These compounds are absorbed from solution by rubber and plastic closures. Nevertheless, **thimerosal** 0.001–0.004% is still used as a preservative of vaccines, antitoxins, and immune sera.

Inorganic silver salts are strongly bactericidal. **Silver nitrate,** 1:1000, has been most commonly used, particularly as a preventive for gonococcal ophthalmitis in newborns. Antibiotic ointments have replaced silver nitrate for this indication. **Silver sulfadiazine** slowly releases silver and is used to suppress bacterial growth in burn wounds (see Chapter 46).

STERILANTS

For many years, pressurized **steam (autoclaving)** at 120°C for 30 minutes has been the basic method for sterilizing instruments and decontaminating materials. When autoclaving is not possible, as with lensed instruments and materials containing plastic and rubber, **ethylene oxide**—diluted with either fluorocarbon or carbon dioxide to diminish explosive hazard—was used at 440–1200 mg/L at 45–60°C with 30–60% relative humidity. The higher concentrations have been used to increase penetration.

Ethylene oxide is classified as a mutagen and carcinogen. The OSHA permissible exposure limit (PEL) for ethylene oxide is 1 ppm calculated as a time-weighted average. Alternative sterilants now being used increasingly include vapor phase hydrogen peroxide, peracetic acid, ozone, gas plasma, chlorine dioxide, formaldehyde, and propylene oxide. Each of these sterilants has potential advantages and problems. Automated peracetic acid systems are being used increasingly for high-level decontamination and sterilization of endoscopes and hemodialyzers because of their effectiveness, automated features, and the low toxicity of the residual products of sterilization.

PRESERVATIVES

Disinfectants are used as preservatives to prevent the overgrowth of bacteria and fungi in pharmaceutical products, laboratory sera and reagents, cosmetic products, and contact lenses. Multi-use vials of medication that may be reentered through a rubber diaphragm, and eye and nose drops, require preservatives. Preservatives should not be irritant or toxic to tissues to which they will be applied, they must be effective in preventing growth of microorganisms likely to contaminate them, and they must have sufficient solubility and stability to remain active.

Commonly used preservative agents include organic acids such as **benzoic acid** and salts, the **parabens,** (alkyl esters of *p*-hydroxybenzoic acid), sorbic acid and salts, phenolic compounds, quaternary ammonium compounds, alcohols, and mercurials such as thimerosal in 0.001–0.004% concentration.

PREPARATIONS AVAILABLE

MISCELLANEOUS ANTIMICROBIAL DRUGS

Colistimethate sodium (Coly-mycin M)
Parenteral: 150 mg for injection
Methenamine hippurate (Hiprex, Urex)
Oral: 1.0 g tablets
Methenamine mandelate (generic)
Oral: 0.5, 1 g tablets; 0.5 g/5 mL suspension
Metronidazole (generic, Flagyl)
Oral: 250, 500 mg tablets; 375 mg capsules; 750 mg extended-release tablets
Parenteral: 5 mg/mL; 500 mg for injection
Mupirocin (Bactroban)
Topical: 2% ointment, cream
Nitrofurantoin (generic, Macrodantin)
Oral: 25, 50, 100 mg capsules, 25 mg/5 mL suspension
Polymyxin B (Polymyxin B Sulfate)
Parenteral: 500,000 units per vial for injection
Ophthalmic: 500,000 units per vial

DISINFECTANTS, ANTISEPTICS, & STERILANTS

Benzalkonium (generic, Zephiran)
Topical: 17% concentrate; 50% solution; 1:750 solution
Benzoyl peroxide (generic)
Topical: 2.5%, 5%, 10% liquid; 5%, 5.5%, 10% lotion; 5%, 10% cream; 2.5%, 4%, 5%, 6%, 10%, 20% gel

Chlorhexidine gluconate (Hibiclens, Hibistat, others)
Topical: 2, 4% cleanser, sponge; 0.5% rinse in 70% alcohol
Oral rinse (Peridex, Periogard): 0.12%
Glutaraldehyde (Cidex)
Instruments: 2.4% solution
Hexachlorophene (pHisoHex)
Topical: 3% liquid; 0.23% foam
Iodine aqueous (generic, Lugol's Solution)
Topical: 2–5% in water with 2.4% sodium iodide or 10% potassium iodide
Iodine tincture (generic)
Topical: 2% iodine or 2.4% sodium iodide in 47% alcohol, in 15, 30, 120 mL and in larger quantities
Nitrofurazone (generic, Furacin)
Topical: 0.2% solution, ointment, and cream
Ortho-phthalaldehyde (Cidex OPA)
Instruments: 0.55% solution
Povidone-iodine (generic, Betadine)
Topical: available in many forms, including aerosol, ointment, antiseptic gauze pads, skin cleanser (liquid or foam), solution, and swabsticks
Silver nitrate (generic)
Topical: 10, 25, 50% solution
Thimerosal (generic, Mersol)
Topical: 1:1000 tincture and solution

REFERENCES

Anonymous: Tinadazole. Med Lett Drugs Ther 2004;46:70.

Bischoff WE et al: Handwashing compliance by health care workers: The impact of introducing an accessible, alcohol-based hand antiseptic. Arch Intern Med 2000;160:1017.

Chambers HF, Winston LG: Mupirocin prophylaxis misses by a nose. Ann Intern Med 2004;140:484.

Gordin FM et al: Reduction in nosocomial transmission of drug resistant bacteria after introduction of an alcohol-based hand-rub. Infect Control Hosp Epidemiol 2005;26:650.

Rutala WA, Weber DJ: New disinfection and sterilization methods. Emerg Infect Dis 2001;7:348.

Widmer AF, Frei R: Decontamination, disinfection, and sterilization. In: Murray PR et al (editors). *Manual of Clinical Microbiology*, 7th ed. American Society for Microbiology, 1999.

Clinical Use of Antimicrobial Agents 51

Harry W. Lampiris, MD, & Daniel S. Maddix, PharmD

The development of antimicrobial drugs represents one of the most important advances in therapeutics, both in the control or cure of serious infections and in the prevention and treatment of infectious complications of other therapeutic modalities such as cancer chemotherapy and surgery. However, evidence is overwhelming that antimicrobial agents are vastly overprescribed in outpatient settings in the United States, and the availability of antimicrobial agents without prescription in many developing countries has—by facilitating the development of resistance—already severely limited therapeutic options in the treatment of life-threatening infections. Therefore, the clinician should first determine whether antimicrobial therapy is warranted for a given patient. The specific questions one should ask include the following:

1. Is an antimicrobial agent indicated on the basis of clinical findings? Or is it prudent to wait until such clinical findings become apparent?
2. Have appropriate clinical specimens been obtained to establish a microbiologic diagnosis?
3. What are the likely etiologic agents for the patient's illness?
4. What measures should be taken to protect individuals exposed to the index case to prevent secondary cases, and what measures should be implemented to prevent further exposure?
5. Is there clinical evidence (eg, from clinical trials) that antimicrobial therapy will confer clinical benefit for the patient?

Once a specific cause is identified based on specific microbiologic tests, the following further questions should be considered:

1. If a specific microbial pathogen is identified, can a narrower-spectrum agent be substituted for the initial empiric drug?
2. Is one agent or a combination of agents necessary?
3. What are the optimal dose, route of administration, and duration of therapy?
4. What specific tests (eg, susceptibility testing) should be undertaken to identify patients who will not respond to treatment?
5. What adjunctive measures can be undertaken to eradicate the infection? For example, is surgery feasible for

removal of devitalized tissue or foreign bodies—or drainage of an abscess—into which antimicrobial agents may be unable to penetrate? Is it possible to decrease the dosage of immunosuppressive therapy in patients who have undergone organ transplantation or to give immunomodulatory drugs or antitoxins to patients with preexisting immune deficiency?

■ EMPIRIC ANTIMICROBIAL THERAPY

Antimicrobial agents are frequently used before the pathogen responsible for a particular illness or the susceptibility to a particular antimicrobial agent is known. This use of antimicrobial agents is called empiric (or presumptive) therapy and is based on experience with a particular clinical entity. The usual justification for empiric therapy is the hope that early intervention will improve the outcome; in the best cases, this has been established by placebo-controlled, double-blind prospective clinical trials. For example, treatment of febrile episodes in neutropenic cancer patients with empiric antimicrobial therapy has been demonstrated to have impressive morbidity and mortality benefits even though the specific bacterial agent responsible for fever is determined for only a minority of such episodes. Conversely, there are many clinical situations in which empiric therapy may not be useful or may actually be harmful. For example, neutropenic patients with fever and pulmonary infiltrates may have a wide variety of causes for their clinical illness, including viruses, bacteria, mycobacteria, fungi, protozoa, and noninfectious disorders. In this setting, it may be more prudent to obtain specimens by sputum culture or via bronchoalveolar lavage early to offer narrow-spectrum therapy based on culture results.

Lastly, there are many clinical entities, such as certain episodes of community-acquired pneumonia, in which it is difficult to identify a specific pathogen. In such cases, a clinical response to empiric therapy may be an important clue to the likely pathogen.

Approach to Empiric Therapy

Initiation of empiric therapy should follow a specific and systematic approach.

A. FORMULATE A CLINICAL DIAGNOSIS OF MICROBIAL INFECTION

Using all available data, the clinician should conclude that there is anatomic evidence of infection (eg, pneumonia, cellulitis, sinusitis).

B. OBTAIN SPECIMENS FOR LABORATORY EXAMINATION

Examination of stained specimens by microscopy or simple examination of an uncentrifuged sample of urine for white blood cells and bacteria may provide important etiologic clues in a very short time. Cultures of selected anatomic sites (blood, sputum, urine, cerebrospinal fluid, stool) and nonculture methods (antigen testing, polymerase chain reaction, serology) may also confirm specific etiologic agents.

C. FORMULATE A MICROBIOLOGIC DIAGNOSIS

The history, physical examination, and immediately available laboratory results (eg, Gram stain of urine or sputum) may provide highly specific information. For example, in a young man with urethritis and a Gram-stained smear from the urethral meatus demonstrating intracellular gram-negative diplococci, the most likely pathogen is *Neisseria gonorrhoeae*. In the latter instance, however, the clinician should be aware that a significant number of patients with gonococcal urethritis have uninformative Gram stains for the organism and that a significant number of patients with gonococcal urethritis harbor concurrent chlamydial infection that is not demonstrated on the Gram-stained smear.

D. DETERMINE THE NECESSITY FOR EMPIRIC THERAPY

Whether or not to initate empiric therapy is an important clinical decision based partly on experience and partly on data from clinical trials. Empiric therapy is indicated when there is a significant risk of serious morbidity if therapy is withheld until a specific pathogen is detected by the clinical laboratory.

In other settings, empiric therapy may be indicated for public health reasons rather than for demonstrated superior outcome of therapy in a specific patient. For example, urethritis in a young sexually active man usually requires treatment for *N gonorrhoeae* and *Chlamydia trachomatis* despite the absence of microbiologic confirmation at the time of diagnosis. Because the risk of noncompliance with follow-up visits in this patient population may lead to further transmission of these sexually transmitted pathogens, empiric therapy is warranted.

E. INSTITUTE TREATMENT

Selection of empiric therapy may be based on the microbiologic diagnosis or a clinical diagnosis without available microbiologic clues. If no microbiologic information is available, the antimicrobial spectrum of the agent or agents chosen must necessarily be broader, taking into account the most likely pathogens responsible for the patient's illness.

Choice of Antimicrobial Agent

Selection from among several drugs depends on **host factors** that include the following: (1) concomitant disease states (eg, AIDS, severe chronic liver disease); (2) prior adverse drug effects; (3) impaired elimination or detoxification of the drug (may be genetically predetermined but more frequently is associated with impaired renal or hepatic function due to underlying disease); (4) age of the patient; and (5) pregnancy status.

Pharmacologic factors include (1) the kinetics of absorption, distribution, and elimination; (2) the ability of the drug to be delivered to the site of infection; (3) the potential toxicity of an agent; and (4) pharmacokinetic or pharmacodynamic interactions with other drugs.

Knowledge of the susceptibility of an organism to a specific agent in a hospital or community setting is important in the selection of empiric therapy. Pharmacokinetic differences among agents with similar antimicrobial spectrums may be exploited to reduce the frequency of dosing (eg, ceftriaxone may be conveniently given once every 24 hours). Finally, increasing consideration is being given to the cost of antimicrobial therapy, especially when multiple agents with comparable efficacy and toxicity are available for a specific infection.

Brief guides to empiric therapy based on presumptive microbial diagnosis and site of infection are given in Tables 51–1 and 51–2.

■ ANTIMICROBIAL THERAPY OF INFECTIONS WITH KNOWN ETIOLOGY

INTERPRETATION OF CULTURE RESULTS

Properly obtained and processed specimens for culture frequently yield reliable information about the cause of infection. The lack of a confirmatory microbiologic diagnosis may be due to the following:

(1) Sample error, eg, obtaining cultures after antimicrobial agents have been administered.

Table 51–1. Empiric antimicrobial therapy based on microbiologic etiology.

Suspected or Proved Disease or Pathogen	Drugs of First Choice	Alternative Drugs
Gram-negative cocci (aerobic)		
Moraxella (Branhamella) catarrhalis	TMP-SMZ,[1] cephalosporin (second- or third-generation)	Erythromycin, quinolone, clarithromycin, azithromycin
Neisseria gonorrhoeae[2]	Ceftriaxone, cefpodoxime	Spectinomycin, cefoxitin
Neisseria meningitidis	Penicillin G	Chloramphenicol, cephalosporin (third-generation)[3]
Gram-negative rods (aerobic)		
E coli, Klebsiella, Proteus	Cephalosporin (first- or second-generation), TMP-SMZ	Quinolone, aminoglycoside
Enterobacter, Citrobacter, Serratia	TMP-SMZ, quinolone, carbapenem	Antipseudomonal penicillin,[4] aminoglycoside,[5] cefepime
Shigella	Quinolone	TMP-SMZ, ampicillin, azithromycin, ceftriaxone
Salmonella	TMP-SMZ, quinolone, cephalosporin (third-generation)	Chloramphenicol, ampicillin
Campylobacter jejuni	Erythromycin or azithromycin	Tetracycline, quinolone
Brucella species	Doxycycline + rifampin or aminoglycoside[5]	Chloramphenicol + aminoglycoside or TMP-SMZ
Helicobacter pylori	Bismuth + metronidazole + tetracycline or amoxicillin	Proton pump inhibitor + amoxicillin or clarithromycin
Vibrio species	Tetracycline	Quinolone, TMP-SMZ
Pseudomonas aeruginosa	Antipseudomonal penicillin + aminoglycoside[5]	Antipseudomonal penicillin + quinolone; cefepime, ceftazidime, imipenem, meropenem or aztreonam ± aminoglycoside
Burkholderia cepacia (formerly *Pseudomonas cepacia*)	TMP-SMZ	Ceftazidime, chloramphenicol
Stenotrophomonas maltophilia (formerly *Xanthomonas maltophilia*)	TMP-SMZ	Minocycline, ticarcillin-clavulanate, quinolone
Legionella species	Azithromycin + rifampin or quinolone + rifampin	Clarithromycin, erythromycin, doxycycline
Gram-positive cocci (aerobic)		
Streptococcus pneumoniae	Penicillin[6]	Doxycycline, ceftriaxone, cefuroxime, quinolones, erythromycin, linezolid, ketolides
Streptococcus pyogenes (group A)	Penicillin, clindamycin	Erythromycin, cephalosporin (first-generation)
Streptococcus agalactiae (group B)	Penicillin (+ aminoglycoside?[5])	Vancomycin
Viridans streptococci	Penicillin	Cephalosporin (first- or third-generation), vancomycin
Staphylococcus aureus		
Beta-lactamase-negative	Penicillin	Cephalosporin (first-generation), vancomycin
Beta-lactamase-positive	Penicillinase-resistant penicillin[7]	As above

(continued)

Table 51–1. Empiric antimicrobial therapy based on microbiologic etiology. (continued)

Suspected or Proved Disease or Pathogen	Drugs of First Choice	Alternative Drugs
Methicillin-resistant	Vancomycin	TMP-SMZ, minocycline, linezolid, daptomycin, tigecycline
Enterococcus species[8]	Penicillin ± aminoglycoside[5]	Vancomycin + aminoglycoside
Gram-positive rods (aerobic)		
Bacillus species (non-*anthracis*)	Vancomycin	Imipenem, quinolone, clindamycin
Listeria species	Ampicillin (± aminoglycoside[5])	TMP-SMZ
Nocardia species	Sulfadiazine, TMP-SMZ	Minocycline, imipenem, amikacin, linezolid
Anaerobic bacteria		
Gram-positive (clostridia, *Peptococcus, Actinomyces, Peptostreptococcus*)	Penicillin, clindamycin	Vancomycin, carbapenems, chloramphenicol
Clostridium difficile	Metronidazole	Vancomycin, bacitracin
Bacteroides fragilis	Metronidazole	Chloramphenicol, carbapenems, beta-lactam–beta-lactamase-inhibitor combinations, clindamycin
Fusobacterium, Prevotella, Porphyromonas	Metronidazole, clindamycin, penicillin	As for *B fragilis*
Mycobacteria		
Mycobacterium tuberculosis	Isoniazid + rifampin + ethambutol + pyrazinamide	Streptomycin, quinolone, amikacin, ethionamide, cycloserine, PAS, linezolid
Mycobacterium leprae		
Multibacillary	Dapsone + rifampin + clofazimine	
Paucibacillary	Dapsone + rifampin	
Mycoplasma pneumoniae	Tetracycline, erythromycin	Azithromycin, clarithromycin, quinolone, ketolide
Chlamydia		
trachomatis	Tetracycline, azithromycin	Clindamycin, ofloxacin
pneumoniae	Tetracycline, erythromycin	Clarithromycin, azithromycin, ketolide
psittaci	Tetracycline	Chloramphenicol
Spirochetes		
Borrelia recurrentis	Doxycycline	Erythromycin, chloramphenicol, penicillin
Borrelia burgdorferi		
Early	Doxycycline, amoxicillin	Cefuroxime axetil, penicillin
Late	Ceftriaxone	
Leptospira species	Penicillin	Tetracycline
Treponema species	Penicillin	Tetracycline, azithromycin, ceftriaxone
Fungi		
Aspergillus species	Voriconazole	Amphotericin B, itraconazole, caspofungin
Blastomyces species	Amphotericin B	Itraconazole, ketoconazole [9]

(continued)

Table 51–1. Empiric antimicrobial therapy based on microbiologic etiology. (continued)

Suspected or Proved Disease or Pathogen	Drugs of First Choice	Alternative Drugs
Candida species	Amphotericin B, caspofungin	Fluconazole, itraconazole, voriconazole, micafungin, anidulafungin
Cryptococcus	Amphotericin B ± flucytosine (5-FC)	Fluconazole
Coccidioides immitis	Amphotericin B	Fluconazole, itraconazole, ketoconazole
Histoplasma capsulatum	Amphotericin B	Itraconazole
Mucoraceae (Rhizopus, Absidia)	Amphotericin B	
Sporothrix schenkii	Amphotericin B	Itraconazole

[1]Trimethoprim-sulfamethoxazole (TMP-SMZ) is a mixture of one part trimethoprim plus five parts sulfamethoxazole.

[2]Quinolones are not recommended for empiric therapy of gonococcal infections acquired in Southeast Asia, Hawaii, and the Pacific Coast of the United States or in male homosexuals in other parts of the United States. Azithromycin 2 g is an alternative agent for the treatment of gonococcal urethritis and cervicitis.

[3]First-generation cephalosporins: cephalothin, cephapirin, or cefazolin for parenteral administration; cephalexin or cephradine for oral administration. Second-generation cephalosporins: cefuroxime, cefamandole, cefonicid for parenteral administration; cefaclor, cefuroxime axetil, cefprozil, ceftibuten for oral administration. Third-generation cephalosporins: cefoperazone, cefotaxime, ceftizoxime, ceftriaxone for parenteral administration; cefixime, cefpodoxime for oral administration.

[4]Antipseudomonal penicillin: carbenicillin, ticarcillin, azlocillin, mezlocillin, piperacillin.

[5]Generally, streptomycin and gentamicin are used to treat infections with gram-positive organisms, whereas gentamicin, tobramycin, and amikacin are used to treat infections with gram-negatives.

[6]See footnote 3 in Table 51–2 for guidelines on the treatment of penicillin-resistant pneumococcal meningitis.

[7]Parenteral nafcillin, oxacillin, or methicillin; oral dicloxacillin, cloxacillin, or oxacillin.

[8]There is no regimen that is reliably bactericidal for vancomycin-resistant enterococcus. Regimens that have been reported to be efficacious include single-drug therapy with chloramphenicol, tetracycline, nitrofurantoin (for urinary tract infection); potential regimens for bacteremia include linezolid, daptomycin + vancomycin, and ampicillin + ciprofloxacin + gentamicin.

[9]Ketoconazole does not penetrate the central nervous system and is unsatisfactory for meningitis.

(2) Noncultivable or slow-growing organisms, (*Histoplasma capsulatum*, bartonella species), in which cultures are often discarded before sufficient growth has occurred for detection.

(3) Requesting *bacterial* cultures when infection is due to other organisms.

(4) Not recognizing the need for special media or isolation techniques (eg, charcoal yeast extract agar for isolation of legionella species, shell-vial tissue culture system for rapid isolation of CMV).

Even in the setting of a classic infectious disease for which isolation techniques have been established for decades (eg, pneumococcal pneumonia, pulmonary tuberculosis, streptococcal pharyngitis), the sensitivity of the culture technique may be inadequate to identify all cases of the disease.

GUIDING ANTIMICROBIAL THERAPY OF ESTABLISHED INFECTIONS

Susceptibility Testing

Testing bacterial pathogens in vitro for their susceptibility to antimicrobial agents is extremely valuable in confirming susceptibility, ideally to a narrow-spectrum nontoxic antimicrobial drug. Tests measure the concentration of drug required to inhibit growth of the organism (**minimal inhibitory concentration [MIC]**) or to kill the organism (**minimal bactericidal concentration [MBC]**). The results of these tests can then be correlated with known drug concentrations in various body compartments. Only MICs are routinely measured in most infections, whereas in infections in which bactericidal therapy is required for eradication of infection (eg, meningitis, endocarditis, sepsis in the granulocytopenic host), MBC measurements occasionally may be useful.

Specialized Assay Methods

A. BETA-LACTAMASE ASSAY

For some bacteria (eg, haemophilus species), the susceptibility patterns of strains are similar except for the production of β-lactamase. In these cases, extensive susceptibility testing may not be required and a direct test for β-lactamase using a chromogenic β-lactam substrate (nitrocephin disk) may be substituted.

Table 51–2. Empiric antimicrobial therapy based on site of infection.

Presumed Site of Infection	Common Pathogens	Drugs of First Choice	Alternative Drugs
Bacterial endocarditis			
Acute	*Staphylococcus aureus*	Vancomycin + gentamicin	Penicillinase-resistant penicillin[1] + gentamicin
Subacute	*Viridans* streptococci, enterococci	Penicillin + gentamicin	Vancomycin + gentamicin
Septic arthritis			
Child	*H influenzae, S aureus,* β-hemolytic streptococci	Ceftriaxone	Ampicillin-sulbactam
Adult	*S aureus,* Enterobacteriaceae	Cefazolin	Vancomycin, quinolone
Acute otitis media, sinusitis	*H influenzae, S pneumoniae, M catarrhalis*	Amoxicillin	Amoxicillin-clavulanate, cefuroxime axetil, TMP-SMZ, ketolide
Cellulitis	*S aureus,* group A streptococcus	Penicillinase-resistant penicillin, cephalosporin (first-generation)[2]	Vancomycin, clindamycin, linezolid
Meningitis			
Neonate	Group B streptococcus, *E coli, Listeria*	Ampicillin + cephalosporin (third-generation)	Ampicillin + aminoglycoside, chloramphenicol, meropenem
Child	*H influenzae,* pneumococcus, meningococcus	Ceftriaxone or cefotaxime ± vancomycin [3]	Chloramphenicol, meropenem
Adult	Pneumococcus, meningococcus	Ceftriaxone, cefotaxime	Vancomycin + ceftriaxone or cefotaxime [3]
Peritonitis due to ruptured viscus	Coliforms, *B fragilis*	Metronidazole + cephalosporin (third-generation), piperacillin-tazobactam	Carbapenem
Pneumonia			
Neonate	As in neonatal meningitis		
Child	Pneumococcus, *S aureus, H influenzae*	Ceftriaxone, cefuroxime, cefotaxime	Ampicillin-sulbactam
Adult (community-acquired)	Pneumococcus, *Mycoplasma, Legionella, H influenzae, S aureus, C pneumoniae,* coliforms	**Outpatient:** Macrolide,[4] amoxicillin, tetracycline **Inpatient:** Macrolide[4] + cephalosporin (third-generation)	**Outpatient:** Ketolide, quinolone **Inpatient:** Doxycycline + piperacillin-tazobactam or ticarcillin-clavulanate, or cefuroxime; quinolone[5]
Septicemia[6]	Any	Vancomycin + cephalosporin (third-generation) or piperacillin-tazobactam or imipenem or meropenem	
Septicemia with granulocytopenia	Any	Antipseudomonal penicillin + aminoglycoside; ceftazidime; cefepime; imipenem or meropenem; consider addition of systemic antifungal therapy if fever persists beyond 5 days of empiric therapy	

[1]See footnote 7, Table 51–1.
[2]See footnote 3, Table 51–1.
[3]When meningitis with penicillin-resistant pneumococcus is suspected, empiric therapy with this regimen is recommended.
[4]Erythromycin, clarithromycin, or azithromycin (an azalide) may be used.
[5]Quinolones used to treat pneumonococcal infections include levofloxacin, moxifloxacin, and gemifloxacin.
[6]Adjunctive immunomodulatory drugs such as drotrecogin-alfa can also be considered for patients with severe sepsis.

B. SYNERGY STUDIES

Synergy studies are in vitro tests that attempt to measure synergistic, additive, indifferent, or antagonistic drug interactions. In general, these tests have not been standardized and have not correlated well with clinical outcome. (See section on Antimicrobial Drug Combinations for details.)

MONITORING THERAPEUTIC RESPONSE: DURATION OF THERAPY

The therapeutic response may be monitored microbiologically or clinically. Cultures of specimens taken from infected sites should eventually become sterile or demonstrate eradication of the pathogen and are useful for documenting recurrence or relapse. Follow-up cultures may also be useful for detecting superinfections or the development of resistance. Clinically, the patient's systemic manifestations of infection (malaise, fever, leukocytosis) should abate and the clinical findings should improve (eg, as shown by clearing of radiographic infiltrates or lessening hypoxemia in pneumonia).

The duration of therapy required for cure depends on the pathogen, the site of infection, and host factors (immunocompromised patients generally require longer courses of treatment). Precise data on duration of therapy exist for some infections (eg, streptococcal pharyngitis, syphilis, gonorrhea, tuberculosis, cryptococcal meningitis in non-AIDS patients). In many other situations, duration of therapy is determined empirically. For serious infections, continuing therapy for 7–10 days after the patient has become afebrile is a good rule of thumb. For recurrent infections (eg, sinusitis, urinary tract infections), longer courses of antimicrobial therapy are frequently necessary for eradication.

Clinical Failure of Antimicrobial Therapy

When the patient has an inadequate clinical or microbiologic response to antimicrobial therapy selected by in vitro susceptibility testing, systematic investigation should be undertaken to determine the cause of failure. Errors in susceptibility testing are rare, but the original results should be confirmed by repeat testing. Drug dosing and absorption should be scrutinized and tested directly using serum measurements, pill counting, or directly observed therapy.

The clinical data should be reviewed to determine whether the patient's immune function is adequate and, if not, what can be done to maximize it. For example, are adequate numbers of granulocytes present and are HIV infection, malnutrition, or underlying malignancy present? The presence of abscesses or foreign bodies should also be considered. Lastly, culture and susceptibility testing should be repeated to determine whether superinfection has occurred with another organism or whether the original pathogen has developed drug resistance.

Table 51–3. Bactericidal and bacteriostatic antibacterial agents.

Bactericidal agents	Bacteriostatic agents
Aminoglycosides	Chloramphenicol
Bacitracin	Clindamycin
Beta-lactam antibiotics	Ethambutol
Daptomycin	Macrolides
Isoniazid	Nitrofurantoin
Ketolides	Novobiocin
Metronidazole	Oxazolidinones
Polymyxins	Sulfonamides
Pyrazinamide	Tetracyclines
Quinolones	Trimethoprim
Rifampin	
Tigecycline	
Vancomycin	

ANTIMICROBIAL PHARMACODYNAMICS

The time course of drug concentration is closely related to the antimicrobial effect at the site of infection and to any toxic effects. Pharmacodynamic factors include pathogen susceptibility testing, drug bactericidal versus bacteriostatic activity, and drug synergism, antagonism, and postantibiotic effects. Together with pharmacokinetics, pharmacodynamic information permits the selection of optimal antimicrobial dosage regimens.

Bacteriostatic versus Bactericidal Activity

Antibacterial agents may be classified as bacteriostatic or bactericidal (Table 51–3). For agents that are primarily bacteriostatic, inhibitory drug concentrations are much lower than bactericidal drug concentrations. In general, cell wall-active agents are bactericidal, and drugs that inhibit protein synthesis are bacteriostatic.

The classification of antibacterial agents as bactericidal or bacteriostatic has limitations. Some agents that are considered to be bacteriostatic may be bactericidal against selected organisms. On the other hand, enterococci are inhibited but not killed by vancomycin, penicillin, or ampicillin used as single agents.

Bacteriostatic and bactericidal agents are equivalent for the treatment of most infectious diseases in immunocompetent hosts. Bactericidal agents should be selected over bacteriostatic ones in circumstances in which local or systemic host defenses are impaired. Bactericidal agents are required for treatment of endocarditis and other endovascular infections, meningitis, and infections in neutropenic cancer patients.

Bactericidal agents can be divided into two groups: agents that exhibit **concentration-dependent killing** (eg, aminoglycosides and quinolones) and agents that exhibit **time-dependent killing** (eg, β-lactams and vancomycin). For drugs whose killing action is concentration-dependent, the rate and extent of killing increase with increasing drug concentrations. Concentration-dependent killing is one of the pharmacodynamic factors responsible for the efficacy of once-daily dosing of aminoglycosides.

For drugs whose killing action is time-dependent, bactericidal activity continues as long as serum concentrations are greater than the MBC. Drug concentrations of time-dependent killing agents that lack a postantibiotic effect should be maintained above the MIC for the entire interval between doses.

Postantibiotic Effect

Persistent suppression of bacterial growth after limited exposure to an antimicrobial agent is known as the postantibiotic effect (PAE). The PAE can be expressed mathematically as follows:

$$PAE = T - C$$

where T is the time required for the viable count in the test (in vitro) culture to increase tenfold above the count observed immediately before drug removal and C is the time required for the count in an untreated culture to increase tenfold above the count observed immediately after completion of the same procedure used on the test culture. The PAE reflects the time required for bacteria to return to logarithmic growth.

Table 51–4. Antibacterial agents with in vitro postantibiotic effects ≥ 1.5 hours.

Against gram-positive cocci	Against gram-negative bacilli
Aminoglycosides	Aminoglycosides
Carbapenems	Carbapenems
Cephalosporins	Chloramphenicol
Chloramphenicol	Quinolones
Clindamycin	Rifampin
Daptomycin	Tetracyclines
Ketolides	Tigecycline
Macrolides	
Oxazolidinones	
Penicillins	
Quinolones	
Rifampin	
Sulfonamides	
Tetracyclines	
Tigecycline	
Trimethoprim	
Vancomycin	

Proposed mechanisms include (1) slow recovery after reversible nonlethal damage to cell structures; (2) persistence of the drug at a binding site or within the periplasmic space; and (3) the need to synthesize new enzymes before growth can resume. Most antimicrobials possess significant in vitro PAEs (≥ 1.5 hours) against susceptible gram-positive cocci (Table 51–4). Antimicrobials with significant PAEs against susceptible gram-negative bacilli are limited to carbapenems and agents that inhibit protein or DNA synthesis.

In vivo PAEs are usually much longer than in vitro PAEs. This is thought to be due to **postantibiotic leukocyte enhancement (PALE)** and exposure of bacteria to subinhibitory antibiotic concentrations. The efficacy of once-daily dosing regimens is in part due to the PAE. Aminoglycosides and quinolones possess concentration-dependent PAEs; thus, high doses of aminoglycosides given once daily result in enhanced bactericidal activity and extended PAEs. This combination of pharmacodynamic effects allows aminoglycoside serum concentrations that are below the MICs of target organisms to remain effective for extended periods of time.

PHARMACOKINETIC CONSIDERATIONS

Route of Administration

Many antimicrobial agents have similar pharmacokinetic properties when given orally or parenterally (ie, tetracyclines, trimethoprim-sulfamethoxazole, quinolones, chloramphenicol, metronidazole, clindamycin, rifampin, linezolid and fluconazole). In most cases, oral therapy with these drugs is equally effective, is less costly, and results in fewer complications than parenteral therapy.

The intravenous route is preferred in the following situations: (1) for critically ill patients; (2) for patients with bacterial meningitis or endocarditis; (3) for patients with nausea, vomiting, gastrectomy, or diseases that may impair oral absorption; and (4) when giving antimicrobials that are poorly absorbed following oral administration.

Conditions That Alter Antimicrobial Pharmacokinetics

Various diseases and physiologic states alter the pharmacokinetics of antimicrobial agents. Impairment of renal or hepatic function may result in decreased elimination. Table 51–5 lists drugs that require dosage reduction in patients with renal or hepatic insufficiency. Failure to reduce antimicrobial agent dosage in such patients may cause toxic side effects. Conversely, patients with burns, cystic fibrosis, or trauma may have increased dosage requirements for selected agents. The pharmacokinetics of antimicrobials are also altered in the elderly, in neonates, and in pregnancy.

Table 51–5. Antimicrobial agents that require dosage adjustment or are contraindicated in patients with renal or hepatic impairment.

Dosage Adjustment Needed in Renal Impairment	Contraindicated in Renal Impairment	Dosage Adjustment Needed in Hepatic Impairment
Acyclovir, amantadine, aminoglycosides, aztreonam, cephalosporins,[1] clarithromycin, cycloserine, daptomycin, didanosine, emtricitabine, ertapenem, ethambutol, famciclovir, fluconazole, flucytosine, foscarnet, ganciclovir, imipenem, lamivudine, meropenem, penicillins,[3] quinolones,[4] rimantadine, stavudine, terbinafine, telithromycin, tenofovir, trimethoprim-sulfamethoxazole, valacyclovir, vancomycin, zalcitabine, zidovudine	Cidofovir, methenamine, nalidixic acid, nitrofurantoin, sulfonamides (long-acting), tetracyclines,[2] voriconazole	Amprenavir, atazanavir, chloramphenicol, clindamycin, erythromycin, fosamprenavir, indinavir, metronidazole, rimantadine, tigecycline

[1]Except cefoperazone and ceftriaxone.
[2]Except doxycycline and possibly minocycline.
[3]Except antistaphylococcal penicillins (eg, nafcillin and dicloxacillin).
[4]Except grepafloxacin and trovafloxacin.

Drug Concentrations in Body Fluids

Most antimicrobial agents are well distributed to most body tissues and fluids. Penetration into the cerebrospinal fluid is an exception. Most do not penetrate uninflamed meninges to an appreciable extent. In the presence of meningitis, however, the cerebrospinal fluid concentrations of many antimicrobials increase (Table 51–6).

Monitoring Serum Concentrations of Antimicrobial Agents

For most antimicrobial agents, the relationship between dose and therapeutic outcome is well established, and serum concentration monitoring is unnecessary for these drugs. To justify routine serum concentration monitoring, it should be established (1) that a direct relationship

Table 51–6. Cerebrospinal fluid (CSF) penetration of selected antimicrobials.

Antimicrobial Agent	CSF Concentration (Uninflamed Meninges) as Percent of Serum Concentration	CSF Concentration (Inflamed Meninges) as Percent of Serum Concentration
Ampicillin	2–3	2–100
Aztreonam	2	5
Cefotaxime	22.5	27–36
Ceftazidime	0.7	20–40
Ceftriaxone	0.8–1.6	16
Cefuroxime	20	17–88
Ciprofloxacin	6–27	26–37
Imipenem	3.1	11–41
Meropenem	0–7	1–52
Nafcillin	2–15	5–27
Penicillin G	1–2	8–18
Sulfamethoxazole	40	12–47
Trimethoprim	< 41	12–69
Vancomycin	0	1–53

exists between drug concentrations and efficacy or toxicity; (2) that substantial interpatient variability exists in serum concentrations on standard doses; (3) that a small difference exists between therapeutic and toxic serum concentrations; (4) that the clinical efficacy or toxicity of the drug is delayed or difficult to measure; and (5) that an accurate assay is available.

In clinical practice, serum concentration monitoring is routinely performed on patients receiving aminoglycosides. Despite the lack of supporting evidence for its usefulness or need, serum vancomycin concentration monitoring is also widespread. Flucytosine serum concentration monitoring has been shown to reduce toxicity when doses are adjusted to maintain peak concentrations below 100 mcg/mL.

MANAGEMENT OF ANTIMICROBIAL DRUG TOXICITY

Owing to the large number of antimicrobials available, it is usually possible to select an effective alternative in patients who develop serious drug toxicity (Table 51–1). However, for some infections there are no effective alternatives to the drug of choice. For example, in patients with neurosyphilis who have a history of anaphylaxis to penicillin, it is necessary to perform skin testing and desensitization to penicillin. It is important to obtain a clear history of drug allergy and other adverse drug reactions. A patient with a documented antimicrobial allergy should carry a card with the name of the drug and a description of the reaction. Cross-reactivity between penicillins and cephalosporins is less than 10%. Cephalosporins may be administered to patients with penicillin-induced maculopapular rashes but should be avoided in patients with a history of penicillin-induced immediate hypersensitivity reactions. The cross-reactivity between penicillins and carbapenems may exceed 50%. On the other hand, aztreonam does not cross-react with penicillins and can be safely administered to patients with a history of penicillin-induced anaphylaxis. For mild reactions, it may be possible to continue therapy with use of adjunctive agents or dosage reduction.

Adverse reactions to antimicrobials occur with increased frequency in several groups, including neonates, geriatric patients, renal failure patients, and AIDS patients. Dosage adjustment of the drugs listed in Table 51–5 is essential for the prevention of adverse effects in patients with renal failure. In addition, several agents are contraindicated in patients with renal impairment because of increased rates of serious toxicity (Table 51–5). See the preceding chapters for discussions of specific drugs.

Polypharmacy also predisposes to drug interactions. Although the mechanism is not known, AIDS patients have an unusually high incidence of toxicity to a number of drugs, including clindamycin, aminopenicillins, and sulfonamides. Many of these reactions, including rash and fever, may respond to dosage reduction or treatment with corticosteroids and antihistamines. Other examples are discussed in the preceding chapters and in Appendix II.

ANTIMICROBIAL DRUG COMBINATIONS

RATIONALE FOR COMBINATION ANTIMICROBIAL THERAPY

Most infections should be treated with a single antimicrobial agent. Although indications for combination therapy exist, antimicrobial combinations are often overused in clinical practice. The unnecessary use of antimicrobial combinations increases toxicity and costs and may occasionally result in reduced efficacy due to antagonism of one drug by another. Antimicrobial combinations should be selected for one or more of the following reasons:

(1) To provide broad-spectrum empiric therapy in seriously ill patients.

(2) To treat polymicrobial infections such as intra-abdominal abscesses. The antimicrobial combination chosen should cover the most common known or suspected pathogens but need not cover all possible pathogens. The availability of antimicrobials with excellent polymicrobial coverage (eg, β-lactamase inhibitor combinations or carbapenems) may reduce the need for combination therapy in the setting of polymicrobial infections.

(3) To decrease the emergence of resistant strains. The value of combination therapy in this setting has been clearly demonstrated for tuberculosis.

(4) To decrease dose-related toxicity by using reduced doses of one or more components of the drug regimen. The use of flucytosine in combination with amphotericin B for the treatment of cryptococcal meningitis in non–HIV-infected patients allows for a reduction in amphotericin B dosage with decreased amphotericin B–induced nephrotoxicity.

(5) To obtain enhanced inhibition or killing. This use of antimicrobial combinations is discussed in the paragraphs that follow.

SYNERGISM & ANTAGONISM

When the inhibitory or killing effects of two or more antimicrobials used together are significantly greater than expected from their effects when used individually, synergism is said to result. Synergism is marked by a fourfold or greater reduction in the MIC or MBC of each drug when used in combination versus when used alone.

The interaction between two antimicrobial agents can be expressed by the fractional inhibitory concentration (FIC) index:

$$FIC_{index} = FIC_A + FIC_B$$

$$FIC_A = \frac{MIC \text{ of drug A in combination}}{MIC \text{ of drug A alone}}$$

$$FIC_B = \frac{MIC \text{ of drug B in combination}}{MIC \text{ of drug B alone}}$$

The fractional bactericidal concentration (FBC) index can be determined by substituting MBCs for MICs in the above equations. Synergism for combinations of two drugs requires an FIC or FBC index of 0.5 or less. Antagonism occurs when the combined inhibitory or killing effects of two or more antimicrobials are significantly less than expected when the drugs are used individually. Antibiotic antagonism is marked by an FIC or FBC index of 4 or more.

Mechanisms of Synergistic Action

The need for synergistic combinations of antimicrobials has been clearly established for the treatment of enterococcal endocarditis. Bactericidal activity is essential for the optimal management of bacterial endocarditis. Penicillin or ampicillin in combination with gentamicin or streptomycin is superior to monotherapy with a penicillin or vancomycin. When tested alone, penicillins and vancomycin are only bacteriostatic against susceptible enterococcal isolates. When these agents are combined with an aminoglycoside, however, bactericidal activity results. The addition of gentamicin or streptomycin to penicillin allows for a reduction in the duration of therapy for selected patients with viridans streptococcal endocarditis. There is some evidence that synergistic combinations of antimicrobials may be of benefit in the treatment of gram-negative bacillary infections in febrile neutropenic cancer patients and in systemic infections caused by *Pseudomonas aeruginosa.*

Other synergistic antimicrobial combinations have been shown to be more effective than monotherapy with individual components. Trimethoprim-sulfamethoxazole has been successfully used for the treatment of bacterial infections and *Pneumocystis jiroveci (carinii)* pneumonia.*
Beta-lactamase inhibitors restore the activity of intrinsically

active but hydrolyzable β-lactams against organisms such as *S aureus* and *Bacteroides fragilis.* Three major mechanisms of antimicrobial synergism have been established:

1. Blockade of sequential steps in a metabolic sequence: Trimethoprim-sulfamethoxazole is the best-known example of this mechanism of synergy (see Chapter 46). Blockade of the two sequential steps in the folic acid pathway by trimethoprim-sulfamethoxazole results in a much more complete inhibition of growth than achieved by either component alone.

2. Inhibition of enzymatic inactivation: Enzymatic inactivation of β-lactam antibiotics is a major mechanism of antibiotic resistance. Inhibition of β-lactamase by β-lactamase inhibitor drugs (eg, sulbactam) results in synergism.

3. Enhancement of antimicrobial agent uptake: Penicillins and other cell wall-active agents can increase the uptake of aminoglycosides by a number of bacteria, including staphylococci, enterococci, streptococci, and *P aeruginosa.* Enterococci are thought to be intrinsically resistant to aminoglycosides because of permeability barriers. Similarly, amphotericin B is thought to enhance the uptake of flucytosine by fungi.

Mechanisms of Antagonistic Action

There are few clinically relevant examples of antimicrobial antagonism. The most striking example was reported in a study of patients with pneumococcal meningitis. Patients who were treated with the combination of penicillin and chlortetracycline had a mortality rate of 79% compared with a mortality rate of 21% in patients who received penicillin monotherapy (illustrating the first mechanism set forth below).

The use of an antagonistic antimicrobial combination does not preclude other potential beneficial interactions. For example, rifampin may antagonize the action of antistaphylococcal penicillins or vancomycin against staphylococci. However, the aforementioned antimicrobials may prevent the emergence of resistance to rifampin.

Two major mechanisms of antimicrobial antagonism have been established:

1. Inhibition of cidal activity by static agents: Bacteriostatic agents such as tetracyclines and chloramphenicol can antagonize the action of bactericidal cell wall-active agents because cell wall-active agents require that the bacteria be actively growing and dividing.

2. Induction of enzymatic inactivation: Some gram-negative bacilli, including enterobacter species, *P aeruginosa, Serratia marcescens,* and *Citrobacter freundii,* possess inducible β-lactamases. Beta-lactam antibiotics such as imipenem, cefoxitin, and ampicillin are potent inducers of β-lactamase production. If an inducing agent is combined with an intrinsically active but hydrolyzable β-lactam such as piperacillin, antagonism may result.

---

*Pneumocystis jiroveci is a fungal organism found in humans (*P carinii* infects animals) that responds to antiprotozoal drugs. See Chapter 53.

NATIONAL RESEARCH COUNCIL (NRC) WOUND CLASSIFICATION CRITERIA

Clean: Elective, primarily closed procedure; respiratory, gastrointestinal, biliary, genitourinary, or oropharyngeal tract not entered; no acute inflammation and no break in technique; expected infection rate ≤ 2%.

Clean contaminated: Urgent or emergency case that is otherwise clean; elective, controlled opening of respiratory, gastrointestinal, biliary, or oropharyngeal tract; minimal spillage or minor break in technique; expected infection rate ≤10%.

Contaminated: Acute nonpurulent inflammation; major technique break or major spill from hollow organ; penetrating trauma less than 4 hours old; chronic open wounds to be grafted or covered; expected infection rate about 20%.

Dirty: Purulence or abscess; preoperative perforation of respiratory, gastrointestinal, biliary, or oropharyngeal tract; penetrating trauma more than 4 hours old; expected infection rate about 40%.

■ ANTIMICROBIAL PROPHYLAXIS

Antimicrobial agents are effective in preventing infections in many settings. Antimicrobial prophylaxis should be used in circumstances in which efficacy has been demonstrated and benefits outweigh the risks of prophylaxis. Antimicrobial prophylaxis may be divided into surgical prophylaxis and nonsurgical prophylaxis.

Surgical Prophylaxis

Surgical wound infections are a major category of nosocomial infections. The estimated annual cost of surgical wound infections in the United States is $1.5 billion.

The National Research Council (NRC) Wound Classification Criteria have served as the basis for recommending antimicrobial prophylaxis. The NRC criteria consist of four classes (see Box: National Research Council (NRC) Wound Classification Criteria).

The Study of the Efficacy of Nosocomial Infection Control (SENIC) identified four independent risk factors for postoperative wound infections: operations on the abdomen, operations lasting more than 2 hours, contaminated or dirty wound classification, and at least three medical diagnoses. Patients with at least two SENIC risk factors who undergo clean surgical procedures are at increased risk of developing surgical wound infections and should receive antimicrobial prophylaxis.

Surgical procedures that necessitate the use of antimicrobial prophylaxis include contaminated and clean-contaminated operations, selected operations in which postoperative infection may be catastrophic such as open heart surgery, clean procedures that involve placement of prosthetic materials, and any procedure in an immunocompromised host. The operation should carry a significant risk of postoperative site infection or cause significant bacterial contamination.

General principles of antimicrobial surgical prophylaxis include the following:

(1) The antibiotic should be active against common surgical wound pathogens; unnecessarily broad coverage should be avoided.

(2) The antibiotic should have proved efficacy in clinical trials.

(3) The antibiotic must achieve concentrations greater than the MIC of suspected pathogens, and these concentrations must be present at the time of incision.

(4) The shortest possible course—ideally a single dose—of the most effective and least toxic antibiotic should be used.

(5) The newer broad-spectrum antibiotics should be reserved for therapy of resistant infections.

(6) If all other factors are equal, the least expensive agent should be used.

The proper selection and administration of antimicrobial prophylaxis is of utmost importance. Common indications for surgical prophylaxis are shown in Table 51–7. Cefazolin is the prophylactic agent of choice for head and neck, gastroduodenal, biliary tract, gynecologic, and clean procedures. Local wound infection patterns should be considered when selecting antimicrobial prophylaxis. The selection of vancomycin over cefazolin may be necessary in hospitals with high rates of methicillin-resistant *S aureus* or *Staphylococcus epidermidis* infections. The antibiotic should be present in adequate concentrations at the operative site before incision and throughout the procedure; initial dosing is dependent on the volume of distribution, peak levels, clearance, protein binding, and bioavailability. Parenteral agents should be administered during the interval beginning 60 minutes before incision; administration up to the time of incision is preferred. In cesarean section, the antibiotic is administered after umbilical cord clamping. If short-acting agents such as cefoxitin are used, doses should be repeated if the procedure exceeds 3–4 hours in duration. Single-dose prophylaxis is effective for most procedures and results in decreased toxicity and antimicrobial resistance.

Table 51–7. Recommendations for surgical antimicrobial prophylaxis.

Type of Operation	Common Pathogens	Drug of Choice
Cardiac (with median sternotomy)	Staphylococci, enteric gram-negative rods	Cefazolin
Noncardiac, thoracic	Staphylococci, streptococci, enteric gram-negative rods	Cefazolin
Vascular (abdominal and lower extremity)	Staphylococci, enteric gram-negative rods	Cefazolin
Neurosurgical (craniotomy)	Staphylococci	Cefazolin
Orthopedic (with hardware insertion)	Staphylococci	Cefazolin
Head and neck (with entry into the oropharynx)	*S aureus*, oral flora	Cefazolin
Gastroduodenal (high-risk patients[1])	*S aureus*, oral flora, enteric gram-negative rods	Cefazolin
Biliary tract (high-risk patients[2])	*S aureus*, enterococci, enteric gram-negative rods	Cefazolin
Colorectal (elective surgery)	Enteric gram-negative rods, anaerobes	Oral erythromycin plus neomycin[3]
Colorectal (emergency surgery or obstruction)	Enteric gram-negative rods, anaerobes	Cefoxitin, cefotetan, or cefmetazole
Appendectomy	Enteric gram-negative rods, anaerobes	Cefoxitin, ceftizoxime, cefotetan, or cefmetazole
Hysterectomy	Enteric gram-negative rods, anaerobes, enterococci, group B streptococci	Cefazolin
Cesarean section	Enteric gram-negative rods, anaerobes, enterococci, group B streptococci	Cefazolin [4]

[1]Gastric procedures for cancer, ulcer, bleeding, or obstruction; morbid obesity; suppression of gastric acid secretion.
[2]Age > 60, acute cholecystitis, prior biliary tract surgery, common duct stones, jaundice, or diabetes mellitus.
[3]In conjunction with mechanical bowel preparation.
[4]Administer immediately following cord clamping.

Improper administration of antimicrobial prophylaxis leads to excessive surgical wound infection rates. Common errors in antibiotic prophylaxis include selection of the wrong antibiotic, administering the first dose too early or too late, failure to repeat doses during prolonged procedures, excessive duration of prophylaxis, and inappropriate use of broad-spectrum antibiotics.

Nonsurgical Prophylaxis

Nonsurgical prophylaxis includes the administration of antimicrobials to prevent colonization or asymptomatic infection as well as the administration of drugs following colonization by or inoculation of pathogens but before the development of disease. Nonsurgical prophylaxis is indicated in individuals who are at high risk for temporary exposure to selected virulent pathogens and in patients who are at increased risk for developing infection because of underlying disease (eg, immunocompromised hosts). Prophylaxis is most effective when directed against organisms that are predictably susceptible to antimicrobial agents. Common indications for nonsurgical prophylaxis are listed in Table 51–8.

Table 51–8. Recommendations for nonsurgical antimicrobial prophylaxis.

Infection to Be Prevented	Indication(s)	Drug of Choice	Efficacy
Anthrax	Suspected exposure	Ciprofloxacin or doxycycline	Proposed effective
Cholera	Close contacts of a case	Tetracycline	Proposed effective
Diphtheria	Unimmunized contacts	Penicillin or erythromycin	Proposed effective
Endocarditis	Dental, oral, or upper respiratory tract procedures[1] in at-risk patients[2]	Amoxicillin or clindamycin	Proposed effective
	Genitourinary or gastrointestinal procedures[3] in at-risk patients[2]	Ampicillin or vancomycin and gentamicin	Proposed effective
Genital herpes simplex	Recurrent infection ($\geq$ 4 episodes per year)	Acyclovir	Excellent
Influenza B	Unvaccinated geriatric patients, immunocompromised hosts, and health care workers during outbreaks	Oseltamivir	Good
Perinatal herpes simplex type 2 infection	Mothers with primary HSV or frequent recurrent genital HSV	Acyclovir	Proposed effective
Group B streptococcal (GBS) infection	Mothers with cervical or vaginal GBS colonization and their newborns with one or more of the following: (a) onset of labor or membrane rupture before 37 weeks' gestation, (b) prolonged rupture of membranes (> 12 hours), (c) maternal intrapartum fever, (d) history of GBS bacteriuria during pregnancy, (e) mothers who have given birth to infants who had early GBS disease or with a history of streptococcal bacteriuria during pregnancy	Ampicillin or penicillin	Excellent
Haemophilus Influenzae type B infection	Close contacts of a case in incompletely immunized children (< 48 months old)	Rifampin	Excellent
HIV infection	Health care workers exposed to blood after needle-stick injury	Zidovudine and lamivudine $\pm$ indinavir or nelfinavir	Good
	Pregnant HIV-infected women who are at $\geq$ 14 weeks of gestation Newborns of HIV-infected women for the first 6 weeks of life, beginning 8–12 hours after birth	Zidovudine	Excellent
Influenza A	Unvaccinated geriatric patients, immunocompromised hosts, and health care workers during outbreaks	Amantadine	Good
Malaria	Travelers to areas endemic for chloroquine-susceptible disease	Chloroquine	Excellent
	Travelers to areas endemic for chloroquine-resistant disease	Mefloquine	Excellent
Meningococcal infection	Close contacts of a case	Rifampin, ciprofaxacin, or ceftriaxone	Excellent
Mycobacterium avium complex	HIV-infected patients with CD4 count < 75/μL	Azithromycin or clarithromycin	Excellent

(*continued*)

Table 51–8. Recommendations for nonsurgical antimicrobial prophylaxis. (continued)

Infection to Be Prevented	Indication(s)	Drug of Choice	Efficacy
Otitis media	Recurrent infection	Amoxicillin	Good
Pertussis	Close contacts of a case	Erythromycin	Excellent
Plague	Close contacts of a case	Tetracycline	Proposed effective
Pneumococcemia	Children with sickle cell disease or asplenia	Penicillin	Excellent
Pneumocystis jiroveci pneumonia (PCP)	High-risk patients (eg, AIDS, leukemia, transplant)	Trimethoprim-sulfamethoxazole	Excellent
Rheumatic fever	History of rheumatic fever or known rheumatic heart disease	Benzathine penicillin	Excellent
Toxoplasmosis	HIV-infected patients with IgG antibody to *Toxoplasma* and CD4 count < 100/μL	Trimethoprim-sulfamethoxazole	Good
Tuberculosis	Persons with positive tuberculin skin tests and one or more of the following: (a) HIV infection, (b) close contacts with newly diagnosed disease, (c) recent skin test conversion, (d) medical conditions that increase the risk of developing tuberculosis, (e) age < 35	Isoniazid, rifampin, or pyrazinamide	Excellent
Urinary tract infections (UTI)	Recurrent infection	Trimethoprim-sulfamethoxazole	Excellent

[1]Prophylaxis is recommended for the following: dental procedures known to induce gingival or mucosal bleeding, tonsillectomy or adenoidectomy, surgical procedures that involve respiratory mucosa, and rigid bronchoscopy.
[2]Risk factors include the following: prosthetic heart valves, previous bacterial endocarditis, congenital cardiac malformations, rheumatic and other acquired valvular dysfunction, and mitral valve prolapse with valvular regurgitation.
[3]Prophylaxis is recommended for the following: surgical procedures that involve intestinal mucosa, sclerotherapy for esophageal varices, esophageal or urethral dilation, biliary tract surgery, cystoscopy, urethral catheterization or urinary tract surgery in the presence of urinary tract infection, prostatic surgery, incision and drainage of infected tissue, vaginal hysterectomy, and vaginal delivery in the presence of infection.

REFERENCES

American Thoracic Society: Guidelines for the management of adults with hospital-acquired, ventilator-associated, and healthcare-associated pneumonia. Am J Respir Crit Care Med 2005;171:388.

Antimicrobial prophylaxis in surgery. Med Lett Drugs Ther 2001;43:92.

Baddour LM et al: Infective endocarditis: Diagnosis, antimicrobial therapy, and management of complications. Circulation 2005; 111:3167.

Blumberg HM et al: American Thoracic Society/Centers for Disease Control and Prevention/Infectious Diseases Society of America: Treatment of tuberculosis. Am J Respir Crit Care Med 2003;167:603.

Bochner BS et al: Anaphylaxis. N Engl J Med 1991;324:1785.

Bratzler DW et al: Antimicrobial prophylaxis for surgery: An advisory statement from the National Surgical Infection Prevention Project. Clin Infect Dis 2004;38:1706.

Classen DC et al: The timing of prophylactic administration of antibiotics and the risk of surgical-wound infection. N Engl J Med 1992;326:281.

Craig WA: Clinical implications of antimicrobial pharmacokinetics. Infect Dis Clin North Am 2003;17:479.

Dajani AS et al: Prevention of bacterial endocarditis. Recommendations by the American Heart Association. JAMA 1997;277:1794.

Gonzales R et al: Principles of appropriate antibiotic use for treatment of acute respiratory tract infections in adults: Background, specific aims, and methods. Ann Intern Med 2001; 134:479.

Jones RN, Pfaller MA: Bacterial resistance: A worldwide problem. Diagn Microbiol Infect Dis 1998;31:379.

Kaye D: Antibacterial therapy and newer agents. Infect Dis Clin North Am 2004;18:401.

Mandell LA et al: Update of practice guidelines for the management of community-acquired pneumonia in immunocompetent adults. Clin Infect Dis 2003;37:1405.

Martone WJ, Nichols RL: Recognition, prevention, surveillance, and management of surgical site infections: Introduction to the problem and symposium overview. Clin Infect Dis 2001; 33(Suppl 2):S67.

National Nosocomial Infections Surveillance (NNIS) System Report. Data Summary from January 1992–June 2001, issued August 2001. Am J Infect Control 2001;29:404.

Sexually transmitted diseases treatment guidelines 2002. Centers for Disease Control and Prevention. MMWR Morb Mortal Wkly Rep 2002;51(RR-6):1.

USPHS/IDSA guidelines for preventing opportunistic infections among HIV-infected persons—2002. MMWR Morb Mortal Wkly Rep 2002;51(RR-8):1.

Introduction to Antiparasitic Chemotherapy

52

Ching Chung Wang, PhD, & Alice Lee Wang, PhD

In its general scientific sense, the term "parasite" includes all of the known infectious agents such as viruses, bacteria, fungi, protozoa, and helminths. In this and the two following chapters, the term is used in a restricted sense to denote the protozoa and helminths. It has been estimated that 3 billion (3×10^9) humans suffer from parasitic infections, plus a much greater number of domestic and wild animals. Although these diseases constitute the most widespread human health problem in the world today, they have for various reasons also been the most neglected.

In theory, the parasitic infections should be relatively easy to treat because the etiologic agents are known in almost all cases. Furthermore, recent advances in cell culture techniques have made possible in vitro cultivation of many of the important parasites. These advances have not only laid to rest the traditional view that parasites somehow depend on a living host for their existence but have also enabled us to study parasites by methods similar to those employed in investigations of bacteria, including biochemistry, molecular biology, and immunologic pharmacology. However, many problems remain to be solved before more effective chemotherapeutic agents will be discovered and made available for all of the parasitic diseases.

TARGETS OF CHEMOTHERAPY

A rational approach to antiparasitic chemotherapy requires comparative biochemical and physiologic investigations of host and parasite to discover differences in essential processes that will permit selective inhibition in the parasite and not in the host. One might expect that the parasite would have many deficiencies in its metabolism associated with its parasitic nature. This is true of many parasites—the oversimplified metabolic pathways are usually indispensable for survival of the parasite and thus represent potential points of vulnerability. However, oversimplified metabolic pathways are not the only opportunity for attack. Although the parasite lives in a metabolically luxurious environment and may become "lazy," the

environment is not entirely friendly and the parasite must have defense mechanisms in order to survive—ie, to defend itself against immunologic attack, proteolytic digestion, etc, by the host. In some instances, necessary nutrients are not supplied to the parasite from the host, although the latter can obtain the same nutrients from the diet. In this situation, the parasite will have acquired the synthetic activity needed for its survival. Finally, the great evolutionary distance between host and parasite has in some cases resulted in sufficient differences among individual enzymes or functional pathways to allow selective inhibition of the parasite. Thus, there can be three major types of targets for chemotherapy of parasitic diseases: (1) unique essential enzymes found only in the parasite; (2) similar enzymes found in both host and parasite but indispensable only for the parasite; and (3) common biochemical functions found in both parasite and host but with different pharmacologic properties. Examples of specific targets and drugs that act on them are summarized in Table 52–1.

ESSENTIAL ENZYMES FOUND ONLY IN PARASITES

These enzymes would appear to be the cleanest targets for chemotherapy. Like enzymes involved in the synthesis of bacterial cell walls (see Chapter 43), inhibition of these enzymes should have no effect on the host. Unfortunately, only a few of these enzymes have been discovered among the parasitic protozoa. Furthermore, their usefulness as chemotherapeutic targets is sometimes limited because of the development of drug resistance.

ENZYMES INDISPENSABLE ONLY IN PARASITES

Because of the many metabolic deficiencies among parasites, there are enzymes whose functions may be essential for the survival of the parasites, but are not indispensable to the host. That is, the host may be able to survive the complete loss of these enzyme func-

842

Table 52–1. Identified targets for chemotherapy in parasites.

Targets	Parasites	Inhibitors
Unique essential enzymes		
Enzymes for dihydropteroate synthesis	Apicomplexa	Sulfones and sulfonamides
Glycolipid synthesis	African trypanosomes	None
Pyruvate:ferrodoxin oxidoreductase	Anaerobic protozoa	Nitroimidazoles
Pyruvate phosphate dikinase	Anaerobic protozoa	None
Nucleoside phosphotransferase	Flagellated protozoa	Allopurinol riboside and formycin B
Trypanothione reductase and peroxidase	Kinetoplastida	Nifurtimox
Indispensable enzymes		
Lanosterol C-14α demethylase	Leishmania and *Trypanosoma cruzi*	Azoles, eg ketoconazole
Purine phosphoribosyl transferase	Protozoa	Allopurinol
Purine nucleoside kinase	*Trichomonas vaginalis* and *Entamoeba histolytica*	None
Ornithine decarboxylase	African trypanosomes	α-Difluoromethylornithine
(S)-Adenosylmethionine decarboxylase	African trypanosomes	Diamidines
Glycolytic enzymes	Kinetoplastida	Glycerol plus salicylhydroxamic acid and suramin
Common indispensable biochemical functions with different pharmacologic properties		
Dihydrofolate reductase-thymidylate synthase bifunctional enzyme	Apicomplexa and Kinetoplastida	Pyrimethamine
Thiamin transporter	Coccidia	Amprolium
Mitochondrial electron transporter	Apicomplexa	4-Hydroxyquinolines and 2-hydroxy-naphthoquinones
Microtubules	Helminth	Benzimidazoles
Nervous synaptic transmission	Helminth and ectoparasite	Levamisole, piperazine, milbemycins, and avermectins

tions by achieving the same result through alternative pathways. This discrepancy opens up opportunities for antiparasitic chemotherapy, although insufficiently selective inhibition of parasite enzymes remains an important safety concern.

INDISPENSABLE BIOCHEMICAL FUNCTIONS FOUND IN BOTH PARASITE & HOST BUT WITH DIFFERENT PHARMACOLOGIC PROPERTIES

In the parasite, these functions have differentiated sufficiently to become probable targets for antiparasitic chemotherapy, not because of the parasitic nature of the organism or its unique environment but, more likely, because of the long evolutionary distances separating the parasite and the host. It is thus difficult to discover these targets through studying metabolic deficiency or special nutritional requirements of the parasite. They have usually been found by investigating the modes of action of some well-established antiparasitic agents discovered by screening methods in the past. More recently, comparison of genome databases between the host and the parasite has become practical. The target may not be a single well-defined enzyme but may include transporters, receptors, cellular structural components, or other specific functions essential for survival of the parasite.

DRUGS WHOSE MECHANISMS HAVE NOT YET BEEN CONCLUSIVELY IDENTIFIED

In spite of considerable progress in defining the mechanisms of action of the drugs listed in Table 52–1, there are still wide gaps in our understanding of several other important antiparasitic agents. These include chloroquine and similar antimalarials, diethylcarbamazine, diloxanide, praziquantel, and others. From the biochemical activities that have been identified for them, it appears that many are capable of binding DNA, some can uncouple oxidative phosphorylation, and some inhibit protein synthesis. These types of activity, which are toxic to the host but could also be involved in the antiparasitic action, may have been preferentially detectable in random screenings routinely used for antiparasitic agents in the past.

REFERENCES

Aronov AM et al: Rational design of selective submicromolar inhibitors of *Tritrichomonas foetus* hypoxanthine-guanine-xanthine phosphoribosyltransferase. Biochemistry 2000;39:4684.

Aronov AM et al: Virtual screening of combinatorial libraries across a gene family, in search of inhibitors of *Giardia lamblia* guanine phosphoribosyltransferase. Antimicrob Agents Chemother 2001;45:2571.

Dan M, Wang AL, Wang CC: Inhibition of pyruvate-ferredoxin oxidoreductase gene expression in *Giardia lamblia* by virus-mediated hammerhead ribozyme. Mol Microbiol 2000; 36:447.

Munagala N, Wang CC: The pivotal role of guanine phosphoribosyltransferase in purine salvage by *Giardia lamblia*. Mol Microbiol 2002;44:1073.

Munagala N, Wang CC: The purine nucleoside phosphorylase from *Trichomonas vaginalis* is a homologue of the bacterial enzyme. Biochemistry 2002;41:10382.

Sarver AE, Wang CC: The adenine phosphoribosyltransferase from *Giardia lamblia* has a unique reaction mechanism and unusual substrate binding properties. J Biol Chem 2002; 277:39973.

Shi W et al: Closed-site complexes of adenine phosphoribosyltransferase from *Giardia lamblia* reveal a mechanism of ribosyl migration. J Biol Chem 2002;277:39981.

Vial HJ: Isoprenoid biosynthesis and drug targeting in the Apicomplexa. Parasitol Today 2000;16:140.

Antiprotozoal Drugs

Philip J. Rosenthal, MD

■ TREATMENT OF MALARIA

Four species of plasmodium cause human malaria: *Plasmodium falciparum, P vivax, P malariae,* and *P ovale.* Although all may cause significant illness, *P falciparum* is responsible for nearly all serious complications and deaths. Drug resistance is an important therapeutic problem, most notably with *P falciparum.*

PARASITE LIFE CYCLE

An anopheline mosquito inoculates plasmodium sporozoites to initiate human infection. Circulating sporozoites rapidly invade liver cells, and exoerythrocytic stage tissue schizonts mature in the liver. Merozoites are subsequently released from the liver and invade erythrocytes. Only erythrocytic parasites cause clinical illness. Repeated cycles of infection can lead to the infection of many erythrocytes and serious disease. Sexual stage gametocytes also develop in erythrocytes before being taken up by mosquitoes, where they develop into infective sporozoites.

In *P falciparum* and *P malariae* infection, only one cycle of liver cell invasion and multiplication occurs, and liver infection ceases spontaneously in less than 4 weeks. Thus, treatment that eliminates erythrocytic parasites will cure these infections. In *P vivax* and *P ovale* infections, a dormant hepatic stage, the hypnozoite, is not eradicated by most drugs, and subsequent relapses can therefore occur after therapy directed against erythrocytic parasites. Eradication of both erythrocytic and hepatic parasites is required to cure these infections.

DRUG CLASSIFICATION

Several classes of antimalarial drugs are available (Table 53–1; Figure 53–1). Drugs that eliminate developing or dormant liver forms are called **tissue schizonticides;** those that act on erythrocytic parasites are **blood schizonticides;** and those that kill sexual stages and prevent transmission to mosquitoes are **gametocides.** No one available agent can reliably effect a **radical cure,** ie, eliminate both hepatic and erythrocytic stages. Few available agents are **causal prophylactic drugs,** ie, capable of pre-

venting erythrocytic infection. However, all effective chemoprophylactic agents kill erythrocytic parasites before they increase sufficiently in number to cause clinical disease.

CHEMOPROPHYLAXIS & TREATMENT

When patients are counseled on the prevention of malaria, it is imperative to emphasize measures to prevent mosquito bites (insect repellents, insecticides, and bed nets), because parasites are increasingly resistant to multiple drugs and no chemoprophylactic regimen is fully protective. Current recommendations from the Centers for Disease Control and Prevention (CDC) include the use of chloroquine for chemoprophylaxis in the few areas infested by only chloroquine-sensitive malaria parasites (principally the Caribbean and Central America west of the Panama Canal), mefloquine or Malarone for most other malarious areas, and doxycycline for areas with a very high prevalence of multidrug-resistant falciparum malaria (principally border areas of Thailand) (Table 53–2). CDC recommendations should be checked regularly (Phone: 877-FYI-TRIP; Internet: www.cdc.gov/travel/), as these may change in response to changing resistance patterns and increasing experience with new drugs. In some circumstances, it may be appropriate for travelers to carry supplies of drugs with them in case they develop a febrile illness when medical attention is unavailable. Regimens for self-treatment should generally include either quinine or artemisinin derivatives. The latter, although not available in the USA, are widely available in other countries. Most authorities do not recommend routine terminal chemoprophylaxis with primaquine to eradicate dormant hepatic stages of *P vivax* and *P ovale* after travel, but this may be appropriate in some circumstances, especially for travelers with major exposure to these parasites.

Treatment of malaria that presents in the USA is straightforward (Table 53–3). Nonfalciparum infections and falciparum malaria from areas without known resistance should be treated with chloroquine. Vivax and ovale malaria should subsequently be treated with primaquine to eradicate liver forms. However, for *P vivax,* chloroquine-resistance is increasingly reported

Table 53–1. Major antimalarial drugs.

Drug	Class	Use
Chloroquine	4-Aminoquinoline	Treatment and chemoprophylaxis of infection with sensitive parasites
Amodiaquine[1]	4-Aminoquinoline	Treatment of infection with some chloroquine-resistant *P falciparum* strains
Quinine	Quinoline methanol	Oral treatment of infections with chloroquine-resistant *P falciparum*
Quinidine	Quinoline methanol	Intravenous therapy of severe infections with *P falciparum*
Mefloquine	Quinoline methanol	Chemoprophylaxis and treatment of infections with *P falciparum*
Primaquine	8-Aminoquinoline	Radical cure and terminal prophylaxis of infections with *P vivax* and *P ovale*
Sulfadoxine-pyrimethamine (Fansidar)	Folate antagonist combination	Treatment of infections with some chloroquine-resistant *P falciparum*
Atovaquone-proguanil (Malarone)	Quinone-folate antagonist combination	Treatment and chemoprophylaxis of *P falciparum* infection
Chlorproguanil-dapsone	Folate antagonist combination	Treatment of multidrug-resistant *P falciparum* in Africa
Proguanil[1]	Folate antagonist	Chemoprophylaxis (with chloroquine)
Doxycycline	Tetracycline	Treatment (with quinine) of infections with *P falciparum*; chemoprophylaxis
Halofantrine [1]	Phenanthrene methanol	Treatment of infections with some chloroquine-resistant *P falciparum*
Lumefantrine[1]	Amyl alcohol	Treatment of *P falciparum* malaria in fixed combination with artemether (Coartem)
Artemisinins[1]	Sesquiterpene lactone endoperoxides	Treatment of infection with multidrug-resistant *P falciparum*

[1]Not available in the USA.

and primaquine may fail to eradicate liver stages. Falciparum malaria from most areas is best treated with oral quinine or intravenous quinidine, in either case plus doxycycline or, for children, clindamycin. Other agents that are generally effective against resistant falciparum malaria include mefloquine and halofantrine, both of which have toxicity concerns at treatment dosages, and the artemisinin derivatives artesunate and artemether (alone or in combination, as discussed below).

CHLOROQUINE

Chloroquine has been the drug of choice for both treatment and chemoprophylaxis of malaria since the 1940s, but its utility against *P falciparum* has been seriously compromised by drug resistance. It remains the drug of choice in the treatment of sensitive *P falciparum* and other species of human malaria parasites.

Chemistry & Pharmacokinetics

Chloroquine is a synthetic 4-aminoquinoline (Figure 53–1) formulated as the phosphate salt for oral use. It is rapidly and almost completely absorbed from the gastrointestinal tract, reaches maximum plasma concentrations in about 3 hours, and is rapidly distributed to the tissues. It has a very large apparent volume of distribution of 100–1000 L/kg and is slowly released from tissues and metabolized. Chloroquine is principally excreted in the urine with an initial half-life of 3–5 days but a much longer terminal elimination half-life of 1–2 months.

Antimalarial Action & Resistance

A. ANTIMALARIAL ACTION

When not limited by resistance, chloroquine is a highly effective blood schizonticide. It is also moderately effective against gametocytes of *P vivax, P ovale,* and *P malariae* but not against those of *P falciparum.* Chloroquine is not active against liver stage parasites.

B. MECHANISM OF ACTION

The mechanism of action remains controversial. Chloroquine probably acts by concentrating in parasite food vacuoles, preventing the polymerization of the hemoglo-

4-AMINOQUINOLINES

Chloroquine

Amodiaquine

8-AMINOQUINOLINE

Primaquine

FOLATE ANTAGONISTS

Sulfadoxine

Pyrimethamine

Proguanil

QUINOLINE METHANOLS

Quinine

Mefloquine

PHENANTHRENE METHANOL

Halofantrine

QUINONE

Atovaquone

ENDOPEROXIDES

Artemisinins
(multiple structures)

Figure 53–1. Structural formulas of antimalarial drugs.

847

Table 53–2. Drugs for the prevention of malaria in travelers.[1]

Drug	Use[2]	Adult Dosage[3]
Chloroquine	Areas without resistant *P falciparum*	500 mg weekly
Malarone	Areas with multidrug-resistant *P falciparum*	1 tablet (250 mg atovaquone/100 mg proguanil) daily
Mefloquine	Areas with chloroquine-resistant *P falciparum*	250 mg weekly
Doxycycline	Areas with multidrug-resistant *P falciparum*	100 mg daily
Primaquine[4]	Terminal prophylaxis of *P vivax* and *P ovale* infections	26.3 mg (15 mg base) daily for 14 days after travel

[1]Recommendations may change, as resistance to all available drugs is increasing. See text for additional information on toxicities and cautions. For additional details and pediatric dosing, see CDC guidelines (phone: 877-FYI-TRIP; http://www.cdc.gov). Travelers to remote areas should consider carrying effective therapy (see text) for use if they develop a febrile illness and cannot reach medical attention quickly.
[2]Areas without known chloroquine-resistant *P falciparum* are Central America west of the Panama Canal, Haiti, Dominican Republic, Egypt, and most malarious countries of the Middle East. Malarone or mefloquine are currently recommended for other malarious areas except for border areas of Thailand, where doxycycline is recommended.
[3]For drugs other than primaquine, begin 1–2 weeks before departure (except 2 days before for doxycycline and Malarone) and continue for 4 weeks after leaving the endemic area (except 1 week for Malarone). All dosages refer to salts.
[4]Screen for G6PD deficiency before using primaquine.

Table 53–3. Treatment of malaria.

Clinical Setting	Drug Therapy[1]	Alternative Drugs
Chloroquine-sensitive *P falciparum* and *P malariae* infections	Chloroquine phosphate, 1 g, followed by 500 mg at 6, 24, and 48 hours –or– Chloroquine phosphate, 1 g at 0 and 24 hours, then 0.5 g at 48 hours	
P vivax and *P ovale* infections	Chloroquine (as above), then (if G6PD normal) primaquine, 26.3 mg daily for 14 days	
Uncomplicated infections with chloroquine-resistant *P falciparum*	Quinine sulfate, 650 mg 3 times daily for 3–7 days *plus one of the following–* Doxycycline, 100 mg twice daily for 7 days –or– Clindamycin, 600 mg twice daily for 7 days –or– Fansidar, three tablets once	Malarone, 4 tablets (total of 1 g atovaquone, 400 mg proguanil) daily for 3 days –or– Mefloquine, 15 mg/kg once or 750 mg, then 500 mg in 6–8 hours –or– Artesunate or artemether, single daily doses of 4 mg/kg on day 0, 2 mg/kg on days 2 and 3, 1 mg/kg on days 4–7 –or– Coartem (coartemether 20 mg, lumefantrine 120 mg), 4 tablets twice daily for 3 days
Severe or complicated infections with *P falciparum*[3]	Quinidine gluconate,[2,3] 10 mg/kg IV over 1–2 hours, then 0.02 mg/kg IV/min –or– 15 mg/kg IV over 4 hours, then 7.5 mg/kg IV over 4 hours every 8 hours	Artesunate,[3] 2.4 mg/kg IV or IM, then 1.2 mg/kg every 12 hours for 1 day, then every day –or– Artemether,[3] 3.2 mg/kg IM, then 1.6 mg/kg/d IM

[1]All dosages are oral and refer to salts unless otherwise indicated. See text for additional information on all agents, including toxicities and cautions. See CDC guidelines (phone: 877-FYI-TRIP; http://www.cdc.gov) for additional information and pediatric dosing.
[2]Cardiac monitoring should be in place during intravenous administration of quinidine.
[3]With all parenteral regimens, change to an oral regimen as soon as the patient can tolerate it.

bin breakdown product, heme, into hemozoin, and thus eliciting parasite toxicity due to the buildup of free heme.

C. RESISTANCE

Resistance to chloroquine is now very common among strains of *P falciparum* and uncommon but increasing for *P vivax*. In *P falciparum,* mutations in a putative transporter, PfCRT, have been correlated with resistance. Chloroquine resistance can be reversed by certain agents, including verapamil, desipramine, and chlorpheniramine, but the clinical value of resistance-reversing drugs is not established.

Clinical Uses

A. TREATMENT

Chloroquine is the drug of choice in the treatment of nonfalciparum and sensitive falciparum malaria. It rapidly terminates fever (in 24–48 hours) and clears parasitemia (in 48–72 hours) caused by sensitive parasites. It is also still used to treat falciparum malaria in many areas with widespread resistance, in particular much of Africa, owing to its safety and low cost and the fact that many partially immune individuals respond to treatment even when infecting parasites are partially resistant to chloroquine. However, other agents are preferred to treat potentially resistant falciparum malaria, especially in nonimmune individuals, and chloroquine is being replaced by other drugs as the standard therapy to treat falciparum malaria in most endemic countries. Chloroquine does not eliminate dormant liver forms of *P vivax* and *P ovale,* and for that reason primaquine must be added for the radical cure of these species.

B. CHEMOPROPHYLAXIS

Chloroquine is the preferred chemoprophylactic agent in malarious regions without resistant falciparum malaria. Eradication of *P vivax* and *P ovale* requires a course of primaquine to clear hepatic stages.

C. AMEBIC LIVER ABSCESS

Chloroquine reaches high liver concentrations and may be used for amebic abscesses that fail initial therapy with metronidazole (see below).

Adverse Effects

Chloroquine is usually very well tolerated, even with prolonged use. Pruritus is common, primarily in Africans. Nausea, vomiting, abdominal pain, headache, anorexia, malaise, blurring of vision, and urticaria are uncommon. Dosing after meals may reduce some adverse effects. Rare reactions include hemolysis in glucose-6-phosphate dehydrogenase (G6PD)-deficient persons, impaired hearing, confusion, psychosis, seizures, agranulocytosis, exfoliative

dermatitis, alopecia, bleaching of hair, hypotension, and electrocardiographic changes (QRS widening, T wave abnormalities). The long-term administration of high doses of chloroquine for rheumatologic diseases (see Chapter 36) can result in irreversible ototoxicity, retinopathy, myopathy, and peripheral neuropathy. These abnormalities are rarely if ever seen with standard-dose weekly chemoprophylaxis, even when given for prolonged periods. Large intramuscular injections or rapid intravenous infusions of chloroquine hydrochloride can result in severe hypotension and respiratory and cardiac arrest. Parenteral administration of chloroquine is best avoided, but if other drugs are not available for parenteral use, it should be infused slowly.

Contraindications & Cautions

Chloroquine is contraindicated in patients with psoriasis or porphyria, in whom it may precipitate acute attacks of these diseases. It should generally not be used in those with retinal or visual field abnormalities or myopathy. Chloroquine should be used with caution in patients with a history of liver disease or neurologic or hematologic disorders. The antidiarrheal agent kaolin and calcium- and magnesium-containing antacids interfere with the absorption of chloroquine and should not be coadministered with the drug. Chloroquine is considered safe in pregnancy and for young children.

AMODIAQUINE

Amodiaquine is closely related to chloroquine, and it probably shares mechanisms of action and resistance with that drug. Amodiaquine has been widely used to treat malaria because of its low cost, limited toxicity, and, in some areas, effectiveness against chloroquine-resistant strains of *P falciparum*. Important toxicities of amodiaquine, including agranulocytosis, aplastic anemia, and hepatotoxicity, have limited use of the drug in recent years. However, recent reevaluation has shown that serious toxicity from amodiaquine is rare, and some authorities now advocate its use as a replacement for chloroquine (especially in combination regimens) in areas with high rates of resistance but limited resources. The World Health Organization lists amodiaquine plus artesunate as a recommended therapy for falciparum malaria in areas with resistance to older drugs and amodiaquine plus sulfadoxine-pyrimethamine as an interim alternative if artemisinin-containing therapies are unavailable. Chemoprophylaxis with amodiaquine is best avoided because of its apparent increased toxicity with long-term use.

QUININE & QUINIDINE

Quinine and quinidine remain first-line therapies for falciparum malaria—especially severe disease—although toxicity may complicate therapy. Resistance to quinine is uncommon but increasing.

Chemistry & Pharmacokinetics

Quinine is derived from the bark of the cinchona tree, a traditional remedy for intermittent fevers from South America. The alkaloid quinine was purified from the bark in 1820, and it has been used in the treatment and prevention of malaria since that time. Quinidine, the dextrorotatory stereoisomer of quinine, is at least as effective as parenteral quinine in the treatment of severe falciparum malaria. After oral administration, quinine is rapidly absorbed, reaches peak plasma levels in 1–3 hours, and is widely distributed in body tissues. The use of a loading dose in severe malaria allows the achievement of peak levels within a few hours. The pharmacokinetics of quinine varies among populations. Individuals with malaria develop higher plasma levels of the drug than healthy controls, but toxicity is not increased, apparently because of increased protein binding. The half-life of quinine also is longer in those with severe malaria (18 hours) than in healthy controls (11 hours). Quinidine has a shorter half-life than quinine, mostly as a result of decreased protein binding. Quinine is primarily metabolized in the liver and excreted in the urine.

Antimalarial Action & Resistance

A. ANTIMALARIAL ACTION

Quinine is a rapidly acting, highly effective blood schizonticide against the four species of human malaria parasites. The drug is gametocidal against *P vivax* and *P ovale* but not *P falciparum*. It is not active against liver stage parasites. The mechanism of action of quinine is unknown.

B. RESISTANCE

Increasing in vitro resistance of parasites from a number of areas suggests that quinine resistance will be an increasing problem. Resistance to quinine is already common in some areas of Southeast Asia, especially border areas of Thailand, where the drug may fail if used alone to treat falciparum malaria. However, quinine still provides at least a partial therapeutic effect in most patients.

Clinical Uses

A. PARENTERAL TREATMENT OF SEVERE FALCIPARUM MALARIA

Quinine dihydrochloride or quinidine gluconate is the treatment of choice for severe falciparum malaria. Quinine can be administered slowly intravenously or, in a dilute solution, intramuscularly, but parenteral preparations of this drug are not available in the USA. Quinidine is now the standard therapy in the USA for the parenteral treatment of severe falciparum malaria. The drug can be administered in divided doses or by continuous intravenous infusion; treatment should begin with a loading dose to rapidly achieve effective plasma concentrations. Because of its cardiac toxicity and the relative unpredictability of its pharmacokinetics, intravenous quinidine should be administered with cardiac monitoring. Therapy should be changed to oral quinine as soon as the patient has improved and can tolerate oral medications.

B. ORAL TREATMENT OF FALCIPARUM MALARIA

Quinine sulfate is appropriate first-line therapy for uncomplicated falciparum malaria except when the infection was transmitted in an area without documented chloroquine-resistant malaria. Quinine is commonly used with a second drug (most often doxycycline or, in children, clindamycin) to shorten quinine's duration of use (usually to 3 days) and limit toxicity. Quinine is less effective than chloroquine against other human malarias and is more toxic, and it is therefore not used to treat infections with these parasites.

C. MALARIAL CHEMOPROPHYLAXIS

Quinine is not generally used in chemoprophylaxis owing to its toxicity, although a daily dose of 325 mg is effective.

D. BABESIOSIS

Quinine is first-line therapy, in combination with clindamycin, in the treatment of infection with *Babesia microti* or other human babesial infections.

Adverse Effects

Therapeutic dosages of quinine and quinidine commonly cause tinnitus, headache, nausea, dizziness, flushing, and visual disturbances, a constellation of symptoms termed **cinchonism.** Mild symptoms of cinchonism do not warrant the discontinuation of therapy. More severe findings, often after prolonged therapy, include more marked visual and auditory abnormalities, vomiting, diarrhea, and abdominal pain. Hypersensitivity reactions include skin rashes, urticaria, angioedema, and bronchospasm. Hematologic abnormalities include hemolysis (especially with G6PD deficiency), leukopenia, agranulocytosis, and thrombocytopenia. Therapeutic doses may cause hypoglycemia through stimulation of insulin release; this is a particular problem in severe infections and in pregnant patients, who have increased sensitivity to insulin. Quinine can stimulate uterine contractions, especially in the third trimester. However, this effect is mild, and quinine and quinidine remain the drugs of choice for severe falciparum malaria even during pregnancy. Intravenous infusions of the drugs may cause thrombophlebitis.

Severe hypotension can follow too-rapid intravenous infusions of quinine or quinidine. Electrocardiographic abnormalities (QT prolongation) are fairly common with intravenous quinidine, but dangerous arrhythmias are uncommon when the drug is administered appropriately in a monitored setting.

Blackwater fever is a rare severe illness that includes marked hemolysis and hemoglobinuria in the setting of quinine therapy for malaria. It appears to be due to a hypersensitivity reaction to the drug, though its pathogenesis is uncertain.

Contraindications & Cautions

Quinine (or quinidine) should be discontinued if signs of severe cinchonism, hemolysis, or hypersensitivity occur. It should be avoided if possible in patients with underlying visual or auditory problems. It must be used with great caution in those with underlying cardiac abnormalities. Quinine should not be given concurrently with mefloquine and should be used with caution in a patient with malaria who has previously received mefloquine chemoprophylaxis. Absorption may be blocked by aluminum-containing antacids. Quinine can raise plasma levels of warfarin and digoxin. Dosage must be reduced in renal insufficiency.

MEFLOQUINE

Mefloquine is effective therapy for many chloroquine-resistant strains of *P falciparum* and against other species. Although toxicity is a concern, mefloquine is one of the recommended chemoprophylactic drugs for use in most malaria-endemic regions with chloroquine-resistant strains.

Chemistry & Pharmacokinetics

Mefloquine hydrochloride is a synthetic 4-quinoline methanol that is chemically related to quinine. It can only be given orally because severe local irritation occurs with parenteral use. It is well absorbed, and peak plasma concentrations are reached in about 18 hours. Mefloquine is highly protein-bound, extensively distributed in tissues, and eliminated slowly, allowing a single-dose treatment regimen. The terminal elimination half-life is about 20 days, allowing weekly dosing for chemoprophylaxis. With weekly dosing, steady-state drug levels are reached over a number of weeks; this interval can be shortened to 4 days by beginning a course with three consecutive daily doses of 250 mg, though this is not standard practice. Mefloquine and acid metabolites of the drug are slowly excreted, mainly in the feces. The drug can be detected in the blood for months after the completion of therapy.

Antimalarial Action & Resistance

A. ANTIMALARIAL ACTION

Mefloquine has strong blood schizonticidal activity against *P falciparum* and *P vivax,* but it is not active against hepatic stages or gametocytes. The mechanism of action of mefloquine is unknown.

B. RESISTANCE

Sporadic resistance to mefloquine has been reported from many areas. At present, resistance appears to be uncommon except in regions of Southeast Asia with high rates of multidrug resistance (especially border areas of Thailand). Mefloquine resistance appears to be associated with resistance to quinine and halofantrine but not with resistance to chloroquine.

Clinical Uses

A. CHEMOPROPHYLAXIS

Mefloquine is effective in prophylaxis against most strains of *P falciparum* and probably all other human malarial species as well. Mefloquine is therefore among the drugs recommended by the CDC for chemoprophylaxis in all malarious areas except for those with no chloroquine resistance (where chloroquine is preferred) and some rural areas of Southeast Asia with a high prevalence of mefloquine resistance. As with chloroquine, eradication of *P vivax* and *P ovale* requires a course of primaquine.

B. TREATMENT

Mefloquine is effective in treating most falciparum malaria. The drug is not appropriate for treating individuals with severe or complicated malaria since quinine and quinidine are more rapidly active and drug resistance is less likely with those agents.

Adverse Effects

Weekly dosing with mefloquine for chemoprophylaxis may cause nausea, vomiting, dizziness, sleep and behavioral disturbances, epigastric pain, diarrhea, abdominal pain, headache, rash, and dizziness. Neuropsychiatric toxicities have received a good deal of publicity, but despite frequent anecdotal reports of seizures and psychosis, a number of controlled studies have found the frequency of serious adverse effects from mefloquine to be no higher than that with other common antimalarial chemoprophylactic regimens. Leukocytosis, thrombocytopenia, and aminotransferase elevations have been reported.

The adverse effects listed above are more common with the higher dosages required for treatment. These effects may be lessened by splitting administration of the drug into two doses separated by 6–8 hours. The incidence of neuropsychiatric symptoms appears to be about ten times more common than with chemoprophylactic dosing, with widely varying frequencies of up to about 50% being reported. Serious neuropsychiatric toxicities (depression, confusion, acute psychosis, or seizures) have been reported in less than one in 1000 treatments, but some authorities believe that these toxicities are actually more common. Mefloquine can also alter cardiac conduction, and arrhythmias and bradycardia have been reported.

Contraindications & Cautions

Mefloquine is contraindicated if there is a history of epilepsy, psychiatric disorders, arrhythmia, cardiac conduction defects, or sensitivity to related drugs. It should not be coadministered with quinine, quinidine, or halofantrine, and caution is required if quinine or quinidine is used to treat malaria after mefloquine chemoprophylaxis. Theoretical risks of mefloquine use must be balanced with the risk of contracting falciparum malaria. The CDC no longer advises against mefloquine use in patients receiving β-adrenoceptor antagonists. Mefloquine is also now considered safe in young children. Available data suggest that mefloquine use is safe throughout pregnancy, although experience in the first trimester is limited. An older recommendation to avoid mefloquine use in those requiring fine motor skills (eg, airline pilots) is controversial. Mefloquine chemoprophylaxis should be discontinued if significant neuropsychiatric symptoms develop.

PRIMAQUINE

Primaquine is the drug of choice for the eradication of dormant liver forms of *P vivax* and *P ovale*.

Chemistry & Pharmacokinetics

Primaquine phosphate is a synthetic 8-aminoquinoline (Figure 53–1). The drug is well absorbed orally, reaching peak plasma levels in 1–2 hours. The plasma half-life is 3–8 hours. Primaquine is widely distributed to the tissues, but only a small amount is bound there. It is rapidly metabolized and excreted in the urine. Its three major metabolites appear to have less antimalarial activity but more potential for inducing hemolysis than the parent compound.

Antimalarial Action & Resistance

A. ANTIMALARIAL ACTION

Primaquine is active against hepatic stages of all human malaria parasites. It is the only available agent active against the dormant hypnozoite stages of *P vivax* and *P ovale*. Primaquine is also gametocidal against the four

human malaria species. Primaquine acts against erythrocytic stage parasites, but this activity is too weak to play an important role. The mechanism of antimalarial action is unknown.

B. RESISTANCE

Some strains of *P vivax* in New Guinea, Southeast Asia, and perhaps Central and South America are relatively resistant to primaquine. Liver forms of these strains may not be eradicated by a single standard treatment with primaquine and may require repeated therapy with increased doses (eg, 30 mg base daily for 14 days) for radical cure.

Clinical Uses

A. THERAPY (RADICAL CURE) OF ACUTE VIVAX AND OVALE MALARIA

Standard therapy for these infections includes chloroquine to eradicate erythrocytic forms and primaquine to eradicate liver hypnozoites and prevent a subsequent relapse. Chloroquine is given acutely, and therapy with primaquine is withheld until the G6PD status of the patient is known. If the G6PD level is normal, a 14-day course of primaquine is given.

B. TERMINAL PROPHYLAXIS OF VIVAX AND OVALE MALARIA

Standard chemoprophylaxis does not prevent a relapse of vivax or ovale malaria, as the hypnozoite forms of these parasites are not eradicated by chloroquine or other available agents. To markedly diminish the likelihood of relapse, some authorities advocate the use of primaquine after the completion of travel to an endemic area.

C. CHEMOPROPHYLAXIS OF MALARIA

Primaquine has been studied as a daily chemoprophylactic agent. Daily treatment with 0.5 mg/kg of base provided good levels of protection against falciparum and vivax malaria. However, potential toxicities of long-term use remain a concern, and primaquine is not routinely recommended for this purpose.

D. GAMETOCIDAL ACTION

A single dose of primaquine (45 mg base) can be used as a control measure to render *P falciparum* gametocytes noninfective to mosquitoes. This therapy is of no clinical benefit to the patient but will disrupt transmission.

E. *PNEUMOCYSTIS JIROVECI* INFECTION

The combination of clindamycin and primaquine is an alternative regimen in the treatment of pneumocystosis, particularly mild to moderate disease. This regimen offers improved tolerance compared with high-dose trimethoprim-sulfamethoxazole or pentamidine, although its efficacy against severe pneumocystis pneumonia is not well studied. (See also page 854.)

Adverse Effects

Primaquine in recommended doses is generally well tolerated. It infrequently causes nausea, epigastric pain, abdominal cramps, and headache, and these symptoms are more common with higher dosages and when the drug is taken on an empty stomach. More serious but rare adverse effects include leukopenia, agranulocytosis, leukocytosis, and cardiac arrhythmias. Standard doses of primaquine may cause hemolysis or methemoglobinemia (manifested by cyanosis), especially in persons with G6PD deficiency or other hereditary metabolic defects.

Contraindications & Cautions

Primaquine should be avoided in patients with a history of granulocytopenia or methemoglobinemia, in those receiving potentially myelosuppressive drugs (eg, quinidine), and in those with disorders that commonly include myelosuppression. It is never given parenterally because it may induce marked hypotension.

Patients should be tested for G6PD deficiency before primaquine is prescribed. When a patient is deficient in G6PD, treatment strategies may consist of withholding therapy and treating subsequent relapses, if they occur, with chloroquine; treating patients with standard dosing, paying close attention to their hematologic status; or treating with weekly primaquine (45 mg base) for 8 weeks. G6PD-deficient individuals of Mediterranean and Asian ancestry are most likely to have severe deficiency, while those of African ancestry usually have a milder biochemical defect. This difference can be taken into consideration in choosing a treatment strategy. In any event, primaquine should be discontinued if there is evidence of hemolysis or anemia. Primaquine should be avoided in pregnancy because the fetus is relatively G6PD-deficient and thus at risk of hemolysis.

ATOVAQUONE

Atovaquone, a hydroxynaphthoquinone (Figure 53–1), was initially developed as an antimalarial and as a component of **Malarone** is recommended for prophylaxis (Table 53-2). It has also been approved by the Food and Drug Administration for the treatment of mild to moderate *P jiroveci* pneumonia.

The drug is only administered orally. Its bioavailability is low and erratic but absorption is increased by fatty food. The drug is heavily protein-bound and has a half-life of 2–3 days. Most of the drug is eliminated unchanged in the feces. The mechanism of action of atovaquone is uncertain. In plasmodia it appears to disrupt mitochondrial electron transport.

Initial use of atovaquone to treat malaria led to disappointing results, with frequent failures apparently due to the selection of resistant parasites during therapy. In contrast, Malarone, a fixed combination of atovaquone (250 mg) and proguanil (100 mg), is highly effective for both the treatment and chemoprophylaxis of falciparum malaria, and it is now approved for both indications in the USA. For chemoprophylaxis, Malarone must be taken daily (Table 53–2). It has an advantage over mefloquine and doxycycline in requiring shorter periods of treatment before and after the period at risk for malaria transmission, but it is more expensive than the other agents. It should be taken with food.

Atovaquone is an alternative therapy for *P jiroveci* infection, though its efficacy is lower than that of trimethoprim-sulfamethoxazole. Standard dosing is 750 mg taken with food three times daily for 21 days. Adverse effects include fever, rash, nausea, vomiting, diarrhea, headache, and insomnia. Serious adverse effects appear to be minimal, although experience with the drug remains limited. Atovaquone has also been effective in small numbers of immunocompromised patients with toxoplasmosis unresponsive to other agents, though its role in this disease is not yet defined.

Malarone is generally well tolerated. Adverse effects include abdominal pain, nausea, vomiting, diarrhea, headache, and rash, and these are more common with the higher dose required for treatment. Reversible elevations in liver enzymes have been reported. The safety of atovaquone in pregnancy is unknown. Plasma concentrations of atovaquone are decreased about 50% by coadministration of tetracycline or rifampin.

INHIBITORS OF FOLATE SYNTHESIS

Inhibitors of enzymes involved in folate metabolism are used, generally in combination regimens, in the treatment and prevention of malaria.

Chemistry & Pharmacokinetics

Pyrimethamine is a 2,4-diaminopyrimidine related to trimethoprim (see Chapter 46). **Proguanil** is a biguanide derivative (Figure 53–1). Both drugs are slowly but adequately absorbed from the gastrointestinal tract. Pyrimethamine reaches peak plasma levels 2–6 hours after an oral dose, is bound to plasma proteins, and has an elimination half-life of about 3.5 days. Proguanil reaches peak plasma levels about 5 hours after an oral dose and has an elimination half-life of about 16 hours. Therefore, proguanil must be administered daily for chemoprophylaxis, whereas pyrimethamine can be given once a week. Pyrimethamine is extensively metabolized before excretion. Proguanil is a prodrug; only its triazine metabolite, cycloguanil, is active. **Fansidar,** a fixed combination of the sulfonamide **sulfadoxine** (500 mg per tablet) and **pyrimethamine** (25 mg per tablet), is well absorbed. Its components display peak plasma levels within 2–8 hours and are excreted mainly by the kidneys. The average half-life of sulfadoxine is about 170 hours.

Antimalarial Action & Resistance

A. ANTIMALARIAL ACTION

Pyrimethamine and proguanil act slowly against erythrocytic forms of susceptible strains of all four human malaria species. Proguanil also has some activity against hepatic forms. Neither drug is adequately gametocidal or effective against the persistent liver stages of *P vivax* or *P ovale*. Sulfonamides and sulfones are weakly active against erythrocytic schizonts but not against liver stages or gametocytes. They are not used alone as antimalarials but are effective in combination with other agents.

B. MECHANISM OF ACTION

Pyrimethamine and proguanil selectively inhibit plasmodial dihydrofolate reductase, a key enzyme in the pathway for synthesis of folate. Sulfonamides and sulfones inhibit another enzyme in the folate pathway, dihydropteroate synthase. As described in Chapter 46 and shown in Figure 46–2, combinations of inhibitors of these two enzymes provide synergistic activity.

C. RESISTANCE

In many areas, resistance to folate antagonists and sulfonamides is common for *P falciparum* and less common for *P vivax*. Resistance is due primarily to mutations in dihydrofolate reductase and dihydropteroate synthase. Because different mutations may mediate resistance to different agents, cross-resistance is not uniformly seen.

Clinical Uses

A. CHEMOPROPHYLAXIS

Chemoprophylaxis with single folate antagonists is no longer recommended because of frequent resistance, but a number of agents are used in combination regimens. The combination of chloroquine (500 mg weekly) and proguanil (200 mg daily) is used as an alternative to mefloquine. This combination has lower efficacy—but also probably less toxicity—than mefloquine. It is anticipated that the efficacy of the combination will continue to decrease as resistance to both chloroquine and proguanil increases. Fansidar and Maloprim (the latter is a combination of pyrimethamine and the sulfone dapsone) are both effective against sensitive parasites with weekly dosing, but they are no longer recommended because of resistance and toxicity.

B. TREATMENT OF CHLOROQUINE-RESISTANT FALCIPARUM MALARIA

Fansidar is commonly used to treat uncomplicated falciparum malaria and it is first-line therapy for this indication in some tropical countries. Advantages of Fansidar in the developing world are relatively low rates of drug resistance and toxicity, ease of administration (a single oral dose), and low cost. However, rates of resistance are increasing. Fansidar is a less optimal regimen than quinine when both drugs are available, especially for nonimmune individuals. It should not be used for severe malaria, as it is slower-acting than other available agents. Fansidar can also be used as an adjunct to quinine therapy to shorten the course of quinine and limit toxicity. Fansidar is not reliably effective in vivax malaria, and its usefulness against *P ovale* and *P malariae* has not been adequately studied. A new antifolate-sulfone combination, chlorproguanil-dapsone, is now available in some countries for the treatment of uncomplicated falciparum malaria in Africa. Chlorproguanil-dapsone is highly effective in regions with fairly high levels of resistance to Fansidar, and its shorter half-life may limit the selection of resistant parasites.

C. PRESUMPTIVE TREATMENT OF FALCIPARUM MALARIA

Fansidar is also used as presumptive therapy for travelers who develop fever while traveling in malaria-endemic regions and who are unable to obtain medical evaluation. Ideally, such patients obtain medical attention as soon as possible after the initiation of therapy to verify the diagnosis and develop an optimal treatment plan. This strategy is increasingly questionable as resistance to Fansidar increases. Alternative presumptive regimens are quinine and mefloquine, which are more toxic but less likely to fail due to drug resistance, or the artemisinin analogs artesunate and artemether, which are not available in the USA.

D. TOXOPLASMOSIS

Pyrimethamine, in combination with sulfadiazine, is first-line therapy in the treatment of toxoplasmosis, including acute infection, congenital infection, and disease in immunocompromised patients. For immunocompromised patients, high-dose therapy is required followed by chronic suppressive therapy. Folinic acid is included to limit myelosuppression. Toxicity from the combination is usually due primarily to sulfadiazine. The replacement of sulfadiazine with clindamycin provides an effective alternative regimen.

E. PNEUMOCYSTOSIS

Pneumocystis jiroveci is the cause of human pneumocystosis and is now recognized to be a fungus, but this organism is discussed in this chapter because it responds to antiprotozoal drugs, not antifungals. (The related species *P carinii* is now recognized to be the cause of animal infections.) First-line therapy of pneumocystosis is trimethoprim plus sulfamethoxazole (see also Chapter 46). Standard treatment includes high-dose intravenous (15–20 mg trimethoprim and 75–100 mg sulfamethoxazole per day in three or four divided doses) or oral (two double-strength tablets every 8 hours) therapy for 21 days. High-dose therapy entails significant toxicity, especially in patients with AIDS. Important toxicities include nausea, vomiting, fever, rash, leukopenia, hyponatremia, elevated hepatic enzymes, azotemia, anemia, and thrombocytopenia. Less common effects include severe skin reactions, mental status changes, pancreatitis, and hypocalcemia. Trimethoprim-sulfamethoxazole is also the standard chemoprophylactic drug for the prevention of *P jiroveci* infection in immunocompromised individuals. Dosing is one double-strength tablet daily or three times per week. The chemoprophylactic dosing schedule is much better tolerated than high-dose therapy in immunocompromised patients, but rash, fever, leukopenia, or hepatitis may necessitate changing to another drug.

Adverse Effects & Cautions

Most patients tolerate pyrimethamine and proguanil well. Gastrointestinal symptoms, skin rashes, and itching are rare. Mouth ulcers and alopecia have been described with proguanil. Fansidar is no longer recommended for chemoprophylaxis because of uncommon but severe cutaneous reactions, including erythema multiforme, Stevens-Johnson syndrome, and toxic epidermal necrolysis. Severe reactions appear to be much less common with single-dose therapy, and use of the drug is justified by the risks associated with falciparum malaria. Rare adverse effects with a single dose of Fansidar are those associated with other sulfonamides, including hematologic, gastrointestinal, central nervous system, dermatologic, and renal toxicity. Maloprim is no longer recommended for chemoprophylaxis because of unacceptably high rates of agranulocytosis. Folate antagonists should be used cautiously in the presence of renal or hepatic dysfunction. Although pyrimethamine is teratogenic in animals, Fansidar has been safely used in pregnancy for therapy and as an intermittent chemoprophylactic regimen to improve pregnancy outcomes. Proguanil is considered safe in pregnancy. With the use of any folate antagonist in pregnancy, folate supplements should be coadministered.

ANTIBIOTICS

A number of antibiotics in addition to the folate antagonists and sulfonamides are modestly active antimalarials. The mechanisms of action of these drugs are unclear. They may inhibit protein synthesis or other functions in two plasmodial prokaryote-like organelles, the mitochondrion and the apicoplast. None of the antibiotics should be used as single agents in the treatment of malaria because their action is much slower than those of standard antimalarials.

Tetracycline and doxycycline (see Chapter 44) are active against erythrocytic schizonts of all human malaria parasites. They are not active against liver stages. Doxycycline is commonly used in the treatment of falciparum malaria in conjunction with quinidine or quinine, allowing a shorter and better-tolerated course of quinine. Doxycycline has also become a standard chemoprophylactic drug, especially for use in areas of Southeast Asia with high rates of resistance to other antimalarials, including mefloquine. Doxycycline side effects include infrequent gastrointestinal symptoms, candidal vaginitis, and photosensitivity. Its safety in long-term chemoprophylaxis has not been extensively evaluated.

Clindamycin (see Chapter 44) is slowly active against erythrocytic schizonts and can be used in conjunction with quinine or quinidine in those for whom doxycycline is not recommended, such as children and pregnant women. Azithromycin (see Chapter 44) also has antimalarial activity and is now under study as an alternative chemoprophylactic drug. Antimalarial activity of fluoroquinolones has been demonstrated, but efficacy for the therapy or chemoprophylaxis of malaria has been suboptimal.

Antibiotics also are active against other protozoans. Tetracycline and erythromycin are alternative therapies for the treatment of intestinal amebiasis. Clindamycin, in combination with other agents, is effective therapy for toxoplasmosis, pneumocystosis, and babesiosis. Spiramycin is a macrolide antibiotic that is used to treat primary toxoplasmosis acquired during pregnancy. Treatment lowers the risk of the development of congenital toxoplasmosis.

HALOFANTRINE & LUMEFANTRINE

Halofantrine hydrochloride, a phenanthrene-methanol related to quinine, is effective against erythrocytic (but not other) stages of all four human malaria species. Oral absorption is variable and is enhanced with food. Because of toxicity concerns, it should not be taken with meals. Plasma levels peak 16 hours after dosing, and the half-life is about 4 days. Excretion is mainly in the feces. The mechanism of action of halofantrine is unknown. The drug is not available in the USA (although it has been approved by the FDA), but it is widely available in malaria-endemic countries.

Halofantrine is rapidly effective against most chloroquine-resistant strains of *P falciparum,* but its use is limited by irregular absorption and cardiac toxicity. Cross-resistance with mefloquine may occur. As treatment for falciparum malaria, halofantrine is given orally in three 500 mg doses at 6-hour intervals, and this course is best repeated in 1 week for nonimmune individuals. Because of toxicity concerns and irregular absorption, halofantrine should not be used for chemoprophylaxis.

Halofantrine is generally well tolerated. The most common adverse effects are abdominal pain, diarrhea, vomiting, cough, rash, headache, pruritus, and elevated liver enzymes. Of greater concern, the drug alters cardiac conduction, with dose-related prolongation of QT and PR intervals. This effect is seen with standard doses and is worsened by prior mefloquine therapy. Rare instances of dangerous arrhythmias and some deaths have been reported. The drug is contraindicated in patients with cardiac conduction defects and should not be used in those who have recently taken mefloquine. The drug is embryotoxic in animal studies and is therefore contraindicated in pregnancy.

Lumefantrine, an aryl alcohol related to halofantrine, is available as a fixed-dose combination with artemether as Coartem in some countries. The half-life of lumefantrine, when used in combination, is 4.5 hours. As with halofantrine, oral absorption is highly variable and improved when the drug is taken with food. Coartem is highly effective in the treatment of falciparum malaria, but it is expensive and requires twice-daily dosing. Despite these limitations, due to its reliable efficacy against falciparum malaria, Coartem has recently been selected as the first-line therapy for malaria in many African countries, although implementation of this change has been slow. Coartem does not appear to cause the cardiac toxicity seen with halofantrine.

ARTEMISININ & ITS DERIVATIVES

Artemisinin (**qinghaosu**) is a sesquiterpene lactone endoperoxide, the active component of an herbal medicine that has been used as an antipyretic in China for over 2000 years. Artemisinin is insoluble and can only be used orally. Analogs have been synthesized to increase solubility and improve antimalarial efficacy. The most important of these analogs are **artesunate** (water-soluble; useful for oral, intravenous, intramuscular, and rectal administration) and **artemether** (lipid-soluble; useful for oral, intramuscular, and rectal administration). Artemisinin and its analogs are rapidly absorbed, with peak plasma levels occurring in 1–2 hours and half-lives of 1–3 hours after oral administration. The compounds are rapidly metabolized to the active metabolite dihydroartemisinin. Drug levels appear to decrease after a number of days of therapy. Dihydroartemisinin is also available as a drug and is under study as combination chemotherapy with piperaquine, a quinoline related to chloro-

quine. None of the artemisinins are available in the USA, but artemether and artesunate are widely available in other countries.

Artemisinin and analogs are very rapidly acting blood schizonticides against all human malaria parasites. Artemisinins have no effect on hepatic stages. Artemisinin resistance is not yet an important problem, but *P falciparum* isolates with diminished in vitro susceptibility to artemether have recently been described. The antimalarial activity of artemisinins may result from the production of free radicals that follows the iron-catalyzed cleavage of the artemisinin endoperoxide bridge in the parasite food vacuole or from inhibition of a parasite calcium ATPase.

Artemisinins—in particular artesunate and artemether—are playing an increasingly important role in the treatment of multidrug-resistant *P falciparum* malaria. They are the only drugs reliably effective against quinine-resistant strains. The efficacy of the artemisinins is limited somewhat by their short plasma half-lives. Recrudescence rates are unacceptably high after short-course therapy, and these drugs are generally best used in conjunction with another agent. Also because of their short-half lives, they are not useful in chemoprophylaxis. In several studies of severe malaria, artemether and artesunate were about as effective as quinine, though mortality from severe malaria remained high. Artesunate has also been effective in the treatment of severe malaria when administered rectally, offering a valuable treatment modality when parenteral therapy is not available.

Artesunate is widely available—although quite expensive—for the treatment of uncomplicated and severe falciparum malaria. It is commonly used in combination with mefloquine to treat highly resistant falciparum malaria in Thailand. Artemether is available alone and as a fixed-dose combination with lumefantrine (see above). In the setting of multidrug resistance, many authorities now advocate combination therapy with an artemisinin as the optimal treatment for falciparum malaria, and current World Health Organization recommendations list artemether plus lumefantrine, artesunate plus amodiaquine, artesunate plus mefloquine, and artesunate plus sulfadoxine plus pyrimethamine as optimal therapies for uncomplicated malaria in regions with resistance to older drugs. However, concerns regarding high cost, limited availability, and potential toxicity remain.

Artemisinins appear to be better tolerated than most antimalarials. The most commonly reported adverse effects have been nausea, vomiting, and diarrhea. Irreversible neurotoxicity has been seen in animals, but only after doses much higher than those used to treat malaria. Artemisinins should be avoided in pregnancy if possible because teratogenicity has been seen in animal studies, but limited inadvertent use in pregnancy has apparently not led to fetal problems.

■ TREATMENT OF AMEBIASIS

Amebiasis is infection with *Entamoeba histolytica*. This organism can cause asymptomatic intestinal infection, mild to moderate colitis, severe intestinal infection (dysentery), ameboma, liver abscess, and other extraintestinal infections. The choice of drugs for amebiasis depends on the clinical presentation (Figure 53–2; Table 53–4).

Treatment of Specific Forms of Amebiasis

A. ASYMPTOMATIC INTESTINAL INFECTION

Asymptomatic carriers generally are not treated in endemic areas but in nonendemic areas they are treated with a luminal amebicide. A tissue amebicidal drug is unnecessary. Standard luminal amebicides are diloxanide furoate, iodoquinol, and paromomycin. Each drug eradicates carriage in about 80–90% of patients

with a single course of treatment. Therapy with a luminal amebicide is also required in the treatment of all other forms of amebiasis.

B. AMEBIC COLITIS

Metronidazole plus a luminal amebicide is the treatment of choice for colitis and dysentery. Tetracyclines and erythromycin are alternative drugs for moderate colitis but are not effective against extraintestinal disease. Dehydroemetine or emetine can also be used, but are best avoided because of toxicity.

C. EXTRAINTESTINAL INFECTIONS

The treatment of choice is metronidazole plus a luminal amebicide. A 10-day course of metronidazole cures over 95% of uncomplicated liver abscesses. For unusual cases in which initial therapy with metronidazole has failed, aspiration of the abscess and the addition of chloroquine to a repeat course of metronidazole should be considered. Dehydroemetine and emetine are toxic alternative drugs.

Figure 53–2. Structural formulas of other antiprotozoal drugs.

Table 53–4. Treatment of amebiasis.[1]

Clinical Setting	Drugs of Choice and Adult Dosage	Alternative Drugs and Adult Dosage
Asymptomatic intestinal infection	Luminal agent: Diloxanide furoate,[2] 500 mg 3 times daily for 10 days *or*– Iodoquinol, 650 mg 3 times daily for 21 days *or*– Paromomycin, 10 mg/kg 3 times daily for 7 days	
Mild to moderate intestinal infection	Metronidazole, 750 mg 3 times daily (or 500 mg IV every 6 hours) for 10 days *or*– Tinidazole, 2 g daily for 3 days *plus*– Luminal agent (see above)	Luminal agent (see above) *plus either*– Tetracycline, 250 mg 3 times daily for 10 days *or*– Erythromycin, 500 mg 4 times daily for 10 days
Severe intestinal infection	Metronidazole, 750 mg 3 times daily (or 500 mg IV every 6 hours) for 10 days *or*– Tinidazole, 2 g daily for 3 days *plus*– Luminal agent (see above)	Luminal agent (see above) *plus either*– Tetracycline, 250 mg 3 times daily for 10 days *or*– Dehydroemetine[3] or emetine,[2] 1 mg/kg SC or IM for 3–5 days
Hepatic abscess, ameboma, and other extraintestinal disease	Metronidazole, 750 mg 3 times daily (or 500 mg IV every 6 hours) for 10 days *or*– Tinidazole, 2 g daily for 5 days *plus*– Luminal agent (see above)	Dehydroemetine[3] or emetine,[2] 1 mg/kg SC or IM for 8–10 days, followed by (liver abscess only) chloroquine, 500 mg twice daily for 2 days, then 500 mg daily for 21 days *plus*– Luminal agent (see above)

[1]Route is oral unless otherwise indicated. See text for additional details and cautions.
[2]Not available in the USA.
[3]Available in the USA only from the Drug Service, CDC, Atlanta (404-639-3670).

METRONIDAZOLE & TINIDAZOLE

Metronidazole, a nitroimidazole (Figure 53–2), is the drug of choice in the treatment of extraluminal amebiasis. It kills trophozoites but not cysts of *E histolytica* and effectively eradicates intestinal and extraintestinal tissue infections. Tinidazole, a related nitroimidazole, appears to have similar activity and a better toxicity profile than metronidazole, and it offers simpler dosing regimens. It has been available in the USA since 2004 and can be substituted for the indications listed below.

Chemistry & Pharmacokinetics

Oral metronidazole and tinidazole are readily absorbed and permeate all tissues by simple diffusion. Intracellular concentrations rapidly approach extracellular levels. Peak plasma concentrations are reached in 1–3 hours. Protein binding of both drugs is low (10–20%); the half-life of unchanged drug is 7.5 hours for metronidazole and 12–14 hours for tinidazole. Metronidazole and

its metabolites are excreted mainly in the urine. Plasma clearance of metronidazole is decreased in patients with impaired liver function.

Mechanism of Action

The nitro group of metronidazole is chemically reduced in anaerobic bacteria and sensitive protozoans. Reactive reduction products appear to be responsible for antimicrobial activity. The mechanism of tinidazole is assumed to be the same.

Clinical Uses

A. AMEBIASIS

Metronidazole or tinidazole is the drug of choice in the treatment of all tissue infections with *E histolytica*. They are not reliably effective against luminal parasites and so must be used with a luminal amebicide to ensure eradication of the infection.

B. Giardiasis

Metronidazole is the treatment of choice for giardiasis. The dosage for giardiasis is much lower—and the drug thus better tolerated—than that for amebiasis. Efficacy after a single treatment is about 90%. Tinidazole is at least equally effective.

C. Trichomoniasis

Metronidazole is the treatment of choice. A single dose of 2 g is effective. Metronidazole-resistant organisms can lead to treatment failures. Tinidazole may be effective against some of these resistant organisms.

Adverse Effects & Cautions

Nausea, headache, dry mouth, or a metallic taste in the mouth occurs commonly. Infrequent adverse effects include vomiting, diarrhea, insomnia, weakness, dizziness, thrush, rash, dysuria, dark urine, vertigo, paresthesias, and neutropenia. Taking the drug with meals lessens gastrointestinal irritation. Pancreatitis and severe central nervous system toxicity (ataxia, encephalopathy, seizures) are rare. Metronidazole has a disulfiram-like effect, so that nausea and vomiting can occur if alcohol is ingested during therapy. The drug should be used with caution in patients with central nervous system disease. Intravenous infusions have rarely caused seizures or peripheral neuropathy. The dosage should be adjusted for patients with severe liver or renal disease. Tinidazole has a similar adverse effect profile, although it appears to be somewhat better tolerated than metronidazole.

Metronidazole has been reported to potentiate the anticoagulant effect of coumarin-type anticoagulants. Phenytoin and phenobarbital may accelerate elimination of the drug, while cimetidine may decrease plasma clearance. Lithium toxicity may occur when the drug is used with metronidazole.

Metronidazole and its metabolites are mutagenic in bacteria. Chronic administration of large doses led to tumorigenicity in mice. Data on teratogenicity are inconsistent. Metronidazole is thus best avoided in pregnant or nursing women, although congenital abnormalities have not clearly been associated with use in humans.

IODOQUINOL

Iodoquinol (diiodohydroxyquin) is a halogenated hydroxyquinoline. It is an effective luminal amebicide that is commonly used with metronidazole to treat amebic infections. Its pharmacokinetic properties are poorly understood. Ninety percent of the drug is retained in the intestine and excreted in the feces. The remainder enters the circulation, has a half-life of 11–14 hours, and is excreted in the urine as glucuronides.

The mechanism of action of iodoquinol against trophozoites is unknown. It is effective against organisms in the bowel lumen but not against trophozoites in the intestinal wall or extraintestinal tissues.

Infrequent adverse effects include diarrhea—which usually stops after several days—anorexia, nausea, vomiting, abdominal pain, headache, rash, and pruritus. The drug may increase protein-bound serum iodine, leading to a decrease in measured ^{131}I uptake that persists for months. Some halogenated hydroxyquinolines can produce severe neurotoxicity with prolonged use at greater than recommended doses. Iodoquinol is not known to produce these effects at its recommended dosage, and this dosage should never be exceeded.

Iodoquinol should be taken with meals to limit gastrointestinal toxicity. It should be used with caution in patients with optic neuropathy, renal or thyroid disease, or nonamebic hepatic disease. The drug should be discontinued if it produces persistent diarrhea or signs of iodine toxicity (dermatitis, urticaria, pruritus, fever). It is contraindicated in patients with intolerance to iodine.

DILOXANIDE FUROATE

Diloxanide furoate is a dichloroacetamide derivative. It is an effective luminal amebicide but is not active against tissue trophozoites. In the gut, diloxanide furoate is split into diloxanide and furoic acid; about 90% of the diloxanide is rapidly absorbed and then conjugated to form the glucuronide, which is promptly excreted in the urine. The unabsorbed diloxanide is the active antiamebic substance. The mechanism of action of diloxanide furoate is unknown.

Diloxanide furoate is considered by many the drug of choice for asymptomatic luminal infections, but it is no longer available in the USA. It is used with a tissue amebicide, usually metronidazole, to treat serious intestinal and extraintestinal infections. Diloxanide furoate does not produce serious adverse effects. Flatulence is common, but nausea and abdominal cramps are infrequent and rashes are rare. The drug is not recommended in pregnancy.

PAROMOMYCIN SULFATE

Paromomycin sulfate is an aminoglycoside antibiotic (see also Chapter 45) that is not significantly absorbed from the gastrointestinal tract. It is used only as a luminal amebicide and has no effect against extraintestinal amebic infections. The small amount absorbed is slowly excreted unchanged, mainly by glomerular filtration. However, the drug may accumulate with renal insufficiency and contribute to renal toxicity. Paromomycin is an effective luminal amebicide that appears to have similar efficacy and probably less toxicity than other agents; in a recent study, it was superior to diloxanide furoate in clearing asymptomatic infections. Adverse effects include occasional abdominal distress and diarrhea. Paromomycin should be avoided in patients with significant renal disease and used with caution in persons with gastrointestinal ulcerations. Parenteral paromomycin is under investigation in the treatment of visceral leishmaniasis.

EMETINE & DEHYDROEMETINE

Emetine, an alkaloid derived from ipecac, and dehydroemetine, a synthetic analog, are effective against tissue trophozoites of *E histolytica,* but because of major toxicity concerns they have been almost completely replaced by metronidazole.

Their use is limited to unusual circumstances in which severe amebiasis warrants effective therapy and metronidazole cannot be used. Dehydroemetine is preferred because of its somewhat better toxicity profile. The drugs should be used for the minimum period needed to relieve severe symptoms (usually 3–5 days).

Emetine and dehydroemetine should be administered subcutaneously (preferred) or intramuscularly (but never intravenously) in a supervised setting. Adverse effects are generally mild when the drugs are used for 3–5 days but increase with prolonged use. Pain and tenderness in the area of injection are frequent, and sterile abscesses may develop. Diarrhea is common. Other adverse effects are nausea, vomiting, muscle weakness and discomfort, and minor electrocardiographic changes. Serious toxicities include cardiac arrhythmias, heart failure, and hypotension. The drugs should not be used in patients with cardiac or renal disease, in young children, or in pregnancy unless absolutely necessary.

■ OTHER ANTIPROTOZOAL DRUGS

See Table 53–5 for a list of drugs used in the treatment of other protozoal infections. Important drugs that are not covered elsewhere in this or other chapters are discussed below.

PENTAMIDINE

Pentamidine has activity against trypanosomatid protozoans and against *P jiroveci,* but toxicity is significant.

Chemistry & Pharmacokinetics

Pentamidine is an aromatic diamidine (Figure 53–2) formulated as an isethionate salt. Pentamidine is only administered parenterally. The drug leaves the circulation rapidly, with an initial half-life of about 6 hours, but it is bound avidly by tissues. Pentamidine thus accumulates and is eliminated very slowly, with a terminal elimination half-life of about 12 days. The drug can be detected in urine 6 or more weeks after treatment. Only trace amounts of pentamidine appear in the central nervous system, so it is not effective against central nervous system African trypanosomiasis. Pentamidine can also be inhaled as a nebulized powder for the prevention of pneumocystosis. Absorption into the systemic circulation after inhalation appears to be minimal. The mechanism of action of pentamidine is unknown.

Clinical Uses

A. PNEUMOCYSTOSIS

Pentamidine is a well-established alternative therapy for pulmonary and extrapulmonary disease caused by *P jiroveci.* The drug has somewhat lower efficacy and greater toxicity than trimethoprim-sulfamethoxazole. The standard dosage is 3 mg/kg/d intravenously for 21 days. Significant adverse reactions are common, and with multiple regimens now available to treat *P jiroveci* infection, pentamidine is best reserved for patients with severe disease who cannot tolerate or fail other drugs.

Pentamidine is also an alternative agent for primary or secondary prophylaxis against pneumocystosis in immunocompromised individuals, including patients with advanced AIDS. For this indication, pentamidine is administered as an inhaled aerosol (300 mg inhaled monthly). The drug is well-tolerated in this form. Its efficacy is very good but clearly less than that of daily trimethoprim-sulfamethoxazole. Because of its cost and ineffectiveness against nonpulmonary disease, it is best reserved for patients who cannot tolerate oral chemoprophylaxis with other drugs.

B. AFRICAN TRYPANOSOMIASIS (SLEEPING SICKNESS)

Pentamidine has been used since 1940 as an alternative to suramin for the early hemolymphatic stage of disease caused by *Trypanosoma brucei* (especially *T brucei gambiense*). The drug can also be used with suramin. Pentamidine should not be used to treat late trypanosomiasis with central nervous system involvement. A number of dosing regimens have been described, generally providing 2–4 mg/kg daily or on alternate days for a total of 10–15 doses. Pentamidine has also been used for chemoprophylaxis against African trypanosomiasis, with dosing of 4 mg/kg every 3–6 months.

C. LEISHMANIASIS

Pentamidine is an alternative to sodium stibogluconate in the treatment of visceral leishmaniasis, although

Table 53–5. Treatment of other protozoal infections.

Organism or Clinical Setting	Drugs of Choice[1]	Alternative Drugs
Babesia species	Clindamycin, 600 mg 3 times daily for 7 days *plus–* Quinine, 650 mg for 7 days	Atovaquone *or* azithromycin
Balantidium coli	Tetracycline, 500 mg 4 times daily for 10 days	Metronidazole, 750 mg 3 times daily for 5 days
Cryptosporidium species	Paromomycin, 500–750 mg 3 or 4 times daily for 10 days	Azithromycin, 500 mg daily for 21 days
Cyclospora cayetanensis	Trimethoprim-sulfamethoxazole, one double-strength tablet 4 times daily for 7–14 days	
Dientamoeba fragilis	Iodoquinol, 650 mg 3 times daily for 20 days	Tetracycline, 500 mg 4 times daily for 10 days *or–* Paromomycin, 500 mg 3 times daily for 7 days
Giardia lamblia	Metronidazole, 250 mg 3 times daily for 5 days *or–* Tinidazole, 2 g once	Furazolidone, 100 mg 4 times daily for 7 days *or–* Albendazole, 400 mg daily for 5 days
Isospora belli	Trimethoprim-sulfamethoxazole, one double-strength tablet 4 times daily for 10 days, then twice daily for 21 days	Pyrimethamine, 75 mg daily for 14 days *plus–* Folinic acid, 10 mg daily for 14 days
Microsporidia	Albendazole, 400 mg twice daily for 20–30 days	
Leishmaniasis Visceral (*L donovani*, *L chagasi*, *L infantum*) or mucosal (*L braziliensis*)	Sodium stibogluconate,[2] 20 mg/kg/d IV or IM for 28 days	Meglumine antimonate[3] *or–* Pentamidine *or–* Amphotericin B *or–* Miltefosine [3]
Cutaneous (*L major*, *L tropica*, *L mexicana*, *L braziliensis*)	Sodium stibogluconate,[2] 20 mg/kg/d IV or IM for 20 days	Meglumine antimonate[2] *or–* Ketoconazole *or–* Pentamidine *or–* Topical or intralesional therapies
Pneumocystis jiroveci, *P carinii*[4]	Trimethoprim-sulfamethoxazole, 15–20 mg trimethoprim component/kg/d IV, or two double-strength tablets every 8 hours for 21 days	Pentamidine *or–* Trimethoprim-dapsone *or–* Clindamycin *plus* primaquine *or–* Atovaquone
Toxoplasma gondii Acute, congenital, immunocompromised	Pyrimethamine *plus* clindamycin *plus* folinic acid	Pyrimethamine *plus* sulfadiazine *plus* folinic acid
Pregnancy	Spiramycin, 3 g daily until delivery	

(*continued*)

Table 53–5. Treatment of other protozoal infections. (continued)

Organism or Clinical Setting	Drugs of Choice[1]	Alternative Drugs
Trichomonas vaginalis	Metronidazole, 2 g once or 250 mg 3 times daily for 7 days *or–* Tinidazole, 2 g once	
Trypanosoma brucei Hemolymphatic	Suramin [2]	Pentamidine *or–* Eflornithine
Advanced CNS disease	Melarsoprol[2]	Eflornithine
Trypanosoma cruzi	Nifurtimox [2] *or–* Benznidizole[3]	

[1]Established, relatively simple dosing regimens are provided. Route is oral unless otherwise indicated. See text for additional information, toxicities, cautions, and discussions of dosing for the more rarely used drugs, many of which are highly toxic.

[2]Available in the USA only from the Drug Service, CDC, Atlanta (404-639-3670).

[3]Not available in the USA.

[4]*P jiroveci* (*carinii* in animals) has traditionally been considered a protozoan because of its morphology and drug sensitivity, but recent molecular analyses have shown it to be most closely related to fungi.

resistance has been reported. The drug has been successful in some cases that have failed therapy with antimonials. The dosage is 2–4 mg/kg intramuscularly daily or every other day for up to 15 doses, and a second course may be necessary. Pentamidine has also shown success against cutaneous leishmaniasis, but it is not routinely used for this purpose.

Adverse Effects & Cautions

Pentamidine is a highly toxic drug, with adverse effects noted in about 50% of patients receiving 4 mg/kg/d. Rapid intravenous administration can lead to severe hypotension, tachycardia, dizziness, and dyspnea, so the drug should be administered slowly (over 2 hours) and patients should be recumbent and monitored closely during treatment. With intramuscular administration, pain at the injection site is common and sterile abscesses may develop.

Pancreatic toxicity is common. Hypoglycemia due to inappropriate insulin release often appears 5–7 days after onset of treatment, can persist for days to several weeks, and may be followed by hyperglycemia. Reversible renal insufficiency is also common. Other adverse effects include rash, metallic taste, fever, gastrointestinal symptoms, abnormal liver function tests, acute pancreatitis, hypocalcemia, thrombocytopenia, hallucinations, and cardiac arrhythmias.

Inhaled pentamidine is generally well-tolerated but may cause cough, dyspnea, and bronchospasm.

SODIUM STIBOGLUCONATE

Pentavalent antimonials, including sodium stibogluconate (pentostam; Figure 53–2) and meglumine antimonate, are generally considered first-line agents for cutaneous and visceral leishmaniasis. The drugs are rapidly absorbed after intravenous (preferred) or intramuscular administration and eliminated in two phases, with short initial (about 2 hour) and much longer terminal (> 24 hour) half-lives. Treatment is given once daily at a dose of 20 mg/kg/d intravenously or intramuscularly for 20 days in cutaneous leishmaniasis and 28 days in visceral and mucocutaneous disease.

The mechanism of action of the antimonials is unknown. Their efficacy against different species may vary, possibly based on local drug resistance patterns. Cure rates are generally quite good, but resistance to sodium stibogluconate is increasing in some endemic areas. Some authorities have advocated initial therapy with other agents (eg, amphotericin B) in areas (such as parts of India) where therapy with sodium stibogluconate is commonly ineffective.

Few adverse effects occur initially, but the toxicity of stibogluconate increases over the course of therapy.

Most common are gastrointestinal symptoms, fever, headache, myalgias, arthralgias, and rash. Intramuscular injections can be very painful and lead to sterile abscesses. Electrocardiographic changes may occur, most commonly T wave changes and QT prolongation. These changes are generally reversible, but continued therapy may lead to dangerous arrhythmias. Thus, the electrocardiogram should be monitored during therapy. Hemolytic anemia and serious liver, renal, and cardiac effects are rare.

NITAZOXANIDE

Nitazoxanide is a nitrothiazolyl-salicylamide prodrug. Nitazoxanide was recently approved in the USA for use against *Giardia lamblia* and *Cryptosporidium parvum*. It is rapidly absorbed and converted to tizoxanide and tizoxanide conjugates, which are subsequently excreted in both urine and feces. The active metabolite, tizoxanide, inhibits the pyruvate:ferredoxin oxidoreductase pathway. Nitazoxanide appears to have activity against metronidazole-resistant protozoal strains and is well tolerated. Unlike metronidazole, nitazoxanide and its metabolites appear to be free of mutagenic effects. Other organisms that may be susceptible to nitazoxanide include *E histolytica, Helicobacter pylori, Ascaris lumbricoides,* several tapeworms, and *Fasciola hepatica.*

The recommended adult dosage is 500 mg twice daily for 3 days.

OTHER DRUGS FOR TRYPANOSOMIASIS & LEISHMANIASIS

Currently available therapies for all forms of trypanosomiasis are seriously deficient in both efficacy and safety. Availability of these therapies is also a concern, as they remain available mainly through donation or nonprofit production by pharmaceutical companies.

A. SURAMIN

Suramin is a sulfated naphthylamine that was introduced in the 1920s. It is the first-line therapy for early hemolymphatic African trypanosomiasis (especially *T brucei gambiense* infection), but because it does not enter the central nervous system, it is not effective against advanced disease. The drug's mechanism of action is unknown. It is administered intravenously and displays complex pharmacokinetics with very tight protein binding. It has a short initial half-life but a terminal elimination half-life of about 50 days. The drug is slowly cleared by renal excretion.

Suramin is administered after a 200 mg intravenous test dose. Regimens that have been used include 1 g on days 1, 3, 7, 14, and 21 or 1 g each week for 5 weeks. Combination therapy with pentamidine may improve efficacy. Suramin can also be used for chemoprophylaxis against African trypanosomiasis. Adverse effects are common. Immediate reactions can include fatigue, nausea, vomiting, and, more rarely, seizures, shock, and death. Later reactions include fever, rash, headache, paresthesias, neuropathies, renal abnormalities including proteinuria, chronic diarrhea, hemolytic anemia, and agranulocytosis.

B. MELARSOPROL

Melarsoprol is a trivalent arsenical that has been available since 1949 and is first-line therapy for advanced central nervous system African trypanosomiasis. After intravenous administration it is excreted rapidly, but clinically relevant concentrations accumulate in the central nervous system within 4 days. Melarsoprol is administered in propylene glycol by slow intravenous infusion at a dosage of 3.6 mg/kg/d for 3–4 days, with repeated courses at weekly intervals if needed. A new regimen of 2.2 mg/kg daily for 10 days had efficacy and toxicity similar to what was observed with three courses over 26 days. Melarsoprol is extremely toxic. The use of such a toxic drug is justified only by the severity of advanced trypanosomiasis and the lack of available alternatives. Immediate adverse effects include fever, vomiting, abdominal pain, and arthralgias. The most important toxicity is a reactive encephalopathy that generally appears within the first week of therapy (in 5–10% of patients) and is probably due to disruption of trypanosomes in the central nervous system. Common consequences of the encephalopathy include cerebral edema, seizures, coma, and death. Other serious toxicities include renal and cardiac disease and hypersensitivity reactions. Failure rates with melarsoprol appear to have increased recently in parts of Africa, suggesting the possibility of drug resistance.

C. EFLORNITHINE

Eflornithine (difluoromethylornithine), an inhibitor of ornithine decarboxylase, is the only new drug registered to treat African trypanosomiasis in the last half-century. It is a second therapy for advanced central nervous system African trypanosomiasis and is less toxic than melarsoprol but not as widely available. The drug had very limited availability until recently, when it was developed for use as a topical depilatory cream, leading to donation of the drug for the treatment of trypanosomiasis. Eflornithine is administered intravenously, and good central nervous system drug levels are achieved. Peak plasma levels are reached rapidly, and the elimination half-life is about 3 hours. The usual regimen is 100 mg/kg intravenously every 6 hours for 7–14 days (14 days was superior for a newly diagnosed infection). An oral formulation is also available and under clinical investigation. Eflornithine appears to be as effective as melarsoprol against advanced *T brucei gambiense* infection, but its efficacy against *T brucei rhodesiense* is limited by drug resistance. Toxicity from eflornithine is significant, but considerably less than that from melarsoprol. Adverse effects include diarrhea, vomiting, anemia, thrombocytopenia, leukopenia, and seizures. These effects are generally reversible. Increased experience with eflornithine and increased availability of the compound in endemic areas may lead to its replacement of suramin, pentamidine, and melarsoprol in the treatment of *T brucei gambiense* infection.

D. NIFURTIMOX

Nifurtimox, a nitrofuran, is the most commonly used drug for American trypanosomiasis (Chagas' disease). Nifurtimox is also under study in the treatment of African trypanosomiasis. Nifurtimox is well absorbed after oral administration and eliminated with a plasma half-life of about 3 hours. The drug is administered at a dose of 8–10 mg/kg/d (divided into three to four doses) orally for 3–4 months in the treatment of acute Chagas' disease. Nifurtimox decreases the severity of acute disease and usually eliminates detectable parasites, but it is often ineffective in fully eradicating infection. Thus, it often fails to prevent progression to the gastrointestinal and cardiac syndromes associated with chronic infection that are the most important clinical consequences of *Trypanosoma cruzi* infection. Efficacy may vary in different parts of South America, possibly related to drug resistance in some areas. Nifurtimox does not appear to be effective in the treatment of chronic Chagas' disease. Toxicity related to nifurtimox is common. Adverse effects include nausea, vomiting, abdominal pain, fever, rash, restlessness, insomnia, neuropathies, and seizures. These effects are generally reversible but often lead to cessation of therapy before completion of a standard course.

E. BENZNIDAZOLE

Benznidazole is an orally administered nitroimidazole that appears to have efficacy similar to that of nifurtimox in the treatment of acute Chagas' disease. Availability of the drug is currently limited. Important toxicities include peripheral neuropathy, rash, gastrointestinal symptoms, and myelosuppression.

F. AMPHOTERICIN

This important antifungal drug (see Chapter 48) is an alternative therapy for visceral leishmaniasis, especially in parts of India with high-level resistance to sodium stibogluconate, but its use is limited in developing countries by difficulty of administration, cost, and toxicity.

G. MILTEFOSINE

Miltefosine is an alkylphosphocholine analog that has recently shown efficacy in the treatment of visceral leishmaniasis. In a recent phase III study, the drug was administered orally with daily doses of 2.5 mg/kg for 28 days and provided excellent clinical results. A 100 mg daily dose is recommended in adults. Vomiting and diarrhea are common but generally short-lived toxicities. Transient elevations in liver enzymes and nephrotoxicity are also seen. The drug should be avoided in pregnancy (or in women who may become pregnant within 2 months of treatment) because of its teratogenic effects. Miltefosine is registered for the treatment of visceral leishmaniasis in India and some other countries, and—considering the serious limitations of other drugs, including parenteral administration, toxicity, and resistance—it may become the treatment of choice for that disease.

Chapter continues on next page.

PREPARATIONS AVAILABLE IN THE USA

Albendazole (Albenza)
    Oral: 200 mg tablets
Atovaquone (Mepron)
    Oral: 750 mg/5 mL suspension
Atovaquone-proguanil (Malarone)
    Oral: 250 mg atovaquone + 100 mg proguanil
    tablets; pediatric 62.5 mg atovaquone + 25
    mg proguanil tablets
Chloroquine (generic, Aralen)
    Oral: 250, 500 mg tablets (equivalent to 150,
    300 mg base, respectively)
    Parenteral: 50 mg/mL (equivalent to 40 mg/
    mL base) for injection
Clindamycin (generic, Cleocin)
    Oral: 75, 150, 300 mg capsules; 75 mg/5 mL
    suspension
    Parenteral: 150 mg/mL for injection
Doxycycline (generic, Vibramycin)
    Oral: 20, 50, 100 mg capsules; 50, 100 mg tablets;
    25 mg/5 mL suspension; 50 mg/5 mL syrup
    Parenteral: 100, 200 mg for injection
Dehydroemetine*
Eflornithine (Ornidyl)
    Parenteral: 200 mg/mL for injection
Halofantrine (Halfan)
    Oral: 250 mg tablets
Iodoquinol (Yodoxin)
    Oral: 210, 650 mg tablets
Mefloquine (generic, Lariam)
    Oral: 250 mg tablets

Melarsoprol (Mel B)*
Metronidazole (generic, Flagyl)
    Oral: 250, 500 mg tablets; 375 mg capsules;
    extended-release 750 mg tablets
    Parenteral: 5 mg/mL
Nifurtimox*
Nitazoxanide (Alinia)
    Oral: 500 mg tablets, powder for 100 mg/5 mL
    oral solution
Paromomycin (Humatin)
    Oral: 250 mg capsules
Pentamidine (Pentam 300, Pentacarinat, pen-
    tamidine isethionate)
    Parenteral: 300 mg powder for injection
    Aerosol (Nebupent): 300 mg powder
Primaquine (generic)
    Oral: 26.3 mg (equivalent to 15 mg base) tablet
Pyrimethamine (Daraprim)
    Oral: 25 mg tablets
Quinidine gluconate (generic)
    Parenteral: 80 mg/mL (equivalent to 50 mg/
    mL base) for injection
Quinine (generic)
    Oral: 260 mg tablets; 200, 260, 325 mg cap-
    sules
Sodium stibogluconate*
Sulfadoxine and pyrimethamine (Fansidar)
    Oral: 500 mg sulfadoxine plus 25 mg py-
    rimethamine tablets
Suramin*
Tinidazole (Tindamax)
    Oral: 250, 500 mg tablets

*Available in the USA only from the Drug Service, CDC, Atlanta (404-639-3670).

REFERENCES

General

Drugs for parasitic infections. Med Lett Drugs Ther 2004;46:1. (Issue available at www.medicalletter.com/freedocs/parasitic.pdf.)

Prevention of malaria. Med Lett Drugs Ther 2005;47:100.

Malaria

Adjuik M et al: Artesunate combinations for treatment of malaria: Meta-analysis. Lancet 2004;363:9.

Baird JK: Effectiveness of antimalarial drugs. N Engl J Med 2005; 352:1565.

Barnes KI et al: Efficacy of rectal artesunate compared with parenteral quinine in initial treatment of moderately severe malaria in African children and adults: A randomised study. Lancet 2004;363:1598.

Dorsey G et al: Sulfadoxine/pyrimethamine alone or with amodiaquine or artesunate for treatment of uncomplicated malaria: A longitudinal randomised trial. Lancet 2002;360:2031.

Guerin PJ et al: Malaria: Current status of control, diagnosis, treatment, and a proposed agenda for research and development. Lancet Infect Dis 2002;2:564.

Lang T, Greenwood B: The development of Lapdap, an affordable new treatment for malaria. Lancet Infect Dis 2003;3:162.

Ling J et al: Randomized, placebo-controlled trial of atovaquone/proguanil for the prevention of *Plasmodium falciparum* or *Plasmodium vivax* malaria among migrants to Papua, Indonesia. Clin Infect Dis 2002;35:825.

Mutabingwa T et al: Chlorproguanil-dapsone for treatment of drug-resistant falciparum malaria in Tanzania. Lancet 2001; 358:1218.

Mutabingwa TK et al: Amodiaquine alone, amodiaquine+sulfadoxine-pyrimethamine, amodiaquine+artesunate, and artemether-lumefantrine for outpatient treatment of malaria in Tanzanian children: A four-arm randomised effectiveness trial. Lancet 2005;365:1474.

Nosten F, Brasseur P: Combination therapy for malaria. Drugs 2002;62:1315.

Olliaro P: Mode of action and mechanisms of resistance for antimalarial drugs. Pharmacol Ther 2001;89:207.

Ridley RG: Medical need, scientific opportunity and the drive for antimalarial drugs. Nature 2002;415:686.

Rosenthal PJ (editor): *Antimalarial Chemotherapy: Mechanisms of Action, Resistance, and New Directions in Drug Discovery.* Humana Press, 2001.

Staedke SG et al: Combination treatments for uncomplicated malaria in Kampala, Uganda: Randomised clinical trial. Lancet 2004;364:1950.

Sulo J et al: Chlorproguanil-dapsone versus sulfadoxine-pyrimethamine for sequential episodes of uncomplicated falciparum malaria in Kenya and Malawi: A randomised clinical trial. Lancet 2002;360:1136.

Winstanley P: Modern chemotherapeutic options for malaria. Lancet Infect Dis 2001;1:242.

Intestinal Protozoal Infections

Blessmann J, Tannich E: Treatment of asymptomatic intestinal *Entamoeba histolytica* infection. N Engl J Med 2002; 347:1384.

Fox LM, Saravolatz LD: Nitazoxanide: A new thiazolide antiparasitic agent. Clin Infect Dis 2005;40:1173.

Haque R et al: Amebiasis. N Engl J Med 2003;348:1565.

Petri WA: Therapy of intestinal protozoa. Trends Parasitol 2003; 19:523.

Other Protozoal Infections

Burchmore RJ et al: Chemotherapy of human African trypanosomiasis. Curr Pharm Des 2002;8:256.

Croft SL, Barrett MP, Urbina JA: Chemotherapy of trypanosomiases and leishmaniasis. Trends Parasitol 2005;21:508.

Guerin PJ et al: Visceral leishmaniasis: Current status of control, diagnosis, and treatment, and a proposed research and development agenda. Lancet Infect Dis 2002;2:494.

Hepburn NC: Management of cutaneous leishmaniasis. Curr Opin Infect Dis 2001;14:151.

Legros D et al: Treatment of human African trypanosomiasis—present situation and needs for research and development. Lancet Infect Dis 2002;2:437.

Murray HW et al: Advances in leishmaniasis. Lancet 2005;366:1561.

Olliaro PL et al: Treatment options for visceral leishmaniasis: A systematic review of clinical studies done in India, 1980–2004. Lancet Infect Dis 2005;5:763.

Sobel JD, Nyirjesy P, Brown W: Tinidazole therapy for metronidazole-resistant vaginal trichomoniasis. Clin Infect Dis 2001; 33:1341.

Sundar S et al: Oral miltefosine for Indian visceral leishmaniasis. N Engl J Med 2002;347:1739.

Urbina JA: Specific treatment of Chagas disease: Current status and new developments. Curr Opin Infect Dis 2001;14:717.

Clinical Pharmacology of the Anthelmintic Drugs

54

Philip J. Rosenthal, MD

CHEMOTHERAPY OF HELMINTHIC INFECTIONS

Table 54–1 lists the major helminthic infections and provides a guide to the drug of choice and alternative drugs for each infection. In the text that follows, these drugs are arranged alphabetically. In general, parasites should be identified before treatment is started.

ALBENDAZOLE

Albendazole, a broad-spectrum oral anthelmintic, is the drug of choice and is approved in the USA for treatment of hydatid disease and cysticercosis. It is also used in the treatment of pinworm and hookworm infections, ascariasis, trichuriasis, and strongyloidiasis, although it is not labeled for these conditions.

Chemistry & Pharmacokinetics

Albendazole is a benzimidazole carbamate. After oral administration, it is erratically absorbed (increased with a fatty meal) and then rapidly undergoes first-pass metabolism in the liver to the active metabolite albendazole sulfoxide. It reaches variable maximum plasma concentrations about 3 hours after a 400 mg oral dose, and its plasma half-life is 8–12 hours. The sulfoxide is mostly protein-bound, distributes well to tissues, and enters bile, cerebrospinal fluid, and hydatid cysts. Albendazole metabolites are excreted in the urine.

Albendazole

Anthelmintic Actions

Benzimidazoles are thought to act against nematodes by inhibiting microtubule synthesis. Albendazole also has larvicidal effects in hydatid disease, cysticercosis, ascariasis, and hookworm infection and ovicidal effects in ascariasis, ancylostomiasis, and trichuriasis.

Clinical Uses

Albendazole is administered on an empty stomach when used against intraluminal parasites but with a fatty meal when used against tissue parasites.

A. ASCARIASIS, TRICHURIASIS, AND HOOKWORM AND PINWORM INFECTIONS

For adults and children older than 2 years of age, the treatment is a single dose of 400 mg orally (repeated for 2–3 days for heavy ascaris infections and in 2 weeks for pinworm infections). These treatments achieve high cure rates for these roundworm infections and marked reduction in egg counts in those not cured.

B. HYDATID DISEASE

Albendazole is the treatment of choice for medical therapy and is a useful adjunct to surgical removal or aspiration of cysts. It is more active against *Echinococcus granulosus* than *E multilocularis*. Dosing is 400 mg twice daily with meals for 1 month or longer. Daily therapy for up to 6 months has been well tolerated. One reported therapeutic strategy is to treat with albendazole and praziquantel, to assess response after 1 month or more, and, depending on the response, to then manage the patient with continued chemotherapy or combined surgical and drug therapy.

C. NEUROCYSTICERCOSIS

Indications for medical therapy for neurocysticercosis are controversial, as anthelmintic therapy is not clearly superior to therapy with corticosteroids alone and may exacerbate neurologic disease. Therapy is probably most

Table 54-1. Drugs for the treatment of helminthic infections.

Infecting Organism	Drug of Choice	Alternative Drugs
Roundworms (nematodes)		
Ascaris lumbricoides (roundworm)	Albendazole[1] or pyrantel pamoate or mebendazole	Piperazine
Trichuris trichiura (whipworm)	Mebendazole or albendazole[1]	Oxantel/pyrantel pamoate[2]
Necator americanus (hookworm); *Ancylostoma duodenale* (hookworm)	Pyrantel pamoate[1] or mebendazole or albendazole[1]	
Strongyloides stercoralis (threadworm)	Ivermectin	Thiabendazole, albendazole[1]
Enterobius vermicularis (pinworm)	Mebendazole or pyrantel pamoate	Albendazole[1]
Trichinella spiralis (trichinosis)	Mebendazole;[1] add corticosteroids for severe infection	Albendazole;[1] add corticosteroids for severe infection
Trichostrongylus species	Pyrantel pamoate[1] or mebendazole[1]	Albendazole[1]
Cutaneous larva migrans (creeping eruption)	Albendazole[1] or ivermectin[1]	Thiabendazole (topical)
Visceral larva migrans	Albendazole[1]	Mebendazole[1]
Angiostrongylus cantonensis	Thiabendazole	Albendazole[1] or mebendazole[1]
Wuchereria bancrofti (filariasis); *Brugia malayi* (filariasis); tropical eosinophilia; *Loa loa* (loiasis)	Diethylcarbamazine[3]	Ivermectin[1]
Onchocerca volvulus (onchocerciasis)	Ivermectin	
Dracunculus medinensis (guinea worm)	Metronidazole[1]	Thiabendazole[1] or mebendazole[1]
Capillaria philippinensis (intestinal capillariasis)	Albendazole[1]	Mebendazole[1] or thiabendazole[1]
Flukes (trematodes)		
Schistosoma haematobium (bilharziasis)	Praziquantel	Metrifonate[2]
Schistosoma mansoni	Praziquantel	Oxamniquine
Schistosoma japonicum	Praziquantel	
Clonorchis sinensis (liver fluke); *Opisthorchis* species	Praziquantel	Albendazole[1]
Paragonimus westermani (lung fluke)	Praziquantel[1]	Bithionol[3]
Fasciola hepatica (sheep liver fluke)	Bithionol[3] or triclabendazole[2]	
Fasciolopsis buski (large intestinal fluke)	Praziquantel[1] or niclosamide[2]	
Heterophyes heterophyes; Metagonimus yokogawai (small intestinal flukes)	Praziquantel[1] or niclosamide[2]	
Tapeworms (cestodes)		
Taenia saginata (beef tapeworm)	Praziquantel[1] or niclosamide[2]	Mebendazole[1,3]
Diphyllobothrium latum (fish tapeworm)	Praziquantel[1] or niclosamide[2]	
Taenia solium (pork tapeworm)	Praziquantel[1] or niclosamide[2]	
Cysticercosis (pork tapeworm larval stage)	Albendazole	Praziquantel[1]
Hymenolepis nana (dwarf tapeworm)	Praziquantel[1]	Niclosamide[2]
Echinococcus granulosus (hydatid disease); *Echinococcus multilocularis*	Albendazole	

[1]Available in the USA but not labeled for this indication.
[2]Not available in the USA but available in some other countries.
[3]Available in the USA only from the Parasitic Disease Drug Service, Parasitic Diseases Branch, Centers for Disease Control and Prevention, Atlanta 30333. Telephone 404-639-3670.

appropriate for symptomatic parenchymal or intraventricular cysts. Corticosteroids are usually given with the anthelmintic drug to decrease inflammation caused by dying organisms. Albendazole is now generally considered the drug of choice over praziquantel because of its shorter course, lower cost, improved penetration into the subarachnoid space, and increased drug levels (as opposed to decreased levels of praziquantel) when administered with corticosteroids. Albendazole is given in a dosage of 400 mg twice a day for up to 21 days.

D. OTHER INFECTIONS

Albendazole is the drug of choice in the treatment of cutaneous larva migrans (400 mg daily for 3 days), visceral larva migrans (400 mg twice daily for 5 days), intestinal capillariasis (400 mg daily for 10 days), microsporidial infections (400 mg twice daily for 2 weeks or longer), and gnathostomiasis (400 mg twice daily for 3 weeks). It also has activity against trichinosis (400 mg twice daily for 1–2 weeks) and clonorchiasis (400 mg twice daily for 1 week). There have been reports of some effectiveness in treatment of opisthorchiasis, toxocariasis, and loiasis and conflicting reports of effectiveness in giardiasis and taeniasis. Albendazole is included in some programs to control lymphatic filariasis, but it appears to be less active than diethylcarbamazine or ivermectin for this purpose.

Adverse Reactions, Contraindications, & Cautions

When used for 1–3 days, albendazole is nearly free of significant adverse effects. Mild and transient epigastric distress, diarrhea, headache, nausea, dizziness, lassitude, and insomnia can occur. In long-term use for hydatid disease, albendazole is well tolerated, but it can cause abdominal distress, headaches, fever, fatigue, alopecia, increases in liver enzymes, and pancytopenia.

Blood counts and liver function studies should be followed during long-term therapy. The drug should not be given to patients with known hypersensitivity to other benzimidazole drugs or to those with cirrhosis. The safety of albendazole in pregnancy and in children younger than 2 years of age has not been established.

BITHIONOL

Bithionol is the drug of choice for the treatment of fascioliasis (sheep liver fluke). An alternative drug, triclabendazole, is not available in the USA.

Bithionol is also an alternative drug in the treatment of pulmonary paragonimiasis.

Pharmacokinetics

After ingestion, bithionol reaches peak blood levels in 4–8 hours. Excretion appears to be mainly via the kidney.

Clinical Uses

For treatment of paragonimiasis and fascioliasis, the dosage of bithionol is 30–50 mg/kg in two or three divided doses, given orally after meals on alternate days for 10–15 doses. For pulmonary paragonimiasis, cure rates are over 90%. For cerebral paragonimiasis, repeat courses of therapy may be necessary.

Adverse Reactions, Contraindications, & Cautions

Adverse effects, which occur in up to 40% of patients, are generally mild and transient, but occasionally their severity requires interruption of therapy. These problems include diarrhea, abdominal cramps, anorexia, nausea, vomiting, dizziness, and headache. Skin rashes may occur after a week or more of therapy, suggesting a reaction to antigens released from dying worms.

Bithionol should be used with caution in children younger than 8 years of age because there has been limited experience in this age group.

DIETHYLCARBAMAZINE CITRATE

Diethylcarbamazine is a drug of choice in the treatment of filariasis, loiasis, and tropical eosinophilia. It has been replaced by ivermectin for the treatment of onchocerciasis.

Chemistry & Pharmacokinetics

Diethylcarbamazine, a synthetic piperazine derivative, is marketed as a citrate salt. It is rapidly absorbed from the gastrointestinal tract; after a 0.5 mg/kg dose, peak plasma levels are reached within 1–2 hours. The plasma half-life is 2–3 hours in the presence of acidic urine but about 10 hours if the urine is alkaline, a Henderson-Hasselbalch trapping effect (see Chapter 1). The drug rapidly equilibrates with all tissues except fat. It is excreted, principally in the urine, as unchanged drug and the N-oxide metabolite. Dosage may have to be reduced in patients with persistent urinary alkalosis or renal impairment.

Anthelmintic Actions

Diethylcarbamazine immobilizes microfilariae and alters their surface structure, displacing them from tissues and making them more susceptible to destruction by host defense mechanisms. The mode of action against adult worms is unknown.

Clinical Uses

The drug should be taken after meals.

A. *WUCHERERIA BANCROFTI, BRUGIA MALAYI, BRUGIA TIMORI,* AND *LOA LOA*

Diethylcarbamazine is the drug of choice for treatment of infections with these parasites because of its efficacy and lack of serious toxicity. Microfilariae of all species are rapidly killed; adult parasites are killed more slowly, often requiring several courses of treatment. The drug is highly effective against adult *L loa*. The extent to which *W bancrofti* and *B malayi* adults are killed is not known, but after appropriate therapy microfilariae do not reappear in the majority of patients.

These infections are treated for 2 or (for *L loa*) 3 weeks, with initial low doses to reduce the incidence of allergic reactions to dying microfilariae. This regimen is 50 mg (1 mg/kg in children) on day 1, three 50 mg doses on day 2, three 100 mg doses (2 mg/kg in children) on day 3, and then 2 mg/kg three times per day to complete the 2–3 week course.

Antihistamines may be given for the first few days of therapy to limit allergic reactions, and corticosteroids should be started and doses of diethylcarbamazine lowered or interrupted if severe reactions occur. Cures may require several courses of treatment.

Diethylcarbamazine may also be used for chemoprophylaxis (300 mg weekly or 300 mg on 3 successive days each month for loiasis; 50 mg monthly for bancroftian and Malayan filariasis).

B. OTHER USES

For tropical eosinophilia, diethylcarbamazine is given orally at a dosage of 2 mg/kg three times daily for 7 days. Diethylcarbamazine is effective in *Mansonella streptocerca* infections, since it kills both adults and microfilariae. Limited information suggests that the drug is not effective, however, against adult *M ozzardi* or *M perstans* and that it has limited activity against microfilariae of these parasites. An important application of diethylcarbamazine has been its use for mass treatment of *W bancrofti* infections to reduce transmission. Weekly or monthly administration regimens have been studied; and, most recently, yearly treatment (with or without ivermectin) markedly reduced reservoirs of infection in Papua New Guinea.

Adverse Reactions, Contraindications, & Cautions

Reactions to diethylcarbamazine, which are generally mild and transient, include headache, malaise, anorexia, weakness, nausea, vomiting, and dizziness. Adverse effects also occur as a result of the release of proteins from dying microfilariae or adult worms. Reactions are particularly severe with onchocerciasis, but diethylcarbamazine is no longer commonly used for this infection, as ivermectin is equally efficacious and less toxic. Reactions to dying microfilariae are usually mild in *W bancrofti*, more intense in *B malayi*, and occasionally severe in *L loa* infections. Reactions include fever, malaise, papular rash, headache, gastrointestinal symptoms, cough, chest pain, and muscle or joint pain. Leukocytosis is common. Eosinophilia may increase with treatment. Proteinuria may also occur. Symptoms are most likely to occur in patients with heavy loads of microfilariae. Retinal hemorrhages and, rarely, encephalopathy have been described.

Between the third and twelfth days of treatment, local reactions may occur in the vicinity of dying adult or immature worms. These include lymphangitis with localized swellings in *W bancrofti* and *B malayi*, small wheals in the skin in *L loa*, and flat papules in *M streptocerca* infections. Patients with attacks of lymphangitis due to *W bancrofti* or *B malayi* should be treated during a quiescent period between attacks.

Caution is advised when using diethylcarbamazine in patients with hypertension or renal disease.

DOXYCYCLINE

This tetracycline antibiotic is described in more detail in Chapter 44. Doxycycline has recently been shown to have significant macrofilaricidal activity against *W bancrofti*, suggesting better activity than any other available drug against adult worms. Activity is also seen against onchocerciasis. Doxycycline acts indirectly, by killing *Wolbachia*, an intracellular bacterial symbiont of filarial parasites. It may prove to be an important drug for filariasis, both for treatment of active disease and in mass chemotherapy campaigns.

IVERMECTIN

Ivermectin is the drug of choice in strongyloidiasis and onchocerciasis. It is also an alternative drug for a number of other helminthic infections.

Chemistry & Pharmacokinetics

Ivermectin, a semisynthetic macrocyclic lactone, is a mixture of avermectin B_{1a} and B_{1b}. It is derived from the soil actinomycete *Streptomyces avermitilis*.

Ivermectin is used only orally in humans. The drug is rapidly absorbed, reaching maximum plasma concentrations 4 hours after a 12 mg dose. The drug has a wide tissue distribution and a volume of distribution of about 50 L. Its half-life is about 16 hours. Excretion of the drug and its metabolites is almost exclusively in the feces.

Anthelmintic Actions

Ivermectin appears to paralyze nematodes and arthropods by intensifying γ-aminobutyric acid (GABA)-

mediated transmission of signals in peripheral nerves. In onchocerciasis, ivermectin is microfilaricidal. It does not effectively kill adult worms but blocks the release of microfilariae for some months after therapy. After a single standard dose, microfilariae in the skin diminish rapidly within 2–3 days, remain low for months, and then gradually increase; microfilariae in the anterior chamber of the eye decrease slowly over months, eventually clear, and then gradually return. With repeated doses of ivermectin, the drug does appear to have a low-level macrofilaricidal action and to permanently reduce microfilarial production.

Clinical Uses

A. Onchocerciasis

Treatment is with a single oral dose of ivermectin, 150 mcg/kg, with water on an empty stomach. Doses are repeated; regimens vary from monthly to less frequent (every 6–12 months) dosing schedules. After acute therapy, treatment is repeated at 12-month intervals until the adult worms die, which may take 10 years or longer. With the first treatment only, patients with microfilariae in the cornea or anterior chamber may be treated with corticosteroids to avoid inflammatory eye reactions.

Ivermectin also now plays a key role in onchocerciasis control. Annual mass treatments have led to major reductions in disease transmission.

B. Strongyloidiasis

Treatment consists of two daily doses of 200 mcg/kg. In immunosuppressed patients with disseminated infection, repeated treatment is often needed, but cure may not be possible. In this case, suppressive therapy—ie, once monthly—may be helpful.

C. Other Parasites

Ivermectin reduces microfilariae in *Brugia malayi* and *M ozzardi* infections but not in *M perstans* infections. It has been used with diethylcarbamazine for the control of *W bancrofti,* but it does not kill adult worms, and whether it offers added benefit is uncertain. In loiasis, although the drug reduces microfilaria concentrations, it can occasionally induce severe reactions. Ivermectin is also effective in controlling scabies, lice, and cutaneous larva migrans and in eliminating a large proportion of ascarid worms.

Adverse Reactions, Contraindications, & Cautions

In strongyloidiasis treatment, infrequent side effects include fatigue, dizziness, nausea, vomiting, abdominal pain, and rashes. In onchocerciasis treatment, the adverse effects are principally from the **Mazotti reaction,** due to killing of microfilariae. The reaction includes fever, head-

ache, dizziness, somnolence, weakness, rash, increased pruritus, diarrhea, joint and muscle pains, hypotension, tachycardia, lymphadenitis, lymphangitis, and peripheral edema. This reaction starts on the first day and peaks on the second day after treatment. The Mazotti reaction occurs in 5–30% of persons and is generally mild, but it may be more frequent and more severe in individuals who are not long-term residents of onchocerciasis-endemic areas. A more intense Mazotti reaction occurs in 1–3% of persons and a severe reaction in 0.1%, including high fever, hypotension, and bronchospasm. Corticosteroids are indicated in these cases, at times for several days. The Mazotti reaction diminishes with repeated dosing. Swellings and abscesses occasionally occur at 1–3 weeks, presumably at sites of adult worms.

Some patients develop corneal opacities and other eye lesions several days after treatment. These are rarely severe and generally resolve without corticosteroid treatment.

It is best to avoid concomitant use of ivermectin and other drugs that enhance GABA activity, eg, barbiturates, benzodiazepines, and valproic acid. Ivermectin should not be used in pregnancy. Safety in children younger than 5 years has not been established.

MEBENDAZOLE

Mebendazole is a synthetic benzimidazole that has a wide spectrum of anthelmintic activity and a low incidence of adverse effects.

Mebendazole

Chemistry & Pharmacokinetics

Less than 10% of orally administered mebendazole is absorbed. The absorbed drug is protein-bound (> 90%), rapidly converted to inactive metabolites (primarily during its first pass in the liver), and has a half-life of 2–6 hours. It is excreted mostly in the urine, principally as decarboxylated derivatives. In addition, a portion of absorbed drug and its derivatives are excreted in the bile. Absorption is increased if the drug is ingested with a fatty meal.

Anthelmintic Actions

Mebendazole probably acts by inhibiting microtubule synthesis; the parent drug appears to be the active form.

Efficacy of the drug varies with gastrointestinal transit time, with intensity of infection, and perhaps with the strain of parasite. The drug kills hookworm, ascaris, and trichuris eggs.

Clinical Uses

In the USA, mebendazole has been approved for use in ascariasis, trichuriasis, and hookworm and pinworm infection. It can be taken before or after meals; the tablets should be chewed before swallowing. For pinworm infection, the dose is 100 mg once, repeated at 2 weeks. For ascariasis, trichuriasis, hookworm, and trichostrongylus infections, a dosage of 100 mg twice daily for 3 days is used for adults and for children older than 2 years of age. Cure rates are 90–100% for pinworm infections, ascariasis, and trichuriasis. Cure rates are lower for hookworm infections, but a marked reduction in the worm burden occurs in those not cured. For intestinal capillariasis, mebendazole is used at a dosage of 400 mg/d in divided doses for 21 or more days. In trichinosis, limited reports suggest efficacy against adult worms in the intestinal tract and tissue larvae. Treatment is three times daily, with fatty foods, at 200–400 mg per dose for 3 days and then 400–500 mg per dose for 10 days. Corticosteroids should be coadministered for severe infections.

Adverse Reactions, Contraindications, & Cautions

Short-term mebendazole therapy for intestinal nematodes is nearly free of adverse effects. Mild nausea, vomiting, diarrhea, and abdominal pain have been reported infrequently. Rare side effects, usually with high-dose therapy, are hypersensitivity reactions (rash, urticaria), agranulocytosis, alopecia, and elevation of liver enzymes.

Mebendazole is teratogenic in animals and therefore contraindicated in pregnancy. It should be used with caution in children younger than 2 years of age because of limited experience and rare reports of convulsions in this age group. Plasma levels may be decreased by concomitant use of carbamazepine or phenytoin and increased by cimetidine. Mebendazole should be used with caution in patients with cirrhosis.

METRIFONATE (TRICHLORFON)

Metrifonate is a safe, low-cost alternative drug for the treatment of *Schistosoma haematobium* infections. It is not active against *S mansoni* or *S japonicum*. It is not available in the USA.

Chemistry & Pharmacokinetics

Metrifonate, an organophosphate compound, is rapidly absorbed after oral administration. Following the standard oral dose, peak blood levels are reached in 1–2 hours; the half-life is about 1.5 hours. Clearance appears to be through nonenzymatic transformation to dichlorvos, its active metabolite. Metrifonate and dichlorvos are well distributed to the tissues and are completely eliminated in 24–48 hours.

Anthelmintic Actions

The mode of action is thought to be related to cholinesterase inhibition. This inhibition temporarily paralyzes the adult worms, resulting in their shift from the bladder venous plexus to small arterioles of the lungs, where they are trapped, encased by the immune system, and die. The drug is not effective against *S haematobium* eggs; live eggs continue to pass in the urine for several months after all adult worms have been killed.

Clinical Uses

In the treatment of *S haematobium,* a single oral dose of 7.5–10 mg/kg is given three times at 14-day intervals. Cure rates on this schedule are 44–93%, with marked reductions in egg counts in those not cured. Metrifonate was also effective as a prophylactic agent when given monthly to children in a highly endemic area, and it has been used in mass treatment programs. In mixed infections with *S haematobium* and *S mansoni*, metrifonate has been successfully combined with oxamniquine.

Adverse Reactions, Contraindications, & Cautions

Some studies note mild and transient cholinergic symptoms, including nausea and vomiting, diarrhea, abdominal pain, bronchospasm, headache, sweating, fatigue, weakness, dizziness, and vertigo. These symptoms may begin within 30 minutes and persist up to 12 hours.

Metrifonate should not be used after recent exposure to insecticides or drugs that might potentiate cholinesterase inhibition. Metrifonate is contraindicated in pregnancy.

NICLOSAMIDE

Niclosamide is a second-line drug for the treatment of most tapeworm infections, but it is not available in the USA.

Chemistry & Pharmacokinetics

Niclosamide is a salicylamide derivative. It appears to be minimally absorbed from the gastrointestinal tract—

neither the drug nor its metabolites have been recovered from the blood or urine.

Niclosamide

Anthelmintic Actions

Adult worms (but not ova) are rapidly killed, presumably due to inhibition of oxidative phosphorylation or stimulation of ATPase activity.

Clinical Uses

The adult dose of niclosamide is 2 g once, given in the morning on an empty stomach. The tablets must be chewed thoroughly and are then swallowed with water.

A. TAENIA SAGINATA (BEEF TAPEWORM), T SOLIUM (PORK TAPEWORM), AND DIPHYLLOBOTHRIUM LATUM (FISH TAPEWRIUM)

A single 2 g dose of niclosamide results in cure rates of over 85% for *D latum* and about 95% for *T saginata*. It is probably equally effective against *T solium*. Cysticercosis is theoretically possible after treatment of *T solium* infections, because viable ova are released into the gut lumen following digestion of segments. However, no such cases of cysticercosis following therapy have been reported.

B. OTHER TAPEWORMS

Most patients treated with niclosamide for *H diminuta* and *Dipylidium caninum* infections are cured with a 7-day course of treatment; a few require a second course. Praziquantel is superior for *Hymenolepis nana* (dwarf tapeworm) infection. Niclosamide is not effective against cysticercosis or hydatid disease.

C. INTESTINAL FLUKE INFECTIONS

Niclosamide can be used as an alternative drug in the treatment of *Fasciolopsis buski*, *Heterophyes heterophyes*, and *Metagonimus yokogawai* infections. The standard dose is given every other day for three doses.

Adverse Reactions, Contraindications, & Cautions

Infrequent, mild, and transitory adverse events include nausea, vomiting, diarrhea, and abdominal discomfort.

The consumption of alcohol should be avoided on the day of treatment and for 1 day afterward.

The safety of the drug has not been established in pregnancy or for children younger than 2 years of age.

OXAMNIQUINE

Oxamniquine is an alternative to praziquantel for the treatment of *S mansoni* infections. It has also been used extensively for mass treatment. It is not effective against *S haematobium* or *S japonicum*.

Pharmacokinetics

Oxamniquine, a semisynthetic tetrahydroquinoline, is readily absorbed orally. Its plasma half-life is about 2.5 hours. The drug is extensively metabolized to inactive metabolites and excreted in the urine—up to 75% in the first 24 hours. Intersubject variations in serum concentration have been noted, which may explain some treatment failures.

Anthelmintic Actions

Oxamniquine is active against both mature and immature stages of *S mansoni* but does not appear to be cercaricidal. The mechanism of action is unknown. Contraction and paralysis of the worms results in detachment from terminal venules in the mesentery and transit to the liver, where many die; surviving females return to the mesenteric vessels but cease to lay eggs.

Strains of *S mansoni* in different parts of the world vary in susceptibility. Oxamniquine has been effective in instances of praziquantel resistance.

Clinical Uses

Oxamniquine is safe and effective in all stages of *S mansoni* disease, including advanced hepatosplenomegaly. In the acute (Katayama) syndrome, treatment results in disappearance of acute symptoms and clearance of the infection. The drug is generally less effective in children, who require higher doses than adults. It is better-tolerated with food.

Optimal dosage schedules vary for different regions of the world. In the Western Hemisphere and western Africa, the adult oxamniquine dosage is 12–15 mg/kg given once. In northern and southern Africa, standard schedules are 15 mg/kg twice daily for 2 days. In eastern Africa and the Arabian peninsula, standard dosage is 15–20 mg/kg twice in 1 day. Cure rates are 70–95%, with marked reduction in egg excretion in those not cured.

In mixed schistosome infections, oxamniquine has been successfully used in combination with metrifonate.

Adverse Reactions, Contraindications, & Cautions

Mild symptoms, starting about 3 hours after a dose and lasting for several hours, occur in more than one third of patients. Central nervous system symptoms (dizziness, headache, drowsiness) are most common; nausea and vomiting, diarrhea, colic, pruritus, and urticaria also occur. Infrequent adverse effects are low-grade fever, an orange to red discoloration of the urine, proteinuria, microscopic hematuria, and a transient decrease in leukocytes. Seizures have been reported rarely.

Since the drug makes many patients dizzy or drowsy, it should be used with caution in patients whose work or activity requires mental alertness (eg, no driving for 24 hours). It should be used with caution in those with a history of epilepsy.

Oxamniquine is contraindicated in pregnancy.

PIPERAZINE

Piperazine is an alternative for the treatment of ascariasis, with cure rates over 90% when taken for 2 days, but it is not recommended for other helminth infections. Piperazine is available as the hexahydrate and as a variety of salts. It is readily absorbed, and maximum plasma levels are reached in 2–4 hours. Most of the drug is excreted unchanged in the urine in 2–6 hours, and excretion is complete within 24 hours.

Piperazine causes paralysis of ascaris by blocking acetylcholine at the myoneural junction; unable to maintain their position in the host, live worms are expelled by normal peristalsis.

For ascariasis, the dosage of piperazine (as the hexahydrate) is 75 mg/kg (maximum dose, 3.5 g) orally once daily for 2 days. For heavy infections, treatment should be continued for 3–4 days or repeated after 1 week.

Occasional mild adverse effects include nausea, vomiting, diarrhea, abdominal pain, dizziness, and headache. Neurotoxicity and allergic reactions are rare.

Piperazine compounds should not be given to women during pregnancy, to patients with impaired renal or hepatic function, or to those with a history of epilepsy or chronic neurologic disease.

PRAZIQUANTEL

Praziquantel is effective in the treatment of schistosome infections of all species and most other trematode and cestode infections, including cysticercosis. The drug's safety and effectiveness as a single oral dose have also made it useful in mass treatment of several infections.

Chemistry & Pharmacokinetics

Praziquantel is a synthetic isoquinoline-pyrazine derivative. It is rapidly absorbed, with a bioavailability of about 80% after oral administration. Peak serum concentrations are reached 1–3 hours after a therapeutic dose. Cerebrospinal fluid concentrations of praziquantel reach 14–20% of the drug's plasma concentration. About 80%

of the drug is bound to plasma proteins. Most of the drug is rapidly metabolized to inactive mono- and poly-hydroxylated products after a first pass in the liver. The half-life is 0.8–1.5 hours. Excretion is mainly via the kidneys (60–80%) and bile (15–35%). Plasma concentrations of praziquantel increase when the drug is taken with a high-carbohydrate meal or with cimetidine; bioavailability is markedly reduced with some antiepileptics (phenytoin, carbamazepine) or with corticosteroids.

Anthelmintic Actions

Praziquantel appears to increase the permeability of trematode and cestode cell membranes to calcium, resulting in paralysis, dislodgement, and death.

In schistosome infections of experimental animals, praziquantel is effective against adult worms and immature stages and it has a prophylactic effect against cercarial infection.

Clinical Uses

Praziquantel tablets are taken with liquid after a meal; they should be swallowed without chewing because their bitter taste can induce retching and vomiting.

A. SCHISTOSOMIASIS

Praziquantel is the drug of choice for all forms of schistosomiasis. The dosage is 20 mg/kg for two (S mansoni and S haematobium) or three (S japonicum and S mekongi) doses at intervals of 4–6 hours. High cure rates (75–95%) are achieved when patients are evaluated at 3–6 months; there is marked reduction in egg counts in those not cured. The drug is effective in adults and children and is generally well tolerated by patients in the hepatosplenic stage of advanced disease. It is not clear, however, whether the drug can be safely or effectively used during the acute stage of the disease (Katayama fever) because release of antigens from dying immature worms may exacerbate symptoms. Increasing evidence indicates rare S mansoni drug resistance, which is treatable with oxamniquine. Effectiveness of the drug for chemoprophylaxis has not been established.

B. CLONORCHIASIS, OPISTHORCHIASIS, AND PARAGONIMIASIS

The dosage of 25 mg/kg three times for 1 day results in nearly 100% cure rates for clonorchiasis and opisthorchiasis, and a 2 day course provides 90–100% cure rates for pulmonary paragonimiasis.

C. TAENIASIS AND DIPHYLLOBOTHRIASIS

A single dose of praziquantel, 5–10 mg/kg, results in nearly 100% cure rates for T saginata, T solium, and D latum infections. Because praziquantel does not kill eggs, it is theoretically possible that larvae of *T solium* released from eggs in the large bowel could penetrate the intestinal wall and give rise to cysticercosis, but this hazard is probably minimal.

D. NEUROCYSTICERCOSIS

Albendazole is now the preferred drug, but when it is not appropriate or available, praziquantel has similar efficacy. Indications are similar to those for albendazole. The praziquantel dosage is 50 mg/kg/d in three divided doses for 14 days or longer. Clinical responses to therapy vary from dramatic improvements of seizures and other neurologic findings to no response and even progression of the disease. Praziquantel—but not albendazole—has diminished bioavailability when taken concurrently with a corticosteroid. Recommendations on corticosteroid use in neurocysticercosis vary.

E. *H NANA*

Praziquantel is the drug of choice for *H nana* infections and the first drug to be highly effective. A single dose of 25 mg/kg is taken initially and repeated in 1 week.

F. HYDATID DISEASE

In hydatid disease, praziquantel kills protoscoleces but does not affect the germinal membrane. Praziquantel is being evaluated as an adjunct with albendazole pre- and postsurgery. In addition to its direct action, praziquantel enhances the plasma concentration of albendazole sulfoxide.

G. OTHER PARASITES

Limited trials at a dosage of 25 mg/kg three times a day for 1–2 days indicate effectiveness of praziquantel against fasciolopsiasis, metagonimiasis, and other forms of heterophyiasis. Praziquantel was not effective for fascioliasis, however, even at dosages as high as 25 mg/kg three times daily for 3–7 days.

Adverse Reactions, Contraindications, & Cautions

Mild and transient adverse effects are common. They begin within several hours after ingestion and may persist for hours to 1 day. Most frequent are headache, dizziness, drowsiness, and lassitude; others include nausea, vomiting, abdominal pain, loose stools, pruritus, urticaria, arthralgia, myalgia, and low-grade fever. Mild and transient elevations of liver enzymes have been reported. Several days after starting praziquantel, low-grade fever, pruritus, and skin rashes (macular and urticarial), sometimes associated with worsened eosinophilia, may occur, probably due to the release of proteins from dying worms rather than direct drug toxicity. The intensity and frequency of adverse effects increase with dosage such that they occur in up to 50% of patients who receive 25 mg/kg three times in 1 day.

In neurocysticercosis, neurologic abnormalities may be exacerbated by inflammatory reactions around dying parasites. Common findings in patients who do not receive corticosteroids, usually presenting during or shortly after therapy, are headache, meningismus, nausea, vomiting, mental changes, and seizures (often accompanied by increased cerebrospinal fluid pleocytosis). More serious findings, including arachnoiditis, hyperthermia, and intracranial hypertension, may also occur. Corticosteroids are commonly used with praziquantel in the treatment of neurocysticercosis to decrease the inflammatory reaction, but this is controversial, and complicated by knowledge that corticosteroids decrease the plasma level of praziquantel up to 50%. Praziquantel is contraindicated in ocular cysticercosis, as parasite destruction in the eye may cause irreparable damage. Some workers also caution against use of the drug in spinal neurocysticercosis.

The safety of praziquantel in children younger than age 4 years is not established, but no specific problems in young children have been documented. Indeed, the drug appears to be better tolerated in children than in adults. Praziquantel increased abortion rates in rats and therefore should be avoided in pregnancy if possible. Because the drug induces dizziness and drowsiness, patients should not drive during therapy and should be warned regarding activities requiring particular physical coordination or alertness.

PYRANTEL PAMOATE

Pyrantel pamoate is a broad-spectrum anthelmintic highly effective for the treatment of pinworm, ascaris, and *Trichostrongylus orientalis* infections. It is moderately effective against both species of hookworm. It is not effective in trichuriasis or strongyloidiasis. Oxantel pamoate, an analog of pyrantel not available in the USA, has been used successfully in the treatment of trichuriasis; the two drugs have been combined for their broad-spectrum anthelmintic activity.

Chemistry & Pharmacokinetics

Pyrantel pamoate is a tetrahydropyrimidine derivative. It is poorly absorbed from the gastrointestinal tract and active mainly against luminal organisms. Peak plasma levels are reached in 1–3 hours. Over half of the administered dose is recovered unchanged in the feces.

Anthelmintic Actions

Pyrantel is effective against mature and immature forms of susceptible helminths within the intestinal tract but not against migratory stages in the tissues or against ova. The drug is a neuromuscular blocking agent that causes release of acetylcholine and inhibition of cholinesterase; this results in paralysis, which is followed by expulsion of worms.

Clinical Uses

The standard dose is 11 mg (base)/kg (maximum, 1 g), given orally once with or without food. For pinworm the dose is repeated in 2 weeks, and cure rates are greater than 95%. The drug is available in the USA without prescription for this indication.

For ascariasis, a single dose yields cure rates of 85–100%. Treatment should be repeated if eggs are found 2 weeks after treatment. For hookworm infections, a single dose is effective against light infections; but for heavy infections, especially with *N americanus,* a 3-day course is necessary to reach 90% cure rates. A course of treatment can be repeated in 2 weeks.

Adverse Reactions, Contraindications, & Cautions

Adverse effects are infrequent, mild, and transient. They include nausea, vomiting, diarrhea, abdominal cramps, dizziness, drowsiness, headache, insomnia, rash, fever, and weakness. Pyrantel should be used with caution in patients with liver dysfunction, because low, transient aminotransferase elevations have been noted in a small number of patients. Experience with the drug in pregnant women and children younger than 2 years of age is limited.

THIABENDAZOLE

Thiabendazole is an alternative to ivermectin for the treatment of strongyloidiasis and cutaneous larva migrans.

Chemistry & Pharmacokinetics

Thiabendazole is a benzimidazole compound. Although it is a chelating agent that forms stable complexes with a number of metals, including iron, it does not bind calcium.

Thiabendazole is rapidly absorbed after ingestion. With a standard dose, drug concentrations in plasma peak within 1–2 hours; the half-life is 1.2 hours. The drug is almost completely metabolized in the liver to the 5-hydroxy form; 90% is excreted in the urine in 48 hours, largely as the glucuronide or sulfonate conjugate. Thiabendazole can also be absorbed from the skin.

Anthelmintic Actions

The mechanism of action of thiabendazole is probably the same as that of other benzimidazoles (see above). The drug has ovicidal effects for some parasites.

Clinical Uses

The standard dosage, 25 mg/kg (maximum, 1.5 g) twice daily, should be given after meals. Tablets should be chewed. For strongyloides infection, treatment is for 2 days. Cure rates are reportedly 93%. A course can be repeated in 1 week if indicated. In patients with hyperinfection syndrome, the standard dose is continued twice daily for 5–7 days. For cutaneous larva migrans, thiabendazole cream can be applied topically or the oral drug can be given for 2 days (although albendazole is less toxic and therefore preferred).

Adverse Reactions, Contraindications, & Cautions

Thiabendazole is much more toxic than other benzimidazoles or ivermectin, so other agents are now preferred for most indications. Common adverse effects include dizziness, anorexia, nausea, and vomiting. Less frequent problems are epigastric pain, abdominal cramps, diarrhea, pruritus, headache, drowsiness, and neuropsychiatric symptoms. Irreversible liver failure and fatal Stevens-Johnson syndrome have been reported.

Experience with thiabendazole is limited in children weighing less than 15 kg. The drug should not be used in pregnancy or in the presence of hepatic or renal disease.

PREPARATIONS AVAILABLE

Albendazole (Albenza, Zentel)
Oral: 200 mg tablets; 100 mg/5 mL suspension
Note: Albendazole is approved in the USA for the treatment of cysticercosis and hydatid disease.

Bithionol (Bitin)
Oral: 200 mg tablets
Note: Bithionol is not marketed in the USA but is available from the Parasitic Disease Drug Service, Centers for Disease Control and Prevention, Atlanta; 404-639-3670.

Diethylcarbamazine (Hetrazan)
Oral: 50 mg tablets
Note: Diethylcarbamazine is no longer marketed in the USA but is available from the Parasitic Disease Drug Service, Centers for Disease Control and Prevention, Atlanta; 404-639-3670.

Ivermectin (Mectizan, Stromectol)
Oral: 3, 6 mg tablets
Note: Ivermectin is approved for use in the USA for the treatment of onchocerciasis and strongyloidiasis. See Chapter 66 for comment on the unlabeled use of drugs.
(continued)

Levamisole (Ergamisol)
    Oral: 50 mg tablets
Mebendazole (generic, Vermox)
    Oral: 100 mg chewable tablets; outside the USA, 100 mg/5 mL suspension
Metrifonate (trichlorfon, Bilarcil)
    Oral: 100 mg tablets
    Note: Metrifonate is not available in the USA.
Niclosamide (Niclocide)
    Oral: 500 mg chewable tablets
    Note: Niclosamide is not available in the USA.
Oxamniquine (Vansil, Mansil)
    Oral: 250 mg capsules; outside the USA, 50 mg/mL syrup
Oxantel pamoate (Quantrel); oxantel/pyrantel pamoate (Telopar)
    Oral: tablets containing 100 mg (base) of each drug; suspensions containing 20 or 50 mg (base) per mL
    Note: Oxantel pamoate and oxantel/pyrantel pamoate are not available in the USA.
Piperazine (generic, Vermizine)
    Oral: piperazine citrate tablets equivalent to 250 mg of the hexahydrate; piperazine cit-rate syrup equivalent to 500 mg of the hexahydrate per 5 mL
Praziquantel (Biltricide; others outside the USA)
    Oral: 600 mg tablets (other strengths outside the USA)
Pyrantel pamoate (Antiminth, Combantrin, Pin-rid, Pin-X)
    Oral: 50 mg (base)/mL suspension; 180 mg tablets; 62.5 mg (base) capsules (available without prescription in the USA)
Suramin (Bayer 205, others)
    Parenteral: ampules containing 0.5 or 1 g powder to be reconstituted as a 10% solution and used immediately
    Note: Suramin is not marketed in the USA but can be obtained from the Parasitic Disease Drug Service, Centers for Disease Control, Atlanta, 404-639-3670.
Thiabendazole (Mintezol)
    Oral: 500 mg chewable tablets; suspension, 500 mg/mL

REFERENCES

Ayles HM et al: A combined medical and surgical approach to hydatid disease: 12 years' experience at the Hospital for Tropical Diseases, London. Ann R Coll Surg Engl 2002;84:100.

Bagheri H et al: Adverse drug reactions to anthelmintics. Ann Pharmacother 2004;38:383.

Bockarie MJ et al: Mass treatment to eliminate filariasis in Papua New Guinea. N Engl J Med 2002;347:1841.

Carpio A: Neurocysticercosis: An update. Lancet Infect Dis 2002; 2:751.

Cioli D, Pica-Mattoccia L: Praziquantel. Parasitol Res 2003;90:S3.

Dayan AD: Albendazole, mebendazole and praziquantel. Review of non-clinical toxicity and pharmacokinetics. Acta Trop 2003; 86:141.

Drugs for parasitic infections. Med Lett Drugs Ther 2004;46:1. Issue available at http://www.medicalletter.com/freedocs/parasitic.pdf

El-On J: Benzimidazole treatment of cystic echinococcosis. Acta Trop 2003;85:243.

Fenwick A et al: Drugs for the control of parasitic diseases: Current status and development in schistosomiasis. Trends Parasitol 2003;19:509.

Ferrari ML et al: Efficacy of oxamniquine and praziquantel in the treatment of *Schistosoma mansoni* infection: A controlled trial. Bull World Health Organ 2003;81:190.

Garcia HH et al: A trial of antiparasitic treatment to reduce the rate of seizures due to cerebral cysticercosis. N Engl J Med 2004; 350:249.

Gardon J et al: Effects of standard and high doses of ivermectin on adult worms of *Onchocerca volvulus*: A randomised controlled trial. Lancet 2002;360:203.

Horton J: Albendazole: A broad spectrum anthelminthic for treatment of individuals and populations. Curr Opin Infect Dis 2002;15:599.

Molyneux DH et al: Mass drug treatment for lymphatic filariasis and onchocerciasis. Trends Parasitol 2003;19:516.

Proano JV et al: Medical treatment for neurocysticercosis characterized by giant subarachnoid cysts. N Engl J Med 2001;345:879

Smego RA Jr, Sebanego P: Treatment options for hepatic cystic echinococcosis. Int J Infect Dis 2005;9:69.

Stephenson I, Wiselka M: Drug treatment of tropical parasitic infections: Recent achievements and developments. Drugs 2000;60:985.

Taylor MJ, Hoerauf A: A new approach to the treatment of filariasis. Curr Opin Infect Dis 2001;14:727.

Taylor MJ et al: Macrofilaricidal activity after doxycycline treatment of *Wuchereria bancrofti*: A double-blind, randomised placebo-controlled trial. Lancet 2005;365:2116.

Tisch DJ, Michael E, Kazura JW: Mass chemotherapy options to control lymphatic filariasis: A systematic review. Lancet Infect Dis 2005;5:514.

Urbani C, Albonico M: Anthelminthic drug safety and drug administration in the control of soil-transmitted helminthiasis in community campaigns. Acta Trop 2003;86:215.

Utzinger J et al: Combination chemotherapy of schistosomiasis in laboratory studies and clinical trials. Antimicrob Agents Chemother 2003;47:1487.

Cancer Chemotherapy

Edward Chu, MD, & Alan C. Sartorelli, PhD

Cancer is a disease characterized by a shift in the control mechanisms that govern cell survival, proliferation, and differentiation. Cells that have undergone neoplastic transformation usually express cell surface antigens that may be of normal fetal type, may display other signs of apparent immaturity, and may exhibit qualitative or quantitative chromosomal abnormalities, including various translocations and the appearance of amplified gene sequences. Such cells proliferate excessively and form local tumors that can compress or invade adjacent normal structures. A small subpopulation of cells within the tumor can be described as **tumor stem cells.** They retain the ability to undergo repeated cycles of proliferation as well as to migrate to distant sites in the body to colonize various organs in the process called **metastasis.** Such tumor stem cells thus can express clonogenic or colony-forming capability. Tumor stem cells are characterized by chromosome abnormalities reflecting their genetic instability, which leads to progressive selection of subclones that can survive more readily in the multicellular environment of the host. Quantitative abnormalities in various metabolic pathways and cellular components accompany this neoplastic progression. The invasive and metastatic processes as well as a series of metabolic abnormalities resulting from the cancer cause illness and eventual death of the patient unless the neoplasm can be eradicated with treatment.

CAUSES OF CANCER

The incidence, geographic distribution, and behavior of specific types of cancer are related to multiple factors, including sex, age, race, genetic predisposition, and exposure to environmental carcinogens. Of these factors, environmental exposure is probably most important. Exposure to ionizing radiation has been well established to be a significant risk factor for a number of cancers, including acute leukemias, thyroid cancer, breast cancer, lung cancer, soft tissue sarcoma, and basal cell skin cancers. Chemical carcinogens (particularly those in tobacco smoke) as well as azo dyes, aflatoxins, asbestos, benzene, and radon have been clearly implicated in cancer induction in humans and animals. Identification of potential carcinogens in the environment has been greatly simplified by the widespread use

ACRONYMS	
ABVD	Doxorubicin (adriamycin), bleomycin, vinblastine, dacarbazine
CHOP	Cyclophosphamide, doxorubicin (hydroxydaunorubicin), vincristine (oncovin), prednisone
CMF	Cyclophosphamide, methotrexate, fluorouracil
COP	Cyclophosphamide, vincristine (oncovin), prednisone
FAC	Fluorouracil, doxorubicin (adriamycin), cyclophosphamide
FEC	Fluorouracil, epirubicin, cyclophosphamide
5-FU	5-Fluorouracil
IFL	Irinotecan, fluorouracil, leucovorin
MP	Melphalan, prednisone
6-MP	6-Mercaptopurine
MOPP	Mechlorethamine, vincristine (oncovin), procarbazine, prednisone
MTX	Methotrexate
PCV	Procarbazine, lomustine, vincristine
PEB	Cisplatin (platinum), etoposide, bleomycin
6-TG	6-Thioguanine
VAD	Vincristine, doxorubicin (adriamycin), dexamethasone

of the Ames test for mutagenic agents. Ninety percent of carcinogens can be shown to be mutagenic with this assay. Ultimate identification of potential human carcinogens, however, requires testing in at least two animal species.

Viruses have been implicated as the etiologic agents of several human cancers. Expression of virus-induced neoplasia probably also depends on additional host and environmental factors that modulate the transformation process. Cellular genes are known that are homologous to the transforming genes of the retroviruses, a family of RNA viruses, and induce oncogenic transformation. These mammalian cellular genes, known as **oncogenes,** have been shown to code for specific growth factors and their receptors and may be amplified (increased number of gene copies) or modified by a single nucleotide in malignant cells. The *bcl*-2 oncogene may be a generalized cell death suppressor gene that directly regulates apoptosis, a pathway of programmed cell death.

Another class of genes, **tumor suppressor genes,** may be deleted or damaged, with resulting neoplastic change. The *p53* gene has been shown to be mutated in up to 50% of all human solid tumors, including liver, breast, colon, lung, cervix, bladder, prostate, and skin. The normal wild form of this gene appears to play an important role in suppressing neoplastic transformation; mutations in this gene place the cell at high risk.

CANCER THERAPEUTIC MODALITIES

In 2005, cancer was the most common cause of death from disease in the USA, causing over 500,000 fatalities. With present methods of treatment, one third of patients are cured with local modalities (surgery or radiation therapy), which are quite effective if the tumor has not metastasized by the time of treatment. Earlier diagnosis might lead to increased cure rates with such local treatment; however, in the remaining cases, early micrometastasis is a characteristic feature of the neoplasm, indicating that a systemic approach such as chemotherapy is required (often along with surgery or radiation) for effective cancer management. At present, about 50% of patients who initially are diagnosed with cancer can be cured. However, chemotherapy is able to cure only about 10–15% of all cancer patients.

Cancer chemotherapy, as currently employed, can be curative in certain disseminated neoplasms that have undergone either gross or microscopic spread by the time of diagnosis. These cancers include germ cell cancer, non-Hodgkin's lymphoma, Hodgkin's disease, and choriocarcinoma as well as childhood cancers such as acute lymphoblastic leukemia, Burkitt's lymphoma, Wilms' tumor, and embryonal rhabdomyosarcoma. In an increasing number of cancers, the use of chemotherapy combined with radiation therapy followed by surgery can increase the cure rate; these include locally advanced bladder cancer, breast cancer, esophageal cancer, head and neck cancer, rectal cancer, and osteogenic sarcoma.

In patients with widespread disseminated disease, chemotherapy provides only palliative rather than curative therapy at present. Effective palliation results in temporary improvement of the symptoms and signs of cancer and enhancement in the overall quality of life. In the past decade, advances in cancer chemotherapy have also begun to provide evidence that chemical control of neoplasia may become a reality for many forms of cancer. This will probably be achieved through a combined-modality approach in which optimal combina-

tions of surgery, radiotherapy, and chemotherapy are used to eradicate both the primary neoplasm and its occult micrometastases before gross spread can be detected on physical or x-ray examination. Use of hormonal agents to modulate tumor growth is playing an increasing role in hormone-responsive tumors thanks to the development of hormone antagonists and partial agonists. Several recombinant biologic agents have been identified as being active for cancer therapy, including certain cytokines.

ANTICANCER DRUG DEVELOPMENT

A major effort to develop anticancer drugs through both empiric screening and rational design of new compounds has been under way for over 3 decades. The drug development program has employed testing in a few well-characterized transplantable animal tumor systems. Simple in vitro assays for measuring drug sensitivity of a battery of human tumor cells augment and shorten the testing program and are used currently as the primary screening tests for new agents. New drugs with potential anticancer activity are subjected to preclinical toxicologic and limited pharmacologic studies in animals as described in Chapter 5. Promising agents that do not have excessive toxicity are then advanced to phase I clinical trials, wherein their pharmacologic and toxic effects are usually tested in patients with advanced cancer. Other features of clinical testing are similar to the procedure for other drugs but may be accelerated.

Under ideal circumstances, anticancer drugs would eradicate cancer cells without harming normal tissues. Unfortunately, no agents currently available are completely devoid of toxicity, and clinical use of these drugs involves a weighing of benefits against toxicity in a search for a favorable therapeutic index.

Classes of drugs that have recently entered clinical development include signal transduction inhibitors, focused on critical signaling pathways essential for cell growth and proliferation; microtubule inhibitors, directed against the mitotic spindle apparatus; differentiation agents, intended to force neoplastic cells past a maturation block to form end-stage cells with little or no proliferative potential; antimetastatic drugs, designed to perturb surface properties of malignant cells and thus reduce their invasive and metastatic potential; antiangiogenic agents, designed to inhibit the formation of tumor vasculature; hypoxic tumor stem cell-specific agents, designed to exploit the greater capacity for reductive reactions in these often therapeutically resistant cells; tumor radiosensitizing and normal tissue radioprotecting drugs, aimed at increased therapeutic effectiveness of radiation therapy; cytoprotective agents, focused on protecting certain normal tissues against the toxic effects of chemotherapy; and biologic response modifiers, which alter tumor-host metabolic and immunologic relationships.

IMPORTANCE OF NEOPLASTIC CELL BURDEN

Patients with widespread cancer may have up to 10^{12} tumor cells throughout the body at the time of diagnosis (Figure 55–1). If tolerable dosing of an effective drug is capable of killing 99.99% (ie, 10^4) of clonogenic tumor cells, treatment would induce a clinical remission of the neoplasm associated with symptomatic improvement. However, there would still be up to 8 "logs" of tumor cells (10^8) remaining in the body, including those that might be inherently resistant to the drug because of tumor heterogeneity. There may also be other tumor cells that reside in pharmacologic sanctuary sites (eg, the central nervous system, testes), where effective drug concentrations may be difficult to achieve. When cell cycle-specific drugs are used, the tumor stem cells must also be in the sensitive phase of the cell cycle (not in G_0). For this reason, scheduling of these agents is particularly important. In common bacterial infections, a three-log reduction in microorganisms might be curative because host resistance factors can eliminate residual bacteria through immunologic and microbicidal mechanisms; however, host mechanisms for eliminating even moderate numbers of cancer cells appear to be generally ineffective.

Combinations of agents with differing toxicities and mechanisms of action are often employed to overcome the limited log kill of individual anticancer drugs. If drugs display nonoverlapping toxicities, they can be used at almost full dosage, and at least additive cytotoxic effects can be achieved with combination chemotherapy; furthermore, subclones resistant to only one of the agents can potentially be eradicated. Some combinations of anticancer drugs also appear to exert true synergism, wherein the effect of the two drugs is greater than additive. The efficacy of combination chemotherapy has now been validated in many human cancers, and combination chemotherapy is now the standard approach to curative treatment of testicular cancer and lymphomas and to palliative treatment of many other tumor types. This important therapeutic approach was first formulated by Skipper and Schabel and described as the log-kill hypothesis (Figure 55–1).

The growth of acute leukemias and aggressive high-grade lymphomas closely follows exponential cell kinetics. In contrast, most human solid tumors do not grow in such a manner; instead, they follow a Gompertzian model of tumor growth and regression. Under Gompertzian kinetics, the growth fraction of the tumor is not constant and peaks when the tumor is about one third of its maximum size.

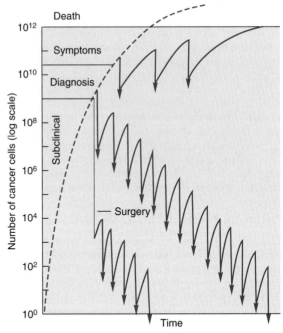

Figure 55–1. The log-kill hypothesis. Relationship of tumor cell number to time of diagnosis, symptoms, treatment, and survival. Three alternative approaches to drug treatment are shown for comparison with the course of tumor growth when no treatment is given *(dashed line)*. In the protocol diagrammed at top, treatment (indicated by the arrows) is given infrequently and the result is manifested as prolongation of survival but with recurrence of symptoms between courses of treatment and eventual death of the patient. The combination chemotherapy treatment diagrammed in the middle section is begun earlier and is more intensive. Tumor cell kill exceeds regrowth, drug resistance does not develop, and "cure" results. In this example, treatment has been continued long after all clinical evidence of cancer has disappeared (1–3 years). This approach has been established as effective in the treatment of childhood acute leukemia, testicular cancers, and Hodgkin's disease. In the treatment diagrammed near the bottom of the graph, early surgery has been employed to remove the primary tumor and intensive adjuvant chemotherapy has been administered long enough (up to 1 year) to eradicate the remaining tumor cells that comprise the occult micrometastases.

IMPORTANCE OF CELL CYCLE KINETICS

Information on cell and population kinetics of cancer cells explains, in part, the limited effectiveness of most available anticancer drugs. A schematic summary of cell cycle kinetics is presented in Figure 55–2. This infor-

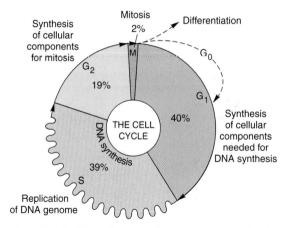

Figure 55–2. The cell cycle and cancer. A conceptual depiction of the cell cycle phases that all cells—normal and neoplastic—must traverse before and during cell division. The percentages given represent the approximate percentage of time spent in each phase by a typical malignant cell; the duration of G_1, however, can vary markedly. Many of the effective anticancer drugs exert their action on cells traversing the cell cycle and are called cell cycle–specific (CCS) drugs (Table 55–1). A second group of agents called cell cycle–nonspecific (CCNS) drugs can sterilize tumor cells whether they are cycling or resting in the G_0 compartment. CCNS drugs can kill both G_0 and cycling cells (although cycling cells are more sensitive).

mation is relevant to the mode of action, indications, and scheduling of **cell cycle–specific (CCS)** and **cell cycle–nonspecific (CCNS)** drugs. Agents falling into these two major classes are summarized in Table 55–1.

In general, CCS drugs are most effective in hematologic malignancies and in solid tumors in which a relatively large proportion of the cells are proliferating or are in the growth fraction. CCNS drugs (many of which bind to cellular DNA and damage these macromolecules) are particularly useful in low growth fraction solid tumors as well as in high growth fraction tumors. In all instances, effective agents sterilize or inactivate tumor stem cells, which are often only a small fraction of the cells within a tumor. Non-stem cells (eg, those that have irreversibly differentiated) are considered sterile by definition and are not a significant component of the cancer problem.

Resistance to Cytotoxic Drugs

A major problem in cancer chemotherapy is the development of cellular drug resistance. Some tumor types, eg, malignant melanoma, renal cell cancer, and brain cancer, exhibit *primary* resistance, ie, absence of response on the

first exposure, to currently available standard agents. The presence of inherent drug resistance is thought to be tightly associated with the genomic instability associated with the development of most cancers. *Acquired* resistance develops in a number of drug-sensitive tumor types. Experimentally, drug resistance can be highly specific to a single drug and usually is based on a change in the genetic apparatus of a given tumor cell with amplification or increased expression of one or more specific genes. In other instances, a multidrug-resistant phenotype occurs—resistance to a variety of natural product anticancer drugs of differing structures developing after exposure to a single agent. This form of multidrug resistance is often associated with increased expression of a normal gene (the *MDR1* gene) for a cell surface glycoprotein (**P-glycoprotein**) involved in drug efflux. This transport molecule requires ATP to expel a variety of foreign molecules (not limited to antitumor drugs) from the cell. It is expressed constitutively in normal tissues such as the epithelial cells of the kidney, large intestine, and adrenal gland as well as in a variety of tumors. Multidrug resistance can be reversed experimentally by calcium channel blockers, such as verapamil, and a variety of other drugs, which inhibit the transporter. Other mecha-

Table 55–1. Cell cycle effects of major classes of anticancer drugs.

Cell Cycle–Specific (CCS) Agents	Cell Cycle–Nonspecific (CCNS) Agents
Antimetabolites	**Alkylating agents**
Capecitabine	Busulfan
Cladribine	Carmustine
Cytarabine	Cyclophosphamide
Fludarabine	Lomustine
5-Fluorouracil (5-FU)	Mechlorethamine
Gemcitabine	Melphalan
6-Mercaptopurine (6-MP)	Thiotepa
Methotrexate (MTX)	**Anthracyclines**
6-Thioguanine (6-TG)	Daunorubicin
Antitumor antibiotic	Doxorubicin
Bleomycin	Epirubicin
Epipodophyllotoxins	Idarubicin
Etoposide	Mitoxantrone
Teniposide	**Antitumor antibiotics**
Taxanes	Dactinomycin
Albumin-bound paclitaxel	Mitomycin
Docetaxel	**Camptothecins**
Paclitaxel	Irinotecan
Vinca alkaloids	Topotecan
Vinblastine	**Platinum analogs**
Vincristine	Carboplatin
Vinorelbine	Cisplatin
	Oxaliplatin

nisms of multiple drug resistance involve overexpression of the **multidrug resistance protein 1 (MRP1),** a member of the ATP-binding cassette transmembrane transporter superfamily that now consists of nine members (MRP1-MRP9). MRP1, the most extensively studied, increases resistance to natural product drugs such as anthracyclines, vinca alkaloids, taxanes, and epipodophyllotoxins by functioning as a drug export pump.

■ I. BASIC PHARMACOLOGY OF CANCER CHEMOTHERAPEUTIC DRUGS

POLYFUNCTIONAL ALKYLATING AGENTS

The major clinically useful alkylating agents (Figure 55–3) have a structure containing a bis(chloroethyl)amine, ethyleneimine, or nitrosourea moiety. Among the bis(chloroethyl)amines, cyclophosphamide, mechlorethamine, melphalan, and chlorambucil are the most useful. Ifosfamide is closely related to cyclophosphamide but has a somewhat different spectrum of activity and toxicity. Thiotepa and busulfan are used for specialized purposes for ovarian cancer and chronic myeloid leukemia, respectively. The major nitrosoureas are carmustine (BCNU), lomustine (CCNU), and semustine (methyl-CCNU). A variety of investigational alkylating agents have been synthesized that link various carrier molecules such as amino acids, nucleic acid bases, hormones, or sugar moieties to a group capable of alkylation; however, successful site-directed alkylation has not been achieved to date.

Mechanism of Action

As a class, the alkylating agents exert their cytotoxic effects via transfer of their alkyl groups to various cellular constituents. Alkylations of DNA within the nucleus probably represent the major interactions that lead to cell death. However, these drugs react chemically with sulfhydryl, amino, hydroxyl, carboxyl, and phosphate groups of other cellular nucleophiles as well. The general mechanism of action of these drugs involves intramolecular cyclization to form an ethyleneimonium ion that may directly or through formation of a carbonium ion transfer an alkyl group to a cellular constituent. In addition to alkylation, a secondary mechanism that occurs with nitrosoureas involves carbamoylation of lysine residues of proteins through formation of isocyanates.

The major site of alkylation within DNA is the N7 position of guanine (Figure 55–4); however, other bases are also alkylated to lesser degrees, including N1 and N3 of adenine, N3 of cytosine, and O6 of guanine, as well as phosphate atoms and proteins associated with DNA. These interactions can occur on a single strand or on both strands of DNA through cross-linking, as most major alkylating agents are bifunctional, with two reactive groups. Alkylation of guanine can result in miscoding through abnormal base pairing with thymine or in depurination by excision of guanine residues. The latter effect leads to DNA strand breakage through scission of the sugar-phosphate backbone of DNA. Cross-linking of DNA appears to be of major importance to the cytotoxic action of alkylating agents, and replicating cells are most susceptible to these drugs. Thus, although alkylating agents are not cell cycle-specific, cells are most susceptible to alkylation in late G_1 and S phases of the cell cycle and express block in G_2.

Drug Resistance

The mechanism of acquired resistance to alkylating agents may involve increased capability to repair DNA lesions, decreased permeability of the cell to the alkylating drug, and increased production of glutathione, which inactivates the alkylating agent through conjugation or through increased glutathione S-transferase activity, which catalyzes the conjugation.

Pharmacologic Effects

Alkylating agents have direct vesicant effects and can damage tissues at the site of injection as well as produce systemic toxicity. Toxicities are generally dose related and occur particularly in rapidly growing tissues such as bone marrow, the gastrointestinal tract, and the reproductive system. After intravenous injection, nausea and vomiting usually occur within 30–60 minutes with mechlorethamine, cyclophosphamide, or carmustine. The emetogenic effects are mediated by the central nervous system and can be reduced by pretreatment with 5-HT$_3$ (serotonin) receptor antagonists such as ondansetron or granisetron.

Cyclophosphamide is inactive in its parent form, and must be activated to cytotoxic forms by liver microsomal enzymes (Figure 55–5). The cytochrome P450 mixed-function oxidase system converts cyclophosphamide to 4-hydroxycyclophosphamide, which is in equilibrium with aldophosphamide. These active metabolites are believed to be delivered by the bloodstream to both tumor and normal tissue, where nonenzymatic cleavage of aldophosphamide to the cytotoxic forms—phosphoramide mustard and acrolein—occurs. The liver appears to be protected through the enzymatic formation of the inactive metabolites 4-ketocyclophosphamide and carboxyphosphamide.

BIS(CHLOROETHYL)AMINES

Where R is:

Cyclophosphamide

Mechlorethamine

Chlorambucil

Melphalan

NITROSOUREAS

Where R is:

— CH₂CH₂Cl

**BCNU
(carmustine)**

**CCNU
(lomustine)**

**Methyl-CCNU
(semustine)**

AZIRIDINES

Thiotepa

Triethylenemelamine

ALKYLSULFONATE

Busulfan

Figure 55–3. Structures of major classes of alkylating agents.

The major toxicities of alkylating agents are outlined in Table 55–2 and discussed below.

Oral administration of alkylating agents has been of great clinical value. Cyclophosphamide, melphalan, chlorambucil, busulfan, and, more recently, temozolomide are those most commonly given via the oral route, and their cytotoxic effects are similar to those observed with parenteral administration. In general, if a tumor is resistant to one alkylating agent, it will be relatively resistant to other agents of this class (though not necessarily to nitrosoureas); however, there are exceptions to this rule depending on the specific tumor. Cyclophosphamide is the most widely used alkylating agent. The oral drug busulfan has a major degree of specificity for the granulocyte series and is therefore of particular value in the treatment of chronic myelogenous leukemia. With all oral alkylating agents, some degree of leukopenia is necessary to provide evidence that the drug has been absorbed adequately. Frequent monitoring of blood counts is essential during administration of these agents

as the development of severe leukopenia or thrombocytopenia necessitates immediate interruption of therapy.

NITROSOUREAS

These drugs appear to be non-cross-resistant with other alkylating agents; all require biotransformation, which occurs by nonenzymatic decomposition, to metabolites with both alkylating and carbamoylating activities. The nitrosoureas are highly lipid-soluble and are able to cross the blood-brain barrier, making them useful in the treatment of brain tumors. Although the majority of alkylations by the nitrosoureas are on the N7 position of guanine in DNA, the critical alkylation responsible for cytotoxicity is on the O6 of guanine, which leads to G-C crosslinks in DNA. After oral administration of lomustine, peak plasma levels of metabolites appear within 1–4 hours; central nervous system concentrations reach 30–40% of the activity present in the plasma. While the initial plasma half-life is approximately 6 hours, a second

Figure 55–4. Mechanism of alkylation of DNA guanine. A bis(chloroethyl)amine forms an ethyleneimonium ion and a carbonium ion that react with a base such as N7 of guanine in DNA, producing an alkylated purine. Alkylation of a second guanine residue, through the illustrated mechanism, results in cross-linking of DNA strands.

Figure 55–5. Cyclophosphamide metabolism.

Table 55–2. Alkylating agents: Dosages and toxicities.

Alkylating Agent	Single-Agent Dosage	Acute Toxicity	Delayed Toxicity
Mechlorethamine (nitrogen mustard)	0.4 mg/kg IV in single or divided doses	Nausea and vomiting	Moderate depression of peripheral blood count; excessive doses produce severe bone marrow depression with leukopenia, thrombocytopenia, and bleeding; alopecia and hemorrhagic cystitis occasionally occur with cyclophosphamide; cystitis can be prevented with adequate hydration; busulfan is associated with skin pigmentation, pulmonary fibrosis, and adrenal insufficiency
Chlorambucil	0.1–0.2 mg/kg/d orally; 6–12 mg/d	Nausea and vomiting	
Cyclophosphamide	3.5–5 mg/kg/d orally for 10 days; 1 g/m^2 IV as single dose	Nausea and vomiting	
Melphalan	0.25 mg/kg/d orally for 4 days every 4–6 weeks	Nausea and vomiting	
Thiotepa (triethylenethio-phosphoramide)	0.2 mg/kg IV for 5 days	Nausea and vomiting	
Busulfan	2–8 mg/d orally; 150–250 mg/course	Nausea and vomiting	
Carmustine (BCNU)	200 mg/m^2 IV every 6 weeks	Nausea and vomiting	Leukopenia, thrombocytopenia, and rarely hepatitis
Lomustine (CCNU)	150 mg/m^2 orally every 6 weeks	Nausea and vomiting	
Altretamine	10 mg/kg/d for 21 days	Nausea and vomiting	Leukopenia, thrombocytopenia, and peripheral neuropathy
Temozolomide	150 mg/m^2 orally for 5 days every 28 days	Nausea and vomiting, headache and fatigue	Leukopenia, thrombocytopenia
Procarbazine	50–200 mg/d orally	Nausea and vomiting	Bone marrow depression, central nervous system depression, leukemogenic
Dacarbazine	300 mg/m^2 daily IV for 5 days	Nausea and vomiting	Bone marrow depression
Cisplatin	20 mg/m^2/d IV for 5 days or 50–70 mg/m^2 as single dose every 3 weeks	Nausea and vomiting	Nephrotoxicity, peripheral sensory neuropathy, ototoxicity, nerve dysfunction
Carboplatin	AUC 5–7 mg x min/mL	Nausea and vomiting	Myelosuppression; rarely: peripheral neuropathy, renal toxicity, and hepatic dysfunction
Oxaliplatin	130 mg/m^2 IV every 3 weeks or 85 mg/m^2 IV every 2 weeks	Nausea and vomiting, laryngopharyngeal dysesthesias	Peripheral sensory neuropathy, diarrhea, myelosuppression, and renal toxicity

half-life is 1–2 days. Urinary excretion appears to be the major route of elimination from the body. One naturally occurring sugar-containing nitrosourea, streptozocin, is interesting because it has minimal bone marrow toxicity. This agent has activity in the treatment of insulin-secreting islet cell carcinoma of the pancreas.

RELATED DRUGS ACTING AS ALKYLATING AGENTS

A variety of other compounds have mechanisms of action that involve alkylation. These include procarbazine, dacarbazine, altretamine (hexamethylmelamine),

cisplatin, and carboplatin. Dosages and major toxicities are listed in Table 55–2.

1. Procarbazine

The oral agent procarbazine is a methylhydrazine derivative, and it is commonly used in combination regimens for Hodgkin's disease, non-Hodgkin's lymphoma, and brain tumors. This drug has leukemogenic, teratogenic, and mutagenic properties.

The precise mechanism of action of procarbazine is uncertain; however, the drug inhibits DNA, RNA, and protein biosynthesis; prolongs interphase; and produces chromosome breaks. Oxidative metabolism of this drug by microsomal enzymes generates azoprocarbazine and H_2O_2, which may be responsible for DNA strand scission. A variety of other drug metabolites are formed that may be cytotoxic. One metabolite is a weak monoamine oxidase (MAO) inhibitor, and adverse effects can occur when procarbazine is given with other MAO inhibitors.

There is an increased risk of secondary cancers in the form of acute leukemia, and the carcinogenic potential of procarbazine is thought to be higher than that of most other alkylating agents.

2. Dacarbazine

Dacarbazine is a synthetic compound that functions as an alkylating agent following metabolic activation by liver microsomal enzymes by oxidative N-demethylation to the monomethyl derivative. This metabolite spontaneously decomposes to 5-aminoimidazole-4-carboxamide, which is excreted in the urine, and diazomethane. The diazomethane generates a methyl carbonium ion that is believed to be the cytotoxic species. Dacarbazine is administered parenterally and is not schedule-dependent. It produces marked nausea, vomiting, and myelosuppression. Its major applications are in melanoma, Hodgkin's disease, and soft tissue sarcomas.

3. Altretamine

Altretamine (Hexamethylmelamine) is structurally similar to triethylenemelamine. It is relatively insoluble and available only in oral form. It is rapidly biotransformed in the liver by demethylation to the pentamethylmelamine and tetramethylmelamine metabolites. This agent is approved for use in ovarian cancer patients who have progressed despite treatment with a regimen based on platinum or an alkylating agent (or both). The main dose-limiting toxicities include nausea, vomiting, and myelosuppression. Neurotoxicity in the form of somnolence, mood changes, and peripheral neuropathy is also observed.

4. Platinum Analogs

Cisplatin (cis-diamminedichloroplatinum [II]) is an inorganic metal complex discovered through the serendipitous observation that neutral platinum complexes inhibited division and induced filamentous growth of *Escherichia coli*. Several platinum analogs have been subsequently synthesized. Although the precise mechanism of action of cisplatin is still undefined, it is thought to exert its cytotoxic effects in the same manner as alkylating agents. It kills cells in all stages of the cell cycle, binds DNA through the formation of intrastrand and interstrand cross-links, and inhibits DNA

synthesis and function. The primary binding site is the N7 position of guanine, but covalent interaction with adenine and cytosine also occurs. The platinum complexes appear to synergize with certain other anticancer drugs. Aggressive hydration with intravenous saline infusion has been shown to significantly reduce the incidence of nephrotoxicity.

Cisplatin

Cisplatin has major antitumor activity in a broad range of solid tumors, including non-small cell and small cell lung cancer, esophageal and gastric cancer, head and neck cancer, and genitourinary cancers, particularly testicular, ovarian, and bladder cancer. When used in combination regimens with vinblastine and bleomycin or etoposide and bleomycin, cisplatin-based therapy has led to the cure of nonseminomatous testicular cancer.

Carboplatin is a second-generation platinum analog that exerts its cytotoxic effects exactly as cisplatin and has activity against the same spectrum of solid tumors. Its main dose-limiting toxicity is myelosuppression, and it has significantly less renal toxicity and gastrointestinal toxicity than cisplatin. Intravenous hydration is not required, and for this reason, carboplatin has now widely replaced cisplatin in combination chemotherapy regimens.

Oxaliplatin is a third-generation diaminocyclohexane platinum analog. Its mechanism of action is identical to that of cisplatin and carboplatin. However, cancer cells that are resistant to cisplatin or carboplatin on the basis of mismatch repair defects are not cross-resistant to oxaliplatin. This agent was originally approved for use as second-line therapy in metastatic colorectal cancer following treatment with the combination of 5-fluorouracil and leucovorin (5-FU/LV)—the FOLFOX regimen. The FOLFOX regimen has now become the most widely used regimen in the first-line treatment of advanced colorectal cancer, and it is now widely used in the adjuvant therapy of stage III colon cancer. Neurotoxicity is dose-limiting and characterized by a peripheral sensory neuropathy. There are two forms of neurotoxicity, an acute form that is often triggered and worsened by exposure to cold, and a chronic form that is dose-dependent. Although this chronic form is cumulative in nature, it tends to be reversible, in sharp contrast to cisplatin-induced neurotoxicity.

ANTIMETABOLITES

The development of drugs with actions on intermediary metabolism of proliferating cells has been important both conceptually and clinically. While biochemical properties unique to all cancer cells have yet to be discovered, neoplastic cells do have a number of quantitative differences in metabolism from normal cells that render them more susceptible to a number of antimetabolites or structural analogs. Many of these agents have been rationally designed and synthesized based on knowledge of critical cellular processes involved in DNA biosynthesis.

Mechanisms of Action

The biochemical pathways that have thus far proved to be most vulnerable to antimetabolites have been those relating to nucleotide and nucleic acid synthesis. In a number of instances, when an enzyme is known to have a major effect on pathways leading to cell replication, inhibitors of the reaction it catalyzes have proved to be useful anticancer drugs.

These drugs and their doses and toxicities are shown in Table 55–3. The principal drugs are discussed below.

METHOTREXATE

Methotrexate (MTX) is a folic acid antagonist that binds to the active catalytic site of dihydrofolate reductase (DHFR), interfering with the synthesis of the reduced form that accepts one-carbon units. Lack of this cofactor interrupts the de novo synthesis of thymidylate, purine nucleotides, and the amino acids serine and methionine, thereby interfering with the formation of DNA, RNA, and key cellular proteins. DHFR binds methotrexate with high affinity, and at pH 6.0, virtually no dissociation of the enzyme-inhibitor complex occurs (inhibition constant about 1 nM). At physiologic pH, reversible competitive kinetics occur (inhibition constant about 1 μM). Intracellular formation of polyglutamate derivatives is critically important for the therapeutic action of methotrexate, and this process is mediated by the enzyme folylpolyglutamate synthase (FPGS). MTX polyglutamates are selectively retained within cancer cells, and they display increased inhibitory effects on enzymes involved in folate metabolism, making them important determinants of the duration of action of methotrexate.

Drug Resistance

Resistance to methotrexate has been attributed to (1) decreased drug transport, (2) decreased formation of cytotoxic MTX polyglutamates, (3) synthesis of increased levels of DHFR through gene amplification, and (4) altered DHFR with reduced affinity for methotrexate. Recent studies have also suggested that decreased accumulation of drug through activation of the multidrug resistance P170 glycoprotein transporter may also result in drug resistance.

Folic acid

Methotrexate

Dosage & Toxicity

Methotrexate is administered by the intravenous, intrathecal, or oral route. Up to 90% of an oral dose is excreted in the urine within 12 hours. The drug is not subject to metabolism, and serum levels are therefore proportionate to dose as long as renal function and hydration status are adequate. Dosages and toxic effects are listed in Table 55–3. The effects of methotrexate can be reversed by administration of the reduced folate leucovorin (5-formyltetrahydrofolate). Leucovorin rescue is generally used in conjunction with high-dose methotrexate therapy to rescue normal cells from undue toxicity and it has also been used in cases of accidental drug overdose.

PEMETREXED

Pemetrexed is a pyrrolopyrimidine antifolate analog with activity in the S phase of the cell cycle. As in the case of MTX, it is transported into the cell via the reduced folate carrier and requires activation by the enzyme FPGS to yield higher polyglutamate forms. While this agent targets DHFR and enzymes involved in de novo purine nucleotide synthesis, its main site of action is via inhibition of thymidylate synthase. At present, this antifolate is approved for use in combination with cisplatin in the treatment of mesothelioma and as a single agent in the second-line therapy of non-small cell lung cancer. The main adverse effects are outlined in Table 55–3 and include myelosuppression, skin rash, mucositis, diarrhea, and fatigue.

Table 55–3. Antimetabolites: Dosages and toxicities.

Chemotherapeutic Agent	Single-Agent Dosage	Delayed Toxicity[1]
Capecitabine	1250 mg/m^2/bid orally for 14 days followed by 1 week of rest. Repeat every 3 weeks.	Diarrhea, hand-and-foot syndrome, myelosuppression, nausea and vomiting
Cladribine	0.09 mg/kg/d for 7 days by continuous IV infusion in sterile saline	Myelosuppression, nausea and vomiting, and immunosuppression
Cytarabine	100 mg/m^2/d for 5–10 days, either by continuous IV infusion or SC every 8 hours.	Nausea and vomiting, bone marrow depression with leukopenia and thrombocytopenia, and cerebellar ataxia
Fludarabine	25 mg/m^2/d for 5 days every 28 days (administer IV over 30 minutes)	Myelosuppression, immunosuppression, fever, myalgias, and arthralgias
5-Fluorouracil	15 mg/kg/d IV for 5 days by 24-hour infusion; 15 mg/kg weekly IV	Nausea, mucositis, diarrhea, bone marrow depression, and neurotoxicity
Gemcitabine	1000 mg/m^2 IV weekly for up to 7 weeks followed by 1 week of rest	Nausea, vomiting, diarrhea, myelosuppression
6-Mercaptopurine	2.5 mg/kg/d orally	Myelosuppression, immunosuppression, and hepatotoxicity
Methotrexate	2.5–5 mg/d orally (Rheumatrex); 10 mg intrathecally (Folex) once or twice weekly	Mucositis, diarrhea, bone marrow depression with leukopenia and thrombocytopenia
Pemetrexed	500 mg/m^2 IV every 3 weeks	Myelosuppression, skin rash, mucositis, diarrhea, and fatigue
6-Thioguanine	2 mg/kg/d orally	Myelosuppression, immunosuppression, and hepatotoxicity

[1]These drugs do not cause acute toxicity.

PURINE ANTAGONISTS

1. 6-Thiopurines

6-Mercaptopurine (6-MP) was the first of the thiopurine analogs found to be effective in cancer therapy. As with other thiopurines, it is inactive in its parent form and must be metabolized by hypoxanthine-guanine phosphoribosyl transferase (HGPRT) to the monophosphate nucleotide 6-thioinosinic acid, which in turn inhibits several enzymes of de novo purine nucleotide synthesis. Significant levels of thioguanylic acid and 6-methylmercaptopurine ribotide (MMPR) are also formed from 6-MP. These metabolites also contribute to its cytotoxic action. 6-MP is used primarily in the treatment of childhood acute leukemia, and a closely related analog, azathioprine, is used as an immunosuppressive agent (see Chapter 56).

6-Thioguanine (6-TG) inhibits several enzymes in the de novo purine nucleotide biosynthetic pathway. Various metabolic lesions result, including inhibition of purine nucleotide interconversion; decrease in intracellular levels of guanine nucleotides, which leads to inhibition of glycoprotein synthesis; interference with the formation of DNA and RNA; and incorporation of thiopurine nucleotides into both DNA and RNA. 6-TG has a synergistic action when used together with cytarabine in the treatment of adult acute leukemia.

Drug Resistance

Resistance to both 6-MP and 6-TG occurs most commonly by decreased expression of the activating enzyme (HGPRT); an alternative mechanism in acute leukemia involves increased expression or activity of the catabolic enzyme alkaline phosphatase, which results in dephosphorylation of thiopurine nucleotides and cellular loss of the resulting ribonucleoside. In addition, increased expression of thiopurine methyltransferase (TMPT) has been observed in thiopurine-resistant acute leukemic cells.

Dosage & Toxicity

6-MP and 6-TG are both given orally (Table 55–3) and excreted mainly in the urine. However, 6-MP is converted to an inactive metabolite (6-thiouric acid) by an oxidation catalyzed by xanthine oxidase, whereas 6-TG requires deamination before it is metabolized by this enzyme. This factor is important because the purine analog allopurinol, a potent xanthine oxidase inhibitor, is frequently used with chemotherapy in hematologic cancers to prevent hyperuricemia after tumor cell lysis. It does so by blocking purine oxidation, allowing excretion of cellular purines that are relatively more soluble than uric acid. Nephrotoxicity and acute gout produced by excessive uric acid are thereby prevented. Simultaneous therapy with allopurinol and 6-MP results in excessive toxicity unless the dose of mercaptopurine is reduced to 25% of the usual level. This effect does not occur with 6-TG, which can be used in full doses with allopurinol.

Hypoxanthine   **6-Mercaptopurine**   **Allopurinol**

Guanine   **6-Thioguanine**

2. Fludarabine

Fludarabine phosphate is rapidly dephosphorylated to 2-fluoro-arabinofuranosyladenosine and then phosphorylated intracellularly by deoxycytidine kinase to the triphosphate. The triphosphate metabolite interferes with the processes of DNA synthesis and DNA repair through inhibition of DNA polymerase-α and DNA polymerase-β. The triphosphate form can also be directly incorporated into DNA, resulting in inhibition of DNA synthesis and function. The diphosphate metabolite of fludarabine inhibits ribonucleotide reductase, leading to inhibition of essential deoxyribonucleotidetriphosphates. Finally, fludarabine induces the process of apoptosis through as yet undetermined mechanisms. Fludarabine is used chiefly in the treatment of low-grade non-Hodgkin's lymphoma and chronic lymphocytic leukemia (CLL). It is given parentally and is excreted primarily in the urine; its dose-limiting toxicity is myelosuppression. In addition, this agent is a potent immunosuppressant with inhibitory effects on CD4 and CD8 T cells. Patients are at increased risk for opportunistic infections, including fungi, herpes, and *Pneumocystis jiroveci.*

3. Cladribine

Cladribine (2-chlorodeoxyadenosine) is a purine nucleoside analog with high specificity for lymphoid cells. Inactive in its parent form, it is initially phosphorylated by deoxycytidine kinase to the monophosphate form and eventually metabolized to the triphosphate form, which can then be incorporated into DNA. The triphosphate metabolite can also interfere with DNA synthesis and DNA repair by inhibiting DNA polymerase-α and DNA-polymerase-β, respectively. Cladribine is indicated for the treatment of hairy cell leukemia, and it also has activity in CLL and low-grade non-Hodgkin's lymphoma. It is normally administered as a single continuous 7-day infusion; under these conditions, it has a very manageable safety profile with the main toxicity consisting of transient myelosuppression. In addition, it has immunosuppressive effects, and a decrease in CD4 and CD8 T cells, lasting for over 1 year, is observed in patients.

PYRIMIDINE ANTAGONISTS

1. 5-Fluorouracil

5-Fluorouracil (5-FU) is a prodrug requiring activation via a complex series of biotransformation reactions to ribosyl and deoxyribosyl nucleotide metabolites. One of these metabolites, 5-fluoro-2'-deoxyuridine-5'-monophosphate (FdUMP), forms a covalently bound ternary complex with the enzyme thymidylate synthase and the reduced folate $N^{5,10}$-methylenetetrahydrofolate, a reaction critical for the de novo synthesis of thymidylate. This results in inhibition of DNA synthesis through "thymineless death." 5-FU is converted to 5-fluorouridine-5'-triphosphate (FUTP), which is then incorporated into RNA, where it interferes with RNA processing and mRNA translation. In addition, 5-FU is converted to 5-fluorodeoxyuridine-5'-triphosphate (FdUTP), which can be incorporated into cellular DNA, resulting in inhibition of DNA synthesis and function. Thus, the cytotoxicity of 5-FU is thought to be the result of the combined effects on both DNA- and RNA-mediated events.

Uracil   **5-FU**

5-FU is normally administered intravenously (Table 55–3) and has a half-life of 10–15 minutes. It is not administered by the oral route because its bioavailability is impaired by the high levels of the breakdown enzyme dihydropyrimidine dehydrogenase present in the gut mucosa. Up to 80–85% of an administered dose of 5-FU is catabolized by this enzyme.

5-FU is the most widely used agent in the treatment of colorectal cancer, both as adjuvant therapy and for advanced disease. In addition, it has activity against a wide variety of solid tumors, including cancers of the breast, stomach, pancreas, esophagus, liver, head and neck, and anus. Its major toxicities are listed in Table 55–3.

2. Capecitabine

Capecitabine is a fluoropyrimidine carbamate prodrug with nearly 70–80% oral bioavailability. It undergoes extensive metabolism in the liver by the enzyme carboxylesterase to an intermediate, 5′-deoxy-5-fluorocytidine. This, in turn, is converted to 5′-deoxy-5-fluorouridine by the enzyme cytidine deaminase. The 5′-deoxy-5-fluorouridine metabolite is then hydrolyzed by thymidine phosphorylase to 5-FU directly in the tumor. The expression of thymidine phosphorylase has been shown to be significantly higher in a broad range of solid tumors than in corresponding normal tissue. Peak plasma levels are achieved in about 1.5 hours, and peak 5-FU levels are reached at 2 hours after oral administration.

Capecitabine is used in the treatment of metastatic breast cancer either as a single agent or in combination with the taxane docetaxel. It is also approved for use in the adjuvant therapy of stage III colon cancer as well as for treatment of metastatic colorectal cancer as monotherapy. At this time, significant efforts are directed at combining this agent with other active cytotoxic agents, including irinotecan or oxaliplatin. The main toxicities of capecitabine include diarrhea and the hand-foot syndrome and are listed in Table 55–3. While myelosuppression, nausea and vomiting, and mucositis can also be observed with this agent, the incidence is significantly less than that seen with intravenous 5-FU.

3. Cytarabine

Cytarabine (cytosine arabinoside, ara-C) is an S phase-specific antimetabolite that is converted by deoxycytidine kinase to the 5′-mononucleotide (ara-CMP). Ara-CMP is further metabolized to the triphosphate ara-CTP, which competitively inhibits DNA polymerase-α and DNA polymerase-β, thereby resulting in blockade of DNA synthesis and DNA repair, respectively. Cytarabine is also incorporated into RNA and DNA. Incorporation into DNA leads to interference with chain elongation and defective ligation of fragments of newly synthesized DNA. The cellular retention time for ara-CTP appears to correlate with its lethality to malignant cells.

After intravenous administration (Table 55–3), the drug is cleared rapidly, with most of an administered dose being deaminated to an inactive form. The ratio of the anabolic enzyme deoxycytidine kinase to the inactivating catalyst cytidine deaminase is important in determining the eventual cytotoxicity of cytarabine.

Cytosine
deoxyriboside

Cytosine
arabinoside
(cytarabine)

In view of cytarabine's S phase specificity, the drug is highly schedule-dependent and must be given either by continuous infusion or every 8–12 hours for 5–7 days. Its activity is limited exclusively to hematologic malignancies, including acute myelogenous leukemia and non-Hodgkin's lymphoma. It has absolutely no activity in solid tumors. The main adverse effects are listed in Table 55–3.

4. Gemcitabine

Gemcitabine is a deoxycytidine analog that is phosphorylated initially by the enzyme deoxycytidine kinase to the monophosphate form and then by other nucleoside kinases to di- and triphosphate nucleotide forms. The antitumor effect is considered to result from two different mechanisms: inhibition of ribonucleotide reductase by gemcitabine diphosphate, which reduces the level of deoxyribonucleoside triphosphates required for DNA synthesis; and incorporation of gemcitabine triphosphate into DNA, leading to inhibition of DNA synthesis and function. Following incorporation of gemcitabine nucleotide, only one additional nucleotide can be added to the growing DNA strand, resulting in chain termination.

Gemcitabine

Gemcitabine was initially approved for use in pancreatic cancer but is now widely used in the treatment of non-small cell lung cancer, bladder cancer, and non-Hodgkin's lymphoma. Myelosuppression in the form of neutropenia is the principal dose-limiting toxicity.

PLANT ALKALOIDS

VINBLASTINE

Vinblastine is an alkaloid derived from the periwinkle plant *Vinca rosea*. Its mechanism of action involves inhibition of tubulin polymerization, which disrupts assembly of microtubules, an important part of the cytoskeleton and the mitotic spindle. This inhibitory effect results in mitotic arrest in metaphase, bringing cell division to a halt, which then leads to cell death. Toxicity includes nausea and vomiting, bone marrow suppression, and alopecia. This agent is also a potent vesicant, and care must be taken in its administration. It has clinical activity in the treatment of Hodgkin's disease, non-Hodgkin's lymphomas, breast cancer, and germ cell cancer. See the section on Clinical Pharmacology, below, and Table 55–4.

Vincristine   **Vinblastine**

VINCRISTINE

Vincristine is an alkaloid derivative of *Vinca rosea* and is closely related in structure to vinblastine. Its mechanism of action is considered to be identical to that of vinblastine in that it functions as a mitotic spindle poison leading to arrest of cells in the M phase of the cell cycle. Despite these similarities to vinblastine, vincristine has a strikingly different spectrum of clinical activity and toxicity.

Vincristine has been effectively combined with prednisone for remission induction in acute lymphoblastic leukemia in children. It is also active in various hematologic malignancies such as Hodgkin's and non-Hodgkin's lymphomas, and multiple myeloma, and in several pediatric

tumors including rhabdomyosarcoma, neuroblastoma, Ewing's sarcoma, and Wilms' tumor. The main dose-limiting toxicity is neurotoxicity, usually expressed as a peripheral sensory neuropathy, although autonomic nervous system dysfunction—with orthostatic hypotension, sphincter problems, and paralytic ileus—cranial nerve palsies, ataxia, seizures, and coma have been observed. While myelosuppression can occur, it is generally milder and much less significant than with vinblastine. The other potential side effect that can develop is the syndrome of inappropriate secretion of antidiuretic hormone (SIADH).

VINORELBINE

Vinorelbine is a semisynthetic vinca alkaloid whose mechanism of action is identical to that of vinblastine and vincristine, ie, inhibition of mitosis of cells in the M phase through inhibition of tubulin polymerization. This agent has activity in non-small cell lung cancer and in breast cancer. Myelosuppression with neutropenia is the dose-limiting toxicity, but nausea and vomiting, transient elevations in liver function tests, neurotoxicity, and SIADH are also reported.

EPIPODOPHYLLOTOXINS

Two compounds, VP-16 (**etoposide**) and a related drug, VM-26 (**teniposide**), are semisynthetic derivatives of podophyllotoxin, which is extracted from the mayapple root *(Podophyllum peltatum)*. Both an intravenous and an oral formulation of etoposide are approved for clinical use in the USA.

Etoposide and teniposide are similar in chemical structure and in their effects—they block cell division in the late S-G$_2$ phase of the cell cycle. Their primary mode of action involves inhibition of topoisomerase II, which results in DNA damage through strand breakage induced by the formation of a ternary complex of drug, DNA, and enzyme. The drugs are water-insoluble and have to be formulated in a Cremophor vehicle for clinical use. These agents are administered via the intravenous route (Table 55–4) and are rapidly and widely distributed throughout the body except for the brain. Up to 90–95% of drug is protein-bound, mainly to albumin. Dose reduction is required in the setting of renal dysfunction. Etoposide has clinical activity in germ cell cancer, small cell and non-small cell lung cancer, Hodgkin's and non-Hodgkin's lymphomas, and gastric cancer and as high-dose therapy in the transplant setting for breast cancer and lymphomas. Teniposide use is limited mainly to acute lymphoblastic leukemia.

CAMPTOTHECINS

The camptothecins are natural products that are derived from the *Camptotheca acuminata* tree, and they inhibit

Table 55–4. Natural product cancer chemotherapy drugs: Dosages and toxicities.

Drug	Single-Agent Dosage	Acute Toxicity	Delayed Toxicity
Bleomycin	Up to 15 units/m^2 IV twice weekly to a total dose of 200–250 units	Allergic reactions, fever, hypotension	Skin toxicity, pulmonary fibrosis, mucositis, alopecia
Dactinomycin (actinomycin D)	0.04 mg/kg IV weekly	Nausea and vomiting	Stomatitis, gastrointestinal tract upset, alopecia, bone marrow depression
Daunorubicin (daunomycin)	30–60 mg/m^2 daily IV for 3 days, or 30–60 mg/m^2 IV weekly	Nausea, fever, red urine (not hematuria)	Cardiotoxicity (see text), alopecia, bone marrow depression
Docetaxel	100 mg/m^2 IV over 1 hour every 3 weeks	Hypersensitivity	Neurotoxicity, fluid retention, neutropenia
Doxorubicin (Adriamycin)	60 mg/m^2 daily IV for 3 days, or 30–60 mg/m^2 IV weekly	Nausea, red urine (not hematuria)	Cardiotoxicity (see text), alopecia, bone marrow depression, stomatitis
Etoposide (VP-16)	50–100 mg/m^2 daily for 5 days	Nausea, vomiting, hypotension	Alopecia, bone marrow depression
Idarubicin	12 mg/m^2 IV daily for 3 days (with cytarabine)	Nausea and vomiting	Bone marrow depression, mucositis, cardiotoxicity
Irinotecan	125 mg/m^2 IV once weekly for 4 weeks; repeat every 6 weeks or 300–350 mg/m^2 IV every 3 weeks	Diarrhea, nausea, vomiting	Diarrhea, bone marrow depression, nausea and vomiting
Mitomycin	20 mg/m^2 IV every 6 weeks	Nausea	Thrombocytopenia, anemia, leukopenia, mucositis
Paclitaxel	130–170 mg/m^2 IV over 3 or 24 hours every 3–4 weeks	Nausea, vomiting, hypotension, arrhythmias, hypersensitivity	Bone marrow depression, peripheral sensory neuropathy
Topotecan	1.5 mg/m^2 IV for 5 days, repeat every 21 days for 4 courses	Nausea and vomiting	Bone marrow depression
Vinblastine	0.1–0.2 mg/kg IV weekly	Nausea and vomiting	Alopecia, loss of reflexes, bone marrow depression
Vincristine	1.5 mg/m^2 IV (maximum: 2 mg weekly)	None	Areflexia, muscle weakness, peripheral neuritis, paralytic ileus, mild bone marrow depression, alopecia
Vinorelbine	30 mg/m^2 IV weekly	Nausea and vomiting	Bone marrow depression, fatigue, constipation, hyporeflexia, paresthesias

the activity of topoisomerase I, the key enzyme responsible for cutting and religating single DNA strands. Inhibition of the enzyme results in DNA damage. **Topotecan** is indicated in the treatment of advanced ovarian cancer as second-line therapy following initial treatment with platinum-based chemotherapy. It is also approved as second-line therapy of small cell lung cancer. The main route of elimination is renal excretion, and dosage must be adjusted in patients with renal impairment.

Irinotecan is a prodrug that is converted mainly in the liver by the carboxylesterase enzyme to the SN-38

metabolite, which is a potent inhibitor of topoisomerase I. In contrast to topotecan, irinotecan and SN-38 are mainly eliminated in bile and feces, and dose reduction is required in the setting of liver dysfunction. Irinotecan was originally approved as second-line monotherapy in patients with metastatic colorectal cancer who had failed fluorouracil-based therapy. It is also approved as first-line therapy when used in combination with 5-FU and leucovorin. Myelosuppression and diarrhea are the two most common adverse events. There are two forms of diarrhea: an early form that occurs within 24 hours after administration and is thought to be a cholinergic event effectively treated with atropine, and a late form that usually occurs 2–10 days after treatment. The late diarrhea can be severe, leading to significant electrolyte imbalance and dehydration in some cases.

TAXANES

Paclitaxel is an alkaloid ester derived from the Pacific yew *(Taxus brevifolia)* and the European yew *(Taxus baccata).* The drug functions as a mitotic spindle poison through high-affinity binding to microtubules with enhancement of tubulin polymerization. This promotion of microtubule assembly by paclitaxel occurs in the absence of microtubule-associated proteins and guanosine triphosphate and results in inhibition of mitosis and cell division.

Paclitaxel has significant activity in a broad range of solid tumors, including ovarian, advanced breast, non-small cell and small cell lung, head and neck, esophageal, prostate, and bladder cancers and AIDS-related Kaposi's sarcoma. It is metabolized extensively by the liver P450 system, and nearly 80% of the drug is excreted in feces via the hepatobiliary route. Therefore, dose reduction is required in the setting of liver dysfunction. The primary dose-limiting toxicities are listed in Table 55–4. Hypersensitivity reactions may be observed in up to 5% of patients, but the incidence can be reduced by premedication with dexamethasone, diphenhydramine, and an H_2 blocker.

A novel albumin-bound paclitaxel formulation (Abraxane) has recently been approved for use in metastatic breast cancer. In contrast to paclitaxel, this formulation is not associated with hypersensitivity reactions, and premedication to prevent such reactions is not required. Moreover, this agent has significantly reduced myelosuppressive effects compared with paclitaxel, and the neurotoxicity that results appears to be more readily reversible than is typically observed with paclitaxel.

Docetaxel is a semisynthetic taxane derived from the European yew tree. Its mechanism of action, metabolism, and elimination are identical to those of paclitaxel. It is approved for use as second-line therapy in advanced breast cancer and non-small cell lung cancer, and it also has major activity in head and neck cancer, small cell lung cancer, gastric cancer, advanced platinum-refractory ovarian cancer, and bladder cancer. Its major toxicities are listed in Table 55–4.

ANTITUMOR ANTIBIOTICS

Screening of microbial products has led to the discovery of a number of growth-inhibiting compounds that have proved to be clinically useful in cancer chemotherapy.

Many of these antibiotics bind to DNA through intercalation between specific bases and block the synthesis of RNA, DNA, or both; cause DNA strand scission; and interfere with cell replication. All of the anticancer antibiotics now being used in clinical practice are products of various strains of the soil microbe *Streptomyces.* These include the anthracyclines, dactinomycin, bleomycin, and mitomycin.

ANTHRACYCLINES

The anthracycline antibiotics, isolated from *Streptomyces peucetius* var *caesius,* are among the most widely used cytotoxic anticancer drugs. The structures of two congeners, **doxorubicin** and **daunorubicin,** are shown below. Several other anthracycline analogs have entered clinical practice, including idarubicin, epirubicin, and mitoxantrone. Daunorubicin was the first agent in this class to be isolated, and it is still used in the treatment of acute myeloid leukemia. Doxorubicin has a broad spectrum of clinical activity against hematologic malignancies and a wide range of solid tumors. The anthracyclines exert their cytotoxic action through four major mechanisms. These are (1) inhibition of topoisomerase II; (2) high-affinity binding to DNA through intercalation, with consequent blockade of the synthesis of DNA and RNA, and DNA strand scission; (3) binding to cellular membranes to alter fluidity and ion transport; and (4) generation of semiquinone free radicals and oxygen free radicals through an iron-dependent, enzyme-mediated reductive process. This free radical mechanism has been established to be the cause of the cardiotoxicity associated with the anthracyclines.

Daunorubicin   **Doxorubicin**

In the clinical setting, anthracyclines are administered via the intravenous route (Table 55–4). The anthracyclines are metabolized extensively in the liver, with reduction and hydrolysis of the ring substituents. The hydroxylated metabolite is an active species, whereas the aglycone is inactive. Up to 50% of drug is eliminated in the feces via biliary excretion, and dose reduction is required in the setting of liver dysfunction. Although anthracyclines are usually administered on an every-3-week schedule, alternative schedules such as low-dose weekly or 72–96 hour continuous infusions have been shown to yield equivalent clinical efficacy with reduced overall toxicity.

Doxorubicin is one of the most important anticancer drugs, with major clinical activity in cancers of the breast, endometrium, ovary, testicle, thyroid, stomach, bladder, liver, and lung; in soft tissue sarcomas; and in several childhood cancers, including neuroblastoma, Ewing's sarcoma, osteosarcoma, and rhabdomyosarcoma. It is also widely used in hematologic malignancies, including acute lymphoblastic leukemia, multiple myeloma, and Hodgkin's and non-Hodgkin's lymphomas. It is generally used in combination with other anticancer agents (eg, cyclophosphamide, cisplatin, and 5-FU), and responses and remission duration tend to be improved with combination regimens as opposed to single-agent therapy. Daunorubicin has a far narrower spectrum of activity than doxorubicin. Daunorubicin has been mainly used for the treatment of acute myeloid leukemia, although there has been a shift in clinical practice toward using idarubicin, an analog of daunorubicin. Its efficacy in solid tumors appears to be limited.

Idarubicin is a semisynthetic anthracycline glycoside analog of daunorubicin, and it is approved for use in combination with cytarabine for induction therapy of acute myeloid leukemia. When combined with cytarabine, idarubicin appears to be more active than daunorubicin in producing complete remissions and in improving survival in patients with acute myelogenous leukemia.

Epirubicin is a doxorubicin analog whose mechanism of action is identical to that of all other anthracyclines. It was initially approved for use as a component of adjuvant therapy of early-stage, node-positive breast cancer but is also used for the treatment of metastatic breast cancer and gastric cancer.

The main dose-limiting toxicity of all anthracyclines is myelosuppression, with neutropenia more commonly observed than thrombocytopenia. In some cases, mucositis is dose-limiting. Two forms of cardiotoxicity are observed. The acute form occurs within the first 2–3 days and presents as arrhythmias and conduction abnormalities, other electrocardiographic changes, pericarditis, and myocarditis. This form is usually transient and in most cases is asymptomatic. The chronic form results in a dose-dependent, dilated cardiomyopathy associated with heart failure. The chronic cardiac toxicity appears to result from increased production of free radicals within the myocardium. This effect is rarely seen at total doxorubicin dosages below 500–550 mg/m². Use of lower weekly doses or continuous infusions of doxorubicin

appear to reduce the incidence of cardiac toxicity. In addition, treatment with the iron-chelating agent dexrazoxane (ICRF-187) is currently approved to prevent or reduce anthracycline-induced cardiotoxicity in women with metastatic breast cancer who have received a total cumulative dose of doxorubicin of 300 mg/m². The anthracyclines can produce a "radiation recall reaction," with erythema and desquamation of the skin observed at sites of prior radiation therapy.

MITOXANTRONE

Mitoxantrone (dihydroxyanthracenedione, DHAD) is an anthracene compound whose structure resembles the anthracycline ring. It binds to DNA to produce strand breakage and inhibits both DNA and RNA synthesis. It is currently used for treatment of advanced, hormone-refractory prostate cancer and low-grade non-Hodgkin's lymphoma. It is also indicated in breast cancer as well as in pediatric and adult acute myeloid leukemias. The plasma half-life of mitoxantrone in patients is approximately 75 hours, and it is predominantly excreted via the hepatobiliary route in feces. Myelosuppression with leukopenia is the dose-limiting toxicity, and mild nausea and vomiting, mucositis, and alopecia also occur. Although the drug is thought to be less cardiotoxic than doxorubicin, both acute and chronic cardiac toxicity are reported. A blue discoloration of the fingernails, sclera, and urine can be observed up to 1–2 days after drug therapy.

DACTINOMYCIN

Dactinomycin is an antitumor antibiotic isolated from a *Streptomyces* organism. It binds tightly to double-stranded DNA through intercalation between adjacent guanine-cytosine base pairs and inhibits all forms of DNA-dependent RNA synthesis, with ribosomal RNA formation being most sensitive to drug action.

Dactinomycin is mainly used to treat pediatric tumors such as Wilms' tumor, rhabdomyosarcoma, and Ewing's sarcoma, but it also has activity against germ cell tumors and gestational trophoblastic disease. As with the anthracyclines, dactinomycin can induce a radiation recall reaction. See Table 55–4 for other toxicities.

MITOMYCIN

Mitomycin (mitomycin C) is an antibiotic isolated from *Streptomyces caespitosus*. It is an alkylating agent that undergoes metabolic activation through an enzyme-mediated reduction to generate an alkylating agent that cross-links DNA. Hypoxic tumor stem cells of solid tumors exist in an environment conducive to reductive reactions and are more sensitive to the cytotoxic actions of mitomycin than normal cells and oxygenated tumor cells. It is active in all phases of the cell cycle, and is the best available drug for use in combination with radiation therapy to attack hypoxic tumor cells. Its main clinical use is in the treatment of squamous cell cancer of the anus in combination with 5-FU and radiation therapy. In addition, it is used in combination chemotherapy for squamous cell carcinoma of the cervix and for breast, gastric, and pancreatic cancer. One special application of mitomycin has been in the intravesical treatment of superficial bladder cancer. Because virtually none of the agent is absorbed systemically, there is little to no systemic toxicity.

The common toxicities are outlined in Table 55–4. The hemolytic-uremic syndrome, manifested as microangiopathic hemolytic anemia, thrombocytopenia, and renal failure, as well as occasional instances of interstitial pneumonitis have been reported.

BLEOMYCIN

Bleomycin is a small peptide that contains a DNA-binding region and an iron-binding domain at opposite ends of the molecule. It acts by binding to DNA, which results in single-strand and double-strand breaks following free radical formation, and inhibition of DNA biosynthesis. The fragmentation of DNA is due to oxidation of a DNA-bleomycin-Fe(II) complex and leads to chromosomal aberrations. Bleomycin is a cell cycle-specific drug that causes accumulation of cells in the G_2 phase of the cell cycle.

Bleomycin is indicated for the treatment of Hodgkin's and non-Hodgkin's lymphomas, germ cell tumor, head and neck cancer, and squamous cell cancer of the skin, cervix, and vulva. In addition, it can be used as a sclerosing agent for malignant pleural effusions and ascites. One advantage of this agent is that it can be given subcutaneously, intramuscularly, or intravenously (Table 55–4). Peak blood levels of bleomycin after intramuscular injection appear within 30–60 minutes. Intravenous injection of similar dosages yields higher peak concentrations and a terminal half-life of about 2.5 hours. Elimination of bleomycin is mainly via renal excretion; dose modification is recommended in the setting of renal dysfunction.

Pulmonary toxicity is dose-limiting for bleomycin and usually presents as pneumonitis with cough, dyspnea, dry inspiratory crackles on physical examination, and infiltrates on chest x-ray. The incidence of pulmonary toxicity is increased in patients older than 70 years of age, in those who receive cumulative doses greater than 400 units, in those with underlying pulmonary disease, and in those who have received prior mediastinal or chest irradiation. In rare cases, pulmonary toxicity can be fatal. Other toxicities are listed in Table 55–4.

HORMONAL AGENTS

ESTROGEN & ANDROGEN INHIBITORS

The antiestrogen **tamoxifen** has proved to be extremely useful for the treatment of both early-stage and metastatic breast cancer. It is also approved as a chemopreventive agent in women at high risk for breast cancer. In addition, this hormonal agent has activity in endometrial cancer. Tamoxifen functions as a competitive partial agonist-inhibitor of estrogen and binds to the estrogen receptors of estrogen-sensitive tumors. However, tamoxifen has a tenfold lower affinity for the estrogen receptor (ER) than does estradiol, indicating the importance of ablation of endogenous estrogen for optimal antiestrogen effect. In addition to its direct antiestrogen effects on tumor cells, tamoxifen also suppresses serum levels of insulin-like growth factor-1 and up-regulates local production of transforming growth factor-beta (TGF-β).

Tamoxifen

Tamoxifen is given orally and is rapidly and completely absorbed. High plasma levels of tamoxifen are obtained within 4–6 hours after oral administration, and the agent has a much longer biologic half-life than estradiol—on the order of 7–14 days. It is extensively metabolized by the liver P450 system, and the main metabolites also possess antitumor activity similar to that of the parent drug. Tamoxifen is well tolerated, and its side effects are generally quite mild (Table 55–5).

Flutamide and **bicalutamide** are nonsteroidal antiandrogen agents that bind to the androgen receptor and inhibit androgen effects. They are administered orally and are rapidly and completely absorbed. At present they are used in combination with radiation therapy for the treatment of early-stage prostate cancer and in the setting of metastatic prostate cancer. Toxicities are listed in Table 55–5.

GONADOTROPIN-RELEASING HORMONE AGONISTS

Leuprolide and **goserelin** are synthetic peptide analogs of naturally occurring gonadotropin-releasing hormone (GnRH, LHRH). They are described in further detail in Chapters 37 and 40. When given as depot prepara-

Table 55–5. Hormonally active agents: Dosages and toxicities.

Drug	Usual Adult Dosage	Acute Toxicity	Delayed Toxicity
Antiandrogen			
Flutamide	250 mg/tid orally	Mild nausea	Hot flushes, transient elevations in liver function tests
Antiestrogen			
Tamoxifen	20 mg/d orally	Transient flare of tumor symptoms	Menopausal symptoms, fluid retention and edema, thromboembolic events, increased incidence of endometrial hyperplasia and cancer
Progestins			
Megestrol acetate	40 mg orally 4 times daily	None	Fluid retention
Adrenocorticosteroids			
Hydrocortisone	40–200 mg/d orally	None	Fluid retention, hypertension, diabetes, increased susceptibility to infection, moon facies
Prednisone	20–100 mg/d orally	None	
Gonadotropin-releasing hormone agonists			
Goserelin acetate	3.6 mg SC monthly	Transient flare of tumor symptoms, pain at injection site	Hot flushes, impotence, gynecomastia
Leuprolide	7.5 mg SC monthly	Transient flare of tumor symptoms, pain at injection site	Hot flushes, impotence, gynecomastia
Aromatase inhibitors			
Aminoglutethimide	250 mg orally twice daily and hydrocortisone 20 mg twice daily	Fatigue, mild nausea	Skin rash, adrenal insufficiency, myelosuppression
Anastrozole	1 mg orally daily	Mild nausea, headache	Fatigue, hot flushes, arthralgias
Exemestane	25 mg orally daily	Mild nausea, headache	Fatigue, hot flushes
Letrozole	2.5 mg orally daily	Mild nausea, headache	Fatigue, hot flushes, arthralgias

tions, these agents lead to a transient release of follicle-stimulating hormone (FSH) and luteinizing hormone (LH) followed by marked inhibition of the release of these gonadotropins. In men, this results in castration levels of testosterone after 2–4 weeks of therapy.

Leuprolide and goserelin are indicated in the treatment of advanced prostate cancer and more recently, these agents have been incorporated as part of neoadjuvant therapy of early-stage prostate cancer. Leuprolide and goserelin are now formulated in long-acting depot forms, which allows for administration at monthly or longer intervals. The main adverse effects include hot flushes, impotence, and gynecomastia. Other toxicities are given in Table 55–5.

AROMATASE INHIBITORS

Aminoglutethimide is a nonsteroidal inhibitor of corticosteroid synthesis at the first step involving the conversion of cholesterol to pregnenolone (see Chapter 39). Aminoglutethimide also inhibits the extra-adrenal synthesis of estrone and estradiol. Aside from its direct effects on adrenal steroidogenesis, aminoglutethimide is an inhibitor of an aromatase enzyme that converts the adrenal androgen androstenedione to estrone (see Figure 40–2). This aromatization of an androgenic precursor into an estrogen occurs in body fat. Since estrogens promote the growth of breast cancer, estrogen synthesis in adipose tissue can be important in breast cancer growth in postmenopausal women.

Aminoglutethimide is primarily used in the treatment of metastatic breast cancer in women whose tumors express significant levels of estrogen or progesterone receptors. It also has activity in hormone-dependent, advanced prostate cancer. Aminoglutethimide is normally administered with hydrocortisone to prevent symptoms of adrenal insufficiency. Hydrocortisone is preferable to dexamethasone because the latter agent accelerates the rate of catabolism of aminoglutethimide. Adverse effects of aminoglutethimide are listed in Table 55–5.

Table 55–6. Miscellaneous anticancer drugs: Dosages and toxicities.

Drug	Usual Dosage	Acute Toxicity	Delayed Toxicity
Arsenic trioxide	0.15 mg/kg/d IV for 60 days as induction therapy; 0.15 mg/kg/d IV for 5 days per week for a total of 5 weeks as consolidation therapy	Headache and lightheadedness	Fatigue, cardiac dysrhythmias, fever, dyspnea, fluid retention and weight gain
Asparaginase	20,000 IU/m^2 daily IV for 5–10 days	Nausea, fever, and allergic reactions	Hepatotoxicity, mental depression, pancreatitis
Bevacizumab	5 mg/kg IV every 2 weeks	Hypertension, infusion reaction	Arterial thromboembolic events, gastrointestinal perforations, wound healing complications
Cetuximab	400 mg/m^2 IV loading dose; 250 mg/m^2 IV weekly	Infustion reaction	Skin rash, interstitial lung disease
Erlotinib	150 mg/d orally	Diarrhea	Skin rash, interstitial lung disease
Gefitinib	250 mg/d orally	Hypertension, diarrhea	Skin rash, interstitial lung disease
Imatinib	400–600 mg/d orally	Nausea and vomiting	Fluid retention with ankle and periorbital edema, diarrhea, myalgias
Hydroxyurea	300 mg/m^2 orally for 5 days	Nausea and vomiting	Bone marrow depression
Mitoxantrone	10–12 mg/m^2 IV every 3–4 weeks	Nausea	Bone marrow depression, occasional cardiac toxicity, mild alopecia
Trastuzumab[1]	4 mg/kg IV loading dose; 2 mg/kg/wk as maintenance	Nausea and vomiting, infusion-related hypersensitivity reaction	Cardiomyopathy, myelosuppression, pulmonary toxicity

[1]This monoclonal antibody is described in Chapter 56: Immunopharmacology.

Anastrozole is a selective nonsteroidal inhibitor of aromatase that has no inhibitory effect on adrenal glucocorticoid or mineralocorticoid synthesis. It is presently approved for first-line treatment of postmenopausal women with metastatic breast cancer that is ER-positive, for treatment of postmenopausal women with metastatic breast cancer that is ER-positive and has progressed while on tamoxifen therapy, and as adjuvant therapy of postmenopausal women with hormone-positive, early-stage breast cancer. **Letrozole** is a nonsteroidal competitive inhibitor of aromatase that is significantly more potent than aminoglutethimide and acts in the same way as anastrozole. It is also indicated for first-line treatment of postmenopausal women with hormone receptor-positive metastatic breast cancer and for second-line treatment of postmenopausal women with advanced breast cancer after progression on tamoxifen therapy. **Exemestane** is a steroid hormonal suicide inhibitor that binds to and irreversibly inactivates aromatase. There appears to be a lack of cross-resistance between exemestane and nonsteroidal aromatase inhibitors. This agent is indicated for the treatment of advanced breast cancer in postmenopausal women whose disease has progressed on tamoxifen therapy. Each of these aromatase inhibitors exhibits a similar side effect profile (Table 55–5, see also Chapter 40).

MISCELLANEOUS ANTICANCER DRUGS (SEE TABLE 55–6)

IMATINIB

Imatinib (STI571; Gleevec) is an inhibitor of the tyrosine kinase domain of the Bcr-Abl oncoprotein and prevents the phosphorylation of the kinase substrate by ATP. It is indicated for the treatment of chronic myelogenous leukemia (CML), a pluripotent hematopoietic stem cell disorder characterized by the t(9:22) Philadelphia chromosomal translocation. This translocation results in the Bcr-Abl fusion protein, the causative agent in CML, and is present in up to 95% of patients with this disease. This agent inhibits other activated receptor tyrosine kinases for platelet-derived growth factor receptor, stem cell factor, and c-kit.

Imatinib is well absorbed orally; it is highly protein-bound in plasma. The drug is metabolized in the liver, and elimination of metabolites occurs mainly in feces via biliary excretion. This agent is approved for use as first-line therapy in chronic phase CML, in blast crisis, and as second-line therapy for chronic phase CML that has progressed on prior interferon-α therapy. Imatinib is effective also for treatment of gastrointestinal stromal tumors expressing the c-kit tyrosine kinase. Dosage and toxicities are listed in Table 55–6.

Dasatinib (Sprycel) is an oral inhibitor of several kinases and is approved for use in CML and Philadelphia chromosome-positive acute lymphoblastic leukemia (ALL).

GROWTH FACTOR RECEPTOR INHIBITORS

1. Cetuximab

The epidermal growth factor receptor (EGFR) is a member of the erb-B family of growth factor receptors, and it is overexpressed in a number of solid tumors. Activation of the EGFR signaling pathway results in downstream activation of several key cellular events involved in cellular growth and proliferation, invasion and metastasis, and angiogenesis. In addition, this pathway inhibits the cytotoxic activity of various anticancer agents and radiation therapy, presumably through suppression of key apoptotic mechanisms, thereby leading to the development of cellular drug resistance.

Cetuximab (IMC-225; Erbitux) is a chimeric monoclonal antibody directed against the extracellular domain of the EGFR, and it is presently approved for use in combination with irinotecan in the refractory setting or as monotherapy in patients who are deemed to be irinotecan-refractory. There is growing evidence that cetuximab can be effectively and safely combined with irinotecan- and oxaliplatin-based chemotherapy in the first-line therapy of metastatic colorectal cancer as well. This agent is also approved for use in combination with radiation therapy in patients with locally advanced head and neck cancer. This agent is well tolerated, with the main adverse effects being an acneiform skin rash and a hypersensitivity infusion reaction. Dosage and toxicities are listed in Table 55–6.

2. Gefitinib & Erlotinib

Gefitinib (ZD1694; Iressa) and **erlotinib** (OSI-774; Tarceva) are small molecule inhibitors of the tyrosine kinase domain associated with the EGFR, and both are approved for use in the treatment of non-small cell lung cancer that is refractory to at least one prior chemotherapy regimen. Dosage and toxicities of both of these agents are listed in Table 55–6. Patients who are nonsmokers and who have a bronchoalveolar histologic subtype appear to be more responsive to these agents. In addition, erlotinib has been approved for use in combination with gemcitabine for the treatment of advanced pancreatic cancer. With respect to toxicity, an acneiform skin rash and diarrhea are the most common adverse effects observed with these small molecules.

3. Bevacizumab

The vascular endothelial growth factor (VEGF) is one of the most critical angiogenic growth factors. The growth of both primary and metastatic tumors requires an intact vasculature; VEGF and the VEGF-signaling pathway therefore represent an attractive target for chemotherapy. Several approaches have been taken to inhibit VEGF signaling; they include inhibition of VEGF interactions with its receptor by targeting either the VEGF ligand with antibodies or soluble chimeric receptors, or by direct inhibition of the VEGF receptor–associated tyrosine kinase activity by small molecule inhibitors.

Bevacizumab (Avastin) is a recombinant humanized monoclonal antibody that targets all forms of VEGF-A. This antibody binds to and prevents VEGF-A from interacting with the target VEGF receptors. Bevacizumab can be safely and effectively combined with 5-FU-, irinotecan-, and oxaliplatin-based chemotherapy in the treatment of metastatic colorectal cancer. Bevacizumab is FDA approved as a first-line treatment for metastatic colorectal cancer in combination with any intravenous fluoropyrimidine-containing regimen. The main adverse effects observed with this agent include hypertension, an increased incidence of arterial thromboembolic events (transient ischemic attack, stroke, angina, and myocardial infarction), wound healing complications and gastrointestinal perforations, and proteinuria. Dosage is given in Table 55–6.

ASPARAGINASE

Asparaginase (L-asparagine amidohydrolase) is an enzyme used to treat childhood acute lymphocytic leukemia. The drug is isolated and purified from bacterial culture for clinical use. It hydrolyzes circulating L-asparagine to aspartic acid and ammonia. Because tumor cells lack asparagine synthetase, they require an exogenous source of L-asparagine. Thus, depletion of L-asparagine results in effective inhibition of protein synthesis. In contrast, normal cells can synthesize L-asparagine and thus are less susceptible to the cytotoxic action of asparaginase. The main adverse effect of this agent is a hypersensitivity reaction manifested by fever, chills, nausea and vomiting, skin rash, and urticaria. Severe cases can present with bronchospasm, respiratory failure, and hypotension. Other toxicities include an increased risk of both clotting and bleeding as a result of alterations in various clotting factors, pancreatitis, and neurologic toxicity with lethargy, confusion, hallucinations, and coma.

HYDROXYUREA

Hydroxyurea is an analog of urea whose mechanism of action involves the inhibition of DNA synthesis by inhibiting the enzyme ribonucleotide reductase, resulting in depletion of deoxynucleoside triphosphate pools. This agent exerts its effects in the S phase of the cell cycle. The drug is administered orally and has nearly 100% oral bioavailability. It is mainly used in chronic myelogenous leukemia and treatment of the blast crisis of acute myeloid leukemia. However, it is also effective as an adjunct with radiation therapy for head and neck cancer and in treating essential thrombocytosis and polycythemia vera. Myelosuppression is the dose-limiting toxicity, but nausea and vomiting, mucositis and diarrhea, headache and increased lethargy, and a maculopapular skin rash with pruritus are also observed.

RETINOIC ACID DERIVATIVES

All-*trans*-retinoic acid (tretinoin) produces remissions in patients with acute promyelocytic leukemia (APL) through the induction of terminal differentiation, in which the leukemic promyelocytes lose their ability to proliferate. APL is associated with a t(15:17) chromosomal translocation, which disrupts the gene for the nuclear receptor-α for retinoic acid and fuses it to a gene called *PML*. This chimeric gene, which expresses aberrant forms of the retinoic acid receptor-α, is present in virtually all patients with promyelocytic leukemia and appears to be responsible for sensitivity to all-*trans*-retinoic acid. This agent is approved for use in APL following progression or relapse with anthracycline-based chemotherapy and for patients in whom anthracycline-based chemotherapy is contraindicated. However, a number of serious adverse events have been observed. They include vitamin A toxicity manifesting as headache, fever, dry skin and mucous membranes, skin rash, pruritus, and conjunctivitis; retinoic acid syndrome with fever, leukocytosis, dyspnea, weight gain, diffuse pulmonary infiltrates, and pleural or pericardial effusions; increased serum cholesterol and triglyceride levels; central nervous system toxicity in the form of dizziness, anxiety, depression, confusion, and agitation; abdominal pain and diarrhea; and transient elevations in liver function tests. This retinoid has also been shown to be teratogenic.

ARSENIC TRIOXIDE

Arsenic trioxide (AS_2O_3) is used for induction of remission in patients with APL with the t(15:17) chromosomal translocation refractory to or relapsed following first-line therapy with all-*trans*-retinoic acid- and anthracycline-based chemotherapy. It functions by inducing differentiation through degradation of the chimeric PML/RAR-α protein. In addition, it induces apoptosis through a mitochondrion-dependent process, resulting in subsequent release of cytochrome C with caspase activation. This drug is administered via the intravenous route, and it is widely distributed in the body. The main toxicities are fatigue, electrocardiographic changes with QT prolongation, arrhythmias, and a syndrome characterized by fever, dyspnea, skin rash, fluid retention, and weight gain.

■ II. CLINICAL PHARMACOLOGY OF CANCER CHEMOTHERAPEUTIC DRUGS

A thorough knowledge of the kinetics of tumor cell proliferation along with an understanding of the pharmacology and mechanism of action of cancer chemotherapeutic agents is important in designing optimal regimens for patients with cancer (Table 55–7). The strategy for developing drug regimens requires a knowledge of the particular characteristics of specific tumors. For example, is there a high growth fraction? Is there a high spontaneous cell death rate? Are most of the cells in G_0? Is a significant fraction of the tumor composed of hypoxic stem cells? Are their normal counterparts under hormonal control? Similarly, knowledge of the pharmacology of specific drugs is important. Are the tumor cells sensitive to the drug? Is the drug cell cycle-specific? Does the drug require activation in certain normal tissue such as the liver (cyclophosphamide), or is it activated in the tumor tissue itself (capecitabine)? Similarly, for some tumor types, knowledge of receptor expression is important. For example, in patients with breast cancer, analysis of the tumor for expression of estrogen or progesterone receptors—or overexpression of HER-2 receptors—is important in guiding therapy. Knowledge of specific pathway abnormalities (eg, EGFR pathway) for intracellular signaling may prove important for the next generation of anticancer drugs.

Drugs that affect cycling cells can often be used most effectively after treatment with a cell cycle-nonspecific agent (eg, alkylating agents); this principle has been tested in a few human tumors with increasing success. Similarly, recognition of true drug synergism (tumor cell kill by the drug combination greater than the additive effects of the individual drugs) or antagonism is important in the design of combination chemotherapeutic programs. The combination of cytarabine with an anthracycline in acute myelogenous leukemia and the use of vinblastine or etoposide along with cisplatin and bleomycin in testicular tumors are good

Table 55–7. Malignancies responsive to chemotherapy.

Diagnosis	Current Treatment of Choice	Other Valuable Agents
Acute lymphocytic leukemia	Induction: vincristine plus prednisone. Remission maintenance: mercaptopurine, methotrexate, and cyclophosphamide in various combinations	Asparaginase, daunorubicin, carmustine, doxorubicin, cytarabine, allopurinol,[1] craniospinal radiotherapy
Acute myelocytic and myelomonocytic leukemia	Combination chemotherapy: cytarabine and mitoxantrone or daunorubicin or idarubicin	Methotrexate, thioguanine, mercaptopurine, allopurinol,[1] mitoxantrone, azacitidine,[2] amsacrine,[2] etoposide
Chronic lymphocytic leukemia	Chlorambucil and prednisone (if indicated), fludarabine	Allopurinol,[1] doxorubicin, cladribine
Chronic myelogenous leukemia	Imatinib, busulfan, or interferon, bone marrow transplantation (selected patients)	Vincristine, mercaptopurine, hydroxyurea, melphalan, interferon, allopurinol[1]
Hodgkin's disease (stages III and IV)	Combination chemotherapy: vinblastine, doxorubicin, dacarbazine, bleomycin	Lomustine, etoposide, ifosfamide, interferon, mechlorethamine, vincristine, procarbazine, prednisone
Non-Hodgkin's lymphoma	Combination chemotherapy: cyclophosphamide, doxorubicin, vincristine, prednisone	Bleomycin, lomustine, carmustine, etoposide, interferon, mitoxantrone, ifosfamide, rituximab
Multiple myeloma	Melphalan plus prednisone or multiagent combination chemotherapy	Cyclophosphamide, vincristine, carmustine, interferon, doxorubicin, epoetin alfa[1]
Macroglobulinemia	Chlorambucil or fludarabine	Prednisone
Polycythemia vera	Busulfan, chlorambucil, or cyclophosphamide	Radioactive phosphorus 32
Carcinoma of adrenal	Mitotane	Suramin[2]
Carcinoma of breast	(1) Adjuvant chemotherapy or tamoxifen after primary breast surgery (2) Combination chemotherapy or hormonal manipulation for late recurrence	Cyclophosphamide, doxorubicin, vincristine, methotrexate, fluorouracil, paclitaxel, mitoxantrone, prednisone,[1] megestrol, androgens,[1] aminoglutethimide, trastuzumab
Carcinoma of cervix	Radiation plus cisplatin (localized), cisplatin, carboplatin (metastatic)	Lomustine, cyclophosphamide, doxorubicin, methotrexate, mitomycin, bleomycin, vincristine, interferon, 13-*cis*-retinoic acid
Carcinoma of colon	Fluorouracil plus leucovorin plus oxaliplatin	Irinotecan
Carcinoma of endometrium	Progestins or tamoxifen	Doxorubicin, cisplatin, carboplatin
Carcinoma of lung	Cisplatin plus taxane	Methotrexate, vincristine, vinblastine, doxorubicin, mitomycin C
Carcinoma of ovary	Cisplatin or carboplatin plus paclitaxel	Cyclophosphamide, doxorubicin, melphalan, fluorouracil, vincristine, altretamine, bleomycin
Carcinoma of pancreas	Gemcitabine	Docetaxel, fluorouracil
Carcinoma of prostate	GnRH agonist plus androgen antagonist	Aminoglutethimide, doxorubicin, cisplatin, prednisone,[1] estramustine, fluorouracil, progestins, suramin[2]
Carcinoma of stomach	Fluorouracil plus cisplatin	Hydroxyurea, lomustine
Carcinoma of testis	Combination chemotherapy: cisplatin, bleomycin, and etoposide	Methotrexate, dactinomycin, plicamycin, vinblastine, doxorubicin, cyclophosphamide, etoposide, ifosfamide plus mesna[1]
Carcinoma of thyroid	Radioiodine (^{131}I), doxorubicin, cisplatin	Bleomycin, fluorouracil, melphalan

(continued)

Table 55–7. Malignancies responsive to chemotherapy. (continued)

Diagnosis	Current Treatment of Choice	Other Valuable Agents
Carcinomas of head and neck	Fluorouracil plus cisplatin, cisplatin plus paclitaxel	Methotrexate, bleomycin, hydroxyurea, doxorubicin, vincristine, vinorelbine
Choriocarcinoma (trophoblastic neoplasms)	Methotrexate alone or etoposide and cisplatin	Vinblastine, mercaptopurine, chlorambucil, doxorubicin
Wilms' tumor	Vincristine plus dactinomycin after surgery and radiotherapy	Methotrexate, cyclophosphamide, doxorubicin
Neuroblastoma	Cyclophosphamide plus doxorubicin and vincristine	Dactinomycin, daunorubicin, cisplatin
Carcinoid	Doxorubicin plus cyclophosphamide, fluorouracil, octreotide	Interferon, dactinomycin, methysergide,[1] streptozocin
Insulinoma	Streptozocin, interferon	Doxorubicin, fluorouracil, mitomycin
Osteogenic sarcoma	Doxorubicin, or methotrexate with leucovorin rescue initiated after surgery	Cyclophosphamide, dacarbazine, interferon, ifosfamide plus mesna[1]
Miscellaneous sarcomas	Doxorubicin plus dacarbazine	Methotrexate, dactinomycin, ifosfamide plus mesna,[1] vincristine, vinblastine
Melanoma	Dacarbazine, cisplatin, temozolomide	Lomustine, hydroxyurea, mitomycin, dactinomycin, interferon, tamoxifen

[1]Supportive agent, not oncolytic.
[2]Investigational agent. Treatment available through qualified investigators and centers authorized by National Cancer Institute and Cooperative Oncology Groups.

examples of true drug synergism against cancer cells but not against normal tissues.

In general, it is preferable to use cytotoxic chemotherapeutic agents in intensive pulse courses every 3–4 weeks rather than to use continuous daily dosage schedules. This schedule allows for maximum effects against neoplastic cell populations with complete hematologic and immunologic recovery between courses rather than leaving the patient continuously suppressed with cytotoxic therapy. This approach reduces adverse effects but does not reduce therapeutic efficacy.

The application of these principles is well illustrated in the current approach to the treatment of acute leukemias, lymphomas, Wilms' tumor, and germ cell testicular cancer.

THE LEUKEMIAS

1. Acute Leukemia

Childhood Leukemia

ALL is the predominant form of leukemia in childhood, and it is the most common form of cancer in children. Children with this disease have a relatively good prognosis. A subset of patients with neoplastic lymphocytes expressing surface antigenic features of T

lymphocytes has a poor prognosis (see Chapter 56). A cytoplasmic enzyme expressed by normal thymocytes, terminal deoxycytidyl transferase (terminal transferase), is also expressed in many cases of ALL. T cell ALL also expresses high levels of the enzyme adenosine deaminase (ADA). This led to interest in the use of the ADA inhibitor pentostatin (deoxycoformycin) for treatment of such T cell cases. Until 1948, the median length of survival in ALL was 3 months. With the advent of the folic acid antagonists, the length of survival was greatly increased. Subsequently, corticosteroids, 6-MP, cyclophosphamide, vincristine, daunorubicin, and asparaginase have all been found to be active against this disease. A combination of vincristine and prednisone plus other agents is currently used to induce remission. Over 90% of children enter complete remission with this therapy with only minimal toxicity. However, circulating leukemic cells often migrate to sanctuary sites located in the brain and testes. The value of prophylactic intrathecal methotrexate therapy for prevention of central nervous system leukemia (a major mechanism of relapse) has been clearly demonstrated. Intrathecal therapy with methotrexate should therefore be considered as a standard component of the induction regimen for children with ALL.

Adult Leukemia

Acute myelogenous leukemia (AML) is the most common leukemia seen in adults. The single most active agent for AML is cytarabine; however, it is best used in combination with an anthracycline, in which case complete remissions occur in about 70% of patients. Idarubicin has now replaced daunorubicin as the preferred anthracycline.

Patients often require intensive supportive care during the period of induction chemotherapy. Such care includes platelet transfusions to prevent bleeding, filgrastim to shorten periods of neutropenia, and antibiotics to combat infections. Younger patients (eg, < age 55) who are in complete remission and have an HLA-matched donor are candidates for allogeneic bone marrow transplantation. The transplant procedure is preceded by high-dose chemotherapy and total body irradiation followed by immunosuppression. This approach may cure up to 35–40% of eligible patients. Patients over age 60 respond less well to chemotherapy, primarily because their tolerance for aggressive therapy and their resistance to infection is lower.

Once remission of AML is achieved, consolidation chemotherapy is required to maintain a durable remission and to induce cure.

2. Chronic Myelogenous Leukemia

Chronic myelogenous leukemia (CML) arises from a chromosomally abnormal hematopoietic stem cell in which a balanced translocation between the long arms of chromosomes 9 and 22, t(9:22), is observed in 90–95% of cases. This translocation results in constitutive expression of the Bcr-Abl fusion oncoprotein with a molecular weight of 210 kDa. The clinical symptoms and course are related to the white blood cell count and its rate of increase. Most patients with white cell counts over 50,000/μL should be treated. The goals of treatment are to reduce the granulocytes to normal levels, to raise the hemoglobin concentration to normal, and to relieve disease-related symptoms. There has been a significant change in the management of this disease. Recently, the signal transduction inhibitor imatinib was approved for use as first-line therapy in previously untreated patients with chronic phase CML. Imatinib is also recommended in patients with chronic phase disease who have failed prior interferon-α therapy. Nearly all patients treated with imatinib exhibit a complete hematologic response, and up to 40–50% of patients will show a complete cytogenetic response. The usual dose for chronic phase disease is 400 mg/d, and an advantage of this drug is that it is given orally. As described previously, this drug is extremely well tolerated and is associated with relatively minor side effects. Other treatment options include interferon-α, busulfan, other oral alkylating agents, and hydroxyurea.

3. Chronic Lymphocytic Leukemia

Patients with early-stage chronic lymphocytic leukemia (CLL) have a relatively good prognosis, and therapy has not changed the course of the disease. However, in the setting of high-risk disease or in the presence of disease-related symptoms, treatment is indicated.

Chlorambucil and cyclophosphamide are the two most widely used alkylating agents for this disease. Chlorambucil is usually administered at a dose of 0.1 mg/kg/d, with close monitoring of blood counts at weekly intervals. It is frequently combined with prednisone, although there is no clear evidence that the combination yields better response rates or survival compared with chlorambucil alone. Cyclophosphamide is usually given in dosages of 1–2 g/m^2 every 3–4 weeks. In most cases, cyclophosphamide is combined with vincristine and prednisone (COP), or it can also be given with these same drugs along with doxorubicin (CHOP). The purine nucleoside analog fludarabine is also effective in treating CLL. This agent can be given alone, in combination with cyclophosphamide and with mitoxantrone and dexamethasone, or combined with the anti-CD20 antibody rituximab.

Monoclonal antibody-targeted therapies are being more widely used in CLL, especially in relapsed or refractory disease. **Alemtuzumab** is a humanized monoclonal antibody directed against the CD52 antigen and is approved for use in CLL that is refractory to alkylating agent or fludarabine therapy. Response rates up to 30–35% are observed, with disease stabilization in another 30% of patients. **Rituximab** is an anti-CD20 antibody that also has documented clinical activity in this setting. This chimeric antibody appears to enhance the antitumor effects of cytotoxic chemotherapy, and is also effective in settings in which resistance to chemotherapy has developed.

THE LYMPHOMAS

1. Hodgkin's Disease

The treatment of Hodgkin's disease has undergone dramatic evolution over the last 30 years. Hodgkin's disease is now recognized as a B cell neoplasm in which the malignant Reed-Sternberg cells have rearranged *VH* genes. In addition, the Epstein-Barr virus genome has been identified in up to 80% of tumor specimens.

Complete staging evaluation is required before a definitive treatment plan can be made. For patients with stage I and stage IIA disease, there has been a significant change in the treatment approach. Initially, these patients were treated with extended-field radiation therapy. However, given the late effects of radiation therapy, which include hypothyroidism and an increased risk of secondary cancers and coronary artery disease, combined-modality therapy with a brief course of combination chemotherapy and involved field radiation therapy is now the recommended approach. The main advance for patients with advanced stage III and IV Hodgkin's disease came with the development of MOPP (mechlorethamine, vincristine, procarbazine, and prednisone) chemotherapy in the 1960s. This regimen resulted initially in high complete response rates—on the order of 80–90%, with cures in up to 60% of patients. More recently, the anthracycline-containing regimen ABVD (doxorubicin, bleomycin, vinblastine, and dacarbazine) has been shown to be more effective and less toxic than MOPP, especially with regard to the incidence of sterility and secondary malignancies. This regimen uses four cycles of ABVD. An alternative regimen, termed Stanford V, utilizes a 12-week course of combination chemotherapy (doxorubicin, vinblastine, mechlorethamine, vincristine, bleomycin, etoposide, and prednisone), followed by involved radiation therapy.

With all these regimens, over 80% of previously untreated patients with advanced Hodgkin's disease (stages III and IV) are expected to go into complete remission, with disappearance of all disease-related symptoms and objective evidence of disease. Approximately 50–60% of all patients with Hodgkin's disease are cured of their disease.

2. Non-Hodgkin's Lymphomas

Over the past 25 years, there has been a dramatic increase in the incidence of non-Hodgkin's lymphoma. This is a heterogeneous disease, and the clinical characteristics of non-Hodgkin's lymphoma subsets are related to the underlying histopathologic features and the extent of disease involvement. In general, the nodular (or follicular) lymphomas have a far better prognosis, with a median survival up to 7 years, compared with the diffuse lymphomas, which have a median survival of about 1–2 years.

Combination chemotherapy is the treatment standard for patients with diffuse non-Hodgkin's lymphoma. The anthracycline-containing regimen CHOP (cyclophosphamide, doxorubicin, vincristine, and prednisone) has been considered the best treatment in terms of initial therapy. Randomized phase III clinical studies have now shown that the combination of CHOP with the anti-CD20 monoclonal antibody rituximab results in improved response rates, disease-free survival, and overall survival compared with CHOP chemotherapy alone.

The nodular follicular lymphomas are low-grade, indolent tumors that tend to present in an advanced stage and are usually confined to lymph nodes, bone marrow, and spleen. This form of non-Hodgkin's lymphomas, when presenting at an advanced stage, is considered incurable, and treatment is generally palliative. To date, there is no evidence that immediate treatment with combination chemotherapy offers clinical benefit over close observation and "watchful waiting" with initiation of chemotherapy at the time of disease symptoms.

MULTIPLE MYELOMA

This plasma cell malignancy is one of the models of neoplastic disease in humans as it arises from a single tumor stem cell. Moreover, the tumor cells produce a marker protein (myeloma immunoglobulin) that allows the total body burden of tumor cells to be quantified. Multiple myeloma principally involves the bone marrow and bone, causing bone pain, lytic lesions, bone fractures, and anemia as well as an increased susceptibility to infection.

Most patients with multiple myeloma are symptomatic at the time of initial diagnosis and require treatment with cytotoxic chemotherapy. Treatment with the combination of the alkylating agent melphalan and prednisone (MP protocol) remains a standard regimen. About 40% of patients respond to the MP combination, and the median remission is on the order of 2–2.5 years. While a host of studies have investigated the efficacy of combinations of multiple alkylating agents, none of these regimens have as yet been shown to be superior to MP.

Melphalan and other alkylating agents should be avoided in patients who are thought to be candidates for high-dose therapy with stem cell transplantation, as prior therapy will affect the success of stem cell harvesting. In this setting, the nonalkylator combination of vincristine, doxorubicin, and dexamethasone (VAD) has been used.

Thalidomide is now a well-established agent for treating refractory or relapsed disease, and about 30% of patients will achieve a response to this therapy. More recently, thalidomide has been used in combination with dexamethasone, and response rates on the order of 65% have been observed. Studies are now under way to directly compare VAD with the combination of thalidomide and dexamethasone. In some patients, especially those with poor performance status, single-agent pulse dexamethasone administered on a weekly basis can be effective in palliating symptoms. The proteosome inhibitor **bortezomib** has been recently approved for use in relapsing or refractory multiple myeloma. This agent is thought to exert its main cytotoxic effects through inhibition of the NF-κB signaling pathway, and further efforts are focused on developing this agent in combination regimens.

BREAST CANCER

1. Stage I & Stage II Disease

The management of primary breast cancer has undergone a remarkable evolution as a result of major efforts at early diagnosis (through encouragement of self-examination as well as through the use of cancer detection centers) and the implementation of combined modality approaches incorporating systemic chemotherapy as an adjuvant to surgery and radiation therapy. Women with stage I disease (small primaries and negative axillary lymph node dissections) are currently treated with surgery alone, and they have an 80% chance of cure.

Women with node-positive disease have a high risk of both local and systemic recurrence. Thus, lymph node status directly indicates the risk of occult distant micrometastasis. In this situation, postoperative use of systemic adjuvant chemotherapy with six cycles of cyclophosphamide, methotrexate, and fluorouracil (CMF protocol) or of fluorouracil, doxorubicin, and cyclophosphamide (FAC) has been shown to significantly reduce the relapse rate and prolong survival. Alternative regimens with equivalent clinical benefit include four cycles of doxorubicin and cyclophosphamide and six cycles of fluorouracil, epirubicin, and cyclophosphamide (FEC). Each of these chemotherapy regimens has benefited women with stage II breast cancer with one to three involved lymph nodes. Women with four or more involved nodes have had limited benefit thus far from adjuvant chemotherapy. Long-term analysis has clearly shown improved survival rates in node-positive premenopausal women who have been treated aggressively with multiagent combination chemotherapy. Preliminary results from three randomized clinical trials suggest that the addition of **trastuzumab,** a monoclonal antibody directed against the HER-2/*neu* receptor, to anthracycline- and taxane-containing adjuvant chemotherapy benefits women with HER-2-overexpressing breast cancer with respect to disease-free and overall survival.

Breast cancer was the first neoplasm shown to be responsive to hormonal manipulation. Tamoxifen is beneficial in postmenopausal women when used alone or when combined with cytotoxic chemotherapy. The present recommendation is to administer tamoxifen for 5 years of continuous therapy after surgical resection. Longer durations of tamoxifen therapy do not appear to add additional clinical benefit. Postmenopausal women who complete 5 years of tamoxifen therapy should be placed on an aromatase inhibitor for at least 2.5 years, although the optimal duration is unknown. In women who have completed 2–3 years of tamoxifen therapy, treatment with an aromatase inhibitor for a total of 5 years of hormonal therapy is now recommended.

Results from several randomized trials for breast cancer have established that adjuvant chemotherapy for premenopausal women and adjuvant tamoxifen for postmenopausal women are of benefit to women with stage I (node-negative) breast cancer. While this group of patients has the lowest overall risk of recurrence after surgery alone (about 35–50% over 15 years), this risk can be further reduced with adjuvant therapy.

2. Stage III & Stage IV Disease

The approach to women with advanced breast cancer remains a major problem, as current treatment options are only palliative. Combination chemotherapy, endocrine therapy, or a combination of both results in overall response rates of 40–50%, with only a 10–20% complete response rate. Breast cancers expressing estrogen receptors (ER) or progesterone receptors (PR), retain the intrinsic hormonal sensitivities of the normal breast— including the growth-stimulatory response to ovarian, adrenal, and pituitary hormones. Patients who show improvement with hormonal ablative procedures also respond to the addition of tamoxifen. The aromatase inhibitors anastrozole and letrozole are now approved as first-line therapy in women with advanced breast cancer whose tumors are hormone-receptor positive. In addition, these agents and exemestane are approved as second-line therapy following treatment with tamoxifen.

Patients with significant visceral involvement of the lung, liver, or brain and those with rapidly progressive disease rarely benefit from hormonal maneuvers, and initial systemic chemotherapy is indicated in such cases. For the 25–30% of breast cancer patients whose tumors express the HER-2/*neu* cell surface receptor, the humanized monoclonal anti-HER-2/*neu* antibody, trastuzumab, is available for therapeutic use alone or in combination with cytotoxic chemotherapy.

Systemic Chemotherapy

About 50–60% of patients with metastatic disease respond to initial chemotherapy. A broad range of anticancer agents have activity in this disease, including the anthracyclines (doxorubicin, mitoxantrone, and epirubicin), the taxanes (docetaxel, paclitaxel, and albumin-bound paclitaxel), navelbine, capecitabine, gemcitabine, cyclophosphamide, methotrexate, and cisplatin. Doxorubicin and the taxanes are the most active cytotoxic drugs. Combination chemotherapy has been found to induce higher and more durable remissions in up to 50–80% of patients, and anthracycline-containing regimens are now considered the standard of care in first-line therapy. With most combination regimens, partial remissions have a median duration of about 10 months and complete remissions have a duration of about 15 months. Unfortunately, only 10–20% of patients achieve complete remissions with any of these regimens, and as noted, complete remissions are usually not long-lasting. The addition of tamoxifen to combination chemotherapy yields only modest additional improvement.

PROSTATE CANCER

Prostate cancer was the second type of cancer shown to be responsive to hormonal manipulation. The treatment of choice for patients with advanced prostate cancer is elimination of testosterone production by the testes either through surgical or chemical castration. Bilateral orchiectomy or estrogen therapy in the form of diethylstilbestrol was previously used as first-line therapy. However, at present, the use of LHRH agonists—including leuprolide and goserelin agonists, alone or in combination with an antiandrogen (eg, flutamide, bicalutamide, or nilutamide)—has become the preferred approach. There appears to be no survival advantage of total androgen blockade using a combination of LHRH agonist and antiandrogen agent compared with single-agent therapy. Hormonal treatment reduces symptoms—especially bone pain—in 70–80% of patients and may cause a significant reduction in the prostate-specific antigen (PSA) level, which is now widely accepted as a surrogate marker for response to treatment in prostate cancer. Although initial hormonal manipulation is able to control symptoms for up to 2 years, patients usually present with progressive disease. Second-line hormonal therapies include aminoglutethimide plus hydrocortisone, the antifungal agent ketoconazole plus hydrocortisone, or hydrocortisone alone.

Unfortunately, nearly all patients with advanced prostate cancer eventually become refractory to hormone therapy. A regimen of mitoxantrone and prednisone is approved in patients with hormone-refractory prostate cancer since it provides effective palliation in those who experience significant bone pain. Estramustine is an antimicrotubule agent that produces an almost 20% response rate as a single agent. However, when used in combination with either etoposide or a taxane such as docetaxel or paclitaxel, response rates are more than doubled to 40–50%. The combination of docetaxel and prednisone was recently shown to confer survival advantage when compared with the mitoxantrone-prednisone regimen, and this combination has now become the standard of care for hormone-refractory prostate cancer.

GASTROINTESTINAL CANCERS

Colorectal cancer is the most common type of gastrointestinal malignancy. Approximately 145,000 new cases are diagnosed each year in the USA; worldwide, there are nearly one million cases diagnosed each year. At the time of initial presentation, only about 40–45% of cases are potentially curable with surgery. Patients presenting with high-risk stage II disease and stage III disease are candidates for adjuvant chemotherapy with an oxaliplatin-based regimen in combination with 5-FU plus leucovorin, or with oral capecitabine and are generally treated for up to 6–8 months following surgical resection. Treatment with this combination regimen reduces the recurrence rate after surgery by 35% in these patients and clearly improves overall patient survival compared with surgery alone. For patients with rectal

carcinoma, surgical adjuvant therapy with protracted intravenous infusion of 5-FU along with pelvic irradiation provides a modest albeit significant improvement in both relapse-free and overall survival.

As a single agent, the topoisomerase I inhibitor irinotecan was initially approved as second-line therapy in patients who were no longer responding to 5-FU-based chemotherapy. The combination of irinotecan, 5-FU, and leucovorin (IFL protocol) when given either in a weekly bolus fashion or via a biweekly infusion schedule has now been shown to provide significant clinical benefit in terms of overall response rates, time to disease progression, and survival when compared with treatment with the combination of 5-FU and leucovorin alone. This regimen is now approved for use in the first-line setting. Oxaliplatin in combination with a biweekly infusion schedule of 5-FU and leucovorin (FOLFOX regimen) is also approved for use in the first-line setting. Recent clinical studies have shown that FOLFOX in combination with the anti-VEGF antibody bevacizumab or with the anti-EGFR antibody cetuximab results in significantly improved response rates with no worsening of the toxicities normally observed with chemotherapy.

The incidence of gastric cancer, esophageal cancer, and pancreatic cancer is much lower than for colorectal cancer, but these malignancies are more aggressive. In most cases, they cannot be completely resected surgically, as most patients present with either locally advanced or metastatic disease at the time of their initial diagnosis. 5-FU-based chemotherapy has been the usual approach for gastroesophageal cancers. Recently, there has been a shift toward incorporating cisplatin-based regimens in combination with either irinotecan or with one of the taxanes, paclitaxel or docetaxel. Response rates of 40–50% are now being reported. In addition, neoadjuvant approaches with combination chemotherapy and radiation therapy prior to surgery appear to have some promise in selected patients. Although gemcitabine is approved for use as a single-agent in metastatic pancreatic cancer, the overall response rate is less than 10%, with no complete responses. Intense efforts are now being placed on incorporating gemcitabine into various combination regimens and on identifying novel agents that target signal transduction pathways thought to be critical for the growth of pancreatic cancer. One such agent is the small molecule inhibitor **erlotinib,** which targets the EGFR-associated tyrosine kinase. This agent was recently approved for use in combination with gemcitabine in locally advanced or metastatic pancreatic cancer.

LUNG CANCER

Lung cancer can be divided into two main histopathologic subtypes, non-small cell and small cell. Non-small cell lung cancer (NSCLC) makes up about 75–80% of all cases of lung cancer, and this group includes adeno-carcinoma, squamous cell cancer, and large cell cancer, while small cell lung cancer (SCLC) makes up the remaining 20–25%. When NSCLC is diagnosed in an advanced stage with metastatic disease, the prognosis is extremely poor, with a median survival of about 8 months. It is clear that prevention (primarily through avoidance of cigarette smoking) and early detection remain the most important means of control. When diagnosed at an early stage, surgical resection can result in patient cure. Moreover, recent studies have shown that adjuvant platinum-based chemotherapy provides a survival benefit in patients with pathologic stage IB, II, and IIIA disease. However, in most cases, distant metastases have occurred at the time of diagnosis. In certain instances, radiation therapy can be offered for palliation of pain, airway obstruction, or bleeding and to treat patients whose performance status would not allow for more aggressive treatments.

In patients with advanced disease, palliative systemic chemotherapy is generally recommended. At this time, for patients with good performance status and those with nonsquamous histology, the combination of the anti-VEGF antibody bevacizumab with carboplatin and paclitaxel has become the treatment of choice. In patients who are deemed not to be candidates for beva-cizumab therapy, a platinum-based chemotherapy regi-men is preferred, although non-platinum regimens may be used as alternatives.

Small cell lung cancer is the most aggressive form of lung cancer, and it is extremely sensitive to platinum-based combination regimens, including cisplatin and etoposide or cisplatin and irinotecan. The topoisomer-ase I inhibitor topotecan is used as second-line mono-therapy in patients who have failed a platinum-based regimen. When diagnosed as limited stage, this disease is potentially curable with a combined modality approach using chemotherapy and radiation therapy.

OVARIAN CANCER

In the majority of patients, this cancer remains occult and becomes symptomatic only after it has already metastasized to the peritoneal cavity. At this stage, it usually presents with malignant ascites. It is important to accurately stage this cancer with laparoscopy, ultra-sound, and CT scanning. Patients with stage I disease appear to benefit from whole-abdomen radiotherapy and may receive additional benefit from combination chemotherapy with cisplatin and cyclophosphamide.

Combination chemotherapy is the standard approach to stage III and stage IV disease. Randomized clinical studies have shown that the combination of paclitaxel and cisplatin provides survival benefit compared with

the previous standard combination of cisplatin plus cyclophosphamide. More recently, carboplatin plus paclitaxel has become the treatment of choice. In patients who present with recurrent disease, the topo-isomerase I inhibitor topotecan, the alkylating agent altretamine, and liposomal doxorubicin are used as sin-gle agent monotherapy.

TESTICULAR CANCER

The introduction of platinum-based combination che-motherapy has made an impressive change in the treat-ment of patients with advanced testicular cancer. At present, chemotherapy is recommended for patients with stage IIC or stage III seminomas and nonsemi-nomatous disease. Over 90% of patients respond to chemotherapy and, depending upon the extent and severity of disease, complete remissions up to 70–80% are observed. Over 50% of patients achieving complete remission are cured with chemotherapy. In patients with good risk features, three cycles of cisplatin, etopo-side, and bleomycin (PEB protocol) or four cycles of cisplatin and etoposide give virtually identical results. In patients with high-risk disease, the combination of cisplatin, etoposide, and ifosfamide can be used as well as etoposide and bleomycin with high-dose cisplatin.

MALIGNANT MELANOMA

Once it has metastasized, malignant melanoma is one of the most difficult neoplasms to treat because it is a rela-tively drug-resistant neoplasm. Dacarbazine, temozolo-mide, and cisplatin are the most active cytotoxic agents for this disease. Biologic agents, including interferon-α and interleukin-2 (IL-2), may have greater activity than traditional anticancer agents, and treatment with high-dose IL-2 has led to cures in a small subset of patients. Several clinical studies are actively investigating the com-bination of biologic therapy with combination chemo-therapy in what have been labeled biochemotherapy regi-mens. Thus far, overall response rates as well as complete response rates appear to be much higher with biochemo-therapy regimens compared with chemotherapy alone. Unfortunately, treatment toxicity also seems to be increased. This approach remains investigational, and further studies are required to determine whether this approach can lead to improved patient survival.

BRAIN CANCER

Chemotherapy has only limited efficacy in the treatment of malignant gliomas. In general, the nitrosoureas, because of their ability to cross the blood-brain barrier, are the most active agents in this disease. Carmustine (BCNU) can be used as a single agent, or lomustine

(CCNU) can be used in combination with procarbazine and vincristine (PCV regimen). In addition, the newer alkylating agent temozolomide has activity in the setting of recurrent disease, and it is approved for this indication. The histopathologic subtype oligodendroglioma has been shown to be especially chemosensitive, and the PCV regimen is the treatment of choice for this disease.

CHORIOCARCINOMA

This rare tumor arises from fetal trophoblastic tissue and was the first metastatic cancer cured with chemotherapy. Single-agent methotrexate produced complete regression of metastatic lesions, resulting in a high percentage of cures. At present, treatment with single-agent methotrexate or dactinomycin is recommended for low-risk disease, while intense combination regimens including methotrexate and leucovorin rescue, etoposide, dactinomycin, vincristine, and cyclophosphamide are recommended for intermediate or high-risk disease.

SECONDARY MALIGNANCIES & CANCER CHEMOTHERAPY

The development of secondary malignancies is a late complication of some types of cancer chemotherapy. The most frequent secondary malignancy is acute myelogenous leu-

kemia (AML). The alkylating agents, procarbazine, etoposide, and ionizing radiation are all considered to be leukemogenic. AML has been observed in up to 15% of patients with Hodgkin's disease who have received radiotherapy plus MOPP chemotherapy and in patients with multiple myeloma, ovarian carcinoma, or breast carcinoma treated with melphalan. The increased risk of AML is observed as early as 2–4 years after the initiation of chemotherapy and peaks at 5 and 9 years. With improvements in the clinical efficacy of various combination chemotherapy regimens resulting in prolonged survival and in some cases actual cure of cancer, the issue of how second cancers may affect long-term survival assumes greater importance. There is already evidence that certain alkylating agents (eg, cyclophosphamide) may be less carcinogenic than others (eg, melphalan). Systematic testing of the carcinogenicity of anticancer drugs in several animal models should allow less toxic agents to be identified and substituted for other more carcinogenic ones in chemotherapy regimens.

PREPARATIONS AVAILABLE

The reader is referred to the manufacturers' literature for the most recent information.

REFERENCES

Books & Monographs

Abbruzzesse JL et al: *Gastrointestinal Oncology.* Oxford Univ Press, 2003.

Chabner BA, Longo DL: *Cancer Chemotherapy and Biotherapy: Principles and Practice,* 4th ed. Lippincott Williams & Wilkins, 2006.

Chu E, DeVita VT Jr: *Cancer Chemotherapy Drug Manual 2006,* 6th ed. Jones & Bartlett, 2006.

DeVita VT Jr, Hellman S, Rosenberg SA: *Cancer: Principles and Practice of Oncology,* 7th ed. Lippincott Williams & Wilkins, 2005.

Frank DA: *Signal Transduction in Cancer.* Kluwer Academic, 2002.

Harris JR et al: *Diseases of the Breast,* 3rd ed. Lippincott Williams & Wilkins, 2004.

Hoskins WJ, Perez CA, Young RC: *Principles and Practice of Gynecologic Oncology,* 4th ed. Lippincott Williams & Wilkins, 2004.

Kantoff PW et al: *Prostate Cancer: Principles and Practice.* Lippincott Williams & Wilkins, 2001.

Kelsen DP et al: *Gastrointestinal Oncology: Principles and Practices.* Lippincott Williams & Wilkins, 2001.

Kufe D et al: Holland Frei *Cancer Medicine,* 7th ed. BC Decker, 2006.

Pass HI et al: *Lung Cancer: Principles and Practice,* 3rd ed. Lippincott Williams & Wilkins, 2004.

Perez CA, Brady LW: *Principles and Practice of Radiation Oncology,* 4th ed. Lippincott Williams & Wilkins, 2003.

Pizzo PA, Poplack AG: *Principles and Practice of Pediatric Oncology,* 5th ed. Lippincott Williams & Wilkins, 2005.

Rosenberg SA: *Principles and Practice of the Biologic Therapy of Cancer,* 3rd ed. Lippincott Williams & Wilkins, 2000.

Articles & Reviews

Abal M, Andreu JM, Barasoain I: Taxanes: Microtubule and centrosome targets, and cell cycle dependent mechanisms of action. Curr Cancer Drug Targets 2003;3:193.

Borst P et al: Mammalian ABC transporters in health and disease. Ann Rev Biochem 2002;71:5370.

Khalil MY, Grandis JR, Shin DM: Targeting epidermal growth factor receptor: Novel therapeutics in the management of cancer. Expert Rev Anticancer Ther 2003;3:367.

Skipper HE et al: Implications of biochemical, pharmacologic, and toxicologic relationships in the design of optimal therapy. Cancer Chemother Rep 1970;54:431.

Immunopharmacology

56

Douglas F. Lake, PhD, Adrienne D. Briggs, MD, & Emmanuel T. Akporiaye, PhD

Agents that suppress the immune system play an important role in preventing the rejection of organ or tissue grafts and in the treatment of certain diseases that arise from dysregulation of the immune response. While precise details of the mechanisms of action of a number of these agents are still obscure, knowledge of the elements of the immune system is useful in understanding their effects. Agents that augment the immune response or selectively alter the balance of various components of the immune system are also becoming important in the management of certain diseases such as cancer, AIDS, and autoimmune or inflammatory diseases. A growing number of other diseases (infections, cardiovascular diseases) may also be candidates for immune manipulation.

■ I. ELEMENTS OF THE IMMUNE SYSTEM

NORMAL IMMUNE RESPONSES

The immune system has evolved to protect the host from invading pathogens and to eliminate disease. At its functioning best, the immune system is exquisitely responsive to invading pathogens while retaining the capacity to recognize self antigens to which it is tolerant. Protection from infection and disease is provided by the collaborative efforts of the innate and adaptive immune systems.

The Innate Immune System

The innate immune system is the first line of defense against an invading pathogen (antigen) and includes physical (eg, skin), biochemical (eg, complement, lysozyme, interferons), and cellular components (neutrophils, monocytes, macrophages, natural killer [NK], and natural killer-T [NKT] cells). An intact skin or mucosa is the first barrier to infection. When this barrier is breached, destruction of the pathogen (eg, bacteria, fungi, parasites) is accomplished by biochemical components such as lysozyme (which breaks down the protec-

ACRONYMS

ADA	Adenosine deaminase
ALG	Antilymphocyte globulin
APC	Antigen-presenting cell
ATG	Antithymocyte globulin
CD	Cluster of differentiation
CSF	Colony-stimulating factor
CTL	Cytotoxic T lymphocyte
DC	Dendritic cell
DTH	Delayed-type hypersensitivity
FKBP	FK-binding protein
HAMA	Human antimouse antibody
HLA	Human leukocyte antigen
IFN	Interferon
IGIV	Immune globulin intravenous
IL	Interleukin
LFA	Leukocyte function-associated antigen
MAB	Monoclonal antibody
MHC	Major histocompatibility complex
NK cell	Natural killer cell
SCID	Severe combined immunodeficiency disease
TCR	T cell receptor
TGF-β	Transforming growth factor-β
TH1, TH2	T helper cell types 1 and 2
TNF	Tumor necrosis factor

tive peptidoglycan cell wall) and the split products arising from complement activation. Complement components (Figure 56–1) enhance macrophage and neutrophil phagocytosis by acting as **opsonins (C3b)** and **chemoattractants (C3a, C5a)** that recruit immune cells to inflammatory sites. The activation of complement eventually leads to pathogen lysis via the generation of a membrane attack complex that creates holes in the membrane and results in leakage of cellular components.

During the inflammatory response triggered by infection, neutrophils and monocytes enter the tissue sites from the peripheral circulation. This cellular influx is mediated by the release and action of **chemoattractant cytokines** (eg, IL-8 [CXCL8], macrophage che-

Figure 56–1. Role of complement in innate immunity. Complement is made up of nine proteins (C1–C9), which are split into fragments during activation. **A:** Complement components (C3a, C5a) attract phagocytes (①) to inflammatory sites (②), where they ingest and degrade pathogens (③). **B:** Complement components C5b, C6, C7, C8, and C9 associate to form a membrane attack complex (MAC) that lyses bacteria, causing their destruction. **C:** Complement component C3b is an opsonin that coats bacteria (①) and facilitates their ingestion (②) and digestion (③) by phagocytes.

motactic protein-1 [MCP-1; CCL2], and macrophage inflammatory protein-1 [MIP-1α; CCL3]) from activated endothelial cells and immune cells (mostly tissue macrophages) at the inflammatory site. It is triggered by the adhesion of cell surface receptors on the immune cells to ligands on the activated endothelial cell surface. If these events occur successfully, the invading pathogen is ingested, degraded, and eliminated, and disease is either prevented or is of short duration.

Natural killer (NK) and **natural killer-T (NKT)** cells recruited to the inflammatory site also contribute to the innate response by secreting interferon–gamma (IFN-γ), which activates resident tissue macrophages and dendritic cells. NK cells are so called because they are able to recognize and destroy virus-infected normal cells as well as tumor cells without prior stimulation. This activity is regulated by so-called "killer cell immu-

noglobulin-like receptors" (KIRs) on the NK cell surface that are specific for major histocompatibility complex (MHC) class I molecules. When NK cells bind self MHC class I proteins (expressed on all nucleated cells), these receptors deliver inhibitory signals, preventing them from killing normal host cells. Tumor cells or virus-infected cells that have down-regulated MHC class I expression do not engage these KIRs, resulting in activation of NK cells and subsequent destruction of the target cell. NK cells kill target cells by releasing cytotoxic granules that induce programmed cell death.

NKT cells express T-cell receptors as well as receptors commonly found on NK cells. NKT cells recognize microbial lipid antigens presented by a unique class of MHC-like molecules known as CD1 and have been implicated in host defense against microbial agents, autoimmune diseases, and tumors.

The Adaptive Immune System

The adaptive immune system is mobilized by cues from the innate response when the innate processes are incapable of coping with an infection. The adaptive immune system has a number of characteristics that contribute to its success in eliminating pathogens. These include the ability to (1) respond to a variety of antigens, each in a specific manner; (2) discriminate between foreign ("non-self") antigens (pathogens) and self antigens of the host; and (3) respond to a previously encountered antigen in a learned way by initiating a vigorous memory response. This adaptive response culminates in the production of **antibodies,** which are the effectors of **humoral immunity;** and the activation of **T lymphocytes,** which are the effectors of **cell-mediated immunity.**

The induction of specific adaptive immunity requires the participation of professional **antigen-presenting cells (APCs),** which include dendritic cells (DC), macrophages, and B lymphocytes. These cells play pivotal roles in the induction of an adaptive immune response because of their capacity to phagocytize or endocytose protein antigens, and enzymatically digest them to generate peptides, which are then loaded onto class I or class II MHC proteins and "presented" to the cell surface T-cell receptor (TCR) (Figure 56–2). CD8 T cells recognize class I-MHC peptide complexes while CD4 T cells recognize class II-MHC peptide complexes. At least two signals are necessary for the activation of T cells. The first signal is delivered following engagement of the TCR with peptide-bound MHC molecules. In the absence of a second signal, the T cells become unresponsive (anergic) or undergo apoptosis. The second signal involves ligation of costimulatory molecules (CD40, CD80 [also known as B7-1], and CD86 [also known as B7-2]) on the antigen-presenting cell to their respective ligands (CD40L for CD40, CD28 for CD80 or CD86). Activation of T cells is regulated via a negative feedback loop involving another molecule known as T-lymphocyte-associated antigen 4 (CTLA-4). Following engagement of CD28 with CD80 or CD86, CTLA-4 in the cytoplasm is mobilized to the cell surface where, because of its higher affinity of binding to CD80 and CD86, it outcompetes or displaces CD28 and results in suppression of T-cell activation and proliferation. This property of CTLA-4 has been exploited as a strategy for sustaining a desirable immune response such as that directed against cancer. A recombinant humanized antibody that binds CTLA-4 (ipilimumab) prevents its association with CD80/CD86. In so doing, the activated state of T cells is sustained. Recently completed vaccine trials in metastatic melanoma patients receiving anti-CTLA-4 antibody reported objective clinical responses in a few of the treated patients. Unfortunately, these beneficial

Figure 56–2. T-cell activation by an antigen-presenting cell requires engagement of the T-cell receptor by the MHC-peptide complex (signal 1) and binding of the co-stimulatory molecules (CD80, CD86) on the dendritic cell to CD28 on the T cell (signal 2). The activation signals are strengthened by CD40/CD40L and ICAM-1/LFA-1 interactions. In a normal immune response, T-cell activation is regulated by T-cell-derived CTLA-4, which binds to CD80 or CD86 with higher affinity than CD28 and sends inhibitory signals to the nucleus of the T cell.

responses were associated with the development of autoimmune toxicity in some patients, raising concern about this approach.

T lymphocytes develop and learn to recognize self and non-self antigens in the thymus; those T cells that bind with high affinity to self antigens in the thymus undergo apoptosis (negative selection), while those that are capable of recognizing foreign antigens in the presence of self MHC molecules are retained and expanded (positive selection) for export to the periphery (lymph nodes, spleen, mucosa-associated lymphoid tissue, peripheral blood), where they become activated after encountering MHC-presented peptides (Figures 56–2 and 56–3).

Studies using murine T-cell clones have demonstrated the presence of two subsets of T helper lymphocytes (**TH1** and **TH2**) based on the cytokines they secrete after activation. This demarcation is not so clear-cut in humans. The TH1 subset characteristically produces interferon-γ (IFN-γ), interleukin-2 (IL-2), and tumor necrosis factor-β (TNF-β) and induces cell-mediated immunity by activation of macrophages, cytotoxic T cells (CTLs), and NK cells. The TH2 subset produces IL-4, IL-5, IL-6, and IL-10 (and sometimes IL-13), which induce B-cell proliferation and differentiation into antibody-secreting plasma cells. IL-10 produced by TH2 cells inhibits cytokine production by TH1 cells via the down-regulation of MHC expression

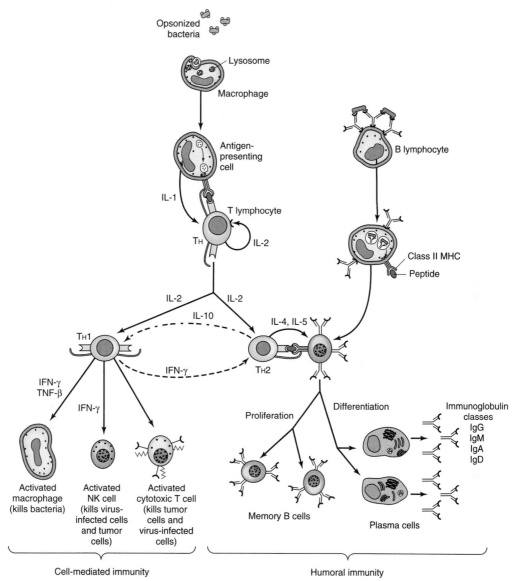

Figure 56–3. Scheme of cellular interactions during the generation of cell-mediated and humoral immune responses (see text). The cell-mediated arm of the immune response involves the ingestion and digestion of antigen by antigen-presenting cells such as macrophages. Activated TH cells secrete IL-2, which causes proliferation and activation of cytotoxic T lymphocytes, and TH1 and TH2 cell subsets. TH1 cells also produce IFN-γ and TNF-β, which can directly activate macrophages and NK cells. The humoral response is triggered when B lymphocytes bind antigen via their surface immunoglobulin. They are then induced by TH2-derived IL-4 and IL-5 to proliferate and differentiate into memory cells and antibody-secreting plasma cells. Regulatory cytokines such as IFN-γ and IL-10 down-regulate TH2 and TH1 responses, respectively.

by APCs. Conversely, IFN-γ produced by TH1 cells inhibits the proliferation of TH2 cells (Figure 56–3). Although these subsets have been well described in vitro, the nature of the antigenic challenge that elicits a TH1 or TH2 phenotype is less clear. Extracellular bacteria typically cause the elaboration of TH2 cytokines, culminating in the production of neutralizing or opsonic antibodies. In contrast, intracellular organisms (eg, mycobacteria) elicit the production of TH1 cytokines, which lead to the activation of effector cells such as macrophages. A less well defined T-cell subset (TH3) has been described that produces transforming growth factor-β (TGF-β), whose numerous functions include down-regulation of proliferation and differentiation of T lymphocytes.

CD8 T lymphocytes recognize endogenously processed peptides presented by virus-infected cells or tumor cells. These peptides are usually nine-amino-acid fragments derived from virus or protein tumor antigens in the cytoplasm and are loaded onto MHC class I molecules (Figure 56–2) in the endoplasmic reticulum. In contrast, class II MHC molecules present peptides (usually 11–22 amino acids) derived from extracellular (exogenous) pathogens to CD4 T helper cells. In some instances, exogenous antigens, upon ingestion by APCs, can be presented on class I MHC molecules to CD8 T cells. This phenomenon is referred to as "cross-presentation" and is thought to be useful in generating effective immune responses against infected host cells that are incapable of priming T lymphocytes. Upon activation, CD8 T cells induce target cell death via lytic granule enzymes ("granzymes"), perforin, and the Fas-Fas ligand (Fas-FasL) apoptosis pathways.

B lymphocytes undergo selection in the bone marrow, during which self-reactive B lymphocytes are clonally deleted while B-cell clones specific for foreign antigens are retained and expanded. The repertoire of antigen specificities by T cells is genetically determined and arises from T-cell *receptor* gene rearrangement while the specificities of B cells arise from *immunoglobulin* gene rearrangement; for both types of cells, these determinations occur prior to encounters with antigen. Upon an encounter with antigen, a mature B cell binds the antigen, internalizes and processes it, and presents its peptide bound to class II MHC to CD4 helper cells, which in turn secrete IL-4 and IL-5. These interleukins stimulate B-cell proliferation and differentiation into memory B cells and antibody-secreting plasma cells. The primary antibody response consists mostly of IgM-class immunoglobulins. Subsequent antigenic stimulation results in a vigorous "booster" response accompanied by class (isotype) switching to produce IgG, IgA, and IgE antibodies with diverse effector functions (Figure 56–3). These antibodies also undergo affinity maturation, which allows them to bind more efficiently to the antigen. With the passage of time, this results in accelerated elimination of microorganisms in subsequent infections. Antibodies mediate their functions by acting as opsonins to enhance phagocytosis and cellular cytotoxicity and by activating complement to elicit an inflammatory response and induce bacterial lysis (Figure 56–4).

ABNORMAL IMMUNE RESPONSES

Whereas the normally functioning immune response can successfully neutralize toxins, inactivate viruses, destroy transformed cells, and eliminate pathogens, inappropriate responses can lead to extensive tissue damage (hypersensitivity) or reactivity against self antigens (autoimmunity); conversely, impaired reactivity to appropriate targets (immunodeficiency) may occur and abrogate essential defense mechanisms.

Hypersensitivity

Hypersensitivity can be classified as antibody-mediated or cell-mediated. Three types of hypersensitivity are antibody-mediated (types I–III), while the fourth is cell-mediated (type IV). Hypersensitivity occurs in two phases: the sensitization phase and the effector phase. Sensitization occurs upon initial encounter with an antigen; the effector phase involves immunologic memory and results in tissue pathology upon a subsequent encounter with that antigen.

A. IMMEDIATE HYPERSENSITIVITY

Immediate, or type I, hypersensitivity is IgE-mediated, with symptoms usually occurring within minutes following the patient's encounter with antigen.

1. Type I–Type I hypersensitivity results from cross-linking of membrane-bound IgE on blood basophils or tissue mast cells by antigen. This cross-linking causes cells to degranulate, releasing substances such as histamine, leukotrienes, and eosinophil chemotactic factor, which induce anaphylaxis, asthma, hay fever, or urticaria (hives) in affected individuals (Figure 56–5). A severe type I hypersensitivity reaction such as systemic anaphylaxis (eg, from insect envenomation, ingestion of certain foods, or drug hypersensitivity) requires immediate medical intervention.

2. Type II–Type II hypersensitivity results from the formation of antigen-antibody complexes between foreign antigen and IgM or IgG immunoglobulins. One example of this type of hypersensitivity is a blood transfusion reaction that can occur if blood is not cross-matched properly. Preformed antibodies bind to red blood cell membrane antigens that activate the complement cascade, generating a membrane attack complex that lyses the transfused red blood cells. In hemolytic disease of the newborn, anti-Rh IgG antibodies pro-

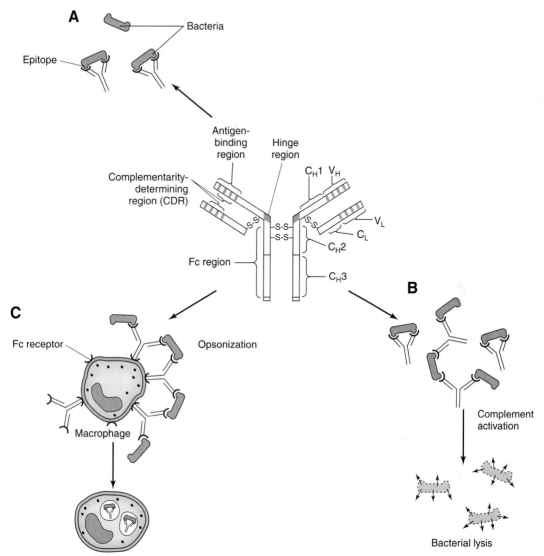

Figure 56–4. Antibody has multiple functions. The prototypical antibody consists of two heavy (H) and two light (L) chains, each subdivided into constant (C_L, C_H) and variable (V_L, V_H) domains. The structure is held together by intra- and interchain disulfide bridges. **A:** The complementarity-determining region (CDR) of the antigen-binding portion of the antibody engages the antigenic determinant (epitope) in a lock and key fashion. **B:** Antigen-antibody complexes activate complement to produce split complement components that cause bacterial lysis. **C:** The Fc portion of antibodies binds to Fc receptors on phagocytes (eg, macrophages, neutrophils) and facilitates uptake of bacteria (opsonization).

duced by an Rh-negative mother cross the placenta, bind to red blood cells of an Rh-positive fetus, and damage them. The disease is prevented in subsequent pregnancies by the administration of anti-Rh antibodies to the mother 24–48 hours after delivery (see Antibodies as Immunosuppressive Agents, below). Type II hypersensitivity can also be drug-induced and may occur during the administration of penicillin to allergic patients. In these patients, penicillin binds to red blood cells or other host tissue to form a neoantigen that evokes production of antibodies capable of inducing complement-mediated red cell lysis. In some circum-

Sensitization phase

Naive B cell

+IL-4,-5

T helper cell

IgE-secreting plasma cell
IgE is specific for allergen

IgE binds IgE Fc
receptors on mast
cells or basophils

Effector phase

Allergen cross-links IgE on mast
cell (or basophil) and triggers
degranulation and release of
pharmacologic mediators

Mediators
Histamine
Serotonin
Leukotrienes
Prostaglandins
Bradykinins
Proteases
Eosinophil chemotactic factor
Neutrophil chemotactic factor

Effects
Smooth muscle contraction
Vasodilation
Increased vascular
permeability
Platelet aggregation
Complement activation
Mucus secretion

Clinical symptoms
Asthma
Hay fever
Skin rashes
Local anaphylaxis
Systemic anaphylaxis

Figure 56–5. Mechanism of type I hypersensitivity. Initial exposure to allergen **(sensitization phase)** leads to production of IgE by plasma cells differentiated from allergen-specific B cells (not shown). The secreted IgE binds IgE-specific receptors (FcεR) on blood basophils and tissue mast cells. Reexposure to allergen leads to cross-linking of membrane-bound IgE **(effector phase).** This cross-linking causes degranulation of cytoplasmic granules and release of mediators that induce vasodilation, smooth muscle contraction, and increased vascular permeability. These effects lead to the clinical symptoms characteristic of type I hypersensitivity.

stances, subsequent administration of the drug can lead to systemic anaphylaxis (type I hypersensitivity).

3. Type III–Type III hypersensitivity is due to the presence of elevated levels of antigen-antibody complexes that deposit on basement membranes in tissues and vessels. Immune complex deposition activates complement to produce components with anaphylatoxic and chemotactic activities (C5a, C3a, C4a) that increase vascular permeability and recruit neutrophils to the site of complex deposition. Complex deposition

and the action of lytic enzymes released by neutrophils can cause skin rashes, glomerulonephritis, and arthritis in these individuals. If patients have type III hypersensitivity against a particular antigen, clinical symptoms usually occur 3 to 4 days after exposure to the antigen.

B. TYPE IV: DELAYED-TYPE HYPERSENSITIVITY

Unlike type I, II, and III hypersensitivities, delayed-type hypersensitivity (DTH) is cell-mediated, and responses occur 2–3 days after exposure to the sensitizing antigen.

Figure 56–6. Mechanism of type IV hypersensitivity (DTH). In the **sensitization phase,** the processed allergen (eg, from poison oak) is presented to CD4 TH1 cells by antigen-presenting cells in association with class II MHC. T cells are induced to express IL-2 receptors and are stimulated to proliferate and differentiate into memory T_{DTH} cells. Secondary contact with antigen triggers the **effector phase,** in which memory T_{DTH} cells release cytokines that attract and activate nonspecific inflammatory macrophages and neutrophils. These cells display increased phagocytic and microbicidal activities and release large quantities of lytic enzymes that cause extensive tissue damage.

DTH is caused by antigen-specific DTH TH1 cells and induces a local inflammatory response that causes tissue damage characterized by the influx of antigen-*non*specific inflammatory cells, especially macrophages. These cells are recruited under the influence of TH1-produced cytokines (Figure 56–6), which chemoattract circulating monocytes and neutrophils, induce myelopoiesis, and activate macrophages. The activated macrophages are primarily responsible for the tissue damage associated with DTH. Although widely considered to be deleterious, DTH responses are very effective in eliminating infections caused by intracellular pathogens such as *Mycobacterium tuberculosis* and *Leishmania* species. Clinical manifestations of DTH include tuberculin and contact hypersensitivities. Tuberculosis exposure is determined using a DTH skin test. Positive responses show erythema and induration caused by accumulation of macrophages and DTH T cells at the site of the tuberculin injection. Poison ivy is the most common cause of contact hypersensitivity, in which pentadecacatechol, the lipophilic chemical in poison ivy, modifies cellular tissue and results in a DTH T-cell response.

Autoimmunity

Autoimmune disease arises when the body mounts an immune response against itself due to failure to distinguish self tissues and cells from foreign (nonself) antigens. This phenomenon derives from the activation of self-reactive T and B lymphocytes that generate cell-mediated or humoral immune responses directed against self antigens. The pathologic consequences of this reactivity constitute several types of autoimmune diseases. Autoimmune diseases are highly complex due to MHC genetics, environmental conditions, infectious entities, and dysfunctional immune regulation. Examples of such diseases include rheumatoid arthritis, systemic lupus erythematosus, multiple sclerosis, and insulin-dependent diabetes mellitus (type 1 diabetes). In rheumatoid arthritis, IgM antibodies (rheumatoid factors) are produced that react with the Fc portion of IgG and may form immune complexes that activate the complement cascade, causing chronic inflammation of the joints and kidneys. In systemic lupus erythematosus, antibodies are made against DNA, histones, red blood cells, platelets, and other cellular components. In multiple sclerosis and type 1 diabetes, cell-mediated autoimmune attack destroys myelin surrounding nerve cells and insulin-producing islet B (beta) cells of the pancreas, respectively. In type 1 diabetes, activated CD4 T_{DTH} cells that infiltrate the islets of Langerhans and recognize self islet B cell peptides are thought to produce cytokines that stimulate macrophages to produce lytic enzymes, which destroy islet B cells. Autoantibodies directed against the islet B cell antigens are produced, but do not contribute significantly to disease.

A number of mechanisms have been proposed to explain autoimmunity:

(1) Exposure of self-reactive T lymphocytes to antigens previously sequestered from the immune system (eg, lens protein, myelin basic protein).

(2) Molecular mimicry by invading pathogens, in which immune responses are directed at antigenic determinants on pathogens that share identical or similar epitopes with normal host tissue. This phenomenon occurs in rheumatic fever following *Streptococcus pyogenes* infection, in which heart damage is thought to arise from an immune response directed against streptococcal antigens shared with heart muscle. The suggested viral etiology of autoimmune diseases has been ascribed to immune responses (both cell-mediated and humoral) directed against virus epitopes that mimic sequestered self antigens.

(3) Inappropriate expression of class II MHC molecules on the membranes of cells that normally do not express class II MHC (eg, islet β cells). Increased expression of MHC II may increase presentation of self peptides to T helper cells, which in turn induce CTL, T_{DTH}, and B-lymphocyte cells that react against self antigens.

Immunodeficiency Diseases

Immunodeficiency diseases result from inadequate function in the immune system; the consequences include increased susceptibility to infections and prolonged duration and severity of disease. Immunodeficiency diseases are either congenitally acquired or arise from extrinsic factors such as bacterial or viral infections or drug treatment. Affected individuals frequently succumb to infections caused by opportunistic organisms of low pathogenicity for the immunocompetent host. Examples of congenitally acquired immunodeficiency disease include X-linked agammaglobulinemia, DiGeorge's syndrome, and severe combined immunodeficiency disease (SCID) due to adenosine deaminase (ADA) deficiency.

X-linked agammaglobulinemia is a disease affecting males that is characterized by a failure of immature B-lymphocytes to mature into antibody-producing plasma cells. These individuals are susceptible to recurrent bacterial infections, although the cell-mediated responses directed against viruses and fungi are preserved. DiGeorge's syndrome is due to failure of the thymus to develop, resulting in diminished T-cell responses (T_{DTH}, CTL), while the humoral response is unaffected.

The ADA enzyme normally prevents the accumulation of toxic deoxy-ATP in cells. Deoxy-ATP is particularly toxic to lymphocytes, and leads to death of T and B cells. Absence of the enzyme therefore results in SCID. Infusion of the purified enzyme (**pegademase,** from bovine sources) and transfer of ADA gene-modified lymphocytes have both been used successfully to treat this disease.

AIDS represents the classic example of immunodeficiency disease caused by extrinsic factors, in this instance the human immunodeficiency virus (HIV). This virus exhibits a strong tropism for CD4 T helper cells; these become depleted, giving rise to increased frequency of opportunistic infections and malignancies in infected individuals. AIDS is also characterized by an imbalance in $T_{H}1$ and $T_{H}2$ cells, and the ratios of cells and their functions are skewed toward $T_{H}2$. This results in hypergammaglobulinemia, loss of cytotoxic lymphocyte activity, and delayed hypersensitivity.

Immunosuppressive agents have proved very useful in minimizing the occurrence or impact of deleterious effects of exaggerated or inappropriate immune responses. Unfortunately, these agents also have the potential to cause disease and to increase the risk of infection and malignancies.

■ II. IMMUNOSUPPRESSIVE AGENTS

GLUCOCORTICOIDS

Glucocorticoids (corticosteroids) were the first hormonal agents recognized as having lympholytic properties. Administration of any glucocorticoid reduces the size and lymphoid content of the lymph nodes and spleen, although it has no toxic effect on proliferating myeloid or erythroid stem cells in the bone marrow.

Glucocorticoids are thought to interfere with the cell cycle of activated lymphoid cells. The details of the mechanism of their action are described in Chapter 39. Glucocorticoids are quite cytotoxic to certain subsets of T cells, but their immunologic effects are probably due to their ability to modify cellular functions rather than to direct cytotoxicity. Although cellular immunity is more affected than humoral immunity, the primary antibody response can be diminished, and with continued use, previously established antibody responses are also decreased. Additionally, continuous administration of corticosteroid increases the fractional catabolic rate of IgG, the major class of antibody immunoglobulins, thus lowering the effective concentration of specific antibodies. Contact hypersensitivity mediated by DTH T cells, for example, is usually abrogated by glucocorticoid therapy.

Glucocorticoids are used in a wide variety of conditions (see Table 56–1). It is thought that the immunosuppressive and anti-inflammatory properties of corticosteroids account for their beneficial effects in diseases like idiopathic thrombocytopenic purpura and rheumatoid arthritis. Glucocorticoids modulate allergic reactions and are useful in the treatment of diseases like asthma or as premedication for other agents (eg, blood products, chemotherapy) that might cause undesirable immune responses. Glucocorticoids are first-line immunosuppressive therapy for both solid organ and hematopoietic stem cell transplant recipients, with variable results. The toxicities of long-term glucocorticoid therapy can be severe and are discussed in Chapter 39.

IMMUNOPHILIN LIGANDS

1. Cyclosporine

Cyclosporine (cyclosporin A, CSA) is an immunosuppressive agent with efficacy in human organ transplantation, in the treatment of graft-versus-host disease after hematopoietic stem cell transplantation, and in the treatment of selected autoimmune disorders. Cyclosporine is a peptide antibiotic that appears to act at an early stage in the antigen receptor-induced differentiation of T cells and blocks their activation. Cyclosporine binds to cyclophilin, a member of a class of intracellular proteins called immunophilins. Cyclosporine and cyclophilin form a complex that inhibits the cytoplasmic phosphatase, calcineurin, which is necessary for the activation of a T-cell-specific transcription factor. This transcription factor, NF-AT, is involved in the synthesis of interleukins (eg, IL-2) by activated T cells. In vitro studies have indicated that cyclosporine inhibits the gene transcription of IL-2, IL-3, IFN-γ, and other factors produced by antigen-stimulated T cells, but it does not block the effect of such factors on primed T cells nor does it block interaction with antigen.

Cyclosporine may be given intravenously or orally, though it is slowly and incompletely absorbed (20–50%). The absorbed drug is primarily metabolized by the P450 3A enzyme system in the liver with resultant multiple drug interactions. This propensity for drug interaction contributes to significant interpatient variability in bioavailability, such that cyclosporine requires individual patient dosage adjustments based on steady-state blood levels and the desired therapeutic ranges for the drug. Cyclosporine ophthalmic solution is now available for severe dry eye syndrome, as well as ocular graft-versus-host disease. Inhaled cyclosporine is being investigated for use in lung transplantation.

Toxicities are numerous and include nephrotoxicity, hypertension, hyperglycemia, liver dysfunction, hyperkalemia, altered mental status, seizures, and hirsutism. Cyclosporine causes very little bone marrow toxicity. While an increased incidence of lymphoma and other cancers (Kaposi's sarcoma, skin cancer) have been observed in transplant recipients receiving cyclosporine, other immunosuppressive agents may also predispose recipients to cancer. Some evidence suggests that tumors may arise after cyclosporine treatment because the drug induces TGF-β, which promotes tumor invasion and metastasis.

Cyclosporine may be used alone or in combination with other immunosuppressants, particularly glucocorticoids. It has been used successfully as the sole immunosuppressant for cadaveric transplants of the kidney, pancreas, and liver, and it has proved extremely useful in cardiac transplants as well. In combination with methotrexate, cyclosporine is a standard prophylactic regimen to prevent graft–versus-host disease after allogeneic stem cell transplants. Cyclosporine has also proved useful in a variety of autoimmune disorders, including uveitis, rheumatoid arthritis, psoriasis, and asthma. Its combination with newer agents is showing considerable efficacy in clinical and experimental settings where effective and less toxic immunosuppression is needed. Newer formulations of cyclosporine have been developed that are improving patient compliance (smaller, better tasting pills), and increasing bioavailability.

2. Tacrolimus

Tacrolimus (FK 506) is an immunosuppressant macrolide antibiotic produced by *Streptomyces tsukubaensis*. It is not chemically related to cyclosporine, but their mechanisms of action are similar. Both drugs bind to cytoplasmic peptidyl-prolyl isomerases that are abundant in all tissues. While cyclosporine binds to cyclophilin, tacrolimus binds to the immunophilin FK-binding protein (FKBP). Both complexes inhibit calcineurin, which is necessary for the activation of the T-cell-specific transcription factor NF-AT.

On a weight basis, tacrolimus is 10–100 times more potent than cyclosporine in inhibiting immune responses. Tacrolimus is utilized for the same indications as cyclosporine, particularly in organ and stem cell transplantation. Multicenter studies in the USA and in Europe indicate that both graft and patient survival are similar for the two drugs. Tacrolimus has been proven to be effective therapy for preventing rejection in solid-organ transplant patients even after failure of standard rejection therapy, including anti-T-cell antibodies. It is now considered a standard prophylactic agent (usually in combination with methotrexate or mycophenolate mofetil) for graft–versus-host disease.

Tacrolimus can be administered orally or intravenously. The half-life of the intravenous form is approximately 9–12 hours. Like cyclosporine, tacrolimus is metabolized primarily by P450 enzymes in the liver, and there is potential for drug interactions. The dosage is determined by trough blood level at steady state. Its toxic effects are similar to those of cyclosporine and include nephrotoxicity, neurotoxicity, hyperglycemia, hypertension, hyperkalemia, and gastrointestinal complaints.

Because of the effectiveness of systemic tacrolimus in some dermatologic diseases, a topical preparation is now available. Tacrolimus ointment is currently used in the therapy of atopic dermatitis and psoriasis.

3. Sirolimus

Sirolimus (rapamycin) is derived from *Streptomyces hygroscopicus,* and binds the immunophilin FKBP-12. Unlike cyclosporine and tacrolimus the sirolimus-FKBP-12 complex does not influence calcineurin activity, nor does it block interleukin (IL-2) production by activated T cells. Sirolimus binds mammalian target of rapamycin (mTOR), inhibiting the cell cycle and proliferation. In vitro, it antagonizes tacrolimus-induced T-cell responses but seems to be synergistic with cyclosporine. Furthermore, it is a potent inhibitor of B-cell proliferation and immunoglobulin production. Sirolimus also inhibits the mononuclear cell proliferative response to colony-stimulating factors and suppresses hematopoietic recovery after myelotoxic treatment in mice.

Sirolimus is available only as an oral drug. It is rapidly absorbed and its elimination is similar to that of cyclosporine and tacrolimus, being a substrate for both cytochrome P450 3A and P-glycoprotein. Significant drug interactions can occur, and the drug level in the blood may need to be monitored.

Sirolimus has been used effectively alone and in combination with other immunosuppressants (corticosteroids, cyclosporine, tacrolimus, and mycophenolate mofetil) to prevent rejection of solid organ allografts. Sirolimus is being investigated as therapy for steroid-refractory acute and chronic graft-versus-host disease in hematopoietic stem cell transplant recipients. Topical sirolimus is also used in some dermatologic disorders and, in combination with cyclosporine, in the management of uveoretinitis. Recently, sirolimus-eluting coronary stents have been shown to reduce restenosis and additional adverse cardiac events in patients with severe coronary artery disease, due to its antiproliferative effects. A derivative of sirolimus, **everolimus,** is a proliferation-signal inhibitor that may be of benefit in decreasing rejection in cardiac transplantation.

Toxicities of sirolimus can include profound myelosuppression (especially thrombocytopenia), hepatotoxicity, diarrhea, hypertriglyceridemia, and headache.

MYCOPHENOLATE MOFETIL

Mycophenolate mofetil (MMF) is a semisynthetic derivative of mycophenolic acid, isolated from the mold *Penicillium glaucum.* In vitro, it inhibits T- and B-lymphocyte responses, including mitogen and mixed lymphocyte responses, probably by inhibition of de novo synthesis of purines. Mycophenolate mofetil is hydrolyzed to mycophenolic acid, the active immunosuppressive moiety; it is synthesized and administered as MMF to enhance bioavailability. Mycophenolate mofetil is used in solid organ transplant patients for refractory rejection and, in combination with prednisone, as an alternative to cyclosporine or tacrolimus in patients who do not tolerate those drugs. Mycophenolate mofetil is used to treat steroid-refractory graft-versus-host disease in hematopoietic stem cell transplant patients. It is also used in combination with tacrolimus or other immunosuppressants as prophylaxis to prevent graft-versus-host disease. Newer immunosuppressant applications for MMF include lupus nephritis, rheumatoid arthritis, and some dermatologic disorders.

Mycophenolate mofetil is available in both oral and intravenous forms. The oral form is rapidly metabolized to mycophenolic acid but not by the cytochrome P450 3A system, though some drug interactions still occur.

Toxicities include gastrointestinal disturbances (nausea and vomiting, diarrhea, abdominal pain) headache, hypertension and reversible myelosuppression (primarily neutropenia).

THALIDOMIDE

Thalidomide is a sedative drug that was withdrawn from the market in the 1960s because of its disastrous teratogenic effects when used during pregnancy. Nevertheless, it has significant immunomodulatory actions and is currently in active use or in clinical trials for over 40 different illnesses. Thalidomide inhibits angiogenesis and has anti-inflammatory and immunomodulatory effects. It inhibits TNF-α, reduces phagocytosis by neutrophils, increases production of IL-10, alters adhesion molecule expression, and enhances cell-mediated immunity via interactions with T cells. The complex actions of thalidomide continue to be studied as its clinical use evolves.

Thalidomide is currently used in the treatment of multiple myeloma at initial diagnosis and for relapsed-refractory disease. Patients generally show signs of response within 2–3 months of starting the drug, with response rates from 20 to 70%. When combined with dexamethasone, the response rates in myeloma are 90% or more in some studies. Many patients have durable responses—up to 12–18 months in refractory disease and even longer in some patients treated at diagnosis. The success of thalidomide in myeloma has lead to numerous clinical trials in other diseases such as myelodysplastic syndrome, acute myelogenous leukemia, and graft-versus-host disease, as well as in solid tumors like colon cancer, renal cell carcinoma, melanoma, and prostate cancer, with variable results to date. Thalidomide has been used for many years in the treatment of some manifestations of leprosy and has been reintroduced in the USA for erythema nodosum leprosum; it is also useful in management of the skin manifestations of lupus erythematosus.

The adverse effect profile of thalidomide is extensive. The most important toxicity is teratogenesis. Because of this effect, thalidomide prescription and use is closely regulated by the manufacturer. Other adverse effects of thalidomide include peripheral neuropathy, constipation, rash, fatigue, hypothyroidism, and increased risk of deep vein thrombosis. Thrombosis is sufficiently frequent, particularly in the myeloma population, that most patients are placed on warfarin when thalidomide treatment is initiated.

Owing to thalidomide's serious toxicity profile, considerable effort has been expended in the development of analogs. Immunomodulatory derivatives of thalidomide are termed **IMiDs.** Some IMiDs are much more potent than thalidomide in regulating cytokines and affecting T-cell proliferation. Lenalidomide is an IMiD that in animal and in vitro studies has been shown to be similar to thalidomide in action, but with less toxicity, especially teratogenicity. Lenalidomide was approved by the Food and Drug Administration in late 2005 as a consequence of trials that showed its effectiveness in the treatment of the myelodysplastic syndrome with the chromosome 5q31 deletion. Several clinical trials using lenalidomide to treat relapsed or refractory myeloma are showing benefits and it is likely to be approved by the FDA for that indication as well.

CC-4047 (Actimid) is another IMiD that is being investigated for the treatment of myelodysplastic syndrome, myeloma, and prostate cancer.

Another group of thalidomide analogs, selective cytokine inhibitory drugs (SelCIDs), are phosphodiesterase type 4 inhibitors with potent anti-TNF-α activity but no T-cell co-stimulatory activity. Several SelCIDs are currently under investigation for clinical use.

CYTOTOXIC AGENTS

1. Azathioprine

Azathioprine is a prodrug of mercaptopurine and, like mercaptopurine, functions as an antimetabolite (see Chapter 55). Although its action is presumably mediated by conversion to mercaptopurine and further metabolites, it has been more widely used than mercaptopurine for immunosuppression in humans. These agents represent prototypes of the antimetabolite group of cytotoxic immunosuppressive drugs, and many other agents that kill proliferative cells appear to work at a similar level in the immune response.

Azathioprine is well absorbed from the gastrointestinal tract and is metabolized primarily to mercaptopurine. Xanthine oxidase splits much of the active material to 6-thiouric acid prior to excretion in the urine. After administration of azathioprine, small amounts of unchanged drug and mercaptopurine are also excreted by the kidney, and as much as a twofold increase in toxicity may occur in anephric or anuric patients. Since much of the drug's inactivation depends on xanthine oxidase, patients who are also receiving allopurinol (see Chapters 36 and 55) for control of hyperuricemia should have the dose of azathioprine reduced to one-fourth to one-third the usual amount to prevent excessive toxicity.

Azathioprine and mercaptopurine appear to produce immunosuppression by interfering with purine nucleic acid metabolism at steps that are required for the wave of lymphoid cell proliferation that follows antigenic stimulation. The purine analogs are thus cytotoxic agents that destroy stimulated lymphoid cells. Although continued messenger RNA synthesis is necessary for sustained antibody synthesis by plasma cells, these analogs appear to have less effect on this process than on nucleic acid synthesis in proliferating cells. Cellular immunity as well as primary and secondary serum antibody responses can be blocked by these cytotoxic agents.

Azathioprine and mercaptopurine appear to be of definite benefit in maintaining renal allografts and may be of value in transplantation of other tissues. These antimetabolites have been used with some success in the management of acute glomerulonephritis and in the renal component of systemic lupus erythematosus. They have also proved useful in some cases of rheumatoid arthritis, Crohn's disease, and multiple sclerosis. The drugs have been of occasional use in prednisone-resistant antibody-mediated idiopathic thrombocytopenic purpura and autoimmune hemolytic anemias.

The chief toxic effect of azathioprine and mercaptopurine is bone marrow suppression, usually manifested as leukopenia, although anemia and thrombocytopenia may occur. Skin rashes, fever, nausea and vomiting, and sometimes diarrhea occur, with the gastrointestinal symptoms seen mainly at higher dosages. Hepatic dysfunction, manifested by very high serum alkaline phosphatase levels and mild jaundice, occurs occasionally, particularly in patients with preexisting hepatic dysfunction.

2. Cyclophosphamide

The alkylating agent cyclophosphamide is one of the most efficacious immunosuppressive drugs available. Cyclophosphamide destroys proliferating lymphoid cells (see Chapter 55) but also appears to alkylate some resting cells. It has been observed that very large doses (eg, > 120 mg/kg intravenously over several days) may induce an apparent specific tolerance to a new antigen if the drug is administered simultaneously with, or shortly after, the antigen. In smaller doses, it has been effective against autoimmune disorders (including systemic lupus erythematosus) and in patients with acquired factor XIII antibodies and bleeding syndromes, autoimmune hemolytic anemia, antibody-induced pure red cell aplasia, and Wegener's granulomatosis.

Treatment with large doses of cyclophosphamide carries considerable risk of pancytopenia and hemorrhagic cystitis and therefore is generally combined with stem cell rescue (transplant) procedures. Although cyclophosphamide appears to induce tolerance for marrow or immune cell grafting, its use does not prevent the subsequent graft-versus-host disease syndrome, which may be serious or lethal if the donor is a poor histocompatibility match (despite the severe immunosuppression induced by high doses of cyclophosphamide). Other adverse effects of cyclophosphamide include nausea, vomiting, cardiac toxicity, and electrolyte disturbances.

3. Leflunomide

Leflunomide is a prodrug of an inhibitor of pyrimidine synthesis (rather than purine synthesis). It is orally active, and the active metabolite has a long half-life of several weeks. Thus, the drug should be started with a loading dose, but it can be taken once daily after reaching steady state. It is approved only for rheumatoid arthritis at present, though studies are underway combining leflunomide with mycophenolate mofetil for a variety of autoimmune and inflammatory skin disorders, as well as preservation of allografts in solid organ transplantation. Leflunomide also appears (from murine data) to have antiviral activity.

Toxicities include elevation of liver enzymes with some risk of liver damage, renal impairment, and teratogenic effects. A low frequency of cardiovascular effects (angina, tachycardia) was reported in clinical trials of leflunomide.

4. Hydroxychloroquine

Hydroxychloroquine is an antimalarial agent with immunosuppressant properties. It is thought to suppress intracellular antigen processing and loading of peptides onto MHC class II molecules by increasing the pH of lysosomal and endosomal compartments, thereby decreasing T-cell activation.

Because of these immunosuppressant activities, hydroxychloroquine is used to treat some autoimmune disorders, eg, rheumatoid arthritis and systemic lupus erythematosus. It has also been used to both treat and prevent graft-versus-host disease after allogeneic stem cell transplantation.

5. Other Cytotoxic Agents

Other cytotoxic agents, including **vincristine, methotrexate,** and **cytarabine** (see Chapter 55), also have immunosuppressive properties. Methotrexate has been used extensively in rheumatoid arthritis (see Chapter 36) and in the treatment of graft-versus-host disease. Although the other agents can be used for immunosuppression, their use has not been as widespread as the purine antagonists, and their indications for immunosuppression are less certain. The use of methotrexate (which can be given orally) appears reasonable in patients with idiosyncratic reactions to purine antagonists. The antibiotic dactinomycin has also been used with some success at the time of impending renal transplant rejection. Vincristine appears to be quite useful in idiopathic thrombocytopenic purpura refractory to prednisone. The related vinca alkaloid **vinblastine** has been shown to prevent mast cell degranulation in vitro by binding to microtubule units within the cell and to prevent release of histamine and other vasoactive compounds. **Pentostatin** is an adenosine deaminase inhibitor primarily used as an antineoplastic agent for lymphoid malignancies, and produces a profound lymphopenia. It is now frequently used for steroid-resistant graft-versus-host disease after allogeneic stem cell transplantation, as well as in preparative regimens prior to those transplants to provide severe immunosuppression to prevent allograft rejection.

IMMUNOSUPPRESSIVE ANTIBODIES

The development of **hybridoma** technology by Milstein and Kohler in 1975 revolutionized the antibody field and radically increased the purity and specificity of antibodies used in the clinic and for diagnostic tests in the laboratory. Hybridomas consist of antibody-forming cells fused to immortal plasmacytoma cells. Hybrid cells that are stable and produce the required antibody can be subcloned for mass culture for antibody production. Large-scale fermentation facilities are now used for this purpose in the pharmaceutical industry.

More recently, molecular biology has been used to develop monoclonal antibodies. Combinatorial libraries of cDNAs encoding immunoglobulin heavy and light chains expressed on bacteriophage surfaces are screened against purified antigens. The result is an antibody fragment with specificity and high affinity for the antigen of interest. This technique has been used to develop antibodies specific for viruses (eg, HIV), bacterial proteins, tumor antigens, and even cytokines. Several antibodies developed in this manner are in clinical trials.

Other genetic engineering techniques involve production of **chimeric** and **humanized** versions of murine monoclonal antibodies in order to reduce their antigenicity and increase the half-life of the antibody in the patient. Murine antibodies administered as such to human patients evoke production of human antimouse antibodies (HAMA), which clear the original murine proteins very rapidly. Humanization involves replacing most of the murine antibody with equivalent human regions while keeping only the variable, antigen-specific regions intact. Chimeric mouse-human antibodies have similar properties with less complete replacement of the murine components. The current naming convention for these engineered substances uses the suffix "umab" or "zumab" for humanized antibodies, and "imab" or "ximab" for chimeric products. These procedures have been successful in reducing or preventing HAMA production for many of the antibodies discussed below.

1. Antilymphocyte & Antithymocyte Antibodies

Antisera directed against lymphocytes have been prepared sporadically for over 100 years. With the advent of human organ transplantation as a therapeutic option, heterologous antilymphocyte globulin (ALG) took on new importance. ALG and antithymocyte globulin (ATG) are now in clinical use in many medical centers, especially in transplantation programs. The antiserum is usually obtained by immunization of large animals such as horses or sheep with human lymphoid cells.

Antilymphocyte antibody acts primarily on the small, long-lived peripheral lymphocytes that circulate between the blood and lymph. With continued administration, "thymus-dependent" lymphocytes from lymphoid follicles are also depleted, as they normally participate in the recirculating pool. As a result of the destruction or inactivation of T cells, an impairment of delayed hypersensitivity and cellular immunity occurs while humoral antibody formation remains relatively intact. ALG and ATG are useful for suppressing certain major compartments (ie, T cells) of the immune system and play a definite role in the management of solid organ and bone marrow transplantation.

Monoclonal antibodies directed against specific antigens such as CD3, CD4, CD25, CD40, IL-2 receptor, and TNF (discussed below) much more selectively influence T-cell subset function. The high specificity of these antibodies improves selectivity and reduces toxicity of the therapy and alters the disease course in several different autoimmune disorders.

In the management of transplants, ALG and monoclonal antibodies can be used in the induction of immunosuppression, in the treatment of initial rejection, and in the treatment of steroid-resistant rejection. There has been some success in the use of ALG and ATG plus cyclosporine to prepare recipients for bone marrow transplantation. In this procedure, the recipient is treated with ALG or ATG in large doses for 7–10 days prior to transplantation of bone marrow cells from the donor. Residual ALG appears to destroy the T cells in the donor marrow graft, and the probability of severe graft-versus-host syndrome is reduced.

The adverse effects of ALG are mostly those associated with injection of a foreign protein obtained from heterologous serum. Local pain and erythema often occur at the injection site (type III hypersensitivity). Since the humoral antibody mechanism remains active, skin-reactive and precipitating antibodies may be formed against the foreign IgG. Similar reactions occur with monoclonal antibodies of murine origin, and reactions thought to be caused by the release of cytokines by T cells and monocytes have also been described.

Anaphylactic and serum sickness reactions to ALG and murine monoclonal antibodies have been observed and usually require cessation of therapy. Complexes of host antibodies with horse ALG may precipitate and localize in the glomeruli of the kidneys. Even more disturbing has been the development of histiocytic lymphomas in the buttock at the site of ALG injection. The incidence of lymphoma as well as other forms of cancer is increased in kidney transplant patients. It appears likely that part of the increased risk of cancer is related to the suppression of a normally potent defense system against oncogenic viruses or transformed cells. The preponderance of lymphoma in these cancer cases is thought to be related to the concurrence of chronic immune suppression with chronic low-level lymphocyte proliferation.

2. Muromonab-CD3

Monoclonal antibodies against T-cell surface proteins are increasingly being used in the clinic for autoimmune disorders and in transplantation settings. Clinical studies have shown that the murine monoclonal antibody **muromonab-CD3** (OKT3) directed against the CD3 molecule on the surface of human thymocytes and mature T cells can also be useful in the treatment of renal transplant rejection. In vitro, muromonab-CD3 blocks killing by cytotoxic human T cells and several other T-cell functions. In a prospective randomized multicenter trial with cadaveric renal transplants, use of muromonab-CD3 (along with lower doses of steroids or other immunosuppressive drugs) proved more effective at reversing acute rejection than did conventional steroid treatment. Muromonab-CD3 is approved for the treatment of renal allograft rejection crises. Several other monoclonal antibodies directed against surface markers on lymphocytes are approved for certain indications (see monoclonal antibody section below), while others are in various stages of development and clinical trials.

3. Immune Globulin Intravenous (IGIV)

A quite different approach to immunomodulation is the intravenous use of polyclonal human immunoglobulin. This immunoglobulin preparation (usually IgG) is prepared from pools of thousands of healthy donors, and no specific antigen is the target of the "therapeutic antibody." Rather, one expects that the pool of different antibodies will have a normalizing effect upon the patient's immune networks.

IGIV in high doses (2 g/kg) has proved effective in a variety of different conditions ranging from immunoglobulin deficiencies to autoimmune disorders to HIV disease to bone marrow transplants. In patients with Kawasaki's disease, it has been shown to be safe and effective, reducing systemic inflammation and preventing coronary artery aneurysms. It has also brought about good clinical responses in systemic lupus erythematosus and refractory idiopathic thrombocytopenic purpura. Possible mechanisms of action of IGIV include a reduction of T helper cells, increase of suppressor T cells, decreased spontaneous immunoglobulin production, Fc receptor blockade, increased antibody catabolism, and idiotypic-anti-idiotypic interactions with "pathologic antibodies." Although its precise mechanism of action is still controversial, IGIV brings undeniable clinical benefit to many patients with a variety of immune syndromes.

4. Rh$_o$(D) Immune Globulin Micro-Dose

One of the earliest major advances in immunopharmacology was the development of a technique for preventing Rh hemolytic disease of the newborn. The technique is based on the observation that a *primary* antibody response to a foreign antigen can be blocked if specific antibody to that antigen is administered passively at the time of exposure to antigen. Rh$_o$(D) immune globulin is a concentrated (15%) solution of human IgG containing a higher titer of antibodies against the Rh$_o$(D) antigen of the red cell.

Sensitization of Rh-negative mothers to the D antigen occurs usually at the time of birth of an Rh$_o$(D)-positive or D^u-positive infant, when fetal red cells may leak into the mother's bloodstream. Sensitization might also occur occasionally with miscarriages or ectopic pregnancies. In subsequent pregnancies, maternal antibody against Rh-positive cells is transferred to the fetus during the third trimester, leading to the development of erythroblastosis fetalis (hemolytic disease of the newborn).

If an injection of Rh$_o$(D) antibody is administered to the mother within 24–72 hours after the birth of an Rh-positive infant, the mother's own antibody response to the foreign Rh$_o$(D)-positive cells is suppressed because the infant's red cells are cleared from circulation before the mother can generate a B-cell response against Rh$_o$(D). Therefore she has no memory B cells that can activate upon subsequent pregnancies with an Rh$_o$(D)-positive fetus.

When the mother has been treated in this fashion, Rh hemolytic disease of the newborn has not been observed in subsequent pregnancies. For this prophylactic treatment to be successful, the mother must be Rh$_o$(D)-negative and D^u-negative and must not already be immunized to the Rh$_o$(D) factor. Treatment is also often advised for Rh-negative mothers who have had miscarriages, ectopic pregnancies, or abortions, when the blood type of the fetus is unknown. ***Note:*** *Rh$_o$(D) immune globulin is administered to the mother and must not be given to the infant.*

The usual dose of Rh$_o$(D) immune globulin is 2 mL intramuscularly, containing approximately 300 mcg anti-Rh$_o$(D) IgG. Adverse reactions are infrequent and consist of local discomfort at the injection site or, rarely, a slight temperature elevation.

5. Hyperimmune Immunoglobulins

Hyperimmune immunoglobulin preparations are IGIV preparations made from pools of selected human or animal donors with high titers of antibodies against particular agents of interest such as viruses or toxins (see also Appendix I). Various hyperimmune IGIVs are available for treatment of respiratory syncytial virus, cytomegalovirus, varicella zoster, human herpesvirus 3, hepatitis B virus, rabies, tetanus, and digoxin overdose. Intravenous administration of the hyperimmune globulins is a passive transfer of high titer antibodies that either reduces risk or reduces the severity of infection. Rabies hyperimmune globulin is injected around the wound and given intravenously. Tetanus hyperimmune globulin is administered intravenously when indicated for prophylaxis. Rattlesnake and coral snake hyperimmune globulins (antivenins) are of equine origin and are effective for North and South American rattlesnakes and some coral snakes (but not Arizona coral snake). Equine and ovine antivenins are available for rattlesnake envenomations, but only equine antivenin is available for coral snake bite. The ovine antivenin is a Fab preparation and is less immunogenic than whole equine IgG antivenins, but retains the ability to neutralize the rattlesnake venom.

MONOCLONAL ANTIBODIES (MABS)

Recent advances in the ability to manipulate the genes of immunoglobulins have resulted in development of a wide array of humanized and chimeric monoclonal antibodies directed against therapeutic targets. The only murine elements of humanized monoclonal antibodies are the complementarity-determining regions in the variable domains of immunoglobulin heavy and light chains. Complementarity-determining regions are primarily responsible for the antigen-binding capacity of antibodies. Chimeric antibodies typically contain antigen-binding murine variable regions and human constant regions. The following are brief descriptions of the engineered antibodies that have been approved by the FDA.

Antitumor MABs

Alemtuzumab is a humanized IgG_1 with a kappa chain that binds to CD52 found on normal and malignant B and T lymphocytes, NK cells, monocytes, macrophages, and a small population of granulocytes. Currently, alemtuzumab is approved for the treatment of B-cell chronic lymphocytic leukemia in patients who have been treated with alkylating agents and have failed fludarabine therapy. Alemtuzumab appears to deplete leukemic and normal cells by direct antibody-dependent lysis. Patients receiving this antibody become lymphopenic and may also become neutropenic, anemic, and thrombocytopenic. As a result patients should be closely monitored for opportunistic infections and hematologic toxicity.

Bevacizumab is a humanized IgG_1 monoclonal antibody that binds to vascular endothelial growth factor (VEGF) and inhibits VEGF from binding to its receptor, especially on endothelial cells. It is an antiangiogenic drug that has been shown to inhibit growth of blood vessels (angiogenesis) in tumors. It is approved for first-line treatment of patients with metastatic colorectal cancer alone or in combination with 5-FU-based chemotherapy. Since bevacizumab is antiangiogenic, it should not be administered until patients heal from surgery. Patients taking the drug should be watched for hemorrhage, gastrointestinal perforations, and wound healing problems.

Cetuximab is a human-mouse chimeric monoclonal antibody that targets epidermal growth factor receptor (EGFR). Binding of cetuximab to EGFR inhibits tumor cell growth by a variety of mechanisms, including decreases in kinase activity, matrix metalloproteinase activity, and growth factor production, and increased apoptosis. It is indicated for use in patients with metastatic colorectal cancer whose tumors overexpress EGFR. Cetuximab may be administered in combination with irinotecan or alone in patients who cannot tolerate irinotecan.

Gemtuzumab is a humanized IgG_4 monoclonal antibody with a kappa light chain specific for CD33, a sialoadhesion protein found on leukemic blast cells in 80–90% of patients with acute myelogenous leukemia (AML). Gemtuzumab alone has some antiblast activity. In the clinical formulation, gemtuzumab is coupled to the cytotoxic agent, ozogamicin, which is a semisynthetic derivative of calicheamicin, an antibiotic with antitumor activity. Internalization of gemtuzumab-ozogamicin by the tumor cell results in release of the cytotoxin from the antibody in the lysosome. Ozogamicin then binds to the minor groove in DNA, causing double-strand breaks and cell death.

Gemtuzumab is approved for the treatment of patients 60 years and older in first relapse with CD33 acute myelogenous leukemia who are not considered candidates for other types of cytotoxic chemotherapy.

Adverse events due to the administration of gemtuzumab-ozogamicin include severe myelosuppression, especially neutropenia, requiring careful hematologic monitoring. Other adverse events associated with gemtuzumab are significant hepatotoxicity and various hypersensitivity reactions.

Rituximab is a chimeric murine-human monoclonal IgG_1 (human Fc) that binds to the CD20 molecule on normal and malignant B lymphocytes and is approved for the therapy of patients with relapsed or refractory low-grade or follicular, B-cell non-Hodgkin's lymphoma. The mechanism of action includes complement-mediated lysis, antibody-dependent cellular cytotoxicity, and induction of apoptosis in the malignant lymphoma cells. This drug appears to be synergistic with chemotherapy (eg, fludarabine, CHOP) for lymphoma (see Chapter 55).

Trastuzumab is a recombinant DNA-derived, humanized monoclonal antibody that binds to the extracellular domain of the human epidermal growth factor receptor HER-2/*neu*. This antibody blocks the natural ligand from binding and down-regulates the receptor. Trastuzumab is approved for the treatment of metastatic breast cancer in patients whose tumors overexpress HER-2/*neu*. As a single agent it induces remission in about 15–20% of patients; in combination with chemotherapy, it increases response rate and duration as well as 1-year survival. Trastuzumab is under investigation for other tumors that express HER-2 (see Chapter 55).

MABs Used to Deliver Isotopes to Tumors

Arcitumomab is a murine $F(ab')_2$ fragment from an anti-carcinoembryonic antigen (CEA) antibody labeled with technetium 99m (^{99m}Tc) that is used for imaging patients with metastatic colorectal carcinoma (immunoscintigraphy) to determine extent of disease. CEA is often upregulated on tumor in patients with gastrointestinal carcinomas. The use of the $F(ab')_2$ fragment decreases the immunogenicity of the agent so that it can be given more than once, unlike other intact murine monoclonal antibodies.

Capromab pendetide is a murine monoclonal antibody specific for prostate specific membrane antigen. It is coupled to isotopic indium (^{111}In) and is used in immunoscintigraphy for patients with biopsy-confirmed prostate cancer and post-prostatectomy in patients with rising prostate specific antibody level to determine extent of disease.

Ibritumomab tiuxetan is an anti-CD20 murine monoclonal antibody labeled with isotopic yttrium (^{90}Y) or ^{111}In. The radiation of the isotope provides the major antitumor activity. Ibritumomab is approved for use in patients with relapsed or refractory low-grade, follicular, or B-cell non-Hodgkin's lymphoma, including patients with rituximab-refractory follicular disease.

It is used in conjunction with rituximab in a two-step therapeutic regimen.

Nofetumomab is a mouse monoclonal antibody coupled to ^{99m}Tc that is used for diagnostic purposes to determine extent of disease and to stage patients with small cell lung cancer. It binds a 40 kD antigen found on many tumor cell types, but also on some normal cells. It is an accurate indicator of extent of disease in biopsy-confirmed small cell lung cancer except in those patients with brain or adrenal metastases.

Tositumomab is another anti-CD20 monoclonal antibody and is complexed with iodine 131 (^{131}I). Tositumomab is used in two-step therapy in patients with CD20-positive, follicular non-Hodgkin's lymphoma whose disease is refractory to rituximab and standard chemotherapy. Toxicities are similar to those for ibritumomab and include severe cytopenias such as thrombocytopenia and neutropenia. Tositumomab should not be administered to patients with greater than 25% bone marrow involvement.

MABs Used as Immunosuppressants and Anti-Inflammatory Agents

A. ANTI-TNF-ALPHA MABs

Adalimumab, etanercept, and infliximab are antibodies that bind TNF-α, a proinflammatory cytokine. Blocking TNF-α from binding to TNF receptors on inflammatory cell surfaces results in suppression of downstream inflammatory cytokines such as IL-1 and IL-6 and adhesion molecules involved in leukocyte activation and migration. An increased risk of lymphoma is common to each of these agents.

Adalimumab is a completely human IgG$_1$ approved for use in rheumatoid arthritis. Like the other anti-TNF-α biologicals, adalimumab blocks the interaction of TNF-α with TNF receptors on cell surfaces; it does not bind TNF-β. Pharmacodynamic studies showed that administration of adalimumab reduced levels of C-reactive protein, erythrocyte sedimentation rate, serum IL-6 and matrix metalloproteinases MMP-1 and MMP-3. In vitro, adalimumab lyses cells expressing TNF-α in the presence of complement. Patients may self-administer single doses of the antibody subcutaneously, every other week. Adalimumab has a serum half-life of two weeks which is increased by 29–44% in patients who are also taking methotrexate.

Etanercept is a dimeric fusion protein composed of human IgG$_1$ constant regions (CH$_2$, CH$_3$, and hinge, but not CH$_1$) fused to the TNF receptor. Etanercept binds to both TNF-α and TNF-β and appears to have effects similar to that of infliximab, ie, inhibition of TNF-α-mediated inflammation, but its half-life is shorter due to its physical form (fusion protein) and the route of injection (subcutaneously, twice weekly). Etanercept is approved for adult RA, polyarticular-course juvenile RA, and psoriatic arthritis. It may be used in combination with methotrexate.

Infliximab is a human-mouse chimeric IgG$_1$ monoclonal antibody possessing human constant (Fc) regions and murine variable regions. Infliximab is currently approved for use in Crohn's disease, ulcerative colitis, rheumatoid arthritis, ankylosing spondylitis, and psoriatic arthritis.

B. ABATACEPT

Abatacept is a recombinant fusion protein composed of the extracellular domain of cytotoxic T-lymphocyte-associated antigen 4 (CTLA-4) fused to human IgG Fc. CTLA-4 is a costimulatory molecule found on T cells that binds to CD80 and CD86 on antigen presenting cells (Figure 56–7). This fusion protein blocks activation of T cells by binding to CD80 or 86 so that CD28 on T cells cannot bind and stimulate the T cell and lead to cytokine release. Abatacept is approved for patients with severe rheumatoid arthritis who have failed other DMARDS (see Chapter 36). Patients should not take other anti-TNF drugs or anakinra while taking abatacept.

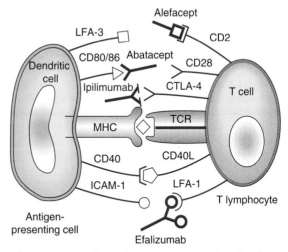

Figure 56–7. Actions of some monoclonal antibodies (dark color). CTLA-4-IgFc fusion protein (CTLA-4-Ig, abatacept) binds to CD80/86 on DC and inhibits T-cell costimulation. Efalizumab blocks CD11a (LFA-1) from binding to ICAM-1, inhibiting T-cell adhesion, migration, and activation. Alefacept inhibits activation of T cells by blocking the interaction of LFA-3 and CD2. T-cell activation can be maintained or restored if CTLA-4 interaction with CD80/86 is blocked using an anti-CTLA-4 antibody (ipilimumab, currently in phase II and III clinical trials); this antibody inhibits CTLA-4 signaling.

C. ALEFACEPT

Alefacept is an engineered protein consisting of the CD2-binding portion of leukocyte-function-associated antigen-3 (LFA-3) fused to a human IgG_1 Fc region (hinge, CH_1, and CH_2), approved for the treatment of plaque psoriasis. It inhibits activation of T cells by binding to cell surface CD2, inhibiting the normal CD2/LFA-3 interaction (Figure 56–7). Treatment of patients with alefacept also results in a dose-dependent reduction of the total number of circulating T cells, including those that predominate in psoriatic plaques. Therefore, T-cell counts of patients receiving alefacept must be monitored, and the drug discontinued if CD4 lymphocyte levels fall below 250 cells/μL.

D. BASILIXIMAB

Basiliximab is a chimeric mouse-human IgG_1 that binds to CD25, the IL-2 receptor alpha chain on activated lymphocytes. It functions as an IL-2 antagonist, blocking IL-2 from binding to activated lymphocytes, and is therefore immunosuppressive. It is indicated for prophylaxis of acute organ rejection in renal transplant patients and is usually used as part of an immunosuppressive regimen that also includes glucocorticoids and cyclosporine A.

E. DACLIZUMAB

Daclizumab is a humanized IgG_1 that binds to the alpha subunit of the IL-2 receptor. Its indications are identical to that of basiliximab, but the mode of administration differs.

F. EFALIZUMAB

Efalizumab is a recombinant humanized anti-CD11a monoclonal antibody approved for the treatment of adult patients with severe psoriasis. Binding of efalizumab to CD11a (the alpha subunit of LFA-1) inhibits the interaction of LFA-1 on all lymphocytes with intercellular adhesion molecule-1 (ICAM-1), thereby inhibiting the adhesion, activation, and migration of lymphocytes into skin (Figure 56–7). Efalizumab is administered by subcutaneous injection.

G. OMALIZUMAB

Omalizumab is an anti-IgE recombinant humanized monoclonal antibody that is approved for the treatment of allergic asthma in adult and adolescent patients whose symptoms are refractory to inhaled corticosteroids (see Chapter 20). The antibody blocks the binding of IgE to the high-affinity Fcε receptor on basophils and mast cells, which suppresses IgE-mediated release of type I allergy mediators such as histamine and leukotrienes. Total serum IgE levels may remain elevated in patients for up to 1 year after administration of this antibody.

Other MABs

Abciximab is a Fab fragment of a murine-human monoclonal antibody that binds to the integrin GPIIb/IIIa receptor on activated platelets and inhibits fibrinogen, von Willebrand factor, and other adhesion molecules from binding to activated platelets, thus preventing their aggregation. See Chapter 34 for additional details.

Palivizumab is a monoclonal antibody that binds to the fusion protein of respiratory syncytial virus, preventing infection in susceptible cells in the airways. It is used in neonates at risk for this viral infection and reduces the frequency of infection and hospitalization by about 50% (see Chapter 49).

■ III. CLINICAL USES OF IMMUNOSUPPRESSIVE DRUGS

Immunosuppressive agents are commonly used in two clinical circumstances: transplantation and autoimmune disorders. The agents used differ somewhat for the specific disorders treated (see specific agents and Table 56–1), as do administration schedules. Because autoimmune disorders are very complex, optimal treatment schedules have yet to be established in many clinical situations.

SOLID ORGAN AND BONE MARROW TRANSPLANTATION

In organ transplantation, tissue typing—based on donor and recipient histocompatibility matching with the human leukocyte antigen (HLA) haplotype system—is required. Close histocompatibility matching reduces the likelihood of graft rejection and may also reduce the requirements for intensive immunosuppressive therapy. Prior to transplant, patients may receive an immunosuppressive regimen, including antithymocyte globulin, muromonab-CD3, daclizumab, or basiliximab. Four types of rejection can occur in a solid organ transplant recipient: **hyperacute, accelerated, acute,** and **chronic.** Hyperacute rejection is due to preformed antibodies against the donor organ, such as anti-blood group antibodies. Hyperacute rejection occurs within hours of the transplant and cannot be stopped with immunosuppressive drugs. It results in rapid necrosis and failure of the transplanted organ. Accelerated rejection is mediated by both antibodies and T cells, but it also cannot be stopped by immunosuppressive drugs. Acute rejection of an organ occurs within days to months and involves mainly cellular immunity. Reversal of acute rejection is usually possible

Table 56–1. Clinical uses of immunosuppressive agents.

Source	Immunosuppressive Agents Used	Response
Autoimmune diseases		
Idiopathic thrombocytopenic purpura (ITP)	Prednisone,[1] vincristine, occasionally cyclophosphamide, mercaptopurine, or azathioprine; commonly high-dose gamma globulin, plasma immunoadsorption or plasma exchange	Usually good
Autoimmune hemolytic anemia	Prednisone,[1] cyclophosphamide, chlorambucil, mercaptopurine, azathioprine, high-dose gamma globulin	Usually good
Acute glomerulonephritis	Prednisone,[1] mercaptopurine, cyclophosphamide	Usually good
Acquired factor XIII antibodies	Cyclophosphamide plus factor XIII	Usually good
Autoreactive tissue disorders (autoimmune diseases)[2]	Prednisone, cyclophosphamide, methotrexate, interferon-α and -β, azathioprine, cyclosporine, infliximab, etanercept, adalimumab	Often good, variable
Isoimmune disease		
Hemolytic disease of the newborn	Rh_o(D) immune globulin	Excellent
Organ transplantation		
Renal	Cyclosporine, azathioprine, prednisone, ALG, OKT3, tacrolimus, basiliximab,[3] daclizumab,[3] sirolimus	Very good
Heart		Good
Liver	Cyclosporine, prednisone, azathioprine, tacrolimus, sirolimus	Fair
Bone marrow	Cyclosporine, cyclophosphamide, prednisone, methotrexate, ALG	Good
Prevention of cell proliferation		
Coronary stents	Sirolimus (impregnated stent)	Good

[1]Drug of choice.
[2]Including systemic lupus erythematosus, rheumatoid arthritis, scleroderma, dermatomyositis, mixed tissue disorder, multiple sclerosis, Wegener's granulomatosis, chronic active hepatitis, lipoid nephrosis, inflammatory bowel disease.
[3]Basiliximab and daclizumab are approved for renal transplant only.

with general immunosuppressive drugs such as azathioprine, mycophenolate mofetil, cyclosporine, tacrolimus, glucocorticoids, cyclophosphamide, methotrexate, and sirolimus. Recently, biologic agents such as anti-CD3 monoclonal antibody have been used to stem acute rejection. Chronic rejection usually occurs months or even years after transplantation. It is characterized by thickening and fibrosis of the vasculature of the transplanted organ, involving both cellular and humoral immunity. Chronic rejection is treated with the same drugs as those used for acute rejection.

Allogeneic hematopoietic stem cell transplantation is a well established treatment for many malignant and nonmalignant diseases. An HLA-matched donor, usually a family member, is located, patients are conditioned with high-dose chemotherapy or radiation therapy, and then donor stem cells are infused. The conditioning regimen is used not only to kill cancer cells in the case of malignant disease, but also to totally suppress the immune system so that the patient does not reject the donor stem cells. As patients' blood counts recover (after reduction by the conditioning regimen) they develop a new immune system that is created from the donor stem cells. Rejection of donor stem cells is uncommon, and can only be treated by infusion of more stem cells from the donor.

Graft-versus-host disease (GVHD), however, is very common, occurring in the majority of patients who receive an allogeneic transplant. Graft-versus-host disease occurs as donor T cells fail to recognize the patient's skin, liver, and gut (usually) as self and attack those tissues. Although patients are given immunosuppressive therapy (cyclosporine, methotrexate, and others) early in the transplant course to help prevent this development, it usually occurs despite these medications. Acute graft-versus-host disease occurs within the first 100 days, and is usually manifested as a skin rash, severe diarrhea, or hepatotoxicity. Additional medications are added, invariably starting with high-dose corticosteroids, and adding drugs such as mycophenolate mofetil, sirolimus, tacrolimus, daclizumab, and others, with variable success rates. Patients generally progress to chronic graft-versus-host disease (after 100 days) and require therapy for variable periods thereafter. Unlike solid organ transplantation, however, stem cell transplant patients generally are able to discontinue immunosuppressive drugs as graft-versus-host disease resolves (generally 1–2 years after their transplant).

AUTOIMMUNE DISORDERS

The effectiveness of immunosuppressive drugs in autoimmune disorders varies widely. Nonetheless, with immunosuppressive therapy, remissions can be obtained in many instances of autoimmune hemolytic anemia, idiopathic thrombocytopenic purpura, type 1 diabetes, Hashimoto's thyroiditis, and temporal arteritis. Improvement is also often seen in patients with systemic lupus erythematosus, acute glomerulonephritis, acquired factor VIII inhibitors (antibodies), rheumatoid arthritis, inflammatory myopathy, scleroderma, and certain other autoimmune states.

Immunosuppressive therapy is utilized in chronic severe asthma, where cyclosporine is often effective and sirolimus is another alternative. Omalizumab (anti-IgE antibody) has recently been approved for the treatment of severe asthma (see previous section). Tacrolimus is currently under clinical investigation for the management of autoimmune chronic active hepatitis and of multiple sclerosis, where IFN-β has a definitive role.

IMMUNOMODULATION THERAPY

The development of agents that modulate the immune response rather than suppress it has become an important area of pharmacology. The rationale underlying this approach is that such drugs may increase the immune responsiveness of patients who have either selective or generalized immunodeficiency. The major potential uses are in immunodeficiency disorders, chronic infectious diseases, and cancer. The AIDS epidemic has greatly increased interest in developing more effective immunomodulating drugs.

Cytokines

The cytokines are a large and heterogeneous group of proteins with diverse functions. Some are immunoregulatory proteins synthesized within lymphoreticular cells and play numerous interacting roles in the function of the immune system and in the control of hematopoiesis. The cytokines that have been clearly identified are summarized in Table 56–2. In most instances, cytokines mediate their effects through receptors on relevant target cells and appear to act in a manner similar to the mechanism of action of hormones. In other instances, cytokines may have antiproliferative, antimicrobial, and antitumor effects.

The first group of cytokines discovered, the interferons (IFNs), were followed by the colony-stimulating factors (CSFs, discussed in Chapter 33). The latter regulate the proliferation and differentiation of bone marrow progenitor cells. Most of the more recently discovered cytokines have been classified as interleukins (ILs) and numbered in the order of their discovery. Cytokines are produced using gene cloning techniques.

Most cytokines (including TNF-α, IFN-γ, IL-2, granulocyte colony-stimulating factor [G-CSF], and granulocyte-macrophage colony-stimulating factor [GM-CSF]) have very short serum half-lives (minutes). The usual subcutaneous route of administration provides slower release into the circulation and a longer duration of action. Each cytokine has its own unique toxicity, but some toxicities are shared. For example, IFN-α, IFN-β, IFN-γ, IL-2, and TNF-α all induce fever, flu-like symptoms, anorexia, fatigue, and malaise.

Interferons are proteins that are currently grouped into three families: **IFN-α, IFN-β,** and **IFN-γ.** The IFN-α and IFN-β families comprise type I IFNs, ie, acid-stable proteins that act on the same receptor on target cells. IFN-γ, a type II IFN, is acid-labile and acts on a separate receptor on target cells. Type I IFNs are usually induced by virus infections, with leukocytes producing IFN-α. Fibroblasts and epithelial cells produce IFN-β. IFN-γ is usually the product of activated T lymphocytes.

IFNs interact with cell receptors to produce a wide variety of effects that depend on the cell and IFN types. IFNs, particularly IFN-γ, display immune-enhancing properties, which include increased antigen presentation and macrophage, NK cell, and cytotoxic T-lymphocyte activation. IFNs also inhibit cell proliferation. In this respect, IFN-α and IFN-β are more potent than IFN-γ. Another striking IFN action is increased expression of MHC molecules on cell surfaces. While all three types of IFN induce MHC class I molecules, only IFN-γ induces class II expression. In glial cells, IFN-β antagonizes this effect and may, in fact, decrease antigen presentation within the nervous system.

IFN-α is approved for the treatment of several neoplasms, including hairy cell leukemia, chronic myelogenous leukemia, malignant melanoma, and Kaposi's sarcoma, and for use in hepatitis B and C infections. It has also shown activity as an anticancer agent in renal cell carcinoma, carcinoid syndrome, and T cell leukemia. IFN-β is approved for use in relapsing-type multiple sclerosis. IFN-γ is approved for the treatment of chronic granulomatous disease and IL-2, for metastatic renal cell carcinoma and malignant melanoma. Numerous clinical investigations of the other cytokines, including IL-1, -3, -4, -6, -11, and -12, are still in progress. Toxicities of IFNs, which include fever, chills, malaise, myalgias, myelosuppression, headache, and depression, can severely restrict their clinical use.

Table 56–2. The cytokines.

Cytokine	Properties
Interferon-α (IFN-α)	Antiviral, oncostatic, activates NK cells
Interferon-β (IFN-β)	Antiviral, oncostatic, activates NK cells
Interferon-γ (IFN-γ)	Antiviral, oncostatic, secreted by and activates or up-regulates TH1 cells, NK cells, CTLs, and macrophages
Interleukin-1 (IL-1)	T cell activation, B cell proliferation and differentiation
Interleukin-2 (IL-2)	T cell proliferation, TH1, NK, and LAK cell activation
Interleukin-3 (IL-3)	Hematopoietic precursor proliferation and differentiation
Interleukin-4 (IL-4)	TH2 and CTL activation, B cell proliferation
Interleukin-5 (IL-5)	Eosinophil proliferation, B cell proliferation and differentiation
Interleukin-6 (IL-6)	HCF, TH2, CTL, and B cell proliferation
Interleukin- 7 (IL-7)	CTL, NK, LAK, and B cell proliferation, thymic precursor stimulation
Interleukin-8 (IL-8)	Neutrophil chemotaxis, proinflammatory
Interleukin-9 (IL-9)	T cell proliferation
Interleukin-10 (IL-10)	TH1 suppression, CTL activation, B cell proliferation
Interleukin-11 (IL-11)	Megakaryocyte proliferation, B cell differentiation
Interleukin-12 (IL-12)	TH1 and CTL proliferation and activation
Interleukin-13 (IL-13)	Macrophage function modulation, B cell proliferation
Interleukin-14 (IL-14)	B cell proliferation and differentiation
Interleukin-15 (IL-15)	TH1, CTL, and NK/LAK activation, expansion of T cell memory pools
Interleukin-16 (IL-16)	T lymphocyte chemotaxis, suppresses HIV replication
Interleukin-17 (IL-17)	Stromal cell cytokine production
Interleukin-18 (IL-18)	Induces TH1 responses
Interleukin-19 (IL-19)	Proinflammatory
Interleukin-20 (IL-20)	Promotes skin differentiation
Interleukin-21 (IL-21)	Promotes proliferation of activated T cells, maturation of NK cells
Interleukin-22 (IL-22)	Regulator of TH2 cells
Interleukin-23 (IL-23)	Promotes proliferation of TH1 memory cells
Interleukin-24 (IL-24)	Induces tumor apoptosis, induces TH1 responses
Interleukin-27 (IL-27)	Stimulates naive CD4 cells to produce IFN-γ
Interleukin-28 and 29 (IL-28, IL-29)	Antiviral, interferon-like properties
Interleukin-30 (IL-30)	p28 subunit of IL-27
Interleukin-31 (IL-31)	Contributes to type I hypersensitivities and TH2 responses
Interleukin-32 (IL-32)	Involved in inflammation
Tumor necrosis factor-α (TNF-α)	Oncostatic, macrophage activation, proinflammatory
Tumor necrosis factor-β (TNF-β)	Oncostatic, proinflammatory, chemotactic
Granulocyte colony-stimulating factor	Granulocyte production
Granulocyte-macrophage colony stimulating factor	Granulocyte, monocyte, eosinophil production
Macrophage colony-stimulating factor	Monocyte production, activation
Erythropoietin (epoetin, EPO)	Red blood cell production
Thrombopoietin (TPO)	Platelet production

HCF, hematopoietic cofactor; LAK, lymphokine-activated killer cell.
Note: Many interleukin activities overlap and are influenced by each other.

TNF-α has been extensively tested in the therapy of various malignancies, but results have been disappointing due to dose-limiting toxicities. One exception is the use of intra-arterial high-dose TNF-α for malignant melanoma and soft tissue sarcoma of the extremities. In these settings, response rates greater than 80% have been noted.

Cytokines have been under clinical investigation as adjuvants to vaccines, and IFNs and IL-2 have shown some positive effects in the response of human subjects to hepatitis B vaccine. IL-12 and GM-CSF have also shown adjuvant effects with vaccines. GM-CSF is of particular interest because it promotes recruitment of professional antigen-presenting cells such as the dendritic cells required for priming naive antigen-specific T-lymphocyte responses. There are some claims that GM-CSF can itself stimulate an antitumor immune response, resulting in tumor regression in melanoma and prostate cancer.

It is important to emphasize that cytokine interactions with target cells often result in the release of a cascade of different endogenous cytokines, which exert their effects sequentially or simultaneously. For example, IFN-γ exposure increases the number of cell surface receptors on target cells for TNF-α. Therapy with IL-2 induces the production of TNF-α, while therapy with IL-12 induces the production of IFN-γ.

Cytokine Inhibitors

A more recent application of immunomodulation therapy involves the use of cytokine inhibitors for inflammatory diseases and septic shock, conditions in which cytokines such as IL-1 and TNF-α are involved in the pathogenesis. Drugs now under investigation include anticytokine monoclonal antibodies, soluble cytokine receptors (soluble forms of IL-1 and TNF-α receptors occur naturally in humans), and the IL-1 receptor antagonist (IL-1Rα), anakinra. Anakinra is a recombinant form of the naturally occurring IL-1 receptor antagonist that prevents IL-1 from binding to its receptor, stemming the cascade of cytokines released if IL-1 were to bind to the IL-1R. Anakinra is approved for use in adult rheumatoid arthritis patients who have failed treatment with one or more disease-modifying antirheumatic drugs. Patients must be carefully monitored if they are also taking an anti-TNF-α drug, have chronic infections, or are otherwise immunosuppressed.

■ IV. IMMUNOLOGIC REACTIONS TO DRUGS & DRUG ALLERGY

The basic immune mechanism and the ways in which it can be suppressed or stimulated by drugs have been dis-

cussed in previous sections of this chapter. Drugs also activate the immune system in undesirable ways that are manifested as adverse drug reactions. These reactions are generally grouped in a broad classification as "drug allergy." Indeed, many drug reactions such as those to penicillin, iodides, phenytoin, and sulfonamides are allergic in nature. These drug reactions are manifested as skin eruptions, edema, anaphylactoid reactions, glomerulonephritis, fever, and eosinophilia.

Drug reactions mediated by immune responses can have several different mechanisms. Thus, any of the four major types of hypersensitivity discussed earlier in this chapter (page 912) can be associated with allergic drug reactions:

- **Type I:** IgE-mediated acute allergic reactions to stings, pollens, and drugs, including anaphylaxis, urticaria, and angioedema. IgE is fixed to tissue mast cells and blood basophils, and after interaction with antigen the cells release potent mediators.
- **Type II:** Drugs often modify host proteins, thereby eliciting antibody responses to the modified protein. These allergic responses involve IgG or IgM in which the antibody becomes fixed to a host cell, which is then subject to complement-dependent lysis or to antibody-dependent cellular cytotoxicity.
- **Type III:** Drugs may cause serum sickness, which involves immune complexes containing IgG and is a multisystem complement-dependent vasculitis that may also result in urticaria.
- **Type IV:** Cell-mediated allergy is the mechanism involved in allergic contact dermatitis from topically applied drugs or induration of the skin at the site of an antigen injected intradermally.

In some drug reactions, several of these hypersensitivity responses may present simultaneously. Some adverse reactions to drugs may be mistakenly classified as allergic or immune when they are actually genetic deficiency states or are idiosyncratic and not mediated by immune mechanisms (eg, hemolysis due to primaquine in glucose-6-phosphate dehydrogenase deficiency, or aplastic anemia caused by chloramphenicol).

IMMEDIATE (TYPE I) DRUG ALLERGY

Type I (immediate) sensitivity allergy to certain drugs occurs when the drug, not capable of inducing an immune response by itself, covalently links to a host carrier protein (hapten). When this happens, the immune system detects the drug-hapten conjugate as "modified self" and responds by generating IgE antibodies specific for the drug-hapten. It is not known why some people mount an IgE response to a drug, while others mount IgG responses. Under the influence of IL-4, IL-5, and IL-13 secreted by TH2 cells, B cells specific for the drug secrete IgE antibody. The mechanism for IgE-mediated immediate hypersensitivity is diagrammed in Figure 56–5.

Fixation of the IgE antibody to high-affinity Fc receptors (FcεRs) on blood basophils or their tissue equivalent (mast cells) sets the stage for an acute allergic reaction. The most important sites for mast cell distribution are skin, nasal epithelium, lung, and gastrointestinal tract. When the offending drug is reintroduced into the body, it binds and cross-links basophil and mast cell-surface IgE to signal release of the mediators (eg, histamine, leukotrienes; see Chapters 16 and 18) from granules. Mediator release is associated with calcium influx and a fall in intracellular cAMP within the mast cell. Many of the drugs that block mediator release appear to act through the cAMP mechanism (eg, catecholamines, glucocorticoids, theophylline), others block histamine release, and still others block histamine receptors. Other vasoactive substances such as kinins may also be generated during histamine release. These mediators initiate immediate vascular smooth muscle relaxation, increased vascular permeability, hypotension, edema, and bronchoconstriction.

Drug Treatment of Immediate Allergy

One can test an individual for possible sensitivity to a drug by a simple scratch test, ie, by applying an extremely dilute solution of the drug to the skin and making a scratch with the tip of a needle. If allergy is present, an immediate (within 10–15 minutes) wheal (edema) and flare (increased blood flow) will occur. However, skin tests may be negative in spite of IgE hypersensitivity to a hapten or to a metabolic product of the drug, especially if the patient is taking steroids or antihistamines.

Drugs that modify allergic responses act at several links in this chain of events. Prednisone, often used in severe allergic reactions, is immunosuppressive; it blocks proliferation of the IgE-producing clones and inhibits IL-4 production by T helper cells in the IgE response, since glucocorticoids are generally toxic to lymphocytes. In the efferent limb of the allergic response, isoproterenol, epinephrine, and theophylline reduce the release of mediators from mast cells and basophils and produce bronchodilation. Epinephrine opposes histamine; it relaxes bronchiolar smooth muscle and contracts vascular muscle, relieving both bronchospasm and hypotension. The antihistamines competitively inhibit histamine, which would otherwise produce bronchoconstriction and increased capillary permeability in the end organ. Glucocorticoids may also act to reduce tissue injury and edema in the inflamed tissue, as well as facilitating the actions of catecholamines in cells that may have become refractory to epinephrine or isoproterenol. Several agents directed toward the inhibition of leukotriene synthesis may be useful in acute allergic and inflammatory disorders (see Chapter 20).

Desensitization to Drugs

When reasonable alternatives are not available, certain drugs (eg, penicillin, insulin) must be used for life-threatening illnesses even in the presence of known allergic sensitivity. In such cases, desensitization can sometimes be accomplished by starting with very small doses of the drug and gradually increasing the dose over a period of hours to the full therapeutic range (see Chapter 43). This practice is hazardous and must be performed under direct medical supervision, as anaphylaxis may occur before desensitization has been achieved. It is thought that slow and progressive administration of the drug gradually binds all available IgE on mast cells, triggering a gradual release of granules. Once all of the IgE on the mast cell surfaces has been bound and the cells have been degranulated, therapeutic doses of the offending drug may be given with minimal further immune reaction. Therefore, a patient is only desensitized during administration of the drug.

AUTOIMMUNE (TYPE II) REACTIONS TO DRUGS

Certain autoimmune syndromes can be induced by drugs. Examples include systemic lupus erythematosus following hydralazine or procainamide therapy, "lupoid hepatitis" due to cathartic sensitivity, autoimmune hemolytic anemia resulting from methyldopa administration, thrombocytopenic purpura due to quinidine, and agranulocytosis due to a variety of drugs. As indicated in other chapters of this book, a number of drugs are associated with type I and type II reactions. In these drug-induced autoimmune states, IgG antibodies bind to drug-modified tissue and are destroyed by the complement system or by phagocytic cells with Fc receptors. Fortunately, autoimmune reactions to drugs usually subside within several months after the offending drug is withdrawn. Immunosuppressive therapy is warranted only when the autoimmune response is unusually severe.

SERUM SICKNESS & VASCULITIC (TYPE III) REACTIONS

Immunologic reactions to drugs resulting in serum sickness are more common than immediate anaphylactic responses, but type II and type III hypersensitivities often overlap. The clinical features of serum sickness include urticarial and erythematous skin eruptions, arthralgia or arthritis, lymphadenopathy, glomerulonephritis, peripheral edema, and fever. The reactions generally last 6–12 days and usually subside once the offending drug is eliminated. Antibodies of the IgM or IgG class are usually involved. The mechanism of tissue injury is immune complex formation and deposition on basement membranes (eg, lung, kidney), followed by complement activation and infiltration of leukocytes, causing tissue destruction. Glucocorticoids are useful in attenuating severe serum sickness reactions to drugs. In severe cases plasmapheresis can be used to remove the offending drug and immune complexes from circulation.

Immune vasculitis can also be induced by drugs. The sulfonamides, penicillin, thiouracil, anticonvulsants, and iodides have all been implicated in the initiation of hypersensitivity angiitis. Erythema multiforme is a relatively mild vasculitic skin disorder that may be secondary to drug hypersensitivity. Stevens-Johnson syndrome is probably a more severe form of this hypersensitivity reaction and consists of erythema multiforme, arthritis, nephritis, central nervous system abnormalities, and myocarditis. It has frequently been associated with sulfonamide therapy. Administration of nonhuman monoclonal or polyclonal antibodies such as rattlesnake antivenin may cause serum sickness.

PREPARATIONS AVAILABLE*

Abatacept (Orencia)
Parenteral: 250 mg/vial lyophilized powder
Abciximab (ReoPro)
Parenteral: 2 mg/mL solution for IV injection
Adalimumab (Humira)
Parenteral: 40 mg/vial for IV injection
Alefacept (Amevive)
Parenteral: 7.5, 15 mg for IV injection
Alemtuzumab (Campath)
Parenteral: 30 mg/3 mL vial for IV injection
Anakinra (Kineret)
Parenteral: 100 mg/mL prefilled glass syringes for SC injection
Antithymocyte globulin (Thymoglobulin)
Parenteral: 25 mg/vial for IV injection
Arcitumomab (CEA-Scan)
Parenteral: 1 mg of arcitumomab mixed with 20-30 mCi of ^{99m}Tc for IV injection
Azathioprine (generic, Imuran)
Oral: 50 mg tablets
Parenteral: 100 mg/vial for IV injection
Basiliximab (Simulect)
Parenteral: 20 mg powder; reconstitute for IV injection
Bevacizumab (Avastin)
Parenteral: 5 mg/kg in 100 mL sodium chloride for injection
Capromab pendetide (Prostascint)
Parenteral: 0.5 mg of Capromab Pendetide mixed with 5 mCi of ^{111}In for IV injection
Cetuximab (Erbitux)
Parenteral: 2 mg/mL in 50 mL vials
Cyclophosphamide (Cytoxan, Neosar)
Oral: 25, 50 mg tablets
Parenteral: 100 mg/mL for injection
Cyclosporine (Sandimmune, Neoral, SangCya)

Oral: 25, 50, 100 mg capsules; 100 mg/mL solution
Parenteral: 50 mg/mL for IV administration
Daclizumab (Zenapax)
Parenteral: 25 mg/5 mL vial for IV infusion
Etanercept (Enbrel)
Parenteral: 25 mg lyophilized powder for SC injection
Gemtuzumab (Mylotarg)
Parenteral: 5 mg powder, reconstitute for injection
Ibritumomab tiuxetan (Zevalin)
Parenteral: 3.2 mg/2 mL for injection
Immune globulin intravenous (IGIV)
(Gamimune, Gammagard, Iveegam, Polygam, others)
Parenteral: 5, 10% solutions; 2.5, 5, 6, 10, 12 g powder for injection
Infliximab (Remicade)
Parenteral: 100 mg lyophilized powder for IV injection
Interferon alpha-2a (Roferon-A)
Parenteral: 3–36 million units powder or solution in vials or prefilled single-use syringes
Interferon alpha-2b (Intron-A)
Parenteral: 3–50 million units/vial
Interferon beta-1a (Avonex, Rebif)
Parenteral: 22, 33, 44 mcg powder for IV injection
Interferon beta-1b (Betaseron)
Parenteral: 0.3 mg powder for SC injection
Interferon gamma-1b (Actimmune)
Parenteral: 100 mcg vials
Interleukin-2 [IL-2, aldesleukin] (Proleukin)
Parenteral: 22 million unit vials
Leflunomide (Arava)
Oral: 10, 20, 100 mg tablets

(continued)

---

*Several drugs discussed in this chapter are available as orphan drugs but are not listed here. Other drugs not listed here will be found in other chapters (see Index).

Lymphocyte immune globulin (Atgam)
Parenteral: 50 mg/mL for injection (in 5 mL ampules)

Methylprednisolone sodium succinate (Solu-Medrol, others)
Parenteral: 40, 125, 500, 1000, 2000 mg powder for injection

Muromonab-CD3 [OKT3] (Orthoclone OKT3)
Parenteral: 5 mg/5 mL ampule for injection

Mycophenolate mofetil (CellCept)
Oral: 250 mg capsules; 500 mg tablets; 200 mg powder for suspension
Parenteral: 500 mg powder; reconstitute for injection

Nofetumomab (Verluma)
Parenteral: kit for coupling ^{99}Tc to nofetumomab Fab fragment for IV infusion (see package insert)

Omalizumab (Xolair)
Parenteral: 202.5 mg; for injection

Pegademase bovine (Adagen)
Parenteral: 250 units/mL for IM injection
Note: Pegademase is bovine adenosine deaminase

Peginterferon alfa-2a (Pegasys)
Parenteral: 180 mcg/mL

Peginterferon alfa-2b (PEG-Intron)
Parenteral: 50, 80, 120, 150 mcg/0.5 mL

Prednisone (generic)
Oral: 1, 2.5, 10, 20, 50 mg tablets; 1, 5 mg/mL solution

Rh₀(D) immune globulin micro-dose (BayRho-D, BayRho-D Mini-Dose, MICRhoGAM, RhoGam, WinRho)
Parenteral: in single-dose and micro-dose vials

Rituximab (Rituxan)
Parenteral: 10 mg/mL for IV infusion

Sirolimus (Rapamune)
Oral: 1 mg tablets; 1 mg/mL solution

Tacrolimus [FK 506] (Prograf)
Oral: 0.5, 1, 5 mg capsules
Parenteral: 5 mg/mL
Topical (Protopic): 0.03%, 0.1% ointment

Thalidomide (Thalomid)
Oral: 50 mg capsules
Note: Thalidomide is labeled for use only in erythema nodosum leprosum in the USA

Tositumomab (Bexxar)
Parenteral: two single-use 225 mg vials, and one 35 mg vial; ^{131}I-labeled tositumomab, 1.1 mg/mL at 5.6 mCi/mL; 0.1, 14 mg/mL

Trastuzumab (Herceptin)
Parenteral: 440 mg powder; reconstitute for IV infusion

REFERENCES

General Immunology

Egen JG, Kuhns MS, Allison JP: CTLA-4: New insights into its biological function and use in tumor immunotherapy. Nature Immunol 2002;3:611.

Goldsby RA et al: *Immunology,* 5th ed. Freeman, 2003.

Janeway C et al: *Immunobiology: The Immune System in Health and Disease,* 6th ed. Current Biology Publications, 2005.

T Helper Cells: T$_H$1 & T$_H$2

Maker AZ et al: Tumor regression and autoimmunity in patients treated with cytotoxic T lymphocyte-associated antigen 4 blockade and interleukin 2: A phase I/II study. Ann Surg Oncol 2005;12:1004.

Phan GQ et al: Cancer regression and autoimmunity induced by cytotoxic T lymphocyte-associated antigen 4 blockade in patients with metastatic melanoma. Proc Natl Acad Sci U S A 2003;100:8372.

Hypersensitivity

Ballow, M: -ximab this and -zumab that! Has the magic bullet arrived in the new millennium of medicine and science? J Allergy Clin Immunol 2005;116:738.

Chiu AM, Kelly KJ: Anaphylaxis: Drug allergy, insect stings, and latex. Immunol Allergy Clin North Am 2005; 25:389.

Martin E et al: Drug hypersensitivity: Insights into pathomechanisms. Allerg Immunol (Paris) 2005;37:207.

Autoimmunity

Arnason BG: Long-term experience with interferon beta-1b (Betaferon) in multiple sclerosis. J Neurol 2005;252(Suppl 3):iii28.

Brown MA: Antibody treatments of inflammatory arthritis. Curr Med Chem 2005;12:2943.

Czaja AJ: Autoimmune liver disease. Curr Opin Gastroenterol 2005;21:293.

Hafler DA et al: Multiple sclerosis. Immunol Rev 2005;204:208.

Weinberg JM et al: Biologic therapy for psoriasis: An update on the tumor necrosis factor inhibitors infliximab, etanercept, and adalimumab, and the T-cell-targeted therapies efalizumab and alefacept. J Drugs Dermatol 2005;4:544.

Immunodeficiency Diseases

Cunningham-Rundles C et al: Molecular defects in T- and B-cell primary immunodeficiency diseases. Nat Rev Immunol 2005;5:880.

DiRenzo M et al: Common variable immunodeficiency: A review. Clin Exp Med 2004;3:211.

Durandy A et al: Immunoglobulin replacement therapy in primary antibody deficiency diseases–maximizing success. Int Arch Allergy Immunol 2005;136:217.

Immunosuppressive Agents

Crane E, List A: Immunomodulatory drugs. Cancer Invest 2005; 23:625.

Gerards AH et al: Cyclosporine A monotherapy versus cyclosporine A and methotrexate combination therapy in patients with early rheumatoid arthritis: A double blind randomised placebo controlled trial. Ann Rheum Dis 2003; 62:291.

McHutchison JG, Fried MW: Current therapy for hepatitis C: Pegylated interferon and ribavirin. Clin Liver Dis 2003; 7:149.

McMurray RW, Harisdangkul V: Mycophenolate mofetil: Selective T cell inhibition. Am J Med Sci 2002;323:194.

Reichenspurner H: Overview of tacrolimus-based immunosuppression after heart or lung transplantation. J Heart Lung Transplant 2005;24:119.

Ribatti D, Vacca A: Therapeutic renaissance of thalidomide in the treatment of haematological malignancies. Leukemia 2005; 19:1525.

Antilymphocyte Globulin & Monoclonal Antibodies

Jolles S et al: Clinical uses of intravenous immunoglobulin. Clin Exp Immunol 2005;142:1.

Jordan SC et al: Current approaches to treatment of antibody-mediated rejection. Pediatr Transplant 2005;9:408.

Nashan B: Antibody induction therapy in renal transplant patients receiving calcineurin-inhibitor immunosuppressive regimens: A comparative review. BioDrugs 2005;19:39.

Weiner LM: Fully human therapeutic monoclonal antibodies. J Immunother 2006;29:1.

Cytokines

Disis ML, Feld JJ: Mechanism of action of interferon and ribavirin in treatment of hepatitis C. Nature 2005;436:967.

Lawson DH: Choices in adjuvant therapy of melanoma. Cancer Control 2005;12:236.

Drug Allergy

Greenberger PA: Drug allergy. J Allergy Clin Immunol 2006; 117(Suppl):S464.

Sicherer SH, Leung DY: Advances in allergic skin disease, anaphylaxis, and hypersensitivity reactions to foods, drugs, and insects. J Allergy Clin Immunol 2005;116:153.

SECTION IX
Toxicology

Introduction to Toxicology: Occupational & Environmental

57

Gabriel L. Plaa, PhD

Humans live in a chemical environment and inhale, ingest, or absorb from the skin many of these chemicals. Toxicology is concerned with the deleterious effects of these chemical agents on all living systems. In the biomedical area, however, the toxicologist is primarily concerned with adverse effects in humans resulting from exposure to drugs and other chemicals as well as the demonstration of safety or hazard associated with their use.

Occupational Toxicology

Occupational toxicology deals with the chemicals found in the workplace. The major emphasis of occupational toxicology is to identify the agents of concern, define the conditions leading to their safe use, and prevent absorption of harmful amounts. Guidelines have been elaborated to establish safe ambient air concentrations for many chemicals found in the workplace. The American Conference of Governmental Industrial Hygienists periodically prepares lists of recommended **threshold limit values (TLVs)** for about 600 such chemicals. These guidelines are reevaluated as new information becomes available.

Environmental Toxicology

Environmental toxicology deals with the potentially deleterious impact of chemicals, present as pollutants of the environment, on living organisms. The term *environment* includes all the surroundings of an individual organism, but particularly the air, soil, and water.

While humans are considered a target species of particular interest, other species are of considerable importance as potential biologic targets.

Air pollution is a product of industrialization, technologic development, and increased urbanization. Humans may also be exposed to chemicals used in the agricultural environment as pesticides or in food processing that may persist as residues or ingredients in food products. The Food and Agriculture Organization and the World Health Organization (FAO/WHO) Joint Expert Commission on Food Additives adopted the term **acceptable daily intake (ADI)** to denote the daily intake of a chemical which, during an entire lifetime, appears to be without appreciable risk. These guidelines are reevaluated as new information becomes available.

Ecotoxicology

Ecotoxicology is concerned with the toxic effects of chemical and physical agents on *populations* and *communities of living organisms* within defined ecosystems; it includes the transfer pathways of those agents and their interactions with the environment. Traditional toxicology is concerned with toxic effects on individual organisms; ecotoxicology is concerned with the impact on populations of living organisms or on ecosystems. It is possible that an environmental event, while exerting severe effects on *individual* organisms, may have no important impact on populations or on an ecosystem. Thus, the terms "environmental toxicology" and "ecotoxicology" are not interchangeable.

BIOACCUMULATION & BIOMAGNIFICATION

If the intake of a long-lasting contaminant by an organism exceeds the latter's ability to metabolize or excrete the substance, the chemical accumulates within the tissues of the organism. This is called **bioaccumulation.**

Although the concentration of a contaminant may be virtually undetectable in water, it may be magnified hundreds or thousands of time as the contaminant passes up the food chain. This is called **biomagnification.**

The biomagnification of polychlorinated biphenyls (PCBs) in the Great Lakes of North America is illustrated by the following residue values available from *Environment Canada,* a report published by the Canadian government, and other sources.

Thus, the biomagnification for this substance in the food chain, beginning with phytoplankton and ending with the herring gull, is nearly 50,000-fold. Domesticated animals and humans may eat fish from the Great Lakes, resulting in PCB residues in these species as well.

Source	PCB Concentration (ppm)[1]	Concentration Relative to Phytoplankton
Phytoplankton	0.0025	1
Zooplankton	0.123	49.2
Rainbow smelt	1.04	416
Lake trout	4.83	1,932
Herring gull	124	49,600

[1]Sources: *Environment Canada, The State of Canada's Environment,* 1991, Government of Canada, Ottawa; and other publications.

TOXICOLOGIC TERMS & DEFINITIONS

Hazard & Risk

Hazard is *the ability of a chemical agent to cause injury in a given situation or setting;* the conditions of use and exposure are primary considerations. To assess hazard, one needs to have knowledge about both the inherent toxicity of the substance and the amounts to which individuals are liable to be exposed. Humans can safely use potentially toxic substances when the necessary conditions minimizing absorption are established and respected.

Risk is defined as *the expected frequency of the occurrence of an undesirable effect* arising from exposure to a chemical or physical agent. Estimation of risk makes use of dose-response data and extrapolation from the observed relationships to the expected responses at doses occurring in actual exposure situations. The quality and suitability of the biologic data used in such estimates are major limiting factors.

Routes of Exposure

The route of entry for chemicals into the body differs in different exposure situations. In the industrial setting, inhalation is the major route of entry. The transdermal route is also quite important, but oral ingestion is a relatively minor route. Consequently, preventive measures are largely designed to eliminate absorption by inhalation or by topical contact. Atmospheric pollutants gain entry by inhalation, whereas for pollutants of water and soil, oral ingestion is the principal route of exposure for humans.

Duration of Exposure

Toxic reactions may differ qualitatively depending on the duration of the exposure. A single exposure—or multiple exposures occurring over 1 or 2 days—represents **acute exposure.** Multiple exposures continuing over a longer period of time represent a **chronic exposure.** In the occupational setting, both acute (eg, accidental discharge) and chronic (eg, repetitive handling of a chemical) exposures may occur, whereas with chemicals found in the environment (eg, pollutants in ground water), chronic exposure is more likely.

ENVIRONMENTAL CONSIDERATIONS

Certain chemical and physical characteristics are known to be important for estimating the potential hazard involved for environmental toxicants. In addition to information regarding effects on different organisms, knowledge about the following properties is essential to predict the environmental impact: The **degradability** of the substance; its **mobility** through air, water, and soil; whether or not **bioaccumulation** occurs; and its transport and **biomagnification** through food chains. (See Box: Bioaccumulation & Biomagnification.) Chemicals that are poorly degraded (by abiotic or biotic pathways) exhibit *environmental persistence* and thus can accumulate. Lipophilic substances tend to bioaccumulate in body fat, resulting in tissue residues. When the toxicant is incorporated into the food chain, biomagnification occurs as one species feeds upon others and concentrates the chemical. The pollutants that have the widest environmental impact are poorly degradable;

Table 57–1. Threshold limit values (TLV) of some common air pollutants and solvents. (NA = none assigned.)

Compound	TLV (ppm)	
	TWA[1]	STEL[2]
Benzene	0.5	2.5
Carbon monoxide	25	NA
Carbon tetrachloride	5	10
Chloroform	10	NA
Nitrogen dioxide	3	5
Ozone	0.05	NA
Sulfur dioxide	2	5
Tetrachloroethylene	25	100
Toluene	50	NA
1,1,1-Trichloroethane	350	450
Trichloroethylene	50	100

[1]TLV-TWA is the concentration for a normal 8-hour workday or 40-hour workweek to which workers may be repeatedly exposed without adverse effects.

[2]TLV-STEL is the maximum concentration that should not be exceeded at any time during a 15-minute exposure period.

are relatively mobile in air, water, and soil; exhibit bioaccumulation; and also exhibit biomagnification.

■ SPECIFIC CHEMICALS

AIR POLLUTANTS

Five major substances account for about 98% of air pollution: carbon monoxide (about 52%), sulfur oxides (about 14%), hydrocarbons (about 14%), nitrogen oxides (about 14%), and particulate matter (about 4%). The sources of these chemicals include transportation, industry, generation of electric power, space heating, and refuse disposal. Sulfur dioxide and smoke resulting from incomplete combustion of coal have been associated with acute adverse effects, particularly among the elderly and individuals with preexisting cardiac or respiratory disease. Ambient air pollution has been implicated as a contributing factor in bronchitis, obstructive ventilatory disease, pulmonary emphysema, bronchial asthma, and lung cancer.

1. Carbon Monoxide

Carbon monoxide (CO) is a colorless, tasteless, odorless, and nonirritating gas, a byproduct of incomplete combustion. The average concentration of CO in the atmosphere is about 0.1 ppm; in heavy traffic, the concentration may exceed 100 ppm. The recommended 2005 threshold limit values (TLV-TWA and TLV-STEL) are shown in Table 57–1.

Mechanism of Action

CO combines reversibly with the oxygen-binding sites of hemoglobin and has an affinity for hemoglobin that is about 220 times that of oxygen. The product formed, carboxyhemoglobin, cannot transport oxygen. Furthermore, the presence of carboxyhemoglobin interferes with the dissociation of oxygen from the remaining oxyhemoglobin, thus reducing the transfer of oxygen to tissues. The brain and the heart are the organs most affected. Normal nonsmoking adults have carboxyhemoglobin levels of less than 1% saturation (1% of total hemoglobin is in the form of carboxyhemoglobin); this level has been attributed to the endogenous formation of CO from heme catabolism. Smokers may exhibit 5–10% saturation, depending on their smoking habits. An individual breathing air containing 0.1% CO (1000 ppm) would have a carboxyhemoglobin level of about 50%.

Clinical Effects

The principal signs of CO intoxication are those of hypoxia and progress in the following sequence: (1) psychomotor impairment; (2) headache and tightness in the temporal area; (3) confusion and loss of visual acuity; (4) tachycardia, tachypnea, syncope, and coma; and (5) deep coma, convulsions, shock, and respiratory failure. There is great variability in individual responses to a given carboxyhemoglobin concentration. Carboxyhemoglobin levels below 15% rarely produce symptoms; collapse and syncope may appear around 40%; above 60%, death may ensue. Prolonged hypoxia and posthypoxic unconsciousness can result in irreversible damage to the brain and the myocardium. The clinical effects may be aggravated by heavy labor, high altitudes, and high ambient temperatures. The presence of cardiovascular disease is considered to increase the risks associated with CO exposure. Delayed neuropsychiatric impairment can occur after poisoning, and the resolution of behavioral consequences can be slow. While CO intoxication is usually thought of as a form of acute toxicity, there is some evidence that chronic exposure to low levels may lead to undesirable effects, including the development of atherosclerotic coronary disease in cigarette smokers. However, convincing experimental evidence is lacking. The fetus may be quite susceptible to the effects of CO exposure.

Treatment

In cases of acute intoxication, removal of the individual from the exposure source and maintenance of respiration is essential, followed by administration of oxygen—the specific antagonist to CO—within the limits of oxygen toxicity. With room air at 1 atm, the elimination half-time of CO is about 320 minutes; with 100% oxygen, the half-time is about 80 minutes; and with hyperbaric oxygen (2–3 atm), the half-time can be reduced to about 20 minutes. Questions still exist about the efficacy of hyperbaric oxygen in the treatment of CO poisoning, and absolute indications for its use have yet to be established.

2. Sulfur Dioxide

Sulfur dioxide (SO_2) is a colorless, irritant gas generated primarily by the combustion of sulfur-containing fossil fuels. The 2005 threshold limit values are given in Table 57–1.

Mechanism of Action

On contact with moist membranes, SO_2 forms sulfurous acid, which is responsible for its severe irritant effects on the eyes, mucous membranes, and skin. It is estimated that approximately 90% of inhaled SO_2 is absorbed in the upper respiratory tract, the site of its principal effect. The inhalation of SO_2 causes bronchial constriction; parasympathetic reflexes and altered smooth muscle tone appear to be involved in this reaction. Exposure to 5 ppm for 10 minutes leads to increased resistance to airflow in most humans. Exposures to 5–10 ppm are reported to cause severe bronchospasm; 10–20% of the healthy young adult population is estimated to be reactive to even lower concentrations. The phenomenon of adaptation to irritating concentrations is a recognized occurrence in workers. Asthmatic individuals are especially sensitive to SO_2.

Clinical Effects & Treatment

The signs and symptoms of intoxication include irritation of the eyes, nose, and throat and reflex bronchoconstriction. If severe exposure has occurred, delayed onset pulmonary edema may be observed. Cumulative effects from chronic low-level exposure to SO_2 are not striking, particularly in humans. Chronic exposure, however, has been associated with aggravation of chronic cardiopulmonary disease. Treatment is not specific for SO_2 but depends on therapeutic maneuvers utilized in the treatment of irritation of the respiratory tract.

3. Nitrogen Oxides

Nitrogen dioxide (NO_2) is a brownish irritant gas sometimes associated with fires. It is formed also from fresh silage; exposure of farmers to NO_2 in the confines of a silo can lead to **silo-filler's disease.** The 2005 threshold limit values are shown in Table 57–1.

Mechanism of Action

NO_2 is a deep lung irritant capable of producing pulmonary edema. The type I cells of the alveoli appear to be the cells chiefly affected on acute exposure. Exposure to 25 ppm is irritating to some individuals; 50 ppm is moderately irritating to the eyes and nose. Exposure for 1 hour to 50 ppm can cause pulmonary edema and perhaps subacute or chronic pulmonary lesions; 100 ppm can cause pulmonary edema and death.

Clinical Effects & Treatment

The signs and symptoms of acute exposure to NO_2 include irritation of the eyes and nose, cough, mucoid or frothy sputum production, dyspnea, and chest pain. Pulmonary edema may appear within 1–2 hours. In some individuals, the clinical signs may subside in about 2 weeks; the patient may then pass into a second stage of abruptly increasing severity, including recurring pulmonary edema and fibrotic destruction of terminal bronchioles (bronchiolitis obliterans). Chronic exposure of laboratory animals to 10–25 ppm NO_2 has resulted in emphysematous changes; thus, chronic effects in humans are of concern. There is no specific treatment for acute intoxication by NO_2; therapeutic measures for the management of deep lung irritation and noncardiogenic pulmonary edema are employed. These measures include maintenance of gas exchange with adequate oxygenation and alveolar ventilation. Drug therapy may include bronchodilators, sedatives, and antibiotics.

4. Ozone

Ozone (O_3) is a bluish irritant gas that occurs normally in the earth's atmosphere, where it is an important absorbent of ultraviolet light. In the workplace, it can occur around high-voltage electrical equipment and around ozone-producing devices used for air and water purification. It is also an important oxidant found in polluted urban air. The effect of low ambient levels of ozone on admission to Ontario, Canada, hospitals for respiratory problems revealed a near-linear gradient between exposure (1-hour level, 20–100 ppb) and response. See Table 57–1 for 2005 threshold limit values.

Clinical Effects & Treatment

O_3 is an irritant of mucous membranes. Mild exposure produces upper respiratory tract irritation. Severe exposure can cause deep lung irritation, with pulmonary edema when inhaled at sufficient concentrations. Ozone penetration in the lung depends on tidal volume; consequently, exercise can increase the amount of ozone reaching the distal lung.

Some of the effects of O_3 resemble those seen with radiation, suggesting that O_3 toxicity may result from the formation of reactive free radicals. The gas causes shallow, rapid breathing and a decrease in pulmonary compliance. Enhanced sensitivity of the lung to bronchoconstrictors is also observed. Exposure around 0.1 ppm for 10–30 minutes causes irritation and dryness of the throat; above 0.1 ppm, one finds changes in visual acuity, substernal pain, and dyspnea. Pulmonary function is impaired at concentrations exceeding 0.8 ppm. Airway hyperresponsiveness and airway inflammation have been observed in humans.

Animal studies indicate that the response of the lung to O_3 is a dynamic one. The morphologic and biochemical changes are the result of both direct injury and secondary responses to the initial damage. Long-term exposure in animals results in morphologic and functional pulmonary changes. Chronic bronchitis, bronchiolitis, fibrosis, and emphysematous changes have been reported in a variety of species exposed to concentrations above 1 ppm. There is no specific treatment for acute O_3 intoxication. Management depends on therapeutic measures utilized for deep lung irritation and noncardiogenic pulmonary edema (see Nitrogen Oxides, above).

SOLVENTS

1. Halogenated Aliphatic Hydrocarbons

These agents find wide use as industrial solvents, degreasing agents, and cleaning agents. The substances include carbon tetrachloride, chloroform, trichloroethylene, tetrachloroethylene (perchloroethylene), and 1,1,1-trichloroethane (methyl chloroform). See Table 57–1 for recommended threshold limit values.

Mechanism of Action & Clinical Effects

In laboratory animals, the halogenated hydrocarbons cause central nervous system depression, liver injury, kidney injury, and some degree of cardiotoxicity. These substances are depressants of the central nervous system in humans, although their relative potencies vary considerably; chloroform is the most potent and was widely used as an anesthetic agent. Chronic exposure to tetrachloroethylene can cause impaired memory and peripheral neuropathy. In 1994, evidence was presented suggesting that 1,1,1-trichloroethane used in some degreasing operations may be associated with peripheral neuropathy. This proposed association requires confirmation because of the widespread use of this agent. Hepatotoxicity is also a common toxic effect that can occur in humans after acute or chronic exposures, the severity of the lesion being dependent on the amount absorbed. Carbon tetrachloride is the most potent of the series in this regard. Nephrotoxicity can occur in humans exposed to carbon tetrachloride, chloroform, and trichloroethylene. With chloroform, carbon tetrachloride, trichloroethylene, and tetrachloroethylene, carcinogenicity has been observed in lifetime exposure studies performed in rats and mice. The potential effects of low-level, long-term exposures in humans are yet to be determined. However, a review of the epidemiologic literature on the occupational exposure of workers to tetrachloroethylene found no association between breast, prostate, skin, or brain cancer and exposure to the agent, while a relationship for cancer of the oral cavity, liver, pancreas, or lung appeared unlikely. Data indicate that the margin of safety for humans is very large with respect to the potential carcinogenic effect of household exposure to chloroform or environmentally relevant concentrations of trichloroethylene.

Treatment

There is no specific treatment for acute intoxication resulting from exposure to halogenated hydrocarbons. Management depends on the organ system involved.

2. Aromatic Hydrocarbons

Benzene is widely used for its solvent properties and as an intermediate in the synthesis of other chemicals. The 2005 recommended threshold limit values are given in Table 57–1. The acute toxic effect of benzene is depression of the central nervous system. Exposure to 7500 ppm for 30 minutes can be fatal. Exposure to concentrations larger than 3000 ppm may cause euphoria, nausea, locomotor problems, and coma; vertigo, drowsiness, headache, and nausea may occur at concentrations ranging from 250 to 500 ppm. No specific treatment exists for the acute toxic effect of benzene.

Chronic exposure to benzene can result in very serious toxic effects, the most significant being an insidious and unpredictable injury to the bone marrow; aplastic anemia, leukopenia, pancytopenia, or thrombocytopenia may occur. Bone marrow cells in early stages of development appear to be most sensitive to benzene. The early symptoms of chronic benzene intoxication may be rather vague (headache, fatigue, and loss of appetite). Epidemiologic data suggest an association between chronic benzene exposure and an increased incidence of leukemia in workers.

Toluene (methylbenzene) does not possess the myelotoxic properties of benzene, nor has it been associated with leukemia. It is, however, a central nervous system depressant. See Table 57–1 for the threshold limit values. Exposure to 800 ppm can lead to severe fatigue and ataxia; 10,000 ppm can produce rapid loss of consciousness. Chronic effects of long-term toluene exposure are unclear because human studies indicating behavioral effects usually concern exposures to several solvents, not toluene alone. In limited occupational studies, however, metabolic interactions and modification of toluene's effects have not been observed in workers also exposed to other solvents.

Table 57–2. Organochlorine insecticides.

Chemical Class	Compounds	Toxicity Rating[1]	ADI[2]
DDT and analogs	Dichlorodiphenyltrichloroethane (DDT)	4	0.005
	Methoxychlor	3	0.1
	Tetrachlorodiphenylethane (TDE)	3	—
Benzene hexachlorides	Benzene hexachloride (BHC; hexachlorocyclohexane)	4	0.008
	Lindane	4	0.008
Cyclodienes	Aldrin	5	0.0001
	Chlordane	4	0.0005
	Dieldrin	5	0.0001
	Heptachlor	4	0.0001
Toxaphenes	Toxaphene (camphechlor)	4	—

[1]Toxicity rating: Probable human oral lethal dosage for class 3 = 500–5000 mg/kg, class 4 = 50–500 mg/kg, and class 5 = 5–50 mg/kg. (See Gosselin et al, 1984.)
[2]ADI = acceptable daily intake (mg/kg/d).

INSECTICIDES

1. Organochlorine Insecticides

These agents are usually classified in four groups: DDT (chlorophenothane) and its analogs, benzene hexachlorides, cyclodienes, and toxaphenes (Table 57–2). They are aryl, carbocyclic, or heterocyclic compounds containing chlorine substituents. The individual compounds differ widely in their biotransformation and capacity for storage in tissues; toxicity and storage are not always correlated. They can be absorbed through the skin as well as by inhalation or oral ingestion. There are, however, important quantitative differences between the various derivatives; DDT in solution is poorly absorbed through the skin, whereas dieldrin absorption from the skin is very efficient.

Human Toxicology

The acute toxic properties of the organochlorine insecticides in humans are qualitatively similar. These agents interfere with inactivation of the sodium channel in excitable membranes and cause rapid repetitive firing in most neurons. Calcium ion transport is inhibited. These events affect repolarization and enhance the excitability of neurons. The major effect is central nervous system stimulation. With DDT, tremor may be the first manifestation, possibly continuing on to convulsions, whereas with the other compounds convulsions often appear as the first sign of intoxication. There is no specific treatment for the acute intoxicated state, management being symptomatic.

Chronic administration of some of these agents to laboratory animals over long periods has resulted in enhanced tumorigenicity; there is no agreement regarding the potential carcinogenic properties of these substances, and extrapolation of these observations to humans is controversial. Evidence of carcinogenic effects in humans has not been established. In a large epidemiologic study, no relationship was observed between the risk of breast cancer and serum levels of DDE, the major metabolite of DDT. Similarly, the results of a case-control study conducted to investigate the relation between DDE and DDT breast adipose tissue levels and breast cancer risk did not support a positive association.

Environmental Toxicology

The organochlorine insecticides are considered persistent chemicals. Degradation is quite slow when compared with other insecticides, and bioaccumulation, particularly in aquatic ecosystems, is well documented. Their mobility in soil depends on the composition of the soil; the presence of organic matter favors the adsorption of these chemicals onto the soil particles, whereas adsorption is poor in sandy soils. Once adsorbed, they do not readily desorb.

Because of their environmental impact, use of the organochlorine insecticides has been largely curtailed in North America and Europe. Some of them are still used, however, in equatorial countries.

2. Organophosphorus Insecticides

These agents, some of which are listed in Table 57–3, are utilized to combat a large variety of pests. They are useful pesticides when in direct contact with insects or

Table 57–3. Organophosphorus insecticides.

Compound	Toxicity Rating[1]	ADI[2]
Azinphos-methyl	5	0.005
Chlorfenvinphos	—	0.002
Diazinon	4	0.002
Dichlorvos	—	0.004
Dimethoate	4	0.01
Fenitrothion	—	0.005
Leptophos	—	—
Malathion	4	0.02
Parathion	6	0.005
Parathion-methyl	5	0.02
Trichlorfon	4	0.01

[1]Toxicity rating: Probable human oral lethal dosage for class 4 = 50–500 mg/kg, class 5 = 5–50 mg/kg, and class 6 = ≤ 5 mg/kg. (See Gosselin et al, 1984.)
[2]ADI = acceptable daily intake (mg/kg/d).

when used as **plant systemics,** where the agent is translocated within the plant and exerts its effects on insects that feed on the plant. Some of these agents are used in human and veterinary medicine as local or systemic antiparasitics (see Chapters 7 and 54). The compounds are absorbed by the skin as well as by the respiratory and gastrointestinal tracts. Biotransformation is rapid, particularly when compared with the rates observed with the chlorinated hydrocarbon insecticides. Current and suggested human inhalation occupational exposure limits for 30 organophosphate pesticides were reviewed by Storm and collaborators in 2000.

Human Toxicology

In mammals as well as insects, the major effect of these agents is inhibition of acetylcholinesterase through phosphorylation of the esteratic site. The signs and symptoms that characterize acute intoxication are due to inhibition of this enzyme and accumulation of acetylcholine; some of the agents also possess direct cholinergic activity. These effects and their treatment are described in Chapters 7 and 8 of this book. Altered neurologic and cognitive function, as well as psychological symptoms of variable duration, have been associated with exposure to high concentrations of these insecticides. Furthermore, there is some indication of an association of low arylesterase activity with neurologic symptom complexes in Gulf War veterans.

In addition to—and independently of—inhibition of acetylcholinesterase, some of these agents are capable of phosphorylating another enzyme present in neural tissue, the so-called **neuropathy target esterase.** This results in development of a delayed neurotoxicity characterized by polyneuropathy, associated with paralysis and axonal degeneration (organophosphorus ester-induced delayed polyneuropathy; OPIDP); hens are particularly sensitive to these properties and have proved very useful for studying the pathogenesis of the lesion and for identifying potentially neurotoxic organophosphorus derivatives. In humans, neurotoxicity has been observed with **triorthocresyl phosphate (TOCP),** a noninsecticidal organophosphorus compound, and is thought to occur with the insecticides dichlorvos, trichlorfon, leptophos, methamidophos, mipafox, and trichloronat. The polyneuropathy usually begins with burning and tingling sensations, particularly in the feet, with motor weakness following a few days later. Sensory and motor difficulties may extend to the legs and hands. Gait is affected, and ataxia may be present. There is no specific treatment for this form of delayed neurotoxicity.

Environmental Toxicology

Organophosphorus insecticides are not considered to be persistent pesticides because they are relatively unstable and break down in the environment. As a class they are considered to have a small impact on the environment in spite of their acute effects on organisms.

3. Carbamate Insecticides

These compounds (Table 57–4) inhibit acetylcholinesterase by carbamoylation of the esteratic site. Thus, they possess the toxic properties associated with inhibition of this enzyme as described for the organophosphorus insecticides. The effects and treatment are described in Chapters 7 and 8. The clinical effects due to carbamates are of shorter duration than those observed with organophosphorus compounds. The range between the doses that cause minor intoxication and those that result in lethality is larger with carbamates than with the organophosphorus agents. Spontaneous reactivation of cholinesterase is more rapid after inhibition by the carbamates. While the clinical approach to carbamate poisoning is similar to that for organophosphates, the use of pralidoxime is not recommended.

The carbamate insecticides are considered to be nonpersistent pesticides and are thought to exert only a small impact on the environment.

4. Botanical Insecticides

Insecticides derived from natural sources include **nicotine, rotenone,** and **pyrethrum.** Nicotine is obtained

Table 57–4. Carbamate insecticides.

Compound	Toxicity Rating[1]	ADI[2]
Aldicarb	6	0.005
Aminocarb	5	—
Carbaryl	4	0.01
Carbofuran	5	0.01
Dimetan	4	—
Dimetilan	4	—
Isolan	5	—
Methomyl	5	—
Propoxur	4	0.02
Pyramat	4	—
Pyrolan	5	—
Zectran	5	—

[1]Toxicity rating: Probable human oral lethal dosage for class 4 = 50–500 mg/kg, class 5 = 5–50 mg/kg, and class 6 = ≤ 5 mg/kg. (See Gosselin et al, 1984.)
[2]ADI = acceptable daily intake (mg/kg/d).

from the dried leaves of *Nicotiana tabacum* and *N rustica.* It is rapidly absorbed from mucosal surfaces; the free alkaloid, but not the salt, is readily absorbed from the skin. Nicotine reacts with the acetylcholine receptor of the postsynaptic membrane (sympathetic and parasympathetic ganglia, neuromuscular junction), resulting in depolarization of the membrane. Toxic doses cause stimulation rapidly followed by blockade of transmission. These actions are described in Chapter 7. Treatment is directed toward maintenance of vital signs and suppression of convulsions.

Rotenone (Figure 57–1) is obtained from *Derris elliptica, D mallaccensis, Lonchocarpus utilis,* and *L urucu.* The oral ingestion of rotenone produces gastrointestinal irritation. Conjunctivitis, dermatitis, pharyngitis, and rhinitis can also occur. Treatment is symptomatic.

Pyrethrum consists of six known insecticidal esters: pyrethrin I (Figure 57–1), pyrethrin II, cinerin I, cinerin II, jasmolin I, and jasmolin II. Synthetic pyrethroids account for about 30% of worldwide insecticide usage. Pyrethrum may be absorbed after inhalation or ingestion; absorption from the skin is not significant. The esters are extensively biotransformed. Pyrethrum insecticides are not highly toxic to mammals. When absorbed in sufficient quantities, the major site of toxic action is the central nervous system; excitation, convulsions, and tetanic paralysis can occur. Voltage-gated sodium, calcium, and chloride channels are con-

sidered targets, as well as peripheral-type benzodiazepine receptors. Symptomatic treatment is usually employed. Anticonvulsants are not consistently effective. The chloride channel agonist, ivermectin, is of use as are pentobarbital and mephenesin. The most frequent injury reported in humans results from the allergenic properties of the substance, especially contact dermatitis. Cutaneous paresthesias have been observed in workers spraying synthetic pyrethroids. Severe occupational exposures to synthetic pyrethroids in China resulted in marked effects on the central nervous system, including convulsions.

HERBICIDES

1. Chlorophenoxy Herbicides

2,4-Dichlorophenoxyacetic acid (2,4-D), 2,4,5-trichlorophenoxyacetic acid (2,4,5-T), and their salts and esters are the major compounds of interest as herbicides used for the destruction of weeds (Figure 57–1). They have been assigned toxicity ratings of 4 or 3, respectively, which place the probable human lethal dosages at 50–500 or 500–5000 mg/kg, respectively.

In humans, 2,4-D in large doses can cause coma and generalized muscle hypotonia. Rarely, muscle weakness and marked hypotonia may persist for several weeks. With 2,4,5-T, coma may occur, but the muscular dysfunction is less evident. In laboratory animals, signs of liver and kidney dysfunction have also been reported. There is limited evidence that occupational exposure to phenoxy herbicides is associated with an increased risk of non-Hodgkin's lymphoma; the evidence for soft-tissue sarcoma, however, is considered equivocal.

The toxicologic profile for these agents, particularly that of 2,4,5-T, has been confusing because of the presence of chemical contaminants (**dioxins**) produced during the manufacturing process (see below). 2,3,7,8-Tetrachlorodibenzo-*p*-dioxin (TCDD) is the most important of these contaminants.

2. Bipyridyl Herbicides

Paraquat is the most important agent of this class (Figure 57–1). Its mechanism of action is said to be similar in plants and animals and involves single-electron reduction of the herbicide to free radical species. It has been given a toxicity rating of 4, which places the probable human lethal dosage at 50–500 mg/kg. Several lethal human intoxications (accidental or suicidal) have been reported. Paraquat accumulates slowly in the lung by an active process and causes lung edema, alveolitis, and progressive fibrosis.

In humans, the first signs and symptoms after oral exposure are attributable to gastrointestinal irritation (hematemesis and bloody stools). Within a few days,

Figure 57–1. Chemical structures of selected herbicides and pesticides.

however, delayed toxicity occurs, with respiratory distress and the development of congestive hemorrhagic pulmonary edema accompanied by widespread cellular proliferation. Hepatic, renal, or myocardial involvement may also be evident. The interval between ingestion and death may be several weeks. Because of the delayed pulmonary toxicity, prompt removal of paraquat from the digestive tract is important. Gastric lavage, the use of cathartics, and the use of adsorbents to prevent further absorption have all been advocated; after absorption, treatment is successful in fewer than 50% of cases. Oxygen should be used cautiously to combat dyspnea or cyanosis, as it may aggravate the pulmonary lesions. Patients require prolonged observation, because the proliferative phase begins 1–2 weeks after ingestion.

ENVIRONMENTAL POLLUTANTS

1. Polychlorinated Biphenyls

The **polychlorinated biphenyls (PCBs, coplanar biphenyls)** have been used in a large variety of applications as dielectric and heat transfer fluids, plasticizers, wax extenders, and flame retardants. Their industrial use and manufacture in the USA was terminated by 1977.

Unfortunately, they persist in the environment. The products used commercially were actually mixtures of PCB isomers and homologs containing 12–68% chlorine. These chemicals are highly stable and highly lipophilic, poorly metabolized, and very resistant to environmental degradation; they bioaccumulate in food chains. Food is the major source of PCB residues in humans.

A serious exposure to PCBs—lasting several months—occurred in Japan in 1968 as a result of cooking oil contamination with PCB-containing transfer medium (Yusho disease). Possible effects on the fetus and on the development of the offspring of poisoned women were reported. It is now known that the contaminated cooking oil contained not only PCBs but also polychlorinated dibenzofurans (PCDFs) and polychlorinated quaterphenyls (PCQs). Consequently, the effects that were initially attributed to the presence of PCBs are now thought to have been largely caused by the other contaminants. Workers occupationally exposed to PCBs have exhibited the following clinical signs: dermatologic problems (chloracne, folliculitis, erythema, dryness, rash, hyperkeratosis, hyperpigmentation), some hepatic involvement, and elevated plasma triglycerides.

The effects of PCBs alone on reproduction and development, as well as their carcinogenic effects, have yet to be established in humans—whether workers or the general population—even though some subjects have been exposed to very high levels of PCBs. Some adverse behavioral effects in infants are reported to have been observed, but the effects were dissimilar. An association between prenatal exposure to PCBs and deficits in childhood intellectual function was described for children born to mothers who had eaten large quantities of contaminated fish. The bulk of the evidence from human studies indicates that PCBs pose little hazard to human health except in situations where food is contaminated with high concentrations of these congeners.

The **polychlorinated dibenzo-p-dioxins (PCDDs),** or **dioxins,** have been mentioned above as a group of congeners of which the most important is **2,3,7,8-tetrachlorodibenzo-p-dioxin (TCDD).** In addition, there is a larger group of dioxin-like compounds, including certain **polychlorinated dibenzofurans (PCDFs)** and **coplanar biphenyls.** While PCBs were used commercially, PCDDs and PCDFs are unwanted by-products that appear in the environment as contaminants because of improperly controlled combustion processes. PCDD and PCDF contamination of the global environment is considered to represent a contemporary problem produced by human activities. Like PCBs, these chemicals are very stable and highly lipophilic. They are poorly metabolized and very resistant to environmental degradation.

In laboratory animals, TCDD administered in suitable doses has produced a wide variety of toxic effects, including a wasting syndrome (severe weight loss accompanied by reduction of muscle mass and adipose tissue), thymic atrophy, epidermal changes, hepatotoxicity, immunotoxicity, effects on reproduction and development, teratogenicity, and carcinogenicity. Fortunately, most of these actions have not been observed in humans. The effects observed in workers involved in the manufacture of 2,4,5-T (and therefore presumably exposed to TCDD) consisted primarily of contact dermatitis and chloracne. In severely TCDD-intoxicated patients, only discrete chloracne may be present.

The presence of TCDD in 2,4,5-T is believed to be largely responsible for other human toxicities associated with the herbicide. There is some epidemiologic evidence indicating an association between occupational exposure to the phenoxy herbicides and an excess incidence of non-Hodgkin's lymphoma. The evidence of an association of increased soft tissue sarcomas with herbicides themselves, however, is considered equivocal. On the other hand, the TCDD contaminant in these herbicides may play a role in soft tissue sarcomas.

2. Endocrine Disruptors

The potential hazardous effects of some chemicals in the environment are receiving considerable attention because of their estrogen-like or antiandrogenic properties. Compounds that affect thyroid function are also of concern. Since 1998, the process of prioritization, screening, and testing of chemicals for such actions has been undergoing worldwide development. These chemicals mimic, enhance, or inhibit a hormonal action. They include a number of plant constituents (phytoestrogens) and some mycoestrogens as well as industrial chemicals, particularly persistent organochlorine agents such as DDT and PCBs. Some brominated flame retardants are now being investigated as possible endocrine disrupters. Concerns exist because of their increasing contamination of the environment, the appearance of bioaccumulation, and their potential for toxicity. In vitro assays alone are unreliable for regulatory purposes, and animal studies are considered indispensable. Modified endocrine responses in some reptiles and marine invertebrates have been observed. In humans, however, a causal relationship between exposure to a specific environmental agent and an adverse health effect due to endocrine modulation has not been established.

REFERENCES

Air Pollution

Burnett RT et al: Effects of low ambient levels of ozone and sulfates on the frequency of respiratory admissions to Ontario hospitals. Environ Res 1994;65:172.

Folinsbee LJ: Human health effects of air pollution. Environ Health Perspect 1993;100:45.

Raub JA et al: Carbon monoxide poisoning—a public health perspective. Toxicology 2000;145:1.

Occupational Toxicology

House RA, Liss GM, Wills MC: Peripheral sensory neuropathy associated with 1,1,1-trichlorethane. Arch Environ Health 1994; 51:196.

Klaassen CD (editor): *Casarett and Doull's Toxicology,* 6th ed. McGraw-Hill, 2001.

Mundt KA, Birk T, Burch MT: Critical review of the epidemiological literature on occupational exposure to perchloroethylene and cancer. Int Arch Occup Environ Health 2003;76:473.

Ukai H et al: Occupational exposure to solvent mixtures: Effects on health and metabolism. Occup Environ Health 1994;51:523.

Environmental Toxicology & Ecotoxicology

Birnbaum LS, Staska DF: Brominated flame retardants: Cause for concern? Environ Health Perspect 2004;112:9.

Crisp TM et al: Environmental endocrine disruption: An effects assessment and analysis. Environ Health Persp 1998;106(Suppl 1):11.

Daston GP, Cook JC, Kavlock RJ: Uncertainties for endocrine disrupters: Our view on progress. Toxicol Sci 2003;74:245.

Degen GH, Bolt HM: Endocrine disruptors: Update on xenoestrogens. Int Arch Occup Environ Health 2000;73:433.

Geusau A et al: Severe 2,3,7,8-tetrachlorodibenzo-*p*-dioxin (TCDD) intoxication: Clinical and laboratory effects. Environ Health Persp 2001;109:865.

Hamm JI, Chen CY, Birnbaum LS: A mixture of dioxin, furans, and non-ortho PCBs based upon consensus toxic equivalency factors produces dioxin-like reproductive effects. Toxicol Sci 2003;74:182.

Jacobson JL, Jacobson SW: Association of prenatal exposure to an environmental contaminant with intellectual function in childhood. J Toxicol Clin Toxicol 2002;40:467.

Kimbrough RD: Polychlorinated biphenyls (PCBs) and human health: An update. CRC Crit Rev Toxicol 1995;25:133.

Lavin AL, Jacobson OF, DeSesso JM: An assessment of the carcinogenic potential of trichloroethylene in humans. Human Ecol Risk Assess 2000;6:575.

Lévesque B et al: Cancer risk associated with household exposure to chloroform. J Toxicol Environ Health A 2002;65:489.

Safe SH: Endocrine disruptors and human health—is there a problem? An update. Environ Health Persp 2000;108:487.

Schecter A: *Dioxins and Health.* Plenum, 1994.

Silberhorn EM, Glauert HP, Robertson LW: Carcinogenicity of polyhalogenated biphenyls: PCBs and PBBs. CRC Crit Rev Toxicol 1990;20:440.

Pesticides & Herbicides

Ecobichon DJ: Our changing perspectives on benefits and risks of pesticides: A historical overview. Neurotoxicology 2000;21:211.

Ecobichon DJ, Joy RM (editors): *Pesticides and Neurological Diseases,* 2nd ed. CRC, 1994.

Haley RW et al: Association of low PON1 type Q (type A) arylesterase activity with neurologic symptom complexes in Gulf War veterans. Toxicol Appl Pharmacol 1999;157:227.

Jorgenson JL: Aldrin and dieldrin: A review of research on their production, environmental deposition and fate, bioaccumulation, toxicology, and epidemiology in the United States. Environ Health Perspect 2001;109(Suppl 1):113.

Krieger N et al: Breast cancer and serum organochlorines: A prospective study among white, black and Asian women. J Natl Cancer Inst 1994;86:589.

Lotti M, Moretto A: Organophosphate-induced delayed polyneuropathy. Toxicol Rev 2005;24:37.

Machemer LD, Pickel M: Carbamate insecticides. Toxicology 1994;91:29.

MacMahon B: Pesticide residues and breast cancer? J Natl Cancer Inst 1994;86:572.

Morrison HI et al: Herbicides and cancer. J Natl Cancer Inst 1992; 84:1866.

Ray DE, Fry JR: A reassessment of the neurotoxicity of pyrethroid insecticides. Pharmacol Ther 2006;111:174.

Sabapathy NN: Quaternary ammonium compounds. Toxicology 1994;91:93.

Soderlund DM et al: Mechanisms of pyrethroid neurotoxicity: Implications for cumulative risk assessment. Toxicology 2002;171:3.

Steenland K et al: Chronic neurological sequelae to organophosphate pesticide poisoning. Am J Public Health 1994;84:731.

Storm JE, Rozman KK, Doull J: Occupational exposure limits for 30 organophosphate pesticides based on inhibition of red blood cell acetylcholinesterase. Toxicology 2000;150:1.

Zheng T et al: DDE and DDT in breast adipose tissue and risk of female breast cancer. Am J Epidemiol 1999;150:453.

Clinical Toxicology

Buckley A et al: Hyperbaric oxygen for carbon monoxide poisoning: A systematic review and critical analysis of the evidence. Toxicol Rev 2005;24:75.

Ellenhorn MJ: *Ellenhorn's Medical Toxicology,* 2nd ed. Lippincott Williams & Wilkins, 1997.

Gosselin RE, Smith RP, Hodge HC: *Clinical Toxicology of Commercial Products,* 5th ed. Williams & Wilkins, 1984.

Kao JW, Nanagas KA: Carbon monoxide poisoning. Emerg Med Clin North Am 2004;22:985.

Olson KR et al (editors): *Poisoning & Drug Overdose,* 5th ed. McGraw-Hill, 2006.

Heavy Metal Intoxication & Chelators

Michael J. Kosnett, MD, MPH

Some metals such as iron are essential for life, while others such as lead are present in all organisms but serve no useful biologic purpose. Some of the oldest diseases of humans can be traced to heavy metal poisoning associated with metal mining, refining, and use. Even with the present recognition of the hazards of heavy metals, the incidence of intoxication remains significant and the need for preventive strategies and effective therapy remains high. When intoxication occurs, chelator molecules (from *chela* "claw"), or their in vivo biotransformation products, may be used to bind the metal and facilitate its excretion from the body. Chelator drugs are discussed in the second part of this chapter.

■ TOXICOLOGY OF HEAVY METALS

LEAD

Lead poisoning is one of the oldest occupational and environmental diseases in the world. Despite its recognized hazards, lead continues to have widespread commercial application, including production of storage batteries, metal alloys, solder, glass, plastics and ceramics. Environmental lead exposure, ubiquitous by virtue of the anthropogenic distribution of lead to air, water, and food, has declined considerably in the past 3 decades as a result of diminished use of lead in gasoline and other applications. While these public health measures, together with improved workplace conditions, have decreased the incidence of serious overt lead poisoning, there remains considerable concern over the effects of low-level lead exposure. Extensive evidence indicates that lead may have subtle subclinical adverse effects on neurocognitive function and on blood pressure at blood lead concentrations once considered "normal" or "safe." Lead serves no useful purpose in the human body. In key target organs such as the developing central nervous system, no safe threshold of lead exposure has been established.

Pharmacokinetics

Inorganic lead is slowly but consistently absorbed via the respiratory and gastrointestinal tracts. Inorganic lead is poorly absorbed through the skin, but organic lead compounds, eg, leaded antiknock gasoline, are well absorbed by this route. Absorption of lead dust via the respiratory tract is the most common cause of industrial poisoning. The intestinal tract is the primary route of entry in nonindustrial exposure (Table 58–1). Absorption via the gastrointestinal tract varies with the nature of the lead compound, but in general, adults absorb about 10–15% of the ingested amount while young children absorb up to 50%. Low dietary calcium, iron deficiency, and ingestion on an empty stomach have all been associated with increased lead absorption.

Once absorbed from the respiratory or gastrointestinal tract, lead is bound to erythrocytes and widely distributed initially to soft tissues such as the bone marrow, brain, kidney, liver, muscle, and gonads; then to the subperiosteal surface of bone; and later to bone matrix. Lead also crosses the placenta and poses a potential hazard to the fetus. The kinetics of lead clearance from the body follows a multicompartment model, composed predominantly of the blood and soft tissues, with a half-life of 1–2 months; and the skeleton, with a half-life of years to decades. Approximately 70% of the lead that is eliminated appears in the urine, with lesser amounts excreted through the bile, skin, hair, nails, sweat, and breast milk. The fraction not undergoing prompt excretion, approximately half of the absorbed lead, may be incorporated into the skeleton, the repository of more than 90% of the body lead burden in most adults. In patients with high bone lead burdens, slow release from the skeleton may elevate blood lead concentrations for years after exposure ceases; and pathologic high bone turnover states such as hyperthyroidism or prolonged immobilization may result in frank lead intoxication. The lead burden in bone has been quantitated using noninvasive x-ray fluorescence, a technique that may provide the best measure of long-term, cumulative lead absorption.

Table 58–1. Toxicology of selected arsenic, lead, and mercury compounds.

	Form Entering Body	Major Route of Absorption	Distribution	Major Clinical Effects	Key Aspects of Mechanism	Metabolism and Elimination
Arsenic	Inorganic arsenic salts	Gastrointestinal, respiratory (all mucosal surfaces), skin	Predominantly soft tissues (highest in liver, kidney). Avidly bound in skin, hair, nails	Cardiovascular: shock, arrhythmias. CNS: encephalopathy, peripheral neuropathy. Gastroenteritis; pancytopenia; cancer (many sites)	Inhibits enzymes; interferes with oxidative phosphorylation; alters cell signaling, gene expression	Methylation. Renal (major); sweat and feces (minor)
Lead	Inorganic lead oxides and salts	Gastrointestinal, respiratory	Soft tissues; redistributed to skeleton (> 90% of adult body burden)	CNS deficits; peripheral neuropathy; anemia; nephropathy; hypertension; reproductive toxicity	Inhibits enzymes; interferes with essential cations; alters membrane structure	Renal (major); feces and breast milk (minor)
	Organic (tetraethyl lead)	Skin, gastrointestinal, respiratory	Soft tissues, especially liver, CNS	Encephalopathy	Hepatic dealkylation (fast) → trialkymetabolites (slow) → dissociation to lead	Urine and feces (major); sweat (minor)
Mercury	Elemental mercury	Respiratory tract	Soft tissues, especially kidney, CNS	CNS: tremor, behavioral (erethism); gingivostomatitis; peripheral neuropathy; acrodynia; pneumonitis (high-dose)	Inhibits enzymes; alters membranes	Elemental Hg converted to Hg^{2+}. Urine (major); feces (minor)
	Inorganic: Hg^+ (less toxic); Hg^{2+} (more toxic)	Gastrointestinal, skin (minor)	Soft tissues, especially kidney	Acute tubular necrosis; gastroenteritis; CNS effects (rare)	Inhibits enzymes; alters membranes	Urine
	Organic: alkyl, aryl	Gastrointestinal, skin, respiratory (minor)	Soft tissues	CNS effects, birth defects	Inhibits enzymes; alters microtubules, neuronal structure	Deacylation. Fecal (alkyl, major); urine (Hg^{2+} after deacylation, minor)

Pharmacodynamics

Lead exerts multisystemic toxic effects that are mediated by multiple modes of action, including inhibition of enzymatic function; interference with the action of essential cations, particularly calcium, iron, and zinc; disturbance of cellular redox status; and alteration of the structure of cell membranes and receptors.

A. NERVOUS SYSTEM

The developing central nervous system of the fetus and young child is the most sensitive target organ for lead's toxic effect. Epidemiologic studies suggest that blood lead concentrations less than 5 mcg/dL may result in subclinical deficits in neurocognitive function in lead-exposed young children, with no demonstrable threshold for a "no effect" level. Hearing acuity may also be diminished. Adults are less sensitive to the central nervous system effects of lead, but at blood lead concentrations in excess of 30 mcg/dL, behavioral and neurocognitive effects may gradually emerge, producing signs and symptoms such as irritability, fatigue, decreased libido, anorexia, sleep disturbance, impaired visual-motor coordination, and slowed reaction time. Headache, arthralgias, and myalgias are also frequent complaints. Tremor occurs but is less common. Lead encephalopathy, usually occurring at blood lead concentrations in excess of 100 mcg/dL, is typically accompanied by increased intracranial pressure and may produce ataxia, stupor, coma, convulsions, and death. Recent studies suggest that lead may accentuate an age-related decline in cognitive function in older adults. There is wide interindividual variation in the magnitude of lead exposure required to cause overt lead-related signs and symptoms.

Peripheral neuropathy may appear after chronic high-dose lead exposure, usually following months to years of blood lead concentrations in excess of 100 mcg/dL. Predominantly motor in character, the neuropathy may present clinically with painless weakness of the extensors, particularly in the upper extremity, resulting in classic wrist-drop. Preclinical signs of lead-induced peripheral nerve dysfunction may be detectable by electrodiagnostic testing.

B. BLOOD

Lead can induce an anemia that may be either normocytic or microcytic and hypochromic. Lead interferes with heme synthesis by blocking the incorporation of iron into protoporphyrin IX and by inhibiting the function of enzymes in the heme synthesis pathway, including aminolevulinic acid dehydratase and ferrochelatase. Within 2–8 weeks after an elevation in blood lead concentration (generally to 30–50 mcg/dL or greater), increases in heme precursors, notably free erythrocyte protoporphyrin or its zinc chelate, zinc protoporphyrin, may be detectable in whole blood. Lead also contributes to anemia by increasing erythrocyte membrane fragility and decreasing red cell survival time. Frank hemolysis may occur with high exposure. The presence of basophilic stippling on the peripheral blood smear, thought to be a consequence of lead inhibition of the enzyme 3′,5′-pyrimidine nucleotidase, is sometimes a suggestive—albeit insensitive and nonspecific—diagnostic clue to the presence of lead intoxication.

C. KIDNEYS

Chronic high-dose lead exposure, usually associated with months to years of blood lead concentrations in excess of 80 mcg/dL, may result in renal interstitial fibrosis and nephrosclerosis. Lead nephropathy may have a latency period of years. Lead may alter uric acid excretion by the kidney, resulting in recurrent bouts of gouty arthritis ("saturnine gout"). Acute high-dose lead exposure sometimes produces transient azotemia, possibly as a consequence of intrarenal vasoconstriction.

D. REPRODUCTIVE ORGANS

High-dose lead exposure is a recognized risk factor for stillbirth or spontaneous abortion. Epidemiologic studies of the impact of low-level lead exposure on reproductive outcome such as low birth weight, preterm delivery, or spontaneous abortion have yielded mixed results. However, a well-designed nested case-control study recently detected an odds ratio for spontaneous abortion of 1.8 (95% CI 1.1–3.1) for every 5 mcg/dL increase in maternal blood lead across an approximate range of 5–20 mcg/dL. In males, blood lead concentrations in excess of 40 mcg/dL have been associated with diminished or aberrant sperm production.

E. GASTROINTESTINAL TRACT

Moderate lead poisoning may cause loss of appetite, constipation, and, less commonly, diarrhea. At high dosage, intermittent bouts of severe colicky abdominal pain ("lead colic") may occur. The mechanism of lead colic is unclear but is believed to involve spasmodic contraction of the smooth muscles of the intestinal wall. In heavily exposed individuals with poor dental hygiene, the reaction of circulating lead with sulfur ions released by microbial action may produce dark deposits of lead sulfide at the gingival margin ("gingival lead lines"). Although frequently mentioned as a diagnostic clue in the past, in recent times this has been a relatively rare sign of lead exposure.

F. CARDIOVASCULAR SYSTEM

Epidemiologic, experimental, and in vitro mechanistic data indicate that lead exposure elevates blood pressure in susceptible individuals. In populations with environmental or occupational lead exposure, blood lead concentration is linked with increases in systolic and diastolic blood pressure. Studies of middle-aged and elderly men and women have identified relatively low levels of lead exposure sustained by the general population to be an independent risk factor for hypertension. Lead can also elevate blood pressure in experimental animals. The effect may be caused by an interaction with calcium-mediated contraction of vascular smooth muscle.

Major Forms of Lead Intoxication

A. INORGANIC LEAD POISONING (TABLE 58–1)

1. Acute—Acute inorganic lead poisoning is uncommon today. It usually results from industrial inhalation of large quantities of lead oxide fumes or, in small children, from ingestion of a large oral dose of lead in lead-based paints or contaminated food or drink. The onset of severe symptoms usually requires several days or weeks of recurrent exposure and presents with signs and symptoms of encephalopathy or colic. Evidence of hemolytic anemia (or anemia with basophilic stippling if exposure has been subacute) and elevated hepatic aminotransferases may be present. The diagnosis of acute inorganic lead poisoning may be difficult, and depending on the presenting symptoms, the condition has sometimes been mistaken for appendicitis, peptic ulcer, pancreatitis, or infectious meningitis. Subacute presentation, featuring headache, fatigue, intermittent abdominal cramps, myalgias, and arthralgias, has often been mistaken for a flu-like viral illness and may not come to medical attention. When there has been recent ingestion of lead-containing paint chips, glazes, or weights, radiopacities may be visible on abdominal radiographs.

2. Chronic—The patient with chronic lead intoxication usually presents with multisystemic findings, including constitutional complaints of anorexia, fatigue, and malaise; neurologic complaints, including headache, difficulty in concentrating, irritability or depressed mood; weakness, arthralgias or myalgias; and gastrointestinal symptoms. Lead poisoning should be strongly suspected in any patient presenting with headache, abdominal pain, and anemia; and less commonly with motor neuropathy, gout, and renal insufficiency. Chronic lead intoxication should be considered in any child with neurocognitive deficits, growth retardation, or developmental delay.

The diagnosis is best confirmed by measuring lead in whole blood. Although this test reflects lead currently circulating in blood and soft tissues and is not a reliable marker of either recent or cumulative lead exposure, most patients with lead-related disease will have blood lead concentrations above the normal range. Average background blood lead concentrations in North America and Europe have declined considerably in recent decades, and the geometric mean blood lead concentration in the United States in 2001–2002 was estimated to be 1.45 mcg/dL. Although predominantly a research tool, the concentration of lead in bone assessed by noninvasive K x-ray fluorescence measurement of lead in bone has been correlated with long-term cumulative lead exposure, and its relationship to numerous lead-related disorders is a subject of ongoing investigation. Measurement of lead excretion in the urine following a single dose of a chelating agent (sometimes called a "chelation challenge test") primarily reflects the lead content of soft tissues and may not be a reliable marker of long-term lead exposure, remote past exposure, or skeletal lead burden.

B. ORGANOLEAD POISONING

Poisoning from organolead compounds is now very rare, in large part due to the worldwide phase-out of tetraethyl and tetramethyl lead as antiknock additives in gasoline. However, organolead compounds such as lead stearate or lead naphthenate are still used in certain commercial processes. Because of their volatility or lipid solubility, organolead compounds tend to be well absorbed through either the respiratory tract or the skin. Organolead compounds predominantly target the central nervous system, producing dose-dependent effects that may include neurocognitive deficits, insomnia, delirium, hallucinations, tremor, convulsions, and death.

Treatment

A. INORGANIC LEAD POISONING

Treatment of inorganic lead poisoning involves immediate termination of exposure, supportive care, and the judicious use of chelation therapy. (Chelation is discussed later in this chapter.) Lead encephalopathy is a medical emergency that requires intensive supportive care. Cerebral edema may improve with corticosteroids and mannitol, and anticonvulsants may be required to treat seizures. Radiopacities on abdominal radiographs may suggest the presence of retained lead objects requiring gastrointestinal decontamination. Adequate urine flow should be maintained, but overhydration should be avoided. Intravenous edetate calcium disodium ($CaNa_2EDTA$) is administered at a dosage of 1000–1500 mg/m²/d (approximately 30–50 mg/kg/d) by continuous infusion for up to 5 days. Some clinicians advocate that chelation treatment for lead encephalopathy be initiated with an intramuscular injection of dimercaprol, followed in 4 hours by concurrent administration of dimercaprol and EDTA. Parenteral chelation is limited to 5 or fewer days, at which time oral treatment with another chelator, succimer, may be instituted. In symptomatic lead intoxication without encephalopathy, treatment may sometimes be initiated with succimer. The end point for chelation is usually resolution of symptoms or return of the blood lead concentration to the premorbid range. In patients with chronic exposure, cessation of chelation may be followed by an upward rebound in blood lead concentration as the lead reequilibrates from bone lead stores.

While most clinicians support chelation for symptomatic patients with elevated blood lead concentrations, the decision to chelate asymptomatic subjects is more controversial. Since 1991, the Centers for Disease Control and Prevention have recommended chelation for all children with blood lead concentrations of 45 mcg/dL or greater. However, a recent randomized, double-blind, placebo-controlled clinical trial of succimer in children with blood lead concentrations between 25 mcg/dL and 44 mcg/dL found no benefit on neurocognitive function or long-term blood lead reduction. Prophylactic use of chelating agents in the workplace should never be a substitute for reduction or prevention of excessive exposure.

B. ORGANIC LEAD POISONING

Initial treatment consists of decontaminating the skin and preventing further exposure. Treatment of seizures requires appropriate use of anticonvulsants. Empiric chelation may be attempted if high blood lead concentrations are present.

ARSENIC

Arsenic is a naturally occurring element in the earth's crust with a long history of use as a constituent of commercial and industrial products, as a component in pharmaceuticals, and as an agent of deliberate poisoning. Recent commercial applications of arsenic include its use in the manufacture of semiconductors, wood preservatives for industrial applications (eg, marine timbers or utility poles), nonferrous alloys, glass, gel-based insecticidal ant baits, and veterinary pharmaceuticals. In some regions of the world, groundwater may contain high levels of arsenic that has leached from natural mineral deposits. Arsenic in drinking water in the Ganges delta of India and Bangladesh is now recognized as one of the world's most pressing environmental health problems. Arsine, a hydride gas with potent hemolytic effects, is manufactured predominantly for use in the semiconductor industry but may also be generated accidentally when arsenic-containing ores come in contact with acidic solutions.

It is of historical interest that Fowler's solution, which contains 1% potassium arsenite, was widely used as a medicine for many conditions from the eighteenth century through the mid-twentieth century. Organic arsenicals were the first pharmaceutical antibiotics[*] and were widely used for the first half of the twentieth century until supplanted by penicillin and other more effective and less toxic agents.

Other organoarsenicals, most notably lewisite (dichloro[2-chlorovinyl]arsine), were developed in the early twentieth century as chemical warfare agents. Arsenic trioxide was reintroduced into the United States Pharmacopeia in 2000 as an orphan drug for the treatment of relapsed acute promyelocytic leukemia and is finding expanded use in experimental cancer treatment protocols (see Chapter 55). Melarsoprol, another triva-

lent arsenical, is used in the treatment of advanced African trypanosomiasis (see Chapter 53).

Pharmacokinetics

Soluble arsenic compounds are well absorbed through the respiratory and gastrointestinal tracts (Table 58–1). Percutaneous absorption is limited but may be clinically significant after heavy exposure to concentrated arsenic reagents. Most of the absorbed inorganic arsenic undergoes methylation, mainly in the liver, to monomethylarsonic acid and dimethylarsinic acid, which are excreted, along with residual inorganic arsenic, in the urine. When chronic daily absorption is less than 1000 mcg of soluble inorganic arsenic, approximately two thirds of the absorbed dose is excreted in the urine. After massive ingestions, the elimination half-life is prolonged. Inhalation of arsenic compounds of low solubility may result in prolonged retention in the lung and may not be reflected by urinary arsenic excretion. Arsenic binds to sulfhydryl groups present in keratinized tissue, and following cessation of exposure, hair, nails, and skin may contain elevated levels after urine values have returned to normal. However, arsenic present in hair and nails as a result of external deposition may be indistinguishable from that incorporated after internal absorption.

Pharmacodynamics

Arsenic compounds are thought to exert their toxic effects by several modes of action. Interference with enzymatic function may result from sulfhydryl group binding by trivalent arsenic or by substitution for phosphate. Inorganic arsenic or its metabolites may induce oxidative stress, alter gene expression, and interfere with cell signal transduction. Although on a molar basis inorganic trivalent arsenic (As^{3+}, arsenite) is generally two to ten times more acutely toxic than inorganic pentavalent arsenic (As^{5+}, arsenate), in vivo interconversion is known to occur, and the full spectrum of arsenic toxicity has occurred after sufficient exposure to either form. Recent studies suggest that the trivalent form of the methylated metabolites (eg, monomethylarsonous acid [MMA^{III}]) may be more toxic than the inorganic parent compounds. Arsine gas is oxidized in vivo and exerts a potent hemolytic effect associated with alteration of ion flux across the erythrocyte membrane; however, it also disrupts cellular respiration in other tissues. Arsenic is a recognized human carcinogen and has been associated with cancer of the lung, skin, and bladder. Marine organisms may contain large amounts of a well-absorbed trimethylated organoarsenic, arsenobetaine, as well as a variety of arsenosugars. Arsenobetaine exerts no known toxic effects when ingested by mam-

---

[*]Paul Ehrlich's "magic bullet" for syphilis (arsphenamine; Salvarsan) was an arsenical.

mals and is excreted in the urine unchanged; arsenosugars are partially metabolized to dimethylarsinic acid.

Major Forms of Arsenic Intoxication

A. Acute Inorganic Arsenic Poisoning

Within minutes to hours after exposure to high doses (tens to hundreds of milligrams) of soluble inorganic arsenic compounds, many systems are affected. Initial gastrointestinal signs and symptoms include nausea, vomiting, diarrhea, and abdominal pain. Diffuse capillary leak, combined with gastrointestinal fluid loss, may result in hypotension, shock, and death. Cardiopulmonary toxicity, including congestive cardiomyopathy, cardiogenic or noncardiogenic pulmonary edema, and ventricular arrhythmias, may occur promptly or after a delay of several days. Pancytopenia usually develops within a week, and basophilic stippling of erythrocytes may be present soon after. Central nervous system effects, including delirium, encephalopathy, and coma, may occur within the first few days of intoxication. An ascending sensorimotor peripheral neuropathy may begin to develop after a delay of 2–6 weeks. This neuropathy may ultimately involve the proximal musculature and result in neuromuscular respiratory failure. Months after an episode of acute poisoning, transverse white striae (Aldrich-Mees lines) may be visible in the nails.

Acute inorganic arsenic poisoning should be considered in an individual presenting with abrupt onset of gastroenteritis in combination with hypotension and metabolic acidosis. Suspicion should be further heightened when these initial findings are followed by cardiac dysfunction, pancytopenia, and peripheral neuropathy. The diagnosis may be confirmed by demonstration of elevated amounts of inorganic arsenic and its metabolites in the urine (typically in the range of several thousand micrograms in the first 2–3 days following acute symptomatic poisoning). Arsenic disappears rapidly from the blood, and except in anuric patients, blood arsenic levels should not be used for diagnostic purposes. Treatment is based on appropriate gut decontamination, intensive supportive care, and prompt chelation with unithiol, 3–5 mg/kg intravenously every 4–6 hours, or dimercaprol, 3–5 mg/kg intramuscularly every 4–6 hours. In animal studies, the efficacy of chelation has been highest when it is administered within minutes to hours after arsenic exposure; therefore, if diagnostic suspicion is high, treatment should not be withheld for the several days to weeks often required to obtain laboratory confirmation. Succimer has also been effective in animal models and has a higher therapeutic index than dimercaprol. However, because it is available in the United States only for oral administration, its use may not be advisable in the initial treatment of

acute arsenic poisoning, when severe gastroenteritis and splanchnic edema may limit absorption by this route.

B. Chronic Inorganic Arsenic Poisoning

Chronic inorganic arsenic poisoning also results in multisystemic signs and symptoms. Overt noncarcinogenic effects may be evident after chronic absorption of more than 500–1000 mcg/d. The time to appearance of symptoms will vary with dose and interindividual tolerance. Constitutional symptoms of fatigue, weight loss, and weakness may be present, along with anemia, nonspecific gastrointestinal complaints, and a sensorimotor peripheral neuropathy, particularly featuring a stocking-glove pattern of dysesthesia. Skin changes—among the most characteristic effects—typically develop after years of exposure and include a "raindrop" pattern of hyperpigmentation, and hyperkeratoses involving the palms and soles. Peripheral vascular disease and noncirrhotic portal hypertension may also occur. Epidemiologic studies suggest a possible link to hypertension, diabetes, and chronic nonmalignant respiratory disease. Cancer of the lung, skin, bladder, and possibly other sites, may appear years after exposure to doses of arsenic that are not high enough to elicit other acute or chronic effects. Administration of arsenite in cancer chemotherapy regimens, often at a daily dose of 10–20 mg for weeks to a few months, has been associated with prolongation of the QT interval on the electrocardiogram and occasionally has resulted in malignant ventricular arrhythmias such as torsade de pointes.

The diagnosis of chronic arsenic poisoning involves integration of the clinical findings with confirmation of exposure. Urinary levels of total arsenic, usually less than 30 mcg/L or 50 mcg/24 h in the general population, may return to normal within days to weeks after exposure ceases. Because it may contain large amounts of nontoxic organoarsenic, all seafood should be avoided for at least 3 days prior to submission of a urine sample for diagnostic purposes. The arsenic content of hair and nails (normally less than 1 ppm) may sometimes reveal past elevated exposure, but results should be interpreted cautiously in view of the potential for external contamination.

C. Arsine Gas Poisoning

Arsine gas poisoning produces a distinctive pattern of intoxication dominated by profound hemolytic effects. After a latent period that may range from 2 hours to 24 hours postinhalation (depending on the magnitude of exposure), massive intravascular hemolysis may occur. Initial symptoms may include malaise, headache, dyspnea, weakness, nausea, vomiting, abdominal pain, jaundice, and hemoglobinuria. Oliguric renal failure, a consequence of hemoglobin deposition in the renal tubules, often appears within 1–3 days. In massive exposures, lethal effects on cellular respiration may occur before renal failure develops. Urinary arsenic levels are elevated but will seldom be available to confirm the diagnosis during the critical period of illness. Intensive supportive care—including exchange transfusion, vigorous hydration, and, in the case of acute renal failure, hemodialysis—is the mainstay of therapy. Currently available chelating agents have not been demonstrated to be of clinical value in arsine poisoning.

MERCURY

Metallic mercury as "quicksilver"—the only metal that is liquid under ordinary conditions—has attracted scholarly and scientific interest from antiquity. In early times it was recognized that the mining of mercury was hazardous to health. As industrial use of mercury became common during the past 200 years, new forms of toxicity were recognized that were found to be associated with various transformations of the metal. In the early 1950s, a mysterious epidemic of birth defects and neurologic disease occurred in the Japanese fishing village of Minamata. The causative agent was determined to be methylmercury in contaminated seafood, traced to industrial discharges into the bay from a nearby factory. In addition to elemental mercury and alkylmercury (including methylmercury), other key mercurials include inorganic mercury salts and aryl mercury compounds, each of which exerts a relatively unique pattern of clinical toxicity.

Mercury is mined predominantly as HgS in cinnabar ore and is then converted commercially to a variety of chemical forms. Key industrial and commercial applications of mercury are found in the electrolytic production of chlorine and caustic soda; the manufacture of electrical equipment, thermometers, and other instruments; fluorescent lamps; dental amalgam; and artisanal gold production. Use in pharmaceuticals and in biocides has declined substantially in recent years, but occasional use in antiseptics and folk medicines is still encountered. Environmental exposure to mercury from the burning of fossil fuels—or the bioaccumulation of methylmercury in fish—remains a concern in some regions of the world. Low-level exposure to mercury released from dental amalgam fillings occurs, but systemic toxicity from this source has not been established.

Pharmacokinetics

The absorption of mercury varies considerably depending on the chemical form of the metal. Elemental mercury is quite volatile and can be absorbed from the lungs (Table 58–1). It is poorly absorbed from the intact gastrointestinal tract. Inhaled mercury is the primary source of occupational exposure. Organic short-chain alkylmercury compounds are volatile and potentially harmful by inhalation as well as by ingestion. Percutaneous absorption of metallic mercury and inorganic mercury can be of clinical concern following massive acute or long-term chronic exposure. Alkylmercury compounds appear to be well absorbed through the skin, and acute contact with a few drops of dimethylmercury has resulted in severe, delayed toxicity. After absorption, mercury is distributed to the tissues within a few hours, with the highest concentration occurring in the kidney. Inorganic mercury is excreted through the urine and the feces. Excretion of inorganic mercury follows a multicomponent model: most is excreted within weeks to months, but a fraction may be retained in the kidneys and brain for years. Following inhalation of elemental mercury vapor, urinary mercury levels decline with a half-life of approximately 1–3 months. Methylmercury, which has a blood and whole body half-life of approximately 50 days, undergoes biliary excretion and enterohepatic circulation, with more than two thirds eventually excreted in the feces. Mercury binds to sulfhydryl groups in keratinized tissue, and, as with lead and arsenic, traces appear in the hair and nails.

Major Forms of Mercury Intoxication

Mercury interacts with sulfhydryl groups in vivo, inhibiting enzymes and altering cell membranes. The pattern of clinical intoxication from mercury depends to a great extent on the chemical form of the metal and the route and severity of exposure.

A. ACUTE

Acute inhalation of elemental mercury vapors may cause chemical pneumonitis and noncardiogenic pulmonary edema. Acute gingivostomatitis may occur, and neurologic sequelae (see below) may also ensue. Acute ingestion of inorganic mercury salts, such as mercuric chloride, can result in a corrosive, potentially life-threatening hemorrhagic gastroenteritis followed within hours to days by acute tubular necrosis and oliguric renal failure.

B. CHRONIC

Chronic poisoning from inhalation of mercury vapor results in a classic triad of tremor, neuropsychiatric disturbance, and gingivostomatitis. The tremor usually begins as a fine intention tremor of the hands, but the face may also be involved, and progression to choreiform movements of the limbs may occur. Neuropsychiatric manifestations, including memory loss, fatigue, insomnia, and anorexia, are common. There may be an insidious change in mood to shyness, withdrawal, and depression along with explosive anger or blushing (a behavioral pattern referred to as **erethism**). Recent studies suggest that low-dose exposure may produce subclinical neurologic effects. Gingivostomatitis, sometimes accompanied by loosening of the teeth, may be reported after high-dose exposure. Evidence of peripheral nerve damage may be detected on electrodiagnostic testing, but overt peripheral neuropathy is rare. Acrodynia is an uncommon idiosyncratic reaction to subacute or chronic mercury exposure and occurs mainly in children. It is characterized by painful erythema of the extremities and may be associated with hypertension, diaphoresis, anorexia, insomnia, irritability or apathy, and a miliarial rash.

Methylmercury intoxication affects mainly the central nervous system and results in paresthesias, ataxia, hearing impairment, dysarthria, and progressive constriction of the visual fields. Signs and symptoms may first appear several weeks or months after exposure begins. Methylmercury is a reproductive toxin. High-dose prenatal exposure to methylmercury may produce mental retardation and a cerebral palsy-like syndrome in the offspring. Low-level prenatal exposures have been associated with a risk of subclinical neurodevelopmental deficits. Dimethylmercury is a rarely encountered but extremely neurotoxic form of organomercury that may be lethal in small quantities.

The diagnosis of mercury intoxication involves integration of the history and physical findings with confirmatory laboratory testing or other evidence of exposure. In the absence of occupational exposure, the urine mercury concentration is usually less than 5 mcg/L, and whole blood mercury is less than 5 mcg/L. In 1990, the Biological Exposure Index (BEI) Committee of the American Conference of Governmental Industrial Hygienists (ACGIH) recommended that workplace exposures should result in urinary mercury concentrations less than 35 mcg per gram of creatinine and end-of-work-week whole blood mercury concentrations less than 15 mcg/L. To minimize the risk of developmental neurotoxicity from methylmercury, the US Environmental Protection Agency and Food and Drug Administration have advised pregnant women, women who might become pregnant, nursing mothers, and young children to avoid consumption of fish with high mercury levels (eg, swordfish), and to limit consumption of fish with lower levels of mercury to no more than 12 ounces (340 g, or two average meals) per week.

Treatment

A. ACUTE EXPOSURE

In addition to intensive supportive care, prompt chelation with oral or intravenous unithiol, intramuscular dimercaprol, or oral succimer may be of value in diminishing nephrotoxicity after acute exposure to inorganic mercury salts. Vigorous hydration may help to main-

tain urine output, but if acute renal failure ensues, days to weeks of hemodialysis or hemodiafiltration in conjunction with chelation may be necessary. Because the efficacy of chelation declines with time since exposure, treatment should not be delayed until the onset of oliguria or other major systemic effects.

B. CHRONIC EXPOSURE

Unithiol and succimer increase urine mercury excretion following acute or chronic elemental mercury inhalation, but the impact of such treatment on clinical outcome is unknown. Dimercaprol has been shown to redistribute mercury to the central nervous system from other tissue sites, and since the brain is a key target organ, dimercaprol should not be used in treatment of exposure to elemental or organic mercury. Limited data suggest that succimer, unithiol, and N-acetyl-L-cysteine (NAC) may enhance body clearance of methylmercury.

■ PHARMACOLOGY OF CHELATORS

Chelating agents are drugs used to prevent or reverse the toxic effects of a heavy metal on an enzyme or other cellular target, or to accelerate the elimination of the metal from the body. Chelating agents are usually flexible molecules with two or more electronegative groups that form stable coordinate-covalent bonds with a cationic metal atom. In some cases, eg, succimer, the parent compound may require in vivo biotransformation to become an active complexing agent. The chelator-metal complexes formed are excreted by the body. Edetate (ethylenediaminetetraacetate, Figure 58–1) is an important example.

The efficiency of the chelator is partly determined by the number of ligand groups on the molecule available for metal binding. The greater the number of these ligand groups, the more stable the metal-chelator complex. Depending on the number of metal-ligand bonds, the complex may be referred to as mono-, bi-, or polydentate. The chelating ligand groups include functional groups such as –OH, –SH, and –NH, which can donate electrons for coordination with the metal. Such bonding effectively prevents interaction of the metal with similar functional groups of enzymes or other proteins, coenzymes, cellular nucleophiles, and membranes.

In addition to removing the target metal that is exerting toxic effects on the body, some chelating agents (such as calcium EDTA used for lead intoxication) may enhance the excretion of essential cations such as zinc or copper. However, this side effect is seldom of clinical sig-

A

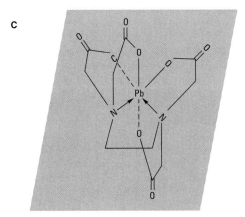

B

C

Figure 58–1. Salt and chelate formation with edetate (ethylenediaminetetraacetate; EDTA). **A:** In a solution of the disodium salt of EDTA, the sodium and hydrogen ions are chemically and biologically available. **B:** In solutions of calcium disodium edetate, calcium is bound by coordinate-covalent bonds with nitrogens as well as by the usual ionic bonds. Calcium ions are effectively removed from solution. **C:** In the lead-edetate chelate, lead is incorporated into five heterocyclic rings. (Modified and reproduced, with permission, from Meyers FH, Jawetz E, Goldfien A: *Review of Medical Pharmacology,* 7th ed. Originally published by Lange Medical Publications. McGraw-Hill, 1980.)

nificance during the limited time frame that characterizes most courses of therapeutic chelation.

In some cases, the metal-mobilizing effect of a therapeutic chelating agent may not only enhance that metal's excretion—a desired effect—but may also redistribute some of the metal to other vital organs. This has been demonstrated for dimercaprol, which redistributes mercury and arsenic to the brain while also enhancing urinary mercury and arsenic excretion. Although several chelating agents have the capacity to mobilize cadmium, their tendency to redistribute cadmium to the kidney and increase nephrotoxicity has negated their therapeutic value in cadmium intoxication.

In most cases, the capacity of chelating agents to prevent or reduce the adverse effects of toxic metals appears to be greatest when they are administered very soon after an acute metal exposure. Use of chelating agents days to weeks after an acute metal exposure ends—or their use in the treatment of chronic metal intoxication—may still be associated with increased metal excretion. However, at that point, the capacity of such enhanced excretion to mitigate the pathologic effect of the metal exposure may be reduced.

The most important chelating agents currently in use in the USA are described below.

DIMERCAPROL (2,3-DIMERCAPTOPROPANOL, BAL)

Dimercaprol (Figure 58–2), an oily, colorless liquid with a strong mercaptan-like odor, was developed in Great Britain during World War II as a therapeutic antidote against poisoning by the arsenic-containing warfare agent lewisite. It thus became known as British anti-Lewisite, or BAL. Because aqueous solutions of dimercaprol are unstable and oxidize readily, it is dispensed in 10% solution in peanut oil and must be administered by intramuscular injection, which is often painful.

In animal models, dimercaprol prevents and reverses arsenic-induced inhibition of sulfhydryl-containing enzymes and, if given soon after exposure, may protect against the lethal effects of inorganic and organic arsenicals. Human data indicate that it can increase the rate of excretion of arsenic and lead and may offer therapeutic benefit in the treatment of acute intoxication by arsenic, lead, and mercury.

Indications & Toxicity

Dimercaprol is FDA-approved as single-agent treatment of acute poisoning by arsenic and inorganic mercury and for the treatment of severe lead poisoning when used in conjunction with edetate calcium disodium (EDTA; see below). Although studies of its metabolism in humans are limited, intramuscularly administered dimercaprol appears to be readily absorbed, metabolized, and excreted by the kidney within 4–8 hours. Animal models indicate that it may also undergo biliary excretion, but the role of this excretory route in humans and other details of its biotransformation are uncertain.

When used in therapeutic doses, dimercaprol is associated with a high incidence of adverse effects, including

Ferroxamine

Dimercaprol   **Succimer**   **Penicillamine**
(2, 3-dimercaptopropanol)   (DMSA)

Figure 58–2. Chemical structures of several chelators. Ferroxamine (ferrioxamine) without the chelated iron is deferoxamine. It is represented here to show the functional groups; the iron is actually held in a caged system. The structures of the in vivo metal-chelator complexes for dimercaprol, succimer, penicillamine, and unithiol (see text), are not known and may involve the formation of mixed disulfides with amino acids. (Modified and reproduced, with permission, from Meyers FH, Jawetz E, Goldfien A: *Review of Medical Pharmacology*, 7th ed. McGraw-Hill, 1980.)

hypertension, tachycardia, nausea, vomiting, lacrimation, salivation, fever (particularly in children), and pain at the injection site. Its use has also been associated with thrombocytopenia and increased prothrombin time—factors that may limit intramuscular injection because of the risk of hematoma formation at the injection site. Despite its protective effects in acutely intoxicated animals, dimercaprol may redistribute arsenic and mercury to the central nervous system, and it is not advocated for treatment of chronic poisoning. Water-soluble analogs of dimercaprol—unithiol and succimer—have higher therapeutic indices and have replaced dimercaprol in many settings.

SUCCIMER (DIMERCAPTOSUCCINIC ACID, DMSA)

Succimer is a water-soluble analog of dimercaprol, and like that agent it has been shown in animal studies to prevent and reverse metal-induced inhibition of sulfhydryl-containing enzymes and to protect against the acute lethal effects of arsenic. In humans, treatment with succimer is associated with an increase in urinary lead excretion and a decrease in blood lead concentration. It may also decrease the mercury content of the kidney, a key target organ of inorganic mercury salts. In the USA, succimer is formulated exclusively for oral use, but intravenous formulations have been used successfully elsewhere. It is absorbed rapidly but somewhat variably after oral administration. Peak blood levels occur at approximately 3 hours. The drug binds in vivo to the amino acid cysteine to form 1:1 and 1:2 mixed disulfides, possibly in the kidney, and it may be these complexes that are the active chelating moieties. The elimination half-time of transformed succimer is approximately 2–4 hours.

Indications & Toxicity

Succimer is currently FDA-approved for the treatment of children with blood lead concentrations greater than 45 mcg/dL, but it is also commonly used in adults. The usual dosage is 10 mg/kg orally three times a day. Oral administration of succimer is comparable to parenteral EDTA in reducing blood lead concentration and has supplanted EDTA in outpatient treatment of patients capable of absorbing the oral drug. However, despite the demonstrated capacity of both succimer and EDTA to enhance lead elimination, their value in reversing established lead toxicity or in otherwise improving therapeutic outcome has yet to be established by a placebo-controlled clinical trial. Based on its protective effects against arsenic in animals and its ability to mobilize mercury from the kidney, succimer has also been used in the treatment of arsenic and mercury poisoning. Succimer has been well tolerated in limited clinical trials. It has a negligible impact on body stores of calcium, iron, and magnesium. It induces a mild increase in urinary excretion of zinc that is of minor or no clinical significance. Gastrointestinal disturbances, including anorexia, nausea, vomiting, and diarrhea, are the most common side effects, occurring in less than 10% of patients. Rashes, sometimes requiring discontinuation of the medication, have been reported in less than 5% of patients. Mild, reversible increases in liver aminotransferases have been noted in 6–10% of patients, and isolated cases of mild to moderate neutropenia have been reported.

EDETATE CALCIUM DISODIUM (ETHYLENEDIAMINETETRAACETIC ACID [EDTA])

Ethylenediaminetetraacetic acid (Figure 58–1) is an efficient chelator of many divalent and trivalent metals in vitro. To prevent potentially life-threatening depletion of calcium, the drug should only be administered as the calcium disodium salt.

EDTA penetrates cell membranes relatively poorly and therefore chelates extracellular metal ions much more effectively than intracellular ions.

The highly polar ionic character of EDTA limits its oral absorption. Moreover, oral administration may increase lead absorption from the gut. Consequently, EDTA should be administered by intravenous infusion. In patients with normal renal function, EDTA is rapidly excreted by glomerular filtration, with 50% of an injected dose appearing in the urine within 1 hour. EDTA mobilizes lead from soft tissues, causing a marked increase in urinary lead excretion and a corresponding decline in blood lead concentration. In patients with renal insufficiency, excretion of the drug—and its metal-mobilizing effects—may be delayed.

Indications & Toxicity

Edetate calcium disodium is indicated chiefly for the chelation of lead, but it may also have utility in poisoning by zinc, manganese, and certain heavy radionuclides. In spite of repeated claims in the alternative medicine literature, EDTA has no demonstrated utility in the treatment of atherosclerotic cardiovascular disease.

Because the drug and the mobilized metals are excreted via the urine, the drug is relatively contraindicated in anuric patients. In such instances, the use of low doses of EDTA in combination with hemodialysis or hemofiltration has been described. Nephrotoxicity from EDTA has been reported, but in most cases this can be prevented by maintenance of adequate urine flow, avoidance of excessive doses, and limitation of a treatment course to 5 or fewer consecutive days. EDTA may result in temporary zinc depletion that is of uncertain clinical significance. Analogs of EDTA, the calcium and zinc disodium salts of diethylenetriaminepentaacetic acid (DTPA), pentetate, have been used for removal ("decorporation") of uranium and certain transuranic radioisotopes, and in 2004 were approved by the FDA for treatment of contamination with plutonium, americium, and curium.

UNITHIOL (DIMERCAPTOPROPANESULFONIC ACID, DMPS)

Unithiol, a dimercapto chelating agent that is a water-soluble analog of dimercaprol, has been available in the official formularies of Russia and other former Soviet countries since 1958 and in Germany since 1976. It has been legally available from compounding pharmacists in the USA since 1999. Unithiol can be administered orally and intravenously. Bioavailability by the oral route is approximately 50%, with peak blood levels occurring in approximately 3.7 hours. Over 80% of an intravenous dose is excreted in the urine, mainly as cyclic DMPS sulfides. The elimination half-time for total unithiol (parent drug and its transformation products) is approximately 20 hours. Unithiol exhibits protective effects against the toxic action of mercury and arsenic in animal models, and it increases the excretion of mercury, arsenic, and lead in humans.

$$\begin{array}{ccc} SH & SH & SO_2H \\ | & | & | \\ CH_2 & - CH - & CH_2 \end{array}$$

Unithiol

Indications & Toxicity

Unithiol has no FDA-approved indications, but experimental studies and its pharmacologic and pharmacodynamic profile suggest that intravenous unithiol offers advantages over intramuscular dimercaprol or oral succimer in the initial treatment of severe acute poisoning by inorganic mercury or arsenic. Aqueous preparations of unithiol (usually 50 mg/mL in sterile water) can be administered at a dose of 3–5 mg/kg every 4 hours by slow intravenous infusion over 20 minutes. If a few days of treatment are accompanied by stabilization of the patient's cardiovascular and gastrointestinal status, it may be possible to change to oral administration at a dose of 4–8 mg/kg every 6–8 hours. Oral unithiol may also be considered as an alternative to oral succimer in the treatment of lead intoxication.

Unithiol has been reported to have a low overall incidence of adverse effects (< 4%). Self-limited dermatologic reactions (drug exanthems or urticaria) are the most commonly reported adverse effects, although isolated cases of major allergic reactions, including erythema multiforme and Stevens-Johnson syndrome, have been reported. Because rapid intravenous infusion may cause vasodilation and hypotension, unithiol should be infused slowly over an interval of 15–20 minutes.

PENICILLAMINE (D-DIMETHYLCYSTEINE)

Penicillamine (Figure 58–2) is a white crystalline, water-soluble derivative of penicillin. D-Penicillamine is less toxic than the L isomer and consequently is the preferred therapeutic form. Penicillamine is readily absorbed from the gut and is resistant to metabolic degradation.

Indications & Toxicity

Penicillamine is used chiefly for treatment of poisoning with copper or to prevent copper accumulation, as in Wilson's disease (hepatolenticular degeneration). It is also used occasionally in the treatment of severe rheumatoid arthritis (see Chapter 36). Its ability to increase urinary excretion of lead and mercury had occasioned its use as outpatient treatment for intoxication with these metals, but succimer, with its stronger metal-mobilizing capacity and lower side effect profile, has generally replaced penicillamine for these purposes.

Adverse effects have been seen in up to one third of patients receiving penicillamine. Hypersensitivity reactions include rash, pruritus, and drug fever, and the drug should be used with extreme caution, if at all, in patients with a history of penicillin allergy. Nephrotoxicity with proteinuria has also been reported, and protracted use of the drug may result in renal insufficiency. Pancytopenia has been associated with prolonged drug intake. Pyridoxine deficiency is a frequent toxic effect of other forms of the drug but is rarely seen with the D form. An acetylated derivative, *N*-acetylpenicillamine, has been used experimentally in mercury poisoning and may have superior metal-mobilizing capacity, but it is not commercially available.

DEFEROXAMINE

Deferoxamine is isolated from *Streptomyces pilosus*. It binds iron avidly but essential trace metals poorly. Furthermore, while competing for loosely bound iron in iron-carrying proteins (hemosiderin and ferritin), it fails to compete for biologically chelated iron, as in microsomal and mitochondrial cytochromes and hemoproteins. Consequently, it is the parenteral chelator of choice for iron poisoning (see Chapters 33 and 59). Deferoxamine plus hemodialysis may also be useful in the treatment of aluminum toxicity in renal failure. Deferoxamine is poorly absorbed when administered orally and may increase iron absorption when given by this route. It should therefore be administered intramuscularly or, preferably, intravenously. It is believed to be metabolized, but the pathways are unknown. The iron-chelator complex is excreted in the urine, often turning the urine an orange-red color.

Rapid intravenous administration may result in hypotension. Adverse idiosyncratic responses such as flushing, abdominal discomfort, and rash have also been observed. Pulmonary complications (eg, acute respiratory distress syndrome) have been reported in some patients undergoing deferoxamine infusions lasting longer than 24 hours, and neurotoxicity and increased susceptibility to certain infections (eg, with *Yersinia enterocolitica*) have been described after long-term therapy of iron overload conditions (eg, thalassemia major).

DEFERASIROX

Deferasirox is a tridentate chelator with a high affinity for iron and low affinity for other metals, eg, zinc and copper. It is orally active and well absorbed. In the circulation it binds iron, and the complex is excreted in the bile. Deferasirox was recently approved for the oral treatment of iron overload caused by blood transfusions, a problem in the treatment of thalassemia and myelodysplastic syndrome.

PRUSSIAN BLUE (FERRIC HEXACYANOFERRATE)

Ferric hexacyanoferrate (insoluble Prussian blue) is a hydrated crystalline compound in which Fe^{II} and Fe^{III} atoms are coordinated with cyanide groups in a cubic lattice structure. Although used as a dark blue commercial pigment for nearly 300 years, it was only 3 decades ago that its potential utility as a pharmaceutical chelator was recognized. Primarily by ion-exchange, and secondarily by mechanical trapping or adsorption, the compound has high affinity for certain univalent cations, particularly cesium and thallium. Used as an oral drug, insoluble Prussian blue undergoes minimal gastrointestinal absorption (< 1%). Because the complexes it forms with cesium or thallium are nonabsorbable, oral administration of the chelator diminishes intestinal absorption or interrupts enterohepatic and enteroenteric circulation of these cations, thereby accelerating their elimination in the feces. In clinical case series, the use of Prussian blue has been associated with a decline in the biologic half-life (ie, in vivo retention) of radioactive cesium and thallium.

Indications & Toxicity

In 2003, the FDA approved Prussian blue for the treatment of contamination with radioactive cesium (^{137}Cs), and for intoxication with thallium salts. Approval was prompted by concern over potential widespread human contamination with radioactive cesium caused by terrorist use of a radioactive dispersal device ("dirty bomb"). The drug is part of the Strategic National Stockpile of pharmaceuticals and medical material maintained by the CDC (http://www.bt.cdc.gov/stockpile/#material) (***Note:*** Although soluble forms of Prussian blue, such as potassium ferric hexacyanoferrate, may have better utility in thallium poisoning, only the insoluble form is currently available as a pharmaceutical.)

Following exposure to ^{137}Cs or thallium salts, the approved adult dosage is 3 g orally three times a day; the corresponding pediatric dosage (2–12 years of age) is 1 g orally three times a day. Serial monitoring of urine and fecal radioactivity (^{137}Cs) and urinary thallium concentrations can guide the recommended duration of therapy. Adjunctive supportive care for possible acute radiation illness (^{137}Cs) or systemic thallium toxicity should be instituted as needed.

Prussian blue has not been associated with significant adverse effects. Constipation, which may occur in some cases, should be treated with laxatives or increased dietary fiber.

PREPARATIONS AVAILABLE

Deferasirox (Exjade)
  Oral: 125, 250, 500 mg tablets
Deferoxamine (Desferal)
  Parenteral: Powder to reconstitute, 500 mg/vial
Dimercaprol (BAL in Oil)
  Parenteral: 100 mg/mL for IM injection
Edetate calcium [calcium EDTA] (Calcium Disodium Versenate)
  Parenteral: 200 mg/mL for injection
Penicillamine (Cuprimine, Depen)
  Oral: 125, 250 mg capsules; 250 mg tablets

Pentetate Calcium Trisodium ([calcium DTPA] and Pentetate Zinc Trisodium [zinc DTPA])
  Parenteral: 200 mg/mL for injection
Prussian Blue (Radiogardase)
  Oral: 500 mg capsules
Succimer (Chemet)
  Oral: 100 mg capsules
Unithiol (Dimaval)
  Bulk powder available for compounding as oral capsules, or for infusion (50 mg/mL)

REFERENCES

Lead

Borja-Aburto VH et al: Blood lead levels measured prospectively and risk of spontaneous abortion. Am J Epidemiol 1999;150:590.

Canfield RL et al: Intellectual impairment in children with blood lead concentrations below 10 μg per deciliter. N Engl J Med 2003;348:1517.

Cheng Y et al: Bone lead and blood lead levels in relation to baseline blood pressure and the prospective development of hypertension. Am J Epidemiol 2001;153:164.

Nash D et al: Blood lead, blood pressure, and hypertension in perimenopausal and postmenopausal women. JAMA 2003;289:1523.

Rogan WJ et al: The effect of chelation therapy with succimer on neuropsychological development in children exposed to lead. N Engl J Med 2001;344:1421.

Third National Report on Human Exposure to Environmental Chemicals. Lead. CDC, 2005. [http://www.cdc.gov/exposurereport/3rd/pdf/results_01.html]

Weisskopf MG et al: Cumulative lead exposure and prospective change in cognition among elderly men. Am J Epidemiol 2004;160:1184.

Arsenic

National Research Council. *Arsenic in Drinking Water: 2001 Update*. National Academy Press, 2001. [http://search.nap.edu/books/0309076293/html/]

Petrick JS et al: Monomethylarsonous acid (MMA[III]) and arsenite: LD50 in hamsters and in vitro inhibition of pyruvate dehydrogenase. Chem Res Toxicol 2001;14:651.

Unnikrishnan D et al: Torsades de pointes in 3 patients with leukemia treated with arsenic trioxide. Blood 2001;97:1514.

von Ehrenstein OS et al: Decrements in lung function related to arsenic in drinking water in West Bengal, India. Am J Epidemiol 2005;162:533.

Mercury

Clarkson TW: The three modern faces of mercury. Environ Health Perspect 2002;110(Suppl 1):11.

EPA web site: [http://www.epa.gov/waterscience/fishadvice/advice.html]

LSRO [Life Sciences Research Office]. *Review and Analysis of the Literature on the Potential Adverse Health Effects of Dental Amalgam*. LSRO: Bethesda, 2004. [http://www.lsro.org/amalgam/frames_amalgam_report.html]

Nierenberg DW et al: Delayed cerebellar disease and death after accidental exposure to dimethylmercury. N Engl J Med 1998; 338:1672.

Rice DC et al: Methods and rationale for derivation of a reference dose for methylmercury by the U.S. EPA. Risk Anal 2003; 23:107.

Third National Report on Human Exposure to Environmental Chemicals. Mercury. CDC, 2005. [http://www.cdc.gov/exposurereport/3rd/pdf/results_01.html]

Chelating Agents

Cremin JD et al: Oral succimer decreases the gastrointestinal absorption of lead in juvenile monkeys. Environ Health Perspect 2001;109:613.

Dargan PI et al: Case report: Severe mercuric sulphate poisoning treated with 2,3-dimercaptopropane-1-sulphonate and haemodiafiltration. Crit Care 2003;7:R1.

Gong Z et al: Determination of arsenic metabolic complex excreted in human urine after administration of sodium 2,3-dimercapto-1-propane sulfonate. Chem Res Toxicol 2002; 15:1318.

Thompson DF, Called ED: Soluble or insoluble prussian blue for radiocesium and thallium poisoning? Ann Pharmacother 2004;38:1509.

Yokel RA et al: Entry, half-life, and desferrioxamine-accelerated clearance of brain aluminum after a single 26Al exposure. Toxicol Sci 2001;64:77.

Management of the Poisoned Patient

Kent R. Olson, MD

Over a million cases of acute poisoning occur in the USA each year, although only a small fraction are fatal. Most deaths are due to intentional suicidal overdose by an adolescent or adult. Childhood deaths due to accidental ingestion of a drug or toxic household product have been markedly reduced in the past 30 years as a result of safety packaging and effective poisoning prevention education.

Even with a serious exposure, poisoning is rarely fatal if the victim receives prompt medical attention and good supportive care. Careful management of respiratory failure, hypotension, seizures, and thermoregulatory disturbances has resulted in improved survival of patients who reach the hospital alive.

This chapter reviews the basic principles of poisoning, initial management, and specialized treatment of poisoning, including methods of increasing the elimination of drugs and toxins.

■ TOXICOKINETICS & TOXICODYNAMICS

The term **toxicokinetics** denotes the absorption, distribution, excretion, and metabolism of toxins, toxic doses of therapeutic agents, and their metabolites. The term **toxicodynamics** is used to denote the injurious effects of these substances on vital function. Although there are many similarities between the pharmacokinetics and toxicokinetics of most substances, there are also important differences. The same caution applies to pharmacodynamics and toxicodynamics.

SPECIAL ASPECTS OF TOXICOKINETICS

Volume of Distribution

The volume of distribution (V_d) is defined as the apparent volume into which a substance is distributed (see Chapter 3). A large V_d implies that the drug is not readily accessible to measures aimed at purifying the

blood, such as hemodialysis. Examples of drugs with large volumes of distribution (> 5 L/kg) include antidepressants, antipsychotics, antimalarials, narcotics, propranolol, and verapamil. Drugs with relatively small volumes of distribution (< 1 L/kg) include salicylate, ethanol, phenobarbital, lithium, valproic acid, and phenytoin (see Table 3–1).

Clearance

Clearance is a measure of the volume of plasma that is cleared of drug per unit time (see Chapter 3). For most drugs the total clearance is the sum of clearances via excretion by the kidneys and metabolism by the liver. In planning detoxification strategy, it is important to know the contribution of each organ to total clearance. For example, if a drug is 95% cleared by liver metabolism and only 5% cleared by renal excretion, even a dramatic increase in urinary concentration of the poison will have little effect on overall elimination.

Overdosage of a drug can alter the usual pharmacokinetic processes, and this must be considered when applying kinetics to poisoned patients. For example, dissolution of tablets or gastric emptying time may be slowed so that absorption and peak toxic effects are delayed. Drugs may injure the epithelial barrier of the gastrointestinal tract and thereby increase absorption. If the capacity of the liver to metabolize a drug is exceeded, more drug will be delivered to the circulation. With a dramatic increase in the concentration of drug in the blood, protein-binding capacity may be exceeded, resulting in an increased fraction of free drug and greater toxic effect. At normal dosage, most drugs are eliminated at a rate proportionate to the plasma concentration (first-order kinetics). If the plasma concentration is very high and normal metabolism is saturated, the rate of elimination may become fixed (zero-order kinetics). This change in kinetics may markedly prolong the apparent serum half-life and increase toxicity.

SPECIAL ASPECTS OF TOXICODYNAMICS

The general dose-response principles described in Chapter 2 are relevant when estimating the potential severity of an intoxication. When considering quantal dose-response data, both the therapeutic index and the over-lap of therapeutic and toxic response curves must be considered. For instance, two drugs may have the same therapeutic index but unequal safe dosing ranges if the slopes of their dose-response curves are not the same. For some drugs, eg, sedative-hypnotics, the major toxic effect is a direct extension of the therapeutic action, as shown by their graded dose-response curve (see Figure 22–1). In the case of a drug with a linear dose-response curve (drug A), lethal effects may occur at ten times the normal therapeutic dose. In contrast, a drug with a curve that reaches a plateau (drug B) may not be lethal at 100 times the normal dose.

For many drugs, at least part of the toxic effect may be quite different from the therapeutic action. For example, intoxication with drugs that have atropine-like effects (eg, tricyclic antidepressants) will reduce sweating, making it more difficult to dissipate heat. In tricyclic antidepressant intoxication, there may also be increased muscular activity or seizures; the body's production of heat is thus enhanced, and lethal hyperpy-rexia may result. Overdoses of drugs that depress the cardiovascular system, eg, β blockers or calcium chan-nel blockers, can profoundly alter not only cardiac function but all functions that are dependent on blood flow. These include renal and hepatic elimination of the toxin and any other drugs that may be given.

■ APPROACH TO THE POISONED PATIENT

HOW DOES THE POISONED PATIENT DIE?

An understanding of common mechanisms of death due to poisoning can help prepare the physician to treat patients effectively. Many toxins depress the central nervous system (CNS), resulting in obtundation or coma. Comatose patients frequently lose their airway protective reflexes and their respiratory drive. Thus, they may die as a result of airway obstruction by the flaccid tongue, aspiration of gastric contents into the tracheobronchial tree, or respiratory arrest. These are the most common causes of death due to overdoses of narcotics and sedative-hypnotic drugs (eg, barbiturates and alcohol).

Cardiovascular toxicity is also frequently encountered in poisoning. Hypotension may be due to depression of cardiac contractility; hypovolemia resulting from vomit-ing, diarrhea, or fluid sequestration; peripheral vascular collapse due to blockade of α-adrenoceptor-mediated

vascular tone; or cardiac arrhythmias. Hypothermia or hyperthermia due to exposure as well as the temperature-dysregulating effects of many drugs can also produce hypotension. Lethal arrhythmias such as ventricular tachy-cardia and fibrillation can occur with overdoses of many cardioactive drugs such as ephedrine, amphetamines, cocaine, digitalis, and theophylline; and drugs not usually considered cardioactive, such as tricyclic antidepressants, antihistamines, and some opioid analogs.

Cellular hypoxia may occur in spite of adequate ven-tilation and oxygen administration when poisoning is due to cyanide, hydrogen sulfide, carbon monoxide, and other poisons that interfere with transport or utili-zation of oxygen. In such patients, cellular hypoxia is evident by the development of tachycardia, hypoten-sion, severe lactic acidosis, and signs of ischemia on the electrocardiogram.

Seizures, muscular hyperactivity, and rigidity may result in death. Seizures may cause pulmonary aspira-tion, hypoxia, and brain damage. Hyperthermia may result from sustained muscular hyperactivity and can lead to muscle breakdown and myoglobinuria, renal failure, lactic acidosis, and hyperkalemia. Drugs and poisons that often cause seizures include antidepres-sants, isoniazid (INH), diphenhydramine, cocaine, and amphetamines.

Other organ system damage may occur after poison-ing and is sometimes delayed in onset. Paraquat attacks lung tissue, resulting in pulmonary fibrosis, beginning several days after ingestion. Massive hepatic necrosis due to poisoning by acetaminophen or certain mush-rooms results in hepatic encephalopathy and death 48–72 hours or longer after ingestion.

Finally, some patients may die before hospitalization because the behavioral effects of the ingested drug may result in traumatic injury. Intoxication with alcohol and other sedative-hypnotic drugs is a frequent contributing factor to motor vehicle accidents. Patients under the influence of hallucinogens such as phencyclidine (PCP) or LSD may die in fights or falls from high places.

■ INITIAL MANAGEMENT OF THE POISONED PATIENT

The initial management of a patient with coma, sei-zures, or otherwise altered mental status should follow the same approach regardless of the poison involved. Attempting to make a specific toxicologic diagnosis only delays the application of supportive measures that form the basis (**"ABCDs"**) of poisoning treatment.

First, the **airway** should be cleared of vomitus or any other obstruction and an oral airway or endotracheal tube inserted if needed. For many patients, simple positioning in the lateral decubitus position is sufficient to move the flaccid tongue out of the airway. **Breathing** should be assessed by observation and oximetry and, if in doubt, by measuring arterial blood gases. Patients with respiratory insufficiency should be intubated and mechanically ventilated. The **circulation** should be assessed by continuous monitoring of pulse rate, blood pressure, urinary output, and evaluation of peripheral perfusion. An intravenous line should be placed and blood drawn for serum glucose and other routine determinations.

At this point, every patient with altered mental status should receive a challenge with concentrated **dextrose,** unless a rapid bedside blood glucose test demonstrates that the patient is not hypoglycemic. Adults are given 25 g (50 mL of 50% dextrose solution) intravenously, children 0.5 g/kg (2 mL/kg of 25% dextrose). Hypoglycemic patients may appear to be intoxicated, and there is no rapid and reliable way to distinguish them from poisoned patients. Alcoholic or malnourished patients should also receive 100 mg of thiamine intramuscularly or in the intravenous infusion solution at this time to prevent Wernicke's syndrome.

The opioid antagonist naloxone may be given in a dose of 0.4–2 mg intravenously. Naloxone will reverse respiratory and CNS depression due to all varieties of opioid drugs (see Chapter 31). It is useful to remember that these drugs cause death primarily by respiratory depression; therefore, if airway and breathing assistance have already been instituted, naloxone may not be necessary. Larger doses of naloxone may be needed for patients with overdose involving propoxyphene, codeine, and some other opioids. The benzodiazepine antagonist flumazenil (see Chapter 22) may be of value in patients with suspected benzodiazepine overdose, but it should not be used if there is a history of tricyclic antidepressant overdose or a seizure disorder, as it can induce convulsions in such patients.

History & Physical Examination

Once the essential initial ABCD interventions have been instituted, one can begin a more detailed evaluation to make a specific diagnosis. This includes gathering any available history and performing a toxicologically oriented physical examination. Other causes of coma or seizures such as head trauma, meningitis, or metabolic abnormalities should be looked for and treated. Some common toxic syndromes are described beginning on page 965.

A. HISTORY

Oral statements about the amount and even the type of drug ingested in toxic emergencies may be unreliable. Even so, family members, police, and fire department or paramedical personnel should be asked to describe the environment in which the toxic emergency occurred and should bring to the emergency department any syringes, empty bottles, household products, or over-the-counter medications in the immediate vicinity of the possibly poisoned patient.

B. PHYSICAL EXAMINATION

A brief examination should be performed, emphasizing those areas most likely to give clues to the toxicologic diagnosis. These include vital signs, eyes and mouth, skin, abdomen, and nervous system.

1. Vital signs—Careful evaluation of vital signs (blood pressure, pulse, respirations, and temperature) is essential in all toxicologic emergencies. Hypertension and tachycardia are typical with amphetamines, cocaine, and antimuscarinic (anticholinergic) drugs. Hypotension and bardycardia are characteristic features of overdose with calcium channel blockers, β blockers, clonidine, and sedative hypnotics. Hypotension with tachycardia is common with tricyclic antidepressants, trazodone, quetiapine, vasodilators, and β agonists. Rapid respirations are typical of salicylates, carbon monoxide, and other toxins that produce metabolic acidosis or cellular asphyxia. Hyperthermia may be associated with sympathomimetics, anticholinergics, salicylates, and drugs producing seizures or muscular rigidity. Hypothermia can be caused by any CNS-depressant drug, especially when accompanied by exposure to a cold environment.

2. Eyes—The eyes are a valuable source of toxicologic information. Constriction of the pupils (miosis) is typical of opioids, clonidine, phenothiazines, and cholinesterase inhibitors (eg, organophosphate insecticides), and deep coma due to sedative drugs. Dilation of the pupils (mydriasis) is common with amphetamines, cocaine, LSD, and atropine and other anticholinergic drugs. Horizontal nystagmus is characteristic of intoxication with phenytoin, alcohol, barbiturates, and other sedative drugs. The presence of both vertical and horizontal nystagmus is strongly suggestive of phencyclidine poisoning. Ptosis and ophthalmoplegia are characteristic features of botulism.

3. Mouth—The mouth may show signs of burns due to corrosive substances, or soot from smoke inhalation. Typical odors of alcohol, hydrocarbon solvents, or ammonia may be noted. Poisoning due to cyanide can be recognized by some examiners as an odor like bitter almonds.

4. Skin—The skin often appears flushed, hot, and dry in poisoning with atropine and other antimuscarinics. Excessive sweating occurs with organophosphates, nicotine, and sympathomimetic drugs. Cyanosis may be caused by hypoxemia or by methemoglobinemia. Icterus may suggest hepatic necrosis due to acetaminophen or *Amanita phalloides* mushroom poisoning.

5. Abdomen—Abdominal examination may reveal ileus, which is typical of poisoning with antimuscarinic, opioid, and sedative drugs. Hyperactive bowel sounds, abdominal cramping, and diarrhea are common in poisoning with organophosphates, iron, arsenic, theophylline, *A phalloides,* and *A muscaria.*

6. Nervous system—A careful neurologic examination is essential. Focal seizures or motor deficits suggest a structural lesion (such as intracranial hemorrhage due to trauma) rather than toxic or metabolic encephalopathy. Nystagmus, dysarthria, and ataxia are typical of phenytoin, carbamazepine, alcohol, and other sedative intoxication. Twitching and muscular hyperactivity are common with atropine and other anticholinergic agents, and cocaine and other sympathomimetic drugs. Muscular rigidity can be caused by haloperidol and other antipsychotic agents, serotonin syndrome, and by strychnine. Seizures are often caused by overdose with antidepressants (especially tricyclic antidepressants and bupropion), cocaine, amphetamines, theophylline, isoniazid, and diphenhydramine. Flaccid coma with absent reflexes and even an isoelectric electroencephalogram may be seen with deep coma due to sedative-hypnotic or other CNS depressant intoxication and may be mistaken for brain death.

Laboratory & Imaging Procedures

A. ARTERIAL BLOOD GASES

Hypoventilation will result in an elevated PCO_2 (hypercapnia) and a low PO_2 (hypoxia). The PO_2 may also be low with aspiration pneumonia or drug-induced pulmonary edema. Poor tissue oxygenation due to hypoxia, hypotension, or cyanide poisoning will result in metabolic acidosis. The PO_2 measures only oxygen dissolved in the plasma and not total blood oxygen content or oxyhemoglobin saturation, and may appear normal in patients with severe carbon monoxide poisoning. Pulse oximetry may also give falsely normal results in carbon monoxide intoxication.

B. ELECTROLYTES

Sodium, potassium, chloride, and bicarbonate should be measured. The anion gap is then calculated by subtracting the measured anions from cations:

$$\text{Anion gap} = (Na^+ + K^+) - (HCO_3^- + Cl^-)$$

Normally the sum of the cations exceeds the sum of the anions by no more than 12–16 mEq/L. A larger-than-expected anion gap is caused by the presence of unmeasured anions (lactate, etc) accompanying metabolic acidosis. This may occur with numerous conditions, such as diabetic ketoacidosis, renal failure, or shock-induced lactic acidosis. Drugs that may induce an elevated anion gap metabolic acidosis (Table 59–1) include aspirin, metformin, methanol, ethylene glycol, isoniazid, and iron.

Alterations in the serum potassium level are hazardous because they can result in cardiac arrhythmias. Drugs

Table 59–1. Examples of drug-induced anion gap acidosis.

Type of Elevation of the Anion Gap	Agents
Organic acid metabolites	Methanol, ethylene glycol, diethylene glycol
Lactic acidosis	Cyanide, carbon monoxide, ibuprofen, isoniazid, metformin, salicylates, valproic acid; any drug-induced seizures, hypoxia, or hypotension

Note: The normal anion gap calculated from $(Na^+ + K^+) - (HCO_3^- + Cl^-)$ is 12–16 mEq/L; calculated from $(Na^+) - (HCO_3^- + Cl^-)$, it is 8–12 mEq/L.

that may cause hyperkalemia despite normal renal function include potassium itself, β blockers, digitalis glycosides, potassium-sparing diuretics, and fluoride. Drugs associated with hypokalemia include barium, β agonists, caffeine, theophylline, and thiazide and loop diuretics.

C. RENAL FUNCTION TESTS

Some toxins have direct nephrotoxic effects; in other cases, renal failure is due to shock or myoglobinuria. Blood urea nitrogen and creatinine levels should be measured and urinalysis performed. Elevated serum creatine kinase (CK) and myoglobin in the urine suggest muscle necrosis due to seizures or muscular rigidity. Oxalate crystals in the urine suggest ethylene glycol poisoning.

D. SERUM OSMOLALITY

The calculated serum osmolality is dependent mainly on the serum sodium and glucose and the blood urea nitrogen and can be estimated from the following formula:

$$2 \times Na^+(meq/L) + \frac{\text{Glucose (mg/dL)}}{18} + \frac{\text{BUN (mg/dL)}}{3}$$

This calculated value is normally 280–290 mOsm/L. Ethanol and other alcohols may contribute significantly to the measured serum osmolality but, since they are not included in the calculation, cause an osmolar gap:

$$\frac{\text{Osmolar}}{\text{gap}} = \frac{\text{Measured}}{\text{osmolality}} - \frac{\text{Calculated}}{\text{osmolality}}$$

Table 59–2 lists the concentration and expected contribution to the serum osmolality in ethanol, methanol, ethylene glycol, and isopropanol poisonings.

E. ELECTROCARDIOGRAM

Widening of the QRS complex duration to greater than 100 milliseconds is typical of tricyclic antidepressant and

Table 59–2. Some substances that cause an osmolar gap.

Substance[1]	Serum Level (mg/dL)	Corresponding Osmolar Gap (mOsm/kg)
Ethanol	350	75
Methanol	80	25
Ethylene glycol	200	35
Isopropanol	350	60

[1]Other substances that can increase the osmolar gap include acetone, mannitol, and magnesium.
Note: Most laboratories use the freezing point method of determining osmolality. However, if the vaporization point method is used, the alcohols may be driven off and their contribution to osmolality will be lost.

quinidine overdoses (Figure 59–1). The QT_c interval may be prolonged to more than 440 milliseconds in many poisonings, including quinidine, tricyclic antidepressants, several newer antidepressants and antipsychotics, lithium, and arsenic (see also http://www.torsades.org/). Variable atrioventricular (AV) block and a variety of atrial and ventricular arrhythmias are common with poisoning by digoxin and other cardiac glycosides. Hypoxemia due to carbon monoxide poisoning may result in ischemic changes on the electrocardiogram.

F. Imaging Findings

A plain film of the abdomen may be useful because some tablets, particularly iron and potassium, may be radiopaque. Chest radiographs may reveal aspiration pneumonia, hydrocarbon pneumonia, or pulmonary edema. When head trauma is suspected, a computed tomography (CT) scan is recommended.

Toxicology Screening Tests

It is a common misconception that a broad toxicology "screen" is the best way to diagnose and manage an acute poisoning. In fact, comprehensive toxicology screening is time-consuming, expensive, and often unreliable. Results of tests may not be available for days. Moreover, many highly toxic drugs such as calcium channel blockers, β blockers, and isoniazid are not included in the screening process. The clinical examination of the patient and selected routine laboratory tests are usually sufficient to generate a tentative diagnosis and an appropriate treatment plan. While screening tests may be helpful in confirming a suspected intoxication or for ruling out intoxication as a cause of apparent brain death, they should not delay needed treatment.

When a specific antidote or other treatment is under consideration, quantitative laboratory testing may be indicated. For example, determination of the acetaminophen serum level is useful in assessing the need for antidotal therapy with acetylcysteine. Serum levels of theophylline, carbamazepine, lithium, salicylates, valproic acid, and other drugs may indicate the need for hemodialysis (Table 59–3).

Decontamination

Decontamination procedures should be undertaken simultaneously with initial stabilization, diagnostic assessment, and laboratory evaluation. Decontamination involves removing toxins from the skin or gastrointestinal tract.

A. Skin

Contaminated clothing should be completely removed and double-bagged to prevent illness in health care pro-

Figure 59–1. Changes in the electrocardiogram in tricyclic antidepressant overdosage. **A:** Slowed intraventricular conduction results in prolonged QRS interval (0.18 s; normal, 0.08 s). **B:** and **C:** Supraventricular tachycardia with progressive widening of QRS complexes mimics ventricular tachycardia. (Reproduced, with permission, from Benowitz NL, Goldschlager N: Cardiac disturbances in the toxicologic patient. In: Haddad LM, Winchester JF [editors]. *Clinical Management of Poisoning and Drug Overdose.* WB Saunders, 1983.)

Table 59–3. Hemodialysis in drug overdose and poisoning.[1]

Hemodialysis may be indicated depending on the severity of poisoning or the blood concentration:
Carbamazepine
Ethylene glycol
Lithium
Methanol
Metformin
Phenobarbital
Salicylate
Theophylline
Valproic acid
Hemodialysis is ineffective or is not useful:
Amphetamines
Antidepressants
Antipsychotic drugs
Benzodiazepines
Calcium channel blockers
Digoxin
Metoprolol and propanolol
Opioids
Many other drugs and poisons

[1]This listing is not comprehensive.

viders and for possible laboratory analysis. Wash contaminated skin with soap and water.

B. Gastrointestinal Tract

Controversy remains regarding the efficacy of gut emptying by emesis or gastric lavage, especially when treatment is initiated more than 1 hour after ingestion. For most ingestions, clinical toxicologists recommend simple administration of activated charcoal to bind ingested poisons in the gut before they can be absorbed. In unusual circumstances, induced emesis or gastric lavage may also be used.

1. Emesis—Emesis can be induced with ipecac *syrup* (never *extract* of ipecac), and this method is sometimes used to treat childhood ingestions at home under telephone supervision of a physician or poison control center personnel. Ipecac should not be used if the suspected intoxicant is a corrosive agent, a petroleum distillate, or a rapidly acting convulsant. Previously popular methods of inducing emesis such as fingertip stimulation of the pharynx, salt water, and apomorphine are ineffective or dangerous and should not be used.

2. Gastric lavage—If the patient is awake or if the airway is protected by an endotracheal tube, gastric lavage may be performed using an orogastric or nasogastric tube. As large a tube as possible should be used. Lavage solutions (usually 0.9% saline) should be at body temperature to prevent hypothermia.

3. Activated charcoal—Owing to its large surface area, activated charcoal can adsorb many drugs and poisons. It is most effective if given in a ratio of at least 10:1 of charcoal to estimated dose of toxin by weight. Charcoal does not bind iron, lithium, or potassium, and it binds alcohols and cyanide only poorly. It does not appear to be useful in poisoning due to corrosive mineral acids and alkali. Recent studies suggest that oral activated charcoal given alone may be just as effective as gut emptying followed by charcoal. Also, other studies have shown that repeated doses of oral activated charcoal may enhance systemic elimination of some drugs (including carbamazepine, dapsone, and theophylline) by a mechanism referred to as "gut dialysis."

4. Cathartics—Administration of a cathartic (laxative) agent may hasten removal of toxins from the gastrointestinal tract and reduce absorption, although no controlled studies have been done. Whole bowel irrigation with a balanced polyethylene glycol-electrolyte solution (GoLYTELY, CoLyte) can enhance gut decontamination after ingestion of iron tablets, enteric-coated medicines, illicit drug-filled packets, and foreign bodies. The solution is administered at 1–2 L/h (500 mL/h in children) for several hours until the rectal effluent is clear.

Specific Antidotes

There is a popular misconception that there is an antidote for every poison. Actually, selective antidotes are available for only a few classes of toxins. The major antidotes and their characteristics are listed in Table 59–4.

Methods of Enhancing Elimination of Toxins

After appropriate diagnostic and decontamination procedures and administration of antidotes, it is important to consider whether measures for enhancing elimination, such as hemodialysis or urinary alkalinization, can improve clinical outcome. Table 59–3 lists intoxications for which dialysis may be beneficial.

A. Dialysis Procedures

1. Peritoneal dialysis—This is a relatively simple and available technique but is inefficient in removing most drugs.

2. Hemodialysis—Hemodialysis is more efficient than peritoneal dialysis and has been well studied. It assists in correction of fluid and electrolyte imbalance and may also enhance removal of toxic metabolites (eg, formate in methanol poisoning, oxalate and glycolate in ethylene glycol poisoning). The efficiency of both peritoneal dialysis and hemodialysis is a function of the molecular weight, water solubility, protein binding, endogenous clearance, and distribution in the body of the specific

Table 59–4. Examples of specific antidotes.

Antidote	Poison(s)	Comments
Acetylcysteine (Acetadote, Mucomyst)	Acetaminophen	Best results if given within 8–10 hours of overdose. Follow liver function tests and acetaminophen blood levels. Acetabate is given intravenously; Mucomyst, orally.
Atropine	Anticholinesterases: organophosphates, carbamates	A test dose of 1–2 mg (for children, 0.05 mg/kg) is given IV and repeated until symptoms of atropinism appear (tachycardia, dilated pupils, ileus). Dose may be doubled every 10–15 minutes, with decrease of secretions as therapeutic end point.
Bicarbonate, sodium	Membrane-depressant cardiotoxic drugs (tricyclic antidepressants, quinidine, etc)	1–2 mEq/kg IV bolus usually reverses cardiotoxic effects (wide QRS, hypotension). Give cautiously in heart failure (avoid sodium overload).
Calcium	Fluoride; calcium channel blockers	Large doses may be needed in severe calcium channel blocker overdose. Start with 15 mg/kg IV.
Deferoxamine	Iron salts	If poisoning is severe, give 15 mg/kg/h IV. Urine may become pink. 100 mg of deferoxamine binds 8.5 mg of iron.
Digoxin antibodies	Digoxin and related cardiac glycosides	One vial binds 0.5 mg digoxin; indications include serious arrhythmias, hyperkalemia.
Esmolol	Theophylline, caffeine, metaproterenol	Short-acting β blocker reverses β_1-induced tachycardia and (possibly) β_2-induced vasodilation. Infuse 25–50 mcg/kg/min IV.
Ethanol	Methanol, ethylene glycol	Ethanol therapy can be started before laboratory diagnosis is confirmed. A loading dose is calculated so as to give a blood level of at least 100 mg/dL (42 g/70 kg in adults).
Flumazenil	Benzodiazepines	Adult dose is 0.2 mg IV, repeated as necessary to a maximum of 3 mg. *Do not give to patients with seizures, benzodiazepine dependence, or tricyclic overdose.*
Fomepizole	Methanol, ethylene glycol	More convenient and easier to use than ethanol. Loading dose 15 mg/kg; repeat every 12 hours.
Glucagon	β blockers	5–10 mg IV bolus may reverse hypotension and bradycardia that was resistant to β-agonist drugs. May cause vomiting.
Naloxone	Narcotic drugs, other opioid derivatives	A specific antagonist of opioids; 1–2 mg initially by IV, IM, or subcutaneous injection. Larger doses may be needed to reverse the effects of overdose with propoxyphene, codeine, or fentanyl derivatives. Duration of action (2–3 hours) may be significantly shorter than that of the opioid being antagonized.
Oxygen	Carbon monoxide	Give 100% by high-flow nonrebreathing mask; use of hyperbaric chamber is controversial.
Physostigmine	Suggested for antimuscarinic anticholinergic agents; not for tricyclic antidepressants	Adult dose is 0.5–1 mg IV slowly. The effects are transient (30–60 minutes), and the lowest effective dose may be repeated when symptoms return. May cause bradycardia, increased bronchial secretions, seizures. Have atropine ready to reverse excess effects. *Do not use for tricyclic antidepressant overdose.*
Pralidoxime (2-PAM)	Organophosphate cholinesterase inhibitors	Adult dose is 1 g IV, which should be repeated every 3–4 hours as needed or preferably as a constant infusion of 250–400 mg/h. Pediatric dose is approximately 250 mg. No proved benefit in carbamate poisoning.

toxin. Hemodialysis is especially useful in overdose cases in which the precipitating drug can be removed and fluid and electrolyte imbalances are present and can be corrected (eg, salicylate intoxication).

B. FORCED DIURESIS AND URINARY pH MANIPULATION

Previously popular but of unproved value, forced diuresis may cause volume overload and electrolyte abnormalities and is not recommended. Renal elimination of a few toxins can be enhanced by alteration of urinary pH. For example, urinary alkalinization is useful in cases of salicylate overdose. Acidification may increase the urine concentration of drugs such as phencyclidine and amphetamines but is not advised because it may worsen renal complications from rhabdomyolysis, which often accompanies the intoxication.

■ COMMON TOXIC SYNDROMES

ACETAMINOPHEN

Acetaminophen is one of the drugs most commonly involved in suicide attempts and accidental poisonings, both as the sole agent and in combination with other drugs. Acute ingestion of more than 150–200 mg/kg (children) or 7 g total (adults) is considered potentially toxic. A highly toxic metabolite is produced in the liver (see Figure 4–4).

Initially, the patient is asymptomatic or has mild gastrointestinal upset (nausea, vomiting). After 24–36 hours, evidence of liver injury appears, with elevated aminotransferase levels and hypoprothrombinemia. In severe cases, fulminant liver failure occurs, leading to hepatic encephalopathy and death. Renal failure may also occur.

The severity of poisoning is estimated from a serum acetaminophen concentration measurement. If the level is greater than 150–200 mg/L approximately 4 hours after ingestion, the patient is at risk for liver injury. (Chronic alcoholics or patients taking drugs that enhance P450 production of toxic metabolites are at risk with lower levels, perhaps as low as 100 mg/L at 4 hours.) The antidote acetylcysteine acts as a glutathione substitute, binding the toxic metabolite as it is being produced. It is most effective when given early and should be started within 8–10 hours if possible. A liver transplant may be required for patients with fulminant hepatic failure.

AMPHETAMINES & OTHER STIMULANTS

Stimulant drugs commonly abused in the USA include methamphetamine ("crank," "crystal"), methylene-dioxymethamphetamine (MDMA, "ecstasy"), and cocaine ("crack") as well as legal substances such as pseudoephedrine (Sudafed) and ephedrine (as such and in the herbal agent *Ma-huang*) (see Chapter 32). Caffeine is often added to dietary supplements sold as "metabolic enhancers" or "fat-burners" and is also sometimes combined with pseudoephedrine in underground pills sold as amphetamine substitutes.

At the doses usually used by stimulant abusers, euphoria and wakefulness are accompanied by a sense of power and well-being. At higher doses, restlessness, agitation, and acute psychosis may occur, accompanied by hypertension and tachycardia. Prolonged muscular hyperactivity can cause dehydration and eventually, hypotension. Seizures and muscle activity may contribute to hyperthermia and rhabdomyolysis. Body temperatures as high as 42°C have been recorded. Hyperthermia can cause brain damage, hypotension, coagulopathy, and renal failure.

Treatment includes general supportive measures as outlined earlier. There is no specific antidote. Seizures and hyperthermia are the most dangerous manifestations and must be treated aggressively. Seizures are usually managed with intravenous benzodiazepines (eg, lorazepam). Temperature is reduced by removing clothing, spraying with tepid water, and encouraging evaporative cooling with fanning. For very high body temperatures (eg, > 40–41°C), neuromuscular paralysis is used to abolish muscle activity quickly.

ANTICHOLINERGIC AGENTS

A large number of prescription and nonprescription drugs, as well as a variety of plants and mushrooms, can inhibit the effects of acetylcholine. Many drugs used for other purposes (eg, antihistamines) also have anticholinergic effects. Many of them have other potentially toxic actions as well—eg, antihistamines such as diphenhydramine can cause seizures; tricyclic antidepressants, which have anticholinergic, quinidine-like, and α-blocking effects, can cause severe cardiovascular toxicity.

The classic anticholinergic syndrome is remembered as "red as a beet" (skin flushed), "hot as a hare" (hyperthermia), "dry as a bone" (dry mucous membranes, no sweating), "blind as a bat" (blurred vision, cycloplegia), and "mad as a hatter" (confusion, delirium). Patients usually have sinus tachycardia, and the pupils are usually dilated (see Chapter 8). Agitated delirium or coma may be present. Muscle twitching is common, but seizures are unusual unless the patient has ingested an antihistamine or a tricyclic antidepressant. Urinary retention is common, especially in older men.

Treatment is largely supportive. Agitated patients may require sedation with a benzodiazepine or an antipsychotic agent (eg, haloperidol). The specific antidote for peripheral and central anticholinergic syndrome is physostigmine, which has a prompt and dramatic effect and is especially useful for patients who are very agitated. It is given in small intravenous doses (0.5–1 mg), with careful monitoring, because it can cause bradycardia and seizures if given too rapidly. Physostigmine should not be given to a patient with suspected tricyclic antidepressant overdose because it can aggravate cardiotoxicity, resulting in heart block or asystole. Catheterization may be needed to prevent excessive distention of the bladder.

ANTIDEPRESSANTS

Tricyclic antidepressants (eg, amitriptyline, desipramine, doxepin, many others; see Chapter 30) are among the most common prescription drugs involved in life-threatening drug overdose. Ingestion of more than 1 g of a tricyclic (or about 15–20 mg/kg) is considered potentially lethal.

Tricyclic antidepressants are competitive antagonists at muscarinic cholinergic receptors, and anticholinergic findings (tachycardia, dilated pupils, dry mouth) are common even at moderate doses. Some tricyclics are also strong α blockers, which can lead to vasodilation. Centrally mediated agitation and seizures may be followed by depression and hypotension. Most importantly, the tricyclics have quinidine-like depressant effects that cause slowed conduction with a wide QRS interval and depressed cardiac contractility. This cardiac toxicity may result in serious arrhythmias (Figure 59–1), including ventricular conduction block and ventricular tachycardia.

Treatment of tricyclic antidepressant overdose includes general supportive care as outlined earlier. Endotracheal intubation and assisted ventilation may be needed. Intravenous fluids are given for hypotension, and dopamine or norepinephrine is added if necessary. Many toxicologists recommend norepinephrine as the initial drug of choice for tricyclic-induced hypotension. The antidote for quinidine-like cardiac toxicity (manifested by a wide QRS complex) is sodium bicarbonate: a bolus of 50–100 mEq (or 1–2 mEq/kg) provides a rapid increase in extracellular sodium that helps overcome sodium channel blockade. *Do not use physostigmine!* Although this agent does effectively reverse anticholinergic symptoms, it can aggravate depression of cardiac conduction and can cause seizures.

Monoamine oxidase inhibitors (eg, tranylcypromine, phenelzine) are a group of older antidepressants that are occasionally used for resistant depression. They can cause severe hypertensive reactions when interacting foods or drugs are taken (see Chapter 9); and they can interact with the selective serotonin reuptake inhibitors (SSRIs).

Newer antidepressants (eg, fluoxetine, paroxetine, citalopram, venlafaxine) are mostly SSRIs and are generally safer than the tricyclic antidepressants and monoamine oxidase inhibitors, although they can cause seizures. Bupropion (not an SSRI) has caused seizures even in therapeutic doses. Some antidepressants have been associated with QT prolongation and torsade de pointes arrhythmia. The SSRIs may interact with each other or especially with monoamine oxidase inhibitors to cause the **serotonin syndrome,** characterized by agitation, muscle hyperactivity, and hyperthermia (see Chapter 16).

ANTIPSYCHOTICS

Antipsychotic drugs include the older phenothiazines and butyrophenones, as well as newer atypical drugs. All of these can cause CNS depression, seizures, and hypotension. Some can cause QT prolongation. The potent dopamine D_2 blockers are also associated with parkinsonian-like movement disorders (dystonic reactions) and in rare cases with the neuroleptic malignant syndrome, characterized by "lead-pipe" rigidity, hyperthermia, and autonomic instability (see Chapters 16 and 29).

ASPIRIN (SALICYLATE)

Salicylate poisoning (see Chapter 36) is a much less common cause of childhood poisoning deaths since the introduction of child-resistant containers and the reduced use of children's aspirin. It still accounts for numerous suicidal and accidental poisonings. Acute ingestion of more than 200 mg/kg is likely to produce intoxication. Poisoning can also result from chronic overmedication; this occurs most commonly in elderly patients using salicylates for chronic pain who become confused about their dosing. Poisoning causes uncoupling of oxidative phosphorylation and disruption of normal cellular metabolism.

The first sign of salicylate toxicity is often hyperventilation and respiratory alkalosis due to medullary stimulation (Figure 59–2). Metabolic acidosis follows, and an increased anion gap results from accumulation of lactate as well as excretion of bicarbonate by the kidney to compensate for respiratory alkalosis. Arterial blood gas testing often reveals this mixed respiratory alkalosis and metabolic acidosis. Body temperature may be elevated due to uncoupling of oxidative phosphorylation. Severe hyperthermia may occur in serious cases. Vomiting and hyperpnea as well as hyperthermia contribute to fluid loss and dehydration. With very severe poisoning, profound metabolic acidosis, seizures, coma, pulmonary edema, and cardiovascular collapse may occur. Absorption of salicylate and signs of toxicity may be delayed after very large overdoses or ingestion of enteric-coated tablets.

General supportive care as described earlier is essential. After massive aspirin ingestions (eg, more than 100 tablets), aggressive gut decontamination is advisable,

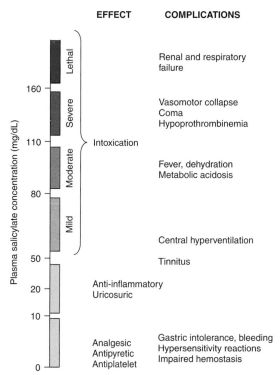

EFFECT **COMPLICATIONS**

Lethal

Renal and respiratory failure

160

Severe

Vasomotor collapse
Coma
Hypoprothrombinemia

110

Intoxication

Moderate

Fever, dehydration
Metabolic acidosis

80

Mild

Central hyperventilation

50

Tinnitus

20

Anti-inflammatory
Uricosuric

10

Analgesic
Antipyretic
Antiplatelet

Gastric intolerance, bleeding
Hypersensitivity reactions
Impaired hemostasis

0

Plasma salicylate concentration (mg/dL)

Figure 59–2. Approximate relationships of plasma salicylate levels to pharmacodynamics and complications. (Modified and reproduced, with permission, from Hollander J, McCary D Jr: *Arthritis and Allied Conditions.* Lea & Febiger, 1972.)

including gastric lavage, repeated doses of activated charcoal, and consideration of whole bowel irrigation. Intravenous fluids are used to replace fluid losses caused by tachypnea, vomiting, and fever. For moderate intoxications, intravenous sodium bicarbonate is given to alkalinize the urine and promote salicylate excretion by trapping the salicylate in its ionized, polar form. For severe poisoning (eg, patients with severe acidosis, coma, and serum salicylate level > 100 mg/dL), emergency hemodialysis is performed to remove the salicylate more quickly and restore acid-base balance and fluid status.

BETA BLOCKERS

In overdose, these drugs block both β_1 and β_2 adrenoceptors; that is, selectivity, if any, is lost at high dosage. The most toxic β blocker is propranolol. As little as two to three times the therapeutic dose can cause serious toxicity. This may be because propranolol has additional properties: At high doses it may cause sodium channel blocking effects similar to those seen with qui-

nidine-like drugs, and it is lipophilic, allowing it to enter the CNS (see Chapter 10).

Bradycardia and hypotension are the most common manifestations of toxicity. Agents with partial agonist activity (eg, pindolol) can cause tachycardia and hypertension. Seizures and cardiac conduction block (wide QRS complex) may be seen with propranolol overdose.

General supportive care should be provided as outlined earlier. The usual measures used to raise the blood pressure and heart rate, such as intravenous fluids, β-agonist drugs, and atropine, are generally ineffective. Glucagon is a useful antidote that—like β agonists—acts on cardiac cells to raise intracellular cAMP but does so through stimulation of glucagon receptors rather than β adrenoceptors. It can improve heart rate and blood pressure when given in high doses (5–20 mg intravenously).

CALCIUM CHANNEL BLOCKERS

Calcium antagonists can cause serious toxicity or death with relatively small overdoses. These channel blockers depress sinus node automaticity and slow AV node conduction (see Chapter 12). They also reduce cardiac output and blood pressure. Serious hypotension is mainly seen with nifedipine and related dihydropyridines, but in severe overdose all of the listed cardiovascular effects can occur with any of the calcium channel blockers.

Treatment requires general supportive care as outlined earlier. Since most ingested calcium antagonists are in a sustained-release form, it may be possible to expel them before they are completely absorbed; initiate whole bowel irrigation and oral activated charcoal as soon as possible, before calcium antagonist-induced ileus intervenes. Calcium, given intravenously in doses of 2–10 g, is a useful antidote for depressed cardiac contractility but less effective for nodal block or peripheral vascular collapse. Other drugs reported to be helpful in managing hypotension associated with calcium channel blocker poisoning include glucagon, vasopressin, epinephrine, and high-dose insulin plus glucose supplementation to maintain euglycemia.

CARBON MONOXIDE & OTHER TOXIC GASES

Carbon monoxide (CO) is a colorless, odorless gas that is ubiquitous because it is created whenever carbon-containing materials are burned (see Table 57–1). Carbon monoxide poisoning is the leading cause of death due to poisoning in the USA. Most cases occur in victims of fires, but accidental and suicidal exposures are also common. Diagnosis and treatment of carbon monoxide poisoning are described in Chapter 57. Many other toxic gases are produced in fires or released in industrial accidents (Table 59–5).

Table 59–5. Characteristics of poisoning with some gases.

Gas	Mechanism of Toxicity	Clinical Features and Treatment
Irritant gases (eg, chlorine, ammonia, sulfur dioxide, nitrogen oxides)	Corrosive effect on upper and lower airways	Cough, stridor, wheezing, pneumonia **Treatment:** Humidified oxygen, bronchodilators
Carbon monoxide	Binds to hemoglobin, reducing oxygen delivery to tissues	Headache, dizziness, nausea, vomiting, seizures, coma **Treatment:** 100% oxygen
Cyanide	Binds to cytochrome, blocks cellular oxygen use	Acidosis, shortness of breath, agitation and tachycardia followed by seizures, coma, hypotension, and death **Treatment:** One cyanide antidote kit consists of nitrites to induce methemoglobinemia (which binds cyanide) and thiosulfate (which hastens conversion of CN^- to less toxic thiocyanate). A newer antidote kit (Cyanokit) consists of concentrated hydroxocobalamin, which directly converts CN^- to cyanocobalamin (Vitamin B_{12})
Hydrogen sulfide	Similar to cyanide	Similar to cyanide. Smell of rotten eggs **Treatment:** No specific antidote
Oxidizing agents (eg, nitrogen oxides)	Can cause methemoglobinemia	Dyspnea, cyanosis (due to brown color of methemoglobin), syncope, seizures, coma **Treatment:** Methylene blue (which hastens conversion back to normal hemoglobin)

CHOLINESTERASE INHIBITORS

Organophosphate and carbamate cholinesterase inhibitors (see Chapter 7) are widely used to kill insects and other pests. Most cases of serious organophosphate or carbamate poisoning result from intentional ingestion by a suicidal person, but poisoning has also occurred at work (pesticide application or packaging) or, rarely, as a result of food contamination or terrorist attack (eg, release of the chemical warfare nerve agent sarin in the Tokyo subway system in 1995).

Stimulation of muscarinic receptors causes abdominal cramps, diarrhea, excessive salivation, sweating, urinary frequency, and increased bronchial secretions (see Chapters 6 and 7). Stimulation of nicotinic receptors causes generalized ganglionic activation, which can lead to hypertension and either tachycardia or bradycardia. Muscle twitching and fasciculations may progress to weakness and respiratory muscle paralysis. CNS effects include agitation, confusion, and seizures. The mnemonic DUMBELS (diarrhea, urination, miosis and muscle weakness, bronchospasm, excitation, lacrimation, and seizures, sweating, and salivation) helps recall the common findings. Blood testing may be used to document depressed activity of red blood cell (acetylcholinesterase) and plasma (butyrylcholinesterase) enzymes, which provide an indirect estimate of synaptic cholinesterase activity.

General supportive care should be provided as outlined above. Extra precautions should be taken to ensure that rescuers and health care providers are not poisoned by exposure to contaminated clothing or skin. This is especially critical for the most potent substances such as parathion or nerve gas agents. Antidotal treatment consists of atropine and pralidoxime (see Chapter 8). Atropine is an effective competitive inhibitor at muscarinic sites but has no effect at nicotinic sites. Pralidoxime given early enough is capable of restoring the cholinesterase activity and is active at both muscarinic and nicotinic sites.

CYANIDE

Cyanide (CN^-) salts and hydrogen cyanide (HCN) are highly toxic chemicals used in chemical synthesis, as rodenticides, formerly as a method of execution, and as agents of suicide or homicide. Hydrogen cyanide gas is formed upon burning of plastics, wool, and many other synthetic and natural products. Cyanide binds readily to cytochrome axidase, leading to cellular hypoxia and lactic acidosis. Symptoms of cyanide poisoning include shortness of breath, agitation, and tachycardia followed by seizures, coma, hypotension, and death. Severe metabolic acidosis is characteristic. Treatment of cyanide poisoning includes rapid administration of activated charcoal (although charcoal binds cyanide poorly, it can reduce absorption) and general supportive care. Two antidote kits are available in the USA (Table 59–5).

DIGOXIN

Digitalis and other cardiac glycosides are found in many plants (see Chapter 13) and in the skin of some toads.

Toxicity may occur as a result of acute overdose or from accumulation of digoxin in a patient with renal insufficiency or one taking a drug that interferes with digoxin elimination. Patients receiving long-term digoxin treatment are often also taking diuretics, which can lead to electrolyte depletion (especially potassium).

Vomiting is common in patients with digitalis overdose. Hyperkalemia may be caused by acute digitalis overdose or severe poisoning, while hypokalemia may be present in patients as a result of long-term diuretic treatment. (Digitalis does not cause hypokalemia.) A variety of cardiac rhythm disturbances may occur, including sinus bradycardia, AV block, atrial tachycardia with block, accelerated junctional rhythm, premature ventricular beats, bidirectional ventricular tachycardia, and other ventricular arrhythmias.

General supportive care should be provided as outlined earlier. Atropine is often effective for bradycardia or AV block. The use of digoxin antibodies (see Chapter 13) has revolutionized the treatment of digoxin toxicity; they should be administered intravenously in the dosage indicated in the package insert. Symptoms usually improve within 30–60 minutes after antibody administration. Digoxin antibodies may also be tried in cases of poisoning by other cardiac glycosides (eg, digitoxin, oleander), although larger doses may be needed due to incomplete cross-reactivity.

ETHANOL & SEDATIVE-HYPNOTIC DRUGS

Overdosage with ethanol and sedative-hypnotic drugs (eg, benzodiazepines, barbiturates, γ-hydroxybutyrate [GHB], carisoprodol [Soma]; see Chapters 22 and 23) occurs frequently because of their common availability and use.

Patients with ethanol or sedative-hypnotic overdose may be euphoric and rowdy ("drunk") or in a state of stupor or coma ("dead drunk"). Comatose patients often have depressed respiratory drive. Depression of protective airway reflexes may result in aspiration of gastric contents. Hypothermia may be present because of environmental exposure and depressed shivering. Ethanol blood levels greater than 300 mg/dL usually cause deep coma, but regular users are often tolerant to the effects of ethanol and may be ambulatory despite even higher levels. Patients with GHB overdose are often deeply comatose for 3–4 hours and then awaken fully in a matter of minutes.

General supportive care should be provided. With careful attention to protecting the airway (including endotracheal intubation) and assisting ventilation, most patients will recover as the drug effects wear off. Hypotension usually responds to body warming if cold, intravenous fluids and, if needed, dopamine. Patients with isolated benzodiazepine overdose may awaken after intravenous flumazenil, a benzodiazepine antagonist. However, this drug is not widely used as empiric ther-

apy for drug overdose because it may precipitate seizures in patients who are addicted to benzodiazepines or who have ingested a convulsant drug (eg, a tricyclic antidepressant). There are no antidotes for ethanol, barbiturates, or most other sedative-hypnotics.

ETHYLENE GLYCOL & METHANOL

These alcohols are important toxins because of their metabolism to highly toxic organic acids (see Chapter 23). They are capable of causing CNS depression and a drunken state similar to ethanol overdose. However, their products of metabolism—formic acid (from methanol) or hippuric, oxalic, and glycolic acids (from ethylene glycol)—cause a severe metabolic acidosis and can lead to coma and blindness (in the case of formic acid) or renal failure (from oxalic acid and glycolic acid). Initially, the patient appears drunk, but after a delay of up to several hours, a severe anion gap metabolic acidosis becomes apparent, accompanied by hyperventilation and altered mental status. Patients with methanol poisoning may have visual disturbances ranging from blurred vision to blindness.

Metabolism of ethylene glycol and methanol to their toxic products can be blocked by inhibiting the enzyme alcohol dehydrogenase with a competing drug. Ethanol is metabolized preferentially by alcohol dehydrogenase, so ethanol can be given orally or intravenously (5% pharmaceutical grade) to a level of approximately 100 mg/dL. Alternatively, the antidote fomepizole—an effective blocker of alcohol dehydrogenase that does not induce ethanol intoxication—can be used.

IRON & OTHER METALS

Iron is widely used in over-the-counter vitamin preparations and is a leading cause of childhood poisoning deaths. As few as 10–12 prenatal multivitamins with iron may cause serious illness in a small child. Poisoning with other metals (lead, mercury, arsenic) is also important, especially in industry. See Chapters 33 and 58 for detailed discussions of poisoning by iron and other metals.

OPIOIDS

Opioids (opium, morphine, heroin, meperidine, methadone, etc) are common drugs of abuse (see Chapters 31 and 32), and overdose is a frequent result of using the poorly standardized preparations sold on the street. See Chapter 31 for a detailed discussion of opioid overdose and its treatment.

RATTLESNAKE ENVENOMATION

In the USA, rattlesnakes are the most common venomous reptiles. Bites are rarely fatal, and 20% do not involve envenomation. However, about 60% of bites cause significant morbidity due to the destructive digestive enzymes found in the venom. Evidence of rattle-snake envenomation includes severe pain, swelling, bruising, hemorrhagic bleb formation, and obvious fang marks. Systemic effects include nausea, vomiting, muscle fasciculations, tingling and metallic taste in the mouth, shock, and systemic coagulopathy with prolonged clotting time and reduced platelet count.

Studies have shown that emergency field remedies such as incision and suction, tourniquets, and ice packs are far more damaging than useful. Avoidance of unnecessary motion, on the other hand, does help to limit the spread of the venom. Definitive therapy relies on intravenous antivenin and should be started as soon as possible.

THEOPHYLLINE

Although it has been largely replaced by inhaled β agonists, theophylline continues to be used for the treatment of bronchospasm by some patients with asthma and bronchitis (see Chapter 20). A dose of 20–30 tablets can cause serious or fatal poisoning. Chronic or subacute theophylline poisoning can also occur as a result of accidental overmedication or use of a drug that interferes with theophylline metabolism (eg, cimetidine, ciprofloxacin, erythromycin; see Chapter 4).

In addition to sinus tachycardia and tremor, vomiting is common after overdose. Hypotension, tachycardia, hypokalemia, and hyperglycemia may occur, probably due to β_2-adrenergic activation. The cause of this activation is not fully understood, but the effects can be ameliorated by the use of β blockers (see below). Cardiac arrhythmias include atrial tachycardias, premature ventricular contractions, and ventricular tachycardia. In severe poisoning (eg, acute overdose with serum level > 100 mg/L), seizures often occur and are usually resistant to common anticonvulsants. Toxicity may be delayed in onset for many hours after ingestion of sustained-release tablet formulations.

General supportive care should be provided. Aggressive gut decontamination should be carried out using repeated doses of activated charcoal and whole bowel irrigation. Propranolol or other β blockers (eg, esmolol) are useful antidotes for β-mediated hypotension and tachycardia. Phenobarbital is preferred over phenytoin for convulsions; most anticonvulsants are ineffective. Hemodialysis is indicated for serum concentrations greater than 100 mg/L and for intractable seizures in patients with lower levels.

REFERENCES

Dart RD (editor): *Medical Toxicology,* 3rd ed. Lippincott Williams & Wilkins, 2004.

Ford M et al (editors): *Clinical Toxicology.* Saunders, 2000.

Goldfrank LR et al (editors): *Goldfrank's Toxicologic Emergencies,* 7th ed. McGraw-Hill, 2002.

Olson KR et al (editors): *Poisoning & Drug Overdose,* 5th ed. McGraw-Hill, 2006.

POISINDEX. (Revised Quarterly.) Thompson/Micromedex.

SECTION X
Special Topics

Special Aspects of Perinatal & Pediatric Pharmacology*

60

Gideon Koren, MD

The effects of drugs on the fetus and newborn infant are based on the general principles set forth in Chapters 1–4 of this book. However, the physiologic contexts in which these pharmacologic laws operate are different in pregnant women and in rapidly maturing infants. At present, the special pharmacokinetic factors operative in these patients are beginning to be understood, whereas information regarding pharmacodynamic differences (eg, receptor characteristics and responses) is still incomplete.

DRUG THERAPY IN PREGNANCY

Pharmacokinetics

Most drugs taken by pregnant women can cross the placenta and expose the developing embryo and fetus to their pharmacologic and teratogenic effects. Critical factors affecting placental drug transfer and drug effects on the fetus include the following: (1) the physicochemical properties of the drug; (2) the rate at which the drug crosses the placenta and the amount of drug reaching the fetus; (3) the duration of exposure to the drug; (4) distribution characteristics in different fetal tissues; (5) the stage of placental and fetal development at the time of exposure to the drug; and (6) the effects of drugs used in combination.

A. LIPID SOLUBILITY

As is true also of other biologic membranes, drug passage across the placenta is dependent on lipid solubility and the degree of drug ionization. Lipophilic drugs tend to diffuse readily across the placenta and enter the fetal circulation. For example, thiopental, a drug commonly used for cesarean sections, crosses the placenta almost immediately and can produce sedation or apnea in the newborn infant. Highly ionized drugs such as succinylcholine and tubocurarine, also used for cesarean sections, cross the placenta slowly and achieve very low concentrations in the fetus. Impermeability of the placenta to polar compounds is relative rather than absolute. If high enough maternal-fetal concentration gradients are achieved, polar compounds cross the placenta in measurable amounts. Salicylate, which is almost completely ionized at physiologic pH, crosses the placenta rapidly. This occurs because the small amount of salicylate that is not ionized is highly lipid-soluble.

B. MOLECULAR SIZE

The molecular weight of the drug also influences the rate of transfer and the amount of drug transferred across the placenta. Drugs with molecular weights of 250–500 can cross the placenta easily, depending upon their lipid solubility and degree of ionization; those with molecular weights of 500–1000 cross the placenta with more difficulty; and those with molecular weights greater than 1000 cross very poorly. An important clinical application of this property is the choice of heparin as an anticoagu-

*Supported by a grant from the Canadian Institutes for Health Research.

lant in pregnant women. Because it is a very large (and polar) molecule, heparin is unable to cross the placenta. Unlike warfarin, which is teratogenic and should be avoided during the first trimester and even beyond (as the brain continues to develop), heparin may be safely given to pregnant women who need anticoagulation. Yet the placenta contains drug transporters, which can carry larger molecules to the fetus. For example, a variety of maternal antibodies cross the placenta and may cause fetal morbidity, as in Rh incompatibility.

C. PLACENTAL TRANSPORTERS

During the last decade, many drug transporters have been identified in the placenta, with increasing recognition of their effects on drug transfer to the fetus. For example, the P-glycoprotein transporter encoded by the *MDR1* gene pumps back into the maternal circulation a variety of drugs, including cancer drugs (eg, vinblastine, doxorubicin) and other agents. Similarly, viral protease inhibitors, which are substrates to P-glycoprotein, achieve only low fetal concentrations—an effect that may increase the risk of vertical HIV infection from the mother to the fetus. The hypoglycemic drug glyburide cannot be measured in umbilical blood despite therapeutic maternal concentrations. Recent work has documented that this agent is effluxed from the fetal circulation by the BCRP transporter as well as by the MRP3 transporter located in the placental brush border membrane.

D. PROTEIN BINDING

The degree to which a drug is bound to plasma proteins (particularly albumin) may also affect the rate of transfer and the amount transferred. However, if a compound is very lipid-soluble (eg, some anesthetic gases), it will not be affected greatly by protein binding. Transfer of these more lipid-soluble drugs and their overall rates of equilibration are more dependent on (and proportionate to) placental blood flow. This is because very lipid-soluble drugs diffuse across placental membranes so rapidly that their overall rates of equilibration do not depend on the free drug concentrations becoming equal on both sides. If a drug is poorly lipid-soluble and is ionized, its transfer is slow and will probably be impeded by its binding to maternal plasma proteins. Differential protein binding is also important since some drugs exhibit greater protein binding in maternal plasma than in fetal plasma because of a lower binding affinity of fetal proteins. This has been shown for sulfonamides, barbiturates, phenytoin, and local anesthetic agents.

E. PLACENTAL AND FETAL DRUG METABOLISM

Two mechanisms help protect the fetus from drugs in the maternal circulation: (1) The placenta itself plays a role both as a semipermeable barrier and as a site of metabolism of some drugs passing through it. Several different types of aromatic oxidation reactions (eg, hydroxylation, N-dealkylation, demethylation) have been shown to occur in placental tissue. Pentobarbital is oxidized in this way. Conversely, it is possible that the metabolic capacity of the placenta may lead to creation of toxic metabolites, and the placenta may therefore augment toxicity (eg, ethanol, benzpyrenes). (2) Drugs that have crossed the placenta enter the fetal circulation via the umbilical vein. About 40–60% of umbilical venous blood flow enters the fetal liver; the remainder bypasses the liver and enters the general fetal circulation. A drug that enters the liver may be partially metabolized there before it enters the fetal circulation. In addition, a large proportion of drug present in the umbilical artery (returning to the placenta) may be shunted through the placenta back to the umbilical vein and into the liver again. It should be noted that metabolites of some drugs may be more active than the parent compound and may affect the fetus adversely.

Pharmacodynamics

A. MATERNAL DRUG ACTIONS

The effects of drugs on the reproductive tissues (breast, uterus, etc) of the pregnant woman are sometimes altered by the endocrine environment appropriate for the stage of pregnancy. Drug effects on other maternal tissues (heart, lungs, kidneys, central nervous system, etc) are not changed significantly by pregnancy, although the physiologic context (cardiac output, renal blood flow, etc) may be altered, requiring the use of drugs that are not needed by the same woman when she is not pregnant. For example, cardiac glycosides and diuretics may be needed for heart failure precipitated by the increased cardiac workload of pregnancy, or insulin may be required for control of blood glucose in pregnancy-induced diabetes.

B. THERAPEUTIC DRUG ACTIONS IN THE FETUS

Fetal therapeutics is an emerging area in perinatal pharmacology. This involves drug administration to the pregnant woman with the fetus as the target of the drug. At present, corticosteroids are used to stimulate fetal lung maturation when preterm birth is expected. Phenobarbital, when given to pregnant women near term, can induce fetal hepatic enzymes responsible for the glucuronidation of bilirubin, and the incidence of jaundice is lower in newborns when mothers are given phenobarbital than when phenobarbital is not used. Before phototherapy became the preferred mode of therapy for neonatal indirect hyperbilirubinemia, phenobarbital was used for this indication. Administration of phenobarbital to the mother was suggested recently as a means of decreasing the risk of intracranial bleeding in preterm infants. However, large randomized studies failed to confirm this effect. Antiarrhythmic drugs have also been given to mothers for treatment of fetal cardiac arrhythmias. Although their efficacy has not yet been established by controlled studies, digoxin, flecainide, procainamide, verapamil, and other antiarrhythmic agents have been shown to be effective in case series. During the last decade it has been shown that maternal use of zidovudine decreases by two thirds transmission of HIV from the mother to the fetus, and use of combinations of three antiretroviral agents can eliminate fetal infection almost entirely (see Chapter 49).

C. PREDICTABLE TOXIC DRUG ACTIONS IN THE FETUS

Chronic use of opioids by the mother may produce dependence in the fetus and newborn. This dependence may be manifested after delivery as a neonatal withdrawal syndrome. A less well understood fetal drug toxicity is caused by the use of angiotensin-converting enzyme inhibitors during pregnancy. These drugs can result in significant and irreversible renal damage in the fetus and are therefore contraindicated in pregnant women. Adverse effects may also be delayed, as in the case of female fetuses exposed to diethylstilbestrol, who may be at increased risk for adenocarcinoma of the vagina after puberty.

D. TERATOGENIC DRUG ACTIONS

A single intrauterine exposure to a drug can affect the fetal structures undergoing rapid development at the time of exposure. Thalidomide is an example of a drug that may profoundly affect the development of the limbs after only brief exposure. This exposure, however, must be at a critical time in the development of the limbs. The thalidomide phocomelia risk occurs during the fourth through the seventh weeks of gestation because it is during this time that the arms and legs develop (Figure 60–1).

1. Teratogenic mechanisms—The mechanisms by which different drugs produce teratogenic effects are poorly understood and are probably multifactorial. For example, drugs may have a direct effect on maternal tissues with secondary or indirect effects on fetal tissues. Drugs may interfere with the passage of oxygen or nutrients through the placenta and therefore have effects on the most rapidly metabolizing tissues of the fetus. Finally, drugs may have important direct actions on the processes of differentiation in developing tissues. For example, vitamin A (retinol) has been shown to have important differentiation-directing actions in normal tissues. Several vitamin A analogs (isotretinoin, etretinate) are powerful teratogens, suggesting that they alter the normal processes of differentiation. Finally, deficiency of a critical substance appears to play a role in some types of abnormalities. For example, folic acid supplementation during pregnancy appears to reduce the incidence of neural tube defects (eg, spina bifida).

Continued exposure to a teratogen may produce cumulative effects or may affect several organs going through varying stages of development. Chronic consumption of high doses of ethanol during pregnancy, particularly during the first and second trimesters, may result in the fetal alcohol syndrome (see Chapter 23). In this syndrome, the central nervous system, growth, and facial development may be affected.

2. Defining a teratogen—To be considered teratogenic, a candidate substance or process should (1) result in a characteristic set of malformations, indicating selectivity for certain target organs; (2) exert its effects at a particular stage of fetal development, ie, during the limited time period of organogenesis of the target organs (Figure 60–1); and (3) show a dose-dependent incidence. Some drugs with known teratogenic or other adverse effects in pregnancy are listed in Table 60–1.

The widely cited Food and Drug Administration system for teratogenic potential (Table 60–2) is an attempt to quantify teratogenic risk from A (safe) to X (definite human teratogenic risk). This system has been criticized as inaccurate and impractical. For example, several drugs have been labeled "X" despite extensive opposite human safety data (eg, oral contraceptives). Diazepam and other benzodiazepines are labeled as "D" despite lack of positive evidence of human fetal risk.

3. Counseling women about teratogenic risk—Since the thalidomide disaster, medicine has been practiced as if every drug were a potential human teratogen when, in fact, fewer than 30 such drugs have been identified, with hundreds of agents proved safe for the unborn. Owing to high levels of anxiety among pregnant women—and because half of the pregnancies in North America are unplanned—every year many thousands of women need counseling about fetal exposure to drugs, chemicals, and radiation. In the Motherisk program in Toronto, thousands of women are counseled every month, and the ability of appropriate counseling to prevent unnecessary abortions has been documented. Clinicians who wish to provide such counsel to pregnant women must ensure that their information is up to date and evidence-based and that the woman understands that the baseline teratogenic risk in pregnancy (ie, the risk of a neonatal abnormality in the absence of any known teratogenic exposure) is about 3%. It is also critical to address the maternal-fetal risks of the untreated condition if a medication is avoided. Recent studies show serious morbidity in women who discontinued selective serotonin reuptake inhibitor therapy for depression in pregnancy.

DRUG THERAPY IN INFANTS & CHILDREN

Physiologic processes that influence pharmacokinetic variables in the infant change significantly in the first

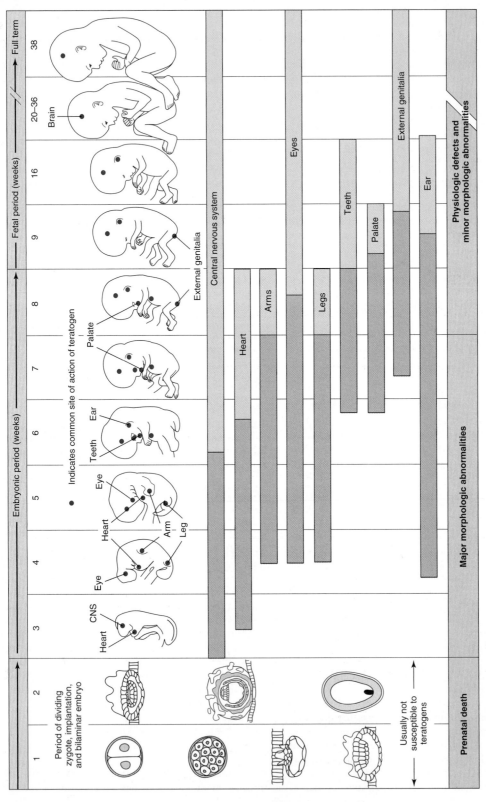

Figure 60-1. Schematic diagram of critical periods of human development. (Reproduced, with permission, from Moore KL: *The Developing Human: Clinically Oriented Embryology*, 4th ed. Saunders, 1988.)

Table 60–1. Drugs with significant adverse effects on the fetus.

Drug	Trimester	Effect
ACE inhibitors	All, especially second and third	Renal damage
Aminopterin	First	Multiple gross anomalies
Amphetamines	All	Suspected abnormal developmental patterns, decreased school performance
Androgens	Second and third	Masculinization of female fetus
Antidepressants, tricyclic	Third	Neonatal withdrawal symptoms have been reported in a few cases with clomipramine, desipramine, and imipramine
Barbiturates	All	Chronic use can lead to neonatal dependence.
Busulfan	All	Various congenital malformations; low birth weight
Carbamazepine	First	Neural tube defects
Chlorpropamide	All	Prolonged symptomatic neonatal hypoglycemia
Clomipramine	Third	Neonatal lethargy, hypotonia, cyanosis, hypothermia
Cocaine	All	Increased risk of spontaneous abortion, abruptio placentae, and premature labor; neonatal cerebral infarction, abnormal development, and decreased school performance
Cyclophosphamide	First	Various congenital malformations
Cytarabine	First, second	Various congenital malformations
Diazepam	All	Chronic use may lead to neonatal dependence
Diethylstilbestrol	All	Vaginal adenosis, clear cell vaginal adenocarcinoma
Ethanol	All	Risk of fetal alcohol syndrome and alcohol-related neurodevelopmental defects
Etretinate	All	High risk of multiple congenital malformations
Heroin	All	Chronic use leads to neonatal dependence
Iodide	All	Congenital goiter, hypothyroidism
Isotretinoin	All	Extremely high risk of CNS, face, ear, and other malformations
Lithium	First	Ebstein's anomaly
Methadone	All	Chronic use leads to neonatal dependence
Methotrexate	First	Multiple congenital malformations
Methylthiouracil	All	Hypothyroidism
Metronidazole	First	May be mutagenic (from animal studies; there is no evidence for mutagenic or teratogenic effects in humans)
Organic solvents	First	Multiple malformations
Misoprostol	First	Möbius sequence
Penicillamine	First	Cutis laxa, other congenital malformations
Phencyclidine	All	Abnormal neurologic examination, poor suck reflex and feeding
Phenytoin	All	Fetal hydantoin syndrome
Propylthiouracil	All	Congenital goiter
Streptomycin	All	Eighth nerve toxicity

(continued)

Table 60–1. Drugs with significant adverse effects on the fetus. (continued)

Drug	Trimester	Effect
Smoking (constituents of tobacco smoke)	All	Intrauterine growth retardation; prematurity; sudden infant death syndrome; perinatal complications
Tamoxifen	All	Increased risk of spontaneous abortion or fetal damage
Tetracycline	All	Discoloration and defects of teeth and altered bone growth
Thalidomide	First	Phocomelia (shortened or absent long bones of the limbs) and many internal malformations
Trimethadione	All	Multiple congenital anomalies
Valproic acid	All	Neural tube defects, cardiac and limb malformations
Warfarin	First	Hypoplastic nasal bridge, chondrodysplasia
	Second	CNS malformations
	Third	Risk of bleeding. Discontinue use 1 month before delivery.

year of life, particularly during the first few months. Therefore, special attention must be paid to pharmacokinetics in this age group. Pharmacodynamic differences between pediatric and other patients have not been explored in great detail and are probably small except for those specific target tissues that mature at birth or immediately thereafter (eg, the ductus arteriosus).

Drug Absorption

Drug absorption in infants and children follows the same general principles as in adults. Unique factors that influence drug absorption include blood flow at the site of administration, as determined by the physiologic status of the infant or child; and, for orally administered drugs, gastrointestinal function, which changes rapidly during the first few days after birth. Age after birth also influences the regulation of drug absorption.

A. BLOOD FLOW AT THE SITE OF ADMINISTRATION

Absorption after intramuscular or subcutaneous injection depends mainly, in neonates as in adults, on the rate of blood flow to the muscle or subcutaneous area injected. Physiologic conditions that might reduce blood flow to these areas are cardiovascular shock, vasoconstriction due to sympathomimetic agents, and heart failure. However, sick preterm infants requiring intramuscular injections may have very little muscle mass. This is further complicated by diminished peripheral perfusion to these areas. In such cases, absorption becomes irregular and difficult to predict, because the drug may remain in the muscle and be absorbed more slowly than expected. If perfusion suddenly improves, there can be a sudden and unpredictable increase in the amount of drug entering the circulation, resulting in

high and potentially toxic concentrations of drug. Examples of drugs especially hazardous in such situations are cardiac glycosides, aminoglycoside antibiotics, and anticonvulsants.

B. GASTROINTESTINAL FUNCTION

Significant biochemical and physiologic changes occur in the neonatal gastrointestinal tract shortly after birth. In full-term infants, gastric acid secretion begins soon after birth and increases gradually over several hours. In preterm infants, the secretion of gastric acid occurs more slowly, with the highest concentrations appearing on the fourth day of life. Therefore, drugs that are partially or totally inactivated by the low pH of gastric contents should not be administered orally.

Gastric emptying time is prolonged (up to 6 or 8 hours) in the first day or so after delivery. Therefore, drugs that are absorbed primarily in the stomach may be absorbed more completely than anticipated. In the case of drugs absorbed in the small intestine, therapeutic effect may be delayed. Peristalsis in the neonate is irregular and may be slow. The amount of drug absorbed in the small intestine may therefore be unpredictable; more than the usual amount of drug may be absorbed if peristalsis is slowed, and this could result in potential toxicity from an otherwise standard dose. Table 60–3 summarizes data on oral bioavailability of various drugs in neonates compared with older children and adults. An increase in peristalsis, as in diarrheal conditions, tends to decrease the extent of absorption, because contact time with the large absorptive surface of the intestine is decreased.

Gastrointestinal enzyme activities tend to be lower in the newborn than in the adult. Activities of α-amylase and other pancreatic enzymes in the duodenum are

Table 60-2. FDA teratogenic risk categories.

Category	Description
A	Controlled studies in women fail to demonstrate a risk to the fetus in the first trimester (and there is no evidence of a risk in late trimesters), and the possibility of fetal harm appears remote.
B	Either animal-reproduction studies have not demonstrated a fetal risk, but there are no controlled studies in pregnant women, or animal-reproduction studies have shown an adverse effect (other than a decrease in fertility) that was not confirmed in controlled studies in women in the first trimester (and there is no evidence of a risk in later trimesters).
C	Either studies in animals have revealed adverse effects on the fetus (teratogenic or embryocidal or other) and there are no controlled studies in women or studies in women and animals are not available. Drugs should be given only if the potential benefit justifies the potential risk to the fetus.
D	There is positive evidence of human fetal risk, but the benefits from use in pregnant women may be acceptable despite the risk (eg, if the drug is needed in a life-threatening situation or for a serious disease for which safer drugs cannot be used or are ineffective).
X	Studies in animals or human beings have demonstrated fetal abnormalities or there is evidence of fetal risk based on human experience or both, and the risk of the use of the drug in pregnant women clearly outweighs any possible benefit. The drug is contraindicated in women who are or may become pregnant.

low in infants up to 4 months of age. Neonates also have low concentrations of bile acids and lipase, which may decrease the absorption of lipid-soluble drugs.

Drug Distribution

As body composition changes with development, the distribution volumes of drugs are also changed. The neonate has a higher percentage of its body weight in the form of water (70–75%) than does the adult (50–60%). Differences can also be observed between the full-term neonate (70% of body weight as water) and the small preterm neonate (85% of body weight as water). Similarly, extracellular water is 40% of body weight in the neonate, compared with 20% in the adult. Most neonates will experience diuresis in the first 24–48 hours of life. Since many drugs are distributed

throughout the extracellular water space, the size (volume) of the extracellular water compartment may be important in determining the concentration of drug at receptor sites. This is especially important for water-soluble drugs (such as aminoglycosides) and less crucial for lipid-soluble agents.

Preterm infants have much less fat than full-term infants. Total body fat in preterm infants is about 1% of total body weight, compared with 15% in full-term neonates. Therefore, organs that generally accumulate high concentrations of lipid-soluble drugs in adults and older children may accumulate smaller amounts of these agents in less mature infants.

Another major factor determining drug distribution is drug binding to plasma proteins. Albumin is the plasma protein with the greatest binding capacity. In general, protein binding of drugs is reduced in the neonate. This has been seen with local anesthetic drugs, diazepam, phenytoin, ampicillin, and phenobarbital. Therefore, the concentration of free (unbound) drug in plasma is increased initially. Because the free drug exerts the pharmacologic effect, this can result in greater drug effect or toxicity despite a normal or even low plasma concentration of total drug (bound plus unbound). Consider a therapeutic dose of a drug (eg, diazepam) given to a patient. The concentration of total drug in the plasma is 300 mcg/L. If the drug is 98% protein-bound in an older child or adult, then 6 mcg/L is the concentration of free drug. Assume that this concentration of free drug produces the desired effect in the patient without producing toxicity. However, if this drug is given to a preterm infant in a dosage adjusted for body weight and it produces a total drug concentration of 300 mcg/L—and protein binding is only 90%—then the free drug concentration will be 30 mcg/L, or five times higher. Although the higher free concentration

Table 60-3. Oral drug absorption (bioavailability) of various drugs in the neonate compared with older children and adults.

Drug	Oral Absorption
Acetaminophen	Decreased
Ampicillin	Increased
Diazepam	Normal
Digoxin	Normal
Penicillin G	Increased
Phenobarbital	Decreased
Phenytoin	Decreased
Sulfonamides	Normal

may result in faster elimination (see Chapter 3), this concentration may be quite toxic initially.

Some drugs compete with serum bilirubin for binding to albumin. Drugs given to a neonate with jaundice can displace bilirubin from albumin. Because of the greater permeability of the neonatal blood-brain barrier, substantial amounts of bilirubin may enter the brain and cause kernicterus. This was in fact observed when sulfonamide antibiotics were given to preterm neonates as prophylaxis against sepsis. Conversely, as the serum bilirubin rises for physiologic reasons or because of a blood group incompatibility, bilirubin can displace a drug from albumin and substantially raise the free drug concentration. This may occur without altering the total drug concentration and would result in greater therapeutic effect or toxicity at normal concentrations. This has been shown to happen with phenytoin.

Drug Metabolism

The metabolism of most drugs occurs in the liver (see Chapter 4). The drug-metabolizing activities of the cytochrome P450-dependent mixed-function oxidases and the conjugating enzymes are substantially lower (50–70% of adult values) in early neonatal life than later. The point in development at which enzymatic activity is maximal depends upon the specific enzyme system in question. Glucuronide formation reaches adult values (per kilogram body weight) between the third and fourth years of life. Because of the neonate's decreased ability to metabolize drugs, many drugs have slow clearance rates and prolonged elimination half-lives. If drug doses and dosing schedules are not altered appropriately, this immaturity predisposes the neonate to adverse effects from drugs that are metabolized by the liver. Table 60–4 demonstrates how neonatal and adult drug elimination half-lives can differ and how the half-lives of phenobarbital and phenytoin decrease as the neonate grows older. The process of maturation must be considered when administering drugs to this age group, especially in the case of drugs administered over long periods.

Another consideration for the neonate is whether or not the mother was receiving drugs (eg, phenobarbital) that can induce early maturation of fetal hepatic enzymes. In this case, the ability of the neonate to metabolize certain drugs will be greater than expected, and one may see less therapeutic effect and lower plasma drug concentrations when the usual neonatal dose is given.

Drug Excretion

The glomerular filtration rate is much lower in newborns than in older infants, children, or adults, and this limitation persists during the first few days of life. Calculated

Table 60–4. Comparison of elimination half-lives of various drugs in neonates and adults.

Drug	Neonatal Age	Neonates $t_{1/2}$ (hours)	Adults $t_{1/2}$ (hours)
Acetamino-phen		2.2–5	0.9–2.2
Diazepam		25–100	40–50
Digoxin		60–70	30–60
Phenobar-bital	0–5 days	200	64–140
	5–15 days	100	
	1–30 months	50	
Phenytoin	0–2 days	80	12–18
	3–14 days	18	
	14–50 days	6	
Salicylate		4.5–11	10–15
Theophylline	Neonate	13–26	5–10
	Child	3–4	

on the basis of body surface area, glomerular filtration in the neonate is only 30–40% of the adult value. The glomerular filtration rate is even lower in neonates born before 34 weeks of gestation. Function improves substantially during the first week of life. At the end of the first week, the glomerular filtration rate and renal plasma flow have increased 50% from the first day. By the end of the third week, glomerular filtration is 50–60% of the adult value; by 6–12 months, it reaches adult values (per unit surface area). Therefore, drugs that depend on renal function for elimination are cleared from the body very slowly in the first weeks of life.

Penicillins, for example, are cleared by preterm infants at 17% of the adult rate based on comparable surface area and 34% of the adult rate when adjusted for body weight. The dosage of ampicillin for a neonate less than 7 days old is 50–100 mg/kg/d in two doses at 12-hour intervals. The dosage for a neonate over 7 days old is 100–200 mg/kg/d in three doses at 8-hour intervals. A decreased rate of renal elimination in the neonate has also been observed with aminoglycoside antibiotics (kanamycin, gentamicin, neomycin, and streptomycin). The dosage of gentamicin for a neonate less than 7 days old is 5 mg/kg/d in two doses at 12-hour intervals. The dosage for a neonate over 7 days old is 7.5 mg/kg/d in three doses at 8-hour intervals. Total body clearance of digoxin is directly dependent upon adequate renal function, and accumulation of digoxin can occur when glomerular filtration is decreased. Since renal function in a sick infant may not improve at the predicted rate during the first weeks and months of life, appropriate adjustments in dosage and dosing schedules may be very difficult. In this situation, adjustments are best made on the basis of plasma drug concentrations determined at intervals throughout the course of therapy.

While great focus is naturally concentrated on the neonate, it is important to remember that toddlers may have *shorter* elimination half-lives of drugs than older children and adults, due probably to *increased* renal elimination and metabolism. For example, the dose per kilogram of digoxin is much higher in toddlers than in adults. The mechanisms for these developmental changes are still poorly understood.

Special Pharmacodynamic Features in the Neonate

The appropriate use of drugs has made possible the survival of neonates with severe abnormalities who would otherwise die within days or weeks after birth. For example, administration of indomethacin (see Chapter 35) causes the rapid closure of a patent ductus arteriosus, which would otherwise require surgical closure in an infant with a normal heart. Infusion of prostaglandin E_1, on the other hand, causes the ductus to remain open, which can be life-saving in an infant with transposition of the great vessels or tetralogy of Fallot (see Chapter 18). An unexpected effect of such infusion has been described. The drug caused antral hyperplasia with gastric outlet obstruction as a clinical manifestation in 6 of 74 infants who received it. This phenomenon appears to be dose-dependent.

PEDIATRIC DOSAGE FORMS & COMPLIANCE

The form in which a drug is manufactured and the way in which the parent dispenses the drug to the child determine the actual dose administered. Many drugs prepared for children are in the form of elixirs or suspensions. **Elixirs** are alcoholic solutions in which the drug molecules are dissolved and evenly distributed. No shaking is required, and unless some of the vehicle has evaporated, the first dose from the bottle and the last dose should contain equivalent amounts of drug. **Suspensions** contain undissolved particles of drug that must be distributed throughout the vehicle by shaking. If shaking is not thorough each time a dose is given, the first doses from the bottle may contain less drug than the last doses, with the result that less than the expected plasma concentration or effect of the drug may be achieved early in the course of therapy. Conversely, toxicity may occur late in the course of therapy, when it is not expected. This uneven distribution is a potential cause of inefficacy or toxicity in children taking phenytoin suspensions. It is thus essential that the prescriber know the form in which the drug will be dispensed and provide proper instructions to the pharmacist and patient or parent.

Compliance may be more difficult to achieve in pediatric practice than otherwise, since it involves not only the parent's conscientious effort to follow directions but also such practical matters as measuring errors, spilling, and spitting out. For example, the measured volume of "teaspoons" ranges from 2.5 to 7.8 mL. The parents should obtain a calibrated medicine spoon or syringe from the pharmacy. These devices improve the accuracy of dose measurements and simplify administration of drugs to children.

When evaluating compliance, it is often helpful to ask if an attempt has been made to give a further dose after the child has spilled half of what was offered. The parents may not always be able to say with confidence how much of a dose the child actually received. The parents must be told whether or not to wake the infant for its every-6-hour dose day or night. These matters should be discussed and made clear, and no assumptions should be made about what the parents may or may not do. Noncompliance frequently occurs when antibiotics are prescribed to treat otitis media or urinary tract infections and the child feels well after 4 or 5 days of therapy. The parents may not feel there is any reason to continue giving the medicine even though it was prescribed for 10 or 14 days. This common situation should be anticipated so the parents can be told why it is important to continue giving the medicine for the prescribed period even if the child seems to be "cured."

Practical and convenient dosage forms and dosing schedules should be chosen to the extent possible. The easier it is to administer and take the medicine and the easier the dosing schedule is to follow, the more likely it is that compliance will be achieved.

Consistent with their ability to comprehend and cooperate, children should also be given some responsibility for their own health care and for taking medications. This should be discussed in appropriate terms both with the child and with the parents. Possible adverse effects and drug interactions with over-the-counter medicines or foods should also be discussed. Whenever a drug does not achieve its therapeutic effect, the possibility of noncompliance should be considered. There is ample evidence that in such cases parents' or children's reports may be grossly inaccurate. Random pill counts and measurement of serum concentrations may help disclose noncompliance. The use of computerized pill containers, which record each lid opening, has been shown to be very effective in measuring compliance.

Because many pediatric doses are calculated—eg, using body weight—rather than simply read from a list, major dosing errors may result from incorrect calculations. Typically, tenfold errors due to incorrect placement of the decimal point have been described. In the case of digoxin, for example, an intended dose of 0.1 mL containing 5 mcg of drug, when replaced by 1.0 mL—which is still a small volume—can result in fatal overdosage. A good rule for avoiding such "decimal point" errors is to use a leading "0" plus decimal point when dealing with doses less than "1" and to avoid using a zero after a decimal point (see Chapter 66).

DRUG USE DURING LACTATION

Despite the fact that most drugs are excreted into breast milk in amounts too small to adversely affect neonatal health, thousands of women taking medications do not breast-feed because of misperception of risk. Unfortunately, physicians contribute heavily to this bias. It is important to remember that formula feeding is associated with higher morbidity and mortality in all socioeconomic groups.

Most drugs administered to lactating women are detectable in breast milk. Fortunately, the concentration of drugs achieved in breast milk is usually low (Table 60–5). Therefore, the total amount the infant would receive in a day is substantially less than what would be considered a "therapeutic dose." If the nursing mother must take medications and the drug is a relatively safe one, she should optimally take it 30–60 minutes after nursing and 3–4 hours before the next feeding. This allows time for many drugs to be cleared from the mother's blood, and the concentrations in breast milk will be relatively low. Drugs for which no data are available on safety during lactation should be avoided or breast-feeding discontinued while they are being given.

Most antibiotics taken by nursing mothers can be detected in breast milk. Tetracycline concentrations in breast milk are approximately 70% of maternal serum concentrations and present a risk of permanent tooth staining in the infant. Isoniazid rapidly reaches equilibrium between breast milk and maternal blood. The concentrations achieved in breast milk are high enough so that signs of pyridoxine deficiency may occur in the infant if the mother is not given pyridoxine supplements.

Most sedatives and hypnotics achieve concentrations in breast milk sufficient to produce a pharmacologic effect in some infants. Barbiturates taken in hypnotic doses by the mother can produce lethargy, sedation, and poor suck reflexes in the infant. Chloral hydrate can produce sedation if the infant is fed at peak milk concentrations. Diazepam can have a sedative effect on the nursing infant, but, most importantly, its long half-life can result in significant drug accumulation.

Opioids such as heroin, methadone, and morphine enter breast milk in quantities potentially sufficient to prolong the state of neonatal narcotic dependence if the drug was taken chronically by the mother during pregnancy. If conditions are well controlled and there is a good relationship between the mother and the physician,

an infant could be breast-fed while the mother is taking methadone. She should not, however, stop taking the drug abruptly; the infant can be tapered off the methadone as the mother's dose is tapered. The infant should be watched for signs of narcotic withdrawal. Although codeine has been believed to be safe, a recent case of neonatal death from opioid toxicity revealed that the mother was an ultra rapid metabolizer of cytochrome 2D6 substrates, producing substantially higher amounts of morphine. Hence, polymorphism in maternal drug metabolism may affect neonatal exposure and safety.

Minimal use of alcohol by the mother has not been reported to harm nursing infants. Excessive amounts of alcohol, however, can produce alcohol effects in the infant. Nicotine concentrations in the breast milk of smoking mothers are low and do not produce effects in the infant. Very small amounts of caffeine are excreted in the breast milk of coffee-drinking mothers.

Lithium enters breast milk in concentrations equal to those in maternal serum. Clearance of this drug is almost completely dependent upon renal elimination, and women who are receiving lithium may expose the infant to relatively large amounts of the drug.

Radioactive substances such as iodinated ^{125}I albumin and radioiodine can cause thyroid suppression in infants and may increase the risk of subsequent thyroid cancer as much as tenfold. Breast-feeding is contraindicated after large doses and should be withheld for days to weeks after small doses. Similarly, breast-feeding should be avoided in mothers receiving cancer chemotherapy or being treated with cytotoxic or immune-modulating agents for collagen diseases such as lupus erythematosus or after organ transplantation.

PEDIATRIC DRUG DOSAGE

Because of differences in pharmacokinetics in infants and children, simple proportionate reduction in the adult dose may not be adequate to determine a safe and effective pediatric dose. The most reliable pediatric dose information is usually that provided by the manufacturer in the package insert. However, such information is not available for the majority of products, even when studies have been published in the medical literature, reflecting the reluctance of manufacturers to label their products for children. Recently, the FDA has moved toward more explicit expectations that manufacturers test their new products in infants and children. Still, most drugs in the common formularies, eg, *Physicians' Desk Reference,* are not specifically approved for children, in part because manufacturers often lack the economic incentive to evaluate drugs for use in the pediatric market.

Most drugs approved for use in children have recommended pediatric doses, generally stated as milligrams per kilogram or per pound. In the absence of explicit pediatric dose recommendations, an approximation can be made

Table 60–5. Drugs often used during lactation and possible effects on the nursing infant.

Drug	Effect on Infant	Comments
Ampicillin	Minimal	No significant adverse effects; possible occurrence of diarrhea or allergic sensitization.
Aspirin	Minimal	Occasional doses probably safe; high doses may produce significant concentration in breast milk.
Caffeine	Minimal	Caffeine intake in moderation is safe; concentration in breast milk is about 1% of total dose taken by mother.
Chloral hydrate	Significant	May cause drowsiness if infant is fed at peak concentration in milk.
Chloramphenicol	Significant	Concentrations too low to cause gray baby syndrome; possibility of bone marrow suppression does exist; recommend not taking chloramphenicol while breast-feeding.
Chlorothiazide	Minimal	No adverse effects reported.
Chlorpromazine	Minimal	Appears insignificant.
Codeine	Minimal	Safe in most cases. Neonatal toxicity described when the mother is ultra rapid 2D6 metabolizer, producing substantially more morphine from codeine.
Diazepam	Significant	Will cause sedation in breast-fed infants; accumulation can occur in newborns.
Dicumarol	Minimal	No adverse side effects reported; may wish to follow infant's prothrombin time.
Digoxin	Minimal	Insignificant quantities enter breast milk.
Ethanol	Moderate	Moderate ingestion by mother unlikely to produce effects in infant; large amounts consumed by mother can produce alcohol effects in infant.
Heroin	Significant	Enters breast milk and can prolong neonatal narcotic dependence.
Iodine (radioactive)	Significant	Enters milk in quantities sufficient to cause thyroid suppression in infant.
Isoniazid (INH)	Minimal	Milk concentrations equal maternal plasma concentrations. Possibility of pyridoxine deficiency developing in the infant.
Kanamycin	Minimal	No adverse effects reported.
Lithium	Significant	Mother should avoid breast-feeding unless levels can be measured.
Methadone	Significant	(See heroin.) Under close physician supervision, breast-feeding can be continued. Signs of opioid withdrawal in the infant may occur if mother stops taking methadone or stops breast-feeding abruptly.
Oral contraceptives	Minimal	May suppress lactation in high doses.
Penicillin	Minimal	Very low concentrations in breast milk.
Phenobarbital	Moderate	Hypnotic doses can cause sedation in the infant.
Phenytoin	Moderate	Amounts entering breast milk are not sufficient to cause adverse effects in infant.
Prednisone	Moderate	Low maternal doses (5 mg/d) probably safe. Doses 2 or more times physiologic amounts (> 15 mg/d) should probably be avoided.
Propranolol	Minimal	Very small amounts enter breast milk.
Propylthiouracil	Significant	Can suppress thyroid function in infant.
Spironolactone	Minimal	Very small amounts enter breast milk.
Tetracycline	Moderate	Possibility of permanent staining of developing teeth in the infant. Should be avoided during lactation.
Theophylline	Moderate	Can enter breast milk in moderate quantities but not likely to produce significant effects.
Thyroxine	Minimal	No adverse effects in therapeutic doses.
Tolbutamide	Minimal	Low concentrations in breast milk.
Warfarin	Minimal	Very small quantities found in breast milk.

Table 60–6. Determination of drug dosage from surface area.[1]

Weight		Approxi- mate Age	Surface Area (m²)	Percent of Adult Dose
(kg)	(lb)			
3	6.6	Newborn	0.2	12
6	13.2	3 months	0.3	18
10	22	1 year	0.45	28
20	44	5.5 years	0.8	48
30	66	9 years	1	60
40	88	12 years	1.3	78
50	110	14 years	1.5	90
60	132	Adult	1.7	102
70	154	Adult	1.76	103

Reproduced, with permission, from Silver HK, Kempe CH, Bruyn HB: *Handbook of Pediatrics*, 14th ed. Originally published by Lange Medical Publications. Copyright © 1983 by the McGraw-Hill Companies, Inc.

[1]For example, if adult dose is 1 mg/kg, dose for 3-month-old infant would be 0.18 mg/kg or 1.1 mg total.

by any of several methods based on age, weight, or surface area. These rules are not precise and shouldz not be used if the manufacturer provides a pediatric dose. When pediatric doses are calculated (either from one of the methods set forth below or from a manufacturer's dose), the pediatric dose should never exceed the adult dose.

Surface Area, Age, & Weight

Calculations of dosage based on age or weight (see below) are conservative and tend to underestimate the required dose. Doses based on surface area (Table 60–6) are more likely to be adequate.

Age (Young's rule):

$$\text{Dose} = \text{Adult dose} \times \frac{\text{Age (years)}}{\text{Age} + 12}$$

Weight (somewhat more precise is Clark's rule):

$$\text{Dose} = \text{Adult dose} \times \frac{\text{Weight (kg)}}{70}$$

or

$$\text{Dose} = \text{Adult dose} \times \frac{\text{Weight (lb)}}{150}$$

In spite of these approximations, only by conducting studies in children can safe and effective doses for a given age group and condition be determined.

REFERENCES

American Heart Association (AHA) guidelines for cardiopulmonary resuscitation (CPR) and emergency cardiovascular care (ECC) of pediatric and neonatal patients: Pediatric basic life support. Circulation. 2005;112(24 Suppl):IV1.

Benitz WE, Tatro DS: *The Pediatric Drug Handbook*, 3rd ed. Year Book, 1995.

Bennett PN: *Drugs and Human Lactation*, 2nd ed. Elsevier, 1996.

Berlin CM Jr: Advances in pediatric pharmacology and toxicology. Adv Pediatr 1997;44:545.

Besunder JB, Reed MD, Blumer JL: Principles of drug biodisposition in the neonate: A critical evaluation of the pharmacokinetic-pharmacodynamic interface. (Two parts.) Clin Pharmacokinet 1988;14:189, 261.

Briggs GG, Freeman RK, Yaffe SJ: *Drugs in Pregnancy and Lactation. A Reference Guide to Fetal and Neonatal Risk*, 6th ed. Williams & Wilkins, 2002.

Gavin PJ, Yogev R: The role of protease inhibitor therapy in children with HIV infection. Paediatr Drugs 2002;4:581.

Gilman JT: Therapeutic drug monitoring in the neonate and paediatric age group: Problems and clinical pharmacologic implications. Clin Pharmacokinet 1990;19:1.

Hansten PD, Horn JR: *Drug Interactions, Analysis and Management*. Facts & Comparisons. [Quarterly.]

Hendrick V et al: Birth outcomes after prenatal exposure to antidepressant medication. Am J Obstet Gynecol 2003;188:812.

Iqbal MM, Sohhan T, Mahmud SZ: The effects of lithium, valproic acid, and carbamazepine during pregnancy and lactation. J Toxicol Clin Toxicol 2001;39:381.

Ito S, Koren G: Fetal drug therapy. Perinat Clin North Am 1994; 21:1.

Koren G: *Medication Safety during Pregnancy and Breastfeeding; A Clinician's Guide*, 4th ed. McGraw Hill, 2006.

Koren G, Klinger G, Ohlsson A: Fetal pharmacotherapy. Drugs 2002;62:757.

Koren G, Pastuszak A: Prevention of unnecessary pregnancy terminations by counseling women on drug, chemical, and radiation exposure during the first trimester. Teratology 1990; 41:657.

Koren G, Pastuszak A, Ito E: Drugs in pregnancy. N Engl J Med 1998;338:1128.

Loebstein R, Koren G: Clinical pharmacology and therapeutic drug monitoring in neonates and children. Pediatr Rev 1998; 19:423.

Neubert D: Reproductive toxicology: The science today. Teratog Carcinog Mutagen 2002;22:159.

Nottarianni LJ: Plasma protein binding of drugs in pregnancy and in neonates. Clin Pharmacokinet 1990;18:20.

Paap CM, Nahata MC: Clinical pharmacokinetics of antibacterial drugs in neonates. Clin Pharmacokinet 1990;19:280.

Peled N et al: Gastric-outlet obstruction induced by prostaglandin therapy in neonates. N Engl J Med 1992;327:505.

Rousseaux CG, Blakely PM: Fetus. In: Haschek WM, Rousseaux CG (editors). *Handbook of Toxicologic Pathology*. Academic Press, 1991.

van Lingen RA et al: The effects of analgesia in the vulnerable infant during the perinatal period. Clin Perinatol 2002; 29:511.

Special Aspects of Geriatric Pharmacology

61

Bertram G. Katzung, MD, PhD

Society has traditionally classified everyone over 65 as "elderly," but most authorities consider the field of geriatrics to apply to persons over 75—even though this too is an arbitrary definition. Furthermore, chronologic age is only one determinant of the changes pertinent to drug therapy that occur in older people. Important changes in responses to some drugs occur with increasing age in many individuals. For other drugs, age-related changes are minimal, especially in the "healthy old." Drug usage patterns also change as a result of the increasing incidence of disease with age and the tendency to prescribe heavily for patients in nursing homes. General changes in the lives of older people have significant effects on the way drugs are used. Among these changes are the increased incidence with advancing age of multiple diseases, nutritional problems, reduced financial resources, and—in some patients—decreased dosing compliance for a variety of reasons. The health practitioner should be aware of the changes in pharmacologic responses that may occur in older people and how to deal with these changes.

PHARMACOLOGIC CHANGES ASSOCIATED WITH AGING

In the general population, measurements of functional capacity of most of the major organ systems show a decline beginning in young adulthood and continuing throughout life. As shown in Figure 61–1, there is no "middle-age plateau" but rather a linear decrease beginning no later than age 45. However, these data reflect the mean and do not apply to every person above a certain age; approximately one third of healthy subjects have no age-related decrease in, for example, creatinine clearance up to the age of 75. Thus, the elderly do not lose specific functions at an accelerated rate compared with young and middle-aged adults but rather accumulate more deficiencies with the passage of time. Some of these changes result in altered pharmacokinetics. For the pharmacologist and the clinician, the most important of these is the decrease in renal function. Other changes and concurrent diseases may alter the pharmacodynamic characteristics of particular drugs in certain patients.

Pharmacokinetic Changes

A. ABSORPTION

There is little evidence for any major alteration in drug absorption with age. However, conditions associated with age may alter the rate at which some drugs are absorbed. Such conditions include altered nutritional habits, greater consumption of nonprescription drugs (eg, antacids, laxatives), and changes in gastric emptying, which is often slower in older persons, especially in older diabetics.

B. DISTRIBUTION

Compared with young adults, the elderly have reduced lean body mass, reduced body water, and increased fat as a percentage of body mass. Some of these changes are shown in Table 61–1. There is usually a decrease in serum albumin, which binds many drugs, especially weak acids. There may be a concurrent *increase* in serum orosomucoid (α-acid glycoprotein), a protein that binds many basic drugs. Thus, the ratio of bound to free drug may be significantly altered. As explained in Chapter 3, these changes may alter the appropriate loading dose of a drug. However, since both the clearance and the effects of drugs are related to the free concentration, the steady-state effects of a maintenance dosage regimen should not be altered by these factors alone. For example, the loading dose of digoxin in an elderly patient with heart failure should be reduced (if used at all) because of the decreased apparent volume of distribution. The maintenance dose may have to be reduced because of reduced clearance of the drug.

C. METABOLISM

The capacity of the liver to metabolize drugs does not appear to decline consistently with age for all drugs. Animal studies and some clinical studies have suggested that certain drugs are metabolized more slowly; some of

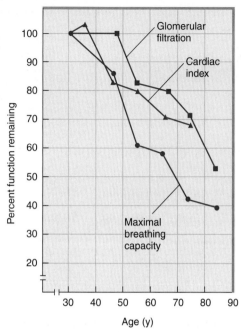

Figure 61–1. Effect of age on some physiologic functions. (Modified and reproduced, with permission, from Kohn RR: *Principles of Mammalian Aging.* Prentice-Hall, 1978.)

these drugs are listed in Table 61–2. The greatest changes are in phase I reactions, ie, those carried out by microsomal P450 systems; there are much smaller changes in the ability of the liver to carry out conjugation (phase II) reactions (see Chapter 4). Some of these

Table 61–1. Some changes related to aging that affect pharmacokinetics of drugs.

Variable	Young Adults (20–30 years)	Older Adults (60–80 years)
Body water (% of body weight)	61	53
Lean body mass (% of body weight)	19	12
Body fat (% of body weight)	26–33 (women) 18–20 (men)	38–45 36–38
Serum albumin (g/dL)	4.7	3.8
Kidney weight (% of young adult)	(100)	80
Hepatic blood flow (% of young adult)	(100)	55–60

Table 61–2. Effects of age on hepatic clearance of some drugs.

Age-Related Decrease in Hepatic Clearance Found	No Age-Related Difference Found
Alprazolam	Ethanol
Barbiturates	Isoniazid
Carbenoxolone	Lidocaine
Chlordiazepoxide	Lorazepam
Chlormethiazole	Nitrazepam
Clobazam	Oxazepam
Desmethyldiazepam	Prazosin
Diazepam	Salicylate
Flurazepam	Warfarin
Imipramine	
Meperidine	
Nortriptyline	
Phenylbutazone	
Propranolol	
Quinidine, quinine	
Theophylline	
Tolbutamide	

changes may be caused by decreased liver blood flow (Table 61–1), an important variable in the clearance of drugs that have a high hepatic extraction ratio. In addition, there is a decline with age of the liver's ability to recover from injury, eg, that caused by alcohol or viral hepatitis. Therefore, a history of recent liver disease in an older person should lead to caution in dosing with drugs that are cleared primarily by the liver, even after apparently complete recovery from the hepatic insult. Finally, malnutrition and diseases that affect hepatic function—eg, heart failure—are more common in the elderly. Heart failure may dramatically alter the ability of the liver to metabolize drugs and may also reduce hepatic blood flow. Similarly, severe nutritional deficiencies, which occur more often in old age, may impair hepatic function.

D. ELIMINATION

Because the kidney is the major organ for clearance of drugs from the body, the age-related decline of renal functional capacity referred to above is very important. The decline in creatinine clearance occurs in about two thirds of the population. It is important to note that this decline is not reflected in an equivalent rise in serum creatinine because the production of creatinine is also reduced as muscle mass declines with age. The practical result of this change is marked prolongation of the half-life of many drugs and the possibility of accumulation to toxic levels if dosage is not reduced in size or frequency. Dosing recommendations for the elderly often include an allowance for reduced renal clearance.

If only the young adult dosage is known for a drug that requires renal clearance, a rough correction can be made by using the Cockcroft-Gault formula, which is applicable to patients from age 40 through age 80:

$$\text{Creatinine clearance (mL/min)} = \frac{(140 - \text{Age}) \times (\text{Weight in kg})}{72 \times \text{Serum creatinine in mg/dL}}$$

For women, the result should be multiplied by 0.85. It must be emphasized that this estimate is, at best, a *population* estimate and may not apply to a particular patient. If the patient has normal renal function (up to one third of elderly patients), a dose corrected on the basis of this estimate will be too low—but a low dose is initially desirable if one is uncertain of the renal function in any patient. If a precise measure is needed, a standard 12- or 24-hour creatinine clearance determination should be obtained. As indicated above, nutritional changes alter pharmacokinetic parameters. A patient who is severely dehydrated (not uncommon in patients with stroke or other motor impairment) may have an additional marked reduction in renal drug clearance that is completely reversible by rehydration.

The lungs are important for the excretion of volatile drugs. As a result of reduced respiratory capacity (Figure 61–1) and the increased incidence of active pulmonary disease in the elderly, the use of inhalation anesthesia is less common and parenteral agents more common in this age group. (See Chapter 25.)

Pharmacodynamic Changes

It was long believed that geriatric patients were much more "sensitive" to the action of many drugs, implying a change in the pharmacodynamic interaction of the drugs with their receptors. It is now recognized that many—perhaps most—of these apparent changes result from altered pharmacokinetics or diminished homeostatic responses. Clinical studies have supported the idea that the elderly are more sensitive to *some* sedative-hypnotics and analgesics. In addition, some data from animal studies suggest actual changes with age in the characteristics or numbers of a few receptors. The most extensive studies show a decrease in responsiveness to β-adrenoceptor agonists. Other examples are discussed below.

Certain homeostatic control mechanisms appear to be blunted in the elderly. Since homeostatic responses are often important components of the total response to a drug, these physiologic alterations may change the pattern or intensity of drug response. In the cardiovascular system, the cardiac output increment required by mild or moderate exercise is successfully provided until at least age 75 (in individuals without obvious cardiac disease), but the increase is the result primarily of increased stroke volume in the elderly and not tachycar-

dia, as in young adults. Average blood pressure goes up with age (in most Western countries), but the incidence of symptomatic orthostatic hypotension also increases markedly. It is thus particularly important to check for orthostatic hypotension on every visit. Similarly, the average 2-hour postprandial blood glucose level increases by about 1 mg/dL for each year of age above 50. Temperature regulation is also impaired, and hypothermia is poorly tolerated in the elderly.

Behavioral & Lifestyle Changes

Major changes in the conditions of daily life accompany the aging process and have an impact on health. Some of these (eg, forgetting to take one's pills) are the result of cognitive changes associated with vascular or other pathology. Others relate to economic stresses associated with greatly reduced income and, possibly, increased expenses due to illness. One of the most important changes is the loss of a spouse.

■ MAJOR DRUG GROUPS

CENTRAL NERVOUS SYSTEM DRUGS

Sedative-Hypnotics

The half-lives of many benzodiazepines and barbiturates increase by 50–150% between age 30 and age 70. Much of this change occurs during the decade from 60 to 70. For many of the benzodiazepines, both the parent molecule and its metabolites (produced in the liver) are pharmacologically active (see Chapter 22). The age-related decline in renal function and liver disease, if present, both contribute to the reduction in elimination of these compounds. In addition, an increased volume of distribution has been reported for some of these drugs. Lorazepam and oxazepam may be less affected by these changes than the other benzodiazepines. In addition to these pharmacokinetic factors, it is generally believed that the elderly vary more in their sensitivity to the sedative-hypnotic drugs on a pharmacodynamic basis as well. Among the toxicities of these drugs, ataxia and other signs of motor impairment should be particularly watched for in order to avoid accidents.

Analgesics

The opioid analgesics show variable changes in pharmacokinetics with age. However, the elderly are often markedly more sensitive to the respiratory effects of these agents because of age-related changes in respiratory function. Therefore, this group of drugs should be used with caution until the sensitivity of the particular patient has been evaluated, and the patient should then be dosed appropriately for full effect. Unfortunately, studies show that opioids are consistently *underutilized* in patients who require strong analgesics for chronic painful conditions such as cancer. There is no justification for underutilization of these drugs, especially in the care of the elderly, and good pain management plans are readily available (see Rabow, 2004; Schug et al, 1992).

Antipsychotic & Antidepressant Drugs

The traditional antipsychotic agents (phenothiazines and haloperidol) have been very heavily used (and probably misused) in the management of a variety of psychiatric diseases in the elderly. There is no doubt that they are useful in the management of schizophrenia in old age, and they are probably useful also in the treatment of some symptoms associated with delirium, dementia, agitation, combativeness, and a paranoid syndrome that occurs in some geriatric patients. However, they are not fully satisfactory in these geriatric conditions, and dosage should not be increased on the assumption that full control is possible. There is no evidence that these drugs have any beneficial effects in Alzheimer's dementia, and on theoretical grounds the antimuscarinic effects of the phenothiazines might be expected to worsen memory impairment and intellectual dysfunction (see below). Much of the apparent improvement in agitated and combative patients may simply reflect the sedative effects of the drugs. When a sedative antipsychotic is desired, a phenothiazine such as thioridazine is appropriate. If sedation is to be avoided, haloperidol is more appropriate. The latter drug has increased extrapyramidal toxicity, however, and should be avoided in patients with preexisting extrapyramidal disease. The phenothiazines, especially older drugs such as chlorpromazine, often induce orthostatic hypotension because of their α-adrenoceptor-blocking effects. They are even more prone to do so in the elderly.

Because of increased responsiveness to all these drugs, dosage should usually be started at a fraction of that used in young adults. The half-lives of some phenothiazines are increased in the geriatric population. Thioridazine's half-life, for example, is more than doubled. Plasma protein binding of fluphenazine is reduced, which results in an increase of the free drug:total drug ratio.

Lithium is often used in the treatment of mania in the aged. Because it is cleared by the kidneys, dosages must be adjusted appropriately and blood levels monitored. Concurrent use of thiazide diuretics reduces the clearance of lithium and should be accompanied by further reduction in dosage and more frequent measurement of lithium blood levels.

Psychiatric depression is thought to be underdiagnosed and undertreated in the elderly. The suicide rate in the over-65 age group (twice the national average) supports this view. Unfortunately, the apathy, flat affect, and social withdrawal of major depression may be mistaken for senile dementia. Clinical evidence suggests that the elderly are as responsive to antidepressants (of all types) as younger patients but are more likely to experience toxic effects. This factor along with the reduced clearance of some of these drugs underlines the importance of careful dosing and strict attention to the appearance of toxic effects. If a tricyclic antidepressant is to be used, a drug with reduced antimuscarinic effects should be selected, eg, nortriptyline or desipramine (see Table 30–2). To minimize autonomic effects, a selective serotonin reuptake inhibitor (SSRI) may be chosen.

Drugs Used in Alzheimer's Disease

Alzheimer's disease is characterized by progressive impairment of memory and cognitive functions and may lead to a completely vegetative state and early death. The biochemical defects responsible for these changes have not been identified, but there is much evidence for a marked decrease in choline acetyltransferase and other markers of cholinergic neuron activity and for changes in brain glutamate, dopamine, norepinephrine, serotonin, and somatostatin activity. Eventually, cholinergic and perhaps other neurons die or are destroyed. Patients with Alzheimer's disease are often exquisitely sensitive to the central nervous system toxicities of drugs with antimuscarinic effects. There is also evidence for abnormal neuronal lipoprotein processing, and one familial form of Alzheimer's disease is strongly associated with an abnormal lipoprotein, apolipoprotein E4.

Many methods of treatment of Alzheimer's disease have been explored. Most attention has been focused on the cholinomimetic drugs because of the evidence for loss of cholinergic neurons noted above. Monoamine oxidase (MAO) type B inhibition with selegiline (L-deprenyl) has been suggested to have some beneficial effects. "Ampakines," substances that facilitate synaptic activity at glutamate AMPA receptors, and nerve growth factors (see Chapter 21), are also under intense study, and one drug that inhibits NMDA glutamate receptors is available (see below). Some evidence suggests that lipid-lowering statins are beneficial. So-called cerebral vasodilators are ineffective.

Tacrine (tetrahydroaminoacridine, THA), a long-acting cholinesterase inhibitor and muscarinic modulator, was the first drug shown to have any benefit in Alzheimer's disease. Tacrine is orally active, enters the central nervous system readily, and has a duration of effect of 6–8 hours. Tacrine blocks both acetylcholinesterase and butyrylcholinesterase and has complex inhibitory effects on M_1, M_2, and nicotinic cholinoceptors. The drug apparently increases the release of acetylcholine from cholinergic nerve endings as well. Finally, tacrine may inhibit MAO, decrease the release of γ-aminobutyric acid, and increase the release of norepinephrine, dopamine, and serotonin from nerve endings. **Donepezil, rivastigmine,** and **galantamine** are newer cholinesterase inhibitors with adequate penetration into the central nervous system and a spectrum of action more limited to indirect cholinomimetic effects than tacrine's. Although the evidence for benefit from cholinesterase inhibitors appears to be robust, the effect is very modest and, at best, only delays further cognitive decline.

Tacrine causes significant adverse effects, including nausea and vomiting, and potentially dangerous hepatic toxicity. The latter is manifested by a reversible increase in serum levels of aspartate or alanine aminotransferase of sufficient magnitude to require dose reduction or withdrawal in 40–50% of patients. Hepatocellular necrosis with jaundice has been reported. The newer drugs appear to be significantly safer than tacrine. The cholinesterase inhibitors should be used with caution in patients receiving other drugs that inhibit cytochrome P450 enzymes (eg, ketoconazole, quinidine; see Chapter 4). Preparations available are listed in Chapter 7.

Excitotoxic activation of glutamate transmission via NMDA receptors has been postulated to contribute to the pathophysiology of Alzheimer's disease. **Memantine** binds to NMDA receptor channels in a use-dependent manner and produces a noncompetitive blockade. This drug may slow progression of the disease. It appears to be better tolerated and less toxic than the cholinesterase inhibitors. Memantine is available as Namenda in 5 and 10 mg oral tablets.

CARDIOVASCULAR DRUGS

Antihypertensive Drugs

As noted previously, blood pressure, especially systolic pressure, increases with age in Western countries and in most cultures in which salt intake is high. In women, the increase is more marked after age 50. The high frequency and sometimes benign course of this form of late-onset systolic hypertension encouraged a conservative approach to its treatment in the past. It is now clear, however, that uncontrolled hypertension leads to the same sequelae in elderly as in younger individuals. Most clinicians believe that hypertension should be treated vigorously in the elderly.

The basic principles of therapy are not different in the geriatric age group from those described in Chapter 11, but the usual cautions regarding altered pharmacokinetics and sensitivity apply. Because of its safety, nondrug therapy (weight reduction in the obese and salt restriction) should be encouraged. Thiazides are a rea-

sonable first step in drug therapy. The hypokalemia, hyperglycemia, and hyperuricemia caused by these agents are more relevant in the elderly because of the higher incidence in these patients of arrhythmias, type 2 diabetes, and gout. Thus, use of low antihypertensive doses—rather than maximum diuretic doses—is important. Calcium channel blockers are effective and safe if titrated to the appropriate response. They are especially useful in patients who also have atherosclerotic angina (see Chapter 12). Beta blockers are potentially hazardous in patients with obstructive airway disease and are considered less useful than calcium channel blockers in older patients unless heart failure is present. Angiotensin-converting enzyme inhibitors are also considered less useful in the elderly unless heart failure or diabetes is present. The most powerful drugs, such as guanethidine and minoxidil, are rarely needed. Every patient receiving antihypertensive drugs should be checked regularly for orthostatic hypotension because of the danger of cerebral ischemia and falls.

Positive Inotropic Agents

Heart failure is a common and particularly lethal disease in the elderly. Fear of this condition may be one reason why physicians overuse cardiac glycosides in this age group. The toxic effects of this drug group are particularly dangerous in the geriatric population, since the elderly are more susceptible to arrhythmias. The clearance of digoxin is usually decreased in the older age group, and while the volume of distribution is often decreased as well, the half-life of this drug may be increased by 50% or more. Because the drug is cleared mostly by the kidneys, renal function must be considered in designing a dosage regimen. There is no evidence that there is any increase in pharmacodynamic sensitivity to the therapeutic effects of the cardiac glycosides; in fact, animal studies suggest a possible decrease in therapeutic sensitivity. On the other hand, as noted above, there is probably an increase in sensitivity to the toxic arrhythmogenic actions. Hypokalemia, hypomagnesemia, hypoxemia (from pulmonary disease), and coronary atherosclerosis all contribute to the high incidence of digitalis-induced arrhythmias in geriatric patients. The less common toxicities of digitalis such as delirium, visual changes, and endocrine abnormalities (see Chapter 13) also occur more often in older than in younger patients.

Antiarrhythmic Agents

The treatment of arrhythmias in the elderly is particularly challenging because of the lack of good hemodynamic reserve, the frequency of electrolyte disturbances, and the high prevalence of severe coronary disease. The clearances of quinidine and procainamide decrease and their half-lives increase with age. Disopyramide should probably be avoided in the geriatric population because its major toxicities—antimuscarinic action, leading to voiding problems in men; and negative inotropic cardiac effects, leading to heart failure—are particularly undesirable in these patients. The clearance of lidocaine appears to be little changed, but the half-life is increased in the elderly. Although this observation implies an increase in the volume of distribution, it has been recommended that the loading dose of this drug be reduced in geriatric patients because of their greater sensitivity to its toxic effects.

Recent evidence indicates that many patients with atrial fibrillation—a very common arrhythmia in the elderly—do as well with simple control of ventricular rate as with conversion to normal sinus rhythm. Of course, measures (such as anticoagulant drugs) should be taken to reduce the risk of thromboembolism in chronic atrial fibrillation.

ANTIMICROBIAL DRUGS

Several age-related changes contribute to the high incidence of infections in geriatric patients. There appears to be a reduction in host defenses in the elderly, manifested in the increase in both serious infections and cancer. This may reflect an alteration in T-lymphocyte function. In the lungs, a major age- and tobacco-dependent decrease in mucociliary clearance significantly increases susceptibility to infection. In the urinary tract, the incidence of serious infection is greatly increased by urinary retention and catheterization in men.

Since 1940, the antimicrobial drugs have contributed more to the prolongation of life than any other drug group because they can compensate to some extent for this deterioration in natural defenses. The basic principles of therapy of the elderly with these agents are no different from those applicable in younger patients and have been presented in Chapter 51. The major pharmacokinetic changes relate to decreased renal function; because most of the β-lactam, aminoglycoside, and fluoroquinolone antibiotics are excreted by this route, important changes in half-life may be expected. This is particularly important in the case of the aminoglycosides, because they cause concentration- and time-dependent toxicity in the kidney and in other organs. For gentamicin, kanamycin, and netilmicin, the half-lives are more than doubled. According to one study, the increase may not be so marked for tobramycin.

ANTI-INFLAMMATORY DRUGS

Osteoarthritis is a very common disease of the elderly. Rheumatoid arthritis is less exclusively a geriatric problem, but the same drug therapy is usually applicable. The basic principles laid down in Chapter 36 and the properties of the anti-inflammatory drugs described there apply fully here.

The nonsteroidal anti-inflammatory agents (NSAIDs) must be used with special care in geriatric patients because they cause toxicities to which the elderly are very susceptible. In the case of aspirin, the most important of these is gastrointestinal irritation and bleeding. In the case of the newer NSAIDs, the most important is renal damage, which may be irreversible. Because they are cleared primarily by the kidneys, these drugs will accumulate more rapidly in the geriatric patient and especially in the patient whose renal function is already compromised beyond the average range for his or her age. A vicious circle is easily set up in which cumulation of the NSAID causes more renal damage, which causes more cumulation. There is no evidence that the COX-2-selective NSAIDs are safer with regard to renal function. Elderly patients receiving high doses of any NSAID should be carefully monitored for changes in renal function.

Corticosteroids are extremely useful in elderly patients who cannot tolerate full doses of NSAIDs. However, they consistently cause a dose- and duration-related increase in osteoporosis, an especially hazardous toxic effect in the elderly. It is not certain whether this drug-induced effect can be reduced by increased calcium and vitamin D intake, but it would seem prudent to consider these agents (and bisphosphonates if osteoporosis is already present) and to encourage frequent exercise in any patient taking corticosteroids.

■ ADVERSE DRUG REACTIONS IN THE ELDERLY

The positive relationship between number of drugs taken and the incidence of adverse reactions to them has been well documented. In long-term care facilities, in which a high fraction of the population is elderly, the average number of prescriptions per patient varies between 6 and 8. Studies have shown that the percentage of patients with adverse reactions increases from about 10% when a single drug is being taken to nearly 100% when ten drugs are taken. Thus, it may be expected that about half of patients in long-term care facilities will have recognized or unrecognized reactions at some time. The overall incidence of drug reactions in geriatric patients is estimated to be at least twice that in the younger population. Reasons for this high incidence undoubtedly include errors in prescribing on the part of the practitioner and errors in drug usage by the patient.

Practitioner errors sometimes occur because the physician does not appreciate the importance of changes in pharmacokinetics with age and age-related diseases. Some errors occur because the practitioner is unaware of incompatible drugs prescribed by other practitioners for the same patient. For example, cimetidine, an H_2-blocking drug heavily prescribed (or recommended in its over-the-counter form) to the elderly, causes a much higher incidence of untoward effects (eg, confusion, slurred speech) in the geriatric population than in younger patients. It also inhibits the hepatic metabolism of many drugs, including phenytoin, warfarin, β blockers, and other agents. A patient who has been taking one of the latter agents without untoward effect may develop markedly elevated blood levels and severe toxicity if cimetidine is added to the regimen without adjustment of dosage of the other drugs. Additional examples of drugs that inhibit liver microsomal enzymes and lead to adverse reactions are described in Chapter 4 and Appendix II.

Patient errors may result from noncompliance for reasons described below. In addition, they often result from use of nonprescription drugs taken without the knowledge of the physician. As noted in Chapters 64 and 65, many over-the-counter agents and herbal medications contain "hidden ingredients" with potent pharmacologic effects. For example, many antihistamines have significant sedative effects and are inherently more hazardous in patients with impaired cognitive function. Similarly, their antimuscarinic action may precipitate urinary retention in geriatric men or glaucoma in the patient with a narrow anterior chamber angle. If the patient is also taking a metabolism inhibitor such as cimetidine, the probability of an adverse reaction is greatly increased. A patient taking an herbal medication containing gingko is more likely to experience bleeding while taking low doses of aspirin.

■ PRACTICAL ASPECTS OF GERIATRIC PHARMACOLOGY

The quality of life in elderly patients can be greatly improved and life span can be prolonged by the intelligent use of drugs. However, there are several practical obstacles to compliance that the prescriber must recognize.

The expense of drugs can be a major disincentive in patients receiving marginal retirement incomes who are not covered or inadequately covered by health insurance. The prescriber must be aware of the cost of the prescription and of cheaper alternative therapies. For example, the monthly cost of arthritis therapy with newer NSAIDs may exceed $100, while that for generic aspirin is about $5 and for ibuprofen, an older NSAID, about $20.

Noncompliance may result from forgetfulness or confusion, especially if the patient has several prescrip-

tions and different dosing intervals. A survey carried out in 1986 showed that the population over 65 years of age accounted for 32% of drugs prescribed in the USA, although these patients represented only 11–12% of the population at that time. Since the prescriptions are often written by several different practitioners, there is usually no attempt to design "integrated" regimens that use drugs with similar dosing intervals for the conditions being treated. Patients may forget instructions regarding the need to complete a fixed duration of therapy when a course of anti-infective drug is being given. The disappearance of symptoms is often regarded as the best reason to halt drug taking, especially if the prescription was expensive.

Noncompliance may also be deliberate. A decision not to take a drug may be based on prior experience with it. There may be excellent reasons for such "intelligent" noncompliance, and the practitioner should try to elicit them. Such efforts may also improve compliance with alternative drugs, because enlisting the patient as a participant in therapeutic decisions tends to increase the motivation to succeed.

Some errors in drug taking are caused by physical disabilities. Arthritis, tremor, and visual problems may all contribute. Liquid medications that are to be measured out "by the spoonful" are especially inappropriate for patients with any type of tremor or motor disability. The use of a pediatric dosing syringe may be helpful in such cases. Because of decreased production of saliva, older patients often have difficulty swallowing large tablets. "Childproof" containers are often "patient-proof" if the patient has arthritis. Cataracts and macular degeneration occur in a large number of patients over 70; therefore, labels on prescription bottles should be large enough for the patient with diminished vision to read, or color-coded if the patient can see but can no longer read.

Drug therapy has considerable potential for both helpful and harmful effects in the geriatric patient. The balance may be tipped in the right direction by adherence to a few principles:

(1) Take a careful drug history. The disease to be treated may be drug-induced, or drugs being taken may lead to interactions with drugs to be prescribed.

(2) Prescribe only for a specific and rational indication. Do not prescribe omeprazole for "dyspepsia."

(3) Define the goal of drug therapy. Then start with small doses and titrate to the response desired. Wait at least three half-lives (adjusted for age) before increasing the dose. If the expected response does not occur at the normal adult dosage, check blood levels. If the expected response does not occur at the appropriate blood level, switch to a different drug.

(4) Maintain a high index of suspicion regarding drug reactions and interactions. Know what other drugs the patient is taking.

(5) Simplify the regimen as much as possible. When multiple drugs are prescribed, try to use drugs that can be taken at the same time of day. Whenever possible, reduce the number of drugs being taken.

REFERENCES

Ancolli-Israel S, Ayalon L: Diagnosis and treatment of sleep disorders in older adults. Am J Geriatr Psychiatry 2006;14:95.

Aronow WS: Drug treatment of systolic and diastolic heart failure in elderly persons. J Gerontol A Biol Med Sci 2005; 60:1597.

Birnbaum LS: Pharmacokinetic basis of age-related changes in sensitivity to toxicants. Annu Rev Pharmacol Toxicol 1991; 31:101.

Chatap G, Giraud K, Vincent JP: Atrial fibrillation in the elderly: Facts and management. Drugs Aging 2002;19:819.

Cockcroft DW, Gault MH: Prediction of creatinine clearance from serum creatinine. Nephron 1976;16:31.

Dergal JM et al: Potential interactions between herbal medicines and conventional drug therapies used by older adults attending a memory clinic. Drugs Aging 2002;19:879.

Docherty JR: Age-related changes in adrenergic neuroeffector transmission. Auton Neurosci 2002;96:8.

Drugs in the elderly. Med Lett Drugs Therap 2006;48:6.

Ferrari AU: Modifications of the cardiovascular system with aging. Am J Geriatr Cardiol 2002;11:30.

Flynn BL, Theeson KA: Pharmacologic management of Alzheimer disease part III: Nonsteroidal anti-inflammatory drugs—emerging protective evidence? Ann Pharmacother 1999;33:840.

Goldberg TH, Finkelstein MS: Difficulties in estimating glomerular filtration rate in the elderly. Arch Intern Med 1987; 147:1430.

Karlsson I: Drugs that induce delirium. Dement Geriatr Cogn Disord 1999;10:412.

Kirby J et al: A systematic review of the clinical and cost-effectiveness of memantine in patients with moderately severe to severe Alzheimer's disease. Drugs Aging. 2006;23:227.

Mangoni AA: Cardiovascular drug therapy in elderly patients: Specific age-related pharmacokinetic, pharmacodynamic and therapeutic considerations. Drugs Aging 2005;22:913.

McLean AJ, LeCouteur DG: Aging biology and geriatric clinical pharmacology. Pharmacol Rev 2004;56:163.

Palmer A: Pharmacotherapy for Alzheimer's disease: Progress and prospects. Trends Pharmacol Sci 2002;23:426.

Rabow MW, Pantilat SZ: Care at the end of life. *Current Medical Diagnosis & Treatment,* 43rd ed, Tierney LM, McPhee SJ, Papadakis MA, eds. McGraw-Hill, 2004

Richards SS, Hendrie HC: Diagnosis, management, and treatment of Alzheimer disease: A guide for the internist. Arch Intern Med 1999;159:789.

Rodriguez EG et al: Use of lipid-lowering drugs in older adults with and without dementia: A community-based epidemiological study. J Am Geriatr Soc 2002;50:1852.

Sawhney R, Sehl M, Naeim A: Physiologic aspects of aging: Impact on cancer management and decision making, part I. Cancer J 2005;11:449.

Schug SA, Dunlap R, Zech D: Pharmacologic management of cancer pain. Drugs 1992;43:44.

Staskin DR: Overactive bladder in the elderly: A guide to pharmacological management. Drugs Aging 2005;22:1013.

Vik SA et al: Medication nonadherence and subsequent risk of hospitalisation and mortality among older adults. Drugs Aging 2006;23:345.

Wade PR: Aging and neural control of the GI tract. I. Age-related changes in the enteric nervous system. Am J Physiol Gastrointest Liver Physiol 2002;283:G489.

Dermatologic Pharmacology

62

Dirk B. Robertson, MD, & Howard I. Maibach, MD

The skin offers a number of special opportunities to the clinician. For example, the topical route of administration is especially appropriate for diseases of the skin, although some dermatologic diseases respond as well or better to drugs administered systemically.

The general pharmacokinetic principles governing the use of drugs applied to the skin are the same as those involved in other routes of drug administration (see Chapters 1 and 3). Although often depicted as a simple three-layered structure, human skin is a complex series of diffusion barriers. Quantitation of the flux of drugs and drug vehicles through these barriers is the basis for pharmacokinetic analysis of dermatologic therapy, and techniques for making such measurements are rapidly increasing in number and sensitivity.

Major variables that determine pharmacologic response to drugs applied to the skin include the following:

(1) Regional variation in drug penetration: For example, the scrotum, face, axilla, and scalp are far more permeable than the forearm and may require less drug for equivalent effect.

(2) Concentration gradient: Increasing the concentration gradient increases the mass of drug transferred per unit time, just as in the case of diffusion across other barriers (see Chapter 1). Thus, resistance to topical corticosteroids can sometimes be overcome by use of higher concentrations of drug.

(3) Dosing schedule: Because of its physical properties, the skin acts as a reservoir for many drugs. As a result, the "local half-life" may be long enough to permit once-daily application of drugs with short systemic half-lives. For example, once-daily application of corticosteroids appears to be just as effective as multiple applications in many conditions.

(4) Vehicles and occlusion: An appropriate vehicle maximizes the ability of the drug to penetrate the outer layers of the skin. In addition, through their physical properties (moistening or drying effects), vehicles may themselves have important therapeutic effects. Occlusion (application of a plastic wrap to hold the drug and its vehicle in close contact with the skin) is extremely effective in maximizing efficacy.

■ DERMATOLOGIC VEHICLES

Topical medications usually consist of active ingredients incorporated in a vehicle that facilitates cutaneous application. Important considerations in selection of a vehicle include the solubility of the active agent in the vehicle; the rate of release of the agent from the vehicle; the ability of the vehicle to hydrate the stratum corneum, thus enhancing penetration; the stability of the therapeutic agent in the vehicle; and interactions, chemical and physical, of the vehicle, stratum corneum, and active agent.

Depending upon the vehicle, dermatologic formulations may be classified as tinctures, wet dressings, lotions, gels, aerosols, powders, pastes, creams, and ointments. The ability of the vehicle to retard evaporation from the surface of the skin increases in this series, being least in tinctures and wet dressings and greatest in ointments. In general, acute inflammation with oozing, vesiculation, and crusting is best treated with drying preparations such as tinctures, wet dressings, and lotions, whereas chronic inflammation with xerosis, scaling, and lichenification is best treated with more lubricating preparations such as creams and ointments. Tinctures, lotions, gels, and aerosols are convenient for application to the scalp and hairy areas. Emulsified vanishing-type creams may be used in intertriginous areas without causing maceration.

Emulsifying agents are used to provide homogeneous, stable preparations when mixtures of immiscible liquids such as oil-in-water creams are compounded. Some patients develop irritation from these agents. Substituting a preparation that does not contain them or using one containing a lower concentration may resolve the problem.

991

■ ANTIBACTERIAL AGENTS

TOPICAL ANTIBACTERIAL PREPARATIONS

Topical antibacterial agents may be useful in preventing infections in clean wounds, in the early treatment of infected dermatoses and wounds, in reducing colonization of the nares by staphylococci, in axillary deodorization, and in the management of acne vulgaris. The efficacy of antibiotics in these topical applications is not uniform. The general pharmacology of the antimicrobial drugs is discussed in Chapters 43–51.

Numerous topical anti-infectives contain corticosteroids in addition to antibiotics. There is no convincing evidence that topical corticosteroids inhibit the antibacterial effect of antibiotics when the two are incorporated in the same preparation. In the treatment of secondarily infected dermatoses, which are usually colonized with streptococci, staphylococci, or both, combination therapy may prove superior to corticosteroid therapy alone. Antibiotic-corticosteroid combinations may be useful in treating diaper dermatitis, otitis externa, and impetiginized eczema.

The selection of a particular antibiotic depends of course upon the diagnosis and, when appropriate, in vitro culture and sensitivity studies of clinical samples. The pathogens isolated from most infected dermatoses are group A β-hemolytic streptococci, *Staphylococcus aureus,* or both. The pathogens present in surgical wounds will be those resident in the environment. Information about regional patterns of drug resistance is therefore important in selecting a therapeutic agent. Prepackaged topical antibacterial preparations that contain multiple antibiotics are available in fixed dosages well above the therapeutic threshold. These formulations offer the advantages of efficacy in mixed infections, broader coverage for infections due to undetermined pathogens, and delayed microbial resistance to any single component antibiotic.

1. Bacitracin & Gramicidin

Bacitracin and gramicidin are peptide antibiotics, active against gram-positive organisms such as streptococci, pneumococci, and staphylococci. In addition, most anaerobic cocci, neisseriae, tetanus bacilli, and diphtheria bacilli are sensitive. Bacitracin is compounded in an ointment base alone or in combination with neomycin, polymyxin B, or both. The use of bacitracin in the anterior nares may temporarily decrease colonization by pathogenic staphylococci. Microbial resistance may develop following prolonged use. Bacitracin-induced contact urticaria syndrome, including anaphylaxis, occurs rarely. Allergic contact dermatitis occurs frequently. Bacitracin is poorly absorbed through the skin, so systemic toxicity is rare.

Gramicidin is available only for topical use, in combination with other antibiotics such as neomycin, polymyxin, bacitracin, and nystatin. Systemic toxicity limits this drug to topical use. The incidence of sensitization following topical application is exceedingly low in therapeutic concentrations.

2. Mupirocin

Mupirocin (pseudomonic acid A) is structurally unrelated to other currently available topical antibacterial agents. Most gram-positive aerobic bacteria, including methicillin-resistant *S aureus,* are sensitive to mupirocin (see Chapter 50). It is effective in the treatment of impetigo caused by *S aureus* and group A β-hemolytic streptococci.

Intranasal mupirocin in Bactroban Nasal ointment for eliminating nasal carriage of *S aureus* may be associated with irritation of mucous membranes caused by the polyethylene glycol vehicle. Mupirocin is not appreciably absorbed systemically after topical application to intact skin.

3. Polymyxin B Sulfate

Polymyxin B is a peptide antibiotic effective against gram-negative organisms, including *Pseudomonas aeruginosa, Escherichia coli,* enterobacter, and klebsiella. Most strains of proteus and serratia are resistant, as are all gram-positive organisms. Topical preparations may be compounded in either a solution or ointment base. Numerous prepackaged antibiotic combinations containing polymyxin B are available. Detectable serum concentrations are difficult to achieve from topical application, but the total daily dose applied to denuded skin or open wounds should not exceed 200 mg in order to reduce the likelihood of neurotoxicity and nephrotoxicity. Hypersensitivity to topically applied polymyxin B sulfate is uncommon.

4. Neomycin & Gentamicin

Neomycin and gentamicin are aminoglycoside antibiotics active against gram-negative organisms, including *E coli,* proteus, klebsiella, and enterobacter. Gentamicin generally shows greater activity against *P aeruginosa* than neomycin. Gentamicin is also more active against staphylococci and group A β-hemolytic streptococci. Widespread topical use of gentamicin, especially in a hospital environment, should be avoided to slow the appearance of gentamicin-resistant organisms.

Neomycin is available in numerous topical formulations, both alone and in combination with polymyxin, bacitracin, and other antibiotics. It is also available as a sterile powder for topical use. Gentamicin is available as an ointment or cream.

Topical application of neomycin rarely results in detectable serum concentrations. However, in the case of gentamicin, serum concentrations of 1–18 mcg/mL are possible if the drug is applied in a water-miscible preparation to large areas of denuded skin, as in burned patients. Both drugs are water-soluble and are excreted primarily in the urine. Renal failure may permit the accumulation of these antibiotics, with possible nephrotoxicity, neurotoxicity, and ototoxicity.

Neomycin frequently causes sensitization, particularly if applied to eczematous dermatoses or if compounded in an ointment vehicle. When sensitization occurs, cross-sensitivity to streptomycin, kanamycin, paromomycin, and gentamicin is possible.

5. Topical Antibiotics in Acne

Several systemic antibiotics that have traditionally been used in the treatment of acne vulgaris have been shown to be effective when applied topically. Currently, four antibiotics are so utilized: clindamycin phosphate, erythromycin base, metronidazole, and sulfacetamide. The effectiveness of topical therapy is less than that achieved by systemic administration of the same antibiotic. Therefore, topical therapy is generally suitable in mild to moderate cases of inflammatory acne.

Clindamycin

Clindamycin has in vitro activity against *Propionibacterium acnes;* this has been postulated as the mechanism of its beneficial effect in acne therapy. Approximately 10% of an applied dose is absorbed, and rare cases of bloody diarrhea and pseudomembranous colitis have been reported following topical application. The hydroalcoholic vehicle and foam formulation (Evoclin) may cause drying and irritation of the skin, with complaints of burning and stinging. The water-based gel and lotion formulations are well tolerated and less likely to cause irritation. Allergic contact dermatitis is uncommon. Clindamycin is also available in a fixed-combination topical gel with benzoyl peroxide (BenzaClin, Duac).

Erythromycin

In topical preparations, the base of erythromycin rather than a salt is used to facilitate penetration. Although the mechanism of action of topical erythromycin in inflammatory acne vulgaris is unknown, it is presumed to be due to its inhibitory effects on *P acnes.* One of the possible complications of topical therapy is the development of antibiotic-resistant strains of organisms, including staphylococci. If this occurs in association with a clinical infection, topical erythromycin should be dis-

continued and appropriate systemic antibiotic therapy started. Adverse local reactions to erythromycin solution may include a burning sensation at the time of application and drying and irritation of the skin. The topical water-based gel is less drying and may be better-tolerated. Allergic hypersensitivity appears to be uncommon. Erythromycin is also available in a fixed combination preparation with benzoyl peroxide (Benzamycin) for topical treatment of acne vulgaris.

Metronidazole

Topical metronidazole is effective in the treatment of acne rosacea. The mechanism of action is unknown, but it may relate to the inhibitory effects of metronidazole on *Demodex brevis* or as an anti-inflammatory agent by direct effect on neutrophil cellular function. Oral metronidazole has been shown to be a carcinogen in susceptible rodent species, and topical use during pregnancy and by nursing mothers and children is therefore not recommended.

Adverse local effects of the water-based gel formulation (MetroGel) include dryness, burning, and stinging. Less drying formulations may be better-tolerated (MetroCream, MetroLotion, and Noritate cream). Caution should be exercised when applying metronidazole near the eyes to avoid excessive tearing.

Sodium Sulfacetamide

Topical sulfacetamide is available alone as a 10% lotion (Klaron) and as a 10% wash (Ovace), and in several preparations in combination with sulfur for the treatment of acne vulgaris and acne rosacea. The mechanism of action is thought to be inhibition of *P acnes* by competitive inhibition of *p*-aminobenzoic acid utilization. Approximately 4% of topically applied sulfacetamide is absorbed percutaneously, and its use is therefore contraindicated in patients having a known hypersensitivity to sulfonamides.

■ ANTIFUNGAL AGENTS

The treatment of superficial fungal infections caused by dermatophytic fungi may be accomplished (1) with topical antifungal agents, eg, clotrimazole, miconazole, econazole, ketoconazole, oxiconazole, sulconazole, ciclopirox olamine, naftifine, terbinafine, butenafine, and tolnaftate; or (2) with orally administered agents, ie, griseofulvin, terbinafine, ketoconazole, fluconazole, and itraconazole. Superficial infections caused by candida species may be treated with topical applications of clotrimazole, miconazole, econazole, ketoconazole, oxiconazole, ciclopirox olamine, nystatin, or amphotericin B. Chronic generalized mucocutaneous candidiasis is responsive to long-term therapy with oral ketoconazole.

TOPICAL ANTIFUNGAL PREPARATIONS

1. Topical Azole Derivatives

The topical imidazoles, which currently include clotrimazole, econazole, ketoconazole, miconazole, oxiconazole, and sulconazole, have a wide range of activity against dermatophytes (epidermophyton, microsporum, and trichophyton) and yeasts, including *Candida albicans* and *Pityrosporum orbiculare*.

Miconazole (Monistat, Micatin) is available for topical application as a cream or lotion and as vaginal cream or suppositories for use in vulvovaginal candidiasis. Clotrimazole (Lotrimin, Mycelex) is available for topical application to the skin as a cream or lotion and as vaginal cream and tablets for use in vulvovaginal candidiasis. Econazole (Spectazole) is available as a cream for topical application. Oxiconazole (Oxistat) is available as a cream and lotion for topical use. Ketoconazole (Nizoral) is available as a cream for topical treatment of dermatophytosis and candidiasis and as a shampoo for the treatment of seborrheic dermatitis. Sulconazole (Exelderm) is available as a cream or solution. Topical antifungal-corticosteroid fixed combinations have recently been introduced on the basis of providing more rapid symptomatic improvement than an antifungal agent alone. Clotrimazole-betamethasone dipropionate cream (Lotrisone) is one such combination.

Once- or twice-daily application to the affected area will generally result in clearing of superficial dermatophyte infections in 2–3 weeks, although the medication should be continued until eradication of the organism is confirmed. Paronychial and intertriginous candidiasis can be treated effectively by any of these agents when applied three or four times daily. Seborrheic dermatitis should be treated with twice-daily applications of ketoconazole until clinical clearing is obtained.

Adverse local reactions to the imidazoles may include stinging, pruritus, erythema, and local irritation. Allergic contact dermatitis appears to be uncommon.

2. Ciclopirox Olamine

Ciclopirox olamine is a synthetic broad-spectrum antimycotic agent with inhibitory activity against dermatophytes, candida species, and *P orbiculare*. This agent appears to inhibit the uptake of precursors of macromolecular synthesis; the site of action is probably the fungal cell membrane.

Pharmacokinetic studies indicate that 1–2% of the dose is absorbed when applied as a solution on the back under an occlusive dressing. Ciclopirox olamine is available as a 1% cream and lotion (Loprox) for the topical treatment of dermatomycosis, candidiasis, and tinea versicolor. The incidence of adverse reactions has been low. Pruritus and worsening of clinical disease have been reported. The potential for delayed allergic contact hypersensitivity appears small.

Topical 8% ciclopirox olamine (Penlac nail lacquer) has been approved for the treatment of mild to moderate onychomycosis of fingernails and toenails. Although well tolerated with minimal side effects, the overall cure rates in clinical trials are less than 12%.

3. Allylamines: Naftifine & Terbinafine

Naftifine hydrochloride and terbinafine (Lamisil) are allylamines that are highly active against dermatophytes but less active against yeasts. The antifungal activity derives from selective inhibition of squalene epoxidase, a key enzyme for the synthesis of ergosterol.

They are available as 1% creams and other forms for the topical treatment of dermatophytosis, to be applied on a twice-daily dosing schedule. Adverse reactions include local irritation, burning sensation, and erythema. Contact with mucous membranes should be avoided.

4. Butenafine

Butenafine hydrochloride (Mentax) is a benzylamine that is structurally related to the allylamines. As with the allylamines, butenafine inhibits the epoxidation of squalene, thus blocking the synthesis of ergosterol, an essential component of the fungal cell membranes. Butenafine is available as a 1% cream to be applied once daily for the treatment of superficial dermatophytosis.

5. Tolnaftate

Tolnaftate is a synthetic antifungal compound that is effective topically against dermatophyte infections caused by epidermophyton, microsporum, and trichophyton. It is also active against *P orbiculare* but not against candida.

Tolnaftate (Aftate, Tinactin) is available as a cream, solution, powder, or powder aerosol for application twice daily to infected areas. Recurrences following cessation of therapy are common, and infections of the palms, soles, and nails are usually unresponsive to tolnaftate alone. The powder or powder aerosol may be used chronically following initial treatment in patients susceptible to tinea infections. Tolnaftate is generally well tolerated and rarely causes irritation or allergic contact sensitization.

6. Nystatin & Amphotericin B

Nystatin and amphotericin B are useful in the topical therapy of *C albicans* infections but ineffective against dermatophytes. Nystatin is limited to topical treatment of cutaneous and mucosal candida infections because of its narrow spectrum and negligible absorption from the gastrointestinal tract following oral administration. Amphotericin B has a broader antifungal spectrum and is used intravenously in the treatment of many systemic mycoses (see Chapter 48) and to a lesser extent in the treatment of cutaneous candida infections.

The recommended dosage for topical preparations of nystatin in treating paronychial and intertriginous candidiasis is application two or three times a day. Oral candidiasis (thrush) is treated by holding 5 mL (infants, 2 mL) of nystatin oral suspension in the mouth for several minutes four times daily before swallowing. An alternative therapy for thrush is to retain a vaginal tablet in the mouth until dissolved four times daily. Recurrent or recalcitrant perianal, vaginal, vulvar, and diaper area candidiasis may respond to oral nystatin, 0.5–1 million units in adults (100,000 units in children) four times daily in addition to local therapy. Vulvovaginal candidiasis may be treated by insertion of 1 vaginal tablet twice daily for 14 days, then nightly for an additional 14–21 days.

Amphotericin B (Fungizone) is available for topical use in cream and lotion form. The recommended dosage in the treatment of paronychial and intertriginous candidiasis is application two to four times daily to the affected area.

Adverse effects associated with oral administration of nystatin include mild nausea, diarrhea, and occasional vomiting. Topical application is nonirritating, and allergic contact hypersensitivity is exceedingly uncommon. Topical amphotericin B is well tolerated and only occasionally locally irritating. Hypersensitivity is very rare. The drug may cause a temporary yellow staining of the skin, especially when the cream vehicle is used.

ORAL ANTIFUNGAL AGENTS

1. Oral Azole Derivatives

Azole derivatives currently available for oral treatment of systemic mycosis include fluconazole (Diflucan), itraconazole (Sporonax), ketoconazole (Nizoral), and others. As discussed in Chapter 48, imidazole derivatives act by affecting the permeability of the cell membrane of sensitive cells through alterations of the biosynthesis of lipids, especially sterols, in the fungal cell.

Ketoconazole was the first imidazole derivative used for oral treatment of systemic mycoses. Patients with chronic mucocutaneous candidiasis respond well to a once-daily dose of 200 mg of ketoconazole, with a median clearing time of 16 weeks. Most patients require long-term maintenance therapy. Variable results have been reported in treatment of chromomycosis.

Ketoconazole has been shown to be quite effective in the therapy of cutaneous infections caused by epidermophyton, microsporum, and trichophyton species. Infections of the glabrous skin often respond within 2–3 weeks to a once-daily oral dose of 200 mg. Palmarplantar skin is slower to respond, often taking 4–6 weeks at a dosage of 200 mg twice daily. Infections of the hair and nails may take even longer before resolving with low cure rates noted for tinea capitis. Tinea versicolor is very responsive to short courses of a once-daily dose of 200 mg.

Nausea or pruritus has been noted in approximately 3% of patients taking ketoconazole. More significant side effects include gynecomastia, elevations of hepatic enzyme levels, and hepatitis. Caution is advised when using ketoconazole in patients with a history of hepatitis. Routine evaluation of hepatic function is advisable for patients on prolonged therapy.

The newer azole derivatives for oral therapy include fluconazole and itraconazole. Fluconazole is well absorbed following oral administration, with a plasma half-life of 30 hours. In view of this long half-life, daily doses of 100 mg are sufficient to treat mucocutaneous candidiasis; alternate-day doses are sufficient for dermatophyte infections. The plasma half-life of itraconazole is similar to fluconazole, with detectable therapeutic concentrations remaining in the stratum corneum for up to 28 days following termination of therapy. Itraconazole has been demonstrated to be effective for the treatment of onychomycosis in a dosage of 200 mg daily taken with food to ensure maximum absorption for 3 consecutive months. Recent reports of heart failure in patients receiving itraconazole for onychomycosis have resulted in recommendations that it not be given for treatment of onychomycosis in patients with ventricular dysfunction. Additionally, routine evaluation of hepatic function is recommended for patients receiving itraconazole for onychomycosis.

Administration of oral azoles with midazolam or triazolam has resulted in elevated plasma concentrations and may potentiate and prolong hypnotic and sedative effects of these agents. Administration with HMG-CoA reductase inhibitors has been shown to cause a significant risk of rhabdomyolysis. *Therefore, administration of the oral azoles with midazolam, triazolam, or HMG-CoA inhibitors is contraindicated.*

2. Griseofulvin

Griseofulvin is effective orally against dermatophyte infections caused by epidermophyton, microsporum, and trichophyton. It is ineffective against candida and *P orbiculare*. Griseofulvin's mechanism of antifungal action is not fully understood, but it is active only against growing cells.

Following the oral administration of 1 g of micronized griseofulvin, drug can be detected in the stratum corneum 4–8 hours later. Reducing the particle size of the medication greatly increases absorption of the drug. Formulations that contain the smallest particle size are labeled "ultramicronized." Ultramicronized griseofulvin achieves bioequivalent plasma levels with half the dose of micronized drug. In addition, solubilizing griseofulvin in polyethylene glycol enhances absorption even further. Micronized griseofulvin is available as 250 mg and 500 mg tablets, and ultramicronized drug is available as 125 mg, 165 mg, 250 mg, and 330 mg tablets and as 250 mg capsules.

The usual adult dosage of the micronized ("microsize") form of the drug is 500 mg daily in single or divided doses with meals; occasionally, 1 g/d is indicated in the treatment of recalcitrant infections. The pediatric dosage is 10 mg/kg of body weight daily in single or divided doses with meals. An oral suspension is available for use in children.

Griseofulvin is most effective in treating tinea infections of the scalp and glabrous (nonhairy) skin. In general, infections of the scalp respond to treatment in 4–6 weeks, and infections of glabrous skin will respond in 3–4 weeks. Dermatophyte infections of the nails respond only to prolonged administration of griseofulvin. Fingernails may respond to 6 months of therapy, whereas toenails are quite recalcitrant to treatment and may require 8–18 months of therapy; relapse almost invariably occurs.

Adverse effects seen with griseofulvin therapy include headaches, nausea, vomiting, diarrhea, photosensitivity, peripheral neuritis, and occasionally mental confusion. Griseofulvin is derived from a penicillium mold, and cross-sensitivity with penicillin may occur. It is contraindicated in patients with porphyria or hepatic failure or those who have had hypersensitivity reactions to it in the past. Its safety in pregnant patients has not been established. Leukopenia and proteinuria have occasionally been reported. Therefore, in patients undergoing prolonged therapy, routine evaluation of the hepatic, renal, and hematopoietic systems is advisable. Coumarin anticoagulant activity may be altered by griseofulvin, and anticoagulant dosage may require adjustment.

3. Terbinafine

Terbinafine (described above) has been shown to be quite effective given orally for the treatment of onychomycosis. Recommended oral dosage is 250 mg daily for 6 weeks for fingernail infections and 12 weeks for toenail infections. Patients receiving terbinafine for onychomycosis should be monitored closely with periodic laboratory evaluations for possible hepatic dysfunction.

■ TOPICAL ANTIVIRAL AGENTS

ACYCLOVIR, VALACYCLOVIR, PENCICLOVIR, & FAMCICLOVIR

Acyclovir, valacyclovir, penciclovir, and famciclovir are synthetic guanine analogs with inhibitory activity against members of the herpesvirus family, including herpes simplex types 1 and 2. Their mechanism of action, indications, and usage in the treatment of cutaneous infections are discussed in Chapter 49.

Topical acyclovir (Zovirax) is available as a 5% ointment; topical penciclovir (Denavir), as a 1% cream for the treatment of recurrent orolabial herpes simplex virus infection in immunocompetent adults. Adverse local reactions to acyclovir and penciclovir may include pruritus and mild pain with transient stinging or burning.

■ IMMUNOMODULATORS

IMIQUIMOD

Imiquimod (Aldara) is an immunomodulator approved for the treatment of external genital and perianal warts in adults, actinic keratoses on the face and scalp, and biopsy-proven primary basal cell carcinomas on the trunk, neck, and extremities. The mechanism of its action is thought to be related to imiquimod's ability to stimulate peripheral mononuclear cells to release interferon-α and to stimulate macrophages to produce interleukins-1, -6, and -8, and tumor necrosis factor-α (TNF-α).

Imiquimod should be applied to the wart tissue three times per week and left on the skin for 6–10 hours prior to washing off with mild soap and water. Treatment should be continued until eradication of the warts is accomplished, but not for more than a total of 16 weeks. Recommended treatment of actinic keratoses consists of twice-weekly applications on the contiguous area of involvement. The cream is removed after approximately 8 hours with mild soap and water. Treatment of superficial basal cell carcinoma consists of five times per week application to the tumor, including a 1 cm margin of surrounding skin, for a 6-week course of therapy.

Percutaneous absorption is minimal, with less than 0.9% absorbed following a single-dose application. Adverse side effects consist of local inflammatory reactions, including pruritus, erythema, and superficial erosion.

TACROLIMUS & PIMECROLIMUS

Tacrolimus (Protopic) and pimecrolimus (Elidel) are macrolide immunosuppressants that have been shown to be of significant benefit in the treatment of atopic dermatitis. Both agents inhibit T-lymphocyte activation and prevent the release of inflammatory cytokines and mediators from mast cells in vitro after stimulation by antigen-IgE complexes. Tacrolimus is available as 0.03% and 0.1% ointments, and pimecrolimus is available as a 1% cream. Both are indicated for short-term and intermittent long-term therapy for mild to moderate atopic dermatitis. Tacrolimus 0.03% ointment and pimecrolimus 1% cream are approved for use in children older than 2 years of age, while all strengths are approved for adult use. Recommended dosing of both agents is twice-daily application to affected skin until clearing is noted. Neither medication should be used with occlusive dressings. The most common side effect of both drugs is a burning sensation in the applied area that improves with continued use. The Food and Drug Administration has added a black box warning to topical tacrolimus and pimecrolimus because of animal tumorgenicity data.

■ ECTOPARASITICIDES

PERMETHRIN

Permethrin is toxic to *Pediculus humanus, Pthirus pubis,* and *Sarcoptes scabiei.* Less than 2% of an applied dose is absorbed percutaneously. Residual drug persists up to 10 days following application.

It is recommended that permethrin 1% cream rinse (Nix) be applied undiluted to affected areas of pediculosis for 10 minutes and then rinsed off with warm water. For the treatment of scabies, a single application of 5% cream (Elimite) is applied to the body from the neck down, left on for 8–14 hours, and then washed off. Adverse reactions to permethrin include transient burning, stinging, and pruritus. Cross-sensitization to pyrethrins or chrysanthemums may occur.

LINDANE
(HEXACHLOROCYCLOHEXANE)

The gamma isomer of hexachlorocyclohexane was commonly called gamma benzene hexachloride, a misnomer, since no benzene ring is present in this compound. Percutaneous absorption studies using a solution of lindane in acetone have shown that almost 10% of a dose applied to the forearm is absorbed, to be subsequently excreted in the urine over a 5-day period. After absorption, lindane is concentrated in fatty tissues, including the brain.

Lindane (Kwell, etc) is available as a shampoo or lotion. For pediculosis capitis or pubis, 30 mL of shampoo is applied to dry hair on the scalp or genital area for 4 minutes and then rinsed off. No additional application is indicated unless living lice are present 1 week after treatment. Then reapplication may be required.

Recent concerns about the toxicity of lindane have altered treatment guidelines for its use in scabies; the current recommendation calls for a single application to the entire body from the neck down, left on for 8–12 hours, and then washed off. Patients should be retreated only if active mites can be demonstrated, and never within 1 week of initial treatment.

Concerns about neurotoxicity and hematotoxicity have resulted in warnings that lindane should be used with caution in infants, children, and pregnant women. The current USA package insert recommends that it not be used as a scabicide in premature infants and in patients with known seizure disorders. California has prohibited the medical use of lindane following evaluation of its toxicologic profile. The risk of adverse systemic reactions to lindane appears to be minimal when it is used properly and according to directions in adult patients. However, local irritation may occur, and contact with the eyes and mucous membranes should be avoided.

CROTAMITON

Crotamiton, *N*-ethyl-*o*-crotonotoluidide, is a scabicide with some antipruritic properties. Its mechanism of action is not known, and studies on percutaneous absorption have not been published.

Crotamiton (Eurax) is available as a cream or lotion. Suggested guidelines for scabies treatment call for two applications to the entire body from the chin down at 24-hour intervals, with a cleansing bath 48 hours after the last application. Crotamiton is an effective agent that can be used as an alternative to lindane. Allergic contact hypersensitivity and primary irritation may occur, necessitating discontinuance of therapy. Application to acutely inflamed skin or to the eyes or mucous membranes should be avoided.

SULFUR

Sulfur has a long history of use as a scabicide. Although it is nonirritating, it has an unpleasant odor, is staining, and is thus disagreeable to use. It has been replaced by more aesthetic and effective scabicides in recent years, but it remains a possible alternative drug for use in infants and pregnant women. The usual formulation is 5% precipitated sulfur in petrolatum.

MALATHION

Malathion is an organophosphate cholinesterase inhibitor that is hydrolyzed by plasma carboxylesterases much faster in humans than in insects, thereby providing a therapeutic advantage in treating pediculosis (see Chapter 7). Malathion is available as a 0.5% lotion (Ovide) that should be applied to the hair when dry; 4–6 hours later, the hair is combed to remove nits and lice.

■ AGENTS AFFECTING PIGMENTATION

HYDROQUINONE, MONOBENZONE, & MEQUINOL

Hydroquinone, monobenzone (Benoquin, the monobenzyl ether of hydroquinone), and mequinol (the monomethyl ether of hydroquinone) are used to reduce hyperpigmentation of the skin. Topical hydroquinone and mequinol usually result in temporary lightening, whereas monobenzone causes irreversible depigmentation.

The mechanism of action of these compounds appears to involve inhibition of the enzyme tyrosinase, thus interfering with the biosynthesis of melanin. In addition, monobenzone may be toxic to melanocytes, resulting in permanent depigmentation. Some percutaneous absorption of these compounds takes place, because monobenzone may cause hypopigmentation at sites distant from the area of application. Both hydroquinone and monobenzone may cause local irritation. Allergic sensitization to these compounds can occur. Prescription combinations of hydroquinone, fluocinolone acetonide, and retinoic acid (Tri-Luma) and mequinol and retinoic acid (Solagé) are more effective than their individual components.

TRIOXSALEN & METHOXSALEN

Trioxsalen and methoxsalen are psoralens used for the repigmentation of depigmented macules of vitiligo. With the recent development of high-intensity long-wave ultraviolet fluorescent lamps, photochemotherapy with oral methoxsalen for psoriasis and with oral trioxsalen for vitiligo has been under intensive investigation.

Psoralens must be photoactivated by long-wavelength ultraviolet light in the range of 320–400 nm (UVA) to produce a beneficial effect. Psoralens intercalate with DNA and, with subsequent UVA irradia-

tion, cyclobutane adducts are formed with pyrimidine bases. Both monofunctional and bifunctional adducts may be formed, the latter causing interstrand crosslinks. These DNA photoproducts may inhibit DNA synthesis. The major long-term risks of psoralen photochemotherapy are cataracts and skin cancer.

■ SUNSCREENS

Topical medications useful in protecting against sunlight contain either chemical compounds that absorb ultraviolet light, called sunscreens, or opaque materials such as titanium dioxide that reflect light, called sunshades. The three classes of chemical compounds most commonly used in sunscreens are p-aminobenzoic acid (PABA) and its esters, the benzophenones, and the dibenzoylmethanes.

Most sunscreen preparations are designed to absorb ultraviolet light in the ultraviolet B (UVB) wavelength range from 280 to 320 nm, which is the range responsible for most of the erythema and tanning associated with sun exposure. Chronic exposure to light in this range induces aging of the skin and photocarcinogenesis. Para-aminobenzoic acid and its esters are the most effective available absorbers in the B region.

The benzophenones include oxybenzone, dioxybenzone, and sulisobenzone. These compounds provide a broader spectrum of absorption from 250 to 360 nm, but their effectiveness in the UVB erythema range is less than that of p-aminobenzoic acid. The dibenzoylmethanes include Parasol and Eusolex. These compounds absorb wavelengths throughout the longer ultraviolet A range, 320 nm to 400 nm, with maximum absorption at 360 nm. Patients particularly sensitive to UVA wavelengths include individuals with polymorphous light eruption, cutaneous lupus erythematosus, and drug-induced photosensitivity. In these patients, dibenzoylmethane-containing sunscreen may provide improved photoprotection. Although not approved by the FDA at this time, terephthalylidene dicamphorsulfuric acid (Mexoryl) appears to provide greater UVA protection than the dibenzoylmethanes.

The sun protection factor (SPF) of a given sunscreen is a measure of its effectiveness in absorbing erythrogenic ultraviolet light. It is determined by measuring the minimal erythema dose with and without the sunscreen in a group of normal people. The ratio of the minimal erythema dose with sunscreen to the minimal erythema dose without sunscreen is the SPF. Fair-skinned individuals who sunburn easily are advised to use a product with an SPF of 15 or greater.

■ ACNE PREPARATIONS

RETINOIC ACID & DERIVATIVES

Retinoic acid, also known as **tretinoin** or *all-trans*-retinoic acid, is the acid form of vitamin A. It is an effective topical treatment for acne vulgaris. Several analogs of vitamin A, eg, 13-*cis*-retinoic acid (isotretinoin), have been shown to be effective in various dermatologic diseases when given orally. Vitamin A alcohol is the physiologic form of vitamin A. The topical therapeutic agent, **retinoic acid,** is formed by the oxidation of the alcohol group, with all four double bonds in the side chain in the *trans* configuration as shown.

Retinoic acid

Retinoic acid is insoluble in water but soluble in many organic solvents. It is susceptible to oxidation, particularly when exposed to light, and ester formation. Topically applied retinoic acid remains chiefly in the epidermis, with less than 10% absorption into the circulation. The small quantities of retinoic acid absorbed following topical application are metabolized by the liver and excreted in bile and urine.

Retinoic acid has several effects on epithelial tissues. It stabilizes lysosomes, increases ribonucleic acid polymerase activity, increases prostaglandin E_2, cAMP, and cGMP levels, and increases the incorporation of thymidine into DNA. Its action in acne has been attributed to decreased cohesion between epidermal cells and increased epidermal cell turnover. This is thought to result in the expulsion of open comedones and the transformation of closed comedones into open ones.

Topical retinoic acid is applied initially in a concentration sufficient to induce slight erythema with mild peeling. The concentration or frequency of application may be decreased if too much irritation occurs. Topical retinoic acid should be applied to dry skin only, and care should be taken to avoid contact with the corners of the nose, eyes, mouth, and mucous membranes. During the first 4–6 weeks of therapy, comedones not previously evident may appear and give the impression that the acne has been aggravated by the retinoic acid. However, with continued therapy, the lesions will clear, and in 8–12 weeks optimal clinical improvement should occur. A timed-release formulation of tretinoin containing microspheres (Retin-A Micro) delivers the medication over time and may be less irritating for sensitive patients.

The effects of tretinoin on keratinization and desquamation offer benefits for patients with photodamaged skin. Prolonged use of tretinoin promotes dermal collagen synthesis, new blood vessel formation, and thickening of the epidermis, which helps diminish fine lines and wrinkles. A specially formulated moisturizing 0.05% cream (Renova) is marketed for this purpose.

The most common adverse effects of topical retinoic acid are erythema and dryness that occur in the first few weeks of use, but these can be expected to resolve with continued therapy. Animal studies suggest that this drug may increase the tumorigenic potential of ultraviolet radiation. In light of this, patients using retinoic acid should be advised to avoid or minimize sun exposure and use a protective sunscreen. Allergic contact dermatitis to topical retinoic acid is rare.

Adapalene (Differin) is a derivative of naphthoic acid that resembles retinoic acid in structure and effects. It is applied as a 0.1% gel once daily. Unlike tretinoin, adapalene is photochemically stable and shows little decrease in efficacy when used in combination with benzoyl peroxide. Adapalene is less irritating than tretinoin and is most effective in patients with mild to moderate acne vulgaris.

Tazarotene (Tazorac) is an acetylenic retinoid that is available as a 0.1% gel and cream for the treatment of mild to moderately severe facial acne. Topical tazarotene should be used by women of childbearing age only after contraceptive counseling. It is recommended that tazarotene should not be used by pregnant women.

ISOTRETINOIN

Isotretinoin (Accutane) is a synthetic retinoid currently restricted to the treatment of severe cystic acne that is recalcitrant to standard therapies. The precise mechanism of action of isotretinoin in cystic acne is not known, although it appears to act by inhibiting sebaceous gland size and function. The drug is well absorbed, extensively bound to plasma albumin, and has an elimination half-life of 10–20 hours.

Most patients with cystic acne respond to 1–2 mg/kg, given orally in two divided doses daily for 4–5 months. If severe cystic acne persists following this initial treatment, after a period of 2 months, a second course of therapy may be initiated. Common adverse effects resemble hypervitaminosis A and include dryness and itching of the skin and mucous membranes. Less common side effects are headache, corneal opacities, pseudotumor cerebri, inflammatory bowel disease, anorexia, alopecia, and muscle and joint pains. These effects are all reversible on discontinuance of therapy. Skeletal hyperostosis has been observed in patients receiving isotretinoin with premature closure of epiphyses noted in children treated with this medication. Lipid abnormalities (triglycerides, high-density lipoproteins) are frequent; their clinical relevance is unknown at present.

Teratogenicity is a significant risk in patients taking isotretinoin; therefore, women of childbearing potential *must* use an effective form of contraception for at least 1 month before, throughout isotretinoin therapy, and for one or more menstrual cycles following discontinuance of treatment. A serum pregnancy test *must* be obtained within 2 weeks before starting therapy in these patients, and therapy should be initiated only on the second or third day of the next normal menstrual period. In the USA health care professionals, pharmacists, and patients must utilize a mandatory registration and followup system.

BENZOYL PEROXIDE

Benzoyl peroxide is an effective topical agent in the treatment of acne vulgaris. It penetrates the stratum corneum or follicular openings unchanged and is converted metabolically to benzoic acid within the epidermis and dermis. Less than 5% of an applied dose is absorbed from the skin in an 8-hour period. It has been postulated that the mechanism of action of benzoyl peroxide in acne is related to its antimicrobial activity against *P acnes* and to its peeling and comedolytic effects.

To decrease the likelihood of irritation, application should be limited to a low concentration (2.5%) once daily for the first week of therapy and increased in frequency and strength if the preparation is well tolerated. Fixed-combination formulations of 5% benzoyl peroxide with 3% erythromycin base (Benzamycin) or 1% clindamycin (BenzaClin) appear to be more effective than individual agents alone.

Benzoyl peroxide is a potent contact sensitizer in experimental studies, and this adverse effect may occur in up to 1% of acne patients. Care should be taken to avoid contact with the eyes and mucous membranes. Benzoyl peroxide is an oxidant and may rarely cause bleaching of the hair or colored fabrics.

AZELAIC ACID

Azelaic acid is a straight-chain saturated dicarboxylic acid that has been demonstrated to be effective in the treatment of acne vulgaris (in the form of Azelex) and acne rosacea (Finacea). Its mechanism of action has not been fully determined, but preliminary studies demonstrate antimicrobial activity against *P acnes* as well as in vitro inhibitory effects on the conversion of testosterone to dihydrotestosterone. Initial therapy is begun with once-daily applications of the 20% cream or 15% gel to the affected areas for 1 week and twice-daily applications thereafter. Most patients experience mild irritation with redness and dryness of the skin during the

first week of treatment. Clinical improvement is noted in 6–8 weeks of continuous therapy.

■ DRUGS FOR PSORIASIS

ACITRETIN

Acitretin (Soriatane), a metabolite of the aromatic retinoid etretinate, is quite effective in the treatment of psoriasis, especially pustular forms. It is given orally at a dosage of 25–50 mg/d. Adverse effects attributable to acitretin therapy are similar to those seen with isotretinoin and resemble hypervitaminosis A. Elevations in cholesterol and triglycerides may be noted with acitretin, and hepatotoxicity with liver enzyme elevations has been reported. Acitretin is more teratogenic than isotretinoin in the animal species studied to date, which is of special concern in view of the drug's prolonged elimination time (more than 3 months) after chronic administration. In cases where etretinate is formed by concomitant administration of acitretin and ethanol, etretinate may be found in plasma and subcutaneous fat for many years.

Acitretin must not be used by women who are pregnant or may become pregnant while undergoing treatment or at any time for at least 3 years after treatment is discontinued. Ethanol must be strictly avoided during treatment with acitretin and for 2 months after discontinuing therapy. Patients must not donate blood during treatment and for 3 years after acitretin is stopped.

TAZAROTENE

Tazarotene (Tazorac) is a topical acetylenic retinoid prodrug that is hydrolyzed to its active form by an esterase. The active metabolite, tazarotenic acid, binds to retinoic acid receptors, resulting in modified gene expression. The precise mechanism of action in psoriasis is unknown but may relate to both anti-inflammatory and antiproliferative actions. Tazarotene is absorbed percutaneously, and teratogenic systemic concentrations may be achieved if applied to more than 20% of total body surface area. Women of childbearing potential must therefore be advised of the risk prior to initiating therapy, and adequate birth control measures must be utilized while on therapy.

Treatment of psoriasis should be limited to once-daily application not to exceed 20% of total body surface area. Adverse local effects include a burning or stinging sensation (sensory irritation) and peeling, erythema, and localized edema of the skin (irritant dermatitis). Potentiation of photosensitizing medication may occur, and patients should be cautioned to minimize sunlight exposure and to use sunscreens and protective clothing.

CALCIPOTRIENE

Calcipotriene (Dovonex) is a synthetic vitamin D_3 derivative that has been shown to be effective in the treatment of plaque-type psoriasis vulgaris of moderate severity. Approximately 6% of the topically applied 0.005% ointment is absorbed through psoriatic plaques, resulting in a transient elevation of serum calcium in fewer than 1% of subjects treated in clinical trials. Improvement of psoriasis was generally noted following 2 weeks of therapy, with continued improvement for up to 8 weeks of treatment. However, fewer than 10% of patients demonstrate total clearing while on calcipotriene as single-agent therapy. Adverse effects include burning, itching, and mild irritation, with dryness and erythema of the treatment area. Care should be taken to avoid facial contact, which may cause ocular irritation.

BIOLOGIC AGENTS

Biologic agents useful in treating adult patients with moderate to severe chronic plaque psoriasis include the T-cell modulators alefacept and efalizumab, and the TNF-α inhibitor etanercept.

1. Alefacept

Alefacept (Amevive) is an immunosuppressive dimeric fusion protein that consists of the extracellular CD2-binding portion of the human leukocyte function antigen-3 linked to the Fc portion of human IgG_1. Alefacept interferes with lymphocyte activation, which plays a role in the pathophysiology of psoriasis, resulting in a reduction in subsets of CD2 T lymphocytes and circulating total CD4 and CD8 T-lymphocyte counts. The recommended dosage is 7.5 mg given once weekly as an intravenous bolus or 15 mg once weekly as an intramuscular injection for a 12-week course of treatment. Patients should have CD4 lymphocyte counts monitored weekly while taking alefacept, and dosing should be withheld if CD4 counts are below 250 cells/μL. The drug should be discontinued if the counts remain below 250 cells/μL for 1 month. Alefacept is an immunosuppressive agent and should not be administered to patients with clinically significant infection. Because of the possibility of an increased risk of malignancy, it should not be administered to patients with a history of systemic malignancy.

2. Efalizumab

Efalizumab (Raptiva) is an immunosuppressive recombinant humanized IgG_1 kappa isotype monoclonal antibody that binds to CD11a subunit of leukocyte function antigen-1. This binding affects the activation, adhesion, and migration of T lymphocytes. The recommended dosage is a single 0.7 mg/kg subcutaneous injection conditioning dose followed by weekly subcutaneous injections of 1 mg/kg not to exceed a maximum single dose of 200 mg. Monitoring of monthly platelet counts is indicated to detect possible severe immune-mediated thrombocytopenia. Efalizumab is an immunosuppressive agent and should not be given concurrently with other immunosuppressive medication.

3. Etanercept

Etanercept (Enbrel) is a dimeric fusion protein consisting of the extracellular ligand-binding portion of the human TNF receptor linked to the Fc portion of human IgG_1. Etanercept binds specifically to TNF-α and -β and blocks interaction with cell surface TNF receptors that play a role in the inflammatory process of plaque psoriasis. The recommended dosage of etanercept is a 50 mg subcutaneous injection given twice weekly for 3 months followed by a maintenance dose of 50 mg weekly. Serious life-threatening infections and sepsis have been reported with the use of etanercept, and concurrent use with other immunosuppressive therapy should be avoided.

■ ANTI-INFLAMMATORY AGENTS

TOPICAL CORTICOSTEROIDS

The remarkable efficacy of topical corticosteroids in the treatment of inflammatory dermatoses was noted soon after the introduction of hydrocortisone in 1952. Since that time, numerous analogs have been developed that offer extensive choices of potencies, concentrations, and vehicles. The therapeutic effectiveness of topical corticosteroids is based primarily on their anti-inflammatory activity. Definitive explanations of the effects of corticosteroids on endogenous mediators of inflammation await further experimental clarification. The antimitotic effects of corticosteroids on human epidermis may account for an additional mechanism of action in psoriasis and other dermatologic diseases associated with increased cell turnover. The general pharmacology of these endocrine agents is discussed in Chapter 39.

Chemistry & Pharmacokinetics

The original topical glucocorticosteroid was hydrocortisone, the natural glucocorticosteroid of the adrenal cortex. The 9α-fluoro derivative of hydrocortisone was active topically, but its salt-retaining properties made it undesirable even for topical use. Prednisolone and methylprednisolone are as active topically as hydrocortisone (Table 62–1). The 9α-fluorinated steroids dexamethasone and betamethasone did not have any advantage over hydrocortisone.

Table 62–1. Relative efficacy of some topical corticosteroids in various formulations.

Concentration in Commonly Used Preparations	Drug	Concentration in Commonly Used Preparations	Drug
Lowest efficacy		**Intermediate efficacy (continued)**	
0.25–2.5%	Hydrocortisone	0.05%	Fluticasone propionate (Cutivate)
0.25%	Methylprednisolone acetate (Medrol)	0.05%	Desonide (Desowen)
0.1%	Dexamethasone[1] (Decaderm)	0.025%	Halcinonide[1] (Halog)
1.0%	Methylprednisolone acetate (Medrol)	0.05%	Desoximetasone[1] (Topicort L.P.)
0.5%	Prednisolone (MetiDerm)	0.05%	Flurandrenolide[1] (Cordran)
0.2%	Betamethasone[1] (Celestone)	0.1%	Triamcinolone acetonide[1]
Low efficacy		0.025%	Fluocinolone acetonide[1]
0.01%	Fluocinolone acetonide[1] (Fluonid, Synalar)	**High efficacy**	
0.01%	Betamethasone valerate[1] (Valisone)	0.05%	Fluocinonide[1] (Lidex)
0.025%	Fluorometholone[1] (Oxylone)	0.05%	Betamethasone dipropionate[1] (Diprosone, Maxivate)
0.05%	Alclometasone dipropionate (Aclovate)	0.1%	Amcinonide[1] (Cyclocort)
0.025%	Triamcinolone acetonide[1] (Aristocort, Kenalog, Triacet)	0.25%	Desoximetasone[1] (Topicort)
0.1%	Clocortolone pivalate[1] (Cloderm)	0.5%	Triamcinolone acetonide[1]
0.03%	Flumethasone pivalate[1] (Locorten)	0.2%	Fluocinolone acetonide[1] (Synalar-HP)
Intermediate efficacy		0.05%	Diflorasone diacetate[1] (Florone, Maxiflor)
0.2%	Hydrocortisone valerate (Westcort)	0.1%	Halcinonide[1] (Halog)
0.1%	Mometasone furoate (Elocon)	**Highest efficacy**	
0.1%	Hydrocortisone butyrate (Locoid)	0.05%	Betamethasone dipropionate in optimized vehicle (Diprolene)[1]
0.1%	Hydrocortisone probutate (Pandel)	0.05%	Diflorasone diacetate[1] in optimized vehicle (Psorcon)
0.025%	Betamethasone benzoate[1] (Uticort)	0.05%	Halobetasol propionate[1] (Ultravate)
0.025%	Flurandrenolide[1] (Cordran)	0.05%	Clobetasol propionate[1] (Temovate)
0.1%	Betamethasone valerate[1] (Valisone)		
0.1%	Prednicarbate (Dermatop)		

[1]Fluorinated steroids.

However, triamcinolone and fluocinolone, the acetonide derivatives of the fluorinated steroids, do have a distinct efficacy advantage in topical therapy. Similarly, betamethasone is not very active topically, but attaching a 5-carbon valerate chain to the 17-hydroxyl position results in a compound over 300 times as active as hydrocortisone for topical use. Fluocinonide is the 21-acetate derivative of fluocinolone acetonide; the addition of the 21-acetate enhances the topical activity about fivefold. Fluorination of the steroid is not required for high potency.

Corticosteroids are only minimally absorbed following application to normal skin; for example, approximately 1% of a dose of hydrocortisone solution applied to the ventral forearm is absorbed. Long-term occlusion with an impermeable film such as plastic wrap is an effective method of enhancing penetration, yielding a tenfold increase in absorption. There is a marked regional anatomic variation in corticosteroid penetration. Compared with the absorption from the forearm, hydrocortisone is absorbed 0.14 times as well through the plantar foot arch, 0.83 times as well through the palm, 3.5 times as well through the scalp, 6 times as well through the forehead, 9 times as well through vulvar skin, and 42 times as well through scrotal skin. Penetration is increased severalfold in the inflamed skin of atopic dermatitis; and in severe exfoliative diseases, such as erythrodermic psoriasis, there appears to be little barrier to penetration.

Experimental studies on the percutaneous absorption of hydrocortisone fail to reveal a significant increase in absorption when applied on a repetitive basis and a single daily application may be effective in most conditions. Ointment bases tend to give better activity to the corticosteroid than do cream or lotion vehicles. Increasing the concentration of a corticosteroid increases the penetration but not to the same degree. For example, approximately 1% of a 0.25% hydrocortisone solution is absorbed from the forearm. A tenfold increase in concentration causes only a fourfold increase in absorption. Solubility of the corticosteroid in the vehicle is a significant determinant of the percutaneous absorption of a topical steroid. Marked increases in efficacy are noted when optimized vehicles are used, as demonstrated by newer formulations of betamethasone dipropionate and diflorasone diacetate.

Table 62–1 groups topical corticosteroid formulations according to approximate relative efficacy. Table 62–2 lists major dermatologic diseases in order of their responsiveness to these drugs. In the first group of diseases, low- to medium-efficacy corticosteroid preparations often produce clinical remission. In the second group, it is often necessary to use high-efficacy preparations, occlusion therapy, or both. Once a remission has been achieved, every effort should be made to maintain the improvement with a low-efficacy corticosteroid.

The limited penetration of topical corticosteroids can be overcome in certain clinical circumstances by the intralesional injection of relatively insoluble corticosteroids, eg, triamcinolone acetonide, triamcinolone diacetate, triamcinolone hexacetonide, and betamethasone acetate-phosphate. When these agents are injected into the lesion, measurable amounts remain in place and are gradually released for 3–4 weeks. This form of therapy is often effective for the lesions listed in Table 62–2 that are generally unresponsive to topical corticosteroids. The dosage of the triamcinolone salts should be limited to 1 mg per treatment site, ie, 0.1 mL of 10 mg/mL suspension, to decrease the incidence of local atrophy (see below).

Adverse Effects

All absorbable topical corticosteroids possess the potential to suppress the pituitary-adrenal axis (see Chapter 39). Although most patients with pituitary-adrenal axis suppression demonstrate only a laboratory test abnormality, cases of severely impaired stress response can occur. Iatrogenic Cushing's syndrome may occur as a result of protracted use of topical corticosteroids in large quanti-

Table 62–2. Dermatologic disorders responsive to topical corticosteroids ranked in order of sensitivity.

Very responsive
Atopic dermatitis
Seborrheic dermatitis
Lichen simplex chronicus
Pruritus ani
Later phase of allergic contact dermatitis
Later phase of irritant dermatitis
Nummular eczematous dermatitis
Stasis dermatitis
Psoriasis, especially of genitalia and face
Less responsive
Discoid lupus erythematosus
Psoriasis of palms and soles
Necrobiosis lipoidica diabeticorum
Sarcoidosis
Lichen striatus
Pemphigus
Familial benign pemphigus
Vitiligo
Granuloma annulare
Least responsive: Intralesional injection required
Keloids
Hypertrophic scars
Hypertrophic lichen planus
Alopecia areata
Acne cysts
Prurigo nodularis
Chondrodermatitis nodularis chronica helicis

ties. Applying potent corticosteroids to extensive areas of the body for prolonged periods, with or without occlusion, increases the likelihood of systemic effects. Fewer of these factors are required to produce adverse systemic effects in children, and growth retardation is of particular concern in the pediatric age group.

Adverse local effects of topical corticosteroids include the following: atrophy, which may present as depressed, shiny, often wrinkled "cigarette paper"-appearing skin with prominent telangiectases and a tendency to develop purpura and ecchymosis; steroid rosacea, with persistent erythema, telangiectatic vessels, pustules, and papules in central facial distribution; perioral dermatitis, steroid acne, alterations of cutaneous infections, hypopigmentation, hypertrichosis; increased intraocular pressure; and allergic contact dermatitis. The latter may be confirmed by patch testing with high concentrations of corticosteroids, ie, 1% in petrolatum, because topical corticosteroids are not irritating. Screening for allergic contact dermatitis potential is performed with tixocortol pivalate, budesonide, and hydrocortisone valerate or butyrate. Topical corticosteroids are contraindicated in individuals who demonstrate hypersensitivity to them. Some sensitized subjects develop a generalized flare when dosed with adrenocorticotropic hormone or oral prednisone.

TAR COMPOUNDS

Tar preparations are used mainly in the treatment of psoriasis, dermatitis, and lichen simplex chronicus. The phenolic constituents endow these compounds with antipruritic properties, making them particularly valuable in the treatment of chronic lichenified dermatitis. Acute dermatitis with vesiculation and oozing may be irritated by even weak tar preparations, which should be avoided. However, in the subacute and chronic stages of dermatitis and psoriasis, these preparations are quite useful and offer an alternative to the use of topical corticosteroids.

The most common adverse reaction to coal tar compounds is an irritant folliculitis, necessitating discontinuance of therapy to the affected areas for a period of 3–5 days. Phototoxicity and allergic contact dermatitis may also occur. Tar preparations should be avoided in patients who have previously exhibited sensitivity to them.

■ KERATOLYTIC & DESTRUCTIVE AGENTS

SALICYLIC ACID

Salicylic acid has been extensively used in dermatologic therapy as a keratolytic agent. The mechanism by which it produces its keratolytic and other therapeutic effects is poorly understood. The drug may solubilize cell surface proteins that keep the stratum corneum intact, thereby resulting in desquamation of keratotic debris. Salicylic acid is keratolytic in concentrations of 3–6%. In concentrations greater than 6%, it can be destructive to tissues.

Salicylic acid

Salicylism and death have occurred following topical application. In an adult, 1 g of a topically applied 6% salicylic acid preparation will raise the serum salicylate level not more than 0.5 mg/dL of plasma; the threshold for toxicity is 30–50 mg/dL. Higher serum levels are possible in children, who are therefore at a greater risk to develop salicylism. In cases of severe intoxication, hemodialysis is the treatment of choice (see Chapter 59). It is advisable to limit both the total amount of salicylic acid applied and the frequency of application. Urticarial, anaphylactic, and erythema multiforme reactions may occur in patients who are allergic to salicylates. Topical use may be associated with local irritation, acute inflammation, and even ulceration with the use of high concentrations of salicylic acid. Particular care must be exercised when using the drug on the extremities of diabetics or patients with peripheral vascular disease.

PROPYLENE GLYCOL

Propylene glycol is used extensively in topical preparations because it is an excellent vehicle for organic compounds. It has recently been used alone as a keratolytic agent in 40–70% concentrations, with plastic occlusion, or in gel with 6% salicylic acid.

Only minimal amounts of a topically applied dose are absorbed through normal stratum corneum. Percutaneously absorbed propylene glycol is oxidized by the liver to lactic acid and pyruvic acid, with subsequent utilization in general body metabolism. Approximately 12–45% of the absorbed agent is excreted unchanged in the urine.

Propylene glycol is an effective keratolytic agent for the removal of hyperkeratotic debris. It is also an effective humectant and increases the water content of the stratum corneum. The hygroscopic characteristics of propylene glycol may help it to develop an osmotic gradient through the stratum corneum, thereby increasing hydration of the outermost layers by drawing water out from the inner layers of the skin.

Propylene glycol is used under polyethylene occlusion or with 6% salicylic acid for the treatment of ichthyosis, palmar and plantar keratodermas, psoriasis, pityriasis rubra pilaris, keratosis pilaris, and hypertrophic lichen planus.

In concentrations greater than 10%, propylene glycol may act as an irritant in some patients; those with eczematous dermatitis may be more sensitive. Allergic contact dermatitis occurs with propylene glycol, and a 4% aqueous propylene glycol solution is recommended for the purpose of patch testing.

UREA

Urea in a compatible cream vehicle or ointment base has a softening and moisturizing effect on the stratum corneum. It has the ability to make creams and lotions feel less greasy, and this has been utilized in dermatologic preparations to decrease the oily feel of a preparation that otherwise might feel unpleasant. It is a white crystalline powder with a slight ammonia odor when moist.

Urea is absorbed percutaneously, although the precise amount absorbed is not well documented. It is distributed predominantly in the extracellular space and excreted in urine. Urea is a natural product of metabolism, and systemic toxicities with topical application do not occur.

Urea allegedly increases the water content of the stratum corneum, presumably as a result of the hygroscopic characteristics of this naturally occurring molecule. Urea is also keratolytic. The mechanism of action appears to involve alterations in prekeratin and keratin, leading to increased solubilization. In addition, urea may break hydrogen bonds that keep the stratum corneum intact.

As a humectant, urea is used in concentrations of 2–20% in creams and lotions. As a keratolytic agent, it is used in 20% concentration in diseases such as ichthyosis vulgaris, hyperkeratosis of palms and soles, xerosis, and keratosis pilaris. Concentrations of 30–50% applied to the nail plate have been useful in softening the nail prior to avulsion.

PODOPHYLLUM RESIN & PODOFILOX

Podophyllum resin, an alcoholic extract of *Podophyllum peltatum,* commonly known as mandrake root or May apple, is used in the treatment of condyloma acuminatum and other verrucae. It is a mixture of podophyllotoxin, α and β peltatin, desoxypodophyllotoxin, dehydropodophyllotoxin, and other compounds. It is soluble in alcohol, ether, chloroform, and compound tincture of benzoin.

Percutaneous absorption of podophyllum resin occurs, particularly in intertriginous areas and from applications to large moist condylomas. It is soluble in lipids and therefore is distributed widely throughout the body, including the central nervous system.

The major use of podophyllum resin is in the treatment of condyloma acuminatum. Podophyllotoxin and its derivatives are active cytotoxic agents with specific affinity for the microtubule protein of the mitotic spindle. Normal assembly of the spindle is prevented, and epidermal mitoses are arrested in metaphase. A 25% concentration of podophyllum resin in compound tincture of benzoin is recommended for the treatment of condyloma acuminatum. Application should be restricted to wart tissue only, to limit the total amount of medication used and to prevent severe erosive changes in adjacent tissue. In treating cases of large condylomas, it is advisable to limit application to sections of the affected area to minimize systemic absorption. The patient is instructed to wash off the preparation 2–3 hours after the initial application, because the irritant reaction is variable. Depending on the individual patient's reaction, this period can be extended to 6–8 hours on subsequent applications. If three to five applications have not resulted in significant resolution, other methods of treatment should be considered.

Toxic symptoms associated with excessively large applications include nausea, vomiting, alterations in sensorium, muscle weakness, neuropathy with diminished tendon reflexes, coma, and even death. Local irritation is common, and inadvertent contact with the eye may cause severe conjunctivitis. Use during pregnancy is contraindicated in view of possible cytotoxic effects on the fetus.

Pure podophyllotoxin (podofilox) is approved for use as a 0.5% podophyllotoxin preparation (Condylox) for application by the patient in the treatment of genital condylomas. The low concentration of podofilox significantly reduces the potential for systemic toxicity. Most men with penile warts may be treated with less than 70 µL per application. At this dose, podofilox is not routinely detected in the serum. Treatment is self administered in treatment cycles of twice-daily application for 3 consecutive days followed by a 4-day drug-free period. Local adverse effects include inflammation, erosions, burning pain, and itching.

FLUOROURACIL

Fluorouracil is a fluorinated pyrimidine antimetabolite that resembles uracil, with a fluorine atom substituted for the 5-methyl group. Its systemic pharmacology is described in Chapter 55. Fluorouracil is used topically for the treatment of multiple actinic keratoses.

Approximately 6% of a topically applied dose is absorbed—an amount insufficient to produce adverse systemic effects. Most of the absorbed drug is metabolized and excreted as carbon dioxide, urea, and α-fluoro-β-alanine. A small percentage is eliminated unchanged in the urine. Fluorouracil inhibits thymidylate synthetase activity, interfering with the synthesis of DNA and, to a lesser extent, RNA. These effects are most marked in atypical, rapidly proliferating cells.

Fluorouracil is available in multiple formulations containing 0.5%, 1%, 2%, and 5% concentrations. The response to treatment begins with erythema and progresses through vesiculation, erosion, superficial ulceration, necrosis, and finally reepithelialization. Fluorouracil should be continued until the inflammatory reaction reaches the stage of ulceration and necrosis, usually in 3–4 weeks, at which time treatment should be terminated. The healing process may continue for 1–2 months after therapy is discontinued. Local adverse reactions may include pain, pruritus, a burning sensation, tenderness, and residual postinflammatory hyperpigmentation. Excessive exposure to sunlight during treatment may increase the intensity of the reaction and should be avoided. Allergic contact dermatitis to fluorouracil has been reported, and its use is contraindicated in patients with known hypersensitivity.

NONSTEROIDAL ANTI-INFLAMMATORY DRUGS

A topical 3% gel formulation of the nonsteroidal anti-inflammatory drug diclofenac (Solaraze) has shown moderate effectiveness in the treatment of actinic keratoses. The mechanism of action is unknown. As with other NSAIDs, anaphylactoid reactions may occur with diclofenac, and it should be given with caution to patients with known aspirin hypersensitivity (see Chapter 36).

AMINOLEVULINIC ACID

Aminolevulinic acid (ALA) is an endogenous precursor of photosensitizing porphyrin metabolites. When exogenous ALA is provided to the cell through topical applications, protoporphyrin IX (PpIX) accumulates in the cell. When exposed to light of appropriate wavelength and energy, the accumulated PpIX produces a photodynamic reaction resulting in the formation of cytotoxic superoxide and hydroxyl radicals. Photosensitization of actinic keratoses using ALA (Levulan Kerastick) and illumination with a blue light photodynamic therapy illuminator (BLU-U) is the basis for ALA photodynamic therapy.

Treatment consists of applying ALA 20% topical solution to individual actinic keratoses followed by blue light photodynamic illumination 14–18 hours later. Transient stinging or burning at the treatment site occurs during the period of light exposure. Patients *must* avoid exposure to sunlight or bright indoor lights for at least 40 hours after ALA application. Redness, swelling, and crusting of the actinic keratoses will occur and gradually resolve over a 3- to 4-week time course.

◼ ANTIPRURITIC AGENTS

DOXEPIN

Topical doxepin hydrochloride 5% cream (Zonalon) may provide significant antipruritic activity when utilized in the treatment of pruritus associated with atopic dermatitis or lichen simplex chronicus. The precise mechanism of action is unknown but may relate to the potent H_1- and H_2-receptor antagonist properties of dibenzoxepin tricyclic compounds. Percutaneous absorption is variable and may result in significant drowsiness in some patients. In view of the anticholinergic effect of doxepin, topical use is contraindicated in patients with untreated narrow-angle glaucoma or a tendency to urinary retention.

Plasma levels of doxepin similar to those achieved during oral therapy may be obtained with topical application; the usual drug interactions associated with tricyclic antidepressants may occur. Therefore, monoamine oxidase inhibitors must be discontinued at least 2 weeks prior to the initiation of doxepin cream. Topical application of the cream should be performed four times daily for up to 8 days of therapy. The safety and efficacy of chronic dosing has not been established. Adverse local effects include marked burning and stinging of the treatment site which may necessitate discontinuation of the cream in some patients. Allergic contact dermatitis appears to be frequent, and patients should be monitored for symptoms of hypersensitivity.

PRAMOXINE

Pramoxine hydrochloride is a topical anesthetic that can provide temporary relief from pruritus associated with mild eczematous dermatoses. Pramoxine is available as a 1% cream, lotion, or gel and in combination with hydrocortisone acetate. Application to the affected area two to four times daily may provide short-term relief of pruritus. Local adverse effects include transient burning and stinging. Care should be exercised to avoid contact with the eyes.

◼ TRICHOGENIC & ANTITRICHOGENIC AGENTS

MINOXIDIL

Topical minoxidil (Rogaine) is effective in reversing the progressive miniaturization of terminal scalp hairs associated with androgenic alopecia. Vertex balding is more responsive to therapy than frontal balding. The mechanism of action of minoxidil on hair follicles is unknown. Chronic dosing studies have demonstrated that the effect of minoxidil is not permanent, and cessation of treatment will lead to hair loss in 4–6 months. Percutaneous absorption of minoxidil in normal scalp is minimal, but possible systemic effects on blood pressure (see Chapter 11) should be monitored in patients with cardiac disease.

FINASTERIDE

Finasteride (Propecia) is a 5α-reductase inhibitor that blocks the conversion of testosterone to dihydrotestosterone (see Chapter 40), the androgen responsible for androgenic alopecia in genetically predisposed men. Oral finasteride, 1 mg/d, promotes hair growth and prevents further hair loss in a significant proportion of men with androgenic alopecia. Treatment for at least 3–6 months is necessary to see increased hair growth or prevent further hair loss. Continued treatment with finasteride is necessary to sustain benefit. Reported (and predictable) adverse effects include decreased libido, ejaculation disorders, and erectile dysfunction, which resolve in most men who remain on therapy and in all men who discontinue finasteride.

There are no data to support the use of finasteride in women with androgenic alopecia. Pregnant women should not be exposed to finasteride either by use or by handling crushed tablets because of the risk of hypospadias developing in a male fetus.

EFLORNITHINE

Eflornithine (Vaniqa) is an irreversible inhibitor of ornithine decarboxylase that catalyzes the rate-limiting step in the biosynthesis of polyamines. Polyamines are required for cell division and differentiation, and inhibition of ornithine decarboxylase affects the rate of hair growth. Eflornithine has been shown to be effective in reducing facial hair growth in approximately 30% of women when applied twice daily for 6 months of therapy. Hair growth was observed to return to pretreatment levels 8 weeks after discontinuation. Local adverse effects include stinging, burning, and folliculitis.

■ ANTINEOPLASTIC AGENTS

Alitretinoin (Panretin) is a topical formulation of 9-*cis*-retinoic acid which is approved for the treatment of cutaneous lesions in patients with AIDS-related Kaposi's sarcoma. Localized reactions may include intense erythema, edema, and vesiculation necessitating discontinuation of therapy. Patients who are applying alitretinoin should not concurrently use products containing deet, a common component of insect repellant products.

Bexarotene (Targretin) is a member of a subclass of retinoids that selectively binds and activates retinoid X receptor subtypes. It is available both in an oral formulation and as a topical gel for the treatment of cutaneous T-cell lymphoma. Teratogenicity is a significant risk for both systemic and topical treatment with bexarotene, and women of childbearing potential must avoid becoming pregnant throughout therapy and for at least 1 month following discontinuation of the drug.

Table 62–3. Antiseborrhea agents.

Active Ingredient	Typical Trade Name
Betamethasone valerate foam	Luxiq
Chloroxine shampoo	Capitrol
Coal tar shampoo	Ionil-T, Pentrax, Theraplex-T, T-Gel
Fluocinolone acetonide shampoo	FS Shampoo
Ketoconazole shampoo	Nizoral
Selenium sulfide shampoo	Selsun, Exsel
Zinc pyrithione shampoo	DHS-Zinc, Theraplex-Z

■ ANTISEBORRHEA AGENTS

Table 62–3 lists topical formulations for the treatment of seborrheic dermatitis. These are of variable efficacy

Table 62–4. Miscellaneous medications and the dermatologic conditions in which they are used.

Drug or Group	Conditions	Comment
Alitretinoin	AIDS-related Kaposi's sarcoma	See also Chapter 49.
Antihistamines	Pruritus (any cause), urticaria	See also Chapter 16.
Antimalarials	Lupus erythematosus, photosensitization	See also Chapter 36.
Antimetabolites	Psoriasis, pemphigus, pemphigoid	See also Chapter 55.
Becaplermin	Diabetic neuropathic ulcers	See also Chapter 41.
Bexarotene	Cutaneous T-cell lymphoma	See also Chapter 55.
Corticosteroids	Pemphigus, pemphigoid, lupus erythematosus, allergic contact dermatoses, and certain other dermatoses	See also Chapter 39.
Cyclosporine	Psoriasis	See also Chapter 56.
Dapsone	Dermatitis herpetiformis, erythema elevatum diutinum, pemphigus, pemphigoid, bullous lupus erythematosus	See also Chapter 47.
Denileukin diftitox	Cutaneous T-cell lymphoma	
Etanercept	Psoriatic arthritis	See also Chapters 36 and 56.
Interferon	Melanoma, viral warts	See also Chapter 56.
Mycophenolate mofetil	Bullous disease	See also Chapter 56.
Thalidomide	Erythema nodosum leprosum	See also Chapters 47 and 56.

and may necessitate concomitant treatment with topical corticosteroids for severe cases.

■ MISCELLANEOUS MEDICATIONS

A number of drugs used primarily for other conditions also find use as oral therapeutic agents for dermatologic conditions. A few such preparations are listed in Table 62–4.

REFERENCES

General

Baran R, Maibach HI: *Cosmetic Dermatology,* 3rd ed. Taylor & Francis, 2005.
Bronaugh R, Maibach HI: *Percutaneous Penetration: Principles and Practices,* 4th ed. Taylor & Francis, 2005.
Wakelin S, Maibach HI: *Systemic Drugs in Dermatology.* Manson, 2004.

Antibacterial, Antifungal, & Antiviral Drugs

Aly R, Beutner K, Maibach HI: *Cutaneous Microbiology.* Marcel Dekker, 1996.
Aly R, Maibach HI: *Atlas of Cutaneous Microbiology.* Saunders, 1999.
James WD: Clinical practice. Acne. N Engl J Med 2005;352:1463.
McClellan KJ et al: Terbinafine. An update of its use in superficial mycoses. Drugs 1999;58:179.

Ectoparasiticides

Elgart ML: A risk-benefit assessment of agents used in the treatment of scabies. Drug Saf 1996;14:386.
Orkin M et al (editors): *Scabies and Pediculosis.* CRC Press, 1990.

Agents Affecting Pigmentation

Engasser PG, Maibach HI: Cosmetics and dermatology: Bleaching creams. J Am Acad Dermatol 1981;5:143.
Stolk LML, Siddiqui AH: Biopharmaceutics, pharmacokinetics, and pharmacology of psoralens. Gen Pharmacol 1988; 19:649.

Retinoids & Other Acne Preparations

Ellis CN et al: Etretinate therapy reduces inpatient treatment of psoriasis. J Am Acad Dermatol 1987;17:787.
Lammer EJ et al: Retinoic acid embryopathy. N Engl J Med 1985; 313:837.
Leyden JJ: Topical treatment of acne vulgaris: Retinoids and cutaneous irritation. J Am Acad Dermatol 1998;38:S1.
Shalita AR et al: Tazarotene gel is safe and effective in the treatment of acne vulgaris. A multicenter, double-blind, vehicle-controlled study. Cutis 1999;63:349.
Thami GP, Sarkar R: Coal tar: Past, present and future. Clin Exp Dermatol 2002;27:99.
Weinstein GD et al: Topical tretinoin for treatment of photodamaged skin. Arch Dermatol 1991;127:659.

Anti-Inflammatory Agents

Brazzini B, Pimpinelli N: New and established topical corticosteroids in dermatology: Clinical pharmacology and therapeutic use. Am J Clin Dermatol 2002;3:47.
Surber C, Maibach HI: *Topical Corticosteroids.* Karger, 1994.
Williams JD, Griffiths CE: Cytokine blocking agents in dermatology. Clin Exp Dermatol 2002 Oct;27:585.

Keratolytic & Destructive Agents

Roenigk H, Maibach HI (editors): *Psoriasis,* 3rd ed. Marcel Dekker, 1998.

Drugs Used in the Treatment of Gastrointestinal Diseases

63

Kenneth R. McQuaid, MD

Many of the drug groups discussed elsewhere in this book have important applications in the treatment of diseases of the gastrointestinal tract and other organs. Other groups are used almost exclusively for their effects on the gut; these are discussed below according to their therapeutic uses.

■ I. DRUGS USED IN ACID-PEPTIC DISEASES

Acid-peptic diseases include gastroesophageal reflux, peptic ulcer (gastric and duodenal), and stress-related mucosal injury. In all these conditions, mucosal erosions or ulceration arise when the caustic effects of aggressive factors (acid, pepsin, bile) overwhelm the defensive factors of the gastrointestinal mucosa (mucus and bicarbonate secretion, prostaglandins, blood flow, and the processes of restitution and regeneration after cellular injury). Over 99% of peptic ulcers are caused by infection with the bacterium *Helicobacter pylori* or by use of nonsteroidal anti-inflammatory drugs (NSAIDs). Drugs used in the treatment of acid-peptic disorders may be divided into two classes: agents that reduce intragastric acidity and agents that promote mucosal defense.

AGENTS THAT REDUCE INTRAGASTRIC ACIDITY

PHYSIOLOGY OF ACID SECRETION

The parietal cell contains receptors for gastrin, histamine (H_2), and acetylcholine (muscarinic, M_3) (Figure 63–1). When acetylcholine or gastrin bind to the parietal cell receptors, they cause an increase in cytosolic calcium, which in turn stimulates protein kinases that stimulate acid secretion from a H^+/K^+ ATPase (the proton pump) on the canalicular surface.

In close proximity to the parietal cells are gut endocrine cells called enterochromaffin-like (ECL) cells. ECL cells have receptors for gastrin and acetylcholine and are the major source for histamine release. Histamine binds to the H_2 receptor on the parietal cell, resulting in activation of adenylyl cyclase, which increases intracellular cyclic adenosine monophosphate (cAMP). cAMP activates protein kinases that stimulate acid secretion by the H^+/K^+ ATPase. In humans, it is believed that the major effect of gastrin upon acid secretion is mediated indirectly through the release of histamine from ECL cells rather than through direct parietal cell stimulation.

ANTACIDS

Antacids have been used for centuries in the treatment of patients with dyspepsia and acid-peptic disorders. They were the mainstay of treatment for acid-peptic disorders until the advent of H_2-receptor antagonists and proton pump inhibitors. They continue to be used commonly by patients as nonprescription remedies for the treatment of intermittent heartburn and dyspepsia.

Antacids are weak bases that react with gastric hydrochloric acid to form a salt and water. Although their principal mechanism of action is reduction of intragastric acidity, they may also promote mucosal defense mechanisms through stimulation of mucosal prostaglandin production. After a meal, approximately 45 mEq/h of hydrochloric acid is secreted. A single dose of 156 mEq of antacid given 1 hour after a meal effectively neutralizes gastric acid for up to 2 hours. However, the acid-neutralization capacity among different proprietary formulations of antacids is highly variable, depending on their rate of dissolution (tablet versus liquid), water solubility, rate of reaction with acid, and the rate of gastric emptying.

Sodium bicarbonate (eg, baking soda, Alka Seltzer) reacts rapidly with HCl to produce carbon dioxide and NaCl. Formation of carbon dioxide results in gastric distention and belching. Unreacted alkali is readily absorbed, potentially causing metabolic alkalosis when given in high doses or to patients with renal insuffi-

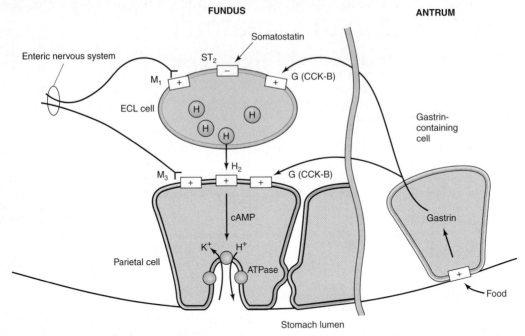

FUNDUS

ANTRUM

Figure 63–1. Schematic diagram of one model of the physiologic control of hydrogen ion secretion by the gastric parietal cell. ECL cell, enterochromaffin-like cell; G(CCK-B), gastrin-cholecystokinin-B receptor; H, histamine; H_2, histamine H_2 receptor; M_1, M_3, muscarinic receptors; ST_2, somatostatin-2 receptor; ATPase, H^+/K^+ ATPase proton pump. Some investigators place histamine receptors—and possibly cholinoceptors—on nearby tissue cells rather than on the parietal cell itself. (Modified and redrawn from Sachs G, Prinz C: Gastric enterochromaffin-like cells and the regulation of acid secretion. News Physiol Sci 1996;11:57, and other sources.)

ciency. Sodium chloride absorption may exacerbate fluid retention in patients with heart failure, hypertension, and renal insufficiency.

Calcium carbonate (eg, Tums, Os-Cal) is less soluble and reacts more slowly than sodium bicarbonate with HCl to form carbon dioxide and $CaCl_2$. Like sodium bicarbonate, calcium carbonate may cause belching or metabolic alkalosis. Calcium carbonate is used for a number of other indications apart from its antacid properties (see Chapter 42). Excessive doses of either sodium bicarbonate or calcium carbonate with calcium-containing dairy products can lead to hypercalcemia, renal insufficiency, and metabolic alkalosis (milk-alkali syndrome).

Formulations containing **magnesium hydroxide** or **aluminum hydroxide** react slowly with HCl to form magnesium chloride or aluminum chloride and water. Because no gas is generated, belching does not occur. Metabolic alkalosis is also uncommon because of the efficiency of the neutralization reaction. Because unabsorbed magnesium salts may cause an osmotic diarrhea and aluminum salts may cause constipation, these

agents are commonly administered together in proprietary formulations (eg, Gelusil, Maalox, Mylanta) to minimize the impact upon bowel function. Both magnesium and aluminum are absorbed and excreted by the kidneys. Hence, patients with renal insufficiency should not take these agents long-term.

All antacids may affect the absorption of other medications by binding the drug (reducing its absorption) or by increasing intragastric pH so that the drug's dissolution or solubility (especially weakly basic or acidic drugs) is altered. Therefore, antacids should not be given within 2 hours of doses of tetracyclines, fluoroquinolones, itraconazole, and iron.

H_2-RECEPTOR ANTAGONISTS

From their introduction in the 1970s until the early 1990s, H_2-receptor antagonists (commonly referred to as H_2 blockers) were the most commonly prescribed drugs in the world (see Clinical Uses). With the recognition of the role of *H pylori* in ulcer disease (which may be treated with appropriate antibacterial therapy) and the advent of proton pump inhibitors, the use of prescription H_2 blockers has declined markedly.

Chemistry & Pharmacokinetics

Four H_2 antagonists are in clinical use: **cimetidine, ranitidine, famotidine,** and **nizatidine** (Figure 63–2). All four agents are rapidly absorbed from the intestine. Cimetidine, ranitidine, and famotidine undergo first-pass hepatic metabolism resulting in a bioavailability of approximately 50%. Nizatidine has little first-pass metabolism and a bioavailability of almost 100%. The serum half-lives of the four agents range from 1.1–4 hours; however, duration of action depends on the dose given (Table 63–1). H_2 antagonists are cleared by a combination of hepatic metabolism, glomerular filtration, and renal tubular secretion. Dose reduction is required in patients with moderate to severe renal (and possibly severe hepatic) insufficiency. In the elderly, there is a decline of up to 50% in drug clearance as well as a significant reduction in volume of distribution.

Pharmacodynamics

The H_2 antagonists exhibit competitive inhibition at the parietal cell H_2 receptor and suppress basal and meal-stimulated acid secretion in a linear, dose-dependent manner (Figure 63–3). They are highly selective and do not affect H_1 or H_3 receptors. The volume of gastric secretion and the concentration of pepsin are also reduced.

H_2 antagonists reduce acid secretion stimulated by histamine as well as by gastrin and cholinomimetic agents through two mechanisms. First, histamine released from ECL cells by gastrin or vagal stimulation is blocked from binding to the parietal cell H_2 receptor. Second, direct stimulation of the parietal cell by gastrin or acetylcholine results in diminished acid secretion in the presence of H_2-receptor blockade. It appears that reduced parietal cell cAMP levels attenuate the intracellular activation of protein kinases by gastrin or acetylcholine.

The potencies of the four H_2-receptor antagonists vary over a 50-fold range (Table 63–1). When given in usual prescription doses however, all of the H_2 antagonists inhibit 60–70% of total 24-hour acid secretion. H_2 antagonists are especially effective at inhibiting nocturnal acid secretion (which depends largely on histamine) but have a modest impact on meal-stimulated acid secretion (which is stimulated by gastrin and acetylcholine as well as histamine). Thus, they block more than 90% of nocturnal acid but only 60–80% of daytime acid secretion. Therefore, nocturnal and fasting intragastric pH is raised to 4–5 but the impact upon the daytime, meal-stimulated pH profile is less. Recommended prescription doses maintain greater than 50% acid inhibition for 10 hours; hence, these drugs are commonly given twice daily. At doses available in over-the-counter formulations, the duration of acid inhibition is less than 6 hours.

Clinical Uses

H_2-receptor antagonists continue to be prescribed commonly. However, due to their superior acid inhibition and safety profile, proton pump inhibitors (see below) are steadily replacing H_2 antagonists for most clinical indications.

A. GASTROESOPHAGEAL REFLUX DISEASE (GERD)

Patients with infrequent heartburn or dyspepsia (fewer than 3 times per week) may take either antacids or intermittent H_2 antagonists. Because antacids provide rapid acid neutralization, they afford faster symptom relief than H_2 antagonists. However, the effect of antacids is short-lived (1–2 hours) compared with H_2 antagonists (6–10 hours). H_2 antagonists may be taken prophylactically before meals in an effort to reduce the likelihood of heartburn. Frequent heartburn is better treated with twice-daily H_2 antagonists; this regimen provides effective symptom control in 50–75% of people (Table 63–1). In patients with erosive esophagitis (approximately half of patients with GERD), H_2 antagonists afford healing in less than 50% of patients. Although higher doses of H_2 antagonists increase healing rates, proton pump inhibitors are preferred.

Figure 63–2. H_2-receptor–blocking drugs.

Table 63–1. Clinical comparisons of H_2-receptor blockers.

Drug	Relative Potency	Dose to Achieve > 50% Acid Inhibition for 10 Hours	Usual Dose for Acute Duodenal or Gastric Ulcer	Usual Dose for Gastroesophageal Reflux Disease	Usual Dose for Prevention of Stress-Related Bleeding
Cimetidine	1	400–800 mg	800 mg HS or 400 mg bid	800 mg bid	50 mg/h continuous infusion
Ranitidine	4–10×	150 mg	300 mg HS or 150 mg bid	150 mg bid	6.25 mg/h continuous infusion or 50 mg IV every 6–8 h
Nizatidine	4–10×	150 mg	300 mg HS or 150 mg bid	150 mg bid	Not available
Famotidine	20–50×	20 mg	40 mg HS or 20 mg bid	20 mg bid	20 mg IV every 12 h

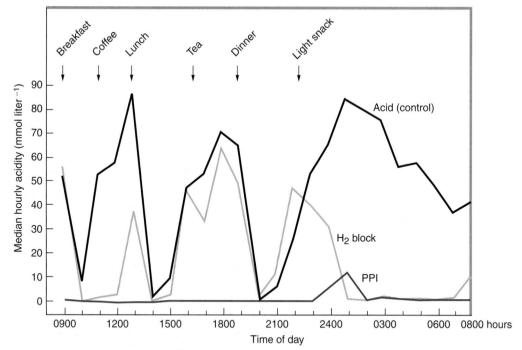

Figure 63–3. Twenty-four hour median intragastric acidity pretreatment (black) and after 1 month of treatment with either ranitidine, 150 mg twice daily (light color, H_2 block), or omeprazole, 20 mg once daily (dark color, PPI). Note that H_2-receptor antagonists have a marked effect upon nocturnal acid secretion but only a modest effect upon meal-stimulated secretion. Proton pump inhibitors markedly suppress meal-stimulated and nocturnal acid secretion. (Redrawn from data in Lanzon-Miller S et al: Twenty-four-hour intragastric acidity and plasma gastrin concentration before and during treatment with either ranitidine or omeprazole. Aliment Pharmacol Ther 1987;1:239.)

B. PEPTIC ULCER DISEASE

Proton pump inhibitors have largely replaced H_2 antagonists in the treatment of peptic ulcer disease. Nocturnal acid suppression by either drug group affords effective ulcer healing in the majority of patients with uncomplicated gastric and duodenal ulcers. Hence, all the agents may be administered once daily at bedtime for acute, uncomplicated ulcers, resulting in ulcer healing rates greater than 80–90% after 6–8 weeks of therapy. For patients with acute peptic ulcers caused by *H pylori*, H_2 antagonists no longer play a significant therapeutic role. For the minority of patients in whom *H pylori* cannot be successfully eradicated, H_2 antagonists may be given daily at bedtime in half of the usual ulcer therapeutic dose to prevent ulcer recurrence (eg, ranitidine, 150 mg; famotidine, 20 mg). For patients with ulcers caused by aspirin or other NSAIDs, H_2 antagonists provide rapid ulcer healing so long as the NSAID is discontinued. If the NSAID must be continued for clinical reasons despite active ulceration, a proton pump inhibitor should be given to promote ulcer healing.

C. NONULCER DYSPEPSIA

H_2 antagonists are commonly used as over-the-counter agents and prescription agents for treatment of intermittent dyspepsia not caused by peptic ulcer. However, benefit compared with placebo has never been convincingly demonstrated.

D. PREVENTION OF BLEEDING FROM STRESS-RELATED GASTRITIS

H_2-receptor antagonists significantly reduce the incidence of bleeding from stress-related gastritis in seriously ill patients in the intensive care unit. H_2 antagonists are given intravenously, either as intermittent injections or continuous infusions. For maximal efficacy, the pH of gastric aspirates should be measured and the doses titrated to achieve a gastric pH higher than 4.

Adverse Effects

H_2 antagonists are extremely safe drugs. Adverse effects occur in fewer than 3% of patients and include diarrhea, headache, fatigue, myalgias, and constipation.

A. CENTRAL NERVOUS SYSTEM

Mental status changes (confusion, hallucinations, agitation) may occur with administration of intravenous H_2 antagonists, especially in patients in the intensive care unit who are elderly or who have renal or hepatic dysfunction. These events may be more common with cimetidine. Mental status changes rarely occur in ambulatory patients.

B. ENDOCRINE EFFECTS

Cimetidine inhibits binding of dihydrotestosterone to androgen receptors, inhibits metabolism of estradiol, and increases serum prolactin levels. When used long-term or in high doses, it may cause gynecomastia or impotence in men and galactorrhea in women. These effects are specific to cimetidine and do not occur with the other H_2 antagonists.

C. PREGNANCY AND NURSING MOTHERS

Although there are no known harmful effects on the fetus, these agents cross the placenta. Therefore, they should not be administered to pregnant women unless absolutely necessary. The H_2 antagonists are secreted into breast milk and may therefore affect nursing infants.

D. OTHER EFFECTS

H_2 antagonists may rarely cause blood dyscrasias. Blockade of cardiac H_2 receptors may cause bradycardia but this is rarely of clinical significance. Rapid intravenous infusion may cause bradycardia and hypotension through blockade of cardiac H_2 receptors; therefore, intravenous injection should be given over 30 minutes. H_2 antagonists rarely cause reversible abnormalities in liver chemistry.

Drug Interactions

Cimetidine interferes with several important hepatic cytochrome P450 drug metabolism pathways, including those catalyzed by CYP1A2, CYP2C9, CYP2D6, and CYP3A4 (see Chapter 4). Hence, the half-lives of drugs metabolized by these pathways may be prolonged. Ranitidine binds 4–10 times less avidly than cimetidine to cytochrome P450. Negligible interaction occurs with nizatidine and famotidine.

H_2 antagonists compete with certain drugs (eg, procainamide) for renal tubular secretion. All of these agents except famotidine inhibit gastric first-pass metabolism of ethanol, especially in women. Although the importance of this is debated, increased bioavailability of ethanol could lead to increased blood ethanol levels.

PROTON PUMP INHIBITORS (PPI)

Since their introduction in the late 1980s, these efficacious acid inhibitory agents have rapidly assumed the major role for the treatment of acid-peptic disorders. They are now among the most widely selling drugs worldwide due to their outstanding efficacy and safety.

Chemistry & Pharmacokinetics

Five proton pump inhibitors are available for clinical use: **omeprazole, lansoprazole, rabeprazole, panto-**

Figure 63–4. Molecular structure of the proton pump inhibitors: omeprazole, lansoprazole, pantoprazole, and the sodium salt of rabeprazole. Omeprazole and esomeprazole have the same chemical structure (see text).

prazole, and **esomeprazole.** All are substituted benzimidazoles that resemble H_2 antagonists in structure (Figure 63–4) but have a completely different mechanism of action. Omeprazole is a racemic mixture of *R*- and *S*-isomers. Esomeprazole is the *S*-isomer of omeprazole. All are available in oral formulations. Esomeprazole, lansoprazole, and pantoprazole are also available in intravenous formulations (Table 63–2).

Proton pump inhibitors are administered as inactive prodrugs. To protect the acid-labile prodrug from rapid destruction within the gastric lumen, oral products are formulated for delayed release as acid-resistant, enteric-coated capsule or tablet formulations. After passing through the stomach into the alkaline intestinal lumen, the enteric coatings dissolve and the prodrug is absorbed. For children or patients with dysphagia or enteral feeding tubes, capsules may be opened and the microgranules mixed with apple or orange juice or mixed with soft foods (eg, applesauce). Lansoprazole is also available as a tablet formulation that disintegrates in the mouth or may be mixed with water and administered via oral syringe or enteral tube. Omeprazole is also available as a non-enteric-coated powder that contains sodium bicarbonate (1680 mg $NaHCO_3$; 460 mg of sodium) to protect the naked (nonenteric coated) drug from acid degradation. When mixed with water and administered on an empty stomach by mouth or enteral tube, this "immediate-release" suspension results in

Table 63–2. Pharmacokinetics of proton pump inhibitors.

Drug	pK_a	Bioavailability (%)	$t_{1/2}$ (h)	T_{max} (h)	Usual Dosage for Peptic Ulcer or GERD
Omeprazole	4	40–65	0.5–1.5	1–3.5	20–40 mg qd
Esomeprazole	4	> 80	1.2–1.5	1.6	20–40 mg qd
Lansoprazole	4	> 80	1.5	1.7	30 mg qd
Pantoprazole	3.9	77	1.0–1.9	2.5–4.0	40 mg qd
Rabeprazole	5	52	1.0–2.0	2.0–5.0	20 mg qd

rapid omeprazole absorption (T_{max} < 30 minutes) and onset of acid inhibition.

The proton pump inhibitors are lipophilic weak bases (pK_a 4–5) and after intestinal absorption diffuse readily across lipid membranes into acidified compartments (such as the parietal cell canaliculus). Within the acidified compartment the prodrug rapidly becomes protonated and is concentrated more than 1000-fold within the parietal cell canaliculus by Henderson-Hasselbalch trapping (see Chapter 1). There, it rapidly undergoes a molecular conversion to the active, reactive thiophilic sulfonamide cation. The sulfonamide reacts with the H^+/K^+ ATPase, forms a covalent disulfide linkage, and irreversibly inactivates the enzyme. The rate of conversion is inversely proportional to the pK_a of the drug.

The pharmacokinetics of available proton pump inhibitors are shown in Table 63–2. Rabeprazole (due to its higher pK_a) or immediate-release omeprazole (due to its rapid release and absorption) may have a slightly faster onset of acid inhibition than other oral formulations. Although differences in pharmacokinetic profiles may affect speed of onset and duration of acid inhibition in the first few days of therapy, they are of little clinical importance with continued daily administration. The bioavailability of all agents is decreased approximately 50% by food; hence, the drugs should be administered on an empty stomach. In a fasting state, only 10% of proton pumps are actively secreting acid and susceptible to inhibition. Proton pump inhibitors should be administered approximately 1 hour before a meal (usually breakfast or dinner), so that the peak serum concentration coincides with the maximal activity of proton pump secretion. The drugs have a short serum half-life of about 1.5 hours; however, the duration of acid inhibition lasts up to 24 hours due to the irreversible inactivation of the proton pump. At least 18 hours are required for synthesis of new H^+/K^+ ATPase pump molecules. Because not all proton pumps are inactivated with the first dose of medication, up to 3–4 days of daily medication are required before the full acid-inhibiting potential is reached. Similarly, after stopping the drug, it takes 3–4 days for full acid secretion to return.

Proton pump inhibitors undergo rapid first-pass and systemic hepatic metabolism and have negligible renal clearance. Dose reduction is not needed for patients with renal insufficiency or mild to moderate liver disease but should be considered in patients with severe liver impairment. Although other proton pumps exist in the body, the H^+/K^+ ATPase appears to exist only in the parietal cell and is distinct structurally and functionally from other H^+ transporting enzymes.

The intravenous formulations of esomeprazole, lansoprazole, and pantoprazole have similar characteristics to the oral drugs. When given to a fasting patient, they inactivate acid pumps that are actively secreting but have no effect on pumps in quiescent, nonsecreting vesicles. Because the half-life of a single injection of the intravenous formulation is short, acid secretion returns several hours later as pumps move from the tubulo-vesicles to the canalicular surface. Thus, in order to provide maximal inhibition during the first 24–48 hours of treatment, the intravenous formulations must be given as a continuous infusion or as repeated bolus injections. The optimal dosing of intravenous proton pump inhibitors to achieve maximal blockade in fasting patients is not yet established.

From a pharmacokinetic perspective, proton pump inhibitors are ideal drugs: they have a short serum half-life, they are concentrated and activated near their site of action, and they have a long duration of action.

Pharmacodynamics

In contrast to H_2 antagonists, proton pump inhibitors inhibit both fasting and meal-stimulated secretion because they block the final common pathway of acid secretion, the proton pump. In standard doses, proton pump inhibitors inhibit 90–98% of 24-hour acid secretion (Figure 63–3). Among commercially available formulations, 40 mg of esomeprazole achieves slightly greater 24-hour gastric acid suppression compared with standard doses of other delayed-release oral proton pump inhibitors (lansoprazole, 30 mg; rabeprazole, 20 mg; omeprazole, 20–40 mg; or pantoprazole 40 mg); however, when administered at equivalent doses there is little difference in clinical efficacy among the different agents. In a crossover study of patients receiving long-term therapy with all five proton pump inhibitors, the mean 24-hour intragastric pH varied from 3.3 (pantoprazole, 40 mg) to 4.0 (esomeprazole, 40 mg) and the mean number of hours the pH was higher than 4 varied from 10.1 (pantoprazole, 40 mg) to 14.0 (esomeprazole, 40 mg).

Clinical Uses

A. GASTROESOPHAGEAL REFLUX DISEASE (GERD)

Proton pump inhibitors are the most effective agents for the treatment of nonerosive and erosive reflux disease, esophageal complications of reflux disease (peptic stricture or Barrett's esophagus), and extraesophageal manifestations of reflux disease. Once-daily dosing provides effective symptom relief and tissue healing in 85–90% of patients; up to 15% of patients require twice-daily dosing.

GERD symptoms recur in over 80% of patients within 6 months after discontinuation of a proton pump inhibitor. For patients with erosive esophagitis or esophageal complications, long-term daily maintenance therapy with a full-dose or half-dose proton pump inhibitor is usually needed. Many patients with nonerosive GERD may be treated successfully with intermittent courses of proton pump inhibitors or H_2 antagonists taken as needed ("on demand") for recurrent symptoms.

In current clinical practice, many patients with symptomatic GERD are treated empirically with medications without prior endoscopy, ie, without knowledge of whether the patient has erosive or nonerosive reflux disease. Empiric treatment with proton pump inhibitors provides sustained symptomatic relief in 70–80% of patients, compared with 50–60% with H_2 antagonists. Due to recent cost reductions, proton pump inhibitors are increasingly being used as first-line therapy for patients with symptomatic GERD.

Sustained acid suppression with twice-daily proton pump inhibitors for at least 3 months is used to treat extraesophageal complications of reflux disease (asthma, chronic cough, laryngitis, and noncardiac chest pain).

B. PEPTIC ULCER DISEASE

Compared with H_2 antagonists, proton pump inhibitors afford more rapid symptom relief and faster ulcer healing for duodenal ulcers and, to a lesser extent, gastric ulcers. All of the pump inhibitors heal more than 90% of duodenal ulcers within 4 weeks and a similar percentage of gastric ulcers within 6–8 weeks.

1. H pylori–associated ulcers—For *H pylori*–associated ulcers, there are two therapeutic goals: heal the ulcer and eradicate the organism. The most effective regimens for *H pylori* eradication are combinations of two antibiotics and a proton pump inhibitor. Proton pump inhibitors promote eradication of *H pylori* through several mechanisms: direct antimicrobial properties (minor) and—by raising intragastric pH—lowering the minimal inhibitory concentrations of antibiotics against *H pylori*. The best treatment regimen consists of a 10–14 day regimen of "triple therapy": a proton pump inhibitor twice daily; clarithromycin, 500 mg twice daily; and amoxicillin, 1 g twice daily. For patients who are allergic to penicillin, metronidazole, 500 mg twice daily, should be substituted for amoxicillin. After completion of triple therapy, the proton pump inhibitor should be continued once daily for a total of 4–6 weeks to ensure complete ulcer healing.

2. NSAID-associated ulcers—For patients with ulcers caused by aspirin or other NSAIDs, either H_2 antagonists or proton pump inhibitors provide rapid ulcer healing so long as the NSAID is discontinued; continued use of the NSAID impairs ulcer healing. Treatment with a once-daily proton pump inhibitor promotes ulcer healing despite continued NSAID therapy.

Proton pump inhibitors are also given to prevent ulcer complications from NSAIDs. Asymptomatic peptic ulceration develops in 10–20% of people taking frequent NSAIDs, and ulcer-related complications (bleeding, perforation) develop in 1–2% of persons per year.

Proton pump inhibitors taken once daily are effective in reducing the incidence of ulcers and ulcer complications in patients taking aspirin or other NSAIDs.

3. Prevention of rebleeding from peptic ulcers—In patients with acute gastrointestinal bleeding due to peptic ulcers, the risk of rebleeding from ulcers that have a visible vessel or adherent clot is increased. Rebleeding in this subset of high-risk ulcers is reduced significantly with use of proton pump inhibitors administered for 3–5 days either as high-dose oral therapy (eg, omeprazole, 40 mg orally twice daily) or as a continuous intravenous infusion. It is believed that an intragastric pH higher than 6 may enhance coagulation and platelet aggregation. The optimal dose of intravenous proton pump inhibitor needed to achieve and maintain this level of near-complete acid inhibition is unknown; however, initial bolus administration (60–80 mg) followed by constant infusion (8 mg/h) commonly is recommended.

C. NONULCER DYSPEPSIA

Proton pump inhibitors have modest efficacy for treatment of nonulcer dyspepsia, benefiting 10–20% more patients than placebo. Despite their increasing use for this indication, superiority to H_2 antagonists (or even placebo) has not been conclusively demonstrated.

D. PREVENTION OF STRESS-RELATED MUCOSAL BLEEDING

Clinically important bleeding from upper gastrointestinal erosions or ulcers occurs in 1–5% of critically ill patients due to mucosal ischemia. Although most critically ill patients have normal or decreased acid secretion, numerous studies have shown that maintaining intragastric pH higher than 4 reduces the incidence of clinically significant bleeding. The only proton pump inhibitor approved by the Food and Drug Administration for reduction of stress-related mucosal bleeding is an oral immediate-release omeprazole formulation, which is administered by nasogastric tube twice daily on the first day, then once daily. In a large controlled trial, nasogastric immediate-release omeprazole had similar efficacy to a continuous intravenous infusion of an H_2 antagonist (cimetidine) in the prevention of stress-related bleeding and superior inhibition of gastric acidity (median pH > 6).

At this time, the optimal agent for the reduction of stress-related mucosal bleeding is uncertain. For patients with nasoenteric tubes, immediate-release omeprazole may be preferred to intravenous H_2 antagonists because of comparable efficacy, lower cost, and ease of administration. For patients without a nasoenteric tube or with significant ileus, intravenous H_2 antagonists are the preferred agents because of their proven efficacy. Although proton pump inhibitors are increasingly used, there are no controlled trials demonstrating efficacy or optimal dosing.

E. GASTRINOMA AND OTHER HYPERSECRETORY CONDITIONS

Patients with isolated gastrinomas are best treated with surgical resection. In patients with metastatic or unresectable gastrinomas, massive acid hypersecretion results in peptic ulceration, erosive esophagitis, and malabsorption. Previously, these patients required vagotomy and extraordinarily high doses of H_2 antagonists, which resulted in suboptimal acid suppression. With proton pump inhibitors, excellent acid suppression can be achieved in all patients. Dosage is titrated to reduce basal acid output to less than 5–10 mEq/h. Typical doses of omeprazole are 60–120 mg/d.

Adverse Effects

A. GENERAL

Proton pump inhibitors are extremely safe. Diarrhea, headache, and abdominal pain are reported in 1–5% of patients, although the frequency of these events is only slightly increased compared with placebo. Proton pump inhibitors do not have teratogenicity in animal models; however, safety during pregnancy has not been established.

B. NUTRITION

Acid is important in releasing vitamin B_{12} from food. A minor reduction in oral cyanocobalamin absorption occurs during proton pump inhibition, potentially leading to subnormal B_{12} levels with prolonged therapy. Acid also promotes absorption of food-bound minerals (iron, calcium, zinc); however, no mineral deficiencies have been reported with proton pump inhibitor therapy.

C. RESPIRATORY AND ENTERIC INFECTIONS

Gastric acid is an important barrier to colonization and infection of the stomach and intestine from ingested bacteria. Increases in gastric bacterial concentrations are detected in patients taking proton pump inhibitors, which is of unclear clinical significance. Some studies have reported an increased risk of both community-acquired respiratory infections and nosocomial pneumonia among patients taking proton pump inhibitors.

A small increased risk of enteric infections may exist in patients taking proton pump inhibitors, especially when traveling in underdeveloped countries. Hospitalized patients may have an increased risk for *Clostridium difficile* infection.

D. POTENTIAL PROBLEMS DUE TO INCREASED SERUM GASTRIN

Gastrin levels are regulated by intragastric acidity. Acid suppression alters normal feedback inhibition so that median gastrin levels rise 1.5- to 2-fold in patients taking proton pump inhibitors. Although gastrin levels remain within normal limits in most patients, they exceed 500 pg/mL (normal, < 100 pg/mL) in 3%. Upon stopping the drug, the levels normalize within 4 weeks.

The rise in serum gastrin levels in patients receiving long-term therapy with proton pump inhibitors has raised two theoretical concerns. First, gastrin is a trophic hormone that stimulates hyperplasia of ECL cells. In female rats given proton pump inhibitors for prolonged periods, gastric carcinoid tumors developed in areas of ECL hyperplasia. Although humans who take proton pump inhibitors for a long time may exhibit ECL hyperplasia in response to hypergastrinemia, carcinoid tumor formation has not been documented. Second, hypergastrinemia increases the proliferative rate of colonic mucosa, potentially promoting carcinogenesis. In humans, hypergastrinemia caused by vagotomy, atrophic gastritis, or Zollinger-Ellison syndrome has not been associated with increased colon cancer risk. At present, routine monitoring of serum gastrin levels is not recommended in patients receiving prolonged proton pump inhibitor therapy.

E. OTHER POTENTIAL PROBLEMS DUE TO DECREASED GASTRIC ACIDITY

Among patients infected with *H pylori*, long-term acid suppression leads to increased chronic inflammation in the gastric body and decreased inflammation in the antrum. Concerns have been raised that increased gastric inflammation may accelerate gastric gland atrophy (atrophic gastritis) and intestinal metaplasia—known risk factors for gastric adenocarcinoma. A special US FDA Gastrointestinal Advisory Committee concluded that there is no evidence that prolonged proton pump inhibitor therapy produces the kind of atrophic gastritis (multifocal atrophic gastritis) or intestinal metaplasia that is associated with increased risk of adenocarcinoma. Routine testing for *H pylori* is no longer recommended in patients who require long-term proton pump inhibitor therapy. Long-term proton pump inhibitor therapy is associated with the development of small benign gastric fundic-gland polyps in a small number of patients, which may disappear after stopping the drug and are of uncertain clinical significance.

Drug Interactions

Decreased gastric acidity may alter absorption of drugs for which intragastric acidity affects drug bioavailability, eg, ketoconazole and digoxin. All proton pump inhibitors are metabolized by hepatic P450 cytochromes, including CYP2C19 and CYP3A4. Due to their short-half lives, clinically significant drug interactions are rare. Omeprazole may inhibit the metabolism of coumadin, diazepam, and phenytoin. Esomeprazole also may decrease metabolism of diazepam. Lansoprazole may enhance clearance of theophylline. Rabeprazole and pantoprazole have no significant drug interactions.

MUCOSAL PROTECTIVE AGENTS

The gastroduodenal mucosa has evolved a number of defense mechanisms to protect itself against the noxious effects of acid and pepsin. Both mucus and epithelial cell-cell tight junctions restrict back diffusion of acid and pepsin. Epithelial bicarbonate secretion establishes a pH gradient within the mucous layer in which the pH ranges from 7 at the mucosal surface to 1–2 in the gastric lumen. Blood flow carries bicarbonate and vital nutrients to surface cells. Areas of injured epithelium are quickly repaired by restitution, a process in which migration of cells from gland neck cells seals small erosions to reestablish intact epithelium. Mucosal prostaglandins appear to be important in stimulating mucus and bicarbonate secretion and mucosal blood flow. A number of agents that potentiate these mucosal defense mechanisms are available for the prevention and treatment of acid-peptic disorders.

SUCRALFATE

Chemistry & Pharmacokinetics

Sucralfate is a salt of sucrose complexed to sulfated aluminum hydroxide. In water or acidic solutions it forms a viscous, tenacious paste that binds selectively to ulcers or erosions for up to 6 hours. Sucralfate has limited solubility, breaking down into sucrose sulfate (strongly negatively charged) and an aluminum salt. Less than 3% of intact drug and aluminum is absorbed from the intestinal tract; the remainder is excreted in the feces.

Pharmacodynamics

A variety of beneficial effects have been attributed to sucralfate, but the precise mechanism of action is unclear. It is believed that the negatively charged sucrose sulfate binds to positively charged proteins in the base of ulcers or erosion, forming a physical barrier that restricts further caustic damage and stimulates mucosal prostaglandin and bicarbonate secretion.

Clinical Uses

Sucralfate is administered in a dosage of 1 g four times daily on an empty stomach (at least 1 hour before meals). At present, its clinical uses are limited. Sucralfate (administered as a slurry through a nasogastric tube) reduces the incidence of clinically significant upper gastrointestinal bleeding in critically ill patients hospitalized in the intensive care unit, although it is slightly less effective than intravenous H_2 antagonists. Sucralfate is still used by many clinicians for prevention of stress-related bleeding because of concerns that acid-inhibitory therapies (antacids, H_2 antagonists, or pro-

ton pump inhibitors) may increase the risk of nosocomial pneumonia.

Adverse Effects

Because it is not absorbed, sucralfate is virtually devoid of systemic adverse effects. Constipation occurs in 2% of patients due to the aluminum salt. Because a small amount of aluminum is absorbed, it should not be used for prolonged periods in patients with renal insufficiency.

Drug Interactions

Sucralfate may bind to other medications, impairing their absorption.

PROSTAGLANDIN ANALOGS

Chemistry & Pharmacokinetics

The human gastrointestinal mucosa synthesizes a number of prostaglandins (see Chapter 18); the primary ones are prostaglandins E and F. **Misoprostol,** a methyl analog of PGE_1, has been approved for gastrointestinal conditions. Following oral administration, it is rapidly absorbed and metabolized to a metabolically active free acid. The serum half-life is less than 30 minutes; hence, it must be administered 3–4 times daily. It is excreted in the urine; however, dose reduction is not needed in patients with renal insufficiency.

Pharmacodynamics

Misoprostol has both acid inhibitory and mucosal protective properties. It is believed to stimulate mucus and bicarbonate secretion and enhance mucosal blood flow. In addition, it binds to a prostaglandin receptor on parietal cells, reducing histamine-stimulated cAMP production and causing modest acid inhibition. Prostaglandins have a variety of other actions, including stimulation of intestinal electrolyte and fluid secretion, intestinal motility, and uterine contractions.

Clinical Uses

Peptic ulcers develop in approximately 10–20% of patients who receive long-term NSAID therapy (see Proton Pump Inhibitors, above). Misoprostol reduces the incidence of NSAID-induced ulcers to less than 3% and the incidence of ulcer complications by 50%. It is approved for prevention of NSAID-induced ulcers in high-risk patients; however, it has never achieved widespread use due to its high adverse effect profile and need for multiple daily dosing. As discussed, proton pump inhibitors may be as effective as and better tolerated than misoprostol for this indication. Cyclooxygenase-2-selective NSAIDs, which may have less gastrointestinal toxicity (see Chapter 36), offer another option for patients at high-risk for NSAID-induced complications.

Adverse Effects & Drug Interactions

Diarrhea and cramping abdominal pain occurs in 10–20% of patients. Because misoprostol stimulates uterine contractions (see Chapter 18), it should not be used during pregnancy or in women of childbearing potential unless they have a negative serum pregnancy test and are compliant with effective contraceptive measures. No significant drug interactions are reported.

COLLOIDAL BISMUTH COMPOUNDS

Chemistry & Pharmacokinetics

The only bismuth compound available in the USA is **bismuth subsalicylate,** a nonprescription formulation containing bismuth and salicylate. In other countries, **bismuth subcitrate** and **bismuth dinitrate** are also available. Bismuth subsalicylate undergoes rapid dissociation within the stomach, allowing absorption of salicylate. Over 99% of the bismuth appears in the stool. Although minimal (< 1%) bismuth is absorbed, it is stored in many tissues and has slow renal excretion. Salicylate (like aspirin) is readily absorbed and excreted in the urine.

Pharmacodynamics

Like sucralfate, bismuth probably coats ulcers and erosions, creating a protective layer against acid and pepsin. It may also stimulate prostaglandin, mucus, and bicarbonate secretion. Bismuth subsalicylate reduces stool frequency and liquidity in acute infectious diarrhea, due to salicylate inhibition of intestinal prostaglandin and chloride secretion. Bismuth has direct antimicrobial effects and binds enterotoxins, accounting for its benefit in preventing and treating traveler's diarrhea. Bismuth compounds have direct antimicrobial activity against *H pylori.*

Clinical Uses

In spite of the lack of comparative trials, nonprescription bismuth compounds are widely used by patients for the nonspecific treatment of dyspepsia and acute diarrhea. Bismuth subsalicylate also is used for the prevention of traveler's diarrhea (30 mL or 2 tablets four times daily).

Bismuth compounds have been used in multidrug regimens for the eradication of *H pylori* infection. In the USA, a "triple therapy" regimen has been used, consisting of bismuth subsalicylate (2 tablets; 262 mg each), tetracycline (500 mg), and metronidazole (250 mg), each taken four times daily for 14 days. Because of the need for four-times daily dosing and the high adverse effect profile, this regimen is no longer used as first-line therapy for *H pylori* eradication (see Proton Pump Inhibitors above). For patients with resistant infections, "quadruple therapy" consisting of a proton pump inhibitor twice daily in addition to the three-drug bismuth-based regimen four times daily for 14 days is highly effective. In Europe, bismuth subcitrate is used instead of bismuth subsalicylate, and treatment for 7–10 days may be sufficient.

Adverse Effects

All bismuth formulations have an excellent safety profile. Bismuth causes blackening of the stool, which may be confused with gastrointestinal bleeding. Liquid formulations may cause harmless darkening of the tongue. Bismuth agents should be used for short periods only and should be avoided in patients with renal insufficiency. Prolonged usage of some bismuth compounds may rarely lead to bismuth toxicity, resulting in encephalopathy (ataxia, headaches, confusion, seizures). However, such toxicity is not reported with bismuth subsalicylate or bismuth citrate. High dosages of bismuth subsalicylate may lead to salicylate toxicity.

■ II. DRUGS STIMULATING GASTROINTESTINAL MOTILITY

Drugs that can selectively stimulate gut motor function (**prokinetic** agents) have significant potential clinical usefulness. Agents that increase lower esophageal sphincter pressures may be useful for GERD. Drugs that improve gastric emptying may be helpful for gastroparesis and postsurgical gastric emptying delay. Agents that stimulate the small intestine may be beneficial for postoperative ileus or chronic intestinal pseudo-obstruction. Finally, agents that enhance colonic transit may be useful in the treatment of constipation. Unfortunately, only a limited number of agents in this group are available for clinical use at this time.

PHYSIOLOGY OF THE ENTERIC NERVOUS SYSTEM

The enteric nervous system (see also Chapter 6) is composed of interconnected networks of ganglion cells and nerve fibers mainly located in the submucosa (submucosal plexus) and between the circular and longitudinal muscle layers (myenteric plexus). These networks give rise to nerve fibers that connect with the mucosa and deep muscle. Although extrinsic sympathetic and para-

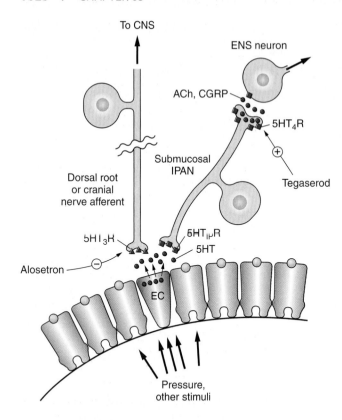

Figure 63–5. Release of serotonin (5-HT) by enterochromaffin (EC) cells from gut distention stimulates submucosal intrinsic primary afferent neurons (IPANs) via 5-HT$_{1P}$ receptors and extrinsic primary afferent neurons via 5-HT$_3$ receptors (5-HT$_{1P}$R, 5-HT$_3$R). Submucosal IPANs activate the enteric neurons responsible for peristaltic and secretory reflex activity. Stimulation of 5-HT$_4$ receptors (5-HT$_4$R) on presynaptic terminals of IPANs enhances release of acetylcholine and calcitonin gene-related peptide (CGRP), promoting reflex activity. ENS, enteric nervous system. (Redrawn from Gershon MD: Serotonin and its implication for the management of irritable bowel syndrome. Rev Gastroenterol Dis 2003;3(Suppl 2):S25.)

sympathetic nerves project onto the submucosal and myenteric plexuses, the enteric nervous system can independently regulate gastrointestinal motility and secretion. Extrinsic primary afferent neurons project via the dorsal root ganglia or vagus nerve to the central nervous system (Figure 63–5). Release of serotonin (5-HT) from intestinal mucosa enterochromaffin (EC) cells stimulates 5-HT$_3$ receptors on the extrinsic afferent nerves, stimulating nausea, vomiting, or abdominal pain. Serotonin also stimulates submucosal 5-HT$_{1P}$ receptors of the intrinsic primary afferent nerves (IPANs), which contain calcitonin gene-related peptide (CGRP) and acetylcholine and project to myenteric plexus interneurons. 5-HT$_4$ receptors on the presynaptic terminals of the IPANs appear to enhance release of CGRP or acetylcholine. The myenteric interneurons are important in controlling the peristaltic reflex, promoting release of excitatory mediators proximally and inhibitory mediators distally. Motilin may stimulate excitatory neurons or muscle cells directly. Dopamine acts as an inhibitory neurotransmitter in the gastrointestinal tract, decreasing the intensity of esophageal and gastric contractions.

Although there are at least 14 serotonin receptor subtypes, 5-HT drug development for gastrointestinal applications to date has focused on **5-HT$_3$-recep-**

tor antagonists and **5-HT$_4$-receptor agonists.** These agents—which have effects upon gastrointestinal motility and visceral afferent sensation—are discussed below under Drugs Used for the Treatment of Irritable Bowel Syndrome and Antiemetic Agents. Other drugs acting on 5-HT receptors are discussed in Chapters 16, 29, and 30.

CHOLINOMIMETIC AGENTS

Cholinomimetic agonists such as **bethanechol** stimulate muscarinic M$_3$ receptors on muscle cells and at myenteric plexus synapses (see Chapter 7). Bethanechol was used in the past for the treatment of GERD and gastroparesis. Due to multiple cholinergic effects and the advent of less toxic agents, it is now seldom used. The acetylcholinesterase inhibitor **neostigmine** can enhance gastric, small intestine, and colonic emptying. Intravenous neostigmine has enjoyed a resurgence in clinical usage for the treatment of hospitalized patients with acute large bowel distention (known as acute colonic pseudo-obstruction or Ogilvie's syndrome). Administration of 2 mg results in prompt colonic evacuation of flatus and feces in the majority of patients. Cholinergic effects include excessive salivation, nausea, vomiting, diarrhea, and bradycardia.

METOCLOPRAMIDE & DOMPERIDONE

Metoclopramide and domperidone are dopamine D_2 receptor antagonists. Within the gastrointestinal tract activation of dopamine receptors inhibits cholinergic smooth muscle stimulation; blockade of this effect is believed to be the primary prokinetic mechanism of action of these agents. These agents increase esophageal peristaltic amplitude, increase lower esophageal sphincter pressure, and enhance gastric emptying but have no effect upon small intestine or colonic motility. Metoclopramide and domperidone also block dopamine D_2 receptors in the chemoreceptor trigger zone of the medulla (area postrema), resulting in potent antinausea and antiemetic action.

Clinical Uses

A. GASTROESOPHAGEAL REFLUX DISEASE (GERD)

Metoclopramide is available for clinical use in the USA; domperidone is available in many other countries. These agents are sometimes used in the treatment of symptomatic GERD but are not effective in patients with erosive esophagitis. Due to the superior efficacy and safety of antisecretory agents in the treatment of heartburn, prokinetic agents are used mainly in combination with antisecretory agents in patients with regurgitation or refractory heartburn.

B. IMPAIRED GASTRIC EMPTYING

These agents are widely used in the treatment of patients with delayed gastric emptying due to postsurgical disorders (vagotomy, antrectomy) and diabetic gastroparesis. Metoclopramide is sometimes administered in hospitalized patients to promote advancement of nasoenteric feeding tubes from the stomach into the duodenum.

C. NONULCER DYSPEPSIA

These agents lead to symptomatic improvement in a small number of patients with chronic dyspepsia.

D. PREVENTION OF VOMITING

Due to their potent antiemetic action, metoclopramide and domperidone are used for the prevention and treatment of emesis (see page 1027).

E. POSTPARTUM LACTATION STIMULATION

Domperidone is sometimes recommended to promote postpartum lactation (see also Adverse Effects).

Adverse Effects

The most common adverse effects of **metoclopramide** involve the central nervous system. Restlessness, drowsiness, insomnia, anxiety, and agitation occur in 10–20% of patients, especially the elderly. Extrapyramidal effects (dystonias, akathisia, parkinsonian features) due to central dopamine receptor blockade occur acutely in 25% of patients given high doses and in 5% of patients receiving long-term therapy. Tardive dyskinesia, sometimes irreversible, has developed in patients treated for a prolonged period with metoclopramide. For this reason, long-term use should be avoided unless absolutely necessary, especially in the elderly. Elevated prolactin levels (caused by both metoclopramide and domperidone) can cause galactorrhea, gynecomastia, impotence, and menstrual disorders.

Domperidone is extremely well tolerated. Because it does not cross the blood-brain barrier to a significant degree, neuropsychiatric and extrapyramidal effects are rare.

MACROLIDES

Macrolide antibiotics such as **erythromycin** directly stimulate motilin receptors on gastrointestinal smooth muscle and promote the onset of a migrating motor complex. Intravenous erythromycin (3 mg/kg) is beneficial in some patients with gastroparesis; however, tolerance rapidly develops. It may be used in patients with acute upper gastrointestinal hemorrhage to promote gastric emptying of blood prior to endoscopy.

CHLORIDE CHANNEL ACTIVATOR

Lubiprostone is a recently approved prostanoic acid derivative labeled for use in chronic constipation. It is reported to act by stimulating chloride channel opening in the intestine. This increases liquid secretion into the intestine and shortens intestinal transit time. The drug also delays gastric emptying, which may cause nausea. No comparative studies with other drugs are available.

◼ III. LAXATIVES

The overwhelming majority of people do not need laxatives, yet they are self-prescribed by a large portion of the population. For most people, intermittent constipation is best prevented with a high fiber diet, adequate fluid intake, regular exercise, and the heeding of nature's call. Patients not responding to dietary changes or fiber supplements should undergo medical evaluation prior to the initiation of long-term laxative treatment. Laxatives may be classified by their major mechanism of action, but many work through more than one mechanism.

BULK-FORMING LAXATIVES

Bulk-forming laxatives are indigestible, hydrophilic colloids that absorb water, forming a bulky, emollient gel that distends the colon and promotes peristalsis. Common preparations include natural plant products **(psyllium, methylcellulose)** and synthetic fibers **(polycarbophil).** Bacterial digestion of plant fibers within the colon may lead to increased bloating and flatus.

STOOL SURFACTANT AGENTS (SOFTENERS)

These agents soften stool material, permitting water and lipids to penetrate. They may be administered orally or rectally. Common agents include **docusate** (oral or enema) or **glycerin suppository.** In hospitalized patients, docusate is commonly prescribed to prevent constipation and minimize straining. **Mineral oil** is a clear, viscous oil that lubricates fecal material, retarding water absorption from the stool. It is used to prevent and treat fecal impaction in young children and debilitated adults. It is not palatable but may be mixed with juices. Aspiration can result in a severe lipid pneumonitis. Long-term use can impair absorption of fat-soluble vitamins (A, D, E, K).

OSMOTIC LAXATIVES

The colon can neither concentrate nor dilute fecal fluid: fecal water is isotonic throughout the colon. Osmotic laxatives are soluble but nonabsorbable compounds that result in increased stool liquidity due to an obligate increase in fecal fluid.

Nonabsorbable Sugars or Salts

These agents may be used for the treatment of acute constipation or the prevention of chronic constipation. **Magnesium oxide (milk of magnesia)** is a commonly used osmotic laxative. It should not be used for prolonged periods in patients with renal insufficiency due to risk of hypermagnesemia. **Sorbitol** and **lactulose** are nonabsorbable sugars that can be used to prevent or treat chronic constipation. These sugars are metabolized by colonic bacteria, producing severe flatus and cramps.

High doses of osmotically active agents produce prompt bowel evacuation (purgation) within 1–3 hours. The rapid movement of water into the distal small bowel and colon leads to a high volume of liquid stool followed by rapid relief of constipation. The most commonly used **purgatives** are **magnesium citrate** and **sodium phosphate.** These hyperosmolar agents may lead to intravascular volume depletion and electrolyte fluctuations; hence they should not be used in patients who are frail, elderly, have renal insufficiency, or have significant cardiac disease.

Balanced Polyethylene Glycol

Lavage solutions containing **polyethylene glycol (PEG)** are used for complete colonic cleansing prior to gas-

trointestinal endoscopic procedures. These balanced, isotonic solutions contain an inert, nonabsorbable, osmotically active sugar (PEG) with sodium sulfate, sodium chloride, sodium bicarbonate, and potassium chloride. The solution is designed so that no significant intravascular fluid or electrolyte shifts occur. Therefore, they are safe for all patients. The solution should be ingested rapidly (4 L over 2–4 hours) to promote bowel cleansing. For treatment or prevention of chronic constipation, smaller doses of PEG powder may be mixed with water or juices (17 g/8 oz) and ingested daily. In contrast to sorbitol or lactulose, PEG does not produce significant cramps or flatus.

STIMULANT LAXATIVES

Stimulant laxatives (cathartics) induce bowel movements through a number of poorly understood mechanisms. These include direct stimulation of the enteric nervous system and colonic electrolyte and fluid secretion. There has been concern that long-term use of cathartics could lead to dependence and destruction of the myenteric plexus, resulting in colonic atony and dilation. More recent research suggests that long-term use of these agents probably is safe in most patients. Cathartics may be required on a long-term basis, especially in patients who are neurologically impaired and in bed-bound patients in long-term care facilities.

Anthraquinone Derivatives

Aloe, senna, and **cascara** occur naturally in plants. These laxatives are poorly absorbed and after hydrolysis in the colon, produce a bowel movement in 6–12 hours when given orally and within 2 hours when given rectally. Chronic use leads to a characteristic brown pigmentation of the colon known as "melanosis coli." There has been some concern that these agents may be carcinogenic, but epidemiologic studies do not suggest a relationship to colorectal cancer.

Diphenylmethane Derivatives

Due to concerns about possible cardiac toxicity, these agents (eg, **phenolphthalein**) were removed from the market.

Castor Oil

This oil is a potent stimulant laxative. It is hydrolyzed in the upper small intestine to ricinoleic acid, a local irritant that stimulates intestinal motility. Formerly used as a purgative to clean the colon before procedures, it is now seldom used.

SEROTONIN 5-HT$_4$-RECEPTOR AGONISTS

Pharmacokinetics & Pharmacodynamics

Tegaserod is a serotonin 5-HT$_4$ partial agonist that resembles serotonin in structure. It has high affinity for 5-HT$_4$ receptors but no appreciable binding to 5-HT$_3$ or dopamine receptors. As discussed earlier, stimulation of 5-HT$_4$ receptors on the presynaptic terminal of submucosal intrinsic primary afferent nerves enhances the release of their neurotransmitters, including calcitonin gene-related peptide, that stimulate second-order enteric neurons to promote the peristaltic reflex (Figure 63–5). These enteric neurons stimulate proximal bowel contraction (via acetylcholine and substance P) and distal bowel relaxation (via nitric oxide and vasoactive intestinal peptide). Tegaserod promotes gastric emptying and enhances small and large bowel transit but has no effect upon esophageal motility. Stimulation of 5-HT$_4$ receptors also activates cAMP-dependent chloride secretion from the colon, leading to increased stool liquidity.

Tegaserod has a bioavailability of only 10%. It should be taken before meals because food further reduces bioavailability by 50%. The drug is metabolized both by gastric acid-catalyzed hydrolysis and hepatic glucuronidation. Approximately 66% of drug is excreted unchanged in the feces and 33% as a metabolite in the urine. It should not be given to patients with severe hepatic or renal impairment.

Clinical Uses

A. CHRONIC CONSTIPATION

Tegaserod is approved for the treatment of patients with chronic constipation. In controlled trials, 40% of patients treated with tegaserod, 2–6 mg twice daily, had a significant increase in the number of spontaneous bowel movements compared with 25% receiving placebo. Responders also reported reduced bloating, straining, and stool hardness, and enhanced satisfaction. The effect of tegaserod on bowel activity is usually noted within 48 hours. Given its high cost, tegaserod should be reserved for patients with chronic constipation who have failed or are intolerant of other less expensive therapies.

B. OTHER USES

The role of tegaserod in the treatment of other gastrointestinal motility disorders, such as nonulcer dyspepsia, gastroparesis, and chronic constipation, is under investigation. The use of tegaserod in the treatment of irritable bowel syndrome is discussed later in the chapter.

Adverse Effects

Tegaserod appears to be an extremely safe agent. Diarrhea occurs in 9% of patients within the first few days of treatment but resolves in the majority of patients. Less than 2% of patients discontinue the drug because of diarrhea. Although it is stated that the drug does not cross the blood-brain barrier (and does not affect central serotonin receptors), headache may occur.

Drug Interactions

Tegaserod has no known effects on cytochrome P450 enzymes and no reported drug interactions.

■ IV. ANTIDIARRHEAL AGENTS

Antidiarrheal agents may be used safely in patients with mild to moderate acute diarrhea. However, they should not be used in patients with bloody diarrhea, high fever, or systemic toxicity because of the risk of worsening the underlying condition. They should be discontinued in patients whose diarrhea is worsening despite therapy. Antidiarrheals are also used to control chronic diarrhea caused by such conditions as irritable bowel syndrome (IBS) or inflammatory bowel disease (IBD).

OPIOID AGONISTS

Opioids have significant constipating effects (see Chapter 31). They increase colonic phasic segmenting activity through inhibition of presynaptic cholinergic nerves in the submucosal and myenteric plexuses and lead to increased colonic transit time and fecal water absorption. They also decrease mass colonic movements and the gastrocolic reflex. Although all opioids have antidiarrheal effects, central nervous system effects and potential for addiction limit the usefulness of most. **Loperamide** is a nonprescription opioid agonist that does not cross the blood-brain barrier and has no analgesic properties or potential for addiction. Tolerance to long-term use has not been reported. It is typically administered in doses of 2 mg taken one to four times daily. **Diphenoxylate** is another opioid agonist that has no analgesic properties in standard doses; however, higher doses have central nervous system effects and prolonged use can lead to opioid dependence. Commercial preparations commonly contain small amounts of atropine to discourage overdosage (2.5 mg diphenoxylate with 0.025 mg atropine). The anticholinergic properties of atropine may contribute to the antidiarrheal action.

COLLOIDAL BISMUTH COMPOUNDS

See the section under Mucosal Protective Agents on page 1018.

KAOLIN & PECTIN

Kaolin is a naturally occurring hydrated magnesium aluminum silicate (attapulgite), and pectin is an indigestible carbohydrate derived from apples. Both appear to act as absorbents of bacteria, toxins, and fluid, thereby decreasing stool liquidity and number. They may be useful in acute diarrhea but are seldom used on a chronic basis. A common commercial preparation is Kaopectate. The usual dose is 1.2–1.5 g after each loose bowel movement (maximum: 9 g/d). Kaolin-pectin formulations are not absorbed and have no significant adverse effects except constipation. They should not be taken within 2 hours of other medications (which they may bind).

BILE SALT–BINDING RESINS

Conjugated bile salts are normally absorbed in the terminal ileum. Disease of the terminal ileum (eg, Crohn's disease) or surgical resection leads to malabsorption of bile salts, which may cause colonic secretory diarrhea. The bile salt-binding resins **cholestyramine** or **colestipol** may decrease diarrhea caused by excess fecal bile acids (see Chapter 35). The usual dose is 4–5 g one to three times daily before meals. Adverse effects include bloating, flatulence, constipation, and fecal impaction. In patients with diminished circulating bile acid pools, further removal of bile acids may lead to an exacerbation of fat malabsorption. These agents bind a number of drugs and reduce their absorption; hence, they should not be given within 2 hours of other drugs.

OCTREOTIDE

Somatostatin is a 14 amino acid peptide that is released in the gastrointestinal tract and pancreas from paracrine cells, D-cells, and enteric nerves as well as from the hypothalamus (see Chapter 37). It is a key regulatory peptide that has many physiologic effects:

1. It inhibits the secretion of numerous hormones and transmitters, including gastrin, cholecystokinin, glucagon, growth hormone, insulin, secretin, pancreatic polypeptide, vasoactive intestinal peptide, and 5-HT.

2. It reduces intestinal fluid secretion and pancreatic secretion.

3. It slows gastrointestinal motility and inhibits gallbladder contraction.

4. It induces direct contraction of vascular smooth muscle, leading to a reduction of portal and splanchnic blood flow.

5. It inhibits secretion of some anterior pituitary hormones.

The clinical usefulness of somatostatin is limited by its short half-life in the circulation (3 minutes) when it is administered by intravenous injection. **Octreotide** is a synthetic octapeptide with actions similar to somatostatin. When administered intravenously, it has a serum half-life of 1.5 hours. It also may be administered by subcutaneous injection, resulting in a 6- to 12-hour duration of action. A longer-acting formulation is available for once-monthly depot intramuscular injection.

Clinical Uses

A. INHIBITION OF ENDOCRINE TUMOR EFFECTS

Two gastrointestinal neuroendocrine tumors (carcinoid, VIPoma) cause secretory diarrhea and systemic symptoms such as flushing and wheezing. For patients with advanced symptomatic tumors that cannot be completely removed by surgery, octreotide decreases secretory diarrhea and systemic symptoms through inhibition of hormonal secretion and may slow tumor progression.

B. OTHER CAUSES OF DIARRHEA

Octreotide inhibits intestinal secretion and has dose-related affects on bowel motility. In low doses (50 mcg subcutaneously) it stimulates motility, whereas at higher doses (eg, 100–250 mcg subcutaneously), it inhibits motility. Octreotide is effective in higher doses for the treatment of diarrhea due to vagotomy or dumping syndrome as well as for diarrhea caused by short bowel syndrome or AIDS. Octreotide has been used in low doses (50 mcg subcutaneously) to stimulate small bowel motility in patients with small bowel bacterial overgrowth or intestinal pseudo-obstruction secondary to scleroderma.

C. OTHER USES

Because it inhibits pancreatic secretion, octreotide may be of value in patients with pancreatic fistula. The role of octreotide in the treatment of pituitary tumors (eg, acromegaly) is discussed in Chapter 37. Octreotide is sometimes used in gastrointestinal bleeding (see below).

Adverse Effects

Impaired pancreatic secretion may cause steatorrhea, which can lead to fat-soluble vitamin deficiency. Alterations in gastrointestinal motility cause nausea, abdominal pain, flatulence, and diarrhea. Due to inhibition of gallbladder contractility and alterations in fat absorption, long-term use can cause formation of sludge or gallstones in over half of patients, which rarely results in the development of acute cholecystitis. Because octreotide alters the balance between insulin, glucagon, and growth hormone, hyperglycemia or, less frequently, hypoglycemia (usually mild) can occur. Prolonged treatment with octreotide may result in hypothyroidism. Octreotide also can cause bradycardia.

V. DRUGS USED IN THE TREATMENT OF IRRITABLE BOWEL SYNDROME

Irritable bowel syndrome (IBS) is an idiopathic chronic, relapsing disorder characterized by abdominal discomfort (pain, bloating, distention, or cramps) in association with alterations in bowel habits (diarrhea, constipation, or both). With episodes of abdominal pain or discomfort, patients note a change in the frequency or consistency of their bowel movements.

Pharmacologic therapies for irritable bowel syndrome are directed at relieving abdominal pain and discomfort and improving bowel function. For patients with predominant diarrhea, antidiarrheal agents, especially loperamide, are helpful in reducing stool frequency and fecal urgency. For patients with predominant constipation, fiber supplements may lead to softening of stools and reduced straining; however, increased gas production may exacerbate bloating and abdominal discomfort. Consequently, osmotic laxatives, especially milk of magnesia, are commonly used to soften stools and promote increased stool frequency.

For the treatment of chronic abdominal pain, low doses of tricyclic antidepressants (eg, amitriptyline or desipramine, 10–50 mg/d) appear to be helpful (see Chapter 30). At these doses, these agents have no effect on mood but may alter central processing of visceral afferent information. The anticholinergic properties of these agents also may have effects on gastrointestinal motility and secretion, reducing stool frequency and liquidity of stools. Finally, tricyclic antidepressants may alter receptors for enteric neurotransmitters such as serotonin, affecting visceral afferent sensation.

Several other agents are available that are specifically intended for the treatment of irritable bowel syndrome.

ANTISPASMODICS (ANTICHOLINERGICS)

Some agents are promoted as providing relief of abdominal pain or discomfort through antispasmodic actions. However, small or large bowel spasm has not been found to be an important cause of symptoms in patients with irritable bowel syndrome. These agents work primarily through anticholinergic activities. Commonly used medications in this class include **dicyclomine** and **hyoscyamine.** These drugs inhibit muscarinic cholinergic receptors in the enteric plexus and on smooth muscle. Efficacy of these agents for relief of abdominal symptoms has never been convincingly demonstrated. At low doses, they have minimal autonomic effects. However, at higher doses they exhibit significant additional anticholinergic effects, including dry mouth, visual disturbances, urinary retention, and constipation. For these reasons, these drugs are infrequently used.

SEROTONIN 5-HT$_3$-RECEPTOR ANTAGONISTS

As discussed earlier, 5-HT$_3$ receptors in the gastrointestinal tract activate visceral afferent pain sensation via extrinsic sensory neurons from the gut to the spinal cord and central nervous system. Inhibition of afferent gastrointestinal 5-HT$_3$ receptors may inhibit unpleasant visceral afferent sensation, including nausea, bloating, and pain. Blockade of central 5-HT$_3$ receptors also reduces the central response to visceral afferent stimulation. In addition, 5-HT$_3$-receptor blockade on the terminals of enteric cholinergic neurons inhibits colonic motility, especially in the left colon, increasing total colonic transit time.

Alosetron is a 5-HT$_3$ antagonist that has been approved for the treatment of patients with severe irritable bowel syndrome with diarrhea (Figure 63–6). Four other 5-HT$_3$ antagonists (ondansetron, granisetron, dolasetron, and palonosetron) have been approved for the prevention and treatment of nausea and vomiting (see Antiemetics); however, their efficacy in the treatment of irritable bowel syndrome has not been determined. The differences between these 5-HT$_3$ antagonists that determine their pharmacodynamic effects have not been well studied.

Pharmacokinetics & Pharmacodynamics

Alosetron is a highly potent and selective antagonist of the 5-HT$_3$ receptor. It is rapidly absorbed from the gastrointestinal tract with a bioavailability of 50–60% and has a plasma half-life of 1.5 hours but a much longer duration of effect. It undergoes extensive hepatic cytochrome P450 metabolism with renal excretion of most metabolites. Alosetron binds with higher affinity and dissociates more slowly from 5-HT$_3$ receptors than other 5-HT$_3$ antagonists, which may account for its long duration of action.

Clinical Uses

Alosetron currently is approved for the treatment of women with severe irritable bowel syndrome in whom diarrhea is the predominant symptom ("diarrhea-predominant IBS"). Efficacy in men has not been established. In a dosage of 1 mg once or twice daily, it reduces IBS-related lower abdominal pain, cramps, urgency, and diarrhea. Approximately 50–60% of patients report adequate relief of pain and discomfort compared

Figure 63–6. Chemical structure of serotonin; the 5-HT$_3$ antagonists ondansetron, granisetron, dolasetron, and alosetron; and the 5-HT$_4$ partial agonist tegaserod.

with 30–40% of patients treated with placebo. It also leads to a reduction in the mean number of bowel movements per day and improvement in stool consistency. This agent has not been evaluated for the treatment of other causes of diarrhea.

Adverse Events

In contrast to the excellent safety profile of other 5-HT$_3$-receptor antagonists, alosetron is associated with rare but serious gastrointestinal toxicity. Constipation occurs in up to 30% of patients with diarrhea-predominant IBS, requiring discontinuation of the drug in 10%. Serious complications of constipation requiring hospitalization or surgery have occurred in 1 of every 1000 patients. Episodes of ischemic colitis—some fatal—have been reported in up to 3 per 1000 patients. Given the seriousness of

these adverse events, alosetron is restricted to women with severe diarrhea-predominant IBS who have not responded to conventional therapies and who have been educated about the relative risks and benefits.

Drug Interactions

Despite being metabolized by a number of CYP enzymes, alosetron does not appear to have clinically significant interactions with other drugs.

SEROTONIN 5-HT$_4$-RECEPTOR AGONISTS

The pharmacology of tegaserod is discussed under Laxatives, above. This agent is approved for the short-term treatment of women with irritable bowel syndrome who have predominant constipation. Controlled studies have demonstrated a modest improvement (approximately 15%) in patient global satisfaction and a reduction in severity of pain and bloating in patients treated with tegaserod, 6 mg twice daily, compared with placebo. Tegaserod also increases the number of bowel movements per week and reduces the hardness of stools. Given the expense of this agent, it should be reserved for patients with moderate to severe symptoms who have failed to respond to standard therapies (ie, fiber supplementation, laxatives). Although its use is approved for up to 12 weeks, long-term therapy may be considered for patients who demonstrate a good response.

■ VI. ANTIEMETIC AGENTS

Nausea and vomiting may be manifestations of a wide variety of conditions, including adverse effects from medications; systemic disorders or infections; pregnancy; vestibular dysfunction; central nervous system infection or increased pressure; peritonitis; hepatobiliary disorders; radiation or chemotherapy; and gastrointestinal obstruction, dysmotility, or infections.

PATHOPHYSIOLOGY

The brainstem vomiting center is located in the lateral medullary reticular formation and coordinates the complex act of vomiting through interactions with cranial nerves VIII and X and neural networks in the nucleus tractus solitarius that control respiratory, salivatory, and vasomotor centers. High concentrations of muscarinic M_1, histamine H_1, and serotonin $5\text{-}HT_3$ receptors have been identified in the vomiting center.

There are five sources of afferent input to the vomiting center:

1. The chemoreceptor trigger zone is located in the fourth ventricle in the area postrema. This is outside the blood-brain barrier and is accessible to emetogenic stimuli in the blood or cerebrospinal fluid. The chemoreceptor trigger zone is rich in dopamine D_2 receptors, serotonin $5\text{-}HT_3$ receptors, neurokinin 1 (NK_1), and opioid receptors.

2. The vestibular system is important in motion sickness via cranial nerve VIII. It is rich in muscarinic and histamine H_1 receptors.

3. Irritation of the pharynx, innervated by the vagus nerve, provokes a prominent gag and retch response.

4. Vagal and spinal afferent nerves from the gastrointestinal tract are rich in $5\text{-}HT_3$ receptors. Irritation of the gastrointestinal mucosa by chemotherapy, radiation therapy, distention, or acute infectious gastroenteritis leads to release of mucosal serotonin and activation of

these receptors, which stimulate vagal afferent input to the vomiting center and chemoreceptor trigger zone.

5. The central nervous system plays a role in vomiting due to psychiatric disorders, stress, and anticipatory vomiting prior to cancer chemotherapy.

Identification of the different neurotransmitters involved with emesis has allowed development of a diverse group of antiemetic agents that have affinity for various receptors. Combinations of antiemetic agents with different mechanisms of action are often used, especially in patients with vomiting due to chemotherapeutic agents.

SEROTONIN $5\text{-}HT_3$ ANTAGONISTS

Pharmacokinetics & Pharmacodynamics

Selective $5\text{-}HT_3$-receptor antagonists have potent antiemetic properties that are mediated mainly through central $5\text{-}HT_3$-receptor blockade in the vomiting center and chemoreceptor trigger zone and blockade of peripheral $5\text{-}HT_3$ receptors on extrinsic intestinal vagal and spinal afferent nerves. The antiemetic action of these agents is restricted to emesis attributable to vagal stimulation (eg, postoperative) and chemotherapy; other emetic stimuli such as motion sickness are poorly controlled.

Four agents are available: **ondansetron, granisetron, dolasetron,** and **palonosetron.** The first three agents (ondansetron, granisetron, and dolasetron, Figure 63–6) have a serum half-life of 4–9 hours and may be administered once daily by oral or intravenous routes. All three drugs have comparable efficacy and tolerability when administered at equipotent doses. Palonosetron is a newer intravenous agent that has greater affinity for the $5\text{-}HT_3$ receptor and a long serum half-life of 40 hours. All four drugs undergo extensive hepatic metabolism and are eliminated by renal and hepatic excretion. However, dose reduction is not required in geriatric patients or patients with renal insufficiency. For patients with hepatic insufficiency, dose reduction may be required with ondansetron.

These agents do not inhibit dopamine or muscarinic receptors. They do not have effects on esophageal or gastric motility but may slow colonic transit.

Clinical Uses

A. CHEMOTHERAPY-INDUCED NAUSEA AND VOMITING

$5\text{-}HT_3$-receptor antagonists are the primary agents for the prevention of acute chemotherapy-induced nausea and emesis. When used alone, these drugs have little or no efficacy for the prevention of delayed nausea and vomiting (ie, occurring > 24 hours after chemotherapy). The drugs are most effective when given as a single dose by intravenous injection 30 minutes prior to administration of chemotherapy in the following doses: ondansetron, 24–32 mg; granisetron, 1 mg; dolasetron, 100 mg; or palonosetron, 0.25 mg. A single oral dose given 1 hour before chemotherapy may be equally effective in the following regimens: granisetron, 2 mg; dolasetron, 100 mg. Ondansetron may be given as a single oral dose (16–24 mg) or as 8 mg every 8–12 hours for 1–2 days. Although 5-HT$_3$-receptor antagonists are effective as single agents for the prevention of chemotherapy-induced nausea and vomiting, their efficacy is enhanced by combination therapy with a corticosteroid (dexamethasone) and NK$_1$ receptor antagonist (see below).

B. POSTOPERATIVE AND POSTRADIATION NAUSEA AND VOMITING

5-HT$_3$-receptor antagonists are used to prevent or treat postoperative nausea and vomiting. Due to adverse effects and increased restrictions on use of other antiemetic agents, 5-HT$_3$-receptor antagonists are increasingly used for this indication. They are also effective in the prevention and treatment of nausea and vomiting in patients undergoing radiation therapy to the whole body or abdomen.

C. OTHER INDICATIONS

The efficacy of 5-HT$_3$-receptor antagonists in the treatment of nausea and vomiting due to acute or chronic medical illness or acute gastroenteritis has not been evaluated.

Adverse Effects

These 5-HT$_3$-receptor antagonists are well-tolerated agents with excellent safety profiles. The most commonly reported adverse effects are headache, dizziness, and constipation. All three agents cause a small but statistically significant prolongation of the QT interval, but this is most pronounced with dolasetron. Although cardiac arrhythmias have not been linked to use of dolasetron, it should not be administered to patients with prolonged QT or in conjunction with other medications that may prolong the QT interval.

Drug Interactions

No significant drug interactions have been reported. All four agents undergo some metabolism by the hepatic cytochrome P450 system but they do not appear to affect the metabolism of other drugs metabolized by these enzyme systems. However, other drugs may reduce hepatic clearance of the 5-HT$_3$-receptor antagonists, altering their half-life.

CORTICOSTEROIDS

Corticosteroids (dexamethasone, methylprednisolone) have antiemetic properties, but the basis for these effects is unknown. The pharmacology of this class of drugs is discussed in Chapter 39. These agents appear to enhance the efficacy of 5-HT$_3$-receptor antagonists for prevention of acute and delayed nausea and vomiting in patients receiving moderately to highly emetogenic chemotherapy regimens. Although a number of corticosteroids have been used, dexamethasone, 8–20 mg intravenously before chemotherapy, followed by 8 mg/d orally for 2–4 days, is commonly administered.

NEUROKININ RECEPTOR ANTAGONISTS

Neurokinin 1 (NK$_1$) receptor antagonists have antiemetic properties that are mediated through central blockade in the area postrema. **Aprepitant** is a highly selective NK$_1$ receptor antagonist that crosses the blood-brain barrier and occupies brain NK$_1$ receptors. It has no affinity for serotonin, dopamine, or corticosteroid receptors.

Pharmacokinetics & Pharmacodynamics

The oral bioavailability is 65%, and the serum half-life is 12 hours. Aprepitant is metabolized by the liver, primarily by the CYP3A4 pathway.

Clinical Uses

Aprepitant is used in combination with 5-HT$_3$-receptor antagonists and corticosteroids for the prevention of acute and delayed nausea and vomiting from highly emetogenic chemotherapeutic regimens. Combined therapy with aprepitant, a 5-HT$_3$-receptor antagonist, and dexamethasone prevents acute emesis in 80–90% of patients compared with less than 70% treated without aprepitant. Prevention of delayed emesis occurs in more than 70% of patients receiving combined therapy versus 30–50% treated without aprepitant. Aprepitant is administered orally for 3 days as follows: 125 mg given 1 hour prior to chemotherapy, followed by 80 mg/d for 2 days after chemotherapy.

Adverse Effects & Drug Interactions

Aprepitant may be associated with fatigue, dizziness, and diarrhea.

The drug is metabolized by CYP3A4 and may inhibit the metabolism of other drugs metabolized by the CYP3A4 pathway, potentially increasing their levels, effects, and toxicity. Several chemotherapeutic agents are metabolized by CYP3A4, including docetaxel, paclitaxel, etoposide, irinotecan, imatinib, vinblastine, and vincristine. Drugs that inhibit CYP3A4 metabolism may significantly increase aprepitant plasma levels (eg, ketoconazole, ciprofloxacin, clarithromycin, nefazodone, ritonavir, nelfinavir, verapamil, and quinidine). Aprepitant decreases the international normalized ratio (INR) in patients taking warfarin.

PHENOTHIAZINES & BUTYROPHENONES

Phenothiazines are antipsychotic agents that can be used for their potent antiemetic and sedative properties (see Chapter 29). The antiemetic properties of phenothiazines are mediated through inhibition of dopamine and muscarinic receptors. Sedative properties are due to their antihistamine activity. The agents most commonly used as antiemetics are **prochlorperazine, promethazine,** and **thiethylperazine.**

Antipsychotic butyrophenones also possess antiemetic properties due to their central dopaminergic blockade (see Chapter 29). The main agent used is **droperidol,** which can be given by intramuscular or intravenous injection. In antiemetic doses, droperidol is extremely sedating. Until recently, it was used extensively for postoperative nausea and vomiting, in conjunction with opiates and benzodiazepines for sedation for surgical and endoscopic procedures, for neuroleptanalgesia, and for induction and maintenance of general anesthesia. Extrapyramidal effects and hypotension may occur. Droperidol may prolong the QT interval, rarely resulting in fatal episodes of ventricular tachycardia including torsade de pointes. Therefore, droperidol should not be used in patients with QT prolongation and should only be used in patients who have not responded adequately to alternative agents.

SUBSTITUTED BENZAMIDES

Substituted benzamides include **metoclopramide** and **trimethobenzamide.** Their primary mechanism of antiemetic action is believed to be dopamine-receptor blockade. Trimethobenzamide also has weak antihistaminic activity. For prevention and treatment of nausea and vomiting, metoclopramide may be given in the relatively high dosage of 10–20 mg orally or intravenously every 6 hours. The usual dose of trimethobenzamide is 250 mg orally, 200 mg rectally, or 200 mg by intramuscular injection. As discussed previously, the principal adverse effects of these central dopamine antagonists are extrapyramidal: restlessness, dystonias, and parkinsonian symptoms.

H$_1$ ANTIHISTAMINES & ANTICHOLINERGICS

The pharmacology of anticholinergic agents is discussed in Chapter 8 and that of H$_1$ antihistaminic agents in Chapter 16. As single agents, these drugs have weak antiemetic activity, although they are particularly useful for the prevention or treatment of motion sickness. Their use may be limited by dizziness, sedation, confusion, dry mouth, cycloplegia, and urinary retention. **Diphenhydramine** and one of its salts, **dimenhydrinate,** are first-generation histamine H$_1$ antagonists that have significant anticholinergic properties. Because of its sedating properties, diphenhydramine is commonly used in conjunction with other antiemetics for treatment of emesis due to chemotherapy. **Meclizine** is an H$_1$ antihistaminic agent with minimal anticholinergic properties that also causes less sedation. It is used for the prevention of motion sickness and treatment of vertigo due to labyrinth dysfunction.

Hyoscine (scopolamine), a prototypic muscarinic receptor antagonist, is one of the best agents for the prevention of motion sickness. However, it has a very high incidence of anticholinergic effects when given orally or parenterally. It is better tolerated as a transdermal patch. Superiority to dimenhydrinate has not been proved.

BENZODIAZEPINES

Benzodiazepines such as lorazepam or diazepam are used prior to the initiation of chemotherapy to reduce anticipatory vomiting or vomiting caused by anxiety. The pharmacology of these agents is presented in Chapter 22.

CANNABINOIDS

Dronabinol is Δ^9-tetrahydrocannabinol (THC), the major psychoactive chemical in marijuana (see Chapter 32). After oral ingestion, the drug is almost completely absorbed but undergoes significant first-pass hepatic metabolism. Its metabolites are excreted slowly over days to weeks in the feces and urine. Like crude marijuana, dronabinol is a psychoactive agent that is used medically as an appetite stimulant and as an antiemetic, but the mechanisms for these effects are not understood. Because of the availability of more effective agents, this drug now is uncommonly used for the prevention of chemotherapy-induced nausea and vomiting. Combination therapy with phenothiazines provides synergistic antiemetic action and appears to attenuate the adverse effects of both agents. Dronabinol is usually administered in a dosage of 5 mg/m^2 prior to chemotherapy and every 2–4 hours as needed. Adverse effects include euphoria, dysphoria, sedation, hallucinations, dry mouth, and increased appetite. It has some autonomic effects that may result in tachycardia, conjunctival injection, and orthostatic hypotension. Dronabinol has no significant drug-drug interactions but may potentiate the clinical effects of other psychoactive agents. **Nabilone** is a closely related THC analog that has been available in other countries and is approved for use in the USA.

■ VII. DRUGS USED TO TREAT INFLAMMATORY BOWEL DISEASE

Inflammatory bowel disease (IBD) comprises two distinct disorders: ulcerative colitis and Crohn's disease. The etiology and pathogenesis of these disorders remains unknown. For this reason, pharmacologic treatment of inflammatory bowel disorders often involves drugs that belong to different therapeutic classes and have different but nonspecific mechanisms of anti-inflammatory action.

AMINOSALICYLATES

Chemistry & Formulations

Drugs that contain **5-aminosalicylic acid (5-ASA)** have been used successfully for decades in the treatment of inflammatory bowel diseases. 5-ASA differs from salicylic acid only by the addition of an amino group at the 5 (meta) position. Aminosalicylates are believed to work topically (not systemically) in areas of diseased gastrointestinal mucosa. Up to 80% of unformulated, aqueous 5-ASA is absorbed from the small intestine and does not reach the distal small bowel or colon in appreciable quantities. To overcome the rapid absorption of 5-ASA from the proximal small intestine, a number of formulations have been designed to deliver 5-ASA to various distal segments of the small bowel or the colon. These include **sulfasalazine, olsalazine, balsalazide,** and various forms of **mesalamine.**

A. Azo Compounds

Sulfasalazine, balsalazide, and olsalazine contain 5-ASA bound by an azo (N=N) bond to an inert compound or to another 5-ASA molecule (Figure 63–7). In sulfasalazine, 5-ASA is bound to sulfapyridine; in balsalazide, 5-ASA is bound to 4-aminobenzoyl-β-alanine; and in olsalazine, two 5-ASA molecules are bound together. The azo structure markedly reduces absorption of the parent drug from the small intestine. In the terminal ileum and colon, resident bacteria cleave the azo bond by means of an azoreductase enzyme, releasing the active 5-ASA. Consequently, high concentrations of active drug are made available in the terminal ileum or colon.

B. Mesalamine Compounds

Other proprietary formulations have been designed that package 5-ASA itself in various ways in order to deliver it to different segments of the small or large bowel. These 5-ASA formulations are known generically as **mesalamine. Pentasa** is a mesalamine formulation that contains time-release microgranules that release 5-ASA throughout the small intestine. **Asacol** has 5-ASA coated in a pH-sensitive resin that dissolves at pH 7 (the pH of the distal ileum and proximal colon). 5-ASA also may be delivered in high concentrations to the rectum and sigmoid colon by means of enema formulations (**Rowasa**) or suppositories (**Canasa**).

Pharmacokinetics & Pharmacodynamics

Although unformulated 5-ASA is readily absorbed from the small intestine, absorption of 5-ASA from the colon is extremely low. In contrast, approximately 20–30% of 5-ASA from current oral mesalamine formulations is systemically absorbed in the small intestine. Absorbed 5-ASA undergoes *N*-acetylation in the gut epithelium and liver to a metabolite that does not possess significant anti-inflammatory activity. The acetylated metabolite is excreted by the kidneys.

Of the azo compounds, 10% of sulfasalazine and less than 1% of balsalazide are absorbed as native compounds. After azoreductase breakdown of sulfasalazine, over 85% of the carrier molecule sulfapyridine is systemically absorbed from the colon. Sulfapyridine undergoes hepatic metabolism (including acetylation) followed by renal excretion. By contrast, after azoreductase breakdown of balsalazide, over 70% of the carrier peptide is recovered intact in the feces and only a small amount of systemic absorption occurs.

The mechanism of action of 5-ASA is not certain. The primary action of salicylate and other NSAIDs is due to blockade of prostaglandin synthesis by inhibition of cyclooxygenase. However, the aminosalicylates have variable effects on prostaglandin production. It is thought that 5-ASA modulates inflammatory mediators derived from both the cyclooxygenase and lipoxygenase pathways. Other potential mechanisms of action of the 5-ASA drugs relate to their ability to interfere with the production of inflammatory cytokines. 5-ASA inhibits the activity of nuclear factor-κB (NF-κB), an important transcription factor for proinflammatory cytokines. 5-ASA may also inhibit cellular functions of natural killer cells, mucosal lymphocytes, and macrophages, and it may scavenge reactive oxygen metabolites.

Clinical Uses

5-ASA drugs induce and maintain remission in ulcerative colitis and are considered to be the first-line agents for treatment of mild to moderate active ulcerative colitis. Their efficacy in Crohn's disease is not as well established, although many clinicians use 5-ASA agents as first-line therapy for mild to moderate disease involving the colon or distal ileum.

The effectiveness of 5-ASA therapy depends in part on achieving high drug concentration at the site of active disease. Thus, 5-ASA suppositories or enemas are useful in patients with ulcerative colitis or Crohn's disease confined to the rectum (proctitis) or distal colon (proctosigmoiditis). In patients with ulcerative colitis or Crohn's colitis that extends to the proximal colon, both the azo compounds and mesalamine formulations are useful. For the treatment of Crohn's disease involving the small bowel, mesalamine compounds, which release 5-ASA in the small intestine, have a theoretic advantage over the azo compounds.

Adverse Effects

Sulfasalazine has a high incidence of adverse effects, most of which are attributable to systemic effects of the sulfa-

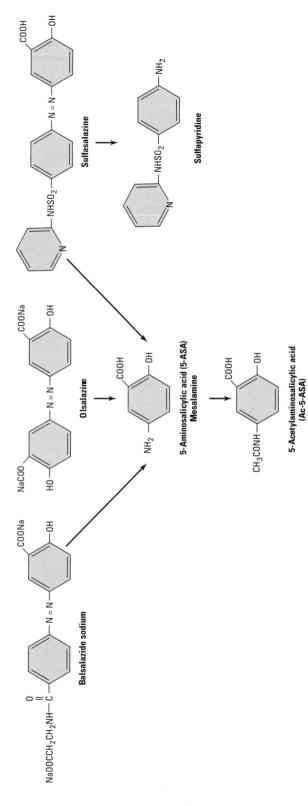

Figure 63–7. Chemical structures of aminosalicylates. Azo compounds (balsalazide, olsalazine, sulfasalazine) are converted by bacterial azoreductase to 5-aminosalicylic acid (mesalamine), the active therapeutic moiety.

pyridine molecule. Slow acetylators of sulfapyridine have more frequent and more severe adverse effects than fast acetylators. Up to 40% of patients cannot tolerate therapeutic doses of sulfasalazine. The most common problems are dose-related and include nausea, gastrointestinal upset, headaches, arthralgias, myalgias, bone marrow suppression, and malaise. Hypersensitivity to sulfapyridine (or, rarely, 5-ASA) can result in fever, exfoliative dermatitis, pancreatitis, pneumonitis, hemolytic anemia, pericarditis, or hepatitis. Sulfasalazine has also been associated with oligospermia, which reverses upon discontinuation of the drug. Sulfasalazine impairs folate absorption and processing; hence, dietary supplementation with 1 mg/d folic acid is recommended.

In contrast to sulfasalazine, other aminosalicylate formulations are well tolerated. In most clinical trials, the frequency of drug adverse events is similar to that in patients treated with placebo. For unclear reasons, olsalazine may stimulate a secretory diarrhea—which should not be confused with active inflammatory bowel disease—in 10% of patients. Rare hypersensitivity reactions may occur with all aminosalicylates but are much less common than with sulfasalazine. Careful studies have documented subtle changes indicative of renal tubular damage in patients receiving high doses of aminosalicylates. Rare cases of interstitial nephritis are reported, particularly in association with high doses of mesalamine formulations; this may be attributable to the higher serum 5-ASA levels attained with these drugs. Sulfasalazine and other aminosalicylates rarely cause worsening of colitis, which may be misinterpreted as refractory colitis.

GLUCOCORTICOIDS

Pharmacokinetics & Pharmacodynamics

In gastrointestinal practice, prednisone and prednisolone are the most commonly used oral glucocorticoids. These drugs have an intermediate duration of biologic activity allowing once-daily dosing.

Hydrocortisone enemas, foam, or suppositories are used to maximize colonic tissue effects and minimize systemic absorption via topical treatment of active inflammatory bowel disease in the rectum and sigmoid colon. Absorption of hydrocortisone is reduced with rectal administration, although 15–30% of the administered dosage is absorbed.

Budesonide is a potent synthetic analog of prednisolone that has high affinity for the glucocorticoid receptor but is subject to rapid first-pass hepatic metabolism (in part by CYP3A4) resulting in low oral bioavailability. A controlled-release oral formulation of budesonide (Entocort) is available that releases the drug in the distal ileum and colon where it is absorbed. The bioavailability of controlled-release budesonide capsules is approximately 10%.

As in other tissues, glucocorticoids inhibit production of inflammatory cytokines (TNF-α, IL-1) and chemokines (IL-8); reduce expression of inflammatory cell adhesion molecules; and inhibit gene transcription of nitric oxide synthase, phospholipase A_2, cyclooxygenase-2, and NF-κB.

Clinical Uses

Glucocorticoids are commonly used in the treatment of patients with moderate to severe active inflammatory bowel disease. Active disease is commonly treated with an initial oral dosage of 40–60 mg/d of prednisone or prednisolone. Higher doses have not been shown to be more efficacious but have significantly greater adverse effects. Once a patient responds to initial therapy (usually within 1–2 weeks), the dosage is tapered to minimize development of adverse effects. In severely ill patients, the drugs are usually administered intravenously.

For the treatment of inflammatory bowel disease involving the rectum or sigmoid colon, rectally administered glucocorticoids are preferred because of their lower systemic absorption.

Oral controlled-release budesonide (9 mg/d) is commonly used in the treatment of mild to moderate Crohn's disease involving the ileum and proximal colon. It appears to be slightly less effective than prednisolone in achieving clinical remission, but has significantly less adverse systemic effects.

Corticosteroids are not useful to maintain disease remission. Other medications such as aminosalicylates or immunosuppressive agents should be used for this purpose.

Adverse Effects

Adverse effects of glucocorticoids are reviewed in Chapter 39.

PURINE ANALOGS: AZATHIOPRINE & 6-MERCAPTOPURINE

Pharmacokinetics & Pharmacodynamics

Azathioprine and 6-mercaptopurine (6-MP) are purine antimetabolites that have immunosuppressive properties (see Chapters 55 and 56).

The bioavailability of azathioprine (80%) is superior to 6-MP (50%). After absorption azathioprine is rapidly converted by a nonenzymatic process to 6-MP. 6-Mercaptopurine subsequently undergoes a complex biotransformation via competing catabolic enzymes (xanthine oxidase and thiopurine methyltransferase) that produce inactive metabolites and anabolic pathways that produce active thioguanine nucleotides. Azathioprine and 6-MP have a serum half-life of less than 2 hours; however, the active 6-thioguanine nucleotides are concentrated in cells resulting in a prolonged half-life of days. The prolonged kinetics of 6-thioguanine nucleotide results in a median delay of 17 weeks before onset of therapeutic benefit from oral azathioprine or 6-MP is observed in patients with inflammatory bowel disease.

The molecular basis for the therapeutic effects of the purine analogs is unknown. Intracellular 6-thioguanine causes inhibition of purine nucleotide metabolism and DNA synthesis and repair, resulting in inhibition of cell division and proliferation, and may promote T-lymphocyte apoptosis.

Clinical Uses

Azathioprine and 6-MP are important agents in the induction and maintenance of remission of ulcerative colitis and Crohn's disease. Although the optimal dose is uncertain, most patients with normal thiopurine-S-methyltransferase (TPMT) activity (see below) are treated with 6-MP, 1–1.5 mg/kg/d, or azathioprine, 2–2.5 mg/kg/d. After 3–6 months of treatment, 50–60% of patients with active disease achieve remission. These agents help maintain remission in up to 80% of patients. Among patients who depend on long-term glucocorticoid therapy to control active disease, purine analogs allow dose reduction or elimination of steroids in the majority.

Adverse Effects

Dose-related toxicities of azathioprine or 6-MP include nausea, vomiting, bone marrow depression (leading to leukopenia, macrocytosis, anemia, or thrombocytopenia), and hepatic toxicity. Routine laboratory monitoring with complete blood count and liver function tests is required in all patients. Leukopenia or elevations in liver chemistries usually respond to medication dose reduction. Severe leukopenia may predispose to opportunistic infections; leukopenia may respond to therapy with granulocyte stimulating factor. Catabolism of 6-MP by TPMT is low in 11% and absent in 0.3% of the population, leading to increased production of active 6-thioguanine metabolites and increased risk of bone marrow depression. TPMT levels can be measured prior to initiating therapy. These drugs should not be administered to patients with absent TPMT activity and should be initiated at lower doses in patients with intermediate activity. Hypersensitivity reactions to azathioprine or 6-MP occur in 5% of patients. These include fever, rash, pancreatitis, diarrhea, and hepatitis.

Although there appears to be an increased risk of lymphoma in transplant recipients receiving long-term 6-MP or azathioprine therapy, it is unclear whether the risk is increased among patients with inflammatory bowel disease. These drugs cross the placenta; however, there are many reports of successful pregnancies in women taking these agents, and the risk of teratogenicity appears to be small.

Drug Interactions

Allopurinol markedly reduces xanthine oxide catabolism of the purine analogs, potentially increasing active 6-thioguanine nucleotides that may lead to severe leukopenia. The dose of 6-MP or azathioprine should be reduced by at least half in patients taking allopurinol.

METHOTREXATE

Pharmacokinetics & Pharmacodynamics

Methotrexate is another antimetabolite that has beneficial effects in a number of chronic inflammatory diseases, including Crohn's disease and rheumatoid arthritis (see Chapter 36), and in cancer (see Chapter 55). Methotrexate may be given orally, subcutaneously, or intramuscularly. Reported oral bioavailability is 50–90% at doses used in chronic inflammatory diseases. Intramuscular and subcutaneous methotrexate exhibit nearly complete bioavailability.

The principal mechanism of action is inhibition of dihydrofolate reductase, an enzyme important in the production of thymidine and purines. At the high doses used for chemotherapy, methotrexate inhibits cellular proliferation. However, at the low doses used in the treatment of inflammatory bowel disease (12–25 mg/wk), the antiproliferative effects may not be evident. Methotrexate may interfere with the inflammatory actions of interleukin-1. It may also stimulate increased release of adenosine, an endogenous anti-inflammatory autacoid. Methotrexate may also stimulate apoptosis and death of activated T lymphocytes.

Clinical Uses

Methotrexate is used to induce and maintain remission in patients with Crohn's disease. Its efficacy in ulcerative colitis is uncertain. To induce remission, patients are treated with 15–25 mg of methotrexate once weekly by subcutaneous injection. If a satisfactory response is achieved within 8–12 weeks, the dose is reduced to 15 mg/wk.

Adverse Effects

At higher dosage, methotrexate may cause bone marrow depression, megaloblastic anemia, alopecia, and mucositis. At the doses used in the treatment of inflammatory bowel disease, these events are uncommon but warrant dose reduction if they do occur. Folate supplementation reduces the risk of these events without impairing the anti-inflammatory action.

In patients with psoriasis treated with methotrexate, hepatic damage is common; however, among patients with inflammatory bowel disease and rheumatoid arthritis, the risk is significantly lower. Renal insufficiency may increase risk of hepatic accumulation and toxicity.

ANTI-TUMOR NECROSIS FACTOR THERAPY

Pharmacokinetics & Pharmacodynamics

A dysregulation of the T helper cell type 1 (TH1) response is present in inflammatory bowel disease, especially Crohn's disease. One of the key proinflammatory cytokines in the TH1 response is tumor necrosis factor-α (TNF-α). **Infliximab** is a chimeric mouse-human monoclonal antibody to human TNF-α that is described in more detail in Chapter 56.

Infliximab is administered as an intravenous infusion. The plasma concentration is linearly proportionate to dose and its elimination follows first-order kinetics. At therapeutic doses of 5–10 mg/kg, the half-life of infliximab is approximately 8–10 days, resulting in plasma disappearance of antibodies over 8–12 weeks.

The biologic activity of TNF-α is mediated by binding of soluble or membrane-bound TNF-α trimers to cell-surface TNF-α receptors. Infliximab binds to soluble TNF-α trimers with high affinity, preventing the cytokine from binding to its receptors. Total serum TNF-α concentrations may actually increase because binding to infliximab slows TNF-α clearance. Infliximab also binds to membrane-bound TNF-α and neutralizes its activity. Furthermore, the Fc portion of human IgG$_1$ region of infliximab promotes complement activation and antibody-mediated apoptosis and cellular cytotoxicity of activated T lymphocytes and macrophages.

Clinical Uses

Infliximab is used in the acute and chronic treatment of patients with moderate to severe Crohn's disease and ulcerative colitis. It leads to symptomatic improvement in two thirds and disease remission in one third of patients with moderately severe or fistulizing Crohn's disease, including patients who have been dependent on glucocorticoids or who have not responded to 6-MP or methotrexate. The median time to clinical response is 2 weeks. Infliximab induction therapy is generally given in a dosage of 5 mg/kg at 0, 2, and 6 weeks. Patients who respond may be treated with repeat infusions every 8 weeks to maintain remission with or without other therapies. Clinical response is maintained in more than 60% of patients with regularly scheduled infusions; however, one third of patients eventually lose response despite higher doses (10 mg/kg) or more frequent infusions. Loss of response in many patients may be due to development of antibodies to infliximab.

Infliximab was recently approved for the treatment of patients with moderate to severe ulcerative colitis who have had inadequate response to mesalamine or corticosteroids. After induction therapy of 5–10 mg/wk at 0, 2, and 6 weeks, 70% of patients had a clinical response and one third were in clinical remission. With continued maintenance infusions every 8 weeks, approximately one half of patients had continued clinical response.

Although infliximab currently is the only anti-TNF agent approved by the FDA for treatment of patients with inflammatory bowel disease, other anti-TNF agents have demonstrated efficacy in large controlled trials. These include **adalimumab** (a fully humanized IgG$_1$ antibody) and **certolizumab** (a polyethylene glycolated Fab fragment of humanized anti-TNF), both of which are administered by subcutaneous injection. It is unknown whether these agents will have similar efficacy to infliximab with reduced complications related to antibody formation.

Adverse Effects

Serious adverse events occur in 6% of patients with infliximab therapy. The most important adverse effect of infliximab therapy is infection due to suppression of the TH1 inflammatory response. Reactivation of latent tuberculosis, with dissemination, has occurred. Before administering infliximab, all patients must undergo purified protein derivative (PPD) testing; prophylactic therapy for tuberculosis is warranted for patients with positive test results. Other infections include pneumonia, sepsis, pneumocystosis, histoplasmosis, listeriosis, and reactivation of hepatitis B.

Antibodies directed at the murine epitope of infliximab develop in approximately one third of patients. These antibodies may attenuate or eliminate the clinical response and increase the likelihood of developing acute or delayed infusion reactions. Antibody development is less likely in patients who receive concomitant therapy with immunomodulators (ie, 6-MP or methotrexate), regularly scheduled infliximab infusions, or preinfusion treatment with corticosteroids (eg, hydrocortisone, 200 mg).

Infliximab infusions result in acute adverse infusion reactions in up to 10% of patients, but discontinuation of the infusion for severe reactions is required in less than 2%. Infusion reactions are more common with the second or subsequent infusions than with the first. Early mild reactions include fever, headache, dizziness, urticaria, or mild cardiopulmonary symptoms that include chest pain, dyspnea, or hemodynamic instability. Reactions to subsequent infusions may be reduced with prophylactic administration of acetaminophen and diphenhydramine. Severe acute reactions, including significant hypotension, shortness of breath, muscle spasms, and chest discomfort, may require treatment with oxygen, epinephrine, and corticosteroids.

A delayed serum sickness-like infusion reaction, which occurs 1–2 weeks after infusion, develops in 1–2% patients who are retreated with infliximab, especially after a prolonged period. These reactions consist of myalgia, arthralgia, jaw tightness, fever, rash, urticaria, and edema. For patients with either acute severe or delayed infusion reactions, the risks and benefits of subsequent infusions must be weighed; pretreatment with acetaminophen, diphenhydramine, and corticosteroids is recommended. Positive antinuclear antibodies and anti-double-stranded DNA develop in a small number of patients. Development of a lupus-like syndrome has been reported that resolved after discontinuation of the drug.

Infliximab may cause severe hepatic reactions leading to acute hepatic failure. Liver enzymes should be monitored routinely.

Lymphoma has developed in patients who were treated with infliximab. However, the observed rates may be similar to those expected in patients with inflammatory bowel disease. Rare cases of multiple sclerosis have been reported. Infliximab may worsen congestive heart failure in patients with cardiac disease.

■ VIII. PANCREATIC ENZYME SUPPLEMENTS

Exocrine pancreatic insufficiency is most commonly caused by cystic fibrosis, chronic pancreatitis, or pancreatic resection. When secretion of pancreatic enzymes falls below 10% of normal, fat and protein maldigestion occur that can lead to steatorrhea, azotorrhea, vitamin malabsorption, and weight loss. Pancreatic enzyme supplements, which contain a mixture of amylase, lipase, and proteases, are the mainstay of treatment for pancreatic enzyme insufficiency. Two major types of preparations in use are **pancreatin** and **pancrelipase.** Pancreatin is an alcohol-derived extract of hog pancreas with relatively low concentrations of lipase and proteolytic enzymes, whereas pancrelipase is an enriched preparation. On a per weight basis, pancrelipase has approximately 12 times the lipolytic activity and more than 4 times the proteolytic activity of pancreatin. Consequently, pancreatin is no longer in common clinical use. Only pancrelipase will be discussed here.

Pancrelipase is available in both nonenteric-coated and enteric-coated preparations. Pancrelipase enzymes are rapidly and permanently inactivated by gastric acids. Therefore, nonenteric-coated preparations (eg, Viokase) should be given concomitantly with acid suppression therapy (proton pump inhibitor or H_2 antagonist) in order to reduce acid-mediated destruction within the stomach. Encapsulated formulations contain acid-resistant microspheres (Creon) or microtablets (Pancrease, Ultrase). Enteric-coated formulations are more commonly used because they do not require concomitant acid suppression therapy.

Pancrelipase preparations are administered with each meal and snack. Formulations are available in sizes containing varying amounts of lipase, amylase, and protease. However, manufacturers' listings of enzyme content do not always reflect true enzymatic activity. Enzyme activity may be listed in international units (IU) or USP units. One IU is equal to 2–3 USP units. Dosing should be individualized according to the age and weight of the patient, the degree of pancreatic insufficiency, and the amount of dietary fat intake. Therapy is initiated at a dose that provides 30,000 IUs (60,000–90,000 USP) of lipase activity in the prandial and postprandial period—a level that is sufficient to reduce steatorrhea to a clinically insignificant level in most cases. Suboptimal response to enteric-coated formulations may be due to poor mixing of granules with food or slow dissolution and release of enzymes. Gradual increase of dose, change to a different formulation, or addition of acid suppression therapy may improve response.

Pancreatic enzyme supplements are well tolerated. The capsules should be swallowed, not chewed, as pancreatic enzymes may cause oropharyngeal mucositis. Excessive doses may cause diarrhea and abdominal pain. The high purine content of pancreas extracts may lead to hyperuricosuria and renal stones. Several cases of colonic strictures were reported in patients with cystic fibrosis who received high doses of pancrelipase with high lipase activity. These high-dose formulations have since been removed from the market.

■ IX. BILE ACID THERAPY FOR GALLSTONES

Ursodiol (ursodeoxycholic acid) is a naturally occurring bile acid that makes up less than 5% of the circulating bile salt pool in humans and a much higher percentage in bears. After oral administration, it is absorbed, conjugated in the liver with glycine or taurine, and excreted in the bile. Conjugated ursodiol undergoes extensive enterohepatic recirculation. The serum half-life is approximately 100 hours. With long-term daily administration, ursodiol constitutes 30–50% of the circulating bile acid pool. A small amount of unabsorbed conjugated or unconjugated ursodiol passes into the colon where it is either excreted or undergoes dehydroxylation by colonic bacteria to lithocholic acid, a substance with potential hepatic toxicity.

Pharmacodynamics

The solubility of cholesterol in bile is determined by the relative proportions of bile acids, lecithin, and cholesterol. Although prolonged ursodiol therapy expands the bile acid pool, this does not appear to be the principal mechanism of action for dissolution of gallstones. Ursodiol decreases the cholesterol content of bile by reducing hepatic cholesterol secretion. Ursodiol also appears to stabilize hepatocyte canalicular membranes, possibly through a reduction in the concentration of other endogenous bile acids or through inhibition of immune-mediated hepatocyte destruction.

Clinical Use

Ursodiol is used for dissolution of small cholesterol gallstones in patients with symptomatic gallbladder disease who refuse cholecystectomy or who are poor surgical candidates. At a dosage of 10 mg/kg/d for 12–24 months, dissolution occurs in up to half of patients with small (< 5–10 mm) noncalcified gallstones. It is also effective for the prevention of gallstones in obese patients undergoing rapid weight loss therapy. Several trials demonstrate that ursodiol 13–15 mg/kg/d is helpful for patients with early-stage primary biliary cirrhosis, reducing liver function abnormalities and improving liver histology.

Adverse Effects

Ursodiol is practically free of serious adverse effects. Bile salt-induced diarrhea is uncommon. Unlike its predecessor, chenodeoxycholate, ursodiol has not been associated with hepatotoxicity.

■ X. DRUGS USED TO TREAT VARICEAL HEMORRHAGE

Portal hypertension most commonly occurs as a consequence of chronic liver disease. Portal hypertension is caused by increased blood flow within the portal venous system and increased resistance to portal flow within the liver. Splanchnic blood flow is increased in patients with cirrhosis due to low arteriolar resistance that is mediated by increased circulating vasodilators and decreased vascular sensitivity to vasoconstrictors. Intrahepatic resistance to blood flow is increased in cirrhosis due to fixed fibrosis within the spaces of Disse and hepatic veins as well as reversible vasoconstriction of hepatic sinusoids and venules. Among the consequences of portal hypertension are ascites, hepatic encephalopathy, and the development of portosystemic collaterals—especially gastric or esophageal varices. Varices can rupture, leading to massive upper gastrointestinal bleeding.

Several drugs are available that reduce portal pressures. These may be used in the short term for the treatment of active variceal hemorrhage or long term to reduce the risk of hemorrhage.

SOMATOSTATIN & OCTREOTIDE

The pharmacology of octreotide is discussed above under Antidiarrheal Agents. In patients with cirrhosis and portal hypertension, intravenous somatostatin (250 mcg/h) or octreotide (50 mcg/h) reduces portal blood flow and variceal pressures; however, the mechanism by which they do so is poorly understood. They do not appear to induce direct contraction of vascular smooth muscle. Their activity may be mediated through inhibition of release of glucagon and other gut peptides that alter mesenteric blood flow. Although data from clinical trials are conflicting, these agents are probably effective in promoting initial hemostasis from bleeding esophageal varices. They are generally administered for 3–5 days.

VASOPRESSIN & TERLIPRESSIN

Vasopressin (antidiuretic hormone) is a polypeptide hormone secreted by the hypothalamus and stored in the posterior pituitary. Its pharmacology is discussed in Chapters 17 and 37. Although its primary physiologic role is to maintain serum osmolality, it is also a potent arterial vasoconstrictor. When administered intravenously by continuous infusion, it causes splanchnic arterial vasoconstriction that leads to reduced splanchnic perfusion and lowered portal venous pressures. Prior to the advent of octreotide, vasopressin was commonly used to treat acute variceal hemorrhage. However, because of its high adverse effect profile, it is no longer used for this purpose. In contrast, for patients with acute gastrointestinal bleeding from small bowel or large bowel vascular ectasias or diverticulosis, vasopressin may be infused—to promote vasospasm—into one of the branches of the superior or inferior mesenteric artery through an angiographically placed catheter. Adverse effects with systemic vasopressin are common. Systemic and peripheral vasoconstriction can lead to hypertension, myocardial ischemia or infarction, or mesenteric infarction. These effects may be reduced by coadministration of nitroglycerin, which may further reduce portal venous pressures (by reducing portohepatic vascular resistance) and may also reduce the coronary and peripheral vascular vasospasm caused by vasopressin. Other common adverse effects are nausea, abdominal cramps, and diarrhea (due to intestinal hyperactivity). Furthermore, the antidiuretic effects of vasopressin promote retention of free water, which can lead to hyponatremia, fluid retention, and pulmonary edema.

Terlipressin is a vasopressin analog that appears to have similar efficacy to vasopressin with fewer adverse effects. Although this agent is available in other countries, it is still undergoing clinical testing in the USA.

BETA-RECEPTOR–BLOCKING DRUGS

The pharmacology of these agents is discussed in Chapter 10. Beta-receptor antagonists reduce portal venous pressures via a decrease in portal venous inflow. This decrease is due to a decrease in cardiac output (β_1 blockade) and to splanchnic vasoconstriction (β_2 blockade) caused by the unopposed effect of systemic catecholamines on α receptors. Thus, nonselective β blockers such as propranolol and nadolol are more effective than selective β_1 blockers in reducing portal pressures. Among patients with cirrhosis and esophageal varices who have not previously had an episode of variceal hemorrhage, the incidence of bleeding among patient treated with nonselective β blockers is 15% compared with 25% in control groups. Among patients with a history of variceal hemorrhage, the likelihood of recurrent hemorrhage is 80% within 2 years. Nonselective β blockers significantly reduce the rate of recurrent bleeding, although a reduction in mortality is unproved.

PREPARATIONS AVAILABLE

ANTACIDS

Aluminum hydroxide gel* (AlternaGEL, others)
Oral: 300, 500, 600 mg tablets; 400, 500 mg capsules; 320, 450, 675 mg/5 mL suspension

Calcium carbonate* (Tums, others)
Oral: 350, 420, 500, 600, 650, 750, 1000, 1250 mg chewable tablets; 1250 mg/5 mL suspension

Combination aluminum hydroxide and magnesium hydroxide preparations*
(Maalox, Mylanta, Gaviscon, Gelusil, others)
Oral: 400 to 800 mg combined hydroxides per tablet, capsule, or 5 mL suspension

H₂ HISTAMINE RECEPTOR BLOCKERS

Cimetidine (generic, Tagamet, Tagamet HB*)
Oral: 200*, 300, 400, 800 mg tablets; 300 mg/5 mL liquid
Parenteral: 300 mg/2 mL, 300 mg/50 mL for injection

Famotidine (generic, Pepcid, Pepcid AC*, Pepcid Complete*)
Oral: 10 mg tablets*, gelcaps*; 10 mg tablet plus calcium carbonate 800 mg and magnesium hydroxide 165 mg*; 20, 40 mg tablets; powder to reconstitute for 40 mg/5 mL suspension
Parenteral: 10 mg/mL for injection

Nizatidine (Axid, Axid AR*)
Oral: 75 mg tablets*; 150, 300 mg capsules

Ranitidine (generic, Zantac, Zantac 75*)
Oral: 75*, 150, 300 mg tablets; 150 mg effervescent tablets; 150, 300 mg capsules; 15 mg/mL syrup
Parenteral: 1, 25 mg/mL for injection

SELECTED ANTICHOLINERGIC DRUGS

Atropine (generic)
Oral: 0.4 mg tablets
Parenteral: 0.05, 0.1, 0.3, 0.4, 0.5, 0.8, 1 mg/mL for injection

Belladonna alkaloids tincture (generic)
Oral: 0.27–0.33 mg/mL liquid

Dicyclomine (generic, Bentyl, others)
Oral: 10, 20 mg capsules; 20 mg tablets; 10 mg/5 mL syrup
Parenteral: 10 mg/mL for injection

Glycopyrrolate (generic, Robinul)
Oral: 1, 2 mg tablets
Parenteral: 0.2 mg/mL for injection

Hyoscyamine (Anaspaz, Levsin, others)
Oral: 0.125, 0.15 mg tablets; 0.375 mg timed-release capsules; 0.125 mg/5 mL oral elixir and solution
Parenteral: 0.5 mg/mL for injection

Methscopolamine (Pamine)
Oral: 2.5, 5 mg tablets

Propantheline (generic, Pro-Banthine)
Oral: 7.5, 15 mg tablets

Scopolamine (generic, Transderm Scop)
Oral: 0.4 mg tablets
Transdermal patch: 1.5 mg/2.5 cm²
Parenteral: 0.4, 1 mg/mL for injection

PROTON PUMP INHIBITORS

Esomeprazole (Nexium)
Oral: 20, 40 mg delayed-release capsules
Parenteral: 20, 40 mg vial powder for IV injection

Omeprazole (Prilosec, Prilosec OTC*, Zegerid)
Oral: 10, 20, 40 mg delayed-release capsules; 20 mg delayed-release tablet*; 20, 40 mg immediate-release powder containing 1680 mg NaHCO₃ for oral suspension

---

*Over-the-counter formulations.

(continued)

Lansoprazole (Prevacid)
Oral: 15, 30 mg delayed-release capsules; 15, 30 mg orally disintegrating tablet containing delayed-release granules; 15, 30 mg delayed-release granules for oral suspension
Parenteral: 30 mg/vial powder for IV injection
Pantoprazole (Protonix)
Oral: 20, 40 mg delayed release tablets
Parenteral: 40 mg/vial powder for IV injection
Rabeprazole (Aciphex)
Oral: 20 mg delayed-release tablets

MUCOSAL PROTECTIVE AGENTS

Misoprostol (Cytotec)
Oral: 100, 200 mcg tablets
Sucralfate (generic, Carafate)
Oral: 1 g tablets; 1 g/10 mL suspension

DIGESTIVE ENZYMES

Pancrelipase (Creon, Lipram, Pancrease MT, Ultrase MT, Viokase)
Oral: Tablets, powder, or delayed-release capsules containing varying amounts of lipase, protease, and amylase activity. See manufacturers' literature for details.

DRUGS FOR MOTILITY DISORDERS & SELECTED ANTIEMETICS

5-HT$_3$-Receptor Antagonists
Alosetron (Lotronex)
Oral: 1 mg tablets
Dolasetron (Anzemet)
Oral: 50, 100 mg tablets
Parenteral: 20 mg/mL for injection
Granisetron (Kytril)
Oral: 1 mg tablets; 2 mg/10 mL oral solution
Parenteral: 0.1, 1 mg/mL for injection
Ondansetron (Zofran)
Oral: 4, 8, 24 mg tablets; 4, 8 mg orally disintegrating tablets; 4 mg/5 mL oral solution
Parenteral: 2 mg/mL, 32 mg/50 mL for IV injection
Palonosetron (Aloxi)
Parenteral: 0.05 mg/mL for injection
Other Motility and Antiemetic Agents
Aprepitant (Emend)
Oral: 80, 125 mg capsules
Dronabinol (Marinol)
Oral: 2.5, 5, 10 mg capsules
Droperidol (Inapsine)
Parenteral: 2.5 mg/mL for IV injection
Metoclopramide (generic, Reglan, others)
Oral: 5, 10 mg tablets; 5 mg/5 mL syrup, 10 mg/mL concentrated solution
Parenteral: 5 mg/mL for injection

Nabilone (Cesamet)
Oral: 1 mg tablets
Prochlorperazine (Compazine)
Oral: 5, 10, 25 mg tablets; 10, 15, 30 mg capsules; 1 mg/mL solution
Rectal: 2.5, 5, 25 mg suppositories
Parenteral: 5 mg/mL for injection
Promethazine (generic, Phenergan, others)
Oral: 10, 13.2, 25, 50 mg tablets; 5, 6.25, 10 mg/5 mL syrup
Rectal: 10, 12.5, 25, 50 mg suppositories
Parenteral: 25, 50 mg/mL for IM or IV injection
Scopolamine (Transderm Scop)
Transdermal patch: 1.5 mg/2.5 cm^2
Tegaserod (Zelnorm)
Oral: 2, 6 mg tablets
Trimethobenzamide (generic, Tigan, others)
Oral: 250, 300 mg capsules
Rectal: 100, 200 mg suppository
Parenteral: 100 mg/mL for injection

SELECTED ANTI-INFLAMMATORY DRUGS USED IN GASTROINTESTINAL DISEASE (SEE ALSO CHAPTER 56)

Balsalazide (Colazal)
Oral: 750 mg capsules
Budesonide (Entocort)
Oral: 3 mg capsules
Hydrocortisone (Cortenema, Cortifoam)
Rectal: 100 mg/60 mL unit retention enema; 90 mg/applicatorful intrarectal foam
Mesalamine (5-ASA)
Oral: Asacol: 400 mg delayed-release tablets; Pentasa: 250 mg controlled-release capsules
Rectal: Rowasa: 4 g/60 mL suspension, 500 mg suppositories; Canasa: 500, 1000 mg suppositories
Methylprednisolone (Medrol Enpack)
Rectal: 40 mg/bottle retention enema
Olsalazine (Dipentum)
Oral: 250 mg capsules
Sulfasalazine (generic, Azulfidine)
Oral: 500 mg tablets and delayed-release enteric-coated tablets
Infliximab (Remicade)
Parenteral: 100 mg powder for injection

SELECTED ANTIDIARRHEAL DRUGS

Bismuth subsalicylate* (Pepto-Bismol, others)
Oral: 262 mg caplets, chewable tablets; 130, 262, 524 mg/15 mL suspension

(continued)

---

*Over-the-counter formulations.

Difenoxin (Motofen)
Oral: 1 mg (with 0.025 mg atropine sulfate) tablets

Diphenoxylate (generic, Lomotil, others)
Oral: 2.5 mg (with 0.025 mg atropine sulfate) tablets and liquid

Kaolin/pectin* (generic, Kaopectate, others)
Oral (typical): 5.85 g kaolin and 260 mg pectin per 30 mL suspension

Loperamide* (generic, Imodium)
Oral: 2 mg tablets, capsules; 1 mg/5 mL liquid

Bulk-Forming Laxatives*

Methylcellulose (generic, Citrucel
Oral: bulk powder, capsules

Psyllium (generic, Serutan, Metamucil, others)
Oral: granules, bulk powder, wafer

Soluble dietary fiber (Benefiber)
Oral: bulk powder, tablets

Other Selected Laxative Drugs

Bisacodyl* (generic, Dulcolax, others)
Oral: 5 mg enteric-coated tablets
Rectal: 10 mg suppositories

Cascara sagrada* (generic)
Oral: 325 mg tablets; 5 mL per dose fluid extract (approximately 18% alcohol)

Castor oil* (generic, others)
Oral: liquid or liquid emulsion

Docusate* (generic, Colace, others)
Oral: 50, 100, 250 mg capsules; 100 mg tablets; 20, 50, 60, 150 mg/15 mL syrup

Glycerin liquid* (Fleet Babylax)
Rectal liquid: 4 mL per applicator
Glycerin suppository (generic, Sani-Supp)

Lactulose (Chronulac, Cephulac)
Oral: 10 g/15 mL syrup

Lubiprostone (Amitiza)
Oral: 24 mcg capsules

Magnesium hydroxide [milk of magnesia, Epsom Salt]* (generic)
Oral: 400, 800 mg/5 mL aqueous suspension

Mineral oil* (generic, others)
Oral: liquid or emulsion

Polycarbophil* (Equalactin, Mitrolan, FiberCon, Fiber-Lax)
Oral: 500, 625 mg tablets; 500 mg chewable tablets

Polyethylene glycol electrolyte solution (Co-Lyte, GoLYTELY, others)
Oral: Powder for oral solution, makes one gallon (approximately 4 L)

Senna* (Senokot, Ex•Lax, others)
Oral: 8.6, 15, 17, 25 mg tablets; 8.8, 15 mg/mL liquid

Drugs That Dissolve Gallstones

Ursodiol (generic, Actigall, URSO)
Oral: 250, 500 mg tablets; 300 mg capsules

REFERENCES

Acid-Peptic Diseases

Bytzer P, O'Morain C: Treatment of Helicobacter pylori. Helicobacter 2005;10(Suppl 1):40.

Capell MS: Clinical presentation, diagnosis, and management of gastroesophageal reflux disease. Med Clin North Am 2005; 89:243.

Chan FK, Leung WK: Peptic-ulcer disease. Lancet 2002;360:933.

Dekel R, Morse C, Fass R: The role of proton pump inhibitors in gastro-oesophageal reflux disease. Drugs 2004;64:277.

Miner P et al: Gastric acid control with esomeprazole, lansoprazole, omeprazole, pantoprazole, and rabeprazole: A five-way crossover study. Am J Gastroenterol 2003;98:2616.

Suerbaum S, Michetti P: Helicobacter pylori infection. N Engl J Med 2002;347:1175.

Wolfe WM, Sachs G: Acid suppression: Optimizing therapy for gastroduodenal ulcer healing, gastroesophageal reflux disease, and stress-related erosive syndrome. Gastroenterology 2000; 118(Suppl 1):S9.

Motility Disorders

Friedenberg FK, Parkman HP: Management of delayed gastric emptying. Clin Gastroenterol Hepatol 2005;3:642.

Galligan JJ, Vanner S: Basic and clinical pharmacology of new promotility agents. Neurogastroenterol Motil 2005;17:643.

Gershon MD: Serotonin receptors and transporters—roles in normal and abnormal gastrointestinal motility. Aliment Pharmacol Ther 2004;20(Suppl 7):3.

Laxatives

American College of Gastroenterology Task Force: An evidence-based approach to the management of chronic constipation in North America. Am J Gastroenterol 2005;100(Suppl 1):S1.

Ramkumar D, Rao SS: Efficacy and safety of traditional medical therapies for chronic constipation: A systematic review. Am J Gastroenterol 2005;100:936.

Antidiarrheal Agents

Camilleri M: Chronic diarrhea: A review of pathophysiology and management for the clinical gastroenterologist. Clin Gastroenterol Hepatol 2004;2:198.

Schiller L: Chronic diarrhea. Gastroenterology 2004;127:287.

Drugs Used for Irritable Bowel Syndrome

American College of Gastroenterology Functional Gastrointestinal Task Force: An evidence-based position statement on the management of irritable bowel syndrome in North America. Am J Gastroenterol 2002;97:S1.

Drossman DA et al: AGA technical review on irritable bowel syndrome. Gastroenterology 2002;123:2108.

Lesbros-Pantoflickova D et al: Meta-analysis: The treatment of irritable bowel syndrome. Aliment Pharmcol Ther 2004;20:1253.

Antiemetic Agents

Aapro M: 5-HT(3)-receptor antagonists in the management of nausea and vomiting in cancer and cancer treatment. Oncology 2005;69:97.

Apfel CC et al: A factorial trial of six interventions for the prevention of postoperative nausea and vomiting. N Engl J Med 2004;350:24.

Hasler WL, Chey WD: Nausea and vomiting. Gastroenterology 2003;125:1860.

Sharma R, Tobin P, Clarke SJ: Management of chemotherapy-induced nausea, vomiting, oral mucositis, and diarrhoea. Lancet Oncol 2005;6:93.

Drugs Used for Inflammatory Bowel Disease

Bebb JR, Scott BB: Systematic review: How effective are the usual treatment for Crohn's disease? Aliment Pharmacol Ther 2004;20:151.

Colombel JF, et al: The safety profile of infliximab in patients with Crohn's disease: The Mayo Clinic experience with 500 patients. Gastroenterology 2004;126:19.

Dubinsky MC: Azathioprine, 6-mercaptopurine in inflammatory bowel disease: Pharmacology, efficacy, and safety. Clin Gastroenterol Hepatol 2004;2:731.

Hanauer S: Aminosalicylates in inflammatory bowel disease. Aliment Pharmacol Ther 2004;20(Suppl 4):60.

Jarnerot G et al: Infliximab as rescue therapy in severe to moderately severe ulcerative colitis: A randomized, placebo-controlled study. Gastroenterolgy 2005;128:1805.

Sandborn WJ et al: Budesonide for maintenance of remission in patients with Crohn's disease in medically induced remission: A predetermined pooled analysis of four randomized, double-blind, placebo-controlled trials. Am J Gastroenterol 2005;100:1780.

Sands B et al: Infliximab maintenance therapy for fistulizing Crohn's disease. N Engl J Med 2004;350:876.

Travis SPL: The management of mild to severe acute ulcerative colitis. Aliment Pharmcol Ther 2004;20(Suppl 4):88.

Vecchi M et al: Diagnosis, monitoring, and treatment of distal colitis. Aliment Pharmacol Ther 2004;17(Suppl 2):2.

Yang YX, Lichetenstein G: Corticosteroids in Crohn's disease. Am J Gastroenterol 2003:97:803.

Pancreatic Enzyme Supplements

Keller J, Layer P: Pancreatic enzyme supplementation therapy. Curr Treat Options Gastroenterol 2003;6:369.

Bile Acids for Gallstone Therapy

Hempfling W, Dilger K, Beuers U: Systematic review: Ursodeoxycholic acid—adverse effects and drug interactions. Aliment Pharmacol Ther 2003;18:963.

Drugs for Portal Hypertension

Bosch J, Garcia-Pagan JC: Prevention of variceal rebleeding. Lancet 2003;361:952.

Comar KM, Sanyal AJ: Portal hypertensive bleeding. Gastroenterol Clin North Am 2003;32:1079.

Gotzsche PC, Hrobjartsson A: Somatostatin analogues for acute bleeding oesophageal varices. Cochrane Database Syst Rev 2005;4(1):CD000193.

Nevens F: A critical comparison of drug therapies in currently used therapeutic strategies for variceal hemorrhage. Aliment Pharmacol Ther 2004;20(Suppl 3):18.

Talwalkar JA, Kamath PS: An evidence-based medicine approach to beta-blocker therapy in patients with cirrhosis. Am J Med 2004;116:759.

Therapeutic & Toxic Potential of Over-the-Counter Agents

64

Robin L. Corelli, PharmD

In the USA, drugs are divided by law into two classes: those restricted to sale by prescription only and those for which directions for safe use by the public can be written. The latter category constitutes the nonprescription or over-the-counter (OTC) drugs. In 2004, the American public spent more than $15 billion on over 100,000 OTC products to medicate themselves for ailments ranging from acne to warts. These products contain approximately 1000 active ingredients in various forms and combinations.

It is apparent that many OTC drugs are no more than "me too" products advertised to the public in ways that suggest significant differences between them. For example, there are over 100 different systemic analgesic products, almost all of which contain aspirin, acetaminophen, nonsteroidal anti-inflammatory drugs (NSAIDs) such as ibuprofen, or a combination of these agents as primary ingredients. They are made different from one another by the addition of questionable ingredients such as caffeine or antihistamines; by brand names chosen to suggest a specific use or strength ("women's," "migraine," "arthritis," "maximum"); or by special dosage formulations (enteric-coated tablets, geltabs, liquids, sustained-release products, powders, seltzers). There is a price attached to all of these features, and in most cases a less expensive generic product can be equally effective. It is probably safe to assume that the public is generally overwhelmed and confused by the wide array of products presented and will probably use those that are most heavily advertised.

Over the past 30 years, the Food and Drug Administration (FDA) has been engaged in a methodical review of OTC ingredients for both safety and efficacy. There have been two major outcomes of this review: (1) Ingredients designated as ineffective or unsafe for their claimed therapeutic use are being eliminated from OTC product formulations (eg, antimuscarinic agents have been eliminated from OTC sleep aids, attapulgite and polycarbophil can no longer be marketed as OTC antidiarrheal products); and (2) agents previously available by prescription only have been made available for OTC use because they were judged by the review panel

to be generally safe and effective for consumer use without medical supervision (Table 64–1). Since the appointment of the Nonprescription Drugs Advisory Committee in 1993, the rate of switches from prescription to OTC status has accelerated. Indeed, more than 700 OTC products contain ingredients and dosages that were available only by prescription less than 30 years ago. Some agents such as docosanol and the nicotine polacrilex lozenge have bypassed the prescription route altogether and have been released directly to the OTC market. Other OTC ingredients previously available in low doses only are now available in higher-strength formulations. Examples of other prescription drugs currently under consideration for OTC reclassification are orlistat for weight loss, and second-generation nonsedating antihistamines (cetirizine, fexofenadine) for relief of allergy and cold symptoms. The prescription to OTC reclassification process is very rigorous, and many agents have not been approved for OTC use. For example, the cholesterol-lowering agents cholestyramine, lovastatin, and pravastatin were denied OTC status on the basis that these agents could not be used safely and effectively in an OTC setting. The advisory committee believed that diagnosis and ongoing management by a health care provider was necessary for the management of hyperlipidemia, a chronic, asymptomatic condition with potentially life-threatening consequences. In a similar recommendation, oral acyclovir for OTC use in the treatment of recurrent genital herpes was not approved because of concerns about misdiagnosis and inappropriate use leading to increased viral resistance.

There are three reasons why it is essential for clinicians to be familiar with the OTC class of products. First, many OTC medications are effective in treating common ailments, and it is important to be able to help the patient select a safe, effective product. Because managed-care practices encourage clinicians to limit the cost of drugs they prescribe, many will begin to recommend effective OTC treatments to their patients, since these drugs are rarely paid for by the insurance plan (Table 64–2). Second, many of the active ingredients

Table 64–1. Selected agents switched from prescription to OTC status by the Food and Drug Administration since 1990.

Ingredient	Indication	Year Ingredient First Switched	Single-Ingredient Product Examples
Systemic agents			
Cimetidine	Acid reducer (H_2 blocker)	1995	Tagamet HB
Clemastine	Antihistamine	1992	Tavist Allergy
Famotidine	Acid reducer (H_2 blocker)	1995	Pepcid AC
Ketoprofen	Analgesic, antipyretic (NSAID)	1995	Orudis KT
Levonorgestrel	Emergency contraceptive	2006	Plan B
Loratadine	Antihistamine	2002	Claritin, Alavert
Naproxen sodium	Analgesic, antipyretic (NSAID)	1994	Aleve
Nicotine transdermal system	Smoking cessation	1996	Nicotrol, Nicoderm CQ
Nicotine polacrilex gum	Smoking cessation	1996	Nicorette
Nizatidine	Acid reducer (H_2 blocker)	1996	Axid AR
Omeprazole	Acid reducer (proton pump inhibitor)	2003	Prilosec OTC
Ranitidine	Acid reducer (H_2 blocker)	1995	Zantac 75
Topical agents			
Butenafine	Antifungal (topical)	2001	Lotrimin Ultra
Butoconazole	Antifungal (vaginal)	1995	Mycelex-3
Clotrimazole	Antifungal (vaginal)	1990	Gyne-Lotrimin, Mycelex-7, Gyne-Lotrimin-3
Cromolyn	Nasal antiallergy	1997	Nasalcrom
Ketoconazole	Dandruff shampoo	1997	Nizoral AD
Miconazole	Antifungal (vaginal)	1991	Monistat-7, Monistat-3
Minoxidil	Hair growth stimulant	1996	Rogaine Regular and Extra Strength For Men, Rogaine For Women
Naphazoline/Antazoline	Ophthalmic decongestant-antihistamine	1994	Vasocon A
Naphazoline/Pheniramine	Ophthalmic decongestant-antihistamine	1994	Naphcon A, Opcon A, Ocuhist
Permethrin	Pediculicide (head lice)	1990	Nix
Terbinafine	Antifungal (topical)	1999	Lamisil AT
Tioconazole	Antifungal (vaginal)	1997	Monistat-1, Vagistat-1

contained in OTC drugs may worsen existing medical conditions or interact with prescription medications. (See Appendix II, Drug Interactions.) Finally, the misuse or abuse of OTC products may actually produce significant medical complications. Phenylpropanolamine, for example, a sympathomimetic previously found in many cold, allergy, and weight control products, was withdrawn from the United States market by the FDA several years ago based on reports that the drug increased the risk of hemorrhagic stroke. Pseudoephedrine, a decongestant contained in numerous OTC cold preparations has been used in the illicit manufac-

Table 64–2. Ingredients of known efficacy for selected OTC classes.

OTC Category	Ingredient and Usual Adult Dosage	Product Examples	Comments
Acid reducers, H₂ antago-nists	Cimetidine, 200 mg once or twice daily	Tagamet HB	These products have been approved for the relief of "heartburn, acid indigestion, and sour stomach." They should not be taken for longer than 2 weeks and are not recommended for children < 12 years of age.
	Famotidine, 10–20 mg once or twice daily	Pepcid AC, Maximum Strength Pepcid AC	
	Nizatidine, 75 mg once or twice daily	Axid AR	
	Ranitidine, 75–150 mg once or twice daily	Zantac 75, Zantac 150	
Acid reducers, (Proton pump inhibitors)	Omeprazole magnesium, 20.6 mg once daily for 14 days	Prilosec OTC	Omeprazole is the first proton pump inhibitor approved for the treatment of frequent heartburn in adults with symptoms of heartburn 2 or more days per week. The product should not be taken for more than 14 days or more often than every 4 months unless directed by a physician. Omeprazole magnesium 20.6 mg is equivalent to 20 mg of omeprazole (prescription strength).
Acne prepara-tions	Benzoyl peroxide, 5%, 10%	Clearasil, Fostex, Oxy-10, various generic	One of the most effective acne preparations. Apply sparingly once or twice daily. Decrease concentration or frequency if excessive skin irritation occurs.
Allergy and "cold" prep-arations	Chlorpheniramine, 4 mg every 4–6 hours; 8–12 mg (extended-release) every 8–12 hours	Chlor-Trimeton Allergy 4 Hour, Chlor-Trimeton Allergy 8 Hour, Chlor-Trimeton Allergy 12 Hour, various generic	Antihistamines alone relieve most symptoms associated with allergic rhinitis or hay fever. Chlorpheniramine, brompheniramine, and clemastine may cause less drowsiness than diphenhydramine. Loratadine, a second-generation antihistamine, is therapeutically comparable to first-generation agents but with a much lower incidence of sedation. Occasionally, symptoms unrelieved by the antihistamine respond to the addition of a sympathomimetic decongestant. OTC sale of products containing pseudoephedrine is restricted (see comments under Decongestants, systemic).
	Clemastine 1.34 mg every 12 hours	Tavist Allergy	
	Diphenhydramine, 25–50 mg every 4–6 hours	Benadryl Allergy, various generic	
	Loratadine (10 mg) every 24 hours	Alavert, Claritin, Tavist ND	
	Brompheniramine (4 mg) with pseudoephedrine (60 mg) every 4–6 hours	Dimetapp Cold & Allergy; various generic	
	Chlorpheniramine (2–4 mg) with pseudo-ephedrine (30–60 mg) every 4–6 hours	Allerest Maximum Strength, Chlor-Trimeton Allergy-D 4 hour, Sudafed Cold & Allergy, various generic	
	Diphenhydramine (25 mg) with pseudoephedrine (60 mg) every 4–6 hours	Benadryl Allergy/Congestion, various generic	
	Loratadine (10 mg with pseudoephedrine (240 mg) every 24 hours	Claritin-D 24 Hour	
	Triprolidine (2.5 mg) with pseudoephedrine (60 mg) every 4–6 hours	Actifed Cold & Allergy, various generic	

(continued)

OTC Category	Ingredient and Usual Adult Dosage	Product Examples	Comments
Analgesics and antipyretics	Acetaminophen, 325–650 mg every 4–6 hours; 650–1300 mg (extended release) every 8 hours	Panadol, Tylenol, Tylenol 8 Hour, various generic	There are numerous product modifications, including the addition of antacids and caffeine; enteric-coated tablets and seltzers; long-acting or extra-strength formulations; and various mixtures of analgesics. None have any substantial advantage over a single-ingredient product. Acetaminophen lacks anti-inflammatory activity but is available as a liquid; this dosage form is used primarily for infants and children who cannot chew or swallow tablets. Do not exceed a total daily acetaminophen dose of 4 g (2 g/d in regular alcohol users). Aspirin should be used cautiously in certain individuals (see text). Use of OTC products containing aspirin, other salicylates, acetaminophen, ibuprofen, naproxen, or ketoprofen may increase the risk of hepatotoxicity and gastrointestinal hemorrhage in individuals who consume 3 or more alcoholic drinks daily. Long-term continuous use of NSAIDs may increase the risk of heart attack or stroke.
	Aspirin, 325–650 mg every 4–6 hours	Bayer Aspirin, Ecotrin, Bufferin, various generic	
	Ibuprofen, 200–400 mg every 4–6 hours (not to exceed 1200 mg daily)	Advil, Motrin IB, various generic	
	Ketoprofen, 12.5 mg every 4–6 hours	Orudis KT	
	Naproxen sodium, 220 mg every 8–12 hours	Aleve, various generic	
Antacids	Magnesium hydroxide and aluminum hydroxide alone or in combination; calcium carbonate, dosage varies; consult product labeling	Amphojel, Maalox, Milk of Magnesia, Mylanta, Tums, various generic	Combinations of magnesium and aluminum hydroxide are less likely to cause constipation or diarrhea and offer high neutralizing capacity. Some preparations include simethicone, an antiflatulent to relieve symptoms of bloating and pressure.
Anthelmintics (pinworm infection)	Pyrantel pamoate, 11 mg/kg (maximum: 1 g)	Antiminth, Pin-X, Reese's Pinworm	Treat all members of the household. Consult physician for children under age 2 years or under 25 lb. Undergarments, pajamas and linens should be washed daily until the infection is resolved. Dose may be repeated in 2 weeks.
Antidiarrheal agents	Bismuth subsalicylate, 524 mg every 30–60 minutes as needed up to 8 doses daily	Kaopectate, Pepto-Bismol, various generic	Antidiarrheals should not be used if diarrhea is accompanied by fever > 101°F or if blood or mucus is present in stool. Bismuth salts can cause dark discoloration of the tongue and stools. Salicylates are absorbed and can cause tinnitus if coadministered with aspirin. Kaolin is an absorbant clay preparation indicated to help firm stools within 24–48 hours. Loperamide, a synthetic opioid acts on intestinal smooth muscle to decrease motility allowing for absorption of water and electrolytes. Poorly penetrates the CNS and has a lower risk of side effects compared to diphenoxylate or opiates. Not considered a controlled substance.
	Kaolin-Pectin, dosage varies, consult product labeling	Various generic	
	Loperamide, 4 mg initially, then 2 mg after each loose stool, not to exceed 8 mg daily	Imodium A-D, various generic	
Antifungal topical preparations	Butenafine, 1% (cream) apply to affected areas once daily	Lotrimin Ultra	Effective for the treatment of tinea pedis (athlete's foot), tinea cruris (jock itch), and tinea corporis (ringworm). Clotrimazole and miconazole also effective against *Candida albicans*.
	Clotrimazole, 1% (cream, solution), apply to affected areas twice daily	Lotrimin AF Cream/Solution, Mycelex OTC	
	Miconazole, 2% (cream, powder, solution), apply to affected areas twice daily	Cruex, Desenex, Lotrimin AF Powder/Spray, Micatin, Zeasorb-AF	
	Terbinafine, 1% (cream, solution, spray), apply to affected areas once daily	Lamisil AT	

(continued)

OTC Category	Ingredient and Usual Adult Dosage	Product Examples	Comments
	Tolnaftate, 1% (cream, powder, spray, solution), apply to affected areas twice daily	Aftate, Tinactin, Ting, various generic	
	Undecylenic acid, 12– 25% (powder, solution) apply to affected areas twice daily	Blis-To-Sol, Elon Dual Defense Anti-Fungal	
Antifungal vaginal preparations	Butoconazole, 2% cream, one applicatorful intravaginally at bedtime for 3 consecutive days	Mycelex-3	Topical vaginal antifungals should only be used for treatment of recurrent vulvovaginal candidiasis in otherwise healthy, nonpregnant women previously diagnosed by a clinician.
	Clotrimazole (1%, 2% vaginal cream, 100 mg, 200 mg tablet); see comments for dosage	Gyne-Lotrimin, Mycelex-7, Gyne-Lotrimin-3, various generic	Insert one applicatorful (1%) or one tablet (100 mg) intravaginally at bedtime for 7 consecutive days. Alternatively: Insert one applicatorful (2%) or one tablet (200 mg), intravaginally at bedtime for 3 consecutive days.
	Miconazole (2%, 4% vaginal cream; 100 mg, 200 mg vaginal suppositories); see comments for dosage	Monistat-7, Monistat-3	Insert one applicatorful intravaginally at bedtime for 7 consecutive days (2%) or 3 consecutive days (4%). Alternatively: insert one suppository intravaginally at bedtime for 7 consecutive days (100 mg) or 3 consecutive days (200 mg).
	Tioconazole, 6.5% vaginal ointment, one applicatorful intravaginally at bedtime (single-dose)	Monistat-1, Vagistat-1	
Anti-inflammatory topical preparations	Hydrocortisone, 0.5% (cream, ointment, lotion), 1% (cream ointment, lotion, spray)	Anusol HC, Cortaid, Cortizone-5, Cortizone-10, various generic	Used to temporarily relieve itching and inflammation associated with minor rashes due to contact or allergic dermatitides, insect bites, and hemorrhoids. Apply sparingly to affected areas two to four times daily.
Antiseborrheal agents	Coal tar, 0.5-5% shampoo, dosage varies; consult product labeling	Denorex, Ionil T Plus, Pentrax 5%, various generic	Tar derivatives inhibit epidermal proliferation and may possess antipruritic and antimicrobial activity.
	Ketoconazole, 1% shampoo, apply every 3–4 days	Nizoral A-D	Synthetic azole antifungal agent with activity versus *Pityrosporum ovale*, a fungus that may cause seborrhea and dandruff. Massage over entire scalp for 3 minutes. Rinse thoroughly and repeat application. Both selenium sulfide and zinc pyrithione are cytostatic agents that decrease epidermal turnover rates. Massage into wet scalp for 2–3 minutes. Rinse thoroughly and repeat application. Selenium sulfide can be irritating to the eyes and skin.
	Pyrithione zinc, 1–2% shampoo, apply once or twice weekly	Head & Shoulders, Sebulon, various generic	
	Selenium sulfide, 1% shampoo, apply once or twice weekly	Head & Shoulders Intensive Treatment, Selsun Blue, various generic	
Antitussives	Codeine, 10–20 mg every 4–6 hours, not to exceed 120 mg in 24 hours (with guaifenesin)	Guiatuss AC, Mytussin AC, various generic	Acts centrally to increase the cough threshold. In doses required for cough suppression, the addictive liability associated with codeine is low. Many codeine-containing antitussive combinations are schedule V narcotics, and OTC sale is restricted in some states.
	Dextromethorphan, 10–20 mg every 4 hours or 30 mg every 6–8 hours	Benylin Adult Formula Cough, Hold DM, Vicks 44 Cough Relief, various generic	Dextromethorphan is a nonopioid congener of levorphanol without analgesic or addictive properties. Often is used with antihistamines, decongestants, and expectorants in combination products.

(continued)

Table 64–2. Ingredients of known efficacy for selected OTC classes. (continued)

OTC Category	Ingredient and Usual Adult Dosage	Product Examples	Comments
Decongestants, topical	Oxymetazoline, 0.05% nasal solution, 2–3 sprays per nostril twice daily	Afrin, Dristan 12 Hour Nasal, Neo-Synephrine 12 Hour, various generic	Topical sympathomimetics are effective for the temporary acute management of rhinorrhea associated with common colds and allergies. Long-acting agents (oxymetazoline and xylometazoline) are generally preferred, though phenylephrine is equally effective. Topical decongestants should not be used for longer than 3 days to prevent rebound nasal congestion.
	Phenylephrine (0.25%, 0.5%, 1%), nasal solution, 2–3 sprays/drops per nostril every 3–4 hours	Neo-Synephrine, various generic	
	Xylometazoline (0.05%, 0.1%), nasal solution, 2–3 sprays/drops per nostril every 8–10 hours	Otrivin	
Decongestants, systemic	Phenylephrine, 10 mg every 4 hours	Sudafed PE, various generic combination products	Oral decongestants have a prolonged duration of action but may cause more systemic effects, including nervousness, excitability, restlessness, and insomnia. Also available in antihistamine, antitussive, expectorant, and analgesic combination products. OTC. Federal regulations established to discourage the illicit manufacture of methamphetamine specify that all drug products containing pseudoephedrine must be stored in locked cabinets or behind the pharmacy counter and can only be sold in limited quanitities to consumers after they provide photo identification and sign a logbook.
	Pseudoephedrine, 60 mg every 4–6 hours or 120 mg (extended release) every 12 hours, or 240 mg (extended-release) every 24 hours	Sudafed, various generic	
Emergency contraceptive	Levonorgestrel, 0.75 mg tablet taken as soon as possible but no later than 72 hours after unprotected sex; repeat dosage 12 hours later	Plan B	OTC sale is limited to women $\geq$ 18 years of age. Prevents ovulation and may inhibit fertilization or implantation.
Expectorants	Guaifenesin, 100–400 mg every 4 hours	Glytuss, Robitussin, various generic	The only OTC expectorant recognized as safe and effective by the FDA. Often used with antihistamines, decongestants, and antitussives in combination products.
Hair growth stimulants	Minoxidil, 2%, 5% solution, apply 1 mL to affected areas of scalp twice daily.	Rogaine for Men, Rogaine for Women, Rogaine Extra Strength for Men	Minoxidil appears to directly stimulate hair follicles resulting in increased hair thickness and reduced hair loss. Treatment for four months or longer may be necessary to achieve visible results. If new hair growth is observed, continued treatment is necessary as hair density returns to pretreatment levels within months following drug discontinuation.
Laxatives	Bulk formers: Polycarbophil, psyllium, and methylcellulose preparations. Dosage varies; consult product labeling	Citrucel, Equalactin, Konsyl, Metamucil, Perdiem, various generic	The safest laxatives for chronic use include the bulk formers and stool softeners. Saline laxatives and stimulants may be used acutely but not chronically (see text). Bulk formers hold water and expand in stool, promoting peristalsis.
	Stool softeners: Docusate sodium, 50–500 mg daily. Docusate calcium, 240 mg daily	Colace, Surfak, various generic	Soften fecal material via detergent action that allows water to penetrate stool.

(continued)

Table 64–2. Ingredients of known efficacy for selected OTC classes. (continued)

OTC Category	Ingredient and Usual Adult Dosage	Product Examples	Comments
	Stimulant laxatives: Bisa-codyl, 5–15 mg daily. Senna, dosage varies, consult product labeling	Correctol, Dulcolax, Ex-Lax, Senokot, various generic	Stimulant laxative actions include direct irritation of intestinal mucosa or stimulation of the myenteric plexus, resulting in peristalsis. These agents may also cause alteration of fluid and electrolyte absorption, resulting in luminal fluid accumulation and bowel evacuation.
Pediculicides (Head lice)	Permethrin 1%	Nix	Instructions for use varies; consult product labeling. Avoid contact with eyes. Comb out nits. Linens, pajamas, combs, and brushes should be washed daily until the infestation is eliminated. Repeat application 7 days later if live nits are still visible.
	Pyrethrins (0.3%) combined with piperonyl butoxide (3–4%)	A-200, RID	
Sleep aids	Diphenhydramine, 25–50 mg at bedtime	Compoz, Nytol, Sominex, various generic	Diphenhydramine and doxylamine are antihistamines with well-documented CNS depressant effects. Because insomnia may be indicative of a serious underlying condition requiring medical attention, patients should consult a physician if insomnia persists continuously for longer than 2 weeks.
	Doxylamine, 25 mg at bedtime	Unisom, various generic	
Smoking cessation aids	Nicotine (transdermal system), dosage varies; consult product labeling	Nicoderm CQ, Nicotrol, various generic	Nicotine replacement products in combination with behavioral support approximately double abstinence rates compared to placebo. Review directions for use carefully, since product strengths vary and self-titration and tapering may be necessary.
	Nicotine polacrilex gum; dosage varies; consult product labeling	Nicorette, various generic	
	Nicotine polacrilex lozenge, dosage varies; consult product labeling	Commit, various generic	

ture of methamphetamine. A general awareness of these products and their formulations will enable clinicians to more fully appreciate the potential for OTC drug-related problems in their patients.

Table 64–2 lists examples of OTC products that may be used effectively to treat common medical problems. The selection of one ingredient over another may be important in patients with certain medical conditions or in patients taking other medications. These are discussed in detail in other chapters. The recommendations listed in Table 64–2 are based on the efficacy of the ingredients and on the principles set forth in the following paragraphs.

(1) Select the product that is simplest in formulation with regard to ingredients and dosage form. In general, single-ingredient products are preferred. Although some combination products contain effective doses of all ingredients, others contain therapeutic doses of some ingredients and subtherapeutic doses of others. Furthermore, there may be differing durations of action among the ingredients, and there is always a possibility that the clinician or patient is unaware of the presence of certain active ingredients in the product. Acetaminophen, for example, is in many cough

and cold preparations; a patient unaware of this may take separate doses of analgesic in addition to that contained in the cold preparation, potentially leading to toxicity.

(2) Select a product that contains a therapeutically effective dose.

(3) Carefully read the product labeling to determine which ingredients are appropriate based on the patient's symptoms and underlying health conditions and whatever is known about the medications the patient is already taking.

(4) Recommend a generic product if one is available.

(5) Be wary of "gimmicks" or advertising claims of specific superiority over similar products.

(6) For children, the dose, dosage form, and palatability of the product are prime considerations.

Certain ingredients in OTC products should be avoided or used with caution in selected patients because they may exacerbate existing medical problems or interact with other medications the patient is taking. Many of the more potent OTC ingredients are hidden in products where their presence would not ordinarily be expected (Table 64–3). Although OTC medications

Table 64–3. Hidden ingredients in OTC products.

Hidden Drug or Drug Class	OTC Class Containing Drug	Product Examples
Alcohol (percent ethanol)	Cough syrups, cold preparations	Cheracol Plus (5%); Comtrex Night Time Maximum Strength (10%); Vicks 44M (10%); Vicks NyQuil Liquid (10%)
	Mouthwashes	Listerine (27%); Scope (19%); Targon Smokers (16%)
Antihistamines	Analgesics	Aspirin Free Anacin PM; Excedrin PM; Extra Strength Bayer PM; Extra Strength Doan's PM; Tylenol PM
	Menstrual products	Midol Maximum Strength Menstrual; Midol Menstrual Complete; Midol Pre-Menstrual Syndrome; Maximum Strength Multi-Symptom Pamprin Menstrual Relief
	Sleep aids	Compoz; Nytol; Sominex; Twilite ; Unisom
Aspirin and other salicylates	Antidiarrheals	Pepto-Bismol (bismuth subsalicylate); Kaopectate (bismuth subsalicylate)
	Cold/allergy preparations	Alka-Seltzer Plus Flu
Caffeine	Analgesics	Anacin; Arthritis Strength BC; BC Powder; Cope; Excedrin Extra Strength; Excedrin Migraine; Goody's Extra Strength Headache Powder
	Menstrual products	Midol Menstrual Complete
	Stimulants	Keep Alert; NoDoz; Vivarin
Local anesthetics (usually benzocaine)	Antitussives/Lozenges	Cepacol Maxium Strength Lozenges; Cylex; Chloraseptic Sore Throat
	Dermatologic preparations	Americaine; Bactine; Dermoplast; Lanacane; Solarcaine
	Hemorrhoidal products	Americaine; Anusol Ointment; Medicone; Tronolane
	Toothache, cold sore, and teething products	Anbesol; Kank-A; Orasept; Orajel; Zilactin-B
Sodium (mg/tablet or as stated)	Analgesics	Alka-Seltzer Original Effervescent Tablet (568); Alka-Seltzer Extra Strength Effervescent Tablet (588); Bromo-Seltzer Granules (959/pre-measured packet)
	Antacids	Alka-Seltzer Original Effervescent Tablet (568); Alka-Seltzer Extra Strength Effervescent Tablet (588); Alka-Seltzer Gold (311); Alka-Seltzer Heartburn Relief (1,150); Bromo-Seltzer Granules (959/pre-measured packet); Citrocarbonate Effervescent Granules (701/teaspoon)
	Laxatives	Fleets Enema (4,439 mg, of which 275–400 mg/enema is absorbed); Fleet Phospho-Soda (554/teaspoon)
Sympathomimetics	Analgesics	Motrin Sinus Headache; Sinarest No Drowsiness; Sine-Aid Sinus Headache Tablets; Sinutab; Tylenol Flu Day Non-Drowsy; Tylenol Sinus Day Non-Drowsy
	Asthma products	Bronkaid Dual Action; Primatene
	Cold/allergy preparations	Advil Flu & Body Ache; Alka-Seltzer Plus Cold; Comtrex Maximum Strength Day and Night Flu; Contac-D Cold; Dimetapp Cold & Allergy; PediaCare Cold & Allergy; Motrin Cold & Sinus; Sudafed; TheraFlu Severe Cold ; Vicks 44M; Vicks DayQuil
	Cough preparations	PediaCare Long Lasting Cough Plus Cold; Robitussin Cold & Cough; Triaminic Cough; Vicks 44D
	Hemorrhoidal products	Hemorid; Preparation H

have standardized label formatting and content requirements that specify the indications for use, dosage, warnings, and active and inactive ingredients contained in the product, many consumers do not carefully read or comprehend this information. Lack of awareness of the ingredients in OTC products and the belief by many physicians that OTC products are ineffective and harmless may cause diagnostic confusion and perhaps interfere with therapy. For example, innumerable OTC products, including analgesics and allergy, cough, and cold preparations, contain sympathomimetics. These agents should be avoided or used cautiously by type 1 diabetics and patients with hypertension, angina, or hyperthyroidism. Aspirin should not be used in children and adolescents for viral infections (with or without fever) because of an increased risk of Reye's syndrome. Aspirin and other NSAIDs should be avoided by individuals with active peptic ulcer disease, certain platelet disorders, and patients taking oral anticoagulants. Cimetidine, an H_2-receptor antagonist, is a well-known inhibitor of hepatic drug metabolism and can increase the blood levels and toxicity of drugs such as phenytoin, theophylline, and warfarin.

Overuse or misuse of OTC products may induce significant medical problems. A prime example is rebound congestion from the regular use of decongestant nasal sprays for more than 3 days. The improper and long-term use of some antacids (eg, aluminum hydroxide) may cause constipation and even impaction in elderly people, as well as hypophosphatemia. Laxative abuse can result in abdominal cramping and fluid and electrolyte disturbances. Insomnia, nervousness, and restlessness can result from the use of sympathomimetics or caffeine hidden in many OTC products (Table 64–3). The long-term use of some analgesics containing large amounts of caffeine may produce rebound headaches, and long-term use of analgesics has been associated with interstitial nephritis. OTC products containing aspirin, other salicylates, acetaminophen, ibuprofen, naproxen, or ketoprofen may increase the risk of hepatotoxicity and gastrointestinal hemorrhage in individuals who consume three or more alcoholic drinks daily. Recent evidence suggests the long-term use of NSAIDs may increase the risk of heart attack or stroke. Furthermore, acute inges-

tion of large amounts of acetaminophen by adults or children can cause serious, and often fatal, hepatotoxicity. Antihistamines may cause sedation or drowsiness, especially when taken concurrently with sedative-hypnotics, tranquilizers, alcohol, or other central nervous system depressants. Finally, antihistamines, local anesthetics, antimicrobial agents, counterirritants, *p*-aminobenzoic acid (PABA) and preservatives contained in a myriad of OTC topical and vaginal products may induce allergic reactions.

There are three major drug information sources for OTC products. *Handbook of Nonprescription Drugs* is the most comprehensive resource for OTC medications; it evaluates ingredients contained in major OTC drug classes and lists the ingredients included in many OTC products. *Nonprescription Drug Therapy* is an annually updated reference that provides detailed OTC product information and patient counseling instructions. *Physicians' Desk Reference for Nonprescription Drugs, Dietary Supplements and Herbs,* a compendium of manufacturers' information regarding OTC products, is published annually but is somewhat incomplete with regard to the number of products included. Any health care provider who seeks more specific information regarding OTC products may find useful the references listed below.

REFERENCES

Brass EP: Changing the status of drugs from prescription to over-the-counter availability. N Engl J Med 2001;345:810.

Consumer Healthcare Products Association Web Page: http://www.chpa-info.org/

Francis SA, Barnett N, Denham M: Switching of prescription drugs to over-the-counter status: Is it a good thing for the elderly? Drugs Aging 2005;22:361.

Handbook of Nonprescription Drugs, 15th ed. American Pharmaceutical Association, 2006.

Nonprescription Drug Therapy: Guiding Patient Self-Care, 4th ed. Facts and Comparisons, 2005.

Physicians' Desk Reference for Nonprescription Drugs, Dietary Supplements and Herbs, 27th ed. Thomson Healthcare, 2006.

US Food and Drug Administration: Center for Drug Evaluation and Research. Over-the-Counter (OTC) Drugs Web Page: http://www.fda.gov/cder/offices/otc/default.htm

Botanicals ("Herbal Medications") & Nutritional Supplements

65

Cathi E. Dennehy, PharmD, & Candy Tsourounis, PharmD

The medical use of botanicals in their natural and unprocessed form undoubtedly began when the first intelligent animals noticed that certain food plants altered particular body functions. Much information exists about the historical use and effectiveness of botanical products. Unfortunately, the quality of this information is extremely variable and much is useless or false. An unbiased and regularly updated compendium of basic and clinical reports regarding botanicals is *Pharmacists Letter/Prescribers Letter Natural Medicines Comprehensive Database* (see references). A useful evidence-based website, www.naturalstandard.com, is available to institutions. Another compendium is the *Report of the German Commission E* (a committee that sets standards for herbal medications in that country). Interest in the endocrine effects and possible nutritional benefits of certain purified chemicals such as glucosamine, melatonin, high-dose vitamins, and minerals has led to a parallel development of consumer demand for such substances.

The alternative medicinal substances are distinguished from similar botanical substances used in traditional medicine (morphine, digitalis, atropine, etc) by virtue of being available without a prescription and, unlike over-the-counter medications, being legally considered dietary supplements rather than drugs (thus avoiding conventional Food and Drug Administration oversight). Among the purified chemicals, glucosamine and melatonin are of significant pharmacologic interest.

This chapter provides an evidence-based approach to the pharmacology and clinical efficacy of several of the commonly used and commercially available botanicals and dietary supplements. Ephedrine, the active principle in Ma-huang, is discussed in Chapter 9.

REGULATORY FACTORS

Dietary supplements (which include vitamins, minerals, cofactors, herbal medications, and amino acids) are not considered over-the-counter drugs in the USA but rather food supplements. In 1994, the United States Congress, influenced by growing "consumerism" as well as strong manufacturer lobbying efforts, passed the Dietary Supplement and Health Education Act (DSHEA). This misguided act prevented adequate FDA oversight of these substances. Thus, DSHEA has allowed a variety of substances with pharmacologic activity—if classified as dietary supplements—to be sold without a prescription or any FDA review of efficacy or safety prior to product marketing. Dietary supplements are governed under Current Good Manufacturing Practice in Manufacturing, Packaging or Holding Human Food (CGMP) regulations. Although administered by the FDA, CGMP regulations are often inadequate to ensure product purity, potency, and other variables such as accurate product identification and appropriate botanical harvesting. Therefore, much of the criticism regarding the dietary supplement industry involves a lack of product purity and variations in potency.

CLINICAL ASPECTS OF THE USE OF BOTANICALS

Many United States consumers have embraced the use of botanicals and other supplements as a "natural" approach to their health care. Unfortunately, misconceptions regarding safety and efficacy of the agents are common, and the fact that a substance can be called "natural" of course does not guarantee its safety. In fact, these products can be adulterated, misbranded, or contaminated either intentionally or unintentionally in a variety of ways. Furthermore, the doses recommended for active botanical substances may be much higher than those considered clinically safe. For example, the doses recommended for several Ma-huang preparations contain three to five times the medically recommended daily dose of the active ingredient, ephedrine—doses that impose significant risks for patients with cardiovascular disease.

Adverse effects have been documented for a variety of botanical medications. Unfortunately, chemical analysis is rarely performed on the products involved. This leads to uncertainty about whether the primary herb or an adulterant caused the adverse effect. In some cases, the chemical constituents of the herb can clearly lead to toxicity. Some of the herbs that should be used cautiously or not at all are listed in Table 65–1.

Table 65–1. Botanical supplements and some associated risks.

Commercial Name, Scientific Name, Plant Parts	Intended Use	Toxic Agents, Effects	Comments
Aconite *Aconitum* species	Analgesic	Alkaloid, cardiac and central nervous system effects	Avoid
Borage *Borago officinalis* Tops, leaves	Anti-inflammatory, diuretic	Pyrrolizidine alkaloids, hepatotoxicity	Avoid
Chaparral *Larrea tridentata* Twigs, leaves	Anti-infective, antioxidant, anticancer	Hepatotoxicity	Avoid
Coltsfoot *Tussilago farfara* Leaves, flower	Upper respiratory tract infections	Pyrrolizidine alkaloids, hepatotoxicity	Avoid ingestion of any parts of plant; leaves may be used topically for anti-inflammatory effects for up to 4–6 weeks
Comfrey *Symphytum* species Leaves and roots	Internal digestive aid, topical for wound healing	Pyrrolizidine alkaloids, hepatotoxicity	Avoid ingestion: topical use should be limited to 4–6 weeks
Ephedra, Ma-huang *Ephedra* species	Diet aid; stimulant; bronchodilator	Central nervous system toxicity, cardiac toxicity	Avoid in patients at risk for stroke, myocardial infarction, uncontrolled blood pressure, seizures, general anxiety disorder
Germander *Teucrium chamaedrys* Leaves, tops	Diet aid	Hepatotoxicity	Avoid
Jin Bu Huan	Analgesic; sedative	Hepatotoxicity	Avoid
Pennyroyal *Mentha pulegium* or *Hedeoma pulegioides* Extract	Digestive aid, induction of menstrual flow, abortifacient	Pulegone and pulegone metabolite, liver failure, renal failure	Avoid
Poke root *Phytolacca americana*	Antirheumatic	Hemorrhagic gastritis	Avoid
Royal jelly *Apis mellifera* (honeybee)	Tonic	Bronchospasm, anaphylaxis	Avoid in patients with chronic allergies or respiratory diseases; asthma, chronic obstructive pulmonary disease, emphysema, atopy
Sassafras *Sassafras albidum* Root bark	Blood thinner	Safrole oil, hepatocarcinogen in animals	Avoid

■ BOTANICAL SUBSTANCES

ECHINACEA (*ECHINACEA PURPUREA*)

Chemistry

The three most widely used species of *Echinacea* are *Echinacea purpurea*, *E pallida*, and *E angustifolia*. The chemical constituents include flavonoids, lipo-philic constituents (eg, alkamides, polyacetylenes), water-soluble polysaccharides, and water-soluble caffeoyl conjugates (eg, echinacoside, chicoric acid, caffeic acid). Within any marketed echinacea formulation, the relative amounts of these components are dependent upon the species used, the method of manufacture, and the plant parts used. The German Commission E has approved two formulations for clinical use: the fresh pressed juice of aerial parts of *E purpurea* and the alcoholic root extract of *E pallida*. *E purpurea* has been the most widely studied in clinical trials. Although the active constituents of echinacea are not completely known, chicoric acid from *E purpurea* and echinacoside from *E pallida* and *E angustifolia*, as well as alkamides and polysaccharides, are most often noted as having immune-modulating properties. Most commercial formulations, however, are not standardized for any particular constituent.

Pharmacologic Effects

A. IMMUNE MODULATION

The effect of echinacea on the immune system is controversial. Human studies using commercially marketed formulations of echinacea have shown increased phagocytosis but not immunostimulation. In vitro, however, *E purpurea* juice increased production of interleukin-1, -6, -10, and tumor necrosis factor-α by human macrophages. Enhanced natural killer cell activity and antibody-dependent cellular toxicity was also observed with *E purpurea* extract in cell lines from both healthy and immunocompromised patients. Studies using the isolated purified polysaccharides from *E purpurea* have also shown cytokine activation. Polysaccharides by themselves, however, are unlikely to accurately reproduce the activity of the entire extract.

B. ANTI-INFLAMMATORY EFFECTS

Certain echinacea constituents have demonstrated anti-inflammatory properties in vitro. Inhibition of cyclooxygenase, 5-lipoxygenase, and hyaluronidase may be involved. In animals, application of *E purpurea* prior to application of a topical irritant reduced both paw and ear edema. There are too few clinical trials in humans to warrant the use of echinacea in wound healing.

C. ANTIBACTERIAL, ANTIFUNGAL, ANTIVIRAL, AND ANTIOXIDANT EFFECTS

Some in vitro studies have reported weak antibacterial, antifungal, antiviral, and antioxidant activity with echinacea constituents. The applicability of these findings to clinical trials is discussed below.

Clinical Trials

Echinacea is most often used to enhance immune function in individuals who have colds and other respiratory tract infections. Older reviews and cold treatment trials reported favorable results for the aerial parts of *E purpurea* in reducing symptoms or time to recovery if the agent was administered within the first 24 hours of a cold. To date, however, most of these trials have contained multiple variables (eg, formulation, dose, duration) that make it difficult to make a clear therapeutic recommendation or ensure reproducible outcomes. At best, symptoms and duration may be reduced by about 25–30%. Recent trials investigating preparations of *E angustifolia* and combinations of echinacea containing *E angustifolia* for cold treatment, however, have failed to find a benefit. Echinacea has also been evaluated as a prophylactic agent in the prevention of upper respiratory tract infection in adults and as a treatment and prophylactic agent for colds in children. These trials have generally reported no effect.

Echinacea has been used investigationally to enhance hematologic recovery following chemotherapy. It has also been used as an adjunct in the treatment of urinary tract and vaginal fungal infections. These indications require further research before they can be accepted in clinical practice. *E purpurea* is ineffective in treating recurrent genital herpes.

Adverse Effects

Flu-like symptoms (eg, fever, shivering, headache, vomiting) have been reported following the intravenous use of echinacea extracts. Adverse effects with oral commercial formulations are minimal and most often include unpleasant taste, gastrointestinal upset, or central nervous system effects (eg, headache, dizziness). Allergic reactions such as rash, acute asthma, and anaphylaxis have been infrequently reported.

Drug Interactions & Precautions

Until the role of echinacea in immune modulation is better defined, this agent should be avoided in patients with immune deficiency disorders (eg, AIDS, cancer), autoimmune disorders (eg, multiple sclerosis, rheumatoid arthritis), and patients with tuberculosis. The German Commission E recommends limiting the chronic use of echinacea to no more than 8 weeks. While there are no reported drug interactions for echinacea, some preparations have a high alcohol content and should not be used with medications known to cause a disulfiram-like reaction. Theoretically echinacea should also be avoided in persons taking immunosuppressant medications (eg, organ transplant recipients).

Dosage

Because of recent negative trials using *E angustifolia* for colds and a lack of clinical trials examining *E pallida*, only the dosing for *E purpurea* is provided here. *E purpurea* freshly pressed juice is given at a dosage of 6–9 mL/d in divided doses two to five times daily. Echinacea is generally taken at the first sign of a cold.

GARLIC (*ALLIUM SATIVUM*)

Chemistry

The pharmacologic activity of garlic involves a variety of organosulfur compounds. The most notable of these is allicin, which is responsible for the characteristic garlic odor.

Pharmacologic Effects

A. CARDIOVASCULAR EFFECTS

In vitro, allicin and related compounds inhibit HMG-CoA reductase, which is involved in cholesterol biosynthesis (see Chapter 35). Several clinical trials have investigated the lipid-lowering potential of garlic. Some have shown significant reductions in cholesterol and others no effect. The most recent meta-analysis suggested a minor (5%) reduction of total cholesterol that was insignificant when dietary controls were in place. Results of a study by the National Center of Complementary and Alternative Medicine (NCCAM) evaluating three different sources of garlic (fresh, powdered, and aged garlic extract) in adults with moderately elevated cholesterol are likely to be published in 2006 and may provide further insight into the efficacy of this botanical for this indication.

Clinical trials report antiplatelet effects (possibly through inhibition of thromboxane synthesis) following garlic ingestion and mixed effects on fibrinolytic activity. These effects in combination with antioxidant effects (eg, increased resistance to low-density lipoprotein oxidation) and reductions in total cholesterol may be beneficial in patients with atherosclerosis. In preliminary trials involving atherosclerotic patients, significant reductions in plaque volume were observed for patients taking garlic versus placebo.

Garlic constituents may affect blood vessel elasticity and blood pressure. Proposed mechanisms include opening of potassium channels in vascular smooth muscle, stimulation of nitric oxide synthesis, and inhibition of angiotensin-converting enzyme. Epidemiologic studies suggest that individuals chronically consuming low doses of garlic (averaging 460 mg/d) may have reductions in aortic stiffness. A meta-analysis of garlic's antihypertensive properties revealed a mild effect with a 7.7 mm Hg decrease in systolic pressure and a 5 mm Hg decrease in diastolic pressure.

B. ENDOCRINE EFFECTS

The effect of garlic on glucose homeostasis does not appear to be significant in persons with diabetes. Certain organosulfur constituents in garlic, however, have demonstrated hypoglycemic effects in nondiabetic animal models.

C. ANTIMICROBIAL EFFECTS

In vitro, allicin has demonstrated activity against some gram-positive and gram-negative bacteria as well as fungi *(Candida albicans)*, protozoa *(Entamoeba histolytica)*, and certain viruses. The primary mechanism involves the inhibition of thiol-containing enzymes needed by these microbes. The antimicrobial effect of garlic has not been extensively studied in clinical trials. Given the availability of effective prescription antimicrobials, the usefulness of garlic in this area appears limited.

D. ANTINEOPLASTIC EFFECTS

In rodent studies, garlic inhibits procarcinogens for colon, esophageal, lung, breast, and stomach cancer, probably by detoxification of carcinogens and reduced carcinogen activation. The evidence for anticarcinogenic properties in vivo is largely epidemiologic. For example, certain populations with high dietary garlic consumption appear to have a reduced incidence of stomach cancer.

Adverse Effects

Following oral ingestion, adverse effects may include nausea (6%), hypotension (1.3%), allergy (1.1%), and bleeding (rare). Breath odor has been reported with an incidence of 20–40% at recommended doses using enteric-coated formulations. Contact dermatitis may occur with the handling of raw garlic.

Drug Interactions & Precautions

Because of reported antiplatelet effects, patients using anticlotting medications (eg, warfarin, aspirin, ibuprofen) should use garlic cautiously. Additional monitoring of blood pressure and signs and symptoms of bleeding is warranted. Garlic may reduce the bioavailability of saquinavir, an antiviral protease inhibitor, but it does not appear to affect the bioavailability of ritonavir.

Dosage

Products should be standardized to contain 1.3% alliin (the allicin precursor) or have an allicin-generating potential of 0.6%. Enteric-coated formulations are recommended to minimize degradation of the active substances. A daily dose of 600–900 mg/d of powdered garlic is most common. This is equivalent to one clove of raw garlic (2–4 g) per day.

GINKGO (*GINKGO BILOBA*)

Chemistry

Ginkgo biloba extract is prepared from the leaves of the ginkgo tree. The most common formulation is prepared by concentrating 50 parts of the crude leaf to prepare one part of extract. The active constituents in ginkgo are flavone glycosides and terpenoids (ie, ginkgolides A, B, C, J, and bilobalide).

Pharmacologic Effects

A. CARDIOVASCULAR EFFECTS

In animal models and some human studies, ginkgo has been shown to increase blood flow and reduce blood viscosity, thus enhancing tissue perfusion. Enhancement of endogenous nitric oxide (see Chapter 19) and antagonism of platelet-activating factor may be involved.

Ginkgo biloba has been studied for its effects on mild to moderate occlusive peripheral arterial disease. Randomized studies involving 120–160 mg of standardized ginkgo leaf extract (EGb761) for up to 6 months have generally reported significant improvements in pain-free walking distance as compared with placebo. Efficacy may be comparable to pentoxyfylline (see Chapter 20) for this indication. (It should be noted that physical conditioning is as effective as pentoxyfylline in improving walking distance.)

B. METABOLIC EFFECTS

Antioxidant and radical-scavenging properties have been observed for the flavonoid fraction of ginkgo as well as some of the terpene constituents. In vitro, ginkgo has demonstrated superoxide dismutase-like activity and superoxide anion- and hydroxyl radical-scavenging properties. It has also demonstrated a protective effect in limiting free radical formation in animal models of ischemic injury and in reducing markers of oxidative stress in patients undergoing coronary artery bypass surgery.

C. CENTRAL NERVOUS SYSTEM EFFECTS

In aged animal models, chronic administration of ginkgo for 3–4 weeks led to modifications in central nervous system receptors and neurotransmitters. Receptor densities increased for muscarinic, α_2, and 5-HT_{1a} receptors and decreased for β adrenoceptors. Increased serum levels of acetylcholine and norepinephrine and enhanced synaptosomal reuptake of serotonin have also been reported. Additional mechanisms that may be involved include reversible inhibition of monoamine (MAO) A and B, reduced corticosterone synthesis, inhibition of amyloid-beta fibril formation, and enhanced GABA levels.

Ginkgo is frequently used to treat cerebral insufficiency and dementia of the Alzheimer type. The term *cerebral insufficiency,* however, includes a variety of manifestations ranging from poor concentration and confusion to anxiety and depression as well as physical complaints such as hearing loss and headache. For this reason, studies evaluating cerebral insufficiency tend to be more inclusive and difficult to assess than trials evaluating dementia. A meta-analysis by the Cochrane Collaboration found that ginkgo showed promising evidence for improvement of cognitive function in patients with cognitive impairment and dementia. The duration of the largest of these studies was 1 year. Recent studies on the effects of ginkgo for memory enhancement in healthy nondemented elderly adults did not show a benefit with 6 weeks of use. Ginkgo is currently under investigation as a prophylactic agent for dementia of the Alzheimer type.

D. MISCELLANEOUS EFFECTS

Ginkgo has been studied for its effects in allergic and asthmatic bronchoconstriction, erectile dysfunction, tinnitus and hearing loss, short-term memory loss in healthy nonelderly adults, and macular degeneration. In all of these conditions, the evidence is insufficient to warrant clinical use at this time.

Adverse Effects

Adverse effects have been reported with a frequency comparable to that of placebo. These include nausea, headache, stomach upset, diarrhea, allergy, anxiety, and insomnia. A few case reports noted bleeding complications in patients using ginkgo. In a few of these cases, the patients were also using either aspirin or warfarin.

Drug Interactions & Precautions

Ginkgo may have antiplatelet properties and should not be used in combination with antiplatelet or anticoagulant medications. A case of an enhanced sedative effect was reported when ginkgo was combined with trazodone. Seizures have been reported as a toxic effect of ginkgo, most likely related to seed contamination in the leaf formulations. Ginkgo seeds are epileptogenic. Ginkgo formulations should be avoided in individuals with preexisting seizure disorders.

Dosage

Ginkgo biloba dried leaf extract should be standardized to contain 24% flavone glycosides and 6% terpene lactones. Products should be concentrated to a 50:1 ratio. The daily dose ranges from 120–240 mg of the dried extract in two or three divided doses. Onset of effect may require 2–4 weeks.

GINSENG

Chemistry

Ginseng botanical preparations may be derived from any of several species of the genus *Panax*. Of these, crude preparations or extracts of *Panax ginseng*, the Chinese or Korean variety, and *P quinquefolium*, the American variety, are most often available to consumers in the United States. The active principles appear to be a dozen or more triterpenoid saponin glycosides called ginsenosides or panaxosides. It is recommended that commercial *P ginseng* formulations be standardized to contain 4–7% ginsenosides.

Other plant materials are commonly sold under the name ginseng but are not from *Panax* species. These include Siberian ginseng (*Eleutherococcus senticosus*) and Brazilian ginseng (*Pfaffia paniculata*). Of these, Siberian ginseng is more widely available in the USA. Siberian ginseng contains eleutherosides but no ginsenosides. Currently, there is no recommended standardization for eleutheroside content in Siberian ginseng products.

Pharmacology

An extensive literature exists on the potential pharmacologic effects of ginsenosides. Unfortunately, the studies differ widely in the species of *Panax* used, the ginsenosides studied, the degree of purification applied to the extracts, the animal species studied, and the measurements used to evaluate the responses. Some of the more commonly reported beneficial pharmacologic effects include modulation of immune function, ergogenic ("energizing") activity, nootropic ("mind-enhancing") activity, antioxidant activity, anti-inflammatory effects, antistress activity (ie, stimulation of pituitary-adrenocortical system), analgesia, vasoregulatory effects, antiplatelet activity, improved glucose homeostasis, and anticancer properties.

Clinical Trials

Ginseng is most often used to help improve physical and mental performance. Unfortunately, the clinical trials are of small sample size and report either an improvement in mental function and physical performance or no effect. Some randomized controlled trials evaluating "quality of life" have claimed significant benefits in some subscale measures of quality of life but rarely in overall composite scores using *P ginseng*. Better results have been observed with *P quinquefolium* in lowering postprandial glucose indices in sub-jects with and without diabetes. Newer trials have shown some immunomodulating benefits of *P quinquefolium* and *P ginseng* in preventing upper respiratory tract infections. Epidemiologic studies have suggested a reduction in several types of cancer with *P ginseng*. Systematic reviews, however, have generally failed to find conclusive evidence for the use of *P ginseng* for any particular condition. Until better clinical studies are published, no recommendation can be made regarding the use of *P ginseng* or *P quinquefolium* for any specific indication.

Adverse Effects

A variety of adverse effects have been reported. Weak estrogenic properties may cause the vaginal bleeding and mastalgia reported by some patients. Central nervous system stimulation (eg, insomnia, nervousness) and hypertension have been reported in patients using high doses (more than 3 g/d) of *P ginseng*. Methylxanthines found in the ginseng plant may contribute to this effect. The German Commission E lists high blood pressure as a contraindication to the use of Siberian ginseng but not *P ginseng*.

Drug Interactions & Precautions

Irritability, sleeplessness, and manic behavior have been reported in psychiatric patients using ginseng in combination with other medications (phenelzine, lithium, neuroleptics). Ginseng should be used cautiously in patients taking any psychiatric, estrogenic, or hypoglycemic medications. Ginseng has antiplatelet properties and should not be used in combination with warfarin. Similar to echinacea, cytokine stimulation has been observed for both *P ginseng* and *P quinquefolium*, necessitating cautious use in individuals who are immunocompromised, are taking immune stimulants or suppressants, or have autoimmune disorders.

Dosing

The German Commission E recommends 1–2 g/d of crude *P ginseng* root or its equivalent. Two hundred milligrams of ginseng extract is equivalent to 1 g of the crude root. Ginsana has been used as a standardized extract in some clinical trials and is available in the USA. Dosing for Siberian ginseng is 2–3 g/d of the crude root.

MILK THISTLE (*SILYBUM MARIANUM*)

Chemistry

The fruit and seeds of the milk thistle plant contain a lipophilic mixture of flavonolignans known as silymarin. Silymarin comprises 2–3% of the dried herb and is composed of three primary isomers, silybin (also known as silybinin or silibinin), silychristin (silichristin), and silydianin (silidianin). Silybin is the most prevalent and potent of the three isomers and accounts for about 50% of the silymarin complex. Products should be standardized to contain 70–80% silymarin.

Pharmacologic Effects

A. LIVER DISEASE

In animal models, milk thistle limits hepatic injury associated with a variety of toxins, including *Amanita* mushrooms, galactosamine, carbon tetrachloride, acetaminophen, radiation, cold ischemia, and ethanol. In vitro studies and some in vivo studies demonstrate that silymarin reduces lipid peroxidation, scavenges free radicals, and enhances glutathione and superoxide dismutase levels. This may contribute to membrane stabilization and reduce toxin entry.

Milk thistle appears to have anti-inflammatory properties. In vitro, silybin strongly and noncompetitively inhibits lipoxygenase and leukotriene formation. Inhibition of leukocyte migration has been observed in vivo and may be a factor when acute inflammation is present. Silymarin also inhibits tumor necrosis factor-α-mediated activation of nuclear factor kappa B (NF-κB), which promotes inflammatory responses. One of the most unusual mechanisms claimed for milk thistle involves an increase in RNA polymerase I activity in nonmalignant hepatocytes but not in hepatoma or other malignant cell lines. By increasing this enzyme's activity, enhanced protein synthesis and cellular regeneration may occur in diseased but not malignant cells. Milk thistle may have a role in hepatic fibrosis. In an animal model of cirrhosis, it reduced collagen accumulation, and in an in vitro model it reduced expression of the profibrogenic cytokine transforming growth factor-β.

It has been suggested that milk thistle may be beneficial in the management of hypercholesterolemia and gallstones. A small trial in humans showed a reduction in bile saturation index and biliary cholesterol concentration. The latter may reflect a reduction in liver cholesterol synthesis. To date, however, there is insufficient evidence to warrant the use of milk thistle for these indications.

B. CHEMOTHERAPEUTIC EFFECTS

Preliminary in vitro and animal studies have been carried out with skin, lung, bladder, colon, tongue, breast, and prostate cancer cell lines. In murine models of skin cancer, silybinin and milk thistle reduced tumor initia-

tion and promotion. It also inhibited cell growth and proliferation by inducing a G_1 cell cycle arrest in cultured human breast and prostate cancer cell lines. However, the use of milk thistle in the treatment of cancer has not yet been adequately studied and should not be recommended to patients.

Clinical Trials

Milk thistle has been used to treat acute and chronic viral hepatitis, alcoholic liver disease, and toxin-induced liver injury in human patients. A recent systematic review of 13 randomized trials involving 915 patients with alcoholic liver disease or hepatitis B or C found no significant reductions in all-cause mortality, liver histology, or complications of liver disease. A significant reduction in liver-related mortality among all trials was documented, but not among trials of better design and controls. It was concluded that the effects of milk thistle in improving liver function or mortality from liver disease are currently poorly substantiated. Until additional well-designed clinical trials (possibly exploring higher doses) can be performed, a clinical effect can be neither supported nor ruled out.

Milk thistle has not been well studied in humans as an antidote following acute exposure to liver toxins. Parenteral silybin, however, is marketed and used in Europe as an antidote in *Amanita phalloides* mushroom poisoning, based on favorable outcomes reported in case-control studies.

Adverse Effects

Milk thistle has rarely been reported to cause adverse effects when used at recommended dosage. In clinical trials, the incidence of adverse effects (eg, gastrointestinal upset, dermatologic, headaches) was comparable to that of placebo.

Drug Interactions, Precautions, & Dosing

There are no reported drug-drug interactions or precautions for milk thistle. Recommended dosage is 280–420 mg/d, calculated as silybin, in three divided doses.

ST. JOHN'S WORT (*HYPERICUM PERFORATUM*)

Chemistry

St. John's wort, also known as hypericum, contains a variety of constituents that may contribute to its pharmacologic activity. Hypericin, a marker of standardization for currently marketed products, was thought to be the primary antidepressant constituent. Recent attention has focused on hyperforin, but a combination of several compounds is probably involved. Commercial formulations are usually prepared by soaking the dried chopped flowers in methanol to create a hydroalcoholic extract that is then dried.

Pharmacologic Effects

A. Anti-Depressant Action

The hypericin fraction was initially reported to have MAO-A and -B inhibitor properties. Later studies found that the concentration required for this inhibition was higher than that which could be achieved with recommended dosages. In vitro studies using the commercially formulated hydroalcoholic extract have shown inhibition of nerve terminal reuptake of serotonin, norepinephrine, and dopamine. While the hypericin constituent did not show reuptake inhibition for any of these systems, a concentrated hyperforin extract did. Chronic administration of the commercial extract has also been shown to significantly down-regulate the expression of cortical β adrenoceptors and up-regulate the expression of serotonin receptors (5-HT$_2$) in a rodent model.

Other effects observed in vitro include opioid sigma receptor binding using the hypericin fraction and GABA receptor binding using the commercial extract. Interleukin-6 production is also reduced in the presence of the extract.

The most systematic review and meta-analysis, which involved 37 randomized controlled trials, demonstrated that St. John's wort is more efficacious than placebo and as efficacious as some prescription antidepressants for mild to moderate depression. Efficacy for more severe depression, however, is still in question. Most trials used doses of St. John's wort ranging from 900 mg/d (for mild to moderate depression) to 1800 mg/d (for severe depression) and lasted 4–8 weeks.

B. Antiviral and Anticarcinogenic Effects

The hypericin constituent of St. John's wort is photolabile and can be activated by exposure to certain wavelengths of visible or ultraviolet A light. Parenteral formulations of hypericin (photoactivated just before administration) have been used investigationally to treat HIV infection (given intravenously) and basal and squamous cell carcinoma (given by intralesional injection). In vitro, photoactivated hypericin inhibits a variety of enveloped and nonenveloped viruses as well as the growth of cells in some neoplastic tissues. Inhibition of protein kinase C and of singlet oxygen radical generation have been proposed as possible mechanisms. The latter could inhibit cell growth or cause cell apoptosis. These studies were carried out using the isolated hypericin constituent of

St. John's wort; the usual hydroalcoholic extract of St. John's wort has not been studied for these indications and should not be recommended for patients with viral illness or cancer.

Adverse Effects

Photosensitization has been reported, and patients should be instructed to wear sunscreen while using this product. Hypomania, mania, and autonomic arousal have also been reported in patients using St. John's wort.

Drug Interactions & Precautions

Inhibition of reuptake of various amine transmitters has been highlighted as a potential mechanism of action for St. John's wort. Drugs with similar mechanisms (ie, antidepressants, stimulants) should be used cautiously or avoided in patients using St. John's wort due to the risk of serotonin syndrome or MAO crisis (see Chapters 16 and 30). This herb may induce hepatic CYP enzymes (3A4, 2C9, 1A2) and the P-glycoprotein drug transporter. This has led to case reports of subtherapeutic levels of numerous drugs, including digoxin, birth control drugs (and subsequent pregnancy), cyclosporine, HIV protease and nonnucleoside reverse transcriptase inhibitors, warfarin, irinotecan, theophylline, and anticonvulsants.

Dosage

The most common commercial formulation of St. John's wort is the dried hydroalcoholic extract. Products should be standardized to 2–5% hyperforin, although most still bear the older standardized marker of 0.3% hypericin. The recommended dosing for mild to moderate depression is 900 mg of the dried extract per day in three divided doses. Onset of effect may take 2–4 weeks. Long-term benefits beyond 12 weeks have not been sufficiently studied.

SAW PALMETTO (*SERENOA REPENS* or *SABAL SERRULATA*)

Chemistry

The active constituents in saw palmetto berries are not well defined. Phytosterols (eg, β-sitosterol), aliphatic alcohols, polyprenic compounds, and flavonoids are all present. Marketed preparations are lipophilic extracts that contain 85–95% fatty acids and sterols.

Pharmacologic Effects

Saw palmetto is most often used in the treatment of benign prostatic hyperplasia (BPH). Enzymatic conversion of testosterone to dihydrotestosterone (DHT) by 5α-reductase is inhibited by saw palmetto in vitro. Specifically, saw palmetto shows a noncompetitive inhibition of both isotypes (I and II) of this enzyme, thereby reducing DHT production. In vitro, saw palmetto also inhibits the binding of DHT to androgen receptors. Additional effects that have been observed in vitro include inhibition of prostatic growth factors, blockade of α_1 adrenoceptors, and inhibition of inflammatory mediators produced by the 5-lipoxygenase pathway.

The clinical pharmacology of saw palmetto in humans is not well defined. One week of treatment in healthy volunteers failed to influence 5α-reductase activity, DHT concentration, or testosterone concentration. Six months of treatment in patients with benign prostatic hyperplasia also failed to affect prostate-specific antigen (PSA) levels, a marker that is typically reduced by enzymatic inhibition of 5α-reductase. In contrast, other researchers have reported a reduction in epidermal growth factor, DHT levels, and estrogen expression after 3 months of treatment in patients with benign prostatic hyperplasia. Results of recent meta-analyses and reviews suggested that saw palmetto is significantly more effective than placebo in alleviating urologic symptoms (eg, peak flow, nocturia, international prostate symptom scores) associated with mild to moderate BPH. Saw palmetto, 320 mg/d, was also shown to have comparable efficacy to 5 mg/d of finasteride (a prescription 5α-reductase inhibitor) and 0.4 mg/d of tamsulosin (a prescription α-blocker) in clinical trials lasting 6 months and 1 year, respectively. In marked contrast, a recent well-controlled, double-blind 1-year study showed no significant effect of saw palmetto on symptoms or objective measures in moderate to severe BPH. The efficacy of saw palmetto in BPH beyond 5 years has not been studied.

Adverse Effects

Adverse effects are rare and reported with an incidence of 1–3%. The most common include gastrointestinal upset, hypertension, decreased libido, abdominal pain, impotence, back pain, urinary retention, and headache. In comparison to tamsulosin and finasteride, saw palmetto is less likely to affect sexual function (eg, ejaculation) in men.

Drug Interactions, Precautions, & Dosing

No drug-drug interactions have been reported for saw palmetto. Because saw palmetto has no effect on the PSA marker, it will not interfere with prostate cancer screening using this test. Recommended dosing of a standardized dried extract (containing 85–95% fatty acids and sterols) is 160 mg orally twice daily. Patients should be instructed that it may take 4–6 weeks for onset of clinical effects.

■ PURIFIED NUTRITIONAL SUPPLEMENTS

COENZYME Q10

Coenzyme Q10, also known as CoQ, CoQ10, and ubiquinone, is found in the mitochondria of many organs, including the heart, kidney, and liver, and in skeletal muscle. After ingestion, the reduced form of coenzyme Q10, ubiquinol, predominates in the systemic circulation. Coenzyme Q10 is a potent antioxidant and may have a role in maintaining healthy muscle function, although the clinical significance of this effect is unknown. Reduced serum levels have been reported in Parkinson's disease.

Clinical Uses

A. HYPERTENSION

Various open label and controlled studies have identified small reductions in systolic and diastolic blood pressure of approximately 10 mm Hg following 10 weeks of therapy. Although this observation appears to be consistent, better designed studies are required.

B. HEART FAILURE

Older studies suggested that coenzyme Q10 was effective as adjunctive therapy in the treatment of heart failure. Current research suggests that the supplement does not alter cardiac function (as determined with Swan-Ganz catheter measurements and echocardiography) in cardiomyopathy patients with class I, II, or III NY Heart Association status. Furthermore, patients with lower than normal endogenous coenzyme Q10 levels do not display subjective or objective improvements in heart failure assessments when given coenzyme Q10 supplements.

C. ISCHEMIC HEART DISEASE

The effects of coenzyme Q10 on coronary artery disease and chronic stable angina are modest but appear promising. Double-blind, placebo-controlled trials have demonstrated that coenzyme Q10 supplementation improved a number of clinical measures in patients with a history of acute myocardial infarction (AMI). Improvements have been observed in lipoprotein a, high-density lipoprotein cholesterol, exercise tolerance, and time to development of ischemic changes on the electrocardiogram during stress tests. In addition, very small reductions in cardiac deaths and rate of reinfarction in patients with previous AMI were reported (absolute risk reduction 1.5%).

D. NEUROLOGIC DISEASES

Coenzyme Q has been reported to slow the progression of early Parkinson's disease when given at high dosage (300–1200 mg/d), although the time to requirement for levodopa treatment was not shortened. Another study indicated that migraine attacks were reduced in frequency at a dosage of 300 mg/d. No benefit was found in the treatment of amyotrophic lateral sclerosis or Huntington's disease.

Adverse Effects

Coenzyme Q10 is well tolerated, rarely leading to any adverse effects at doses as high as 3000 mg/d. In clinical trials gastrointestinal upset, anorexia, and nausea have been reported. Cases of maculopapular rash and thrombocytopenia have very rarely been observed. Other rare adverse effects include irritability, dizziness, and headache.

Drug Interactions

Coenzyme Q10 shares a structural similarity with vitamin K, and an interaction has been observed between coenzyme Q10 and warfarin. Coenzyme Q10 supplements may decrease the effects of warfarin therapy. This combination should be avoided or very carefully monitored.

A reduction in endogenous coenzyme Q10 levels has been observed in patients beginning HMG-CoA reductase inhibitors. The clinical significance of this reduction is currently unknown, and the long-term effects of coenzyme Q10 supplementation in patients taking HMG-CoA reductase inhibitors has not been studied clinically. Anecdotal evidence has suggested that adding coenzyme Q10 to HMG-CoA reductase inhibitor therapy may help to prevent the rare adverse effect of myopathy, which can ultimately progress to rhabdomyolysis. Clinical trials are needed to confirm this effect.

Dosage

As a dietary supplement, 30 mg of coenzyme Q10 is adequate to replace low endogenous levels. For neural or cardiac effects, typical doses are 100–600 mg/d given in two or three divided doses. These therapeutic doses increase endogenous levels to 2–3 mcg/mL (normal for healthy adults, 0.7–1 mcg/mL).

GLUCOSAMINE

Glucosamine is found in human tissue, is a substrate for the production of articular cartilage, and also serves as a cartilage nutrient. Glucosamine is commercially derived from crabs and other crustaceans. As a dietary supplement, glucosamine is primarily used for pain associated with knee osteoarthritis.

Pharmacologic Effects & Clinical Uses

Endogenous glucosamine is used for the production of glycosaminoglycans and other proteoglycans in articular cartilage. In osteoarthritis, the rate of production of new cartilage is exceeded by the rate of degradation of existing cartilage. Supplementation with glucosamine is thought to increase the supply of the necessary glycosaminoglycan building blocks, leading to better maintenance and strengthening of existing cartilage.

Many clinical trials have been conducted on the effects of both oral and intra-articular administration of glucosamine. Early studies demonstrated significant improvements in overall mobility, range of motion, and strength in patients with osteoarthritis. Some recent evidence has shown mixed results, with both positive and negative trials. One meta-analysis found an overall moderate effect in knee osteoarthritis improvement, although study limitations may have overestimated treatment benefits. However, the most recent large double-blind trial, which compared glucosamine, chondroitin sulfate, the combination, and placebo, found no benefit for this therapy. It is possible that specific subgroups may benefit from glucosamine. More research is needed to better define the specific patient populations that stand to benefit from glucosamine.

Adverse Effects

Glucosamine is very well tolerated. In clinical trials, mild diarrhea and nausea were occasionally reported. Cross allergenicity in people with shellfish allergies is a potential concern; however, this is unlikely if the formulation has been adequately manufactured and purified.

Drug Interactions & Precautions

There are no known drug interactions with glucosamine.

Dosage

The dosage used most often in clinical trials is 500 mg three times daily or 1500 mg once daily. Glucosamine does not have direct analgesic effects, and improvements, if any, may not be observed for 1–2 months. Although all salt forms of glucosamine (sulfate and hydrochloride) should dissolve and be available for absorption, there is some evidence that the sulfate formulation may be superior clinically.

MELATONIN

Melatonin, a serotonin derivative produced by the pineal gland and some other tissues (see also Chapter 16), is believed to be responsible for regulating sleep-wake cycles. Release coincides with darkness; it typically begins around 9 PM and lasts until about 4 AM. Melatonin release is suppressed by daylight. Melatonin has also been studied for a number of other functions, including contraception, protection against endogenous oxidants, prevention of aging, and treatment of depression, HIV infection, and a variety of cancers. Currently, melatonin is most often administered to prevent jet lag and to induce sleep.

Pharmacologic Effects & Clinical Uses

A. Jet Lag

Jet lag, a disturbance of the sleep-wake cycle, occurs when there is a disparity between the external time and the traveler's endogenous circadian clock (internal time). The internal time regulates not only daily sleep rhythms but also body temperature and many metabolic systems. The synchronization of the circadian clock relies on light as the most potent "zeitgeber" (time giver).

Jet lag is especially common among frequent travelers and airplane cabin crews. Typical symptoms of jet lag may include daytime drowsiness, insomnia, frequent awakenings, and gastrointestinal upset. Clinical studies with administration of melatonin have reported subjective reduction in daytime fatigue, improved mood, and a quicker recovery time (return to normal sleep patterns, energy, and alertness). Unfortunately, many of these studies were characterized by inconsistencies in dosing, duration of therapy, and time of drug administration. In addition to melatonin, maximizing exposure to daylight on arrival at the new destination can aid in resetting the internal clock.

B. Insomnia

Melatonin has been studied in the treatment of various sleep disorders, including insomnia and delayed sleep-phase syndrome. It has been shown to improve sleep onset, duration, and quality when administered to healthy volunteers, suggesting a pharmacologic hypnotic effect. Melatonin has also been shown to increase rapid-eye-movement (REM) sleep.

Clinical studies in patients with sleep disorders have shown that oral melatonin supplementation may alter sleep architecture. Subjective improvements in sleep quality and improvements in sleep onset and sleep duration have been reported. However, the significance of these findings is impaired by many study limitations.

Patients older than 65 years of age tend to suffer from sleep maintenance insomnia; melatonin serum levels have been reported to be low in these patients. Elderly patients with sleep maintenance insomnia who received immediate-release and sustained-release melatonin had improved sleep onset time. They did not, however, experience an improvement in sleep maintenance or total sleep time.

C. Female Reproductive Function

Melatonin receptors have been identified in granulosa cell membranes, and significant amounts of melatonin have been detected in ovarian follicular fluid. Melatonin has been associated with midcycle suppression of luteinizing hormone surge and secretion. This may result in partial inhibition of ovulation. Nightly doses of melatonin (75–300 mg) given with a progestin through days 1–21 of the menstrual cycle resulted in lower mean luteinizing hormone levels. Therefore, melatonin should not be used by women who are pregnant or attempting to conceive. Furthermore, melatonin supplementation may decrease prolactin release in women and therefore should be used cautiously or not at all while nursing.

D. Male Reproductive Function

In healthy men, chronic melatonin administration (≥ 6 months) decreased sperm quality, possibly by aromatase inhibition in the testes. Until more is known, melatonin should not be used by couples who are actively trying to conceive.

Adverse Effects

Melatonin appears to be well tolerated and is often used in preference to over-the-counter "sleep-aid" drugs. Although melatonin is associated with few adverse effects, some next-day drowsiness has been reported as well as tachycardia, depression, vivid dreams, and headache. Sporadic case reports of movement disorders and psychoses have also appeared.

Drug Interactions

Melatonin drug interactions have not been formally studied. Various studies, however, suggest that melatonin concentrations are altered by a variety of drugs, including nonsteroidal anti-inflammatory drugs, antidepressants, β-adrenoceptor agonists and antagonists, scopolamine, and sodium valproate. The relevance of these effects is unknown. Melatonin is metabolized by CYP450 1A2 and may interact with other drugs that either inhibit or induce the 1A2 isoenzyme.

Dosage

A. Jet Lag

The optimal timing and dose of melatonin have not been established. Current information suggests 5–8 mg of the immediate-release formulation given on the evening of departure and for 1–3 nights after arrival at the new destination. Exposure to daylight at the new time zone is also important to regulate the sleep-wake cycle.

B. Insomnia

Doses of 0.3–10 mg of the immediate-release formulation orally given once nightly have been tried. The lowest effective dose should be used first and may be repeated in 30 minutes up to a maximum of 10–20 mg. Sustained-release formulations may be used but currently do not appear to offer any advantages over the immediate-release formulations. Sustained-release formulations are also more costly.

REFERENCES

General

Blumenthal M et al: *Herbal Medicine: Expanded Commission E Monograph.* American Botanical Council. Integrative Medicine Communications, 2000.

De Smet PA: Herbal remedies. N Engl J Med 2002;347:2046.

Jellin JM et al: *Pharmacist's Letter/Prescriber's Letter Natural Medicines Comprehensive Database,* 4th ed. Therapeutic Research Faculty, 2006.

www.naturalstandard.com. (Evidence-based compendium authored by academics, available to institutions.)

Coenzyme Q10

Berman M et al: Coenzyme Q10 in patients with end-stage heart failure awaiting cardiac transplantation: A randomized, placebo-controlled study. Clin Cardiol 2004;27:295.

Hodgson JM et al: Coenzyme Q10 improves blood pressure and glycaemic control: A controlled trial in subjects with type 2 diabetes. Eur J Clin Nutr 2002;56:1137.

Khatta M et al: The effect of coenzyme Q10 in patients with congestive heart failure. Ann Intern Med 2000;132:636.

Schults CW et al: Effects of coenzyme Q10 in early Parkinson's disease: Evidence of slowing of the functional decline. Arch Neurol 2002;59:1541.

Singh RB et al: Effect of coenzyme Q10 on risk of atherosclerosis in patients with recent myocardial infarction. Mol Cell Biochem 2003;246:75.

Echinacea

Goel V et al: Efficacy of a standardized echinacea preparation (Echinalin™) for the treatment of the common cold: A randomized double-blind, placebo-controlled trial. J Clin Pharm Therapeutics 2004;29:75.

Melchart D et al: Echinacea for preventing and treating the common cold. Cochrane Database Syst Rev 2006;1:CD000530.

Taylor JA et al: Efficacy and safety of echinacea in treating upper respiratory tract infections in children (a randomized controlled trial). JAMA 2003;290:2824.

Turner RB et al: An evaluation of *Echinacea angustifolia* in experimental rhinovirus infections. N Engl J Med 2005;353:341.

Garlic

Ackermann RT et al: Garlic shows promise for improving some cardiovascular risk factors. Arch Intern Med 2001;161:813.

Khanum F et al: Anticarcinogenic properties of garlic: A review. Crit Rev Food Sci Nutr 2004;44:479.

Stevinson C, Pittler MH, Ernst E: Garlic for treating hypercholesterolemia. A meta-analysis of randomized clinical trials. Ann Intern Med 2000;133:420.

Ginkgo

Ahlemeyer B et al: Neuroprotective effects of *Ginkgo biloba* extract. Cell Mol Life Sci 2003;60:1779.

Horsch S et al: *Gingko biloba* special extract EGb761 in the treatment of peripheral arterial occlusive disease (PAOD)—a review based on randomized controlled studies. Int J Clin Pharmacol Ther 2004;42:63.

Ginseng

Coleman CI et al: The effects of Panax ginseng on quality of life. J Clin Pharm Therapeut 2003;28:5.

Predy GN et al: Efficacy of an extract of North American ginseng containing poly-furanosyl-pyranosyl-saccharides for preventing upper respiratory tract infections: A randomized controlled trial. Can Med Assoc J 2005;173:1043.

Yun TK: Experimental and epidemiological evidence on non-organ specific cancer preventative effect of Korean ginseng and identification of active compounds. Mutat Res 2003;523-524:63.

Glucosamine

Clegg D et al: Glucosamine, chondroitin sulfate, and the two in combination for painful knee osteoarthritis. N Engl J Med 2006;354:795.

McAlindon T et al: Effectiveness of glucosamine for symptoms of knee osteoarthritis: Results from an internet-based randomized double-blind controlled trial. Am J Med 2004;117:643.

Milk Thistle

Jacobs BP et al: Milk thistle for the treatment of liver disease: A systematic review and meta-analysis. Am J Med 2002;113:506.

Rambaldi A et al: Milk thistle for alcoholic and/or hepatitis B or C virus liver diseases. Cochrane Database Syst Rev 2005;2:CD003620.

Singh RP et al: Mechanisms and preclinical efficacy of silibinin in preventing skin cancer. Eur J Cancer 2005;41:1969.

St. John's Wort

Butterweck V: Mechanism of action of St. John's wort in depression: What is known? CNS Drugs 2003;17:539.

Hypericum Depression Trial Study Group: Effect of *Hypericum perforatum* (St John's wort) in major depressive disorder. JAMA 2002;287:1807.

Linde K et al: St. John's wort for depression—meta-analysis of randomised controlled trials. Br J Psychiatry 2005;186:99.

Szegedi A et al: Acute treatment of moderate to severe depression with hypericum extract WS 5570 (St. John's wort): Randomised controlled double blind non-inferiority trial versus paroxetine. BMJ 2005;330:503.

Saw Palmetto

Bent S et al: Saw palmetto for benign prostatic hyperplasia. N Engl J Med 2006;354:557.

Boyle P et al: Updated meta-analysis of clinical trials of *Serenoa repens* extract in the treatment of symptomatic benign prostatic hypertrophy. BJU International 2004;93:751.

Raynaud JP et al: Inhibition of type 1 and type 2 5α-reductase activity by free fatty acids, active ingredients in Permixon®. J Steroid Biochem Molec Biol 2002;82:233.

Melatonin

Baskett JJ et al: Does melatonin improve sleep in older people? A randomised crossover trial. Age Ageing 2003;32:164.

Petrie K et al: A double-blind trial of melatonin as a treatment for jet lag in international cabin crew. Biol Psychiatry 1993; 33:526.

Rational Prescribing & Prescription Writing

Paul W. Lofholm, PharmD, & Bertram G. Katzung, MD, PhD

66

Once a patient with a clinical problem has been evaluated and a diagnosis has been reached, the practitioner can often select from a variety of therapeutic approaches. Medication, surgery, psychiatric treatment, radiation, physical therapy, health education, counseling, further consultation, and no therapy are some of the options available. Of these options, drug therapy is by far the one most frequently chosen. In most cases, this requires the writing of a prescription. A written prescription is the prescriber's order to prepare or dispense a specific treatment—usually medication—for a specific patient. When a patient comes for an office visit, the physician or other authorized health professional prescribes medications 67% of the time, and an average of one prescription per office visit is written because more than one prescription may be written at a single visit.

In this chapter, a plan for prescribing is presented. The physical form of the prescription, common prescribing errors, and legal requirements that govern various features of the prescribing process are then discussed. Finally, some of the social and economic factors involved in prescribing and drug use are described.

RATIONAL PRESCRIBING

Like any other process in health care, writing a prescription should be based on a series of rational steps.

(1) Make a specific diagnosis: Prescriptions based merely on a desire to satisfy the patient's psychological need for some type of therapy are often unsatisfactory and may result in adverse effects. A specific diagnosis, even if it is tentative, is required to move to the next step. For example, in a 35-year-old woman with symmetric joint stiffness, pain, and inflammation that are worse in the morning and not associated with a history of infection, a diagnosis of rheumatoid arthritis would be considered. This diagnosis and the reasoning underlying it should be shared with the patient.

(2) Consider the pathophysiologic implications of the diagnosis: If the disorder is well understood, the prescriber is in a much better position to offer effective therapy. For example, increasing knowledge about the mediators of inflammation makes possible more effective use of NSAIDs and other agents used in rheumatoid arthritis. The patient should be provided with the appropriate level and amount of information about the pathophysiology. Many pharmacies and disease-oriented public and private agencies (eg, American Heart Association, American Cancer Society, Arthritis Foundation) provide information sheets suitable for patients.

(3) Select a specific therapeutic objective: A therapeutic objective should be chosen for each of the pathophysiologic processes defined in the preceding step. In a patient with rheumatoid arthritis, relief of pain by reduction of the inflammatory process is one of the major therapeutic goals that identifies the drug groups which will be considered. Arresting the course of the disease process in rheumatoid arthritis is a different therapeutic goal that might lead to consideration of other drug groups and prescriptions.

(4) Select a drug of choice: One or more drug groups will be suggested by each of the therapeutic goals specified in the preceding step. Selection of a drug of choice from among these groups follows from a consideration of the specific characteristics of the patient and the clinical presentation. For certain drugs, characteristics such as age, other diseases, and other drugs being taken are extremely important in determining the most suitable drug for management of the present complaint. In the example of the patient with probable rheumatoid arthritis, it would be important to know whether the patient has a history of aspirin intolerance or ulcer disease, whether the cost of medication is an especially important factor and the nature of the patient's insurance coverage, and whether there is a need for once-daily dosing. Based on this information, a drug would probably be selected from the nonsteroidal anti-inflammatory group. If the patient is intolerant of aspirin and does not have ulcer disease but does have a need for low-cost treatment, ibuprofen or naproxen would be a rational choice.

(5) Determine the appropriate dosing regimen: The dosing regimen is determined primarily by the pharmacokinetics of the drug in that patient. If the patient is known to have disease of the organs required for elimination of the drug selected, adjustment of the average regimen is needed. For a drug such as ibuprofen, which is eliminated mainly by the kidneys, renal function should be assessed. If renal function is normal, the half-life of ibuprofen (about 2 hours) requires administration three or four times daily. The dose suggested in this book, drug handbooks, and the manufacturer's literature is 400–800 mg four times daily.

(6) Devise a plan for monitoring the drug's action and determine an end point for therapy: The prescriber should be able to describe to the patient the kinds of drug effects that will be monitored and in what way, including laboratory tests (if necessary) and signs and symptoms that the patient should report. For conditions that call for a limited course of therapy (eg, most infections), the duration of therapy should be made clear so that the patient does not stop taking the drug prematurely and understands why the prescription probably need not be renewed. For the patient with rheumatoid arthritis, the need for prolonged—perhaps indefinite—therapy should be explained. The prescriber should also specify any changes in the patient's condition that would call for changes in therapy. For example, in the patient with rheumatoid arthritis, development of gastrointestinal bleeding would require an immediate change in drug therapy and a prompt workup of the bleeding. Major toxicities that require immediate attention should be explained clearly to the patient.

(7) Plan a program of patient education: The prescriber and other members of the health team should be prepared to repeat, extend, and reinforce the information transmitted to the patient as often as necessary. The more toxic the drug prescribed, the greater the importance of this educational program. The importance of informing and involving the patient in each of the above steps must be recognized, as shown by experience with teratogenic drugs (see Chapter 60). Many pharmacies routinely provide this type of information with each prescription filled, but the prescriber must not assume that this will occur.

THE PRESCRIPTION

Although a prescription can be written on any piece of paper (as long as all of the legal elements are present), it usually takes a specific form. A typical printed prescription form for outpatients is shown in Figure 66–1.

In the hospital setting, drugs are prescribed on a particular page of the patient's hospital chart called the **physician's order sheet (POS)** or **chart order.** The contents of that prescription are specified in the medical staff rules by the hospital's Pharmacy and Therapeutics Committee. The patient's name is typed or written on the form;

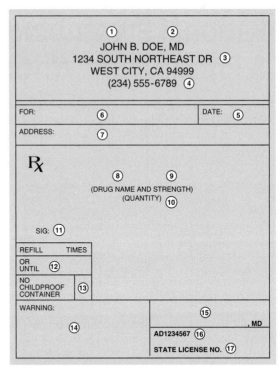

Figure 66-1. Common form of outpatient prescription. Circled numbers are explained in the text.

therefore, the orders consist of the name and strength of the medication, the dose, the route and frequency of administration, the date, other pertinent information, and the signature of the prescriber. If the duration of therapy or the number of doses is not specified (which is often the case), the medication is continued until the prescriber discontinues the order or until it is terminated as a matter of policy routine, eg, a stop-order policy.

A typical chart order might be as follows:

11/13/06
10:30 a.m.

(1) Ampicillin 500 mg IV q6h × 5 days
(2) Aspirin 0.6 g per rectum q6h prn temp over 101

[Signed] Janet B. Doe, MD

Thus, the elements of the hospital chart order are equivalent to the central elements (5, 8–11, 15) of the outpatient prescription.

Elements of the Prescription

The first four elements (see circled numerals in Figure 66–1) of the outpatient prescription establish the identity of the prescriber: name, license classification (ie, professional degree), address, and office telephone number. Before dispensing a prescription, the pharmacist must establish the prescriber's bona fides and should be able to contact the prescriber by telephone if any questions arise. Element [5] is the date the prescription was written. It should be near the top of the prescription form or at the beginning (left margin) of the chart order. Since the order has legal significance and usually has some temporal relationship to the date of the patient-prescriber interview, a pharmacist should refuse to fill a prescription without verification by telephone if too much time has elapsed since its writing.

Elements [6] and [7] identify the patient by name and address. The patient's name and full address should be clearly spelled out.

The body of the prescription contains the elements [8] to [11] that specify the medication, the strength and quantity to be dispensed, the dosage, and complete directions for use. When writing the drug name (element [8]), either the brand name (proprietary name) or the generic name (nonproprietary name) may be used. Reasons for using one or the other are discussed below. The strength of the medication [9] should be written in metric units. However, the prescriber should be familiar with both systems now in use: metric and apothecary. For practical purposes, the following approximate conversions are useful:

> **1 grain (gr) = 0.065 grams (g), often rounded to 60 milligrams (mg)**
> **15 gr = 1 g**
> **1 ounce (oz) by volume = 30 milliliters (mL)**
> **1 teaspoonful (tsp) = 5 mL**
> **1 tablespoonful (tbsp) = 15 mL**
> **1 quart (qt) = 1000 mL**
> **1 minim = 1 drop (gtt)**
> **20 drops = 1 mL**
> **2.2 pounds (lb) = 1 kilogram (kg)**

The strength of a solution is usually expressed as the quantity of solute in sufficient solvent to make 100 mL; for instance, 20% potassium chloride solution is 20 grams of KCl per deciliter (g/dL) of final solution. Both the concentration and the volume should be explicitly written out.

The quantity of medication prescribed should reflect the anticipated duration of therapy, the cost, the need for continued contact with the clinic or physician, the potential for abuse, and the potential for toxicity or overdose. Consideration should be given also to the standard sizes in which the product is available and whether this is the initial prescription of the drug or a repeat prescription or refill. If 10 days of therapy are required to effectively cure a streptococcal infection, an appropriate quantity for the full course should be prescribed. Birth control pills are often prescribed for 1

year or until the next examination is due; however, some patients may not be able to afford a year's supply at one time; therefore, a 3-month supply might be ordered, with refill instructions to renew three times or for 1 year (element [12]). Some third-party (insurance) plans limit the amount of medicine that can be dispensed—often to only a month's supply. Finally, when first prescribing medications that are to be used for the treatment of a chronic disease, the initial quantity should be small, with refills for larger quantities. The purpose of beginning treatment with a small quantity of drug is to reduce the cost if the patient cannot tolerate it. Once it is determined that intolerance is not a problem, a larger quantity purchased less frequently is sometimes less expensive.

The directions for use (element [11]) must be both drug-specific and patient-specific. The simpler the directions, the better; and the fewer the number of doses (and drugs) per day, the better. Patient noncompliance (also known as nonadherence, failure to adhere to the drug regimen) is a major cause of treatment failure. To help patients remember to take their medications, prescribers often give an instruction that medications be taken at or around mealtimes and at bedtime. However, it is important to inquire about the patient's eating habits and other lifestyle patterns, because many patients do not eat three regularly spaced meals a day.

The instructions on how and when to take medications, the duration of therapy, and the purpose of the medication must be explained to each patient both by the prescriber and by the pharmacist. (Neither should assume that the other will do it.) Furthermore, the drug name, the purpose for which it is given, and the duration of therapy should be written on each label so that the drug may be identified easily in case of overdose. An instruction to "take as directed" may save the time it takes to write the orders out but often leads to noncompliance, patient confusion, and medication error. The directions for use must be clear and concise to avoid toxicity and to obtain the greatest benefits from therapy.

Although directions for use are no longer written in Latin, many Latin apothecary abbreviations (and some others included below) are still in use. Knowledge of these abbreviations is essential for the dispensing pharmacist and often useful for the prescriber. Some of the abbreviations still used are listed in Table 66–1.

Note: It is always safer to write out the direction without abbreviating.

Elements [12] to [14] of the prescription include refill information, waiver of the requirement for childproof containers, and additional labeling instructions (eg, warnings such as "may cause drowsiness," "do not drink alcohol"). Pharmacists put the name of the medication on the label unless directed otherwise by the prescriber, and some medications have the name of the drug stamped or

Table 66–1. Abbreviations used in prescriptions and chart orders.

ABBREVIATION	EXPLANATION	ABBREVIATION	EXPLANATION
$\bar{a}$	before	PR	per rectum
ac	before meals	prn	when needed
agit	shake, stir	q	every
Aq	water	qam, om	every morning
Aq dest	distilled water	qd (do not use)	every day (write "daily")
bid	twice a day	qh, q1h	every hour
$\bar{c}$	with	q2h, q3h, etc	every 2 hours, every
cap	capsule		3 hours, etc
D5W, D$_5$W	dextrose 5% in water	qhs	every night at bedtime
dil	dissolve, dilute	qid	four times a day
disp, dis	dispense	qod (do not use)	every other day
elix	elixir	qs	sufficient quantity
ext	extract	rept, repet	may be repeated
g	gram	Rx	take
gr	grain	$\bar{s}$	without
gtt	drops	SC, SQ	subcutaneous
h	hour	sid (veterinary)	once a day
hs	at bedtime	Sig, S	label
IA	intra-arterial	sos	if needed
IM	intramuscular	$\bar{ss}$, ss	one-half
IV	intravenous	stat	at once
IVPB	IV piggyback	sup, supp	suppository
kg	kilogram	susp	suspension
mEq, meq	milliequivalent	tab	tablet
mg	milligram	tbsp, T (do not use)	tablespoon (always write out
mcg, μg (do not use)	microgram (always write		"15 mL")
	out "microgram")	tid	three times a day
no	number	tr, tinct	tincture
non rep	do not repeat	tsp (do not use)	teaspoon (always write out
OD	right eye		"5 mL")
OS, OL	left eye	U (do not use)	units (always write out "units")
OTC	over-the-counter	vag	vaginal
OU	both eyes	i, ii, iii, iv, etc	one, two, three, four, etc
$\bar{p}$	after	ʒ (do not use)	dram (in fluid measure, 3.7 mL)
pc	after meals	℥ (do not use)	ounce (in fluid measure, 29.6 mL)
PO	by mouth		

imprinted on the tablet or capsule. Pharmacists must place the expiration date for the drug on the label. If the patient or prescriber does not request waiver of childproof containers, the pharmacist or dispenser must place the medication in such a container. Pharmacists may not refill a prescription medication without authorization from the prescriber. Prescribers may grant authorization to renew prescriptions at the time of writing the prescription or over the telephone. Elements [15] to [17] are the prescriber's signature and other identification data.

PRESCRIBING ERRORS

All prescription orders should be legible, unambiguous, dated (and timed in the case of a chart order), and signed clearly for optimal communication between prescriber, pharmacist, and nurse. Furthermore, a good prescription or chart order should contain sufficient information to permit the pharmacist or nurse to discover possible errors before the drug is dispensed or administered.

Several types of prescribing errors are particularly common. These include errors involving omission of needed information; poor writing perhaps leading to errors of drug dose or timing; and prescription of drugs that are inappropriate for the specific situation.

Omission of Information

Errors of omission are common in hospital orders and may include instructions to "resume pre-op meds," which assumes that a full and accurate record of the "pre-op meds" is available; "continue present IV fluids," which fails to state exactly what fluids are to be given, in what volume, and over what time period; or "continue eye drops," which omits mention of which eye is to be treated as well as the drug, concentration, and frequency of administration. Chart orders may also fail to discontinue a prior medication when a new one is begun; may fail to state whether a regular or long-acting form is to be used; may fail to specify a strength or notation for long-acting forms; or may authorize "as needed" (prn) use that fails to state what conditions will justify the need.

Poor Prescription Writing

Poor prescription writing is traditionally exemplified by illegible handwriting. However, other types of poor writing are common and often more dangerous. One of the most important is the misplaced or ambiguous decimal point. Thus ".1" is easily misread as "1," a tenfold overdose, if the decimal point is not unmistakably clear. This danger is easily avoided by always preceding the decimal point with a zero. On the other hand, appending an unnecessary zero after a decimal point increases the risk of a tenfold overdose, because "1.0 mg" is easily misread as "10 mg," whereas "1 mg" is not. The slash or virgule ("/") was traditionally used as a substitute for a decimal point. This should be abandoned because it is too easily misread as the numeral "1." Similarly, the abbreviation "U" for units should never be used because "10U" is easily misread as "100"; the word "units" should *always* be written out. Doses in micrograms should *always* have this unit written out because the abbreviated form ("μg") is very easily misread as "mg," a 1000-fold overdose! Orders for drugs specifying only the number of dosage units and not the total dose required should not be filled if more than one size dosage unit exists for that drug. For example, ordering "one ampule of furosemide" is unacceptable because furosemide is available in ampules that contain 20, 40, or 100 mg of the drug. The abbreviation "OD" should be used (if at all) only to mean "the right eye"; it has been used for "every day" and has caused inappropriate administration of drugs into the eye. Similarly, "Q.D." or "QD" should not be used because it is often read as "QID," resulting in four daily doses instead of one. Acronyms such as "ASA" (aspirin), "5-ASA" (5-aminosalicylic acid), "6MP" (6-mercaptopurine), etc, should not be used; drug names should be written out. Unclear handwriting can be lethal when drugs with similar names but very different effects are available, eg, acetazolamide and acetohexamide, methotrexate and metolazone. In this situation, errors are best avoided by noting the indication for the drug in the body of the prescription, eg, "acetazolamide, for glaucoma."

Inappropriate Drug Prescriptions

Prescribing an inappropriate drug for a particular patient results from failure to recognize contraindications imposed by other diseases the patient may have, failure to obtain information about other drugs the patient is taking (including over-the-counter drugs), or failure to recognize possible physicochemical incompatibilities between drugs that may react with each other. Contraindications to drugs in the presence of other diseases or pharmacokinetic characteristics are listed in the discussions of the drugs described in this book. The manufacturer's package insert usually contains similar information. Some of the important drug interactions are listed in Appendix II of this book as well as in package inserts.

Physicochemical incompatibilities are of particular concern when parenteral administration is planned. For example, certain insulin preparations should not be mixed. Similarly, the simultaneous administration of antacids or products high in metal content may compromise the absorption of many drugs in the intestine, eg, tetracyclines. The package insert and the *Handbook on Injectable Drugs* (see References) are good sources for this information.

COMPLIANCE

Compliance (sometimes called adherence) is the extent to which patients follow treatment instructions. There are four types of noncompliance leading to medication errors.

(1) The patient fails to obtain the medication. Some studies suggest that one third of patients never have their prescriptions filled. Some patients leave the hospital without obtaining their discharge medications, whereas others leave the hospital without having their prehospitalization medications resumed. Some patients cannot afford the medications prescribed.

(2) The patient fails to take the medication as prescribed. Examples include wrong dosage, wrong frequency of administration, improper timing or sequencing of administration, wrong route or technique of administration, or taking medication for the wrong purpose. This usually results from inadequate communication between the patient and the prescriber and the pharmacist.

(3) The patient prematurely discontinues the medication. This can occur, for instance, if the patient incorrectly assumes that the medication is no longer needed because the bottle is empty or symptomatic improvement has occurred.

(4) The patient (or another person) takes medication inappropriately. For example, the patient may share a medication with others for any of several reasons.

Several factors encourage noncompliance. Some diseases cause no symptoms (eg, hypertension); patients with these diseases therefore have no symptoms to remind them to take their medications. Patients with painful conditions, such as arthritis, may continually change medications in the hope of finding a better one. Characteristics of the therapy itself can limit the degree of compliance; patients taking a drug once a day are much more likely to be compliant than those taking a drug four times a day. Various patient factors also play a role in compliance. Patients living alone are much less likely to be compliant than married patients of the same age. Packaging may also be a deterrent to compliance—elderly arthritic patients often have difficulty opening their medication containers. Lack of transportation as well as various social or personal beliefs about medications are likewise barriers to compliance.

Strategies for improving compliance include enhanced communication between the patient and health care team members; assessment of personal, social, and economic conditions (often reflected in the patient's lifestyle); development of a routine for taking medications (eg, at mealtimes if the patient has regular meals); provision of systems to assist taking medications (ie, containers that separate drug doses by day of the week, or medication alarm clocks that remind patients to take their medications); and mailing of refill reminders by the pharmacist to patients taking drugs chronically. The patient who is likely to discontinue a medication because of a perceived drug-related problem should receive instruction about how to monitor and understand the effects of the medication. Compliance can often be improved by enlisting the patient's active participation in the treatment.

LEGAL FACTORS (USA)

The United States government recognizes two classes of drugs: (1) over-the-counter (OTC) drugs and (2) those that require a prescription from a licensed prescriber (Rx Only). OTC drugs are those that can be safely self-administered by the layman for self-limiting conditions and for which appropriate labels can be written for lay comprehension. Half of all drug doses consumed by the American public are OTC drugs.

Physicians, dentists, podiatrists, and veterinarians—and, in some states, specialized pharmacists, nurses, physician's assistants, and optometrists—are granted authority to prescribe dangerous drugs (those bearing the federal legend statement, "Rx Only") on the basis of their training in diagnosis and treatment (see Box: Who May Prescribe?). Pharmacists are authorized to dispense prescriptions pursuant to a prescriber's order provided that the medication order is appropriate and rational for the patient. Nurses are authorized to administer medications to patients subject to a prescriber's order (Table 66–2).

Prescription drugs are controlled by the United States Food and Drug Administration as described in Chapter 5. The federal legend statement as well as the package insert is part of the packaging requirements for all prescription drugs. The package insert is the official brochure setting forth the indications, contraindications, warnings, and dosing for the drug.

The prescriber, by writing and signing a prescription order, controls who may obtain prescription drugs. The pharmacist may purchase these drugs, but they may be dispensed only on the order of a legally qualified prescriber. Thus, a **prescription** is actually three things: the **physician's order in the patient's chart,** the **written order to which the pharmacist refers** when dispensing, and the patient's **medication container with a label affixed.**

WHO MAY PRESCRIBE?

The right to prescribe drugs has traditionally been the responsibility of the physician, dentist, podiatrist, or veterinarian. Prescribing now includes—in a number of states and in varying degrees—pharmacists, nurse practitioners, nurse midwives, physician's assistants, and optometrists (see Table 66–2). The development of large health maintenance organizations has greatly strengthened this movement because it offers these extremely powerful economic bodies a way to reduce their expenses.

The primary organizations controlling the privilege of prescribing in the USA are the state boards, under the powers delegated to them by the state legislatures. As indicated in Table 66–2, many state boards have attempted to reserve some measure of the primary responsibility for prescribing to physicians by requiring that the ancillary professional work with or under a physician according to a specific protocol. In the state of California, this protocol must include a statement of the training, supervision, and documentation requirements of the arrangement and must specify referral requirements, limitations to the list of drugs that may be prescribed (ie, a formulary), and a method of evaluation by the supervising physician. The protocol must be in writing and must be periodically updated (See reference: An Explanation of the Scope of RN Practice, 1994).

Table 66–2. Prescribing authority of certain allied health professionals in selected states.

State	Pharmacists	Nurse Practitioners	Physician's Assistants	Optometrists
California	Yes, under protocol[1]; must be trained in clinical practice	Yes[2]	Yes, under protocol[1]	Yes; limited to certain drug classes
Florida	Yes, according to state formulary; protocol not required	Yes[2]	Yes[2]	Yes; limited to certain drug classes
Michigan	Yes, under protocol; must be specially qualified by education, training, or experience	Yes; do not need physician supervision	Yes[2]	Yes; limited to certain drug classes
Mississippi	Yes, under protocol in an institutional setting	Yes,[2] under narrowly specified conditions	No	Yes; limited to certain drug classes
Nevada	Yes, under protocol, within a licensed medical facility	Yes[2]	Yes[2]	Yes; limited to certain drug classes
New Mexico	Yes, under protocol, must be "pharmacist clinician"	Yes; do not need physician supervision	Yes[2]	Yes; limited to certain drug classes
North Dakota	Yes, under protocol in an institutional setting	Yes; do not need physician supervision	Yes	Yes; limited to certain drug classes
Oregon	Yes, under guidelines set by the state board	Yes; do not need physician supervision	Yes[2]	Yes; limited to certain drug classes
Texas	Yes, under protocol set for a particular patient in an institutional setting	Yes; do not need physician supervision	Yes	Yes; limited to certain drug classes
Washington	Yes, under guidelines set by the state board	Yes; do not need physician supervision	Yes[2]	Yes; limited to certain drug classes

[1]Under protocol: see Box: Who May Prescribe.
[2]In collaboration with or under the supervision of a physician.

Whereas the federal government controls the drugs and their labeling and distribution, the state legislatures control who may prescribe drugs through their licensing boards, eg, the Board of Medical Examiners. Prescribers must pass examinations, pay fees, and—in the case of some states and some professions—meet other requirements for relicensure such as continuing education. If these requirements are met, the prescriber is licensed to order dispensing of drugs.

The federal government and the states further impose special restrictions on drugs according to their perceived potential for abuse (Table 66–3). Such drugs include opioids, hallucinogens, stimulants, depressants, and anabolic steroids. Special requirements must be met when these drugs are to be prescribed. The Controlled Drug Act requires prescribers and dispensers to register with the Drug Enforcement Agency (DEA), pay a fee, receive a personal registration number, and keep records of all controlled drugs prescribed or dispensed. Every time a controlled drug is prescribed, a valid DEA number must appear on the prescription blank.

Prescriptions for substances with a high potential for abuse (schedule II) cannot be refilled. Prescriptions for schedule III, IV, and V drugs can be refilled, but there is a five-refill maximum, and in no case may the prescription be refilled after 6 months from the date of writing. Schedule II drug prescriptions may not be transmitted over the telephone, and some states require a special state-issued prescription blank. These restrictive prescribing laws are intended to limit the amount of drugs of abuse that are made available to the public.

Unfortunately, the inconvenience occasioned by these laws—and an unwarranted fear by medical professionals themselves regarding the risk of patient tolerance and addiction—continues to hamper adequate treatment of patients with terminal conditions. This has been shown to be particularly true in children and elderly patients with cancer. *There is no excuse for inadequate treatment of pain in a terminal patient; not only is addiction irrelevant in such a patient, it is actually uncommon in patients who are being treated for*

Table 66–3. Classification of controlled substances. (See Inside Front Cover for examples.)

Schedule	Potential for Abuse	Other Comments
I	High	No accepted medical use; lack of accepted safety as drug.
II	High	Current accepted medical use. Abuse may lead to psychologic or physical dependence.
III	Less than I or II	Current accepted medical use. Moderate or low potential for physical dependence and high potential for psychologic dependence.
IV	Less than III	Current accepted medical use. Limited potential for dependence.
V	Less than IV	Current accepted medical use. Limited dependence possible.

pain (see Chapter 31). Some states have recognized the underutilization of pain medications in the treatment of pain associated with chronic and terminal conditions. California, for example, has enacted an "intractable pain treatment" act that reduces the difficulty of renewing prescriptions for opioids. Under the provisions of this act, upon receipt of a copy of the order from the prescriber, eg, by fax, a pharmacist may write a prescription for a Schedule II substance for a patient under hospice care or living in a skilled nursing facility or in cases in which the patient is expected to live less than 6 months, provided that the prescriber countersigns the order (by fax); the word "exemption" with regulatory code number is written on a typical prescription, thus providing easier access for the terminally ill.

Labeled & Unlabeled Uses of Drugs

In the USA, the FDA approves a drug only for the specific uses proposed and documented by the manufacturer in its New Drug Application (see Chapter 5). These approved (labeled) uses or indications are set forth in the package insert that accompanies the drug. For a variety of reasons, these labeled indications may not include all the conditions in which the drug might be useful. Therefore, a clinician may wish to prescribe the agent for some other, unapproved (unlabeled) clinical condition, often on the basis of adequate or even compelling scientific evidence. Federal laws governing

FDA regulations and drug use place no restrictions on such unapproved use.*

Even if the patient suffers injury from the drug, its use for an unlabeled purpose does not in itself constitute "malpractice." However, the courts may consider the package insert labeling as a complete listing of the indications for which the drug is considered safe unless the clinician can show that other use is considered safe by competent expert testimony.

SOCIOECONOMIC FACTORS

Generic Prescribing

Prescribing by generic name offers the pharmacist flexibility in selecting the particular drug product to fill the order and the patient a potential savings if there is price competition. The brand name of a popular sedative is, for example, *Valium*, manufactured by Roche. The generic (public nonproprietary) name of the same chemical substance adopted by United States Adopted Names (USAN) and approved by the Food and Drug Administration (FDA) is *diazepam*. All diazepam drug products in the USA meet the pharmaceutical standards expressed in *United States Pharmacopeia (USP)*. However, there are several manufacturers, and prices vary greatly. For some drugs in common use, the difference in cost between the trade-named product and generic products varies from less than twofold to more than 100-fold.

In most states and in most hospitals, pharmacists have the option of supplying a generically equivalent drug product even if a proprietary name has been specified in the order. If the prescriber wants a particular brand of drug product dispensed, handwritten instruction to "dispense as written" or words of similar meaning are required. Some government-subsidized health care programs and many third-party insurance payers *require* that pharmacists dispense the cheapest generically equivalent product in the inventory (generic substitution). However, the principles of drug product selection by private pharmacists do not permit substituting one therapeutic agent for another (therapeutic substitution)—ie, dispensing trichlormethiazide for hydrochlorothiazide would not be permitted without the prescriber's permission even though these two diuretics may be considered pharmacodynamically equivalent. Pharmacists within managed care organizations may follow different policies; see below.

---

*"Once a product has been approved for marketing, a physician may prescribe it for uses or in treatment regimens or patient populations that are not included in the approved labeling. Such 'unapproved' or, more precisely, 'unlabeled' uses may be appropriate and rational in certain circumstances, and may, in fact, reflect approaches to drug therapy that have been extensively reported in medical literature."—FDA Drug Bull 1982;12:4.

It should not be assumed that every generic drug product is as satisfactory as the trade-named product, although most generics are satisfactory. Bioavailability—the effective absorption of the drug product—varies between manufacturers and sometimes between different lots of a drug produced by the same manufacturer. In the case of a very small number of drugs, which usually have a low therapeutic index, poor solubility, or a high ratio of inert ingredients to active drug content, a specific manufacturer's product may give more consistent results. In the case of life-threatening diseases, the advantages of generic substitution may be outweighed by the clinical urgency so that the prescription should be filled as written.

In an effort to codify bioequivalence information, the FDA publishes *Approved Drug Products with Therapeutic Equivalence Evaluations,* with monthly supplements, commonly called "the Orange Book." The book contains listings of multisource products in one of two categories: Products given a code beginning with the letter "A" are considered bioequivalent to a reference standard formulation of the same drug and to all other versions of that product with a similar "A" coding. Products not considered bioequivalent are coded "B." Of the approximately 8000 products listed, 90% are coded "A." Additional code letters and numerals are appended to the initial "A" or "B" and indicate the approved route of administration and other variables.

Mandatory drug product selection on the basis of price is common practice in the USA because third-party payers (insurance companies, health maintenance organizations, etc) enforce money-saving regulations. If outside a managed care organization, the prescriber can sometimes override these controls by writing "dispense as written" on a prescription that calls for a brand-named product. However, in such cases, the patient may have to pay the difference between the dispensed product and the cheaper one.

Within most managed care organizations, formulary controls have been put in place that force the selection of less expensive medications whenever they are available. In a managed care environment, the prescriber often selects the drug group rather than a specific agent, and the pharmacist dispenses the formulary drug from that group. For example, if a prescriber in such an organization decides that a patient needs a thiazide diuretic, the pharmacist automatically dispenses the single thiazide diuretic carried on the organization's formulary. As noted below, the choice of drugs for the organization's formulary may change from time to time, depending on negotiation of prices and rebates with different manufacturers.

THE COST OF PRESCRIPTIONS

The cost of prescriptions has risen dramatically in the last several decades. The average price for a single prescription in the USA in 2004 was $55. In the California Medicaid Sector, the average charge was over $80, with generic products being under $40 per prescription and brand-name products over $140. This rise is occasioned by new technology, marketing costs, and stockholder expectations. The pharmaceutical industry typically posts double-digit profits annually whereas the retail business sector shows a 3% profit. The cost to the patient for many new drugs such as statins exceeds $1000 per year. The cost of some therapeutic antibody products (MABs) is more than $10,000 per year. Pharmaceuticals tend to be the highest out-of-pocket health-related cost because other health care services are covered by health insurance, whereas prescriptions often are not.

Because of public and political pressure resulting from this problem, the US Congress enacted the Medicare Modernization Act in 2003 establishing the Medicare Part D plan. This voluntary prescription plan provides for partial payment by private medical insurance companies for some prescriptions for patients who are MediCare-eligible. Unfortunately, the complexity of the legislation and the resulting confusing insurance plans with gaps in coverage, formulary and quantity limits, and the favored economic treatment given the pharmaceutical industry, prevent this plan from solving the high drug cost problem.

High drug costs have caused payers and consumers alike to do without or seek alternative sources. Because the Canadian government has done a better job in controlling drug prices, their prices for the same drug are less than those in the United States. This fact has caused a number of United States citizens to purchase their drugs "off-shore" for "personal use" in quantities up to a 3-month supply—at substantial savings, often as much as 50%. However, there is no assurance that these drugs are what they are purported to be or that they will be delivered in a timely manner—or that there is a traditional doctor-pharmacist-patient relationship and the safeguards that such a relationship offers.

Without a true universal health care program, the cost of drugs in the USA will continue to be subject to the negotiating power (or lack thereof) of the purchasing group—insurance company, hospital consortium, HMO, small retail pharmacy, etc. Thus far, only the US Veterans Administration system and the larger HMOs have proved strong enough to control costs through bulk purchases of drugs and serious negotiation of prices with manufacturers. Until new legislation gives other organizations the same power to negotiate, or pricing policies are made more equitable, no real solution to the drug cost problem can be expected.

Other Cost Factors

The private pharmacy bases its charges on the cost of the drug plus a fee for providing a professional service. Each time a prescription is dispensed, there is a fee. The prescriber controls the frequency of filling prescriptions by authorizing refills and specifying the quantity to be dispensed. Thus, the prescriber can save the patient money by prescribing standard sizes (so that drugs do not have to be repackaged) and, when chronic treatment is involved, by ordering the largest quantity consistent with safety, expense, and third-party plan. Optimal prescribing for cost savings often involves consultation between the prescriber and the pharmacist. Because of continuing increases in the wholesale prices of drugs in the USA, prescription costs have risen dramatically over the past 3 decades (see Box: The Cost of Prescriptions).

REFERENCES

An explanation of the scope of RN practice including standardization procedures. Board of Registered Nursing, State of California, August 1994.

Avorn J: Part "D" for "Defective"—The Medicare Drug Benefit Chaos. N Engl J Med 2006;354:1339.

California Business and Professions Code, Chapter 9, Division 2, Pharmacy Law. Department of Consumer Affairs, Sacramento, California, 2006.

Do we pay too much for prescriptions? Consumer Reports 1993; 58:668.

Hendrickson R (editor): *Remington's Practice and Science of Pharmacy.* Advanced Concepts Institute, 2005.

Jerome JB, Sagan P: The USAN nomenclature system. JAMA 1975;232:294.

Lesar TS, Briceland L, Stein DS: Factors related to errors in medication prescribing. JAMA 1997;277:312.

Schnipper JL et al: Role of pharmacist counseling in preventing adverse drug events after hospitalization. Arch Intern Med 2006;166:565.

Shulman SR: The broader message of Accutane. Am J Public Health 1989;79:1565.

Trissel LA: *Handbook on Injectable Drugs,* 13th ed. American Society of Hospital Pharmacists, 2005. (With supplements.)

Use of approved drugs for unlabeled indications. FDA Drug Bull 1982;12:4.

WHO Drug Action Committee: *Model Guide to Good Prescribing.* WHO, 1994.

Appendix I: Vaccines, Immune Globulins, & Other Complex Biologic Products

Harry W. Lampiris, MD, & Daniel S. Maddix, PharmD

Vaccines and related biologic products constitute an important group of agents that bridge the disciplines of microbiology, infectious diseases, immunology, and immunopharmacology. A listing of the most important preparations is provided here. The reader who requires more complete information is referred to the sources listed at the end of this appendix.

■ ACTIVE IMMUNIZATION

Active immunization consists of the administration of antigen to the host to induce formation of antibodies and cell-mediated immunity. Immunization is practiced to induce protection against many infectious agents and may utilize either inactivated (killed) materials or live attenuated agents (Table I–1). Desirable features of the ideal immunogen include complete prevention of disease, prevention of the carrier state, production of prolonged immunity with a minimum of immunizations, absence of toxicity, and suitability for mass immunization (eg, cheap and easy to administer). Active immunization is generally preferable to passive immunization—in most cases because higher antibody levels are sustained for longer periods of time, requiring less frequent immunization, and in some cases because of the development of concurrent cell-mediated immunity. However, active immunization requires time to develop and is therefore generally inactive at the time of a specific exposure (eg, for parenteral exposure to hepatitis B, concurrent hepatitis B IgG [passive antibodies] and active immunization are given to prevent illness).

Current recommendations for routine active immunization of children are given in Table I–2.

■ PASSIVE IMMUNIZATION

Passive immunization consists of transfer of immunity to a host using preformed immunologic products. From a practical standpoint, only immunoglobulins have been utilized for passive immunization, since passive administration of cellular components of the immune system has been technically difficult and associated with graft-versus-host reactions. Products of the cellular immune system (eg, interferons) have also been used in the therapy of a wide variety of hematologic and infectious diseases (see Chapter 56).

Passive immunization with antibodies may be accomplished with either animal or human immunoglobulins in varying degrees of purity. These may contain relatively high titers of antibodies directed against a specific antigen or, as is true for pooled immune globulin, may simply contain antibodies found in most of the population. Passive immunization is useful for (1) individuals unable to form antibodies (eg, congenital agammaglobulinemia); (2) prevention of disease when time does not permit active immunization (eg, postexposure); (3) for treatment of certain diseases normally prevented by immunization (eg, tetanus); and (4) for treatment of conditions for which active immunization is unavailable or impractical (eg, snakebite).

Complications from administration of *human* immunoglobulins are rare. The injections may be moderately painful and rarely a sterile abscess may occur at the injection site. Transient hypotension and pruritus occasionally occur with the administration of intravenous immune globulin (IVIG) products, but generally are mild. Individuals with certain immunoglobulin deficiency states (IgA deficiency, etc) may occasionally develop hypersensitivity reactions to immune globulin

(continued on page 1077)

Table I–1. Materials commonly used for active immunization in the United States.[1]

Vaccine	Type of Agent	Route of Administration	Primary Immunization	Booster[2]	Indications
Diphtheria-tetanus-acellular pertussis (DTaP)	Toxoids and inactivated bacterial components	Intramuscular	See Table I–2		1. For all children 2. Booster every 10 years in adolescents and adults
Haemophilus influenzae type b conjugate (Hib)	Bacterial polysaccharide conjugated to protein	Intramuscular	One dose (see Table I–2 for childhood schedule)	Not recommended	1. For all children 2. Asplenia and other at-risk conditions
Hepatitis A	Inactivated virus	Intramuscular	One dose (administer at least 2–4 weeks before travel to endemic areas)	At 6–12 months for long-term immunity	1. Travelers to hepatitis A endemic areas 2. Homosexual and bisexual men 3. Illicit drug users 4. Chronic liver disease or clotting factor disorders 5. Persons with occupational risk for infection 6. Persons living in, or relocating to, endemic areas 7. Household and sexual contacts of individuals with acute hepatitis A
Hepatitis B	Inactive viral antigen, recombinant	Intramuscular (subcutaneous injection is acceptable in individuals with bleeding disorders)	Three doses at 0, 1, and 6 months (see Table I–2 for childhood schedule)	Not routinely recommended	1. For all infants 2. Preadolescents, adolescents, and young adults 3. Persons with occupational, lifestyle, or environmental risk 4. Hemophiliacs 5. Hemodialysis patients 6. Postexposure prophylaxis
Influenza, inactivated	Inactivated virus or viral components	Intramuscular	One dose. (Children ≤ 12 years of age should receive split virus vaccine only; children < 9 who are receiving influenza vaccine for the first time should receive two doses administered at least 1 month apart)	Yearly with current vaccine	1. Adults ≥ 50 years of age 2. Persons with high risk conditions (eg, asthma) 3. Health care workers and others in contact with high-risk groups 4. Residents of nursing homes and other residential chronic care facilities 5. All children aged 6–23 months

Vaccine	Type	Route	Primary Dosing	Revaccination	Indications
Influenza, live attenuated	Live virus	Intranasal	Split dose in each nostril. Children aged 5–8 who are receiving influenza vaccine for the first time should receive two doses administered 6–10 weeks apart	Yearly with current vaccine	Healthy persons aged 5–49 years who desire protection against influenza
Measles	Live virus	Subcutaneous	Two doses at least 1 month apart	None	1. Adults and adolescents born after 1956 without a history of measles or live virus vaccination on or after their first birthday 2. Postexposure prophylaxis in unimmunized persons
Measles-mumps-rubella (MMR)	Live virus	Subcutaneous	See Table I-2	None	For all children
Meningococcal conjugate vaccine	Bacterial polysaccharides conjugated to diphtheria toxoid	Intramuscular	One dose	Every 2–3 years if there is continuing high risk of exposure	1. All adolescents 2. Preferred over polysaccharide vaccine in persons aged 11–55 years
Meningococcal polysaccharide vaccine	Bacterial polysaccharides of serotypes A/C/Y/W-135	Subcutaneous	One dose	Every 5 years if there is continuing high risk of exposure	1. Military recruits 2. Travelers to areas with epidemic meningococcal disease 3. Individuals with asplenia, complement deficiency, or properdin deficiency 4. Control of outbreaks in closed or semi-closed populations 5. College freshmen who live in dormitories 6. Microbiologists who are routinely exposed to isolates of *Neisseria meningitidis*
Mumps	Live virus	Subcutaneous	One dose	None	Adults born after 1956 without a history of mumps or live virus vaccination on or after their first birthday
Pneumococcal conjugate vaccine	Bacterial polysaccharides conjugated to protein	Intramuscular or subcutaneous	See Table I-2	None	
Pneumococcal polysaccharide vaccine	Bacterial polysaccharides of 23 serotypes	Intramuscular or subcutaneous	One dose	Repeat after 5 years in patients at high risk	1. Adults ≥ 65 years of age 2. Persons at increased risk for pneumococcal disease or its complications

(continued)

Table I–1. Materials commonly used for active immunization in the United States.[1] (continued)

Vaccine	Type of Agent	Route of Administration	Primary Immunization	Booster[2]	Indications
Poliovirus vaccine, inactivated (IPV)	Inactivated viruses of all three serotypes	Subcutaneous	See Table I–2 for childhood schedule. Adults: Two doses 4 to 8 weeks apart, and a third dose 6 to 12 months after the second	One-time booster dose for adults at increased risk of exposure	1. For all children 2. Previously unvaccinated adults at increased risk for occupational or travel exposure to polioviruses
Rabies	Inactivated virus	Intramuscular (IM) or intradermal (ID)	**Preexposure:** Three doses (IM or ID) at days 0, 7, and 21 or 28 **Postexposure:** Five-doses (IM only) at days 0, 3, 7, 14, and 28	Serologic testing every 6 months to 2 years in persons at high risk	1. **Preexposure** prophylaxis in persons at risk for contact with rabies virus 2. **Postexposure** prophylaxis (administer with rabies immune globulin)
Rubella	Live virus	Subcutaneous	One or two doses (at least 28 days apart)	None	Adults born after 1956 without a history of rubella or live virus vaccination on or after their first birthday
Tetanus-diphtheria (Td or DT)[3]	Toxoids	Intramuscular	Two doses 4–8 weeks apart, and a third dose 6–12 months after the second	Every 10 years or a single booster at age 50[4]	1. All adults who have not been immunized as children 2. Postexposure prophylaxis if > 5 years has passed since last dose
Typhoid, Ty21a oral	Live bacteria	Oral	Four doses administered every other day	Four doses every 5 years	Risk of exposure to typhoid fever
Varicella	Live virus	Subcutaneous	Two doses 4–8 weeks apart in persons past their 13th birthday. (See Table I–2 for childhood schedule.)	Unknown	1. For all children 2. Persons past their 13th birthday without a history of varicella infection or immunization 3. Postexposure prophylaxis in susceptible persons
Yellow Fever	Live virus	Subcutaneous	One dose 10 years to 10 days before travel	Every 10 years	1. Laboratory personnel who may be exposed to yellow fever virus 2. Travelers to areas where yellow fever occurs

[1]Dosages for the specific product, including variations for age, are best obtained from the manufacturer's package insert.

[2]One dose unless otherwise indicated.

[3]Td = Tetanus and diphtheria toxoids for use in persons ≥ 7 years of age (contains less diphtheria toxoid than DPT and DT). DT = Tetanus and diphtheria toxoids for use in persons < 7 years of age (contains the same amount of diphtheria toxoid as DPT).

[4]Diphtheria/acellular pertussis/tetanus vaccine was licensed in the USA in 2005 and may be used instead of DT booster in selected individuals.

Table I–2. Recommended routine childhood immunization schedule.[1]

Age	Immunization	Comments
Birth to 2 months	Hepatitis B vaccine (HBV)	**Infants born to seronegative mothers:** Administration should begin at birth, with the second dose administered at least 4 weeks after the first dose. **Infants born to seropositive mothers:** Should receive the first dose within 12 hours after birth (with hepatitis B immune globulin), the second dose at 1–2 months of age, and the third dose at 6 months of age.
2 months	Diphtheria and tetanus toxoids and acellular pertussis vaccine (DTaP), inactivated poliovirus vaccine (IPV), *Haemophilus influenzae* type b conjugate vaccine (Hib)[2], pneumococcal conjugate vaccine (PCV)	
1–4 months	HBV	The second dose should be given at least 4 weeks after the first dose.
4 months	DTaP, Hib[2], IPV, PCV	
6 months	DTaP, Hib[2], PCV	
6–18 months	HBV, IPV	The third dose of HBV should be given at least 16 weeks after the first dose and at least 8 weeks after the second dose, but not before age 6 months.
6–23 months	Influenza, split virus vaccine	Two doses ≥ 1 month apart are recommended for children ≤ 9 years who are receiving influenza vaccine for the first time.
12–15 months	Measles-mumps-rubella vaccine (MMR), Hib[2], PCV	
12–18 months	DTaP at 15–18 months, varicella vaccine	DTaP may be given as early as age 12 months. Varicella vaccine is recommended at any visit after the first birthday for susceptible children. Susceptible children ≥ 13 years of age should receive two doses given at least 4 weeks apart.
2–18 years	Hepatitis A vaccine	Two doses ≥ 6 months apart. For children and adolescents in selected states and regions and for certain groups, consult your local public health authority.
4–6 years	DTaP IPV, MMR	The second dose of MMR should be routinely administered at 4–6 years of age but may be given during any visit if at least 4 weeks have elapsed since administration of the first dose. The second dose should be given no later than age 11–12 years.
11–12 years	Diphtheria and tetanus toxoids and acellular pertussis vaccine (DTaP)	Vaccination is recommended if at least 5 years has elapsed since administration of the last dose of DTaP. Routine booster doses of DTaP should be given every 10 years thereafter.
12–16 years	Meningococcal conjugate vaccine	One dose is recommended. Repeat every 2–3 years if continuing high risk of exposure

[1]Adapted from MMWR Morb Mortal Wkly Rep 2002;31:31.
[2]Three Hib conjugate vaccines are available for use: (a) oligosaccharide conjugate Hib vaccine (HbOC), (b) polyribosylribitol phosphate-tetanus toxoid conjugate (PRP-T), and (c) *Haemophilus influenzae* type b conjugate vaccine (meningococcal protein conjugate) (PRP-OMP). Children immunized with PRP-OMP at 2 and 4 months of age do not require a dose at 6 months of age.

that may limit therapy. Conventional immune globulin contains aggregates of IgG; it will cause severe reactions if given intravenously. However, if the passively administered antibodies are derived from *animal* sera, hypersensitivity reactions ranging from anaphylaxis to serum sickness may occur. Highly purified immunoglobulins, especially from rodents or lagomorphs, are the least likely to cause reactions. To avoid anaphylactic reactions, tests for hypersensitivity to the animal serum must be performed. If an alternative preparation is not available and administration of the specific antibody is deemed essential, desensitization can be carried out.

Antibodies derived from human serum not only avoid the risk of hypersensitivity reactions but also have a much longer half-life in humans (about 23 days for IgG antibodies) than those from animal sources (5–7 days or less). Consequently, much smaller doses of human antibody can be administered to provide therapeutic concentrations for several weeks. These advantages point to the desirability of using human antibodies for passive protection whenever possible. Materials available for passive immunization are summarized in Table I–3.

■ LEGAL LIABILITY FOR UNTOWARD REACTIONS

It is the physician's responsibility to inform the patient of the risk of immunization and to employ vaccines and antisera in an appropriate manner. This may require skin testing to assess the risk of an untoward reaction. Some of the risks described above are, however, currently unavoidable; on the balance, the patient and society are clearly better off accepting the risks for routinely administered immunogens (eg, influenza and tetanus vaccines).

Manufacturers should be held legally accountable for failure to adhere to existing standards for production of biologicals. However, in the present litigious atmosphere of the USA, the filing of large liability claims by the statistically inevitable victims of good public health practice has caused many manufacturers to abandon efforts to develop and produce low-profit but medically valuable therapeutic agents such as vaccines. Since the use and sale of these products are subject to careful review and approval by government bodies such as the Surgeon General's Advisory Committee on Immunization Practices and the Food and Drug Administration, "strict product liability" (liability without fault) may be an inappropriate legal standard to apply when rare reactions to biologicals, produced and administered according to government guidelines, are involved.

■ RECOMMENDED IMMUNIZATION OF ADULTS FOR TRAVEL

Every adult, whether traveling or not, should be immunized with tetanus toxoid and should also be fully immunized against poliomyelitis, measles (for those born after 1956), and diphtheria. In addition, every traveler must fulfill the immunization requirements of the health authorities of the countries to be visited. These are listed in *Health Information for International Travel*, available from the Superintendent of Documents, United States Government Printing Office, Washington, DC 20402. A useful website is www.cdc.gov/travel/vaccinat.htm. *The Medical Letter on Drugs and Therapeutics* also offers periodically updated recommendations for international travelers (see *Treatment Guidelines from The Medical Letter*, 2006;4:25). Immunizations received in preparation for travel should be recorded on the International Certificate of Immunization. *Note:* Smallpox vaccination is not recommended or required for travel in any country.

Table I–3. Materials available for passive immunization.[1]

Indication	Product	Dosage	Comments
Black widow spider bite	Antivenin (*Latrodectus mactans*), equine	One vial (6000 units) IV or IM.	For persons with hypertensive cardiovascular disease or age < 16 or > 60 years.
Bone marrow transplantation	Immune globulin (intravenous)[2]	500 mg/kg IV on days 7 and 2 prior to transplantation and then once weekly through day 90 after transplantation.	Prophylaxis to decrease the risk of infection, interstitial pneumonia, and acute graft-versus-host disease in adults undergoing bone marrow transplantation.
Botulism	Botulism antitoxin (trivalent, types A, B, and E), equine	Consult the CDC.[3]	Treatment and prophylaxis of botulism. Available from the CDC.[3] Ten to 20 percent incidence of serum reactions.
Chronic lymphocytic leukemia (CLL)	Immune globulin (intravenous)[2]	400 mg/kg IV every 3–4 weeks. Dosage should be adjusted upward if bacterial infections occur.	CLL patients with hypogammaglobulinemia and a history of at least one serious bacterial infection.

(continued)

Table I–3. Materials available for passive immunization.[1] (continued)

Indication	Product	Dosage	Comments
Cytomegalovirus (CMV)	Cytomegalovirus immune globulin (intravenous)	Consult the manufacturer's dosing recommendations.	Prophylaxis of CMV infection in bone marrow, kidney, liver, lung, pancreas, heart transplant recipients.
Diphtheria	Diphtheria anti-toxin, equine	20,000–120,000 units IV or IM depending on the severity and duration of illness.	Early treatment of respiratory diphtheria. Available from the CDC.[3] Anaphylactic reactions in ≥ 7% of adults and serum reactions in ≥ 5–10% of adults.
Hepatitis A	Immune globulin (intramuscular)	**Preexposure prophylaxis:** 0.02 mL/kg IM for anticipated risk of ≤ 3 months, 0.06 mL/kg for anticipated risk of > 3 months, repeated every 4–6 months for continued exposure. **Postexposure:** 0.02 mL/kg IM as soon as possible after exposure up to 2 weeks.	Preexposure and postexposure hepatitis A prophylaxis. The availability of hepatitis A vaccine has greatly reduced the need for preexposure prophylaxis.
Hepatitis B	Hepatitis B immune globulin (HBIG)	0.06 mL/kg IM as soon as possible after exposure up to 1 week for percutaneous exposure or 2 weeks for sexual exposure. 0.5 mL IM within 12 hours after birth for perinatal exposure.	Postexposure prophylaxis in nonimmune persons following percutaneous, mucosal, sexual, or perinatal exposure. Hepatitis B vaccine should also be administered.
HIV-infected children	Immune globulin (intravenous)[2]	400 mg/kg IV every 28 days.	HIV-infected children with recurrent serious bacterial infections or hypogammaglobulinemia.
Kawasaki disease	Immune globulin (intravenous)[2]	400 mg/kg IV daily for 4 consecutive days within 4 days after the onset of illness. A single dose of 2 g/kg IV over 10 hours is also effective.	Effective in the prevention of coronary aneurysms. For use in patients who meet strict criteria for Kawasaki disease.
Measles	Immune globulin (intramuscular)	**Normal hosts:** 0.25 mL/kg IM. **Immunocompromised hosts:** 0.5 mL/kg IM (maximum 15 mL for all patients).	Postexposure prophylaxis (within 6 days after exposure) in nonimmune contacts of acute cases.
Idiopathic thrombocyto-penic purpura (ITP)	Immune globulin (intravenous)[2]	Consult the manufacturer's dosing recommendations for the specific product being used.	Response in children with ITP is greater than in adults. Corticosteroids are the treatment of choice in adults, except for severe pregnancy-associated ITP.
Primary immuno-deficiency disorders	Immune globulin (intravenous)[2]	Consult the manufacturer's dosing recommendations for the specific product being used.	Primary immunodeficiency disorders include specific antibody deficiencies (eg, X-linked agammaglobulinemia) and combined deficiencies (eg, severe combined immunodeficiencies).
Rabies	Rabies immune globulin	20 IU/kg. The full dose should be infiltrated around the wound and any remaining volume should be given IM at an anatomic site distant from vaccine administration.	Postexposure rabies prophylaxis in persons not previously immunized with rabies vaccine. Must be combined with rabies vaccine.

(continued)

Table I–3. Materials available for passive immunization.[1] (continued)

Indication	Product	Dosage	Comments
Respiratory syncytial virus (RSV)	Palivizumab	15 mg/kg IM once prior to the beginning of the RSV season and once monthly until the end of the season.	For use in infants and children younger than 24 months with chronic lung disease or a history of premature birth (≤ 35 weeks' gestation).
	RSV immune globulin	750 mg/kg IV once prior to the beginning of the RSV season and once monthly until the end of the season.	As for palivizumab. Palivizumab is preferred for selected high-risk children, but RSV-IGIV may be preferred for selected high-risk children.
Rubella	Immune globulin (intramuscular)	0.55 mL/kg IM.	Nonimmune pregnant women exposed to rubella who will not consider therapeutic abortion. Administration does not prevent rubella in the fetus of an exposed mother.
Snake bite (coral snake)	Antivenin *(Micrurus fulvius),* equine	At least 3–5 vials (30–50 mL) IV initially within 4 hours after the bite. Additional doses may be required.	Neutralizes venom of eastern coral snake and Texas coral snake. Serum sickness occurs in almost all patients who receive > 7 vials.
Snake bite (pit vipers)	Antivenin (Crotalidae) polyvalent, equine	The entire dose should be given within 4 hours after the bite by the IV or IM route (1 vial = 10 mL): Minimal envenomation: 2–4 vials Moderate envenomation: 5–9 vials Severe envenomation: 10–15 vials Additional doses may be required.	Neutralizes the venom of rattlesnakes, copperheads, cottonmouths, water moccasins, and tropical and Asiatic crotalids. Serum sickness occurs in almost all patients who receive > 7 vials.
	Antivenin (Crotalidae) polyvalent immune Fab, ovine	An initial dose of 4–6 vials should be infused intravenously over 1 hour. The dose should be repeated if initial control is not achieved. After initial control, 2 vials should be given every 6 hours for up to 3 doses.	For the management of minimal to moderate North American crotalid envenomation.
Tetanus	Tetanus immune globulin	**Postexposure prophylaxis:** 250 units IM. For severe wounds or when there has been a delay in administration, 500 units is recommended. **Treatment:** 3000–6000 units IM.	Treatment of tetanus and postexposure prophylaxis of nonclean, nonminor wounds in inadequately immunized persons (less than two doses of tetanus toxoid or less than three doses if wound is more than 24 hours old).
Vaccinia	Vaccinia immune globulin	Consult the CDC.[3]	Treatment of severe reactions to vaccinia vaccination, including eczema vaccinatum, vaccinia necrosum, and ocular vaccinia. Available from the CDC.[3]
Varicella	Varicella-zoster immune globulin	**Weight (kg)** / **Dose (units)** ≤ 10 / 125 IM 10.1–20 / 250 IM 20.1–30 / 375 IM 30.1–40 / 500 IM > 40 / 625 IM	**Postexposure prophylaxis** (preferably within 48 hours but no later than within 96 hours after exposure) in susceptible immunocomprised hosts, selected pregnant women, and perinatally exposed newborns.

[1]Passive immunotherapy or immunoprophylaxis should always be administered as soon as possible after exposure. Prior to the administration of animal sera, patients should be questioned and tested for hypersensitivity.

[2]See the following references for an analysis of additional uses of intravenously administered immune globulin: Ratko TA et al: Recommendations for off-label use of intravenously administered immunoglobulin preparations. JAMA 1995;273:1865; and Dalakas MC: Intravenous immune globulin therapy for neurologic diseases. Ann Intern Med 1997;126:721.

[3]Centers for Disease Control and Prevention, 404-639-3670 during weekday business hours; 404-639-2888 during nights, weekends, and holidays (emergency requests only).

REFERENCES

Ada G: Vaccines and vaccination. N Engl J Med 2001;345:1042.

Advice for travelers. Med Lett Drugs Ther 2002;44:33.

Avery RK: Immunizations in adult immunocompromised patients: Which to use and which to avoid. Cleve Clin J Med 2001; 68:337.

CDC Website: www.cdc.gov/travel/vaccinat.htm.

Dennehy PH: Active immunization in the United States: Developments over the past decade. Clin Micro Rev 2001;14:872.

Gardner P, Peter G: Vaccine recommendations: Challenges and controversies. Infect Dis Clin North Am 2001;15:1.

Gardner P et al: Guidelines for quality standards for immunization. Clin Infect Dis 2002;35:503.

General recommendations on immunization. Recommendations of the Advisory Committee on Immunization Practices (ACIP) and the American Academy of Family Physicians (AAFP). MMWR Morb Mortal Wkly Rep 2002;51(RR-2):1.

Keller MA, Stiehm ER: Passive immunity in prevention and treatment of infectious diseases. Clin Microbiol Rev 2000; 13:602.

Recommended adult immunization schedule—United States, October 2004–September 2005. MMWR Morb Mortal Wkly Rep 2004;53:Q1.

Recommended childhood and adolescent immunization schedule—United States, 2005. MMWR Morb Mortal Wkly Rep 2005;63:Q1.

Appendix II: Important Drug Interactions & Their Mechanisms

John R. Horn, PharmD, FCCP

One of the factors that can alter the response to drugs is the concurrent administration of other drugs. There are several mechanisms by which drugs may interact, but most can be categorized as pharmacokinetic (absorption, distribution, metabolism, excretion), pharmacodynamic, or combined interactions. Knowledge of the mechanism by which a given drug interaction occurs is often clinically useful, since the mechanism may influence both the time course and the methods of circumventing the interaction. Some important drug interactions occur as a result of two or more mechanisms.

Pharmacokinetic Mechanisms

The gastrointestinal **absorption** of drugs may be affected by concurrent use of other agents that (1) have a large surface area upon which the drug can be adsorbed, (2) bind or chelate, (3) alter gastric pH, (4) alter gastrointestinal motility, or (5) affect transport proteins such as P-glycoprotein. One must distinguish between effects on absorption *rate* and effects on *extent* of absorption. A reduction in only the absorption rate of a drug is seldom clinically important, whereas a reduction in the extent of absorption will be clinically important if it results in subtherapeutic serum levels.

The mechanisms by which drug interactions alter drug **distribution** include (1) competition for plasma protein binding, (2) displacement from tissue binding sites, and (3) alterations in local tissue barriers, eg, P-glycoprotein inhibition in the blood-brain barrier. Although competition for plasma protein binding can increase the free concentration (and thus the effect) of the displaced drug in plasma, the increase will be transient owing to a compensatory increase in drug disposition. The clinical importance of protein binding displacement has been overemphasized; current evidence suggests that such interactions are unlikely to result in adverse effects. Displacement from tissue binding sites would tend to transiently increase the blood concentration of the displaced drug.

The **metabolism** of drugs can be stimulated or inhibited by concurrent therapy. Induction (stimulation) of cytochrome P450 isozymes in the liver and small intestine can be caused by drugs such as barbiturates, bosentan, carbamazepine, efavirenz, nevirapine, phenytoin, primidone, rifampin, rifabutin, and St. John's wort. Enzyme inducers can also increase the activity of phase II metabolism such as glucuronidation. Enzyme induction does not take place quickly; maximal effects usually occur after 7–10 days and require an equal or longer time to dissipate after the enzyme inducer is stopped. Rifampin, however, may produce enzyme induction after only a few doses. Inhibition of metabolism generally takes place more quickly than enzyme induction and may begin as soon as sufficient tissue concentration of the inhibitor is achieved. However, if the half-life of the affected drug is long, it may take a week or more to reach a new steady-state serum concentration. Drugs that may inhibit cytochrome P450 metabolism of other drugs include amiodarone, androgens, atazanavir, chloramphenicol, cimetidine, ciprofloxacin, clarithromycin, cyclosporine, delavirdine, diltiazem, diphenhydramine, disulfiram, enoxacin, erythromycin, fluconazole, fluoxetine, fluvoxamine, substances in grapefruit juice, indinavir, isoniazid, itraconazole, ketoconazole, metronidazole, mexiletine, miconazole, nefazodone, omeprazole, paroxetine, propoxyphene, quinidine, ritonavir, sulfamethizole, verapamil, voriconazole, zafirlukast, and zileuton.

The **renal excretion** of active drug can also be affected by concurrent drug therapy. The renal excretion of certain drugs that are weak acids or weak bases may be influenced by other drugs that affect urinary pH. This is due to changes in ionization of the drug, as described in Chapter 1 under Ionization of Weak Acids and Weak Bases; the Henderson-Hasselbalch Equation. For some drugs, active secretion into the renal tubules is an important elimination pathway. The ABC transporter P-glycoprotein is involved in active tubular secretion of some drugs, and inhibition of this transporter can inhibit renal elimination with attendant increase in serum drug concentrations.

Pharmacodynamic Mechanisms

When drugs with similar pharmacologic effects are administered concurrently, an additive or synergistic response is usually seen. The two drugs may or may not act on the same receptor to produce such effects. Conversely, drugs with opposing pharmacologic effects may reduce the response to one or both drugs. Pharmacodynamic drug interactions are relatively common in clinical practice, but adverse effects can usually be minimized if one understands the pharmacology of the drugs involved. In this way, the interactions can be anticipated and appropriate countermeasures taken.

Combined Toxicity

The combined use of two or more drugs, each of which has toxic effects on the same organ, can greatly increase the likelihood of organ damage. For example, concurrent administration of two nephrotoxic drugs can produce kidney damage even though the dose of either drug alone may have been insufficient to produce toxic-ity. Furthermore, some drugs can enhance the organ toxicity of another drug even though the enhancing drug has no intrinsic toxic effect on that organ.

PREDICTABILITY OF DRUG INTERACTIONS

The designations listed in Table II–1 will be used here to *estimate* the predictability of the drug interactions. These estimates are intended to indicate simply whether or not the interaction will occur and do not always mean that the interaction is likely to produce an adverse effect. Whether the interaction occurs and produces an adverse effect or not depends upon (1) the presence or absence of factors that predispose to the adverse effects of the drug interaction (diseases, organ function, dose of drugs, etc) and (2) awareness on the part of the prescriber, so that appropriate monitoring can be ordered or preventive measures taken.

Table II–1. Important drug interactions.

HP = Highly predictable. Interaction occurs in almost all patients receiving the interacting combination.	
P = Predictable. Interaction occurs in most patients receiving the combination.	
NP = Not predictable. Interaction occurs only in some patients receiving the combination.	
NE = Not established. Insufficient data available on which to base estimate of predictability.	

Drug or Drug Group	Properties Promoting Drug Interaction	Clinically Documented Interactions

Alcohol	Chronic alcoholism results in enzyme induction. Acute alcoholic intoxication tends to inhibit drug metabolism (whether person is alcoholic or not). Severe alcohol-induced hepatic dysfunction may inhibit ability to metabolize drugs. Disulfiram-like reaction in the presence of certain drugs. Additive central nervous system depression with other central nervous system depressants.	**Acetaminophen:** [NE] Increased formation of hepatotoxic acetaminophen metabolites (in chronic alcoholics).
		Acitretin: [P] Increased conversion of acitretin to etretinate (teratogenic).
		Anticoagulants, oral: [NE] Increased hypoprothrombinemic effect with acute alcohol intoxication.
		Central nervous system depressants: [HP] Additive or synergistic central nervous system depression.
		Insulin: [NE] Acute alcohol intake may increase hypoglycemic effect of insulin (especially in fasting patients).
		Drugs that may produce a disulfiram-like reaction:
		    Cephalosporins: [NP] Disulfiram-like reactions noted with cefamandole, cefoperazone, cefotetan, and moxalactam.
		    Chloral hydrate: [NP] Mechanism not established.
		    Disulfiram: [HP] Inhibits aldehyde dehydrogenase.
		    Metronidazole: [NP] Mechanism not established.
		    Sulfonylureas: [NE] Chlorpropamide is most likely to produce a disulfiram-like reaction; acute alcohol intake may increase hypoglycemic effect (especially in fasting patients).

Allopurinol	Inhibits hepatic drug-metabolizing enzymes.	**Anticoagulants, oral:** [NP] Increased hypoprothrombinemic effect. **Azathioprine:** [P] Decreased azathioprine detoxification resulting in increased azathioprine toxicity. **Mercaptopurine:** [P] Decreased mercaptopurine metabolism resulting in increased mercaptopurine toxicity.

(continued)

Table II–1. Important drug interactions. (continued)

HP = Highly predictable. Interaction occurs in almost all patients receiving the interacting combination.	
P = Predictable. Interaction occurs in most patients receiving the combination.	
NP = Not predictable. Interaction occurs only in some patients receiving the combination.	
NE = Not established. Insufficient data available on which to base estimate of predictability.	

Drug or Drug Group	Properties Promoting Drug Interaction	Clinically Documented Interactions
Antacids	Antacids may adsorb drugs in gastrointestinal tract, thus reducing absorption. Antacids tend to speed gastric emptying, thus delivering drugs to absorbing sites in the intestine more quickly. Some antacids (eg, magnesium hydroxide with aluminum hydroxide) alkalinize the urine somewhat, thus altering excretion of drugs sensitive to urinary pH.	**Digoxin:** [NP] Decreased gastrointestinal absorption of digoxin. **Iron:** [P] Decreased gastrointestinal absorption of iron with calcium-containing antacids. **Itraconazole:** [P] Reduced gastrointestinal absorption of itraconazole due to increased pH (itraconazole requires acid for absorption). **Ketoconazole:** [P] Reduced gastrointestinal absorption of ketoconazole due to increased pH (ketoconazole requires acid for absorption). **Quinolones:** [HP] Decreased gastrointestinal absorption of ciprofloxacin, norfloxacin, enoxacin (and probably other quinolones). **Salicylates:** [P] Increased renal clearance of salicylates due to increased urine pH; occurs only with large doses of salicylates. **Sodium polystyrene sulfonate:** [NE] Binds antacid cation in gut, resulting in metabolic alkalosis. **Tetracyclines:** [HP] Decreased gastrointestinal absorption of tetracyclines. **Thyroxine:** [NP] Reduced gastrointestinal absorption of thyroxine.
Anticoagulants, oral	Metabolism inducible. Susceptible to inhibition of metabolism by CYP2C9. Highly bound to plasma proteins. Anticoagulation response altered by drugs that affect clotting factor synthesis or catabolism.	*Drugs that may increase anticoagulant effect:* **Acetaminophen:** [NE] Impaired synthesis of clotting factors. **Amiodarone:** [P] Inhibits anticoagulant metabolism. **Anabolic steroids:** [P] Alter clotting factor disposition? **Chloramphenicol:** [NE] Decreased dicumarol metabolism (probably also warfarin). **Cimetidine:** [HP] Decreased warfarin metabolism. **Ciprofloxacin:** [NP] Decreased anticoagulant metabolism? **Clofibrate:** [P] Mechanism not established. **Danazol:** [NE] Impaired synthesis of clotting factors? **Dextrothyroxine:** [P] Enhances clotting factor catabolism? **Disulfiram:** [P] Decreased warfarin metabolism. **Erythromycin:** [NP] Probably inhibits anticoagulant metabolism. **Fluconazole:** [P] Decreased warfarin metabolism. **Gemfibrozil:** [NE] Mechanism not established. **Lovastatin:** [NE] Probably decreased anticoagulant metabolism. **Metronidazole:** [P] Decreased warfarin metabolism. **Miconazole:** [NE] Decreased warfarin metabolism. **Nonsteroidal anti-inflammatory drugs:** [P] Inhibition of platelet function, gastric erosions; some agents increase hypoprothrombinemic response (unlikely with diclofenac, ibuprofen, or naproxen). **Propafenone:** [NE] Probably decreased anticoagulant metabolism. **Quinidine:** [NP] Additive hypoprothrombinemia. **Salicylates:** [HP] Platelet inhibition with aspirin but not with other salicylates; [P] large doses have hypoprothrombinemic effect. **Sulfinpyrazone:** [NE] Inhibits warfarin metabolism. **Sulfonamides:** [NE] Inhibit warfarin metabolism; displace protein binding. **Thyroid hormones:** [P] Enhance clotting factor catabolism. **Trimethoprim-sulfamethoxazole:** [P] Inhibits warfarin metabolism; displaces from protein binding. **Voriconazole:** [NP] Decreased warfarin metabolism. *See also* Alcohol; Allopurinol.

Table II–1. Important drug interactions. (continued)

HP = Highly predictable. Interaction occurs in almost all patients receiving the interacting combination.
P = Predictable. Interaction occurs in most patients receiving the combination.
NP = Not predictable. Interaction occurs only in some patients receiving the combination.
NE = Not established. Insufficient data available on which to base estimate of predictability.

Drug or Drug Group	Properties Promoting Drug Interaction	Clinically Documented Interactions
Anticoagulants, oral (*continued*)	(See preceding page.)	*Drugs that may decrease anticoagulant effect:* **Aminoglutethimide:** [P] Enzyme induction. **Barbiturates:** [P] Enzyme induction. **Carbamazepine:** [P] Enzyme induction. **Cholestyramine:** [P] Reduces absorption of anticoagulant. **Glutethimide:** [P] Enzyme induction. **Nafcillin:** [NE] Enzyme induction. **Phenytoin:** [NE] Enzyme induction; anticoagulant effect may increase transiently at start of phenytoin therapy due to protein-binding displacement. **Primidone:** [P] Enzyme induction. **Rifabutin:** [P] Enzyme induction. **Rifampin:** [P] Enzyme induction. **St. John's wort:** [NE] Enzyme induction. *Effects of anticoagulants on other drugs:* **Hypoglycemics, oral:** [P] Dicumarol inhibits hepatic metabolism of tolbutamide and chlorpropamide. **Phenytoin:** [P] Dicumarol inhibits metabolism of phenytoin.
Antidepressants, tricyclic and heterocyclic	Inhibition of amine uptake into postganglionic adrenergic neuron. Antimuscarinic effects may be additive with other antimuscarinic drugs. Metabolism inducible. Susceptible to inhibition of metabolism by CYP2D6 and other CYP450 enzymes.	**Barbiturates:** [P] Increased antidepressant metabolism. **Bupropion:** [NE] Decreased antidepressant metabolism. **Carbamazepine:** [NE] Enhanced metabolism of antidepressants. **Cimetidine:** [P] Decreased antidepressant metabolism. **Clonidine:** [P] Decreased clonidine antihypertensive effect. **Guanadrel:** [P] Decreased uptake of guanadrel into sites of action. **Guanethidine:** [P] Decreased uptake of guanethidine into sites of action. **Monoamine oxidase inhibitors:** [NP] Some cases of excitation, hyperpyrexia, mania, and convulsions, especially with serotonergic antidepressants such as clomipramine and imipramine, but many patients have received combination without ill effects. **Quinidine:** [NE] Decreased antidepressant metabolism. **Rifampin:** [P] Increased antidepressant metabolism. **Selective serotonin reuptake inhibitors (SSRIs):** [P] Fluoxetine and paroxetine inhibit CYP2D6 and decrease metabolism of antidepressants metabolized by this enzyme (eg, desipramine). Citalopram, sertraline, and fluvoxamine are only weak inhibitors of CYP2D6, but fluvoxamine inhibits CYP1A2 and CYP3A4 and thus can inhibit the metabolism of antidepressants metabolized by these enzymes. **Sympathomimetics:** [P] Increased pressor response to norepinephrine, epinephrine, and phenylephrine.
Azole antifungals	Inhibition of CYP3A4 (itraconazole = ketoconazole > voriconazole > fluconazole). Inhibition of CYP2C9 (fluconazole, voriconazole). Susceptible to enzyme inducers (itraconazole,	**Barbiturates:** [P] Increased metabolism of itraconazole, ketoconazole, voriconazole. **Calcium channel blockers:** [P] Decreased calcium channel blocker metabolism. **Carbamazepine:** [P] Decreased carbamazepine metabolism. **Cisapride:** [NP] Decreased metabolism of cisapride; possible ventricular arrhythmias.

(continued)

Table II–1. Important drug interactions. (continued)

HP = Highly predictable. Interaction occurs in almost all patients receiving the interacting combination.		
P = Predictable. Interaction occurs in most patients receiving the combination.		
NP = Not predictable. Interaction occurs only in some patients receiving the combination.		
NE = Not established. Insufficient data available on which to base estimate of predictability.		

Drug or Drug Group	Properties Promoting Drug Interaction	Clinically Documented Interactions
Azole antifungals (*continued*)	ketoconazole, voriconazole). Gastrointestinal absorption pH-dependent (itraconazole, ketoconazole). Inhibition of P-glycoprotein (itraconazole, ketoconazole).	**Cyclosporine:** [P] Decreased metabolism of cyclosporine. **Digoxin:** [NE] Increased gastrointestinal absorption and decreased renal excretion of digoxin with itraconazole and ketoconazole. **H$_2$-receptor antagonists:** [NE] Decreased absorption of itraconazole and ketoconazole. **HMG CoA reductase inhibitors:** Decreased metabolism of lovastatin, simvastatin, and, to a lesser extent, atorvastatin. **Phenytoin:** [P] Decreased metabolism of phenytoin with fluconazole and probably voriconazole. **Pimozide:** [NE] Decreased pimozide metabolism. **Proton pump inhibitors:** [P] Decreased absorption of itraconazole and ketoconazole. **Rifampin:** [P] Increased metabolism of itraconazole, ketoconazole, and voriconazole. *See also* Antacids; Anticoagulants, oral.
Barbiturates	Induction of hepatic microsomal drug-metabolizing enzymes. Additive central nervous system depression with other central nervous system depressants.	**Beta-adrenoceptor blockers:** [P] Increased β-blocker metabolism. **Calcium channel blockers:** [P] Increased calcium channel blocker metabolism. **Central nervous system depressants:** [HP] Additive central nervous system depression. **Corticosteroids:** [P] Increased corticosteroid metabolism. **Cyclosporine:** [NE] Increased cyclosporine metabolism. **Delavirdine:** [P] Increased delavirdine metabolism. **Doxycycline:** [P] Increased doxycycline metabolism. **Estrogens:** [P] Increased estrogen metabolism. **Methadone:** [NE] Increased methadone metabolism. **Phenothiazine:** [P] Increased phenothiazine metabolism. **Protease inhibitors:** [NE] Increased protease inhibitor metabolism. **Quinidine:** [P] Increased quinidine metabolism. **Sirolimus:** [NE] Increased sirolimus metabolism. **Tacrolimus:** [NE] Increased tacrolimus metabolism. **Theophylline:** [NE] Increased theophylline metabolism; reduced theophylline effect. **Valproic acid:** [P] Decreased phenobarbital metabolism. *See also* Anticoagulants, oral; Antidepressants, tricyclic.
Beta-adrenoceptor blockers	Beta-blockade (especially with nonselective agents such as propranolol) alters response to sympathomimetics with β-agonist activity (eg, epinephrine). Beta-blockers that undergo extensive first-pass metabolism may be affected by drugs capable of altering this process. Beta-blockers may reduce hepatic blood flow.	*Drugs that may increase β-blocker effect:* **Cimetidine:** [P] Decreased metabolism of β-blockers that are cleared primarily by the liver, eg, propranolol. Less effect (if any) on those cleared by the kidneys, eg, atenolol, nadolol. *Drugs that may decrease β-blocker effect:* **Enzyme inducers:** [P] Barbiturates, phenytoin, and rifampin may enhance β-blockers metabolism; other enzyme inducers may produce similar effects. **Nonsteroidal anti-inflammatory drugs:** [P] Indomethacin reduces antihypertensive response; other prostaglandin inhibitors probably also interact. *Effects of β-blockers on other drugs:* **Clonidine:** [NE] Hypertensive reaction if clonidine is withdrawn while patient is taking propranolol.

(*continued*)

Table II–1. Important drug interactions. (continued)

| HP = Highly predictable. Interaction occurs in almost all patients receiving the interacting combination. |
| P = Predictable. Interaction occurs in most patients receiving the combination. |
| NP = Not predictable. Interaction occurs only in some patients receiving the combination. |
| NE = Not established. Insufficient data available on which to base estimate of predictability. |

Drug or Drug Group	Properties Promoting Drug Interaction	Clinically Documented Interactions
Cyclosporine	Metabolism inducible. Susceptible to inhibition of metabolism by CYP3A4. (Tacrolimus and sirolimus appear to have similar interactions.)	**Aminoglycosides:** [NE] Possible additive nephrotoxicity. **Amphotericin B:** [NE] Possible additive nephrotoxicity. **Androgens:** [NE] Increased serum cyclosporine. **Barbiturates:** [P] Increased cyclosporine metabolism. **Carbamazepine:** [P] Increased cyclosporine metabolism. **Clarithromycin:** [P] Decreased cyclosporine metabolism. **Diltiazem:** [NE] Decreased cyclosporine metabolism. **Erythromycin:** [NE] Decreased cyclosporine metabolism. **Lovastatin:** [NE] Myopathy and rhabdomyolysis noted in patients taking lovastatin and cyclosporine. **Nefazodone:** [P] Decreased cyclosporine metabolism. **Phenytoin:** [NE] Increased cyclosporine metabolism. **Pimozide:** [NE] Decreased pimozide metabolism. **Rifampin:** [P] Increased cyclosporine metabolism. **Ritonavir:** [P] Decreased cyclosporine metabolism. **St. John's wort:** [NE] Increased cyclosporine metabolism. **Verapamil:** [NE] Decreased cyclosporine metabolism. *See also* Azole antifungals, Barbiturates; Calcium channel blockers.
Digitalis glycosides	Digoxin susceptible to inhibition of gastrointestinal absorption. Digitalis toxicity may be increased by drug-induced electrolyte imbalance (eg, hypokalemia). Digitoxin metabolism inducible. Renal excretion of digoxin susceptible to inhibition.	*Drugs that may increase digitalis effect:* **Amiodarone:** [P] Reduced renal digoxin excretion leads to increased plasma digoxin concentrations. **Clarithromycin:** [NE] Reduced renal excretion of digoxin. **Diltiazem:** [P] Increased plasma digoxin (usually 20–30%) due to reduced renal and nonrenal clearance. **Erythromycin:** [NE] Reduced renal excretion of digoxin. **Itraconazole:** [NE] Reduced renal excretion of digoxin. **Potassium-depleting drugs:** [P] Increased likelihood of digitalis toxicity. **Propafenone:** [P] Increased plasma digoxin levels. **Quinidine:** [HP] Reduced digoxin excretion; displacement of digoxin from tissue binding sites; digitoxin may also be affected. **Spironolactone:** [NE] Decreased renal digoxin excretion and interference with some serum digoxin assays. **Verapamil:** [P] Increased plasma digoxin levels. *Drugs that may decrease digitalis effect:* **Kaolin-pectin:** [P] Decreased gastrointestinal digoxin absorption. **Penicillamine:** [NE] Decreased plasma digoxin. **Rifampin:** [NE] Increased metabolism of digitoxin and possibly digoxin. **Sulfasalazine:** [NE] Decreased gastrointestinal digoxin absorption. *See also* Antacids; Azole antifungals; Bile acid–binding resins.
Disulfiram	Inhibits hepatic microsomal drug-metabolizing enzymes. Inhibits aldehyde dehydrogenase.	**Benzodiazepines:** [P] Decreased metabolism of chlordiazepoxide and diazepam but not lorazepam and oxazepam. **Metronidazole:** [NE] Confusion and psychoses reported in patients receiving this combination; mechanisms unknown. **Phenytoin:** [P] Decreased phenytoin metabolism. *See also* Alcohol; Anticoagulants, oral.

(continued)

1090 / APPENDIX II

Table II–1. Important drug interactions. (continued)

HP = Highly predictable. Interaction occurs in almost all patients receiving the interacting combination.		
P = Predictable. Interaction occurs in most patients receiving the combination.		
NP = Not predictable. Interaction occurs only in some patients receiving the combination.		
NE = Not established. Insufficient data available on which to base estimate of predictability.		

Drug or Drug Group	Properties Promoting Drug Interaction	Clinically Documented Interactions
Estrogens	Metabolism inducible. Enterohepatic circulation of estrogen may be interrupted by alteration in bowel flora (eg, due to antibiotics).	**Ampicillin:** [NP] Interruption of enterohepatic circulation of estrogen; possible reduction in oral contraceptive efficacy. Some other oral antibiotics may have a similar effect. **Corticosteroids:** [P] Decreased metabolism of corticosteroids leading to increased corticosteroid effect. **Diazepam:** [NE] Decreased diazepam metabolism. **Griseofulvin:** [NE] Possible inhibition of oral contraceptive efficacy; mechanism unknown. **Phenytoin:** [NP] Increased estrogen metabolism; possible reduction in oral contraceptive efficacy. **Primidone:** [NP] Increased estrogen metabolism; possible reduction in oral contraceptive efficacy. **Rifabutin:** [NP] Increased estrogen metabolism; possible reduction in oral contraceptive efficacy. **Rifampin:** [NP] Increased estrogen metabolism; possible reduction in oral contraceptive efficacy. **St. John's wort:** [NE] Increased estrogen metabolism; possible reduction in oral contraceptive efficacy. *See also* Barbiturates; Carbamazepine.
HMG-CoA reductase inhibitors	Lovastatin, simvastatin, and, to a lesser extent, atorvastatin are susceptible to CYP3A4 inhibitors; lovastatin, simvastatin, and, to a lesser extent, atorvastatin are susceptible to CYP3A4 inducers; increased risk of additive myopathy risk with other drugs that can cause myopathy.	**Clarithromycin:** [P] Decreased statin metabolism. **Clofibrate:** [NP] Increased risk of myopathy. **Diltiazem:** [NE] Decreased statin metabolism. **Cyclosporine:** [P] Decreased statin metabolism. **Erythromycin:** [P] Decreased statin metabolism. **Gemfibrozil:** [NP] Increased plasma lovastatin and simvastatin. **Nefazodone:** [NE] Decreased statin metabolism. **Ritonavir:** [NE] Decreased statin metabolism. **Verapamil:** [NE] Decreased statin metabolism. *See also* Azole antifungals.
Iron	Binds with drugs in gastrointestinal tract, reducing absorption.	**Methyldopa:** [NE] Decreased methyldopa absorption. **Quinolones:** [P] Decreased absorption of ciprofloxacin. **Tetracyclines:** [P] Decreased absorption of tetracyclines; decreased efficacy of iron. **Thyroid hormones:** [P] Decreased thyroxine absorption. *See also* Antacids.
Levodopa	Levodopa degraded in gut prior to reaching sites of absorption. Agents that alter gastrointestinal motility may alter degree of intraluminal degradation. Antiparkinsonism effect of levodopa susceptible to inhibition by other drugs.	**Clonidine:** [NE] Inhibits antiparkinsonism effect. **Monoamine oxidase inhibitors:** [P] Hypertensive reaction (carbidopa prevents the interaction). **Papaverine:** [NE] Inhibits antiparkinsonism effect. **Phenothiazines:** [P] Inhibits antiparkinsonism effect. **Phenytoin:** [NE] Inhibits antiparkinsonism effect. **Pyridoxine:** [P] Inhibits antiparkinsonism effect (carbidopa prevents the interaction). *See also* Antimuscarinics.

Table II–1. Important drug interactions. (continued)

HP = Highly predictable. Interaction occurs in almost all patients receiving the interacting combination.	
P = Predictable. Interaction occurs in most patients receiving the combination.	
NP = Not predictable. Interaction occurs only in some patients receiving the combination.	
NE = Not established. Insufficient data available on which to base estimate of predictability.	

Drug or Drug Group	Properties Promoting Drug Interaction	Clinically Documented Interactions
Lithium	Renal lithium excretion sensitive to changes in sodium balance. (Sodium depletion tends to cause lithium retention.) Susceptible to drugs enhancing central nervous system lithium toxicity.	**ACE inhibitors:** [NE] Probable reduced renal clearance of lithium; increased lithium effect. **Angiotensin II receptor blockers:** [NE] Probable reduced renal clearance of lithium; increased lithium effect. **Diuretics (especially thiazides):** [P] Decreased excretion of lithium; furosemide may be less likely to produce this effect than thiazide diuretics. **Haloperidol:** [NP] Occasional cases of neurotoxicity in manic patients, especially with large doses of one or both drugs. **Methyldopa:** [NE] Increased likelihood of central nervous system lithium toxicity. **Nonsteroidal anti-inflammatory drugs:** [NE] Reduced renal lithium excretion (except sulindac and salicylates). **Theophylline:** [P] Increased renal excretion of lithium; reduced lithium effect.
Monoamine oxidase inhibitors (MAOIs)	Increased norepinephrine stored in adrenergic neuron. Displacement of these stores by other drugs may produce acute hypertensive response. MAOIs have intrinsic hypoglycemic activity.	**Anorexiants:** [P] Hypertensive episodes due to release of stored norepinephrine (benzphetamine, diethylpropion, mazindol, phendimetrazine, phentermine). **Antidiabetic agents:** [P] Additive hypoglycemic effect. **Buspirone:** [NE] Possible serotonin syndrome; avoid concurrent use. **Dextromethorphan:** [NE] Severe reactions (hyperpyrexia, coma, death) have been reported. **Guanethidine:** [P] Reversal of the hypotensive action of guanethidine. **Mirtazapine:** [NE] Possible serotonin syndrome; avoid concurrent use. **Narcotic analgesics:** [NP] Some patients develop hypertension, rigidity, excitation; meperidine may be more likely to interact than morphine. **Nefazodone:** [NE] Possible serotonin syndrome; avoid concurrent use. **Phenylephrine:** [P] Hypertensive episode, since phenylephrine is metabolized by monoamine oxidase. **Selective serotonin reuptake inhibitors (SSRIs):** [P] Fatalities have occurred due to serotonin syndrome; SSRIs are contraindicated in patients taking MAOIs. **Sibutramine:** [NE] Possible serotonin syndrome; avoid concurrent use. **Sympathomimetics (indirect-acting):** [HP] Hypertensive episode due to release of stored norepinephrine (amphetamines, ephedrine, isometheptene, phenylpropanolamine, pseudoephedrine). **Tramadol:** [NE] Possible serotonin syndrome; avoid concurrent use. **Venlafaxine:** [NE] Possible serotonin syndrome; avoid concurrent use. *See also* Antidepressants, tricyclic and heterocyclic; Levodopa.
Nonsteroidal anti-inflammatory drugs (NSAIDs)	Prostaglandin inhibition may result in reduced renal sodium excretion, impaired resistance to hypertensive stimuli, and reduced renal lithium excretion. Most NSAIDs inhibit	**ACE inhibitors:** [P] Decreased antihypertensive response. **Furosemide:** [P] Decreased diuretic, natriuretic, and antihypertensive response to furosemide. **Hydralazine:** [NE] Decreased antihypertensive response to hydralazine. **Methotrexate:** [NE] Possible increase in methotrexate toxicity (especially with anticancer doses of methotrexate).

(continued)

Table II–1. Important drug interactions. (continued)

HP = Highly predictable. Interaction occurs in almost all patients receiving the interacting combination.		
P = Predictable. Interaction occurs in most patients receiving the combination.		
NP = Not predictable. Interaction occurs only in some patients receiving the combination.		
NE = Not established. Insufficient data available on which to base estimate of predictability.		

Drug or Drug Group	Properties Promoting Drug Interaction	Clinically Documented Interactions
Nonsteroidal anti-inflammatory drugs (*continued*)	platelet function; may increase likelihood of bleeding due to other drugs that impair hemostasis. Most NSAIDs are highly bound to plasma proteins. Phenylbutazone may inhibit hepatic microsomal drug metabolism (also seems to act as enzyme inducer in some cases). Phenylbutazone may alter renal excretion of some drugs.	**Phenytoin:** [P] Decreased hepatic phenytoin metabolism. **Triamterene:** [NE] Decreased renal function noted with triamterene plus indomethacin in both healthy subjects and patients. *See also* Anticoagulants, oral; Beta-adrenoceptor blockers; Lithium.

Phenytoin	Induces hepatic microsomal drug metabolism. Susceptible to inhibition of metabolism by CYP2C9 and, to a lesser extent, CYP2C19.	*Drugs whose metabolism is stimulated by phenytoin:*
		  Corticosteroids: [P] Decreased serum corticosteroid levels.
		  Doxycycline: [P] Decreased serum doxycycline levels.
		  Methadone: [P] Decreased serum methadone levels; withdrawal symptoms.
		  Mexiletine: [NE] Decreased serum mexiletine levels.
		  Quinidine: [P] Decreased serum quinidine levels.
		  Theophylline: [NE] Decreased serum theophylline levels.
		  Verapamil: [NE] Decreased serum verapamil levels.
		See also Calcium channel blockers, Cyclosporine, Estrogens.
		Drugs that inhibit phenytoin metabolism:
		  Amiodarone: [P] Increased serum phenytoin; possible reduction in serum amiodarone.
		  Capecitabine: [NE] Increased serum phenytoin.
		  Chloramphenicol: [P] Increased serum phenytoin.
		  Felbamate: [P] Increased serum phenytoin.
		  Fluorouracil: [NE] Increased serum phenytoin.
		  Fluvoxamine: [NE] Increased serum phenytoin.
		  Isoniazid: [NP] Increased serum phenytoin; problem primarily with slow acetylators of isoniazid.
		  Miconazole: [P] Increased serum phenytoin.
		  Ticlopidine: [NP] Increased serum phenytoin.
		See also Azole antifungals, Cimetidine; Disulfiram.
		Drugs that enhance phenytoin metabolism:
		  Rifampin: [P] Decreased serum phenytoin levels.

Pimozide	Susceptible to CYP3A4 inhibitors; may exhibit additive effects with other agents that prolong QT$_c$ interval.	**Clarithromycin:** [NE] Decreased pimozide metabolism. **Erythromycin:** [NE] Decreased pimozide metabolism **Nefazodone:** [NE] Decreased pimozide metabolism. *See also* Azole antifungals, Cyclosporine.
Potassium-sparing diuretics (amiloride, spironolactone, triamterene)	Additive effects with other agents increasing serum potassium concentration. May alter renal excretion of substances other than potassium (eg, digoxin, hydrogen ions).	**ACE inhibitors:** [NE] Additive hyperkalemic effect. **Potassium supplements:** [P] Additive hyperkalemic effect; especially a problem in presence of renal impairment. *See also* Digitalis glycosides; Nonsteroidal anti-inflammatory drugs.

(continued)

Table II–1. Important drug interactions. (continued)

HP = Highly predictable. Interaction occurs in almost all patients receiving the interacting combination.
P = Predictable. Interaction occurs in most patients receiving the combination.
NP = Not predictable. Interaction occurs only in some patients receiving the combination.
NE = Not established. Insufficient data available on which to base estimate of predictability.

Drug or Drug Group	Properties Promoting Drug Interaction	Clinically Documented Interactions
Probenecid	Interference with renal excretion of drugs that undergo active tubular secretion, especially weak acids. Inhibition of glucuronide conjugation of other drugs.	**Clofibrate:** [P] Reduced glucuronide conjugation of clofibric acid. **Methotrexate:** [P] Decreased renal methotrexate excretion; possible methotrexate toxicity. **Penicillin:** [P] Decreased renal penicillin excretion. **Salicylates:** [P] Decreased uricosuric effect of probenecid (interaction unlikely with less than 1.5 g of salicylate daily).
Quinidine	Metabolism inducible. Inhibits CYP2D6. Renal excretion susceptible to changes in urine pH. Additive effects with other agents that prolong the QT_c interval.	**Acetazolamide:** [P] Decreased renal quinidine excretion due to increased urinary pH; elevated serum quinidine. **Amiodarone:** [NE] Increased serum quinidine levels; mechanism not established. **Kaolin-pectin:** [NE] Decreased gastrointestinal absorption of quinidine. **Rifampin:** [P] Increased hepatic quinidine metabolism. **Thioridazine:** [NE] Decreased thioridazine metabolism; additive prolongation of QT_c interval. *See also* Anticoagulants, oral; Antidepressants, tricyclic; Barbiturates; Cimetidine; Digitalis glycosides; Phenytoin.
Quinolone antibiotics	Susceptible to inhibition of gastrointestinal absorption. Some quinolones inhibit CYP1A2.	**Caffeine:** [P] Ciprofloxacin, enoxacin, pipedemic acid, and to a lesser extent, norfloxacin, inhibit caffeine metabolism. **Sucralfate:** [HP] Reduced gastrointestinal absorption of ciprofloxacin, norfloxacin, and probably other quinolones. **Theophylline:** [P] Ciprofloxacin, enoxacin, and, to a lesser extent, norfloxacin inhibit theophylline metabolism; gatifloxacin, levofloxacin, lomefloxacin, ofloxacin, and sparfloxacin appear to have little effect. *See also* Antacids; Anticoagulants, oral.
Rifampin	Induction of hepatic microsomal drug-metabolizing enzymes.	**Corticosteroids:** [P] Increased corticosteroid hepatic metabolism; reduced corticosteroid effect. **Mexiletine:** [NE] Increased mexiletine metabolism; reduced mexiletine effect. **Sulfonylurea hypoglycemics:** [P] Increased hepatic metabolism of tolbutamide and probably other sulfonylureas metabolized by the liver (including chlorpropamide). **Theophylline:** [P] Increased theophylline metabolism; reduced theophylline effect. *See also* Anticoagulants, oral; Azole antifungals; Beta-adrenoceptor blockers; Calcium channel blockers; Cyclosporine; Digitalis glycosides; Estrogens.
Salicylates	Interference with renal excretion of drugs that undergo active tubular secretion. Salicylate renal excretion dependent on urinary pH when large doses of salicylate used. Aspirin (but not other salicylates) interferes with platelet function. Large doses of salicylates have intrinsic hypoglycemic activity. Salicylates may displace drugs from plasma protein binding sites.	**Carbonic anhydrase inhibitors:** [NE] Increased acetazolamide serum concentrations; increased salicylate toxicity due to decreased blood pH. **Corticosteroids:** [P] Increased salicylate elimination; possible additive toxic effect on gastric mucosa. **Heparin:** [NE] Increased bleeding tendency with aspirin, but probably not with other salicylates. **Methotrexate:** [P] Decreased renal methotrexate clearance; increased methotrexate toxicity (primarily at anticancer doses). **Sulfinpyrazone:** [HP] Decreased uricosuric effect of sulfinpyrazone (interaction unlikely with less than 1.5 g of salicylate daily). *See also* Antacids; Anticoagulants, oral; Probenecid.

(continued)

Table II-1. Important drug interactions. (continued)

HP = Highly predictable. Interaction occurs in almost all patients receiving the interacting combination.
P = Predictable. Interaction occurs in most patients receiving the combination.
NP = Not predictable. Interaction occurs only in some patients receiving the combination.
NE = Not established. Insufficient data available on which to base estimate of predictability.

Drug or Drug Group	Properties Promoting Drug Interaction	Clinically Documented Interactions
Theophylline	Susceptible to inhibition of hepatic metabolism by CYP1A2. Metabolism inducible.	**Benzodiazepines:** [NE] Inhibition of benzodiazepine sedation. **Diltiazem:** [P] Decreased theophylline metabolism. **Clarithromycin:** [NE] Decreased theophylline metabolism. **Erythromycin:** [P] Decreased theophylline metabolism. **Fluvoxamine:** [P] Decreased theophylline metabolism. **Smoking:** [HP] Increased theophylline metabolism. **Tacrine:** [P] Decreased theophylline metabolism. **Ticlopidine:** [NE] Decreased theophylline metabolism. **Troleandomycin:** [P] Decreased theophylline metabolism. **Verapamil:** [P] Decreased theophylline metabolism. **Zileuton:** [P] Decreased theophylline metabolism. *See also* Barbiturates; Carbamazepine; Cimetidine; Lithium; Phenytoin; Quinolones; Rifampin.

REFERENCES

Asberg A: Interactions between cyclosporin and lipid-lowering drugs: Implications for organ transplant recipients. Drugs 2003;63:367.

Blanchard N et al: Qualitative and quantitative assessment of drug-drug interaction potential in man, based on Ki, IC50 and inhibitor concentration. Curr Drug Metab 2004;5:147.

deMaat MM et al: Drug interactions between antiretroviral drugs and comedicated agents. Clin Pharmacokinet 2003;42:223.

Doucet J et al: Drug-drug interactions related to hospital admissions in older adults: A prospective study of 1000 patients. J Am Geriatr Soc 1996;44:944.

DuBuske LM: The role of P-glycoprotein and organic anion-transporting polypeptides in drug interactions. Drug Saf 2005;28:789.

Egger SS et al: Potential drug-drug interactions in the medication of medical patients at hospital discharge. Eur J Clin Pharmacol 2003;58:773.

Hansten PD: Understanding drug interactions. Science & Medicine 1998;5:16.

Hansten PD, Horn JR: *Drug Interactions Analysis and Management.* Facts & Comparisons. [Quarterly.]

Hansten PD, Horn JR: *The Top 100 Drug Interactions. A Guide to Patient Management.* H&H Publications, 2006.

Juurlink DN et al: Drug-drug interactions among elderly patients hospitalized for drug toxicity. JAMA 2003;289:1652.

Kim RB (editor): *The Medical Letter Handbook of Adverse Interactions.* Medical Letter, 2003.

Levy RH et al (editors): *Metabolic Drug Interactions.* Lippincott Williams & Wilkins, 2000.

Lin JH, Yamazaki M: Role of P-glycoprotein in pharmacokinetics: Clinical implications. Clin Pharmacokinet 2003;42:59.

Riesenman C: Antidepressant drug interactions and the cytochrome P450 system: A critical appraisal. Pharmacotherapy 1995;15:84S.

Tatro DS (editor): *Drug Interaction Facts.* Facts & Comparisons. [Quarterly.]

Williamson EM: Drug interactions between herbal and prescription medicines. Drug Saf 2003;26:1075.

Index

Note: Page numbers in boldface type indicate major discussions. A *t* following a page number indicates tabular material and an *i* following a page number indicates an illustration. Most drugs are listed under their generic names. Insofar as possible, when a drug trade name is listed, page numbers are for preparations available. For further detail, refer to the generic name provided.